Bates' Guide to Physical Examination and History Taking

Fourteenth Edition

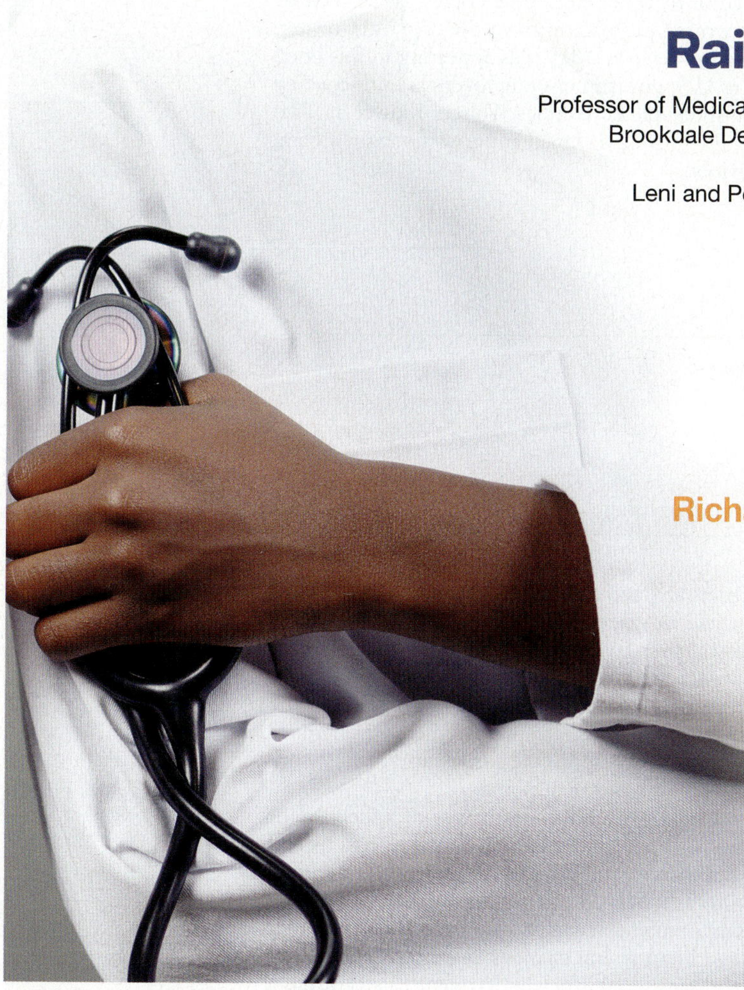

Lead Author and Editor

Rainier P. Soriano, MD

Professor of Medical Education, Geriatrics and Palliative Medicine
Brookdale Department of Geriatrics and Palliative Medicine
Senior Associate Dean for Curricular Affairs
Leni and Peter W. May Department of Medical Education
Icahn School of Medicine at Mount Sinai
New York, New York

Co-Editors

Peter G. Szilagyi, MD, MPH

Distinguished Professor of Pediatrics
David Geffen School of Medicine at UCLA
Los Angeles, California

Richard Hoffman, MD, MPH, FACP

Emeritus Professor
Department of Medicine
University of Iowa Carver College of Medicine
Iowa City, Iowa

Editor Emeritus

Lynn S. Bickley, MD, FACP

Clinical Professor of Internal Medicine
University of New Mexico School of Medicine
Albuquerque, New Mexico

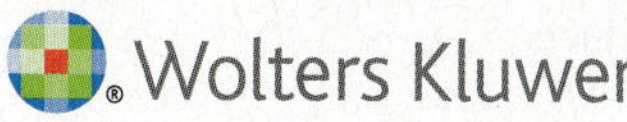

Philadelphia • Baltimore • New York • London
Buenos Aires • Hong Kong • Sydney • Tokyo

Acquisitions Editor: Matt Hauber
Development Editor: Deborah Bordeaux
Senior Editorial Coordinator: Sean Hanrahan
Editorial Assistant: Parisa Saranj
Marketing Manager: Kirsten Watrud
Senior Production Project Manager: Catherine Ott
Manager, Graphic Arts & Design: Stephen Druding
Art Director, Illustration: Jennifer Clements
Illustrator: Body Scientific International
Photographer: Mike Stog at DesignWorksVisualMedia
Media Production: Liz Simmons Thibodeau at Thibodeau Media Group
Manufacturing Coordinator: Margie Orzech
Prepress Vendor: Aptara, Inc.

Fourteenth edition

9 8 7 6 5 4 3 2 1

Printed in Mexico

Library of Congress Cataloging-in-Publication Data

North American ISBN-13: 978-1-9752-1834-8
International ISBN-13: 978-1-9752-1839-3

Cataloging-in-Publication data available on request from Publisher

---

shop.lww.com

QUADM0525

To Lynn Bickley, whose dedication to the art and science of physical diagnosis has inspired generations of clinicians and laid the foundation for countless students; it is an honor to continue your legacy.

Faculty Contributors

George A. Alba, MD
Assistant Professor of Medicine
Division of Pulmonary and Critical Care Medicine
Massachusetts General Hospital
Harvard Medical School
Boston, Massachusetts

Cara A. Brown, MD, AEMUS-FPD, FACEP
Assistant Professor
Director, Advanced Emergency Ultrasound Fellowship
Department of Emergency Medicine
Icahn School of Medicine at Mount Sinai
New York, New York

Christopher T. Doughty, MD
Assistant Professor of Neurology
Harvard Medical School
Brigham and Women's Hospital
Boston, Massachusetts

Nicola A. Feldman, MD, MS
Resident Physician
Boston Combined Residency Program in Pediatrics
Boston Children's Hospital and Boston Medical Center
Boston, Massachusetts

Rocco M. Ferrandino, MD, MSCR
Assistant Professor
Department of Otolaryngology-Head and Neck Surgery
University of Washington
Seattle, Washington

Raisa Gao, MD, FACOG
Vice Chair
Department of Obstetrics and Gynecology
Huntington Hospital
Northwell Health
Assistant Professor
Donald and Barbara Zucker School of Medicine at Hofstra
Hempstead, New York

Sarah M. Gustafson, MD
Associate Clinical Professor
Division of Pediatric Hospital Medicine
David Geffen School of Medicine at UCLA
Los Angeles, California

Michael L. Herscher, MD
Associate Professor of Medicine and Medical Education
Division of Hospital Medicine
Mount Sinai Hospital
Icahn School of Medicine at Mount Sinai
New York, New York

Alexander R. Lloyd, MD
PM&R Sports Medicine Physician
Assistant Program Director, Sports Medicine Fellowship
Rehabilitation and Performance Medicine
Providence Swedish
Seattle, Washington

Christopher C. Lo, MD
Orbital and Oculofacial Plastic Surgery
Medical Director
Eyesthetica
Los Angeles, California

Stephen A. McCullough, MD
Assistant Professor of Clinical Medicine
Division of Cardiology
Weill Cornell Medicine
New York Presbyterian Hospital
New York, New York

Bret P. Nelson, MD, AEMUS-FPD, FACEP
Professor, Department of Emergency Medicine
System Vice Chair, Education
Chief, Emergency Ultrasound Division
Department of Emergency Medicine
Icahn School of Medicine at Mount Sinai
New York, New York

Matthew E. Pollard, MD
Reproductive Urology
Regional Medical Director, Vice President of Quality and Clinical Excellence
Posterity Health, PC
Nashville, Tennessee

Bess M. Storch, MD
Assistant Professor
Department of Emergency Medicine
Mount Sinai West-Morningside Hospitals
Department of Medical Education
Icahn School of Medicine at Mount Sinai
New York, New York

Preface

I am excited to introduce the fourteenth edition of *Bates' Guide to Physical Examination and History Taking*, a trusted resource that has guided generations of health care learners in developing the essential skills of patient assessment. This edition continues to evolve alongside the practice of medicine, integrating modern diagnostic techniques while preserving the core principles of clinical reasoning and physical diagnosis that remain at the heart of patient care.

The comprehensive updates introduced in the thirteenth edition continue here, reflecting advancements in clinical education, patient care, and medical technology. With input from active clinicians and experienced educators, this edition responds to the changing needs of students and instructors across health care disciplines, ensuring it remains relevant, accessible, and clinically practical. A key focus of this edition is enhancing the usability and clinical application of the physical examination chapters, with refinements that help learners bridge the gap between textbook knowledge and real-world patient care.

This edition expands the **structured health history questions** to provide clearer guidance on how to ask effective, clinically relevant questions and interpret patient responses in ways that inform diagnosis and management. These revisions emphasize the connection between patient narratives, clinical reasoning, and differential diagnosis, helping learners move beyond memorization toward a deeper understanding of history-taking as a critical diagnostic tool. **Discussions of common symptoms** have also been refined, providing a stronger foundation for assessing patient complaints by integrating key historical features, physical exam findings, and considerations for differential diagnosis. Rather than presenting symptoms in isolation, this approach reinforces how clinicians analyze and synthesize information in practice. In addition, recognizing that many patients present with medical devices or prior surgical interventions that require **modifications to standard examination techniques**, this edition includes specific guidance on how to adapt the physical exam in these cases. These updates ensure that learners develop a flexible, patient-centered approach that accounts for real-world complexities in clinical assessment.

New content includes a dedicated chapter on **Point-of-Care Ultrasound (POCUS)** and updates to **Clinical Documentation and Presentation**, equipping learners with the tools to integrate technology-assisted diagnostics and effective communication into clinical workflows. The **Older Adults chapter**, now structured around the **Geriatric 5Ms framework**, provides a comprehensive approach to assessing aging patients, reinforcing the importance of age-specific considerations in physical diagnosis.

Beyond structural and content updates, terminology throughout the text has been refined to ensure clarity, accuracy, and consistency with modern medical language. Where historical medical terms and eponyms are still in use, they have been carefully retained for continuity while ensuring that descriptions are as precise and clinically useful as possible. The **Health Promotion and Counseling** sections have also been expanded, emphasizing patient-centered communication, disease prevention strategies, and clinical reasoning in primary care and specialty settings.

With these updates, the fourteenth edition of *Bates' Guide to Physical Examination and History Taking* remains a cornerstone resource in health care education, equipping students, educators, and practicing clinicians with the knowledge and skills necessary for effective, evidence-based, and compassionate patient care. This edition upholds the highest standards in medical training, ensuring that future health care professionals are well prepared to integrate clinical knowledge, physical exam skills, and patient communication into their practice.

R.P. Soriano, MD
Lead Author and Editor

New Content and Features

The fourteenth edition introduces several new features and expanded content designed to enhance clinical learning and patient assessment skills. These updates improve both usability and content depth, ensuring that learners gain a strong foundation in physical examination, clinical reasoning, and diagnostic techniques.

Layout and Design Enhancements:

- The streamlined double-column layout for Unit 1 has been introduced to improve readability, allowing for a cleaner and more focused presentation of foundational content. Units 2 and 3 retain the familiar two-column layout, providing continuity and maintaining the traditional structure that many readers appreciate.

- We have revamped the overall layout to make navigation easier, ensuring that you can find the information you need quickly and efficiently. This improved design enhances your study experience by reducing the time spent searching for key topics.

- With new, high-quality images added throughout the book provide greater visual clarity, reinforcing important physical examination techniques and clinical findings. These images are designed to support and enhance the textual content, making complex concepts more intuitive.

- Additional tables have been incorporated to organize information more clearly. These tables help distill complex data into easily digestible formats, aiding in quicker comprehension and retention of critical facts.

Refinements in Language and Clinical Terminology:

- Language and terminology have been refined to ensure clarity, precision, and accessibility, reflecting best practices in clinical communication while maintaining consistency with modern health care education standards.

Enhancements to Regional Physical Examination Chapters:

- The inclusion of common symptoms with high-yield health history questions is aimed at enhancing clinical reasoning-focused interviews. These structured questions guide learners in asking the right questions during patient assessments, ultimately improving diagnostic accuracy.

- New sections on high-yield Point-of-Care Ultrasound (POCUS) techniques in selected regional physical examination chapters provide essential skills for modern diagnostic practices. Learning these techniques alongside time-honored physical exam skills will give learners a competitive edge in clinical settings and develop a more comprehensive diagnostic approach.

- We have added new tables on physical examination modifications for patients with clinical devices. These tables offer practical guidance on adapting exams for patients with special needs, ensuring comprehensive, patient-centered, and sensitive care.

- The new clinical reasoning–focused interpretation of sample documentations in regional chapters will help learners understand how to effectively document findings and think critically about assessments. This skill is crucial for developing accurate patient records and improving overall patient care.

- Updated recommendations in the Health Promotion and Counseling sections ensure you have access to the latest guidelines and best practices for patient care. Staying current with these recommendations is vital for providing the best possible advice and treatment to patients.

Specific Chapter Revisions and Additions:

- The addition of new chapters on POCUS and Documentation and Presentation expands the scope of the textbook, providing learners with essential modern techniques and skills that are increasingly important in clinical practice.

- The Genitourinary (GU) content has been reorganized, and the Musculoskeletal (MSK) chapter has been split, allowing for a more detailed and focused presentation of each area. This reorganization allows for a deeper understanding of each area, enhancing overall clinical knowledge and application.

- The introduction of the 5Ms framework in the Older Adults chapter enhances health history and assessment for older patients, offering a comprehensive approach to evaluating and managing geriatric care. This framework ensures a thorough and holistic approach to geriatric care, which is crucial given the aging population.

These updates and enhancements ensure that the fourteenth edition remains a comprehensive and indispensable resource for clinical skills training and education. With these improvements, learners will be well equipped to succeed in their clinical studies and future careers, confident in their ability to perform thorough physical examinations, apply clinical reasoning, and provide high-quality patient care.

ORGANIZATION

The book comprises three units: *Foundations of Health Assessment*, *Regional Examinations*, and *Special Populations*.

Unit 1, Foundations of Health Assessment, focuses on essential skills and knowledge required for the clinical encounter. This unit with nine chapters begins with foundational skills crucial to the clinical setting, followed by effective interviewing, communication, and interpersonal skills. The subsequent chapters cover the health history, physical examination, and the processes of clinical reasoning, assessment, and planning. In addition, this unit includes new chapters on clinical documentation and presentation, as well as the basic principles and techniques of point-of-care ultrasound. Health maintenance and screening are also addressed, along with evaluating clinical evidence, ensuring a comprehensive foundation for effective patient assessment and clinical decision making.

Unit 2, Regional Examinations, covers comprehensive regional examinations from head to toe. This unit with 18 chapters begins with an overview of the general survey, vital signs, and pain assessment, followed by cognition, behavior, and mental status. Subsequent chapters detail the examination of the skin, hair, and nails; head and neck; eyes; ears and nose; throat and oral cavity; thorax and lungs; cardiovascular system; and peripheral vascular system. The unit continues with the examination of the breasts and axillae, abdomen, anus and rectum, and the pelvis and genitourinary system, with separate chapters for different anatomical structures. The musculoskeletal system is covered in two chapters, focusing on the neck, shoulders, and upper extremities, and the lumbosacral spine, hip, and lower extremities, respectively. The unit concludes with a detailed examination of the nervous system. Each chapter includes a review of relevant anatomy and physiology, common symptoms encountered in the health history, detailed descriptions and images of examination techniques, a sample written record, comparative tables of abnormalities, and extensive references from recent clinical literature. Important topics for health promotion and counseling are now placed at the end of each chapter to facilitate a more focused understanding of these complex issues.

Unit 3, Special Populations, addresses health assessments across different stages of life, including three chapters on children (infancy through adolescence), pregnant individuals, and older adults.

ADDITIONAL RESOURCES

Bates' Pocket Guide to Physical Examination and History Taking

As a practical companion to *Bates' Guide to Physical Examination and History Taking, 14th Edition*, we highly recommend the *Bates' Pocket Guide to Physical Examination and History Taking, 10th Edition*. Together, these two resources are designed to support learners at every stage—whether laying the groundwork in the classroom or applying knowledge in real-time clinical settings.

The full textbook delivers comprehensive, in-depth instruction on examination techniques, clinical reasoning, and foundational principles of patient care. It is best suited for structured study, offering the detail and context needed to build lasting understanding and clinical confidence.

The Pocket Guide complements this by serving as a concise, accessible reference at the bedside or point of care. Its compact format makes it ideal for quick consultation during clinical encounters, while its clear summaries, updated algorithms, and new illness scripts help reinforce core concepts and support diagnostic reasoning in the moment. The continued inclusion of clinical algorithms reflects their enduring value and the consistently strong feedback from learners and clinicians alike.

Used together, the textbook and Pocket Guide form a dynamic and integrated learning system—helping learners bridge the gap between knowledge and practice with clarity, confidence, and ease.

Bates' Videos

The Bates' video series is an essential adjunct for mastering the many techniques of physical examination. Comprehensive videos bring clinical skills to life through clear, structured demonstrations organized into three integrated collections:

Physical Examination Series: This core series features 18 volumes of head-to-toe and systems-based physical examination videos. Updated and reorganized for clarity and consistency, each video emphasizes relevant anatomy, step-by-step examination techniques, and common pathologic findings. Learners observe experienced clinicians performing regional exams and applying techniques such as inspection, palpation, percussion, and auscultation—across both general and special populations.

Communication and Interpersonal Skills Series: This 27-video series highlights the essential human side of clinical practice. Learners watch clinicians demonstrate foundational communication and interpersonal skills, from building rapport and gathering information to navigating difficult conversations. These skills are critical for effective, compassionate care and will serve as a lifelong foundation for professional growth.

OSCE Clinical Skills Series: Designed to strengthen clinical reasoning and exam readiness, this series includes 15 realistic, scenario-based patient encounters that mirror Objective Structured Clinical Examinations (OSCEs). Each video features a student evaluating a patient with a common presenting problem—such as chest pain, sore throat, or abdominal pain—interspersed with guiding questions and key teaching points. These videos help learners apply their knowledge in context and prepare for both formative assessments and real-world patient care.

Students are encouraged to use the textbook, pocket guide, and video series together as a cohesive learning system—studying the textbook to build foundational knowledge, using the pocket guide to support clinical application, and revisiting the videos to visually reinforce key techniques. Engaging with these resources repeatedly and at different stages of learning helps solidify understanding, sharpen skills, and build confidence in both the classroom and clinical environment.

The Bates' video series is available via Lippincott® Connect as the *Bates' Visual Guide to Physical Examination*. Purchase *Bates' Guide to Physical Examination and History Taking*, Lippincott® Connect version with Videos, for access to the videos, assessment, and other dynamic resources that enhance your learning.

Bates' Visual Guide to Physical Examination is available for purchase by institutions and enables seamless, concurrent access for all students, with options for institutions to subscribe to the full range of videos or select collections. Each video has a unique, stable URL that instructors can provide in their Learning Management Systems for easy student access.

Acknowledgments

Bates' Guide to Physical Examination and History Taking has always been a collaborative effort driven by a singular goal: to honor and support the lifelong learner—student, teacher, and practitioner—in mastering the evolving art and science of clinical medicine. This fourteenth edition continues this tradition, bringing together contributions from a diverse group of dedicated professionals committed to excellence in physical diagnosis and patient care. With this edition, *Dr. Rainier P. Soriano* assumes the role of lead author and editor, building on the solid foundation established by previous editions. He brings a deep commitment to integrating traditional physical examination with evolving best practices in clinical teaching.

Profound appreciation is extended to *Dr. Lynn S. Bickley*, who skillfully led the guide from the seventh through the thirteenth editions. Her vision and clarity helped shape generations of learners. Gratitude is also owed to *Dr. Peter L. Szilagyi*, whose contributions since the eighth edition have greatly enriched the content, and to *Dr. Richard M. Hoffman*, whose expertise since the twelfth edition has significantly advanced the integration of clinical evidence and health promotion strategies throughout the guide.

This edition also benefited greatly from the insights and contributions of a number of expert reviewers and advisors—active clinicians and educators who embody the intersection of bedside skills and clinical teaching. Their feedback ensures that the content remains accurate, relevant, and grounded in real-world practice. The contributions of the following esteemed colleagues are gratefully acknowledged: *George A. Alba, MD; Cara A. Brown, MD; Christopher T. Doughty, MD; Nicola A. Feldman, MD, MS; Rocco M. Ferrandino, MD, MSCR; Raisa Gao, MD; Sarah M. Gustafson, MD; Michael L. Herscher, MD; Alexander R. Lloyd, MD; Christopher C. Lo, MD; Stephen A. McCullough, MD; Bret P. Nelson, MD; Matthew E. Pollard, MD;* and *Bess M. Storch, MD.*

The production of the *Bates' Guide to Physical Examination and History Taking*, fourteenth edition is a complex endeavor requiring extraordinary coordination and meticulous attention to detail. Special thanks go to Freelance Development Editor *Kelly Horvath*, whose editorial precision and dedication brought coherence and excellence to every chapter. Additional heartfelt acknowledgments go to Development Editor *Deborah Bordeaux*, who has guided the development of the content; Senior Editorial Coordinator *Sean Hanrahan*, who has managed the editorial process; Marketing Manager *Kirsten Watrud*, and Production Project Manager *Catherine Ott* at Wolters Kluwer, whose oversight ensured the successful execution of every phase. Gratitude is also extended to Manager of Graphic Arts & Design *Stephen Druding*, Art Director of Illustration *Jennifer Clements* at Wolters Kluwer, and the team at *Body Scientific International*, for their creation of updated, high-quality illustrations; to photographer *Mike Stog* at DesignWorksVisualMedia and to *Liz*

Simmons Thibodeau and her crew at Thibodeau Media Group, who have delivered exceptional photography and high-quality media production; and to *Aptara* for their expert handling of the digital production process. Finally, and most importantly, heartfelt thanks to Acquisitions Editor *Matt Hauber*, whose leadership and vision have ensured that the *Bates* suite of teaching materials continues to meet the evolving needs of today's learners and educators.

The talent, insight, and dedication of all those involved in this edition uphold the long-standing tradition of excellence that has made the *Bates' Guide to Physical Examination and History Taking*, reaffirming its role as the premier resource in the teaching and learning of clinical skills.

Contents

List of Tables

CHAPTER 26 Musculoskeletal System: Lumbosacral Spine, Hips, and Lower Extremities 841

CHAPTER 27 Nervous System 899

CHAPTER 28 Children: Infancy Through Adolescence 995

CHAPTER 29 Pregnant Persons 1121

UNIT 1

Foundations of Health Assessment

CHAPTER 1

Foundational Skills Essential to the Clinical Encounter

> *"The ritual of one individual coming to another and telling [them] things that [they] would not tell [their] preacher or rabbi; and then, incredibly, on top of that, disrobing and allowing touch... I think our skills in examining a patient have to be worthy of that kind of trust."*
>
> —Abraham Verghese, MD, A Doctor's Touch, TEDGlobal, 2011.

THE CLINICAL ENCOUNTER

As you begin your clinical training, you'll learn a range of essential skills that will deepen your patient relationships and enhance your ability to provide care. A *clinical skill* is any discrete act within the overall process of patient care.[1] Clinical skills are the singular elements that constitute clinical competence. Through the purposeful selection and integration of these individual skillful acts during the patient encounter, you will lay the foundation for high-quality clinical care.

Your clinical skills will evolve over time as you develop your professional relationship with each patient, take their clinical history, perform a mental and physical examination, conduct tests and procedures, and provide diagnostic and therapeutic interventions.[2] To become a skilled clinician, you will need to integrate contemporary biomedical knowledge into your patient care in a professional and culturally sensitive manner.[2] As a student, you will gradually move from passive observation to active patient assessment, gaining confidence and expertise with each encounter. You will also need to commit to ongoing practice and honest self-assessment in order to continuously improve your skills.

The initial chapters in this unit will introduce you to the essentials of the clinical encounter, with a focus on establishing trust, which is the foundation of the therapeutic alliance with patients (Fig. 1-1). Initially, you will focus on gathering information, but with experience and empathic listening, you will learn to allow the patient's story to unfold in its most authentic and detailed form. By mastering these skills and building caring patient relationships based on mutual trust and respect, you will reap the timeless rewards of the clinical professions. These are the fundamental features of all clinical care.[2]

Chapter Content Guide

- Approach to the Clinical Encounter
- Structure and Sequence of the Clinical Encounter
- Disparities in Health Care
- Other Major Considerations

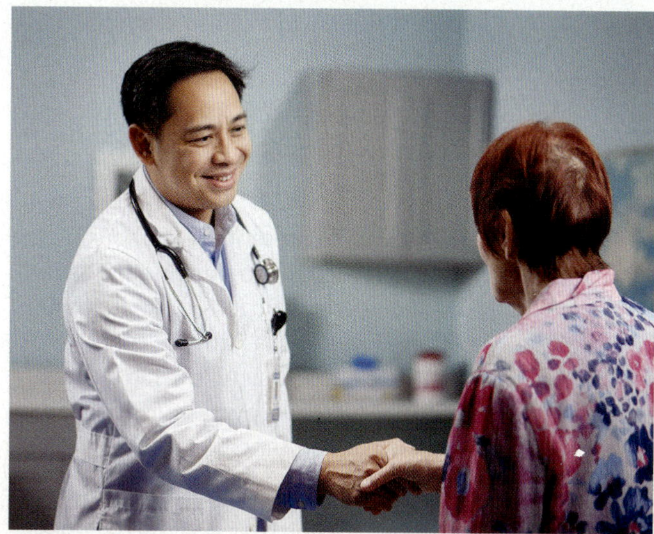

FIGURE 1-1. Therapeutic alliance between clinician and patient.

APPROACH TO THE CLINICAL ENCOUNTER

The clinical encounter involves both the clinician and the patient and can be approached in two ways: *clinician-centered* and *patient-centered*. The former approach prioritizes acquiring details about symptoms and disease, potentially neglecting the personal dimensions of illness.[3,4] In contrast, the patient-centered approach values patients' expressions of personal concerns and emotions and considers the patient's perspective of illness.

The *disease/illness distinction model* helps to clarify the distinct but complementary perspectives of the clinician and the patient (Box 1-1).[5] A successful clinical interview must incorporate both the clinician's and the patient's perspectives of reality, disease, and illness.[3]

Research indicates that integrating both clinician-centered and patient-centered approaches in a clinical encounter leads to a more comprehensive understanding of the patient's illness and enables clinicians to convey qualities of respect, empathy, humility, and sensitivity.[3,7] This merged approach has been shown to be more satisfying for both patients and clinicians and more effective in achieving desired health outcomes.[8,9] By incorporating both perspectives in your clinical encounters, you can gain a more well-rounded view of the patient's problems from both your own and their point of view. Achieving a balance between these two essential components is critical for conducting an effective clinical interview in a patient encounter.

Box 1-1. Disease/Illness Distinction Model

Disease	Explanation used by the clinician to organize symptoms, leading to a clinical diagnosis
Illness	Construct that explains how the patient experiences the disease, including its impact on relationships, function, and overall well-being

For example, when a patient presents with a sore throat, the clinician may focus on identifying the cause of the symptoms, such as streptococcal pharyngitis or allergies to penicillin. However, the patient's concerns may extend beyond the physical symptoms to include worries about pain, difficulty swallowing, missing work, or even the fear of developing cancer.

These divergent concerns illustrate the importance of incorporating both the clinician's and the patient's perspectives into the clinical interview.[3,6]

STRUCTURE AND SEQUENCE OF THE CLINICAL ENCOUNTER

In general, an effective clinical encounter moves through a logical sequence (Box 1-2).[10] In this chapter, we focus on the behaviors related to the initiation and closure of the clinical encounter as well as the exploration of the patient's perspectives of their illness. An illustrative example of this framework is the enhanced *Calgary–Cambridge Guides* (Fig. 1-2), which describes the structure and timeline of the clinical encounter and highlight the need to elicit information regarding both the biomedical disease process and the patient's perspective. They also include a place for the physical examination. The structure includes five major steps: *initiating the session, information gathering, physical examination, explaining and planning*, and *closing the session*.[11–13]

Box 1-2. General Structure and Sequence of the Clinical Encounter

1. Initiating the encounter
   - Setting the stage/preparation
   - Greeting the patient and establishing initial rapport
2. Gathering information
   - Initiating information gathering
   - Exploring patient's perspective of illness
   - Exploring biomedical perspective of disease including relevant background and context
3. Performing the physical examination
4. Explaining and planning
   - Provide correct amount and type of information
   - Negotiate plan of action
   - Shared decision making
5. Closing the encounter

Note: Two additional frameworks occur as continuous threads throughout the sequence—namely, building the relationship and structuring the interview (see Fig. 1-2).

Source: Adapted from Kurtz S, Silverman J, Benson J, Draper J. Marrying content and process in clinical method teaching: enhancing the Calgary–Cambridge guides. *Acad Med.* 2003;78(8):802–809; van de Poel K, Vanagt E, Schrimpf U, Gasiorek J. *Communication Skills for Foreign and Mobile Medical Professionals*. Springer; 2013:xvii, 145; de Haes H, Bensing J. Endpoints in medical communication research, proposing a framework of functions and outcomes. *Patient Educ Couns.* 2009;74(3):287–294.

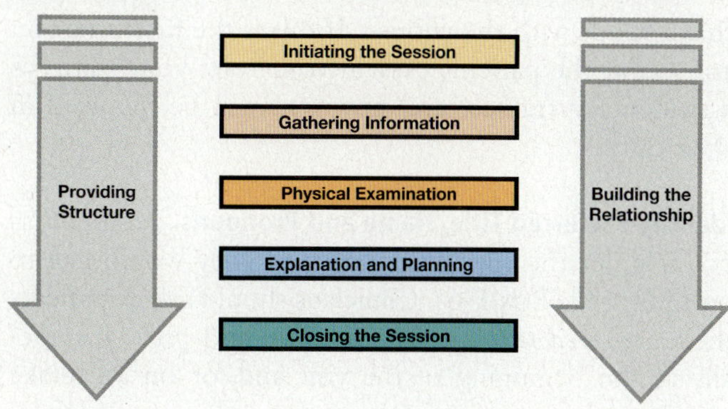

FIGURE 1-2. Enhanced Calgary–Cambridge Guides: Structure and timeline of the clinical encounter. (Reproduced with permission from Kurtz S, Silverman J, Benson J, Draper J. Marrying content and process in clinical method teaching: enhancing the Calgary–Cambridge guides. *Acad Med.* 2003;78[8]:802–809.)

Stage 1: Initiating the Encounter

This is the stage of relationship-building with your patient. Fostering the patient–clinician relationship is critical because without a good relationship, none of the other goals of the clinical encounter can be pursued in an optimal manner.[14] Respect, trust, and rapport are necessary components of a burgeoning therapeutic relationship.

Set the Stage. To start, set the stage and prepare for the interview. Check your appearance, make sure the patient is comfortable, and create an environment that is conducive to sharing personal information. Each interview has its own rhythm and sequence, so mastering the steps described is essential. Also, reflect on any biases you may have that could color your reactions to the patient and the therapeutic alliance you need to create. See Racism and Bias, p. 11.

Adjust the Environment. Adjust the environment to ensure effective communication with your patient. Even in challenging settings like a two-bedded hospital room or a busy emergency department, improving communication is worth the effort. Use privacy curtains or move to an empty room to create a more confidential setting.

Consider factors like cultural background and individual preferences about interpersonal space. Choose a distance that allows for good eye contact and clear conversation, pull up a chair, and sit at eye level with the patient to facilitate communication. Move any physical barriers out of the way to create an open and welcoming environment (Fig. 1-3).

Be mindful of arrangements that may convey disrespect, such as interviewing a patient who is already positioned for a pelvic exam or talking through a bathroom door. Ensure that any computer monitors are positioned so as not to obstruct your view of the patient or hide your face from them. Lighting is another essential consideration. Create a private and welcoming environment to help facilitate effective communication and build a positive rapport with your patient.

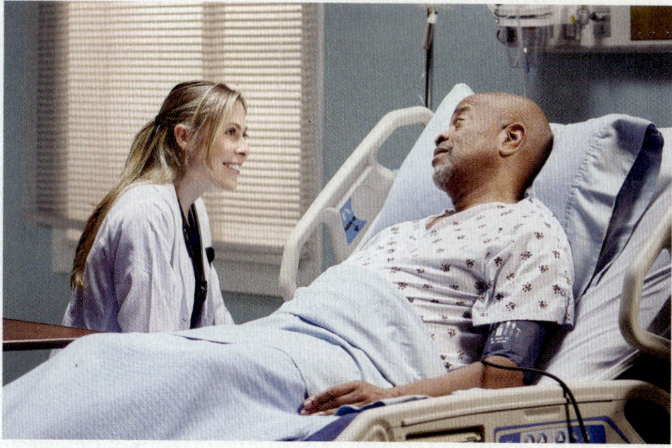

FIGURE 1-3. Move physical barriers out of the way and be at eye level.

Review the Clinical Record. Before seeing the patient, review the clinical record (Fig. 1-4). It will provide important background information and suggest areas to explore during the visit. Review identifying data such as age, gender, address, and insurance as well as the Patient Problem List, medications, and allergies.

The clinical record usually contains past diagnoses and treatments, but making your assessment based on what you learn during the visit is important. Keep in mind that the clinical record is compiled from many observers,

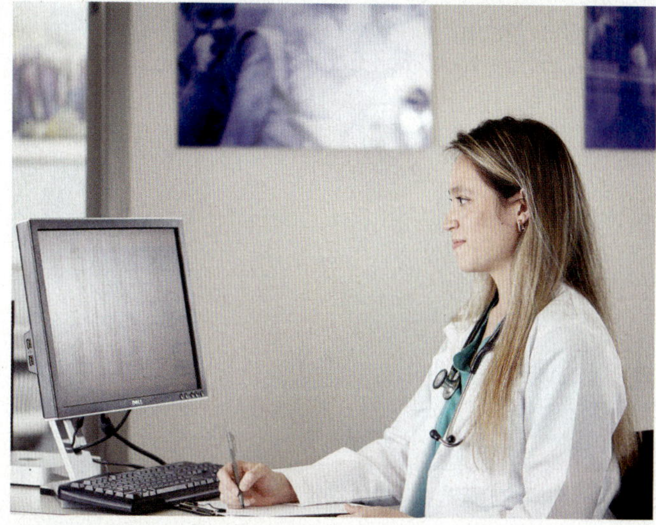

FIGURE 1-4. Review the health record before the clinical encounter.

and data may be incomplete or even contradict what the patient tells you. Reconcile any discrepancies in the record for the patient's care. Be aware of potential problems that may arise from documentation mismatches, especially as electronic health records are being developed to include preferred names and gender pronouns. Address any issues related to this or other sensitive topics that may arise during the visit. Being thorough in your review of the clinical record allows you to provide the best possible care for your patient.

Set Your Agenda. Before speaking with the patient, clarify your goals for the interview. A student goal may be completing a comprehensive history, whereas for an advanced trainee or clinician, goals range from assessing a new concern to treatment follow-up. Regardless, balancing clinician-centered and patient-centered goals is essential, as is considering the agendas of the patient, their family, and health care agencies. Taking a few minutes to think about your goals will help you align your priorities with the patient's agenda.[15]

Greet the Patient and Establish Initial Rapport. The initial moments of your encounter lay the foundation for your ongoing relationship. How you greet the patient and other visitors in the room, provide for the patient's comfort, and arrange the physical setting, all shape the patient's first impressions (Fig. 1-5). Relating effectively with patients is among the most valued skills of clinical care. For the patient, "a feeling of connectedness . . . of being deeply heard and understood . . . is the very heart of healing."[16] For the clinician, this deeper relationship enriches the rewards of patient care.[17–19] Suggestions on how to establish rapport with specific patient populations are shown in Box 1-3.

As you begin, *welcome the patient by introducing yourself*, giving your own first and last name. If possible, shake hands with the patient. If this is the first time you are seeing the patient, explain your role, your status as a student or trainee, and how you will be involved in their care.

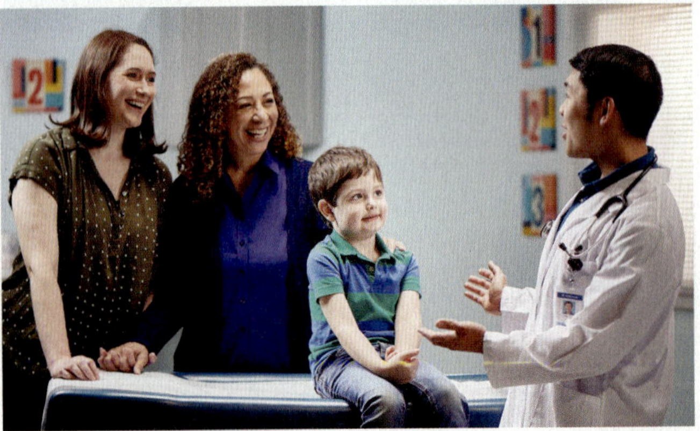

FIGURE 1-5. Greeting the patient and establishing rapport.

Identify Preferred Title, Name and Pronouns. As much as possible, let the patient dictate how they would like to be addressed (Box 1-6). Clinicians should ask all patients their *preferred titles*, *preferred name*, and *pronouns*, ideally at the beginning of the visit and/or on an intake questionnaire.

Preferred Title. Titles include Mr., Mrs., Ms., or honorifics such as Professor or Doctor. This not only provides valuable information about the patient's identity but is also important in establishing rapport and showing respect, especially if you are seeing the patient for the first time and promotes a welcoming environment.

Preferred Name. The name may be a nickname (e.g., "Pat" for "Patrick"), use of a middle name, or some other name altogether. After stating your name, ask the patient what name they would like you to use. Except with children or adolescents, avoid first names until you have specific permission. Calling a patient *"dear," "sweetie,"* or overly familiar names can depersonalize and demean them.[21]

If you are unsure how to pronounce the patient's name, do not be afraid to ask. You can say, *"I am afraid of mispronouncing your name. Could you say it for me?"* Then repeat it to make sure you heard it correctly. For patients who identify as transgender and gender nonbinary, the preferred name may match their affirmed gender and be different than their given name, which may have matched their sex assigned at birth.[20]

Pronouns. When asking patients about their pronouns, it can be helpful to share your own pronouns with patients, asking: *"Which gender pronouns do you use?"* (Box 1-7). For example, *"I use . . . he and him/she and hers/they and theirs."* Some of your patients may use *gender-neutral pronouns* or *inclusive pronouns*. These are pronouns that are not associated with a particular gender. They are used by individuals who do not identify as strictly male or female or who prefer not to be referred to as he/him or she/her. Some examples include *they/them*, *ze/hir*, *xe/xem*, and *ey/em*. These pronouns are used to promote inclusivity and respect for individuals who identify outside of the gender binary.

To show respect and avoid making patients feel disrespected or invalidated, it's crucial to use the correct title, name, and pronoun they have provided. Misgendering

Box 1-3. Approach to Establishing Rapport with Specific Populations

Population	Recommendations
Newborns and Infants (birth to 30 days; 1 month to 1 year) 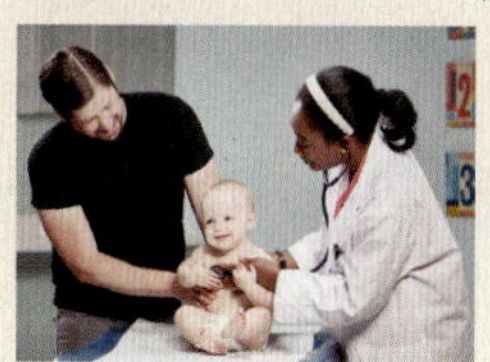	■ Building rapport is still important even though newborns and infants are unable to communicate like older children. ■ Congratulate the family on their newborn, encourage caregivers to feed the newborn either while talking or before the encounter to keep the newborn calm, and focus on the caregivers to ask about their well-being. ■ Take advantage of opportunities to obtain quick screening questions about family health topics.
Young and School-Age Children (1 to 4 years; 5 to 10 years)[22–25] 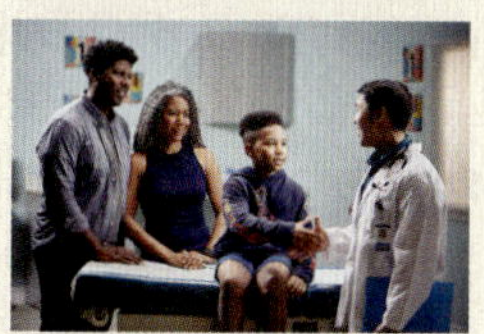	■ To begin the encounter with a child patient and their family, introduce yourself first, then engage the child with play to build rapport and manage their mood. ■ While the child is playing, obtain the health history from the caregiver, asking for confirmation or elaboration as necessary. ■ For school-age children, familiarize yourself with "kid culture" and ask age-appropriate questions to facilitate engagement.
Adolescents[26–28] 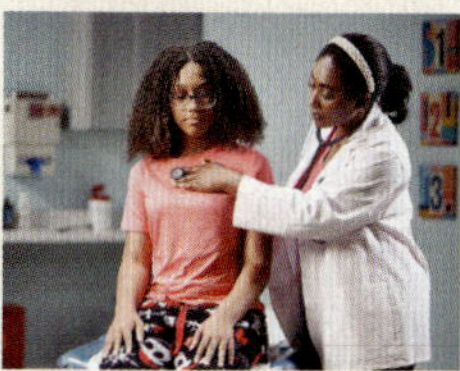	■ When interacting with adolescent patients, prioritize their confidentiality and trust while ensuring family members and caregivers feel comfortable and heard. ■ Use open-ended questions, provide ample opportunities for adolescents to share their concerns, and acknowledge the importance of their privacy. ■ Inform the family that they will have an opportunity to speak with you but first spend time alone with the adolescent patient without any family members present.
Older Adults[21] 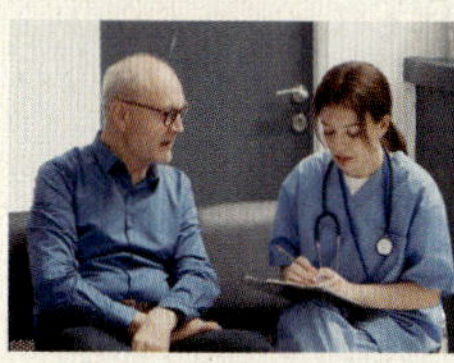	■ When interacting with older adult patients, elicit their preferred way of being addressed and adjust the environment to put them at ease. ■ Provide a well-lit, moderately warm setting with minimal background noise, chairs with arms, and ample space for safe navigation, particularly if using an assistive device. ■ Allow time for open-ended questions, reminiscing, and include family and caregivers, especially when cognitive impairment is present.
Patients with Physical and Sensory Disabilities 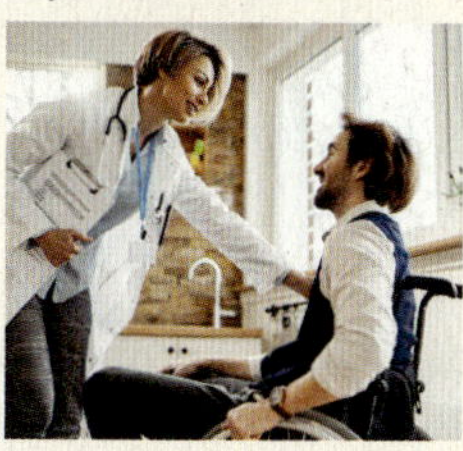	■ When referring to patients with disabilities, use "people-first" language (e.g., *person who is blind, person who uses a wheelchair, person with hearing loss*) unless they specify otherwise. ■ Always presume that patients with physical and/or sensory disabilities are competent to manage their medical care and avoid making assumptions about what assistance they may require. ■ Speak directly with the patient, not to an aide or companion, and refrain from asking whether they are accompanied if they entered the room alone (Box 1-4).
Lesbian, Gay, Bisexual, Transgender, Queer + (LGBTQ+) Adults[29–32] 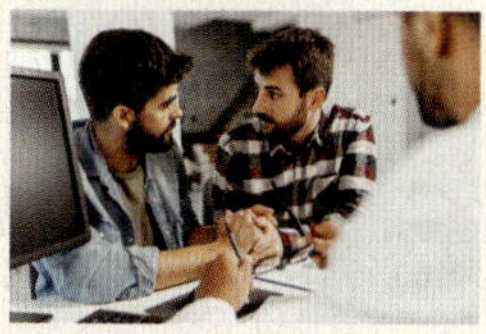	■ When working with LGBTQ+ patients, recognize that they may experience anxiety related to acceptance and discomfort in disclosing their sexual behaviors and identity. ■ Expand your knowledge and clinical skills in gay, lesbian, and transgender health and engage with available resources. ■ Prepare to answer questions about fertility and transgender issues such as hormonal therapy and gender-affirming procedures and be open to discussing these topics with patients (Box 1-5).

Box 1-4. Establishing Rapport with Patients with Physical and Sensory Disabilities

- Based on 2023 global population estimates, more than 1.3 billion people (16% of the world's population) are estimated to live with some form of disability.[89]
- In the United States, the overall rate of people with disabilities in 2021 was estimated as 13.5% of the population.[90]

Patients Who Are Blind or Have Low Vision

- Always verbally identify yourself when you approach and introduce other people in the room.
- Do not leave without letting the patient know.
- Ask before you help. Always ask how the patient would like to be assisted.
- Be prepared to provide written materials in an auditory, tactile, or electronic format of the patient's preference (audio file, Braille, large print).
- Explain what is about to happen before beginning the encounter and ask if the patient has any questions.
- Tell the patient where personal effects (clothes and other belongings) are in the room and do not move them without telling the patient.
- Staff should be welcoming and describe the physical environment (doors, steps, ramps, bathroom location, etc.).
- Never distract or touch a service animal without asking the owner.

Patients Who Are Hard of Hearing

- Ask how best to communicate.
- Be prepared to give written materials as long as they are not the primary form of communication.
- Inform patients that sign language interpreting and real-time captioning services are available.
- If requested, promptly provide sign language interpreting or real-time captioning service for effective communication.
- Do not talk at a distance from the patient or from another room.
- Look directly at the patient when speaking so your mouth is visible.
- Speak normally and clearly. Do not shout, exaggerate mouth movements, or speak rapidly.
- Minimize background noise and glare.

Patients Who Are Deaf

- Ask how best to communicate.
- Inform patients that sign language interpreting and real-time captioning services are available.
- If requested, promptly provide sign language interpreting or real-time captioning service for effective communication.
- Do not use family members to interpret.
- Address the patient, not the interpreter.
- Be prepared to give written materials as long as they are not the primary form of communication.

Patients Who Use Wheelchairs

- Make sure there is a path of access to the room.
- Respect personal space, including wheelchair and assistive devices.
- Do not propel the wheelchair unless asked to do so.
- Provide accessible equipment as needed.
- Assist as needed, such as by clearing obstacles from the path of travel or helping patients transfer to equipment if accessible equipment is unavailable.
- Do not separate patients from their wheelchairs.

Source: Reprinted with permission from Access to Medical Care: Adults with Physical Disabilities (Project Director: Marsha Saxton, PhD). World Institute on Disability; 2016. Accessed June 16, 2023. https://worldinstituteondisabilityblog.files.wordpress.com/2016/01/access-to-medical-care-curriculum-pdf-format.pdf

Box 1-5. Lesbian, Gay, Bisexual, and Transgender Health

Several recent surveys provide some of the first national data sets on the lesbian, gay, bisexual, and transgender (LGBT) population.

- For the first time, in 2013, the National Health Interview Survey included a measure of sexual orientation: in the 2018 report, a sample of around 27,000 adults, 1.6% identified as gay or lesbian, 1.0% identified as bisexual, and 1.6% responded either other or did not know. Most gay and lesbian respondents were ages 18 to 44 years, with a higher percentage of bisexual respondents ages 18 to 44 years.[91]
- In 2012, the Gallup Daily Tracking Survey initiated the largest single study of the distribution of the LGBT population in the United States.[92,93] The Survey added an LGBT identity question that generated 120,000 responses: 3.4% answered "yes" when asked if they identify as LGBT. Of those identifying as LGBT, 53% were female and 6.4% were ages 18 to 29 years. Nearly 13% were in a domestic partnership or living with a partner. Non-Whites were more likely to identify as LGBT: African American 4.6%, Asians 4.3%, Hispanics 4.9%, and non-Hispanic White 3.2%.
- The 2013 American Community Survey of the United States Census Bureau reported more than 726,000 same-sex couple households; 34% had same-sex spouses.[94]
- In its 2011 report on LGBT health disparities, the Institute of Medicine called for better measures of health care disparities among the diverse LGBT subpopulations to elucidate their differing health behaviors and health care needs.[95]
- LGBT patients have higher rates of depression, suicide, anxiety, drug use, sexual victimization, and risk of infection with HIV and sexually transmitted infections.[96,97]
- One-third (33%) of transgender individuals who saw a health care provider in the past year reported having at least one negative experience related to being transgender, such as *"being refused treatment, verbally harassed, or physically or sexually assaulted, or having to teach the provider about transgender people in order to get appropriate care, with higher rates for people of color and people with disabilities."*[98]
- The Institute of Medicine has stated that barriers to accessing quality health care for LGBT adults are "a lack of providers who are knowledgeable about LGBT health needs as well as a fear of discrimination in health care settings."[95]

a patient can lead to feelings of alienation, dysphoria, or disrespect. While it's not always possible to avoid mistakes, a simple apology can go a long way. Instead of over-apologizing, say something like, "*I apologize for using the wrong pronoun [or preferred name]. I did not mean to disrespect you.*" It can be tempting to overstate how badly you feel about making a mistake, but that

Box 1-6. Obtaining Patients' Preferred Method of Address

Example:

Student: *"Good morning. I am Susannah Velasquez, a third-year clinical student. I am part of the clinical team taking care of you. I'm here to help make sure we're meeting your needs. Are you Richard Clarkson?"*
Patient: *"Yes, that's me."*
Student: *"Thank you. How would you like me to address you?"*
Patient: *"You can call me Mr. Clarkson."* Or, *"Richard is fine."*

Box 1-7. Obtaining Patients' Gender Pronouns

Example:

Student: *"Good morning. I am Susannah Velasquez, a third-year clinical student. I am part of the clinical team taking care of you and will assist them figure out how we can best help you. Are you Richard Clarkson?"*
Patient: *"Yes."*
Student: *"How would you like me to address you?"*
Patient: *"You can call me Mr. Clarkson."* Or, *"Richard is fine."*
Student: *"It is a pleasure to meet you, Mr. Clarkson. Please feel free to call me Susie. May I ask you a few more background questions before we start?"*
Patient: *"Sure."*
Student: *"In our effort to promote an inclusive and respectful environment, we like to use each other's correct pronouns. The pronouns I prefer when others refer to me are 'she' and 'her'. How about you? What pronouns do you prefer?"*
Patient: *"I use 'he' and 'him,' I guess."*

Box 1-8. Steps in Stage 2: Gathering Information

Steps	Description
Initiate information gathering	After establishing rapport, ask the patient about their chief complaint or presenting problem(s), taking notes during the interview to ensure nothing is missed (Box 1-9).
Establish the agenda for the patient encounter[33]	Ask open-ended questions to encourage patients to discuss all of their concerns, not just clinical ones. You should identify all concerns and ask about missed ones to prioritize them.
Invite the patient's story[33]	Encourage patients to share their stories in their own words using an open-ended approach, actively listening without interrupting or injecting new information to prevent bias.
Gather information about the patient's perspective of illness	Explore the patient's perspective on their illness by using different types of questions to uncover their feelings, ideas, the effect on their function, and expectations (Box 1-10).
Identify and respond to the patient's emotional cues[34,35]	Check for emotional cues and feelings by asking about them, as visits tend to be longer when you miss emotional cues. See Box 1-11 for suggested techniques.
Gather information by exploring the biomedical perspective	The health history format is a structured framework for gathering and organizing patient information in written or verbal form. It focuses one's attention on the specific kinds of information clinicians need to obtain, facilitates clinical reasoning, and standardizes communication with other health care providers.
Gather important background information and context[36]	Learn about the patient's life circumstances, emotional health, perception of health care, health behaviors, and access to and utilization of health care to strengthen the therapeutic alliance and improve health outcomes.

might make the misgendered patient feel more awkward and inclined to comfort you, which is not appropriate.

Stage 2: Gathering Information

This stage has two functions: *gathering* and *providing information* (Box 1-8).[14] Clinicians gather information from patients regarding symptoms, experiences, and expectations to establish a diagnosis and treatment plan. Simultaneously, patients require information to comprehend their health issues, mitigate uncertainties, and support their coping mechanisms. This phase lays the groundwork for shared decision making later in the clinical encounter.

To explore the patient's perspective, use different types of questions. A mnemonic for the patient's perspective on the illness is *FIFE—Feelings, Ideas, effect on Function, and Expectations* (Box 1-12). The combination of concerns and expectations has been shown to have a major influence on the patient's decision to seek help from a clinician.

Box 1-9. A Note about Taking Notes

- Jot down or type short phrases, specific dates, or words; but do not let note-taking or the keyboard and computer screen distract you from the patient.
- Maintain good eye contact (Fig. 1-6). If the patient is talking about sensitive or disturbing material, put down your pen or move away from the keyboard.
- For patients who find note taking uncomfortable, explore their concerns and explain your need to make an accurate record.
- When using an electronic health record, face the patient directly as you elicit the patient's story, maintaining good eye contact and observing nonverbal behaviors; turn to the screen only after engaging the patient in the goals for the visit.
- Look up at the patient as often as possible, readjusting your screen and position if needed.[99]

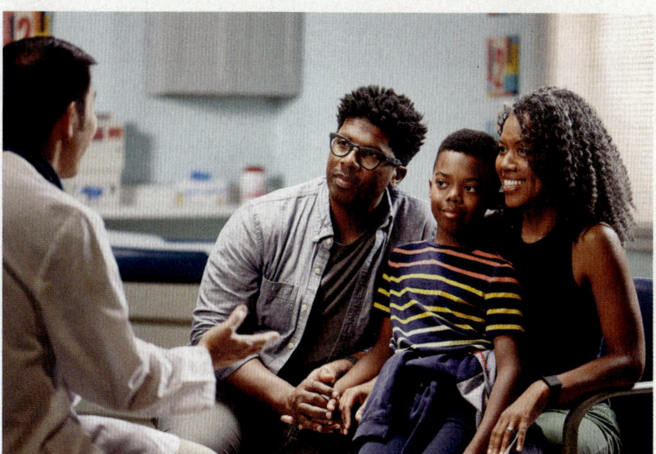

FIGURE 1-6. Maintain good eye contact.

Stage 3: Performing the Physical Examination

The physical examination also enhances your relationship with the patient. Physical findings denote the presence or absence of disease and an opportunity for you to learn more about your patient's outlook and condition. Since the physical examination almost always follows the history, it provides an avenue for the patient to talk about deeper fears or more serious issues. Maintain your patient's comfort throughout, avoid embarrassment, and demonstrate facility with the skills of physical examination to enhance the patient's satisfaction with the clinical encounter.[37]

Box 1-10. Clues to the Patient's Perspective on Illness

- Direct statement(s) by the patient of explanations, emotions, expectations, and effects of the illness
- Expression of feelings about the illness without naming the illness
- Attempts to explain or understand symptoms
- Speech clues (e.g., repetition, prolonged reflective pauses)
- Sharing a personal story
- Behavioral clues indicative of unidentified concerns, dissatisfaction, or unmet needs such as reluctance to accept recommendations, seeking a second opinion, or early return appointment

Source: Lang F, Floyd MR, Beine KL. Clues to patients' explanations and concerns about their illnesses. A call for active listening. *Arch Fam Med.* 2000;9(3):222–227.

Box 1-11. Responding to Emotional Cues Using NURSE Statements[100,101]

Learn to respond attentively to emotional cues using techniques like reflection, feedback, and "continuers" that convey support. A mnemonic for responding to emotional cues is NURSE:

Name: *"That sounds like a scary experience"*

Understand or legitimize: *"It's understandable that you feel that way"*

Respect: *"You've done better than most people would with this"*

Support: *"I will continue to work with you on this"*

Explore: *"How else were you feeling about it?"*

Source: Communication: what do patients want and need? *J Oncol Pract.* 2008;4(5):249–253; Pollak KI, Arnold RM, Jeffreys AS, et al. Oncologist communication about emotion during visits with patients with advanced cancer. *J Clin Oncol.* 2007;25(36):5748–5752.

Stage 4: Explaining and Planning

This stage includes the elaboration of the patient's chief concerns from the disease and illness perspectives. Your goal is to assess and respond to the patient's needs for information. To achieve a shared understanding, make it easy for the patient to understand and remember your explanations and encourage mutual discussion rather than one-way communication. This will allow your patients to understand shared clinical decision making, determine how much they want to be involved, and hopefully increase their commitment to the plans made.

Box 1-12. Exploring the Patient's Perspective (F-I-F-E)[3,6]

- The patient's **F**eelings, including fears or concerns, about the problem
- The patient's **I**deas about the nature and the cause of the problem
- The effect of the problem on the patient's life and **F**unction
- The patient's **E**xpectations of the disease, of the clinician, or of health care, often based on prior personal or family experiences

Source: Fortin AH VI, Dwamena FC, Frankel RM, Smith RC. *Smith's Patient-Centered Interviewing: An Evidence-Based Method.* 3rd ed. McGraw-Hill Medical; 2012; Mauksch L, Farber S, Greer HT. Design, dissemination, and evaluation of an advanced communication elective at seven U.S. medical schools. *Acad Med.* 2013;88(6):843–851.

Provide Useful Information and Verify Patient Understanding.[38–40] Studies show that patients forget up to 80% of the clinical information provided during office visits, with nearly half of the information retained being incorrect. To verify the patient's understanding of the plan of care, the *"teach-back" technique* can be used, in which the patient is asked to explain the plan of care in their own words. The *"show-me" method* can also be used to confirm that patients can follow specific instructions (Box 1-13).

Negotiate the Plan of Action through Shared Decision Making.[41,42] Interactive history taking creates a shared understanding of the patient's issues, serving as a basis for further evaluation and treatment planning. *Shared decision making* involves a three-step process of introducing choices, exploring patient preferences, and moving to a decision while checking for readiness and offering additional time if needed. This approach promotes optimal therapy, treatment adherence, and patient satisfaction. It may be necessary to explain recommendations multiple times to ensure the patient understands and agrees with the proposed plan.

Stage 5: Closing the Encounter

Ending the interview or visit can be challenging since patients often have numerous questions and feel engaged if the clinician has done their job well. Inform the patient of the approaching end to allow for any final questions, but avoid bringing up a new topic during the last few minutes, unless it concerns a life-threatening issue. Instead, assure the patient of your interest and arrange to address the issue at a future time. Reaffirming your commitment to the patient's health shows involvement and esteem. Summarizing the mutual plans developed with the patient before leaving the room and asking if they have any questions about what was discussed is helpful.

Self-reflection or mindfulness is crucial in developing clinical empathy. *Mindfulness* involves being purposefully and nonjudgmentally attentive to your own experience, thoughts, and feelings.[43] Given patients' diverse backgrounds, being consistently respectful and open to individual differences is an ongoing challenge in clinical care. Since clinicians bring their values, assumptions, and biases to every encounter, looking inward is necessary to understand how our expectations and reactions impact our behavior and communication. Self-reflection is a continuous part of professional development in clinical work that brings personal awareness to patient care and is one of the most rewarding aspects of it.[44,45]

Box 1-13. Teach-Back Method

- **Plan your approach.** Think about how you will ask your patient to teach back the information. An example would be: *"We covered a lot today and I want to make sure that I explained things clearly. So, let's review what we discussed. Can you please describe the three things you agreed to do to help you control your diabetes?"*
- **"Chunk and Check."** Don't wait until the end of the visit to initiate teach-back. Chunk out information into small segments and have your patient teach it back. Repeat several times during a visit.
- **Clarify and check again.** If teach-back uncovers a misunderstanding, explain things again using a different approach. Ask patients to teach-back again until they are able to correctly describe the information in their own words. If they parrot your words back to you, they may not have understood.
- **Start slowly and use consistently.** At first, you may want to try teach-back with the last patient of the day. Once you are comfortable with the technique, use teach-back with everyone, every time!
- **Practice.** It will take a little time, but once it is part of your routine, teach-back can be done without awkwardness and does not lengthen a visit.
- **Use the *show-me* method.** When prescribing new medicines or changing a dose, research shows that even when patients correctly say when and how much medicine they will take, many will make mistakes when asked to demonstrate the dose.
- **Use handouts along with teach-back.** Write down key information to help patients remember instructions at home. Point out important information by reviewing written materials to reinforce your patients' understanding. You can allow patients to refer to handouts when using teach-back, but make sure they use their own words and are not reading the material back verbatim.

Source: Use the Teach-Back Method: Tool #5. Content last reviewed September 2020. Agency for Healthcare Research and Quality. Accessed June 16, 2023. https://www.ahrq.gov/health-literacy/improve/precautions/tool5.html

DISPARITIES IN HEALTH CARE

Disparities in risks of disease, morbidity, and mortality are marked and broadly documented across different population groups, reflecting inequities in health care access, income level, type of insurance, educational level,

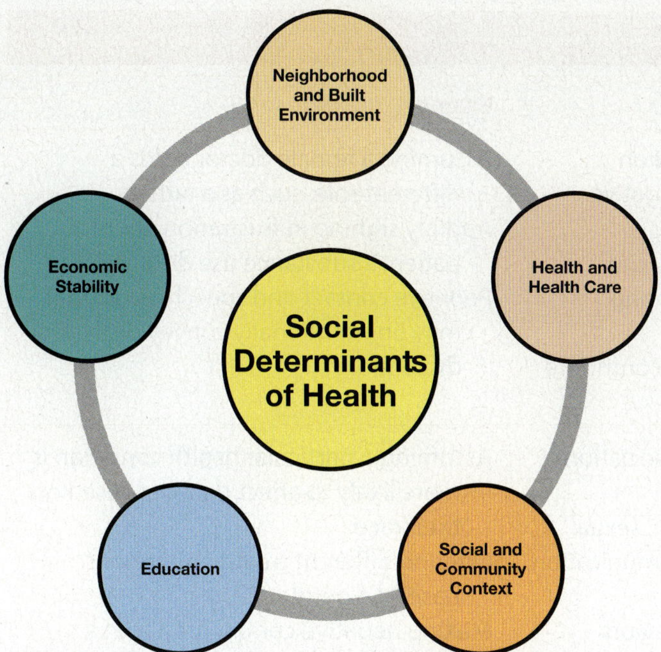

FIGURE 1-7. Social determinants of health. (Adapted from HealthyPeople2030 at https://www.healthypeople.gov.)

language proficiency, and provider decision making.[45,46] This section focuses on important factors that potentiate unequal treatment in the clinical encounter and approaches to help mitigate them.

Social Determinants of Health

Health is significantly affected by the social environment, also known as the *social determinants of health (SDOH)*. The World Health Organization (WHO) defines SDOH as "the conditions in which people are born, grow, work, live, and age, and the wider set of forces and systems shaping the conditions of daily life" (Fig. 1-7). This includes economic policies and systems, development agendas, social norms, social policies, and political systems.[48] In short, these are the social, economic, and political factors that impact the health of individuals and populations (Box 1-14).[47] More than their genetic susceptibilities, patients' health is often influenced by SDOH such as stress, early life, social exclusion, working conditions, unemployment, social support, addiction, healthy food, and transportation policies. Evidence supports addressing social determinants of health to improve patient health and reduce inequities (Box 1-15).[49]

Box 1-14. Key Social Health Determinant Domains

- **Economic stability** (employment, food insecurity, housing instability, poverty)
- **Education access and quality** (early childhood education and development, enrollment in higher education, high school graduation, language, and literacy)
- **Social and community context** (civic participation, discrimination, incarceration, social cohesion)
- **Health care access and quality** (access to health care, access to primary care, health literacy)
- **Neighborhood and built environment** (access to foods that support healthy eating patterns, crime and violence, environmental conditions, quality of housing)

Source: Healthy People 2030, U.S. Department of Health and Human Services, Office of Disease Prevention and Health Promotion. Accessed June 16, 2023. https://health.gov/healthypeople/objectives-and-data/social-determinants-health

Racism and Bias

Research indicates that implicit clinician biases can negatively impact patient encounters and contribute to health care disparities among different demographic groups.[51] Unconscious mental processes help sort and organize patterns to improve cognitive efficiency, leading to implicit biases formed by society's exposure to imagery, values, media, and emotions depicting stereotypes associated with different demographic groups. Addressing implicit bias in clinical encounters requires understanding its cognitive origins and acknowledging its relation to explicit bias (Box 1-16).[53]

Several skills are available that clinicians can use to mitigate the impact of bias in their clinical encounters (Box 1-17).

Box 1-15. Addressing Social Determinants of Health

Level of Interventions	Sample Actions
Patient level	Identify social challenges Offer culturally safe services Help patients access benefits and support services
Practice level	Use patient navigators to ensure care is accessible to those most in need
Community level	Partner with local organizations Engage in health planning Improve environments for health

Box 1-16. Types of Bias

Type of Bias	Description	Example Scenarios
Implicit Bias	Unconscious evaluation of a person based on perceived group identity, leading to negative associations[50] Can negatively impact patient encounters and contribute to health care disparities among different demographic groups Can manifest in nonverbal behaviors and contribute to institutional bias	Assuming a female doctor holds a different role, such as a nurse Audibly sighing in frustration about a patient's substance use disorder Poor eye contact and speech errors that may unintentionally convey distrust or discomfort
Explicit Bias	Conscious decision based on beliefs or associations regarding group identity Patient characteristics such as race, gender, sexual orientation, and age can influence communication, diagnostic decision making, treatment recommendations, and nonverbal behaviors	Assuming a particular health condition is more likely to affect patients based on their race. Offering different treatment options based on gender Making negative comments about a patient's age or sexual orientation
Institutional Bias	Refers to the aggregation of implicit biases that lead to a structural system of privilege[52–56] Misallocates care for marginalized groups	Limiting access to care for certain demographic groups Offering unequal treatment options based on social identities Disregarding patient symptoms or concerns based on assumptions linked to identity

Box 1-17. Skills and Practices to Mitigate Bias in Your Clinical Encounters[55,56,102]

Reflect on patterns of emotion and behavior.	Pay attention to how you feel and how you behave around patients of different identities. The patterns you recognize may reflect biases that impact your interactions with patients as well as your clinical reasoning. Being aware of these biases is the first step in reducing their impact on patient care.
Pause before starting an encounter and prepare for potential triggers of bias	Once you are aware of your potential biases, pay attention to situations that may trigger them. Simply being aware of a bias can help minimize its effect. You may take deliberate actions to reduce the impact of your biases.
Generate alternative hypotheses for biases anchored in behavior	Many biases are anchored in clinician assumptions about observed patient behavior (nonadherence, substance use, etc.). Make it a habit to consider what structural forces (socioeconomic status, race/racism, homophobia, etc.) impact patient behaviors, and how they can challenge assumptions you make about patients.
Practice universal communication and interpersonal skills	Often, clinicians will not recognize when a bias is at play in a clinical encounter. The foundational communication and interpersonal skills described in this book (see Chapter 2, Interviewing, Communication, and Interpersonal Skills, p. 21) can reduce the impact of such truly unconscious biases on the way you interact with patients.
Explore your patients' identities	Many biases are anchored in clinician assumptions about patient identities. By simply asking patients to clarify what their identities mean to them, clinicians can dismantle their assumptions and better understand their patients. Many approaches to exploring patient identities are presented in this book (see pp. 52–53).

Explore your patients' experiences of bias	Clinical encounters are influenced by patients' prior experiences of implicit and explicit bias in their health care. Exploring and understanding these experiences can help you be a better partner with your patients. "Unfortunately, many of my patients have had negative experiences with health care. What have been your experiences with health care?"

Source: Burgess DJ, Fu SS, van Ryn M. Why do providers contribute to disparities and what can be done about it? *J Gen Intern Med.* 2004;19(11):1154–1159; Stone J, Moskowitz GB. Non-conscious bias in medical decision making: what can be done to reduce it? *Med Educ.* 2011;45(8):768–776; van Ryn M, Burgess DJ, Dovidio JF, et al. The impact of racism on clinician cognition, behavior, and clinical decision making. *Du Bois Rev.* 2011;8(1):199–218.

Cultural Humility

Cultural humility helps clinicians acknowledge and respect patients' individuality, mitigate implicit bias, and promote empathy. It involves self-reflection and critique as lifelong learners, examining cultural beliefs and systems to locate points of dissonance or synergy that contribute to patients' health outcomes.[57,58] To moderate disparities in health care, clinicians should engage in self-reflection, critical thinking, and cultural humility as they experience diversity in their clinical practices.[59–61] This process calls for clinicians to address power imbalances in communication with patients and maintain mutually respectful partnerships with patients and communities (Box 1-18).[62–66]

Box 1-18. Three Dimensions of Cultural Humility

Self-Awareness

Cultural humility begins with examining our own cultural identity, values, and biases. Overcoming biases, which are natural, but can influence our perceptions of others, is crucial.

For example, a clinician who grew up in a culture that stigmatizes mental health issues may need to challenge their own biases when working with a patient who is seeking treatment for depression. The clinician should recognize their own biases and strive to understand and respect the patient's cultural beliefs and values around mental health.

Respectful Communication

To provide culturally sensitive care, you should let patients lead the conversation about their unique cultural perspectives. Specific questions and an open, respectful attitude can elicit important information. You should be mindful of assumptions and acknowledge your own biases. Learning about a patient's culture can broaden understanding of their needs, but you should avoid stereotyping and research the life experiences of individuals in ethnic or racial groups in their area. Talking to different healers can also expand your knowledge.

For example, a clinician treating a patient from a culture that values natural remedies may need to ask specific questions about the remedies the patient is using and how they fit into the patient's overall treatment plan. The clinician should avoid making assumptions about the effectiveness or safety of these remedies and instead seek to understand the patient's cultural beliefs and values regarding health care.

Collaborative Partnerships

You can promote better health outcomes by cultivating self-awareness and empathy, building collaborative relationships with patients through respectful communication and openness to diverse perspectives. You should validate patients' emotions, remain flexible in treatment planning, and re-examine your own assumptions about clinical care. Success of care is determined by the patient's engagement and investment in your treatment plan.

For example, a clinician may need to collaborate with a patient from a culture that values community involvement in health care decisions. The clinician should be willing to engage with the patient's community and involve them in the patient's treatment plan. The clinician should also be willing to re-examine their own assumptions about what constitutes effective health care and work with the patient to develop a plan that reflects the patient's beliefs and values. The success of the plan will depend on whether the patient feels engaged and invested in the treatment.

Box 1-19. 5Rs of Cultural Humility

	Aim	Ask
Reflection	Clinicians will approach every encounter with humility and understanding that there is always something to learn from everyone.	What did I learn from each person in that encounter?
Respect	Clinicians will treat every person with the utmost respect and strive to preserve dignity at all times.	Did I treat everyone involved in that encounter respectfully?
Regard	Clinicians will hold every person in their highest regard, be aware of, and not allow unconscious biases to interfere in any interactions.	Did unconscious biases drive this interaction?
Relevance	Clinicians will expect cultural humility to be relevant and apply this practice to every encounter.	How was cultural humility relevant in this encounter?
Resiliency	Clinicians will embody the practice of cultural humility to enhance personal resiliency and global compassion.	How was my personal resiliency affected by this interaction?

Source: The 5Rs of Cultural Humility. Reprinted with permission from Society of Hospital Medicine. Accessed June 16, 2023. https://www.hospitalmedicine.org/practice-management/the-5-rs-of-cultural-humility/

The 5Rs of Cultural Humility *(reflection, respect, regard, relevance, and resiliency)* is a coaching tool (Box 1-19) that provides clinicians with a concise framework with specific aims and asks to incorporate skills identified at reducing implicit biases in health care.[67]

OTHER MAJOR CONSIDERATIONS

Other Major Considerations

- Spirituality
- Medical Ethics
- Decisional Capacity
- Approach to a Clinical Ethical Dilemma

Spirituality

Spirituality and religion are sometimes used interchangeably, but it is important to differentiate the two. *Spirituality* is a broader concept that encompasses religion, focusing on universal themes such as meaning, purpose, transcendence, and connection with others. It refers to the way individuals seek and express meaning and purpose and experience their connectedness to the moment, self, others, nature, and the significant and sacred.[68] *Religion*, on the other hand, involves specific beliefs, practices, texts, and rituals common to a community in relation to something larger than themselves, such as God, the holy, the transcendent, or a higher power.

Respecting patients' religious and spiritual beliefs is essential in culturally competent care. Box 1-20 provides questions to assess spirituality's role in health decisions and coping, while Box 1-21 outlines respectful practices for discussing beliefs in clinical settings.

Medical Ethics

While many clinicians have a general sense of right and wrong, the complexity and uncertainty of clinical situations require a more comprehensive set of ethical principles to guide decision making (Box 1-22).

Medical ethics is a subdiscipline of applied ethics, which itself is a subdiscipline of philosophy. It has an ancient heritage, typically traced back to the Hippocratic Oath, which includes principles such as beneficence, confidentiality, and nonmaleficence. However, this oath also reflected a paternalistic approach to medicine, which remained dominant as the profession became more formalized in the 18th century.[76,77]

In the 20th century, there were several events that challenged this dominant ethic of paternalism. Court decisions such as Schloendorff versus Society of New York Hospital established the need for clinicians to obtain informed consent from patients before treatment.[78] Additionally, revelations of physician misconduct, such as the Nazi doctors and the U.S. Tuskegee Syphilis study, led to a further reassessment of medical ethics.[79,80]

Box 1-20. Guiding Questions in Assessing the Role of Spirituality in Your Patient

- What values guide your patient's health care decisions?
  - Does your patient consult a religious/spiritual leader before making important health care decisions?
  - Does your patient have particular religious/spiritual concerns about blood products or porcine implants?
- How do patient spiritual beliefs and practices influence how they cope with their illness and care for themselves?[103]
  - Is there a significant community involved who may aid them while they are sick?
  - Is there a spiritual practice such as yoga or meditation that may aid them in their healing?
- Does your patient have spiritual struggle or distress and need a referral to a chaplain?
  - *Spiritual struggle* is defined as "...tensions, conflicts, and questions over sacred matters within oneself, with others, and with God."[104] Examples include feeling abandoned by God or one's religious community, a belief that the universe is out to get you, or doubts about one's fundamental beliefs and values.
  - Spiritual struggle has been shown to increase depressive symptoms, emotional distress, and risk of mortality while decreasing physical health, quality of life, and recovery of independence in daily activities.[105]

Box 1-21. Do's and Don'ts for Religious and Spiritual Beliefs in Clinical Encounters

Don't assume that patients are religious.	In the United States, 27% of adults identify as "spiritual, but not religious."[70,71]
Don't assume that patients are not religious.	Nearly 75% of U.S. adults identify as religious.[72]
Don't assume that you know what religion or spirituality means to the patient.	Patients often customize their beliefs and practices, so taking a spiritual history is important.
Don't assume that religion or spirituality has no effect on health.	Religion and spirituality can be social determinants of health and impact health outcomes positively or negatively. For example, Seventh-Day Adventists who follow a vegetarian diet for religious reasons live an average of 10 years longer than most Americans. On the other hand, medically ill older adult patients who feel that God has abandoned them have an increased risk of death.[73–75]
Do take a spiritual history.	Ask patients about their spiritual or religious beliefs, practices, and community involvement to understand how they may affect their health and health care decisions.
Do use nonjudgmental language.	Avoid imposing your beliefs on the patient or making assumptions. Use open-ended questions to encourage patients to share their beliefs and experiences.
Do be respectful of the patient's beliefs.	Show empathy and understanding toward their religious or spiritual practices and support their autonomy in making health care decisions that align with their beliefs.
Do be aware of resources available.	Accessing resources like chaplains or spiritual advisors can help provide additional support to patients.

Box 1-22. Core Values of Medical Ethics

- ***Nonmaleficence*** *("first, do no harm")* directive that health care professionals should avoid causing harm to patients and minimize the negative effects of treatments.
- ***Beneficence*** dictum that clinicians are to act for the patients' good by preventing or treating disease.
- ***Respect for autonomy*** commitment to accept the choices patients with decisional capacity make about which treatments to undergo, including to reject treatment. The addition of this value to medical ethics changed the clinician–patient relationship from a paternalistic one to a more collaborative one.
- ***Decisional capacity*** ability to make an autonomous choice that clinicians should respect.[83]
- ***Confidentiality*** duty to prevent the disclosure of patients' personal information to parties who are not authorized to learn that information.
- ***Informed consent*** principle that clinicians must elicit patients' voluntary and informed authorization to test or treat them for illness or injury. Because patients cannot consent to treatment without knowing what they are being treated for, this principle also encompasses the responsibility to inform patients of diagnoses, prognoses, and treatment alternatives.
- ***Truth telling*** value that clinicians should disclose information beyond that required by informed consent that may be relevant to patients (e.g., the number of similar procedures a physician has performed).
- ***Justice*** value that all patients with similar medical needs should receive similar medical treatment and should be treated fairly by clinicians.

As a response, there was a "bioethics revolution" in the mid-20th century, led by philosophers and theologians, which retained the older principles of Hippocratic and professional values, while also establishing respect for patient autonomy as a core value of medicine. This respect for autonomy empowered patients to make health choices that reflect their own views of what is good for them. Respect for autonomy, along with beneficence, nonmaleficence, and justice, became established as the common core of health care ethics and are now incorporated into most professional codes for health care providers.[81,82]

Decisional Capacity

Capacity and competence are two distinct concepts in health care. *Capacity* is a clinical designation that clinicians can assess, while *competence* is a judicial determination that only a court can make. Determining a patient's capacity to make informed health care decisions is important, and it involves assessing their ability to communicate a choice, understand relevant information, appreciate the situation and its consequences, and reason about treatment options (Box 1-23).[83]

Box 1-23. Elements of Decisional Capacity

Patients must have the ability to:

- Understand the relevant information about proposed diagnostic tests or treatment
- Appreciate their situation (including their underlying values and current clinical situation)
- Use reason to make a decision
- Communicate their choice

Source: Sessums LL, Zembrzuska H, Jackson JL. Does this patient have medical decision-making capacity? *JAMA.* 2011;306(4):420–427.

If a patient lacks capacity, identifying a health care proxy or surrogate decision maker is necessary, and this role may be assumed by a spouse or family member if the patient has not designated one. Importantly, decisional capacity is both temporal and situational and can fluctuate depending on the patient's condition and the complexity of the decision at hand.[84,85]

Approach to a Clinical Ethical Dilemma

Medical ethics is a crucial aspect of every clinical encounter with patients, even though it may not always be explicitly considered. As students, you will be exposed to ethical challenges that you may encounter in your future practice as clinicians. While adhering to ethical values becomes a natural part of clinical practice through training, some complex cases may require explicit and critical reflection to determine the ethical course of action. In such situations, heuristics can provide guidance on how to approach ethical dilemmas (Box 1-24).[86–88] While these practical methods may not guarantee an optimal or perfect solution, they can help achieve an immediate goal and lead to a satisfactory solution in situations where finding an optimal one is impossible or impractical.

Box 1-24. How to Resolve a Clinical Ethical Dilemma

Step	Description
1	Formulate an ethics question that summarizes the challenge they face in an ethically complex clinical situation.
2	Collect all of the information that clinicians believe is relevant to the case, including clinical information, patient's goals, preferences, cultural or religious commitments, financial resources, and interests and concerns of other stakeholders.
3	Identify the ethical principles and guidelines, including laws, institutional policies, and ethics concepts, that would guide the clinician's conduct in the case.
4	Reflect on how the relevant principles identified in the prior step would guide their conduct in the case and clarify the ethical dilemma if there is any.
5	Evaluate the different options and decide which ethical concept is the most important in the case and follow its guidance.
6	Make an action plan on how to communicate the decision and plan how to implement the ethical course of action. Enlist institutional support from an ethics consultant or committee and other services, such as social work services, if necessary.

REFERENCES

1. Athreya BH. *Handbook of Clinical Skills: A Practical Manual.* World Scientific Publishing Co.; 2010.
2. AAMC Task Force On the Clinical Skills Education of Medical Students. *Recommendations for Clinical Skills Curricula for Undergraduate Medical Education.* Association of American Medical Colleges; 2005. Accessed June 16, 2023. https://store.aamc.org/downloadable/download/sample/sample_id/174
3. Fortin AH VI, Dwamena FC, Frankel RM, Smith RC. *Smith's Patient-Centered Interviewing: An Evidence-Based Method.* 3rd ed. The McGraw-Hill Companies, Inc; 2012.
4. Smith RC. An evidence-based infrastructure for patient-centered interviewing. In: Frankel RM, Quill TE, McDaniel SH, eds. *The Biopsychosocial Approach: Past, Present, and Future.* University of Rochester Press; 2003:148.
5. Kleinman A, Eisenberg L, Good B. Culture, illness, and care: clinical lessons from anthropologic and cross-cultural research. *Ann Intern Med.* 1978;88(2):251–258.
6. Mauksch L, Farber S, Greer HT. Design, dissemination, and evaluation of an advanced communication elective at seven U.S. medical schools. *Acad Med.* 2013;88(6):843–851.
7. Haidet P, Paterniti DA. "Building" a history rather than "taking" one: a perspective on information sharing during the medical interview. *Arch Intern Med.* 2003;163(10):1134–1140.
8. Stewart M, Brown JB, Weston WW, McWhinney IR, McWilliam CL, Freeman TR. *Patient-Centered Medicine: Transforming the Clinical Method.* 2nd ed. Radcliffe Medical Press Ltd; 2003.
9. Atlas SJ, Grant RW, Ferris TG, Chang Y, Barry MJ. Patient-physician connectedness and quality of primary care. *Ann Intern Med.* 2009;150(5):325–335.
10. van de Poel K, Vanagt E, Schrimpf U, Gasiorek J. *Communication Skills for Foreign and Mobile Medical Professionals.* Springer; 2013.
11. Kurtz S, Silverman J, Benson J, Draper J. Marrying content and process in clinical method teaching: enhancing the Calgary–Cambridge guides. *Acad Med.* 2003;78(8):802–809.
12. Kurtz S, Silverman J, Draper J. *Teaching and Learning Communication Skills in Medicine.* 2nd ed. Radcliffe Medical Press; 1998.
13. Kurtz SM, Silverman JD. The Calgary–Cambridge Referenced Observation Guides: an aid to defining the curriculum and organizing the teaching in communication training programmes. *Med Educ.* 1996;30(2):83–89.
14. de Haes H, Bensing J. Endpoints in medical communication research, proposing a framework of functions and outcomes. *Patient Educ Couns.* 2009;74(3):287–294.
15. Tomsik PE, Witt AM, Raddock ML, et al. How well do physician and patient visit priorities align? *J Fam Pract.* 2014;63(8):E8–E13.
16. Suchman AL, Matthews DA. What makes the patient-doctor relationship therapeutic? Exploring the connexional dimension of medical care. *Ann Intern Med.* 1988;108(1):125–130.
17. Matthews DA, Suchman AL, Branch WT Jr. Making "connexions": enhancing the therapeutic potential of patient-clinician relationships. *Ann Intern Med.* 1993;118(12):973–977.
18. Larson EB, Yao X. Clinical empathy as emotional labor in the patient-physician relationship. *JAMA.* 2005;293(9):1100–1106.
19. Krasner MS, Epstein RM, Beckman H, et al. Association of an educational program in mindful communication with burnout, empathy, and attitudes among primary care physicians. *JAMA.* 2009;302(12):1284–1293.
20. Deutsch MB, Buchholz D. Electronic health records and transgender patients–practical recommendations for the

collection of gender identity data. *J Gen Intern Med.* 2015; 30(6):843–847.
21. Makoul G, Zick A, Green M. An evidence-based perspective on greetings in medical encounters. *Arch Intern Med.* 2007;167(11):1172–1176.
22. Meiri N, Ankri A, Hamad-Saied M, Konopnicki M, Pillar G. The effect of medical clowning on reducing pain, crying, and anxiety in children aged 2–10 years old undergoing venous blood drawing–a randomized controlled study. *Eur J Pediatr.* 2016;175(3):373–379.
23. Meiri N, Ankri A, Ziadan F, et al. Assistance of medical clowns improves the physical examinations of children aged 2–6 years. *Isr Med Assoc J.* 2017;19(12):786–791.
24. Damm L, Leiss U, Habeler U, Ehrich J. Improving care through better communication: understanding the benefits. *J Pediatr.* 2015;166(5):1327–1328.
25. Drutz JE, White-Satcher D. The pediatric physical examination: general principles and standard measurements. *UpToDate.* 2023. Accessed November 5, 2024. www.uptodate.com/contents/the-pediatric-physical-examination-general-principles-and-standard-measurements
26. Berlan ED, Bravender T. Confidentiality, consent, and caring for the adolescent patient. *Curr Opin Pediatr.* 2009; 21(4):450–456.
27. Gilbert AL, Rickert VI, Aalsma MC. Clinical conversations about health: the impact of confidentiality in preventive adolescent care. *J Adolesc Health.* 2014;55(5):672–677.
28. Lewis Gilbert A, McCord AL, Ouyang F, et al. Characteristics associated with confidential consultation for adolescents in primary care. *J Pediatr.* 2018;199:79–84.e1.
29. Friedman MR, Dodge B, Schick V, et al. From bias to bisexual health disparities: attitudes toward bisexual men and women in the United States. *LGBT Health.* 2014;1(4):309–318.
30. Polek CA, Hardie TL, Crowley EM. Lesbians' disclosure of sexual orientation and satisfaction with care. *J Transcult Nurs.* 2008;19(3):243–249.
31. Durso LE, Meyer IH. Patterns and predictors of disclosure of sexual orientation to healthcare providers among lesbians, gay men, and bisexuals. *Sex Res Social Policy.* 2013;10(1):35–42.
32. Strutz KL, Herring AH, Halpern CT. Health disparities among young adult sexual minorities in the U.S. *Am J Prev Med.* 2015;48(1):76–88.
33. Beckman HB, Frankel RM. The effect of physician behavior on the collection of data. *Ann Intern Med.* 1984;101(5): 692–696.
34. Jackson JL, Passamonti M, Kroenke K. Outcome and impact of mental disorders in primary care at 5 years. *Psychosom Med.* 2007;69(3):270–276.
35. Lang F, Floyd MR, Beine KL. Clues to patients' explanations and concerns about their illnesses. A call for active listening. *Arch Fam Med.* 2000;9(3):222–227.
36. Behforouz HL, Drain PK, Rhatigan JJ. Rethinking the social history. *N Engl J Med.* 2014;371(14):1277–1279.
37. Robbins JA, Bertakis KD, Helms LJ, Azari R, Callahan EJ, Creten DA. The influence of physician practice behaviors on patient satisfaction. *Fam Med.* 1993;25(1):17–20.
38. Agency for Healthcare Research and Quality. Use the Teach-Back Method: Tool #5. Content last reviewed September 2020. Accessed June 16, 2023. https://www.ahrq.gov/health-literacy/improve/precautions/tool5.html
39. Kripalani S, Jackson AT, Schnipper JL, Coleman EA. Promoting effective transitions of care at hospital discharge: a review of key issues for hospitalists. *J Hosp Med.* 2007;2(5): 314–323.
40. Kemp EC, Floyd MR, McCord-Duncan E, Lang F. Patients prefer the method of "tell back-collaborative inquiry" to assess understanding of medical information. *J Am Board Fam Med.* 2008;21(1):24–30.
41. Barry MJ, Edgman-Levitan S. Shared decision making–pinnacle of patient-centered care. *N Engl J Med.* 2012; 366(9):780–781.
42. Elwyn G, Frosch D, Thomson R, et al. Shared decision making: a model for clinical practice. *J Gen Intern Med.* 2012;27(10):1361–1367.
43. Epstein RM. Mindful practice. *JAMA.* 1999;282(9):833–839.
44. Beach MC, Roter D, Korthuis PT, et al. A multicenter study of physician mindfulness and health care quality. *Ann Fam Med.* 2013;11(5):421–428.
45. Institute of Medicine (US) Committee on Understanding and Eliminating Racial and Ethnic Disparities in Health Care. Smedley BD, Stith AY, Nelson AR, eds. *Unequal Treatment: Confronting Racial and Ethnic Disparities in Health Care.* National Academies Press (US); 2003.
46. *National Healthcare Disparities Report, 2013.* Agency for Healthcare Research and Quality; 2014. https://archive.ahrq.gov/research/findings/nhqrdr/nhdr13/index.html
47. Lucyk K, McLaren L. Taking stock of the social determinants of health: a scoping review. *PLoS One.* 2017;12(5):e0177306.
48. Wilkinson R, Marmot M, eds. *Social Determinants of Health: The Solid Facts.* 2nd ed., World Health Organization; 2003. Accessed November 5, 2024. https://iris.who.int/handle/10665/326568
49. Andermann A; CLEAR Collaboration. Taking action on the social determinants of health in clinical practice: a framework for health professionals. *CMAJ.* 2016;188(17–18):E474–E483.
50. FitzGerald C, Hurst S. Implicit bias in healthcare professionals: a systematic review. *BMC Med Ethics.* 2017;18(1):19.
51. *Racial Disparities in Health Care: Confronting Unequal Treatment, Hearing Before the Subcommittee on Criminal Justice, Drug Policy and Human Resources of the Committee on Government Reform.* Second Session. U.S. Government Printing Office; 2002. https://www.govinfo.gov/content/pkg/CHRG-107hhrg86436/pdf/CHRG-107hhrg86436.pdf
52. Chapman EN, Kaatz A, Carnes M. Physicians and implicit bias: how doctors may unwittingly perpetuate health care disparities. *J Gen Intern Med.* 2013;28(11):1504–1510.
53. Gordon HS, Street RL Jr, Sharf BF, Souchek J. Racial differences in doctors' information-giving and patients' participation. *Cancer.* 2006;107(6):1313–1320.
54. Penner LA, Blair IV, Albrecht TL, Dovidio JF. Reducing racial health care disparities: a social psychological analysis. *Policy Insights Behav Brain Sci.* 2014;1(1):204–212.
55. Burgess DJ, Fu SS, van Ryn M. Why do providers contribute to disparities and what can be done about it? *J Gen Intern Med.* 2004;19(11):1154–1159.
56. Stone J, Moskowitz GB. Non-conscious bias in medical decision making: what can be done to reduce it? *Med Educ.* 2011;45(8):768–776.
57. Tervalon M, Murray-García J. Cultural humility versus cultural competence: a critical distinction in defining physician training outcomes in multicultural education. *J Health Care Poor Underserved.* 1998;9(2):117–125.

58. Tervalon M. Components of culture in health for medical students' education. *Acad Med.* 2003;78(6):570–576.
59. Like RC. Educating clinicians about cultural competence and disparities in health and health care. *J Contin Educ Health Prof.* 2011;31(3):196–206.
60. Boutin-Foster C, Foster JC, Konopasek L. Viewpoint: physician, know thyself: the professional culture of medicine as a framework for teaching cultural competence. *Acad Med.* 2008;83(1):106–111.
61. Teal CR, Street RL. Critical elements of culturally competent communication in the medical encounter: a review and model. *Soc Sci Med.* 2009;68(3):533–543.
62. Smith WR, Betancourt JR, Wynia MK, et al. Recommendations for teaching about racial and ethnic disparities in health and health care. *Ann Intern Med.* 2007;147(9):654–665.
63. Embedding cultural diversity and cultural and linguistic competence: a guide for UCEDD curricula and training activities. Georgetown University Center for Child and Human Development; District of Columbia's University Center for Excellence in Developmental Disabilities; 2017. Accessed June 16, 2023. https://gucchd.georgetown.edu/resources.php
64. Juarez JA, Marvel K, Brezinski KL, Glazner C, Towbin MM, Lawton S. Bridging the gap: a curriculum to teach residents cultural humility. *Fam Med.* 2006;38(2):97–102.
65. Labib MA, Abou-Al-Shaar H, Cavallo C. Minimally invasive cranial neurosurgery in the 21st century. *J Neurosurg Sci.* 2018;62(6):615–616.
66. Jacobs EA, Rolle I, Ferrans CE, Whitaker EE, Warnecke RB. Understanding African Americans' views of the trustworthiness of physicians. *J Gen Intern Med.* 2006;21(6):642–647.
67. Masters C, Robinson D, Faulkner S, Patterson E, McIlraith T, Ansari A. Addressing biases in patient care with the 5Rs of cultural humility, a clinician coaching tool. *J Gen Intern Med.* 2019;34(4):627–630.
68. Puchalski C, Ferrell B, Virani R, et al. Improving the quality of spiritual care as a dimension of palliative care: the report of the Consensus Conference. *J Palliat Med.* 2009; 12(10):885–904.
69. Whitley R. Religious competence as cultural competence. *Transcult Psychiatry.* 2012;49(2):245–260.
70. Lipka M, Gecewicz C. More Americans now say they're spiritual but not religious. Pew Research Center; 2017. https://www.pewresearch.org/fact-tank/2017/09/06/more-americans-now-say-theyre-spiritual-but-not-religious/
71. Oppenheimer M. When some turn to church, others go to CrossFit. *New York Times.* November 27, 2015. https://www.nytimes.com/2015/11/28/us/some-turn-to-church-others-to-crossfit.html
72. Pew Research Center. Religious landscape study. https://www.pewforum.org/religious-landscape-study
73. Idler EL, ed. *Religion as a Social Determinant of Public Health.* Oxford University Press; 2014.
74. Fraser GE, Shavlik DJ. Ten years of life: is it a matter of choice? *Arch Intern Med.* 2001;161(13):1645–1652.
75. Pargament KI, Koenig HG, Tarakeshwar N, Hahn J. Religious struggle as a predictor of mortality among medically ill elderly patients: a 2-year longitudinal study. *Arch Intern Med.* 2001;161(15):1881–1885.
76. Baker RB, McCullough LB. What is the history of medical ethics? In: Baker RB, McCullough LB, eds. *The Cambridge World History of Medical Ethics.* Cambridge University Press; 2009:3–15.
77. McCullough LB. Contributions of ethical theory to pediatric ethics: pediatricians and parents as co-fiduciaries of pediatric patients. In: Miller G, ed. *Pediatric Bioethics.* Cambridge University Press; 2010:11–21.
78. *Schloendorff v. Society of the New York Hospital,* 105 NE 92 (211 NY 125 1914).
79. White BD, Shelton WN, Rivais CJ. Were the "pioneer" clinical ethics consultants "outsiders"? For them, was "critical distance" that critical? *Am J Bioeth.* 2018;18(6):34–44.
80. Fox RC, Swazey JP. *Observing Bioethics.* Oxford University Press; 2008.
81. Baker R. *Before Bioethics: A History of American Medical Ethics from the Colonial Period to the Bioethics Revolution.* Oxford University Press; 2013.
82. Jonsen AR. *The Birth of Bioethics.* Oxford University Press; 1998.
83. Appelbaum PS. Clinical practice. Assessment of patients' competence to consent to treatment. *N Engl J Med.* 2007; 357(18):1834–1840.
84. Sessums LL, Zembrzuska H, Jackson JL. Does this patient have medical decision-making capacity? *JAMA.* 2011;306(4): 420–427.
85. Joint Centre for Bioethics. Aid to Capacity Evaluation (ACE). University of Toronto, 2003. Accessed June 16, 2023. https://jcb.utoronto.ca/wp-content/uploads/2021/03/ace.pdf
86. *Core Competencies for Healthcare Ethics Consultation.* American Society for Bioethics and Humanities; 2011.
87. Shamoo AE, Resnik DB. *Responsible Conduct of Research.* 2nd ed. Oxford University Press; 2009.
88. DeLamater JD, Myers DJ. *Social Psychology.* 7th ed. Cengage Learning; 2010.
89. World Health Organization. Disability and Health. *World Health Organization,* 2023. Accessed November 5, 2024. www.who.int/news-room/fact-sheets/detail/disability-and-health
90. Institute on Disability, University of New Hampshire. *2023 Disability Statistics Annual Report.* ERIC. Accessed November 5, 2024. https://eric.ed.gov/?id=ED628657
91. Ward BW, Dahlhamer JM, Galinsky AM, Joestl SS. Sexual orientation and health among U.S. adults: national health interview survey, 2013. *Natl Health Stat Report.* 2014;(77): 1–10.
92. Gates GJ. Demographics and LGBT health. *J Health Soc Behav.* 2013;54(1):72–74.
93. Ahmad F, Hogg-Johnson S, Stewart DE, Skinner HA, Glazier RH, Levinson W. Computer-assisted screening for intimate partner violence and control: a randomized trial. *Ann Intern Med.* 2009;151(2):93–102.
94. United States Census Bureau. Same-Sex Couple Households: Characteristics by Sex of Spouses or Partners. *United States Census Bureau.* Accessed November 5, 2024. https://www.census.gov/data/tables/time-series/demo/same-sex-couples/ssc-house-characteristics.html
95. Institute of Medicine (US) Committee on Lesbian, Gay, Bisexual, and Transgender Health Issues and Research Gaps and Opportunities. *The Health of Lesbian, Gay, Bisexual, and Transgender People: Building a Foundation for Better Understanding.* National Academies Press (US); 2011. https://www.ncbi.nlm.nih.gov/books/NBK64806/
96. Tomczyk S, Bennett NM, Stoecker C, et al; Centers for Disease Control and Prevention (CDC). Use of 13-valent pneumococcal conjugate vaccine and 23-valent pneumococcal

polysaccharide vaccine among adults aged ≥65 years: recommendations of the Advisory Committee on Immunization Practices (ACIP). *MMWR Morb Mortal Wkly Rep.* 2014;63(37):822–825.

97. Centers for Disease Control and Prevention. 6440: National Health Interview Survey, 2022. *CDC Blogs.* Accessed November 5, 2024. https://blogs.cdc.gov/nchs/2022/05/25/6440/
98. James SE, Herman JL, Rankin S, Keisling M, Mottet L, Anafi M. *The Report of the 2015 U.S. Transgender Survey.* National Center for Transgender Equality; 2016. Accessed June 16, 2023. https://transequality.org/sites/default/files/docs/usts/USTS-Full-Report-Dec17.pdf
99. Ventres W, Kooienga S, Vuckovic N, Marlin R, Nygren P, Stewart V. Physicians, patients, and the electronic health record: an ethnographic analysis. *Ann Fam Med.* 2006;4(2):124–131.
100. Communication: what do patients want and need? *J Oncol Pract.* 2008;4(5):249–253.
101. Pollak KI, Arnold RM, Jeffreys AS, et al. Oncologist communication about emotion during visits with patients with advanced cancer. *J Clin Oncol.* 2007;25(36):5748–5752.
102. van Ryn M, Burgess DJ, Dovidio JF, et al. The impact of racism on clinician cognition, behavior, and clinical decision making. *Du Bois Rev.* 2011;8(1):199–218.
103. Puchalski C, Romer AL. Taking a spiritual history allows clinicians to understand patients more fully. *J Palliat Med.* 2000;3(1):129–137.
104. Exline JJ, Rose ED. Religious and spiritual struggles. In: Paloutzian RF, Park CL, eds. *Handbook of the Psychology of Religion and Spirituality.* 1st ed. Guilford Press; 2005:380–398.
105. Fitchett G, Risk JL. Screening for spiritual struggle. *J Pastoral Care Counsel.* 2009;63(1–2):4-1-12.

CHAPTER

2

Interviewing, Communication, and Interpersonal Skills

Choosing to enter the health care professions is a significant decision, often driven by the desire to foster effective, healing relationships—a cornerstone of patient care.[1] This chapter delves into the essential techniques of therapeutic interviewing, skills that require continual refinement throughout your career. Such skills are not innate; they necessitate diligent practice and constructive feedback from mentors to enhance your proficiency. As you gain experience, you will become adept at selecting the most appropriate techniques to navigate the complex dynamics of human behavior within patient relationships.

Chapter 1 introduced the concept that clinical interviewing transcends a mere exchange of questions and answers. It demands a nuanced sensitivity to patients' emotional and behavioral signals (Fig. 2-1). This approach allows you to weave together a patient's narrative in a way that is both dynamic and responsive to their cues, emotions, and concerns.[2]

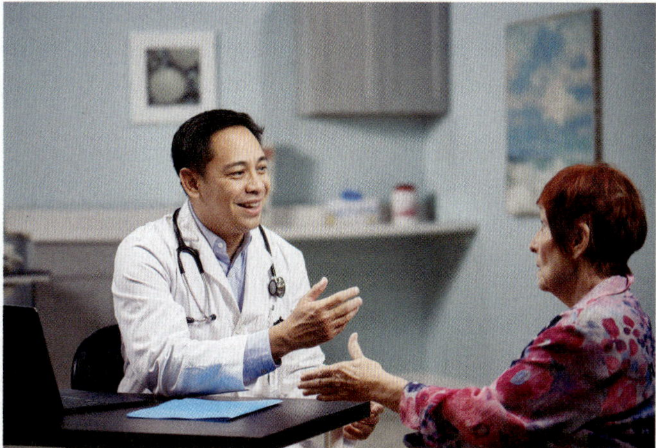

FIGURE 2-1. The interviewing process using effective communication skills.

Chapter 1 also highlighted that the competencies required for effective interviewing diverge significantly from those used in compiling a health history. While the health history format is crucial for categorizing a patient's medical story into relevant sections (present, past, and family health), it serves a different purpose from the interview process. The interview is about building a connection and understanding, whereas the health history provides a structured overview of the patient's medical background. As you explore the art of skilled interviewing in this chapter, appreciate the distinct yet complementary roles of these two aspects.

See Chapter 3, Health History, for the format of the health history, pp. 47–61.

Chapter Content Guide

- Organizing Patient–Clinician Communication Strategies
- Establishing the Foundation of Communication
- Building the Interaction
- Strengthening the Relationship
- Addressing Sensitive Topics
- Practicing Legal and Ethical Communication
- Using Advanced Communication Strategies
- Navigating Complex Discussions
- Encouraging Patient Self-Efficacy
- Enhancing Interprofessional Communication
- Managing Challenging Patient Situations and Behaviors
- Being Patient-Centered in Computerized Clinical Settings
- Learning Communication Skills from Standardized Patients

ORGANIZING PATIENT–CLINICIAN COMMUNICATION STRATEGIES

Communication skills refer to the ability to convey information effectively and efficiently in various contexts. These skills include listening, speaking, observing, empathizing, and using diplomacy and tact. Communication skills encompass the capacity to engage in meaningful interaction with others. They are fundamental to successful relationships, both personal and professional.

You may recall that the clinical encounter has a structure and sequence: *initiating the session, information gathering, physical examination, explaining and planning,* and *closing the session.*[3–5] In this section, we will consider the global communication and interpersonal techniques that can be used across all stages of the clinical encounter.

This chapter is organized to reflect the progression of a typical patient–clinician encounter, highlighting foundational communication skills, building rapport, addressing sensitive topics, and navigating through complex discussions and ethical considerations.

At the outset, **establishing the foundation of communication** focuses on initiating the interaction through active or attentive listening and empathic responses. These initial steps are crucial for building trust and understanding, setting the stage for a more in-depth exploration of the patient's concerns.

As the interaction progresses, the focus shifts to **building the interaction** through guided questioning and specific techniques aimed at eliciting detailed information from the patient. This segment ensures that the clinician gathers comprehensive data necessary for accurate diagnosis and treatment planning.

The **strengthening the relationship** section explores enhancing the patient–clinician relationship through summarization, transitions, validation, partnering, and empowering the patient. These strategies emphasize the importance of collaboration and shared decision-making in the therapeutic process.

Addressing sensitive topics and ethical considerations acknowledges the challenges of broaching sensitive subjects and the complexities of informed consent and working with medical interpreters. This part underscores the significance of ethical communication in maintaining patient dignity and autonomy.

Finally, **advanced communication strategies** and **navigating complex discussions** cover the delivery of serious news and advance care planning, while **encouraging patient self-efficacy** focuses on motivational interviewing (MI) as a technique to foster behavior change for improved health outcomes.

This structured approach to patient–clinician communication aims to enhance the effectiveness of clinical encounters, ensuring that patients feel heard, understood, and actively involved in their care.

ESTABLISHING THE FOUNDATION OF COMMUNICATION

Active (Attentive) Listening

Active listening or *attentive listening* lies at the heart of the patient interview. It involves several specific skills that enhance, guide, and structure your interaction. It involves intently focusing on the patient's messages, empathizing with their emotional state, and using both verbal and nonverbal cues to encourage them to share more about their feelings and concerns. Through active listening, you can connect with the patient on various levels of their experience, which requires practice.[6] It is common to become preoccupied with your next question or potential diagnoses, leading to a loss of focus on the patient's narrative. Therefore, concentrate on both what the patient is explicitly saying and the unspoken cues their body language may reveal, as these can sometimes convey a message that differs from their words.

BUILDING THE INTERACTION

Guided Questioning

Several strategies can help you gather more information without disrupting the patient's narrative flow. The objective is to enable comprehensive communication, allowing the patient to express themselves fully in their own words, without interruptions. With guided questions, you demonstrate ongoing interest in the patient's emotions and revelations (Box 2-1).[7] This approach prevents questions that might predetermine the direction of the conversation or inadvertently silence the patient. A series of "yes–no" questions can make the patient feel constrained and passive, resulting in a notable loss of detail. Guided questioning is a more effective way to capture the entirety of the patient's story.

By strategically using a variety of questioning techniques, clinicians can navigate the complexities of patient narratives, uncovering vital information that might otherwise remain obscured.

Box 2-1. Techniques of Guided Questioning

- Moving from open-ended to focused questions
- Using questioning that elicits a graded response
- Asking a series of questions, one at a time
- Offering multiple choices for answers
- Clarifying what the patient means
- Encouraging with continuers
- Using echoing/repetition

Moving from Open-Ended to Focused Questions. After inviting patients to share their story in their own words using open-ended questions, your questions become more focused, homing in on specific aspects of the patient's experience. This gradual narrowing of focus helps clinicians gather comprehensive data, while allowing patients to express themselves fully (Fig. 2-2).

Start with a genuinely open-ended inquiry that does not imply a specific answer. An effective sequence might look like this:

- *"Describe your chest discomfort."* (Pause)
- *"What more can you tell me?"* (Pause)
- *"Where exactly did you feel it?"* (Pause) *"Please show me."*
- *"Did you feel it anywhere else?"* (Pause) *"Did the sensation move?"* (Pause) *"Which arm did it move to?"*

Steer clear of *leading questions* that suggest a particular answer or response, such as: *"Has your pain been getting better?"* or *"You haven't noticed any blood in your stools, have you?"* Asking, *"Does your pain feel like pressure?"* may lead to a simple *"Yes"* that cuts short the opportunity for the patient to provide a detailed description of their experience. Instead, use a more neutral prompt like, *"Please describe your pain,"* to encourage a comprehensive response.

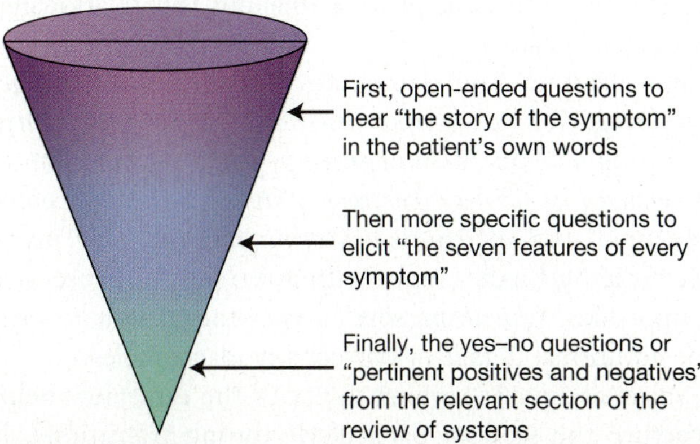

FIGURE 2-2. Guided questioning from open-ended to more focused questions.

Questioning that Elicits a Graded Response. Rather than settling for binary answers, this approach seeks to quantify experiences or symptoms, providing a richer, more nuanced understanding of the patient's condition.

Ask questions that require a graded response, providing deeper insight into the patient's condition, rather than a yes–no answer. For example, asking *"How many steps can you climb before feeling short of breath?"* is more informative than the straightforward *"Do you get short of breath climbing stairs?"*

Asking a Series of Questions, One at a Time. This clear, methodical approach prevents overwhelming the patient, ensuring that each question is given the attention it deserves and that answers are as informative as possible.

Be sure to ask one question at a time. Bundling inquiries such as, *"Any history of tuberculosis, diabetes, asthma, heart conditions, or high blood pressure in your family?"* might simply elicit a *"No"* due to confusion. Instead, frame your questions clearly, for example: *"Do you have any of the following health issues?"* Make sure to pause and establish eye contact before listing each condition individually. This approach helps maintain clarity and encourages more accurate responses.

Offering Multiple Choices for Answers. Sometimes, patients need help in describing their symptoms. By providing a range of options, clinicians can help patients better articulate their experiences, leading to more accurate and detailed responses.

To minimize bias, present multiple-choice options when asking questions. For example, inquire about the nature of pain by asking, *"Which of the following words best describes your pain: aching, sharp, pressing, burning, shooting, or something else?"* This method can be applied broadly; nearly every specific question can offer a choice between two alternatives, such as asking, *"Is your cough accompanied by phlegm, or is it dry?"* This approach encourages more precise responses and helps in gathering detailed information without leading the patient.

Clarifying What the Patient Means. This critical step ensures that the clinician's understanding aligns with the patient's intent, avoiding misinterpretations that could lead to misguided conclusions.

Phrases like *"Could you explain what you mean by 'the flu'?"* or *"You mentioned you were acting like your mother. Can you elaborate on that?"* are essential for this purpose. Taking the time to request such details conveys your genuine interest in comprehending the patient's story, which not only reassures them but also strengthens the therapeutic relationship.

Encouraging with Continuers. Nonverbal cues and verbal affirmations signal that you are engaged and interested, encouraging the patient to delve deeper into their narrative.

Even without speaking, your posture and gestures (*nonverbal encouragements*), as well as simple verbal affirmations (*neutral utterances*), can motivate the patient to share more. A pause, a nod, or maintaining attentive and relaxed silence signals to the patient to proceed. Leaning in, establishing eye contact, and using phrases such as *"Uh-huh," "Go on,"* or *"I'm listening"* all contribute to fostering an environment where the patient feels encouraged to continue their narrative.

Echoing (Repetition). This simple yet powerful technique reflects the patient's own words back to them, prompting further elaboration and demonstrating a genuine interest in their story. For instance, consider the following exchange:

- Patient: *"The pain got worse and started to spread."* (Pause)
- Response: *"Spread?"* (Pause)
- Patient: *"Yes, it moved to my shoulder and traveled down my left arm to my fingers. It was so severe I feared for my life."* (Pause)
- Response: *"Feared for your life?"*
- Patient: *"Yes, it reminded me of the pain my father experienced during his heart attack, which made me worry I was undergoing the same ordeal."*

Using this reflective technique not only uncovers the pain's location and intensity but also its significance to the patient. This approach avoids skewing the narrative or disrupting the patient's thought process.

STRENGTHENING THE RELATIONSHIP

Empathic Responses

Empathic responses play a crucial role in building patient rapport and fostering healing.[8,9] *Empathy* is often described as the ability to put yourself in the patient's shoes, to genuinely feel their pain as if it were your own, and to offer support in a compassionate manner.[10] It entails a readiness to share in the patient's suffering, an integral aspect of the healing process.[11] As patients communicate with you, they might reveal emotions through their words or facial expressions that they have not fully recognized themselves. Recognizing these unspoken feelings is key to understanding their health issues.

To effectively express empathy, first acknowledge the patient's emotions, then actively seek and engage with the emotional aspects of their experience.[12,13] Initially, delving into these emotions may feel uncomfortable, but such empathic engagement is vital for building deeper trust. When you pick up on subtle cues of unvoiced emotions, whether through facial expressions, tone of voice, behaviors, or their words, gently probe with questions like, *"How do you feel about that?"* or *"It seems like this is troubling you; can you tell me more?"*

Be aware that a patient's feelings may not always align with your initial perceptions. For example, assuming that a parent's death is solely a source of grief might overlook the patient's relief from a burdensome relationship. Instead, asking open-ended questions like, *"You've lost your father. What has that experience been like for you?"* encourages the patient to share their true feelings, avoiding assumptions on your part. Empathy can also be expressed nonverbally, such as by placing a hand on the patient's arm or offering tissues to a crying patient. Demonstrating your concern helps uncover vital aspects of the patient's experience.

Once the patient has opened up about their feelings, respond with understanding and acceptance. Your replies can be simple, yet profound, statements like, *"I can't imagine how difficult this must be for you," "That sounds very upsetting,"* or *"You must be feeling very sad."* For a response to truly be empathic, it must resonate with what the patient is feeling, conveying that you are genuinely sharing in their emotional experience.

Summarization

Summarizing the patient's story during the interview fulfills multiple objectives. It demonstrates that you have been listening attentively and clarifies what you understand and what you still need to learn. It allows for the correction of any misunderstandings and organizes the clinical reasoning process, making the relationship more collaborative.

For example, you might say, *"Let me ensure I've got everything. You've mentioned a cough for the last 3 days, worsening at night, accompanied by yellow phlegm. You've experienced no fever or shortness of breath, but you've noted congestion and difficulty breathing through your nose."* Encouraging further input with a thoughtful pause or a prompt like, *"Anything else?"* invites the patient to provide additional details or correct any inaccuracies.

Summarizing at various stages of the interview helps structure the session, particularly during transitions. It aids in organizing your clinical thoughts and sharing your diagnostic process with the patient, fostering a more collaborative relationship. Additionally, this strategy is beneficial for guiding clinicians, especially when they are uncertain about the next question to ask.

Transitions

Signposting or clearly stating when the interview is moving to a new topic or phase helps prepare the patient and reduces anxiety, facilitating a smoother interaction.

As you transition from taking the patient's history to conducting the physical examination, use concise transitional phrases to guide the patient, such as, *"I will now ask you some questions about your previous health."* Clearly communicate the next steps to ensure the patient knows what to expect. For example, you might say, *"Before we proceed to review your medications, is there anything else you'd like to share about your past health issues?"* When moving to the physical examination, inform the patient politely, *"We will now begin the physical examination. I'll leave the room for a moment. Please change into this gown."* This approach helps maintain a smooth and respectful flow of the consultation, ensuring the patient feels informed and comfortable with the process.

Validation

Validating the patient's emotional experience, especially in the context of distressing events or diagnoses, affirms their feelings as legitimate and understandable, enhancing trust and rapport.

A patient involved in a car accident, even without physical injuries, may experience significant distress. Acknowledging their feelings with a statement such as, *"It must have been frightening to be in that accident. Car accidents can be deeply unsettling, highlighting our vulnerability. It's completely natural that you're feeling upset,"* validates their emotions as both legitimate and understandable.

Partnering

Demonstrating a commitment to a lasting relationship offers patients the reassurance of ongoing care and support, an aspect that is especially comforting in hospital environments or throughout long-term treatment. This assurance of support is critical, particularly for students working in hospital settings, as it significantly impacts patient comfort and trust.

For instance, saying, *"I'm here for you, and we'll navigate this together,"* or *"We're committed to providing you continuous care and support at every step,"* can profoundly convey your dedication to their well-being and foster a strong sense of partnership.

Empowering the Patient

The relationship between clinician and patient is fundamentally unequal. As a student, you might initially feel inexperienced, but this feeling evolves as you gain more clinical expertise. On the other hand, patients often encounter vulnerabilities due to pain, anxiety about symptoms, or the overwhelming nature of accessing health care. Factors such as gender, ethnicity, race, and socioeconomic status further intensify this imbalance of power. Nevertheless, recognize that patients bear the ultimate responsibility for their own health care.[14] Empowering patients by encouraging them to ask questions, voice their concerns, and critically evaluate your recommendations significantly increases the likelihood that they will follow your advice, adopt healthier lifestyles, or adhere to prescribed medication regimens.[12]

Box 2-2 outlines strategies for equalizing the power dynamic with your patients. While many of these techniques have been addressed, emphasizing the importance of patients taking charge of their health is a key principle worth reiterating.

Reassurance

When patients are anxious or upset, offering quick reassurance like *"Don't worry. Everything is going to be alright"* might seem helpful, but for clinicians, such assurances can be premature and counterproductive. In some cases, they might even mislead and hinder further communication. Patients could interpret these reassurances as a sign of the clinician's discomfort with anxiety or an underestimation of their distress.

The first step to effective reassurance is simply identifying and acknowledging the patient's feelings. Saying something like, *"You seem upset today,"* can foster a connection and show empathy. Genuine reassurance should follow the completion of the interview, physical examination, and any necessary lab tests. At this juncture,

Box 2-2. Empowering the Patient: Techniques for Sharing Power

- Evoke the patient's perspective.
- Convey interest in the person, not just the problem.
- Follow the patient's leads.
- Elicit and validate emotional content.
- Share information with the patient, especially at transition points during the visit.
- Make your clinical reasoning transparent to the patient.
- Reveal the limits of your knowledge.

explaining your findings and addressing concerns directly is more impactful. Reassurance becomes meaningful and appropriate when the patient feels their issues are understood and actively managed.

ADDRESSING SENSITIVE TOPICS

In the upcoming chapters, you will discover how clinicians navigate discussions on a range of sensitive issues. Engaging in conversations about topics like alcohol or drug use, sexual practices, death, financial worries, racial and ethnic biases, domestic violence, mental health, physical abnormalities, and bowel function can be challenging, especially for those new to the field or when dealing with unfamiliar patients. Such discussions are often hindered by societal norms, even for experienced clinicians, as these subjects may provoke strong reactions stemming from personal, cultural, and societal beliefs.

To effectively address these sensitive subjects, several strategies can enhance your comfort and proficiency (Box 2-3). We recommend engaging with both clinical and general literature on these topics, discussing your concerns with peers and mentors, participating in courses designed to explore your emotional responses, and reflecting on your own experiences. Maximizing these resources is crucial. Observing seasoned clinicians handle these conversations and practicing their techniques can also be invaluable. As you gain experience, you will find your ability to discuss these topics with ease and sensitivity improves over time.

Box 2-3. Guidelines for Broaching Sensitive Topics[15]

- **Embrace nonjudgmental engagement:** The cornerstone principle is maintaining a nonjudgmental stance. Your objective is to learn from your patient and facilitate their journey toward improved health. Demonstrating acceptance is paramount to achieving this aim.
- **Clarify the purpose of your inquiries:** To mitigate patient anxiety, communicate the rationale behind your questions. For instance, you might tell a patient, *"In order to provide you with the best possible care, I need to ask some questions regarding your sexual health and practices."*
- **Identify and use appropriate opening questions:** Begin discussions on sensitive topics with carefully chosen questions, and understand the specific information required for a comprehensive assessment and collaborative planning.
- **Acknowledge your own discomfort:** Recognize and admit any personal discomfort you may feel about the topic. Ignoring these feelings can lead to avoidance of the subject, which is counterproductive.

van de Poel K, Vanagt E, Schrimpf U, Gasiorek J. *Communication Skills for Foreign and Mobile Medical Professionals.* Springer; 2013.

PRACTICING LEGAL AND ETHICAL COMMUNICATION

Informed Consent

A patient's consent to a procedure or treatment is more than simply signing a form. *Informed consent* involves a comprehensive communication process where a clinician thoroughly educates a patient about the risks, benefits, and alternatives associated with a procedure or intervention. This educational dialogue is crucial for ensuring that patients make informed decisions regarding their health care.[16] Box 2-4 describes the required elements for documentation of the informed consent discussion.

Clinicians bear both a legal and ethical obligation to adhere to this consent process meticulously, ensuring that no critical details are omitted.

Recognizing that each patient's situation is unique is key to obtaining informed consent. Variables such as personal circumstances, cultural background, and cognitive abilities can significantly influence decision-making capabilities. It is imperative to confirm that the patient has the *decisional capacity.* If doubts arise, consultation with the designated health care proxy becomes necessary. Effective communication involves using simple, nonpatronizing language and avoiding medical jargon. Using the teach-back method can be invaluable in gauging the patient's comprehension of the information.

See Chapter 1, Foundational Skills Essential to the Clinical Encounter for further discussion of the teach-back method, p. 10.

Providing additional resources for the patient to explore independently, like brochures, websites, or videos, can further aid in their understanding. Engaging in an open dialogue by encouraging questions and being available for follow-up discussions is fundamental.

Every patient with decisional capacity retains the right to either consent to or decline procedures or treatments once fully informed.

See determination of decisional capacity in Chapter 1, Foundational Skills Essential to the Clinical Encounter, p. 16.

Box 2-4. Essential Elements for Informed Consent Documentation

Element	Description	Sample Statements
Nature of the procedure or treatment	Clear explanation of what the patient should expect	*"This procedure involves..." "It's designed to..." "You can expect..."*
Risks and benefits	Honest discussion about the potential outcomes and the likelihood of success or complications	*"While many patients experience improvement, there are risks such as..." "The benefits include..."*
Reasonable alternatives	Information on other viable options, including opting for no treatment	*"Apart from this procedure, other options include... including the option of not undergoing any treatment at this time."*
Risks and benefits of alternatives	Comparison to help the patient understand their choices fully	*"Comparing this to the alternatives, the risks are... However, the benefits might be..."*
Assessment of patient understanding	Verification that the patient grasps the implications of their decisions based on the information provided	*"Do you feel you understand the differences between...?" "What are your thoughts on the risks and benefits I discussed?"*

Collaborating with a Medical Interpreter

A few words in the language that is most comfortable for your patient may enhance rapport, but they are no substitute for the full story. Even fluent speakers might miss subtle meanings in specific words. Likewise, relying on family members for translation can breach confidentiality and result in distorted or incomplete information. Key details may be lost as lengthy explanations are condensed. The best solution is a "*cultural navigator*": a neutral interpreter skilled in both the relevant languages and cultures. Nonetheless, even professionals might not fully understand the nuances of all subcultures.[17,18]

When working with an interpreter, start by building a connection and outlining the key information needed (Box 2-5). Ask that the interpreter translate everything without summarizing. To aid clarity, pose questions that are concise and direct. Clearly define your objectives for each part of the patient's history. Before starting, arrange the seating to maintain direct eye contact with the patient, which fosters a more personal connection. Speak directly to the patient, using "you" instead of referring to them in the third person, and position the interpreter to minimize the need to turn your head.

With linguistic diversity on the rise, clinicians increasingly rely on interpretation technologies to bridge the gap between languages and cultures. Box 2-6 provides a comparative overview of the current technologic solutions available for medical interpretation, highlighting their distinctive features and optimal use cases.

USING ADVANCED COMMUNICATION STRATEGIES

Appropriate Verbal Communication

As clinicians, we must be careful in *what* we say as well as *how* we say it. The effectiveness of the clinical encounter rests on the use of appropriate language. This can also enhance patient rapport and lead to a satisfying patient–clinician relationship.

Use Understandable Language. Using simple and clear language is key when talking to patients, no matter how much they know about health. Use easy-to-understand words (avoiding medical terms and abbreviations) and short sentences, and stick to the most important information.

For example, instead of, *"Does the pain radiate?"* ask, *"Does the pain move anywhere?"* If you use a word that is not understood, explain it in a way that is easier to understand. Also, choose specific and clear words over vague ones like "*a little bit*," "*common*," or "*rare*."

Box 2-5. Guidelines for Working with an Interpreter: "INTERPRET"

I	**Introductions:** Make sure to introduce all the individuals in the room. During the introduction, include what role each individual will play.
N	**Note goals:** Note the goals of the interview. What is the diagnosis? What will the treatment entail? Will there be any follow-up?
T	**Transparency:** Let the patient know that everything said will be interpreted throughout the session.
E	**Ethics:** Use qualified interpreters (not family members or children) when conducting an interview. Qualified interpreters allow the patient to maintain autonomy and make informed decisions about their care.
R	**Respect beliefs:** Patients with limited English proficiency (LEP) may have cultural beliefs that need to be considered as well. The interpreter may be able to serve as a cultural broker and help explain any cultural beliefs that may exist.
P	**Patient focus:** The patient should remain the focus of the encounter. Providers should interact with the patient and not the interpreter. Make sure to ask and address any questions the patient may have before ending the encounter. If you do not have trained interpreters on staff, the patient may not be able to call in with questions.
R	**Retain control:** As the provider, you must remain in control of the interaction and not let the patient or the interpreter take over the conversation.
E	**Explain:** Use simple language and short sentences when working with an interpreter. This will ensure that comparable words can be found in the second language and that all the information can be conveyed clearly.
T	**Thanks:** Thank the interpreter and the patient for their time. On the chart, note that the patient needs an interpreter and who served as interpreter.

Source: Administration for Children and Families. U.S. Department of Health and Human Services. INTERPRET tool: working with interpreters in cultural settings. Accessed March 17, 2024. https://www.acf.hhs.gov/sites/default/files/documents/otip/hhs_clas_interpret_tool.pdf

Always communicate clearly with all patients, no matter their education, wealth, or cultural background.

Remember, even with clear language, patients can feel overwhelmed if they get too much information at once. During visits, focus on one to three main points and repeat them often. A good way to make sure patients understand and engage in their care is by using the *"Ask Me Three" method*. This encourages patients to ask three important questions in each visit.[20]

1. What is my main problem?
2. What do I need to do?
3. Why is it important for me to do this?

Modifying this approach to "Tell Them Three" can also help clinicians keep their message focused and simple. Another approach to make sure your patient understands you is the teach-back method.[21,22] Keep in mind that "teach back" is not a test of the patient's knowledge but a test of how well you explained things in a manner your patient understands.

See Chapter 1, Foundational Skills Essential to the Clinical Encounter for further discussion of the teach-back method, p. 10.

Use Nonstigmatizing Language. It is important to use language that respects and affirms the individual's dignity during clinical interactions. Sometimes, we might inadvertently use phrases or terms in the clinical setting that could feel dehumanizing to the patient, perpetuating stigma and marginalization instead of fostering a supportive environment.[23] The language we choose should mirror the full spectrum of human identity, recognizing each person's potential for change and growth. Words that carry unintended stigma can alienate patients, deter them from seeking necessary support or treatment, and reinforce harmful stereotypes.[24]

For instance, instead of asking, *"Do you still consider yourself a drug addict?"* or *"Are you wheelchair bound?"*

Box 2-6. Comparative Overview of Medical Interpretation Technologies

Technology	Description	Ideal Use Cases
Telephonic interpretation	Provides interpretation services over the phone, connecting health care providers and patients with interpreters remotely[19]	Quick access to interpreters, especially for less commonly spoken languages, anonymity required situations, and when video or in-person interpretation is not feasible
Video remote interpreting (VRI)	Video conferencing tools provide real-time interpreting services, allowing interpreters to see and respond to nonverbal cues	Situations requiring visual communication, such as physical examinations, and when in-person interpreters are not available
Digital translation tools	Artificial intelligence–powered applications offering instant textual translations (such tools are constantly improving in accuracy but should be used with caution)	Quick, basic exchanges or preliminary understanding when human interpreters are unavailable, with a note on the potential for inaccuracies
Remote simultaneous interpretation (RSI)	Offers real-time interpreting with minimal delay through headphones, traditionally used in conferences, adapted for medical use	Complex discussions or procedures involving multiple nonnative speakers, facilitating smoother conversation flow without typical consecutive interpreting interruptions
Multilingual patient portals	Online platforms providing access to personal health records, appointment scheduling, and communication with providers in multiple languages	Enhancing patient engagement and understanding by offering accessible health information and services in the patient's preferred language
Augmented reality (AR) for sign language	Innovative use of AR technology to project sign language interpretation into the visual field, making information accessible for deaf or hard-of-hearing patients	Improving accessibility and communication in health care settings for patients with hearing impairments, especially where sign language interpreters are not available

consider phrasing these questions as "*Do you still see yourself as someone who has struggled with substance use?*" or "*Do you use a wheelchair daily?*"

A key strategy in avoiding stigmatizing language is adopting a *"people-first" approach*. Labeling someone a "drug abuser," for example, suggests that the individual's identity is the problem. A more supportive approach would be to say, "person who uses drugs" or "person with a substance use disorder," which acknowledges the issue without defining the person by it. This subtle shift in language can make a significant difference in how individuals perceive themselves and their ability to seek help and heal (Box 2-7).[25]

Appropriate Nonverbal Communication

As you attentively observe your patient, be mindful that the patient is also observing you. Whether consciously or not, you communicate messages through your words and actions. Your posture, gestures, eye contact, and tone of voice all significantly contribute to showing your level of interest, attention, acceptance, and understanding (Fig. 2-3).

The skilled interviewer appears calm and composed, even under time constraints. Patients can detect when you are distracted; therefore, mastering the ability to concentrate fully on the patient is vital. Patients are keenly aware of any signs of disapproval, embarrassment, impatience, or boredom as well as actions that may seem patronizing, stereotypical, critical, or dismissive. Maintaining professionalism demands balance and the practice of "unconditional positive regard" to foster therapeutic relationships.[26]

Both clinicians and patients engage in continuous nonverbal communication, offering essential insights into their emotions. Being attuned to these nonverbal signals enhances your ability to understand the patient

Box 2-7. Examples of Stigmatizing and Corresponding Nonstigmatizing Language

Ex-offender, thug, criminal, ex-felon, ex-con, convict, inmate, offender, felon, prisoner	Person who was/is incarcerated, formerly incarcerated person	Emphasizes the person beyond their past actions or the justice system's labels, recognizing their humanity first and foremost
Parolee, probationer	Person on parole, a person on probation	Focuses on the individual's current status without reducing their identity to that status, fostering a more neutral and respectful approach
Drug abuser, addict, junkie	Person who uses/injects drugs, a person with an addiction	Avoids derogatory terms that imply moral failing, focusing instead on the condition as a health issue, which encourages a more compassionate perspective
Schizophrenic, depressive	Person who has been diagnosed with schizophrenia or depression	Acknowledges the diagnosis without letting it define the individual, promoting an understanding that they are more than their mental health condition
AIDS or HIV patient, suffering from HIV, AIDS victim	Person living with HIV, a person living with AIDS	Shifts from defining individuals by their condition to recognizing their resilience and life beyond the diagnosis, removing implications of passivity or victimhood
Prostitute, hooker, street walker	Sex worker, a person who is involved in transactional or survival sex	Uses terms that respect the agency of individuals in their work or situation, moving away from judgmental and stigmatizing language
Rape victim	Sexual assault survivor, a rape survivor	Highlights the individual's resilience and survival, moving the focus away from victimhood to strength and recovery
Handicapped, disabled	People with disabilities	Puts the person first, recognizing them as individuals with disabilities rather than defining them by their disabilities
Normal, healthy, whole, or typical people	People without disabilities	Avoids implying that people with disabilities are abnormal or incomplete, promoting inclusivity and equality
Dwarf, a midget	Person of short stature, little person	Uses respectful and preferred terminology that avoids historical pejoratives and focuses on the individual, not their physical characteristics
Confined to a wheelchair; wheelchair bound	Person who uses a wheelchair or a mobility chair	Highlights the wheelchair as a tool for mobility rather than a constraint, recognizing the autonomy and mobility of the person using it

Source: People First Language. Texas Council for Developmental Disabilities. Accessed September 21, 2024. https://tcdd.texas.gov/wp-content/uploads/2021/06/People-First-Language.pdf

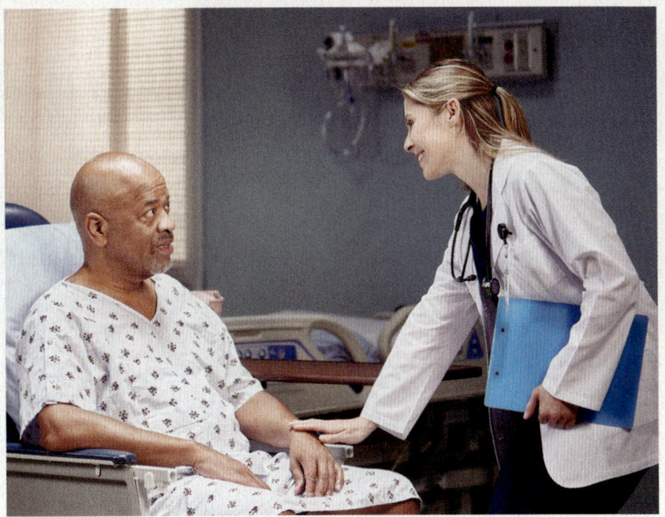

FIGURE 2-3. Nonverbal behaviors can convey empathy.

better and to effectively convey your own messages. Pay careful attention to nonverbal cues like *eye contact, facial expressions, posture, head movements, the space between you,* and the *positioning of limbs.* Recognize that while some nonverbal expressions are universal, others are culturally specific.

Mirroring the patient's posture can reflect a connection, while adjusting your own posture to align with the patient's may deepen rapport. Approaching the patient or offering a comforting touch, such as a hand on the shoulder, can express empathy and assist the patient in managing distressing emotions. Indeed, nonverbal communication may even surpass verbal interaction in expressing empathy[27] and is often the main medium for showing feelings.[28] The first step in using this powerful method is to observe nonverbal behaviors and become consciously aware of them (Box 2-8).

NAVIGATING COMPLEX DISCUSSIONS

Disclosing Serious News

The complex task of disclosing serious news to patients such as illnesses with poor survival outcomes, disease recurrence, or failure of treatments requires advanced communication skills. In addition to the verbal component of actually giving the serious news, it also requires

Box 2-8. Forms of Nonverbal Communication

Body orientation and proximity[29]	■ How you orient your body and the physical distance you maintain from a patient can signal your engagement and willingness to connect.
Gaze orientation (eye contact) toward patients[a,30,31]	■ Maintaining appropriate eye contact demonstrates your focus and concern for what the patient is sharing.
Head nodding with facial animation[a,32]	■ Nodding in response to patient statements, combined with expressive facial gestures, validates the patient's feelings and encourages them to continue sharing.
Head nodding with gesture[a,33]	■ Accompanying nods with gestures can underscore understanding and agreement, enhancing the communicative exchange.
Posture	■ An open, relaxed posture invites trust and openness, while a closed posture may suggest disinterest or discomfort.
Tone and use of voice	■ The tone, pitch, and speed of your speech can greatly affect how your message is received, conveying empathy, urgency, or calm as needed.
Use of silence	■ Strategic pauses can give patients the time to reflect and express themselves more fully, indicating that you value their thoughts.
Use of touch (*haptics*)	■ Appropriate, gentle touch can communicate support and compassion, breaking down barriers and soothing anxieties.

[a]Found in studies to be correlated with increasing patient rapport with clinician.

responding to patients' emotional reactions, shared decision-making, the stress created by patients' expectations, the involvement of multiple family members, and how to provide hope despite a bleak situation.[34] The SPIKES protocol for disclosing serious news has been recommended to guide clinicians due to the complexity of these interactions that can often create serious communication issues. The six-step protocol: **S**etting up the interview, assessing the patient's **P**erception, obtaining the patient's **I**nvitation, giving **K**nowledge and information to the patient, addressing the patient's **E**motions with empathic responses, and **S**trategy and **S**ummary (Box 2-9).[34,35]

Advance Care Planning

In general, encourage any adult, but especially adults who are older or chronically ill, to have an *advance directive* and establish a *health care proxy* or *health care power of attorney* who can act as the patient's health decision maker. Part of this process involves conducting a "*values history*" during the interview (Box 2-10). This aims to understand what the patient values in life, what gives their life meaning, and under what circumstances they would find life no longer worth living.

Engage in conversations about how they spend their days, their pleasures, and what they look forward

Box 2-9. SPIKES: Six-Step Protocol for Delivering Bad News

Steps	Information
1: **S**etting up the interview	■ Ensure privacy to create a comfortable environment. ■ Include family members or significant others, as appropriate. ■ Sit down to signal your full attention and to physically level with the patient. ■ Establish a personal connection to build rapport. ■ Manage your time and minimize interruptions to maintain focus, indicating readiness with statements like, *"Let me take a moment to ensure everything is in order."*
2: Assessing the patient's **P**erception	■ Use open-ended questions to understand the patient's view of their medical situation, such as, *"What are your thoughts following the biopsy?"* or *"How do you interpret the need for the MRI?"*
3: Obtaining the patient's **I**nvitation	■ Clarify the patient's desire for information. The key is not if they want to know, but how much detail they seek. Ask, for example, *"If the results are serious, would you prefer to know all the details?"*
4: Giving **K**nowledge and information to the patient	■ Tailor the delivery of information to the patient's level of understanding and desire for detail. ■ Begin with a gentle warning, like *"Unfortunately, I have some bad news,"* to brace the patient. ■ Allow a pause after delivering the main information to let the patient process the news. ■ Use clear, straightforward language, avoiding medical jargon.
5: Addressing the patient's **E**motions with **E**mpathic responses	■ Anticipate an emotional response first and foremost. ■ Recognize and validate these feelings openly with responses like, *"I can see this is very distressing for you,"* or *"It's clear this wasn't the news you were hoping for. I'm truly sorry."*
6: **S**trategy and **S**ummary	■ Confirm that the patient has understood the information shared. Only then, discuss the next steps, ensuring they are ready for this discussion. ■ Offer support and clarify any questions, suggesting, *"Is there anything specific I can do to help right now?"* or *"Let's talk about what comes next and make sure you're comfortable with our plan."*

Sources: Baile WF, Buckman R, Lenzi R, Glober G, Beale EA, Kudelka AP. SPIKES-A six-step protocol for delivering bad news: application to the patient with cancer. *Oncologist*. 2000;5(4):302–311; VitalTalk. *Serious News*. Accessed March 17, 2024. https://www.vitaltalk.org/guides/serious-news/

Box 2-10. Values History Interview Guide

Aspect of Care	Questions for Patients
Life-sustaining treatment	*"How do you feel about life-sustaining treatments in situations of severe illness? What's important to you in making such decisions?"*
Pain management	*"In managing serious illness, would you prioritize pain management over extending life, especially if it affects your alertness or lifespan? Can you share your thoughts on this?"*
Personal interactions	*"What aspects of dignity, respect, and communication are most important to you when receiving health care?"*
End-of-life care	*"Could you share your preferences regarding end-of-life care? For instance, do you have a preference for being at home, if possible?"*
Organ donation	*"What are your views on organ donation? Is this something you would consider, and under what conditions?"*
Spiritual/religious beliefs	*"Do your spiritual or religious beliefs play a role in your health care decisions? How can we respect these beliefs in your care plan?"*
Independence	*"How important is it for you to maintain independence during treatment? Are there any treatments you would decline if they might diminish your independence?"*

to (Fig. 2-4). When a patient expresses concerns, like not wanting to be a burden, delve deeper by asking them to elaborate. Explore any worries they may have regarding their illness, pain, or treatment preferences, and offer information and support to address these concerns. Discuss the patient's religious or spiritual beliefs to make informed health care decisions together.

Remember, patients nearing the end of their life may not always want to discuss their illness at every meeting, nor share their feelings with everyone. If they prefer light, social interaction, honor that choice. Simple acts of kindness, such as smiling, a gentle touch, asking about their family, commenting on current events, or sharing light humor can show your care and attention.

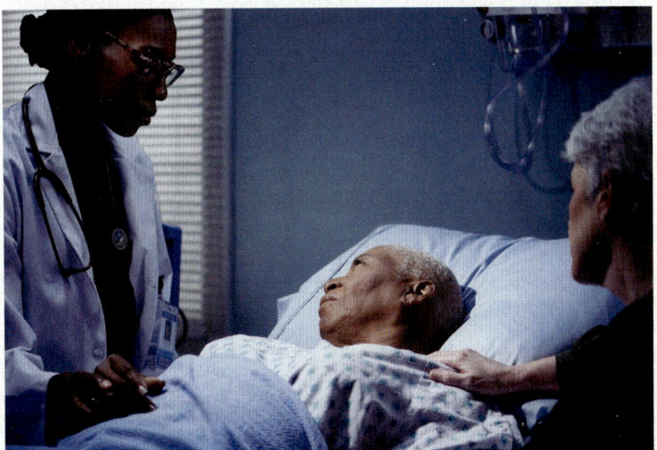

FIGURE 2-4. Learn how to improve the care of dying patients.

Facilitating discussions about end-of-life treatment is a key responsibility. Neglecting to address these decisions is considered a significant oversight in clinical care. The nature of these discussions can depend on the patient's health status and setting. For terminally ill or frail patients expected to live less than a year, completing a *Physician Orders for Life Sustaining Treatment (POLST)* or *Medical Orders for Life-Sustaining Treatment (MOLST)* form is recommended.[36,37]

The POLST/MOLST form, which exists at various levels of implementation in the United States, is an actionable medical order form that tells others the patient's medical treatment preferences.[38] Creating these orders involves detailed conversations about the patient's values, beliefs, and care goals, alongside the health care professional's insights into the diagnosis, prognosis, and treatment options. This collaborative process ensures that the patient's wishes are clearly understood and respected.[36]

In acute hospital settings, discussions about how to handle cardiac or respiratory emergencies, including *Do Not Resuscitate (DNR)* orders or allowing natural death, are essential. These conversations might be challenging, especially without an established relationship with the patient or if the patient has misconceptions

Box 2-11. Key Strategies of Motivational Interviewing

Strategy	Description
Express empathy	Create a supportive and understanding environment. Accept patients' feelings and perspectives without judgment to build rapport and trust, which is crucial for motivating change.
Develop discrepancy	Help patients recognize the gap between their current behaviors and the healthier behaviors they aspire to. This can make the reasons for change more apparent and compelling.
Roll with resistance	Instead of arguing or confronting directly, listen to patients' concerns and preferences, maintaining an open dialogue that respects their autonomy.
Support self-efficacy	Encourage belief in the ability to change by discussing past successes, strategies to overcome obstacles, and affirming their right to choose their health path.
Identify and enhance motivation	Engage patients in exploring their motivations for change. Use open-ended questions to help them articulate their own reasons for wanting to improve health or behaviors.
Plan for change	Collaborate on a specific, actionable plan once a patient is ready to make a change. Set achievable goals and discuss strategies for dealing with potential challenges.

about their illness or the effectiveness of resuscitation, often influenced by unrealistic media portrayals. Ask about the patient's previous experiences with death and their understanding of cardiopulmonary resuscitation (CPR). Educating patients on the realistic outcomes of CPR, particularly for those with chronic conditions or advanced age, and reassuring them that their comfort, pain management, and spiritual needs will be prioritized, are integral parts of this discussion.

ENCOURAGING PATIENT SELF-EFFICACY

Motivational Interviewing (MI)

MI is a critical tool in the health care provider's toolkit, especially useful during patient consultations that conclude with the need for lifestyle or behavioral changes. Such changes might include adopting a healthier diet, increasing physical activity, quitting smoking or alcohol, following medication schedules more closely, or applying specific self-management techniques. MI is particularly effective in improving health outcomes for patients dealing with substance overuse issues, but its principles can be applied broadly across a range of behavioral health challenges.[39] At its core, MI is a collaborative, patient-centered form to elicit and strengthen motivation for change. It engages with patients in a way that respects their autonomy and empowers them to discover their personal reasons for making health-related changes, rather than prescribing actions they should take.

Box 2-11 lists key components and steps involved in MI, which can help you implement this approach effectively.

For further discussion of MI, see Chapter 7, Health Maintenance and Screening, pp. 130-132.

ENHANCING INTERPROFESSIONAL COMMUNICATION

As a trainee in the clinical environment, you will often find yourself caring for patients with other trainees and clinicians from various fields such as medicine, nursing, dentistry, advanced practice nursing, social work, podiatry, and rehabilitation therapists (Fig. 2-5). Working as a team using effective communication is key to providing efficient, quality care that leads to excellence in patient outcomes.[40] Collaboration between disciplines is also critical in minimizing the risk of errors in patient care.[41] However, many barriers can obstruct this team-based approach (Box 2-12).[42–44] Mutual respect is essential for interprofessional communication because it helps facilitate a positive environment for setting shared goals, creating collaborative plans, making decisions, and sharing responsibilities.[45]

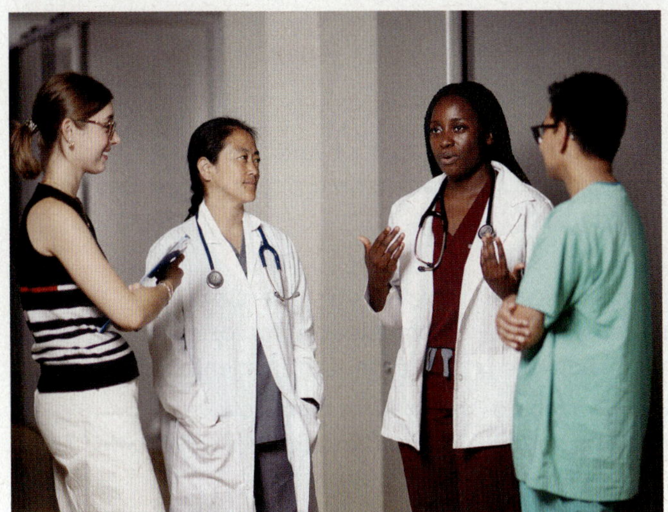

FIGURE 2-5. Effective communication between disciplines is key to patient safety.

Box 2-13 outlines prominent frameworks for improving interprofessional communication. Each framework provides unique strategies and tools to improve interprofessional communication and collaboration, aiming to enhance patient care and outcomes by fostering a culture of teamwork and mutual respect among health care professionals from different disciplines.

One of the tools to improve interprofessional communication and teamwork is the SBAR (**S**ituation-**B**ackground-**A**ssessment-**R**ecommendation), a shared mental model that provides a clear, concise, and organized framework for communication between clinicians. This tool facilitates active listening (Box 2-14) and provides all interprofessional team members a constructive and standardized approach to openly discuss patient issues they may have, especially around patient safety.[46]

MANAGING CHALLENGING PATIENT SITUATIONS AND BEHAVIORS

As you spend time inviting patient stories, you will find that some patients are more difficult to interview than others. Clinicians may find it challenging to care for people who are silent, while finding those who are assertive to be more demanding. Being aware of your reactions helps develop your clinical skills. Your success in eliciting the history from different types of patients grows with experience, but takes into account your own stressors, such as fatigue, mood, and overwork. Self-care is also vital in caring for others. Even if a patient is challenging, *always remember the importance of listening to the patient and clarifying their concerns.*

Learning how to communicate effectively with different types of patients is crucial. Box 2-15 focuses on the specific communication skills you will need to connect with various patients effectively. Whether it is offering support to silent patients, managing conversations with talkative ones, or providing reassurance to those who are anxious, understanding how to adjust your communication approach is key.

Box 2-12. Strategies to Overcome Barriers to Interprofessional Communication

Barrier	Description and Adaptation
Diverse skill sets and knowledge	■ Variations in backgrounds lead to different patient care approaches. ■ Adaptation: Participate in interprofessional simulations to appreciate diverse expertise.
Different professional identities	■ Strong discipline-specific identities can hinder a unified care perspective. ■ Adaptation: Engage in multidisciplinary projects to value each role.
Lack of interprofessional cultural competence	■ Not understanding other professions' roles impedes teamwork. ■ Adaptation: Attend cultural competence workshops to foster collaboration.
Perceived power differentials	■ Hierarchical dynamics can silence lower-ranking team members. ■ Adaptation: Practice assertive communication in role-playing to voice contributions equally.
Profession-centric role models	■ Emphasis on discipline excellence over teamwork reinforces silos. ■ Adaptation: Seek mentors who exemplify interprofessional collaboration.

Box 2-13. Frameworks for Enhancing Interprofessional Communication in Health Care

Framework	How It Works	Description
Interprofessional Education Collaborative (IPEC) Competencies	Focuses on developing core competencies across four domains: values/ethics, roles/responsibilities, interprofessional communication, and teams/teamwork	Prepares health professions students for integrated team-based care
Canadian Interprofessional Health Collaborative (CIHC) Framework	Outlines competencies in six domains essential for interprofessional collaboration, including role clarification and team functioning	Provides a set of national competencies for fostering effective teamwork and patient-centered care
Four Cs Model	Emphasizes communication, cooperation, coordination, and collaboration as key components for effective interprofessional teamwork	Enhances teamwork and communication among health care professionals
TeamSTEPPS®	Offers strategies and tools focusing on leadership, situation monitoring, mutual support, and communication to enhance team performance and patient safety	Evidence-based framework designed to improve patient safety and quality through better communication and teamwork

Sources: IPEC Core Competencies for Interprofessional Collaborative Practice: Version 3 (2023). Interprofessional Education Collaborative (IPEC). https://www.ipecollaborative.org/ipec-core-competencies. Accessed March 17, 2024. Canadian Interprofessional Health Collaborative (CIHC) framework. Canadian Interprofessional Health Collaborative (CIHC) framework. https://www.mcgill.ca/ipeoffice/ipe-curriculum/cihc-framework. Accessed March 17, 2024. TeamSTEPPS (July 2023). Agency for Healthcare Research and Quality, Rockville, MD. https://www.ahrq.gov/teamstepps-program/index.html. Accessed March 17, 2024.

Box 2-14. SBAR: Tool to Facilitate Interprofessional Communication

SBAR	Examples
Situation (a concise statement of the problem)	*"I am…I am calling because…" "I have a patient who is…"*
Background (pertinent and brief information related to the situation)	*"The patient was admitted on…because of…"*
Assessment (analysis and considerations of options — what you found/think)	*"I think this patient is likely having a…"*
Recommendation (action requested/ recommended — what you want)	*"Let us transfer…" "Let us monitor and then…"*

Source: Institute for Healthcare Improvement. SBAR Tool: Situation-Background-Assessment-Recommendation. 2017. ihi.org/resources/Pages/Tools/SBARToolkit.aspx. Accessed March 17, 2024.

Box 2-15. Communication Approaches Based on Specific Patient-Centered Clinical Situations

Patient Type	Key Considerations and Strategies	Communication Skills and Techniques
Patient who is silent	▪ Silence can have many meanings (thought collection, trust evaluation). ▪ Clinicians should be attentive, respectful, and encourage continuation when ready. ▪ Watching for nonverbal cues is crucial. ▪ Comfort with silence can be therapeutic. ▪ Directly address if silence may be due to clinician's approach or oversight of symptoms.	*Silent support:* Use nonverbal cues to show attentiveness, and use open-ended questions to encourage dialogue.

Patient Type	Key Considerations and Strategies	Communication Skills and Techniques
Patient who is talkative	■ Allow the patient free reign initially while listening carefully. ■ Focus on what seems most important to the patient and show interest by asking relevant questions. ■ Learn to set limits and structure the interview to gain valuable information. ■ Summarize patient concerns to validate them and then focus on specific issues. ■ Avoid showing impatience and prepare the patient for a follow-up visit if necessary.	*Active listening and structuring:* Practice active listening while guiding the conversation to remain focused on relevant topics.
Patient with a confusing narrative	■ Keep differential diagnoses in mind when assessing confusing stories. ■ Use skills of guiding, clarification, and summarizing to construct a coherent story. ■ Focus on the patient's perspective and guide the interview into a psychosocial assessment for patients presenting with multiple symptoms. ■ Transition to mental status examination if necessary, focusing on consciousness, orientation, memory, and understanding. ■ Seek information from other sources if the patient cannot provide their own history.	*Clarification and summarizing:* Use clarification techniques and summarize information to achieve a coherent understanding.
Patient with emotional lability	■ Crying signals strong emotions; pause, probe gently, or respond with empathy. ■ Offer a tissue, wait for recovery, and make supportive remarks. ■ Learn to accept displays of emotion to support patients effectively.	*Empathetic response:* Show empathy and patience, allowing space for emotions while gently guiding the conversation.
Patient who is angry or aggressive[47]	■ Acknowledge justified anger and try to make amends. ■ Accept angry feelings without retreating or reciprocating. ■ Validate feelings without reinforcing negative criticism (Fig. 2-6). ■ Maintain a calm, nonconfrontational stance and suggest moving to a private area if needed. ■ Listen carefully to understand the root of the anger.	*De-escalation techniques:* Use calming language, validate feelings, and maintain a nonthreatening posture to de-escalate aggression.

(continued)

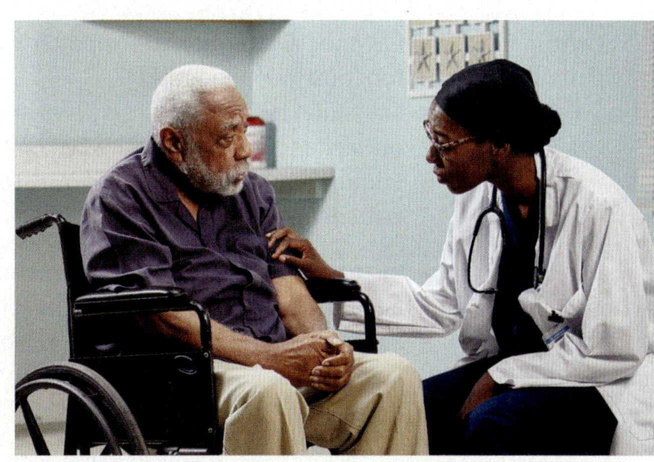

FIGURE 2-6. Validate the patient's feelings.

Box 2-15. Communication Approaches Based on Specific Patient-Centered Clinical Situations (*Continued*)

Patient Type	Key Considerations and Strategies	Communication Skills and Techniques
Patient exhibiting overly friendly behavior	■ Recognize and manage your feelings to maintain professionalism. ■ Set clear professional boundaries. ■ Leave and find a chaperone if necessary. ■ Evaluate and avoid sending misleading signals. ■ *Any* inappropriate physical contact or romantic involvement with patients is *unethical* keep your relationship with the patient within professional bounds and seek help if you need it.[48–51]	*Boundary setting:* Communicate boundaries clearly and maintain professional demeanor at all times.
Patient who is discriminatory	■ Assess the situation and decide whether to continue care or seek help. ■ Cultivate a therapeutic alliance with the patient with supervisor support.[52] ■ Discriminatory patient behavior should be named and processed appropriately, since such interactions with patients can undermine your resilience. ■ Address discriminatory behavior directly with your supervisor.[53] ■ Establish a supportive learning environment and receive training on handling discrimination. ■ You should be empowered to state your discomfort with continuing an encounter with a discriminatory patient to your supervisor.	*Assertive communication:* Address discriminatory remarks directly while maintaining professionalism and seeking support if needed.
Patient with hearing loss	■ Determine the patient's preferred communication method. ■ Use certified American sign language interpreters or written communication as needed. ■ Ensure the environment is conducive to effective communication (eliminate background noise, face the patient, etc.).[54,55]	*Adapted communication:* Use visual aids, sign language interpreters, or written methods to ensure understanding.
Patient with low or impaired vision	■ Establish contact and explain who you are and the purpose of your visit. ■ Orient the patient to the surroundings. ■ Adjust lighting if necessary and encourage the use of glasses. ■ Rely more on verbal explanations.	*Verbal guidance and description:* Use detailed verbal explanations and guide the patient through the clinical process with clear, descriptive language.
Patient with limited intelligence	■ Pay special attention to the patient's school record and ability to function independently. ■ Transition to the mental status examination for deeper understanding if needed. ■ Engage family or caregivers for history but show interest in the patient first.	*Simplified language and visual aids:* Use simple, clear language and visual aids to enhance understanding.
Patient burdened by personal problems	■ Instead of giving direct advice, encourage the patient to discuss alternatives and the pros and cons of each. ■ Let the patient talk through the problem, offering a therapeutic listening ear.	*Supportive listening:* Listen and encourage the patient to explore their feelings and options.

Patient Type	Key Considerations and Strategies	Communication Skills and Techniques
Patient who is nonadherent	■ Recognize factors leading to nonadherence such as cognitive abilities, emotional status, and socioeconomic conditions.[56,57] ■ Employ strategies for better adherence like informational handouts and positive feedback.[58]	*Motivational interviewing:* Explore and resolve ambivalence toward treatment.
Patient with low literacy	■ Assess reading ability and comfort with health forms discreetly. ■ Be sensitive and do not confuse literacy with intelligence.[59] ■ Explore reasons for impaired literacy and provide suitable support.	*Clear and simple communication:* Use plain language and ensure the patient understands the instructions through verbal confirmation.
Patient with low health literacy	■ Health literacy involves the ability to navigate the health care environment effectively. ■ Tailor communication to enhance the patient's ability to understand health information and make informed decisions.[60]	*Teach-back method:* Confirm the patient's understanding of health information.
Patient with limited language proficiency	■ Utilize qualified interpreters and ensure communication is culturally and linguistically appropriate.[61] ■ Learning to work with interpreters effectively is crucial for optimal patient care.[62–66]	*Use of interpreters and cultural sensitivity:* Work effectively with interpreters and show sensitivity to cultural differences.
Patient with a terminal illness or who is dying	■ Engage in open discussions about preferences for care and understand the stages of grief.[67,68] ■ Provide support and ensure excellent communication with patients nearing the end of their lives.[68–70] ■ There are overlapping and sometimes prolonged phases of anticipatory grief and bereavement (Box 2-16).[71]	*Compassionate communication:* Offer support and understanding during difficult conversations.

Box 2-16. Kübler–Ross Model: Five Stages of Grief[72,73]

Stage	Description
Denial	The initial stage where individuals may refuse to accept the reality of their situation, often as a defense mechanism.
Anger	Feelings of frustration, resentment, or rage toward oneself, others, or the circumstances surrounding the loss or illness.
Bargaining	Attempts to negotiate or make deals in an effort to postpone or mitigate the inevitable outcome, often with a higher power.
Depression	Deep feelings of sadness, hopelessness, and despair as the individual begins to confront the reality of their situation.
Acceptance	The final stage marked by a sense of peace, calm, and understanding of the situation, allowing for greater emotional resolution.

BEING PATIENT-CENTERED IN COMPUTERIZED CLINICAL SETTINGS

In modern clinical practice, the widespread adoption of the electronic health record (EHR) marks a significant change.[74] The presence of a computer during a clinical encounter transforms the traditional dyadic patient–clinician interaction into a triadic one (Fig. 2-7).[75]

Negative communication behaviors associated with EHR use include interruptions in patient and clinician speech, increased gaze shifts and multitasking episodes, and limited sharing of the computer screen with patients.[76,77] Numerous strategies and techniques have been identified to help clinicians maintain rapport with patients and mitigate the negative impact of EHRs on communication in computerized settings, as outlined in Box 2-17.[78,79]

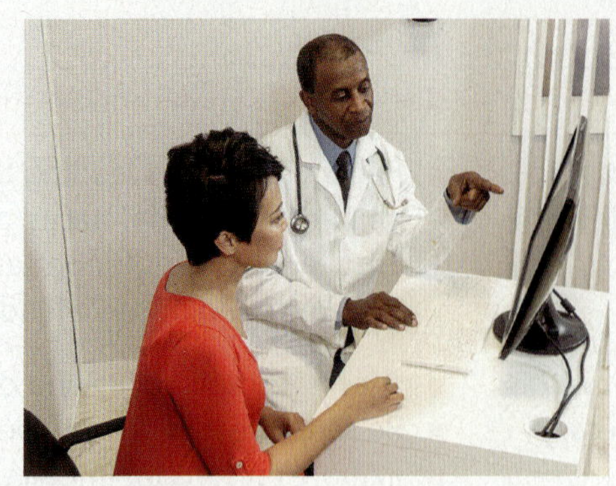

FIGURE 2-7. Visually sharing EHR information using the screen with the patient.

Box 2-17. Strategies to Maintain Patient-Centeredness in Computerized Clinical Settings

Area of Focus	Enhanced Guidelines
Making pre-visit preparations	Ensure familiarity with the patient's medical history before they enter the room, focusing on the patient rather than the screen during the consultation.
Initiating the visit	Begin each session by addressing the patient's immediate concerns and establishing a connection before interacting with the electronic health record (EHR).
Optimizing physical layout for engagement	Adjust the computer's position or modify seating to create a clinician–patient–computer triangle that facilitates open communication.[80]
Maintaining engagement during the consultation	Keep body and gaze oriented toward the patient to ensure they feel acknowledged while interacting with the EHR. Communicate continuously to avoid silence and explain the use of the computer.
Involving the patient	Make the EHR a collaborative tool by showing the screen to the patient and involving them in the charting process, enhancing transparency and trust. See Figure 2-7 for visual guidance.
Balancing technology and personal interaction	Strategically choose moments to shift attention fully to the patient, particularly during critical conversations about their care, signaling these transitions clearly.
Using time efficiently	Utilize natural pauses, such as when a patient is preparing to leave or during a physical exam, to update the EHR, optimizing time for both patient and provider.
Recording post-visit documentation	Complete detailed notes in the patient's electronic record after the visit concludes to maximize face-to-face engagement during their appointment.

Sources: Modified from Crampton NH, Reis S, Shachak A. Computers in the clinical encounter: a scoping review and thematic analysis. *J Am Med Inform Assoc*. 2016;23(3):654–665; Biagioli FE, Elliot DL, Palmer RT, et al. The electronic health record objective structured clinical examination: assessing student competency in patient interactions while using the electronic health record. *Acad Med*. 2017;92(1):87–91.

LEARNING COMMUNICATION SKILLS FROM STANDARDIZED PATIENTS

Reflecting on Sir William Osler's timeless wisdom, *"it is a safe rule to have no teaching without a patient for a text, and the best teaching is that taught by the patient himself" (1905)*.[81] Although clinical training has traditionally relied on patient contact, often alternative approaches to using "real" patients augment clinical learning for many reasons: patients with conditions required for learning who are unavailable, patients with unpredictable behavior, or patients in situations that may be inappropriate.

Standardized patients (*SPs*) offer consistent portrayals of clinical cases with predictable behaviors, enabling students to practice skills in a controlled environment. They fill the gap when real patients with specific conditions are unavailable or when unpredictable behavior or inappropriate situations arise. In addition to serving as teaching and assessment tools, SPs can evaluate student performance and provide constructive feedback.[82] SPs are particularly valuable in training students in both simple and complex communication skills, offering diverse scenarios for learning and assessment, as highlighted in Box 2-18.[83,84–86]

Box 2-18. Tips for Making the Most Out of Learning from Standardized Patients

Take the standardized patient (SP) encounter seriously.	Treat the SP as you would a real patient to maximize the learning experience. Respect their role and dedication to helping you improve your clinical skills.
Trust your "patient."	Understand that SPs meticulously prepare for scenarios and aim to guide rather than obstruct your learning. Trust their responses as part of the structured learning process.
Ask specific questions.	Practice formulating precise questions to elicit detailed responses from SPs, aligning with the expectations of your training program. This approach enhances efficiency during assessments.
Make your "patient" comfortable.	Prioritize the comfort of SPs during interactions, mirroring how you would approach real patient encounters. Seek permission before any physical examinations and demonstrate kindness throughout.
Build a connection.	Cultivate patience, empathy, and authenticity to establish rapport with SPs, fostering open communication and a more enriching learning experience.
Keep your cool.	Remain composed when faced with challenging scenarios presented by SPs, practicing assertiveness and emotional control to manage difficult situations effectively.
Summarize the encounter.	Conclude the interview with a brief recap of key points discussed to demonstrate attentive listening and provide opportunities for clarification.
Enjoy the experience.	Embrace SP encounters as valuable learning opportunities, allowing you to explore new approaches and learn from mistakes in a supportive environment.

Source: Modified from Brown E. Eight Tips for Standardized Patient Encounters. Accessed March 17, 2024. https://www.codeblueessays.com/standardized-patient/

REFERENCES

1. Matthews DA, Suchman AL, Branch WT Jr. Making "connexions": enhancing the therapeutic potential of patient-clinician relationships. *Ann Intern Med.* 1993;118(12):973–977.
2. Haidet P. Jazz and the 'art' of medicine: improvisation in the medical encounter. *Ann Fam Med.* 2007;5(2):164–169.
3. Kurtz S, Silverman J, Benson J, Draper J. Marrying content and process in clinical method teaching: enhancing the Calgary-Cambridge guides. *Acad Med.* 2003;78(8):802–809.
4. Kurtz S, Silverman J, Draper J. *Teaching and Learning Communication Skills in Medicine.* 2nd ed. Radcliffe Publishing Ltd; 1998.
5. Kurtz SM, Silverman JD. The Calgary-Cambridge Referenced Observation Guides: an aid to defining the curriculum and organizing the teaching in communication training programmes. *Med Educ.* 1996;30(2):83–89.
6. Coulehan JL, Block MR. *The Medical Interview: Mastering Skills for Clinical Practice.* 5th ed. F.A. Davis Company; 2005.
7. Fortin AH VI, Dwamena FC, Frankel RM, Smith RC. *Smith's Patient-Centered Interviewing: An Evidence-Based Method.* 3rd ed. The McGraw-Hill Companies, Inc; 2012.
8. Halpern J. Empathy and patient-physician conflicts. *J Gen Intern Med.* 2007;22(5):696–700.
9. Halpern J. What is clinical empathy? *J Gen Intern Med.* 2003; 18(8):670–674.
10. Buckman R, Tulsky JA, Rodin G. Empathic responses in clinical practice: intuition or tuition? *CMAJ.* 2011;183(5):569–571.
11. Egnew TR. Suffering, meaning, and healing: challenges of contemporary medicine. *Ann Fam Med.* 2009;7(2):170–175.
12. Batt-Rawden SA, Chisolm MS, Anton B, Flickinger TE. Teaching empathy to medical students: an updated, systematic review. *Acad Med.* 2013;88(8):1171–1177.
13. Epner DE, Baile WF. Difficult conversations: teaching medical oncology trainees communication skills one hour at a time. *Acad Med.* 2014;89(4):578–584.
14. Lipkin M Jr, Putnam SM, Lazare A, eds. *The Medical Interview: Clinical Care, Education, and Research.* Springer-Verlag; 1995.
15. van de Poel K, Vanagt E, Schrimpf U, Gasiorek J. *Communication Skills for Foreign and Mobile Medical Professionals.* Springer; 2013.
16. Shah P, Thornton I, Turrin D, Hipskind JE. *Informed Consent.* In: StatPearls [Internet]. Treasure Island (FL): StatPearls Publishing; 2024.
17. Gregg J, Saha S. Communicative competence: a framework for understanding language barriers in health care. *J Gen Intern Med.* 2007;22(Suppl 2):368–370.
18. Saha S, Fernandez A. Language barriers in health care. *J Gen Intern Med.* 2007;22(Suppl 2):281–282.
19. Eissa M, Patel AA, Farag S, et al. Awareness and attitude of university students about screening and testing for hemoglobinopathies: case study of the Aseer Region, Saudi Arabia. *Hemoglobin.* 2018;42(4):264–268.
20. Tervalon M, Murray-García J. Cultural humility versus cultural competence: a critical distinction in defining physician training outcomes in multicultural education. *J Health Care Poor Underserved.* 1998;9(2):117–125.
21. Kripalani S, Jackson AT, Schnipper JL, Coleman EA. Promoting effective transitions of care at hospital discharge: a review of key issues for hospitalists. *J Hosp Med.* 2007;2(5):314–323.
22. Kemp EC, Floyd MR, McCord-Duncan E, Lang F. Patients prefer the method of "tell back-collaborative inquiry" to assess understanding of medical information. *J Am Board Fam Med.*2008;21(1):24–30.
23. Ashford RD, Brown AM, Curtis B. Substance use, recovery, and linguistics: The impact of word choice on explicit and implicit bias. *Drug Alcohol Depend.* 2018;189:131–138.
24. Kelly JF, Wakeman SE, Saitz R. Stop talking 'dirty': clinicians, language, and quality of care for the leading cause of preventable death in the United States. *Am J Med.* 2015;128(1):8–9.
25. Ashford RD, Brown AM, McDaniel J, Curtis B. Biased labels: an experimental study of language and stigma among individuals in recovery and health professionals. *Subst Use Misuse.* 2019;54(8):1376–1384.
26. Makoul G, Zick A, Green M. An evidence-based perspective on greetings in medical encounters. *Arch Intern Med.* 2007; 167(11):1172–1176.
27. Brugel S, Postma-Nilsenová M, Tates K. The link between perception of clinical empathy and nonverbal behavior: the effect of a doctor's gaze and body orientation. *Patient Educ Couns.* 2015;98(10):1260–1265.
28. Graves JR, Robinson JD. Proxemic behavior as a function of inconsistent verbal and nonverbal messages. *J Couns Psychol.* 1976;23(4):333–338.
29. Buller DB, Street RL Jr. Physician-patient relationships. In: Feldman RS, ed. *Applications of Nonverbal Behavior Theories and Research.* Lawrence Erlbaum Associates, Inc; 1992: 119–141.
30. van Dulmen AM, Verhaak PF, Bilo HJ. Shifts in doctor-patient communication during a series of outpatient consultations in non-insulin-dependent diabetes mellitus. *Patient Educ Couns.* 1997;30(3):227–237.
31. Verhaak PF. Detection of psychologic complaints by general practitioners. *Med Care.* 1988;26(10):1009–1020.
32. Duggan AP, Bradshaw YS, Swergold N, Altman W. When rapport building extends beyond affiliation: communication overaccommodation toward patients with disabilities. *Perm J.* 2011;15(2):23–30.
33. Weinberger M, Greene JY, Mamlin JJ. The impact of clinical encounter events on patient and physician satisfaction. *Soc Sci Med E.* 1981;15(3):239–244.
34. Baile WF, Buckman R, Lenzi R, Glober G, Beale EA, Kudelka AP. SPIKES—a six-step protocol for delivering bad news: application to the patient with cancer. *Oncologist.* 2000;5(4):302–311.
35. Rosenzweig MQ. Breaking bad news: a guide for effective and empathetic communication. *Nurse Pract.* 2012;37(2):1–4.
36. POLST form. National POLST. Accessed March 18, 2024. https://polst.org/form-patients/
37. Moss AH, Ganjoo J, Sharma S, et al. Utility of the "surprise" question to identify dialysis patients with high mortality. *Clin J Am Soc Nephrol.* 2008;3(5):1379–1384.
38. MOLST: Medical Orders for Life-Sustaining Treatment. New York State Department of Health; 2022. Accessed March 18, 2024. https://www.health.ny.gov/professionals/patients/patient_rights/molst/docs/general_instructions_and_glossary.pdf
39. Cole S, Bogenschutz M, Hungerford D. Motivational interviewing and psychiatry: use in addiction treatment, risky drinking and routine practice. *FOCUS.* 2011;9(1):42–54.
40. Scotten M, Manos EL, Malicoat A, Paolo AM. Minding the gap: interprofessional communication during inpatient and post discharge chasm care. *Patient Educ Couns.* 2015;98(7):895–900.

41. Edwards S, Siassakos D. Training teams and leaders to reduce resuscitation errors and improve patient outcome. *Resuscitation.* 2012;83(1):13–15.
42. Pecukonis E, Doyle O, Bliss DL. Reducing barriers to interprofessional training: promoting interprofessional cultural competence. *J Interprof Care.* 2008;22(4):417–428.
43. Whitehead C. The doctor dilemma in interprofessional education and care: how and why will physicians collaborate? *Med Educ.* 2007;41(10):1010–1016.
44. Gilbert JH. Interprofessional learning and higher education structural barriers. *J Interprof Care.* 2005;19(Suppl 1):87–106.
45. Winnipeg Regional Health Authority. (n.d.). *Competency 5: Interprofessional Communication.* https://professionals.wrha.mb.ca/nursing/tools/clinical-education/. Accessed September 22, 2024.
46. TeamSTEPPS. Agency for Healthcare Research and Quality. Accessed March 18, 2024. http://teamstepps.ahrq.gov/
47. Markowitz JC, Milrod BL. The importance of responding to negative affect in psychotherapies. *Am J Psychiatry.* 2011; 168(2):124–128.
48. American College of Obstetricians and Gynecologists Committee on Ethics. ACOG Committee Opinion no. 373: sexual misconduct. *Obstet Gynecol.* 2007;110(2 Pt 1):441–444.
49. Nadelson C, Notman MT. Boundaries in the doctor-patient relationship. *Theor Med Bioeth.* 2002;23(3):191–201.
50. Gabbard GO, Nadelson C. Professional boundaries in the physician-patient relationship. *JAMA.* 1995;273(18):1445–1449.
51. McMurray RJ, Clarke OW, Barrasso JA, et al. Sexual misconduct in the practice of medicine. *JAMA.* 1991;266(19):2741–2745.
52. Dvir Y, Moniwa E, Crisp-Han H, Levy D, Coverdale JH. Survey of threats and assaults by patients on psychiatry residents. *Acad Psychiatry.* 2012;36(1):39–42.
53. Whitgob EE, Blankenburg RL, Bogetz AL. The discriminatory patient and family: strategies to address discrimination towards trainees. *Acad Med.* 2016;91(11):S64–S69.
54. World Health Organization. *Deafness and hearing loss.* Published February 2, 2024. Accessed March 18, 2024. https://www.who.int/news-room/fact-sheets/detail/deafness-and-hearing-loss.
55. Barnett S, Klein JD, Pollard RQ Jr, et al. Community participatory research with deaf sign language users to identify health inequities. *Am J Public Health.* 2011;101(12):2235–2238.
56. Jin J, Sklar GE, Min Sen Oh V, Chuen Li S. Factors affecting therapeutic compliance: a review from the patient's perspective. *Ther Clin Risk Manag.* 2008;4(1):269–286.
57. Vermeire E, Hearnshaw H, Van Royen P, Denekens J. Patient adherence to treatment: three decades of research. A comprehensive review. *J Clin Pharm Ther.* 2001;26(5):331–342.
58. Athreya BH. *Handbook of Clinical Skills: A Practical Manual.* World Scientific Publishing Co.; 2010.
59. National Center for Education Statistics. National Assessment of Adult Literacy (NAAL). U.S. Department of Education; 2005. Accessed March 18, 2024. https://nces.ed.gov/naal/
60. Berkman ND, Sheridan SL, Donahue KE, Halpern DJ, Crotty K. Low health literacy and health outcomes: an updated systematic review. *Ann Intern Med.* 2011;155(2):97–107.
61. Ryan C. *Language Use in the United States: 2011: American Community Survey Reports.* United States Census Bureau; 2013. https://www2.census.gov/library/publications/2013/acs/acs-22/acs-22.pdf
62. Karliner LS, Jacobs EA, Chen AH, Mutha S. Do professional interpreters improve clinical care for patients with limited English proficiency? A systematic review of the literature. *Health Serv Res.* 2007;42(2):727–754.
63. Thompson DA, Hernandez RG, Cowden JD, Sisson SD, Moon M. Caring for patients with limited English proficiency: are residents prepared to use medical interpreters? *Acad Med.* 2013;88(10):1485–1492.
64. Schyve PM. Language differences as a barrier to quality and safety in health care: the Joint Commission perspective. *J Gen Intern Med.* 2007;22(Suppl 2):360–361.
65. Jacobs EA, Sadowski LS, Rathouz PJ. The impact of an enhanced interpreter service intervention on hospital costs and patient satisfaction. *J Gen Intern Med.* 2007;22(Suppl 2): 306–311.
66. Hardt E, Jacobs EA, Chen A. Insights into the problems that language barriers may pose for the medical interview. *J Gen Intern Med.* 2006;21(12):1357–1358.
67. *Clinical Practice Guidelines for Quality Palliative Care,* 4th ed. National Consensus Project for Quality Palliative Care; 2013. https://www.nationalcoalitionhpc.org/ncp/
68. Dy SM, Aslakson R, Wilson RF, et al. Closing the quality gap: revisiting the state of the science (vol. 8: improving health care and palliative care for advanced and serious illness). *Evid Rep Technol Assess (Full Rep).* 2012;(208.8):1–249.
69. Bakitas M, Lyons KD, Hegel MT, et al. Effects of a palliative care intervention on clinical outcomes in patients with advanced cancer: the Project ENABLE II randomized controlled trial. *JAMA.* 2009;302(7):741–749.
70. Casarett D, Pickard A, Bailey FA, et al. Do palliative consultations improve patient outcomes? *J Am Geriatr Soc.* 2008; 56(4):593–599.
71. Maciejewski PK, Zhang B, Block SD, Prigerson HG. An empirical examination of the stage theory of grief. *JAMA.* 2007;297(7):716–723.
72. Kübler-Ross E. *On Death and Dying.* Scribner; 1997.
73. Palliative care. World Health Organization. Accessed March 18, 2024. https://www.who.int/cancer/palliative/definition/en/
74. Swinglehurst D, Roberts C, Greenhalgh T. Opening up the 'black box' of the electronic patient record: a linguistic ethnographic study in general practice. *Commun Med.* 2011; 8(1):3–15.
75. Margalit RS, Roter D, Dunevant MA, Larson S, Reis S. Electronic medical record use and physician-patient communication: an observational study of Israeli primary care encounters. *Patient Educ Couns.* 2006;61(1):134–141.
76. Biagioli FE, Elliot DL, Palmer RT, et al. The electronic health record objective structured clinical examination: assessing student competency in patient interactions while using the electronic health record. *Acad Med.* 2017;92(1):87–91.
77. Alkureishi MA, Lee WW, Lyons M, et al. Impact of electronic medical record use on the patient-doctor relationship and communication: a systematic review. *J Gen Intern Med.* 2016;31(5):548–560.
78. Crampton NH, Reis S, Shachak A. Computers in the clinical encounter: a scoping review and thematic analysis. *J Am Med Inform Assoc.* 2016;23(3):654–665.
79. LoSasso AA, Lamberton CE, Sammon M, et al. Enhancing student empathetic engagement, history-taking, and communication skills during electronic medical record use in patient care. *Acad Med.* 2017;92(7):1022–1027.
80. Morrow JB, Dobbie AE, Jenkins C, Long R, Mihalic A, Wagner J. First-year medical students can demonstrate EHR-specific communication skills: a control-group study. *Fam Med.* 2009;41(1):28–33.
81. Berlan ED, Bravender T. Confidentiality, consent, and caring for the adolescent patient. *Curr Opin Pediatr.* 2009;21(4):450–456.

82. Ker JS, Dowie A, Dowell J, et al. Twelve tips for developing and maintaining a simulated patient bank. *Med Teach.* 2005; 27(1):4–9.
83. Cleland JA, Abe K, Rethans JJ. The use of simulated patients in medical education: AMEE Guide No 42. *Med Teach.* 2009; 31(6):477–486.
84. Haist SA, Wilson JF, Pursley HG, et al. Domestic violence: increasing knowledge and improving skills with a four-hour workshop using standardized patients. *Acad Med.* 2003; 78(10 Suppl):S24–S26.
85. Haist SA, Griffith C III, Hoellein AR, Talente G, Montgomery T, Wilson JF. Improving students' sexual history inquiry and HIV counseling with an interactive workshop using standardized patients. *J Gen Intern Med.* 2004;19(5 Pt 2):549–553.
86. Halbach JL, Sullivan L. To err is human 5 years later. *JAMA.* 2005;294(14):1758–1759; author reply 1759.

CHAPTER

3

Health History

HEALTH HISTORY

The clinical interview in a patient encounter is a conversation with a purpose, undertaken with a set of goals and priorities (Fig. 3-1).[1] In Chapter 1, Foundational Skills Essential to the Clinical Encounter, we discussed how each stage of the clinical encounter has a corresponding purpose and unfolds in a logical sequence.[2–4] In Chapter 2, Interviewing, Communication, and Interpersonal Skills, we focused on describing the fundamental communication and interpersonal techniques you can use throughout the interview to achieve therapeutic alliance with the patient (the *process*, or flow of the patient's history). In this chapter, we will focus on how to structure the *content* of the health history, starting with the *format of the health history*. This is the important framework for organizing the patient's story into various categories pertinent to their present, past, and family health. By knowing the content and relevance of the different components of the comprehensive health history, you are able to select the elements most pertinent to the visit and shared goals for the patient's health.

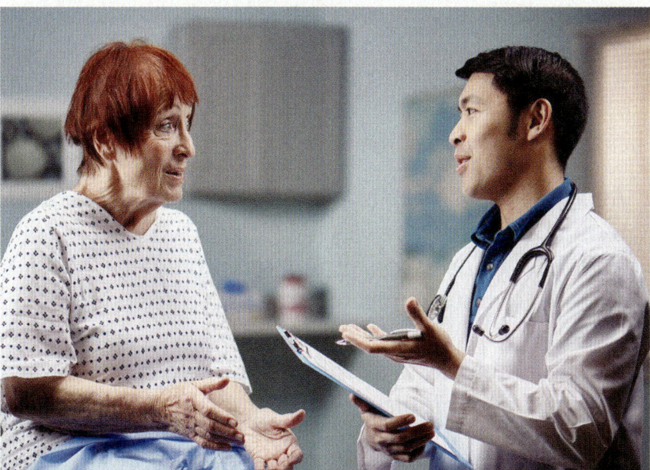

FIGURE 3-1. The clinical interview is a conversation with a purpose.

We have intentionally introduced you to the process of eliciting historical information before focusing on the specific information you need to gather in the clinical encounter. Often, especially for a novice student, pursuing specific information about the patient's symptoms, from the presenting problem to the patient's social and occupational history, leads to sacrificing the relational skills that you use to respond effectively to patient cues, feelings, and concerns.[5] So be mindful of keeping your interview patient-centered as you learn and practice obtaining the information related to the format of the health history.

See Chapter 6, Clinical Documentation and Oral Presentation, for the format for documenting the various health history information gathered in the clinical encounter, pp. 99–100.

Chapter Content Guide

- Health History
  - Different Kinds of Health Histories
  - Determining the Scope of Your Patient Assessment: Comprehensive or Focused?
  - Subjective versus Objective Data
- Components of the Adult Health History
  - Initial Patient Information
  - Gather Information about the Patient's:
    - Chief Concern or Presenting Concern
    - History of Present Illness
    - Past Medical History
    - Family History
    - Personal and Social History
    - Review of Systems
- Recording Your Findings
- Modification of the Clinical Interview for Various Clinical Settings

Different Kinds of Health Histories

The scope and detail of the history depends on the patient's needs and concerns, your goals for the encounter, and the clinical setting (inpatient or outpatient, the amount of time available, primary care or subspecialty).

- For new patients, in most settings, you will do a *comprehensive health history*.
- For patients seeking care for specific concerns, for example, cough or painful urination, a more limited interview tailored to that specific problem may be indicated; this is sometimes known as a *focused* or *problem-oriented history*.
- For patients seeking care for ongoing or chronic problems, focusing on the patient's self-management, response to treatment, functional capacity, and quality of life is most appropriate.[6]
- Patients frequently schedule health maintenance visits with the more focused goals of keeping up screening examinations or discussing concerns about smoking, weight loss, or sexual behavior.
- A specialist may need a more comprehensive history to evaluate a problem with numerous possible causes.

Determining the Scope of Your Patient Assessment: Comprehensive or Focused?

At the outset of each clinical encounter, you will face the common questions, "How much should I do?" and "Should my assessment be comprehensive or focused?" For patients you are seeing for the first time in the office or hospital, you will usually choose to conduct a *comprehensive assessment*, which includes all the elements of the health history and the complete physical examination. In many situations, a more flexible *focused* or *problem-oriented assessment* is appropriate, particularly for patients you know well returning for routine care, or those with specific "urgent care" concerns like sore throat or knee pain. You will adjust the scope of your health history and physical examination to the situation at hand, keeping several factors in mind: the magnitude and severity of the patient's problems; the need for thoroughness; the clinical setting including whether inpatient or outpatient, primary or subspecialty care; and the time available, among others. Skill in all the components of a comprehensive assessment allows you to select the elements that are most pertinent to the patient's concerns yet meet clinical standards for best practice and diagnostic accuracy.

As outlined in Box 3-1, the comprehensive patient assessment does more than assess body systems. It is a source of fundamental and personalized knowledge about the patient that strengthens the clinician–patient relationship.[7] Most people seeking care have specific worries or symptoms. The comprehensive examination provides a more complete basis for assessing these concerns and answering patient questions. For the focused patient assessment, you will select the methods relevant to thorough assessment of the targeted problem. The patient's symptoms, age, and health history help determine the scope of the focused examination, as does your knowledge of disease patterns.

See Chapter 5, Clinical Reasoning, for discussion of the process that underlies and guides clinical decisions, pp. 85–92.

Box 3-1. Patient Assessment: Comprehensive or Focused?

Comprehensive Patient Assessment	Focused Patient Assessment
▪ Appropriate for new patients in the office or hospital ▪ Provides fundamental and personalized knowledge about the patient ▪ Strengthens the clinician–patient relationship ▪ Helps identify or rule out physical causes related to patient concerns ▪ Provides a baseline for future assessments ▪ Creates a platform for health promotion through education and counseling ▪ Develops proficiency in the essential skills of physical examination	▪ Appropriate for established patients, especially during routine or urgent care visits ▪ Addresses focused concerns or symptoms ▪ Assesses symptoms restricted to a specific body system ▪ Applies examination methods relevant to assessing the concern or problem as thoroughly and carefully as possible

Subjective versus Objective Data

As you acquire the techniques of history taking and physical examination, remember the important differences between *subjective information* and *objective information*. Subjective information includes *symptoms*, which are health concerns that the patient conveys to you. Examples include sore throat, headache, or pain. It also includes feelings, perceptions, and concerns obtained from the clinical interview. An example of objective information is the physical examination findings or *signs* you detect during the examination. All laboratory and diagnostic testing results are also considered objective information. For example, "chest pain" as relayed by the patient is subjective information while "tenderness on palpation of anterior chest" observed on physical examination is objective. Knowing these differences helps you group together the different types of patient information. These distinctions are equally important for organizing written and oral presentations about patients into a logical and understandable format. The clinical record from the chief concern (CC) through the review of systems is considered subjective information, whereas all physical examination, laboratory information, and test data are objective information.

See the format of the health history on pp. 107–109.

COMPONENTS OF THE ADULT HEALTH HISTORY

This section will highlight the key components related to your patient's health history (Box 3-2).

Box 3-2. Components of the Adult Health History

Identifying patient information including source of information	■ *Identifying data*—such as patient's initials, age, and gender ■ *Source of the history*—usually the patient, but it can be a family member, caregiver or friend, or the clinical record
Chief concern(s)	■ Primary symptom or concern causing the patient to seek care ■ It may be one or two concerns and rarely more than that
History of present illness	■ Amplifies the chief concern; describes the chronology of events as to how each symptom developed ■ Includes patient's thoughts and feelings about the illness ■ Includes the presence or absence of relevant patient's symptoms, called "*pertinent positives and negatives*" (see p. 50)
Past medical history	■ Lists *adult illnesses* with dates for events in at least four categories: medical, surgical, obstetric/gynecologic, and psychiatric ■ May list *childhood illnesses* ■ Includes *health maintenance practices* such as immunizations, screening tests, lifestyle issues, and home safety ■ May include *medications* and *allergies*
Family history	■ Outlines age and health, or age and cause of death, of siblings, parents, and grandparents ■ Includes presence or absence of specific illnesses in family, such as hypertension, diabetes, or type of cancer
Personal and social history	■ Includes any history of *tobacco, alcohol,* or *recreational drug use* ■ Describes *sexual history* ■ Describes *educational level, family of origin, current household, personal interests,* and *lifestyle*
Review of systems	■ Documents presence or absence of common symptoms related to each of the major body systems

As you learned in Chapter 1, Foundational Skills Essential to the Clinical Encounter, when you talk with patients, the health history rarely emerges in this order. The interview is more fluid; you will closely follow the patient's cues to elicit their narrative of illness, provide empathy, and strengthen rapport. You will quickly learn where to fit different aspects of the patient's story into the more formal format of the oral presentation and written record. You will transform the patient's language and story into the components of the health history familiar to all members of the health care team. This restructuring organizes your clinical reasoning and provides a foundation for your expanding clinical expertise. As you begin your clinical journey, review the components of the adult health history.

See Chapter 28, Children: Infancy Through Adolescence, for the comprehensive history and examination of infants, children, and adolescents, pp. 995–1120.

Initial Patient Information

Identifying Personal Data. Identifying data includes obtaining the patient's full name, preferred name and/or title, and pronouns. Importantly, a person's assigned sex at birth determines their risk for certain conditions, but gender identity and expression may also play a role in a person's health care needs.[8] Additional information includes the patient's age, which can help determine age-related risk factors for certain conditions, as well as other demographic information such as ancestry/ethnicity, and primary language.

Date and Time of History. The date is always important. Also be sure to take note of the time you evaluate the patient, especially in urgent, emergent, or hospital settings.

Source of Information. The *source of information* can be the patient, a family member or friend, a consultant, or the clinical record. Although the *reliability* of a patient's history is important for diagnosis and treatment, decisions indicating it should be done carefully and objectively, keeping in mind the potential biases and challenges in interpretation. Despite our best intentions, we may unconsciously harbor biases that can influence our judgment. Labeling a patient's history as unreliable might inadvertently be more influenced by these biases than by objective facts, and this can potentially lead to inconsistencies in documentation, potential stigmatization, and could discourage patients from being forthcoming in future interactions.

Gather Information about the Patient's Chief Concern or Presenting Concern

The *chief concern* (CC) or *presenting concern*, refers to the primary issue or condition that prompted the patient to seek medical attention. The CC serves as the starting point for information gathering, as it prompts you to ask follow-up questions to better understand the patient's symptoms and medical history. Patients typically present with one CC and other accompanying minor symptoms. For example, a patient may report chest pain with accompanying palpitations and shortness of breath.

To gather information about the patient's CCs, you should conduct a thorough interview while taking detailed notes to ensure no important details are missed. Begin with an open-ended question, such as "*What brings you in today?*" to encourage the patient to provide a detailed response. Establishing rapport with the patient and creating a safe, nonjudgmental environment that encourages the patient to openly discuss their concerns is important.

Gather Information about the Patient's History of Present Illness

The *history of present illness (HPI)* is a clear, concise, and chronologic description of the problems prompting the patient's visit. At its core, the HPI is the story of the patient's problem. It reveals the patient's responses to their symptoms and the effect that the illness has had on their life. By gathering this information, you will be able to better understand the patient's medical history and symptoms, which will guide the course of treatment and improve patient outcomes. During the HPI, you will characterize the CC fully by describing its attributes (Box 3-3).

To prevent bias, invite the patient to tell their story[9] and actively listen to their concerns without interrupting or injecting new information. An open-ended approach encourages patients to share all of their concerns, not just clinical ones. Identify all concerns and ask about missed ones to prioritize them.

Elaborate on the Chief Concern with Attention to Chronology. In the HPI, the CC should be well characterized by its attending attributes. This set of attributes works particularly well for pain-based symptoms but may also be used, with some modification, to describe CCs such as shortness of breath, cough, or diarrhea. Helpful mnemonics are available to assist you in remembering these attributes (Box 3-4).

Box 3-3. Attributes of a Chief Concern

Attribute	Description	Examples
Location	Where in/on the body the problem, symptom, or pain occurs or moves to other areas	■ *"Where did the pain start?"* ■ *"Does your pain move anywhere?"*
Quality	Adjective describing the type of problem, symptom, or pain	■ *"Can you describe the pain for me?"* ■ *"Tell me how you feel when you . . .* (use the patient's words about the quality of the pain)"
Quantity or severity	Patient's nonverbal actions or verbal description as to the degree or extent of the problem, symptom, or pain: pain scale 0–10, comparison of the current problem, symptom, or pain to previous experiences	■ *"On a scale of 1–10, with 10 being the worst possible pain, how would you rate your pain? At its worst? At its best?"* ■ *"How would you characterize the severity of your shortness of breath—mild, moderate, or severe?"* ■ *"Overall, has the pain been getting better, worse, or staying the same?"*
Timing including:	When the problem, symptom, or pain started	
■ **Onset**	Setting where it occurs; what actions or circumstances cause the problem, symptom, or pain to occur, worsen, or improve	■ *"When did this start?" "Tell me what you were doing when this started?" "Was anything unusual going on in your life when this started?"*
■ **Duration**	How long the problem, symptom, or pain have been present, or how long they last	■ *"How long does the headache last?"*
■ **Frequency**	How often the problem, symptom, or pain occur	■ *"How often did you vomit yesterday?"* ■ *"Is the dizziness more frequent today?"*
Modifying factors	Actions or activities taken to improve the problem, symptom, or pain and their outcome	■ *"Does anything make it worse?* ■ *"Does anything make it better?"*
Associated manifestations	Other signs or symptoms that occur when the problem, symptom, or pain occur	■ *"Do you get nauseous when you are dizzy?"* ■ *"Are there any other things that happen when you are experiencing this problem?"*

Pay particular attention to the clarity of the story by noting the timing of symptoms.

One method to maintain clarity of the patient's story is to anchor each event to a timeline or its chronology. For example, "*Two days prior to hospitalization*, the patient developed multiple episodes of watery nonbloody diarrhea. This is *followed a day later* by two episodes of nonbloody vomiting. *Six hours prior to hospitalization*, the patient developed severe epigastric pain...." Try to avoid common mistakes such as inconsistent time anchors: "*On June 12th*, the patient started to develop ... *then 3 days prior to admission* ... *then on Monday*...." Try to keep the time anchors consistent to make it easier to follow each event's timeline.

See Chapter 5, Clinical Reasoning, for the process of clinical reasoning, pp. 85–92.

Ask about Accompanying Symptoms. Asking about additional symptoms that may help you generate a list of possible causes (*differential diagnosis*) to explain the patient's problem or condition is also important. This list will include the *most likely* and, at times, the *most serious* causes, even if less likely. When clinicians obtain a health

Box 3-4. Helpful Mnemonics for Characterizing the Chief Concern

OPQRST	OLD CARTS
■ **O**nset ■ **P**recipitating and **P**alliating factors ■ **Q**uality ■ **R**egion or **R**adiation ■ **S**everity ■ **T**iming or **T**emporal characteristics	■ **O**nset ■ **L**ocation ■ **D**uration ■ **C**haracter ■ **A**ggravating or **A**lleviating factors ■ **R**adiation ■ **T**iming ■ **S**etting

history, they are continually generating possible explanations in their minds, allowing the patient's answers to direct the logical use of additional probing questions. This process of probing with questions is similar to testing a hypothesis. With each question, the list of probable diagnoses (or hypotheses) is pared down until a few likely choices are left from a formerly longer list of diagnostic possibilities.

In this step, you should describe any symptoms brought up during the encounter that you believe may be related to the CC, termed *pertinent positives.* Pertinent positives are "symptoms or signs that you would expect to find if a possible cause for a patient's problem were true, which then supports this diagnosis."[10] For instance if a patient describes shortness of breath as their CC, and this is accompanied by palpitations and intense facial flushing, it may point to several potential diagnoses. These could include conditions such as panic attack, anxiety, hyperthyroidism, anaphylaxis (severe allergic reaction), a lung infection, or even a heart attack.

Ask about Pertinent Absent Symptoms. You also note the absence of any symptoms related to your differential diagnosis, termed *pertinent negatives.* Pertinent negatives are "expected symptoms or signs that are not present, facts that you would expect to find if a possible cause for a patient's problem were true, which then weaken this diagnosis by their absence."[10] In the example of a patient with shortness of breath, what if the patient does not exhibit signs of fever, doesn't have a cough that produces sputum, and isn't experiencing chest pain? Additionally, there's no known history of coronary artery disease. The absence of these symptoms and medical history are referred to as "pertinent negatives." For instance, a lung infection typically presents with fever and a productive cough, while a heart attack is commonly associated with chest pain, especially in individuals with a history of coronary artery disease. Given these pertinent negatives, the likelihood of diagnoses like lung infection or heart attack becomes less probable for this patient.

The pertinent positives and especially the pertinent negatives clarify the possible causes of the patient's condition as well as eliminate other less likely possibilities based on the patient's story. You may find this stage of gathering information to be challenging because it requires clinical experience and exposure as well as medical knowledge. In due time, you will learn the appropriate lines of questioning pertinent for a particular CC and its more commonly occurring causes.

Ask Additional Pertinent Information. Here you should note any additional facts pertinent to the CC, regardless of where they are typically asked (Box 3-2). For example, if your patient has a fever and cough who you believe has pneumonia (lung infection), you may want to ask about the patient's smoking history. For a patient with fever and weight loss who you think may have tuberculosis (TB), you may want to ask for any history of living in a shelter for individuals who are unhoused and possibly in close contact with persons with pulmonary TB. These two facts would typically be asked in the social history section of the clinical interview, but they are asked in the HPI section because they may have an impact on the evolving list of possible causes of the CC.

Concluding the HPI section of the clinical interview by asking how and why the patient came to seek medical attention is often helpful. For example, the patient may have sought help from their primary clinician because fevers did not resolve with acetaminophen or because they were brought to the ER by ambulance when they nearly passed out on the subway. Responses to this concluding question give insight into the severity of the condition as well as the patient's motivations for seeking care.

Gather Information about the Patient's Past Medical History

The *past medical history (PMH)* includes all of the patient's medical problems, whether they are currently active or remote, that may be contributing to the patient's current symptoms. A query about the patient's general state of health may also be included here. You may ask: *"Over your lifetime, how would you describe your health status?"*

Childhood Illnesses. Ask patients about illnesses such as measles, rubella, mumps, whooping cough, chickenpox, rheumatic fever, scarlet fever, and polio. Also, ask about any chronic childhood illnesses such as asthma or diabetes mellitus.

Adult Illnesses. Ask the patient to provide information in each of the four areas:

- *Medical*: Ask about illnesses such as diabetes, high blood pressure, heart attack, hepatitis, asthma, human immunodeficiency virus (HIV), seizures, arthritis, TB, and cancer as well as time frame and hospitalizations.
- *Surgical:* Ask dates and types of operations or procedures. If they are unable to recall the name of the operation or procedure, ask why it was performed (*indication*).
- *Obstetric/Gynecologic:* Ask about obstetric history, menstrual history, methods of contraception, and sexual function.
- *Psychiatric:* Ask about any illnesses such as depression, anxiety, and suicidal ideations/attempts, including time frame, diagnoses, hospitalizations, and treatments (Box 3-5).

Health Maintenance. Ask about immunizations and screening tests. For *immunizations,* find out whether the patient has received vaccines for tetanus, pertussis, diphtheria, polio, measles, rubella, mumps, influenza, varicella, hepatitis B virus (HBV), human papillomavirus (HPV), meningococcal disease, *Haemophilus influenzae* type B, pneumococci, and herpes zoster. For *screening tests,* review tuberculin tests, Pap smears, mammograms, stool tests for occult blood, colonoscopy, and cholesterol tests, together with results and when they were last performed.

Allergies. Ask for any allergies the patient has, including drug allergies, food allergies, and environmental allergies. Allergies can cause a wide range of symptoms and can be potentially life-threatening, so identifying and avoiding any allergens that may be contributing to the patient's symptoms is important. Often, your patient may report an "allergy" to a medication when it was instead a side effect. For example, a patient may report a penicillin allergy that was actually nausea after taking a penicillin-based antibiotic in the past. This may negatively impact future decisions about administering antibiotics by limiting possible alternatives.

Try to differentiate whether the patient has a true allergic reaction, an adverse drug reaction, or a side effect of a medication. An *adverse drug reaction* is any "noxious and unintended response to a drug which occurs at doses normally used in humans for prophylaxis, diagnosis, or therapy of disease or for the modification of physiologic function."[11] An *allergy* is an adverse drug reaction mediated by an immune response (e.g., generalized rash, wheezing, or appearance of hives). A *side effect* is an expected and known effect of a drug that is not the intended therapeutic outcome (e.g., nausea, constipation).

Box 3-5. Mental Health

- Cultural constructs of mental and physical illness vary widely, leading to differences in social acceptance and attitudes. Think how easy it is for patients to talk about diabetes and take insulin compared with discussing schizophrenia and using psychotropic medications.
- Ask open-ended questions initially. *"Have you ever had any problem with emotional or mental illnesses?"* Then move to more specific questions such as *"Have you ever seen a counselor or psychotherapist?" "Have you ever taken medication for a mental health condition?" "Have you ever been hospitalized for an emotional or mental health problem?" "What about members of your family?"*
- For patients with depression or thought disorders such as schizophrenia, take a careful history of their symptoms and course of illness. Watch for mood changes or symptoms such as fatigue, unusual tearfulness, appetite or weight changes, insomnia, and vague somatic problems.
- Two validated screening questions for depression are: *"Over the past 2 weeks, have you felt down, depressed, or hopeless?"* and *"Over the past 2 weeks, have you felt little interest or pleasure in doing things?"*[55]
- If the patient seems depressed, always ask about suicide: *"Have you ever thought about hurting yourself or ending your life?"* As with chest pain, you must evaluate severity—both depression and angina are potentially lethal.
- Many patients with psychotic disorders like schizophrenia are living in the community and can tell you about their diagnoses, symptoms, hospitalizations, and current medications. Investigate whether their symptoms and level of function are stable and review their support systems and plan of care.

Medication History. Medications should be carefully asked about, including name, dose, route, and frequency of use. Also ask about nonprescription or over-the-counter (OTC) medications, vitamins, mineral or herbal supplements, eye drops, suppositories, patches, creams or ointments, oral contraceptives, home remedies, and medicines borrowed from family members or friends. This can help identify any potential drug interactions or side effects that may be contributing to the patient's symptoms. Ask patients to bring in all medications, so that you can see exactly what they take (Fig. 3-2).

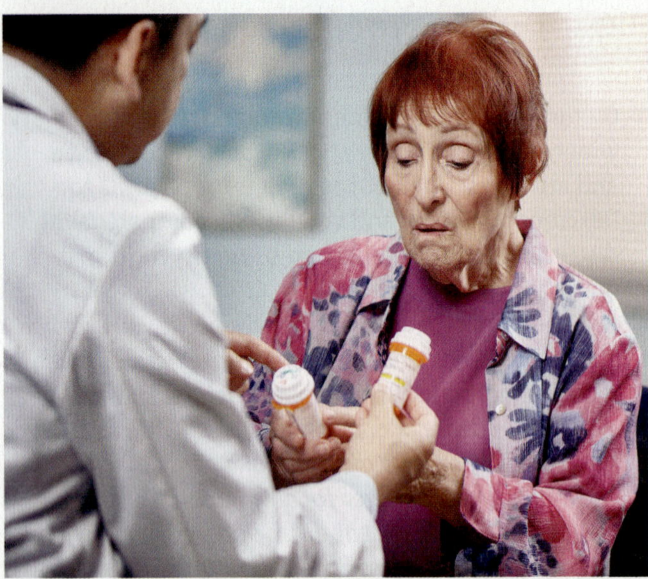

FIGURE 3-2. Reviewing and reconciling patient's medications.

Gather Information about the Patient's Family History

Ask about your patient's *family history*, their health information as well as that of their immediate relatives. Note the ages and health, or ages and causes of death, of each immediate relative including parents, grandparents, siblings, children, and grandchildren. Information about the health of your patient's immediate family members can help identify any hereditary or genetic conditions that may be contributing to their symptoms.

Some examples of conditions to ask about include:

- Cardiovascular disease (heart attacks, strokes, high blood pressure)
- Cancer (breast cancer, colon cancer, prostate cancer)
- Diabetes
- Autoimmune disorders (rheumatoid arthritis, lupus, multiple sclerosis)
- Inherited conditions (cystic fibrosis, sickle cell anemia, hemophilia)
- Mental health conditions (depression, anxiety, bipolar disorder)

Gather Information about the Patient's Personal and Social History

The patient's *personal history,* which is included in the social history, captures their personality and interests, coping style, strengths, and concerns. It attempts to personalize your relationship with the patient and builds rapport. This personal history may include:

Box 3-6. Basic and Instrumental Activities of Daily Living

Basic ADLs	Instrumental ADLs
■ Ambulating	■ Using the telephone
■ Feeding	■ Shopping
■ Dressing	■ Preparing food
■ Toileting	■ Housekeeping
■ Personal hygiene or grooming	■ Doing laundry
■ Transferring	■ Using transportation
	■ Taking medicine
	■ Managing money

- Sexual orientation and gender identification (SOGI)
- Place of birth and personal environmental map
- Occupation and education
- Significant relationships including safety in those relationships
- Home environment including family and household composition
- Important life experiences such as military service, job history, financial situation, and retirement
- Leisure activities
- Sexuality
- Spirituality
- Social support systems
- Baseline level of function, that is, activities of daily living (ADLs), is particularly important in older adults or persons with disabilities (Box 3-6).

Other parts of the *social history* include tobacco, recreational drug, and alcohol use. It also includes lifestyle habits that promote health or create risk: *exercise and nutrition* including frequency of exercise; usual daily food intake; dietary supplements or restrictions; and use of coffee, tea, and other caffeinated beverages as well as *safety measures* including use of seat belts, helmets, sunblock, presence of smoke detectors, firearms, and other devices related to specific hazards in the patient's environment.

Sexual Orientation and Gender Identity. Discussing SOGI touches a vital and multifaceted core of your patients' lives (Box 3-7). Reflect on any biases you may have so that they do not interfere with professional responses to your patients' disclosures and concerns. A supportive nonjudgmental approach is essential for exploring your patients' health and well-being.[12] Asking patients

Box 3-7. Terminology and Definitions

Term	Definition
Assigned sex	Sex designated at birth, typically based on external genitalia
Sexual orientation	Person's physical, romantic, and/or emotional attraction to another person of a specific gender or genders
Gender identity	Individual's internal sense of being male, female, or something else; this is not necessarily visible to others
Gender expression	External manifestations of gender, expressed through a person's name, pronouns, clothing, haircut, behavior, voice, and/or body characteristics
Transgender (trans)	Person whose gender identity and/or expression differs from the cultural expectations of the sex they were assigned at birth
Transgender man (transman)	Transgender individual who currently or lives as a man
Transgender woman (transwoman)	Transgender individual who currently or lives as a woman
Cisgender	Person whose gender identity, expression, or behavior is the same as those typically associated with assigned sex at birth
Nonbinary	Individual who identifies as neither entirely male nor entirely female Other terms include *genderqueer, agender, bigender*, and more All refer to an experience of gender that is not simply male or female
Transition	Period when a person begins living as the gender with which they identify rather than the gender they were assigned at birth, which often includes changing their first name and dressing and grooming differently May or may not also include medical and legal aspects, including taking hormones, having surgery, and changing identity documents (e.g., driver's license, Social Security record) to reflect gender identity

Adapted with permission from the Advocates for Trans Equality. Transgender 101. Accessed September 22, 2024. https://transequality.org/trans-101

their SOGI will enable you to provide relevant, specific, and compassionate care that is patient centered and grounded in appropriate language.

Some questions may need to be asked at every visit, as SOGI can be fluid, especially in adolescents, and clinicians should recall that many patients may have sexual encounters that may not be predicted by their declared orientation.[13] Clinicians should not assume the sexual orientation or gender identity of patients is the same as prior visits or is based on behavior, appearance, or genders of partners. For example, many males do not identify as gay but have same-sex partners, and one study found that 81% of females with same-sex attraction also report having sexual experiences with males.[14] Instead, you should ask open-ended questions and use language that is inclusive, allowing your patient to decide when and what to disclose.

Sample questions:

- *"How would you describe your sexual orientation?"* The range of responses can include heterosexual or straight, lesbian, gay, bisexual, pansexual, queer, and questioning, among others.
- Continue with *"How would you describe your gender identity?"* Responses include male, female, transgender, transmale, transfemale, genderqueer, gender nonbinary, unsure or questioning, or even "prefer not to answer."
- *"What is the sex on your original birth certificate?"* This question helps elicit further gender history when asked as a follow-up to gender identity and will give the clinician a sense of which organs the patient may have in order to help guide sexually transmitted infection (STI) and cancer screening recommendations.

Familial and Social Relationships. Social relationships have short- and long-term effects on mental health, health behavior, and physical health.[15] Many studies provide evidence that social ties influence health behaviors that promote health and prevent illness (e.g., exercise, consuming nutritionally balanced diets, adherence to medical regimens) and those that undermine health (e.g., smoking, excessive weight gain, heavy drug use, heavy alcohol consumption).[15,16] Ask about parents, children, partners, friends, acquaintances, and distant relatives. Seek those that your patient identifies as providing *social support*, which refers to the emotionally sustaining qualities of relationships, or to those who provide a sense that the patient is loved, cared for, and listened to.[17,18]

Detecting Threatening Relationships. While social relationships are the central source of emotional support for most patients, they can also be stressful, overburdening, strained, conflicted, or abusive, which then undermine the patient's health (Box 3-8).[15] Experts recommend beginning with normalizing statements such as "*Because abuse is common in many of my patients' lives, I've begun to ask about it routinely.*" Disclosure is more likely when probing questions lead and then in-depth direct questions follow. "*Are you in a relationship where you have been hit or threatened?*" with a pause to encourage the patient to respond. If the patient says no, continue with "*Has anyone ever treated you badly or made you do things you don't want to do?*" or "*Is there anyone you are afraid of?*" or "*Have you ever been hit, kicked, punched, or hurt by someone you know?*" Following disclosure, empathic validating and nonjudgmental responses are critical but currently occur less than half the time.

When you suspect abuse, spending part of the visit alone with the patient is important. You can use the transition to the physical examination as a reason to ask others to leave the room. If the patient is also resistant, do not force the situation, potentially placing the patient, who may be experiencing abuse, in jeopardy.

Box 3-8. Clues to Physical and Sexual Abuse

Be alert to the unspoken clues to abuse, often present in the growing numbers of victims of human sex trafficking in the United States and internationally, estimated at 50,000 women and children annually in the United States alone.[56,57]

- Injuries that are unexplained, seem inconsistent with the patient's story, are concealed by the patient, or cause embarrassment
- Delay in getting treatment for trauma
- History of repeated injuries or "accidents"
- Presence of alcohol or drug abuse in patient or partner
- Partner tries to dominate the visit, will not leave the room, or seems unusually anxious or solicitous
- Pregnancy at a young age; multiple partners
- Repeated vaginal infections and sexually transmitted infections
- Difficulty walking or sitting due to genital/anal pain
- Vaginal lacerations or bruises
- Fear of the pelvic examination or physical contact
- Fear of leaving the examination room

See Chapter 7, Health Maintenance and Screening, for discussion of intimate partner violence and domestic abuse, p. 126; Chapter 29, Pregnant Persons, for intimate partner violence during pregnancy, pp. 1145–1146.

Alcohol History. Learning about your patient's *patterns* of alcohol consumption, not just their average levels of consumption, is important. "*Tell me about your use of alcohol*" is an opening query that avoids the easy yes-no response. Positive answers to two additional questions are highly suspicious for problem-drinking: "*Have you ever had a drinking problem?*" and "*When was your last drink?*" especially if the night before.[19]

The widely used screening questions are the *CAGE* questions about ***C***utting down, ***A***nnoyance when criticized, ***G***uilty feelings, and ***E***ye openers.[20] Two or more affirmative answers to the CAGE Questionnaire suggest lifetime alcohol overuse and dependence alcohol use disorders (AUDs) and have a sensitivity that ranges from 43% to 94% and specificity ranging from 70% to 96%.[21,22] A more preferred and well-validated short screening test is the *Alcohol Use Disorders Identification Test-Concise (AUDIT-C)*.[23] It identifies not just the harmful drinkers detected by the CAGE, but also hazardous drinkers, who have not yet reached that level of harm and who may respond better to interventions aimed at reducing their consumption.[24] If you detect misuse, ask about blackouts (loss of memory about events during drinking), seizures, accidents or injuries while drinking, job problems, and conflict in personal relationships.

See Chapter 7, Health Maintenance and Screening, for further discussion of screening for alcohol misuse, pp. 126–127.

Tobacco Use History. Determine tobacco use, including the type (smoking, chewing). Examples: "*Do you smoke?*" "*Have you ever smoked?*" "*What do you smoke?*" "*How many cigarettes per day? For how many years?*" "*Do you* *chew tobacco?"* Cigarettes are often reported in *pack-years*. It is a way to measure the amount a person has smoked over a period of time. It is calculated by multiplying the number of packs of cigarettes smoked per day by the number of years the person has smoked.[25] For example, a person who has smoked 1½ packs a day for 12 years has an 18–pack-year history. If someone has quit, note for how long and note as a former smoker.

See Chapter 7, Health Maintenance and Screening, for further discussion of screening for tobacco misuse, pp. 127–128.

Recreational Drug Use History. The National Institute on Drug Abuse recommends first asking a highly sensitive and specific single question: *"How many times in the past year have you used a recreational drug or used a prescription medication for nonclinical reasons?"*[26,27] If the response is positive, ask specifically about nonclinical use of recreational and prescription drugs: *"In your lifetime, have you ever used marijuana; cocaine; prescription stimulants; methamphetamines; sedatives or sleeping pills; hallucinogens like lysergic acid diethylamide (LSD), ecstasy, or mushrooms; street opioids like heroin or opium; prescription opioids like fentanyl, oxycodone, or hydrocodone; or other substances?"* For those answering yes, a series of further questions is recommended.[26]

See Chapter 7, Health Maintenance and Screening, for further discussion of screening for substance use disorders, pp. 125–126.

Sexual History. Exploring the sexual history can be lifesaving. Sexual behaviors determine risks for pregnancy, STIs, and HIV; good interviewing helps prevent or reduce these risks and promote and maintain health.[28,29] Sexual practices may be directly related to the patient's symptoms and integral to both diagnosis and treatment. Many patients express their concerns more freely when you ask about *sexual health*. In addition, sexual dysfunction may result from medications or clinical issues that can be readily corrected. Answering questions about sexual health may be uncomfortable for some patients, particularly if they have experienced judgment or discrimination. Acknowledging and validating these feelings and experiences and providing reassurance that all patients are asked these questions, can help build an environment of understanding and respect.

You can elicit the sexual history at multiple points in the interview. If the CC involves genitourinary symptoms, include questions about sexual health as part of expanding and clarifying the patient's story. For patients with vaginas, you can ask these questions during the obstetric/gynecologic section of the PMH. You can include the sexual history in discussions about health maintenance or in the social history as you explore lifestyle issues and important relationships. In a comprehensive history, you can also ask about sexual practices during the review of systems. Do not forget to cover the sexual history in older patients and patients living with disabilities or chronic illnesses.

An orienting sentence or two are often helpful. *"To help me take better care of you, I need to ask you some questions about your sexual health and practices"* or *"I routinely ask all patients about their sexual function."* For more specific concerns, you might state, *"To figure out why you have this discharge and what we should do, I need to ask some questions about your sexual activity."* If you are straightforward, the patient is more likely to follow your lead.

In order to broach this sensitive topic using appropriate, direct but also sensitive questioning, using a sexual history script that includes questions about sexual problems or concerns is often helpful.[30] Students have reported that having a written script improves ease of learning sexual history–taking skills.[31] The most common sexual history script is the *5 Ps (partners, practices, protection from STIs, past history of STIs, and prevention of pregnancy)* from the Centers for Disease Control and Prevention (CDC) that outlines the important elements of a sexual risk assessment (Box 3-9).[32,33] It has been recommended that a sixth "P" for "plus" be added. *The "plus" should encompass an assessment of trauma, violence, sexual satisfaction, sexual health concerns/problems, and support for gender identity and sexual orientation.*[30]

These questions are designed to help patients reveal their concerns. Note that these questions make no assumptions about marital status, sexual orientation, or attitudes about pregnancy or contraception. Listen to each of the patient's responses, and invite additional history as indicated. To elicit information about sexual behaviors, you will need to ask more specific and focused questions.

Refer to genitalia with explicit words. Choose words that are understandable and explain what you mean. Be aware to avoid referring to body parts with language that might increase a patient's discomfort with how they now identify, especially for transgender and gender nonbinary patients. For example, transmasculine patients may use the term *"front hole"* or *"bottom"* to describe the vagina and *"chest"* rather than breasts. You should attempt to refer to body parts with gender-neutral language whenever possible, or, better yet, ask the patient what terms they use for their own body parts and then use those terms throughout the visit.[34] Inquire about the use of toys or other objects for sex. If a patient is engaging in anal sex, a clinician should clarify if they are engaging in insertive ("top") or receptive ("bottom") penetration or both.

See SOGI questions in the Social History section on p. 52.

Box 3-9. Sexual History: Five Ps+

General	■ *"Do you have any specific concerns or questions we can start with, about your sexual health or sexual practices?"*
Partners	■ *"When was the last time you had intimate physical contact with someone?" "Did that contact include sexual intercourse?"* The term "sexually active" can be ambiguous. ■ *"What are the genders of your sexual partners?"* Asking broad open-ended questions with gender-neutral terms validates the wide diversity of sex and gender and allows the patient to provide a more accurate representation of their history, instead of asking "Do you have sex with men, women, or both?" Patients may have same-sex partners, yet not consider themselves gay, lesbian, or bisexual. Some gay and lesbian patients have had opposite-sex partners. ■ *"How many sexual partners have you had in the last 6 months? In the last 5 years? In your lifetime?"* These questions make it easy for the patient to acknowledge multiple partners. ■ Ask, *"Have you had any new partners in the past 6 months?"* If patients question why this information is important, explain that new partners or multiple partners over a lifetime can raise the risk for sexually transmitted infections (STIs).
Practices	■ *"How do you have sex?"* or *"What kinds of sex are you having?* (e.g., oral sex, vaginal sex, anal sex, sharing sex toys)" ■ *"What parts of your body do you use for sex?"* or *"What body parts go where, when you are sexually active?"* (penis, mouth, anus, vagina, hands, toys, and other objects)
Protection from sexually transmitted infections	■ *"What do you do to protect yourself from HIV and STIs ?"* ■ Ask about routine use of condoms. *"Can you tell me when you use condoms? With which partners?"* are open-ended questions that do not presume an answer. If never: *"There are a lot of reasons why people don't use condoms. Can you tell me why you are not using them for sex?"* ■ Ask all patients, *"Do you have any concerns about HIV infection or AIDS?"* since infection can occur in the absence of risk factors.
Past history of sexually transmitted infections	■ *"Have you ever had a sexually transmitted infection* (e.g., gonorrhea, chlamydia, herpes, genital warts, syphilis)?" If yes: *"What kind have you had?" "When did you have it?" "How were you treated/what medications did you take?"* ■ *"Have you ever been tested for any (other) STIs?"* If yes: *"When and what were the test results?"*
Pregnancy plans	■ For all patients: *"Do you have any plans or desires to have (more) children?"* ■ For opposite sex partners: *"Are you concerned about getting pregnant or getting your partner pregnant?" "Are you doing anything to prevent yourself or your partner from getting pregnant?" "Do you want information on birth control?" "Do you have any questions or concerns about pregnancy prevention?"*
Plus	■ The "plus" should encompass an assessment of trauma, violence, sexual satisfaction, sexual health concerns/problems, and support for sexual orientation and gender identity (SOGI).

Sources: U.S. Department of Health and Human Services: Centers for Disease Control and Prevention. *Taking a Sexual History: A Guide to Taking a Sexual History. CDC Publication 99–8445.* Centers for Disease Control and Prevention; 2005. Accessed June 16, 2024. https://www.cdc.gov/std/treatment/sexualhistory.pdf; National LGBT Health Education Center. Taking routine histories of sexual health: a system-wide approach for health centers. Accessed June 16, 2024. https://www.lgbthealtheducation.org/publication/taking-routine-histories-of-sexual-health-a-system-wide-approach-for-health-centers; and Rubin ES, Rullo J, Tsai P, et al. Best practices in North American Pre-Clinical Medical Education in sexual history taking: consensus from the summits in medical education in sexual health. *J Sex Med.* 2018;15:1414–1425.

Spiritual History. Taking a spiritual history is a process of interviewing patients to better understand their spiritual and/or religious needs and resources.[35] Many patients would like their clinicians to ask about their religious and/or spiritual beliefs,[36–41] yet many do not.[42] Inquiring about a patient's spirituality can convey compassion and hope and increase a patient's sense of being understood by their clinicians.[41]

Your role is to conduct a spiritual history as part of your comprehensive health history in the personal and social history portions. A spiritual history may be taken as part of a new patient visit, annual examination, or a follow-up visit. Keep it patient-centered and listen actively.[43] Several formats for spiritual histories exist including FICA©, HOPE, and Open Invite.[44] The most widely used is the *FICA© Spiritual Tool*, which is an acronym for **F**aith, Belief, Meaning; **I**mportance and **I**nfluence; **C**ommunity and **A**ddress (Box 3-10).[35,43,45] Use FICA© as a guide for opening up a discussion about spiritual issues.[45]

If spiritual struggle is identified, then a referral should be made to a hospital chaplain. *Chaplains* are members of the interdisciplinary team who are specially trained to provide spiritual care to patients of any religion, spirituality, or none at all. Chaplains conduct comprehensive spiritual assessments of patients' spiritual needs, hopes, and resources; develop care plans aligned with the physician's overall plan; and intervene to address patients' spiritual needs.

Summary of Social History. Box 3-11 summarizes several questions you can ask your patient regarding the various

Box 3-10. FICA© Spiritual Tool

THE GW INSTITUTE FOR
SPIRITUALITY & HEALTH

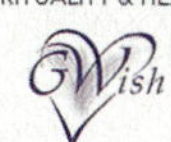

FICA Spiritual History Tool©*

The acronym FICA can help to structure questions for healthcare professionals who are taking a spiritual history.

***

F – Faith, Belief, Meaning

"Do you consider yourself to be spiritual?" or "Is spirituality something important to you?"
"Do you have spiritual beliefs, practices, or values that help you to cope with stress, difficult times, or what you are going through right now?" (contextualize to visit)
"What gives your life meaning?"

I – Importance and Influence

"What importance does spirituality have in your life?"
"Has your spirituality influenced how you take care of yourself, particularly regarding your health?"
"Does your spirituality affect your healthcare decision making?

C – Community

"Are you part of a spiritual community?"
"Is your community of support to you and how?" For people who don't identify with a community consider asking "Is there a group of people you really love or who are important to you?"
(Communities such as churches, temples, mosques, family, groups of like-minded friends, or yoga or similar groups can serve as strong support systems for some patients.)

A - Address/Action in Care

"How would you like me, as your healthcare provider, to address spiritual issues in your healthcare?"
(With newer models, including the diagnosis of spiritual distress, "A" also refers to the "Assessment and Plan" for patient spiritual distress, needs and or resources within a treatment or care plan.

* Adapted from Puchalski C, Romer AL. Taking a spiritual history allows clinicians to understand patients more fully. *J Palliat Med.* 2000;3(1):129–137.

Box 3-11. Social History: Sample Questions

Social History Domain	Sample Questions
Sexual orientation and gender identity: These questions are essential for understanding an individual's self-identification in terms of sexuality and gender. They help in ensuring that health care and other services are tailored to the individual's unique needs.	■ *How would you describe your sexual orientation?* ■ *How would you describe your gender identity?* ■ *What is the sex on your original birth certificate?*
Personal geographic map: Geographic information can provide insights into potential environmental exposures, cultural influences, and access to resources.	■ *Where were you born?* ■ *How long have you lived in the United States? In New York?* ■ *Where do you currently live?*
Significant relationships: Questions in this domain are key to understanding an individual's support system, relational dynamics, and potential sources of stress or support.	■ *Do you have a life partner, spouse, significant other?* ■ *Do you have any children?* ■ *Are there times in your relationship that you felt afraid or unsafe?*
Local support systems: Understanding who an individual lives with or spends time with can offer insights into their daily routines, support systems, and potential challenges.	■ *Who lives with you at home?* ■ *Are there friends or family nearby?* ■ *With whom do you spend your day?*
Work History/Occupation: Job-related questions can reveal potential occupational hazards, sources of stress, and factors affecting mental and physical well-being.	■ *Are you currently working?* ■ *What kind of jobs have you had in the past?* ■ *Have you ever held more than one job at a time?* ■ *What did you do before you retired? Is that what you have always done?* ■ *Tell me what that job is like for you. What are your hours like?* ■ *Do you feel secure in your job?* ■ *Do you think anything at work is making you feel sick or affecting your symptoms?*
Education: This helps clinicians understand the individual's educational background, which might be correlated with health literacy, access to resources, and more.	■ *What is the highest level of school that you have completed?* ■ *Where did you go to school?*
Lifestyle and Activities of Daily Living: These questions paint a picture of an individual's daily routines, capacities, and potential barriers to care.	■ *What do you do when you are not working or going to school?* ■ *Can you walk me through a typical day?* ■ *Do you travel?* ■ *How do you get around the house?* ■ *Do you need help with dressing or bathing?* ■ *How do you travel outside of your home?*
Nutrition: This is a key determinant of health. Understanding dietary habits can offer insights into potential health risks and areas for intervention.	■ *Tell me about your eating habits.* ■ *Do you eat fresh fruits and vegetables?* ■ *Do you maintain the same weight?* ■ *Are you happy with your weight?* ■ *What do you eat on a typical day?* ■ *Do you cook at home? Do you eat out?*

Social History Domain	Sample Questions
Exercise: This is a key determinant of health. Understanding physical activity levels can offer insights into potential health risks and areas for intervention.	■ *Do you get a chance to exercise?* ■ *Do you exercise regularly?* ■ *How often do you exercise?* ■ *What form of exercise do you enjoy?*
Substance Use (Alcohol, Tobacco, Illicit Drugs): Substance use questions are crucial for identifying potential health risks, dependencies, and areas for intervention.	■ *Tell me about your use of alcohol.* ■ *Have you ever had a drinking problem?* ■ *When was your last drink?* ■ *Do you smoke?* ■ *Have you ever smoked?* ■ *What do you smoke?* ■ *How many cigarettes per day? For how many years? Do you chew tobacco?* ■ *How many times in the past year have you used an illegal drug or used a prescription medication for nonclinical reasons?*
Safety measures: Safety-related questions can uncover risks in the home or in an individual's daily life that might require intervention.	■ *Have you ever been seriously injured? (How?) How about anyone that you know?* ■ *Do you always wear a seat belt?* ■ *Do you own a firearm? Does someone you live with own a firearm? How do you keep it safely stored?* ■ *Where do you keep your medications? Cleaning materials?* ■ *How do you protect yourself from the sun?*
Spirituality: Understanding an individual's spiritual beliefs can provide insights into their values, sources of strength, and potential conflicts with medical treatments.	■ *What is your faith or belief?* ■ *Do you consider yourself spiritual or religious?* ■ *What things do you believe that give your life meaning and purpose?* ■ *Are you active in your faith community?* ■ *Are you a part of a religious or spiritual community? Do you have access to what you need/want to apply your faith/beliefs?* ■ *Do any of your beliefs conflict with your medical treatments?*
Sexual history: Questions in this domain can help identify risks, concerns, or areas where education might be beneficial.	■ *Do you have any specific concerns or questions we can start with, about your sexual health or sexual practices?* ■ *When was the last time you had intimate physical contact with someone?* ■ *How do you have sex?* ■ *What are the genders of your sexual partners?*

sections of the social history. In time, you will learn to intersperse these questions throughout the interview to make the patient feel more at ease and enhance rapport.

Review of Systems

The *review of systems* questions may uncover problems or symptoms that you or the patient may have overlooked, particularly in areas unrelated to the HPI. This is an inquiry method called *scanning*[10] in which you ask patients questions regarding dysfunctions in different organ systems. These "yes-no" questions should come at the end of the interview. This section of the health history is useful when your clinical reasoning process has run aground. By going over the review of systems, you may uncover supporting facts that may generate new possibilities for your patient's problems.

Prepare the patient by saying, "*The next part of the history may feel like a lot of questions, but it is important to make sure we have not missed anything. I would just like you to answer yes or no to each question.*" Think about asking a series of questions going from "head to toe." Start with a fairly general question as you address each of the different systems, then shift to more specific questions about systems that may be of concern. Examples of starting questions are, "*How are your ears and hearing?*" "*How about your lungs and breathing?*" "*Any trouble with your heart?*" "*How is your digestion?*" "*How about your bowels?*"

Understanding and using review of systems questions may seem challenging at first (Box 3-12). Keep your

Box 3-12. Review of Systems

For each regional system, ask: *"Have you ever had any . . .?"*

- **General:** Usual weight, recent weight change; weakness, fatigue, or fever
- **Skin:** Rashes, lumps, sores, itching, dryness, changes in color; changes in hair or nails; changes in size or color of moles
- **Head, Eyes, Ears, Nose, Throat (HEENT):**
  - *Head:* Headache, head injury, dizziness, lightheadedness
  - *Eyes:* Vision, glasses or contact lenses, pain, redness, excessive tearing, double or blurred vision, spots, specks, flashing lights, glaucoma, cataracts
  - *Ears:* Hearing, tinnitus, vertigo, earaches, infection, discharge; if hearing is decreased, use or nonuse of hearing aids
  - *Nose and sinuses:* Frequent colds, nasal stuffiness, discharge, or itching, hay fever, nosebleeds, sinus trouble
  - *Throat (or mouth and pharynx):* Condition of teeth and gums, bleeding gums, dentures, if any, and how they fit, sore tongue, dry mouth, frequent sore throats, hoarseness
- **Neck:** Swollen glands, goiter, lumps, pain, or stiffness in the neck
- **Breasts:** Lumps, pain, or discomfort, nipple discharge
- **Respiratory:** Cough, sputum (color, quantity; presence of blood or *hemoptysis*), shortness of breath (*dyspnea*), wheezing, pain with a deep breath (*pleuritic pain*)
- **Cardiovascular:** "Heart trouble"; high blood pressure; rheumatic fever; heart murmurs; chest pain or discomfort; palpitations; shortness of breath; need to use pillows at night to ease breathing (*orthopnea*); need to sit up at night to ease breathing (*paroxysmal nocturnal dyspnea*); swelling in the hands, ankles, or feet (*edema*)
- **Gastrointestinal:** Trouble swallowing, heartburn, appetite, nausea; bowel movements, stool color and size, change in bowel habits, pain with defecation, rectal bleeding or black or tarry stools, hemorrhoids, constipation, diarrhea; abdominal pain, food intolerance, excessive belching or passing of gas; jaundice, liver, or gallbladder trouble
- **Peripheral Vascular:** Intermittent leg pain with exertion (*claudication*); leg cramps; varicose veins; past clots in the veins; swelling in calves, legs, or feet; color change in fingertips or toes during cold weather; swelling with redness or tenderness
- **Urinary:** Frequency of urination, polyuria, nighttime urination (*nocturia*), urgency, burning or pain during urination, blood in the urine (*hematuria*), urinary infections, kidney or flank pain, kidney stones, ureteral colic, suprapubic pain, incontinence; in males, reduced caliber or force of the urinary stream, hesitancy, dribbling

- **Genital:**
  - Hernias, discharge from or sores on the penis, testicular pain or masses, scrotal pain or swelling, history of sexually transmitted infections (STIs) and their treatments; sexual interest (*libido*), function, satisfaction
  - Menstrual regularity, frequency, and duration of periods, amount of bleeding; bleeding between periods or after intercourse, dysmenorrhea, premenstrual tension; menopausal symptoms, postmenopausal bleeding; vaginal discharge, itching, sores, lumps, STIs and treatments; sexual interest, satisfaction, any problems, including pain during intercourse (*dyspareunia*)
- **Musculoskeletal:** Muscle or joint pain, stiffness, arthritis, gout, backache (if present, describe location of affected joints or muscles, any swelling, redness, pain, tenderness, stiffness, weakness, or limitation of motion or activity; include timing of symptoms, e.g., morning or evening, duration, and any history of trauma); neck or low back pain; joint pain with systemic symptoms such as fever, chills, rash, anorexia, weight loss, or weakness
- **Psychiatric:** Nervousness, tension, mood, including depression, memory change, suicidal ideation, suicide plans or attempts
- **Neurologic:** Changes in mood, attention, or speech; changes in orientation, memory, insight, or judgment; headache, dizziness, vertigo, fainting, blackouts; weakness, paralysis, numbness, or loss of sensation, tingling or "*pins and needles*," tremors or other involuntary movements, seizures
- **Hematologic:** Anemia, easy bruising, or bleeding
- **Endocrine:** Heat or cold intolerance, excessive sweating, excessive thirst (*polydipsia*), hunger (*polyphagia*), or urine output (*polyuria*)

technique flexible. The need for additional questions will vary depending on the patient's age, concerns, and general state of health and your clinical judgment.

Recall the discussion of the role of pertinent positives and negatives in establishing the differential diagnosis, p. 50.

Some experienced clinicians ask questions about the review of systems during the physical examination, asking about the ears, for example, as they examine them. If the patient has only a few symptoms, this combination can be efficient. If multiple symptoms are present, however, this can disrupt the flow of both the history and the examination, and necessary note-taking becomes awkward.

RECORDING YOUR FINDINGS

Your goal is to produce a clear, concise, but comprehensive report that documents key findings and communicate your assessment in a succinct format to clinicians, consultants, and other members of the health care team. For guidance on documenting the health history details you've collected, refer to Chapter 6, Clinical Documentation and Oral Presentation.

MODIFICATION OF THE CLINICAL INTERVIEW FOR VARIOUS CLINICAL SETTINGS

You will encounter patients in a variety of clinical settings ranging from ambulatory clinics to inpatient wards to busy emergency rooms. So far, we have discussed conducting health history interviews in ideal situations: quiet, with unlimited time, and with minimal distractions. As you may know, the realities of patient encounters are far from ideal. Box 3-13 provides guidance on adapting your physical examination techniques for these diverse settings.

Box 3-13. Modification of the Clinical Interview for Various Clinical Settings

Clinical Setting	Key Points
Ambulatory Care Clinic	This setting is ideal for health history, especially for beginners. Quiet, private rooms with minimal distractions. Patients are mobile with low-acuity chief concerns (CCs). Patients might provide information more readily. Focus on the CC, chronic issues, and routine health care maintenance.
Emergency Care	This setting can be challenging due to patient acuity, fast pace, and 24/7 operations. Ensure patient stability before a detailed interview.[46,47] Prioritize symptoms of potential life-threatening conditions.[46,47] Interviews might be interrupted for tests or procedures you may have to complete your interview at a later time. If a patient is incapacitated, obtain a history from other reliable sources.[47,48]
Intensive Care Unit (ICU)	Many patients have limited communication abilities. Information often comes from family, other clinicians, or electronic health records.[48,49] On the first visit, focus on events leading to intensive care. If the patient can communicate, gather details on treatment preferences and life-sustaining interventions.[48,49]
Nursing Home	Patients are referred to as *residents* as they live there temporarily or permanently.[50,51] Some are undergoing rehabilitation; others are long-term residents. Common issues include dementia, hearing loss, and vision loss. First, try to obtain a history from the resident. Confirm information if cognitive dysfunction is suspected. Include details on activities of daily living (ADLs), both basic (BADLs) and more instrumental (IADLs).[50] Do not feel pressured to get all of the health history at once, as multiple visits can be done.[50]
Home	Care for chronically ill patients and those with functional impairments that make it difficult to leave home without supportive devices or another person's help (*home-limited status*).[52,53] Focus on the patient's functional level and impact on overall health. Evaluate the environment for hazards, cleanliness, food availability, and medication status. Check if patient has friends or family nearby as potential resources.[54]

REFERENCES

1. Walker HK, Hall WD, Hurst JW. *Clinical Methods: The History, Physical and Laboratory Examinations.* 3rd ed. Butterworths; 1990.
2. Kurtz S, Silverman J, Benson J, Draper J. Marrying content and process in clinical method teaching: enhancing the Calgary-Cambridge guides. *Acad Med.* 2003;78(8): 802–809.
3. Kurtz S, Silverman J, Draper J. *Teaching and Learning Communication Skills in Medicine.* 2nd ed. Radcliffe Publishing Ltd; 1998.
4. Kurtz SM, Silverman JD. The Calgary-Cambridge Referenced Observation Guides: an aid to defining the curriculum and organizing the teaching in communication training programmes. *Med Educ.* 1996;30(2):83–89.
5. Haidet P. Jazz and the 'art' of medicine: improvisation in the medical encounter. *Ann Fam Med.* 2007;5(2):164–169.
6. Wagner EH, Austin BT, Von Korff M. Organizing care for patients with chronic illness. *Milbank Q.* 1996;74(4):511–544.
7. Makoul G, Zick A, Green M. An evidence-based perspective on greetings in medical encounters. *Arch Intern Med.* 2007; 167(11):1172–1176.
8. Deutsch MB, Buchholz D. Electronic health records and transgender patients–practical recommendations for the collection of gender identity data. *J Gen Intern Med.* 2015;30(6): 843–847.
9. Beckman HB, Frankel RM. The effect of physician behavior on the collection of data. *Ann Intern Med.* 1984;101(5): 692–696.
10. Barrows HS, Pickell GC. *Developing Clinical Problem-Solving Skills: A Guide to More Effective Diagnosis and Treatment.* W.W. Norton & Company, Inc; 1991.
11. Nebeker JR, Barach P, Samore MH. Clarifying adverse drug events: a clinician's guide to terminology, documentation, and reporting. *Ann Intern Med.* 2004;140(10):795–801.
12. Barbara AM, Chaim G, Doctor F, Centre for Addiction and Mental Health. *Asking the Right Questions, 2: Talking with Clients About Sexual Orientation and Gender Identity in Mental Health, Counselling and Addiction Settings.* Rev. ed. Centre for Addiction and Mental Health; 2007. Accessed September 22, 2024. https://central.bac-lac.gc.ca/.item?id=9780888685414&op=pdf&app=Library
13. Marcell AV, Burstein GR. Sexual and reproductive health care services in the pediatric setting. *Pediatrics.* 2017;140(5): e20172858.
14. Diamant AL, Schuster MA, McGuigan K, Lever J. Lesbians' sexual history with men: implications for taking a sexual history. *Arch Intern Med.* 1999;159(22):2730–2736.
15. Umberson D, Montez JK. Social relationships and health: a flashpoint for health policy. *J Health Soc Behav.* 2010; 51(1 Suppl):S54–S66.
16. Umberson D, Crosnoe R, Reczek C. Social relationships and health behavior across life course. *Annu Rev Sociol.* 2010;36: 139–157.
17. Cohen S. Social relationships and health. *Am Psychol.* 2004; 59(8):676–684.
18. Uchino BN. *Social Support and Physical Health: Understanding the Health Consequences of Relationships.* Yale University Press; 2004. Accessed June 16, 2023. www.jstor.org/stable/j.ctt1nq4mn
19. Cyr MG, Wartman SA. The effectiveness of routine screening questions in the detection of alcoholism. *JAMA.* 1988; 259(1):51–54.
20. Mayfield D, McLeod G, Hall P. The CAGE questionnaire: validation of a new alcoholism screening instrument. *Am J Psychiatry.* 1974;131(10):1121–1123.
21. Moyer VA. Screening and behavioral counseling interventions in primary care to reduce alcohol misuse: U.S. Preventive Services Task Force recommendation statement. *Ann Intern Med.* 2013;159(3):210–218.
22. Ewing JA. Detecting alcoholism. The CAGE questionnaire. *JAMA.* 1984;252(14):1905–1907.
23. Friedmann PD. Clinical practice. Alcohol use in adults. *N Engl J Med.* 2013;368(4):365–373.
24. McCusker MT, Basquille J, Khwaja M, Murray-Lyon IM, Catalan J. Hazardous and harmful drinking: a comparison of the AUDIT and CAGE screening questionnaires. *QJM.* 2002;95(9):591–595.
25. NCI dictionary of cancer terms: pack year. National Cancer Institute. Accessed June 16, 2023. https://www.cancer.gov/publications/dictionaries/cancer-terms/def/pack-year
26. *Screening for Drug Use in General Medical Settings: Resource Guide.* National Institute on Drug Abuse; 2012. https://nida.nih.gov/sites/default/files/resource_guide.pdf
27. Smith PC, Schmidt SM, Allensworth-Davies D, Saitz R. A single-question screening test for drug use in primary care. *Arch Intern Med.* 2010;170(13):1155–1160.
28. Coverdale JH, Balon R, Roberts LW. Teaching sexual history-taking: a systematic review of educational programs. *Acad Med.* 2011;86(12):1590–1595.
29. Shindel AW, Ando KA, Nelson CJ, Breyer BN, Lue TF, Smith JF. Medical student sexuality: how sexual experience and sexuality training impact U.S. and Canadian medical students' comfort in dealing with patients' sexuality in clinical practice. *Acad Med.* 2010;85(8):1321–1330.
30. Rubin ES, Rullo J, Tsai P, et al. Best practices in North American pre-clinical medical education in sexual history taking: consensus from the summits in medical education in sexual health. *J Sex Med.* 2018;15(10):1414–1425.
31. O'Keefe R, Tesar CM. Sex talk: what makes it hard to learn sexual history taking? *Fam Med.* 1999;31(5):315–316.
32. *A guide to taking a sexual history.* Centers for Disease Control and Prevention. Accessed 2023. https://www.cdc.gov/std/treatment/SexualHistory.htm
33. *Taking Routine Histories of Sexual Health: A System-Wide Approach for Health Centers.* National Association of Community Health Centers; National LGBT Health Education Center; 2015. Accessed June 16, 2023. https://www.lgbthealtheducation.org/publication/taking-routine-histories-of-sexual-health-a-system-wide-approach-for-health-centers/
34. Samuel L, Zaritsky E. Communicating effectively with transgender patients. *Am Fam Physician.* 2008;78(5):648, 650.
35. Puchalski CM, Ferrell B. *Making Health Care Whole: Integrating Spirituality into Patient Care.* Templeton Press; 2010.
36. Banin LB, Suzart NB, Guimarães FAG, Lucchetti ALG, de Jesus MA, Lucchetti G. Religious beliefs or physicians' behavior: what makes a patient more prone to accept a physician to address his/her spiritual issues? *J Relig Health.* 2014;53(3):917–928.
37. Ehman JW, Ott BB, Short TH, Ciampa RC, Hansen-Flaschen J. Do patients want physicians to inquire about their spiritual or religious beliefs if they become gravely ill? *Arch Intern Med.* 1999;159(15):1803–1806.

38. King DE, Bushwick B. Beliefs and attitudes of hospital inpatients about faith healing and prayer. *J Fam Pract.* 1994; 39(4):349–352.
39. Kristeller JL, Zumbrun CS, Schilling RF. 'I would if I could': how oncologists and oncology nurses address spiritual distress in cancer patients. *Psychooncology.* 1999;8(5):451–458.
40. MacLean CD, Susi B, Phifer N, et al. Patient preference for physician discussion and practice of spirituality. *J Gen Intern Med.* 2003;18(1):38–43.
41. McCord G, Gilchrist VJ, Grossman SD, et al. Discussing spirituality with patients: a rational and ethical approach. *Ann Fam Med.* 2004;2(4):356–361.
42. Rasinski KA, Kalad YG, Yoon JD, Curlin FA. An assessment of US physicians' training in religion, spirituality, and medicine. *Med Teach.* 2011;33(11):944–945.
43. FICA Spiritual History Tool©. *GW Institute for Spirituality & Health (GWish).* https://gwish.smhs.gwu.edu/programs/patient-research/monitoring-effectiveness-fica-tool
44. Saguil A, Phelps K. The spiritual assessment. *Am Fam Physician.* 2012;86(6):546–550.
45. Puchalski C, Romer AL. Taking a spiritual history allows clinicians to understand patients more fully. *J Palliat Med.* 2000; 3(1):129–137.
46. Ellis G, Marshall T, Ritchie C. Comprehensive geriatric assessment in the emergency department. *Clin Interv Aging.* 2014; 9:2033–2043.
47. Linzer M, Yang EH, Estes NA III, Wang P, Vorperian VR, Kapoor WN. Clinical guideline: diagnosing syncope. Part 1: value of history, physical examination, and electrocardiography. *Ann Intern Med.* 1997;126(12):989–996.
48. Hamill-Ruth RJ, Marohn ML. Evaluation of pain in the critically ill patient. *Crit Care Clin.* 1999;15(1):35–54.
49. Gélinas C, Fillion L, Puntillo KA. Item selection and content validity of the Critical-Care Pain Observation Tool for non-verbal adults. *J Adv Nurs.* 2009;65(1):203–216.
50. King MS, Lipsky MS. Evaluation of nursing home patients. A systematic approach can improve care. *Postgrad Med.* 2000; 107(2):201–215.
51. Kanter SL. The nursing home as a core site for educating residents and medical students. *Acad Med.* 2012;87(5): 547–548.
52. Smith KL, Ornstein K, Soriano T, Muller D, Boal J. A multidisciplinary program for delivering primary care to the underserved urban homebound: looking back, moving forward. *J Am Geriatr Soc.* 2006;54(8):1283–1289.
53. Ornstein KA, Leff B, Covinsky KE, et al. Epidemiology of the homebound population in the United States. *JAMA Intern Med.* 2015;175(7):1180–1186.
54. Josephson KR, Fabacher DA, Rubenstein LZ. Home safety and fall prevention. *Clin Geriatr Med.* 1991;7(4):707–731.
55. U.S. Preventive Services Task Force. Screening for depression: recommendations and rationale. *Ann Intern Med.* 2002; 136(10):760–764.
56. Hossain M, Zimmerman C, Abas M, Light M, Watts C. The relationship of trauma to mental disorders among trafficked and sexually exploited girls and women. *Am J Public Health.* 2010;100(12):2442–2449.
57. Logan TK, Walker R, Hunt G. Understanding human trafficking in the United States. *Trauma Violence Abuse.* 2009; 10(1):3–30.

CHAPTER 4

Physical Examination

ROLE OF THE PHYSICAL EXAMINATION IN THE ERA OF TECHNOLOGY

Careful physical examination and skilled health history taking have long served as the foundational pillars of clinical practice, historically relied on to discern the underlying causes of a patient's symptoms (Fig. 4-1). Even in today's emergency and resource-poor clinical settings, the patient's narrative and physical examination findings remain paramount.

The landscape of clinical practice has been redefined by the emergence of new resources and technologies, which have not only enhanced but, at times, seemed to supplant classic clinical skills.[1,2] Diagnostic technologies have significantly expanded our ability to identify anatomic and physiologic abnormalities, augmenting our clinical capabilities.[1] However, these advanced tools should complement rather than replace careful physical examination in reaching a diagnosis. The integration of information gleaned from these technologies with findings from physical examinations is essential for clinicians to optimize diagnostic accuracy.[3] Overreliance on tests can potentially compromise patient care, mirroring the pitfalls of overreliance on bedside evaluation.[4]

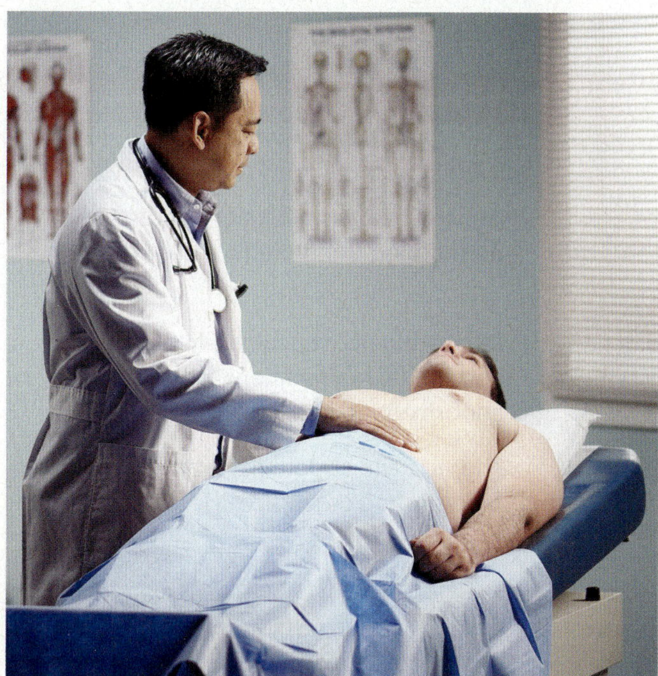

FIGURE 4-1. Art of the physical examination.

The central question is not whether physical examination alone surpasses technology, but, rather, whether clinicians achieve better patient outcomes by combining both approaches instead of relying on one exclusively.[4] Recent studies have begun to view physical examination findings as diagnostic tests themselves, validating their value by identifying their test characteristics.[5,6] Many of these physical examination signs are now evaluated akin to any other diagnostic test, assessing their validity and capacity to either confirm or exclude a disease.[2]

With time, the *rational clinical examination* is anticipated to refine diagnostic decision making, particularly as national competencies and best teaching practices for physical examination skills continue to evolve.[7,8] Meanwhile, the physical examination offers intangible benefits, including enhanced communication with patients,[8] fostering a unique therapeutic relationship, facilitating more accurate diagnoses, and enabling more targeted assessments and care plans.[2,7,9]

Chapter Content Guide

- Conducting Cardinal Techniques of Examination
- Beginning the Physical Examination
- Performing a Head-to-Toe Physical Examination
- Adapting the Physical Examination: Specific Patient Conditions
- Recording Your Findings

CONDUCTING CARDINAL TECHNIQUES OF EXAMINATION

The core of the physical examination is built on four fundamental techniques of examination: *inspection, palpation, percussion,* and *auscultation* (Box 4-1). These techniques form the foundation of your diagnostic approach.

Insonation, a technique that uses the strategic application of sound waves, represents a pivotal advancement in the realm of examination techniques. Central to the practice of point-of-care ultrasound (POCUS), its effectiveness is explored in greater detail in later sections. Additionally, you will explore techniques like instructing patients to lean forward for clearer detection of aortic regurgitation murmurs and using patellar ballottement to identify joint effusion. These methods enhance the diagnostic process, providing a more detailed and nuanced approach to patient evaluation.

Auscultating Through Clothing in Clinical Practice

Auscultation through clothing in clinical settings has sparked controversy and confusion among medical trainees. Traditionally, clinical education emphasizes the necessity of direct skin contact during auscultation to ensure diagnostic accuracy. However, learners often observe their teachers and supervisors auscultating through clothing in practice, creating a discrepancy between what is taught and what is observed. This divergence can be perplexing for beginners, necessitating a clear understanding of when and how this approach might be appropriately used without compromising patient care.

Considerations for Auscultation Through Clothing in Clinical Settings. Despite the conventional practice of auscultation requiring direct skin contact, clinical settings sometimes dictate auscultating through clothing. This practice, while seemingly straightforward, demands careful consideration of its advantages and limitations to maintain diagnostic precision.

Advantages of Auscultation Through Clothing

- *Efficiency in clinical practice:* In certain contexts, particularly during routine or follow-up examinations in which no significant changes in chest pathology are anticipated, auscultating through clothing can expedite the process, allowing for efficient patient management.
- *Patient comfort and dignity:* Recognizing and respecting patient comfort and privacy is paramount. Opting to auscultate through clothing can alleviate discomfort or embarrassment for patients, fostering a more reassuring examination environment.
- *Adaptability in clinical practice:* Evidence and experience suggest that with careful technique, lung sounds can be adequately assessed through light clothing. This flexibility is valuable, illustrating the diverse approaches within clinical practice.

Box 4-1. Cardinal Techniques of Examination

Technique	Description	Application in Physical Examination
Inspection	Close observation of the patient's appearance, behavior, and movements; includes assessments of mood, skin conditions, symmetry, and gait	General health status, signs of disease in dermatology, neurology, and cardiology
Palpation	Uses tactile pressure from the palmar fingers or finger pads to assess skin texture, lymph nodes, pulses, organ sizes, and joint conditions	Dermatologic, musculoskeletal, and abdominal examinations for structural abnormalities
Percussion	Involves using one finger to tap quickly on another finger that is pressed against the surface body surface to generate sounds indicating the presence of fluid, air, or organ size	Thoracic and abdominal exams to assess fluid, air, and organ sizes via sound quality
Auscultation	Uses a stethoscope to detect heart, lung, and bowel sounds, focusing on characteristics like pitch and intensity	Cardiovascular, respiratory, and gastrointestinal exams for diagnostic insights via sound analysis

Limitations of Auscultation Through Clothing

- *Potential for diagnostic inaccuracy:* The primary concern with auscultating through clothing is the possibility of attenuated or altered sounds, which could lead to misinterpretation or oversight of critical clinical signs.
- *Introduction of acoustic artifacts:* The interaction between the stethoscope and clothing may produce extraneous noises, potentially mimicking pathologic sounds or obscuring genuine auditory signals, complicating the diagnostic process.
- *Compromise on comprehensive examination:* Sole reliance on this method may restrict the thoroughness of physical examinations. Essential components such as inspection and percussion might be compromised, limiting the clinician's ability to perform a full assessment.
- *Variable influence of clothing:* The type and thickness of clothing can markedly affect sound transmission. Dense or layered fabrics may significantly hinder the process compared to lighter, single-layer materials.

As you progress in your clinical education, cultivating the ability to navigate these complexities with informed judgment and sensitivity to patient needs will be essential.

BEGINNING THE PHYSICAL EXAMINATION

Before starting the adult physical examination, allocate time for preparation (Box 4-2). This preparation extends beyond gathering equipment; it involves a thoughtful consideration of your approach to the patient, your professional demeanor, and strategies to ensure the patient's comfort and relaxation. Take a moment to reflect on these aspects, ensuring that you are poised to engage with the patient effectively. Additionally, review measures aimed at promoting the patient's physical comfort and make necessary adjustments to the environment to optimize their experience.

Box 4-2. Steps in Beginning the Physical Examination

1. Reflect on your approach to the patient.
2. Optimize the examination environment.
3. Prepare your equipment.
4. Enhance the patient's comfort.
5. Observe standard and universal precautions.
6. Optimize the sequence, scope, and positioning of examination

Reflecting on Your Approach

When meeting the patient, introduce yourself as a student and maintain a calm, organized presence. It is okay to feel inexperienced and to forget parts of the examination; if needed, simply cover these areas later. Inform the patient if you plan to spend more time on certain exams, like listening to their heart, assuring them it does not imply something is wrong. To avoid alarming the patient, forewarn them by saying something like, *"I'd like to spend some extra time listening to your heart and the heart sounds, but this doesn't mean I hear anything wrong."* Acknowledge that patients may feel anxious during exams, feeling exposed and concerned about findings. Your thorough, yet efficient, approach, combined with flexibility and gentle technique, can ease their discomfort and foster positive interactions.

Optimizing the Examination Environment

Create a comfortable examination setting by adjusting the bed height for easy access and repositioning the patient as necessary. Good lighting and a quiet environment are crucial; use natural light, overhead lights, or a penlight as needed, and manage any distractions. A conducive environment improves the examination quality and patient experience.

Preparing Your Equipment

Ensuring that you have the necessary equipment on hand is essential for conducting a thorough physical examination. The equipment required for performing a standard examination is outlined in Box 4-3. The growing importance of POCUS means having portable ultrasound devices ready. Check each item for proper function, like stethoscope diaphragms for integrity and otoscope bulbs for brightness, and ensure a stock of disposable items like gloves and alcohol swabs. Proper equipment preparation prevents delays and promotes an effective examination process.

Enhancing Patient Comfort

Ensuring patient comfort during examinations is not just a courtesy but a cornerstone of effective health care. Enhancing your patient's comfort involves a holistic approach that addresses physical, emotional, and environmental factors to create a reassuring and safe

Box 4-3. Tools of the Trade: Instruments and Supplies for the Physical Examination

Tool/Instrument	Description and Parts	Physical Examination Use
Stethoscope Eartip Binaural Binaural spring Tubing Acoustic valve stem Diaphragm (over) Chest piece Bell	Features ear tips designed for a snug and comfortable fit, connected by an adjustable metal band. It includes thick-walled tubing, ideally ~30 cm in length, to maximize sound transmission. The instrument also has a *bell for low-frequency* sounds and a *diaphragm for high-frequency sounds*, with a mechanism for easy switching between the two.	Used across multiple specialties, including cardiology for heart sounds, pulmonology for lung sounds, and gastroenterology for bowel sounds. The bell is used for low-frequency sounds, while the diaphragm is for higher-frequency sounds, allowing for a comprehensive assessment of internal body sounds.
Sphygmomanometer 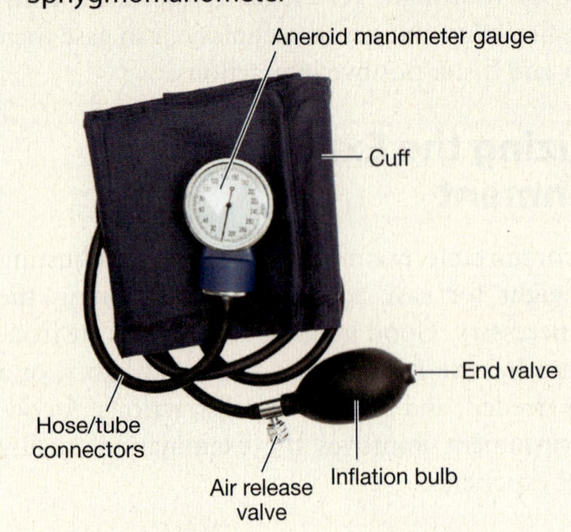	Includes a cuff designed to inflate and constrict blood flow, alongside an aneroid or digital display for blood pressure readings. Modern sphygmomanometers are typically digital, facilitating quicker and more reliable measurements.	Vital for measuring blood pressure, a fundamental aspect of nearly every physical examination. Digital models offer ease of use and improved accuracy, making them essential in detecting hypertension or hypotension across a wide range of clinical settings.
Ophthalmoscope 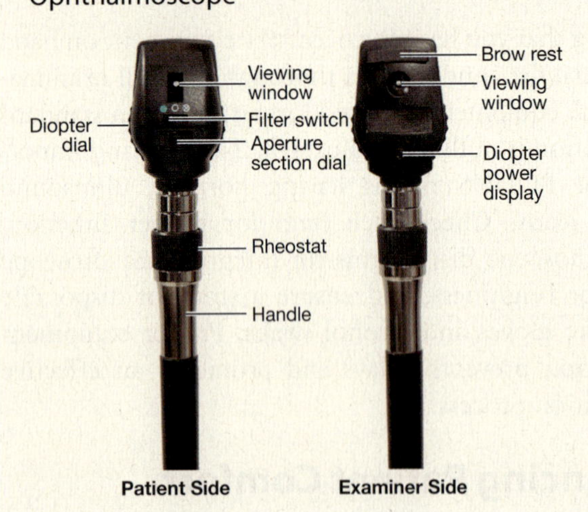	Equipped with a light source and several lenses, enabling the examiner to view the interior structures of the eye, including the retina, optic nerve, and blood vessels.	Used in the eye exam, particularly the fundus, to diagnose conditions such as glaucoma, diabetic retinopathy, and age-related macular degeneration. Its ability to inspect the internal structures of the eye makes it indispensable in ophthalmology.

Tool/Instrument	Description and Parts	Physical Examination Use
Visual acuity card/chart (e.g., Snellen chart) 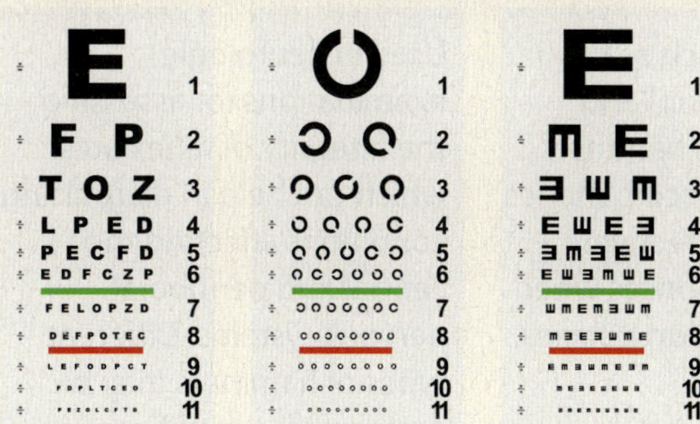	Features rows of letters or symbols in decreasing sizes and is used to measure the sharpness of vision.	Used in vision screening to identify refractive errors and other visual acuity problems. It helps in diagnosing conditions like myopia (nearsightedness), hyperopia (farsightedness), and astigmatism, and is a standard tool in primary care and ophthalmology examinations.
Otoscope 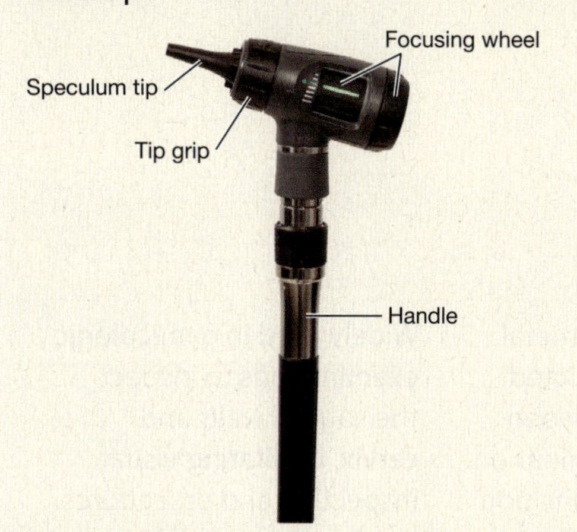	Includes a light source and a magnifying lens for viewing the external auditory canal and tympanic membrane. Advanced models allow for *pneumatic otoscopy*, which involves changing air pressure to assess the mobility of the tympanic membrane.	Used for the ear exam, particularly for detecting infections, blockages, or damage to the ear canal and tympanic membrane. Pneumatic otoscopy is especially useful in pediatric examinations to assess eardrum mobility, aiding in the diagnosis of conditions like otitis media.
Tuning forks 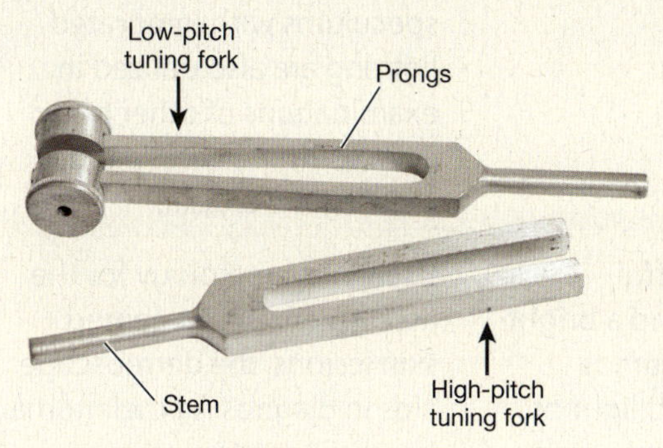	Produce a pure tone when struck, commonly used at 512 Hz and 128 Hz frequencies, to assess auditory function and vibratory sensation respectively.	Used in neurologic and audiometric examinations to evaluate hearing acuity and sensory nerve function. They are essential for conducting tests like the Weber and Rinne tests for auditory function and for assessing vibratory sense in the diagnosis of peripheral neuropathies.
Digital thermometer 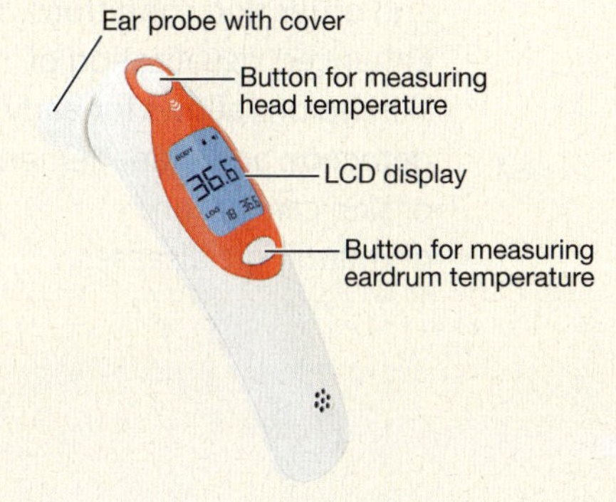	Uses electronic sensors to measure body temperature. They can be applied orally, rectally, under the armpit, or in the ear (tympanically).	Used in assessing body temperature; critical for diagnosing fever or monitoring hypothermia. The choice of measurement site can vary based on patient age, clinical setting, and specific conditions, with digital thermometers providing quick and accurate readings.

(*continued*)

Box 4-3. Tools of the Trade: Instruments and Supplies for the Physical Examination (*Continued*)

Tool/Instrument	Description and Parts	Physical Examination Use
Neurologic reflex hammer 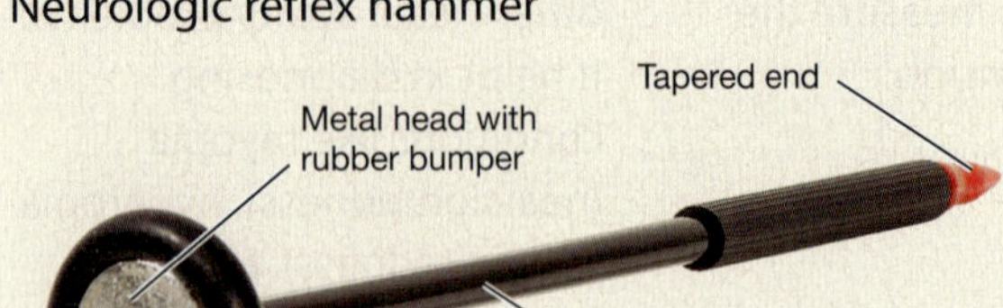 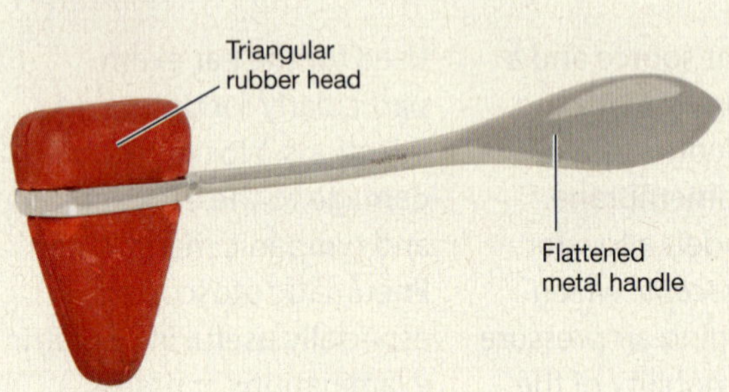 	Includes types such as the Queens Square (top) and Thomas (bottom) hammers, designed with specific shapes and weights to effectively elicit muscle responses when testing deep tendon reflexes.	Used in neurologic examinations for assessing the integrity of reflex arcs, which can help in diagnosing conditions affecting the central and peripheral nervous systems. Different types of hammers may be preferred for specific reflex assessments.
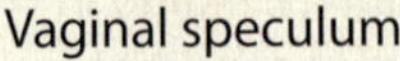 Vaginal speculum 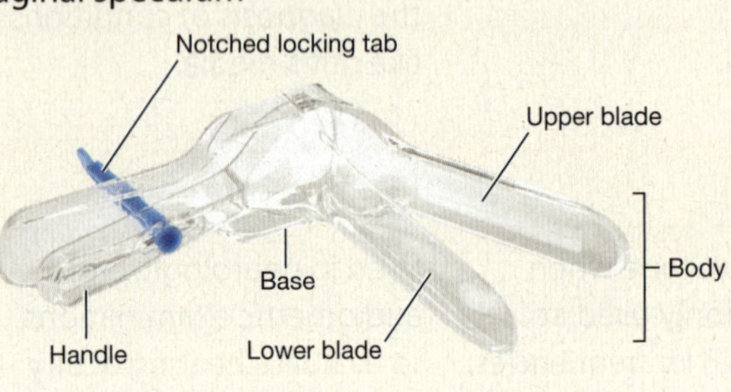 	Traditionally made of metal but now often constructed from plastic; used to widen body cavities for examination. Modern designs may include attachments for fiber-optic light sources to improve visibility.	Widely used in gynecologic examinations to inspect the vaginal walls and cervix, facilitating visual inspection and procedures like Pap smears and human papillomavirus testing. Plastic speculums with integrated lighting are also utilized in examinations of other body cavities where access and visibility are crucial.
Dermoscope 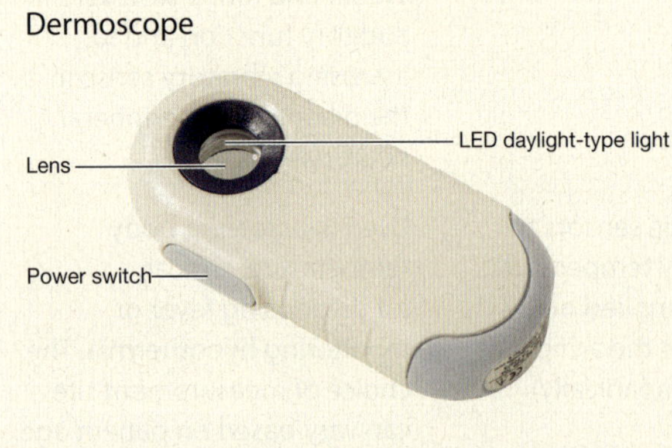 	Combines a powerful magnifying lens and a bright light source, sometimes including polarized light or fluid interfaces, to examine skin lesions with enhanced detail.	Used in dermatology for the assessment of pigmented skin lesions, the dermoscope aids in diagnosing melanoma, basal cell carcinoma, squamous cell carcinoma, and other skin conditions. Enhanced visualization of skin lesions allows for early detection and management of skin cancers and dermatologic diseases.

Tool/Instrument	Description and Parts	Physical Examination Use
Portable ultrasound machine 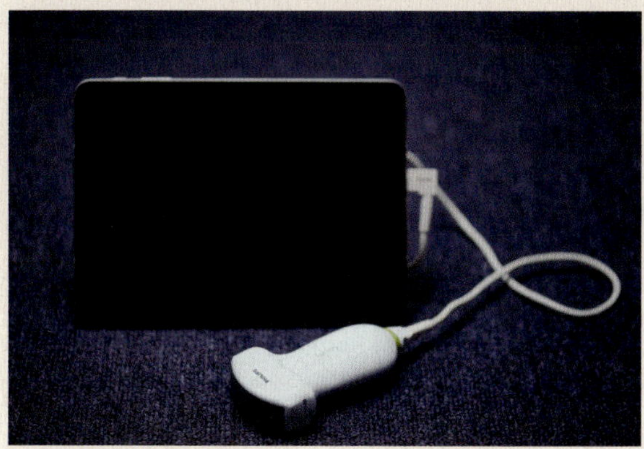	A compact and mobile device that utilizes ultrasound technology to create images of internal body structures. It can be easily transported and used in various clinical settings for real-time imaging.	Employed across numerous medical specialties for diagnostic purposes, including obstetrics for fetal health assessment, cardiology for evaluating heart conditions, and emergency medicine for rapid assessment of internal injuries or conditions. Its portability allows for bedside diagnostics, improving patient care.

Additional supplies:

- *Sampling equipment for cytologic and bacteriologic studies:* Used to collect cells or bacteria samples from the body for laboratory analysis, aiding in the diagnosis of infections, cancers, and other conditions.
- *Cotton swabs, or other disposable objects:* Used for testing light touch sensation and two-point discrimination; used in neurologic exams to assess sensory nerve function, including the ability to feel light touch and differentiate between two closely spaced points.
- *Tongue depressor:* Used to hold down the tongue to examine the mouth and throat for signs of infection, inflammation, or other abnormalities.
- *Ruler or a flexible tape measure, preferably marked in centimeters:* Used to measure the size of wounds, lesions, or other physical features as well as for assessing body growth and development in children.
- *Disposable face mask:* Used by health care providers to prevent the spread of infectious agents during patient interactions, especially important in preventing the transmission of respiratory infections.
- *Disposable gown:* Used by health care providers to protect themselves and their clothing from contamination during examinations or procedures.
- *Gloves and lubricant for oral, vaginal, and rectal examinations:* Used to protect both the patient and health care provider from the transmission of infections during intimate examinations, while lubricant improves patient comfort.
- *Light source:* Used to illuminate dark or internal areas during examinations, such as the throat, nasal passages, ears, and during procedures requiring enhanced visibility.
- *Timepiece with a second hand (timer):* Used to time various aspects of the physical examination, such as heart rate, respiratory rate, and other timed tests.
- *Hand sanitizer:* Used for infection control, allowing health care providers to quickly disinfect their hands between patient contacts.
- *Paper and pen or pencil:* Used for documenting findings during the physical examination; important for maintaining accurate patient records.
- *Access via computer or mobile device to the electronic health record (EHR):* Used to access and update patient medical records digitally, facilitating the integration of examination findings with the patient's overall health information.

Image sources: The following images are used with permission from Shutterstock: stethoscope (Paul Maguire), sphygmomanometer (LeventeGyori), ophthalmoscope, Snellen chart (tuulijumala), otoscope, tuning forks (Duntrune Studios), thermometer (doomu), and vaginal speculum (New Africa). All other images were created for this book by Wolters Kluwer.

Box 4-4. Best Practices for Patient Comfort and Privacy During Physical Examinations

Ensuring patient privacy and comfort	Your role as a clinician grants you unique access to a patient's body, requiring a deep respect for their privacy and modesty. This involves closing doors, drawing curtains, and washing hands before the examination to convey respect for the patient's vulnerability.
Observing and responding to patient needs	Stay alert to the patient's feelings and any signs of discomfort during the examination. Use their facial expressions as cues to ask about their well-being, adjusting the environment (e.g., bed angle, pillows, blankets) as needed to ensure their comfort.
Positioning and draping	Proper patient positioning and draping are essential for an effective examination and the examiner's comfort. Learning the correct techniques for each examination segment maximizes patient comfort without compromising diagnostic goals.
Providing clear instructions	Communicate clearly and courteously with the patient at each examination step, setting expectations and reducing anxiety. Inform the patient of what to expect, especially if a procedure might cause embarrassment or discomfort.
Keeping the patient informed	Engage with the patient about their findings and address any questions or concerns they might have. This keeps them involved in their care and helps build trust.
Concluding the examination	Share your general impressions with the patient and what they can expect moving forward. Ensure their safety by returning the environment to its original state, such as lowering the bed to prevent falls and raising the bedrails. Before leaving, practice good hygiene by washing your hands, cleaning your equipment, and properly disposing of waste materials to conclude the examination on a note of care and professionalism.

atmosphere. Box 4-4 provides a structured overview of the key aspects involved in ensuring patient comfort and privacy during medical examinations, highlighting the importance of sensitivity, clear communication, and attentive care throughout the process.

Observing Standard and Universal Precautions

The Centers for Disease Control and Prevention (CDC) has published a series of guidelines aimed at safeguarding both patients and health care providers from the transmission of infectious diseases. All clinicians who perform patient examinations should familiarize themselves with and adhere to these recommendations, accessible on the CDC's website. The guidelines encompass protocols for both Standard Precautions, Contact Precautions specific to methicillin-resistant *Staphylococcus aureus* (MRSA), and Universal Precautions (Box 4-5).[10–14] The following fluids are considered potentially infectious: all blood and other body fluids containing visible blood, semen, and vaginal secretions and cerebrospinal, synovial, pleural, peritoneal, pericardial, and amniotic fluids.

The three primary transmission-based precautions outlined in Box 4-7—*contact, droplet,* and *airborne precautions*—cover the main strategies for preventing the spread of infectious agents in health care settings based on the mode of transmission of the pathogen. These are designed to supplement standard precautions, which are applied to the care of all patients regardless of their diagnosis or presumed infection status.

Included is *reverse isolation (protective isolation)*. While the latter three are primarily aimed at preventing the spread of infectious diseases from an infected patient to others (health care workers, visitors, and other patients), reverse isolation serves an opposite function and is designed to protect a specific group of patients from infections present in their environment (e.g., patients with decreased immune systems).

OPTIMIZING THE SEQUENCE, SCOPE, AND POSITIONING OF EXAMINATION

Optimizing your examination strategy involves a nuanced approach that includes choosing between comprehensive and focused exams, and carefully considering sequence, scope, and positioning. This tailored process ensures that your patient's specific needs are met with attention to comfort, dignity, and efficiency.

Box 4-5. Comparative Overview of Precautionary Measures: Standard, MRSA, and Universal Precautions

Category	Standard Precautions	MRSA Precautions	Universal Precautions
Principle	Based on the assumption that all blood, body fluids, secretions, excretions (except sweat), nonintact skin, and mucous membranes may contain transmissible infectious agents	Focuses on preventing the transmission of multidrug-resistant organisms, especially MRSA and vancomycin-resistant enterococcus (VRE)[10]	Aimed at preventing health care workers' exposure to bloodborne pathogens, including HIV and hepatitis B virus (HBV)
Application	Apply to all patients, regardless of their diagnosis or presumed infection status, in any health care setting	Specific to environments and situations where MRSA or VRE transmission is a concern	Applies to all situations with the potential for exposure to bloodborne pathogens
Key components	■ Hand hygiene (Fig. 4-2 and Box 4-6) ■ Use of personal protective equipment (PPE) such as gloves, gowns, and eye protection (Fig. 4-3) ■ Safe injection practices ■ Safe handling of potentially contaminated equipment or surfaces ■ Respiratory hygiene and cough etiquette ■ Patient isolation criteria ■ Precautions for handling equipment, toys, solid surfaces, and laundry ■ Regular cleaning of white coats, scrub suits, and stethoscopes[15,16]	■ Hand hygiene upon entering and exiting the patient's room ■ Use of PPE, such as gloves and gowns ■ Patient isolation: Single room or cohorting with others infected with the same organism ■ Dedicated or disposable equipment for each patient ■ Environmental cleaning and disinfection of high-touch surfaces ■ Minimizing patient transport to essential purposes only ■ Proper handling of contaminated laundry and waste	■ Immunization with HBV vaccine ■ Use of protective barriers (gloves, gowns, aprons, masks, protective eyewear) ■ Precautions for safe injections and prevention of injuries from needlesticks, scalpels, and other sharp instruments ■ Immediate reporting of injury from sharp instruments
Infectious agents	All patients may carry infectious agents	Focus on multidrug-resistant organisms	Specifically targets bloodborne pathogens (e.g., HIV, HBV)
Fluids considered potentially infectious	Assumes all blood, body fluids (except sweat), secretions, excretions, nonintact skin, and mucous membranes may contain transmissible infectious agents	Within the context of multidrug-resistant organism precautions	All blood and body fluids containing visible blood, semen, vaginal secretions, and several other specific body fluids (cerebrospinal, synovial, pleural, peritoneal, pericardial, amniotic)

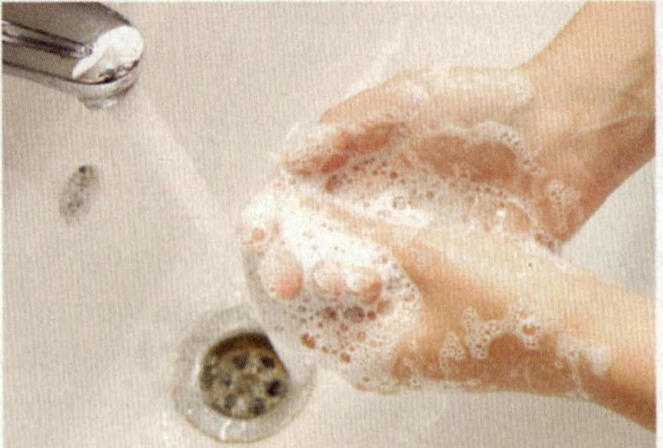

FIGURE 4-2. Observing proper standard precautions with handwashing.

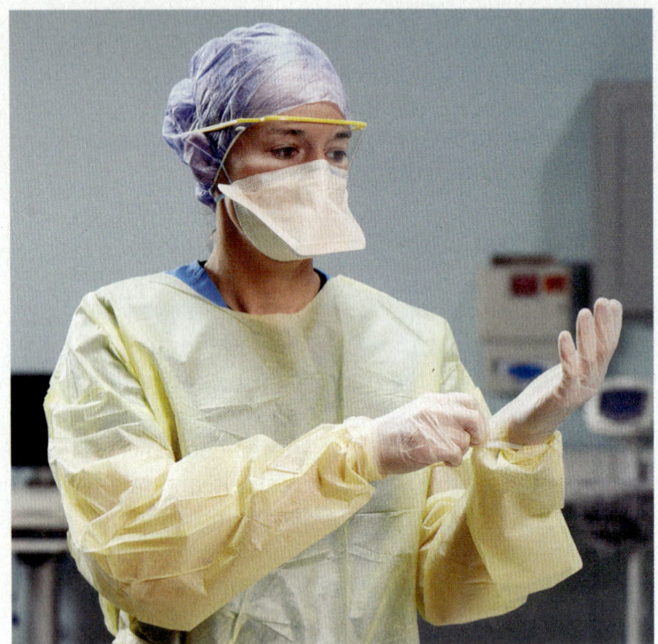

FIGURE 4-3. Personal protective equipment (PPE).

Box 4-6. Hand Hygiene Guidance in Health Care Settings

Health care personnel should use an alcohol-based hand rub or wash with soap and water for the following clinical indications:

- Immediately before touching a patient
- Before performing an aseptic task (e.g., placing an indwelling device) or handling invasive medical devices
- Before moving from work on a soiled body site to a clean body site on the same patient
- After touching a patient or the patient's immediate environment
- After contact with blood, body fluids, or contaminated surfaces
- Immediately after glove removal

Unless hands are visibly soiled, an alcohol-based hand rub is preferred over soap and water in most clinical situations due to evidence of better compliance compared to soap and water. Hand rubs are generally less irritating to hands and, in the absence of a sink, are an effective method of cleaning hands.

Source: CDC. *Hand Hygiene in Healthcare Settings*. January 29, 2020. Accessed March 19, 2024. https://www.cdc.gov/handhygiene/providers/guideline.html

Box 4-7. Transmission-Based Precautions in Patient Care Facilities

		Type of Personal Protective Equipment Required			
Type of Precaution	**Description**	**Gloves**	**Gown**	**Mask**	**Respirator Mask**
Contact precautions	Conditions that can be contracted through touching or contact such as MRSA and *Clostridioides difficile*.	✓	✓		
Droplet precautions	Conditions spread through respiratory secretions from the mouth, nose, and lungs, especially when coughing or sneezing. Droplets usually travel only ~3 ft. (e.g., influenza, whooping cough); COVID-19 droplets can travel beyond 6 ft.	✓	✓	✓	

Type of Precaution	Description	Type of Personal Protective Equipment Required			
		Gloves	Gown	Mask	Respirator Mask
Airborne precautions	Conditions that can spread through the air over long distances such as tuberculosis and chickenpox. Patients are also placed in a *negative pressure room* designed to prevent contaminated air from escaping.	✓	✓		✓
Reverse or protective isolation	Used to protect patients with weakened immune systems (e.g., from chemotherapy) from germs carried by staff or visitors.	✓	✓	✓	

Source: CDC. *Guideline for Isolation Precautions: Preventing Transmission of Infectious Agents in Healthcare Settings* (2007). Updated September 2024. Accessed October 3, 2024. https://www.cdc.gov/infection-control/media/pdfs/guideline-isolation-h.pdf

Sequence of Examination

A well-structured sequence not only streamlines your examination but also minimizes patient discomfort and maximizes the efficiency of your diagnostic process. Starting with less invasive procedures and gradually moving to more detailed examinations can help maintain patient comfort. For instance, you may want to start with observing your patient's general appearance and checking their vital signs before proceeding to more focused examinations. This allows you to gather essential information without immediate intrusion. Review the proposed physical examination sequence in the Head-to-Toe section (pp. 78–80), which meets the three goals of patient comfort, minimal changes in positioning, and efficiency.

Positioning of Examination

Each part of the examination may require different positions, such as sitting, supine, or lateral recumbent, to best access and evaluate the area of interest. Effective positioning, combined with strategic examination sequencing, reduces the need for unnecessary changes, thereby minimizing patient exertion and enhancing the examination flow. Box 4-8 offers guidance on optimal positioning for various components of the examination. Likewise, employing effective draping techniques at appropriate times throughout the examination respects patient dignity and contributes to a comfortable and secure environment (Box 4-9).

Scope of Examination

Determining whether a comprehensive or focused examination is necessary should be based on the patient's presenting symptoms, history, and specific health concerns (Box 4-10). A *comprehensive exam* is thorough and evaluates the patient in a holistic manner, ideal for annual check-ups or when your patient presents with complex or multisystem issues. In contrast, a *focused exam* is targeted to a specific problem or area of concern, suitable for follow-up visits or when you are addressing a particular symptom. Your strategic choice significantly impacts your subsequent steps, ensuring that your examination is both appropriate and efficient.

PERFORMING A HEAD-TO-TOE PHYSICAL EXAMINATION

A head-to-toe examination is a systematic approach that ensures a thorough and efficient assessment of the patient. Starting at the head and moving toward the feet, this methodical process allows you to maintain an organized flow, reducing the risk of missing important signs or symptoms.

Box 4-11 provides a structured approach that ensures moving seamlessly from one section to the next while keeping the patient's comfort in mind. The order and depth of examination may be adapted based on the patient's presenting concerns and health history. Flexibility within this structured approach allows for focused assessments that address your patient's specific needs while ensuring a comprehensive evaluation.

Box 4-8. Common Patient Positioning for Physical Examinations and Indications

Position	Description	Purpose/Use
Standing 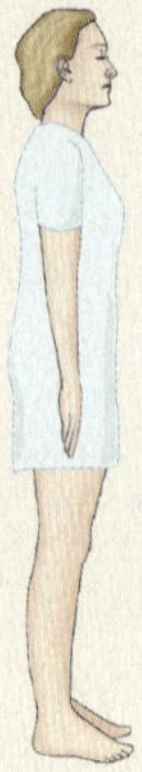	Patient stands upright with weight evenly distributed on both feet.	Used for assessing posture, gait, and lower extremity strength. Can also be used for certain orthopedic and neurologic examinations.
Sitting 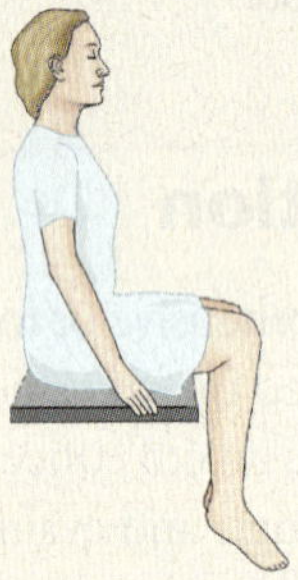	Patient sits on the edge of the examination table or chair, feet dangling or on a stool.	Used for examining the head, neck, chest, and upper extremities. Ideal for respiratory, cardiovascular, and neurologic examinations.
Supine 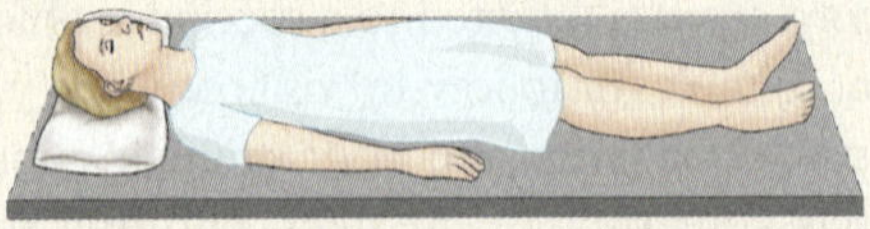	Patient lies flat on their back with legs extended.	Facilitates the examination of the abdomen, heart, and the lower extremities. Allows for relaxation of abdominal muscles.
Prone 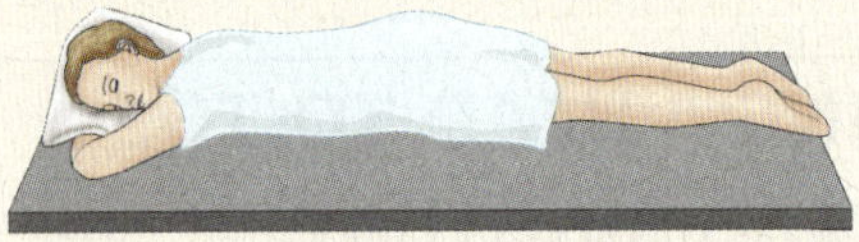	Patient lies flat on their stomach with the head turned to one side.	Primarily used for the examination of the back and to assess hip joint mobility.
Lithotomy 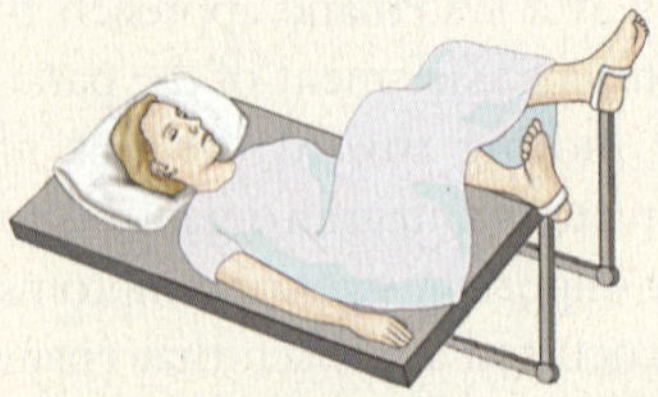	Patient lies on their back with hips and knees flexed, thighs apart and externally rotated, feet in foot rests.	Essential for gynecologic examinations and procedures, as well as rectal exams.
Lateral recumbent 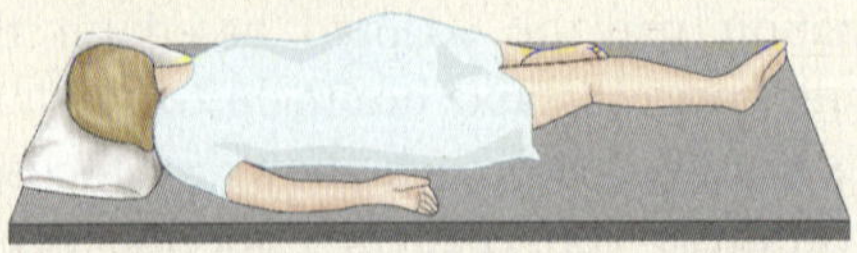	Patient lies on their left side with the right knee flexed toward the chest and the left knee slightly bent.	Provides optimal exposure for examining the rectum and the anus. Also used for sigmoidoscopy and as a position to reduce prolapsed rectal tissue.

Position	Description	Purpose/Use
Dorsal recumbent 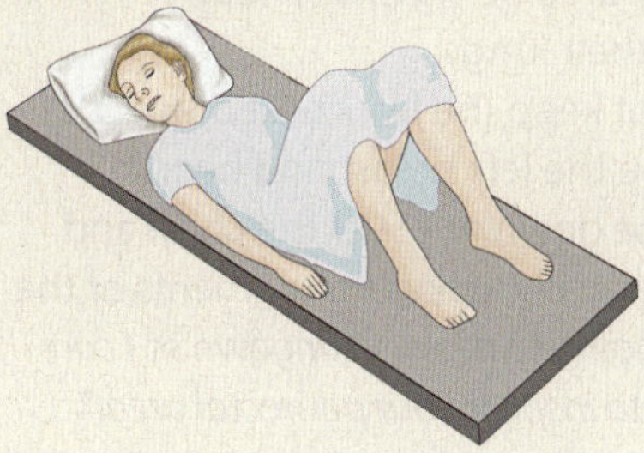	Patient lies on their back with knees bent and feet flat on the examination table.	Used to reduce tension in the abdominal muscles during abdominal assessment. Can be used for patients who have difficulty maintaining the supine position.
Standard Fowler's 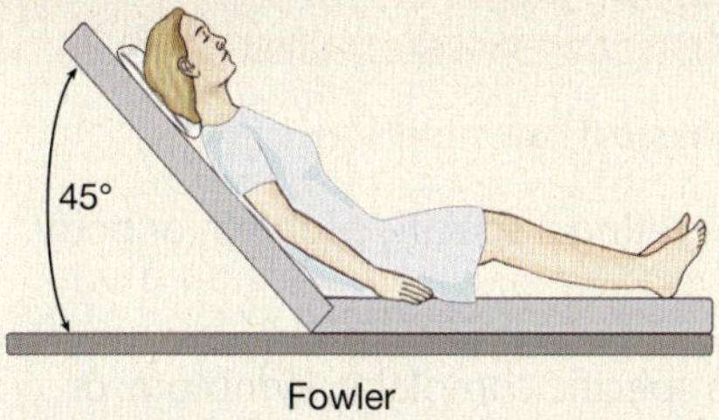	Patient sits partially upright (at a 45°–60° angle) with legs either bent or hanging off the table.	Facilitates breathing and is used in cardiovascular and respiratory examinations. It is also used for patients experiencing difficulty in breathing.
Semi-Fowler's 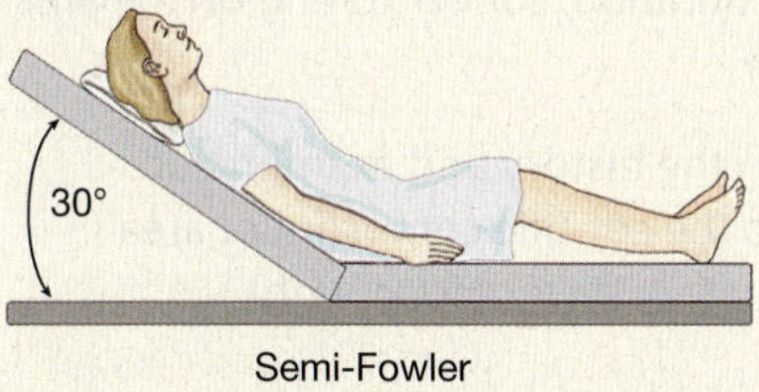	Patient sits or lies in a semi-upright position (~30°–45°) with legs extended or slightly bent.	Promotes lung expansion, facilitates breathing, and aids in reducing the risk of aspiration in patients with dysphagia or those at risk of reflux.
High-Fowler's 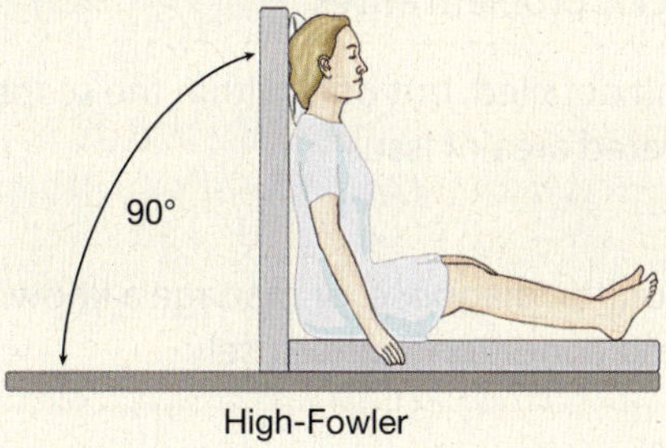	Patient sits or lies in an elevated position (>45°) with legs extended or slightly bent.	Maximizes lung expansion and facilitates breathing. Often used in patients with respiratory distress, congestive heart failure, or undergoing mechanical ventilation.
Trendelenburg 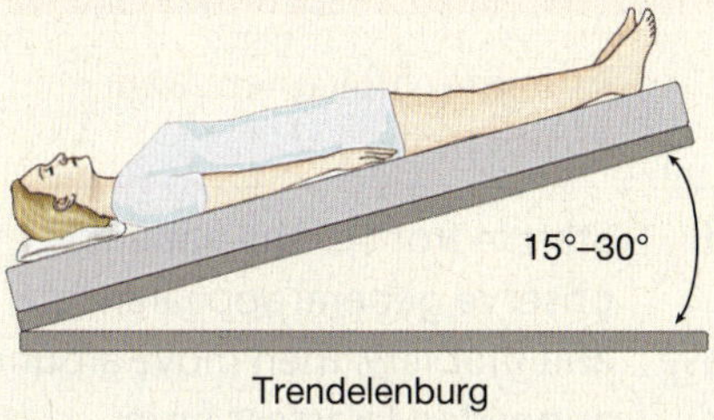	Patient lies on their back with the body tilted so that their head is lower than their feet.	Rarely used in routine exams but can be used in emergency situations to improve circulation or for specific surgical procedures.

Image sources: The first seven images are modified with permission from Taylor C, Lillis C, Lynn P. *Fundamentals of Nursing: The Art and Science of Person-Centered Care*. 8th ed. Wolters Kluwer; 2015. Figures 25-2-1 through 25-2-7. All remaining images were created for this book by Wolters Kluwer.

Box 4-9. Tips for Draping the Patient

- Thoughtful draping preserves the patient's modesty and helps you focus on the area being examined.
- With the patient sitting, for example, untie the gown in back to better listen to their lungs.
- For the breast examination, with the patient supine, uncover the right breast but keep the left chest draped. Drape the right chest again, then uncover the left chest and proceed to examine the left breast and heart.
- For the abdominal examination, only the abdomen should be exposed. Adjust the gown to cover the chest and place the sheet or drape at the inguinal level. To help the patient prepare for potentially awkward segments of the examination, briefly describe your plans before starting, for example, *"Now I am going to move your gown so I can check the pulse in your groin area,"* or *"Because you mentioned irritation, I am going to inspect your perirectal area."*

Box 4-10. Differences Between Comprehensive and Focused Physical Examinations

Feature	Comprehensive Physical Examination	Focused Physical Examination
Scope	Broad and general, covering multiple body systems	Narrow, targeting a specific problem or body system
Purpose	To get an overall view of the patient's health and to screen for potential diseases	To assess a specific complaint, symptom, or diagnosed condition
Time	Usually takes longer, as it involves a detailed check of the whole body	Shorter in duration, concentrating on the area of concern
Components	Includes patient history, vital signs, and examination of all major body systems (e.g., cardiovascular, respiratory, gastrointestinal, neurologic)	Focuses on the history and examination relevant to the specific complaint or area (e.g., respiratory system for cough)
Indications	During an initial visit, annual physicals, or for patients not seen for a long time	In follow-up visits for ongoing issues, or when a new specific problem arises
Detail level	Comprehensive, involving a thorough examination and often more general screening tests	Specific and detailed, but only within the scope of the targeted area or issue
Outcome	Can lead to the identification of previously undiagnosed conditions or risk factors	Aims to monitor, diagnose, or manage a known or suspected condition more closely

Box 4-11. Suggested Comprehensive (Head-to-Toe) Physical Examination Sequence

Organ/System	Physical Examination Considerations	Patient Positioning	Examiner Movement and Positioning
General survey	Observe overall appearance, health status, build, sexual development, posture, motor activity, gait, dress, grooming, personal hygiene, odors, facial expressions, manner, affect, and reactions. Measure height and weight, assess awareness or consciousness.	Have the patient stand or sit comfortably, ensuring they are at ease and fully accessible for observation.	Start in front of the patient to observe general appearance and mobility, then move around as needed to assess from different angles.

Organ/System	Physical Examination Considerations	Patient Positioning	Examiner Movement and Positioning
Vital signs	Measure blood pressure, pulse, respiratory rate, and body temperature.	Seat the patient comfortably with their arm supported at heart level for blood pressure measurement.	Stand to the patient's side, where you can easily access the arm for blood pressure and palpate the pulse at the wrist.
Skin	Inspect and palpate the skin across all body regions for moisture, dryness, temperature, and lesions. Note characteristics of hair and nails.	Position the patient as needed to expose different areas of the skin, ensuring privacy and comfort.	Move around the patient to thoroughly inspect and palpate all accessible skin surfaces, adjusting your position as you proceed with the examination.
Head and neck	*Head:* Examine scalp, skull, and face. *Neck:* Inspect and palpate cervical lymph nodes, trachea, and thyroid.	Patient remains seated.	Begin in front of the patient to examine the head, then move to either side or behind for neck palpation, maintaining an efficient flow.
Eyes	Assess visual acuity, visual fields, alignment, eyelids, sclera, conjunctiva, cornea, iris, lens, pupils, light reaction, and extraocular movements. Use an ophthalmoscope for ocular fundi.	Patient should be seated with eyes at examiner's eye level.	Remain in front of the patient, adjusting your position slightly as needed for direct eye contact and use of instruments like the ophthalmoscope.
Ears and nose	*Ears:* Inspect auricles, canals, drums, check auditory acuity, perform Weber and Rinne tests. *Nose:* Examine external nose, nasal mucosa, septum, turbinates, and sinuses.	Patient remains seated.	For the ear examination, move to the side or slightly behind the patient. For the nose, stand in front of the patient, adjusting as needed for a clear view.
Throat and oral cavity	Inspect lips, oral mucosa, gums, teeth, tongue, palate, tonsils, and pharynx.	Patient remains seated, asked to open their mouth and possibly stick out their tongue.	Stay in front of the patient, using a light source to illuminate the oral cavity for a thorough inspection.
Posterior thorax and lungs	Inspect and palpate the spine and upper back muscles. Chest inspection, palpation, percussion, and auscultation for breath sounds.	Patient can be seated or standing, depending on comfort and ability.	Begin behind the patient for the back inspection, then continue with palpation, percussion, and auscultation of the lungs.
Breasts and axillae	Inspect and palpate the breasts and axillae for lumps, skin changes, or nipple discharge.	Position the patient sitting for visual inspection, then lying down for palpation.	Start in front of the patient for visual inspection, then move to the side for palpation, ensuring access to both the breasts and axillae.
Anterior thorax and lungs	Inspect, palpate, and percuss the chest. Auscultate for breath sounds and adventitious sounds.	Have the patient seated or lying down, with the chest exposed.	Position yourself in front of the patient for inspection and palpation, moving around to the side as necessary for auscultation.

(*continued*)

Box 4-11. Suggested Comprehensive (Head-to-Toe) Physical Examination Sequence (*Continued*)

Organ/System	Physical Examination Considerations	Patient Positioning	Examiner Movement and Positioning
Cardiovascular system	Observe jugular venous distention, palpate carotid pulses, inspect and palpate the precordium, auscultate heart sounds and murmurs.	Position the patient semi-reclined for jugular observation, then lying down for the precordial examination.	Start at the patient's right side for jugular venous pressure observation, then adjust as needed for palpation and auscultation, moving around the patient efficiently.
Abdomen	Inspect, auscultate, percuss, and palpate the abdomen for bowel sounds, organ size, masses, and tenderness.	Patient should lie down with their abdomen exposed, knees slightly bent or a pillow under the knees to relax abdominal muscles.	Stand on the patient's right side to perform the examination in sequence from inspection to palpation, maintaining a position that allows for gentle and precise movements.
Lower extremities	Examine for edema, discoloration, ulcers, varicose veins, palpate pulses, assess musculoskeletal and nervous system functions.	Start with the patient lying down; have them stand for examination of venous system and gait assessment.	Move around the patient as needed, from the bedside for palpation and sensory examination to assisting and observing the patient standing for musculoskeletal and gait assessment.
Nervous system	(Optional) Assess mental status, cranial nerves, motor and sensory systems, and reflexes.	Patient is seated or lying down, depending on the component being assessed.	Adapt your position based on the examination phase, from sitting opposite the patient for mental status to moving alongside for reflex testing.
Musculoskeletal system	(Optional) Examine muscle strength and joint range of motion, and check for any deformities or abnormalities.	Various positions as needed for specific joint or muscle group examination.	Position yourself for optimal access to the area being examined, moving as necessary to apply appropriate examination techniques.
Genitourinary system: penis, scrotum, and prostate	(Optional) Inspect and palpate the penis, testicles, scrotum, and check for hernias. Perform a rectal examination to assess the prostate.	Initially standing for external examination, then lying down for a rectal examination.	For the external exam, stand in front of the patient. For rectal exams, position yourself behind the patient.
Genitourinary system: vulva, vagina, uterus, and adnexa	(Optional) Examine the external genitalia, perform speculum examination of the vagina and cervix, obtain Pap smear, and perform bimanual palpation of the uterus and adnexa. Perform a rectal examination if indicated.	Lying down in the lithotomy position for external and internal examination.	Sit or stand at the end of the examination table, adjusting your position as needed for speculum insertion and bimanual examination.

As you review the following chapters, note that clinicians vary in where they place different segments of the examination, especially examinations of the musculoskeletal and nervous systems. You will also quickly see that some segments of the examination are best assessed when the patient is sitting, such as the head and neck and thorax and lungs, whereas others are best obtained with the patient supine, such as the cardiovascular and abdominal examinations.

With practice, you will develop your own sequence of examination, keeping the need for thoroughness and patient comfort in mind. At first, you may need notes to remind you what to look for, but, over time, this sequence will become habitual and remind you to return to segments of the examination you may have skipped, helping you to be complete.

For more detailed information on examining each specific organ system, including nuanced techniques and interpretations of findings, refer to the individual chapters dedicated to each system.

ADAPTING THE PHYSICAL EXAMINATION: SPECIFIC PATIENT CONDITIONS

As you progress through your training, you may need to modify your physical examination due to the patient's clinical status, which, in turn, may dictate changes in your sequence of examination. Box 4-12 provides an overview of considerations and modifications necessary for physical examinations across different patient types, ensuring you can adapt your approach to meet the needs of each individual patient effectively.

For the approach and modification of clinical skills for specific patient populations, see Chapter 28, Children: Infancy Through Adolescence, pp. 995–1120; Chapter 29, Pregnant Persons, pp. 1121–1157; and Chapter 30, Older Adults, pp. 1158–1194.

Box 4-12. Physical Examination Modifications for Specific Patient Types

Patient Type	Considerations	Specific Physical Examination Modifications
Patient prescribed bed rest	■ Must abstain from weight bearing or certain activities post injury or surgery ■ At risk of developing pressure injuries, especially in sacral area	■ *Anterior examination:* Limited to head, neck, and chest with patient lying supine ■ *Posterior examination:* If safe, patient can roll over for posterior chest auscultation and skin examination, especially the sacral area
Patient who uses a wheelchair	■ Clinicians often examine patients in wheelchairs, sometimes omitting parts of the exam[17] ■ At risk for pressure injuries at major pressure points due to prolonged sitting	■ *Seated examinations:* Cardiovascular, pulmonary, head, and neck exams with patient in wheelchair ■ *Transfer for examination:* Abdominal exams require transfer to examination table or bed ■ *Skin examination:* Inspect for pressure injuries at pressure points like sacrum, heels, calves, elbows, and spine
Patient recovering from a procedure	■ Postsurgery patients may have difficulty following commands due to anesthesia effects ■ Movement may be restricted; confirm restrictions with clinician	■ *Surgical site and dressing:* Focus on cleanliness, dryness, and signs of healing or infection ■ *Abdominal area:* Check for return of bowel function ■ *Peripheral vascular/neurologic exams:* Assess for specific postoperative complications
Patient with obesity	■ Challenges in examination due to adipose tissue obscuring areas. ■ Increased risk for disorders like cardiovascular diseases and diabetes mellitus due to fat distribution[18,19]	■ *Fat distribution and body folds:* Examine for skin breakdown and infection ■ *Lower extremities:* Inspect for skin breakdown, swelling, or vascular changes ■ *Breast, cardiovascular, and pulmonary examinations:* Essential due to associations with diseases like breast cancer, heart failure, and hypoventilation[18,19]

(continued)

Box 4-12. Physical Examination Modifications for Specific Patient Types (*Continued*)

Patient Type	Considerations	Specific Physical Examination Modifications
Patient experiencing pain	■ Need to balance assessing physical findings with potential for exacerbating pain ■ Pain can elevate blood pressure and heart rate[20–22]; nonverbal or comatose patients can still experience pain	■ *Observation:* Look for signs of distress ■ *Pain management:* Consider controlling pain before starting the exam ■ *Examination adjustments:* Use pain characteristics to guide which maneuvers to perform or adjust ■ *Nonverbal/comatose patient:* Note vital signs, facial expressions, signs of agitation, and withdrawal for pain assessment and management
Patient requiring special precautions	■ Special PPE required when examining patients with an infection or at risk for infection, may limit examination capabilities	■ *Auscultation and palpation limitations:* Adjust examination techniques or omit as required by PPE limitations, document accordingly

RECORDING YOUR FINDINGS

Recall that your goal is to produce a clear, concise, but comprehensive report that documents key findings and communicates your assessment in a succinct format to clinicians, consultants, and other members of the health care team (see Box 6-3. Checklist to Ensure a Quality Clinical Record, p. 98). Study documentation of the physical examination findings (Box 4-13). Note the standard format of the clinical record from General Survey to Neurologic Examination. Additional sample documentation can also be found Chapter 6, Clinical Documentation and Oral Presentation, pp. 107–109 and in each of the Unit 2 regional chapters.

Box 4-13. Sample Patient Note: Physical Examination

Physical Examination

General Survey: RS is a middle-aged individual with a short stature and higher body weight, who is animated and responds quickly to questions. Her hair is well groomed. Her color is good, and she lies flat without discomfort.

Vital signs: Height (without shoes) 157 cm (5′2″). Weight (dressed) 65 kg (143 lb). BMI 26. BP 164/98 mm Hg right arm, supine; 160/96 mm Hg left arm, supine; 152/88 mm Hg right arm, supine with wide cuff. Heart rate (HR) 88 and regular, respiratory rate (RR) 18/min, Temperature (tympanic) 36 °C (98.6 °F).

Skin: Palms cold and moist, but color good. Scattered cherry angiomas over upper trunk. Nails without clubbing, or cyanosis.

Head, Eyes, Ears, Nose, Throat (HEENT): Head: Hair of average texture. Scalp without lesions, normocephalic/atraumatic (NC/AT). *Eyes:* Vision 20/30 in each eye. Visual fields full by confrontation. Conjunctiva pink; sclera white. Pupils 4 mm constricting to 2 mm, round, regular, equally reactive to light. Extraocular movements intact. Disc margins sharp, without hemorrhages, exudates. No arteriolar narrowing or A-V nicking. *Ears:* Cerumen partially obscures right tympanic membrane (TM); left canal clear, TM with good cone of light. Acuity good to whispered voice. Weber midline. AC > BC. *Nose:* Mucosa pink, septum midline. No sinus tenderness. *Mouth:* Oral mucosa pink. Dentition good. Tongue midline. Tonsils absent. Pharynx without exudates.

Neck: Neck supple. Trachea midline. Thyroid isthmus barely palpable, lobes not felt.

Lymph nodes: No cervical, axillary, or epitrochlear nodes.

Thorax and lungs: Thorax symmetric with good excursion. Lungs resonant on percussion. Breath sounds vesicular with no added sounds. Diaphragms descend 4 cm bilaterally.

Cardiovascular: Jugular venous pressure 3 cm above the sternal angle, with head of the examining table raised to 30°. Carotid upstrokes brisk, without bruits. Apical impulse discrete and tapping, barely palpable in the 5th left interspace, 8 cm lateral to the midsternal line. Good S_1, S_2; no S_3 or S_4. A 2/6 medium-pitched midsystolic murmur at the 2nd second right interspace; does not radiate to the neck. No diastolic murmurs.

Breasts: Pendulous, symmetric. No masses; nipples without discharge.

Abdomen: Protuberant. Well-healed scar, right lower quadrant. Bowel sounds active. No tenderness or masses. Liver span 7 cm in right midclavicular line; edge smooth, palpable 1 cm below right costal margin (RCM). Spleen not felt. No costovertebral angle tenderness (CVAT).

Genitalia: External genitalia without lesions. Mild cystocele at introitus on straining. Vaginal mucosa pink. Cervix pink, parous, and without discharge. Uterus anterior, midline, smooth, not enlarged. Adnexa not palpated due to patient body habitus and poor relaxation. No cervical or adnexal tenderness. Pap smear taken. Rectovaginal wall intact.

Rectal: No external hemorrhoids, with tight sphincter tone, rectal vault without masses. Stool brown, negative for occult blood.

Extremities: Warm and without edema. Calves supple, nontender.

Peripheral vascular: Trace edema at both ankles. No varicosities in lower extremities. No stasis pigmentation or ulcers. Pulses (2+ = brisk, or normal):

	Radial	Femoral	Popliteal	Dorsalis Pedis	Posterior Tibial
Right	2+	2+	2+	2+	2+
Left	2+	2+	2+	2+	2+

Musculoskeletal: No joint deformities or swelling on inspection and palpation. Good range of motion in hands, wrists, elbows, shoulders, spine, hips, knees, ankles.

Neurologic: Mental Status: Alert and cooperative. Thought processes are coherent and insight is good. Oriented to person, place, and time. *Cranial nerves:* II to XII intact. *Motor:* Good muscle bulk and tone. *Strength:* 5/5 bilaterally in deltoids, biceps, triceps, hand grips, iliopsoas, hamstrings, quadriceps, tibialis anterior, and gastrocnemius. *Cerebellar:* rapid alternating movement (RAMs) and point-to-point movements intact. Gait stable, fluid. *Sensory:* Pinprick, light touch, position sense, vibration, and stereognosis intact. Romberg negative. *Reflexes:*

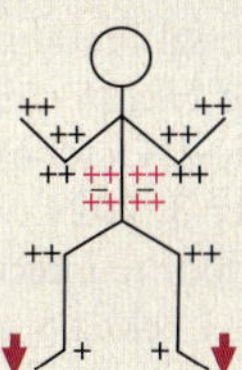

REFERENCES

1. Zoneraich S, Spodick DH. Bedside science reduces laboratory art. Appropriate use of physical findings to reduce reliance on sophisticated and expensive methods. *Circulation.* 1995; 91(7):2089–2092.
2. Elhassan M. Physical examination checklist for medical students: can less be more? *Int J Med Educ.* 2017;8:227–228.
3. Patel N, Ngo E, Paterick TE, Chandrasekaran K, Tajik J. Should doctors still examine patients? *Int J Cardiol.* 2016; 221:55–57.
4. Elder A, Chi J, Ozdalga E, Kugler J, Verghese A. A piece of my mind. The road back to the bedside. *JAMA.* 2013;310(8): 799–800.
5. Herrle SR, Corbett EC Jr, Fagan MJ, Moore CG, Elnicki DM. Bayes' theorem and the physical examination: probability assessment and diagnostic decision making. *Acad Med.* 2011;86(5):618–627.
6. McGee SR. *Evidence-Based Physical Diagnosis.* 3rd ed. Elsevier/Saunders; 2012.
7. Mookherjee S, Pheatt L, Ranji SR, Chou CL. Physical examination education in graduate medical education—a systematic review of the literature. *J Gen Intern Med.* 2013;28(8): 1090–1099.
8. Smith MA, Burton WB, Mackay M. Development, impact, and measurement of enhanced physical diagnosis skills. *Adv Health Sci Educ Theory Pract.* 2009;14(4):547–556.
9. Verghese A, Horwitz RI. In praise of the physical examination. *BMJ.* 2009;339:b5448.
10. Siegel JD, Rhinehart E, Jackson M, Chiarello L, and the Healthcare Infection Control Practices Advisory Committee, 2007 Guideline for Isolation Precautions: Preventing Transmission of Ifnectious Agents in Healthcare Settings, June 2007. Updated May 15, 2024. Accessed October 3, 2024. https://stacks.cdc.gov/view/cdc/156043
11. National Center for Emerging and Zoonotic Infectious Diseases (U.S.). Division of Healthcare Quality Promotion. Guide to infection prevention for outpatient settings: minimum expectations for safe care, 2014. Accessed October 3, 2024. https://stacks.cdc.gov/view/cdc/25622/
12. Centers for Disease Control and Prevention. Hand hygiene in healthcare settings. Accessed October 3, 2024. http://www.cdc.gov/handhygiene/
13. Centers for Disease Control and Prevention. Methicillin-resistant *Staphylococcus aureus* (MRSA): preventing infections

in healthcare. Centers for Disease Control and Prevention. Accessed October 3, 2024. https://www.cdc.gov/mrsa/healthcare/inpatient.html
14. Centers for Disease Control and Prevention. "Bloodborne Infectious Diseases: Universal Precautions." *National Institute for Occupational Safety and Health (NIOSH)*, U.S. Department of Health & Human Services, October 6, 2020, Updated April 23, 2024. Accessed October 3, 2024. www.cdc.gov/niosh/healthcare/risk-factors/bloodborne-infectious-diseases.html
15. Bearman G, Bryant K, Leekha S, et al. Healthcare personnel attire in non-operating-room settings. *Infect Control Hosp Epidemiol.* 2014;35(2):107–121.
16. Treakle AM, Thom KA, Furuno JP, Strauss SM, Harris AD, Perencevich EN. Bacterial contamination of health care workers' white coats. *Am J Infect Control.* 2009;37(2):101–105.
17. Pharr JR. Accommodations for patients with disabilities in primary care: a mixed methods study of practice administrators. *Glob J Health Sci.* 2013;6(1):23–32.
18. Greenway F. Clinical evaluation of the obese patient. *Prim Care.* 2003;30(2):341–356.
19. Blackburn GL, Kanders BS. Medical evaluation and treatment of the obese patient with cardiovascular disease. *Am J Cardiol.* 1987;60(12):55G–58G.
20. Hamill-Ruth RJ, Marohn ML. Evaluation of pain in the critically ill patient. *Crit Care Clin.* 1999;15(1):35–54.
21. Manfredi PL, Breuer B, Meier DE, Libow L. Pain assessment in elderly patients with severe dementia. *J Pain Symptom Manage.* 2003;25(1):48–52.
22. Gélinas C, Fillion L, Puntillo KA. Item selection and content validity of the Critical-Care Pain Observation Tool for non-verbal adults. *J Adv Nurs.* 2009;65(1):203–216.

CHAPTER 5

Clinical Reasoning

DEVELOPING A DIFFERENTIAL DIAGNOSIS: MASTERING CLINICAL REASONING

On completing the patient's history and physical examination (PE), you enter the pivotal phase of developing a *differential diagnosis*. This step requires you to apply rigorous clinical reasoning to sift through your findings and compile a list of possible causes for the patient's issues. The breadth of this list mirrors your degree of uncertainty regarding the underlying cause of the problem at hand. It should commence with the most probable cause but also encompass alternative diagnoses, especially those with significant risks if left unrecognized and untreated. You are tasked with assigning likelihoods to these diagnoses based on how plausible you deem them as explanations for the patient's condition.

The concept of clinical reasoning might appear elusive, even enigmatic, to novices. Seasoned clinicians often process information swiftly, with minimal apparent conscious deliberation, and it may prove challenging for some to articulate the rationale underpinning their clinical judgments. As a proactive learner, you are encouraged to seek clarification from educators and practicing clinicians on the nuances of their clinical reasoning and decision-making processes. As you gain experience, your clinical reasoning will begin from the moment you meet the patient, rather than at the visit's end. This is critical, as the majority of diagnoses can be determined on the basis of your clinical assessment.[1,2] Keep these considerations in mind as you evaluate your initial patients, consistently aiming to elucidate their concerns and identify the relevant findings, challenges, and diagnoses.[3,4]

Chapter Content Guide

CLINICAL REASONING PROCESS

Kahneman introduces the concept of *"dual processing"* in decision making, outlining two distinct thought systems.[5] *System 1*, or the *intuitive system*, operates quickly and automatically, relying on mental shortcuts known as *heuristics*. These shortcuts are habitual response patterns that are challenging to alter. *System 2*, or the *hypothetico-deductive system*, on the other hand, involves a more deliberate and controlled thought process, employing logic and probabilities to reach conclusions. This system requires significantly more time and cognitive effort, making it resource-intensive.[6]

Cognitive psychology research has demonstrated that clinicians integrate elements of both systems in clinical problem-solving.[7–14] These approaches are not exclusive; clinicians adapt and combine different reasoning strategies depending on the scenario (Fig. 5-1).

BASIC STRUCTURE OF THE CLINICAL REASONING PROCESS

The clinical reasoning process begins with collecting data from the patient,[10,15] including historical information,

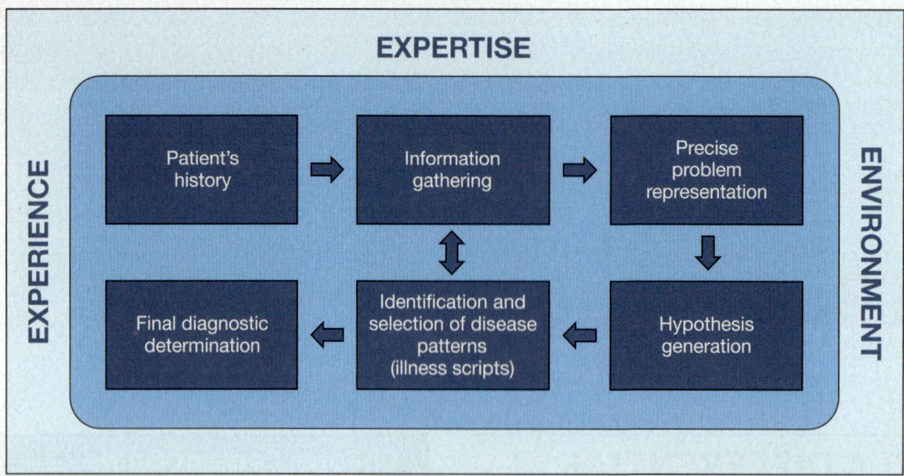

FIGURE 5-1. Key elements of the clinical diagnostic reasoning process.

PE findings, and any initial diagnostic and laboratory tests. This also encompasses data acquired from other clinicians and the patient's previous health records, topics extensively discussed in earlier chapters. The subsequent step involves organizing and interpreting this information to create a precise and relevant *problem representation*, documented in the clinical record as the *summary statement*.[10]

From this problem representation, you then generate, prioritize, and test a list of potential diagnoses until identifying a working diagnosis that best matches your patient's issue. This working diagnosis serves as the foundation for devising your patient's treatment plan.

The basic structure is:

- Step 1: Gather initial patient information
- Step 2: Organize and interpret clinical information
- Step 3: Synthesize clinical information and develop the problem representation
- Step 4: Generate hypotheses
- Step 5: Test hypotheses and establish a working diagnosis
- Step 6: Plan the diagnostic and treatment strategy

Step 1: Gathering Initial Patient Information

Chapters 3, Health History, and 4, Physical Examination extensively cover information gathering through health interviews and PEs. Beyond these, you may access additional data pre- and postclinical encounters, including prior health records and input from individuals familiar with the patient. This broad scope of information encompasses elicited patient symptoms, observed signs during examination, and any available laboratory or other reports (Box 5-1).

Use a methodical and organized approach to ensure thorough identification of all abnormal and unexpected findings. With advancing clinical reasoning skills, this identification process becomes more immediate, occurring in real time during patient encounters. Nonetheless, revisiting data postencounter remains a critical practice to catch any overlooked abnormalities. After assembling a list of abnormal findings, the next step involves organizing them to narrow down potential causes.

Step 2: Organizing and Interpreting Clinical Information

Determining if clinical data represent a single problem or multiple issues can be complex, especially when faced with extensive lists of symptoms, signs, and possible explanations. One strategy involves segmenting observations into distinct clusters and examining each cluster individually (Box 5-2). Identifying differentiating and key clinical features within these clusters can facilitate this process. Experienced clinicians typically have the ability to instantly and intuitively organize patient information into relevant findings.[10] As a beginner, you might benefit from adopting one or several specific approaches to tackle this challenge.

Note that while age is undoubtedly a significant variable, its utility may be limited for novice clinicians. Relying heavily on age can inadvertently narrow the scope of potential diagnoses, potentially overlooking atypical presentations of diseases that occur across different age groups.

Box 5-1. Initial Patient Information Collection Sources

Source of Information	Data Collected
Patient's health interview	Includes details on the chief concern, history of present illness, past medical and family history, social milieu, and a complete review of systems to capture nuanced information on symptoms, lifestyle, and familial health patterns.
Physical examination	Encompasses vital signs thorough inspection, palpation, percussion, and auscultation across body systems to identify physical signs indicative of health issues.
Prior health records	Critical review of historical health documents to understand the patient's previous health issues, treatments received, surgeries undergone, and outcomes of past medical interventions, establishing a baseline for current health status.
Comments from others	Supplementary insights from family members, caregivers, and health care professionals provide external observations on the patient's symptoms, behaviors, and general well-being.
Diagnostic and other reports	Current and relevant laboratory test results, imaging studies, and other diagnostic procedures provide objective, quantifiable data essential for confirming diagnoses or guiding further investigation into the patient's condition.

Box 5-2. Techniques for Clustering Observations for Individualized Analysis

Approach	Description	Examples
Anatomic location	Information is organized by anatomical location, from specific structures to broader regions, aiding in identifying the problem's source. However, some symptoms, though unrelated anatomically, may stem from a common case.	■ Scratchy throat and an erythematous inflamed posterior pharynx localize the problem to the pharynx. ■ Headache leads to the structures of the skull and brain. ■ Chest pain can originate from various areas like the coronary arteries or musculoskeletal components.
Timing of symptoms	Symptom timing is analyzed against the natural history of diseases to distinguish between separate conditions and stages of the same disease.	■ A yellow penile discharge followed 3 weeks later by a painless penile ulcer suggests two problems: gonorrhea and primary syphilis. ■ A penile ulcer followed in 6 weeks by a maculopapular skin rash and generalized lymphadenopathy suggests two stages of the same problem: primary and secondary syphilis.
Involvement of different body systems	Symptoms and signs are categorized by body system to assess whether they suggest a single disease or multiple conditions, necessitating knowledge of disease patterns.	■ High blood pressure, sustained apical impulse, and retinal hemorrhages grouped under "cardiovascular disease with hypertensive retinopathy," separate from another group for the same patient's mild fever, left lower quadrant tenderness, and diarrhea.
Developing pattern recognition	Novice clinicians are encouraged to actively seek correlations among diverse symptoms and signs, gradually mastering the skill of linking seemingly unrelated manifestations through pattern recognition, a skill that improves with experience.	■ Symptoms like cough, hemoptysis, and weight loss with a long history of smoking suggest lung cancer. ■ Acute chest pain accompanied by hemoptysis, tachycardia, and unilateral leg swelling could indicate a pulmonary embolus.

Step 3: Synthesizing Clinical Information and Developing the Problem Representation

As you gather and organize clinical information during a patient encounter, you are simultaneously synthesizing this data to create a *problem representation*—your evolving understanding of the clinical scenario. This representation typically includes the patient's initial information (chief concern, epidemiology, risk factors), key findings from the history and PE, and diagnostic test results. In your clinical documentation, this is referred to as the *summary statement*. The problem representation becomes increasingly detailed with the addition of new data (Box 5-3).[17]

Box 5-3. Case Example: Development of a Problem Representation

Part 1: A 57-year-old male arrives at the emergency room with a chief concern of chest pain for the past 2 hours.

- Identifying the acute onset of chest pain in a middle-aged adult immediately raises concern for cardiac conditions. The specificity of age and symptom onset is crucial for prioritizing initial assessments and interventions.
- *Initial problem representation:* "A 57-year-old male with acute onset of chest pain."

Part 2: The patient reports that the pain, located centrally behind the sternum, began suddenly while shoveling snow. It was moderately severe, lasting 1 to 2 minutes, and accompanied by shortness of breath (SOB). He has a 35-year history of smoking one pack of cigarettes daily and has previously been diagnosed with congestive heart failure (CHF).

- This information adds significant depth to our understanding, highlighting risk factors (smoking, CHF) that elevate the concern for ischemic heart disease. The nature of the pain and its association with exertion further point to a cardiovascular origin, prompting considerations beyond the initial symptom of chest pain.
- *Updated problem representation:* "A 57-year-old male with CHF and a 35-pack-year smoking history presenting with acute, severe, exertional, retrosternal chest pain and associated SOB."

Part 3: On physical examination (PE), the patient demonstrated a new S_3 gallop, crackles at both lung bases, and swelling of both legs.

- The PE findings of a new S_3 gallop, bibasilar crackles, and bilateral edema significantly contribute to the clinical picture, reinforcing the likelihood of a cardiac issue, potentially acute heart failure, or ischemic heart disease exacerbation. These findings underscore the importance of integrating specific physical signs with the patient's history to refine the problem representation and guide toward a differential diagnosis.
- *Refined problem representation:* "A 57-year-old male with CHF and a 35-pack-year smoking history presenting with acute, severe, exertional, retrosternal chest pain and associated SOB. PE reveals a new S_3 gallop, bibasilar crackles, and bilateral lower extremity edema."

Consideration of differential diagnosis: The patient's presentation and findings lead to the consideration of acute coronary syndrome (ACS) as a primary differential diagnosis, given the risk factors, symptoms, and physical signs. However, differential considerations should also briefly entertain and rule out noncardiac causes for chest pain, such as pulmonary embolism or musculoskeletal pain, although they are less likely with the given presentation.

Source: Weinstein A, Gupta S, Pinto-Powell R, et al. Diagnosing and remediating clinical reasoning difficulties: a faculty development workshop. *MedEdPORTAL*. 2017;13:10650.

This is an important step in the clinical reasoning process. The development of a well-developed and concise problem representation guides a clinician in generating a hypothesis and developing the differential diagnosis. This summary rarely contains unnecessary data and rarely leaves out any significant data. An accurate problem representation helps activate appropriate illness scripts (see Box 5-7, p. 92).

Step 4: Generating Hypotheses by Searching for the Probable Cause of the Findings

For early learners facing unfamiliar or complex clinical situations, adopting a structured, step-by-step approach is essential to minimize cognitive errors (Box 5-4).

Box 5-4. Approaches to Searching for Probable Causes of the Findings

Approach	Description	Examples
Generate an exhaustive list.	Gather every piece of information available, asking every possible question to help arrive at the diagnosis. List both pathologic and pathophysiologic processes spanning diseases of specific body systems or structures as well as disruptions in biologic functions (Boxes 5-5 and 5-6).[17,23]	Pathologic examples include heart failure and migraine headaches, while psychopathologic instances include mood disorders such as depression.
Select the most specific and critical findings to support your hypothesis.	Identify clues that are characteristic of the diagnoses (*defining features*) or features unique to disease (*discriminating feature*) (Fig. 5-2).[10]	Symptoms like severe headache, nausea, vomiting, confusion, papilledema, and neck stiffness point more to increased intracranial pressure than gastrointestinal issues.
Match findings against all causative conditions (*illness scripts*).	Use clinical patterns to evoke previously assimilated knowledge, aligning the patient's presentation with established illness scripts encountered in practice (Box 5-7).[14]	Envision diagnosing acute appendicitis in an emergency room setting, guided by classic symptoms and signs such as right lower quadrant pain, anorexia, and vomiting with tenderness to palpation on exam.
Eliminate diagnostic possibilities.	Exclude diagnostic considerations that fail to encapsulate the patient's specific presentation.	Bifrontal, throbbing headache accompanied by nausea and vomiting would lead away from cluster headaches as this would be an uncharacteristic presentation.
Weigh competing possibilities and select the most likely diagnosis.	Consider the fit between the patient's presentation and typical cases, including statistical probability and patient demographics.	In evaluating back pain, consider osteoarthritis or metastatic prostate cancer for a 70-year-old individual, but these would be unlikely in a 25-year-old individual with similar symptoms.
Give special attention to potentially life-threatening conditions.	Systematically rule out life-threatening conditions as part of the differential diagnosis process to ensure critical conditions are promptly identified and addressed.	Prioritize ruling out critical conditions such as meningococcal meningitis, pulmonary embolism, or subdural hematoma based on clinical evidence and evaluations.

On identifying each problem or related group of issues, you should formulate a clinical hypothesis. This requires leveraging your entire breadth of knowledge and experience as well as engaging in extensive reading. Consulting clinical literature at this stage is particularly valuable, aligning with the ongoing pursuit of evidence-based decision making and practice.[18–22] At first, your hypotheses might lack specificity, but they will progress according to the extent of your knowledge and the data at hand.

Box 5-5. Memory Aids for Generating Differential Diagnosis (Exhaustive Method)

Tom G. Prince, MD, Psychiatrist, General Hospital	VINDICATE
Toxin/**T**rauma including medications	**V**ascular
Oncologic	**I**nfectious
Musculoskeletal/rheumatologic	**N**eoplastic
Gastrointestinal	**D**rug related
Pulmonary	**I**nflammatory/**I**diopathic/**I**atrogenic
Renal	**C**ongenital
Infectious	**A**utoimmune/**A**llergic
Neurologic	**T**rauma/**T**oxic
Cardiovascular	**E**ndocrine/metabolic
Endocrine	
Metabolic/genetic	
Dermatologic	
Psychiatric	
Genitourinary/gynecologic	
Hematologic	

Source: Collins RD. Dynamic Differential Diagnosis. J.B. Lippincott; 1981.

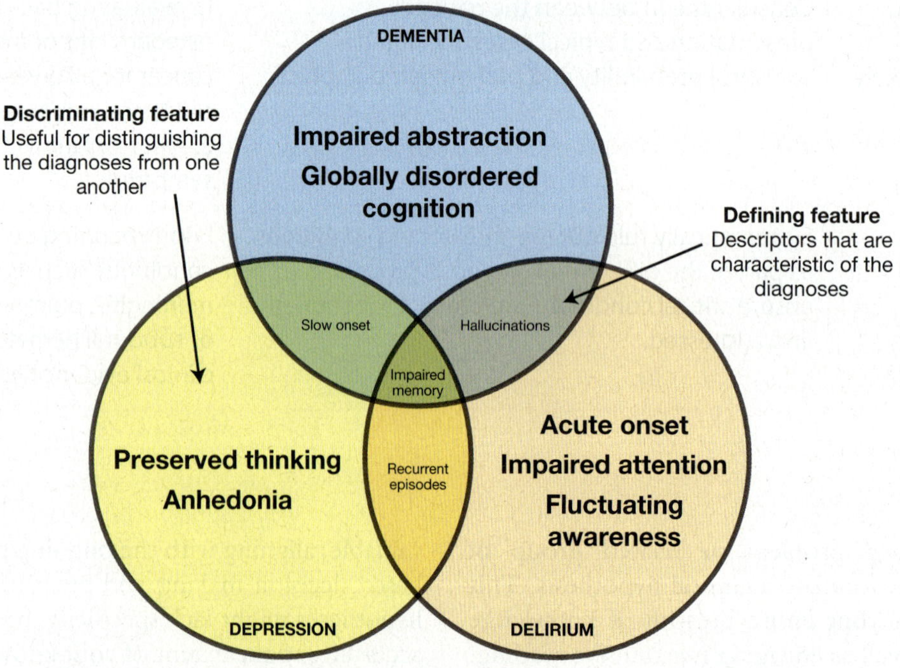

FIGURE 5-2. Defining and discriminating features: memory impairment.

Box 5-6. Application of the VINDICATE Mnemonic in a 57-Year-Old Previously Healthy Individual Presenting with Altered Mental Status for 3 Days

Vascular	▪ *Stroke (ischemic or hemorrhagic):* vascular events are a significant concern in this age group ▪ *Transient ischemic attack (TIA):* can present with transient neurologic deficits that may alter mental status
Infectious	▪ *Meningitis:* even in the absence of fever, can present with altered mental status ▪ *Encephalitis:* consider particularly if signs of focal neurologic deficits or seizures
Neoplastic	▪ *Brain tumors:* primary or metastatic tumors can present suddenly with bleeding or rapid growth.
Drug related	▪ *Prescription medication side effects or interactions:* consider especially if the patient recently started new medications. ▪ *Accidental poisoning or overdose*
Inflammatory/**I**diopathic/**I**atrogenic	▪ *Autoimmune encephalitis:* consider if signs of systemic autoimmune disorders ▪ *Sarcoidosis:* can involve the central nervous system (CNS) and present with nonspecific symptoms like altered mental status
Congenital	▪ Less likely in a previously healthy 57-year-old person without relevant history
Autoimmune/**A**llergic	▪ Autoimmune conditions such as vasculitis or systemic lupus erythematosus affecting the CNS
Trauma/**T**oxic	▪ *Subdural hematoma:* important to consider, especially if history of recent head trauma, even minor ▪ *Toxic exposure:* relevant in the context of occupational exposures or environmental toxins.
Endocrine/metabolic	▪ *Hypo- or hyperthyroidism:* can present subtly with cognitive changes. ▪ *Hyponatremia:* common in older adults, can cause significant changes in mental status.

Step 5: Testing Hypotheses and Establishing a Working Diagnosis

Once you have formulated a hypothesis regarding the patient's issue, validate it through additional history, PEs, or diagnostic tests to confirm or eliminate your initial diagnosis. For straightforward conditions, like a common cold or hives, further testing might not be necessary.

Define the problem as precisely as the data allows. At times, you might identify a diagnosis without an apparent underlying explanation, such as an "unknown cause of tension headache." Other instances allow for more specific definitions based on anatomy, disease process, or etiology, like "pneumococcal bacterial meningitis" or "hypertensive heart disease with heart failure." Symptoms may remain unexplained, necessitating simple descriptions such as "fatigue."

Step 6: Planning the Diagnostic and Treatment Strategy

Building on the working diagnosis, your strategy should cover diagnostic tests, treatments, patient education, medication adjustments, referrals, and follow-ups. Successful planning hinges on strong interpersonal skills, understanding the patient's life context, and ensuring their active participation in care decisions (Fig. 5-3). Involving the patient in decision making is crucial, grounded in evidence-based medicine that balances clinical evidence, judgment, and patient values.[16] This collaborative approach fosters better treatment adherence and satisfaction, recognizing that multiple valid care options may exist. Discuss and agree on the care plan with the patient before proceeding, ensuring their engagement and consent.

Box 5-7. Example: Illness Script for Acute Coronary Syndrome[10]

The elements of an illness script often include a disease's pathophysiology, epidemiology, time course, salient symptoms and signs, diagnostics, and treatment.[24]

Epidemiology or pathophysiology	Acute coronary syndrome (ACS) primarily affects older adults. Key risk factors include diabetes, hypertension, dyslipidemia, a family history of cardiovascular disease, and tobacco use. Pathophysiologically, ACS is commonly caused by rupture of an atherosclerotic plaque leading to thrombosis and subsequent myocardial ischemia.
Time course	ACS is characterized by a sudden-onset symptoms that develop rapidly and typically persist for several minutes to hours, indicating the acute nature of the condition.
Clinical presentation	Patients typically experience chest pain that intensifies to a peak, often described as dull, and located substernally, with potential radiation to the arms or shoulders. Accompanying symptoms include diaphoresis, shortness of breath, nausea, and vomiting. Tachycardia may be observed during physical examination.
Diagnostic studies	Diagnosis is supported by elevated cardiac biomarkers. Electrocardiogram (ECG) findings may show ST elevation or depression and T-wave changes. An echocardiogram can reveal regional wall motion abnormalities indicative of myocardial ischemia or infarction. Coronary angiography may be used for definitive diagnosis and to guide treatment decisions.
Management/treatment	Immediate management often involves revascularization techniques such as percutaneous coronary intervention (PCI) or thrombolytic therapy, depending on the clinical scenario. Medication management typically includes antiplatelets, β-blockers, statins, and angiotensin-converting enzyme inhibitors to reduce myocardial demand and prevent further ischemic events.

Source: Bowen JL. Educational strategies to promote clinical diagnostic reasoning. *N Engl J Med*. 2006;355(21):2217–2225.

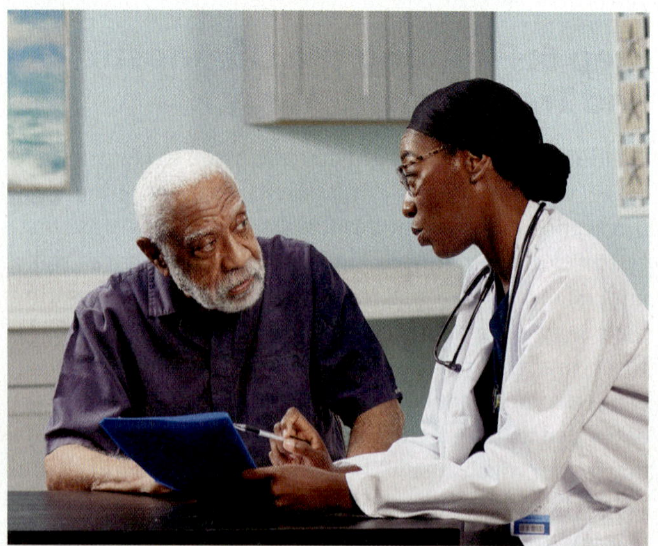

FIGURE 5-3. Successful planning needs empathy and patient involvement.

CLINICAL DIAGNOSTIC ERRORS

While learning the process of clinical reasoning, consider common sources of error in this process.[17,25–27] Box 5-8 describes common sources of cognitive error in clinical reasoning.[28,29] An awareness of the cognitive processes used to make decisions can reduce the likelihood of poor decisions.[29] You should be vigilant for these errors and follow several general rules to improve your decision-making process (Box 5-9).

CLINICAL REASONING: DOCUMENTATION

While all of your clinical documentation of the health history and PE is a reflection of your data-gathering skills,

Box 5-8. Common Types of Clinical Cognitive Errors

Cognitive Error	Description	Vignette
Anchoring bias	Tendency to perceptually lock onto salient features in the patient's initial presentation too early in the diagnostic process and failure to adjust in light of later information	Clinician "locks onto" a patient's description of an aura that precedes her headaches as indicative of a migraine and fails to recognize red flags of increased intracranial pressure that should prompt neuroimaging for this patient.
Availability heuristic	Assumption that a diagnosis is more likely, or more frequently occurring, if it more readily comes to mind	Clinician who has recently seen several patients with acute appendicitis does not consider ovarian torsion in an adolescent girl presenting with acute right lower quadrant abdominal pain.
Confirmation bias	Seeking supportive evidence for a diagnosis at the exclusion of more persuasive information refuting it	Clinician makes a presumptive diagnosis of an upper respiratory infection in a well-appearing patient presenting with cough, rhinorrhea, and fever and does not consider pneumonia even after finding asymmetric chest wall excursion and dullness to chest percussion on examination.
Diagnostic momentum	Prioritizing a diagnosis made by prior clinicians, discounting evidence of alternative explanations	Clinician does not consider acute myocardial infarction in a patient who was recently diagnosed with acid reflux in the setting of similar symptoms.
Framing effect	Interpretation of information is influenced heavily by the way in which the information is presented (*framed*)	Patient is presented as having *"frequent ER visits for asthma exacerbation in the setting of medication nonadherence."* The clinician fails to explore structural forces that drive medication adherence and fails to explore alternative causes of the current exacerbation.
Representation error	Failure to take prevalence into account when estimating the probability of a diagnosis	Clinician who often sees older patients places diverticular bleed high on their differential diagnosis when evaluating rectal bleeding in an adolescent patient.
Visceral bias	Visceral arousal (negative and positive feelings toward patients) leads to poor diagnostic decisions	Clinician assumes that a patient who is unhoused will not be able to manage a complicated treatment plan and prescribes a simpler, less optimal plan, without discussing the options with the patient.

Sources: Croskerry P. The importance of cognitive errors in diagnosis and strategies to minimize them. *Acad Med*. 2003;78(8):775–780; Weinstein A, Gupta S, Pinto-Powell R, et al. Diagnosing and remediating clinical reasoning difficulties: a faculty development workshop. *MedEdPORTAL*. 2017;13:10650.

Box 5-9. Suggested Rules for Good Decision Making[7,29]

- Slow down.
- Be aware of base rate of disease for items on your differential diagnosis.
- Consider what data is truly relevant.
- Actively seek alternative diagnoses.
- Ask questions to disprove, rather than confirm, your current hypothesis.
- Remember you are often wrong. Consider the immediate implications of this.

Sources: Kassirer JP, Wong JB, Kopelman RI. *Learning Clinical Reasoning*. 2nd ed. Wolters Kluwer Health/Lippincott Williams & Wilkins; 2010; Klein JG. Five pitfalls in decisions about diagnosis and prescribing. *BMJ*. 2005;330(7494):781–783.

the *summary statement, assessment*, and *plan* represent the most robust reflection of your clinical reasoning and data synthesis skills. For detailed guidance on documenting and presenting your assessment and plan, including the creation of your problem representation (summary statement) and compiling a problem list, refer to Chapter 6, Clinical Documentation and Oral Presentation.

REFERENCES

1. Hampton JR, Harrison MJ, Mitchell JR, Prichard JS, Seymour C. Relative contributions of history-taking, physical examination, and laboratory investigation to diagnosis and management of medical outpatients. *Br Med J*. 1975;2(5969): 486–489.
2. Peterson MC, Holbrook JH, Von Hales D, Smith NL, Staker LV. Contributions of the history, physical examination, and laboratory investigation in making medical diagnoses. *West J Med*. 1992;156(2):163–165.
3. McGee SR. *Evidence-Based Physical Diagnosis*. 3rd ed. Elsevier/Saunders; 2012.
4. Schneiderman H, Peixoto AJ. *Bedside Diagnosis: An Annotated Bibliography of Literature on Physical Examination and Interviewing*. 3rd ed. American College of Physicians; 1997.
5. Kahneman D. *Thinking, Fast and Slow*. Farrar, Straus and Giroux; 2011.
6. Cabrera D, Thomas JF, Wiswell JL, et al. Accuracy of 'My Gut Feeling:' comparing System 1 to System 2 decision-making for acuity prediction, disposition and diagnosis in an academic emergency department. *West J Emerg Med*. 2015; 16(5):653–657.
7. Kassirer J, Wong J, Kopelman R. *Learning Clinical Reasoning*. 2nd ed. Lippincott Williams & Wilkins; 2010.
8. Kassirer JP. Teaching clinical reasoning: case-based and coached. *Acad Med*. 2010;85(7):1118–1124.
9. Norman GR, Eva KW. Diagnostic error and clinical reasoning. *Med Educ*. 2010;44(1):94–100.
10. Bowen JL. Educational strategies to promote clinical diagnostic reasoning. *N Engl J Med*. 2006;355(21):2217–2225.
11. Coderre S, Mandin H, Harasym PH, Fick GH. Diagnostic reasoning strategies and diagnostic success. *Med Educ*. 2003; 37(8):695–703.
12. Elstein AS, Schwartz A. Clinical problem solving and diagnostic decision making: selective review of the cognitive literature. *BMJ*. 2002;324(7339):729–732.
13. Norman G. Research in clinical reasoning: past history and current trends. *Med Educ*. 2005;39(4):418–427.
14. Mengel MB, Fields SA. *Introduction to Clinical Skills: A Patient-Centered Textbook*. Plenum Publishing Corporation; 1997.
15. Barrows HS, Pickell GC. *Developing Clinical Problem-Solving Skills: A Guide to More Effective Diagnosis and Treatment*. W.W. Norton & Company, Inc; 1991.
16. Barry MJ, Edgman-Levitan S. Shared decision making–pinnacle of patient-centered care. *N Engl J Med*. 2012;366(9): 780–781.
17. Weinstein A, Gupta S, Pinto-Powell R, et al. Diagnosing and remediating clinical reasoning difficulties: a faculty development workshop. *Med Ed Portal*. 2017;13:10650.
18. Sackett DL. A primer on the precision and accuracy of the clinical examination. *JAMA*. 1992;267(19):2638–2644.
19. Simel DL, Rennie D. *The Rational Clinical Examination: Evidence-Based Clinical Diagnosis*. McGraw-Hill Companies, Inc; 2009.
20. Guyatt G, Rennie D, Meade MO, Cook DJ. *Users' Guides to the Medical Literature: A Manual for Evidence-Based Clinical Practice*. 2nd ed. McGraw Hill Professional; 2008.
21. Fletcher RH, Fletcher SW, Fletcher GS. *Clinical Epidemiology: The Essentials*. 5th ed. Lippincott Williams & Wilkins; 2014.
22. Straus SE, Richardson WS, Glasziou P, Haynes RB. *Evidence-Based Medicine: How to Practice and Teach EBM*. 3rd ed. Churchill Livingstone; 2005.
23. Collins RD. *Dynamic Differential Diagnosis*. Lippincott Williams & Wilkins; 1981.
24. Schmidt HG, Rikers RM. How expertise develops in medicine: knowledge encapsulation and illness script formation. *Med Educ*. 2007;41(12):1133–1139.
25. Croskerry P. When I say . . . cognitive debiasing. *Med Educ*. 2015;49(7):656–657.
26. Croskerry P, Singhal G, Mamede S. Cognitive debiasing 1: origins of bias and theory of debiasing. *BMJ Qual Saf*. 2013; 22:ii58–ii64.
27. Croskerry P, Singhal G, Mamede S. Cognitive debiasing 2: impediments to and strategies for change. *BMJ Qual Saf*. 2013;22:ii65–ii72.
28. Croskerry P. The importance of cognitive errors in diagnosis and strategies to minimize them. *Acad Med*. 2003;78(8): 775–780.
29. Klein JG. Five pitfalls in decisions about diagnosis and prescribing. *BMJ*. 2005;330(7494):781–783.

CHAPTER

6

Clinical Documentation and Oral Presentation

Chapter Content Guide

- Navigating Communication in Health Care
- Documenting History and Physical Examination Notes
- Conducting Oral Presentations for New Patients
- Documenting Progress Notes
- Addressing Special Considerations in Clinical Documentation

NAVIGATING COMMUNICATION IN HEALTH CARE

Effective communication is an essential skill for all health care professionals in ensuring high-quality patient care. Clinicians must be able to accurately convey patient histories, physical examination (PE) results, diagnostic findings, and care plans to colleagues. This communication takes two primary forms: *written documentation* ("notes") and *oral presentations.*[1]

Written Documentation in Electronic Health Records

When writing notes in the electronic health record (EHR), the goal is to create a clear, concise, and comprehensive report that effectively communicates your key findings and assessment to other members of the health care team (Fig. 6-1). The key to effective EHR documentation lies in the thoughtful organization of information, language precision, and judicious inclusion of relevant details.

As a student, you may prefer to err on the side of detail, enhancing your descriptive abilities, clinical vocabulary, and documentation effectiveness. This practice lays a strong foundation for clinical observation and reasoning. As you progress, the realities of clinical practice, including time constraints and workload demands, necessitate a more streamlined approach. However, even concise notes must still provide robust evidence from the health histories, PEs, and diagnostic findings to support all concerns or diagnoses. This evolution in documentation style reflects not just a response to external pressures but a maturation of clinical judgment. Embrace this process as an ongoing journey, in which each note you write not only contributes to patient care but also to your development as a health care professional.

Remember, EHR documentation is not just record-keeping but a pivotal exercise in clinical communication, critical thinking, and professional growth. Using EHR features effectively, such as templates and smart phrases, can further enhance the quality and efficiency of your notes, making them invaluable tools for the entire health care team.[2]

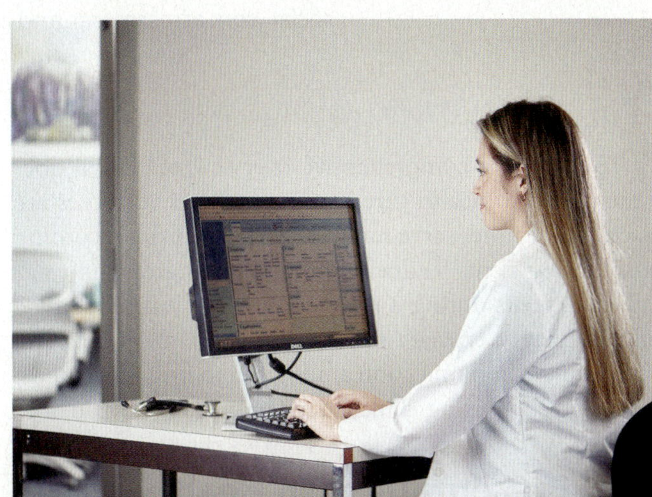

FIGURE 6-1. Documenting a patient encounter in the electronic health record.

Box 6-1. Types of Patient Notes in the Clinical Setting

Type of Note	Description	Alternative Names
History and Physical Examination Note	Written when a patient is admitted to the hospital or for the first visit in the outpatient setting; includes the patient's health history and the findings from the physical examination	Admission Note, Initial Assessment
Progress Note	Written daily during a patient's hospital stay to update the team on what is happening that day or for subsequent outpatient visits	Follow-up Note, Daily Note
Discharge Summary	Completed on the day of discharge from the hospital; summarizes the patient's hospital course, management, and further recommended management for a seamless transition back to their primary care provider	Handover Summary, Release Note
Procedure Note	Describes a surgical or bedside procedure	Operative Note, Intervention Note
Event Note	Describes a particular event of interest, such as a behavioral altercation or the receipt of a home medication list	Incident Report, Observation Note
Transfer-of-Care Note	Written when a patient is transferred within the hospital (e.g., from an intensive care unit to a medical-surgical floor)	Handoff Note, Transfer Note
Consultation Note	Written by a specialist or consultant who was asked to evaluate the patient; provides their expert opinion and recommendations	Specialist Note, Referral Note
Multidisciplinary Team Meeting Note	Summarizes discussions and decisions made during meetings involving various health care professionals focused on a patient's care plan	MDT Note, Team Conference Note
Allied Health Note	Documents observations, interventions, and responses in their respective fields; includes nursing staff's care, pharmaceutical care adjustments and monitoring, and social work assessments and plans	Nursing Records, Care Note, Pharmacist's Note, Medication Management Note, Psychosocial Note, Support Plan

To provide a comprehensive overview of clinical documentation in health care settings, a variety of notes are used. These notes serve multiple purposes, from recording initial assessments to documenting ongoing care and significant events during a patient's hospital stay. Each type of note plays a crucial role in ensuring continuity of care, facilitating communication among health care team members, and supporting clinical decision making (Box 6-1).

Oral Presentations in Health Care

Oral presentations are equally important, often serving as the primary channel for communication among health care providers to exchange information. They not only play a critical role in streamlining patient care and enhancing its efficiency but also act as an engaging platform for learning, sharing knowledge, and showcasing clinical decision-making skills.[3] These presentations vary in format and content, depending on the audience, setting, and specific objectives (Box 6-2). From discussing new patient admissions to coordinating care at discharge, each type of oral presentation serves a unique role in the patient care continuum.

Like written notes, the essence of oral presentations is to succinctly convey your critical findings and the rationale behind your assessments and plans. However, oral

Box 6-2. Types of Oral Patient Presentations in the Clinical Setting

Type of Oral Presentation	Description	Alternative Names
Case Presentation	Detailed report of a patient's history, symptoms, examination findings, diagnosis, and treatment plan; often presented during clinical rounds or meetings	Patient Report, Clinical Presentation
Morning Report	Oral presentation given typically in the morning, summarizing the overnight admissions, significant events, or challenging cases and is an educational opportunity for discussion and learning	Handover Report, Morning Handover
Admission Presentation	Given when a new patient is admitted, highlighting the reasons for admission, initial findings, and proposed management plan	Initial Presentation, Admission Summary
Discharge Presentation	Outlines the patient's hospital course, treatment received, response to treatment, discharge medications, and follow-up plan	Discharge Summary, Discharge Report
Procedure Briefing	Brief, preprocedure presentation on the patient's background, reason for the procedure, and expected outcome	Preprocedure Brief, Procedure Overview
Postprocedure Debrief	Summary given after a procedure detailing what was done, findings, any complications, and postprocedure care	Procedure Summary, Postop Debrief
Consult Presentation	Presented to a specialist or consulting physician, detailing the patient's case, to seek advice or a second opinion on management	Specialist Consult, Referral Presentation
Multidisciplinary Team (MDT) Presentation	Focuses on complex cases that require input from various health care professionals to form a comprehensive care plan	Team Huddle, MDT Report
Handoff Presentation	Oral report given during the transition of care, such as shift changes, to ensure the continuity of care; includes patient status, recent changes, and pending tasks	Shift Handoff, Change of Shift Report
Transfer Presentation	Given when a patient is being transferred from one department to another or from one health care facility to another, focusing on the reason for transfer, patient's condition, and care plan	Interdepartmental Transfer, Facility Transfer

presentations demand an even more selective approach to information sharing. In your clinical interactions, patients often provide more information than what is directly relevant to their care. Your written notes should capture only the clinically pertinent details. Similarly, when it comes to oral presentations, the challenge is to refine this information further, ensuring you highlight only what is essential to the patient's immediate health concerns or condition. This process involves a careful selection of facts, ensuring that your presentation remains focused and impactful, avoiding the trap of overelaboration on nonessential details, such as an exhaustive family history that does not pertain to the immediate clinical situation.[4] This process of distillation is key to maintaining focus and relevance in both your documentation and communication (Fig. 6-2).

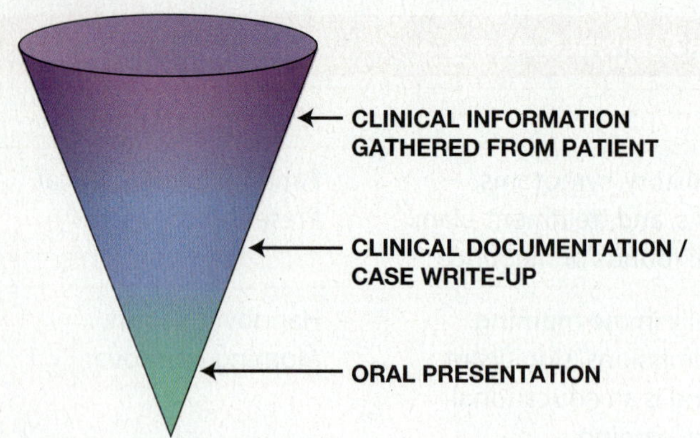

FIGURE 6-2. Reducing information to the essentials.

DOCUMENTING HISTORY AND PHYSICAL EXAMINATION NOTES

The history and physical examination (H&P) note is most appropriate for documenting a patient's initial admission to the hospital (Box 6-3). As you explore its components, refer to the detailed example of a full H&P outlined in Table 6-1.

Initial Information

Your EHR will typically automatically populate certain standard information, such as the date and time the note is created, the patient's name, and the patient's age. Always review and update this auto-populated information to ensure its accuracy.

Source and Reliability

When documenting the source of information, which can vary from the patient to family members, or clinical records, assess and note the reliability of these sources. When describing the source's reliability with descriptors like *"good," "fair,"* or *"poor,"* you should enhance this assessment with brief justifications, for instance, noting *"altered mental status"* or inconsistencies in the patient's account. This practice promotes a deeper understanding of the context and reliability of your information.

Chief Concern

The *chief concern* (*CC*) should succinctly capture the patient's main issue using a short phrase and a time descriptor, such as *"Epigastric pain ×3 months."* When multiple concerns are present, prioritize and document based on the predominance or patient emphasis. Utilizing the patient's own words can add valuable insight

Box 6-3. Checklist to Ensure a Quality Clinical Record

Is the organization clear?

Make sure each piece of information is in the appropriate section; for example, keep the "subjective" items of the history in the HPI and do not let them stray into the physical examination.

Does the included information contribute directly to the assessment?

Spell out the supporting evidence, both positive and negative, for each problem or diagnosis. Make sure there is sufficient detail to support your differential diagnosis and plan. At the same time, avoid excess detail that is irrelevant to your assessment and makes the relevant information more difficult to find.

Are there overgeneralizations or omissions of important data?

Remember that any information not recorded is information lost. No matter how vividly you can recall clinical details today, you will probably not remember them in a few months. If you only record "Neurologic examination negative," anyone reading your note (including your future self) will not know, for example, if you specifically checked all the reflexes.

Are clear descriptions or images included whenever possible?

To ensure accurate evaluations and future comparisons, describe findings fully. For example, write "1 cm × 1 cm lymph node" rather than "pea-sized lymph node." In addition, images add greatly to the clarity of the record. If possible, take a picture of the finding, then upload to the EHR.

Is the tone neutral and professional?

Particularly when documenting frustrating interactions, be objective. Rather than, "Patient rude and abusive to staff!" document the specific comments the patient made, if necessary. Hostile, disapproving, or inflammatory language may damage your relationship with the patient or prove difficult to defend in a legal setting.

into their experience and should be considered, especially if they convey the concern in a unique or particularly expressive manner.

History of Present Illness

Structuring the history of present illness (HPI) is one of the most daunting tasks for any beginning student but is central to understanding the patient's current condition. Focus on using the standard framework described in Box 6-4, ensuring that someone reading your HPI will understand what is happening with your patient, organizing the events leading up to your clinical interview in chronologic order, and writing concisely and clearly.

Opening Statement. Begin with an *opening statement* that lays the groundwork for the reader to begin thinking of potential causes of the patient's condition. This initial statement should provide the patient's age, the CC, and relevant historical information that may suggest possible causes of the CC.

Example 1: *"JM, a 48-year-old cisgender man with poorly controlled diabetes mellitus, presents with 3 days of fever."* This statement suggests to the clinician that JM's fever might be related to complications from his diabetes, such as an infected diabetic foot ulcer.

Example 2: *"RP, a 23-year-old transgender man who recently traveled to Mexico, reports a month-long low-grade fever and night sweats."* This hints at the possibility of an infectious disease common to Mexico.

Keep in mind that simple opening statements like these, which highlight only the historical elements relevant to the CC, are uncommon in practice. Typically, clinicians compose a concise "one-liner" in the opening statement that encapsulates the patient's health history while also drawing attention to the details most relevant to the CC. Effective strategies to underscore the critical components involve prioritizing the most pertinent health conditions and integrating the CC seamlessly into the narrative. This approach ensures a focused yet thorough overview right from the start. To modify the earlier examples:

Revised Example 1: *"JM is a 48-year-old cisgender man with diabetes mellitus, chronic kidney disease, hyperlipidemia, and coronary artery disease with stent placement in 2024, presenting with 3 days of fever in the setting of worsening control of his diabetes."*

Revised Example 2: *"RP is a 23-year-old transgender man with hypertension and scoliosis, presenting with a month of low-grade fever and night sweats following recent travel to Mexico."*

You should develop the practice of incorporating the patient's chronic conditions into the opening statement,

Box 6-4. Suggested Alternative Templates for Documenting the History of Present Illness

HPI template for CC that represents an exacerbation of a chronic illness:

- Opening statement: CC in light of the patient's clinical context
- Description of the chronic illness
- Diagnosis or symptom
- When diagnosed
- Presence or absence of complications
- Treatments
- Recent symptom control prior to this exacerbation
- Elaboration of the CC
- Pertinent accompanying symptoms and absent symptoms
- Additional pertinent information
- Concluding statement: how the patient got to the care site

CC: Shortness of breath × 4 hours

HPI: AJ is a 28-year-old cisgender woman with a history of asthma presenting with shortness of breath since this morning in the setting of cat hair exposure. AJ was diagnosed with asthma at age 8 years and usually gets asthma attacks every 2–3 months. She is usually triggered by exposure to allergens such as dust and smoke or, sometimes, by changes in temperature. Each attack is characterized by sudden-onset shortness of breath described as "gasping for air." During attacks, she takes her albuterol inhaler, and the attacks almost always subside. In addition to the albuterol inhaler, she also uses a low-dose inhaled corticosteroid daily. She is not on chronic systemic steroids. She has not been to the emergency room or intubated for her asthma attacks. This morning, while visiting a client at their home, she suddenly felt short of breath, similar to prior asthma attacks. She felt like she was gasping for air, and her breathing felt labored. She also noticed that her client has cats as pets. She used her albuterol inhaler several times, but the shortness of breath persisted and actually became worse. She denies any fever, runny nose, palpitations, or chest pain. She asked her client to call emergency services and was promptly brought in via ambulance to the emergency room.

(*continued*)

Box 6-4. Suggested Alternative Templates for Documenting the History of Present Illness (*Continued*)

HPI template for an encounter with no CC:

- Opening statement: statement of the patient's past medical problems
- Status report of the patient's chronic conditions
- Current treatment and response
- Prior relevant labs/studies
- Presence or absence of complications
- Pertinent symptoms—present and absent
- Concluding statement: how the patient got to the care site

CC: Checkup

HPI: EL is a 72-year-old cisgender woman with hypertension, osteoarthritis, and constipation presenting to the clinic for follow-up of her chronic conditions. She was last seen 3 months ago and today reports no concerns.

She has hypertension diagnosed 12 years ago and controlled well on hydrochlorothiazide. Her blood pressures at home are typically 110 s/80 s. She has never had a myocardial infarction or stroke. She reports that she has not had any recent chest pain, palpitations, headaches, loss of consciousness, dizziness, or leg swelling.

She also has osteoarthritis diagnosed 10 years ago involving her shoulders and knees. She takes acetaminophen on occasion for pain with prompt relief. She also does yoga and tai chi at a local senior center and says that they also help with the pain. Her last lumbosacral x-ray, taken after a fall after slipping while trying to get on a bus 3 years ago, showed diffuse osteoarthritic changes. She reports that she has not fallen recently or had any pain elsewhere.

EL also has constipation and takes senna on occasion. She usually has regular bowel movements daily without any straining or blood in the stools.

EL was called in to the clinic for her regularly scheduled follow-up visit.

as other providers may overlook them if they are not listed until later in the note. The opening statement often includes the patient's gender identity (Box 6-5).

Elaboration of Chief Concern with Attention to Chronology. Next, provide the details about the CC that you obtained during the interview (Box 6-6).

Box 6-5. Inclusion of Gender Identity in the Opening Statement

Traditionally, the HPI of a note or oral presentation includes the patient's gender identity (e.g., *"DP is a 48-year-old cisgender man…"* or *"NT is an 8-year-old girl…"*) as a frame for their presentation. Most providers continue to use this convention.

However, as we strive to create health care environments that are more inclusive of diverse identities, including diverse gender identities, some experts have suggested omission of gender identity in notes and presentations if it is irrelevant to the patient's presentation.[5] Goals include facilitating person-first language, avoiding bias, and focusing on the essential elements of the case. Examples of applications of this strategy include[5]:

- Stating relevant physiologic or anatomic considerations rather than using gender identity as a proxy: *"A 32-year-old pregnant patient at 37 weeks' gestation…"* instead of *"A 32-year-old cisgender woman at 37 weeks' gestation…"*
- Providing the specific context needed when gender identity is relevant to the case: *"A 41-year-old cisgender man presents with inability to conceive…"*
- Completely omitting gender identity when it is entirely irrelevant to the patient's presentation: *"A 6-year-old with a history of asthma…"* instead of *"A 6-year-old boy with a history of asthma…"*

One method to maintain clarity of the patient's story is to anchor each event to a consistent timeline. "*Two days prior to hospitalization*, the patient began experiencing multiple episodes of watery nonbloody diarrhea, which was *followed a day later* by two episodes of nonbloody vomiting. Then, *6 hours prior to hospitalization*, the patient reported severe epigastric pain." This approach ensures a coherent story flow.

Try to avoid mixing time references, such as specific dates with relative times: *"On June 12, the patient started to develop…then 3 days prior to admission…then on Monday…."* This can lead to confusion and disrupt the narrative's continuity.

Pertinent Accompanying Symptoms and Absent Symptoms. When documenting symptoms related to the CC, describe both present symptoms (*pertinent positives*) and the absence of expected symptoms (*pertinent negatives*).

Pertinent Positives. Pertinent positives "help to make the argument for a particular diagnosis, using the classic signs

Box 6-6. Framework for Elaborating the Chief Concern in the HPI

Feature	Description	Examples
Location	Identify the specific area(s) impacted by the concern, including side (left, right), bilateral/unilateral, and specific anatomical regions (anterior, posterior, upper, lower). Describe if the condition is widespread, localized, stationary, moving, or radiates to other areas.	▪ Localized pain on the right side ▪ Widespread rash ▪ Moving discomfort in the upper abdomen
Quality	Describe the nature of the concern using appropriate descriptors. For symptoms like pain, use terms such as "dull," "sharp," "throbbing," etc. For other concerns, use descriptors like "heavy," "light," "frequent," "rare," etc. Note any changes over time.	▪ Sharp pain ▪ Heavy breathing ▪ Intermittent cough
Quantity or severity	Quantify the concern, such as rating pain on a scale from 1 to 10, describing the intensity of symptoms, or estimating the volume of discharge.	▪ Pain rated 8/10 ▪ Moderate dizziness ▪ Half a cup of bloody discharge
Timing	Detail the onset, duration, and frequency of the concern.	▪ *Onset:* 3 hours ago ▪ *Duration:* For the past week ▪ *Frequency:* Daily
Setting	Mention the circumstances under which the issue either worsens or improves.	▪ Worse when standing ▪ Improved with rest ▪ Aggravated by eating
Modifying factors	Document any actions that have alleviated or exacerbated the concern.	▪ Relieved with acetaminophen ▪ No change with ibuprofen
Effects on daily life	Describe how the issue affects the patient's daily activities and well-being.	▪ Unable to attend school ▪ Creating tension at home ▪ Impacting work

and symptoms of the disease. The more of these classic findings are present, the more likely the diagnosis."[6] For example, in a patient presenting with shortness of breath: *"...The patient also had an episode of palpitations described as her 'heart racing really fast' for less than a minute followed by intense facial flushing."* adds weight to a specific diagnostic consideration.

Pertinent Negatives. Conversely, pertinent negatives "help to rule out alternatives to the leading diagnosis while also showing that a thorough differential diagnosis has been considered" and include "both the expected positives that are *not* present" and "findings that, *by their absence*, help to rule out alternative diagnoses."[6] In this same example regarding a patient with shortness of breath: *"...She has not had any fever or cough. No chest pain, nausea, or vomiting. She has no prior history of coronary artery disease."* Including this information shows your reader that you have thought about possible causes of the patient's shortness of breath, such as pneumonia or myocardial infarction, and have deemed them less likely based on the patient's presentation.

Incorporating both pertinent positives and negatives into your documentation provides a comprehensive overview, guiding the diagnostic process by highlighting relevant findings and dismissing unrelated conditions.

Additional Pertinent Information. Here you should note any additional facts pertinent to the CC, regardless of where they are typically documented in the note. For instance, a patient's smoking history is vital if you suspect pneumonia, while a history of living in a homeless shelter could be crucial for a patient you believe might have tuberculosis. These two facts would typically be documented in the social history, but they are included in the HPI for these patients because they have an impact on the evolving list of possible causes of the CC. To avoid redundancy, reference these details in the social history by noting *"as per HPI"* unless further elaboration is needed.

Often, it is helpful to conclude your HPI with an explanation of how and why the patient sought medical care. For example: *"The patient sought care from their primary doctor after fevers persisted despite taking acetaminophen."* or *"The patient was rushed to the ER by ambulance after nearly fainting on the train."*

This approach to structuring the HPI, including both specific and general information relevant to the CC, is adaptable for various clinical scenarios, from single acute concerns to more complex cases. For guidance on customizing this format to fit different types of CCs, refer back to Box 6-4 and the comprehensive example in Box 6-11.

Prior Health History

The information you gathered in the clinical encounter is organized into distinct sections for clarity and thoroughness, as described in Box 6-7. Continue to refer to the complete example in Box 6-11.

Box 6-7. Documentation of Patient's Prior Health History

Section	Description	Examples
Allergies	Document all known allergies, including reactions to medications, foods, and environmental triggers. Detail the nature of each allergic reaction.	▪ *Medication: Penicillin causes rash.* ▪ *Food: Peanuts cause anaphylaxis.* ▪ *Environmental: Pollen causes sneezing and itchy eyes.*
Medications	List every medication the patient is currently taking, specifying the dosage and frequency. This includes prescription drugs, over-the-counter medications, vitamins, and supplements. For as-needed medications, note the usage frequency to gauge symptom management.	▪ *Lisinopril 10 mg daily for hypertension.* ▪ *Vitamin D 500 IU daily.* ▪ *Ibuprofen 400 mg as needed for pain, approximately twice a week.*
Past medical history (PMH)	Record all chronic conditions and significant acute illnesses that required hospitalization, along with the dates or years of these episodes. Mild illnesses that resolved on their own or were treated outside a hospital setting may be omitted unless directly relevant to the current chief concern.	▪ *Diabetes mellitus diagnosed in 2010.* ▪ *Hospitalized for pneumonia in March 2015.* ▪ *Mild seasonal allergies, not typically relevant.*
Past surgical history (PSH)	Include a list of all surgical procedures the patient has undergone, noting the year of each surgery.	▪ *Appendectomy in 2001.* ▪ *Knee arthroscopy in 2018.*
Obstetric/ gynecologic (OB/GYN) history	For patients with a uterus, detail gravidity and parity, including the number of pregnancies, deliveries (with a breakdown of term and preterm), miscarriages or abortions before 20 weeks' gestation, and living children. Further OB/GYN details might include age at menarche or menopause, date of the last menstrual period, and any significant gynecologic conditions or obstetric complications.	▪ *Gravida 3, Para 2: One term delivery, one preterm delivery, one miscarriage* (see Chapter 29, Pregnant Persons, pp. 1128–1129 for details on this system) ▪ *Menarche at age 12, menopause at age 51.* ▪ *Last menstrual period: April 1, 2024.*
Psychiatric history	Document any psychiatric conditions diagnosed in the past, along with treatments that have been tried.	▪ *Diagnosed with major depressive disorder in 2018, treated with sertraline.*
Health maintenance	Confirm whether the patient's vaccinations are current. Record the dates and results of recent health maintenance screenings relevant to the patient's age and health status, such as colonoscopies, Pap smears, mammograms, and lipid profiles.	▪ *Immunizations up to date.* ▪ *Colonoscopy in 2023: Normal* ▪ *Pap smear in 2024: Normal.* ▪ *Mammogram in 2024: Benign findings.*

Family History

Include significant chronic conditions in the patient's immediate relatives, such as parents, siblings, grandparents, and children. Also, include conditions in more distant relatives if they are directly relevant to the patient's current health concerns. You can also consider including pertinent negatives but limit them to those that are relevant to the patient's current presentation (e.g., *"No family history of autoimmune disease"* for a patient being evaluated for possible chronic autoimmune thyroiditis). While a comprehensive pedigree might not be necessary for every patient, in cases in which genetic factors are under consideration, a genetic counselor can create a detailed pedigree and incorporate it into the EHR as part of the patient's broader health record.

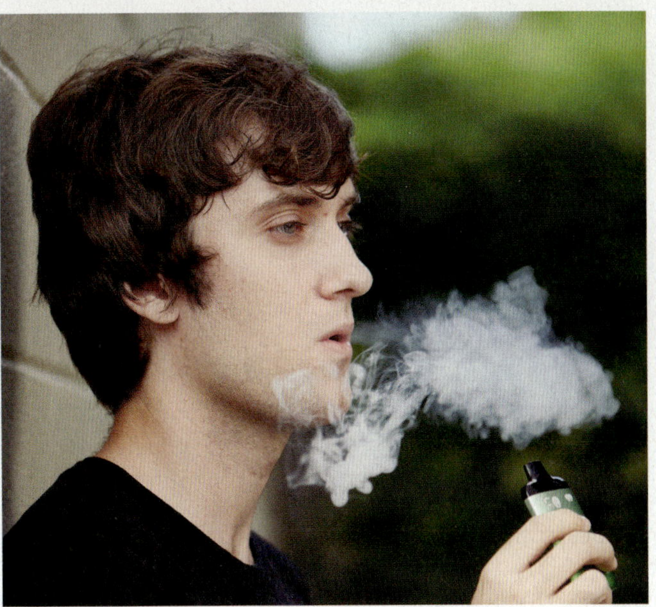

FIGURE 6-3. Vaping.

Social History

The social history section of your notes can be extensive, reflecting the wide range of information you collect about your patient's lifestyle and background. Begin this section with background personal information about your patient, such as their origin and their current residence. Then include important details of their daily life such as occupation, spiritual beliefs, living situation, social support networks, safety in relationships, exercise routines, diet, and safety practices (e.g., seatbelt usage and firearm storage). For older adults or patients with disabilities, detail any assistance they require carrying out activities of daily living. (See Chapter 3, Health History, Box 3-6, p. 52).

Certain elements of the social history are often essential to a patient's health and should be documented in detail. Any *alcohol use* should be described with the type of alcohol used, quantity and frequency of use, and its influence on daily functioning, if present. Clarity is key: *"rare"* alcohol use might mean once a year to one person and once a day to another; elicit a specific response from your patient so you can document *"One glass of wine per year"* versus *"One shot of whiskey per day."* *Tobacco use* documentation should include the number of pack-years, current quantity of use, or how long ago the patient quit as well as details regarding vaping practices. This should encompass the type of devices used, frequency of use, and the duration of vaping habits (Fig. 6-3). *Recreational drug use*, which may include prescription medications not prescribed to the patient, should specify types of substances used, injection or other use practices, and effects on daily functioning. *Sexual history* should include sexual orientation, number of partners, contraceptive use, history of sexually transmitted infections, and any other information gleaned from the interview.

Box 6-8 organizes the social history into specific documentation details, providing clear examples for each domain to guide you in collecting comprehensive and relevant information from your patients.

Review of Systems

Include in this section any symptoms, whether present or absent, that were discussed during the review of systems (ROS) portion of your encounter. Organize the information by each system for clarity. Start with constitutional symptoms then proceed in a head-to-toe sequence. Common practice is to denote absent symptoms with "(−)" and present symptoms with "(+)," followed by the lists of symptoms.

Remember that you do not need to restate information you wrote in the HPI, opting for *"as per HPI"* if needed. For example, for a patient whose CC is fever, and this symptom has been thoroughly explored in the HPI, you might note in the ROS, *"Constitutional: (−) weight loss, weight gain, fatigue, (+) fever as per HPI."*

Also remember that symptoms uncovered in the ROS that you think are relevant to the CC should be documented in the HPI. Refer to Chapter 3, Health History for specific ROS questioning techniques, and consult Box 6-11 for a complete ROS documentation example.

Physical Examination

Like the ROS, the PE should be documented by system, starting with the patient's general appearance and vital

Box 6-8. Documentation of Patient's Social History

Documentation Details	Documentation Examples
Sexual orientation and gender identity	■ *Sexual orientation:* Bisexual ■ *Gender identity:* Genderqueer ■ *Sex on original birth certificate:* Female
Personal geographic map	■ *Born in:* São Paulo, Brazil ■ *Time in the United States:* 10 years. ■ *Current residence:* New York City
Significant relationships	■ *Partner status:* Married for 15 years ■ *Children:* Two, ages 5 and 8 ■ *Safety:* Feels safe in relationship
Local support systems	■ *Living situation:* Lives with spouse and two children ■ *Nearby support: Close to extended family* ■ *Daily company:* Spends days with coworkers and family
Work history/occupation	■ *Employment:* Nurse ■ *Past jobs:* Retail ■ *Job security:* Feels secure in current position
Education	■ *Highest level completed:* Bachelor's degree in nursing ■ *Schooling location:* Florida
Lifestyle and activities of daily living	■ *Daily routine:* Works 9:00 AM–5:00 PM, cooks dinner, weekend hiking ■ *Mobility:* Uses cane for walking longer distances ■ *Assistance needed:* Requires help with heavy lifting
Nutrition	■ *Eating habits:* Vegetarian, eats mostly home-cooked meals ■ *Weight management:* Maintains a consistent weight; wishes to lose 10 lb ■ *Dining:* Eats out once a week
Exercise	■ *Physical activity:* Jogs three times a week ■ *Exercise preference:* Yoga and swimming
Substance use	■ *Alcohol:* Drinks socially, one glass of wine per week ■ *Tobacco:* Smoked 10 years; quit 5 years ago ■ *Illicit drugs:* None
Safety measures	■ *Injuries:* Broke an arm in a biking accident in 2024 ■ *Seatbelt use:* Always wears a seatbelt ■ *Firearm storage:* No firearms in the home
Spirituality	■ *Beliefs:* Practices Buddhism ■ *Community involvement:* Active in local meditation center ■ *Treatment conflicts:* None
Sexual history	■ *Concerns:* Questions about contraception ■ *Intimacy frequency:* Once a week ■ *Partners' genders:* Male

signs and moving to a detailed head-to-toe assessment. Provide a concise but clear and thorough summary for each system examined. For systems possibly related to the CC, you will provide more details captured in the PE. For example, for a patient presenting with possible stroke, ensure to include a full assessment using the National Institutes of Health Stroke Scale[7] documented in their neurologic examination section. Additional detailed documentation specific to each system can be found in each of the corresponding regional chapters.

Some parts of the PE may not be performed during a particular encounter, in which case, simply document that part as *"Not done."* For example, conducting pelvic and rectal examinations for a patient consulting about ear pain would typically be unnecessary unless the examination uncovers additional health concerns that warrant such assessments. Refer to Box 6-11 for an example of documentation of a complete PE.

Assessment and Plan

While your clinical documentation of the health history and PE is primarily a reflection of your data gathering skills, the *Summary Statement*, *Assessment*, and *Plan* represent the most robust reflection of your clinical reasoning skills. It involves carefully selecting and grouping pertinent information, analyzing its significance, and interpreting the patient's condition, including its management. This is often the most valuable part of your note for other health care professionals, as it succinctly communicates your diagnostic impression of the patient's problem and details the specific actions that are being taken or are in progress for diagnosis and treatment.

Summary Statement. Start your assessment and plan (A&P) with two to three sentences that succinctly encapsulate your understanding of the patient's problem. This summary statement should distill the salient information and defining features of the case to argue in favor of your working diagnosis, going beyond merely repeating data. It should include the patient's demographic information; notable medical history relevant to the CC; the CC itself with its clinical context; and limited, carefully selected historical information, PE findings, and laboratory or other results that most directly support your working diagnosis. The goal is to guide the reader toward the main diagnosis you have in mind by aligning the patient's story with common characteristics of that illness (*illness script*).

For example: *"JL, a 57-year-old cisgender man with hypertension and a 35 pack-year smoking history, presents with acute, severe, exertional, retrosternal pain accompanied by shortness of breath. His examination is notable for a new S_3 gallop, bibasilar crackles, and bilateral lower extremity edema."*

This description highlights the patient's cardiovascular risk factors, the anginal qualities of the chest pain, and the abnormal PE findings indicative of acute-onset heart failure, suggesting the illness script for myocardial infarction.

Effective summary statements often use *semantic qualifiers*, precise descriptive terms that help delineate the diagnosis by providing a clear, contrasting description of the condition. Typically, they are opposing descriptors that can be used to compare and contrast diagnostic considerations (Box 6-9). Studies have shown that successful diagnosticians use semantic qualifiers more frequently.[8]

In the previous example, notice several semantic qualifiers, including *"acute," "severe," "exertional," "new," "bibasilar," and "bilateral."* These terms not only

Box 6-9. Examples of Semantic Qualifiers

Concepts	Semantic Qualifiers
Duration	Acute, chronic Old, new Progressive, regressive
Intensity	Mild, severe Sharp, dull
Occurrence	Constant, intermittent Sporadic, frequent
Location	Diffuse, localized Unilateral, bilateral Radiating, localized
Activity	At rest, exertional
Sensation	Tender, nontender
Depth	Deep, superficial
Association	Associated, unassociated
Position/behavior	Positional, nonpositional
Effect/response	Exacerbating, alleviating
Initiation/resolution	Onset, resolution

enhance the problem's portrayal but also guide the differential diagnosis toward the most probable cause.

Prioritized Problem List. Following the summary statement, make a prioritized list of all the patient's problems addressed during the clinical encounter, ranging from known diagnoses to symptoms, and psychosocial factors. Your list should showcase your ability to critically analyze and synthesize your findings, cohesively grouping related symptoms under a single problem whenever possible. For instance, if a patient reports both chest pain and shortness of breath and you think these two are interrelated, they should be combined into one comprehensive problem, rather than listed separately. A well-articulated problem should be specific (e.g., "*Headache*" or "*Type 2 diabetes mellitus*") rather than vaguely referencing an organ system (e.g., "*Neuro/pain*"). This methodical organization aids in creating focused and effective assessments and plans for each problem, facilitating targeted patient care.

Corresponding Individual Assessments and Plans. Once you have created your problem list, provide an A&P for each identified problem. Prioritize each problem, offering a differential diagnosis that highlights evidence supporting or contesting potential causes, and outline a corresponding strategy for intervention.

In general, an A&P can be *diagnostic*, *therapeutic*, or both (Box 6-10). For symptoms lacking a definitive cause, such as anorexia or fatigue, detail a concise differential diagnosis—specifying which conditions are more or less probable based on your analysis—and delineate the investigative steps intended to ascertain a definitive diagnosis. Incorporate therapeutic measures when applicable, like prescribing pain relief while investigating the underlying cause of discomfort. In cases of established diagnoses or ongoing conditions, evaluate the current status, focusing on symptom management, potential complications, and treatment compliance, and propose a plan for ongoing care.

In the context of inpatient care, the last entry on your problem list should address *disposition*, identifying any factors hindering discharge, like the need for further diagnostic work or placement considerations. Regular updates on this aspect are crucial to strategize timely discharge planning.

For outpatient encounters, *health maintenance* often concludes the list, serving as a reminder to monitor and manage routine health checks based on the patient's health history, and to schedule any necessary screenings.

For a comprehensive illustration of a fully developed A&P, see Box 6-11, which provides an example tailored to a new patient's needs.

Box 6-10. Annotated Example of Diagnostic and Therapeutic Assessment and Plan

Assessment/Plan: A 62-year-old male with diabetes mellitus and hypertension, who was recently on a long flight, presents with acute exertional chest pain. On examination, the patient is tachycardic but without leg edema.

This is the summary statement.

1. Chest pain

The patient's known cardiovascular risk factors of hypertension and diabetes mellitus, and the acute onset and exertional nature of the chest pain make this diagnosis most likely. Pulmonary embolism is less likely as the patient has no evidence of shortness of breath or unilateral leg swelling; however, the patient has tachycardia and recently took a long flight.

This is an example of a *diagnostic assessment*. You should provide supporting evidence for the likelihood of each item in your differential diagnosis.

Plan:

- Request for an ECG and serial troponin levels to evaluate acute coronary syndrome.
- Request for D-dimer. As this patient has low probability for a pulmonary embolism, a negative D-dimer would likely rule out this diagnosis as the cause of the patient's chest pain.

This is an example of a *diagnostic plan*. You should provide rationale for evaluating each item in your differential diagnosis.

2. Diabetes mellitus, type 2

- The diabetes is currently poorly controlled, with a hemoglobin A_{1c} of 9.0%, on metformin 1,000 mg twice a day. He reports excellent adherence to this medication without any side effects.

This is an example of a *therapeutic assessment*. You should provide the clinical status of the chronic condition or a known diagnosis.

Plan:

- After discussion with the patient, a long-acting insulin will be started, as the addition of a second oral agent is unlikely to bring his hemoglobin A_{1c} to goal. Educate patient on the use of the insulin pen and possible complications. Excellent teach back.

This is an example of a *therapeutic plan*. You should provide rationale for the management of chronic condition or known diagnosis moving forward.

Box 6-11. Example of a History and Physical: Patient MN

Source: Patient

CC: Acute worsening of chronic headache with neurologic symptoms ×3 days

HPI: MN, a 54-year-old cisgender woman with a history of intermittent headaches and controlled hypertension, presents to the emergency department with a 3-day history of severe headache. Unlike her usual headache episodes, these headaches are described as unrelenting, peaking at 9 out of 10 in severity, localized to the frontal area with new-onset photophobia, and not relieved by her usual coping mechanisms (sleep, damp cool towel) or acetaminophen. MN also reports new associated symptoms including blurred vision, slurred speech, and right-sided weakness. Her functional status has declined, rendering her unable to perform daily activities or work. In addition, she experiences persistent nausea and has vomited several times since the onset of these symptoms. Given her mother's history of a stroke preceding death, MN is particularly alarmed. Due to this, she decided to come to the ER today.

Allergies: Ampicillin (rash), no environmental or food allergies.

Medications: Lisinopril 10 mg daily, multivitamin daily, acetaminophen 325 mg to 650 mg as needed for headaches (about once a week).

PMH: Hypertension, hospitalized for pyelonephritis (2020).

PSH: Tonsillectomy (1981), appendectomy (1988).

OB/GYN history: G3P3-0-0-3 with spontaneous vaginal deliveries. Menarche at age 12. Last menstrual period 6 months ago.

Psychiatric history: Brief consultation with a therapist approximately 10 years ago for episodes of low mood, no formal diagnosis.

Health maintenance: Immunizations up to date. Last Pap smear in 2022 with co-testing normal. Last mammogram in 2024 was reported as normal. No colonoscopy or other colon cancer screening conducted. Uncertain about HIV screening.

Family history: Father deceased at age 43 in a car accident. Mother died at age 67 from a stroke, had a history of headaches. One brother (age 61) with hypertension; another brother (age 58) with mild arthritis; a sister who died in infancy of unknown cause. Daughter (age 33) with migraine headaches; son (age 31) with headaches; another son (age 27) is well. No family history of epilepsy, subarachnoid hemorrhage, or brain tumor syndromes.

Social history: MN was born and raised in Las Cruces and moved to Española after marrying at 19. Identifies as a cisgender female. Completed high school and an apprenticeship in welding, has been working as a welder since. Husband died suddenly from a heart attack 4 years ago. She moved to an apartment to save money and live closer to her daughter. Lives alone, feels safe in her home, keeps a loaded handgun in an unlocked dresser. Daughter's husband has a problem with alcohol, contributing to MN's stress. Does not often discuss family problems, stating a preference to keep them private. Raised Catholic, faith is important but has not attended church since husband's death. Reports no current spiritual support system. Diet is high in carbohydrates, and she does not get much exercise. Current smoker, 1 pack per day since age 18 (36 pack-years). Consumes wine rarely (one glass three to four times a year). No recreational drug use. Not sexually active currently, no history of STIs.

ROS:

- Constitutional: (−) weight loss, (−) weight gain, (−) fatigue, (−) fevers, (−) chills, (−) night sweats
- Skin: (−) rash, (−) jaundice
- HEENT: (+) headache as per HPI, (−) change in vision, (−) change in hearing, (−) lymphadenopathy
- Respiratory: (−) cough, (−) shortness of breath
- Cardiovascular: (−) chest pain, (−) palpitations
- Gastrointestinal: (+) nausea, (+) vomiting, (−) anorexia, (−) dysphagia, (−) abdominal pain, (−) diarrhea, (+) occasional constipation with hard stools for 2–3 days when feeling especially tense
- Genitourinary: (+) occasional urinary incontinence when coughing, (−) hematuria, (−) dysuria, (−) urinary frequency, (−) dyspareunia

(continued)

Box 6-11. Example of a History and Physical: Patient MN (*Continued*)

- Hematologic: (–) easy bruising, (–) bleeding
- Endocrine: (–) polyuria, (–) polydipsia, (–) cold intolerance, (–) heat intolerance
- Musculoskeletal: (–) joint pain, (–) myalgias
- Neurologic: For this hospitalization, important to update based on current findings: (+) right-sided weakness (new), (+) slurred speech (new), (–) numbness, (–) paresthesia, (–) dizziness
- Psychiatric: (–) low mood, (–) anhedonia, (+) anxiety as per social history

PE:

- General appearance: MN is alert but appears distressed and uncomfortable due to pain. She is lying in bed and is occasionally grimacing.
- Vital signs: BP: 178/102 mm Hg, HR: 88 bpm, RR: 16/min, Temp: 98.9 °F (37.2 °C), oxygen saturation is 99% on room air.
- Skin: Warm and well-perfused. No rash, erythema, or jaundice. Scattered cherry angiomas noted over the upper trunk. No signs of cyanosis or nail clubbing.
- Head, eyes, ears, nose, throat (HEENT): Head is normocephalic and atraumatic. Eyes: Pupils are equally round and reactive to light, but there is noted photophobia. Extraocular movements intact. No conjunctival injection or pallor. Fundoscopic exam shows sharp optic disc margins bilaterally. Ears: External canals clear, tympanic membranes intact. Nose: Mucous membranes are moist, no sinus tenderness. Throat: Oropharynx is moist without erythema or exudates. Tonsils absent.
- Neck: Supple, no lymphadenopathy or thyroid enlargement palpable.
- Cardiovascular: Heart rate and rhythm are regular, S_1 and S_2 heard, no murmurs, rubs, or gallops noted on auscultation. No jugular venous distension or peripheral edema.
- Respiratory: Lungs are clear to auscultation bilaterally, with no wheezes, crackles, or rhonchi. No increased work of breathing.
- Abdomen: Soft, nontender, and nondistended. Bowel sounds are present and normal in all quadrants. No hepatosplenomegaly or masses palpable.
- Musculoskeletal: No joint swelling or deformities. Full range of motion in all extremities. Good muscle bulk and tone.
- Neurologic: Patient is alert and oriented to person, place, and time. Cranial nerves II–XII are intact, except for mild right-sided facial droop. Motor examination reveals 4/5 strength in right upper and lower extremities, compared to 5/5 on the left. Sensory exam is intact to light touch and pinprick throughout. Reflexes are 2+ and symmetric in both upper and lower extremities. Coordination tests (finger-to-nose, heel-to-shin) are normal. Gait could not be assessed due to patient's discomfort and neurologic deficits.

A&P: MN, a 54-year-old cisgender woman with a history of intermittent, stress-related headaches, now presents with acute, severe, frontal headaches with associated photophobia, blurred vision, slurred speech, and right-sided weakness, diverging markedly from her usual headache pattern. The examination highlights focal neurologic deficits and controlled hypertension.

1. **Severe headache with neurologic deficits:** The most likely cause to consider is a cerebrovascular event. This could either be an ischemic stroke or a hemorrhagic stroke. These conditions are particularly concerning given MN's acute change in neurologic function, including speech difficulties, blurred vision, and unilateral weakness. A subarachnoid hemorrhage (SAH) must also be considered given the sudden onset of a severe headache, especially considering the rapid development of her neurologic deficits. Though less likely given MN's symptomatology and the absence of fever or meningeal irritation, CNS infections like meningitis or encephalitis could theoretically present with severe headache and neurologic signs. Similarly, a brain tumor or other mass lesions could manifest similarly, but these are typically associated with a more gradual onset of symptoms rather than the acute presentation observed in MN.
   - Immediate neuroimaging is warranted to assess for acute abnormalities.
   - Consult neurology for further evaluation and management.

- Start IV hydration, analgesics for headache management, and antiemetics for nausea.
- Monitor closely for changes in neurologic status.

2. **Hypertension:** Blood pressure on admission was 178/102 mm Hg, indicating poorly controlled hypertension possibly contributing to her acute presentation.
   - Start IV antihypertensive medication (labetalol or nicardipine) to gradually lower blood pressure to prevent further neurologic compromise.
   - Continue monitoring of blood pressure
   - Monitor neurologic status and renal function
3. **Social stressors:** Include providing emotional support to daughter whose husband may have alcohol use problem, financial constraints since husband's death, and spiritual duress with lack of social and spiritual support.
   - Once stable, plan to address these through multidisciplinary team including social work and psychology to provide support and resources for stress management and coping strategies.
4. **Tobacco use:** 1 pack per day for 36 years. Currently precontemplative for smoking cessation in setting of multiple life stressors (as per outpatient note).
   - Referral to a smoking cessation program will be made for follow-up after discharge
5. **Disposition:** The patient was admitted to the neurology stroke unit for immediate management of her acute neurologic symptoms and severe headache, suggestive of a potential stroke. The hospital course is aimed at stabilizing her condition, conducting a thorough diagnostic evaluation, and initiating appropriate treatment based on the findings.
   - Plan for a multidisciplinary team discussion to evaluate rehabilitation needs based on the patient's progress and recovery from the acute event.
   - Upon stabilization and prior to discharge, reassess home environment safety.

CONDUCTING ORAL PRESENTATIONS FOR NEW PATIENTS

When delivering an oral presentation, your aim is to refine and present only the information that pertains directly to the patient's current health concerns. Introducing a patient to your team, especially if they are newly admitted to the hospital or attending their first clinic visit, requires you to provide a comprehensive background (Fig. 6-4). This ensures the team has a full understanding of the patient's situation, demanding a level of detail that balances thoroughness with brevity. Although this type of presentation might be longer to ensure completeness, maintaining conciseness is crucial to keep your audience engaged.

One survey of clinician-educators showed that, on average, faculty expected student presentations of new inpatients to take 9.9 minutes[4]—a short window that emphasizes the importance of a focused and efficient presentation. You are encouraged to adapt the structure and tips provided in Box 6-12, while also considering other established presentation frameworks.[3,9]

DOCUMENTING PROGRESS NOTES

The *SOAP note* is the most widely adopted structure for progress notes.[10] This format offers a systematic way to summarize patient encounters, starting with the patient's account (*Subjective*), followed by clinical findings and

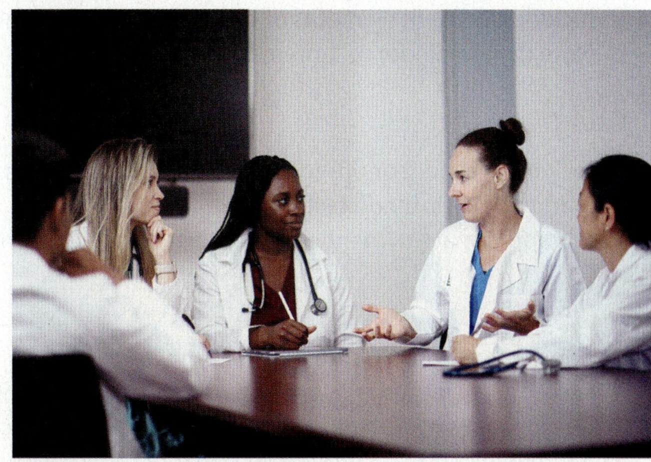

FIGURE 6-4. Orally presenting a patient to the clinical team.

Box 6-12. Guideline for Oral Patient Presentation: New Patient

Make a convincing case for the important problems, the differential, and the plan. Make it structured, organized, and targeted, as it should take only 3–5 minutes.

Opening Statement

- Briefly state the CC and why the patient was admitted.
- Include pointed and relevant historical information.

Source

- If indicated, briefly note if/why the patient cannot give reliable history.
- Note any information sources beside the patient.
- Unless you comment on the source, the patient will be assumed to be reliable.

Present Illness

- Use your differential diagnosis as a guide for what to include.
- Consider starting with: *"…usual state of health until…."*
- Be chronologically organized and clear without analyzing.
- Remember the attributes of a CC.
- Include elements of past history (with supporting studies and therapeutic interventions), medications, family history, social history (including psychosocial factors) that specifically contribute to the present illness.
- Include pertinent positives and negatives so the listener better understands your differential diagnosis.
- Only include ER course if it significantly affects/alters triage or immediate treatment decisions prior to the patient's coming to your care.

Other History

- Include important PMH (with supporting history/data).
- Exclude minor diagnoses without impact on current care.
- Include important medications with doses of relevant ones. Omit unimportant medications.
- List allergies.
- Include focused family and social histories and an ROS. Do not repeat previously stated information.

Physical Examination

- Always include general appearance and specific vitals.
- Include pertinent elements of examination and any abnormal findings.
- Note the remainder as "unremarkable."

Labs/Data

- Include pertinent or otherwise significant labs/studies.
- Start with basic blood tests first.
- It is appropriate to mention other tests as being "normal."

Synthesis

- Consider beginning with: *"And in summary,…."*
- Assess and synthesize, avoid regurgitating information.
- Demonstrate your thinking about the patient-specific differential diagnosis.
- If multiple issues are present, weave together or discuss lesser issues in problem list.

Enumerated Problem List

- Start with the most important problem first.
- Use the most specific label for the problem you can.
- Avoid labeling a problem solely by its organ system.
- Include your understanding of the cause of the problem.
- Include a diagnostic and/or therapeutic specific plan for addressing it.

Source: Modified from Green EH, Hershman W, DeCherrie L, Greenwald J, Torres-Finnerty N, Wahi-Gururaj S. Developing and implementing universal guidelines for oral patient presentation skills. *Teach Learn Med.* 2005;17(3):263–267. Reprinted by permission of Taylor & Francis Ltd. http://www.tandfonline.com

test results (*Objective*), then the health care provider's diagnosis or *Assessment*, and concluding with the diagnostic and/or treatment *Plan*.

Despite its popularity, alternatives like the *Patient-Centered Medical Record (PCMR)* have been proposed to address some of SOAP's limitations (Box 6-13).[11] For instance, labeling patient narratives as "subjective" might suggest they are less reliable, overlooking that all data, including "objective" findings, involve a degree of interpretation by the health care provider. The PCMR emphasizes the patient's narrative and preferences, integrates clinical findings, builds a mutual understanding of the health issue, and collaborates on the care plan, highlighting a more holistic and patient-centered approach.

Box 6-13. Comparing Documentation Approaches: SOAP Note versus Patient-Centered Medical Record for Hypertension Management

SOAP Component	SOAP Note Example	PCMR Component	PCMR Example
Subjective	*Reports feeling generally well, with occasional headaches. Consistent adherence to medication, but no home blood pressure monitoring.*	Patient's story	*Expresses satisfaction with the treatment plan and concern about occasional headaches, questioning their relation to hypertension or medication.*
Objective	*Blood pressure is 138/88 mm Hg in the clinic. Physical exam unremarkable. Lab tests show normal kidney function and electrolytes.*	Health care findings	*Clinical measurements show blood pressure generally under control with occasional borderline high readings. Lab work indicates no adverse effects from medication.*
Assessment	*Hypertension moderately controlled. Occasional borderline high readings noted. Good medication adherence with no signs of secondary effects.*	Shared understanding	*Discussion between provider and patient on the potential nonrelation of headaches to blood pressure. Agreement on the unlikely direct link but decision to monitor.*
Plan	*Continue current antihypertensive medication. Recommend home blood pressure monitoring and logging. Schedule follow-up in 3 months. Discuss lifestyle modifications for blood pressure control.*	Collaborative plan	*Decision to maintain current medication dose, with patient undertaking regular home monitoring. Commitment to lifestyle changes with provided resources. Follow-up scheduled to reassess and potentially adjust the care plan.*

Box 6-14. Structuring SOAP Notes for Follow-Up Patient Visits

Section	Examples
Subjective (S)	
■ Start with a concise "one-liner" summarizing the patient's PMH, reason for presentation, and the purpose of the current follow-up. ■ Update with new information shared by the patient since the last visit. ■ Exclude comprehensive past history details unless there are relevant changes.	*JM, a 48-year-old cisgender man with diabetes mellitus, chronic kidney disease, hyperlipidemia, and coronary artery disease (stent placed in 2023) admitted for 3 days of fever in the setting of worsening control of his diabetes, diagnosed with pneumonia and now on day 2 of broad-spectrum antibiotics.*
Objective (O)	
■ Begin with general appearance and vital signs. ■ Document relevant physical exam findings focused on the patient's current condition. ■ Include recent lab results and other tests, summarizing or quoting significant changes or findings.	*Physical exam shows reduced crackles in the lung fields compared to yesterday, indicating improvement in pneumonia. Latest labs show a WBC count reduced to 9.2 from 15 on admission. BMP results from this morning are stable with a notable potassium of 5.5.*
Assessment (A)	
■ Provide a summary statement with relevant updates since the last encounter, reflecting on the patient's condition. ■ Then, discuss each problem in your prioritized problem list, focusing on updates in diagnostic considerations or the status of chronic issues.	*JM is a 48-year-old cisgender man with a complex PMH notable for poorly controlled diabetes who was admitted for acute-onset fever and found to have an infected diabetic foot ulcer. He is now on day 2 of broad-spectrum antibiotics and clinically improving with resolution of fevers, still awaiting blood culture results.*
Plan (P)	
■ Detail the diagnostic and/or therapeutic plan for each problem discussed in the Assessment. ■ Focus on changes or continuations in treatment and any anticipated next steps in care.	*Problem #1: Infected diabetic foot ulcer:* *JM shows clinical improvement on antibiotics with fever resolved, awaiting further blood culture results. Continue current treatment and reassess in 48 hours.*

Nonetheless, due to its widespread use and utility in organizing patient information efficiently, we will focus on structuring SOAP notes for returning patients here (Box 6-14).

Ensure you regularly update each progress note by meticulously reviewing the information: delete outdated details, incorporate new data, and adjust the organization as necessary to accurately reflect the latest management plan. Your A&P section should mirror the current state of your patient's care. In addition, clearly indicate any improvement or resolution of issues, such as noting *"Diaper rash, resolved"* for a patient whose condition has been successfully treated. This approach guarantees that the A&P provides a precise and current overview of the patient's status and care strategy. Box 6-14 provides a detailed example of a follow-up progress note using the SOAP format, based on the initial H&P note documented in Box 6-6.

ADDRESSING SPECIAL CONSIDERATIONS IN CLINICAL DOCUMENTATION

As you become more accustomed to the note structure, you will gradually start composing notes for patients in your institution's EHR. During this transition, consider the various factors influencing your utilization of the EHR, as outlined in Table 6-1.

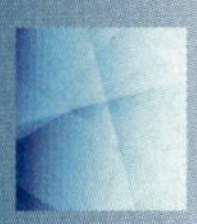

TABLE 6-1. Special Considerations in Clinical Documentation

Factor	What to Consider
Digitization of the medical record	■ Electronic health records (EHRs) are now widespread, and you are unlikely to work in a setting that relies primarily on paper charts. ■ Benefits include the ability to share patient data across locations, improved communication among providers, clearer information exchange, better adherence to guidelines, and reduced medical errors.[12] EHRs are powerful tools for clinical decision support, providing timely prompts to enhance care quality (e.g., reminding a provider to order a flu vaccine if the patient is due). ■ Pitfalls include the risk of plagiarism through a "copy-and-paste" culture, loss of focus on key clinical data, reduced patient-centeredness during interactions, and a generic, automated approach to diagnosis and care.[13] ■ As a novice, be cautious when using efficiency features (e.g., checkboxes, templates, note forwarding) to avoid including incorrect, misleading, or outdated information.
Billing	■ Since 1995, the federal government has regulated the documentation required for reimbursement via the Evaluation & Management (E&M) Guidelines.[14] ■ Many EHRs were developed to help providers meet these guidelines, leading to "note bloat" and clinician burnout as providers "overdocument" to avoid audit risks.[14] ■ The E&M Guidelines frequently change, so you should stay updated on what is required for reimbursement and ensure these elements are present in your notes. ■ For instance, starting in 2021, the guidelines no longer require a specific scope of history and exam documentation; instead, they focus on the complexity and time spent on medical decision-making.[15] ■ Since 2018, medical student notes can be used for billing purposes.[16] Therefore, it is crucial for students to include required elements, which can also enhance learning through increased supervisor feedback.[17]
Patient access to notes	■ As of 2021, the 21st Century Cures Act mandates that patients must have immediate and free access to their health information in the EHR.[18] ■ Through patient portals, patients can view the notes you write and may also see test results immediately—sometimes even before the provider has reviewed them. ■ Providers can block a patient's access to notes only if they believe it could result in harm to the patient or others, or if they need to protect another individual's health information (e.g., a parent's information in a child's record).[18] ■ Potential benefits of patient access include better understanding of their health, improved communication and collaboration with providers, greater patient empowerment, and increased provider accountability.[19] ■ However, potential downsides include patient distress from seeing bad news before it is discussed, confusion from medical jargon, a compromise in the quality or purpose of notes, and an increased workload for providers.[19]

(*continued*)

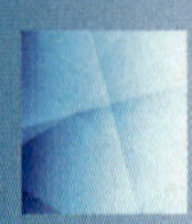

TABLE 6-1. Special Considerations in Clinical Documentation *(Continued)*

Factor	What to Consider
Patient problem list	■ Most EHRs allow you to create a "patient problem list" that exists outside individual clinical notes and includes all of the patient's significant health issues. ■ This is different from the "problem list" documented in the assessment and plan (A&P) of a specific note, which only addresses the issues relevant to that particular encounter. ■ Each entry in the problem list can represent a symptom, diagnosis, or past health event, such as a hospital admission or surgery. ■ Update the "patient problem list" at every visit by adding new problems or revising existing ones with details like the date of onset, test results, treatment responses, and current status. ■ For future encounters, the list provides a quick summary of the patient's medical history, prompts a review of ongoing issues the patient may not mention, and helps track follow-up needs or missing actions.
Use of artificial intelligence (AI)	■ AI tools, such as "digital scribes," can leverage speech recognition and natural language processing to convert patient-provider interactions into clinical notes. ■ Potential benefits include improved efficiency, reduced documentation workload for providers, and an intuitive interface that requires minimal training. ■ However, risks include inaccurate information that could harm patients, technical issues (such as difficulty distinguishing speakers or filtering ambient noise), and potential medicolegal consequences.[20] ■ One study involving ChatGPT-4 found it generated more detailed and higher-quality histories of present illnesses (HPIs), but 36% of its notes contained erroneous or "hallucinated" information.[21]

REFERENCES

1. *Core Entrustable Professional Activities for Entering Residency: Curriculum Developers' Guide.* Association of American Medical Colleges; 2014. Accessed March 18, 2024. https://store.aamc.org/downloadable/download/sample/sample_id/63/
2. Bowker D, Torti J, Goldszmidt M. Documentation as composing: how medical students and residents use writing to think and learn. *Adv Health Sci Educ Theory Pract.* 2023;28(2):453–475.
3. Green EH, Hershman W, DeCherrie L, Greenwald J, Torres-Finnerty N, Wahi-Gururaj S. Developing and implementing universal guidelines for oral patient presentation skills. *Teach Learn Med.* 2005;17(3):263–267.
4. Green EH, DeCherrie L, Fagan MJ, Sharpe BA, Hershman W. The oral case presentation: what internal medicine clinician-teachers expect from clinical clerks. *Teach Learn Med.* 2011;23(1):58–61.
5. Baecher-Lind L, Sutton JM, Bhargava R, et al; Association of Professors of Gynecology and Obstetrics Undergraduate Medical Education Committee. Strategies to create a more gender identity inclusive learning environment in preclinical and clinical medical education. *Acad Med.* 2023;98(12):1351–1355.
6. Packer CD. Chapter 5: Pertinent positives and negatives. In: *Presenting Your Case: A Concise Guide for Medical Students.* Springer Nature Switzerland AG; 2019:57. Accessed March 18, 2024.
7. NIH Stroke Scale. National Institute of Neurological Disorders and Stroke. Updated June 12, 2023. Accessed March 18, 2024. https://www.ninds.nih.gov/health-information/public-education/know-stroke/health-professionals/nih-stroke-scale
8. Bordage G. Prototypes and semantic qualifiers: from past to present. *Med Educ.* 2007;41(12):1117–1121.
9. Edwards JC, Brannan JR, Burgess L, Plauche WC, Marier RL. Case presentation format and clinical reasoning: a strategy for teaching medical students. *Med Teach.* 1987;9(3):285–292.
10. Donnelly WJ. Viewpoint: patient-centered medical care requires a patient-centered medical record. *Acad Med.* 2005;80(1):33–38.
11. Donnelly WJ, Brauner DJ. Why SOAP is bad for the medical record. *Arch Intern Med.* 1992;152(3):481–484.
12. Shachak A, Reis S. The impact of electronic medical records on patient-doctor communication during consultation: a narrative literature review. *J Eval Clin Pract.* 2009;15(4):641–649.
13. Hartzband P, Groopman J. Off the record–avoiding the pitfalls of going electronic. *N Engl J Med.* 2008;358(16):1656–1658.
14. Basch P, Smith JRL. CMS payment policy, E&M Guideline reform, and the prospect of electronic health record optimization. *Appl Clin Inform.* 2018;9(4):914–918.
15. AAPC Thought Leadership Team. 2023 E/M coding changes. American Academy of Professional Coders. Updated April 27, 2023. Accessed March 18, 2024. https://www.aapc.com/resources/evaluation-management-coding-changes-2023
16. Department of Health & Human Services, Centers for Medicare & Medicaid Services. *CMS Manual System, Pub 100–04 Medicare Claims Processing.* 2018. Accessed March 18, 2024. https://www.cms.gov/Regulations-and-Guidance/Guidance/Transmittals/2018Downloads/R4068CP.pdf
17. Stevens LA, Pageler NM, Hahn JS. Improved medical student engagement with EHR documentation following the 2018 Centers for Medicare and Medicaid billing changes. *Appl Clin Inform.* 2021;12(3):582–588.
18. U.S. federal rule mandates open notes. OpenNotes. Updated November 10, 2023. Accessed March 18, 2024. https://www.opennotes.org/onc-federal-rule/
19. Kelly MM, Smith CA, Hoonakker PLT, et al. Stakeholder perspectives in anticipation of sharing physicians' notes with parents of hospitalized children. *Acad Pediatr.* 2021;21(2):259–264.
20. Avendano JP, Gallagher DO, Hawes JD, et al. Interfacing with the electronic health record (EHR): a comparative review of modes of documentation. *Cureus.* 2022;14(6):e26330.
21. Baker HP, Dwyer E, Kalidoss S, Hynes K, Wolf J, Strelzow JA. ChatGPT's ability to assist with clinical documentation: a randomized controlled trial. *J Am Acad Orthop Surg.* 2024;32(3):123–129.

CHAPTER

7

Health Maintenance and Screening

CONCEPT OF PREVENTIVE CARE

Advances in preventive health care in the past 50 years have resulted in a tremendous decline in the incidence of debilitating common illnesses. Increasing knowledge and acceptance of health maintenance and disease prevention measures by patients have greatly facilitated and improved health care delivery by clinicians. As you proceed through your training, you will realize that many clinical conditions are largely preventable. Counseling your patients to eat a healthy diet, exercise regularly, avoid tobacco and illicit drugs, limit alcohol, avoid unsafe sexual practices, and receive preventive services such as cancer screenings and vaccinations are just a few examples of ways you can help them maintain and promote their overall health and well-being. The promotion of health, as the World Health Organization (WHO) has stated in its *Ottawa Charter for Health Promotion*, "enables patients to increase their control over, and improve, their health."[1] See the discussion of the Determinants of Health in Chapter 1, Foundational Skills Essential to the Clinical Encounter, pp. 10–11.

Chapter Content Guide

- Guideline Recommendations
- Screening
- Behavioral Counseling
- Immunization
- Screening Guidelines for Adults
- Counseling Guidelines for Adults
- Immunization Guidelines for Adults
- Preventive Care in Special Populations
- Disease-Specific Recommendations

Throughout this book you will find health promotion recommendations based on guidelines issued by professional organizations such as the U.S. Preventive Services Task Force (USPSTF), an independent, volunteer panel of experts in prevention and evidence-based medicine who base their recommendations on a rigorous review of existing peer-reviewed evidence and decision models.[2,3] USPSTF guidelines consider the quality of the evidence, assess the balance of benefits and harms of the preventive service, and rate the strength of the recommendation. There are various preventive health care strategies (Box 7-1).[4] *Primary prevention* are interventions designed to prevent disease which include immunizations, chemoprevention, surgery, and behavioral counseling. This chapter also discusses recommendations for *secondary prevention*, which are interventions (screening tests) designed to find disease or disease processes at an early stage when the patient has not yet manifested any signs or symptoms (*asymptomatic*) of the condition (Box 7-1).

GUIDELINE RECOMMENDATIONS

Guidelines are practice recommendations issued by professional organizations that should be rigorously developed and trustworthy.[5] There are many ways to rate the strength of recommendations; we will highlight the approach of the USPSTF.

United States Preventive Services Task Force Approach

Grade. The USPSTF assigns 1 of 5 ratings to its recommendations as well as a level of certainty regarding net benefit (Boxes 7-2 and 7-3). The USPSTF tracks the medical literature and performs periodic systematic

Box 7-1. Preventive Health Care Strategies

Prevention Type	Target Population	Examples
Primary prevention: prevent a disease from ever occurring by limiting risk exposure or increasing immunity	Healthy individuals or susceptible populations	■ Immunizations to prevent infectious diseases ■ Tobacco cessation programs to prevent lung and other types of cancers ■ Needle exchange programs to prevent the spread of infectious diseases among injection drug users ■ Micronutrient supplementation to prevent nutritional deficiencies
Secondary prevention: detect diseases early in their subclinical stage, allowing for interventions that prevent progression	Healthy-appearing individuals with subclinical forms of disease	■ Pap smear for early detection of cervical cancer ■ Mammography for early detection of breast cancer ■ Colonoscopies for early detection of colon cancer ■ Blood pressure screening for early detection of hypertension
Tertiary prevention: reduce the severity of the disease and improve quality of life through management and rehabilitation	Symptomatic patients with established disease	■ Occupational and physical therapy in burn patients to improve function and reduce disability ■ Cardiac rehab post-myocardial infarction to prevent further heart disease ■ Diabetic foot care to prevent complications from diabetes
Quaternary prevention: protect individuals from medical interventions that are likely to cause more harm than good, focusing on the ethical aspect of medical treatments	Patients with illness but without the disease; individuals at risk of overmedicalization	■ Minimizing treatment in radiologic incidentalomas to avoid unnecessary interventions ■ Rethinking the use of antiarrhythmic drugs post-myocardial infarction due to increased mortality despite reduced arrhythmias ■ Reevaluating hormone replacement therapy due to increased risk of breast cancer, stroke, and failure in reducing cardiovascular mortality

Box 7-2. U.S. Preventive Services Task Force Ratings: Grade Definitions and Implications for Practice[6]

Grade	Definition	Suggestions for Practice
A	The USPSTF recommends the service. There is high certainty that the net benefit is substantial.	Offer or provide this service.
B	The USPSTF recommends the service. There is high certainty that the net benefit is moderate or there is moderate certainty that the net benefit is moderate to substantial.	Offer or provide this service.
C	The USPSTF recommends selectively offering or providing this service to individual patients based on professional judgment and patient preferences. There is at least moderate certainty that the net benefit is small.	Offer or provide this service for selected patients depending on individual circumstances.

(*continued*)

Box 7-2. U.S. Preventive Services Task Force Ratings: Grade Definitions and Implications for Practice[6] (*Continued*)

Grade	Definition	Suggestions for Practice
D	The USPSTF recommends against the service. There is moderate or high certainty that the service has no net benefit or that the harms outweigh the benefits.	Discourage the use of this service.
I	The USPSTF concludes that the current evidence is insufficient to assess the balance of benefits and harms of the service. Evidence is lacking, of poor quality, or conflicting, and the balance of benefits and harms cannot be determined.	If the service is offered, patients should understand the uncertainty about the balance of benefits and harms.

Source: Reprinted with permission from Grade Definitions After July 2012 & Levels of Certainty Regarding Net Benefit. (Last reviewed October 2018). U.S. Preventive Services Task Force (USPSTF). Rockville, MD. https://www.uspreventiveservicestaskforce.org/uspstf/about-uspstf/methods-and-processes/grade-definitions#july2012

evidence syntheses and decision models to determine whether its recommendations need to be updated.

Certainty. *Certainty* is defined as the "likelihood that the USPSTF assessment of the net benefit of a preventive service is correct." The *net benefit* is defined as benefit minus harm of the preventive service as implemented in a general, primary care population (see Box 7-3).

SCREENING

Screening is testing to identify asymptomatic patients with early-stage disease or precursors to disease who could benefit from early intervention. Some of the criteria for considering whether to implement a screening program, based on a monograph by the WHO and subsequently

Box 7-3. U.S. Preventive Services Task Force Levels of Certainty Regarding Net Benefit[6]

Level of Certainty	Description
High	The available evidence usually includes consistent results from well-designed, well-conducted studies in representative primary care populations. These studies assess the effects of the preventive service on health outcomes. This conclusion is therefore unlikely to be strongly affected by the results of future studies.
Moderate	The available evidence is sufficient to determine the effects of the preventive service on health outcomes, but confidence in the estimate is constrained by such factors as: ■ Number, size, or quality of individual studies ■ Inconsistency of findings across individual studies ■ Limited generalizability of findings to routine primary care practice ■ Lack of coherence in the chain of evidence As more information becomes available, the magnitude or direction of the observed effect could change, and this change may be large enough to alter the conclusion.
Low	The available evidence is insufficient to assess effects on health outcomes. Evidence is insufficient because of: ■ Limited number or size of studies ■ Important flaws in study design or methods ■ Inconsistency of findings across individual studies ■ Gaps in the chain of evidence ■ Findings not generalizable to routine primary care practice ■ Lack of information on important health outcomes More information may allow estimation of effects on health outcomes.

Source: Reprinted with permission from U.S. Preventive Services Task Force (USPSTF). Grade Definitions After July 2012 & Levels of Certainty Regarding Net Benefit. Last reviewed October 2018. https://www.uspreventiveservicestaskforce.org/uspstf/about-uspstf/methods-and-processes/grade-definitions#july2012

Box 7-4. When Does It Make Sense to Consider Screening for a Disease or Condition?

- It causes substantial public health burden.
- Natural history is well understood and there is recognized latent or early symptomatic stage.
- Screening tests are available, acceptable, and accurate.
- Treatment for patients with clinically detected disease is available, acceptable, and more effective when delivered at the time of screening diagnosis.
- Screening programs are cost effective.
- Net health benefits of screening outweigh the harms.

Box 7-5. Benefits and Harms of Screening[11]

Benefits	Harms
■ Mortality rate reduction ■ Morbidity rate reduction ■ Reassurance	■ False-positive results that can cause anxiety and lead to additional testing ■ Overdiagnosis of low-risk disease that will never cause any clinical problems ■ False reassurance from false-negative tests ■ Pain or discomfort from diagnostic tests ■ Incidental findings leading to additional tests and treatments ■ Complications from treating disease

Source: McCaffery KJ, Jacklyn GL, Barratt A, et al. Recommendations about screening. In: Guyatt G, Rennie D, Meade MO, Cook DJ, eds. *Users' Guides to the Medical Literature: A Manual for Evidence-Based Clinical Practice*. 3rd ed. McGraw-Hill Education; 2015.

modified by others, are shown in the Box 7-4.[7–9] Most screening programs target common diseases that have substantial morbidity and mortality, such as cancers, diabetes, chronic viral infections, substance abuse, and cardiovascular disease. Occasionally, screening programs also target rare diseases, such as phenylketonuria in newborns, because detection is based on a simple blood test and avoiding dietary products with phenylalanine can prevent disease complications.[10]

For a screening program to be considered effective, there should be a sufficiently long period of opportunity where disease can be detected at an early stage and during which interventions can be more effective and/or simpler to deliver compared to when the disease is clinically detected. Screening tests should be widely accessible; acceptable to patients in terms of safety, convenience, and cost; and accurate. Effective treatments for the disease, once clinically detected, should be widely available and acceptable to patients. Chapter 8, Evaluating Clinical Evidence, provides more information about test accuracy, addressing topics such as sensitivity, specificity, predictive values, likelihood ratios, and test reliability, which are important for evaluating the efficacy of screening tests and ensuring that screening programs achieve their intended outcomes.

In determining whether to recommend a screening program, organizations such as the USPSTF weigh the evidence for benefit and harm (Box 7-5). The strongest evidence comes from *randomized trials* in which patients are randomly assigned to receive either screening or usual care and followed—often for many years—to look for differences in disease survival. *Observational studies,* which compare outcomes between patients who receive screening and those who do not, are subject to important biases and are not considered to be a valid measure of screening effectiveness.[11]

The Health Promotion and Counseling Sections throughout the textbook that focus on *screening* are shown in Box 7-6.

BEHAVIORAL COUNSELING

One of the most important skills of an effective clinician is being able to help patients make behavioral changes. You can support a healthy lifestyle by counseling patients to exercise and follow healthy diets and to avoid unhealthy habits related to tobacco, alcohol, drugs, and unsafe sexual practices. However, changing behaviors is difficult, and an important first step is to understand where patients are in terms of thinking about change.

Stages of Behavioral Change Model

A useful model characterizing patients who should be adopting healthy behaviors or stopping unhealthy behaviors

Box 7-6. Health Promotion and Counseling Sections: Screening

Screening	Book Section
Abdominal aortic aneurysm	Chapter 19, Peripheral Vascular System, pp. 567–568
Abuse of vulnerable adults including elderly	Chapter 30, Older Adults, pp. 1187–1189
Alcohol use	Chapter 7, Health Maintenance and Screening, pp. 126–127
Breast cancer	Chapter 20, Breasts and Axillae, pp. 595–598 Chapter 30, Older Adults, pp. 1185–1187
Cardiovascular risk factors (family history of premature cardiovascular disease, cigarette smoking, unhealthy diet, physical inactivity, obesity, hypertension, dyslipidemias, diabetes mellitus)	Chapter 7, Health Maintenance and Screening, pp. 129–130 Chapter 18, Cardiovascular System, pp. 516–521 Chapter 27, Nervous System, pp. 962–963
Cervical cancer	Chapter 24, Pelvis and Genitourinary System: Vulva, Vagina, Uterus, and Adnexa, pp. 759–760 Chapter 30, Older Adults, pp. 1185–1187
Colorectal cancer	Chapter 21, Abdomen, pp. 653–654 Chapter 30, Older Adults, pp. 1185–1187
Depression	Chapter 11, Cognition, Behavior, and Mental Status, pp. 218–219 Chapter 29, Pregnant Persons, p. 1144
Prediabetes and type 2 diabetes	Chapter 7, Health Maintenance and Screening, pp. 129–130
Glaucoma	Chapter 14, Eyes, p. 344
Hearing impairment	Chapter 30, Older Adults, p. 924
Hearing loss	Chapter 15, Ears and Nose, pp. 382–383
Hepatitis B Hepatitis C	Chapter 21, Abdomen, pp. 651–653
HIV infection	Chapter 7, Health Maintenance and Screening, p. 129 Chapter 29, Pregnant Persons, pp. 1141–1142
Hypertension	Chapter 18, Cardiovascular System, pp. 517–518
Intimate partner violence	Chapter 7, Health Maintenance and Screening, p. 126 Chapter 29, Pregnant Persons, pp. 1145–1146
Lower extremity peripheral artery disease	Chapter 19, Peripheral Vascular System, p. 567
Lung cancer	Chapter 17, Thorax and Lungs, pp. 451–452 Chapter 30, Older Adults, pp. 1185–1187
Neurocognitive disorders: dementia and delirium	Chapter 11, Cognition, Behavior, and Mental Status, pp. 220–222 Chapter 30, Older Adults, pp. 1173–1175

Screening	Book Section
Obstructive sleep apnea	Chapter 17, Thorax and Lungs, pp. 453–454
Osteoporosis	Chapter 26, Musculoskeletal System: Lumbosacral Spine, Hips, and Lower Extremities, pp. 890–892
Prenatal screenings (Rh[D] incompatibility, bacteriuria, iron deficiency, genetic and aneuploidy)	Chapter 29, Pregnant Persons, pp. 1142–1144, 1146
Prostate cancer	Chapter 23, Pelvis and Genitourinary System: Penis, Scrotum, and Prostate, pp. 712–713 Chapter 30, Older Adults, pp. 1185–1187
Sexually transmitted infections including chlamydia, gonorrhea, and syphilis	Chapter 7, Health Maintenance and Screening, pp. 128–129
Skin cancer including melanoma	Chapter 12, Skin, Hair, and Nails, pp. 269–270 Chapter 30, Older Adults, pp. 1185–1187
Stroke risk factors (atrial fibrillation, asymptomatic carotid artery stenosis)	Chapter 27, Nervous System, pp. 963–964
Substance use disorders, including misuse of prescription and illicit drugs	Chapter 7, Health Maintenance and Screening, pp. 125–126
Suicide risk	Chapter 11, Cognition, Behavior, and Mental Status, pp. 219–220
Thyroid cancer Thyroid dysfunction	Chapter 13, Head and Neck, pp. 314–315
Tobacco use	Chapter 7, Health Maintenance and Screening, pp. 127–128
Tuberculosis	Chapter 17, Thorax and Lungs, pp. 452–453
Visual impairment	Chapter 14, Eyes, p. 344
Weight (unhealthy)	Chapter 10, General Survey, Vital Signs, and Pain, pp. 192–194 Chapter 29, Pregnant Persons, pp. 1147–1148

is Prochaska and DiClemente's *Transtheoretical or Stages of Behavioral Change Model,* as shown in Figure 7-1.[12,13] In this model, behavior change is conceptualized as a process that unfolds over time, progressing through five stages: *precontemplation*, *contemplation*, *preparation*, *action*, and *maintenance* (Box 7-7). Patients do not always move through the stages of change in a linear manner and may recycle, depending on their level of motivation and self-efficacy. For example, patients in the maintenance stage work hard to practice a new and healthier behavior but may revert back to their old behaviors (*relapse*).[14] Try to identify where your patient is on this continuum and tailor your interventions to their readiness and self-efficacy to make lifestyle changes.

Structured Counseling Models: Five As and FRAMES

Following this initial assessment of a patient's readiness to change, the next step is to use structured interviewing approaches such as the *five As* (*ask*, *advise*, *assess*, *assist*, and *arrange*) and *FRAMES* (*feedback about personal risk*,

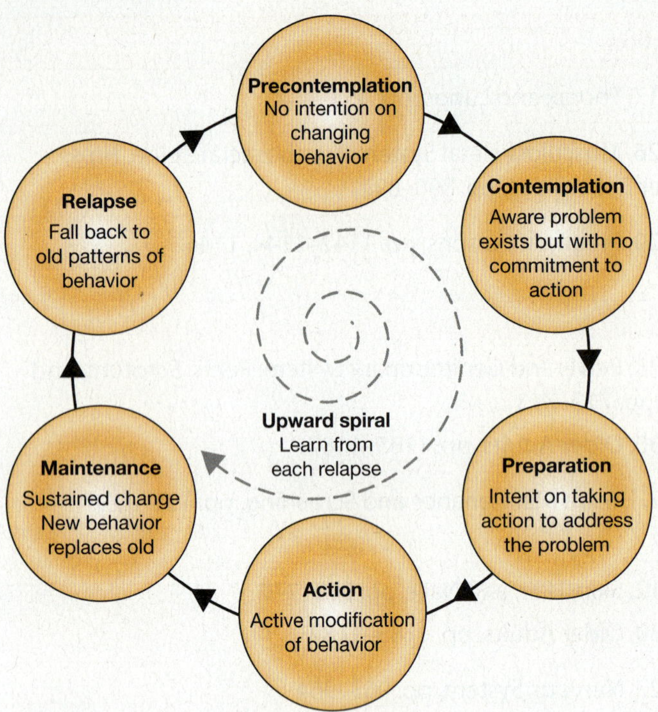

FIGURE 7-1. Transtheoretical model for behavioral change. (Adapted with permission from Prochaska JO, DiClemente CC. Stages and processes of self-change of smoking: toward an integrative model of change. *J Consult Clin Psychol.* 1983;51(3):390–395. Copyright © 1983 American Psychological Association.)

responsibility of patient, *advice to change*, *menu of options*, *empathetic style*, *promote self-efficacy*) to effectively facilitate behavioral change (Box 7-8).[15]

Despite the inherent challenges of changing established behaviors, structured frameworks enable clinicians to provide tailored advice, encourage personal responsibility, and enhance motivation. This methodical approach ensures that interventions are not only patient centered but also adaptable to the individual's specific stage of readiness and personal circumstances, thereby increasing the likelihood of successful behavioral change.

The Health Promotion and Counseling Sections on *counseling* for various conditions and diseases are found in this chapter and throughout the book (Box 7-9).

IMMUNIZATION

Vaccines, a cornerstone of public health, have significantly contributed to preventing and controlling infectious disease outbreaks. *Immunization* denotes the process of inducing or providing immunity by administering an immunobiologic. Immunization can be active or passive. *Active immunization* involves the administration of antigens in the form of vaccines to stimulate the body's immune system to develop immunity over time. In contrast, *passive*

Box 7-7. Transtheoretical Model for Behavioral Change[12–14]

Stage	Description	Statement
Precontemplation	Patients have no intention to change behavior in the foreseeable future. They are often unaware of their problems.	*"I do not think that I need to change any behaviors."*
Contemplation	Patients are aware that a problem exists and are seriously thinking about overcoming it. No commitment has been made to take action.	*"I'm concerned about my behavior, but not ready to make any changes now."*
Preparation	Patients have expressed intention to take action soon and are reporting small behavioral changes.	*"I'm ready to change my behavior now."*
Action	Patients modify their behavior to overcome their problems for a period from 1 day to 6 months.	*"I'm changing my behavior now."*
Maintenance	Patients continue their action for behavioral change (usually >6 months) and work to prevent relapse.	*"I've changed my behavior."*
Relapse[a]	Cessation of behavioral changes and patients revert to old behavior.	*"I've returned to my old behavior."*

[a]Not a stage itself, but rather the "return from action or maintenance to an earlier stage."

Sources: Prochaska JO, DiClemente CC. Stages and processes of self-change of smoking: toward an integrative model of change. *J Consult Clin Psychol.* 1983;51(3):390–395; Prochaska JO, Velicer WF. The transtheoretical model of health behavior change. *Am J Health Promot.* 1997;12(1):38–48; Prochaska JO. Assessing how people change. *Cancer.* 1991;67(3 Suppl):805–807.

Box 7-8. Comparison of Counseling Models: 5 As and FRAMES

Step	5 As Approach	5 As Example Dialogue	FRAMES Approach	FRAMES Example Dialogue
1	**Ask:** Initiates dialogue by nonjudgmentally inquiring about the individual's behavior, opening a discussion on health-related practices.	*"Can you tell me about your current exercise routine?"*	**Feedback:** Provides specific information about the effects of the individual's behavior on their health, aiming to increase awareness.	*"Based on your check-up, your current alcohol consumption is affecting your liver health."*
2	**Advise:** Offers clear, specific advice on the benefits of making a health-related change, tailored to the individual's situation.	*"Increasing your physical activity can significantly reduce health risks like diabetes and heart disease."*	**Responsibility:** Emphasizes the individual's personal responsibility for their health and the decision to change their behavior.	*"It's important to recognize that only you can decide to make this change for your health."*
3	**Assess:** Evaluates the individual's readiness and willingness to change their behavior, considering their current stage of change.	*"How do you feel about making a change to your exercise habits?"*	**Advice:** After establishing a foundation of feedback and responsibility, provides direct, nonjudgmental advice to encourage change.	*"Cutting down on your drinking could improve your health and personal relationships."*
4	**Assist:** Offers support by helping to identify actionable steps and strategies for overcoming obstacles to change.	*"Let's work together to set realistic exercise goals and identify potential challenges."*	**Menu of options:** Presents a range of options for behavior change, allowing the individual to choose strategies that they feel will work best for them.	*"There are several strategies we can explore to help you reduce drinking, such as…"*
5	**Arrange:** Sets up a system of follow-up support to monitor and discuss progress, ensuring ongoing motivation and accountability.	*"I'd like to schedule a follow-up visit to discuss your progress. How does that sound?"*	**Empathy:** Acknowledges and validates the individual's feelings and challenges, demonstrating understanding and compassion.	*"I understand that this change can be challenging, and it's okay to have mixed feelings about it."*
6			**Self-efficacy:** Focuses on enhancing the individual's confidence in their ability to change, reinforcing their belief in their own capabilities.	*"You've made significant changes before; I believe you have the strength to do this too."*

Source: Searight R. Realistic approaches to counseling in the office setting. *Am Fam Physician*. 2009;79(4):277–284.

Box 7-9. Health Promotion and Counseling Sections: Counseling

Counseling	Book Section
Alcohol use (unhealthy)	Chapter 7, Health Maintenance and Screening, p. 130 Chapter 29, Pregnant Persons, pp. 1146–1147
Blood pressure	Chapter 18, Cardiovascular System, pp. 519–521
Breast cancer (*BRCA*-related cancer)	Chapter 20, Breasts and Axillae, p. 597
Cardiovascular risk factor modification (healthful diet and physical activity)	Chapter 18, Cardiovascular System, pp. 519–521
Exercise and physical activity	Chapter 18, Cardiovascular System, pp. 519–521 Chapter 29, Pregnant Persons, pp. 1147–1148
Fall prevention	Chapter 30, Older Adults, pp. 1189–1190
Health supervision visits for newborns and infants up to 12 months Health supervision visits for children ages 1–4 years Health supervision visits for children ages 5–10 years Health supervision visits for children ages 11–18 years	Chapter 28, Children: Infancy Through Adolescence, pp. 1044–1045, 1083–1085, and 1100–1101
Optimal weight	Chapter 10, General Survey, Vital Signs, and Pain, pp. 192–194 Chapter 29, Pregnant Persons, pp. 1147–1148
Oral health	Chapter 16, Throat and Oral Cavity, p. 404
Perinatal depression Prenatal supplementation (multivitamins, minerals, folic acid, iron)	Chapter 29, Pregnant Persons, pp. 1148–1150
Sexual practices to prevent sexually transmitted infections and HIV/AIDS	Chapter 7, Health Maintenance and Screening, pp. 131–132
Skin cancer including melanoma	Chapter 12, Skin, Hair, and Nails, pp. 268–269
Tobacco misuse	Chapter 7, Health Maintenance and Screening, pp. 130–131 Chapter 29, Pregnant Persons, pp. 1146–1147

immunization involves the direct transfer of antibodies to an individual, offering immediate but temporary protection against diseases. Although often used interchangeably, the terms *vaccination* and *immunization* are not synonymous because the administration of a vaccine cannot be equated automatically with developing adequate immunity in the individual.[16]

The benefits of immunization extend beyond preventing specific infectious diseases. Vaccines against human papillomavirus (HPV) and hepatitis B may also reduce the risk of developing cancer, showcasing the broader preventive potential of vaccines. Benefits of immunization are also not limited to the vaccinated individual but also include promotion of *herd immunity* for the population at large, including nonimmunized persons and those with waning immunity or who may not have fully responded to prior vaccination. This protective effect not only benefits those who are vaccinated but also provides a shield for nonimmunized individuals, those with waning immunity, and individuals who may not have fully responded to vaccination. For example, diseases like smallpox have been eradicated, and polio and measles have seen drastic reductions in incidence in regions with high vaccination coverage.

The recommendations for *immunization* are found in this chapter and the regional examination chapters throughout this book (Box 7-10).

Box 7-10. Health Promotion and Counseling Sections: Immunizations

Immunization	Book Section
COVID-19 vaccine	Chapter 7, Health Maintenance and Screening, p. 133
Hepatitis A (HepA) vaccine	Chapter 7, Health Maintenance and Screening, p. 135 Chapter 29, Pregnant Persons, p. 1149
Hepatitis B (HepB) vaccine	Chapter 7, Health Maintenance and Screening, p. 135 Chapter 29, Pregnant Persons, pp. 1140–1141
Human papilloma virus (HPV) vaccine	Chapter 7, Health Maintenance and Screening, pp. 134–135 Chapter 24, Pelvis and Genitourinary System: Vulva, Vagina, Uterus, and Adnexa, pp. 759–760
Influenza vaccine: inactivated (IIV), recombinant (RIV) or live attenuated (LAIV)	Chapter 7, Health Maintenance and Screening, p. 132
Measles, mumps, rubella (MMR) vaccine Pneumococcal vaccine: conjugated (PCV15, PCV20, and PCV21) and polysaccharide (PPSV23)	Chapter 7, Health Maintenance and Screening, pp. 132–133 Chapter 29, Pregnant Persons, p. 1149
Respiratory syncytial virus (RSV) vaccine	Chapter 7, Health Maintenance and Screening, p. 133
Tetanus/diphtheria (Td) or Tetanus/diphtheria/pertussis (Tdap) vaccine Varicella (VAR) vaccine Zoster vaccine: recombinant (RZV) or live (ZVL)	Chapter 7, Health Maintenance and Screening, p. 134 Chapter 29, Pregnant Persons, p. 1149

SCREENING GUIDELINES FOR ADULTS

Screening Guidelines

- Screening for substance use disorders, including misuse of prescription and illicit drugs
- Screening for intimate partner violence in females of reproductive age
- Screening for unhealthy alcohol use
- Screening for tobacco use
- Screening for sexually transmitted infections: syphilis, chlamydia, and gonorrhea
- Screening for human immunodeficiency virus
- Screening for prediabetes and type 2 diabetes

Screening for Substance Use Disorders, Including Misuse of Prescription and Illicit Drugs

Substance use disorders are characterized by "impairment caused by the recurrent use of alcohol or other drugs (or both), including health problems, disability, and failure to meet major responsibilities at work, school, or home" (Box 7-11).[17] The National Institute on Drug Abuse (NIDA) supports using the Tobacco, Alcohol, Prescription Medication, and Other Substance Use (TAPS) tool.[19,20] This is a four-item screening for tobacco use, alcohol use, prescription medication misuse, and illicit drug use.

- The prescription medication misuse question is: "In the past 12 months, how often have you used any prescription medications just for the feeling, more than prescribed, or that were not prescribed for you?"
- The illicit drug use question is: "In the past 12 months, how often have you used any drugs, including marijuana, cocaine or crack, heroin, methamphetamine (crystal meth), hallucinogens, or ecstasy/MDMA?"

For those who screen positive, additional questions categorize risk severity according to each substance class.

Box 7-11. Facts About Substance Use Disorders

- The 2021 National Survey on Drug Use and Health report (NSDUH)[17] estimated that 61.2 million Americans ages 12 and older had illicit drug use during the past year, including:
  - 52.5 million people who used marijuana
  - 8.7 million people who misused prescription pain medications
  - 14.3 million people who misused prescription psychotherapeutic drugs, including tranquilizers, sedatives, and stimulants
  - 4.8 million people who used cocaine, 1.1 million people who used heroin, and 2.5 million people who used methamphetamine
- An estimated 24.0 million people met *Diagnostic and Statistical Manual of Mental Disorders-5* criteria for having a drug use disorder in the past year.
- Drug overdoses accounted for 106,699 deaths in 2021, with more than three-fourths involving opioids.[18]
- Opioid-related death rates have been increasing in recent years, particularly due to synthetic opioids contaminated with fentanyl and fentanyl analogs.[18]

Results from the tool can be used to guide referrals for substance use disorder treatment.

The USPSTF issued a grade B recommendation in 2020 to ask adults ages 18 and older about unhealthy drug use "when services for accurate diagnosis, effective treatment, and appropriate care can be offered or referred."[21] Evidence was insufficient to issue a recommendation on screening for adolescents (I statement).

Screening for Intimate Partner Violence in Females of Reproductive Age

Intimate partner violence (IPV) is a common problem in the United States, though often undetected (Box 7-12). The USPSTF defines *intimate partner violence* as the "physical violence, sexual violence, psychological aggression (including coercive tactics, such as limiting access to financial resources), or stalking by a romantic or sexual partner, including spouses, boyfriends, girlfriends, dates, and casual 'hookups'."[25]

Box 7-12. Facts about Intimate Partner Violence

- The U.S. Centers for Disease Control and Prevention (CDC) reports that almost 1 in 2 U.S. women and >40% of U.S. men experience IPV during their lifetime.[22]
- Overall, 33% of women experienced severe physical violence during their lifetime, compared to 25% of men.
- Homicide is the fifth leading cause of death for women ages 20–44.[23] The CDC's National Violent Death Reporting System analyzed homicide data on women aged ≥18 years in 2003–2014. Almost half of all female homicides (49.2%) with known circumstances were IPV-related.[24]

Screening for IPV can begin with general "normalizing" questions: "Because abuse is common in many people's lives, I've begun to ask about it routinely. Are there times in your relationships that you feel unsafe or afraid?" "Have you ever been hit, kicked, punched, or hurt by someone you know?"

The USPSTF recommends several screening instruments, including the Humiliation, Afraid, Rape, Kick (HARK); Hurt, Insult, Threaten, Scream (HITS); Extended-HITS (E-HITS); Partner Violence Screen (PVS); and Woman Abuse Screening Tool (WAST). The sensitivity of these tests ranged from 64% to 87%, while specificity ranged from 80% to 95%. Effective interventions following screen-detected IPV include ongoing delivery of support services such as counseling and home visits. The USPSTF has issued a grade B recommendation to screen for IPV among women of reproductive age and refer those screening positive to support services.[25] See Chapter 29, Pregnant Persons for intimate partner violence during pregnancy, pp. 1145–1146.

Screening for Unhealthy Alcohol Use

Unhealthy alcohol use encompasses a spectrum of behaviors, ranging from risky drinking that can lead to health problems to alcohol dependence or overuse (Box 7-13). The USPSTF issued a grade B recommendation in 2018 to screen adults, including pregnant women, for "unhealthy alcohol use and provide persons engaged in risky or hazardous drinking with brief behavioral counseling interventions."[27]

Box 7-13. Facts About Unhealthy Alcohol Use[17,26]

- The 2021 National Survey on Drug Use and Health (NSDUH) estimated that more than 133 million Americans aged 12 years and older had consumed alcohol in the past 30 days.
- Of these, 16.3 million people were identified as engaging in heavy drinking, and 60.0 million people were identified as engaging in binge drinking.
- An estimated 29.5 million Americans met the criteria for alcohol use disorder.
- Each year, more than 140,000 U.S. deaths are attributed to excessive alcohol use.

Sources: Substance Abuse and Mental Health Services Administration. Key Substance Use and Mental Health Indicators in the United States: Results from the 2021 National Survey on Drug Use and Health 2022. https://www.samhsa.gov/data/report/2021-nsduh-annual-national-report; Centers for Disease Control and Prevention. Alcohol and Public Health: Alcohol-Related Disease Impact (ARDI). Accessed January 11, 2024. https://nccd.cdc.gov/DPH_ARDI/Default/

Box 7-14. Definitions of Drinking Levels for Adults[31]

Standard Drink Equivalents: One standard drink is equivalent to 12 oz of regular beer or wine cooler, 8 oz of malt liquor, 5 oz of wine, or 1.5 oz of 80-proof spirits.

	Women	Men
Moderate drinking	≤1 drink/day	≤2 drinks/day
Unsafe drinking levels (increased risk for developing an alcohol use disorder)[a]	>3 drinks/day and >7 drinks/wk	>4 drinks/day and >14 drinks/wk
Binge drinking[b]	≥4 drinks on one occasion	≥5 drinks on one occasion

[a]Pregnant persons and those with health problems that could be worsened by drinking; should not drink any alcohol.

[b]Brings blood alcohol level to 0.08 g/dL (g%), usually within 2 hours.

Source: National Institute on Alcohol Abuse and Alcoholism. Helping Patients Who Drink Too Much: A Clinician's Guide. National Institute on Alcohol Abuse and Alcoholism, National Institutes of Health, U.S. Department of Health & Human Services. Accessed January 13, 2024. https://www.issup.net/files/2017-07/Helping%20Patients%20Who%20Drink%20Too%20Much%20A%20Clinician%E2%80%99s%20Guide.pdf

If your patient reports drinking alcoholic beverages, you can begin to assess for unhealthy alcohol use (Box 7-14) by asking some simple screening questions.

- The *Single Alcohol Screening Question (SASQ)* asks "How many times in the past year have you had five or more drinks in a day (men) or four or more drinks in a day (women)?"[28] The SASQ has a sensitivity ranging from 0.73 to 0.88 for detecting unhealthy alcohol use with a specificity ranging from 0.74 to 1.00.[27]
- The *Alcohol Use Disorders Identification Test-Consumption (AUDIT-C)* questionnaire asks about how often the person drinks alcohol, how many standard alcohol drinks are consumed on a typical day, and how often the person consumes six or more drinks on one occasion.[29] The AUDIT-C, which is scored from 0 to 12, has sensitivities ranging from 0.73 to 1.00, using cutoffs of ≥3 (women) or ≥4 (men). The corresponding specificities range from 0.28 to 0.94.[27]
- The widely used *CAGE* tool, which asks about **C**utting down, **A**nnoyance when criticized, **G**uilty feelings, and **E**ye-openers, is best at detecting alcohol dependence.[30]

Patients with positive screens for unhealthy alcohol use should be further assessed, including asking about *blackouts* (loss of memory for events during drinking), seizures, accidents or injuries while drinking, job loss, marital conflict, legal problems, and drinking while driving or operating machinery. Clinicians will need to address the appropriate care strategies for patients with confirmed unhealthy alcohol use.

Screening for Tobacco Use

Smokers are more likely than nonsmokers to develop cardiovascular disease, emphysema, and lung cancer (Box 7-15).[35] In addition to respiratory tract cancers, smoking can cause cancers of the bladder, cervix, colon and rectum, kidney, oropharynx, larynx, esophagus, stomach, liver, and pancreas as well as acute myeloid leukemia. Smoking is associated with developing diabetes, cataracts, and rheumatoid arthritis and increases risk of infertility, preterm birth, low birth weight, and sudden infant death syndrome. About half of all long-term smokers die of smoking-related diseases, losing an average of 10 years of life.

The USPSTF has made a grade A recommendation to ask all adults, particularly pregnant patients, about their tobacco use and providing behavioral interventions

Box 7-15. Facts About Tobacco Use[17,32–34]

- Despite declining smoking rates over the past several decades, an estimated 61.2 million (22%) of U.S. persons ages 12 years or older were currently using tobacco products or nicotine vaping in 2021, including 43.6 million (15.6%) who were smoking cigarettes.
- The use of tobacco products decreased from 2011–2020 among high school students (15.8–4.6%) and among middle school students (4.3–1.6%).
- However, electronic cigarettes, also known as "e-cigs," "vapes," or "electronic nicotine delivery systems (ENDS)," have become the most frequently used tobacco product among youth, many of whom use two or more tobacco products.
- Cigarette smoking causes more than 480,000 deaths in the United States each year, nearly one-fifth of all deaths.
- Nonsmokers exposed to smoke have increased risk of lung cancer, ear and respiratory infections, and asthma.

Sources: Substance Abuse and Mental Health Services Administration. *Key Substance Use and Mental Health Indicators in the United States: Results from the 2021 National Survey on Drug;* Centers for Disease Control and Prevention. Health Effects of Cigarette Smoking. Accessed January 13, 2024. https://www.cdc.gov/tobacco/data_statistics/fact_sheets/health_effects/effects_cig_smoking/

Centers for Disease Control and Prevention. Trends in Tobacco Use Among Youth. Accessed January 13, 2024. https://www.cdc.gov/tobacco/data_statistics/fact_sheets/fast_facts/trends-in-tobacco-use-among-youth.html

Centers for Disease Control and Prevention. About E-Cigarettes (Vapes). Accessed January 11, 2024. (https://www.cdc.gov/tobacco/e-cigarettes/about.html)

and/or pharmacotherapy for tobacco cessation to all who are using tobacco.[36]

Secondhand smoke is also an important health risk, causing heart disease, stroke, and lung cancer among other health care problems.[37] Ask nonsmokers about exposure to secondhand smoke and tobacco use by other persons in the household or workplace.

Screening for Sexually Transmitted Infections: Syphilis, Chlamydia, and Gonorrhea

Screening for sexually transmitted infections (STIs) such as syphilis, chlamydia, and gonorrhea is a crucial component of public health efforts to control the spread of these infections and to prevent their serious long-term health consequences (Box 7-16). Early detection through screening is key because many STIs, including these three, can be asymptomatic in their initial stages, meaning individuals may not know they are infected. Without screening, these infections can silently progress to more serious health issues, such as infertility; pelvic inflammatory disease; increased risk of human immunodeficiency virus (HIV) transmission; and, for pregnant persons, risks to the health of the unborn child.

Box 7-16. Facts About Chlamydia, Gonorrhea, and Syphilis[38–41]

- More than 26 million new cases of STIs were estimated to occur in the U.S. population in 2018, including nearly 4 million chlamydia infections, 1.6 million gonorrhea infections, and 146,000 syphilis infections. In recent years, rates of all three infections have been increasing.
- Almost half of these cases occurred in persons ages 15–24 years.
- These figures likely underestimate the true national burden of STIs; many cases of gonorrhea, chlamydia, and syphilis are unreported, and mandatory reporting is not required for infections such as HPV, trichomoniasis, and genital herpes.

Sources: Centers for Disease Control and Prevention. National Overview of STDs, 2021. Accessed January 13, 2024. https://www.cdc.gov/std/statistics/2021/overview.htm

Kreisel KM, Spicknall IH, Gargano JW, et al. sexually transmitted infections among us women and men: prevalence and incidence estimates, 2018. *Sex Transm Dis*. 2021;48(4):208–214.

Screening for Syphilis Infection. The USPSTF issued a grade A recommendation for screening high-risk nonpregnant adults and adolescents for syphilis infection.[42] Risk factors including being a man who has sex with men, being infected with HIV or other STI, using illicit drugs, and having a history of incarceration or commercial sex work. The USPSTF issued a grade A recommendation for screening all pregnant patients for syphilis infection.[43]

Screening for Chlamydia and Gonorrhea. The USPSTF issued a grade B recommendation for chlamydia and gonorrhea screening in sexually active females ages 24 years and younger and for females ages 25 and older who are at increased risk for infection.[44] *Increased risk*

is defined as having a previous or current STI, new or multiple sex partners, a sex partner with an STI, inconsistent condom use when not in a mutually monogamous relationship, and a history of transactional sex or incarceration. Nucleic acid amplification tests (NAATs) performed on urine and swabbed specimens are recommended for screening. Screening can be repeated at a subsequent encounter following a negative test if the patient reports new or persistent risk factors. Evidence is insufficient to make a recommendation for sexually active males (I statement).

The Centers for Disease Control and Prevention (CDC) recommends chlamydia and gonorrhea screening annually for all sexually active females ages younger than 25 years and older females with risk factors such as new or multiple sex partners or a sex partner infected with an STI.[45] Chlamydia, gonorrhea, and syphilis screening are recommended at least once a year for all sexually active gay, bisexual, and other men who have sex with men (MSM). MSM is a term used to describe a behavior rather than a sexual orientation or identity. It focuses on sexual actions and is used to study, track, and address HIV/AIDS among this population without necessarily considering the individuals' self-identified sexual orientation (such as gay, bisexual, or heterosexual). MSM who have multiple or anonymous partners should be screened more frequently for STIs (i.e., at 3- to 6-month intervals).

Screening for Human Immunodeficiency Virus

Despite advances in detection and treatment, HIV infection remains a significant public health threat, particularly for younger Americans, MSM, and people who inject drugs (Box 7-17).

Identifying early HIV infection and initiating antiretroviral therapy (ART) decreases the risk of progressing to AIDS. Treatment also reduces the risk of transmitting HIV to uninfected sex partners and for perinatal transmission. Current screening recommendations are summarized in Box 7-18.

Screening for Prediabetes and Type 2 Diabetes

Diabetes is associated with increased risk for ischemic heart disease, stroke, end-stage kidney disease, fatty liver disease, lower extremity amputations, and blindness (Box 7-19). Risk factors for type 2 diabetes include being overweight or having obesity; being age 35 years or older; having a family history of diabetes; not being physically active; having a history of gestational diabetes or prediabetes; or belonging to a racial or ethnic group such as African American, Hispanic or Latino, American Indian or Alaska Native, or Pacific Islander.[50]

The USPSTF issued a grade B recommendation to screen adults who are overweight (BMI 25–29.9 kg/m^2) or obese (BMI ≥30 kg/m^2), ages 35 to 70 years for prediabetes and type 2 diabetes.[51] Earlier screening can be considered for populations at higher risk for diabetes. The USPSTF found "adequate evidence" for the effectiveness of behavioral or pharmacologic interventions on health outcomes for newly diagnosed diabetes and "convincing evidence" for the benefit of lifestyle interventions in preventing the progression of prediabetes to type 2 diabetes. Acceptable screening tests include HbA_{1c}, fasting plasma glucose, and the oral glucose tolerance test.

Box 7-17. Facts About Human Immunodeficiency Virus/Acquired Immune Deficiency Syndrome[38–41]

- In 2021, 32,100 people in the United States were diagnosed with an HIV infection.
- At highest risk for HIV infection are MSM (86% of new infections among males) and African American (40% of new infections), and Hispanics/Latino people (29% of new infections); People who inject drugs represent 8% of new HIV infections.
- More than 1.2 million Americans ages ≥13 years are currently infected with HIV, although up to 13% remain undiagnosed. About three-quarters of those currently living with HIV are receiving some form of HIV care, and about two-thirds are virally suppressed. Most HIV transmission occurs among people who are HIV-positive and either unaware of their status or not receiving medical care.
- More than 700,000 Americans have died with an AIDS diagnosis.

Sources: Centers for Disease Control and Prevention. HIV Surveillance Supplemental Report: Estimated HIV Incidence and Prevalence in the United States, 2017–2021. Accessed January 13, 2024. (https://stacks.cdc.gov/view/cdc/149080)

Centers for Disease Control and Prevention. Monitoring Selected National HIV Prevention and Care Objectives by Using HIV Surveillance Data—United States and 6 Territories and Freely Associated States, 2022. Accessed January 13, 2024. (https://www.cdc.gov/hiv-data/nhss/national-hiv-prevention-and-care-outcomes.html)

Box 7-18. Summary: Screening Recommendations for Human Immunodeficiency Virus

- The USPSTF gives a grade A recommendation for HIV screening of adolescents and adults ages 15–65 years and for screening all pregnant persons.[46] Screening is also recommended for younger adolescents and older adults who are at increased risk for infection.
- The CDC recommends universal HIV testing for adolescents and adults ages 13–64 years in health care settings and prenatal testing of all pregnant patients.[47]
- The CDC recommends an opt-out approach to HIV testing—notifying the patient verbally or in writing that testing will be performed unless the patient declines. Separate written consent is not required.[47]
- Patients and prospective sex partners should be tested before beginning a new sexual relationship.[47]
- One-time testing for low-risk patients is reasonable, but at least an annual testing is recommended for high-risk groups, defined as MSM; individuals with multiple sexual partners; people with past or current injection drug use; persons who exchange sex for money or drugs; and sex partners of people who are living with HIV, are bisexual, or use injection drugs. Patients beginning treatment for tuberculosis and those with any STIs or those requesting STI testing should be tested for coinfection with HIV.[47,48]

Box 7-19. Facts About Prediabetes and Type 2 Diabetes

- The CDC estimated in 2021 that 38.1 million persons ages ≥18 years in the United States (14.7% of the adult population) had diabetes, although nearly one-quarter were undiagnosed.[49]
- In 2021, nearly 8 million adult hospital discharges listed diabetes as a diagnosis, and diabetes was the eighth leading cause of death in the United States.[49]
- Another 97.6 million persons ages ≥18 years (38.0% of the adult population) had prediabetes, based on a hemoglobin A_{1c} level (HbA_{1c}) of 5.7–6.4% or fasting blood plasma glucose levels of 100–125 mg/dL.[49]
- Increased HbA_{1c}, body mass index (BMI), and waist circumference are associated with progressing from prediabetes to type 2 diabetes.[50]

COUNSELING GUIDELINES FOR ADULTS

Counseling Guidelines

- Counseling for unhealthy alcohol use
- Counseling for tobacco smoking cessation
- Counseling on sexually transmitted infections

Counseling for Unhealthy Alcohol Use

The USPSTF issued a grade B recommendation advising primary care clinicians to provide behavioral counseling interventions to adults with unhealthy alcohol use.[27] The USPSTF identified many effective behavioral interventions, which varied by elements (feedback, motivational interviewing, drinking diaries, cognitive behavioral therapy, and action plans on alcohol use), delivery method (in-person, web-based, one-on-one, group), frequency (most involved ≤4 sessions), and intensity (most involved ≤2 hours of contact time).[30]

One commonly used approach that has been shown to effectively reduce alcohol use and alcohol-related complications is the *Screening, Brief Intervention, and Referral to Treatment (SBIRT) program.*[52] This program is designed to be administered in a series of encounters conducted by practitioners who are not experts in substance abuse to reduce and prevent harm for those with non-dependent alcohol use. Brief interventions target people at low risk for unhealthy alcohol use by educating them about the harms of exceeding drinking limits and, if applicable, identifying any links between alcohol use and other health problems. Motivational techniques are used to help those at moderate to high risk for unhealthy alcohol use to reduce their alcohol intake or to seek additional treatment, particularly those with a high-risk screening result.

Other government publications also provide useful guidance for counseling and treating patients with unhealthy alcohol use, including the National Institute of Alcohol Abuse and Alcoholism publications, "Helping Patients Who Drink Too Much: A Clinician's Guide"[31] and "Medication for the Treatment of Alcohol Use Disorder: A Brief Guide."[53]

Counseling for Tobacco Smoking Cessation

Counseling for tobacco smoking cessation aims to address both the physical addiction to nicotine and the

Box 7-20. Fact Sheet on Smoking Cessation Behaviors

- Most adults who smoke cigarettes want to quit.
- More than half of the adults who smoke cigarettes report having made a quit attempt in the past year.
- Fewer than 1 in 10 adults who smoke cigarettes succeed in quitting each year.
- Out of every 9 adults who smoke cigarettes and saw a health professional during the past year, 4 did not receive advice to quit.
- Less than one-third of adults who smoke cigarettes use cessation counseling or medications approved for cessation by the U.S. Food and Drug Administration when trying to quit smoking.
- More than 3 out of 5 adults who have ever smoked cigarettes have quit.
- About two-thirds of youths who use tobacco report wanting to quit, and nearly two-thirds report trying to quit in the past year.

Modified from: Centers for Disease Control and Prevention. Smoking Cessation: Fast Facts. Accessed March 12, 2024. https://www.cdc.gov/tobacco/data_statistics/fact_sheets/cessation/smoking-cessation-fast-facts/index.html. Accessed March 12, 2024. Additional resources: US Department of Health and Human Services' websites, BeTobaccoFree (https://betobaccofree.hhs.gov/quit-now/index.html), and SmokeFreeWomen (https://women.smokefree.gov/pregnancy-motherhood).

psychological aspects of quitting smoking. It can significantly increase the chances of successfully quitting by providing smokers with strategies to cope with cravings, develop healthier habits, and manage withdrawal symptoms (Box 7-20).

The USPSTF recommends (grade A) that clinicians ask all adult patients about tobacco use, advise tobacco cessation for tobacco users, and provide behavioral interventions and pharmacotherapy to all nonpregnant adults who use tobacco.[36] Pregnant persons should be similarly screened and advised to stop using tobacco products and be offered behavioral support (grade A). The evidence is insufficient (I statement) to make recommendations about pharmacotherapy for pregnant persons. Use the "5 As" framework or the stages-of-change model to assess readiness to quit using tobacco products (see Boxes 7-7 and 7-8).[36]

The most commonly used pharmacotherapies are nicotine replacement therapies (NRTs), including patches, gum, lozenges, inhalers, and nasal spray as well varenicline and bupropion hydrochloride sustained release.[36] Combining multiple types of NRT has additive benefits, and combining pharmacotherapy with behavioral counseling is more effective than either modality alone.

Effective behavioral interventions include minimal and intensive individual or group counseling sessions led by clinicians or other types of primary care providers; telephone counseling sessions led by trained professionals (National Smoking Cessation Hotline: 1-800-QUIT NOW); and tailored, print-based self-help material or self-help tools delivered by apps, web, and mobile interventions.[54,55] Motivational interviewing techniques may be helpful for patients who are not yet ready to quit smoking, but evidence is limited.[56]

E-cigarettes may benefit nonpregnant adults who smoke if used to completely replace the use of all tobacco products, but there are many potential harms; e-cigarettes are not considered safe for youths, young adults, and pregnant persons.[34] The USPSTF concluded that evidence was insufficient to make a recommendation about using e-cigarettes for tobacco cessation (I statement).[36]

Counseling on Sexually Transmitted Infections

The USPSTF issued a grade B recommendation supporting behavioral counseling for all sexually active adolescents and for adults who are at increased risk for STIs, including HIV/AIDS.[57] Adults at increased risk are described in the section on Screening for STIs (p. 128) and Screening for HIV (p. 129). The USPSTF noted that behavioral counseling can reduce the risk of acquiring an STI; effective interventions should "provide information on common STIs and STI transmission; assess the person's risk for acquiring STIs; aim to increase motivation or commitment to safer sex practices; and provide training in condom use, communication about safer sex, problem solving, and other pertinent skills." The CDC recommends using condoms, reducing the number of sex partners, getting vaccinations for hepatitis B and HPV, practicing mutual monogamy, and abstinence.[58]

Clinicians must master the skills of eliciting the sexual history and asking frank but tactful questions about sexual practices. Key information includes the patient's sexual orientation, the number of partners in the past month, and any history of past STIs (see also pp. 55–56). As you counsel patients, encourage them to seek prompt attention for any genital lesions or penile discharge. Highlight risky behaviors such as not using condoms, particularly when engaging in anal intercourse; having multiple sexual partners; concomitant use of alcohol and drugs, which may be associated with disinhibition; and engaging in sexual intercourse while being treated for an STI.

Box 7-21. Essential Guidelines for Safe Condom Use

Key instructions should include:

- Use a new condom with each act of sex.
- Apply the condom before any sexual contact occurs.
- Use only water-based lubricants with the condom.
- If the condom breaks during sex, stop immediately, and, during withdrawal, hold onto the condom to prevent it from slipping off.

Correct use of external (male) condoms is highly effective in preventing the transmission of HIV, HPV, and other STIs (Box 7-21).[59]

Standard recommendations for preventing HIV infection include choosing less risky sexual behaviors, getting treated for injection drug use and using sterile equipment, getting HIV tests with partners, and using condoms correctly. Using pre-exposure prophylaxis (PrEP) medications is another recommended strategy for preventing HIV infection (see p. 135).

IMMUNIZATION GUIDELINES FOR ADULTS

Immunization Guidelines

- Influenza vaccine
- Pneumococcal vaccine
- Respiratory syncytial virus vaccine
- COVID-19 vaccine
- Mpox vaccine
- Varicella vaccine
- Herpes zoster vaccine
- Tetanus, diphtheria, pertussis vaccine
- Human papillomavirus vaccine
- Hepatitis A vaccine
- Hepatitis B vaccine

Influenza Vaccine

Influenza can cause substantial morbidity and mortality; the flu season usually begins during the late fall and can last into the spring, peaking between December and February. The number of annual deaths related to influenza varies depending on the virus type and subtype, ranging from 25,000 to over 50,000 between the 2012 to 2013 and 2019 to 2020 flu seasons.[60] During that time, many hundreds of thousands of people were hospitalized. However, mortality and hospitalizations were dramatically lower during the 2020 to 2021 and 2021 to 2022 flu seasons, likely due to behavioral interventions to prevent transmission of SARS-CoV-2 virus. Mortality and hospitalizations subsequently increased to prepandemic levels.

Box 7-22. Summary of 2024 CDC Influenza Vaccine Recommendations—Adults and Children

Annual vaccination is recommended for all people ages ≥6 months, especially the following groups[61]:

- Adults and children with chronic pulmonary disease (including asthma); cardiovascular disease (except isolated hypertension); renal, hepatic, neurologic, hematologic, or metabolic disorders (including diabetes mellitus); persons who are immunosuppressed due to any cause; and people with severe obesity
- Adults ages ≥50 years
- People who are pregnant or will be pregnant during flu season
- Residents of nursing homes and long-term care facilities
- American Indian and Alaska Native people
- Health care personnel
- Household contacts and caregivers of children ages <5 years (especially infants ages <6 months), adults ages ≥50 years, and those with clinical conditions that place them at higher risk for flu complications

The CDC Advisory Committee on Immunization Practices (ACIP) updates its recommendations for vaccination annually (Box 7-22). Two types of vaccine are available.[61] The "flu shot" is an inactivated vaccine containing killed virus, which comes in a standard dose for those younger than age 65 years and a high dose for those 65 years and older. A nasal-spray vaccine, containing attenuated live viruses, is approved only for healthy people between ages 2 to 49 years. Because flu viruses mutate from year to year, each vaccine contains three to four vaccine strains and is modified yearly.

Pneumococcal Vaccine

Streptococcal pneumonia causes pneumonia, bacteremia, and meningitis. The estimated mortality rate from invasive pneumococcal disease is around 10%.[62] However, the introduction of the 7-valent pneumococcal vaccination for infants and children in 2000 has directly and indirectly (through herd immunity) reduced pneumococcal infections among children and adults.

Recommend *pneumococcal vaccines* to adults aged 50 years and older and to those aged 19 to 64 years who are at increased risk of pneumococcal pneumonia. Adults aged 50 years and older who have never been vaccinated for pneumococcal pneumonia can receive one dose of PCV21, PCV20 (conjugated vaccine) or one dose of PCV15 (conjugated vaccine) followed by one dose of PPSV23 (polysaccharide vaccine) at least 1 year later. As shown in Box 7-23, adults 19 to 64 years old with certain risk conditions have multiple options depending on whether they have chronic health conditions or immunocompromising conditions and their previous vaccine history (including PPSV23, PCV13, PCV15, PCV20, or PCV21). Because the vaccine schedules, which include options for PCV15, PCV20, PCV21, and PPSV23, are complicated, you should refer to the ACIP adult immunization schedule[63] or download the free CDC mobile app: http://www.cdc.gov/vaccines/vpd/pneumo/hcp/pneumoapp.html.

Box 7-23. Medical Conditions in Which Pneumococcal Vaccination Is Recommended at Ages 19–64 Years[64]

Risk Group	Medical Condition
People who are immunocompetent	Chronic heart disease Chronic lung disease Diabetes mellitus Cerebrospinal fluid leak Cochlear implant Alcoholism Chronic liver disease, cirrhosis Cigarette smoking
People with functional or anatomic asplenia	Sickle cell disease Congenital or acquired asplenia
People who are immunocompromised	Congenital or acquired immunodeficiency HIV infection Chronic renal failure Nephrotic syndrome Leukemia Lymphoma Hodgkin disease Generalized malignancy Iatrogenic immunosuppression Solid organ transplants Multiple myeloma

Source: Centers for Disease Control and Prevention. Pneumococcal Vaccine Recommendations. Accessed November 16, 2024. https://www.cdc.gov/pneumococcal/hcp/vaccine-recommendations/index.html

Respiratory Syncytial Virus Vaccine

Respiratory syncytial virus (RSV) causes seasonal epidemics of respiratory illness that can lead to hospitalizations and death among older adults.[65] The U.S. Food and Drug Administration (FDA) licensed two RSV vaccines in 2023. The ACIP recommends a single dose of an RSV vaccine for adults aged 75 years and older. For adults aged 60 to 74, vaccination is recommended based on shared decision-making.[63] Persons most likely to benefit from vaccination are those at risk for severe respiratory disease due to underlying chronic medical conditions; residents in nursing homes or other long-term care facilities; and those who are frail or advanced in age. One dose of maternal RSV vaccine is also recommended during weeks 32 through 36 of pregnancy.

COVID-19 Vaccine

A global outbreak of COVID-19, caused by the severe acute respiratory syndrome coronavirus 2 (SARS-CoV-2), began in late 2019. More than 800 million cases of COVID-19 have been reported to the WHO with nearly 7 million deaths.[66] COVID-19 vaccines became available in late 2020. The ACIP now recommends that individuals aged 6 months and older receive the 2024–2025 COVID-19 vaccine, regardless of their previous vaccination history.[63] Adults aged 65 years and older, as well as those who are moderately or severely immunocompromised, are advised to receive a second dose six months after their initial dose. Additional doses for moderately or severely immunocompromised individuals may be considered based on shared clinical decision-making with their healthcare provider.

Mpox Vaccine

A global outbreak of Mpox (formerly known as Monkeypox) infections occurred in 2022. The viral infection, related to smallpox, is characterized by painful firm or rubbery lesions that often occur in the genital, anorectal area, or mouth along with fever, chills, headaches, and myalgias.[67] More severe dermatologic and systemic complications, including death, can occur among those with immune deficiencies. Persons at high risk for Mpox are those who are gay, bisexual, and other MSM and transgender or nonbinary people who in the past 6 months have had a new diagnosis of at least one STI, more than one sex partner, sex at a commercial sex venue, or sex in association with a large public event in a geographic area where Mpox vaccine is occurring. The ACIP recommends administering a two-dose series of Mpox vaccine 28 days apart for at-risk persons.[63] The vaccine is also recommended for sexual partners of at-risk persons.

Varicella Vaccine

Varicella infection, or *chickenpox*, usually occurs in childhood and causes an itchy rash. Infections can also occur in adults, particularly patients who are immunocompromised who are at risk for disseminated disease. Before the varicella vaccination program was implemented in the United States in 1996, an average of 4 million cases and 100 to 150 deaths occurred each year.[68] Annual varicella incidence and mortality rates subsequently declined by 97% and 87%, respectively.

A two-dose series of varicella vaccine is recommended for adolescents ages 13 years and older and adults, particularly health care personnel, who were previously unvaccinated and/or have no evidence of immunity.[63,69] Live vaccines should not be given to pregnant patients or people who have a very weakened immune system, which includes people with HIV infection and a CD4 count less than 200.

Herpes Zoster Vaccine

Herpes zoster, known as *shingles*, which results from reactivation of latent varicella (chickenpox) virus infection within the sensory ganglia, usually causes painful unilateral vesicular rashes in a dermatomal distribution.[70] The lifetime risk of herpes zoster infection is about 1 in 3 and is higher for females than for males. Up to 1 in 4 adults experience complications following infection, including *postherpetic neuralgia* (persistent pain in the area of the rash), bacterial skin infections, ophthalmic complications, cranial and peripheral neuropathies, encephalitis, pneumonitis, and hepatitis. Herpes zoster risk is increased in immunocompromised persons including those with cancer, HIV, bone marrow or organ transplantation, and immunosuppressive therapies. Increasing age is also strongly associated with developing both herpes zoster infection and postherpetic neuralgia.

To mitigate the risk of herpes zoster and its severe sequelae, such as postherpetic neuralgia, the administration of the recombinant zoster vaccine (RZV) is advised for adults ages 50 years and older. This recommendation includes those who have previously experienced shingles or have received the older zoster vaccine live (ZVL). The RZV should be delivered in two doses, spaced 2 to 6 months apart.[63]

The RZV effectively reduces the short-term risks for zoster and postherpetic neuralgia in adults ages 50 years and older. RZV can be used in persons who are immunocompromised.[71]

Tetanus, Diphtheria, Pertussis Vaccine

About 30 cases of tetanus are reported each year in the United States with fewer than 10 deaths.[72] The infection is caused by the anaerobic bacterium *Clostridium tetani*, which enters the body through broken skin. *Tetanus*, or *"lockjaw"* is a neurologic disorder that causes intense painful muscle contractions that can affect swallowing and breathing.

Diphtheria is caused by *Corynebacterium diphtheriae* and is usually spread through respiratory droplets.[73] The infection causes a "pseudomembrane" of dead respiratory tissue that can extend throughout the respiratory tract. Complications can include pneumonia, myocarditis, neurologic toxicities, and kidney failure. A common and deadly childhood disease in the pre-vaccine era, only 14 cases of diphtheria were reported in the United States from 1996 through 2018.*Pertussis*, or *"whooping cough,"* is a contagious respiratory disease caused by *Bordetella pertussis*.[74] In the pre-vaccine era, pertussis was a major cause of infant and child mortality. In 2017, the CDC reported about 19,000 cases, although only 72 deaths occurred from 2012 through 2017. Vaccination has dramatically reduced the number of cases of these diseases; most deaths occur in infants who were too young to be vaccinated.

A single dose of tetanus, diphtheria, and pertussis (Tdap) vaccine is recommended for persons ages 11 to 18.[63,75] Persons ages 19 years and older who never received Tdap should receive a single dose, regardless of when they last received a tetanus (Td) vaccine. A Tdap or Td vaccine booster should be offered every 10 years. Pregnant persons should receive a Tdap vaccine during every pregnancy.

Human Papillomavirus Vaccine

HPV is the most common STI in the United States.[76] Approximately half of new infections occur among persons ages 15 to 24 years. HPV is associated with cervical, vulvar, vaginal, penile anal and oropharyngeal cancers.

Recommend that patients begin a vaccination series between the ages of 9 and 14 years with the 9-valent HPV vaccine, which protects against the HPV types most likely to cause cancer and anogenital warts.[63] All individuals up to age 26 are recommended to complete either a two- or three-dose vaccine series depending on their age at initial vaccination or the presence of immunocompromising conditions. Shared clinical decision-making is recommended for adults aged 27 to 45 years who have not initiated or completed a vaccine series. The discussion should address the risks of acquiring a new HPV infection. For further discussion of HPV and HPV vaccine benefits, see Chapter 24, Pelvis and Genitourinary System: Vulva, Vagina, Uterus, and Adnexa, pp. 759–760.

For people assigned male at birth, the HPV vaccine can prevent HPV-related diseases such as genital warts, anal cancer, and penile cancer, lower the risk of oropharyngeal cancers, and potentially reduce HPV transmission to their sexual partners.

Hepatitis A Vaccine

Recommend a hepatitis A vaccine series for individuals at risk for infection, including those with chronic liver disease or HIV infection, men who have sex with men (MSM), people who use injection or non-injection drugs, unhoused persons, travelers to countries with high or intermediate rates of endemic hepatitis A, and close personal contacts of an international adoptee within the first 60 days after the adoptee's arrival from a country with high or intermediate endemic rates of hepatitis A.[63] Persons not at risk but wanting protection from hepatitis A infection should also be vaccinated. For further discussion of viral hepatitis A, see Chapter 21, Abdomen, p. 651.

Hepatitis B Vaccine

Recommend routine vaccination for individuals aged 19 through 59 years.[63] Vaccination is optional for those ages 60 years and older without risk factors for hepatitis B; shared decision making, though, is recommended for unvaccinated persons with diabetes. Vaccination is recommended for those ages 60 years and older at risk for hepatitis B infection, including those with chronic liver disease, HIV infection, sexual exposure risk, current or recent injection drug use, percutaneous or mucosal risk for exposure to blood, incarceration, and travel in countries with high or intermediate endemic hepatitis B. For further discussion of viral hepatitis B, see Chapter 21, Abdomen, pp. 651–652.

PREVENTIVE MEDICATION GUIDELINES

Prevention of Human Immunodeficiency Virus Infection: Pre-exposure Prophylaxis

In addition to behavioral strategies for preventing HIV infections among HIV-negative persons, a pharmacologic option is PrEP. The FDA has approved several medications to prevent HIV, including two oral medication and a long-acting injectable medication.[77] Preventive medications have been consistently shown to significantly reduce the risk of acquiring HIV among high-risk populations.[78] In 2023, the USPSTF issued a grade A recommendation to prescribe PrEP to adults and adolescents weighing at least 35 kg who are at increased risk of acquiring HIV.[79] They advise clinicians to routinely obtain a sexual activity and drug use history for all patients.

Persons eligible for PrEP include those who are sexually active adolescents and adults who have HIV-positive sexual partners, history of an STI within the past 6 months, inconsistent or no condom use with partners of unknown HIV status, engage in transactional sex, transgender women, persons who inject drugs and have a drug-injecting partner with HIV or who shared equipment, and persons who request PrEP.

PREVENTIVE CARE IN SPECIAL POPULATIONS

Screening, counseling, and immunization recommendations for children, older adults, and pregnant persons are found in Unit 3, Special Populations (pp. 995–1194).

DISEASE-SPECIFIC RECOMMENDATIONS

To provide context to the various diseases and conditions, screening and prevention recommendations are found in the individual regional chapters.

REFERENCES

1. Potvin L, Jones CM. Twenty-five years after the Ottawa Charter: the critical role of health promotion for public health. *Can J Public Health.* 2011;102(4):244–248.
2. U. S. Preventive Services Task Force. Task force at a glance. Accessed January 10, 2024. https://www.uspreventiveservicestaskforce.org/uspstf/about-uspstf/task-force-at-a-glance
3. U. S. Preventive Services Task Force. Use of decision models in the development of evidence-based clinical preventive services recommendations. https://www.uspreventiveservicestaskforce.org/uspstf/about-uspstf/methods-and-processes/use-decision-models-development-evidence-based-clinical-preventive-services-recommendations
4. Kisling LA, Das JM. Prevention Strategies. Accessed January 10, 2024. https://www.statpearls.com/point-of-care/27736
5. Institute of Medicine. *Clinical Practice Guidelines We Can Trust.* National Academies Press; 2011.

6. U. S. Preventive Services Task Force. Grade definitions. Accessed January 10, 2024. https://www.uspreventiveservicestaskforce.org/uspstf/about-uspstf/methods-and-processes/grade-definitions
7. Wilson JMG, Jungner G. *Principles and Practice of Screening for Disease*. World Health Organization; 1968.
8. Andermann A, Blancquaert I, Beauchamp S, Dery V. Revisiting Wilson and Jungner in the genomic age: a review of screening criteria over the past 40 years. *Bull World Health Organ*. 2008;86(4):317–319.
9. Harris R, Sawaya GF, Moyer VA, Calonge N. Reconsidering the criteria for evaluating proposed screening programs: reflections from 4 current and former members of the U.S. Preventive services task force. *Epidemiol Rev*. 2011;33:20–35.
10. Opladen T, Lopez-Laso E, Cortes-Saladelafont E, et al. Consensus guideline for the diagnosis and treatment of tetrahydrobiopterin (BH(4)) deficiencies. *Orphanet J Rare Dis*. 2020; 15(1):126.
11. McCaffery KJ, Jacklyn GL, Barratt A, et al. Chapter 28: Recommendations about screening. In: Guyatt G, Rennie D, Meade MO, Cook DJ, eds. *Users' Guides to the Medical Literature: A Manual for Evidence-Based Clinical Practice*. 3rd ed. McGraw-Hill Education; 2015.
12. Prochaska JO, DiClemente CC. Stages and processes of self-change of smoking: toward an integrative model of change. *J Consult Clin Psychol*. 1983;51(3):390–395.
13. Prochaska JO, Velicer WF. The transtheoretical model of health behavior change. *Am J Health Promot*. 1997;12(1):38–48.
14. Prochaska JO. Assessing how people change. *Cancer*. 1991; 67(3 Suppl):805–807.
15. Searight R. Realistic approaches to counseling in the office setting. *Am Fam Physician*. 2009;79(4):277–284.
16. Centers for Disease Control and Prevention. Vaccines & immunizations. Glossary. Accessed January 10, 2024. https://www.cdc.gov/vaccines/terms/glossary.html#v
17. Substance Abuse and Mental Health Services Administration. *Key substance use and mental health indicators in the United States: Results from the 2021 National Survey on Drug Use and Health*. 2022. https://www.samhsa.gov/data/report/2021-nsduh-annual-national-report
18. Ahmad FB, Cisewski JA, Rossen LM, Sutton P. Provisional drug overdose death counts. National Center for Health Statistics. 2024.
19. National Institute on Drug Abuse. TAPS. tobacco, alcohol, prescription medication, and other substance use tool. U.S. Department of Health and Human Services. Accessed January 11, 2024. https://nida.nih.gov/taps2/
20. McNeely J, Wu LT, Subramaniam G, et al. Performance of the Tobacco, Alcohol, Prescription Medication, and Other Substance Use (TAPS) tool for substance use screening in primary care patients. *Ann Intern Med*. 2016;165(10):690–699.
21. U. S. Preventive Services Task Force, Krist AH, Davidson KW, Mangione CM, et al. Screening for unhealthy drug use: US Preventive Services Task Force recommendation statement. *JAMA*. 2020;323(22):2301–2309.
22. Leemis RW, Friar N, Khatiwada S, et al. *The National Intimate Partner and Sexual Violence Survey: 2016/2017 Report on Intimate Partner Violence*. 2022. Accessed January 11, 2024. https://www.cdc.gov/violenceprevention/pdf/nisvs/nisvsreportonipv_2022.pdf
23. Centers for Disease Control and Prevention. Leading causes of death-females—All races and origins-United States, 2017. Accessed January 11, 2024. https://www.cdc.gov/women/lcod/2017/all-races-origins/index.htm
24. Petrosky E, Ertl A, Sheats KJ, Wilson R, Betz CJ, Blair JM. Surveillance for violent deaths - National Violent Death Reporting System, 34 states, four California counties, the District of Columbia, and Puerto Rico, 2017. *MMWR Surveill Summ*. 2020;69(8):1–37.
25. U. S. Preventive Services Task Force, Curry SJ, Krist AH, Owens DK, et al. Screening for intimate partner violence, elder abuse, and abuse of vulnerable adults: US Preventive Services Task Force final recommendation statement. *JAMA*. 2018;320(16):1678–1687.
26. Centers for Disease Control and Prevention. Alcohol and Public Health: Alcohol-Related Disease Impact (ARDI). Accessed January 11, 2024. https://nccd.cdc.gov/DPH_ARDI/Default/Default.aspx
27. U. S. Preventive Services Task Force, Curry SJ, Krist AH, Owens DK, et al. Screening and behavioral counseling interventions to reduce unhealthy alcohol use in adolescents and adults: US Preventive Services Task Force recommendation statement. *JAMA*. 2018;320(18):1899–1909.
28. Smith PC, Schmidt SM, Allensworth-Davies D, Saitz R. A single-question screening test for drug use in primary care. *Arch Intern Med*. 2010;170(13):1155–1160.
29. Bush K, Kivlahan DR, McDonell MB, Fihn SD, Bradley KA. The AUDIT alcohol consumption questions (AUDIT-C): an effective brief screening test for problem drinking. Ambulatory Care Quality Improvement Project (ACQUIP). Alcohol Use Disorders Identification Test. *Arch Intern Med*. 1998;158(16):1789–1795.
30. O'Connor EA, Perdue LA, Senger CA, et al. Screening and behavioral counseling interventions to reduce unhealthy alcohol use in adolescents and adults: updated evidence report and systematic review for the US Preventive Services Task Force. *JAMA*. 2018;320(18):1910–1928.
31. National Institute on Alcohol Abuse and Alcoholism. *Helping patients who drink too much: a clinician's guide*. National Institute on Alcohol Abuse and Alcoholism, National Institutes of Health, U.S. Department of Health & Human Services. 2005. Accessed January 13, 2024. https://www.issup.net/files/2017-07/Helping%20Patients%20Who%20Drink%20Too%20Much%20A%20Clinician%E2%80%99s%20Guide.pdf
32. Centers for Disease Control and Prevention. Health effects of cigarette smoking. 2005. Accessed January 13, 2024. https://www.cdc.gov/tobacco/data_statistics/fact_sheets/health_effects/effects_cig_smoking/
33. Centers for Disease Control and Prevention. Trends in tobacco use among youth. Accessed January 13, 2024. https://www.cdc.gov/tobacco/data_statistics/fact_sheets/fast_facts/trends-in-tobacco-use-among-youth.html
34. Centers for Disease Control and Prevention. About E-Cigarettes (Vapes). Accessed January 11, 2024. https://www.cdc.gov/tobacco/e-cigarettes/about.html
35. U.S. Department of Health and Human Services. *The Health Consequences of Smoking-50 Years of Progress. A Report of the Surgeon General*. U.S. Department of Health and Human Services, Centers for Disease Control and Prevention, National Center for Chronic Disease Prevention and Health Promotion, Office on Smoking and Health; 2014.
36. U. S. Preventive Services Task Force, Krist AH, Davidson KW, Mangione CM, et al. Interventions for tobacco smoking cessation in adults, including pregnant persons: US

Preventive Services Task Force recommendation statement. *JAMA*. 2021;325(3):265–279.

37. Centers for Disease Control and Prevention. Health problems caused by secondhand smoke. Accessed January 13, 2024. https://www.cdc.gov/tobacco/secondhand-smoke/health.html
38. Centers for Disease Control and Prevention. National overview of STDs, 2021. Accessed January 13, 2024. https://stacks.cdc.gov/view/cdc/109048
39. Kreisel KM, Spicknall IH, Gargano JW, et al. Sexually transmitted infections among US women and men: prevalence and incidence estimates, 2018. *Sex Transm Dis*. 2021;48(4):208–214.
40. Centers for Disease Control and Prevention. HIV Surveillance Supplemental Report: Estimated HIV Incidence and Prevalence in the United States, 2017–2021. Accessed January 13, 2024. https://stacks.cdc.gov/view/cdc/149080
41. Centers for Disease Control and Prevention. Monitoring Selected National HIV Prevention and Care Objectives by Using HIV Surveillance Data—United States and 6 Territories and Freely Associated States, 2022. Accessed January 13, 2024. https://www.cdc.gov/hiv-data/nhss/national-hiv-prevention-and-care-outcomes.html
42. U. S. Preventive Services Task Force, Mangione CM, Barry MJ, Nicholson WK, et al. Screening for syphilis infection in nonpregnant adolescents and adults: US Preventive Services Task Force reaffirmation recommendation statement. *JAMA*. 2022;328(12):1243–1249.
43. U. S. Preventive Services Task Force, Curry SJ, Krist AH, Owens DK, et al. Screening for syphilis infection in pregnant women: US Preventive Services Task Force reaffirmation recommendation statement. *JAMA*. 2018;320(9):911–917.
44. U. S. Preventive Services Task Force, Davidson KW, Barry MJ, Mangione CM, et al. Screening for chlamydia and gonorrhea: US Preventive Services Task Force recommendation statement. *JAMA*. 2021;326(10):949–956.
45. Centers for Disease Control and Prevention. Which STD tests should I get? Accessed January 13, 2024. https://www.cdc.gov/sti/about/which-std-tests-should-i-get.html
46. U. S. Preventive Services Task Force, Owens DK, Davidson KW, Krist AH, et al. Screening for HIV Infection: US Preventive Services Task Force Recommendation Statement. *JAMA*. 2019;321(23):2326–2336.
47. Branson BM, Handsfield HH, Lampe MA, et al; Centers for Disease Control and Prevention (CDC). Revised recommendations for HIV testing of adults, adolescents, and pregnant women in health-care settings. *MMWR Recomm Rep*. 2006;55(RR-14):1–17; quiz CE1-4.
48. DiNenno EA, Prejean J, Irwin K, et al. Recommendations for HIV screening of gay, bisexual, and other men who have sex with men–United States, 2017. *MMWR Morb Mortal Wkly Rep*. 2017;66(31):830–832.
49. Centers for Disease Control and Prevention. National Diabetes Statistics Report. Estimates of Diabetes and Its Burden in the United States. Accessed January 8, 2024. https://stacks.cdc.gov/view/cdc/85309
50. National Institute of Diabetes and Digestive and Kidney Diseases. *Risk Factors for Type 2 Diabetes*. National Institutes of Health. Accessed January 8, 2024. https://www.niddk.nih.gov/health-information/diabetes/overview/risk-factors-type-2-diabetes
51. U. S. Preventive Services Task Force, Davidson KW, Barry MJ, Mangione CM, et al. Screening for prediabetes and type 2 diabetes: US Preventive Services Task Force recommendation statement. *JAMA*. 2021;326(8):736–743.
52. Substance Abuse and Mental Health Services Administration. Resources for Screening, Brief Intervention, and Referral to Treatment (SBIRT). Accessed January 13, 2024. https://www.samhsa.gov/sbirt/resources
53. U.S. Department of Health and Human Services. *Medication for the Treatment of Alcohol Use Disorder: A Brief Guide*. 2015. https://store.samhsa.gov/sites/default/files/sma15-4907.pdf
54. Patel MS, Patel SB, Steinberg MB. Smoking cessation. *Ann Intern Med*. 2021;174(12):ITC177–ITC192.
55. Centers for Disease Control and Prevention. Quit smoking. Accessed January 11, 2024. https://www.cdc.gov/tobacco/campaign/tips/quit-smoking/index.html
56. Lindson N, Thompson TP, Ferrey A, Lambert JD, Aveyard P. Motivational interviewing for smoking cessation. *Cochrane Database Syst Rev*. 2019;7(7):CD006936.
57. U. S. Preventive Services Task Force, Krist AH, Davidson KW, Mangione CM, et al. Behavioral counseling interventions to prevent sexually transmitted infections: US Preventive Services Task Force recommendation statement. *JAMA*. 2020;324(7):674–681.
58. Centers for Disease Control and Prevention. How to Prevent STIs. Accessed January 13, 2024. https://www.cdc.gov/sti/prevention/index.html
59. Centers for Disease Control and Prevention. Condom Use: An Overview. Accessed January 13, 2024. https://www.cdc.gov/condom-use/
60. Centers for Disease Control and Prevention. Disease burden of flu. Accessed January 11, 2024. https://www.cdc.gov/flu/about/burden/
61. Grohskopf LA, Alyanak E, Ferdinands JM, et al. Prevention and control of seasonal influenza with vaccines: recommendations of the advisory committee on immunization practices–United States, 2023–24 influenza season. *MMWR Recomm Rep*. 2023;72(1):1–25.
62. Gierke R, McGee L, Beall B, Pilishivili T. Chapter 11: Pneumococcal. *Centers for Disease Control and Prevention*. Accessed January 11, 2024. https://www.cdc.gov/vaccines/pubs/surv-manual/chpt11-pneumo.html
63. Recommended adult immunization schedule for ages 19 years or older, United States 2024. *JAAPA*. 2024;37(1):1–13.
64. Centers for Disease Control and Prevention. Pneumococcal vaccination: summary of who and when to vaccinate. Accessed January 9, 2024. https://www.cdc.gov/vaccines/vpd/pneumo/hcp/who-when-to-vaccinate.html
65. Melgar M, Britton A, Roper LE, et al. Use of respiratory syncytial virus vaccines in older adults: recommendations of the advisory committee on immunization practices–United States, 2023. *MMWR Morb Mortal Wkly Rep*. 2023;72(29):793–801.
66. World Health Organization. WHO COVID-19 dashboard. Accessed January 8, 2024. https://data.who.int/dashboards/covid19/
67. Centers for Disease Control and Prevention. Mpox. Information for healthcare professionals. Accessed January 6 2024. https://www.cdc.gov/poxvirus/mpox/clinicians/index.html
68. Lopez A, Leung J, Schmid S, Marin M. Chapter 17: Varicella. *Centers for Disease Control and Prevention*. Accessed January 11, 2024. https://www.cdc.gov/vaccines/pubs/surv-manual/chpt17-varicella.html

69. Centers for Disease Control and Prevention. Chapter 17: Varicella. Accessed January 11, 2024. https://www.cdc.gov/vaccines/vpd/varicella/hcp/recommendations.html
70. Centers for Disease Control and Prevention. Clinical Overview of Shingles (Herpes Zoster). Accessed January 11, 2024. https://www.cdc.gov/shingles/hcp/clinical-overview/
71. Centers for Disease Control and Prevention. Shingles. About the vaccine. Accessed January 11, 2024. https://www.cdc.gov/vaccines/vpd/shingles/hcp/shingrix/about-vaccine.html
72. Blain A, Tiwari TSP. Chapter 16: Tetanus. Centers for Disease Control and Prevention. Accessed January 11, 2024. https://www.cdc.gov/vaccines/pubs/surv-manual/chpt16-tetanus.html
73. Acosta AM, Bampoe VD. Chapter 1: Diphtheria. Centers for Disease Control and Prevention. Accessed January 11, 2024. https://www.cdc.gov/vaccines/pubs/surv-manual/chpt01-dip.html
74. Blain A, Skoff T, Cassiday MS, Tondella ML, Acosta A. Chapter 10: Pertussis. Centers for Disease Control and Prevention. Accessed January 11, 2024. https://www.cdc.gov/vaccines/pubs/surv-manual/chpt10-pertussis.html
75. Havers FP, Moro PL, Hunter P, Hariri S, Bernstein H. Use of tetanus toxoid, reduced diphtheria toxoid, and acellular pertussis vaccines: updated recommendations of the Advisory Committee on Immunization Practices–United States, 2019. *MMWR Morb Mortal Wkly Rep.* 2020;69(3):77–83.
76. Meites E, Gee J, Unger E, Markowitz L. Chapter 11: Human Papillomavirus. Centers for Disease Control and Prevention. Accessed January 11, 2024. https://www.cdc.gov/vaccines/pubs/pinkbook/hpv.html
77. HIVinfo.NIH.gov. HIV Prevention: Pre-exposure prophylaxis (PrEP). Accessed January 8, 2024. https://hivinfo.nih.gov/understanding-hiv/fact-sheets/pre-exposure-prophylaxis-prep
78. Chou R, Spencer H, Bougatsos C, Blazina I, Ahmed A, Selph S. Preexposure prophylaxis for the prevention of HIV: updated evidence report and systematic review for the US Preventive Services Task Force. *JAMA.* 2023;330(8):746–763.
79. U. S. Preventive Services Task Force, Barry MJ, Nicholson WK, Silverstein M, et al. Preexposure prophylaxis to prevent acquisition of HIV: US Preventive Services Task Force recommendation statement. *JAMA.* 2023;330(8):736–745.

CHAPTER

8

Evaluating Clinical Evidence

INTRODUCTION

Clinical decision making requires integrating clinical expertise, patient preferences, and the best available clinical evidence (Fig. 8-1).[1] Acquiring skills for each of these components is essential for excellence in patient care. You will develop your clinical expertise as you practice your clinical discipline, enabling you to make diagnoses and identify potential interventions more efficiently. You will also begin to learn how to incorporate your patients' individualized preferences, concerns, and expectations into those health decisions. Finally, you will learn to identify and appraise the best sources of available evidence to inform your clinical practice.[2] Throughout the regional examination chapters, you will encounter evidence about using elements of the history and physical examination (PE) to support diagnostic reasoning. This chapter provides you with foundational knowledge of the criteria utilized to evaluate that clinical evidence.

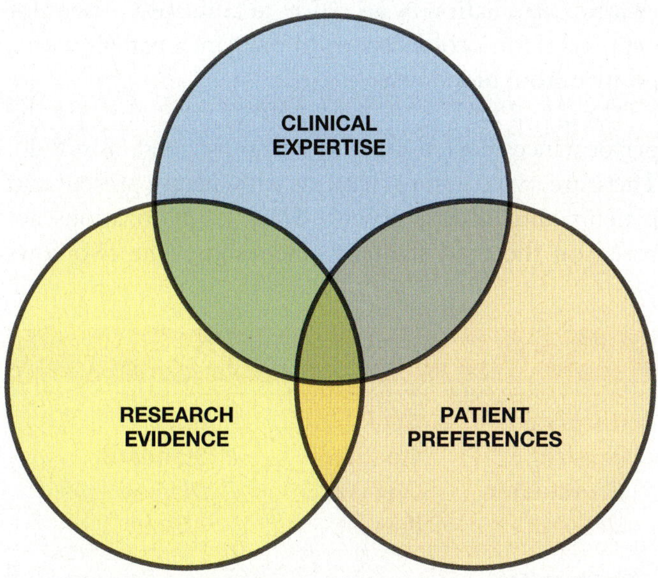

FIGURE 8-1. Evidence-based clinical practice Venn diagram. (Adapted from Haynes RB, Sackett DL, Gray JM, Cook DJ, Guyatt GH. Transferring evidence from research into practice: 1. The role of clinical care research evidence in clinical decisions. *ACP J Club.* 1996;125(3):A14–A16.)

Chapter Content Guide

USING ELEMENTS OF THE HISTORY AND PHYSICAL EXAMINATION AS DIAGNOSTIC TESTS

As discussed in Chapter 5, Clinical Reasoning, the process of diagnostic reasoning begins with generating a list of potential causes for the patient's problems (*differential diagnosis*). As you conduct your history and PE, you will consider the likelihood that these various diagnoses can explain your patient's problems with the goal of determining the need to perform additional testing or to initiate treatment.[3]

Key elements from the health history, especially those discussed in the history of present illness (e.g., precordial chest pain, a vertiginous sensation of dizziness, or orthopnea), are used in this initial step in the diagnostic reasoning process. This is also true for the findings in the PE elicited through the classic techniques of inspection, palpation, percussion, and auscultation or through special maneuvers.

An example illustrating how elements in the history and PE are used to support diagnostic reasoning follows.

> The patient is a 43-year-old female presenting to the emergency room with an acute episode of right upper quadrant (RUQ) abdominal pain. The pain is described as a being steady and severe, has lasted for over 4 hours, and developed about an hour after eating a fatty meal. She reports nausea, vomiting, and anorexia.

Studies evaluating the predictive value of elements of the history suggest that the location and onset of this patient's pain and symptoms increase the likelihood of this being *acute cholecystitis* (inflammation of the gallbladder).[4,5] However, your list of possible causes also includes diagnoses such as biliary colic, acute cholangitis, and hepatitis.

> On PE, she has a temperature of 38 °C (100.8 °F), her blood pressure is 145/90 mm Hg, her pulse is 110 beats per minute, and she appears uncomfortable. She is not jaundiced but has RUQ tenderness without rebound and a positive Murphy sign (suggestive of acute cholecystitis).[4,5]

The presence or absence of jaundice and rebound tenderness has not been consistently found to be significantly associated with acute cholecystitis.[4,5] However, fever, RUQ tenderness, and a positive Murphy sign increase the likelihood of acute cholecystitis. Nonetheless, you still need to consider the other diagnoses in your list. (See Chapter 21, Abdomen for a discussion of the Murphy sign, pp. 641–642.)

> Laboratory studies show an elevated white blood cell count and normal liver function tests, including transaminases, bilirubin, and alkaline phosphatase.

These results make the diagnosis of acute hepatitis unlikely, although they do not substantially alter the likelihood of having acute cholecystitis. Indeed, no single element of the history, PE, or lab results is sufficient to help you cross the *treatment threshold* for acute cholecystitis. Because the suspicion for a gallbladder problem is high, the next step in this case is visually confirming the diagnosis with imaging.

> The RUQ bedside ultrasound shows gallstones and gallbladder wall thickening. The sonographic Murphy sign is positive. These results confirm the diagnosis of acute cholecystitis, and the patient will be admitted for antibiotics and surgery to remove her gallbladder.

You can turn to the clinical literature to determine *quantitatively* how a diagnostic test—any information in the health history and PE as well as lab tests, radiographic imaging, and procedures—can revise the probabilities of the possible causes for a patient's condition (*differential diagnosis*). Two concepts in evaluating diagnostic tests are the *validity* of the findings and the *reproducibility* of the test results.

EVALUATING DIAGNOSTIC TESTS: VALIDITY

The initial step in evaluating a diagnostic test is to determine whether it provides valid results. *Does the test accurately identify whether a patient has a disease (or condition)?* This involves comparing the test against an appropriate *gold (reference) standard* test, which is the best measure of whether a patient has disease. This could be a biopsy to evaluate a lung nodule, a structured psychiatric examination by an expert to evaluate a patient for depression, or a colonoscopy to evaluate a patient with a positive stool blood test.

The *2 × 2 table* is the basic format for evaluating the performance characteristics of a diagnostic test (Box 8-1). There are two columns: patients with disease present and patients with disease absent. These categorizations are based on the gold standard test results. The two rows

Box 8-1. Setting Up the 2 × 2 Table

History or Physical Examination Element	Gold Standard: Disease Present	Gold Standard: Disease Absent
Present (test positive)	a True positive	b False positive
Absent (test negative)	c False negative	d True negative

correspond to the presence of the element of history and PE of interest (positive) or its absence (negative). The four cells (a, b, c, d) would then correspond to true positives, false positives, false negatives, and true negatives, respectively.[6]

Sensitivity and Specificity

The first test statistics to estimate are *sensitivity* and *specificity* (Box 8-2). Knowing the sensitivity and specificity of a test does not necessarily help you make clinical decisions because these statistics are based on knowing whether the patient has disease. However, there are two exceptions. A negative result from a test with a high sensitivity (i.e., a very low false-negative rate) usually excludes disease. This is represented by the mnemonic SnNOUT—a **Sn**sitive test with a **N**egative result rules **OUT** disease. Conversely, a positive result in a test with high specificity (e.g., a very low false-positive rate) usually indicates disease. This is represented by the mnemonic SpPIN—a **Sp**ecific test with a **P**ositive result rules **IN** disease.[7]

An example of clinically applying these statistics is with a patient presenting with acute low back pain. If you suspect that the likely cause of a patient's low back pain is a herniated lumbosacral disc, you may want to perform PE maneuvers that could bolster your diagnosis. One maneuver is called the *straight-leg raise test* with a sensitivity of about 92%.[8] Conversely, the specificity of this maneuver is about 28%. In contrast, another maneuver is the *crossed straight-leg raise test*, which has a sensitivity of only about 28% for detecting a herniated disk, but a specificity of about 90%. Thus, the presence of a positive crossed straight-leg test on PE makes your diagnosis more likely, while a negative straight-leg raise on PE makes the diagnosis less likely.

Unfortunately, most single PE maneuvers and elements of the history lack either a high sensitivity or a high specificity.

Box 8-2. Sensitivity and Specificity

Sensitivity is the probability that a person with disease has a positive test. This is represented as a/(a + c) in the Disease Present column of the 2 × 2 table.

Sensitivity is also known as the true positive rate.

Specificity is the probability that a nondiseased person has a negative test, represented as d/(b + d) in the Disease Absent column of the 2 × 2 table.

Specificity is also known as the true negative rate.

Box 8-3. Predictive Values

The **positive predictive value (PPV)** is the probability that a person with a positive test has the disease, represented as a/(a + b) from the first (test positive) row in the 2 × 2 table.

The **negative predictive value (NPV)** is the probability that a person with a negative test does not have the disease, represented as d/(c + d) in the second (test negative) row in the 2 × 2 table.

Predictive Values

The typical clinical scenario faced by clinicians involves determining whether a person has a disease based on a test result that is either positive or negative. *How useful is the test result in telling us whether the disease is present or absent?* This is called the *predictive value,* and it links the sensitivity and specificity of the test with how commonly the disease occurs in the population (*prevalence*). Predictive values can be *positive* or *negative* (Box 8-3).[9]

Prevalence of Disease

Although the predictive value statistics seem intuitively useful, they will vary substantially according to the *prevalence of disease* (i.e., the proportion of patients in the "Disease Present" column). The prevalence is based on the characteristics of the patient population and the clinical setting. For example, the prevalence of many diseases will usually be higher among older patients and among patients being seen in specialist clinics or at referral hospitals.

Let us see how variability in the prevalence of a disease modifies the predictive values of diagnostic tests. For example, we have findings from a PE maneuver that could inform you of the presence or absence of a disease (Box 8-4). It has a sensitivity of 90% and specificity of 90%. The box shows the 2 × 2 table for performing this maneuver in a patient population of 1,000, in which the disease prevalence (proportion of subjects that have the disease) is 10%:

$$\text{Sensitivity} = a/(a + c) = 90/100 \text{ or } 90\%;$$
$$\text{Specificity} = d/(b + d) = 810/900 = 90\%$$

The PPV calculated from the test positive row of the table would be 90/180 = 50%. This means that half of the people with a positive test have disease.

Box 8-4. Predictive Values: Prevalence of 10% with Sensitivity and Specificity = 90%

	Disease Present	Disease Absent	Total
Test positive	a **90**	b **90**	**180**
Test negative	c **10**	d **810**	**820**
Total	**100**	**900**	**1,000**

However, if the sensitivity and specificity of the diagnostic test remained the same, but prevalence of the disease was only 1%, the cells would look very different (Box 8-5).

$$\text{Sensitivity} = a/(a + c) = 9/10 \text{ or } 90\%;$$
$$\text{Specificity} = d/(b + d) = 891/990 = 90\%$$

Now the PPV calculated from the test positive row of the table would be only 9/108 = 8.3%.

The consequence is that the great majority of positive test results in the *low prevalence* population are *false positives*—meaning most of the persons will not have disease. However, to know whether persons who had a positive diagnostic test (false positives) have disease, clinicians may need to perform further diagnostic tests, which can be invasive, expensive, and potentially harmful. This has implications for patient safety and resource allocation because clinicians want to limit the number of healthy persons who undergo unnecessary diagnostic tests.

The example shows that predictive values will not necessarily provide sufficient guidance for evaluating diagnostic tests across populations with differing disease prevalence.

Box 8-5. Predictive Values: Prevalence of 1% with Sensitivity and Specificity = 90%

	Disease Present	Disease Absent	Total
Test positive	a **9**	b **99**	**108**
Test negative	c **1**	d **891**	**892**
Total	**10**	**990**	**1,000**

Likelihood Ratios

Fortunately, there are other ways to evaluate the performance of a diagnostic test—again, elements of the history and PE, laboratory tests, radiographic imaging, and procedures—that can account for the varying disease prevalence observed in different patient populations.

One way uses *likelihood ratio* (*LR*) statistics, defined as the probability of obtaining a given test result in a person with a health condition divided by the probability of obtaining a given test result in a healthy patient.[6] The LR tells us how much a test result changes the probability of having the disease of interest before the diagnostic test is performed (*pre-test disease probability*) to the probability of having the disease of interest after the diagnostic test is performed and its findings known (*post-test disease probability*). The pretest probability is the *prevalence* of the disease in the population.

In the simplest case, we will assume that the test result is either positive or negative. Therefore, the *LR for a positive test* is the ratio of getting a positive test result in a person with a health condition divided by the probability of getting a positive test result in a healthy person.[10] From the 2 × 2 table, we see that this is the same as saying the ratio of the true-positive rate (sensitivity) over the false-positive rate (1 – specificity). A higher value (much >1) indicates that a positive test is much more likely to be coming from a person with a health condition than from a healthy person, increasing our confidence that a person with a positive result has disease.

The *LR for a negative test* is the ratio of the probability of getting a negative test result in a person with a health condition divided by the probability of getting a negative test result in a healthy person.[10] From the 2 × 2 table, we see that this is the same as saying the ratio of the false-negative rate (1 – sensitivity) divided by the true-negative rate (specificity). A lower value (much <1) indicates that the negative test is much more likely to be coming from a healthy person than from a person with a health condition, increasing our confidence that a person with a negative result does not have disease.

The magnitude of the LR indicates how strongly a given test result will raise (rule in) or lower (rule out) the likelihood of disease.[6] Box 8-6 shows how to interpret LRs based on how much a test result changes the pre- to posttest probabilities for disease.

APPLYING CONCEPTS TO EVALUATING ABDOMINAL PAIN

The acute cholecystitis example on p. 143 used general terms to describe whether an element of the history, PE,

Box 8-6. Interpreting Likelihood Ratios

Likelihood Ratios[a]	Effect on Pre- to Post-test Probability
LRs >10 or <0.1	Generate large changes
LRs 5–10 or 0.1–0.2	Generate moderate changes
LRs 2–5 and 0.5–0.2	Generate small (sometimes important) changes
LRs 1–2 and 0.5–1	Alter the probability to a small degree (rarely important)

[a]*LRs >1* are associated with positive results and an increased probability for disease. *LRs <1* are associated with negative results and a decreased probability of disease. A test with an *LR of 1* provides no additional information about the probability of disease.

or lab or imaging finding made the diagnosis more or less likely. However, each of these elements can be evaluated for their performance as a diagnostic test. Box 8-7 shows the LRs for the presence or absence of various elements from the history and PE.[11]

Figure 8-2 shows how the presence or absence of physical findings can alter the probability for diagnosis. Elements of the history and lab and imaging study results can also be used to revise probabilities.

APPLYING CONCEPTS TO SCREENING TESTS

Throughout the book, you will find recommendations for health promotion interventions, especially screening and prevention. These recommendations are based on

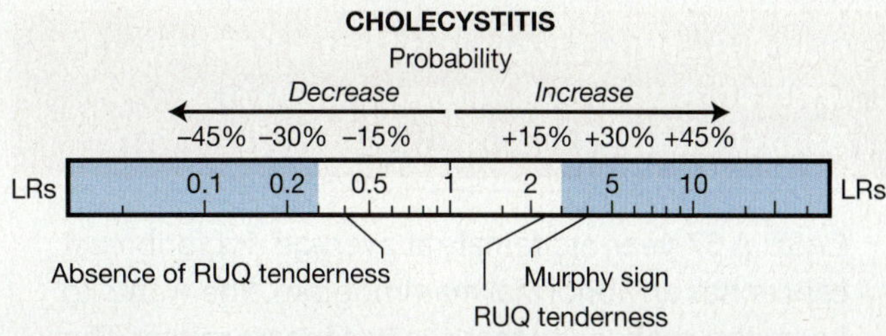

FIGURE 8-2. Revising probabilities for acute cholecystitis. (Adapted with permission of Elsevier Science & Technology Journals from McGee S, ed. Abdominal pain and tenderness. In: *Evidence-Based Physical Diagnosis.* 5th ed. Elsevier; 2022:433–442; permission conveyed through Copyright Clearance Center, Inc.)

evidence from the clinical literature that can be evaluated according to criteria presented in this chapter. We will show how LRs can be used to revise probabilities for disease with the example of breast cancer screening (Box 8-8).

Fagan Nomogram

The Fagan nomogram provides a simple way to use LRs for revising probabilities (Fig. 8-3).[12] With this nomogram, you read the pre-test probabilities from the line on the left, then take a straight edge and draw a line from the pre-test probability through the LR in the middle line, and then read the post-test probability on the line on the right (Box 8-9).

Natural Frequencies

Using frequency statements is perhaps a more intuitive alternative to LRs for determining how a test result will change the probability of disease.[13] Natural frequencies represent the joint frequency of two events, such as the number of patients with disease and the number who have a positive test result.

Box 8-7. Likelihood Ratios of Physical Examination Signs for Diagnosing Cholecystitis in Adult Patients with Abdominal Pain or Suspected Cholecystitis

Finding	Sensitivity (%)	Specificity (%)	Likelihood Ratio if Finding is: Present	Likelihood Ratio if Finding is: Absent
Fever	29–44	37–83	NS	NS
RUQ tenderness	0–98	1–97	2.4	0.4
Murphy sign	8–97	48–98	3.9	0.5
RUQ mass	2–23	70–99	NS	NS

NS, not significant.

Adapted with permission of Elsevier Science & Technology Journals from McGee S, ed. Abdominal pain and tenderness. In: *Evidence-Based Physical Diagnosis*. 5th ed. Elsevier; 2022:433–442; permission conveyed through Copyright Clearance Center, Inc.

Box 8-8. How Likely Is It that a Patient with an Abnormal Mammogram Has Breast Cancer?

CASE: A 57-year-old female at average risk for breast cancer has an abnormal mammogram. She wants to know the probability that she has breast cancer. The literature states that the baseline risk (prevalence) is 1%, the sensitivity of mammography is 90%, and the specificity is 91%. *What will you tell her?*

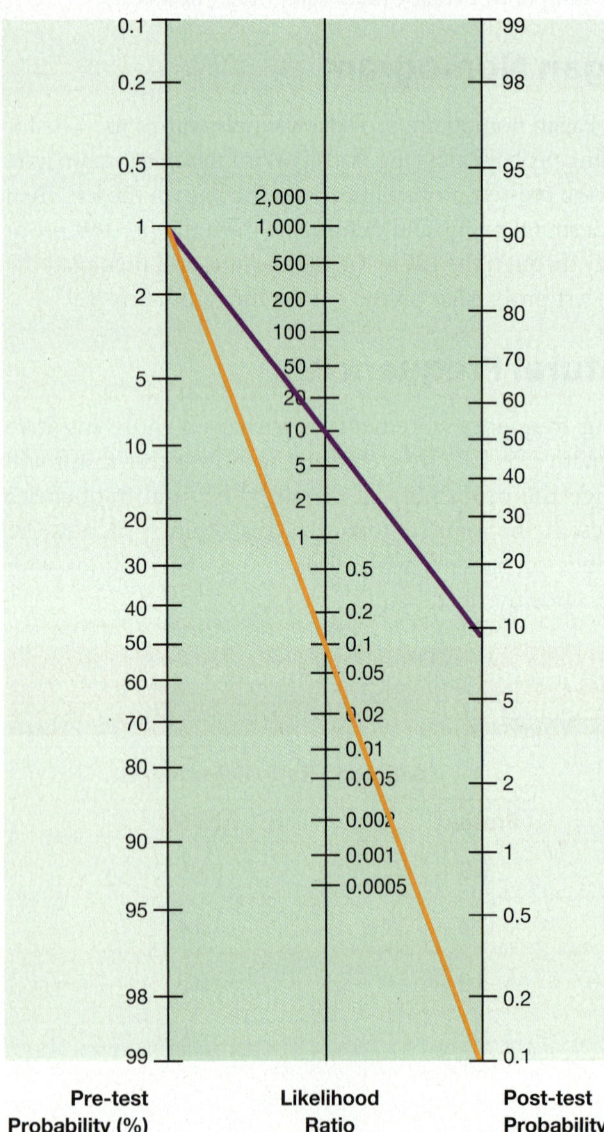

FIGURE 8-3. Fagan nomogram.

Box 8-9. Using the Fagan Nomogram to Answer the Mammography Question

- The pre-test probability (prevalence) = 1%, and the likelihood for a positive test (sensitivity/[1 – specificity]) would be 90%/9% = 10.
- The blue line corresponds to the case of a positive test with a post-test probability of ~9%.
- If the mammogram result was negative (red line), the LR for a negative test ([1 – sensitivity]/specificity) would be 10%/91% = 0.11, and the post-test probability for breast cancer would be 0.1%.

Start by taking a large number of people (e.g., 100 or 1,000, depending on the prevalence) and break the number down into natural frequencies (i.e., how many of the people have disease, how many with disease will test positive, how many without disease will test positive).

We begin by creating a 2 × 2 table based on a population of 1,000 females (Box 8-10). The 1% prevalence means that 10 patients will have breast cancer. The sensitivity of 90% means that 9 of the patients with breast cancer will have an abnormal mammogram. The specificity of 91% means that 89 of the 990 females without breast cancer will still have an abnormal mammogram. The probability that a patient with an abnormal mammogram will have breast cancer is 9/(9 + 89) = ~9%.

EVALUATING DIAGNOSTIC TESTS: REPRODUCIBILITY

Another characteristic of a diagnostic test is *reproducibility*.[14] An important aspect of evaluating diagnostic elements of the health history or PE is determining the reproducibility of the findings for diagnosing a clinical disorder.

Box 8-10. Using Natural Frequencies to Answer the Mammography Question

Mammogram Result	Breast Cancer	No Breast Cancer	Total
Positive	9	89	**98**
Negative	1	901	**902**
	10	**990**	**1,000**

Adapted from Gigerenzer G. What are natural frequencies? *BMJ.* 2011;343:d6386.

For example, when two clinicians perform the Murphy sign on a patient suspected as having acute cholecystitis, they may not always agree on the presence of this finding. This raises the question of whether this finding is useful for diagnosing the clinical disorder of acute cholecystitis. By chance, if many patients are being examined, there will be a certain amount of agreement in the findings between the two clinicians. *Understanding whether there is agreement well beyond chance*, though, is important in knowing whether the finding is useful enough to support clinical decision making.

Box 8-11. Interpreting Kappa Values

Value of Kappa	Strength of Agreement
<0.20	Poor
0.21–0.40	Fair
0.41–0.60	Moderate
0.61–0.80	Good
0.81–1.00	Excellent

Kappa Score

The *kappa score* measures the amount of agreement that occurs beyond chance.[14] In Figure 8-4, the total possible agreement for any clinical judgment as to the presence of a finding is 100%. However, say that the agreement between observers for a given abnormal PE finding based on chance alone is 50%. In our example, the abnormal finding is a positive Murphy sign. If our two clinicians agree 75% of the time whether the patient suspected of having acute cholecystitis has a positive Murphy sign, this means that the actual observer agreement *beyond* chance is 25%.

Because the *potential* agreement beyond chance is 50%, the kappa level is then calculated as 25%/50% = 0.5, which indicates moderate agreement. Box 8-11 shows how to interpret kappa values.

The degree of agreement for routinely elicited findings can be quite variable; for example, kappa values were 0.18 for clinicians detecting an S_3 gallop on cardiac auscultation using computerized phonocardiograms as a gold standard[15] and 0.87 for intensive care unit nurses in assessing the presence of extensive skin mottling over the knee (sign of sepsis).[16]

Precision

In the context of reproducibility, *precision* refers to being able to apply the same test to the same unchanged person and obtain the same results.[17] Precision is often used

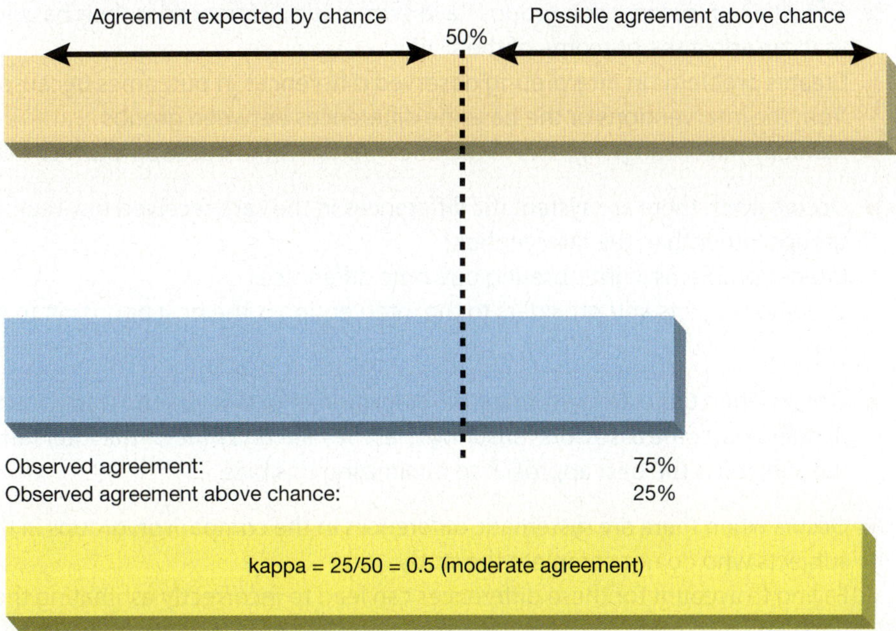

FIGURE 8-4. Kappa scores. (Reprinted with permission from McGinn T, Wyer PC, Newman TB, et al. Tips for learners of evidence-based medicine: 3. Measures of observer variability [kappa statistic]. *CMAJ*. 2004;171: 1369–1373.)

when referring to laboratory tests. For example, when measuring a troponin level for cardiac ischemia, clinicians might use a particular cutoff level to decide whether to admit a patient to a coronary care unit. If the test results are imprecise, this could lead to admitting a patient without ischemic heart disease or sending a patient home with an ischemic event. A statistical test used to characterize precision is the *coefficient of variation,* defined as the standard deviation divided by the mean value. Lower values indicate greater precision.

CRITICALLY APPRAISING THE CLINICAL EVIDENCE

Throughout this book, you will find health promotion sections that make recommendations based on guidelines issued by professional organizations such as those produced by the U.S. Preventive Services Task Force (USPSTF).[18] During your health care training, you must learn the process of *critically appraising* the clinical literature in order to be able to interpret new studies, recommendations, and guidelines as they appear throughout your professional career.

A widely accepted process for critically appraising the clinical literature has been developed by The Evidence Based Working Group.[2] These experts in epidemiology created a rigorous and standardized approach for evaluating studies. This approach has been applied to a wide range of clinical topics, including therapeutic and prevention trials, diagnostic tests, meta-analysis, cost-effectiveness analyses, and practice guidelines. This approach asks three basic questions:

1. Are the results valid (can you believe them)?
2. What are the results (magnitude and precision)?
3. How can you apply the results to patient care (generalizability)?

Are the Results Valid?

Understanding Bias. When evaluating study results, a thorough understanding of *bias* (a systematic error in conducting a study that threatens the validity of the results) is necessary. Studies with a low risk of bias provide the most valid evidence for clinical decision making and health promotion interventions. Important sources of bias in clinical studies evaluating interventions are shown in Box 8-12.

Box 8-12. Types of Biases Affecting Evidence

Selection bias[19]	■ Occurs when comparison groups have systematic differences in their baseline characteristics that can affect the outcome of the study ■ Creates problems in interpreting observed differences in outcomes because they could result from the interventions or the baseline differences between groups ■ Randomly allocating subjects to the intervention is the best approach to minimizing this bias
Performance bias[20]	■ Occurs when there are systematic differences in the care received between comparison groups (other than the intervention) ■ Creates problems in interpreting outcome differences ■ Blinding subjects and providers to the intervention is the best approach to minimizing this bias
Ascertainment bias[21]	■ Occurs when there are systematic differences in efforts to diagnose or ascertain an outcome ■ Blinding outcome assessors (ensuring that they are unaware of the intervention received by the subject) is the best approach to minimizing this bias
Attrition bias[22]	■ Occurs when there are systematic differences in the comparison groups in the number of subjects who do not complete the study ■ Failing to account for these differences can lead to incorrectly estimating the effectiveness of an intervention ■ Using an intention-to-treat analysis, where all analyses consider all subjects who were assigned to a comparison group, regardless of whether they received or completed the intervention, can minimize this bias

Box 8-13. 2 × 2 Table for Evaluating Studies of Treatment or Prevention

	Event Occurred	No Event	Total
Experimental group	a	b	a + b
Control group	c	d	c + d

What Are the Results?

Assessing Performance of a Treatment or Prevention Intervention. We have discussed the results found in studies of diagnostic tests. Guidelines for health promotion are usually based on clinical trials of interventions. Results from these studies are also calculated from a 2 × 2 table, in which the columns correspond to whether the subject developed the outcome, and the rows correspond to whether the subject received (or was exposed to) the intervention (Box 8-13). The statistics used to characterize the performance of a treatment or prevention intervention include *relative risks*, *relative risk differences* (can be a reduction or increase, reflecting benefit or harm), *absolute risk differences* (can be a reduction or increase, reflecting benefit or harm), *numbers needed to treat*, and *numbers needed to harm* (Box 8-14).[9]

Box 8-15. 2 × 2 Table for Evaluating Lung Cancer Screening: NELSON Trial[23]

Screening Test	Lung Cancer Death	No Lung Cancer Death	Total
Low-dose computed tomography (LDCT)	24	976	1,000
No screening	32	968	1,000

Source: de Koning HJ, van der Aalst CM, de Jong PA, et al. Reduced lung-cancer mortality with volume CT screening in a randomized trial. *N Engl J Med.* 2020;382(6):503–513.

Calculating these statistics from the 2 × 2 table begins with determining probabilities for outcomes (Box 8-14).

An example of these calculations is based on the results from the Dutch–Belgian lung cancer screening trial (Nederlands–Leuvens Longkanker Screenings Onderzoek [NELSON]), which compared screening to detect lung cancer with low-dose computed tomography (LDCT) against no screening.[23] The outcome of interest (event) was death from lung cancer. After four rounds of screening (over 5.5 years) and with 10 years of follow-up, the LDCT (experimental) group had an event rate of 0.024, while the no screening (control) group had an event rate of 0.032 (Box 8-15).

Box 8-14. Statistics Used to Characterize the Performance of a Treatment or Prevention Intervention

Experimental event rate (EER)	■ Probability that an intervention subject had the outcome is described by a/(a + b) from row 1 (experimental group)
Control event rate (CER)	■ Probability that a control subject had the outcome is c/(c + d) from row 2 (control group)
Relative risk (RR)	■ Probability of an outcome in the intervention group compared to the probability of an outcome in the control group, is expressed as the EER/CER
Relative risk difference	■ Defined as CER − EER/CER × 100% or 100%, the RR, which describes the proportion of baseline risk that is reduced/increased by the therapy
Absolute risk difference	■ Difference in outcome rates between the comparisons groups, is expressed by the CER − EER
Number needed to treat (NNT)	■ Reciprocal of the absolute risk difference (reported as a fraction) and is the number of subjects who need to be treated over a specific time period to prevent one outcome; if the intervention increases the risk for a bad outcome, this statistic becomes the *number needed to harm (NNH)*

The relative risk of dying from lung cancer with LDCT screening compared to no screening was 0.024/0.032 = 0.75, or 75%. The relative risk reduction is 1 – 0.77 = 0.25, or 25%, meaning that the risk of a lung cancer death among the LDCT group was 25% lower than in the no-screening group. LDCT led to a reduction in lung cancer deaths, so we use the absolute risk reduction, which is reported as a decimal: 0.032 – 0.024 = 0.008. The reciprocal of this value (1/0.008) gives us a *number needed to screen* of 125—meaning that for every 125 persons receiving an LDCT instead of no screening, there was 1 fewer lung cancer death. The number needed to screen is always based on a specific time period, so we would say that we need to screen 125 patients four times over 5.5 years with LDCT compared to no screening to prevent 1 lung cancer death after 10 years.

How Can You Apply the Results to Patient Care?

Generalizability. The final point to consider when evaluating the quality of the literature is whether the results are generalizable (e.g., whether the study results can be applied to your patients).

To make this determination, you need to first look at the *demographics of the study subjects* (e.g., age, gender, race/ethnicity, socioeconomic status, clinical conditions). Then, you need to determine whether the demographics are *similar enough* to your patient to make the results applicable. You also need to determine whether the *intervention is feasible* in your setting. *Do you have the clinical expertise, technology, and capacity to offer the intervention?* Most importantly, you need to consider the *range of potential benefits and harm* associated with the intervention and decide whether the intervention is acceptable for your patients.

COMMUNICATING CLINICAL EVIDENCE TO PATIENTS

Health care providers must be able to effectively communicate evidence on prognosis, treatments, diagnostic testing, and prevention to help patients understand their risks and options. How we frame information can often lead to poor-quality patient decisions. In one study, respondents were given information on three different screening tests for unspecified cancers.[24] In fact, the benefits were identical, except that they were expressed differently. When the benefit of the test was presented in the form of *relative risk reduction*, 80% of people said they would likely accept the test. When the same information was presented in the form of *absolute risk reduction* and *number needed to treat*, only 53% and 43%, respectively, responded positively.

Clinicians should strive to present information to reduce framing effects and encourage informed shared decision making.[25] Several approaches for these discussions include the *five As* (*ask*, *advise*, *assess*, *assist*, and *arrange*) and *FRAMES* (*feedback about personal risk*, *responsibility of patient*, *advice to change*, *empathetic style*, *promote self-efficacy*) as discussed in Chapter 7, Health Maintenance and Screening, pp. 121–123.[26] Decision aids, which provide support for patients facing treatment or prevention decisions, increase knowledge, improve communication with clinicians, and increase confidence in making a decision.[27]

REFERENCES

1. Haynes RB, Sackett DL, Gray JM, Cook DJ, Guyatt GH. Transferring evidence from research into practice: 1. The role of clinical care research evidence in clinical decisions. Editorial. *ACP J Club*. 1996;125(3):A14–A16.
2. Guyatt G, Rennie D, Meade M, Cook DJ. *Users' Guides to the Medical Literature: A Manual for Evidence-Based Clinical Practice*. 3rd ed. McGraw-Hill Education; 2015.
3. Richardson WS, Wilson M. Chapter 16: The process of diagnosis. In: Guyatt G, Rennie D, Meade M, Cook DJ, eds. *Users' Guides to the Medical Literature: A Manual for Evidence-Based Clinical Practice*. 3rd ed. McGraw-Hill Education; 2015.
4. Jain A, Mehta N, Secko M, et al. History, physical examination, laboratory testing, and emergency department ultrasonography for the diagnosis of acute cholecystitis. *Acad Emerg Med*. 2017;24(3):281–297.
5. Trowbridge RL, Rutkowski NK, Shojania KG. Does this patient have acute cholecystitis? *JAMA*. 2003;289(1):80–86.
6. Furukawa TA, Strauss SE, Bucher HC, Thomas A, Guyatt G. Chapter 18: Diagnostic tests. In: Guyatt G, Rennie D, eds. *Users' Guides to the Medical Literature: A Manual for Evidence-Based Clinical Practice*. 3rd ed. McGraw-Hill Education; 2015.
7. Centre for Evidence-Based Medicine. SpPin and SnNout. Accessed January 15, 2024. https://www.cebm.ox.ac.uk/resources/ebm-tools/sppin-and-snnout
8. van der Windt DA, Simons E, Riphagen II, et al. Physical examination for lumbar radiculopathy due to disc herniation in patients with low-back pain. *Cochrane Database Syst Rev*. 2010;(2):CD007431.
9. Strauss SE, Glasziou P, Richardson WS, Haynes RB. *Evidence-Based Medicine. How to Practice and Teach EBM*. 5th ed. Elsevier; 2019.
10. Centre for Evidence-Based Medicine. Likelihood ratios. Accessed January 15, 2024. https://www.cebm.ox.ac.uk/resources/ebm-tools/likelihood-ratios
11. McGee S. Abdominal pain and tenderness. In: McGee S, ed. *Evidence-Based Physical Diagnosis*. 5th ed. Philadelphia, PA: Elsevier; 2022:433.

REFERENCES

12. Fagan TJ. Nomogram for Bayes theorem. *N Engl J Med.* 1975;293:257.
13. Gigerenzer G. What are natural frequencies? *BMJ.* 2011;343:d6386.
14. McGinn T, Guyatt G, Cook R, Korenstein D, Meade M. Chapter 19.3: Measuring agreement beyond chance. In: Guyatt G, Rennie D, Meade M, Cook DJ, eds. *Users' Guides to the Medical Literature: A Manual for Evidence-Based Clinical Practice.* 2nd ed. McGraw-Hill Education; 2015.
15. Lok CE, Morgan CD, Ranganathan N. The accuracy and interobserver agreement in detecting the 'gallop sounds' by cardiac auscultation. *Chest.* 1998;114(5):1283–1288.
16. Coudroy R, Jamet A, Frat JP, et al. Incidence and impact of skin mottling over the knee and its duration on outcome in critically ill patients. *Intensive Care Med.* 2015;41(3):452–459.
17. Sackett DL, Haynes RB, Guyatt GH, Tugwell P, eds. Clinical Epidemiology: *A Basic Science for Clinical Medicine.* 2nd ed. Boston, MA: Little, Brown and Company; 1991.
18. U.S. Preventive Services Task Force. Recommendation topics. Accessed January 15, 2024. https://www.uspreventiveservicestaskforce.org/uspstf/recommendation-topics
19. Catalog of Bias Collaboration, Nunan D, Bankhead C, Aronson JK. Catalogue of Bias. Selection bias. Accessed January 16, 2024. https://catalogofbias.org/biases/selection-bias/
20. Catalog of Bias Collaboration, Banerjee A, Pluddemann A, O'Sullivan J, Nunan D. Catalogue of Bias. Performance bias. Accessed January 16, 2024. https://catalogofbias.org/biases/performance-bias/
21. Catalog of Bias Collaboration, Spencer EA, Brassey J. Catalogue of Bias. Ascertainment bias. Accessed January 16, 2024. https://catalogofbias.org/biases/ascertainment-bias/
22. Catalog of Bias Collaboration, Bankhead C, Aronson JK, Nunan D. Catalogue of Bias Attrition bias. Accessed January 16, 2024. https://catalogofbias.org/biases/attrition-bias/#preventive
23. de Koning HJ, van der Aalst CM, de Jong PA, et al. Reduced lung-cancer mortality with volume CT screening in a randomized trial. *N Engl J Med.* 2020;382(6):503–513.
24. Sarfati D, Howden-Chapman P, Woodward A, Salmond C. Does the frame affect the picture? A study into how attitudes to screening for cancer are affected by the way benefits are expressed. *J Med Screen.* 1998;5(3):137–40.
25. Epstein RM, Alper BS, Quill TE. Communicating evidence for participatory decision making. *JAMA.* 2004;291(19):2359–2366.
26. Searight R. Realistic approaches to counseling in the office setting. *Am Fam Physician.* 2009;79(4):277–284.
27. Stacey D, LégaréF, Lewis K, et al. Decision aids for people facing health treatment or screening decisions. *Cochrane Database Syst Rev.* 2017;4:CD001431.

CHAPTER

9

Basic Principles and Techniques: Point-of-Care Ultrasound

POINT-OF-CARE ULTRASOUND

In recent years, point-of-care ultrasound (POCUS) has emerged as a revolutionary tool in clinical medicine, significantly augmenting the traditional physical examination (PE) techniques that have been the cornerstone of patient assessment for centuries (Fig. 9-1). This advanced technology brings a new dimension to bedside evaluation, enabling clinicians to gain real-time visual insights into the patient's anatomy and physiology.

Traditionally, PEs have relied on the four basic techniques of inspection, palpation, percussion, and auscultation. These methods, while fundamental, often provide limited information and can sometimes lead to ambiguity in clinical diagnosis. POCUS, by contrast, offers a dynamic and immediate visual understanding of the patient's internal state, allowing for a more accurate and comprehensive assessment.

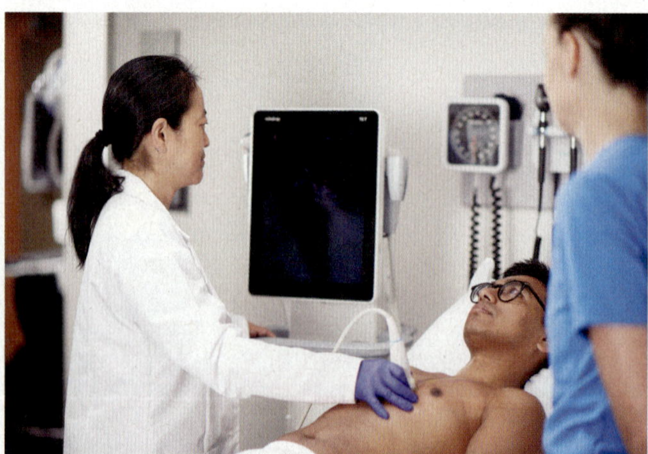

FIGURE 9-1. Point-of-care ultrasound (POCUS).

In modern health care, POCUS has become indispensable, enhancing diagnostic accuracy and patient care across a wide spectrum of clinical environments. Its ability to provide rapid and precise insights is invaluable in various settings, allowing for quick and effective decision-making. Moreover, POCUS's portability and noninvasive nature make it an ideal tool for bedside examination. It complements PE techniques by providing visual confirmation of clinical suspicions, ruling out pathologies, or guiding further diagnostic testing. This synergy of traditional and modern approaches not only enriches the clinician–patient interaction but also fosters a more holistic understanding of patient health.

Goal of the Chapter

The primary goal of this chapter is to introduce the basic POCUS terminology and techniques, particularly focusing on those that are both easy to perform *and* have equivalent PE findings through traditional methods (Boxes 9-1 and 9-2). This strategic approach aims to demonstrate how POCUS can effectively complement and reinforce findings obtained from conventional PE methods. The content has been meticulously curated to ensure you gain a foundational understanding of how POCUS can be applied across a variety of clinical scenarios.

Importantly, while theoretical knowledge provides a solid foundation, the mastery of POCUS skills is greatly enhanced through practical, hands-on practice. Engaging with the ultrasound machine directly by participating in courses or rotations specifically focused on POCUS is highly recommended for developing your proficiency in this innovative technique.

Box 9-1. Glossary of Key Terms in Point-of-Care Ultrasound

Term	Definition
Acoustic coupling gel	Medium applied between the ultrasound transducer and skin to reduce acoustic impedance and improve image quality.
Acoustic impedance	Property of a medium affecting the transmission and reflection of ultrasound waves, depending on its density
Anechoic	Refers to a structure that does not produce echoes and appears black on an ultrasound image, typically representing fluid or blood
B-mode (brightness mode)	Standard ultrasound imaging mode that produces two-dimensional grayscale images showing structural details
Calipers/measure	Tools used to measure structures on the ultrasound image
Depth	Control on the ultrasound machine that adjusts the depth of the field of view
Doppler modes	Techniques in ultrasound that measure and visualize blood flow; includes color Doppler and pulsed-wave Doppler
Echogenicity	Property of a tissue to reflect ultrasound waves, which determines its appearance on an ultrasound image; categorized into various types
Endocavitary transducer	High-frequency probe with a sector-shaped image and small curved footprint, used for gynecologic, obstetric, and intraoral imaging
Gain	Setting on the ultrasound machine that adjusts the brightness of the returning echoes, affecting image contrast
Hyperechoic	Describes structures that produce strong echoes and appear bright or white on the ultrasound, such as bones, gallstones, or pleura
Hypoechoic	Indicates medium echo-producing structures that appear in varying shades of gray, like solid organs or tissues
Isoechoic	Describes areas with similar echogenicity to each other
Knobology	Study of the controls and settings of an ultrasound machine to optimize image quality
Linear transducer	High-frequency probe with a rectangular image and long narrow footprint, used for soft tissue, musculoskeletal, and procedural guidance imaging
M-mode (motion mode)	Captures motion over time, useful for visualizing moving structures like heart valves or pleura
Phased array transducer	Low-frequency probe with a sector-shaped image and small footprint, suitable for cardiac and abdominal imaging
Piezoelectric crystals	Components in an ultrasound probe that vibrate to generate ultrasound waves when electrical signals are applied
Point-of-care ultrasound (POCUS)	Bedside ultrasound technique that provides real-time visual information about anatomy and pathophysiology during a clinical examination
Probe movements	Ways to manipulate the ultrasound probe include rocking, fanning, rotating, sliding, sweeping, and pressure

(continued)

Box 9-1. Glossary of Key Terms in Point-of-Care Ultrasound (*Continued*)

Term	Definition
Transducer (probe)	Device that converts electrical energy into mechanical energy (sound) and vice versa, used in ultrasound to create and capture images
Curvilinear transducer	Low-frequency probe with a sector-shaped image and large curved footprint, used for abdominal imaging.
Ultrasound transducer types	Describes different types of probes like curvilinear, phased array, linear, and endocavitary, each with specific uses

Box 9-2. Clinical Correlation of Physical Examination with Point-of-Care Ultrasound Findings

Pathology	Traditional PE Technique and Findings	POCUS Technique	POCUS Findings	Chapter Section
Cellulitis	Inspection: redness, warmth, and sometimes swelling Palpation: tenderness and skin warmth	Patient position: supine Transducer probe: linear probe Imaging mode: B-mode	Appears as "cobblestoning"; note that pitting edema can sometimes mimic cellulitis on ultrasound	Chapter 12, Skin, Hair, and Nails, pp. 265–267
Abscess	Palpation: defined fluid collection with tenderness	Patient position: supine Transducer probe: linear probe Imaging mode: B-mode	Characterized by a defined anechoic or heterogeneous fluid collection that swirls with pressure, often with posterior acoustic enhancement	Chapter 12, Skin, Hair, and Nails, pp. 265–267
Congestive heart failure (CHF) (pulmonary edema)	Inspection: signs of respiratory distress, including increased work of breathing Palpation: increased chest wall movement due to labored breathing Auscultation: crackles (rales) in the lungs	Patient position: supine Transducer probe: curvilinear probe Imaging mode: B-mode	B-lines and pleural effusion	Chapter 17, Thorax and Lungs, pp. 448–449
Left ventricular systolic function (LVSF)	Palpation: displaced apical impulse and a laterally displaced point of maximal impulse (PMI) Auscultation: abnormal heart sounds like S_3 or S_4	Patient position: left lateral decubitus Transducer probe: phased array (cardiac) probe Imaging mode: M-mode, two-dimensional, Doppler	Reduced LVSF may show decreased left ventricular contractility and abnormal wall motion.	Chapter 18, Cardiovascular System, pp. 514–516

Pathology	Traditional PE Technique and Findings	POCUS Technique	POCUS Findings	Chapter Section
Nonpalpable peripheral pulses	Palpation: strength and regularity of peripheral pulses Absent or diminished pulses may indicate vascular compromise	Patient position: comfortable position Transducer probe: linear probe with color/ spectral Doppler Imaging mode: color/ spectral Doppler	Visualizes peripheral arteries and assesses blood flow; can identify pulsations or the absence of pulsations in the arteries	Chapter 19, Peripheral Vascular System, pp. 563–564
Deep vein thrombosis (DVT)	Inspection: may show unilateral limb swelling, and palpation may detect tenderness and warmth in the affected area Auscultation: not typically used for DVT assessment	Patient position: supine Transducer probe: linear probe with compression ultrasound Imaging mode: compression ultrasound	Can visualize deep veins to identify thrombi; DVT may show anechoic intraluminal filling defects in the veins	Chapter 19, Peripheral Vascular System, pp. 564–566
Liver enlargement	Palpation: palpable liver edge during abdominal palpation	Patient position: supine Transducer probe: curvilinear probe, adjust the ultrasound machine settings for optimal liver size measurement and pattern visualization	Measures liver size and compare it to normal; a "starry night" pattern may be visible in hepatitis or a nodular appearance in cirrhosis	Chapter 21, Abdomen, pp. 645–646
Gallbladder pathology	Palpation: positive Murphy sign (pain on inspiration during palpation of the RUQ)	Patient position: supine Transducer probe: curvilinear probe Imaging mode: B-mode	Visualizes gallstones, sonographic Murphy sign, thickened gallbladder wall, and pericholecystic fluid	Chapter 21, Abdomen, pp. 646–648
Bladder volume	Inspection: suprapubic fullness Percussion: tympanic sound over an enlarged bladder	Patient position: supine Transducer probe: curvilinear probe Imaging mode: B-mode with Doppler	Enlarged bladder depicted as an anechoic walled fluid collection in the suprapubic area	Chapter 24, Pelvis and Genitourinary System: Vulva, Vagina, Uterus, and Adnexa, pp. 757–758
Knee joint effusion	Inspection: joint swelling Palpation: fluid accumulation in the knee joint Percussion: can indicate increased fluid content	Patient position: supine Transducer probe: linear probe with Doppler capability Imaging mode: B-mode with Doppler	Can confirm the presence of knee joint effusion, which appears as an anechoic fluid collection near the joint space with no color flow or blood flow	Chapter 26, Musculoskeletal System: Back, Hips, and Lower Extremities, pp. 889–890

The landscape of ultrasound technology is constantly evolving, marked by enhancements in cost-efficiency, portability, and image quality. This ongoing development parallels the improvements seen in traditional diagnostic tools such as stethoscopes, sphygmomanometers, ophthalmoscopes, and otoscopes. Staying rooted in the principles of the scientific method while actively refining your clinical skills enables you to effectively incorporate these advancing technologies into your emerging clinical practice.

As we continue to witness rapid advancements in ultrasound technology, the role and significance of POCUS in clinical settings is set to expand further, promising a new era in the art and science of PE, promising enhanced diagnostic capabilities and a more comprehensive approach to patient care.

Enhancing Clinical Assessment: Insonation

In clinical practice, traditional assessment of organ systems has predominantly relied on techniques like inspection, palpation, percussion, and auscultation. Complementing these, this chapter introduces an essential addition to your diagnostic toolkit: *insonation*, a central aspect of POCUS. Central to the effective use of POCUS is the establishment of focused, binary clinical questions. These are straightforward inquiries that yield clear yes or no answers, such as: Is there a pericardial effusion? Are there gallstones? Is hydronephrosis present?

Employing such binary questions is a powerful strategy for supporting a specific hypothesis about a diagnosis or for narrowing down differential diagnoses. The operator-dependent nature of ultrasound underscores the need for skillful application. By concentrating on precise clinical questions and applying POCUS techniques under expert supervision, along with consistent guidance and feedback, you can refine your POCUS skills efficiently and effectively.

SOUND WAVES AND ULTRASOUND BASICS

Acquiring a basic understanding of acoustic physics is crucial for mastering POCUS imaging techniques. *Acoustic physics* explains how sound waves behave and interact with various mediums. In this section, we will explore these principles to understand how ultrasound machines use sound waves to create detailed internal images.

Sound Waves

Sound is a form of mechanical energy, and sound waves are generated by variations in pressure within a medium, such as body tissues. These variations create regions of high pressure (*compressions*) and low pressure (*rarefactions*) that move through the medium. Sound waves are measured in *hertz (Hz)*, representing the number of waves passing a point per second. Audible sound falls in the range of 20 Hz to 20,000 Hz, while ultrasound refers to frequencies above 20,000 Hz, typically in the range of 2 million to 20 million Hz.[1]

Acoustic Impedance in Ultrasound Imaging

The propagation speed of sound varies with the medium; it is fastest in bones and progressively slower in soft tissues, fluids, and gases. This variation affects sound wave transmission and reflection, a concept known as *acoustic impedance.*[2] It plays a pivotal role in ultrasound image quality.

High acoustic impedance, encountered when sound waves travel from soft tissue to denser structures like bone, leads to increased reflection and decreased transmission of these waves. This scenario often complicates image acquisition, as more sound waves are bounced back rather than passing through the tissues.

Conversely, *low acoustic impedance* occurs when sound waves move through materials with similar densities, such as from soft tissue through organs like the liver and kidney. In this case, there is less reflection and more transmission of sound waves, allowing better visualization of deeper structures.

The key to optimized ultrasound imaging lies in finding appropriate *acoustic windows*. These are areas in the body where the tissue density is akin to liquid, facilitating smoother sound wave transmission. Identifying and using these windows, such as the liver or bladder, is crucial for obtaining clear images. Specific windows suitable for each organ system will be detailed in respective chapters. Without finding and optimizing these acoustic windows, achieving a clear and accurate view can be challenging.

ULTRASOUND EQUIPMENT AND TECHNIQUE

Ultrasound Transducers

A *transducer* converts one form of energy to another. The ultrasound transducer, or *probe*, converts electrical energy into mechanical energy (i.e., sound) which is

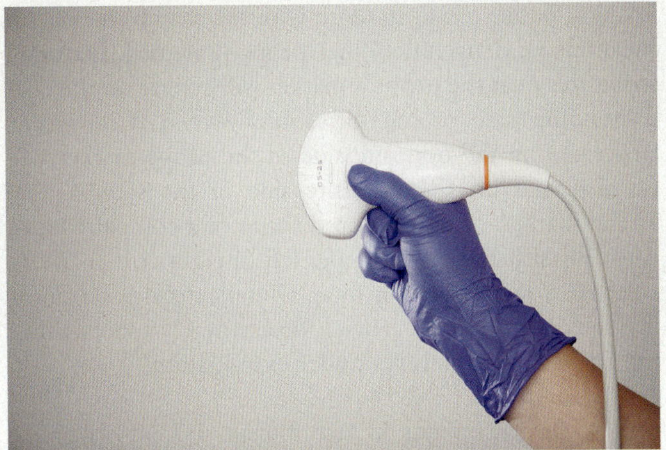

FIGURE 9-2. Ultrasound transducer.

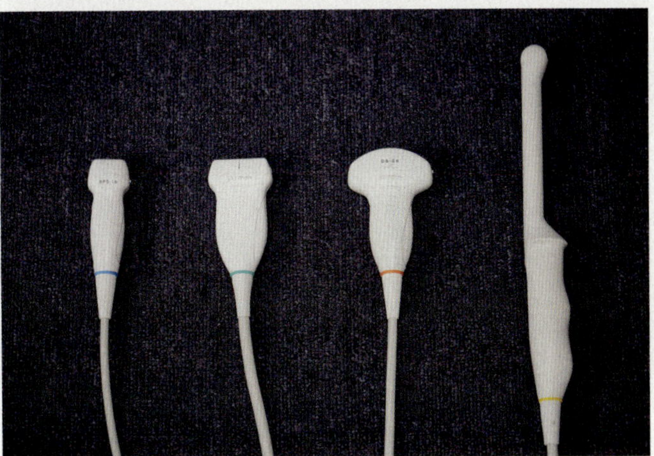

FIGURE 9-3. Common ultrasound probes used in POCUS. From left to right, phased array, linear, curvilinear, endocavitary.

directed into the patient's body. The sound waves that bounce back from the body are then transformed back into electrical signals to create an image (Fig. 9-2). This process is accomplished through *piezoelectric crystals* in the probe. These crystals vibrate at high speeds when electrical signals pass through them, generating ultrasound waves. The machine constantly emits and receives these waves, creating the images you see on the ultrasound screen.[1,2]

The choice of transducer depends on the specific body region being examined: high-frequency probes are optimal for superficial structures, whereas low-frequency probes are more suitable for deeper organs.[3] To facilitate effective sound transmission and reduce signal loss, an *acoustic coupling gel* is applied between the probe and the skin. It also facilitates movement of the probe on the skin and improves patient comfort.[4] Each probe has an area called the *footprint* that is typically a darker color and softer than the probe casing and will contact the gel on the skin.[5]

There are four commonly used types of probes in POCUS: phased array, curvilinear, linear, and endocavitary (Fig. 9-3).[1] Mastery in probe handling, including proper orientation and technique, is essential for generating accurate images (Box 9-3).

Box 9-3. Ultrasound Probe Specifications and Their Impact on Advanced Clinical Examination Techniques

Probe Type	Frequency	Characteristics	Applications in Clinical Examination
Curvilinear	Low	Wide sector-shaped image with a large, curved footprint for deep penetration	Suitable for general abdominal imaging, enhancing visualization of deep organs and structures, often replacing the need for deep palpation
Phased Array	Low	Sector-shaped image with a small footprint for fine intercostal use	Ideal for cardiac imaging, especially echocardiography, offering detailed views of heart structures; enhances pediatric abdominal exams where space is limited
Linear	High	Rectangular image with a high definition, long, narrow, and flat footprint for precise imaging	Essential for superficial soft tissue, musculoskeletal imaging, and procedural guidance; offers high-resolution images that can replace traditional palpation and inspection methods
Endocavitary	High	Sector-shaped image with a small, curved footprint for high-resolution imaging in confined spaces	Provides detailed imaging for gynecologic and obstetric examinations, enhancing or replacing bimanual exams and improving intraoral imaging beyond standard visual inspection

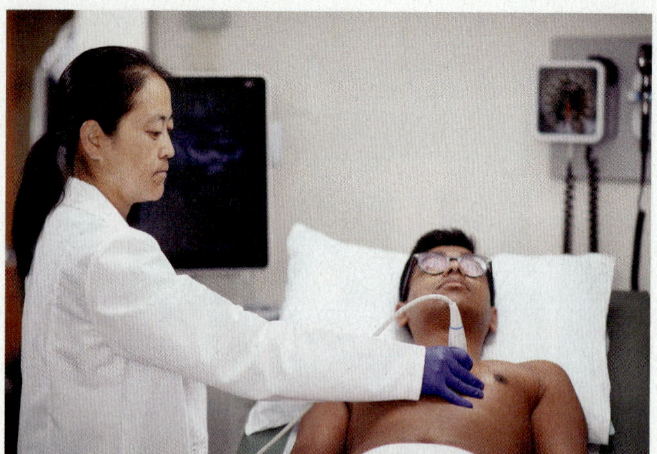

FIGURE 9-4. Proper positioning for POCUS imaging.

Image Acquisition

Beginning POCUS imaging calls for precision in both technique and positioning. These essential steps, starting from positioning to the final probe manipulation, ensure clarity and precision.

Step 1: Properly Position Yourself. To start POCUS imaging, position yourself as you would for a standard PE, facing both the patient and the ultrasound machine monitor (Fig. 9-4). Ensure you have a clear view of both the patient and the screen throughout the procedure. Hold the ultrasound probe firmly in your dominant hand. Familiarize yourself with the fundamental movements of the probe, as precise manipulation is essential for accurately evaluating anatomical structures.

Step 2: Hold the Probe Effectively. Ensure the probe is stable in your hand and can rest comfortably against the patient's body (Fig. 9-5). Adopt a grip similar to how you would hold a pencil or an otoscope for precision and control. Position your thumb, index, and middle finger around the neck of the probe to secure a firm grip, aiding in maneuvering the probe with precision. In addition, extend and rest your fourth and fifth fingers against the patient's body. This technique not only stabilizes the probe during scanning but also helps in maintaining steady contact without applying excessive pressure, critical for producing clear and accurate ultrasound images.[4] Remember, the stability of your hand and the probe directly impacts the quality of the images obtained, so practice this grip to ensure proficiency in probe handling.

Step 3: Probe and Screen Orientation. Each ultrasound probe comes with an orientation marker, typically a raised dot or an indentation. This marker is essential for accurate imaging because it must align with the screen marker on the ultrasound machine. When properly aligned, anatomic structures near the probe's marker will appear on the corresponding side of the ultrasound screen. Conversely, structures on the opposite side of the probe marker will be displayed on the opposite side of the screen. The screen marker, often a colored shape or a company logo, is usually situated in the upper left or right corner of the screen as you face the machine. Understanding and aligning these markers are crucial for accurately representing the anatomical structures under examination.[3,4]

Step 4: Obtain Images in Two Planes. When obtaining ultrasound images, you should capture both transverse and sagittal planes to accurately represent a three-dimensional structure in two-dimensional imaging.[3,4] For transverse views, align the probe marker with the screen marker to achieve a short-axis view. Typically, this entails orienting the probe marker toward the patient's right side as you face the ultrasound screen.

For sagittal views, turn the probe marker cephalad, along the long axis of the body. During most examinations, the patient will be in a supine position. Adhering to these directional conventions ensures that the ultrasound images are analogous to computed tomography scan images, in which the left side of the screen corresponds to the patient's right side, and vice versa for axial images.

In sagittal imaging, the patient's head is usually displayed on the left side of the screen, with their feet on

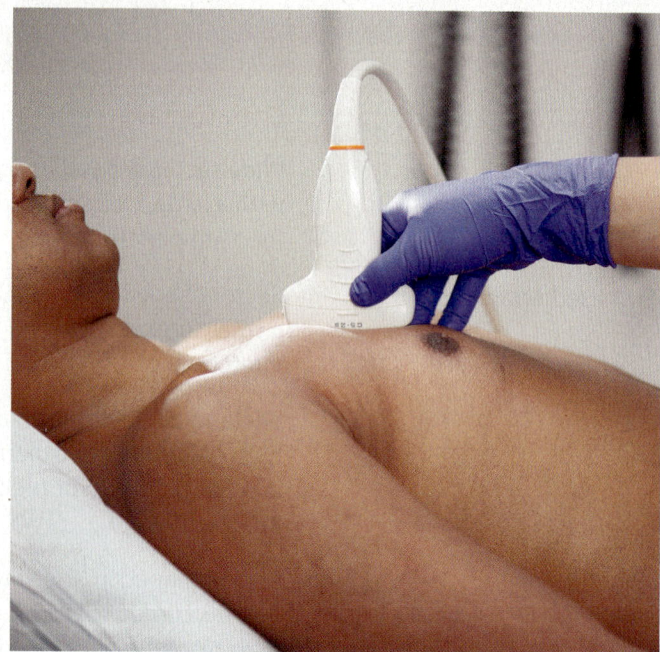

FIGURE 9-5. Hand position for holding an ultrasound probe.

the right. These conventions, including any exceptions, are elaborated in the relevant organ system chapters for specific examinations.

Step 5: Manipulate the Probe. In ultrasound imaging, probe manipulation is confined to three spatial dimensions.[6,7] To ensure uniform communication and technique, specific terms are used to describe each movement (Box 9-4). These movements are categorized based on whether they occur in a fixed location (rocking, fanning, rotating) or involve repositioning the probe (sliding, sweeping, applying pressure).

Box 9-4. Ultrasound Probe Movements

Category	Movement	Description	Purpose
Fixed-position movements	Rocking 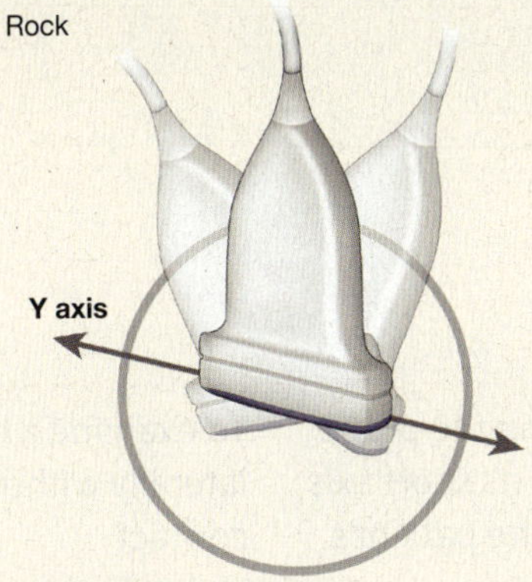	Tilting the probe side to side along its long axis	To view different angles of the same area without changing the probe's position
	Fanning 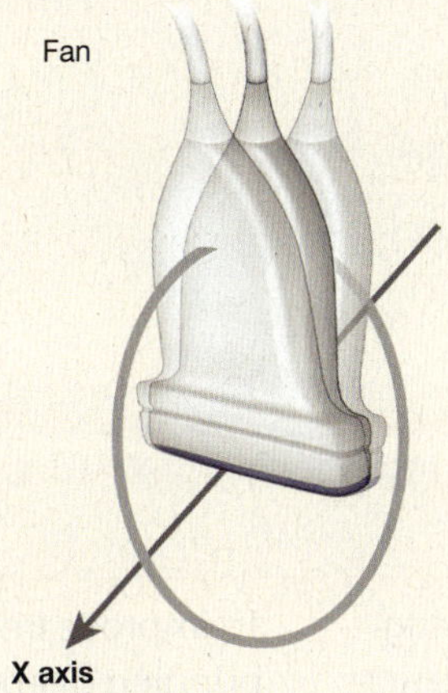	Tilting the probe side to side along its short axis	To broaden the scanned area across the region of interest while keeping the probe steady
	Rotating 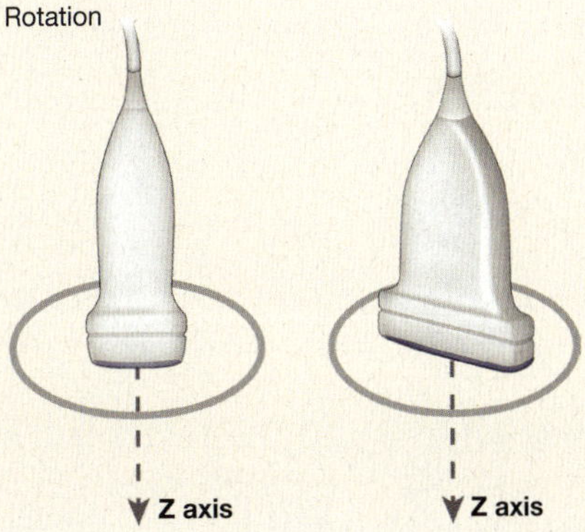	Twisting the probe around its own axis, clockwise or counterclockwise	To change the orientation of the scan plane for a comprehensive examination

(continued)

Box 9-4. Ultrasound Probe Movements (*Continued*)

Category	Movement	Description	Purpose
Repositioning movements	Sliding 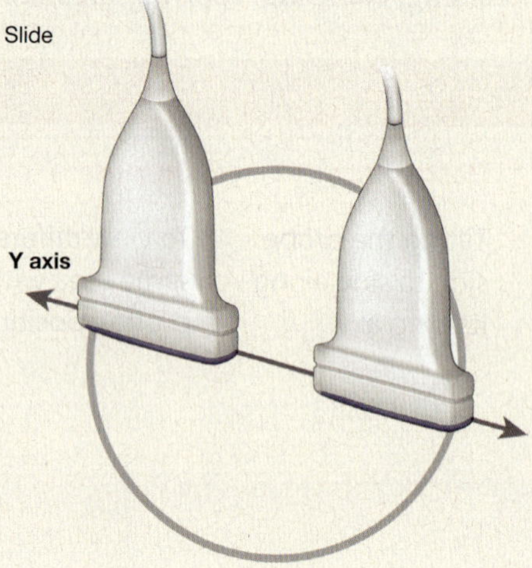 Slide Y axis	Moving the probe along its long axis across the patient's body	To explore a larger area while maintaining constant contact with the skin
	Sweeping 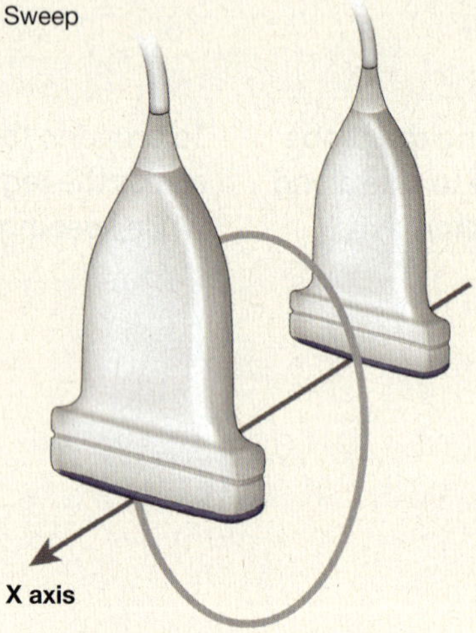 Sweep X axis	Moving the probe along its short axis over the patient's body	To examine a broader area laterally without losing skin contact
	Applying pressure 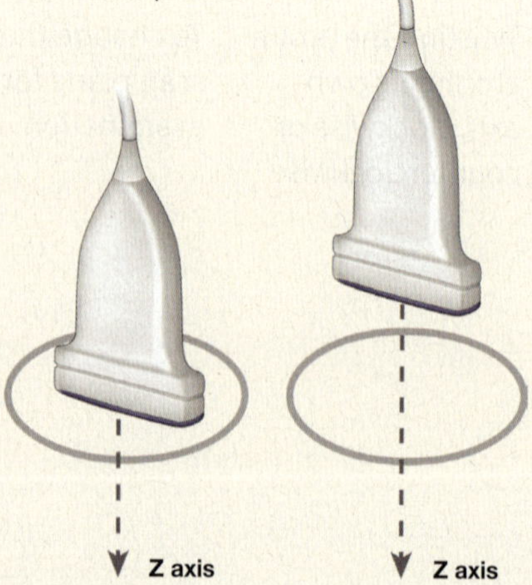 Pressure/compression Z axis Z axis	Gently pressing the probe against the patient's body	To improve image clarity by bringing deeper structures closer or reducing obstructions

UNDERSTANDING IMAGING MODES

Ultrasound machines offer various imaging modes to suit different diagnostic needs in POCUS. The three most commonly used modes are B-mode, M-mode, and Doppler mode. Each mode has specific applications and advantages in clinical examinations (Box 9-5).

B-Mode (Brightness Mode)

B-mode, or *brightness mode*, is the foundational imaging mode in POCUS. It is primarily used for producing two-dimensional grayscale images that provide detailed structural information.

The key to interpreting these images lies in understanding *echogenicity*, which refers to how bright or dark structures appear on the screen. This brightness corresponds to the amplitude of sound waves reflected back to the transducer, offering insights into the composition of tissues. Structures that reflect more sound waves appear brighter (*hyperechoic*), while those that reflect fewer waves appear darker (*anechoic* or *hypoechoic*). B-mode is versatile and invaluable in general examinations, particularly effective in identifying masses, fluid collections, and structural abnormalities across various organs and tissues (Box 9-6 and Fig. 9-6).

M-Mode (Motion Mode)[1,4]

M-mode, or *Motion mode*, brings a dynamic aspect to ultrasound imaging. It is uniquely suited for visualizing and analyzing motion, especially within the heart. In M-mode, a single line is selected from a B-mode image, and the motion along this line is tracked and displayed over time. This technique creates a time-motion graph that provides a detailed view of the moving structures, like the fluttering of heart valves, motion of heart walls, or sliding of pleura. This capability makes M-mode an essential tool in cardiac or lung motion assessments, allowing clinicians to observe and measure movement. (Fig. 9-7). By translating these

Box 9-5. Ultrasound Imaging Modes[1,4,5]

Ultrasound Mode	Description	Application in Clinical Examination
B-mode (brightness mode)	■ Produces two-dimensional grayscale images for detailed structural information ■ Echogenicity describes the brightness based on reflected sound waves	General examination of organs and tissues; identification of masses, fluid collections, and structural abnormalities
M-mode (motion mode)	■ Visualizes motion over time by following a single line from a B-mode image ■ Useful for tracking movement of structures like heart valves or lung sliding	Assessment of cardiac or lung function, particularly valvular movements or lung motion.
Doppler mode: color	■ Uses visual color (red and blue) to indicate flow direction toward or away from the probe ■ Color scale is in the upper left of the screen	Evaluates direction and velocity of blood flow but cannot assess flow perpendicular to the probe
Doppler mode: pulsed wave	■ Uses waveforms and acoustics to determine if flow is going toward or away from the probe ■ Arterial waveforms are pulsatile, individual peaks while venous waveforms are continuous and band-like ■ Plots echo velocities along a baseline ■ Flow toward the probe is above the baseline and flow away is below the baseline	Determines blood flow direction and velocity; effective for assessing arterial and venous waveforms

Sources: Au A, Zwank M. Physics and Technical Facts for the Beginner. Accessed January 15, 2024. https://www.acep.org/sonoguide/basic/ultrasound-physics-and-technical-facts-for-the-beginner/; Noble VE, Nelson B. *Manual of emergency and critical care ultrasound*. 2nd ed. Cambridge medicine. Cambridge University Press; 2011:xi, 346 pages; Dinh V. Ultrasound Machine Basics-Knobology, Probes, and Modes. Accessed January 15, 2024. https://www.pocus101.com/ultrasound-machine-basics-knobology-probes-and-modes/

Box 9-6. Echogenicity Types in Ultrasound Imaging: B-Mode[1,3,4]

Echogenicity	Characteristics	Examples
Anechoic	Characterized by minimal returning echoes, appearing black on the screen Indicates areas where ultrasound waves pass freely, like fluid-filled spaces	Commonly seen in structures like simple cysts, the urinary bladder, and blood vessels
Hyperechoic	Exhibits strong echoes, appearing bright or white Indicates denser tissues that reflect more sound waves	Bones, tendons, and the pericardium, which are denser compared to surrounding tissues
Hypoechoic	Shows medium-strength echoes, appearing as shades of gray Relative term comparing tissues that are less echogenic than others	Used to describe solid organs or tissues like the liver and kidneys, which are less dense than bones but denser than fluid-filled structures

Sources: Au A, Zwank M. Physics and Technical Facts for the Beginner. Accessed January 15, 2024. https://www.acep.org/sonoguide/basic/ultrasound-physics-and-technical-facts-for-the-beginner/; Loukas M, Burns D. *Essential Ultrasound Anatomy*. Wolters Kluwer; 2020:xi, 275 pages; Noble VE, Nelson B. *Manual of Emergency and Critical Care ultrasound*. 2nd ed. Cambridge medicine. Cambridge University Press; 2011:xi, 346 pages.

movements into a traceable and interpretable pattern, M-mode offers a deeper understanding of cardiac or lung function and anomalies.

Doppler Modes, Color, and Pulsed Wave

Doppler modes in ultrasound imaging capitalize on the *Doppler effect*, which is a change in frequency or wavelength of sound waves as they reflect off moving objects. This principle is similar to the changing pitch of a siren as an ambulance approaches and then moves away from a listener.

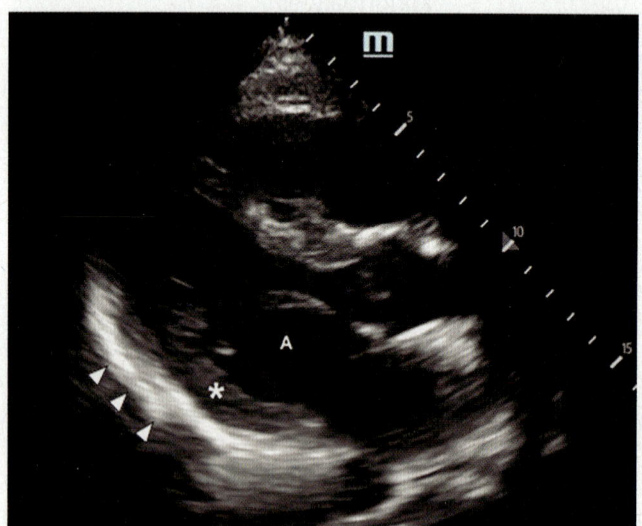

FIGURE 9-6. Echogenicity. In this parasternal long view of the heart, note the hypoechoic myocardium (*) is defined relative to the black, anechoic blood (A) and hyperechoic pericardium (arrowheads). Different areas with the same echogenicity are referred to as being isoechoic with each other.

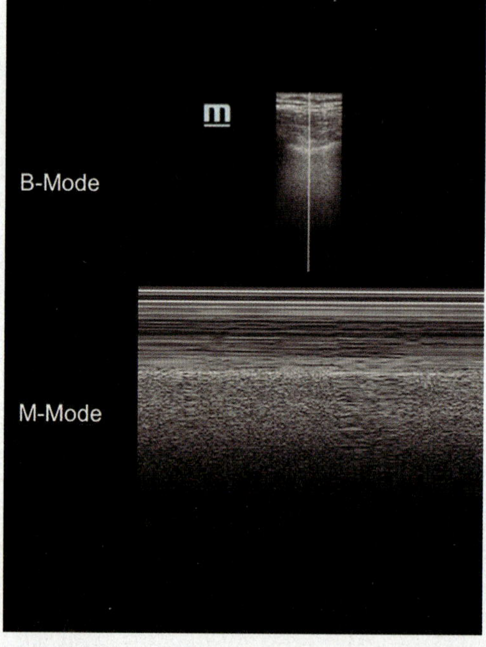

FIGURE 9-7. M-mode. In this image, evaluating lung sliding, the echoes returning along the line in the top B-mode image are plotted over time thus creating the M-mode image. Within the M-mode, the straight lines correspond to a minimally moving object (the chest wall) and the grainy area corresponds to the lung sliding. M-mode is useful in visualizing rapidly moving objects and in detailing motion with a still image.

This mode is divided into two primary types. *Color Doppler* uses colors (typically red and blue) to represent the direction of blood flow relative to the probe, employing the mnemonic "BART" (Blue Away, Red Toward the transducer) to aid in interpretation. This visual representation is invaluable for evaluating blood flow direction and velocity, particularly in cardiac and vascular examinations.

On the other hand, *pulsed-wave Doppler* provides a more quantitative assessment of blood flow. It uses waveforms to display the velocity of blood flow, distinguishing between arterial (pulsatile) and venous (continuous) flow patterns. This mode is crucial for a detailed analysis of blood flow characteristics in various clinical scenarios, from assessing heart valve functions to detecting vascular abnormalities (Fig. 9-8).

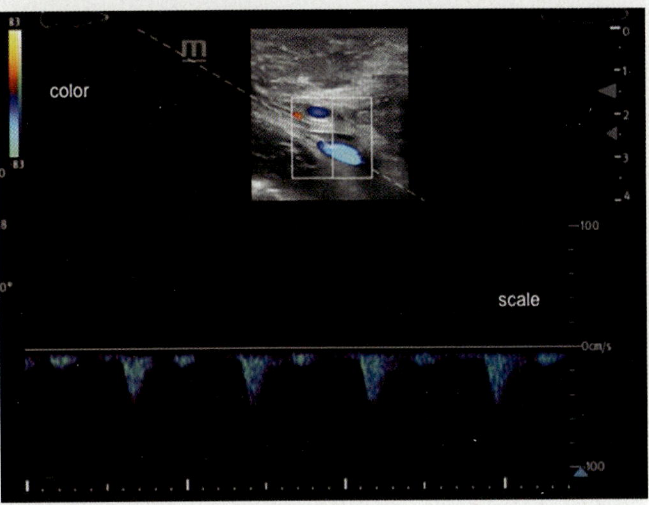

FIGURE 9-8. Color and pulsed-wave Doppler. Note the color scale in the upper left corner, where red/yellow is the flow toward the probe and blue is the flow away from the probe. The right lower scale represents the velocity of flow, which is measured using pulsed-wave Doppler.

ULTRASOUND IMAGE OPTIMIZATION ("KNOBOLOGY")

After applying the probe with a sufficient amount of gel and directing sound into the body through an effective acoustic window (like a fluid-rich structure, such as a full bladder or the liver), it is important to optimize the ultrasound machine's settings.

Machine Settings and Adjustments

Most ultrasound machines are equipped with organ-specific presets that automatically adjust settings like depth and gain for optimal imaging of particular organs. While presets provide a quick starting point, manual adjustments tailor the imaging to specific patient conditions and anatomical variations. Developing a good understanding of when and how to adjust these settings manually is a key skill in POCUS (Box 9-7).

The details of optimizing images for specific organ systems and examinations are thoroughly covered in the respective organ system chapters. Understanding these settings and how to adjust them is essential for acquiring high-quality ultrasound images and making accurate clinical assessments.

Box 9-7. Common Ultrasound Imaging Settings[5]

Setting	Description	Examples
Depth	Adjusts the penetration of ultrasound waves Target anatomy should be centered on the screen, neither too deep nor too shallow	Peripheral veins may be just a few centimeters deep, whereas cardiac views might require depths of 10–15 cm
Gain	Controls the brightness of the image by adjusting the intensity of returning echoes Aim for a balance, where the image has a spectrum from black (low echo) to white (high echo) to delineate tissue differences effectively	Lower the gain to distinguish blood within a vessel (appearing black) from the surrounding tissue (gray) Ideal image should not be overly bright (overgained) or too dark (undergained)
Calipers/ measure	Used for precise measurement of structures on the screen, ensuring accurate size assessment of anatomical features	Measure the liver, bladder size, or the thickness of the gallbladder wall for accurate diagnosis

Source: Dinh V. Ultrasound Machine Basics-Knobology, Probes, and Modes. Accessed January 15, 2024. https://www.pocus101.com/ultrasound-machine-basics-knobology-probes-and-modes/

REFERENCES

1. Au A, Zwank M. Physics and Technical Facts for the Beginner. Sonoguide. Accessed January 15, 2024. https://www.acep.org/sonoguide/basic/ultrasound-physics-and-technical-facts-for-the-beginner/
2. Middleton WD, Hertzberg BS. *Ultrasound: The Requisites.* 3rd ed. Elsevier; 2016;xv, 612.
3. Loukas M, Burns D. *Essential Ultrasound Anatomy.* Wolters Kluwer; 2020:xi, 275.
4. Noble VE, Nelson B. *Manual of Emergency and Critical Care Ultrasound.* 2nd ed. Cambridge University Press; 2011;xi: 346.
5. Dinh V. Ultrasound Machine Basics-Knobology, Probes, and Modes. Pocus 101. Accessed January 15, 2024. https://www.pocus101.com/ultrasound-machine-basics-knobology-probes-and-modes/
6. Alberta Sono. Transducer Manipulation. Accessed January 15, 2024. https://www.albertasono.ca/sonology/transducer-manipulation/
7. Bahner DP, Blickendorf JM, Bockbrader M, et al. Language of transducer manipulation: codifying terms for effective teaching. *J Ultrasound Med.* 2016;35(1):183–188.

UNIT 2 Regional Examinations

CHAPTER 10

General Survey, Vital Signs, and Pain

HEALTH HISTORY: GENERAL APPROACH

This chapter focuses on patient concerns collectively known as *constitutional symptoms*. These symptoms, commonly accompanying various diseases, are often not confined to just one specific organ system; instead, they broadly affect a patient's "constitution," or their physical state with regard to vitality, health, and strength.[1] Examples include *fatigue*, *weakness*, *fever*, *chills*, *night sweats*, *weight loss or weight gain*, and *pain*. Regularly asking patients about these symptoms allows for proactive diagnosis and treatment. Even if the exact cause remains elusive, implementing robust strategies to manage such symptoms can greatly improve the patient's quality of life.[2]

Common or Concerning Symptoms

- Fatigue and weakness
- Fever and night sweats
- Weight change
- Pain

Fatigue and Weakness

Fatigue, often described by patients as a profound sense of weariness or energy loss, can manifest in statements like, "I struggle to start my day," or "I'm exhausted by the time I start work." Although fatigue is a natural response to heavy work, prolonged stress, and emotional distress, understanding the context in which it arises is important. Fatigue unrelated to such situations requires further investigation.

Use open-ended questions to encourage the patient to fully describe what they are experiencing. Taking an insightful psychosocial history, understanding sleep habits, and conducting a detailed review of systems often provides valuable cues to the root cause of fatigue (Box 10-1).

Weakness is different from fatigue. It denotes a demonstrable loss of muscle power and is discussed with other neurologic symptoms in Chapter 27, Nervous System, pp. 912–914.

Box 10-1. Fatigue: High-Yield Health History Questions

Domain	Questions	Rationale
Duration and Onset	*When did the fatigue start?* *Was it sudden or gradual?*	Acute presentations often align with sudden illnesses or disruptions, while chronic issues tend to manifest gradually. *Sudden onset:* Acute infections like mononucleosis, recent blood loss leading to anemia *Gradual onset:* Chronic diseases such as hypothyroidism, malignancies, or chronic fatigue syndrome
Severity and Pattern	*How do you rate your fatigue on a scale of 1–10?* *Is it constant or does it come and go?*	The intensity and pattern can hint at the systemic impact and potential triggers. *Constant:* Chronic diseases, ongoing mental health issues *Intermittent*: Factors like circadian rhythm disturbances, periodic exertion, or intermittent stressors
Associated Symptoms	*Any weight changes? Any fever, night sweats, or lymphadenopathy?* *Any sleep disturbances or snoring?*	Symptoms accompanying fatigue can point to systemic conditions. *Weight loss:* Malignancies, hyperthyroidism *Fever/night sweats:* Tuberculosis, lymphomas, chronic infections *Snoring*: Sleep apnea, leading to nonrestorative sleep
Lifestyle	*How is your sleep routine?* *What is your diet like?* *Any recent changes in activity levels or stress?*	Lifestyle choices can be primary causes or exacerbate underlying conditions. *Poor sleep*: Poor sleep hygiene, insomnia *Poor diet:* Iron-deficiency anemia from dietary insufficiency *Increased stress:* Occupational burnout, high cortisol levels
Psychosocial	*How is your mood lately?* *Feeling stressed or anxious?* *Any recent losses or life changes?*	Mental health is intrinsically tied to fatigue. *Low mood*: Major depressive disorder, dysthymia *High stress*: Generalized anxiety disorder *Recent loss*: Bereavement, major life adjustments leading to adjustment disorders

Causes include **hematologic disorders** (e.g., anemia, where decreased hemoglobin levels impair oxygen delivery to tissues, leading to symptoms like pallor and shortness of breath), **cardiac causes** (e.g., heart failure, result in inadequate blood circulation and subsequent tissue hypoxia, manifesting as fatigue even with minimal exertion), **chronic kidney disease** (by failing to adequately excrete waste products, can induce a state of chronic fatigue and weakness), **neurologic disorders** (e.g., multiple sclerosis or myasthenia gravis directly affect nerve or muscle function, leading to muscle weakness and fatigue), **sleep disorders** (obstructive sleep apnea, where interrupted breathing leads to poor sleep quality and daytime tiredness), and **mental health disorders** (e.g., depression and anxiety can manifest physically, often presenting with persistent fatigue and lack of energy).

Domain	Questions	Rationale
Medical History	*Any history of cardiac, pulmonary, renal, or liver diseases?* *Previous diagnoses of anemia or endocrine disorders?*	Underlying chronic conditions may manifest or exacerbate fatigue. *Cardiac history*: Reduced cardiac output in heart failure *Pulmonary history*: Reduced oxygenation in chronic obstructive pulmonary disease, asthma *Renal history*: Electrolyte imbalances in chronic kidney disease

Fever and Night Sweats

Fever refers to an abnormal elevation in body temperature (see p. 183 for definitions of normal) and is the body's responses to various internal and external triggers. Find out if the patient has measured their own temperature. Focus on the timing of the illness and its associated symptoms (Box 10-2). Be aware that recent ingestion of aspirin, acetaminophen, corticosteroids, and nonsteroidal anti-inflammatory drugs may mask fever and affect the temperature recorded during the clinical encounter.

General causes include **bacterial**, **viral**, and **fungal infections** (e.g., tuberculosis and endocarditis that may present with prolonged fever and drenching night sweats), **inflammatory disorders** (e.g., in rheumatoid arthritis and systemic lupus erythematosus, the body's immune response results in fever and other systemic symptoms), **malignancies** (cancers, notably lymphomas, can present with intermittent or persistent fever and profound night sweats), **medications** (certain antibiotics and *antipyretics*, intended to reduce fever, can paradoxically induce fever and exacerbate night sweats as side effects).

Box 10-2. Fever and Night Sweats: High-Yield Health History Questions

Domain	Questions	Rationale
Duration and Onset	*When did the symptoms start?* *Were they sudden or gradual?*	Understanding the timeline can help distinguish between acute and chronic conditions. *Sudden onset*: Influenza, acute bacterial infections *Gradual onset:* Tuberculosis, lymphoma
Associated Symptoms	*Any weight loss?* *Any cough or shortness of breath?* *Any joint pains or rashes?*	Concomitant symptoms can help narrow down potential etiologies. *Weight loss and cough:* Tuberculosis, lung cancer *Joint pains/rashes:* Rheumatologic conditions like systemic lupus erythematosus and rheumatoid arthritis
Exposure History	*Recent travel?* *Exposure to sick contacts?* *Any animal exposures?*	Understanding potential exposures can hint at specific infectious agents or environmental factors. *Travel to endemic areas:* Malaria, typhoid *Sick contacts:* Viral infections, streptococcal infections

(*continued*)

Box 10-2. Fever and Night Sweats: High-Yield Health History Questions (*Continued*)

Domain	Questions	Rationale
Medical History	*Any previous diagnoses of chronic diseases?* *Are your immunizations up to date?* *Any history of similar symptoms or recurrent fevers?*	Past medical events might provide clues to current conditions or hint at recurrent issues. *Chronic diseases:* HIV leading to opportunistic infections *Recurrent fevers:* Familial Mediterranean fever, cyclic neutropenia
Medication and Substance Use	*Any new medications started recently?* *Are you using any over-the-counter medications, supplements, or illicit drugs?*	Some medications and substances can induce fevers or mimic infectious symptoms. *New medications:* Drug fever from antibiotics, antiepileptics *Illicit drugs:* Fevers associated with certain substances like cocaine or amphetamines

Weight Change

Weight change, whether a gain or loss, can be indicative of underlying medical, psychological, or lifestyle factors. *Weight loss* is defined as unintentional loss of 5% or more of usual body weight over a period of 6 to 12 months (or less). *Weight gain* occurs when caloric intake exceeds caloric expenditure over time and typically results in increased body fat. Objective guidelines for weight gain are less standardized than for weight loss. However, rapid, unintended weight gain over a short period can be concerning. Weight gain can also reflect abnormal accumulation of body fluids, particularly when the gain is very rapid.

If weight gain or loss appears to be a problem, ask about the magnitude, speed, and context of weight fluctuations. A thorough clinical evaluation to identify potential causes or contributing factors is warranted (Box 10-3).

Patients with a body mass index (BMI) of $\geq$25 kg/m^2 to 29 kg/m^2 are defined as *overweight;* those with a BMI $\geq$30 kg/m^2 are considered *obese*. For these patients, plan a thorough assessment to avert the many associated risks of morbidity and mortality.

Pain

The International Association for the Study of Pain defines *pain* as "an unpleasant sensory and emotional experience associated with, or resembling that associated with, actual or potential tissue damage." The experience of pain is complex and multifactorial. Pain involves sensory, emotional, and

Box 10-3. Weight Change: High-Yield Health History Questions

Domain	Questions	Rationale
Duration and Onset	*When did you notice the weight change?* *Was it intentional or unintentional?*	Understanding the onset can help distinguish between acute and chronic conditions. *Rapid loss:* Overactive thyroid, malignancy, acute illness *Rapid gain:* Fluid retention due to heart failure, kidney disease, or medication side effect
Associated Symptoms	*Any changes in appetite?* *Fatigue, palpitations, or heat intolerance?* *Changes in bowel habits or swelling in extremities?*	Additional symptoms can guide the differential diagnosis. *Appetite and fatigue:* Hyperthyroidism, diabetes *Bowel changes:* Inflammatory bowel disease, colorectal cancer
Lifestyle and Diet	*Any changes in eating habits or diet?* *Any new medications, supplements, or herbal products?* *Any alcohol or drug use?*	Lifestyle factors might be the primary cause or exacerbate underlying issues. *Diet changes:* Eating disorders, malnutrition *Medication use:* Steroids leading to weight gain, some antidepressants
Psychosocial	*Any recent stress, depression, or anxiety?* *Have there been changes in work, relationships, or daily routines?*	Mental health and life events can significantly affect weight. *Stress/Depression:* Can lead to weight loss (reduced appetite) or weight gain (comfort eating) *Life changes:* New job, divorce, bereavement affecting daily routines and eating habits
Medical History	*Any history of thyroid issues, diabetes, or gastrointestinal problems?* *Any previous surgeries, especially involving the gastrointestinal tract?*	Underlying conditions or interventions might be the root cause. *Thyroid issues:* Hyperthyroidism leading to weight loss, hypothyroidism causing weight gain *Surgeries:* Malabsorption postgastrectomy

Causes associated with *weight gain* include **endocrine disorders** (hypothyroidism in which decreased thyroid hormone levels lead to a reduced basal metabolic rate and clinical manifestations like lethargy and cold intolerance), **Cushing syndrome** (resulting from prolonged exposure to glucocorticoids, either from endogenous sources like adrenal tumors or exogenous steroid therapy, presenting with features like central obesity and moon facies), **medications** (certain antidepressants, antipsychotics, and corticosteroids can induce weight gain due to appetite stimulation or metabolic changes), and **lifestyle factors** (e.g., caloric excess and reduced physical activity).

Causes associated with *weight loss* encompass **endocrine disorders (hyperthyroidism** in which elevated thyroid hormone levels increase basal metabolic rate, leading to clinical features like tremors and heat intolerance), **uncontrolled diabetes mellitus** (persistent hyperglycemia due to insulin deficiency or resistance, presenting with polyuria, polydipsia, and polyphagia), **gastrointestinal (GI) disorders** (Crohn's and celiac disease impair nutrient absorption and may manifest with diarrhea and abdominal pain), and **malignancies** (cancers, particularly GI or pulmonary origins, can present with cachexia and a constellation of systemic symptoms).

cognitive processing but may lack a specific physical etiology.[3] Adopt a multidisciplinary, measurement-based approach to assessing pain, carefully listening to the patient's story and being mindful of the many features of pain and its contributing factors.[4,5] Elicit the full history of the patient's pain, tailoring your approach to each patient's unique experience (Box 10-4).

See Chapter 3, Health History, for discussion of Attributes of a Symptom, p. 49. See section on Acute and Chronic Pain, pp. 185–188, for an approach to assessment.

Causes include *neuropathic pain* such as in **diabetic neuropathy** (prolonged hyperglycemia injures nerve fibers, presenting with tingling or burning sensations) and **post-herpetic neuralgia** (persistent pain after an outbreak of shingles, characterized by sharp, electric-like pain); *musculoskeletal pain* such as in **osteoarthritis** (joint degeneration leads to pain on movement) and **rheumatoid arthritis** (autoimmune disorder in which the body's immune response targets joint linings, resulting in painful joint inflammation); *visceral pain* like **angina** (stemming from myocardial ischemia, often described as a squeezing or pressure-like sensation) and **inflammatory pain** (due to tissue damage and inflammation, as seen in conditions like appendicitis or pancreatitis, presenting with sharp, localized pain). **Medications** and **therapeutic interventions** (certain chemotherapy agents causing neuropathic pain and postsurgical pain) can also be implicated in the onset and exacerbation of pain syndromes.

Box 10-4. Pain: High-Yield Health History Questions

Domain	Questions	Rationale
Location and Radiation	*Where is the pain located?* *Does it radiate or move to any other area?*	Pinpointing the location can help identify the affected organ or tissue. *Chest pain radiating to arm:* Myocardial infarction *Right lower quadrant pain:* Appendicitis
Character and Quality	*How would you describe the pain (e.g., sharp, dull, burning, throbbing)?* *Does it come and go, or is it constant?*	The nature of pain can hint at its etiology. *Burning pain:* Neuralgia, gastric ulcer *Throbbing pain:* Migraine, abscess
Duration and Onset	*When did the pain start?* *Was it sudden or gradual?* *How long does each episode last?*	Acute vs. chronic onset can help identify the potential cause. *Sudden severe pain:* Kidney stone, gallstone *Gradual pain:* Arthritis, cancer
Aggravating and Relieving Factors	*What makes the pain worse (e.g., movement, pressure, eating)?* *What makes it better (e.g., rest, medication)?*	These can help narrow down the diagnosis and potential interventions. *Pain with movement:* Musculoskeletal injury *Pain relieved by eating:* Duodenal ulcer
Associated Symptoms	*Any swelling, redness, or warmth in the area?* *Any numbness, tingling, or weakness?* *Other systemic symptoms like fever or fatigue?*	Additional symptoms can guide the differential diagnosis. *Pain with redness and warmth:* Cellulitis, gout *Pain with numbness and tingling:* Nerve impingement, neuropathy

PHYSICAL EXAMINATION: GENERAL APPROACH

The skills of observation begin with the opening moments of the patient encounter. The best clinicians continually sharpen their powers of observation and description of the encounter. As you talk with and examine a patient, heighten your focus on their mood, build, and behavior. These details enrich and deepen your emerging clinical impression. Your goal is to describe the patient's distinguishing features so clearly that colleagues could spot that patient in a crowd of strangers, avoiding clichés like "middle-aged gentleman" and uninformative statements such as "in no acute distress."

TECHNIQUES OF EXAMINATION

Key Components of the General Survey, Vital Signs, and Pain Assessment

- Perform a general survey.
- Measure height and weight.
- Measure blood pressure using a sphygmomanometer.
- Examine arterial pulses for rate and rhythm.
- Observe respiratory rate, rhythm, depth, and effort.
- Measure core body temperature.
- Assess acute and chronic pain.
- Consider health disparities in pain.

Perform a General Survey

The *general survey* is the initial assessment of a patient's appearance, height, and weight and begins from the very first moments of interaction. However, these observations truly come into focus during the physical examination (PE).

Several factors influence a patient's body habitus, including their socioeconomic status, nutrition, genetic makeup, level of physical activity, emotional state, early-life illnesses, gender, geographical environment, and generational influences. Notably, nutritional status plays a pivotal role in determining various characteristics examined during the general survey. This includes attributes like height, weight, blood pressure (BP), posture, alertness, facial coloration, dental health, nail bed color, and muscle mass, among others (Box 10-5). Therefore, routinely assessing height, weight, BMI, and potential obesity risk is crucial for every patient you see in your clinical practice.

See Chapter 11, Cognition, Behavior, and Mental Status, pp. 206–207, Chapter 12, Skin, Hair, and Nails, pp. 254–257; Chapter 27, Nervous System, Level of Consciousness, pp. 953–956, Table 27-9, Tremors and Involuntary Movements, pp. 982–983 and Table 27-3, Abnormalities of Gait and Posture, p. 969.

Each of these observations can prompt questions or hypotheses, shaping the direction of your ongoing assessment. However, remaining conscious of potential implicit biases is imperative. Our perceptions and interpretations can sometimes be unintentionally influenced by deep-seated beliefs or stereotypes. Continually self-reflect and ensure that any judgments made are

Box 10-5. General Survey: Key Observational Indicators

Category	Observation/Assessment Details
Apparent state of health	Try to make a general judgment based on observations throughout the encounter. Is the patient acutely or chronically ill, frail, or fit and robust?
Level of consciousness	Is the patient awake, alert, and responsive to you and others in the environment? If not, promptly assess the level of consciousness.
Apparent state of discomfort or distress	Does the patient show signs of cardiac or respiratory distress, pain, anxiety, or depression? Is clutching of the chest, pallor, diaphoresis, labored breathing, wheezing, or coughing seen? Is wincing, diaphoresis, protectiveness of a painful area, grimacing, or an unusual posture favoring one limb or region of the body seen? Are facial expressions or fidgeting seen?
Skin color and obvious lesions	Inspect for changes in skin color, scars, plaques, or nevi. Pallor, cyanosis, jaundice, rashes, bruises, or mottling of the extremities should be pursued.
Dress, grooming, and personal hygiene	How is the patient dressed? Is it suitable for the temperature and weather? Is it clean and appropriate for the setting? Excess clothing may reflect various conditions or personal lifestyle preferences.
Facial expression	Observe facial expression at rest, during conversation, interactions, and physical examination. Note eye contact. Decreased eye contact may be culture-specific or suggest anxiety, fear, or sadness.[54] Watch for signs of medical conditions or emotional states.
Odors of the body and breath	Odors can offer diagnostic clues, like fruity odor of diabetes or the scent of alcohol.
Posture, gait, and motor activity	Assess the patient's preferred posture, any restlessness, frequency of position changes, involuntary motor activity, and quality of the gait. Various postures and gait patterns can indicate specific medical conditions.

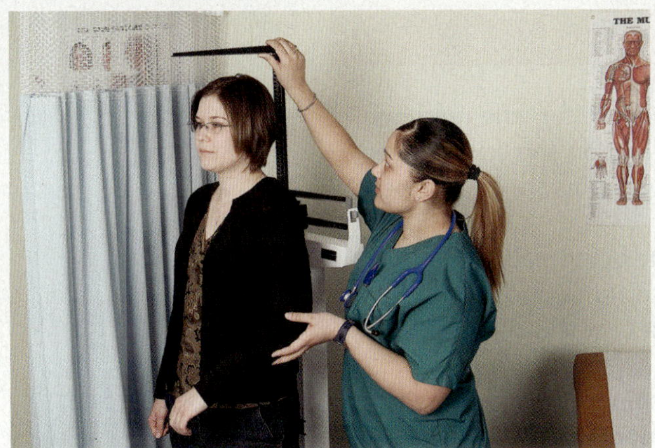

FIGURE 10-1. Measuring the height using a stadiometer. (Reprinted with permission from Springhouse. *Lippincott's Visual Encyclopedia of Clinical Skills.* Wolters Kluwer Health/Lippincott Williams & Wilkins; 2009:232.)

evidence-based and not influenced by your biases. Such self-awareness promotes equitable care and helps maintain trust in your emerging patient–provider relationship.

Measure Height and Weight

Height and weight are fundamental in nutrition screening as well as interventions that may arise from treatment including accurate drug dosage, body fluid gain or loss, and fluid requirements (Figs. 10-1 and 10-2).[6] Use proper technique with appropriate equipment that is regularly calibrated to ensure accuracy (Boxes 10-6 and 10-7).

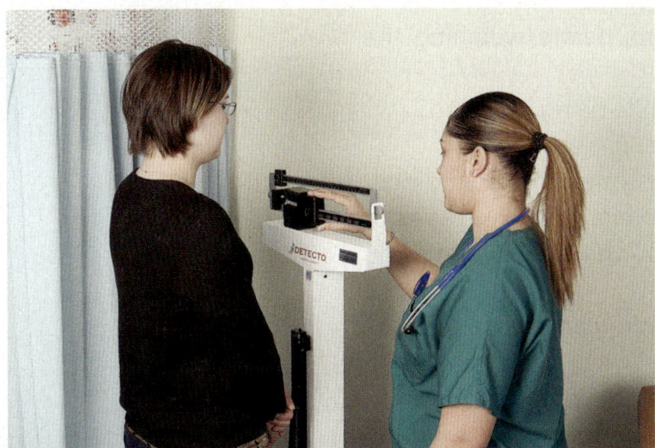

FIGURE 10-2. Measuring the weight using a standing scale. (Reprinted with permission from Springhouse. *Lippincott's Visual Encyclopedia of Clinical Skills.* Wolters Kluwer Health/Lippincott Williams & Wilkins; 2009:232.)

Box 10-6. Determining Patient Height[55]

- **Stadiometers** are devices specifically designed for the accurate measurement of height. Ask the patient to stand on the stadiometer, facing forward as tall and straight as possible with arms hanging loosely at their sides.
- The patient's feet should be flat on the baseplate of the stadiometer and positioned slightly apart, in line with the hips, to aid balance.
- The patient's knees should be straight, and their buttocks and shoulders should touch the stadiometer.
- Ensure the patient's head is in the midline position—an imaginary line from the center of the earhole to the lower border of the eye socket.
- Bring the headplate down onto the head, ensuring it rests on the crown of the head (i.e., the top back half).
- Read the measurement. Your eyes should be level with the counter/pointer, and the measurement read to the nearest 1 mm.
- Record the measurement and assist the patient off the stadiometer.
- If you are making repeated measurements on the same individual on different days, measure at the same time of day if possible. Throughout the day, height decreases due to compression of the spine.

Source: *Procedure for Measuring Adult Height*. NIHR Southampton Biomedical Research Centre; 2014. Accessed October 29, 2023. https://www.uhs.nhs.uk/Media/Southampton-Clinical-Research/Procedures/BRCProcedures/Procedure-for-adult-height.pdf

Box 10-7. Determining Patient Weight[56]

- Ask the patient to remove footwear and outdoor garments as appropriate. If weighing a patient with a stoma or catheter bag, ensure it is emptied beforehand.
- Ensure the scales are balanced, or display zero, before weighing the patient.
- The patient should remain as still as possible while being weighed.
- Monitor to ensure that:
  - Clothing is not touching any fixed part of the scales or surroundings.
  - Body weight is not supported on an object (e.g., a walking stick or wall), and the patient's feet are not placed on the floor (when using chair scales).
- Once the scales register a weight, record the reading on the scales in the appropriate documentation.
- Once accurate weight is recorded, assist the patient to move away from the weighing scale. Ensure that they are dressed appropriately and comfortable at the end of procedure.
- When monitoring periodical weight change, ensure the patient always wears clothing of similar weight.

Source: *Good Practice Guideline—For Accurate Body Weight Measurement Using Weighing Scales in Adults and Children*. National Nurses Nutrition Group. Accessed October 29, 2023. https://nnng.org.uk/wp-content/uploads/2013/10/Good-Practice-Guidelines-Accurate-Body-Weight-Measurement-Final.pdf

Calculate the BMI. Use your measurements of height and weight to determine *body mass index (BMI)*.

To determine BMI, choose the method best suited to your practice. Use a standard BMI table or the electronic medical record software, which commonly shows BMI automatically.[7] You can also calculate the BMI as shown below with the weight in kilograms and height in meters.

$$\text{BMI} = \frac{\text{Weight (kg)}}{\text{Height (m}^2\text{)}}$$

Conversion formulas: 1 lb = 0.45 kg; 1 in = 2.54 cm; 100 cm = 1 m.

Then classify the BMI according to national guidelines (Box 10-8).

Importantly, although BMI provides a simple and easy-to-calculate metric and is a useful tool for population-level risk assessment, it has limitations (Box 10-9). Therefore, other factors like waist circumference, dietary habits, physical activity, and overall health should be taken into account when evaluating an individual's health risks.

Assess Vital Signs

The vital signs—*blood pressure, heart rate, respiratory rate,* and *temperature*—provide critical initial information that often influences the tempo and direction of your evaluation. If already recorded by office or hospital staff, review vital signs promptly at the outset of the encounter. If they are abnormal, you will often retake them yourself during the visit. Learn the techniques that ensure accuracy when you measure vital signs, described in the pages to follow.

See Chapter 18, Cardiovascular System, Table 18-3, Abnormalities of the Arterial Pulse and Pressure Waves, p. 524.

Measure Blood Pressure

The accuracy of BP measurements varies according to how these measurements are taken. Office screening with manual and automated cuffs remains common, but elevated readings increasingly require confirmation with home and ambulatory monitoring (Box 10-10).

See Out-of-Office and Self-Monitoring of Blood Pressure, pp. 189–191.

The "ABC QUES" mnemonic is a useful tool for remembering the key steps and considerations when measuring BP and helps in obtaining a more accurate and reliable BP measurement (Box 10-11 and Fig. 10-3).

Prepare the Patient and the Setting. The examining room should be quiet and comfortably warm. The patient should be seated comfortably, with their back supported and legs uncrossed. The patient should avoid smoking, caffeine, or exercise for 30 minutes prior to measurement (Box 10-12). They should rest for 5 minutes prior to measuring the BP.[8]

Select the Appropriate Blood Pressure–Measuring Device (Sphygmomanometer). Measure the BP using a *sphygmomanometer*. Take the time to ensure that your BP measurement will be accurate. Proper technique is important and reduces the inherent variability arising from the patient or examiner, the equipment, and the procedure itself.[9] The BP measurement techniques that follow mostly apply to the use of manual sphygmomanometers.

See Chapter 4, Physical Examination, Box 4-3, Tools of the Trade: Instruments and Supplies for the Physical Examination, pp. 68–71.

To detect BP, an accurate instrument is essential. No matter which device you use, all measuring instruments should be routinely calibrated using international protocols for accuracy and continued reliable use in clinical settings.[10,11] Two types are currently used to measure BP: manual or digital sphygmomanometers (Box 10-13).

Box 10-8. World Health Organization Classification for Body Mass Index[12]

Category	BMI (kg/m²)	Potential Implications
Underweight	<18.5	Can be associated with malnutrition, weakened immune function, increased risk of infections, osteoporosis, and anemia May also indicate underlying medical conditions or eating disorders
Normal	18.5–24.9	Generally associated with a lower risk of chronic diseases compared to other categories Suggests a balanced ratio of weight to height
Overweight	25.0–29.9	Increased risk for various conditions like cardiovascular diseases, type 2 diabetes, and certain cancers Lifestyle interventions often recommended to prevent progression to obesity
Obesity class I	30.0–34.9	Increased risk of chronic conditions such as hypertension, type 2 diabetes, cardiovascular diseases, sleep apnea, and certain types of cancer Weight management and lifestyle changes typically advised
Obesity class II	35.0–39.9	Even greater risk of chronic conditions compared to class I Medical interventions, including surgery, may be considered along with lifestyle changes
Obesity class III	≥40	Also known as "severe" or "morbid" obesity Associated with a very high risk of health problems, including heart disease, stroke, type 2 diabetes Medical supervision is crucial, and aggressive treatment options, including bariatric surgery, might be considered

Box 10-9. Evaluation of Body Mass Index: Recognized Limitations

Limitation	Description
Fat vs. Muscle Differentiation[57]	Body mass index (BMI) does not account for muscle mass, potentially classifying muscular individuals as overweight or obese.
Fat Distribution[58]	Two people with the same BMI can have different fat distributions, with some areas posing more health risks than others.
Health Indication[59]	Someone with a "normal" BMI could still have health issues, while someone with a higher BMI might be perfectly healthy.
Ethnic Variations[60]	BMI cut-off points might not be suitable for all ethnic groups.
Age, Bone Density, and Other Factors[61]	Elderly patients might have lost muscle and bone mass, so their BMI might not reflect the same health risks as for younger people.

Box 10-10. In-Office Methods for Measuring Blood Pressure

Method	Features
Auscultatory office blood pressure with aneroid or mercury blood pressure	▪ Common, inexpensive ▪ Subject to patient anxiety ("white coat hypertension"), observer technique, cuff recalibration every 6 months ▪ Requires measurements over several visits ▪ Ambulatory or home monitoring needed to detect masked hypertension ▪ Single measurements with sensitivity and specificity of 75% compared to ambulatory monitoring[9]
Automated oscillometric office blood pressure	▪ Requires optimal patient positioning, cuff size and placement, and device calibration ▪ Takes multiple measurements over short period ▪ Requires confirmatory measurements to reduce misdiagnosis. ▪ Comparable sensitivity and specificity to manual measurements[9]

Box 10-11. "ABC QUES" Mnemonic for Blood Pressure Measurement Positioning

Arm supported at heart level	Aligning the arm with the heart ensures hydrostatic pressures do not affect the reading, which can occur if the arm is above or below heart level.
Bare arm for cuffs	Clothing can interfere with the cuff's ability to evenly compress the artery and may lead to a falsely high or low reading.
Correct cuff size and placement is vital	A cuff that is too tight may yield a reading that is falsely high, whereas a cuff that is too loose or large can give a falsely low reading. The cuff should encircle at least 80% of the arm without overlapping.
Quiet at rest and during the measurement	Noise and conversation can increase sympathetic nervous system activity, potentially increasing blood pressure. A quiet environment promotes relaxation and a more accurate reading.
Uncrossed legs	Crossing legs can increase venous return and vascular resistance, potentially leading to a higher reading. Keeping legs uncrossed and flat on the floor maintains normal blood flow.
Empty bladder	A full bladder can raise blood pressure temporarily due to discomfort and sympathetic nervous system activation, possibly leading to an overestimation of the blood pressure.
Supported back and feet	Proper support helps the patient maintain a consistent position without activating muscles that could influence the reading due to increased stress or effort.

Source: AMA Ed Hub. *BP Measurement Essentials: Student Edition;* 2023. Accessed October 21, 2023. https://edhub.ama-assn.org/ama-cvd-prevention-education/interactive/18594970.

Select the Correct Size Blood Pressure Cuff. Using a cuff that fits the patient's arm is critical because the BP cuff works by compressing the brachial artery in the patient's arm. When the cuff is inflated, it blocks the flow of blood through the artery. If the BP cuff is too small (narrow), it will compress the brachial artery more than it should, which will give a falsely high BP reading. If the BP cuff is too large (wide), it will not compress the brachial artery enough, which will give a falsely low BP reading.

Follow the guidelines outlined here for selecting the correct size (Box 10-14).

- The standard cuff is 12 × 23 cm, appropriate for arm circumferences up to 28 cm.
- The width of the inflatable bladder of the cuff should be about 40% of upper arm circumference (about 12–14 cm in the average adult).
- The length of the inflatable bladder should be about 80% of upper arm circumference (almost long enough to encircle the arm).

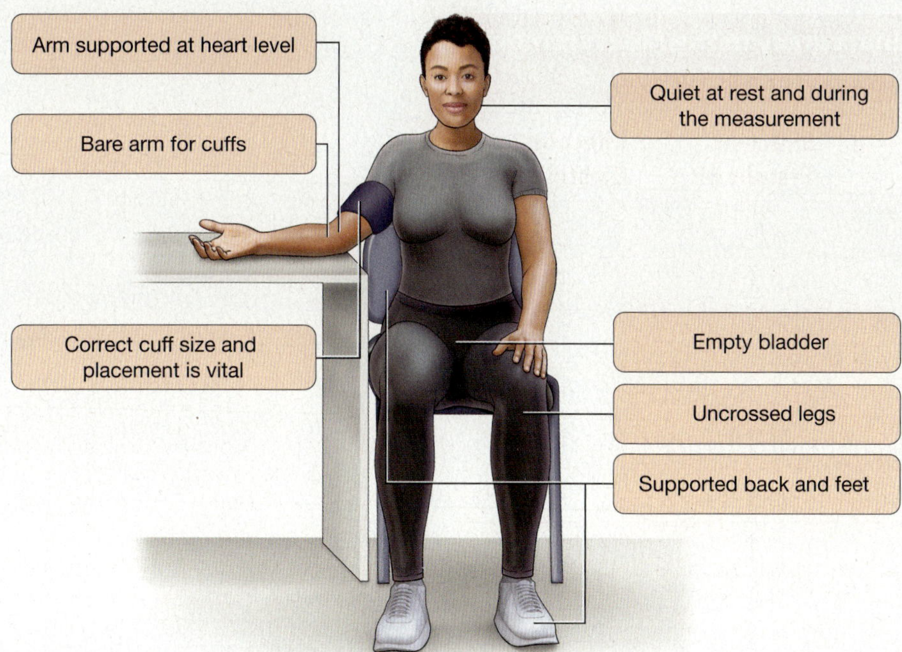

FIGURE 10-3. Need some cues to easily remember how to position a patient for blood pressure readings? Think of "ABC QUES"! (From AMA Ed Hub. *BP Measurement Essentials: Student Edition;* 2023. Accessed October 21, 2023. https://edhub.ama-assn.org/ama-cvd-prevention-education/interactive/18594970.)

Position the Arm and Cuff Appropriately. The arm selected should be free of clothing, fistulas for dialysis, or lymphedema from axillary node dissection or radiation therapy. Palpate the brachial artery to confirm a viable pulse and position the patient's arm so that the brachial artery, at the antecubital crease, is at heart level; their palm should be facing up. This is because the hydrostatic

Box 10-12. Potential Sources of Inaccuracy in the Measurement of Adult Blood Pressure in Clinical Settings[62]

	Effect on Systolic BP	Effect on Diastolic BP
Patient-Related Factors		
Acute meal ingestion	↓	↓
Acute alcohol ingestion	↓	↓
Acute caffeine use	↑	↑
Acute nicotine use or exposure	↑	↑
Bladder distention	↑	↑
Cold exposure	↑	↑
Paretic arm	↑	↑
White coat effect	↑	↑

(*continued*)

Box 10-12. Potential Sources of Inaccuracy in the Measurement of Adult Blood Pressure in Clinical Settings[62] (*Continued*)

	Effect on Systolic BP	Effect on Diastolic BP
Procedure-Related Factors		
Insufficient rest period	↑	↑
Legs crossed at knees	↑	↑
Unsupported arm	↑	↑
Arm lower than heart level	↑	↑
Talking during measurement	↑	↑
Incorrect smaller cuff size	↑	↑
Incorrect larger cuff size	↓	↓
Stethoscope under cuff	↑	↓
Fast cuff deflation rate (>3 mm Hg/sec)	↑	↓
Unsupported back	No effect	↑
Excessive pressure on stethoscope head	No effect	↑

Source: Kallioinen N, Hill A, Horswill MS, Ward HE, Watson MO. Sources of inaccuracy in the measurement of adult patients' resting blood pressure in clinical settings: a systematic review. *J Hypertens*. 2017;35(3):421–441.

Box 10-13. Comparison of Blood Pressure Measurement Devices

Type of Sphygmomanometer	Description
Manual: Mercury	Stethoscope required to auscultate both the systolic and diastolic pressures Considered the gold standard Replaced in most clinical settings due to safety concerns from accidental glass column breakage
Manual: Aneroid	Stethoscope required to auscultate both the systolic and diastolic pressures Uses mechanical parts to transmit the pressure in the cuff to a dial Can be knocked out of calibration easily; should be recalibrated every 6 months for accuracy[63]
Digital	Does not require a stethoscope; systolic and diastolic pressures calculated electronically Uses oscillometric technique to measure blood pressure[14]

Box 10-14. Cuff Recommendations Based on Arm Circumference for Blood Pressure Measurement

Arm Circumference	Recommended Cuff and Method
Large arm circumference	Use a cuff 16 cm in width.[28] If the upper arm is short despite a large circumference, use a thigh cuff or a very long cuff.
Arm circumference >50 cm and not amenable to thigh cuff	Wrap an appropriately sized cuff around the forearm, hold the forearm at heart level, and feel for the radial pulse.[64]
Very small arm circumference	Consider using a pediatric cuff. Other options include using a Doppler probe at the radial artery or an oscillometric device.

pressure of the blood changes with the position of the arm. If the patient's arm is below heart level, the BP reading will be too high. If the patient's arm is above heart level, the BP reading will be too low.

If the patient is seated, rest the arm on a table a little above their waist or roughly level with the fourth interspace at its junction with the sternum; if the patient is standing, try to support their arm at the midchest level.

With the arm at the appropriate level, center the inflatable bladder over the brachial artery. The lower border of the cuff should be about 2.5 cm above the antecubital crease. Secure the cuff snugly. Slightly flex the patient's arm at the elbow.

Palpate the Radial Pulse to Estimate the Systolic Blood Pressure. To decide how high to raise the cuff pressure, first estimate the systolic blood pressure (SBP) by palpating the radial artery.[12]

To palpate the radial pulse, place your index and middle fingers on the inside of the patient's wrist, below the thumb. You should feel the pulse pulsating under your fingertips. Inflate the sphygmomanometer cuff until the pulse disappears. Then, slowly deflate the cuff and listen for the *Korotkoff sounds* with a stethoscope. The SBP is the first Korotkoff sound that you hear (see Box 10-15). Use this value as your *target level* for subsequent inflations to minimize patient discomfort from unnecessarily high cuff pressures. Deflate the cuff promptly and completely and wait for 15 to 30 seconds.

Importantly, palpating the radial pulse is not a substitute for taking a BP measurement with a sphygmomanometer. However, it can be a helpful tool for getting a rough estimate of the SBP and for ensuring that the sphygmomanometer cuff is inflated to the appropriate pressure. This palpatory technique also avoids the occasional error caused by an *auscultatory gap*—a silent interval that may be present between the systolic and the diastolic pressures (Fig. 10-4).

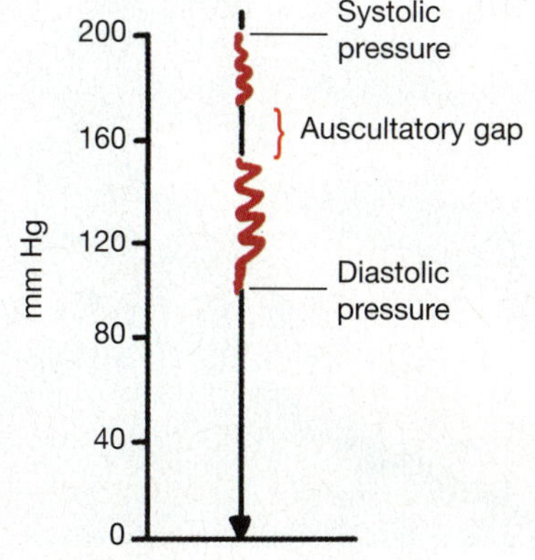

FIGURE 10-4. Auscultatory gap.

An auscultatory gap is associated with arterial stiffness and atherosclerotic disease.[13] An unrecognized auscultatory gap may lead to serious underestimation of SBP or overestimation of diastolic blood pressure (DBP).

Box 10-15. Korotkoff Sounds in Blood Pressure Measurement

Phase	Description	Corresponding Blood Pressure
Phase I	First appearance of clear tapping sounds, produced by blood starting to flow through the previously occluded brachial artery	Systolic blood pressure
Phase II	Sounds become softer with a possible swishing quality due to turbulent blood flow	–
Phase III	Return of sharper, crisper sounds similar to those in phase I	–
Phase IV	Sounds become muffled with a soft blowing quality	Diastolic blood pressure (in children)
Phase V	Complete disappearance of sounds	Diastolic blood pressure (in adults)

Position the Stethoscope Diaphragm or Bell Over the Brachial Artery. Now place the diaphragm (bell) of your stethoscope lightly over the brachial artery, taking care to make an air seal with the full rim (Fig. 10-5). There should be a 2- to 3-cm space for the stethoscope between the lower end of the cuff and the antecubital fossa.[14]

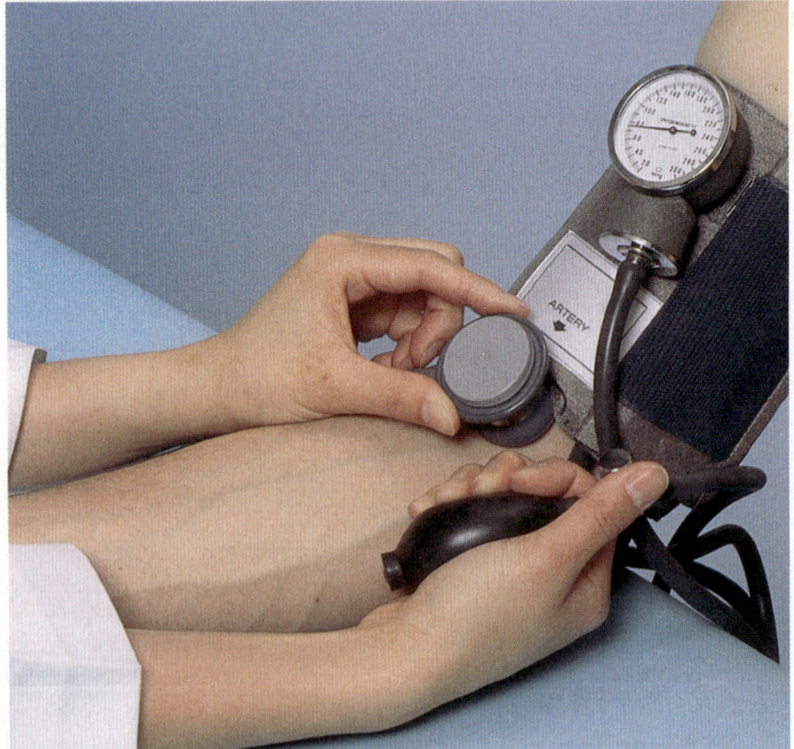

FIGURE 10-5. Properly positioned arm and stethoscope over the brachial artery.

Inflate the Cuff Rapidly to Target Level Followed by Gradual Deflation. Inflate the cuff again rapidly to the target level, and then deflate the cuff slowly at a rate no faster than 2 to 3 mm Hg/s. Avoid slow or repetitive inflations of the cuff because the resulting venous congestion can cause false readings.

Venous congestion makes the sounds less audible and may produce artificially low systolic and high diastolic pressures.

Identify the Systolic and Diastolic Blood Pressures. Begin by listening for the initial faint, repetitive tapping known as the *Korotkoff sounds* (Box 10-15). These sounds will gradually grow louder for a minimum of two consecutive beats, indicating the SBP (phase I). Avoid using the upward movements of the needle or the rise of the mercury column on the manometer to determine the systolic pressure.

Subsequently, for a brief period (phases II and III; see Box 10-15), these sounds soften and take on a swishing characteristic. They may later become clearer, matching or even surpassing the intensity of phase I.

Continue deflating the cuff at a steady pace. The sounds will eventually become muffled (phase IV) and then vanish completely (phase V). To ensure the exact point of disappearance, keep listening as the pressure decreases by another 10 to 20 mm Hg before quickly releasing all the pressure from the cuff. Typically, the point of disappearance (phase V) is just a few mm Hg below where the sounds become muffled. This point offers the most accurate estimation of the DBP (Fig. 10-6).

Occasionally, as in aortic regurgitation, the sounds never disappear. If the difference is 10 mm Hg or greater, record both figures (e.g., 154/80/68).

When you hear weak Korotkoff sounds, consider erroneous stethoscope placement, failure to make full skin contact with the bell, and venous engorgement of the patient's arm from repeated inflations of the cuff. If you cannot hear Korotkoff sounds at all, alternative methods using a Doppler probe or direct arterial pressure tracings may be necessary.

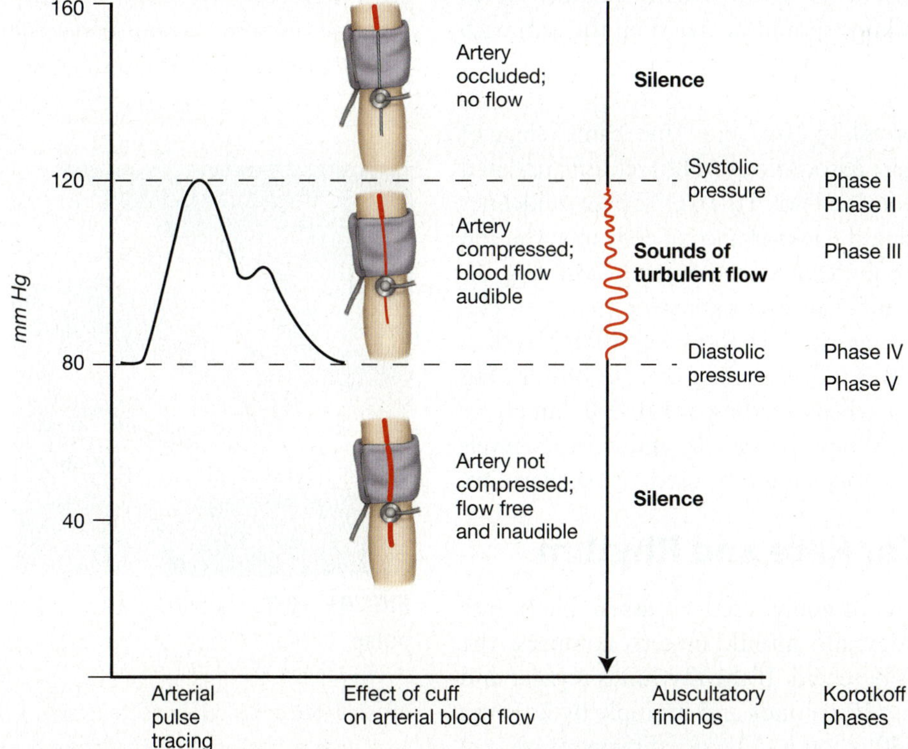

FIGURE 10-6. Auscultating systolic (phase I) and diastolic (phase V) Korotkoff sounds.

Box 10-16. Blood Pressure Categories for Adults (2017 ACC/AHA)[65]

Category[a]	Systolic (mm Hg)		Diastolic (mm Hg)
Normal	<120	and	<80
Elevated	120–129	and	<80
Stage 1 hypertension	130–139	or	80–89
Stage 2 hypertension	≥140	or	≥90

ACC, American College of Cardiology; AHA, American Heart Association.

Patients with systolic blood pressure and diastolic blood pressure in two categories should be designated to the higher blood pressure (BP) category.

[a]BP indicates blood pressure (based on an average of ≥2 careful readings obtained on ≥2 occasions).

Source: Whelton PK, Carey RM, Aronow WS, et al. 2017 ACC/AHA/AAPA/ABC/ACPM/AGS/APhA/ASH/ASPC/NMA/PCNA guideline for the prevention, detection, evaluation, and management of high blood pressure in adults: executive summary: a report of the American College of Cardiology/American Heart Association Task Force on Clinical Practice Guidelines. *Hypertension*. 2018;71(6):1269–1324. Copyright © 2017 by the American College of Cardiology Foundation and the American Heart Association, Inc.

Read both the systolic and the diastolic levels. *Wait for at least 1 minute and repeat.* Average your readings. The first reading in a series is usually the highest. Additional readings should be taken if the difference between the first two is >5 mm Hg.[14]

Normally, differences in pressure measurements of 5 mm Hg and sometimes up to 10 mm Hg may occur on the arms of the same patient. Measure BP in both arms at least once. Subsequent readings should be made on the arm with the higher pressure.

A pressure difference of >10 to 15 mm Hg occurs in subclavian steal syndrome, supravalvular aortic stenosis, and aortic dissection and should be investigated.

Classify Blood Pressure as Normal or Abnormal. In 2017, the American College of Cardiology (ACC) and the American Heart Association (AHA) released updated guidelines on the management of hypertension (Box 10-16).[15] These guidelines revised the classification of BP, emphasizing the importance of early intervention even at lower levels of BP elevation. The guidelines recommend classifying BP into several categories, with a particular focus on the risks associated with elevated BP levels. BP in adults should be categorized as normal if SBP is less than 120 mm Hg **and** DBP is less than 80 mm Hg.[9] A reading of 130/80 mm Hg or higher is considered *stage 1 hypertension*, while a reading of 140/90 mm Hg or higher is considered *stage 2 hypertension*. When the systolic and diastolic levels fall into different categories, the *higher* category should be used for classification.

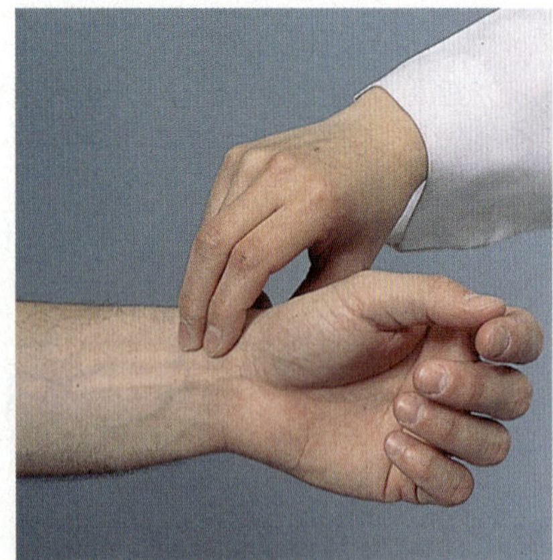

FIGURE 10-7. Palpating the radial pulse.

Examine Arterial Pulses for Rate and Rhythm

Assess Pulse Rate. The radial pulse is commonly used to assess heart rate (Fig. 10-7). With the pads of your index and middle fingers, compress the radial artery until a maximal pulsation is detected. If the rhythm is regular and the rate seems normal, count the rate for 30 seconds and multiply by 2. If the rate is unusually fast or slow, count for 60 seconds. The usual range of normal is 60 to 90 to 100 beats/min.[22]

An elevated resting heart rate is associated with increased risk of cardiovascular disease and mortality.[23]

Assess Pulse Rhythm. Begin by palpating the radial pulse. Is the rhythm regular or irregular? If there are any irregularities, assess the rhythm at the cardiac apex by listening with your stethoscope. If irregular, try to identify a pattern: (1) Do early beats appear in a basically regular rhythm? (2) Does the irregularity vary consistently with respiration? (3) Is the rhythm totally irregular? Always check an electrocardiogram (ECG) to identify the type of rhythm.

See Chapter 18, Cardiovascular System, Table 18-1, Selected Heart Rates and Rhythms, p. 522, and Table 18-2, Selected Irregular Rhythms, p. 523.

Premature beats of low amplitude may not be transmitted to the peripheral pulses, leading to underestimates of the heart rate.

Observe Respiratory Rate, Rhythm, Depth, and Effort

Assess Respiratory Rate. Count the number of respirations in 1 minute either by visual inspection or by subtly listening over the patient's trachea with your stethoscope during your examination of the head and neck or chest. Normally, adults take approximately 12 to 20 breaths/min in a quiet, regular pattern.

A respiratory rate <12 or >25 breaths/min while resting is considered abnormal.

Assess Respiratory Rhythm. Watch the patient's chest or abdomen rise and fall consistently over time. Note if the intervals between breaths are regular (evenly spaced) or irregular (varying intervals).

Prolonged expiration is common in chronic obstructive pulmonary disease.

Observe Depth of Breathing. Assess the amplitude of each breath. Does the chest or abdomen move a small amount (shallow) or a large amount (deep)? Compare the depth of each breath is consistent or if there are variations.

Observe Effort of Breathing. Inquire if the patient feels any discomfort or difficulty while breathing. Look for signs of increased effort such as flaring nostrils, use of neck or facial muscles, or pursed-lip breathing. Place your hand on the patient's chest or back. Notice if you can feel any vibrations or grunting with each breath, indicating strain.

Measure Core Body Temperature

The core body temperature, measured internally, is approximately 37 °C (98.6 °F) and fluctuates approximately 1 °C over the course of the day. It is lowest in the early morning and highest in the afternoon and evening. Females have a wider range of normal temperature than males.[24]

Fever, or **pyrexia**, refers to an elevated body temperature. **Hyperpyrexia** refers to extreme elevation in temperature, above 41.1 °C (106 °F).

Hypothermia refers to an abnormally low temperature, below 35 °C (95 °F) rectally. The chief cause is exposure to cold. Other causes include reduced movement as in paralysis, interference with vasoconstriction from sepsis or excess alcohol, starvation, hypothyroidism, and hypoglycemia. Older adults are especially susceptible to hypothermia and also less likely to develop fever.

Although the research gold standard for core body temperature is the blood temperature in the pulmonary artery,[25–27] clinical practice relies on noninvasive oral, rectal, axillary, tympanic membrane, and temporal artery measurements (Box 10-17).[28] Tympanic membrane and temporal artery temperatures use infrared thermometry. Axillary temperatures take 5 to 10 minutes to register and are considered less accurate.

Box 10-17. Comparison of Temperature Measurement Methods and Procedures

Measurement Method	Description/Procedure
Oral temperature	For electronic: Insert thermometer under tongue and position the tip as far back as possible on either side of the frenulum linguae (Fig. 10-8). Watch for digital readout (usually in about 10 seconds). Hot or cold liquids and smoking can alter the temperature reading; delay measurement for 10–15 minutes. Oral temperatures are generally lower than the core body temperature and are 0.4 °C–0.5 °C (0.7 °F–0.9 °F) lower than rectal temperatures. They are also 1 °C (1.8 °F) higher than axillary temperatures.
Rectal temperature	Ask the patient to lie on one side with their hips flexed. Use a rectal thermometer with a stubby tip, lubricate it, and insert 3–4 cm into the anal canal toward the umbilicus (Fig. 10-9). Remove after 3 minutes and read. Alternatively, use an electronic thermometer and wait about 10 seconds for the digital readout.
Tympanic membrane temperature	The tympanic membrane shares blood supply with the hypothalamus, where temperature regulation occurs. Ensure the external auditory canal is free of cerumen. Stabilize the patient's head; pull their ear appropriately and position the probe (Fig. 10-10). Wait 2–3 seconds for the digital reading. Accurate readings require direct access to the tympanic membrane. Tympanic temperatures can be more variable than oral or rectal measurements.
Temporal artery temperature	Uses the location of the temporal artery near the skin surface of the forehead, cheek, and behind earlobes. Place the probe against the center of the forehead; depress the scanning button; and brush the device across the patient's forehead, down their cheek, and behind an earlobe (Fig. 10-11). Read the display, recording the highest temperature. Combined forehead and behind-the-ear contact is more accurate than scanning only the forehead.

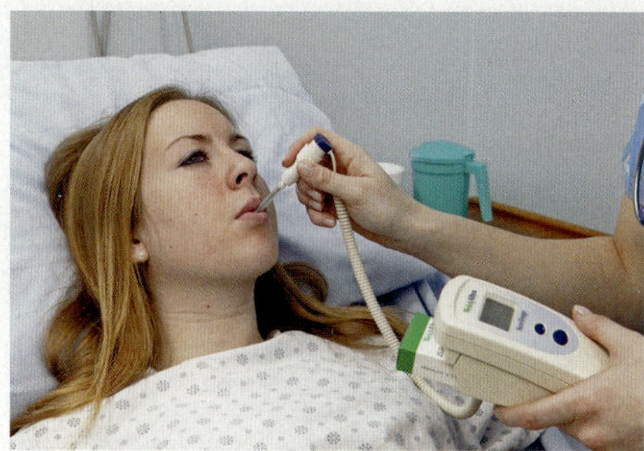

FIGURE 10-8. Taking the oral temperature using an electronic thermometer. (Reprinted with permission from Taylor C, Lillis C, Lynn P. *Fundamentals of Nursing: The Art and Science of Person-Centered Nursing Care.* 8th ed. Wolters Kluwer; 2015:605. Figure 24-1-2.)

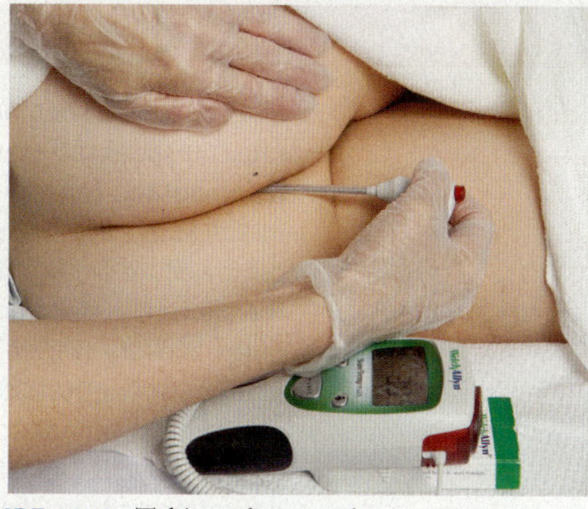

FIGURE 10-9. Taking the rectal temperature using an electronic thermometer. (Reprinted with permission from Craven RF, Hirnle CJ, Henshaw C. *Fundamentals of Nursing: Human Health and Function.* 8th ed. Wolters Kluwer; 2017:354.)

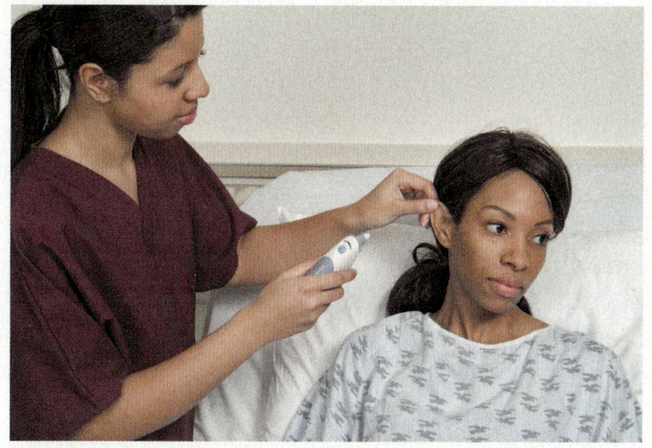

FIGURE 10-10. Taking the tympanic temperature using a tympanic thermometer. (Reprinted with permission from Springhouse. *Lippincott's Visual Encyclopedia of Clinical Skills.* Wolters Kluwer Health/Lippincott Williams & Wilkins; 2009:519.)

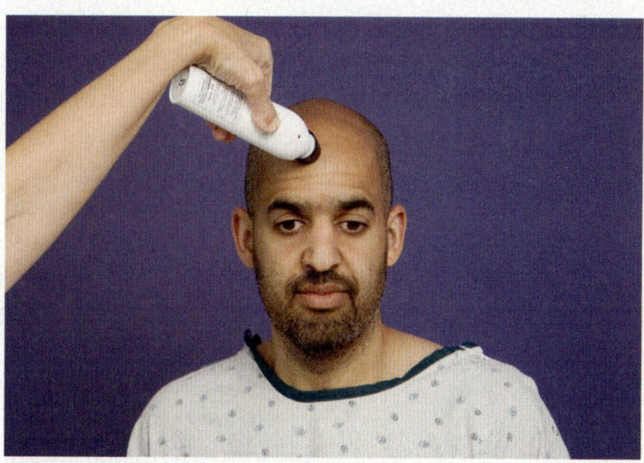

FIGURE 10-11. Taking the temporal temperature using a temporal thermometer. (Reprinted with permission from Lynn P. *Taylor's Clinical Nursing Skills: A Nursing Process Approach.* 5th ed. Wolters Kluwer; 2019:46. Figure 2-9.)

Assess for Acute and Chronic Pain

Characterize the Type of Pain. *Acute pain* is "the normal, predicted physiologic response to an adverse chemical, thermal, or mechanical stimulus" that typically lasts less than 3 to 6 months and is commonly associated with surgery, trauma, and acute illness."[29,30] It may also be a useful and life-sustaining function (protective function). Symptoms can last hours, days, or weeks but gradually resolve as the injured tissues heal.

Chronic pain is defined in several ways: pain not associated with cancer or other medical conditions that persists for more than 3 to 6 months, pain lasting more than 1 month beyond the course of an acute illness or injury, or pain recurring at intervals of months or years. Chronic pain is the leading cause of disability and impaired performance at work.

Depressive, somatoform, and anxiety disorders affect patients' coping strategies and have to be identified in order to effectively treat acute pain, in particular, chronic pain.[31]

Box 10-18. Types of Pain[4,68]

Nociceptive (somatic) pain	■ Linked to tissue damage to the skin, musculoskeletal system, or viscera (visceral pain), but the sensory nervous system is intact, as in arthritis or spinal stenosis. It can be acute or chronic. It is mediated by the afferent A-delta and C-nerve fibers of the sensory system. The involved afferent nociceptors can be sensitized by inflammatory mediators and modulated by both psychological processes and neurotransmitters like endorphins, histamines, acetylcholine, serotonin, norepinephrine, and dopamine. ■ It is usually described as *dull, pressing, pulling, throbbing, boring, spasmodic,* or *colicky.*
Neuropathic pain	■ A direct consequence of a lesion or disease affecting the somatosensory system. Over time, neuropathic pain may become independent of the inciting injury. It may persist even after healing from the initial injury has occurred. Mechanisms postulated to evoke neuropathic pain include central nervous system brain or spinal cord injury from stroke or trauma; peripheral nervous system disorders causing entrapment or pressure on spinal nerves, plexuses, or peripheral nerves; and referred pain syndromes with increased or prolonged pain responses to inciting stimuli. These triggers appear to induce changes in pain signal processing through "neuronal plasticity," leading to pain that persists beyond healing from the initial injury. ■ It is often described as *electric shock-like, stabbing, burning,* or *"pins and needles."*

Source: Institute of Medicine; Board on Health Sciences Policy; Committee on Advancing Pain Research, Care, and Education. *Relieving Pain in America: A Blueprint for Transforming Prevention, Care, Education, and Research (2011).* Accessed October 21, 2023. https://www.nap.edu/catalog/13172/relieving-pain-in-america-a-blueprint-for-transforming-prevention-care

Review the summary of types of pain to aid in your diagnosis and management (Box 10-18).

Assess Pain Severity. Use a consistent method to assess pain severity. Three scales are common (Box 10-19): the Visual Analog Scale (VAS), the Numeric Rating Scale (NRS), and the Wong–Baker FACES® Pain Rating Scale.

Box 10-19. Scales for Pain Assessment

Visual Analog Scale (VAS)	Horizontal line with verbal descriptive anchors at each end to express the extremes of pain Patients mark the point on the line that best corresponds to their symptom severity
Numeric Rating Scale (NRS)	Numerical ratings from 0–10; 0 indicates the absence of pain, whereas 10 represents the most intense pain possible Patient indicates the number that corresponds to their pain intensity (Fig. 10-12)
Wong–Baker FACES® Pain Rating Scale	Used by children and patients with language barriers or cognitive impairment Six faces depict different expressions, ranging from happy to extremely upset; each face is assigned a numerical rating between 0 (smiling) and 10 (crying)[31] Patients point to the picture that best represents the degree and intensity of their pain (Fig. 10-13)
Faces Pain Scale–Revised (FPS-R)	Developed by the International Association for the Study of Pain[69] Another commonly used scale for pain assessment
Other Multidimensional Tools	Tools like the Brief Pain Inventory and the McGill Pain Questionnaire Provide a more detailed assessment but take longer to administer[70]

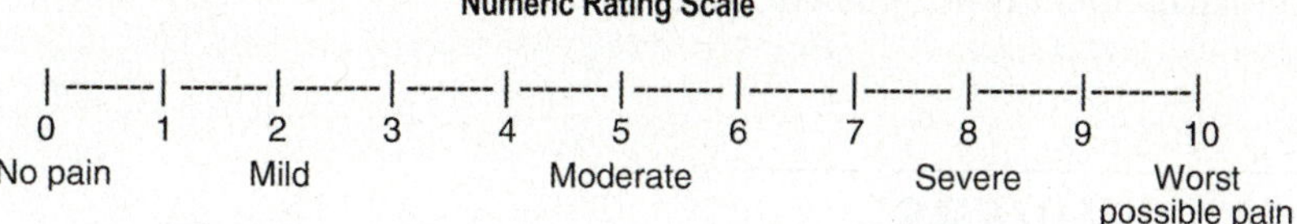

FIGURE 10-12. Numeric Rating Scale (NRS). (From Fishman SM, Ballantyne JC, Rathmell JP. *Bonica's Management of Pain*. 4th ed. Wolters Kluwer Health/Lippincott Williams & Wilkins; 2009:1590. The Partners Against Pain website no longer exists.)

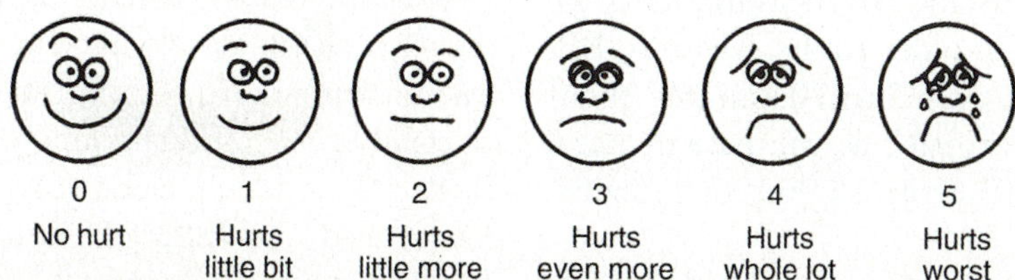

FIGURE 10-13. Wong-Baker FACES® Pain Rating Scale. (Copyright © 1983 Wong-Baker FACES Foundation. www.WongBakerFACES.org. Used with permission. Originally published in *Whaley & Wong's Nursing Care of Infants and Children*. © Elsevier Inc.)

The use of questionnaires, pain diaries, and analogue scales to complement history and PE are part of the essential documentation for every pain treatment plan.[32]

Consider Health Disparities in Pain

Health disparities in pain assessment, treatment, and delivery of care have been a persistent and concerning issue. These disparities manifest in a variety of ways, notably through differences in treatment based on race, ethnicity, and socioeconomic status. African American and Hispanic patients, for instance, have been found to receive lower doses of analgesics in emergency rooms compared to their White counterparts. Similarly, disparities are also evident in the use of analgesics for conditions such as cancer, postoperative recovery, and low back pain.[4] Such differences in care can lead to prolonged suffering, complications, and a general distrust in the health care system.

Numerous studies point toward several underlying reasons for these disparities. Clinician-held stereotypes, whether conscious or unconscious, can influence clinician judgment and decision-making processes. Language barriers further exacerbate the issue, as patients with limited English proficiency might not effectively communicate their pain, leading to undertreatment. In addition, unconscious biases in clinicians can inadvertently result in different treatment strategies. These biases might be rooted in cultural misunderstandings, lack of diversity training, or simply unawareness.[33]

See the Institutes of Medicine report, Unequal Treatment: Confronting Racial and Ethnic Disparities in Health Care, 2002.[34]

As future members of the health care community, you must critically evaluate these disparities and actively work toward solutions. Self-assess your communication styles and constantly strive for improvement. By seeking out information, staying updated with best practice standards, and actively engaging in patient education, we can bridge the gap in pain management disparities.

Patient empowerment is another essential strategy. Encouraging your patients to voice their concerns, pain levels, and treatment expectations can provide valuable insights and improve treatment outcomes. Collaboration between health care providers and community leaders can also pave the way for culturally sensitive care, ensuring that pain management is not just effective but also equitable.

SPECIAL TECHNIQUES AND MANEUVERS

Measure Orthostatic Blood Pressures

Interpret relatively low levels of BP in the light of past readings and the patient's clinical state. If indicated, perform orthostatic BP measurements to assess *orthostatic* or *postural hypotension*, common in older adults. Measure BP in two positions—*supine* after the patient is resting from 3 to 10 minutes, then within 3 minutes once the patient *stands up*. Normally, as the patient rises from the horizontal to the standing position, SBP drops slightly or remains unchanged, whereas DBP rises slightly.

Orthostatic hypotension is a sustained reduction in SBP of ≥20 mm Hg or in DBP of ≥10 mm Hg within 3 minutes of standing.[16–18] Causes include drugs, moderate or severe blood loss, prolonged bed rest, and diseases of the autonomic nervous system.

Special Patient-Related Situations

BP measurement, while straightforward in most cases, can present unique challenges and variations depending on various conditions and scenarios. Some

Box 10-20. Characteristics of Special Blood Pressure Conditions

Condition	Definition
White coat hypertension	Defined as BP ≥140/90 in medical settings and mean awake ambulatory readings <135/85 Reported in up to 20% of patients with elevated office BP Attributed to a conditioned anxiety response Considered clinically significant when office SBP/DBPs are >20/10 mm Hg higher than home or ambulatory BP monitoring SBP/DBPs[20,21,66]
Masked hypertension	Defined as office BP <140/90 but an elevated daytime BP of >135/85 on home or ambulatory testing More serious condition Untreated adults with masked hypertension, an estimated 10% to 30% of the general population, have an increased risk of cardiovascular disease and end-organ damage[20,21] Consider home or ambulatory BP monitoring
Concurrent arrhythmias	Irregular rhythms produce variations in BP, leading to unreliable measurements Ignore the effects of an occasional premature contraction; for frequent premature contractions or atrial fibrillation, determine the average of several observations and note that measurements are approximate Ambulatory monitoring for 2–24 hours recommended[64]

BP, blood pressure; DBP, diastolic blood pressure; SBP, systolic blood pressure.

patients may experience unusual BP readings in clinical settings, while others may have discrepancies between office measurements and readings taken elsewhere. Understanding these distinct BP phenomena is crucial for accurate diagnosis and appropriate management (Box 10-20).

Other examination techniques that use BP measurements as clinical assessments are discussed in their individual regional examination chapters (e.g., ankle–brachial index, p. 557, pulsus paradoxus, p. 498, and pulsus alternans, p. 498).

Out-of-Office and Self-Monitoring of Blood Pressure

Self-monitoring of BP refers to the regular measurement of BP by a patient outside the clinic setting. When done at home, it is called *home blood pressure monitoring (HBPM). Ambulatory blood pressure monitoring (ABPM),* on the other hand, is used to obtain out-of-office BP readings at preset intervals, usually programmed to obtain readings over a period of 24 hours while patients go about

Box 10-21. Out-of-Office Methods for Measuring Blood Pressure

Method	Features
Home blood pressure monitoring (HBPM)	■ Accurate automated device applied by patient, easy to use, less expensive than ambulatory monitoring ■ Acceptable alternative if ambulatory monitoring not feasible; more predictive of cardiovascular risk than office measurements[20] ■ Requires patient education for accurate technique, repeated measurements (two morning, two evening readings daily for 1 week); nighttime readings not recorded[20] ■ Detects *white coat hypertension*—present in 20%[20] ■ Detects *masked hypertension*—present in 10%[20] ■ Sensitivity 85%, specificity 62% compared to ambulatory monitoring[67]
Ambulatory blood pressure monitoring (ABPM)	■ Automated; clinical and research "gold standard" ■ Provides 24-hour average BPs and averages of daytime (awake), nighttime (asleep), systolic, and diastolic BPs ■ Shows whether nocturnal BP "dips" (normal) or stays elevated (a cardiovascular disease risk factor) ■ More expensive; may not be covered by insurance

their normal daily activities. Although ABPM is generally accepted as the best out-of-office measurement method, HBPM is often a more practical approach in clinical practice (Box 10-21).[19] Typically, a clinic BP of 140/90 mm Hg (hypertension) corresponds to:

- Home BP: 135/85 mm Hg[20]
- Ambulatory BP[21]
  - 24-hour average: 130/80 mm Hg
  - Daytime (awake) average: 135/85 mm Hg
  - Nighttime (asleep) average: 120/70 mm Hg

Both ABPM and HBPM typically provide BP estimates that can be helpful for confirmation and management of hypertension (Box 10-22). If you recommend out-of-office BP monitoring, advise your patients how to choose the best upper arm cuff for home use and have it recalibrated. Let them know that wrist and finger monitors are popular but less accurate. SBP increases in more distal arteries, whereas DBP falls, and hydrostatic effects introduce errors due to differences in position relative to the heart. Patient education about the correct use of home monitors is essential. Make sure patients understand all the steps needed to ensure accurate readings at home, as detailed in this section.

Box 10-22. Corresponding Blood Pressure Values in mm Hg for Clinic, Home, Daytime, Nighttime, and 24-Hour Ambulatory Measurements[65]

Clinic	HBPM	Daytime ABPM	Nighttime ABPM	24-Hour ABPM
120/80	120/80	120/80	100/65	115/75
130/80	130/80	130/80	110/65	125/75
140/90	135/85	135/85	120/70	130/80
160/100	145/90	145/90	140/85	145/90

ABPM, ambulatory blood pressure monitoring; HBPM, home blood pressure monitoring.

Source: Whelton PK, Carey RM, Aronow WS, et al. 2017 ACC/AHA/AAPA/ABC/ACPM/AGS/APhA/ASH/ASPC/NMA/PCNA guideline for the prevention, detection, evaluation, and management of high blood pressure in adults: executive summary: a report of the American College of Cardiology/American Heart Association Task Force on Clinical Practice Guidelines. *Hypertension*. 2018;71(6):1269–1324. Copyright © 2017 by the American College of Cardiology Foundation and the American Heart Association, Inc.

RECORDING YOUR FINDINGS

Your write-up of the PE begins with a general description of the patient's appearance, based on the general survey. Note that initially you may use sentences to describe your findings; later you will use phrases. Choose vivid and graphic adjectives, as if you are painting a picture in words. Avoid overused terms such as "well developed," "well nourished," or "in no acute distress," because they are too general and may not truly capture the unique attributes of the patient in front of you. Record the vital signs taken at the time of your examination rather than earlier in the day. The style below contains phrases appropriate for most examination write-ups.

Recording the General Survey and Vital Signs

"Mrs. Cortez is a young, healthy-appearing woman, well-groomed, fit, and cheerful. Height is 5 ft 4 in; weight, 135 lb; BMI, 24; BP, 120/80, right and left arms; HR, 72 and regular; RR, 16; temperature, 37.5 °C."

OR

"Mr. Robinson is an elderly man who looks pale and chronically ill. He is alert, with good eye contact but unable to speak more than two or three words at a time due to shortness of breath. He has intercostal muscle retraction when breathing and sits upright in bed. He is thin, with diffuse muscle wasting. Height is 6 ft 2 in; weight, 175 lb; BP, 160/95, right arm; HR, 108 and irregular; RR, 32 and labored; temperature, 101.2 °F."

This is suggestive of a patient with a potential chronic illness (like chronic obstructive pulmonary disease, or congestive heart failure) that might be acutely exacerbated.

The practice of dissecting PE documentation into detailed components exemplifies how your clinical observations can offer pivotal clues for diagnosis. This process highlights specific findings and nuances that might otherwise be overlooked, directly contributing to the accuracy and efficiency of the diagnostic process. The findings in Mr. Robinson's case suggest several clinical concerns:

- *Appearance of being pale and chronically ill:* This may indicate chronic disease, anemia, or malnutrition.
- *Difficulty speaking due to shortness of breath:* This is a sign of respiratory distress, possibly due to lung disease, heart failure, or severe infection.
- *Intercostal muscle retraction when breathing:* This is a sign of severe respiratory distress, often seen in conditions like severe asthma, pneumonia, and other severe lung pathologies.
- *Sitting upright in bed:* This position, often adopted to ease breathing, suggests severe respiratory distress or heart failure.
- *Diffuse muscle wasting:* This indicates chronic illness, possibly malnutrition, chronic obstructive pulmonary disease, or cancer.
- *Vital signs:* The elevated BP (BP 160/95), tachycardia (HR 108 and irregular), tachypnea (RR 32 and labored), and fever (temperature 101.2 °F) suggest a state of physiologic stress, possibly due to infection, heart failure, or other systemic illnesses.

Overall, Mr. Robinson's presentation is concerning for a *serious, potentially life-threatening condition*, likely involving a combination of respiratory, cardiac, and possibly infectious processes.

HEALTH PROMOTION AND COUNSELING: EVIDENCE AND RECOMMENDATIONS

Important Topics for Health Promotion and Counseling

- Achieving optimal weight

Other related topics are addressed in more detail in the following sections:

- Healthy Diet and Physical Activity (Chapter 18, Cardiovascular System, p. 519)
- Excessive Dietary Sodium (Chapter 18, Cardiovascular System, p. 521)

Note that in the following section, the terms "men," "women," "male," and "female" are used as they were in the original research to accurately represent the study populations and findings. While we recognize the importance of inclusivity in language, retaining these terms is essential for maintaining the fidelity and context of the information presented.

Achieving Optimal Weight

Definitions and Epidemiology. The BMI measurement, which is calculated by dividing weight in kilograms by height in meters squared, has been used to classify excess weight based on risk of cardiovascular disease (CVD).[35–37] As stated earlier, overweight is defined as BMI of 25.0 to 29.9 kg/m^2, while obesity is defined by a BMI ≥30 kg/m^2.

Obesity is further categorized as class 1 (30.0–34.9 kg/m^2), class II (35.0–39.9 kg/m^2), and class III, also referred to as severe obesity (BMI ≥40 kg/m^2).

Epidemiologic data on obesity are generally based on the BMI.[38] In the United States, National Health and Nutrition Survey (NHANES) data for 2017 through March 2020 (before the COVID-19 pandemic) estimated an age-adjusted prevalence of overweight or obesity among adults ages ≥20 years of just over 70%. About 2 in 5 adults were obese, with similar prevalence for men and women, and 1 in 11 adults had severe obesity. More than a third of U.S. children and adolescents ages 2 to 19 years were overweight or obese, and about 1 in 5 were obese. Compared to the most recent NHANES data, the age-adjusted prevalence of obesity among adults (1 in 3) and severe obesity (1 in 20) was substantially lower in 1999 to 2000. The prevalence of obesity among children and adolescents has increased by about 50% in the past few decades.[39]

Elevated BMI has been associated with a number of metabolic health problems, including CVD, type 2 diabetes mellitus, fatty liver disease, chronic kidney disease, and cancer as well as higher all-cause mortality.[35,40,41] Mechanical effects of obesity contribute to obstructive sleep apnea and osteoarthritis, and obesity is associated with depression, anxiety, and social isolation. Obesity-related health care costs are substantial, particularly among those with severe obesity. An analysis of U.S. data estimated the annual medical expenditures due to excess body weight to be $173 billion.[42]

Screening and Interventions. In 2018, the U.S. Preventive Services Task Force (USPSTF) issued a grade B recommendation for clinicians to offer intensive, multicomponent behavioral weight loss interventions to patients with a BMI ≥30 kg/m^2, reinforcing an earlier grade B recommendation to screen all adults for obesity.[41,43] However, BMI does not measure body composition (body muscle and fat content) and may misleadingly overestimate health risks in those with muscular physiques and underestimate health risks in older patients and those who have lost muscle mass.[35,40] Furthermore, because the cardiovascular risk attributed to BMI varies across populations, BMI may underestimate risk in Asian individuals and overestimate risk in Black individuals. Women have higher adiposity than men, but this does not confer increased risk for diabetes or CVD. Combining an annual waist circumference measurement, which estimates abdominal (visceral) obesity, with BMI may be the best approach for assessing cardiovascular risk, particularly for patients with BMI >35 kg/m^2.[44] A waist circumference of ≥40 cm in men and ≥35 cm in women is considered elevated.

When counseling patients about their weight, educate them that moderate weight loss of 5% to 10% is considered clinically important because it is associated with a reduced risk for type 2 diabetes, obstructive sleep apnea, and CVD.[40]

Lifestyle Modifications, Pharmacotherapy Interventions, and Bariatric Procedures for Weight Loss. An influential 2013 guideline published by the American Heart Association/American College of Cardiology/The Obesity Society (AHA/ACC/TOS) emphasized that comprehensive lifestyle interventions should address dietary strategies for weight loss, prescribe exercise, and incorporate behavioral strategies for achieving and maintaining weight loss.[45] Reducing caloric intake is the cornerstone of any weight-loss strategy. Specific dietary recommendations include increasing consumption of fruits, vegetables, legumes, whole grains, and nuts and decreasing energy intake from total fats and sugars.[40] Many structured diets, including commercial weight loss programs, can be helpful; however, you should consider your patient's preferences in selecting a dietary plan because adherence is more important than diet composition in achieving weight loss.[46] Meal-replacement diets and intermittent fasting may also be effective strategies. You should advise your patients to engage in moderate-intensity physical activity, including aerobic exercise and resistance training, for at least 150 minutes weekly. Periodically monitoring food intake, activity levels, and weight may help individuals to achieve and maintain weight loss. While acknowledging that primary care clinicians can offer behavioral interventions, the USPSTF found the strongest evidence support for high-intensity, multidisciplinary interventions of 1 to 2 years duration that helped participants achieve and maintain a ≥5% weight loss.[41]

The USPSTF evidence synthesis evaluated medications currently approved at the time by the Food and Drug Administration (FDA), including liraglutide, orlistat, naltrexone/bupropion, phentermine, and topiramate.[47] The FDA has been approving medications as adjuncts to lifestyle modifications for those with a BMI ≥30 kg/m^2 and ≥27 kg/m^2 with weight-related complications.[48] Pharmacotherapy used with lifestyle modifications was more effective than lifestyle modifications alone in achieving and maintaining weight loss. Recent evidence suggests that newer medications, particularly subcutaneous semaglutide, a glucagon-like peptide 1 (GLP-1) receptor agonist, and tirzepatide, a dual-acting GLP-1 agonist and gastric inhibitory polypeptide (GIP) receptor agonist, are much more effective than earlier drugs in achieving weight loss.[49,50] The USPSTF is currently updating its recommendations for weight loss interventions.

Metabolic and bariatric surgery, which has seen many technologic advances and increased use since the AHA/ACC/TSO guideline, is also an option for those with severe obesity, BMI 30.0 to 34.9 kg/m^2 with diabetes, and BMI 30.0 to 34.9 kg/m^2 and an inadequate response to behavioral interventions or pharmacotherapy.[51] The Roux-en-Y gastric bypass and sleeve gastrectomy, the most commonly performed treatments, can improve clinical outcomes for obesity-related comorbidities, including diabetes, obstructive sleep apnea, hypertension, dyslipidemia, and osteoarthritis as well as reduce cancer risk.[52] Other procedures and devices endorsed by the American Society for Metabolic and Bariatric Surgery include laparoscopic gastric banding and intragastric balloons.[53]

REFERENCES

1. "Constitution". Merriam-Webster. Accessed October 29, 2023. https://www.merriam-webster.com/dictionary/constitution
2. Cunningham WE, Shapiro MF, Hays RD, et al. Constitutional symptoms and health-related quality of life in patients with symptomatic HIV disease. *Am J Med.* 1998;104(2):129–136.
3. IASP Terminology. International Association for the Study of Pain. Accessed October 29, 2023. http://www.iasp-pain.org/Education/Content.aspx?ItemNumber=1698#Pain
4. Institute of Medicine; Board on Health Sciences Policy; Committee on Advancing Pain Research, Care, and Education. *Relieving Pain in America: A Blueprint for Transforming Prevention, Care, Education, and Research.* The National Academies Press; 2011. Accessed October 29, 2023. https://www.nap.edu/catalog/13172/relieving-pain-in-america-a-blueprint-for-transforming-prevention-care
5. Washington State Agency Medical Directors' Group. *Interagency Guideline on Opioid Dosing for Chronic Non-Cancer Pain: An Educational Aid to Improve Care and Safety With Opioid Treatment: 2010 Update.* Washington Department of Health; 2010. Accessed October 29, 2023. https://www.agencymeddirectors.wa.gov
6. Clarkson DM. Patient weighing: standardisation and measurement. *Nurs Stand.* 2012;26(29):33–37.
7. Body mass index tables 1 and 2. National Heart, Lung, and Blood Institute. Accessed October 29, 2023. https://www.nhlbi.nih.gov/health/educational/lose_wt/BMI/bmi_tbl.htm
8. Buchanan S, Orris P, Karliner J. Alternatives to the mercury sphygmomanometer. *J Public Health Policy.* 2011;32(1):107–120.
9. James PA, Oparil S, Carter BL, et al. 2014 evidence-based guideline for the management of high blood pressure in adults: report from the panel members appointed to the Eighth Joint National Committee (JNC 8). *JAMA.* 2014;311(5):507–520.
10. O'Brien E, Asmar R, Beilin L, et al; European Society of Hypertension Working Group on Blood Pressure Monitoring. European Society of Hypertension recommendations for conventional, ambulatory and home blood pressure measurement. *J Hypertens.* 2003;21(5):821–848.
11. O'Brien E, Pickering T, Asmar R, et al; Working Group on Blood Pressure Monitoring of the European Society of Hypertension. Working Group on Blood Pressure Monitoring

of the European Society of Hypertension International Protocol for validation of blood pressure measuring devices in adults. *Blood Press Monit.* 2002;7(1):3–17.

12. *Clinical Guidelines on the Identification, Evaluation, and Treatment of Overweight and Obesity in Adults: The Evidence Report.* National Institutes of Health; National Heart, Lung, and Blood Institute; 1998. Accessed October 29, 2023. https://www.nhlbi.nih.gov/files/docs/guidelines/ob_gdlns.pdf
13. Cavallini MC, Roman MJ, Blank SG, Pini R, Pickering TG, Devereux RB. Association of the auscultatory gap with vascular disease in hypertensive patients. *Ann Intern Med.* 1996;124(10):877–883.
14. Smith L. New AHA recommendations for blood pressure measurement. *Am Fam Physician.* 2005;72(7):1391–1398.
15. Whelton PK, Carey RM, Aronow WS, et al. 2017 ACC/AHA/AAPA/ABC/ACPM/AGS/APhA/ASH/ASPC/NMA/PCNA guideline for the prevention, detection, evaluation, and management of high blood pressure in adults: a report of the American College of Cardiology/American Heart Association Task Force on Clinical Practice Guidelines. *Hypertension.* 2018;71(6):e13–e115.
16. Freeman R. Clinical practice. Neurogenic orthostatic hypotension. *N Engl J Med.* 2008;358(6):615–624.
17. Carlson JE. Assessment of orthostatic blood pressure: measurement technique and clinical applications. *South Med J.* 1999;92(2):167–173.
18. Freeman R, Wieling W, Axelrod FB, et al. Consensus statement on the definition of orthostatic hypotension, neurally mediated syncope and the postural tachycardia syndrome. *Clin Auton Res.* 2011;161(1–2):46–48.
19. Piper MA, Evans CV, Burda BU, Margolis KL, O'Connor E, Whitlock EP. Diagnostic and predictive accuracy of blood pressure screening methods with consideration of rescreening intervals: a systematic review for the U.S. Preventive Services Task Force. *Ann Intern Med.* 2015;162(3):192–204.
20. Pickering TG, Miller NH, Ogedegbe G, Krakoff LR, Artinian NT, Goff D; American Heart Association; American Society of Hypertension; Preventive Cardiovascular Nurses Association. Call to action on use and reimbursement for home blood pressure monitoring: executive summary: a joint scientific statement from the American Heart Association, American Society of Hypertension, and Preventive Cardiovascular Nurses Association. *Hypertension.* 2008;52(1):1–9.
21. O'Brien E, Parati G, Stergiou G, et al; European Society of Hypertension Working Group on Blood Pressure Monitoring. European Society of Hypertension position paper on ambulatory blood pressure monitoring. *J Hypertens.* 2013;31(9):1731–1768.
22. Mason JW, Ramseth DJ, Chanter DO, Moon TE, Goodman DB, Mendzelevski B. Electrocardiographic reference ranges derived from 79,743 ambulatory subjects. *J Electrocardiol.* 2007;40(3):228–234.
23. Aladin AI, Whelton SP, Al-Mallah MH, et al. Relation of resting heart rate to risk for all-cause mortality by gender after considering exercise capacity (the Henry Ford exercise testing project). *Am J Cardiol.* 2014;114(11):1701–1706.
24. Sund-Levander M, Forsberg C, Wahren LK. Normal oral, rectal, tympanic and axillary body temperature in adult men and women: a systematic literature review. *Scand J Caring Sci.* 2002;16(2):122–128.
25. Jefferies S, Weatherall M, Young P, Beasley R. A systematic review of the accuracy of peripheral thermometry in estimating core temperatures among febrile critically ill patients. *Crit Care Resusc.* 2011;13(3):194–199.
26. Lawson L, Bridges EJ, Ballou I, et al. Accuracy and precision of noninvasive temperature measurement in adult intensive care patients. *Am J Crit Care.* 2007;16(5):485–496.
27. McCallum L, Higgins D. Measuring body temperature. *Nurs Times.* 2012;108(45):20–22.
28. Weber MA, Schiffrin EL, White WB, et al. Clinical practice guidelines for the management of hypertension in the community: a statement by the American Society of Hypertension and the International Society of Hypertension. *J Hypertens.* 2014;32(1):3–15.
29. Federation of State Medical Boards of the United States, Inc. *Model Guidelines for the Use of Controlled Substances in the Management of Pain.* 1998.
30. Zeller JL, Burke AE, Glass RM. JAMA patient page. Acute pain treatment. *JAMA.* 2008;299(1):128.
31. Keller S, Bann CM, Dodd SL, Schein J, Mendoza TR, Cleeland CS. Validity of the brief pain inventory for use in documenting the outcomes of patients with noncancer pain. *Clin J Pain.* 2004;20(5):309–318.
32. Committee on Education of the EFIC (European Federation of IASP Chapters). *The Pain Management Core Curriculum for European Medical Schools.* European Pain Federation; 2013. Accessed October 29, 2023. https://www.europeanpainfederation.eu/wp-content/uploads/2016/12/Core-CurriculumPainManagement-EFIC-June-2013_FINAL.pdf
33. Green CR, Anderson KO, Baker TA, et al. The unequal burden of pain: confronting racial and ethnic disparities in pain. *Pain Med.* 2003;4(3):277–294.
34. Institute of Medicine; Board on Health Sciences Policy; Committee on Understanding and Eliminating Racial and Ethnic Disparities in Health Care; Smedley BD, Stith AY, Nelson AR, eds. *Unequal Treatment: Confronting Racial and Ethnic Disparities in Health Care.* The National Academies Press; 2003.
35. Tsao CW, Aday AW, Almarzooq ZI, et al; American Heart Association Council on Epidemiology and Prevention Statistics Committee and Stroke Statistics Subcommittee. Heart Disease and Stroke Statistics-2023 Update: a report from the American Heart Association. *Circulation.* 2023;147(8):e93–e621.
36. Obesity: preventing and managing the global epidemic. Obesity: preventing and managing the global epidemic. Report of a WHO consultation. *World Health Organ Tech Rep Ser.* 2000;894:i–xii, 1–253.
37. Prospective Studies Collaboration, Whitlock G, Lewington S, Sherliker P, et al. Body-mass index and cause-specific mortality in 900 000 adults: collaborative analyses of 57 prospective studies. *Lancet.* 2009;373(9669):1083–1096.
38. Stierman B, Afful J, Carroll MD, et al. National Health and Nutrition Examination Survey 2017-March 2020 prepandemic data files—development of files and prevalence estimates for selected health outcomes. *National Health Statistics Reports.* 2021;58. https://stacks.cdc.gov/view/cdc/106273
39. Hales CM, Carroll MD, Fryar CD, Ogden CL. Prevalence of obesity among adults and youth: United States, 2015–2016. *NCHS Data Brief.* 2017;(288):1–8.
40. Tsai AG, Bessesen DH. Obesity. *Ann Intern Med.* 2019;170(5):ITC33–ITC48.
41. US Preventive Services Task Force, Curry SJ, Krist AH, Owens DK, et al. Behavioral weight loss interventions to prevent obesity-related morbidity and mortality in adults: US Preventive

Services Task Force Recommendation Statement. *JAMA.* 2018;320(11):1163–1171.
42. Ward ZJ, Bleich SN, Long MW, Gortmaker SL. Association of body mass index with health care expenditures in the United States by age and sex. *PLoS One.* 2021;16(3):e0247307.
43. Moyer VA; U.S. Preventive Services Task Force. Screening for and management of obesity in adults: U.S. Preventive Services Task Force recommendation statement. *Ann Intern Med.* 2012;157(5):373–378.
44. Arnett DK, Blumenthal RS, Albert MA, et al. 2019 ACC/AHA guideline on the primary prevention of cardiovascular disease: a report of the American College of Cardiology/American Heart Association Task Force on clinical practice guidelines. *Circulation.* 2019;140(11):e596–e646.
45. Jensen MD, Ryan DH, Apovian CM, et al; American College of Cardiology/American Heart Association Task Force on Practice Guidelines; Obesity Society. 2013 AHA/ACC/TOS guideline for the management of overweight and obesity in adults: a report of the American College of Cardiology/American Heart Association Task Force on Practice Guidelines and The Obesity Society. *Circulation.* 2014;129(25 Suppl 2):S102–S138.
46. Johnston BC, Kanters S, Bandayrel K, et al. Comparison of weight loss among named diet programs in overweight and obese adults: a meta-analysis. *JAMA.* 2014;312(9):923–933.
47. LeBlanc ES, Patnode CD, Webber EM, Redmond N, Rushkin M, O'Connor EA. Behavioral and pharmacotherapy weight loss interventions to prevent obesity-related morbidity and mortality in adults: updated evidence report and systematic review for the US Preventive Services Task Force. *JAMA.* 2018;320(11):1172–1191.
48. Administration; FaD. WEGOVY (semaglutide) injection, for subcutaneous use. US Food and Drug Administration (FDA) approved product information. Accessed September 7, 2023. https://www.accessdata.fda.gov/drugsatfda_docs/label/2022/215256s005lbl.pdf
49. Wilding JPH, Calanna S, Kushner RF. Once-weekly semaglutide in adults with overweight or obesity. Reply. *N Engl J Med.* 2021;385(1):e4.
50. Garvey WT, Frias JP, Jastreboff AM, et al; SURMOUNT-2 investigators. Tirzepatide once weekly for the treatment of obesity in people with type 2 diabetes (SURMOUNT-2): a double-blind, randomised, multicentre, placebo-controlled, phase 3 trial. *Lancet.* 2023;402(10402):613–626.
51. Eisenberg D, Shikora SA, Aarts E, et al. 2022 American Society for Metabolic and Bariatric Surgery (ASMBS) and International Federation for the Surgery of Obesity and Metabolic Disorders (IFSO): Indications for Metabolic and Bariatric Surgery. *Surg Obes Relat Dis.* 2022;18(12):1345–1356.
52. Arterburn DE, Telem DA, Kushner RF, Courcoulas AP. Benefits and risks of bariatric surgery in adults: a review. *JAMA.* 2020;324(9):879–887.
53. American Society for Metabolic and Bariatric Surgery. AMSBS Endorsed Procedures and FDA Approved Devices. Accessed September 7, 2023. https://asmbs.org/resources/endorsed-procedures-and-devices
54. Fernández-Dols J-M, Russell JA, eds. *The Science of Facial Expression.* Oxford University Press; 2017.
55. *Procedure for Measuring Adult Height.* NIHR Southampton Biomedical Research Centre; 2014. Accessed October 29, 2023. https://www.uhs.nhs.uk/Media/Southampton-Clinical-Research/Procedures/BRCProcedures/Procedure-for-adult-height.pdf
56. *Good Practice Guideline—For Accurate Body Weight Measurement Using Weighing Scales in Adults and Children.* National Nurses Nutrition Group. Accessed October 29, 2023. https://nnng.org.uk/wp-content/uploads/2013/10/Good-Practice-Guidelines-Accurate-Body-Weight-Measurement-Final.pdf
57. Gallagher D, Visser M, Sepúlveda D, Pierson RN, Harris T, Heymsfield SB. How useful is body mass index for comparison of body fatness across age, sex, and ethnic groups? *Am J Epidemiol.* 1996;143(3):228–239.
58. Després JP, Lemieux I. Abdominal obesity and metabolic syndrome. *Nature.* 2006;444(7121):881–887.
59. Lavie CJ, McAuley PA, Church TS, Milani RV, Blair SN. Obesity and cardiovascular diseases: implications regarding fitness, fatness, and severity in the obesity paradox. *J Am Coll Cardiol.* 2014;63(14):1345–1354.
60. WHO Expert Consultation. Appropriate body-mass index for Asian populations and its implications for policy and intervention strategies. *Lancet.* 2004;363(9403):157–163.
61. Siervo M, Bunn D, Prado CM, Hooper L. Accuracy of prediction equations for serum osmolarity in frail older people with and without diabetes. *Am J Clin Nutr.* 2014;100(3):867–876.
62. Kallioinen N, Hill A, Horswill MS, Ward HE, Watson MO. Sources of inaccuracy in the measurement of adult patients' resting blood pressure in clinical settings: a systematic review. *J Hypertens.* 2017;35(3):421–441.
63. Murray A. In praise of mercury sphygmomanometers: appropriate sphygmomanometer should be selected. *BMJ.* 2001;322(7296):1248–1249.
64. Pickering TG, Hall JE, Appel LJ, et al. Recommendations for blood pressure measurement in humans and experimental animals: part 1: blood pressure measurement in humans: a statement for professionals from the Subcommittee of Professional and Public Education of the American Heart Association Council on High Blood Pressure Research. *Circulation.* 2005;111(5):697–716.
65. Whelton PK, Carey RM, Aronow WS, et al. 2017 ACC/AHA/AAPA/ABC/ACPM/AGS/APhA/ASH/ASPC/NMA/PCNA guideline for the prevention, detection, evaluation, and management of high blood pressure in adults: executive summary: a report of the American College of Cardiology/American Heart Association Task Force on Clinical Practice Guidelines. *Hypertension.* 2018;71(6):1269–1324.
66. Myers MG, Godwin M, Dawes M, et al. Conventional versus automated measurement of blood pressure in primary care patients with systolic hypertension: randomised parallel design controlled trial. *BMJ.* 2011;342:d286.
67. Hodgkinson J, Mant J, Martin U, et al. Relative effectiveness of clinic and home blood pressure monitoring compared with ambulatory blood pressure monitoring in diagnosis of hypertension: systematic review. *BMJ.* 2011;342:d3621.
68. Haanpää M, Attal N, Backonja M, et al. NeuPSIG guidelines on neuropathic pain assessment. *Pain.* 2011;152(1):14–27.
69. Faces pain scale—Revised. International Association for the Study of Pain. Accessed October 29, 2023. http://www.iasp-pain.org/Education/Content.aspx?ItemNumber=1519&navItemNumber=577
70. Bieri D, Reeve RA, Champion DG, Addicoat L, Ziegler JB. The faces pain scale for the self-assessment of the severity of pain experienced by children: development, initial validation, and preliminary investigation for ratio scale properties. *Pain.* May 1990;41(2):139–150.

CHAPTER

11

Cognition, Behavior, and Mental Status

ANATOMY AND PHYSIOLOGY

The origins of psychiatric symptoms are less clearly defined compared to symptoms in other major body systems, such as the heart's conduction system or the gastrointestinal tract's digestion process. This ambiguity arises from the intricate nature of the human brain, complicating the task of identifying the exact sources of mental disorders. Nonetheless, advances in neuroscience have illuminated the roles specific brain areas play in these disorders.

The *central nervous system (CNS)* comprises the *brain* and *spinal cord.* While the spinal cord is crucial for motor and sensory functions, it plays a smaller role in mental disorders. The brain is further divided into the *cerebrum* (cerebral hemispheres), which includes *cortical structures* (frontal, temporal, parietal, and occipital lobes) and *subcortical structures* (fornix, cingulate cortex, basal ganglia, and basal forebrain), the *diencephalon* (consisting of the thalamus, epithalamus, subthalamus, and hypothalamus), the *cerebellum*, and the *brainstem*, which is made up of the midbrain, pons, and medulla.[1]

See the anatomy of the nervous system in greater detail in Chapter 27, Nervous System, Anatomy and Physiology, pp. 899–908.

Deep within the CNS, clusters of *neurons*, or *nuclei*, organized as *modulatory systems*, synthesize *neurotransmitters* that are crucial for higher-level CNS functions (Box 11-1, Figs. 11-1 to 11-4).[2]

The CNS is composed of intricate pathways (also known as circuits and networks) that link its diverse structures. These networks handle vast amounts of information and execute coordinated functions. Due to the complexity of these networks, pinpointing specific brain areas responsible for mental disorders or symptoms is difficult. An illness might arise from multiple deficits within a network. Current research on these networks is ongoing and has not yet provided a complete picture.[1]

See Table 11-2. Neurocircuitry of Mental Disorders, p. 225

In this chapter, the term "mental disorder" is used, aligning with the terminology primarily adopted by the *Diagnostic and Statistical Manual of Mental Disorders*, Fifth Edition (*DSM-5*). The *DSM-5* serves as the main diagnostic reference for mental health professionals in the United States and categorizes various conditions under this term.[3]

Box 11-1. Overview of Diffuse Modulatory Systems in the Central Nervous System

System Type	Origin	Description and Functions
Serotonergic diffuse modulatory system **FIGURE 11-1.** (Reprinted with permission from Bear MF, Connors BW, Paradiso MA. *Neuroscience: Exploring the Brain*. 4th ed. Wolters Kluwer; 2016. Figure 15-13.)	Raphe nuclei	Clustered along the brainstem's midline, projects throughout the central nervous system (CNS) Make serotonin that regulates mood, arousal, and cognition
Norepinephrine diffuse modulatory system 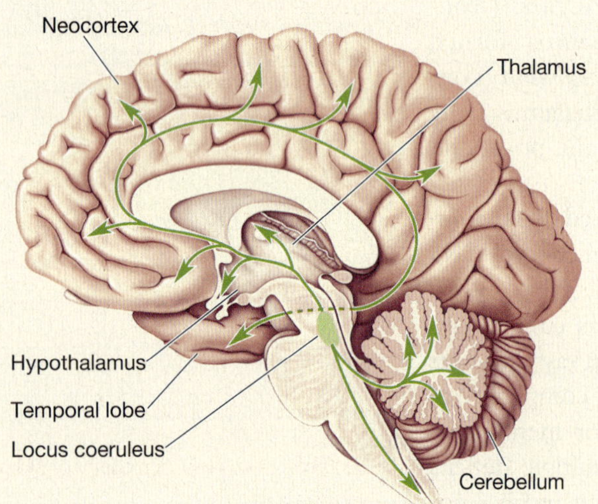 **FIGURE 11-2.** (Reprinted with permission from Bear MF, Connors BW, Paradiso MA. *Neuroscience: Exploring the Brain*. 4th ed. Wolters Kluwer; 2016. Figure 15-12.)	Locus coeruleus	Small cluster of neurons projects extensively across the CNS Produces norepinephrine, which manages mood, arousal, attention, and cognition

System Type	Origin	Description and Functions
Dopaminergic diffuse modulatory system 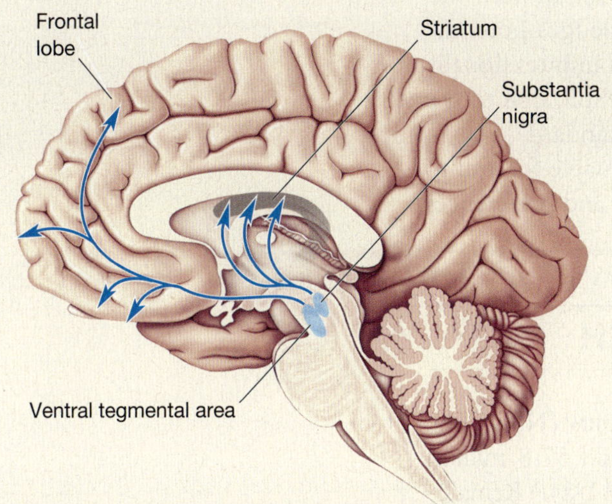 **FIGURE 11-3.** (Reprinted with permission from Bear MF, Connors BW, Paradiso MA. *Neuroscience: Exploring the Brain*. 4th ed. Wolters Kluwer; 2016. Figure 15-14.)	Substantia nigra and ventral tegmental area	Located closely in the midbrain, they project to the striatum and limbic/frontal cortical regions Make dopamine for mood, arousal, cognition, and motor control
Cholinergic diffuse modulatory system 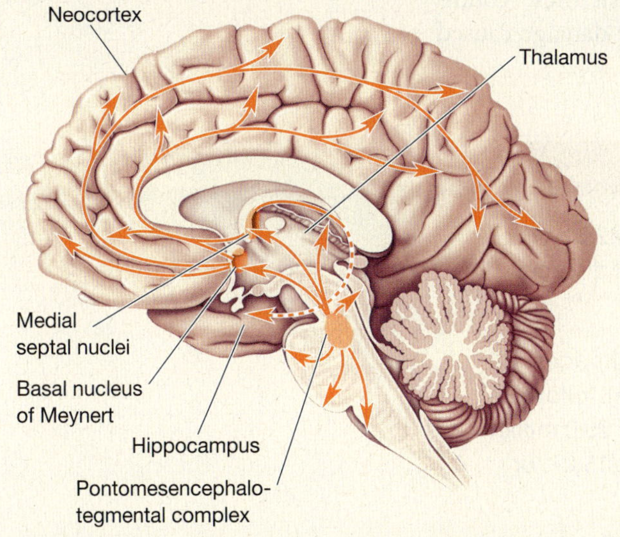 **FIGURE 11-4.** (Reprinted with permission from Bear MF, Connors BW, Paradiso MA. *Neuroscience: Exploring the Brain*. 4th ed. Wolters Kluwer; 2016. Figure 15-1.)	Basal forebrain and brainstem	Medial septal nuclei and basal nucleus of Meynert project broadly on the cerebral cortex Primary CNS center for acetylcholine production regulating sleep, arousal, and attention

Note: Low levels of serotonin, norepinephrine, and dopamine have been associated with depressive symptoms. Low concentrations of serotonin with high levels of norepinephrine have been associated with anxiety symptoms. Too much dopamine with low concentrations of serotonin in certain areas of the brain lead to symptoms of psychosis and mania. Dementia is notable for low concentration levels of acetylcholine.[2]

While "mental disorder" is the standard terminology within clinical and academic contexts of the *DSM-5*, in broader public health and advocacy settings, the phrase "mental health condition" is often used to emphasize health and to diminish stigma. Nevertheless, recognize that different terms, like "mental illness," "psychiatric disorder," and "psychological disorder," might hold varied connotations for distinct audiences. The *DSM-5* acknowledges potential misconceptions tied to the term "mental disorder," as it could unintentionally imply a stark division between mental and physical ailments. Still, due to the manual's clinical and diagnostic focus, this term remains its standard.

When engaging in mental health discussions, it's always valuable for you to prioritize person-first language and be attuned to the context and preferences of the intended audience.

HEALTH HISTORY: GENERAL APPROACH

Based on the 2021 National Survey on Drug Use and Health (NSDUH), released in 2023, approximately 22.8% of U.S. adults—around 57.8 million people—experienced a mental disorder in the past year (Box 11-2).[4] Remaining attentive to potential signs of mental disorders and detrimental behaviors is vital.[5,6] Regrettably, these signs are frequently overlooked, leading to issues such as poor medication adherence, loss of interest in regular activities, and challenges in performing daily tasks. Additionally, certain clinical conditions might obscure mental disorders, necessitating a sensitive approach and a detailed mental status examination when appropriate. Early identification is essential since mental disorders can strain family ties, affect employment status, and potentially lead to disability. A significant stigma surrounds patients with mental disorders[7]; therefore, it's imperative to emphasize that these conditions are legitimate and treatable, a step that helps combat the damage caused by stigma.

Box 11-2. Mental Illness Among Adults[25]

Overall adults	Among adults ages ≥18 years in 2023, 22.8% (or 58.7 million people) had any mental disorder in the past year.
By age group	Incidence is highest among young adults ages 18 to 25 years (31.9% or 8.3 million people), followed by adults aged 26 to 49 years (28.1% or 29.0 million people), then by adults ages ≥50 years (15.0% or 17.7 million people).
By ethnicity/race	Adults identifying as multiracial (34.9%) were more likely to report having experienced a mental disorder in the past year compared with White (23.9%), Black (21.4%), Hispanic (20.7%), Native Hawaiian or Other Pacific Islander (18.1%), and Asian adults (16.4%).

Source: Substance Abuse and Mental Health Services Administration. Key Substance Use and Mental Health Indicators in the United States: Results from the 2023 National Survey on Drug Use and Health 2024. https://www.samhsa.gov/data/report/2023-nsduh-annual-national-report. Accessed September 25, 2024.

Common or Concerning Symptoms

- Anxiety and excessive worrying
- Depressed mood
- Memory problems
- Medically unexplained symptoms

Anxiety and Excessive Worrying

Anxiety disorders include generalized anxiety disorder (GAD), social phobia, panic disorder, posttraumatic stress disorder (PTSD), and acute stress disorder.[8–11] These are among the most common mental disorders, with lifetime prevalence rates as high as 31%, yet the chronic and disabling nature of these conditions is often seriously underestimated.[12] Common risk factors in patients with anxiety and related disorders include family history of anxiety,[11] personal history of anxiety or mood disorder,[13,14] childhood stressful life events or trauma,[15,16] being female,[12,17] chronic medical illness,[13,18] and behavioral inhibition (Box 11-3).[4,19]

Box 11-3. Anxiety and Excessive Worrying: High-Yield Health History Questions

Domain	Questions	Rationale
Psychiatric history	*Have you been diagnosed with any mental disorders?* *Have you ever been hospitalized for a psychiatric condition?*	Anxiety disorders, such as generalized anxiety disorder,[3] panic disorder,[125] and social anxiety disorder, are common mental disorders that may cause excessive worrying and anxiety. Other mental disorders, such as major depressive disorder (MDD) and posttraumatic stress disorder (PTSD), may also cause anxiety symptoms.
Family psychiatric history	*Does anyone in your family have a history of mental disorders?* *If so, what type of disorder, and who in your family is affected?*	Anxiety disorders can run in families, indicating a genetic predisposition to the condition.[11,13,14] Other mental disorders that may cause anxiety, such as bipolar disorder or schizophrenia, also have a genetic component.

(continued)

Common causes and factors include **generalized anxiety disorder (GAD)** (chronic disorder characterized by prolonged and excessive worry about various aspects of life, often disproportionate to the situation), **panic disorder** (recurrent, unexpected panic attacks accompanied by intense fear and physical symptoms, leading to persistent worry about future episodes), **phobias** (intense, irrational fears of specific objects or situations, inducing significant anxiety when encountered or anticipated), and **posttraumatic stress disorder (PTSD)** (stemming from exposure to traumatic events, which manifests as intrusive memories, heightened arousal, avoidance behaviors, and persistent anxiety). **External stressors** (events or situations, such as financial difficulties or relationship issues) can amplify feelings of worry and anxiety.

Box 11-3. Anxiety and Excessive Worrying: High-Yield Health History Questions (*Continued*)

Domain	Questions	Rationale
Current symptoms	*Are you experiencing excessive worry or nervousness?* *Do you have physical symptoms such as sweating, trembling, or racing heartbeat?*	These symptoms are common in anxiety disorders such as generalized anxiety disorder (GAD), panic disorder, and social anxiety disorder.[126] Other mental disorders, such as obsessive-compulsive disorder and PTSD, may also cause anxiety symptoms.
Duration of symptoms	*How long have you been experiencing these symptoms?* *Do your symptoms come and go, or are they present all the time?*	Acute anxiety may be related to a specific event or situation, whereas chronic anxiety disorders persist for months or years.
Triggers	*Are there specific situations or triggers that cause your anxiety symptoms?* *If so, what are they?*	Patients with social anxiety disorder may experience anxiety in social situations, while patients with panic disorder may experience panic attacks triggered by specific situations or events.[15,16]
Impact on daily life	*Is your anxiety affecting your ability to work or perform daily activities? Have you been avoiding certain situations because of anxiety?*	Patients with GAD may have difficulty concentrating or making decisions, while patients with agoraphobia may avoid leaving their homes due to anxiety.

Depressed Mood

Assessing depression can sometimes be difficult, as patients may be reluctant to share their symptoms with providers or may not recognize that they are struggling with depression. However, screening for depression is crucial since depression is a treatable risk factor for suicide. Several high-yield questions may help to clarify depressive symptoms and rule out potential causes (Box 11-4).

See Screening for Depression, pp. 218-219.

Box 11-4. Depressed Mood: High-Yield Health History Questions

Domain	Questions	Rationale
Psychiatric history	*Have you ever been diagnosed with depression or another mental disorder?* *Have you ever attempted suicide or had thoughts of suicide?*	Major depressive disorder (MDD) is the most common mental disorder that causes a depressed mood.[12] Other disorders that may cause a depressed mood include bipolar disorder, dysthymia, and seasonal affective disorder. Patients with a history of suicide attempts or thoughts of suicide are at increased risk for depressive disorders.
Family psychiatric history	*Does anyone in your family have a history of depression or other mental disorders?* *If so, what type of disorder, and who in your family is affected?*	Family history is an important risk factor for depression, and a positive family history may indicate a genetic predisposition to the disorder. Other mental disorders that may cause a depressed mood include bipolar disorder and schizophrenia.
Current symptoms	*Have you been feeling sad, hopeless, or empty? Have you lost interest in activities that you used to enjoy?*	These symptoms are common in MDD and can help diagnose the condition. Other mental disorders that may cause a depressed mood include bipolar disorder and dysthymia.
Duration of symptoms	*How long have you been experiencing these symptoms?* *Have you experienced these symptoms in the past?*	Patients with bipolar disorder may experience alternating episodes of depression and mania, whereas patients with dysthymia may experience a chronic low mood for ≥2 years.[12]
Suicidal ideation	*Have you had thoughts of hurting yourself or ending your life?* *Do you have a plan for how you would hurt yourself?*	Patients with bipolar disorder and borderline personality disorder are at increased risk for suicide attempts.
Impact on daily life	*Is your depression affecting your ability to work or perform daily activities?* *Have you been avoiding certain situations or activities because of depression?*	Patients with MDD may have difficulty concentrating or making decisions, while patients with agitated depression may be irritable and have difficulty sleeping.

Prominent causes and factors include **major depressive disorder (MDD)** (prolonged periods of sadness, hopelessness, and loss of interest in previously enjoyed activities, often accompanied by physical symptoms), **dysthymia** or **persistent depressive disorder** (chronic depression with milder symptoms lasting ≥2 years), **bipolar disorder** (condition marked by alternating episodes of mania and depression, affecting mood, energy, and activity levels), **seasonal affective disorder** (depression related to changes in seasons, typically manifesting during fall and winter months), and **medication** or **substance-induced depression** (mood changes as a result of certain medications such as propranolol, clonidine, prednisone, recreational drugs, or alcohol).

Memory Problems

In the *DSM-5*, both *delirium* and *dementia* are categorized under the umbrella of *neurocognitive disorders.* This classification was based on consultations with expert groups.[3] Dementia is designated as a *major neurocognitive disorder.* A milder form of cognitive impairment, "*mild neurocognitive disorder,*" can be applicable to younger individuals with impairment due to traumatic brain injuries or HIV infection. Despite these changes, the *DSM-5* retains the term "dementia" because of its widespread clinical usage. Tables within this chapter offer clear definitions of each cognitive domain, presenting symptoms in relation to everyday activities and associated assessments. Through a careful inquiry into the onset, frequency, associated symptoms, and possible triggers, you can form a cohesive picture of your patient presenting with memory problems (Box 11-5).

See Table 11-3, Neurocognitive Disorders: Delirium and Dementia, p. 226.

Box 11-5. Memory Problems: High-Yield Health History Questions

Domain	Questions	Rationale
Medical history	*Have you been diagnosed with any medical conditions, such as hypertension or diabetes?* *Have you had any recent infections or illnesses?*	Certain medical conditions, such as hypothyroidism, vitamin B12 deficiency, and infections such as meningitis or encephalitis, can cause memory problems.
Medication history	*What medications are you currently taking, including over-the-counter and herbal remedies?* *Have you started or stopped any medications recently?*	Medications that can cause memory problems as a side effect include benzodiazepines, anticholinergics, and certain antidepressants.
Lifestyle factors	*How much sleep are you getting each night?* *Do you drink alcohol, and if so, how much?*	Sleep deprivation can interfere with the consolidation of memories, while excessive alcohol consumption can cause memory impairment and affect cognitive function.
Type of memory problem	*Are you having trouble remembering recent events, or is your memory loss primarily for events that happened a long time ago?* *Are you having difficulty with short-term, long-term memory, or both?*	Difficulty with short-term memory may be indicative of a concussion, while difficulty with long-term memory may be indicative of Alzheimer disease (AD) or other forms of dementia.

Key underlying causes and conditions include **Alzheimer disease (AD)** (progressive neurodegenerative disorder leading to deterioration in memory and cognitive functions), **vascular dementia** (memory problems resulting from reduced blood flow to the brain, often due to strokes or other vascular events), **medication side effects** (especially benzodiazepines, anticholinergics, and opioids, which can impair cognitive functions, leading to memory lapses), **alcohol use disorder** (excessive and prolonged alcohol consumption can result in memory gaps and cognitive decline), **vitamin deficiencies** (especially vitamin B_{12}, can affect memory and cognition), and **depression** (can manifest as decreased concentration, decision-making challenges, and memory problems).

Domain	Questions	Rationale
Duration and progression	*How long have you been experiencing memory problems? Have your memory problems been getting worse over time?*	AD or other forms of dementia may have a gradual onset and worsen over time.
Associated symptoms	*Are you having trouble with language or speech?* *Are you experiencing any changes in mood or behavior?*	AD and depression can be associated with other cognitive or psychiatric symptoms, such as difficulty with language or speech, changes in mood or behavior, or confusion.

Medically Unexplained Symptoms

See Table 11-4, Somatic Symptoms and Related Disorders, p. 227.

Physical symptoms account for roughly 50% of office visits. Of these, about 25% of patients present with persistent and recurring symptoms that defy straightforward assessment and show no improvement. According to studies,[20,21] approximately 30% of these symptoms are medically unexplained.

Patients with these medically unexplained symptoms constitute a diverse group. Their conditions range from specific impairments to behaviors that align with the *DSM-5* criteria for mood and somatic symptom disorders.[21,22] Notably, while anxiety and depression are the most common mental disorders in the broader population, many of these patients do not report such symptoms. Instead, they emphasize their physical concerns. Approximately one-third of physical symptoms remain unexplained. Among patients with depression, two-thirds present primarily with physical problems. Half of these individuals report multiple unexplained or somatic symptoms.[21]

Functional disorders, which encompass conditions like **fibromyalgia** (widespread pain throughout the body accompanied by fatigue, sleep disturbances, and often tenderness in specific areas when pressure is applied) and **chronic fatigue syndrome** (**CFS**) **(**marked by persistent, unexplained fatigue that does not improve with rest)**,** often overlap in symptoms and certain objective abnormalities.

Infections, immune system issues, and hormonal imbalances have been considered as potential triggers. A review of 53 studies found overlap rates between fibromyalgia and CFS ranging from 34% to 70%.[23]

Failure to recognize the combination of physical symptoms, functional syndromes, and common mental disorders—anxiety, depression, unexplained and somatoform symptoms, and substance abuse—adds to the burden of patient undertreatment and poor quality of life.

PHYSICAL EXAMINATION: GENERAL APPROACH

Assessing mental health is both intricate and challenging. As students, you must meticulously evaluate changes in mental health, looking for potential pathologic and pharmacologic causes. The patient's personality, psychodynamics, family history, life experiences, and cultural background are significant factors to consider in your assessments. When you gather findings from the patient's health history and physical examination, use them to determine which parts of the formal mental status examination require further exploration.

The mental status examination is crucial for understanding a patient's mental health. Additionally, it is vital for evaluating the nervous system and serves as the introductory segment of the nervous system write-up. As you progress in your studies and training, you will learn to describe the patient's mood, speech, behavior, and cognition. Moreover, linking these observations to examinations of the cranial nerves, motor and sensory systems, and reflexes is a skill you will hone over time.

See Chapter 27, Nervous System, pp. 919–920 and Recording Your Findings, pp. 960–962.

While the format of the mental status examination in the following section offers a structured approach to making observations, it is not meant to be a rigid guide. Being adaptable in your assessments is important, but thoroughness should always be a priority. In certain situations, the order of your assessments is crucial. For instance, if a patient shows signs of impaired consciousness, attention, comprehension, or speech, these deficits should be prioritized. If a patient cannot provide a reliable health history, assessing most other mental functions becomes more challenging, emphasizing the need to look into acute causes.

TECHNIQUES OF EXAMINATION

Key Components of the Mental Status Examination

- Assess appearance and behavior, including level of consciousness.
- Assess speech and language.
- Assess mood.
- Assess thought process and perceptions.
- Assess insight and judgment.
- Assess cognitive function.
- Assess higher cognitive functions.

The mental status examination consists of six components: *appearance and behavior; speech and language; mood; thoughts and perceptions; insight and judgment; and cognitive function.* Each of these components is discussed in the following sections.

Assess Appearance and Behavior Including Level of Consciousness

Integrate the observations you have made throughout the history and physical examination, including the following aspects (Box 11-6). Also note the patient's level of consciousness (Box 11-7). Avoid using terms that lack precision, such as "sleepy," "out of it," "sluggish," or "groggy."

Box 11-6. Assessment Criteria for Patient Appearance and Behavior

Aspect	Description	Notes
Level of consciousness	Assessing the level of consciousness is a fundamental step in evaluating a patient's neurologic status. This pertains to how alert and attentive a person is to their surroundings and stimuli and checks if the patient is awake, alert, understands questions as well as how they respond.	If the patient doesn't respond to your inquiries, escalate the stimulus, as described in Box 11-7.
Posture and motor behavior	Evaluating a patient's posture and motor behavior is essential in understanding their neurologic and psychological state. This refers to how a patient positions themself and how they move. Observations consider pace, range, nature of movements, and any changes.	Look for tense posture, restlessness, and more. Observe for signs like poor eye contact of psychosis, or the expansive movements of a manic episode.
Dress, grooming, and personal hygiene	Evaluating these aspects provides critical insights into their self-care and can be an indicator of mental and emotional well-being. This checks the patient's attire, its condition, and how well-maintained it is. Grooming aspects like hair, nails, teeth, and skin are noted.	Grooming and hygiene may deteriorate in conditions like depression. Excessive attention to grooming may indicate obsessive-compulsive disorder. One-sided neglect can result from specific lesions.
Facial expression	Facial expressions are indicators of a patient's emotional state and cognitive processes. Observing the range and appropriateness of emotions displayed on a patient's face is essential.	Note expressions of anxiety, depression, and others. Facial immobility might indicate parkinsonism.
Manner, affect, and relationship to people and things	Assess the patient's affect through observable behaviors that express feelings or emotions through voice, facial expression, and demeanor. *Affect* is the external representation of inner emotional state. Check if it is appropriate to the topics being discussed.	Watch for signs like the hostility of paranoia, the elation of mania, or the flat affect of schizophrenia. Be aware of signs like hallucinations that can occur in conditions like schizophrenia or alcohol withdrawal.

Box 11-7. Levels of Consciousness

Level	Patient Response
Alert	The alert patient has eyes open, looks at you when spoken to in a *normal tone of voice*, and responds fully and appropriately to stimuli.
Lethargy	The lethargic patient appears drowsy but opens the eyes when spoken to in a *loud voice* and looks at you, responds to questions, and then falls asleep.
Obtundation	The obtunded patient opens the eyes when *tactile* stimulus is applied and looks at you but responds to you slowly and is somewhat confused.
Stupor	The stuporous patient arouses only after *painful* stimuli. Verbal responses are slow or even absent. The patient lapses into an unresponsive state when the stimulus ceases.
Coma	A comatose patient remains unarousable with eyes closed. There is no evident response to inner need or external stimuli.

Assess Speech and Language

Language is the complex symbolic system for expressing, receiving, and comprehending words; as with consciousness, attention, and memory, language is essential for assessing other mental functions. Throughout the interview, note characteristics of the patient's speech (Box 11-8).

Depression can cause slow speech, while mania may lead to louder, faster speech. Dysarthria relates to articulation issues, aphasia to language disorders, and dysphonia to voice changes. For a detailed overview, refer to Chapter 27, Nervous System, Table 27-2, Disorders of Speech, p. 968.

Watch for abnormalities in spontaneous speech, such as hesitancies, disrupted inflections like monotones, **circumlocutions** where phrases replace forgotten words, and **paraphasias** where words are malformed, incorrect, or invented.

If the patient's speech lacks meaning or fluency, proceed with further testing as outlined in Box 11-9. Check for deficits in vision, hearing, intelligence, and education that may affect responses.

See Chapter 27, Nervous System, Table 27-2, Disorders of Speech, p. 968.

Box 11-8. Assessment of Speech and Language Characteristics

Aspect	Description	Representative Questions
Quantity	The amount of speech produced by the patient, which may be too much or too little depending on the underlying condition.	*Are you finding yourself talking more than usual?* *Are you finding it hard to talk as much as you used to?*
Rate and volume	The speed and loudness of speech, which may be too fast or too slow, and too loud or too soft.	*Are you having difficulty speaking at a normal speed?* *Do you feel like you're speaking too loudly or too softly?*
Articulation of words	The clarity and precision of speech, which may be affected by difficulty pronouncing certain sounds or words.	*Are you having difficulty pronouncing certain sounds or words?* *Do you feel like your speech is slurred or unclear?*
Fluency	The smoothness and flow of speech, which may be affected by stuttering or hesitations.	*Are you having difficulty speaking fluently?* *Are you experiencing any hesitations or repetitions when speaking?*

Box 11-9. Testing for Aphasia

Word comprehension	Ask the patient to follow a one-stage command, such as "Point to your nose." Try a two-stage command: "Point to your mouth, then your knee."
Repetition	Ask the patient to repeat a phrase of one-syllable words (the most difficult repetition task): "No ifs, ands, or buts."
Naming	Ask the patient to name the parts of a watch.
Reading comprehension	Ask the patient to read a paragraph aloud.
Writing	Ask the patient to write a sentence.

Note: These questions are designed to identify the type of aphasia. There are two common types:

Expressive (Broca) *aphasia* is characterized by preserved comprehension and slow, nonfluent speech. For example: A person is trying to say, "*I took my dog for a walk*," but instead says, "*I…I…walk dog.*" The person knows what they want to say but struggles to find the right words. Their speech might be halting, and they might omit small words like "is," "and," or "the."

Receptive (Wernicke) *aphasia* is marked by impaired comprehension despite fluent speech. For example, a person hears the question, "*How are you today?*" and responds with, "*Happy green the to sky.*" The person speaks using real words, and the speech is fluent in rhythm and rate. However, the words are put together in a nonsensical sequence, making them difficult to understand.

Assess Mood

Mood is the pervasive and sustained emotion that colors a person's perception of the world. *Affect* refers to the external expression of a person's emotional state, which can be observed through their facial expressions, tone of voice, and other observable behaviors. These terms are often confused. Simply, affect is to mood as weather is to climate.

Ask the patient to describe their mood, including usual mood level and fluctuations related to life events. If you suspect depression, assess its severity and any risk of suicide (Box 11-10).

It is your responsibility to ask directly about suicidal thoughts. This may be the only way to uncover suicidal ideation and plans that would launch immediate intervention and treatment. Studies show that asking at-risk individuals if they are suicidal does not increase suicides or suicidal thoughts.[24] Approach these questions with sensitivity and empathy (Box 11-11). Patients might be more forthcoming when they feel understood and safe.

Assess Thought Process and Perceptions

Thought process refers to the logic, organization, coherence, and relevance of a patient's thoughts as they pertain to specific goals. It essentially describes *how* people think. *Perceptions* refer to how individuals interpret sensory information from their environment. It is the individual's awareness and understanding of reality, often through senses like hearing or seeing. For clarity, while thought process is about the flow and organization of ideas,

Box 11-10. Assessment of Mood Characteristics

Aspect	Description	Representative Questions
Current mood	Patient's present emotional state (e.g., happy, sad, angry)	*How are you feeling right now?* *Would you describe your current mood for me?*
Duration	Length of time the patient has been experiencing the current mood or emotional state	*How long have you been feeling this way?*
Intensity	Depth or strength of the emotional state	*On a scale of 1 to 10, how intense would you say your emotions are right now?*
Fluctuation	Changes in mood or how frequently the mood shifts	*How often does your mood change? Do you have sudden mood swings?*
Triggers	External or internal factors that influence or lead to a change in mood	*Are there specific things or events that make you feel better or worse?*
Impact on daily life	How the mood or emotional state affects the patient's daily activities and relationships	*How has your mood affected your daily activities or relationships with others?*

Box 11-11. Assessment of Suicidal Thoughts

Aspect	Description	Representative Questions
Presence of thoughts	Identifying if the patient has any thoughts of wanting to harm themself or end their life	*Have you had thoughts of hurting yourself or ending your life?*
Frequency	How often these thoughts occur	*How often do you have these thoughts?*
Intensity	Depth or strength of these thoughts	*On a scale of 1 to 10, how strong are these thoughts when they occur?*
Plans	Whether the patient has considered specific methods or made any preparations	*Have you thought about how you would do it?* *Have you taken any steps toward this?*
Means	Availability of tools or resources the patient might consider using	*Do you have access to the things you would need to carry out these thoughts?*
Previous attempts	Any past incidents in which the patient tried to hurt themself or take their life	*Have you ever acted on these thoughts in the past?*
Protective factors	Elements in the patient's life that make them reconsider or avoid acting on their suicidal thoughts	*What stops you or holds you back from acting on these thoughts?*

perceptions focus on interpreting external sensory input. You should determine if your patient might be experiencing distortions in reality, such as hallucinations. Assess your patient's thought processes throughout the interview (Boxes 11-12 to 11-15).

Box 11-12. Assessment of Thought Process Characteristics

Aspect	Description	Representative Questions
Thought content	Content of a patient's thoughts, including their beliefs, attitudes, and values; patients with thought content problems may have delusions, hallucinations, or obsessive thoughts that affect their behavior and functioning	*Do you believe that anyone is trying to harm you?* *Have you been hearing voices or seeing things that other people don't?*
Perception	How a patient perceives and interprets their environment; patients with perception problems may have distorted perceptions of reality, such as seeing or hearing things that are not actually present	*Are you feeling like your surroundings are distorted or not real?* *Are you seeing or hearing things that other people don't?*
Insight	Degree to which a patient is aware of their mental state and condition; patients with insight problems may be unaware of their symptoms or the need for treatment	*Do you think that you might have a mental health problem? Do you feel like your behavior or thinking is unusual or problematic?*
Judgment	Ability to make sound decisions and solve problems; patients with judgment problems may make impulsive or irrational decisions or have difficulty weighing the risks and benefits of different options	*Can you describe a difficult decision you've had to make recently and how you approached it?* *Do you feel like you make good decisions and choices in your life?*

Patients with psychotic disorders often lack self-awareness, especially in neurologic cases affecting the parietal lobe. Judgment is compromised in conditions like delirium and dementia. Factors like mood disorders, education, and cultural values further influence judgment.

Box 11-13. Variations and Abnormalities in Thought Processes[3]

	Description	Example
Blocking	Sudden interruption of speech in midsentence or before the idea is completed, attributed to "losing the thought"; blocking occurs in healthy people	Mid-sentence, a person might say, *"I was walking to the… uh…"* and then pause, unable to continue the thought.
Circumstantiality	Mildest thought disorder, consisting of speech with unnecessary detail, indirection, and delay in reaching the point; some topics may have a meaningful connection; many people without mental disorders have circumstantial speech	When asked where they went over the weekend, a person might describe the weather, the outfit they chose, the history of the place, and finally conclude with their destination.
Clanging	Speech with choice of words based on sound, rather than meaning, as in rhyming and punning	*"I heard the bell, tell, fell, well, sell."*
Confabulation	Fabrication of facts or events in response to questions, to fill in the gaps from impaired memory	When asked about a recent trip they never took, a person might invent details about places, people, and events.
Derailment (loosening of associations)	Tangential speech with shifting topics that are loosely connected or unrelated; patient is unaware of the lack of association.	"I like apples. The car is fast. Did you see the blue shoes? My uncle is tall."
Echolalia	Repetition of the words and phrases of others	Clinician: *"How are you today?"* Patient: *"How are you today?"*
Flight of ideas	Almost continuous flow of accelerated speech with abrupt changes from one topic to the next; changes are based on understandable associations, plays on words, or distracting stimuli, but ideas are not well connected	*"I need to buy apples, but the store is so far, far like the stars, stars are in movies, movies have popcorn."*

Blocking may be striking in schizophrenia.

Circumstantiality occurs in people with obsessions.

Clanging occurs in schizophrenia and manic episodes.

Confabulation is seen in Korsakoff syndrome.

Derailment is seen in schizophrenia, manic episodes, and other psychotic disorders.

Echolalia occurs in manic episodes and schizophrenia.

Flight of ideas is most frequently noted in manic episodes.

	Description	Example
Incoherence	Speech that is incomprehensible and illogical, with lack of meaningful connections, abrupt changes in topic, or disordered grammar or word use Flight of ideas, when severe, may produce incoherence	*"Apples blue run happiness under for why."*
Neologisms	Invented or distorted words, or words with new and highly idiosyncratic meanings	*"I enjoy flibberflop during the summertime."*
Perseveration	Persistent repetition of words or ideas	Clinician: *"What did you eat for breakfast?"* Patient: *"Toast."* Clinician: *"What color is your shirt?"* Patient: *"Toast."*

Incoherence is seen in severe psychotic disturbances (usually schizophrenia).

Neologisms are observed in schizophrenia, psychotic disorders, and aphasia.

Perseveration occurs in schizophrenia and other psychotic disorders.

Source: American Psychiatric Association. *Diagnostic and Statistical Manual of Mental Disorders: DSM-5*. 5th ed. American Psychiatric Association; 2013.

Box 11-14. Abnormalities of Thought Content[3]

Anxieties	Apprehensive anticipation of future danger or misfortune accompanied by feelings of worry, distress, and/or somatic symptoms of tension
Compulsions	Repetitive behaviors that the person feels driven to perform in response to an obsession, aimed at preventing or reducing anxiety or a dreaded event or situation; these behaviors are excessive and unrealistically connected to the provoking stimulus
Delusions	False fixed personal beliefs that are not amenable to change in light of conflicting evidence; types of delusions include: ■ Persecutory ■ Grandiose ■ Jealous ■ Erotomanic—the belief that another person is in love with the individual ■ Somatic—involves bodily functions or sensations. ■ Unspecified—includes delusions of reference without a prominent persecutory or grandiose component, or the belief that external events, objects, or people have a particular and unusual personal significance (e.g., commands from the radio or television)

Compulsions, obsessions, phobias, and anxieties often occur in anxiety disorders. See the *DSM-5*.[3]

Delusions and feelings of unreality or depersonalization are often associated with psychotic disorders. For official diagnostic criteria, see the *DSM-5*.[3]

Delusions may also occur in delirium, severe mood disorders, and dementia.

(continued)

Box 11-14. Abnormalities of Thought Content[3] (*Continued*)

Depersonalization	Sense that one's self or identity is different, changed, unreal; lost; or detached from one's mind or body
Derealization	Sense that the environment is strange, unreal, or remote
Obsessions	Recurrent persistent thoughts, images, or urges experienced as intrusive and unwanted that the person tries to ignore, suppress, or neutralize with other thoughts or actions (e.g., performing a compulsive behavior)
Phobias	Persistent irrational fears accompanied by a compelling desire to avoid the provoking stimulus

Source: American Psychiatric Association. *Diagnostic and Statistical Manual of Mental Disorders: DSM-5*. 5th ed. American Psychiatric Association; 2013.

Box 11-15. Abnormalities of Perception[3]

Hallucinations	Perception-like experiences that seem real but, unlike illusions, lack actual external stimulation. The person may or may not recognize the experiences as false. Hallucinations may be auditory, visual, olfactory, gustatory, tactile, or somatic. False perceptions associated with dreaming, falling asleep, and awakening are not classified as hallucinations.
Illusions	These are misinterpretations of real external stimuli, such as mistaking rustling leaves for the sound of voices.

Hallucinations may occur in delirium, dementia (less commonly), posttraumatic stress disorder, schizophrenia, and substance use.

Illusions may occur in grief reactions, delirium, acute and posttraumatic stress disorders, and schizophrenia.

Source: American Psychiatric Association. *Diagnostic and Statistical Manual of Mental Disorders: DSM-5*. 5th ed. American Psychiatric Association; 2013.

Assess Cognitive Function

Cognition refers to the mental processes involved in gaining knowledge and comprehension. Assess cognitive function, which includes *orientation*, *attention*, and *memory* (remote, recent, new learning). See Box 11-16.

Tests of Cognitive Function. Testing helps you distinguish between patients with life-long intellectual impairment (whose information and vocabulary are limited) from those with mild or moderate neurocognitive disorders (whose information and vocabulary are generally well preserved). The *Digit Span*, *Serial 7s*, and *Spelling Backward* are all tests of cognitive function and can help assess your patient's ability to concentrate and process information. These tests can be adapted to your patient's level of education and familiarity with numerical and linguistic sequences and can provide insight into potential underlying causes of poor cognitive performance (Box 11-17).

Box 11-16. Assessment of Cognitive Functions Characteristics

Aspect	Description	Representative Questions
Orientation	Ability to know where one is, what time it is, and other basic information about the world; patients with orientation problems may be confused or disoriented, and may have difficulty with memory	*Do you know where you are right now?* *What day of the week is it today?*
Attention	Ability to focus and sustain attention on a task; patients with attention problems may be easily distracted or have difficulty with tasks that require sustained focus, such as reading or working on a project	*Are you able to focus and concentrate on a task for a sustained period?* *Do you find yourself getting easily distracted or losing focus?*
Recent memory	Ability to remember events or information that occurred recently, such as in the past few hours or days; patients with recent memory problems may have difficulty recalling recent events or conversations	*Can you tell me what you had for breakfast this morning?* *Do you remember what you did yesterday afternoon?*
Remote memory	Ability to remember events or information from the distant past, such as childhood or early adulthood; patients with remote memory problems may have difficulty recalling past events or experiences	*Can you tell me about a vacation you took when you were younger?* *What was your first job like?*
New learning ability	Ability to learn and remember new information; patients with new learning ability problems may have difficulty learning new things and may have difficulty with memory recall	*Are you able to learn and remember new information? How have you found your ability to remember new things compared to the past?*

Box 11-17. Cognitive Function Tests

Test	Description	Questions	Causes of Poor Performance
Digit Span	Test of a patient's ability to concentrate by reciting a series of digits and asking the patient to repeat them back; the series starts with two digits and increases in length if the patient responds correctly and ends after a second failure in a single series. The test is then repeated in reverse order.	*Can you repeat the series of digits that I'm about to say to you?* *Can you repeat the digits in reverse order?*	Delirium, dementia, intellectual disability, performance anxiety
Serial 7s	Instruct the patient to start from 100 and subtract 7 repeatedly. The test measures the effort required and the speed and accuracy of the responses.	*Can you start from 100 and subtract 7 repeatedly?*	Delirium, late-stage of dementia, intellectual disability, anxiety, depression, and educational level
Spelling Backward	The patient is given a five-letter word and is asked to spell it backward.	*Can you spell this five-letter word backward for me?*	Delirium, dementia, intellectual disability, anxiety, depression, and educational level

Assess Higher Cognitive Functions

Higher cognitive functions are assessed by vocabulary, fund of information, abstract thinking, calculations, and construction of objects that have two or three dimensions (Box 11-18).

Box 11-18. Assessment of Higher Cognitive Functions Characteristics

Aspect	Description	Representative Questions
Information	Ability to recall and understand basic information, such as current events or personal history; patients with information problems may have difficulty with general knowledge or memory recall	*Can you tell me the name of the current president/prime minister? Do you remember where you were born?*
Vocabulary	Ability to use and understand language; patients with vocabulary problems may have difficulty with word finding or understanding complex language	*Are you having difficulty finding the right word to express yourself?* *Do you find it difficult to understand metaphors or abstract language?*
Calculating ability	Ability to perform mathematical calculations; patients with calculating ability problems may have difficulty with simple arithmetic or complex mathematical reasoning.	*Can you tell me what is 7 × 8?* *If something costs 78 cents, and you give the salesperson 1 dollar, how much change should you get back?*
Abstract thinking	Ability to understand abstract concepts and relationships; patients with abstract thinking problems may have difficulty with problem-solving or understanding metaphors	Proverbs: *Can you explain the meaning of the saying "don't count your chickens before they hatch"?* *Can you solve this problem: "If Mary has two apples and John has three apples, how many apples do they have together?"*
Constructional ability	Ability to perceive and reproduce visual-spatial information; patients with constructional ability problems may have difficulty with tasks such as drawing, copying a design, or assembling objects.	*Can you copy this simple design?* (Figs. 11-5 and 11-6 are examples) *Can you draw a clock face complete with numbers and hands?* (Figs. 11-7 and 11-8 are examples)

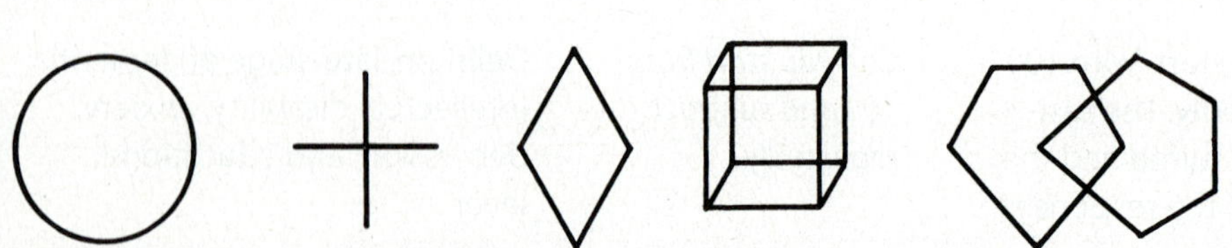

FIGURE 11-5. Ask the patient to copy these figures (starting from the left) on a piece of paper.

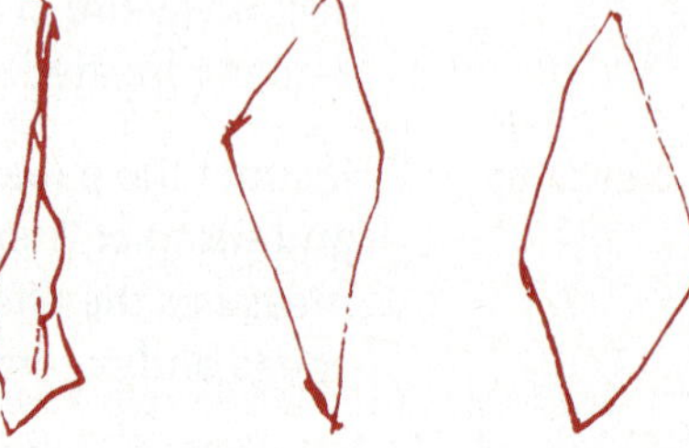

FIGURE 11-6. From left to right: poor, fair, and good attempts of drawn shapes.

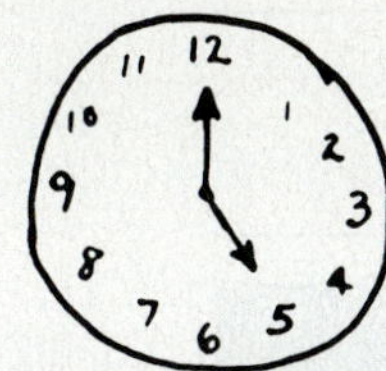

FIGURE 11-7. Patient-drawn clock face, with hands and numbers, rated as excellent.

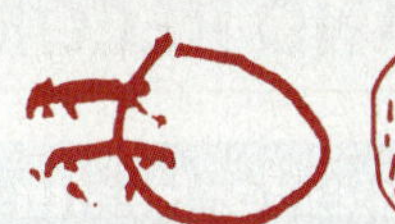
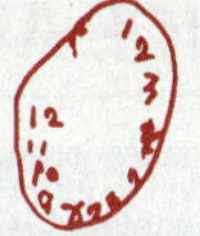

FIGURE 11-8. From left to right: poor, fair, and good attempts of clock face drawings.

RECORDING YOUR FINDINGS

Recording Behavior and Mental Status

"***Mental Status:*** The patient is alert, well-groomed, and cheerful. Speech is fluent and words are clear. Thought processes are coherent, insight is good. The patient is oriented to person, place, and time. Serial 7s accurate; recent and remote memory intact. Calculations intact."

OR

"***Mental Status:*** The patient appears sad and displays signs of fatigue, with wrinkled clothing. Speech is slow, and the words come out mumbled. While the thought processes are coherent, the patient demonstrates limited insight into current life challenges. The patient is oriented to person, place, and time. Tests for cognitive functions such as digit span, serial 7s, and calculations are accurate, but with delayed responses. The clock drawing test is executed well."

The description suggests that the patient may be experiencing symptoms consistent with depression or a mood disorder.

By dissecting physical examination documentation into its detailed parts, we see a clear example of how thorough clinical observations provide critical diagnostic clues. The described findings in the mental status examination highlight the following important clues:

- *Appearance of sadness and fatigue:* This is commonly observed in depression.
- *Wrinkled clothing:* This can indicate a lack of attention to personal care, often seen in depressive states.
- *Slow, mumbled speech:* This suggests psychomotor retardation, a symptom frequently associated with depression.
- *Coherent thought processes but limited insight:* This reflects an ability to think logically, yet a diminished capacity to understand or acknowledge the full extent of their life challenges, often seen in depressive states.
- *Orientation intact:* This indicates no gross cognitive impairment.
- *Accurate but delayed responses in cognitive testing:* This suggests the patient's cognitive functions are intact but may be hindered by decreased psychomotor speed, often seen in depression.
- *Adequate performance on clock drawing test:* This indicates preserved visuospatial ability and executive function, which are typically not impaired in uncomplicated cases of depression.

Overall, the patient's presentation is consistent with symptoms of *depression*, characterized by mood disturbance, slowed thought and speech, and reduced insight, yet with preserved basic cognitive functions.

HEALTH PROMOTION AND COUNSELING: EVIDENCE AND RECOMMENDATIONS

Important Topics for Health Promotion and Counseling

- Screening for depression
- Screening for anxiety disorders
- Assessing for suicide risk
- Screening for neurocognitive disorders
- Screening for substance use disorder, including misuse of alcohol, tobacco, and prescription drugs; see Chapter 7, Health Maintenance and Screening, pp. 125–127

In the following section, both traditional terms like "men," "women," "male," and "female" and inclusive terms such as "individuals assigned female at birth" and "individuals assigned male at birth" are used. This approach balances inclusivity with the need to accurately represent the original research.

Mental disorders impose a substantial burden of suffering.[25] About 1 in 5 U.S. adults (57.8 million) experienced mental disorder in 2021, with about 1 in 20 (14.1 million) experiencing serious mental disorder (schizophrenia, MDD, or bipolar disorder). Depression and anxiety, which frequently overlap, are a common cause of hospitalization in the United States. Mental disorders are associated with increased risks for chronic medical conditions, decreased life expectancy, disability, substance use, and suicide. For many adolescents and adults, the COVID-19 pandemic adversely affected mental health, even among those with no history of mental disorder.[25]

In 2021 U.S. data, about 10% of individuals who used drugs in the past year reported using drugs "a little more or much more" during the pandemic, while about 15% of individuals who consumed alcohol in the past year reported a similar increase. Among adults ages ≥18 years in 2021, a minority of those who had thoughts of suicide (16%), made a suicide plan (14%), or attempted suicide (16%) in the past year did so because of the pandemic.

See Chapter 3, Health History, pp. 54–55.

Screening for Depression

About 21 million adult Americans (8.3%) reported a major depressive episode in 2021; the prevalence was highest among adults ages 18 to 25 years (18.6%).[25] Major depressive episodes were reported nearly twice as often by individuals assigned female at birth (10.3%) than individuals assigned male at birth (6.2%); about 13% of individuals with a recent live birth reported postpartum depressive symptoms.[26] Symptoms of depression can include depressed mood, low self-esteem, loss of pleasure in daily activities (anhedonia), fatigue, sleep disorders, weight loss, psychomotor changes, difficulty concentrating or making decisions, and thoughts of death.[27] Look carefully for symptoms of depression in vulnerable patients, especially those with the risk factors of older age, female sex, chronic illness, low socioeconomic status, history of adverse childhood events, recent stressful events, recent childbirth, and other psychiatric disorders including substance use disorder. A personal or family history of depression also places patients at risk.

See discussions of depression in older adults in Chapter 30, Older Adults, p. 1175 and postpartum depression in Chapter 29, Pregnant Persons, p. 1144.

The U.S. Preventive Services Task Force (USPSTF) issued a grade B recommendation in 2021 to screen adults for depression in clinical settings where patients who screen positive "are appropriately diagnosed and treated with evidence-based care or referred to a setting that can provide the necessary care."[28] The USPSTF also issued a grade B recommendation to screen adolescents ages 12 to 18 years for depression, but concluded that evidence was insufficient to recommend screening for children ages ≤11 years (I statement).[29] For adults, responding yes to two simple questions about mood and anhedonia has a sensitivity of 91% and a specificity of 67% for detecting major depression and appears to be as effective as using more detailed instruments.[30]

See Table 11-5, Screening for Depression: Geriatric Depression Scale, p. 228, and Table 11-6, Screening for Depression: Patient Health Questionnaire (PHQ-9), pp. 229–230.

- "*Over the past 2 weeks, have you felt down, depressed, or hopeless?*" Screens for depressed mood.
- "*Over the past 2 weeks, have you felt little interest or pleasure in doing things?*" Screens for anhedonia.

A single screening question, "*Do you often feel sad or depressed?*" has a sensitivity of 69% and specificity of 90%.[31] All positive screening tests warrant further evaluation to confirm the diagnosis.

Screening for Anxiety Disorders

Anxiety disorders are characterized by chronic excessive anxiety and worry that can be accompanied by symptoms of restlessness, easy fatigue, difficulty concentrating, irritability, muscle tension, or sleep disturbances.[3,32,33] Anxiety disorders are common; in the 2019 National Health Interview survey, 6.1% of U.S. adults reported experiencing moderate or severe anxiety within the previous 2 weeks.[34] Anxiety is associated with reduced health-related quality of life, decreased work productivity, and higher health care utilization and costs. Recognize the risk factors for anxiety, including marital status (widowed or divorced), female sex, low socioeconomic status, stressful life events, smoking and alcohol use, comorbid psychiatric disorders, and family history.

A widely used screening test is the GAD scale.[33,35] The GAD-7 is a self-reported scale that has sensitivities ranging from 67% to 89% and specificities ranging from 82% to 95% for detecting a GAD, depending upon the cut-offs. A two-item version (GADS-2), which uses only the first two GAD-7 items, also has adequate sensitivity and specificity for detecting GAD. A positive screening test warrants further evaluation to confirm the diagnosis. Both psychological and pharmacologic interventions have been shown to reduce anxiety symptoms.

See Table 11-7, Screening for Anxiety Disorders: GAD-7, p. 237.

The USPSTF issued a grade B recommendation to screen for anxiety in adults ages 19 to 64 years, including pregnant and postpartum patients.[33] Evidence was insufficient to recommend screening those aged ≥65 years (I statement). The USPSTF also issued a grade B recommendation to screen children and adolescents ages 8 to 18 years for anxiety.[36] Evidence was insufficient to recommend screening younger children (I statement).

Assessing for Suicide Risk. Suicide ranked as the 11th leading cause of death in the United States in 2021, accounting for nearly 48,000 deaths (1.4% of all deaths).[25,37,38] Suicide risk is associated with age, sex, race, and ethnicity. Most deaths occur among those ages 45 to 64 years, although suicide is the second leading cause of death among people ages 10 to 14 years and 20 to 34 years. Annually, more than 14 suicides occur per 100,000 population; rates have been stable since 2018.[39] Suicide rates are highest among adults aged 85 and older, adults aged 25 to 34, and White individuals assigned male at birth. While individuals assigned male at birth have suicide rates nearly four times higher than those assigned female at birth, those assigned female at birth are nearly twice as likely to attempt suicide.[40] Firearms or hanging are more commonly used by individuals assigned male at birth, while poisoning is more commonly used by individuals assigned female at birth.[41] Overall, non-Hispanic White individuals account for about 90% of all suicides, though American Indian/Alaska Native individuals aged 25 to 44 have the highest suicide rate among any racial or ethnic group. Suicide risk is also higher among veterans; rural populations; and people identifying as lesbian, gay, bisexual, or transgender.[42,43] An estimated 25 attempts are made for each death by suicide, with a ratio of 4 to 1 among older adults and ratios of 100 to 200 to 1 among young adults. In 2021, about 13% of both adolescents ages 12 to 17 years and young adults ages 18 to 25 years reported serious thoughts about suicide in the previous year. Additionally, 3.4% of the adolescents and 2.7% of the young adults reported a suicide attempt.

Despite the public health burden of suicide, the USPSTF found insufficient evidence to assess the balance of benefits and harms of routinely screening either adults or children and adolescents for suicide risk (I statement).[28,29] However, the USPSTF advised clinicians to use their judgment, based on patient circumstances, to determine whether to screen for suicide risk.

Screening for Neurocognitive Disorders

Dementia. *Dementia* is "a decline in two or more cognitive capacities that causes impairment in function but not alertness or attention."[44] In the *DSM-5*, dementia is classified as a *major neurocognitive disorder.*[3] Dementia can affect the cognitive domains of complex attention, executive function, learning and memory, language, perceptual motor function, and social cognition and cause functional declines severe enough to interfere with activities of daily living. The major dementia syndromes include AD, vascular dementia, frontotemporal dementia, dementia with Lewy bodies, Parkinson disease with dementia, and dementia of mixed etiology.[45] AD, the predominant form, affects 10% of Americans age >65 years, or roughly 6.7 million people; almost two-thirds are women. By 2060, nearly 14 million Americans are expected to have AD. The strongest risk factors for AD are advancing age, family history, and genetics, particularly the gene mutation apolipoprotein (APOE) ε4 and trisomy 21 in Down syndrome. However, an estimated 40% of dementias are associated with modifiable risk factors, including midlife obesity, physical inactivity, tobacco use, hearing impairment, excess alcohol consumption, and social isolation.[46]

Diagnosing AD is challenging because clinicians must exclude delirium, depression, mild cognitive impairment, and medications as explanations for changes in cognition and function.[44] Box 11-19 highlights distinguishing features between age-related cognitive decline, mild cognitive impairment, and AD.

The *Mini-Mental State Examination* is the best-known screening test for dementia but is now copyrighted for commercial use, so is less accessible. Recommended screening tests now include the *Mini-Cog, the Montreal Cognitive Assessment (MoCA),* and the *St. Louis University Mental Status Exam (SLUMS),* as shown in Tables 11-8 to 11-10, pp. 232–234.

The Mini-Cog has a sensitivity and specificity of 76% and 73%, respectively, and can be administered in about 3 to 5 minutes.[47] The MoCA has a sensitivity

Box 11-19. Spectrum of Cognitive Decline

Cognitive Decline	Description	Characteristics
Age-related cognitive decline	Normal part of aging, characterized by a slight decline in cognitive function, such as memory and processing speed	No significant interference with daily activities
Mild cognitive impairment (MCI)	Mild decline in cognitive function from a previous level of performance, but without significant interference with daily activities[3,127,128]	May include difficulty with memory, attention, or problem-solving Alzheimer disease (AD) develops at a higher frequency in MCI patients, progressing to AD at a reported rate of 6% to 15% per year[129,130]
Major neurocognitive disorder (dementia)	Substantial decline in cognitive function from a previous level of performance, with significant interference with daily activities	May include difficulty with memory, attention, language, problem-solving, and judgment

Specific Types of Dementia[129,131]

Type of Dementia	Description	Characteristics
Alzheimer disease	Most common type of dementia, characterized by a progressive decline in cognitive function due to the buildup of amyloid plaques and tau tangles in the brain	May include difficulty with memory, attention, language, problem-solving, and judgment
Vascular dementia	Dementia caused by damage to the blood vessels in the brain	May include difficulty with memory, attention, processing speed, and executive function
Dementia with Lewy bodies	Dementia characterized by the presence of Lewy bodies in the brain, which are also found in Parkinson disease	May include difficulty with memory, attention, visual hallucinations, and movement problems

Sources: Markwick A, Zamboni G, de Jager CA. Profiles of cognitive subtest impairment in the Montreal Cognitive Assessment (MoCA) in a research cohort with normal Mini-Mental State Examination (MMSE) scores. *J Clin Exp Neuropsychol*. 2012;34(7):750–757; Rabins PV, Blass DM. In the Clinic. Dementia. *Ann Intern Med*. 2014;161(3):ITC1–ITC16.

and specificity of 90% and 60%, respectively, and takes 10 minutes to administer.[48] Although less widely studied than other screening tests, SLUMS, which can be administered in 7 minutes, has been reported to have a sensitivity and specificity of 93% and 96%, respectively.[49] While highlighting the accuracy of screening tests for detecting dementia, the USPSTF issued an I statement on screening community-dwelling adults ages ≥65 years for cognitive impairment.[50] The USPSTF noted that screening tests were less accurate for detecting cognitive impairment and found insufficient evidence regarding whether pharmacologic or nonpharmacologic interventions could benefit patients with mild to moderate cognitive impairment.

Delirium. *Delirium*, a multifactorial syndrome, is an acute confusional state marked by sudden onset; fluctuating course; inattention; and, at times, changing levels of consciousness.[51] Risk for developing delirium depends on both predisposing conditions that increase susceptibility and the immediate precipitating factors. Predisposing conditions include cognitive impairment, multiple comorbidities, polypharmacy, hearing or visual impairment, mental disorder, substance use disorders, and having poor functional status.

See Table 11-3, Neurocognitive Disorders: Delirium and Dementia, p. 226.

Delirium is common in hospitalized older patients, particularly with severe illnesses and following elective and high-risk surgeries. Intensive care unit admissions requiring mechanical ventilation are associated with a high incidence of delirium regardless of age. Even though delirium is associated with poor patient outcomes, more than 50% of cases are undetected.

The *Confusion Assessment Method (CAM)* (Box 11-20) is recommended for screening at-risk patients.[52] The CAM instrument can quickly and accurately detect delirium at the bedside. Multicomponent interventions by interdisciplinary teams that target key clinical risk factors for delirium, including cognitive impairment and disorientation, sleep deprivation, immobility, visual impairment, hearing impairment, pain, infection, poor nutrition, dehydration, polypharmacy, and prescription of psychoactive drugs can reduce the incidence of delirium.[53,54]

Box 11-20. The Confusion Assessment Method (CAM) Diagnostic Algorithm[132]

Diagnosing delirium requires features 1 and 2 AND either 3 or 4.

1. **Acute change in mental status and fluctuating course:**
   Is there evidence of an acute change in cognition from baseline? Does the abnormal behavior fluctuate during the day?
2. **Inattention:**
   Does the patient have difficulty focusing attention?
3. **Disorganized thinking:**
   Does the patient have rambling or irrelevant conversations, unclear or illogical flow of ideas, or unpredictable switching from subject to subject?
4. **Abnormal level of consciousness:**
   Is the patient anything besides alert—hyperalert, lethargic, stuporous, or comatose?

Source: Wong CL, Holroyd-Leduc J, Simel DL, Straus SE. Does this patient have delirium? Value of bedside instruments. *JAMA*. 2010;304(7):779–786.

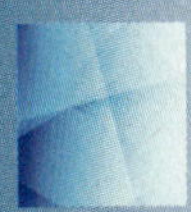

TABLE 11-1. Central Nervous System Structures and Mental Disorders

Structure	Roles	Clinical Manifestations of Dysfunction
Cortical Structures		
Parietal lobe	Involved in visuospatial sense, attention, and movement[1,55]	Deficits in parietal lobe function have been associated with attention-deficit/hyperactivity disorder (ADHD), obsessive–compulsive disorder (OCD), and schizophrenia.[56–59]
Temporal lobe: primary auditory cortex	Responsible for auditory processing	In schizophrenia, the primary auditory cortex activates even in the absence of sound, which often result in the experience of *auditory hallucinations*.[59,60]
Temporal lobe: hippocampus	Critical to memory and learning[61–63] High concentrations of cortisol receptors in the hippocampus	Hippocampus dysfunction may contribute to cognitive impairment in Alzheimer disease (AD) and schizophrenia.[64,65] Major depressive disorder (MDD) and posttraumatic stress disorder (PTSD) both cause significant increases of cortisol, which may cause memory and cognitive problems seen in these disorders.[66–69] Hippocampus dysfunction is also thought to contribute to anxiety symptoms.[63]
Temporal lobe: amygdala	Involved in the cortical processes that cause emotions Fight-or-flight response, or fear response, is activated through the amygdala	In PTSD, the amygdala is often hyperactivated and cannot be easily turned off.[69] People with PTSD often startle easily and struggle with anxiety or panic. Excess amygdala activity is also seen in people with bipolar disorder, which is thought to contribute to irritability and labile mood.[70]
Frontal lobe	Vital to executive function (which includes memory, cognition, behavioral control, and attention) and emotions	Dysfunction has been associated with most mental disorders, including bipolar disorder, schizophrenia, ADHD, MDD, OCD, PTSD, and AD.[71–83]
Subcortical Structures		
Cingulate cortex	Manages attention, emotion, and memory[72,81–89]	Dysfunction is seen in people with ADHD, OCD, generalized anxiety disorder (GAD), MDD, and schizophrenia.[84,85,90–95]
Basal Forebrain		
Nucleus basalis of Meynert	Major center for acetylcholine production in the central nervous system, which helps to regulate sleep, arousal, and attention[96]	Dysfunction contributes to cognitive deficits in neurocognitive disorders.
Nucleus accumbens	Vital to the functioning of the reward pathway[68]	Excess activation is commonly seen in substance use disorders.[97]

(*continued*)

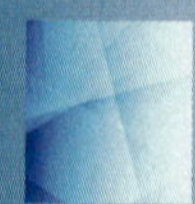

TABLE 11-1. Central Nervous System Structures and Mental Disorders *(Continued)*

Structure	Roles	Clinical Manifestations of Dysfunction
Basal ganglia	Works with the nucleus accumbens to control reward	Dysfunction is seen in substance use disorders,[68,97] OCD, MDD, ADHD, schizophrenia, and bipolar disorder.[68,98–100]
Epithalamus: pineal gland	Produces melatonin, which regulates sleep[1]	Dysfunction contributes to sleep disturbances in MDD, OCD, PTSD, and AD.[72–83]
Epithalamus: habenula	Helps regulate reproductive behavior, pain, nutrition, sleep, stress, and learning[101,102]	Increased activity in the habenula can cause anhedonia in depression.[103] Decreased habenula activity is associated with psychosis and substance use disorders.[104]
Hypothalamus	Periods of increased stress associated with increased activity of the hypothalamic–pituitary–adrenal axis and increased release of corticotropin-releasing factor, which causes cortisol (a steroid hormone) release	Increased cortisol can cause depressive symptoms.[105]
Mammillary bodies	Crucial in memory	Damage to the mammillary bodies is seen in vitamin B_1 (thiamine) deficiency in people with alcohol use disorder. This may lead to *Wernicke–Korsakoff syndrome*, a condition characterized by severe memory impairment.[1]
Cerebellum	Regulates motor coordination and motor learning	Alcohol use impairs cerebellar function, which can cause *ataxia*, or a loss of motor coordination.[106]

Note: Based on current research, the occipital lobe does not play as significant a role in mental disorders as do other cortical and subcortical structures.

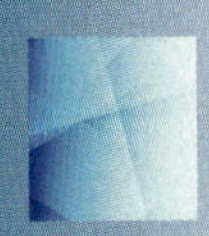

TABLE 11-2. Neurocircuitry of Mental Disorders

System/Network	Central Nervous System Structures Involved	Role When Activated	Mental Disorder
Limbic system	Hippocampus, amygdala, fornix, hypothalamus, thalamus, mammillary bodies, frontal lobes, temporal lobes, and cingulate gyrus	Responsible for experience of emotion as well as empathy[1,107,108]	Dysfunction seen in the vast majority of mental disorders, including but not limited to schizophrenia, major depressive disorder (MDD), bipolar disorder, anxiety, and posttraumatic stress disorder (PTSD)[109–113]
Fear network (subdivision of the limbic system)	Thalamus, frontal lobes, and amygdala		Dysfunction seen in anxiety, PTSD, and bipolar disorder[69,70]
Attention network	Frontal lobes and parietal lobes	Responsible for controlling attention	Dysfunction seen in persons with attention-deficit/hyperactivity disorder (ADHD)[58]
Salience network	Connections between the amygdala, basal ganglia, temporal lobes, and the cingulate cortex	Involved in monitoring internal states (homeostasis, emotion, pain) and external states (body position, environment); activity here has been associated with self-awareness, social behavior, and communication	Dysfunction associated with schizophrenia, mood disorder, anxiety, dementia, and substance use[114,115]
Reward network	Composed of the amygdala, hippocampus, frontal lobes, cingulate cortex, brainstem, basal forebrain, and basal ganglia	Causes a pleasurable feeling of reward and contributes to the learning	Dysfunction occurs in substance use disorders and ADHD[1,58]
Default mode network	Frontal lobes, cingulate cortex, parietal lobes, and temporal lobes	Involved in rest and internal awareness	Dysfunction seen in schizophrenia and MDD, leading to delusions and negative thoughts, respectively[116]
Executive network	Frontal lobes and cingulate cortex	Responsible for memory and planning	Dysfunction has been associated with numerous mental disorders, including PTSD, MDD, and schizophrenia[117]

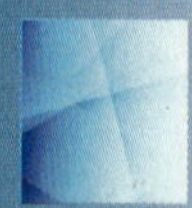

TABLE 11-3. Neurocognitive Disorders: Delirium and Dementia

Delirium and dementia are common and important disorders that affect multiple aspects of mental status. Both have many possible causes. Some clinical features of these two conditions and their effects on mental status are compared below. A delirium may be superimposed on dementia.

	Delirium	Dementia
Clinical Features		
Onset	Acute	Insidious
Course	Fluctuating, with lucid intervals; worse at night	Slowly progressive
Duration	Hours to weeks	Months to years
Sleep/wake cycle	Always disrupted	Sleep fragmented
General clinical illness or drug toxicity	Either or both present	Often absent, especially in Alzheimer disease
Mental Status		
Level of consciousness	Disturbed; person less alert to clearly aware of the environment and less able to focus, sustain, or shift attention	Usually normal until late in the course of the illness
Behavior	Activity often abnormally decreased (somnolence) or increased (agitation, hypervigilance)	Normal to slow; may become inappropriate
Speech	May be hesitant, slow, or rapid, incoherent	Difficulty in finding words, aphasia
Mood	Fluctuating, labile, from fearful or irritable to normal or depressed	Often flat, depressed
Thought processes	Disorganized, may be incoherent	Impoverished. Speech gives little information
Thought content	Delusions common, often transient	Delusions may occur
Perceptions	Illusions, hallucinations, most often visual	Hallucinations may occur
Judgment	Impaired, often to a varying degree	Increasingly impaired over the course of the illness
Orientation	Usually disoriented, especially for time. A known place may seem unfamiliar.	Fairly well maintained, but becomes impaired in the later stages of illness
Attention	Fluctuates, with inattention. Person easily distracted, unable to concentrate on selected tasks	Usually unaffected until late in the illness
Memory	Immediate and recent memory impaired	Recent memory and new learning especially impaired
Examples of Cause	Delirium tremens (due to withdrawal from alcohol) Uremia Acute hepatic failure Acute cerebral vasculitis Atropine poisoning	*Reversible:* Vitamin B_{12} deficiency, thyroid disorders *Irreversible:* Alzheimer disease, vascular dementia (from multiple infarcts), dementia due to head trauma

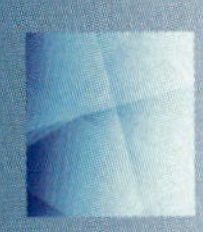

TABLE 11-4. Somatic Symptom and Related Disorders

Type of Disorder	Diagnostic Features
Somatic symptom disorder	Symptoms either very distressing or result in significant disruption of functioning as well as excessive and disproportionate thoughts, feelings, and behaviors related to those symptoms; symptoms should be specific if with predominant pain
Illness anxiety disorder	Preoccupation with having or acquiring a serious illness, whereas somatic symptoms, if present, are only mild in intensity
Conversion disorder	Syndrome of symptoms of deficits mimicking neurologic or medical illness in which psychological factors are judged to be of etiologic importance
Psychological factors affecting other medical conditions	Presence of one or more clinically significant psychological or behavioral factors that adversely affect a medical condition by increasing the risk for suffering, death, or disability
Factitious disorder	Falsification of physical or psychological signs or symptoms, or induction of injury or disease, associated with identified deception; individual presents themself as ill, impaired, or injured even in the absence of external rewards
Other Related Disorders or Behaviors	
Body dysmorphic disorder	Preoccupation with one or more perceived defects or flaws in physical appearance that are not observable or appear only slight to others
Dissociative disorder	Disruption of and/or discontinuity in the normal integration of consciousness, memory, identity, emotion, perception, body representation, motor control, and behavior

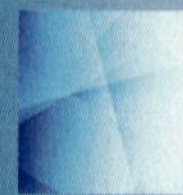

TABLE 11-5. Screening for Depression: Geriatric Depression Scale (Short Form)[118–121]

Administration

Ask the patient 15 questions for how they felt over the past week. Instruct the patient to respond either YES or NO. You may also ask the patient to complete the form using the self-rated form.

Scoring

Answers indicating depression are in bold; score 1 point for each one selected. Maximum score = 15; 0–4 = normal, depending on age, education, complaints; 5–8 = mild; 9–11 = moderate; 12–15 = severe

Choose the best answer for how you have felt over the past week:

1. Are you basically satisfied with your life? YES / **NO**
2. Have you dropped many of your activities and interests? **YES** / NO
3. Do you feel that your life is empty? **YES** / NO
4. Do you often get bored? **YES** / NO
5. Are you in good spirits most of the time? YES / **NO**
6. Are you afraid that something bad is going to happen to you? **YES** / NO
7. Do you feel happy most of the time? YES / **NO**
8. Do you often feel helpless? **YES** / NO
9. Do you prefer to stay at home, rather than going out and doing new things? **YES** / NO
10. Do you feel you have more problems with memory than most? **YES** / NO
11. Do you think it is wonderful to be alive now? YES / **NO**
12. Do you feel pretty worthless the way you are now? **YES** / NO
13. Do you feel full of energy? YES / **NO**
14. Do you feel that your situation is hopeless? **YES** / NO
15. Do you think that most people are better off than you are? **YES** / NO

Sources: Brink TL, Yesavage JA, Lum O, Heersema PH, Adey M, Rose TL. Screening tests for geriatric depression. *Clinical Gerontologist.* 1982;1(1):37–43.
Yesavage JA, Brink TL, Rose TL, et al. Development and validation of a geriatric depression screening scale: a preliminary report. *J Psychiatr Res.* 1982;17(1):37–49.
Sheikh JI, Yesavage JA. Geriatric Depression Scale (GDS): recent evidence and development of a shorter version. *Clinical Gerontologist.* 1986;5(1–2):165–173.
Sheikh JI, Yesavage JA, Brooks JO 3rd, et al. Proposed factor structure of the Geriatric Depression Scale. *Int Psychogeriatr.* 1991;3(1):23–28.

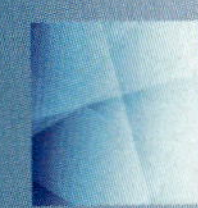

TABLE 11-6. Screening for Depression: Patient Health Questionnaire (PHQ-9)[15,122]

Administration

The PHQ-9 should be completed by the patient and scored by a staff person or clinician.

Scoring

Count the number (#) of boxes checked in a column. Multiply that number by the value indicated below, then add the subtotal to produce a total score. The possible range is 0–27. Use the table below to interpret the PHQ-9 score.

- Not at all (#) _____ × 0 = _____
- Several days (#) _____ × 1 = _____
- More than half the days (#) _____ × 2 = _____
- Nearly every day (#) _____ × 3 = _____

Total score: _____

Total Score	Depression Severity	Proposed Treatment Action
0–4	None–Minimal	None
5–9	Mild	Watchful waiting; repeat PHQ-9 at follow-up
10–14	Moderate	Treatment plan, consider counseling, follow up, and/or pharmacotherapy
15–19	Moderately severe	Active treatment with pharmacotherapy and/or psychotherapy
20–27	Severe	Immediate initiation of pharmacotherapy and, if severe impairment or poor response to therapy, expedited referral to a mental health specialist for psychotherapy, and/or collaborative management

(continued)

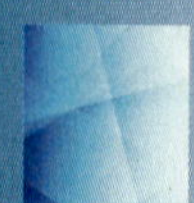

TABLE 11-6. Screening for Depression: Patient Health Questionnaire (PHQ-9)[15,122] *(Continued)*

Patient Health Questionnaire (PHQ-9)

Nine Symptom Depression Checklist

Name: ______________________ **Date:** ______________________

Over the *last 2 weeks*, how often have you been bothered by any of the following problems? (Please circle your answer.)

	Not at All	**Several Days**	**More than Half the Days**	**Nearly Every Day**
1. Little interest or pleasure in doing things	0	1	2	3
2. Feeling down, depressed, or hopeless	0	1	2	3
3. Trouble falling or staying asleep, or sleeping too much	0	1	2	3
4. Feeling tired or having little energy	0	1	2	3
5. Poor appetite or overeating	0	1	2	3
6. Feeling bad about yourself—or that you are a failure or have let yourself or your family down	0	1	2	3
7. Trouble concentrating on things, such as reading the newspaper or watching television	0	1	2	3
8. Moving or speaking so slowly that other people could have noticed. Or the opposite—being so fidgety or restless that you have been moving around a lot more than usual	0	1	2	3
9. Thoughts that you would be better off dead or of hurting yourself in some way	0	1	2	3

Add Columns, ______ + ______ + ______

Total Score*, ______ *Score is for healthcare provider incorporation

10. If you circled *any* problems, how *difficult* have these problems made it for you to do your work, take care of things at home, or get along with other people? (Please circle your answer.)	**Not Difficult at All**	**Somewhat Difficult**	**Very Difficult**	**Extremely Difficult**

A score of: 0–4 is considered non-depressed; 5–9 mild depression; 10–14 moderate depression; 15–19 moderately severe depression; and 20–27 severe depression.

PHQ-9 is adapted from PRIME ME TODAY™.

Note: Perform suicide risk assessment in patients who respond positively to item 9 "Thoughts that you would be better off dead or of hurting yourself in some way."

Additional information on administering the PHQ-2 and PHQ-9 can be found at: www.phqscreeners.com. (Copyright © 1999 Pfizer Inc. All rights reserved. Reproduced with permission. PRIME-MD© is a trademark of Pfizer Inc.)

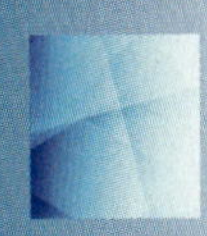

TABLE 11-7. Screening for Anxiety Disorders: GAD-7[33,35]

Administration

- The GAD-7 can be administered to individuals ages ≥18 years.
- It can be self-administered or administered by a health care professional or other trained individual.
- The GAD-7 should be administered in a quiet and private setting.
- The individual should be instructed to read each item carefully and answer it honestly based on their experiences over the past 2 weeks.
- There are no right or wrong answers to the GAD-7 items.
- Note that the GAD-7 is a screening tool and is not intended to be used for diagnosis.

Over the past 2 weeks, how often have you been bothered by the following problems?

Item	Not at All	Several Days	More than Half the Days	Nearly Every Day
Feeling nervous, anxious, or on edge	0	1	2	3
Not being able to stop or control worrying	0	1	2	3
Worrying too much about different things	0	1	2	3
Trouble relaxing	0	1	2	3
Being so restless that it is hard to sit still	0	1	2	3
Becoming easily annoyed or irritable	0	1	2	3

COLUMN TOTALS ______ + ______ + ______ + ______ =

TOTAL SCORE: ________

Scoring

- To score the GAD-7, add up the scores for all seven items.
- Each item is scored on a 4-point scale from 0 (not at all) to 3 (nearly every day).
- The total score can range from 0 to 21.

Interpretation

- A score of 10 or higher suggests a diagnosis of GAD.
- A score of 5 to 9 suggests mild anxiety.
- A score of 10 to 14 suggests moderate anxiety.
- A score of 15 to 21 suggests severe anxiety.

Sources: U. S. Preventive Services Task Force, Barry MJ, Nicholson WK, et al. Screening for Anxiety Disorders in Adults: US Preventive Services Task Force Recommendation Statement. *JAMA*. 2023;329(24):2163–2170.

Spitzer RL, Kroenke K, Williams JB, Lowe B. A brief measure for assessing generalized anxiety disorder: the GAD-7. *Arch Intern Med*. 2006;166(10):1092–1097.

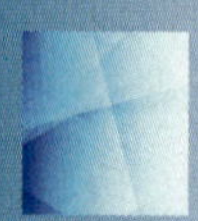

TABLE 11-8. Screening for Dementia: Mini-Cog[123]

Administration

The test is administered as follows:

1. Instruct the patient to listen carefully to and remember three unrelated words and then to repeat the words.
2. Instruct the patient to draw the face of a clock, either on a blank sheet of paper or on a sheet with the clock circle already drawn on the page. After the patient puts the numbers on the clock face, ask them to draw the hands of the clock to read a specific time.
3. Ask the patient to repeat the three previously stated words.

Scoring

Give 1 point for each recalled word after the clock drawing test (CDT) distractor.

Patients recalling none of the three words are classified as demented (score = 0).

Patients recalling all three words are classified as nondemented (score = 3).

Patients with intermediate word recall of one to two words are classified based on the CDT (abnormal = demented; normal = nondemented).

Note: The CDT is considered normal if all numbers are present in the correct sequence and position, and the hands readably display the requested time.

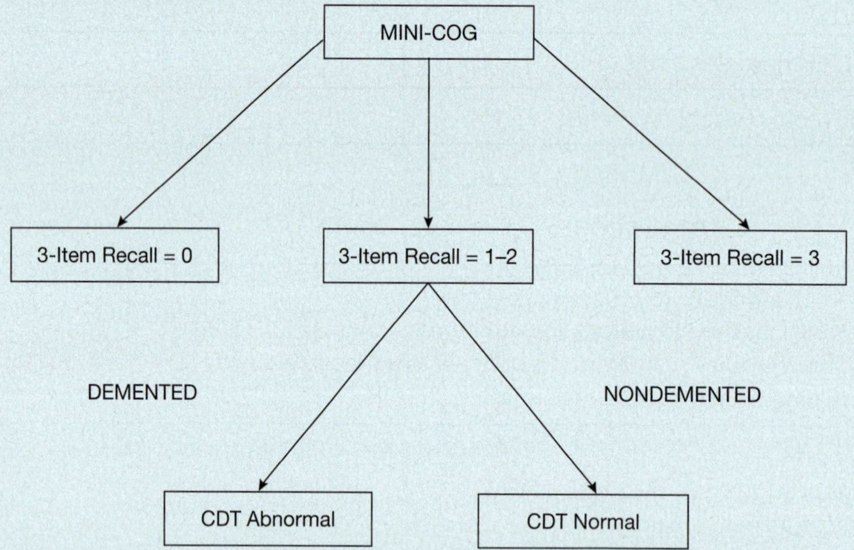

Source: Borson S, Scanlan JM, Chen P, Ganguli M. The Mini-Cog as a screen for dementia: validation in a population-based sample. *J Am Geriatr Soc*. 2003; 51(10):1451–1454.

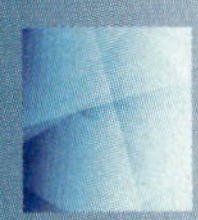

TABLE 11-9. Screening for Dementia: Montreal Cognitive Assessment (MoCA)[124]

Administration

The Montreal Cognitive Assessment (MoCA) was designed as a rapid screening instrument for mild cognitive dysfunction. It assesses different cognitive domains: attention and concentration, executive functions, memory, language, visuoconstructional skills, conceptual thinking, calculations, and orientation. Time to administer the MoCA is approximately 10 minutes.

Scoring

Sum all subscores listed on the right-hand side. Add one point for an individual who has 12 years or fewer of formal education, for a possible maximum of 30 points. A final total score of 26 and above is considered normal.

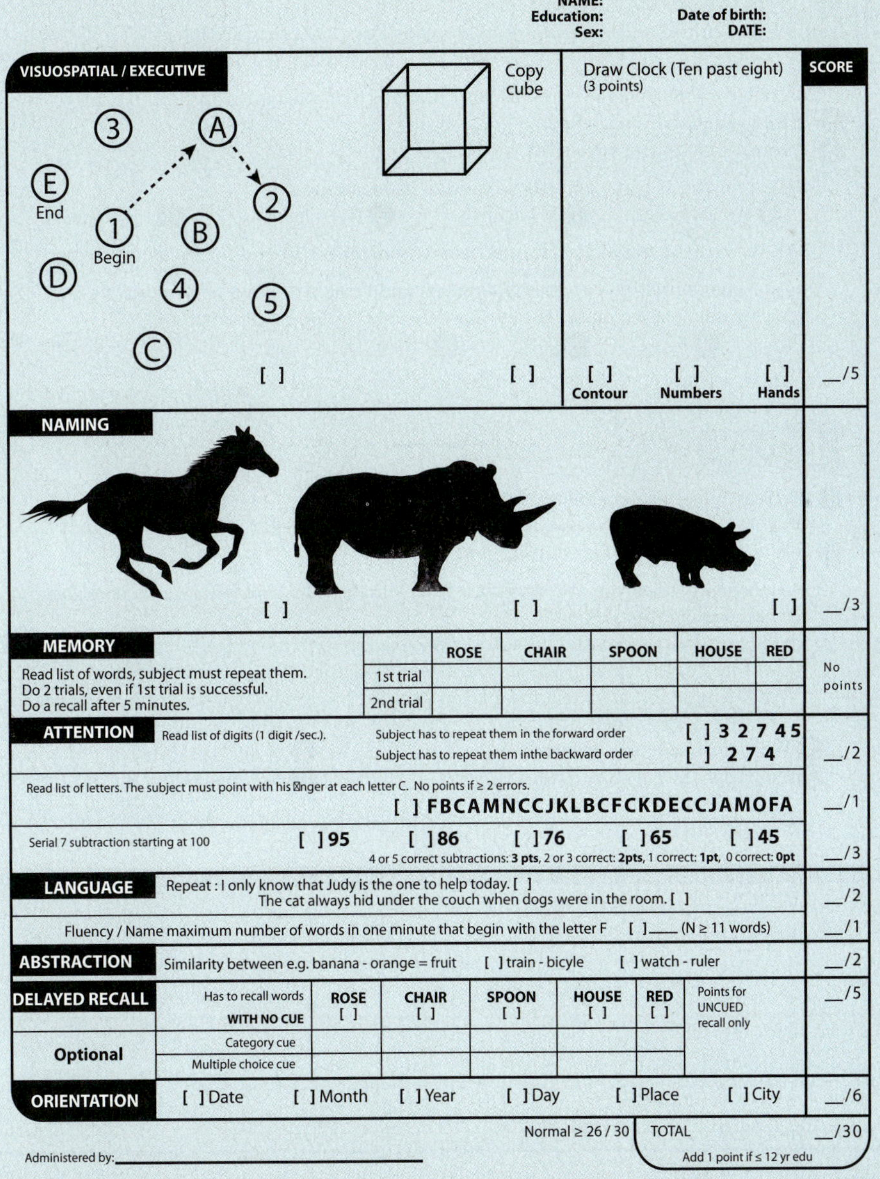

NAME:
Education: Date of birth:
Sex: DATE:

		SCORE
VISUOSPATIAL / EXECUTIVE	(Trail: 1 Begin, A, 2, B, 3, C, 4, D, 5, E End) [ ] — Copy cube [ ] — Draw Clock (Ten past eight) (3 points) [ ] Contour [ ] Numbers [ ] Hands	__/5
NAMING	[ ] [ ] [ ]	__/3
MEMORY	Read list of words, subject must repeat them. Do 2 trials, even if 1st trial is successful. Do a recall after 5 minutes.	No points
ATTENTION	Read list of digits (1 digit /sec.). Subject has to repeat them in the forward order [ ] 3 2 7 4 5; Subject has to repeat them inthe backward order [ ] 2 7 4	__/2
	Read list of letters. The subject must point with his finger at each letter C. No points if ≥ 2 errors. [ ] FBCAMNCCJKLBCFCKDECCJAMOFA	__/1
	Serial 7 subtraction starting at 100 [ ] 95 [ ] 86 [ ] 76 [ ] 65 [ ] 45 — 4 or 5 correct subtractions: **3 pts**, 2 or 3 correct: **2pts**, 1 correct: **1pt**, 0 correct: **0pt**	__/3
LANGUAGE	Repeat : I only know that Judy is the one to help today. [ ] The cat always hid under the couch when dogs were in the room. [ ]	__/2
	Fluency / Name maximum number of words in one minute that begin with the letter F [ ]___ (N ≥ 11 words)	__/1
ABSTRACTION	Similarity between e.g. banana - orange = fruit [ ] train - bicyle [ ] watch - ruler	__/2
DELAYED RECALL	Has to recall words WITH NO CUE: ROSE [ ] CHAIR [ ] SPOON [ ] HOUSE [ ] RED [ ] — Points for UNCUED recall only	__/5
ORIENTATION	[ ] Date [ ] Month [ ] Year [ ] Day [ ] Place [ ] City	__/6

Memory trials:

	ROSE	CHAIR	SPOON	HOUSE	RED
1st trial					
2nd trial					

Delayed recall, optional:

Optional	ROSE	CHAIR	SPOON	HOUSE	RED
Category cue					
Multiple choice cue					

Normal ≥ 26 / 30 TOTAL __/30
Add 1 point if ≤ 12 yr edu

Administered by:______________________

Copies are available at www.mocatest.org.

Source: Nasreddine ZS, Phillips NA, Bédirian V, et al. The Montreal Cognitive Assessment, MoCA: a brief screening tool for mild cognitive impairment. *J Am Geriatr Soc*. 2005;53(4):695–699.

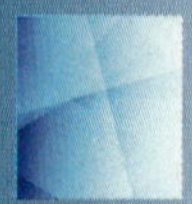

TABLE 11-10. Screening for Cognitive Impairment and Dementia: Saint Louis University Mental Status Exam (SLUMS)

VAMC

SLUMS EXAMINATION

Questions about this assessment tool? E-mail aging@slu.edu

Name________________________ Age__________

Is the patient alert?__________ Level of education__________________

__/1 ❶ **1. What day of the week is it?**

__/1 ❶ **2. What is the year?**

__/1 ❶ **3. What state are we in?**

4. Please remember these five objects. I will ask you what they are later.

Apple Pen Tie House Car

5. You have $100 and you go to the store and buy a dozen apples for $3 and a tricycle for $20.

❶ **How much did you spend?**

__/3 ❷ **How much do you have left?**

6. Please name as many animals as you can in one minute.

__/3 ⓪ 0-4 animals ❶ 5-9 animals ❷ 10-14 animals ❸ 15+ animals

__/5 **7. What were the five objects I asked you to remember? 1 point for each one correct.**

8. I am going to give you a series of numbers and I would like you to give them to me backwards. For example, if I say 42, you would say 24.

__/2 ⓪ 87 ❶ 648 ❶ 8537

9. This is a clock face. Please put in the hour markers and the time at ten minutes to eleven o'clock.

❷ Hour markers okay

__/4 ❷ Time correct

❶ **10. Please place an X in the triangle.**

__/2 ❶ **Which of the above figures is largest?**

11. I am going to tell you a story. Please listen carefully because afterwards, I'm going to ask you some questions about it.

Jill was a very successful stockbroker. She made a lot of money on the stock market. She then met Jack, a devastatingly handsome man. She married him and had three children. They lived in Chicago. She then stopped work and stayed at home to bring up her children. When they were teenagers, she went back to work. She and Jack lived happily ever after.

❷ **What was the female's name?** ❷ **What work did she do?**

__/8 ❷ **When did she go back to work?** ❷ **What state did she live in?**

_______ **TOTAL SCORE**

SCORING		
HIGH SCHOOL EDUCATION		LESS THAN HIGH SCHOOL EDUCATION
27-30	NORMAL	25-30
21-26	MILD NEUROCOGNITIVE DISORDER	20-24
1-20	DEMENTIA	1-19

CLINICIAN'S SIGNATURE ____________ DATE ________ TIME ________

SH Tariq, N Tumosa, JT Chibnall, HM Perry III, and JE Morley. The Saint Louis University Mental Status (SLUMS) Examination for detecting mild cognitive impairment and dementia is more sensitive than the Mini-Mental Status Examination (MMSE) - A pilot study. *Am J Geriatr Psych* 14:900-10, 2006.

Source: Tariq SH, Tumosa N, et al. SLU Mental Status Examination for detecting MCI & dementia is more sensitive than the Mini-Mental Status Examination—a pilot study. *Am J Geriatr Psych*. 2006;14:900–910. https://www.slu.edu/medicine/internal-medicine/geriatric-medicine/aging-successfully/pdfs/slums_form.pdf

REFERENCES

1. Purves D, Augustine GJ, Fitzpatrick D, et al. *Neuroscience.* 4th ed. Sinauer Associates, Inc.; 2008.
2. Stahl SM. *Stahl's Essential Psychopharmacology: Neuroscientific Basis and Practical Applications.* 4th ed. Cambridge University Press; 2013.
3. American Psychiatric Association. *Diagnostic and Statistical Manual of Mental Disorders: DSM-5.* 5th ed. American Psychiatric Association; 2013.
4. Substance Abuse and Mental Health Services Administration. *Key Substance Use and Mental Health Indicators in the United States: Results from the 2017 National Survey on Drug Use and Health.* Center for Behavioral Health Statistics and Quality, Substance Abuse and Mental Health Services Administration; 2018. Accessed November 11, 2018. https://www.samhsa.gov/data/
5. Olfson M, Kroenke K, Wang S, Blanco C. Trends in office-based mental health care provided by psychiatrists and primary care physicians. *J Clin Psychiatry.* 2014;75(3):247–253.
6. Lorenzetti RC, Jacques CHM, Donovan C, Cottrell S, Buck J. Managing difficult encounters: understanding physician, patient, and situational factors. *Am Fam Physician.* 2013; 87(6):419–425.
7. Oexle N, Corrigan PW. Understanding mental illness stigma toward persons with multiple stigmatized conditions: implications of intersectionality theory. *Psychiatr Serv.* 2018;69(5): 587–589.
8. Kroenke K, Spitzer RL, Williams JB, Löwe B. An ultra-brief screening scale for anxiety and depression: the PHQ-4. *Psychosomatics.* 2009;50(6):613–621.
9. Spitzer RL, Kroenke K, Williams JB, Löwe B. A brief measure for assessing generalized anxiety disorder: the GAD-7. *Arch Intern Med.* 2006;166(10):1092–1097.
10. Kroenke K, Spitzer RL, Williams JB, Monahan PO, Löwe B. Anxiety disorders in primary care: prevalence, impairment, comorbidity, and detection. *Ann Intern Med.* 2007;146(5): 317–325.
11. Löwe B, Gräfe K, Zipfel S, et al. Detecting panic disorder in medical and psychosomatic outpatients: comparative validation of the Hospital Anxiety and Depression Scale, the Patient Health Questionnaire, a screening question, and physicians' diagnosis. *J Psychosom Res.* 2003;55(6):515–519.
12. Kessler RC, Chiu WT, Demler O, Merikangas KR, Walters EE. Prevalence, severity, and comorbidity of 12-month DSM-IV disorders in the National Comorbidity Survey Replication. *Arch Gen Psychiatry.* 2005;62(6):617–627.
13. Conradt M, Cavanagh M, Franklin J, Rief W. Dimensionality of the Whiteley Index: assessment of hypochondriasis in an Australian sample of primary care patients. *J Psychosom Res.* 2006;60(2):137–143.
14. Pilowsky I. Dimensions of hypochondriasis. *Br J Psychiatry.* 1967;113(494):89–93.
15. Spitzer RL, Kroenke K, Williams JB. Validation and utility of a self-report version of PRIME-MD: the PHQ primary care study. *JAMA.* 1999;282(18):1737–1744.
16. Compton WM, Thomas YF, Stinson FS, Grant BF. Prevalence, correlates, disability, and comorbidity of DSM-IV drug abuse and dependence in the United States: results from the national epidemiologic survey on alcohol and related conditions. *Arch Gen Psychiatry.* 2007;64(5):566–576.
17. Hepner KA, Rowe M, Rost K, et al. The effect of adherence to practice guidelines on depression outcomes. *Ann Intern Med.* 2007;147(5):320–329.
18. Gunderson JG. Clinical practice. Borderline personality disorder. *N Engl J Med.* 2011;364(21):2037–2042.
19. *Mental illness.* National Institute of Mental Health. Accessed November 11, 2018. http://www.nimh.nih.gov/health/statistics/prevalence/any-mental-illness-ami-among-adults.shtml
20. Kroenke K. Patients presenting with somatic complaints: epidemiology, psychiatric comorbidity and management. *Int J Methods Psychiatr Res.* 2003;12(1):34–43.
21. Kroenke K. The interface between physical and psychological symptoms. *Prim Care Companion J Clin Psychiatry.* 2003; 5(Suppl 7):11–18.
22. Dwamena FC, Lyles JS, Frankel RM, Smith RC. In their own words: qualitative study of high-utilising primary care patients with medically unexplained symptoms. *BMC Fam Pract.* 2009;10:67.
23. Aaron LA, Buchwald D. A review of the evidence for overlap among unexplained clinical conditions. *Ann Intern Med.* 2001;134(9 Pt 2):868–881.
24. Mathias CW, Michael Furr R, Sheftall AH, Hill-Kapturczak N, Crum P, Dougherty DM. What's the harm in asking about suicidal ideation? *Suicide Life Threat Behav.* 2012;42(3): 341–351.
25. Substance Abuse and Mental Health Services Administration. *Key Substance Use and Mental Health Indicators in the United States: Results from the 2021 National Survey on Drug Use and Health 2022.* https://www.samhsa.gov/data/report/2021-nsduh-annual-national-report
26. Bauman BL, Ko JY, Cox S, et al. Vital signs: postpartum depressive symptoms and provider discussions about perinatal depression – United States, 2018. *MMWR Morb Mortal Wkly Rep.* 2020;69(19):575–581.
27. McCarron RM, Shapiro B, Rawles J, Luo J. Depression. *Ann Intern Med.* 2021;174(5):ITC65–ITC80.
28. U. S. Preventive Services Task Force, Barry MJ, Nicholson WK, et al. Screening for depression and suicide risk in adults: US Preventive Services Task Force Recommendation Statement. *JAMA.* 2023;329(23):2057–2067.
29. U. S. Preventive Services Task Force, Mangione CM, Barry MJ, et al. Screening for depression and suicide risk in children and adolescents: US Preventive Services Task Force Recommendation Statement. *JAMA.* 2022;328(15):1534–1542.
30. O'Connor EA, Perdue LA, Coppola EL, Henninger ML, Thomas RG, Gaynes BN. Depression and suicide risk screening: Updated evidence report and systematic review for the US Preventive Services Task Force. *JAMA.* 2023;329(23): 2068–2085.
31. Mahoney J, Drinka TJ, Abler R, et al. Screening for depression: single question versus GDS. *J Am Geriatr Soc.* 1994; 42(9):1006–1008.
32. DeMartini J, Patel G, Fancher TL. generalized anxiety disorder. *Ann Intern Med.* 2019;170(7):ITC49–ITC64.
33. U. S. Preventive Services Task Force, Barry MJ, Nicholson WK, et al. Screening for anxiety disorders in adults: US Preventive Services Task Force Recommendation Statement. *JAMA.* 2023;329(24):2163–2170.
34. Terlizzi EP, Villarroel MA. Symptoms of generalized anxiety disorder among adults: United States, 2019. *NCHS Data Brief.* 2020;(378):1–8.

35. Spitzer RL, Kroenke K, Williams JB, Lowe B. A brief measure for assessing generalized anxiety disorder: the GAD-7. *Arch Intern Med.* 2006;166(10):1092–1097.
36. U. S. Preventive Services Task Force, Mangione CM, Barry MJ, et al. Screening for Anxiety in children and adolescents: US Preventive Services Task Force Recommendation Statement. *JAMA.* 2022;328(14):1438–1444.
37. Drapeau CW, McIntosh JL. *U.S.A. suicide: 2021 Offical final data. Suicide Awareness Voices of Education (SAVE).* Accessed August 12, 2023. https://save.org/about-suicide/suicide-statistics
38. Centers for Disease Control and Prevention. *Facts About Suicide. Accessed* August 11, 2023. https://www.cdc.gov/suicide/facts/index.html
39. Garnett MF, Curtin SC. *Suicide mortality in the United States, 2001-2021. NCHS Data Brief no 464. National Center for Health Statistics.* https://stacks.cdc.gov/view/cdc/125705
40. Bommersbach TJ, Rosenheck RA, Petrakis IL, Rhee TG. Why are women more likely to attempt suicide than men? Analysis of lifetime suicide attempts among US adults in a nationally representative sample. *J Affect Disord.* 2022;311:157–164.
41. Schrijvers DL, Bollen J, Sabbe BG. The gender paradox in suicidal behavior and its impact on the suicidal process. *J Affect Disord.* 2012;138(1-2):19–26.
42. Centers for Disease Control and Prevention. *Disparities in suicide.* Accessed August 12, 2023. https://www.cdc.gov/suicide/facts/disparities-in-suicide.html
43. Erlangsen A, Jacobsen AL, Ranning A, Delamare AL, Nordentoft M, Frisch M. Transgender identity and suicide attempts and mortality in Denmark. *JAMA.* 2023;329(24):2145–2153.
44. Oh ES, Rabins PV. Dementia. *Ann Intern Med.* 2019;171(5):ITC33–ITC48.
45. Alzheimer's Association. *2023 Alzheimer's Disease Facts and Figures.* Alzheimer's Association; 2023. https://www.alz.org/media/Documents/alzheimers-facts-and-figures.pdf
46. Livingston G, Huntley J, Sommerlad A, et al. Dementia prevention, intervention, and care: 2020 report of the Lancet Commission. *Lancet.* 2020;396(10248):413–446.
47. Seitz DP, Chan CC, Newton HT, et al. Mini-cog for the detection of dementia within a primary care setting. *Cochrane Database Syst Rev.* 2021;7(7):CD011415.
48. Davis DH, Creavin ST, Yip JL, Noel-Storr AH, Brayne C, Cullum S. Montreal Cognitive Assessment for the detection of dementia. *Cochrane Database Syst Rev.* 2021;7(7):CD010775.
49. Cummings-Vaughn LA, Chavakula NN, Malmstrom TK, Tumosa N, Morley JE, Cruz-Oliver DM. Veterans Affairs Saint Louis University Mental Status examination compared with the Montreal Cognitive Assessment and the Short Test of Mental Status. *J Am Geriatr Soc.* 2014;62(7):1341–1346.
50. U. S. Preventive Services Task Force, Owens DK, Davidson KW, et al. Screening for cognitive impairment in older adults: US Preventive Services Task Force Recommendation Statement. *JAMA.* 2020;323(8):757–763.
51. Mattison MLP. Delirium. *Ann Intern Med.* 2020;173(7):ITC49–ITC64.
52. Shi Q, Warren L, Saposnik G, Macdermid JC. Confusion assessment method: a systematic review and meta-analysis of diagnostic accuracy. *Neuropsychiatr Dis Treat.* 2013;9:1359–1370.
53. Greer N, Rossom RC, Anderson P, et al. *Delirium: Screening, Prevention, and Diagnosis—A Systematic Review of the Evidence.* Department of Veterans Affairs; 2011. https://www.ncbi.nlm.nih.gov/books/NBK82554/
54. Khan A, Boukrina O, Oh-Park M, Flanagan NA, Singh M, Oldham M. Preventing delirium takes a village: systematic review and meta-analysis of delirium preventive models of care. *J Hosp Med.* 2019;14(9):558–564.
55. Yang Y, Cui Y, Sang K, et al. Ketamine blocks bursting in the lateral habenula to rapidly relieve depression. *Nature.* 2018;554(7692):317–322.
56. Hugdahl K, Løberg E-M, Nygård M. Left temporal lobe structural and functional abnormality underlying auditory hallucinations in schizophrenia. *Front Neurosci.* 2009;3(1):34–45.
57. Olabi B, Ellison-Wright I, McIntosh AM, Wood SJ, Bullmore E, Lawrie SM. Are there progressive brain changes in schizophrenia? A meta-analysis of structural magnetic resonance imaging studies. *Biol Psychiatry.* 2011;70(1):88–96.
58. Lenet AE. Shifting focus: from group patterns to individual neurobiological differences in attention-deficit/hyperactivity disorder. *Biol Psychiatry.* 2017;82(9):e67–e69.
59. Li B, Mody M. Cortico-striato-thalamo-cortical circuitry, working memory, and obsessive-compulsive disorder. *Front Psychiatry.* 2016;7:78.
60. Ikuta T, DeRosse P, Argyelan M, et al. Subcortical modulation in auditory processing and auditory hallucinations. *Behav Brain Res.* 2015;295:78–81.
61. Eichenbaum H. The hippocampus and declarative memory: cognitive mechanisms and neural codes. *Behav Brain Res.* 2001;127(1–2):199–207.
62. Ofen N, Kao Y-C, Sokol-Hessner P, Kim H, Whitfield-Gabrieli S, Gabrieli JD. Development of the declarative memory system in the human brain. *Nat Neurosci.* 2007;10(9):1198–1205.
63. Bannerman DM, Rawlins JN, McHugh SB, et al. Regional dissociations within the hippocampus–memory and anxiety. *Neurosci Biobehav Rev.* 2004;28(3):273–283.
64. Hampel H, Bürger K, Teipel SJ, Bokde ALW, Zetterberg H, Blennow K. Core candidate neurochemical and imaging biomarkers of Alzheimer's disease. *Alzheimers Dement.* 2008;4(1):38–48.
65. Campbell S, Macqueen G. The role of the hippocampus in the pathophysiology of major depression. *J Psychiatry Neurosci.* 2004;29(6):417–426.
66. Joëls M. Functional actions of corticosteroids in the hippocampus. *Eur J Pharmacol.* 2008;583(2–3):312–321.
67. Karl A, Schaefer M, Malta LS, Dörfel D, Rohleder N, Werner A. A meta-analysis of structural brain abnormalities in PTSD. *Neurosci Biobehav Rev.* 2006;30(7):1004–1031.
68. Kempton MJ, Salvador Z, Munafò MR, et al. Structural neuroimaging studies in major depressive disorder. Meta-analysis and comparison with bipolar disorder. *Arch Gen Psychiatry.* 2011;68(7):675–690.
69. Bremner JD. Traumatic stress: effects on the brain. *Dialogues Clin Neurosci.* 2006;8(4):445–461.
70. Chen C-H, Suckling J, Lennox BR, Ooi C, Bullmore ET. A quantitative meta-analysis of fMRI studies in bipolar disorder. *Bipolar Disord.* Feb 2011;13(1):1–15.
71. Gusnard DA, Akbudak E, Shulman GL, Raichle ME. Medial prefrontal cortex and self-referential mental activity: relation to a default mode of brain function. *Proc Natl Acad Sci U S A.* 2001;98(7):4259–4264.

REFERENCES

72. Meyer-Lindenberg AS, Olsen RK, Kohn PD, et al. Regionally specific disturbance of dorsolateral prefrontal-hippocampal functional connectivity in schizophrenia. *Arch Gen Psychiatry.* 2005;62(4):379–386.
73. Pia L, Tamietto M. Unawareness in schizophrenia: neuropsychological and neuroanatomical findings. *Psychiatry Clin Neurosci.* 2006;60(5):531–537.
74. Potkin SG, Turner JA, Brown GG, et al. Working memory and DLPFC inefficiency in schizophrenia: the FBIRN study. *Schizophr Bull.* 2009;35(1):19–31.
75. Bush G. Attention-deficit/hyperactivity disorder and attention networks. *Neuropsychopharmacology.* 2010;35(1):278–300.
76. Keener MT, Phillips ML. Neuroimaging in bipolar disorder: a critical review of current findings. *Curr Psychiatry Rep.* 2007;9(6):512–520.
77. Koenigs M, Grafman J. The functional neuroanatomy of depression: distinct roles for ventromedial and dorsolateral prefrontal cortex. *Behav Brain Res.* 2009;201(2):239–243.
78. Schmidt CK, Khalid S, Loukas M, Tubbs RS. Neuroanatomy of anxiety: a brief review. *Cureus.* 2018;10(1):e2055.
79. Maia TV, Cooney RE, Peterson BS. The neural bases of obsessive-compulsive disorder in children and adults. *Dev Psychopathol.* 2008;20(4):1251–1283.
80. Aupperle RL, Allard CB, Grimes EM, et al. Dorsolateral prefrontal cortex activation during emotional anticipation and neuropsychological performance in posttraumatic stress disorder. *Arch Gen Psychiatry.* 2012;69(4):360–371.
81. Kaufman LD, Pratt J, Levine B, Black SE. Executive deficits detected in mild Alzheimer's disease using the antisaccade task. *Brain Behav.* 2012;2(1):15–21.
82. Kringelbach ML. The human orbitofrontal cortex: linking reward to hedonic experience. *Nat Rev Neurosci.* 2005;6(9): 691–702.
83. Etkin A, Wager TD. Functional neuroimaging of anxiety: a meta-analysis of emotional processing in PTSD, social anxiety disorder, and specific phobia. *Am J Psychiatry.* 2007;164(10): 1476–1488.
84. Leech R, Sharp DJ. The role of the posterior cingulate cortex in cognition and disease. *Brain.* 2014;137(1):12–32.
85. Mayberg HS, Liotti M, Brannan SK, et al. Reciprocal limbic-cortical function and negative mood: converging PET findings in depression and normal sadness. *Am J Psychiatry.* 1999; 156(5):675–682.
86. Hamani C, Mayberg H, Stone S, Laxton A, Haber S, Lozano AM. The subcallosal cingulate gyrus in the context of major depression. *Biol Psychiatry.* 2011;69(4):301–308.
87. Maddock RJ, Garrett AS, Buonocore MH. Remembering familiar people: the posterior cingulate cortex and autobiographical memory retrieval. *Neuroscience.* 2001;104(3): 667–676.
88. Maddock RJ, Garrett AS, Buonocore MH. Posterior cingulate cortex activation by emotional words: fMRI evidence from a valence decision task. *Hum Brain Mapp.* 2003;18(1): 30–41.
89. Bush G, Frazier JA, Rauch SL, et al. Anterior cingulate cortex dysfunction in attention-deficit/hyperactivity disorder revealed by fMRI and the Counting Stroop. *Biol Psychiatry.* 1999;45(12):1542–1552.
90. McGovern RA, Sheth SA. Role of the dorsal anterior cingulate cortex in obsessive-compulsive disorder: converging evidence from cognitive neuroscience and psychiatric neurosurgery. *J Neurosurg.* 2017;126(1):132–147.
91. Milad MR, Furtak SC, Greenberg JL, et al. Deficits in conditioned fear extinction in obsessive-compulsive disorder and neurobiological changes in the fear circuit. *JAMA Psychiatry.* 2013;70(6):608–618.
92. McClure EB, Monk CS, Nelson EE, et al. Abnormal attention modulation of fear circuit function in pediatric generalized anxiety disorder. *Arch Gen Psychiatry.* 2007;64(1):97–106.
93. Fornito A, Yücel M, Dean B, Wood SJ, Pantelis C. Anatomical abnormalities of the anterior cingulate cortex in schizophrenia: bridging the gap between neuroimaging and neuropathology. *Schizophr Bull.* 2009;35(5):973–993.
94. Mundy P. Annotation: the neural basis of social impairments in autism: the role of the dorsal medial-frontal cortex and anterior cingulate system. *J Child Psychol Psychiatry.* 2003; 44(6):793–809.
95. Goard M, Dan Y. Basal forebrain activation enhances cortical coding of natural scenes. *Nat Neurosci.* 2009;12(11): 1444–1449.
96. Di Chiara G, Bassareo V, Fenu S, et al. Dopamine and drug addiction: the nucleus accumbens shell connection. *Neuropharmacology.* 2004;47(1):227–241.
97. Aylward EH, Reiss AL, Reader MJ, Singer HS, Brown JE, Denckla MB. Basal ganglia volumes in children with attention-deficit hyperactivity disorder. *J Child Neurol.* 1996; 11(2):112–115.
98. Perez-Costas E, Melendez-Ferro M, Roberts RC. Basal ganglia pathology in schizophrenia: dopamine connections and anomalies. *J Neurochem.* 2010;113(2):287–302.
99. Welter ML, Burbaud P, Fernandez-Vidal S, et al. Basal ganglia dysfunction in OCD: subthalamic neuronal activity correlates with symptoms severity and predicts high-frequency stimulation efficacy. *Transl Psychiatry.* 2011;1(5):e5.
100. Maletic V, Raison C. Integrated neurobiology of bipolar disorder. *Front Psychiatry.* 2014;5:98.
101. Andres KH, von Düring M, Veh RW. Subnuclear organization of the rat habenular complexes. *J Comp Neurol.* 1999; 407(1):130–150.
102. Matsumoto M, Hikosaka O. Lateral habenula as a source of negative reward signals in dopamine neurons. *Nature.* 2007;447(7148):1111–1115.
103. Hikosaka O. The habenula: from stress evasion to value-based decision-making. *Nat Rev Neurosci.* 2010;11(7):503–513.
104. Luo J. Effects of ethanol on the cerebellum: advances and prospects. *Cerebellum.* 2015;14(4):383–385.
105. Ropper AH, Samuels MA, Klein JP. *Adams and Victor's Principles of Neurology.* 10th ed. McGraw-Hill Education; 2014.
106. Phan KL, Wager T, Taylor SF, Liberzon I. Functional neuroanatomy of emotion: a meta-analysis of emotion activation studies in PET and fMRI. *Neuroimage.* 2002;16(2):331–348.
107. Tamminga CA, Thaker GK, Buchanan R, et al. Limbic system abnormalities identified in schizophrenia using positron emission tomography with fluorodeoxyglucose and neocortical alterations with deficit syndrome. *Arch Gen Psychiatry.* 1992;49(7):522–530.
108. Pandya M, Altinay M, Malone DA Jr, Anand A. Where in the brain is depression? *Curr Psychiatry Rep.* 2012;14(6): 634–642.
109. Blond BN, Fredericks CA, Blumberg HP. Functional neuroanatomy of bipolar disorder: structure, function, and connectivity in an amygdala-anterior paralimbic neural system. *Bipolar Disord.* 2012;14(4):340–355.

110. Martin EI, Ressler KJ, Binder E, Nemeroff CB. The neurobiology of anxiety disorders: brain imaging, genetics, and psychoneuroendocrinology. *Psychiatr Clin North Am.* 2009; 32(3):549–575.
111. Sherin JE, Nemeroff CB. Post-traumatic stress disorder: the neurobiological impact of psychological trauma. *Dialogues Clin Neurosci.* 2011;13(3):263–278.
112. Menon V. Salience network. In: Toga AW, ed. *Brain Mapping: An Encyclopedic Reference.* Elsevier; 2015:597–611.
113. Taylor KS, Seminowicz DA, Davis KD. Two systems of resting state connectivity between the insula and cingulate cortex. *Hum Brain Mapp.* 2009;30(9):2731–2745.
114. Whitfield-Gabrieli S, Ford JM. Default mode network activity and connectivity in psychopathology. *Annu Rev Clin Psychol.* 2012;8:49–76.
115. Yehuda R, Hoge CW, McFarlane AC, et al. Post-traumatic stress disorder. *Nat Rev Dis Primers.* 2015;1:15057.
116. Manoliu A, Meng C, Brandl F, et al. Insular dysfunction within the salience network is associated with severity of symptoms and aberrant inter-network connectivity in major depressive disorder. *Front Hum Neurosci.* 2013;7:930.
117. Manoliu A, Riedl V, Zherdin A, et al. Aberrant dependence of default mode/central executive network interactions on anterior insular salience network activity in schizophrenia. *Schizophr Bull.* 2014;40(2):428–437.
118. Brink TL, Yesavage JA, Lum O, Heersema PH, Adey M, Rose TL. Screening tests for geriatric depression. *Clinical Gerontologist.* 1982;1(1):37–43.
119. Yesavage JA, Brink TL, Rose TL, et al. Development and validation of a geriatric depression screening scale: a preliminary report. *J Psychiatr Res.* 1982;17(1):37–49.
120. Sheikh JI, Yesavage JA. Geriatric Depression Scale (GDS): recent evidence and development of a shorter version. *Clinical Gerontologist.* 1986;5(1–2):165–173.
121. Sheikh JI, Yesavage JA, Brooks JO 3rd, et al. Proposed factor structure of the Geriatric Depression Scale. *Int Psychogeriatr.* 1991;3(1):23–28.
122. Kroenke K, Spitzer RL, Williams JB. The Patient Health Questionnaire-2: validity of a two-item depression screener. *Med Care.* 2003;41(11):1284–1292.
123. Borson S, Scanlan JM, Chen P, Ganguli M. The Mini-Cog as a screen for dementia: validation in a population-based sample. *J Am Geriatr Soc.* 2003;51(10):1451–1454.
124. Nasreddine ZS, Phillips NA, Bédirian V, et al. The Montreal Cognitive Assessment, MoCA: a brief screening tool for mild cognitive impairment. *J Am Geriatr Soc.* 2005;53(4):695–699.
125. Mancini C, Van Ameringen M, Pipe B, et al. Development and validation of self-report psychiatric screening tool: MACSCREEN. Presented at: Anxiety Disorders Association of American 23rd Annual Conference; March 27–30, 2003; Toronto, Canada.
126. Connor KM, Kobak KA, Churchill LE, Katzelnick D, Davidson JR. Mini-SPIN: a brief screening assessment for generalized social anxiety disorder. *Depress Anxiety.* 2001; 14(2):137–140.
127. Lin JS, O'Connor E, Rossom RC, et al. *Screening for Cognitive Impairment in Older Adults: An Evidence Update for the U.S. Preventive Services Task Force.* Agency for Healthcare Research and Quality (US); 2013. Accessed November 12, 2018. http://www.ncbi.nlm.nih.gov/books/NBK174643/
128. Albert MS, DeKosky ST, Dickson D, et al. The diagnosis of mild cognitive impairment due to Alzheimer's disease: recommendations from the National Institute on Aging-Alzheimer's Association workgroups on diagnostic guidelines for Alzheimer's disease. *Alzheimers Dement.* 2011;7(3): 270–279.
129. Markwick A, Zamboni G, de Jager CA. Profiles of cognitive subtest impairment in the Montreal Cognitive Assessment (MoCA) in a research cohort with normal Mini-Mental State Examination (MMSE) scores. *J Clin Exp Neuropsychol.* 2012;34(7):750–757.
130. Peters ME, Rosenberg PB, Steinberg M, et al. Neuropsychiatric symptoms as risk factors for progression from CIND to dementia: the Cache County Study. *Am J Geriatr Psychiatry.* 2013;21(11):1116–1124.
131. Rabins PV, Blass DM. In the clinic. Dementia. *Ann Intern Med.* 2014;161(3):ITC1–ITC16.
132. Wong CL, Holroyd-Leduc J, Simel DL, Straus SE. Does this patient have delirium? Value of bedside instruments. *JAMA.* 2010;304(7):779–786.

CHAPTER 12

Skin, Hair, and Nails

ANATOMY AND PHYSIOLOGY

Skin

The *skin*, the heaviest single organ, comprises about 16% of body weight and spans an area of around 1.2 to 2.3 m^2. It has three layers: the epidermis, dermis, and subcutaneous tissues (Fig. 12-1).

For a more comprehensive representation of dermatologic diversity, we recommend the Inclusive Dermatology Atlas from the University of New Mexico: https://hsc.unm.edu/medicine/departments/dermatology/inclusive-dermatology/gallery.html.

The outermost layer, the *epidermis*, is a thin, avascular, keratinized epithelium with two layers: an outer stratum corneum of dead keratinized cells and an inner cellular layer, including the stratum basale and stratum spinosum or malpighian layer, where melanin and keratin form. Migration from inner to outer layers takes roughly a month.

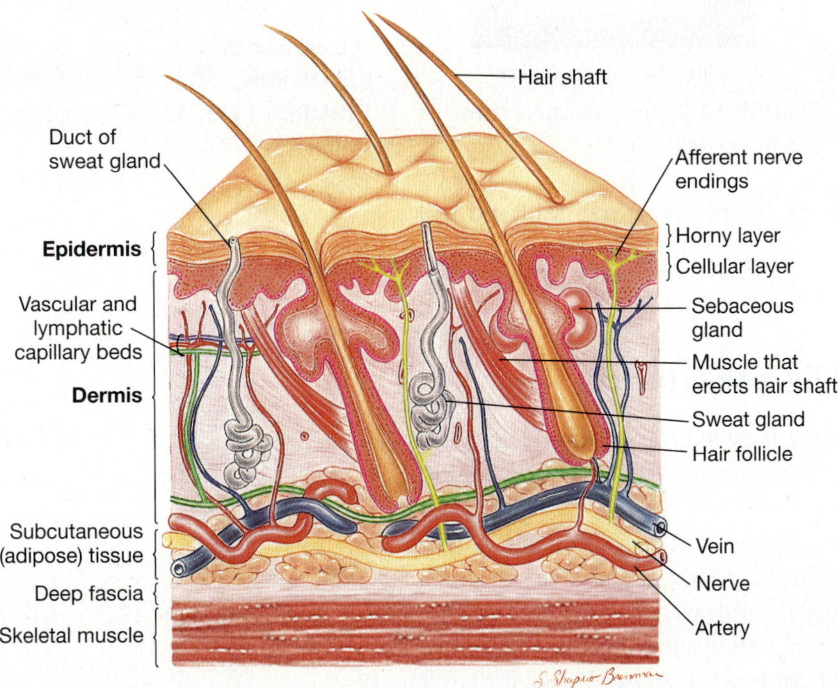

FIGURE 12-1. Structure of skin and subcutaneous tissue.

The *epidermis* relies on the vascularized dermis for nourishment. The dermis contains interconnecting collagen and elastic fibers and houses epidermal appendages like *pilosebaceous glands, sweat glands, hair follicles*, and most cutaneous nerve terminals. The dermis merges with subcutaneous fatty tissue, or *adipose tissue*, at its base.

Normal skin color is influenced by melanin levels, vascular structures, hemodynamics, and carotene and bilirubin changes. *Melanin*, a brown pigment, is genetically determined and increased by sun exposure. *Hemoglobin*, a bright red pigment, carries oxygen as *oxyhemoglobin* in arteries and capillaries, reddening the skin. *Deoxyhemoglobin*, a darker bluish pigment, circulates in veins after oxygen is released to tissues. Light scattering through skin and blood vessels makes veins appear bluer and less red than venous blood.

Pallor may indicate anemia.

Cyanosis, manifested as a bluish hue, may suggest reduced oxygen levels in the blood or diminished blood flow due to cold conditions.

Carotene, a yellow pigment, is found in the subcutaneous fat and heavily keratinized areas such as the palms and soles. *Bilirubin*, a yellow-brown pigment, arises from the breakdown of heme in the red blood cells.

Jaundice, characterized by a yellow tint to the skin, arises from elevated bilirubin levels.

Hair

Adults have two hair types: *vellus hair*, which is short, fine, inconspicuous, and relatively unpigmented, and *terminal hair*, which is coarser, thicker, conspicuous, and typically pigmented. Scalp hair and eyebrows are examples of terminal hair.

Nails

Nails protect the fingertips and toes. The firm, rectangular, and usually curved *nail plate* gets its pink color from the vascular nail bed to which it is firmly attached (Figs. 12-2 and 12-3). The whitish moon, or *lunula*, and the free edge of the nail plate are visible features. About one fourth of the nail plate, the *nail root*, is covered by the proximal nail fold. The *cuticle* extends from the fold and functions as a seal, protecting the space between the fold and the plate from external moisture. Lateral *nail folds* cover the sides of the nail plate. The angle between the proximal nail fold and nail plate is typically <180 degrees.

FIGURE 12-2. Surface structures of the fingernail.

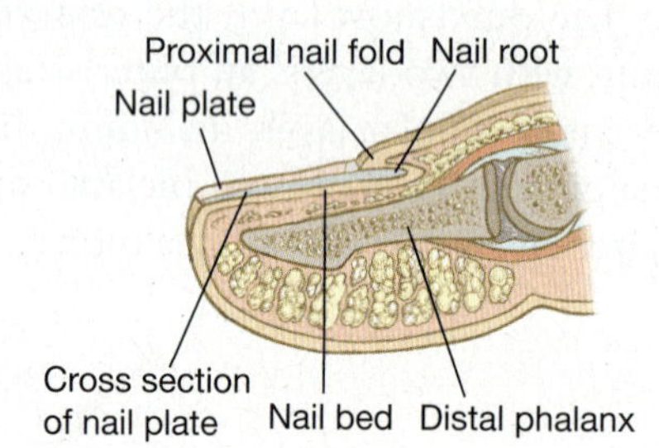

FIGURE 12-3. Cross-section of fingertip.

Fingernails grow approximately 0.1 mm daily, while toenails grow more slowly.

Pilosebaceous Glands and Sweat Glands

Pilosebaceous glands, or oil glands, produce a fatty substance that is secreted onto the skin surface through hair follicles. These glands are present on all skin surfaces except for the palms and soles.

Sweat glands come in two types: eccrine and apocrine. *Eccrine sweat glands* are widely distributed, open directly onto the skin surface, and help control body temperature through sweat production. In contrast, *apocrine sweat glands* are primarily located in the axillary and genital regions and typically open into hair follicles. Bacterial decomposition of apocrine sweat is responsible for adult body odor.

HEALTH HISTORY: GENERAL APPROACH

Diagnosing skin diseases requires a comprehensive health history and physical examination (PE), focusing on symptoms like itching or pain. A detailed history refines your diagnostic possibilities, informs further investigations, and aids optimal management. Key information you should obtain includes the disease's duration, evolution, periodicity, and previous episodes. A thorough interview is crucial for gathering this information, especially when lesions are not visible.[1] Your patient's medical history is important, as systemic diseases can have skin manifestations. In addition, factors like diet, cosmetics, chemicals, sunlight, medications, and travel may be relevant to dermatologic conditions.

See Table 12-10. Systemic Diseases and Associated Skin Findings, pp. 292–293.

Common or Concerning Symptoms

- Skin lesions
- Rashes and itching (pruritus)
- Hair loss or alopecia
- Nail changes

Skin Lesions

A skin *lesion*, an all-encompassing term, is any single area of altered skin. It may be solitary or multiple. Look for skin lesions suggesting melanoma, basal cell carcinoma (BCC), or squamous cell carcinoma (SCC) throughout the skin examination regardless of the patient's skin color. Detecting skin cancer at an early stage can increase the likelihood of successful treatment. You must ask questions and gather detailed information if a suspicious lesion is identified to ensure appropriate care and management for your patient (Box 12-1).

Typical skin lesions include **acne** (pimples or red bumps, often with whiteheads or blackheads, typically caused by blocked hair follicles), **eczema** (red, itchy skin patches often stemming from an overactive immune response or external irritants), **moles** (brownish spots or growths on the skin, usually harmless but can sometimes signal skin cancer), and **infections** (may be caused by bacteria, viruses, or fungi that lead to redness, swelling, and sometimes pus).

Box 12-1. Skin Lesions: High-Yield Health History Questions

Domain	Questions	Rationale
Onset and duration	*When did you first notice the skin lesion(s)?* *How long have they been present?*	This helps determine whether the skin condition is *acute* (e.g., contact dermatitis), *subacute* (e.g., drug eruption), or *chronic* (e.g., psoriasis, eczema), which can help narrow down the possible causes.
Location and distribution	*Where are the skin lesions located?* *Are they localized or widespread?*	Certain conditions tend to appear in specific body areas or follow certain patterns, such as psoriasis (elbows, knees), tinea corporis (annular lesions), and shingles (dermatomal distribution).

(*continued*)

Box 12-1. Skin Lesions: High-Yield Health History Questions (*Continued*)

Domain	Questions	Rationale
Symptoms and associated factors	*Are the skin lesions itchy, painful, or associated with any other symptoms?* *Have you noticed any triggers or factors that worsen or improve the condition?*	Itchiness is common in eczema and hives, while pain can be associated with shingles or cellulitis; sun exposure in systemic lupus erythematosus or food allergens in hives worsens the conditions.

Rashes and Itching (Pruritus)

A *rash* is a widespread eruption of lesions. When patients present with a rash, inquire about itching (*pruritus*), which is the most important symptom when assessing rashes. Understanding the presence and severity of itching can provide valuable insights into the nature and potential causes of the rash (Box 12-2).

Box 12-2. Rash: High-Yield Health History Questions

Domain	Questions	Rationale
Onset and duration	*When did the rash first appear?* *Has it changed or spread since then?*	Can help to identify potential triggers, such as medications or allergens, and assess whether the rash is acute or chronic, guiding the diagnostic process
Location	*Where did the rash first appear?* *Where is it currently located on the body?*	Can suggest certain conditions (e.g., a rash in skin folds may suggest candidiasis or inverse psoriasis) and help to differentiate between similar-looking rashes
Associated symptoms	*Are there any other symptoms or discomfort associated with the rash, such as pain, fever, or joint swelling?*	Can help narrow potential diagnoses and recognize systemic involvement, such as in vasculitis and systemic lupus erythematosus (SLE)

Common underlying causes include **allergic reactions** (responses to substances like pollen, certain foods, or insect bites that lead to red, itchy spots), **dermatitis** (inflammation of the skin, often caused by irritants or allergens, resulting in red, itchy, and sometimes scaly patches), **fungal infections** (conditions like athlete's foot or ringworm, which produce itchy, scaling patches), and **systemic diseases** (liver disease or kidney failure can manifest as itching or rashes on the skin).

Domain	Questions	Rationale
Triggers	*Have you noticed any factors that seem to trigger or worsen the rash, such as exposure to certain substances, foods, or environmental factors?*	Can help pinpoint potential allergens, irritants, or other factors contributing to the rash, which can be crucial in diagnosing conditions like contact dermatitis or atopic dermatitis
Medical history	*Do you have any personal or family history of skin conditions, allergies, or autoimmune diseases?*	History of atopy, allergies, or autoimmune diseases can increase the likelihood of certain diagnoses, such as eczema, psoriasis, and SLE and help guide further investigations
Treatments and medications	*Have you tried any treatments for the rash?* *Are you currently taking any medications, including over-the-counter or herbal remedies?*	Can help assess their effectiveness and guide further management, while recognizing potential drug-related causes of the rash

Hair Loss or Alopecia

Alopecia, commonly known as hair loss, can stem from a wide range of causes, ranging from genetic factors to external influences. Determining its precise cause is essential for effective treatment. Refer to Box 12-3 for a set of high-yield questions that can assist you in identifying potential origins.

Box 12-3. Alopecia: High-Yield Health History Questions

Domain	Questions	Rationale
Onset	*When did you first notice your hair loss?*	This helps differentiate between *sudden* (e.g., alopecia areata, telogen effluvium) or *gradual* (e.g., androgenetic alopecia, traction alopecia) hair loss and assess the progression and urgency.
Pattern	*Is your hair loss localized or diffuse, and is it in a specific pattern?*	*Localized hair loss:* suggests alopecia areata, tinea capitis, or scarring alopecia. *Diffuse hair loss:* may indicate telogen effluvium, anagen effluvium, or nutritional deficiencies; *specific patterns* can point to androgenetic or traction alopecia.

(continued)

Common reasons include **androgenic alopecia** (commonly known as male or female pattern baldness, often hereditary and follows a predictable pattern), **telogen effluvium** (temporary hair shedding often after a significant stressor, such as surgery, childbirth, or severe illness), **alopecia areata** (an autoimmune condition in which the body's own immune system attacks hair follicles, resulting in round, bald patches), and **traction alopecia** (hair loss caused by tight hairstyles that pull at the hair over time).

Box 12-3. Alopecia: High-Yield Health History Questions (*Continued*)

Domain	Questions	Rationale
Severity	*How would you rate the severity of your hair loss?*	More severe hair loss might suggest significant underlying causes (e.g., autoimmune diseases, hormonal imbalances).
Scalp symptoms	*Have you experienced any itching, pain, or redness on your scalp?*	Itching, redness, or pain may point to tinea capitis, seborrheic dermatitis, scarring alopecia, or other inflammatory scalp conditions contributing to hair loss.
Triggers	*Can you identify any triggers or events that may have contributed to your hair loss (e.g., stress, recent illness, medications, hair styling practices)?*	Stress or illness suggests telogen effluvium; medications can cause anagen effluvium or drug-induced hair loss; hair styling practices may lead to traction alopecia or trichotillomania.
Medical history	*Do you have a history of thyroid disease, autoimmune disorders, or a family history of hair loss?*	Thyroid disease can cause hair loss; autoimmune disorders can affect hair growth; family history may indicate androgenetic alopecia or hereditary predisposition to certain types of hair loss.

Nail Changes

Alterations in nail color, texture, or shape may signal underlying systemic diseases or localized nail disorders. For precise diagnosis and appropriate care, investigate further with specific questions, as detailed in Box 12-4.

See Table 12-9, pp. 290–291 for common nail changes such as onychomycosis, habit tic deformity, and melanonychia.

Frequent causes include **onychomycosis** (fungal infection of the nails, typically leading to thickening, discoloration, and crumbling of the nail), **trauma** (physical injuries to the nails, which can cause discoloration like "black nails" from impacts or separation of the nail plate), **psoriasis** (skin condition that can also affect the nails, producing pitting, thickening, or separation from the nail bed), and **nutritional deficiencies** (lack of certain nutrients can manifest as ridges, white spots, or brittle nails).

Box 12-4. Nail Changes: High-Yield Health History Questions

Domain	High-Yield Health History Questions	Rationale
General health	*Have you experienced any recent weight loss, fatigue, or fever?*	Nail changes can reflect overall health; asking about general health symptoms such as weight loss, fatigue, and fever can help identify systemic issues that may be affecting nail health, such as infection, autoimmune disorders, or malignancy.

Domain	High-Yield Health History Questions	Rationale
Nutritional status	*Have you had any changes in your diet or experienced issues with nutrient absorption?*	Nutritional deficiencies, such as iron, zinc, or biotin, can cause nail changes; asking about dietary habits or nutrient absorption issues (e.g., due to gastrointestinal disorders) can reveal potential nutritional causes for nail changes.
Medications	*Are you currently taking any medications, including over-the-counter drugs, supplements, or herbal remedies?*	Some medications (e.g., chemotherapy drugs, retinoids, antifungal medications, anti-malarial, tetracycline) and supplements (e.g., vitamin A, selenium, or biotin) can cause nail changes, either due to direct effects or interactions with other drugs.
Underlying conditions	*Have you been exposed to any chemicals or substances, either at work or in your daily life, that could affect your nails?*	Iron-deficiency anemia can cause spoon-shaped nails (koilonychia) or pale nail beds; psoriasis can cause nail pitting, thickening, discoloration, and onycholysis; and both hypothyroidism and hyperthyroidism can cause nail changes, such as brittle nails, ridges, or onycholysis.
Occupational/ environmental exposure	*Can you identify any triggers or events that may have contributed to your hair loss (e.g., stress, recent illness, medications, hair styling practices)?*	Occupational and environmental exposures, such as chemicals or repetitive trauma, can cause nail changes.
Family history	*Is there a history of nail disorders or related medical conditions in your family?*	Some nail disorders can have a genetic component, and a family history of nail disorders or related medical conditions can suggest a possible hereditary cause.

DESCRIBING SKIN LESIONS

Using specific terminology is crucial for describing skin lesions and rashes, including elements like number, size, color, shape, texture, primary lesion, location, and configuration. For instance, seborrheic keratosis can be described as "Multiple 5-mm to 2-cm tan to brown, oval, stuck-on, flat-topped verrucous plaques on the back and abdomen, following skin tension lines."

To screen moles for melanomas, clinicians use the *ABCDE-EFG method* (see Box 12-5 and Table 12-6), assessing:

- **A**symmetry (of one side of mole compared to the other)
- **B**order irregularity especially if ragged, notched, or blurred
- **C**olor variations (more than two colors, especially blue-black, white, or red)
- **D**iameter >6 mm
- **E**volving or changing rapidly in size, symptoms, or morphology
- **E**levation
- **F**irmness to palpation
- **G**rowth (progressive) over several weeks

Review the ABCDE-EFG method and photographs in Box 12-5, pp. 246–247 and Table 12-6, Brown Lesions: Melanoma and Its Mimics, pp. 281–284, which provide additional helpful identifiers and comparisons of benign brown lesions with melanoma (Fig. 12-4). Also see discussion of screening for skin cancers in the Health Promotion and Counseling section, pp. 268–270.

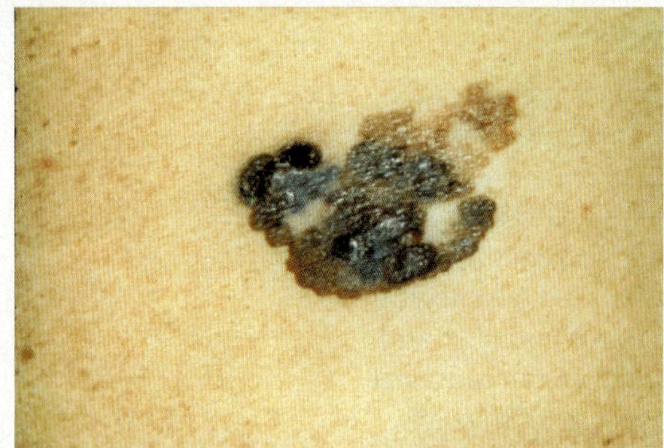

FIGURE 12-4. Melanoma with all the classic features of the ABCD method: **A**symmetry, **B**order irregularity, **C**olor variation, and **D**iameter >6 mm. (Reprinted with permission from DeVita VT, Lawrence TS, Rosenberg SA. *DeVita, Hellman, and Rosenberg's Cancer: Principles & Practice of Oncology.* 11th ed. Wolters Kluwer; 2019. Figure 92.3, part C.)

Box 12-5. The ABCDE-EFG Method

The **ABCDE** method has been used for many years to teach clinicians and patients about features suspicious for melanoma.[36]

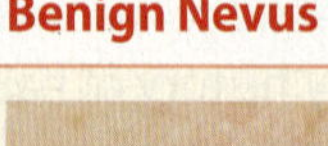

	Melanoma	Benign Nevus
Asymmetry of one side of mole compared to the other	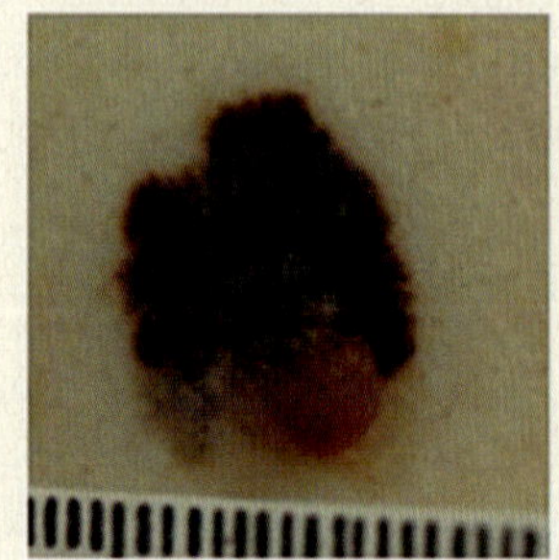	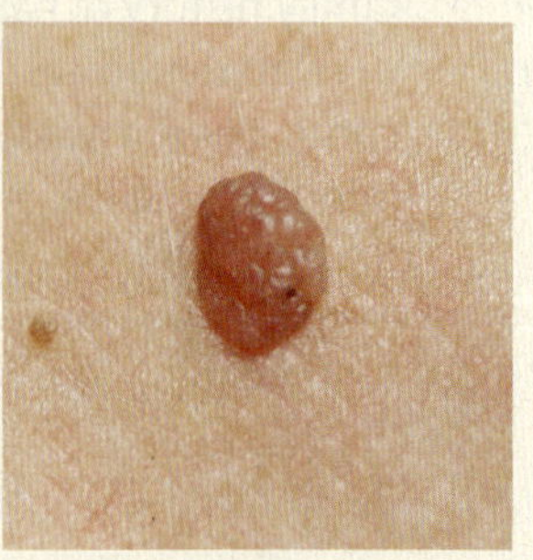

	Melanoma	Benign Nevus	
Border irregularity especially if ragged, notched, or blurred	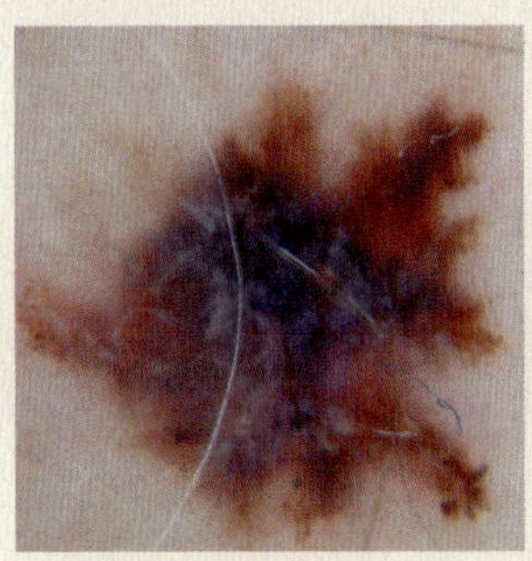	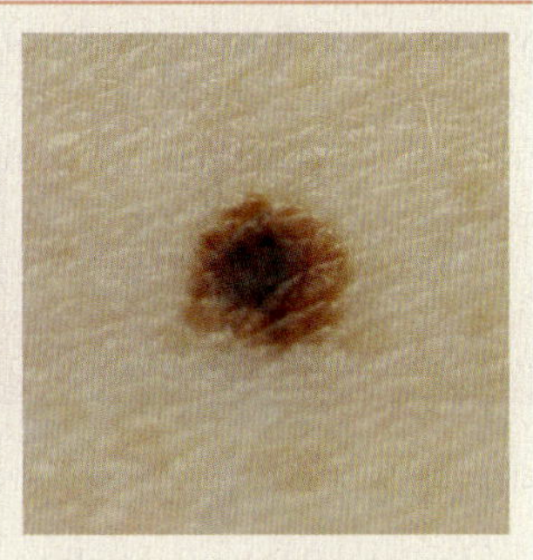	
Color variations more than two colors, especially blue-black, white (loss of pigment due to regression), or red (inflammatory reaction to abnormal cells)	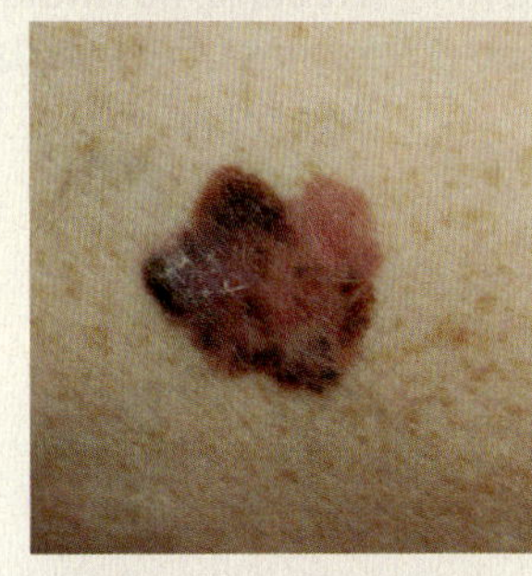	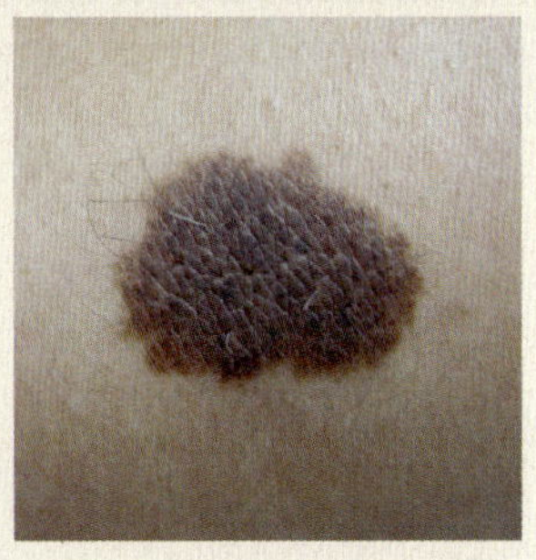	Except for a homogeneous blue color in a blue nevus, blue or black color within a larger pigmented lesion is especially concerning for melanoma.
Diameter >6 mm approximately the size of a pencil eraser	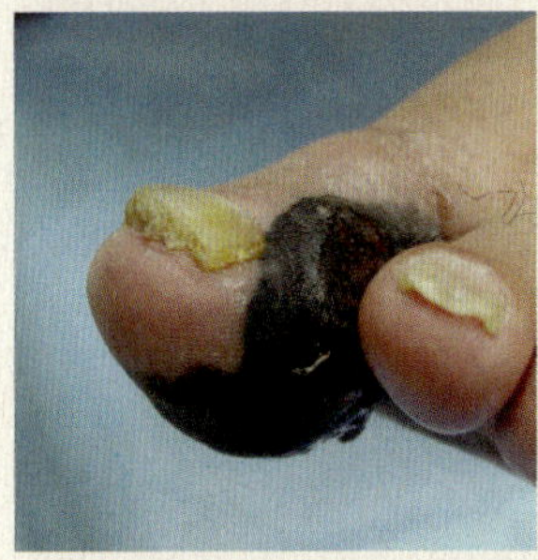	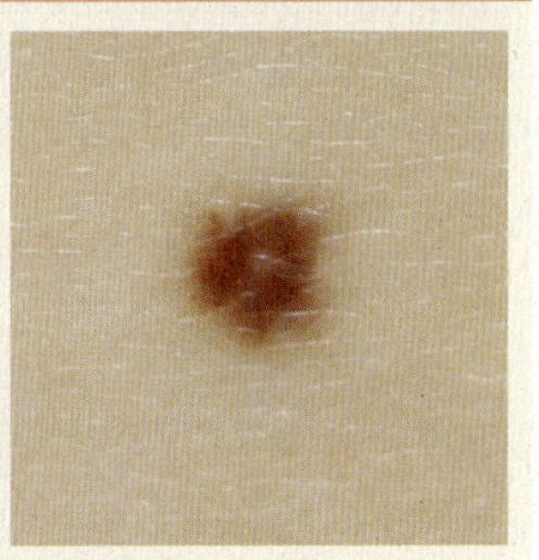	Early melanomas may be <6 mm, and many benign lesions are >6 mm.
Evolving or changing rapidly in size, symptoms, or morphology	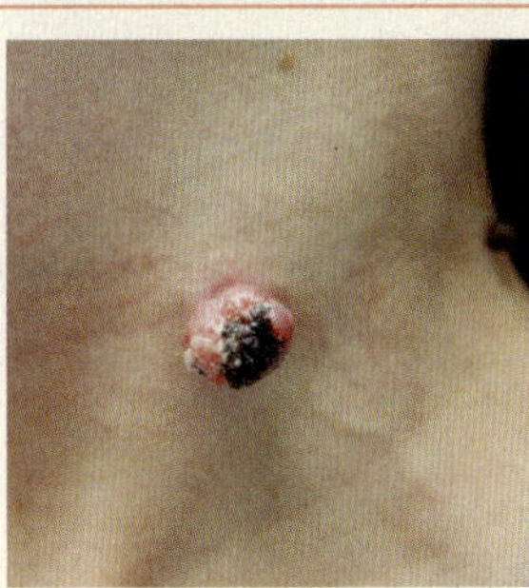	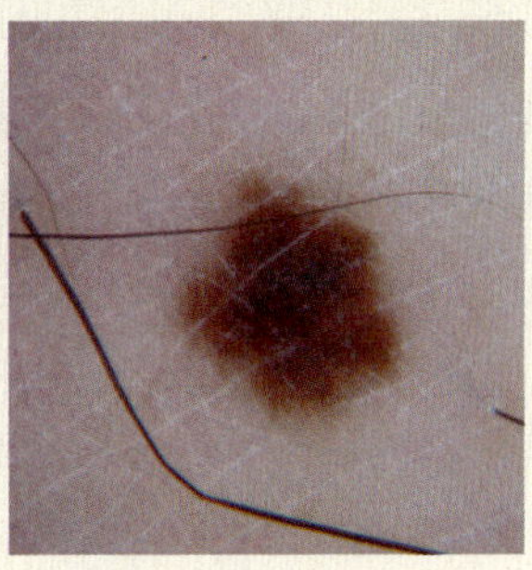	Evolution is the most sensitive of these criteria. A reliable history of change may prompt biopsy of a benign-appearing lesion.

Some have suggested adding **EFG** to help detect aggressive nodular melanomas.[40]
Elevated
Firm to palpation
Growing progressively over several weeks

Primary Lesions

Primary skin lesions are those that develop as a direct result of, and therefore are most characteristic of, the disease process. Review the descriptions of these primary lesions so you can identify these in your patients (Box 12-6 and Figs. 12-5 to 12-13). Primary lesions may be flat, raised, or fluid filled.

Box 12-6. Dermatologic Classification and Examples of Skin Lesions

Type of Lesion	Description	Examples
FIGURE 12-5. Macule.	Circumscribed flat area of change in color of the skin <1 cm in diameter	Freckles, flat moles, port-wine stains, rashes of rickettsial infections, rubella, and measles[41]
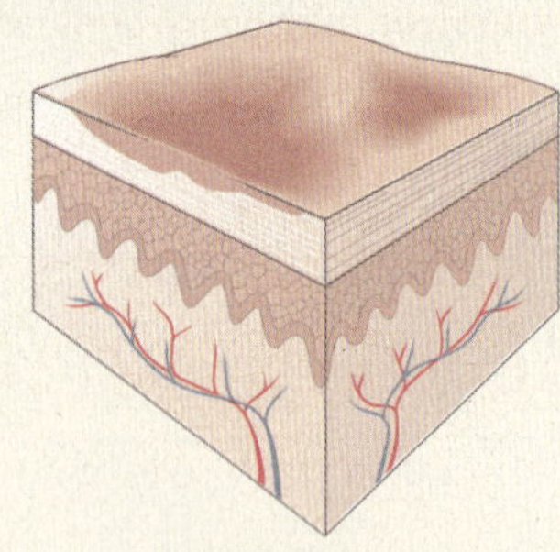 **FIGURE 12-6.** Patch.	Circumscribed flat area of change in color of the skin >1 cm in diameter	Café-au-lait macule present from birth or develop during childhood and can be associated with certain genetic conditions, such as neurofibromatosis type 1[41]
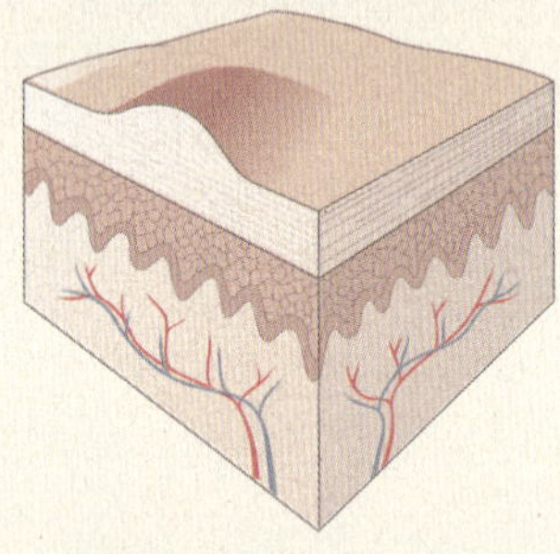 **FIGURE 12-7.** Papule.	Small solid elevation of the skin <1 cm in diameter	Nevi, warts, lichen planus, insect bites, seborrheic keratoses, actinic keratoses, some lesions of acne, and skin cancers[41]
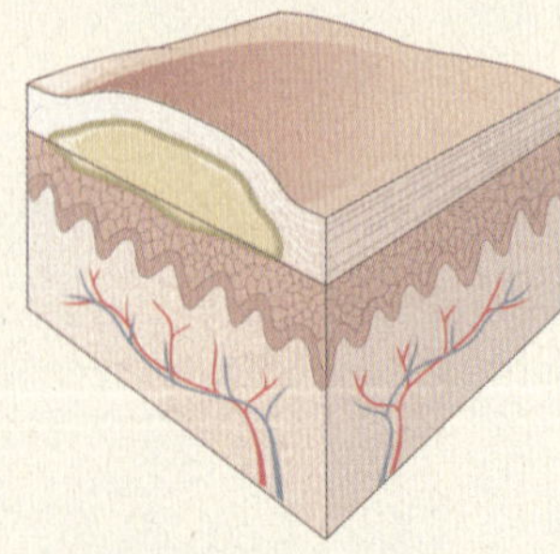 **FIGURE 12-8.** Plaque.	Large flatter elevation of the skin, sometimes formed by papules coalescing	Lesions of psoriasis and granuloma annulare[41]

Type of Lesion	Description	Examples
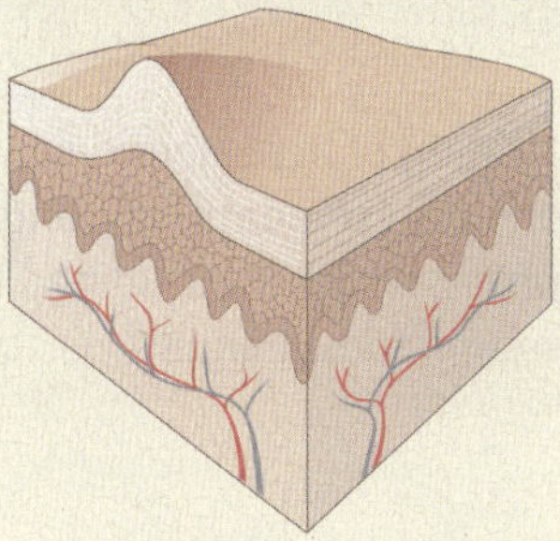 **FIGURE 12-9.** Nodule.	Solid elevation of the skin >1 cm in diameter that usually extends into the deeper skin layers	Cysts, lipomas, and fibromas[41]
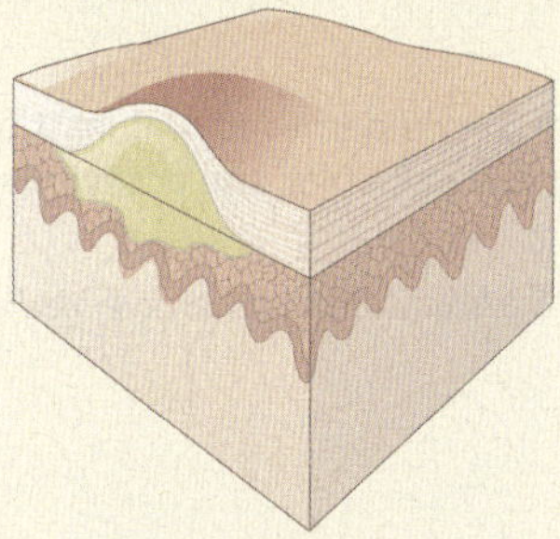 **FIGURE 12-10.** Pustule.	Small, circumscribed elevation of the epidermis filled with purulent fluid	Common in bacterial infections and folliculitis[41]
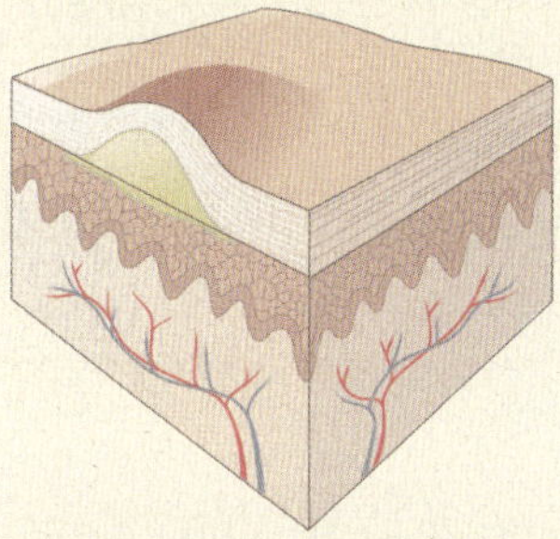 **FIGURE 12-11.** Vesicle.	Small, circumscribed elevation of the epidermis containing clear fluid <1 cm in diameter	Characteristic of herpes infections, acute allergic contact dermatitis, and some autoimmune blistering disorders such as dermatitis herpetiformis[41]
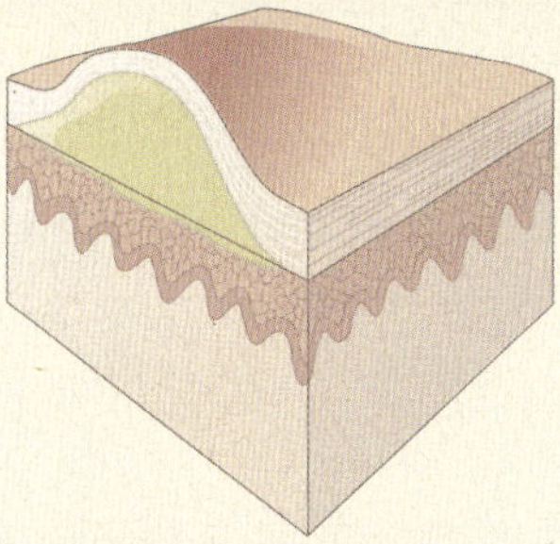 **FIGURE 12-12.** Bulla.	Circumscribed elevation of the epidermis containing clear fluid >1 cm in diameter	Classic autoimmune bullous diseases include pemphigus vulgaris and bullous pemphigoid[41]

(continued)

Box 12-6. Dermatologic Classification and Examples of Skin Lesions (*Continued*)

Type of Lesion	Description	Examples
FIGURE 12-13. Wheal.	Circumscribed, raised lesion consisting of dermal edema, also known as hives or urticaria; typically last <24 hours	Common manifestation of hypersensitivity to drugs; stings or bites; autoimmunity; and, less commonly, physical stimuli including temperature, pressure, and sunlight[41]

Other primary lesions include **erosions** (loss of epidermal or mucosal epithelium), **ulcers** (deeper loss of the epidermis and at least the upper dermis), **petechiae** (nonblanchable punctate foci of hemorrhage), **purpuras** (nonblanchable, raised, and palpable), and **ecchymoses** (nonblanchable larger areas or purpuras).

Figures 12-5 to 12-13 are modified with permission from Kronenberger J, Ledbetter J. *Lippincott Williams & Wilkins' Comprehensive Medical Assisting*. 5th ed. Wolters Kluwer; 2016. Figure 28-2.

Other Features of Skin Lesions

As you begin to learn to assess and describe skin lesions, the goal is to provide a comprehensive and accurate description. Box 12-7 provides a guide for accurately describing skin lesions.

Box 12-7. Clinical Assessment Criteria for Skin Lesions

Feature	Description
Size	■ Measure the lesion with a ruler in millimeters or centimeters. For oval lesions, measure in the long axis, then perpendicular to the axis ■ For example: 3 mm oval lesion (as in basal cell carcinoma)
Number	■ Determine if the lesion is solitary or multiple. Record the number of lesions and estimate the total number of the specific lesion type ■ For example: single lesion on the cheek (as in seborrheic keratosis); 20 papules on the back (as in acne)
Distribution	■ Describe how the skin lesions are scattered or spread out. Note the affected body parts, the pattern or symmetry, and whether lesions are confined to sun-exposed or protected skin ■ For example: randomly distributed across the torso (as in urticaria); symmetrically located on both forearms (as in psoriasis)

Psoriasis often affects the scalp, extensor surfaces of the elbows and knees, umbilicus, and the gluteal cleft.

Lichen planus often affects wrists, forearms, genitals, and lower legs.

Feature	Description
Configuration	■ Describe the shape of single lesions and the arrangement of groups of lesions. Some descriptive terms: ▪ Linear or striate (straight line) ▪ Annular (ring-like, with central clearing) ▪ Nummular or discoid (coin-shaped, no central clearing) ▪ Target, bull's eye, or iris (rings with central duskiness) ▪ Serpiginous or gyrate (having linear, branched, and curving elements) ■ For example: annular lesion with central clearing (as in tinea corporis); linear arrangement of papules (as in allergic contact dermatitis)
Texture	■ Palpate the lesion to determine its texture, whether it is smooth, fleshy, verrucous, or scaly ■ For example: smooth, raised lesion (as in cyst); verrucous or warty surface (as in verruca vulgaris or common wart)
Color	■ Describe the color of the lesion, being as specific as possible. Use a color wheel for reference, if needed. For red lesions, check if they are blanchable or nonblanchable ■ For example: light brown macule (as in melasma), red nonblanching papule (as in purpura)

Vitiligo may be patchy and isolated or may group around the distal extremities and face, particularly the eyes and mouth.

Discoid lupus erythematosus has characteristic lesions on sun-exposed facial skin, especially the forehead, nose, and ears.

Hidradenitis suppurativa involves skin containing many apocrine glands, including the axillae, groin, and under the breasts.

Examples are herpes zoster with unilateral and dermatomal vesicles, herpes simplex with grouped vesicles or pustules on an erythematous base, tinea pedis with annular lesions; and poison ivy allergic contact dermatitis with linear lesions.

Scaling can be greasy, like seborrheic dermatitis or seborrheic keratoses, dry and fine like tinea pedis, or hard and keratotic like actinic keratoses or SCC.

Blanchable lesions are erythematous and suggest inflammation. *Nonblanching* (because blood has extravasated out from the capillaries into the surrounding tissues) lesions such as petechiae, purpuras, and vascular structures (cherry angiomas, vascular malformations) are not erythematous but are bright red, purple, or violaceous.

See Tables 12-4 to 12-6 for rough, pink, and brown lesions and their mimics, pp. 278–284.

See Table 12-1, Describing Primary Skin Lesions: Flat, Raised, and Fluid-Filled, pp. 271–274; Table 12-2, Additional Primary Lesions: Pustules, Furuncles, Nodules, Cysts, Wheals, Burrows, pp. 275–276; and Table 12-3, Dermatology Safari: Benign Skin Lesions, p. 277. See Table 12-7, Vascular and Purpuric Lesions of the Skin, pp. 285–286.

PHYSICAL EXAMINATION: GENERAL APPROACH

When skin lesions are seen, inspect and palpate all lesions. Learn to describe each lesion accurately, using the terminology specified previously. Changing moles, a history of skin cancer, and other risk factors all warrant a full-body skin examination.

Skin Examination Setup

Lighting, Equipment, and Dermoscopy. Make sure there is adequate lighting. Good overhead ambient lighting or natural light from windows is usually adequate. You may wish to add a strong light source if the room is dark. You will also need a small ruler or tape measure. In addition, a small magnifying glass allows you to examine lesions more closely. These tools help you document important features of skin lesions, such as size, shape, color, and texture.

The use of a *dermoscope* is an increasingly useful office practice for deciding whether a melanocytic lesion is benign or malignant. This handheld device provides cross-polarized or unpolarized light to visualize patterns of pigmentation or vascular structures (Fig. 12-14).

With adequate clinician training, use of dermoscopy improves the sensitivity and specificity of differentiating melanomas from benign lesions.[2,3]

Patient Positioning. Standard and alternative techniques for positioning patients during a skin exam aim to ensure both patient comfort and thorough examination of all body areas (Box 12-8). Considering patient privacy, comfort, and modesty during a skin exam is essential. Use drapes or sheets to cover areas not being examined, and always explain each step of the examination process to your patient.

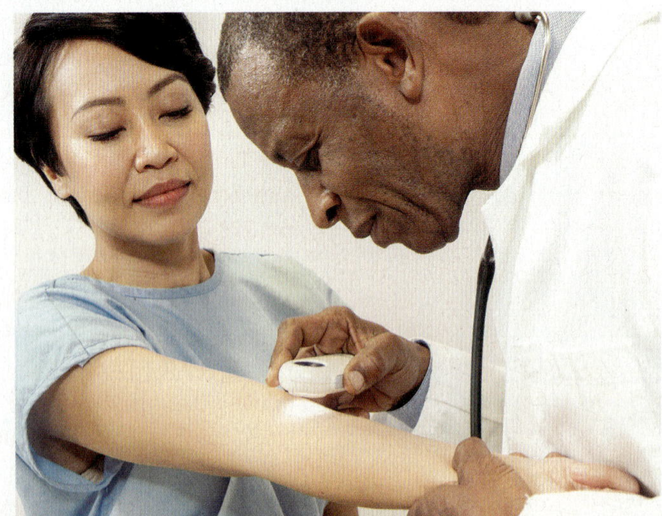

FIGURE 12-14. Using a dermoscope to examine skin lesions.

Box 12-8. Standard and Alternative Techniques for Positioning Patients During a Skin Examination

Position	Description	Areas Examined	Example Skin Conditions
Seated	Patient sits on the examination table; clinician examines their head, neck, face, arms, and hands.	Head, neck, face, arms, hands	Acne, rosacea, eczema, psoriasis
Supine	Patient lies on their back on the examination table; clinician examines their chest, abdomen, legs, and feet.	Chest, abdomen, legs, feet	Tinea corporis, vitiligo, melanoma
Prone	Patient lies on their stomach on the examination table; clinician examines the back, buttocks, and posterior legs.	Back, buttocks, posterior legs	Psoriasis, seborrheic keratosis
Standing	Patient stands while the clinician examines their entire body.	Entire body	Basal cell carcinoma, skin cancer
Left lateral decubitus (formerly Sims)	Patient lies on their side with the upper leg flexed at the hip and knee; clinician has better access to skin folds and hard-to-reach areas, such as the inner thighs, groin, and perianal region.	Inner thighs, groin, perianal region	Hidradenitis suppurativa, intertrigo
Lithotomy	Patient lies on their back with their legs bent at the knees and supported in stirrups; clinician examines the perianal area and genitals.	Perianal area, genitals	Genital warts, herpes, vulvar lesions
Modified positions	Clinician modifies standard positions to accommodate patients with mobility issues or physical limitations, which may involve the use of pillows, blankets, or specialized equipment to support the patient.	Varies based on patient needs and comfort	Conditions affecting patients with limited mobility

See Table 12-11. Acne Vulgaris—Primary and Secondary Lesions, p. 294.

Patient Gown. Ask your patient to change into a gown with the opening in the back and clothes removed except for underwear. This is the first requirement for the skin examination (Fig. 12-15). Ask permission to expose the area to be examined before moving the gown to see each area. You may say, "I'd like to separate the gown to look at your back now. Is that okay?" Do this for every part of the body. Also ask if the patient would like to have a chaperone present, especially when examination of the genital areas is anticipated.

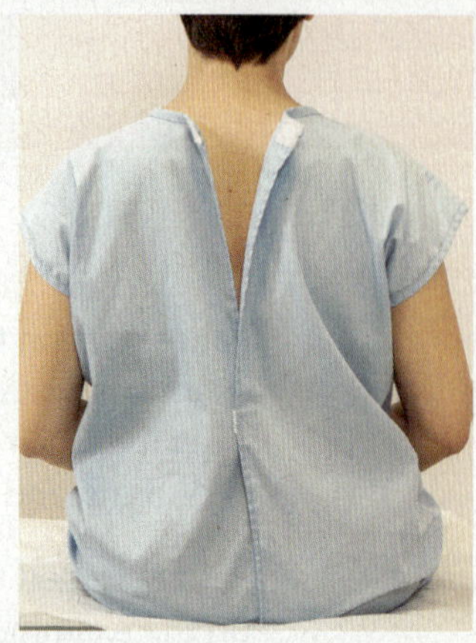

FIGURE 12-15. Patient's gown should open in the back.

Handwashing. Before beginning the examination, ensure your hands are thoroughly cleaned. When palpating lesions, assess for texture, firmness, and scaliness. Dermatologists often recommend hand sanitizers since they tend to be less drying than soap and water and can reduce the risk of irritant contact dermatitis. Let the patient know that this step in hand cleansing is crucial for both hygiene and facilitating a meticulous examination. Use gloves when examining wounds or potentially contagious skin lesions to protect both you and your patient. A professional yet compassionate touch can be therapeutic, especially for individuals living with conditions that can carry stigma, such as psoriasis.

See section on Universal Precautions in Chapter 4, pp. 72–75.

TECHNIQUES OF EXAMINATION

Key Components of the Full-Body Skin Examination

- Examine the hair and scalp—seated.
- Examine the head and neck—seated.
- Examine the upper back—seated.
- Examine the shoulders, arms, and hands—seated.
- Examine the chest and abdomen—seated.
- Examine the anterior thighs and legs—seated.
- Examine the feet and toes—seated.
- Examine the lower back, posterior thighs and legs—standing.
- Integrate a full-body skin examination.

Examine the Hair and Scalp—Seated

Plan to examine the skin in the same order every time, so you are less likely to skip part of the examination. With the *patient seated* on the examining table, stand in front of the patient and adjust the table to a comfortable height. Start by examining the *hair* and *scalp* (Fig. 12-16). Note the distribution, texture,

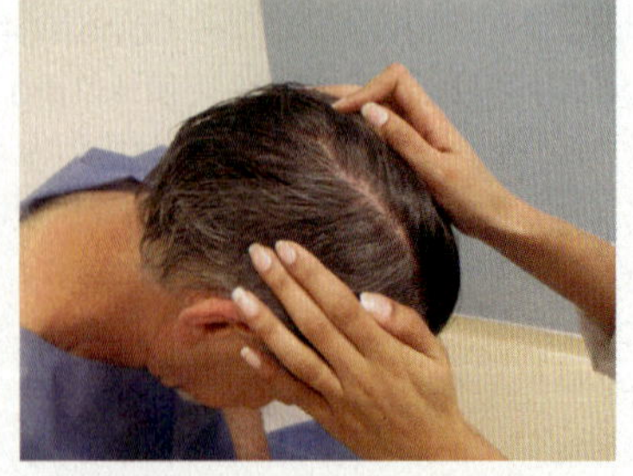

FIGURE 12-16. Parting the hair to expose the scalp.

Alopecia can be diffuse, patchy, or total. Male and female pattern hair loss is normal with aging. Focal patches may be lost suddenly in alopecia areata.[4] Refer scarring alopecia to a dermatologist.

and quantity of hair. Then, using your fingers or a cotton-tipped applicator, separate the hair to examine the scalp from one side to the other.

Sparse hair is seen in hypothyroidism; fine, silky hair in hyperthyroidism. See Table 12-8, Hair Loss, pp. 287–289.

Examine the Head and Neck—Seated

Now inspect the *head* and *neck,* including the forehead, eyes (including eyelids, conjunctivae, and sclerae), nose, ears, cheeks, lips, oral cavity, and chin (Figs. 12-17 to 12-19). Examination should also include inspection of terminal hair of the eyebrows, eyelashes, and beard.

Look for signs of BCC on the face. See Table 12-5, Pink Lesions: Basal Cell Carcinoma and Its Mimics, pp. 279–280.

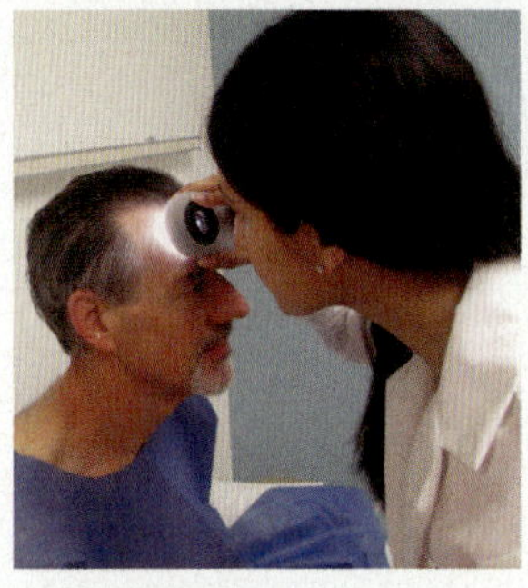

FIGURE 12-17. Inspecting a lesion in the forehead with a dermoscope.

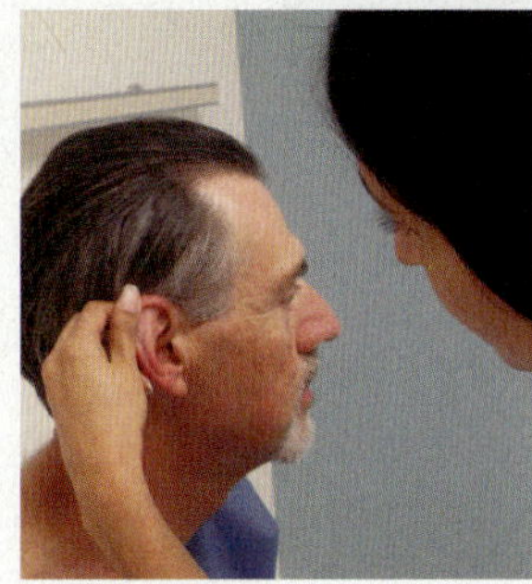

FIGURE 12-18. Inspecting the face and ears.

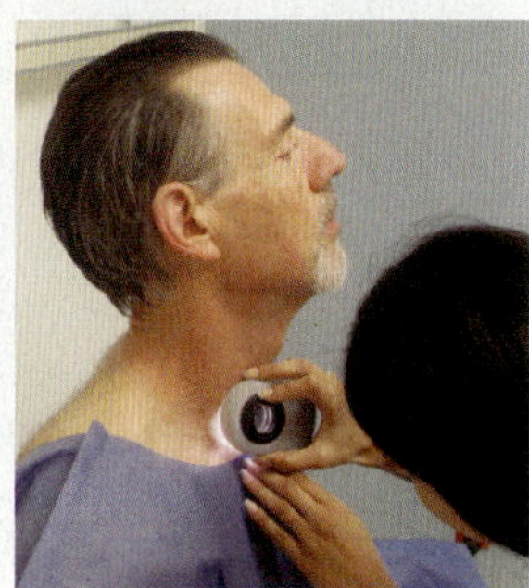

FIGURE 12-19. Inspecting an anterior neck lesion with a dermoscope.

Examine the Upper Back—Seated

Now ask the patient to lean forward, ask permission before opening their gown, and then inspect their upper back (Fig. 12-20).

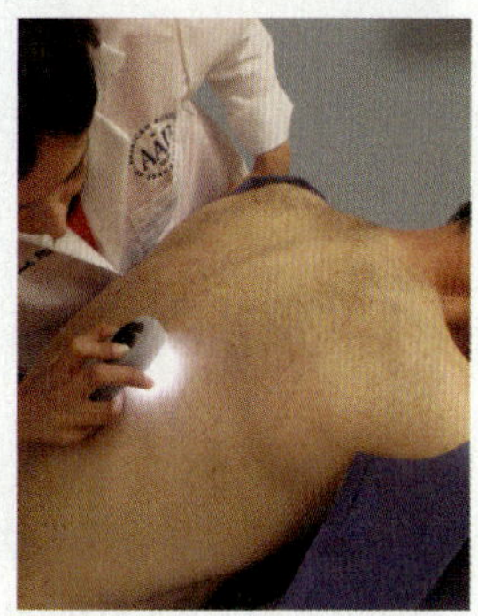

FIGURE 12-20. Inspecting a lesion in the back with the patient leaning forward.

Examine the Shoulders, Arms, and Hands—Seated

Now inspect the *shoulders, arms, and hands* (Fig. 12-21). Inspect and palpate the fingernails (Fig. 12-22). Note their color, shape, and any lesions. Longitudinal bands of pigment are normal in people with darker skin.

See Table 12-9, Findings in or Near the Nails, pp. 290–291.

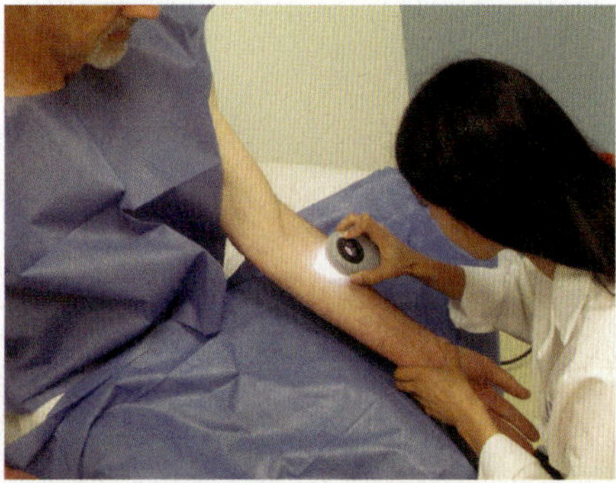

FIGURE 12-21. Inspecting an arm lesion with a dermoscope.

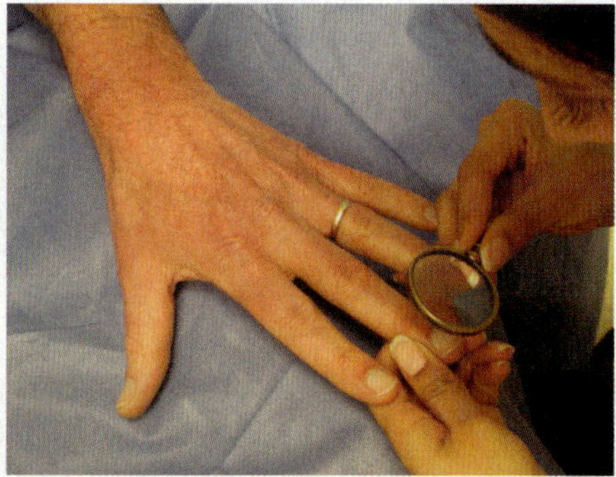

FIGURE 12-22. Inspecting the hands with a magnifying lens and palpating the fingernails.

Examine the Chest and Abdomen—Seated

Now inspect the *chest* and *abdomen*, preparing the patient by saying, "Let's look at your upper chest and then your stomach area" (Fig. 12-23). The patient will generally help by lowering or raising their gown to expose these areas and covering up when you are finished (Fig. 12-24). You may want to inspect the axillae at this point or integrate them later in the examination of the breasts.

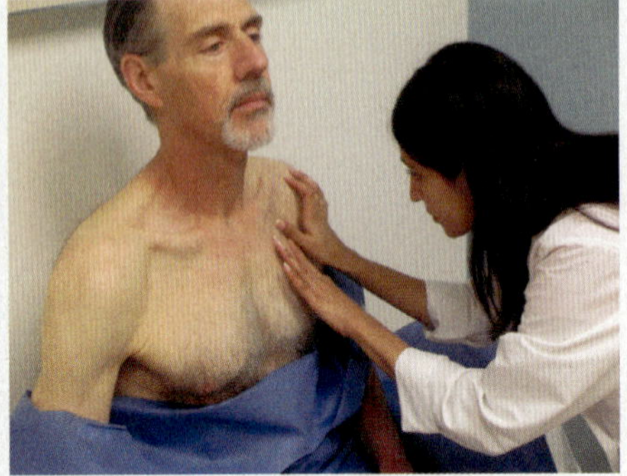

FIGURE 12-23. Inspecting the anterior chest.

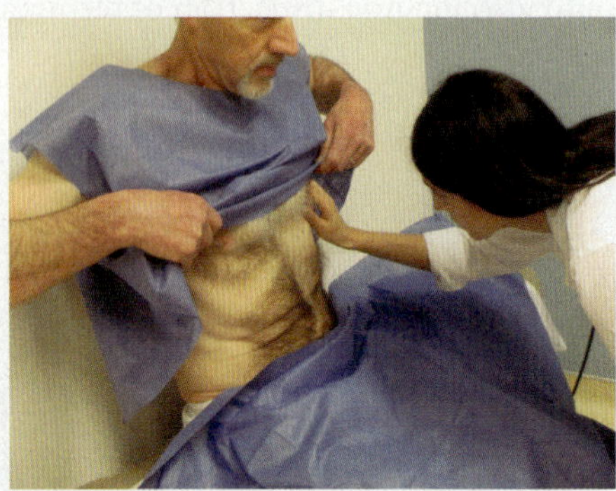

FIGURE 12-24. Inspecting the abdomen.

Examine the Anterior Thighs and Legs—Seated

Now let the patient know that you will be inspecting their *anterior thighs* and *legs* (Fig. 12-25). You and the patient can work together to expose the skin in these areas.

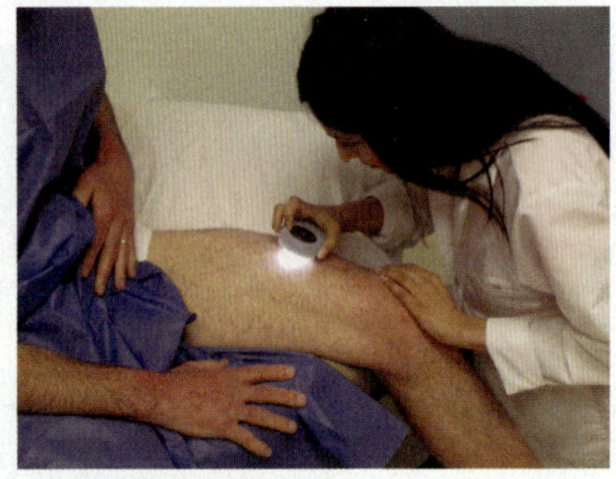

FIGURE 12-25. Inspecting a thigh lesion with a dermoscope.

Examine the Feet and Toes—Seated

Now move down to the *feet* and *toes* (Fig. 12-26). Inspect and palpate the *toenails* and inspect the *soles* and areas between the toes (Figs. 12-27 and 12-28).

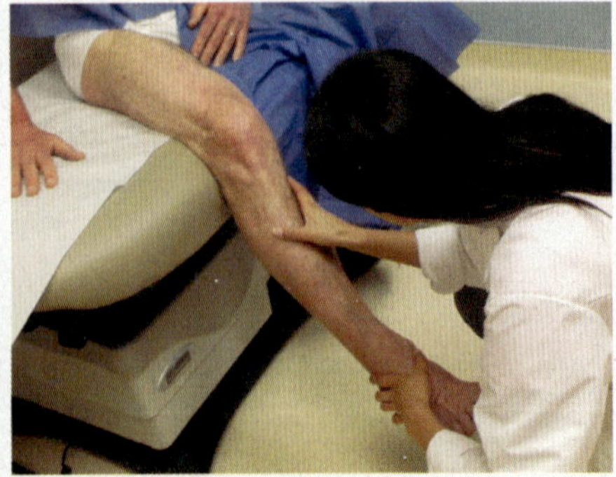

FIGURE 12-26. Inspecting the anterior legs.

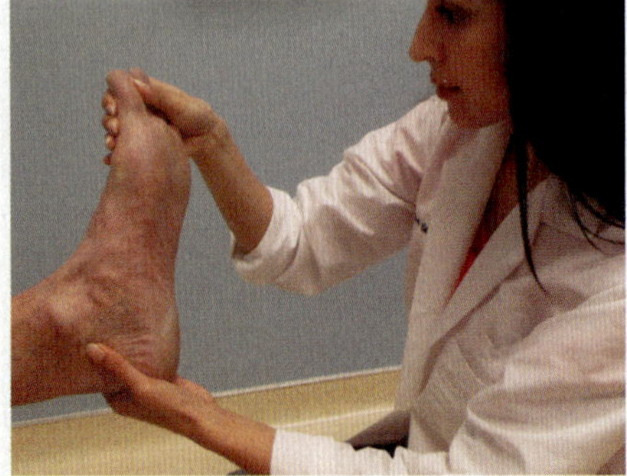

FIGURE 12-27. Inspecting the soles and heels of the feet.

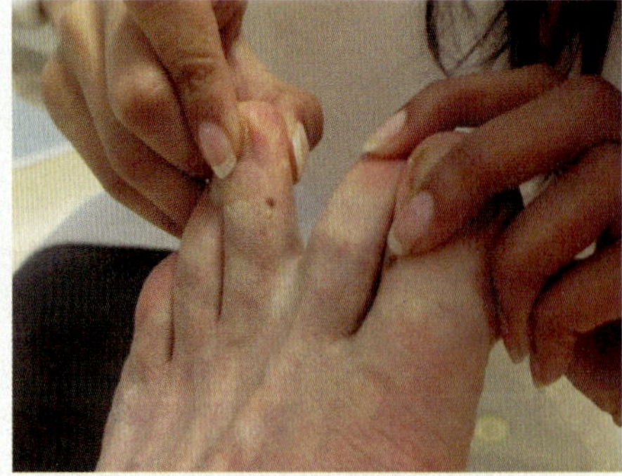

FIGURE 12-28. Inspecting the interdigital areas between toes.

Examine the Lower Back, Posterior Thighs, and Legs—Standing

Now ask the patient to stand so that you can inspect their *lower back* and *posterior legs* (Figs. 12-29 and 12-30). If needed, ask the patient to uncover their buttocks (Fig. 12-31).

Examination of the *breasts* and *genitalia* may be saved for last. These examinations are described in other chapters. Remember to consider patient comfort, modesty, and use of a chaperone during these examinations. Examination should also include inspection of the *axilla* and hair in the *pubic area*.

See Chapter 20, Breasts and Axillae, pp. 584–592; Chapter 23, Pelvis and Genitourinary System: Penis, Scrotum, and Prostate, pp. 701–704; and Chapter 24, Pelvis and Genitourinary System: Vulva, Vagina, Uterus, and Adnexa, pp. 747–750.

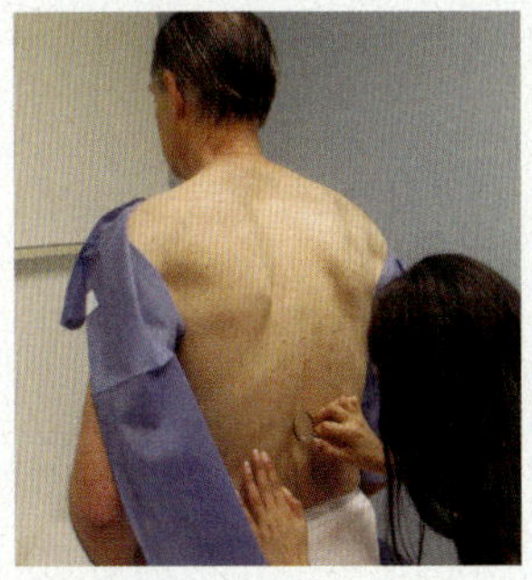

FIGURE 12-29. Inspecting lower back with the patient standing.

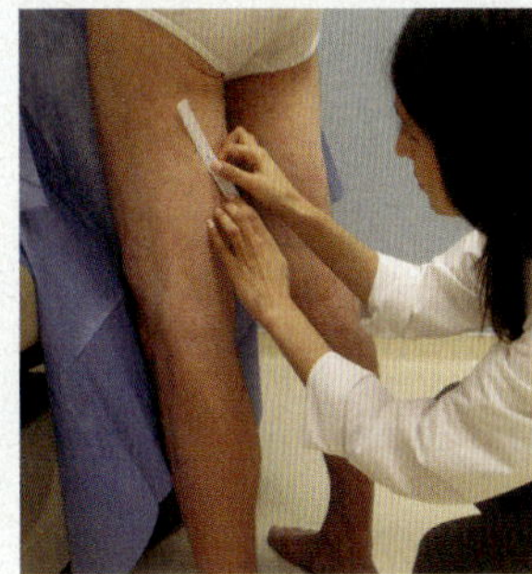

FIGURE 12-30. Determining the size of a lesion with a tape measure in the posterior thigh.

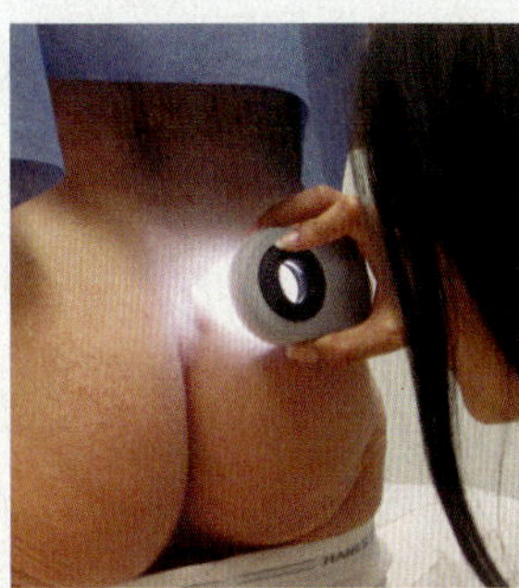

FIGURE 12-31. Inspecting a lesion in the gluteal area.

Integrate a Full-Body Skin Examination

Integrate a full-body skin examination into your routine PE to detect melanomas and other skin cancers more effectively, especially in hard-to-see areas like the back and posterior legs. This integrated approach saves time and enables early detection, making treatment easier. During your training, implement this method with patients in both outpatient and inpatient settings. Focus on documenting skin features that are present rather than what is absent.

SPECIAL TECHNIQUES AND MANEUVERS

Instructing the Patient in Skin Self-Examination

The American Academy of Dermatology (AAD) recommends regular self-examination of the skin using the techniques illustrated in Box 12-9. The patient will need a full-length mirror, a handheld mirror, and a well-lit room that provides privacy. Teach the patient the ABCDE-EFG method for assessing moles. Help them to identify melanomas by looking at photographs of benign and malignant nevi on easy-to-access websites, handouts, or tables in this chapter.

Review the ABCDE-EFG criteria on pp. 246–247.

Box 12-9. Patient Instructions for Skin Self-Examination[35]

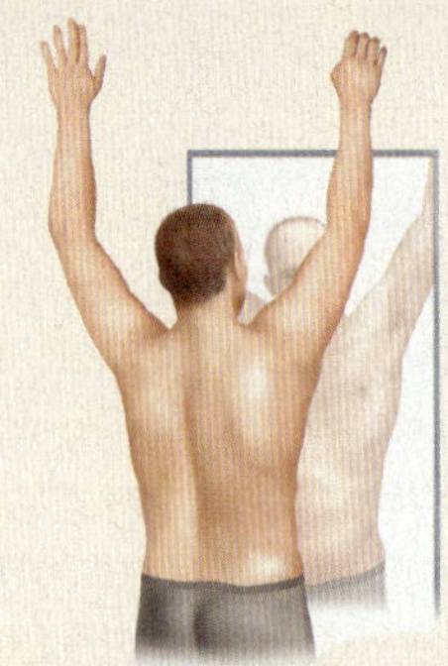

Examine your body front and back in the mirror, then look at right and left sides with your arms raised.

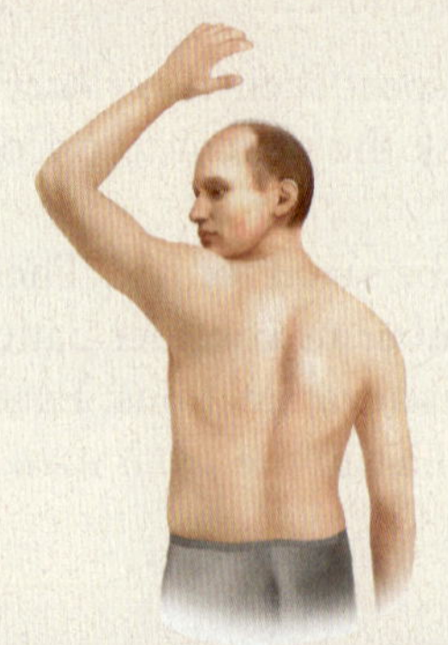

Bend your elbows and look carefully at forearms, underarms, and palms.

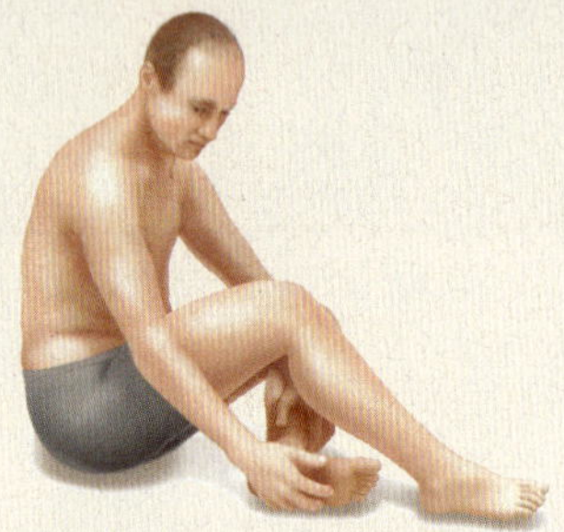

Look at the backs of your legs and feet, the spaces between your toes, and the soles.

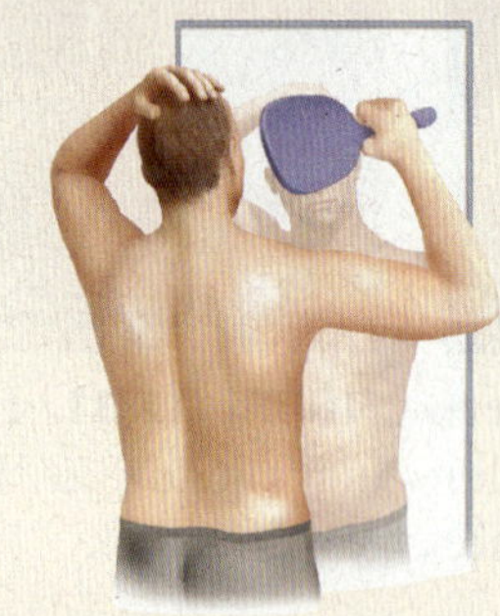

Examine the back of your neck and scalp with a hand mirror. Part your hair for a closer look.

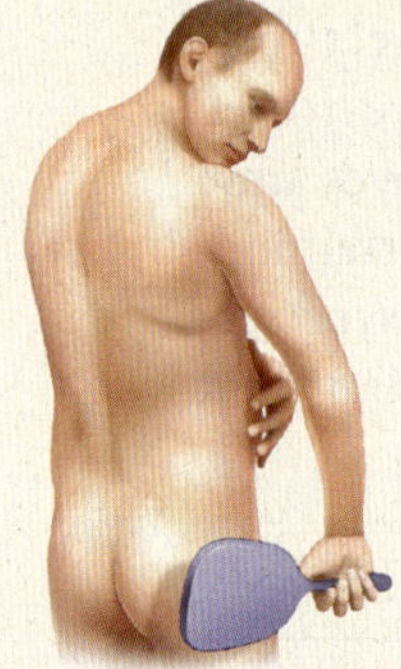

Finally, check your back and buttocks with a hand mirror.

Source: American Cancer Society medical and editorial content team. How to Do a Skin Self-Exam. American Cancer Society. Accessed August 1, 2023. https://www.cancer.org/cancer/risk-prevention/sun-and-uv/skin-exams.html

Examining the Patient with Hair Loss

Based on the patient's history, start by examining the hair to determine the overall pattern of hair loss or hair thinning. Inspect the *scalp* for erythema, scaling, pustules, tenderness, bogginess, and scarring. Look at the width of the hair part in various sections of the scalp.

To examine the hair for shedding from the roots, perform a *hair pull test* by gently grasping 50 to 60 hairs with your thumb and index and middle fingers, pulling firmly away from the scalp (Fig. 12-32). If all the hairs have telogen bulbs, the most likely diagnosis is *telogen effluvium*.

To examine the hair for fragility, perform the *tug test* by holding a group of hairs in one hand, pulling along the hair shafts with the other; any breakage is abnormal (Fig. 12-33). Most (97%) hair loss is nonscarring, but any scarring, namely shiny spots without any hair follicles on close examination with a magnifying glass, should prompt referral to dermatology for scalp biopsy.

Possible internal causes of diffuse nonscarring hair shedding are iron-deficiency anemia, hyper- and hypothyroidism.

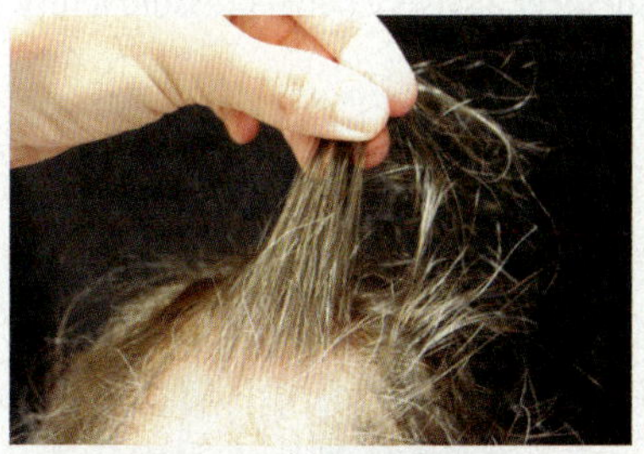

FIGURE 12-32. Examining the hair for shredding from the roots (hair pull test).

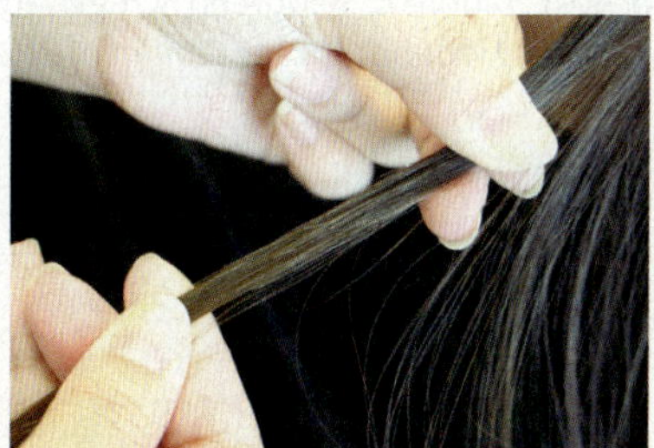

FIGURE 12-33. Examining the hair for fragility (tug test).

Evaluating the Patient Who Is Confined to a Bed

People confined to a bed, particularly those who are emaciated, elderly, or neurologically impaired, are highly prone to skin damage and ulceration. *Pressure injuries* or *ulcers* arise from prolonged compression that cuts off blood flow to the skin and from shear forces due to body movements. For instance, sliding down in bed or being dragged rather than lifted can distort soft tissues and obstruct arteries. Friction and moisture heighten the risk of abrasions and sores. Pressure injuries are classified using staging systems that detail tissue loss and injury appearance caused by pressure and/or shear (Box 12-10).[5]

See Table 12-13, Pressure Injuries, pp. 296–297.

To assess vulnerable patients, carefully examine the skin overlying the sacrum, buttocks, greater trochanters, knees, and heels. Turn the patient to one side for optimal examination of the lower back and gluteal area. Inspect for skin breaks and injuries and check any pressure injuries for infection signs such as drainage, odor, cellulitis, or necrosis.

Box 12-10. Revised Pressure Injury Staging System[5]

The revised staging system uses the term *injury* instead of *ulcer* and denotes stages using Arabic numerals rather than Roman numerals (Fig. 12-34).

- **Stage 1:** Intact skin with a localized area of non-blanchable erythema, which may appear as deeper tones like purple, blue, or darker than the surrounding skin in darkly pigmented individuals.
- **Stage 2:** Partial-thickness loss of skin with exposed dermis
- **Stage 3:** Full-thickness skin loss, in which adipose (fat) is visible in the ulcer and granulation tissue and rolled wound edges, is often present
- **Stage 4:** Full-thickness skin and tissue loss with exposed or directly palpable fascia, muscle, tendon, ligament, cartilage, or bone in the ulcer
- **Unstageable:** Full-thickness skin and tissue loss in which the extent of tissue damage within the ulcer cannot be confirmed because it is obscured by *slough* or *eschar*
- **Deep tissue pressure injury:** Persistent nonblanchable deep red, maroon, or purple discoloration

Source: Edsberg LE, Black JM, Goldberg M, McNichol L, Moore L, Sieggreen M. Revised national pressure ulcer advisory panel pressure injury staging system: revised pressure injury staging system. *J Wound Ostomy Continence Nurs*. 2016;43(6):585–597.

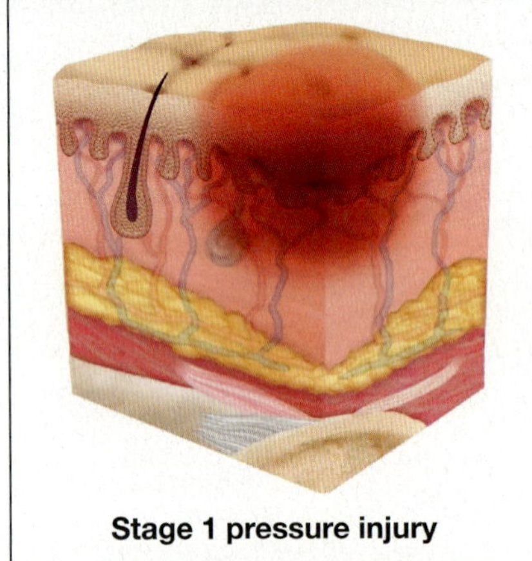
Stage 1 pressure injury

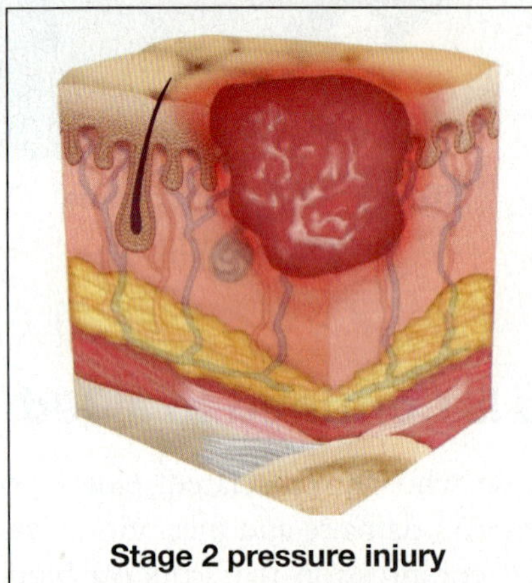
Stage 2 pressure injury

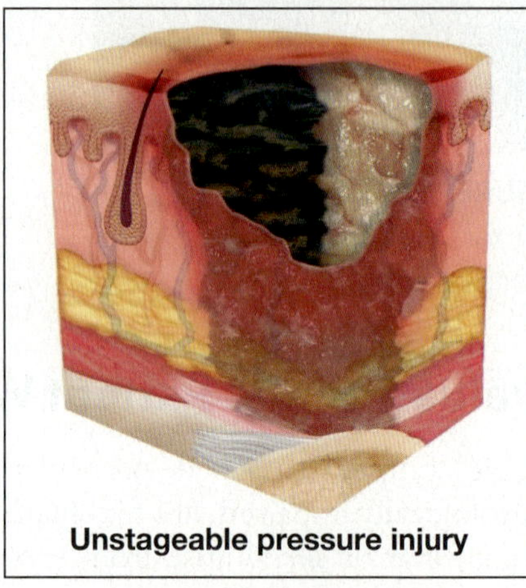
Unstageable pressure injury

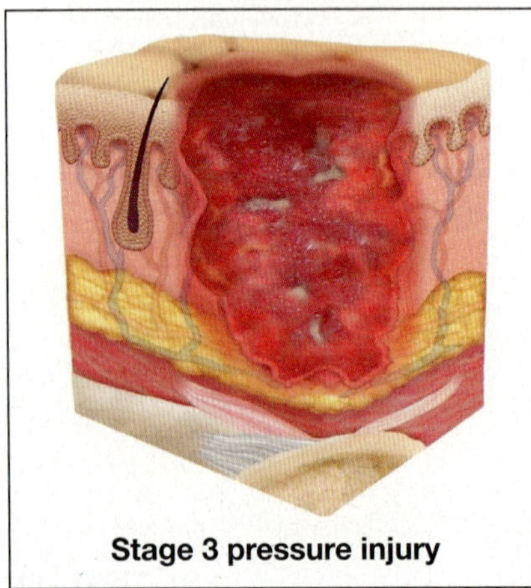
Stage 3 pressure injury

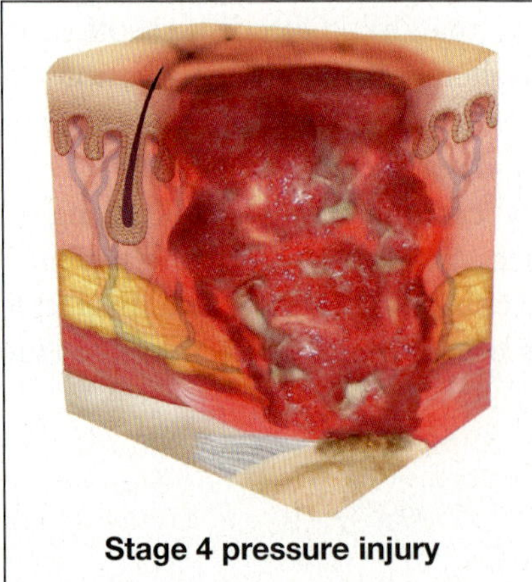
Stage 4 pressure injury

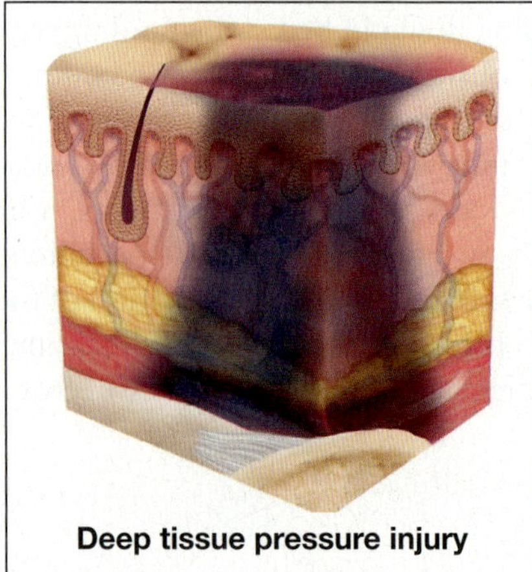
Deep tissue pressure injury

FIGURE 12-34. Pressure injury stages. (Modified with permission from Nettina SM. *Lippincott Manual of Nursing Practice*. 11th ed. Wolters Kluwer; 2019. Figure 9-3.)

Modifications in Physical Examinations: Best Practices for Specialized Patient Populations

Devices like implantable continuous glucose monitors (CGMs) and insulin pumps have transformed the way you can monitor and care for your patients, providing real-time glucose information and precise insulin administration. However, during your routine skin examinations, being mindful of these devices is essential. Carefully inspect the skin around them to ensure its health, the device's proper functioning, and your patient's comfort. In addition, you must familiarize yourself with these devices to prevent unintentional damage or cause discomfort to your patient. For a detailed guide on these devices and how to modify your approach during a skin examination, refer to Box 12-11.

Box 12-11. Skin Examination in the Presence of Medical Devices, Conditions, or Procedures

	Implantable Continuous Glucose Monitor	Insulin Pump
Device/condition	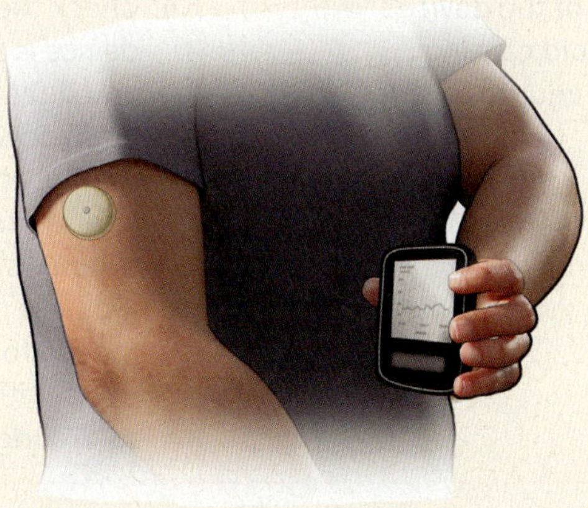 Small sensor implanted under the skin that measures interstitial glucose levels at regular intervals and transmits the readings to a receiving device	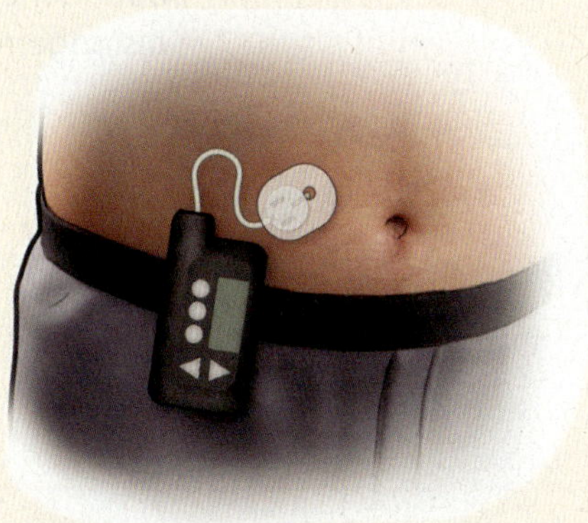 Delivers precise doses of insulin continuously or in boluses via a cannula placed under the skin
General indication	Continuous monitoring of glucose levels in patients with diabetes, aiding in better glucose management	Insulin delivery for patients with diabetes who require intensive insulin therapy; acts as an alternative to multiple daily injections of insulin by syringes or a pen
General location	Typically inserted in the subcutaneous tissue of the upper arm or abdomen	Often worn on the belt, in a pocket, or with special clips; infusion set (subcutaneous cannula, tubing, adhesive mount) is typically positioned on the subcutaneous tissue of the abdomen or thigh

(*continued*)

Box 12-11. Skin Examination in the Presence of Medical Devices, Conditions, or Procedures (*Continued*)

	Implantable Continuous Glucose Monitor	Insulin Pump
Modification to the physical exam	1. Visually inspect the general area around the device for discoloration, scars, or signs of trauma 2. Examine the specific site of the device for erythema, swelling, or discharge, which might indicate infection or irritation 3. With gloved hands, palpate gently around the device site, feeling for any subcutaneous nodules or induration; avoid direct pressure over the device 4. Ask the patient if they experience any pain or discomfort as you palpate, which may suggest underlying issues 5. Always be aware of the device's boundaries to avoid causing dislodgement or injury	1. Identify the location of the insulin pump's infusion set on the skin 2. Visually inspect the skin around the infusion set for signs of irritation, such as redness, swelling, or skin breakdown 3. Gently palpate around the infusion site, feeling for signs of subcutaneous leakage of insulin or any hardened areas, which might suggest *lipohypertrophy*; avoid pressing directly over the infusion set 4. Check the adhesive area (where the device is attached to the skin) for any signs of allergic reactions or skin breakdown 5. Inquire about the patient's cleaning and site rotation routine to ensure optimal skin health 6. If device needs to be temporarily moved for a thorough examination, do so with utmost care, ensuring not to dislodge the infusion set

RECORDING YOUR FINDINGS

Documenting your PE findings thoroughly in your clinical notes aids in diagnostic determination and hypothesis testing. Over time, you typically will refine your documentation style to shorter, standardized phrases reflecting your professional growth.

Recording the Skin, Hair, and Nail Examination

"Skin warm and dry. Nails without clubbing or cyanosis. Approximately 20 brown, round macules on upper back, chest, and arms; are all symmetric in pigmentation, none suspicious. No rash, petechiae, or ecchymoses."

OR

"Marked facial pallor, and circumoral cyanosis. Palms cold and moist. Cyanosis in nail beds of fingers and toes. Numerous palpable purpuras on lower legs bilaterally."

OR

"Scattered stuck-on verrucous plaques on back and abdomen. More than 30 small round brown macules with symmetric pigmentation on back, chest, and arms. Single 1.2 × 1.6 cm asymmetric dark brown and black plaque with erythematous, uneven border, on left upper arm."

OR

"Facial plethora. Skin icteric. Many telangiectatic mats on chest and abdomen. Single 5-mm pearly papule with rolled border on left zygomatic cheek. Nails with clubbing but no cyanosis."

Analyzing PE documentation in detail highlights how nuanced clinical observations can be instrumental in revealing essential clues for accurate diagnoses.

The first PE findings described indicate several observations about the patient's skin condition:

- *Skin warm and dry:* This is generally a normal finding. It indicates that the patient does not have a fever or excessive moisture (sweat) on their skin, which could suggest an infection or other systemic condition.
- *Nails without clubbing or cyanosis:* The absence of these signs is a positive indication of normal respiratory and circulatory function.
- *Brown, round macules on upper back, chest, and arms:* The description of these as brown and symmetric suggests they might be benign lesions. The key here is that they are symmetric in pigmentation, and none are suspicious, which typically means they are uniform in color and borders.
- *No rash, petechiae, or ecchymoses:* Their absence suggests that there are no acute skin infections, bleeding disorders, or physical trauma.

Overall, these findings suggest a skin condition that is likely *benign*, with no immediate signs of systemic illness, infection, or significant dermatologic disease.

The symptoms described in the second PE note suggest a more concerning clinical picture:

- *Marked facial pallor and circumoral cyanosis:* Facial pallor can indicate anemia or poor blood circulation, while circumoral cyanosis suggests a lack of oxygenation in the blood. This combination often points to cardiovascular or respiratory issues that are affecting blood oxygen levels.
- *Palms cold and moist:* This can be a sign of poor circulation or a response to stress or shock. It can also indicate an autonomic nervous system response in which blood flow is reduced to the extremities.
- *Cyanosis in nail beds of fingers and toes:* Similar to circumoral cyanosis, this finding indicates poor oxygenation of the blood. When present in the extremities, it can be a sign of peripheral vasoconstriction, respiratory dysfunction, or cardiac issues.
- *Numerous palpable purpuras on lower legs bilaterally:* Palpable purpuras are often a sign of vasculitis. This can be associated with autoimmune diseases, infections, and drug reactions. Their presence on both lower legs reinforces the likelihood of a systemic issue.

The combination of these findings could point to a variety of *systemic diseases* including severe respiratory or cardiac conditions, a systemic vasculitic process, or other systemic diseases.

The third PE note description suggests a mix of possibly benign and potentially concerning skin findings:

- *Scattered stuck-on verrucous plaques on back and abdomen:* These plaques are likely to be seborrheic keratoses, which are common, benign, wart-like growths that appear "stuck on" the skin. They are generally harmless and more frequently seen in older adults.
- *More than 30 small round brown macules with symmetric pigmentation on back, chest, and arms:* These sound like benign pigmented lesions, such as freckles, lentigines, or nevi (moles). The key observation here is their symmetry in pigmentation, which usually indicates a benign nature but could warrant monitoring for any changes.
- *Single 1.2 × 1.6 cm asymmetric dark brown and black plaque with erythematous and uneven border on left upper arm:* This particular lesion is concerning. The asymmetry in color (dark brown and black) and the uneven, erythematous border are features that align with the ABCDE (Asymmetry, Border irregularity, Color variation, Diameter, and Evolving) criteria used to identify melanoma, a serious form of skin cancer. The size of the lesion (>1 cm) also raises concern.

The described skin findings include benign features like *seborrheic keratoses* and *symmetrical macules*, but the presence of an asymmetric, irregularly bordered, and variably pigmented plaque raises concern for potential *melanoma*.

The findings described in the fourth PE note suggest a combination of findings that could be associated with various medical conditions:

- *Facial plethora:* Plethora is often associated with increased blood flow or increased red blood cells. It can be seen in conditions such as polycythemia vera and Cushing syndrome, and can be a reaction to medications or alcohol.
- *Skin icteric:* Icterus, or jaundice, is typically due to elevated bilirubin levels, which can be a sign of liver or gallbladder disease or hemolysis.
- *Many telangiectatic mats on chest and abdomen:* Telangiectatic mats are networks of small, dilated blood vessels. They can occur due to genetic conditions, like hereditary hemorrhagic telangiectasia, or be associated with liver disease, aging, or sun damage.
- *Single 5-mm pearly papule with rolled border on left zygomatic cheek:* A pearly appearance and a rolled border are characteristic features of BCC.
- *Nails with clubbing but no cyanosis:* Nail clubbing often indicates long-term low oxygen levels in the blood. It can be associated with lung diseases, heart disease, gastrointestinal conditions, and other systemic diseases. The absence of cyanosis is a positive sign.

This patient presents with facial redness, jaundice, dilated blood vessels on the chest and abdomen, a suspicious skin lesion on the cheek suggestive of *basal cell carcinoma*, and nail clubbing, suggesting a combination of *liver pathology*, *vascular issues*, and potential *skin cancer*.

POINT-OF-CARE ULTRASOUND EXAMINATION

In a dermatologic assessment, the skin's surface provides vital clues. However, with the integration of **point-of-care ultrasound** (**POCUS**), you can now explore beyond the superficial layers. This powerful tool offers a noninvasive glimpse into the deeper structures of the skin, aiding in differentiating conditions like cellulitis from abscesses and detecting foreign bodies. As you navigate through this section, recognize our primary goal: emphasizing the supplemental value of POCUS in dermatologic evaluations. While we underscore its advantages, note that we will not explore into the intricate procedural steps of POCUS.

Distinguishing Between Cellulitis and Abscess

Physical Examination. Skin and soft tissue infections (SSTIs) are frequently encountered in clinical settings, accounting for around 35 million visits between 2006 and 2010.[6] Two common SSTIs are *cellulitis* and *abscess*; however, the clinical exam for differentiating between them can be challenging due to overlapping clinical signs such as erythema and warmth (Box 12-12). Complications like pain and induration can further impede an accurate clinical assessment, potentially masking a deep-seated abscess. While cellulitis typically necessitates antibiotic therapy, abscesses often require an incision and drainage (I&D). Therefore, identifying the need for invasive management is of the utmost importance, especially in pediatric patients, for whom an unnecessary I&D can cause increased stress or pain.[7,8]

POCUS has been shown to be highly effective in distinguishing between cellulitis and abscess and improving equivocal PE findings in both pediatric

Box 12-12. Comparison of Physical Examination Findings: Cellulitis vs. Abscess

Feature	Cellulitis	Abscess
Appearance	Red, swollen area	Red, swollen lump
Tenderness	Yes	Yes
Warmth	Yes	Yes
Pain	Yes	Yes, often more intense
Pus	No (or not typically seen)	Yes (central pocket of pus)
Induration (hardening)	Yes	Yes, especially around the lump
Fluctuance (liquid feeling)	No	Yes (feeling of liquid under pressure)
Fever	Possible, if severe	Possible, especially if not drained

and adult patients.[7,9–11] Ultrasound of SSTIs can be easily performed by novices with limited training, making it ideal as an adjunct to the PE.[7,12] Overall, POCUS for SSTIs improves equivocal PE findings and can change management decisions[7,11]

Ultrasound Technique

Basic Ultrasound Setup	
Patient positioning	Supine
Probe	Linear probe
Ultrasound setting	"Superficial" or "MSK" setting, B-mode

POCUS evaluation for SSTIs[8,13–15] is performed with the patient in a supine position. The study is performed with the linear probe. The higher-frequency probe is useful for evaluating superficial structures. The ultrasound machine is set to the "superficial" or "MSK" preset.

When examining an SSTI with ultrasound, ensure that you apply a generous amount of gel. This action reduces pressure on the sensitive infected area. Your main attention should be directed to two primary scanning planes: the *transverse* and *sagittal* (Box 12-13).

- Carefully inspect the skin's sublayers for signs of fluid accumulations. If you encounter a fluid pocket, apply gentle pressure. This technique helps determine if the fluid inside shifts, a characteristic known as the "*squish sign*" and which suggests the presence of pus.

  Always use the color Doppler over these fluid regions and the surrounding area (Box 12-14). This step is vital to ensure that you are not mistakenly identifying a blood vessel as an infection pocket. It also serves as a safety precaution to pinpoint any blood vessels you should avoid if considering an I&D.
- Before embarking on any procedure, assess the depth and breadth of the possible abscess. This gives you a clearer understanding of what to expect.

Box 12-13. Ultrasound Probe Placement for Skin and Soft Tissue Infections

View	Procedure
Transverse view	■ Place the ultrasound probe with its marker directed to the patient's right side, right over the infection. ■ Slide the probe vertically, from top to bottom. ■ Make a mental comparison between the infected and normal tissue.
Sagittal view	■ Rotate the probe 90 degrees from its transverse position, with the marker now facing the patient's head. ■ Slide the probe horizontally, moving from the outer side toward the center of the body.

Box 12-14. Images in Soft Tissue Ultrasound

Normal	Note the clearly demarcated layers of tissue, muscle, and bone (Fig. 12-35)
Cellulitis	Note the "cobblestone" appearance due to fluid tracking between subcutaneous tissue and fat (Fig. 12-36)
Abscess	Discrete anechoic or hypoechoic fluid collection often with internal echogenicity, irregular borders, but no internal color flow (Fig. 12-37)

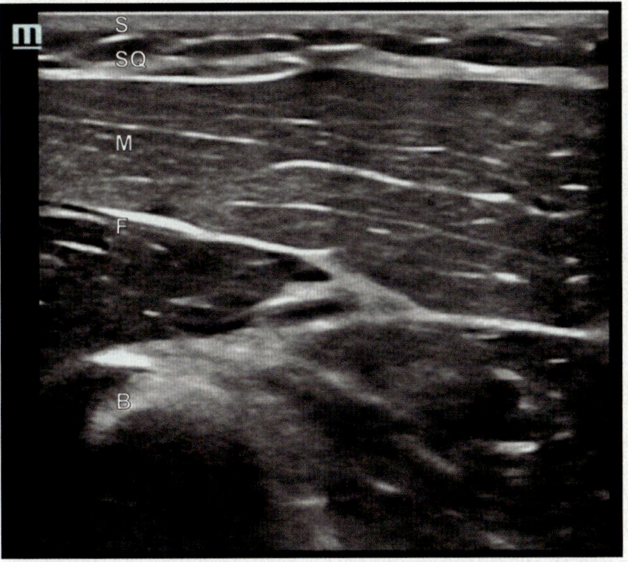

FIGURE 12-35. Normal soft tissue and bone. S, skin; SQ, subcutaneous tissue; M, muscle; F, fascial layer; B, bone.

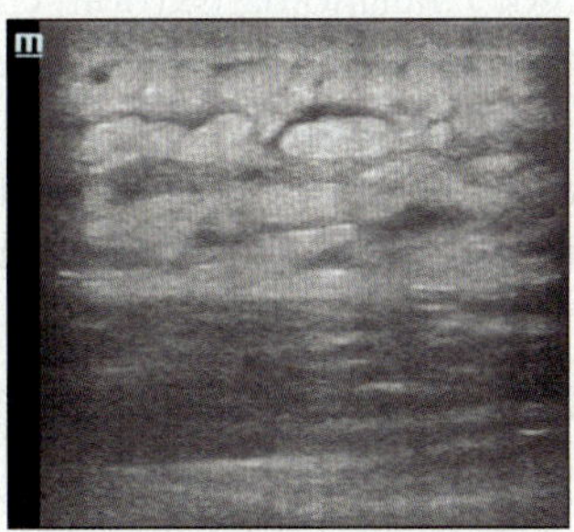

FIGURE 12-36. Cellulitis.

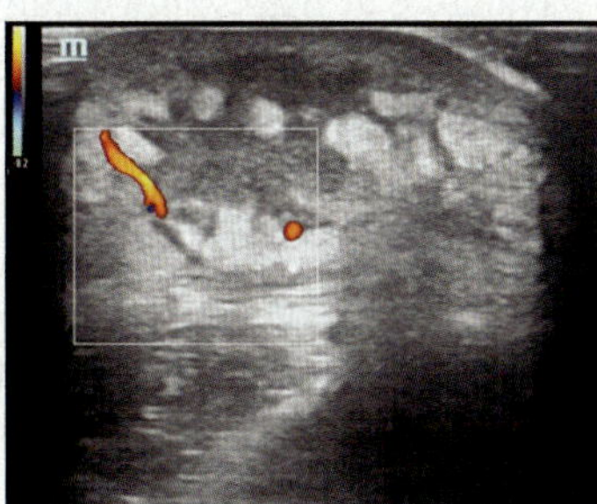

FIGURE 12-37. Abscess with color Doppler.

HEALTH PROMOTION AND COUNSELING: EVIDENCE AND RECOMMENDATIONS

Important Topics for Health Promotion and Counseling

- Skin cancer epidemiology
- Skin cancer prevention
- Clinician skin cancer screening
- Skin self-examination

In the following section, both traditional terms like "men," "women," "male," and "female" and inclusive terms such as "individuals assigned female at birth" and "individuals assigned male at birth" are used. This approach balances inclusivity with the need to accurately represent the original research.

Skin Cancer Epidemiology

Skin cancers are the most commonly diagnosed cancers in the United States, with a lifetime risk estimated to be about one in five.[16] The most common skin cancer is BCC, followed by SCC, and then melanoma. More than 3 million Americans are diagnosed each year with a nonmelanoma skin cancer,[17] and nearly 100,000 were diagnosed with melanoma in 2023.[18] Melanoma is the fifth most frequently diagnosed cancer. The estimated lifetime risk of being diagnosed with melanoma is 1 in 45 (2.2%), with the highest risk observed in non-Hispanic Whites (3.0%). Individuals assigned male at birth have a risk of 2.6% compared to 1.7% for those assigned female at birth.[19] Nonmelanoma skin cancers are rarely fatal, causing only about 2,000 deaths each year.[17] Although melanoma accounts for just 1% of skin cancers, it is the most lethal, causing an estimated 7,990 deaths in 2023.[20]

For discussion and examples of types of skin cancers, turn to Table 12-4, Rough Lesions: Actinic Keratoses, Squamous Cell Carcinoma, and Their Mimics on p. 278, Table 12-5, Pink Lesions: Basal Cell Carcinoma and Its Mimics, pp. 279–280, and Table 12-6, Brown Lesions: Melanoma and Its Mimics, pp. 281–284.

Sun and ultraviolet (UV) radiation exposure are the strongest risk factors for developing nonmelanoma skin cancer.[21] People with light-colored eyes, fair skin, freckling, or skin that burns easily with sun exposure are most at risk; other risk factors include receiving immunosuppressive therapy after organ transplantation and arsenic exposure. Melanoma risk factors are listed in Box 12-15. The *Melanoma Risk Assessment Tool*, developed by the National Cancer Institute, is available at http://www.cancer.gov/melanomarisktool. This tool assesses an individual's 5-year risk of developing melanoma based on geographic location, gender, race, age, history of blistering sunburns, complexion, number and size of moles, freckling, and sun damage. The tool is not intended for individuals with a personal history of skin cancer or a family history of melanoma.

Skin Cancer Prevention

Avoiding Ultraviolet Radiation and Tanning Beds. Increasing lifetime sun exposure correlates directly with increasing risk of skin cancer. The best defense against skin cancer is to avoid UV radiation exposure by limiting time in the sun, avoiding midday sun, using sunscreen, and wearing sun-protective clothing with long sleeves and hats with wide brims. Advise patients to avoid indoor tanning, especially children, teens, and young adults.

Signs of chronic sun damage include numerous *solar lentigines* on the shoulders and upper back, many melanocytic nevi, solar elastosis (yellow, thickened skin with bumps, wrinkles, or furrowing), cutis rhomboidalis nuchae (leathery thickened skin on the posterior neck), and actinic purpura. See Table 12-12, Signs of Sun Damage, on p. 295.

Box 12-15. Risk Factors for Melanoma

- Personal or family history of previous melanoma
- ≥50 common moles
- Atypical or large moles, especially if dysplastic
- Red or light hair
- *Solar lentigines* (acquired brown macules on sun-exposed areas)
- Freckles (inherited brown macules)
- Ultraviolet radiation from heavy sun exposure, sunlamps, or tanning booths
- Light eye or skin color, especially skin that freckles or burns easily
- Severe blistering sunburns in childhood
- Immunosuppression from human immunodeficiency virus (HIV) or organ transplantation
- Personal history of nonmelanoma skin cancer

The International Agency for Research on Cancer has classified UV-emitting tanning devices as "carcinogenic to humans."[22] Ever use of sunbeds is associated with an increased risk for all skin cancers, particularly among those using sunbeds before age 35 years.[23] The risk for melanoma increases with each additional tanning session. The U.S. Preventive Services Task Force (USPSTF) has issued a grade B recommendation supporting behavioral counseling to minimize UV radiation exposure in fair-skinned people aged 6 months to 24 years.[24] The USPSTF suggested considering risk factors for skin cancer in selectively counseling fair-skinned adults aged 24 years and older (grade C recommendation).

Use of indoor tanning beds, especially before age 35 years, increases risk of melanoma by as much as 75%.[25]

Regular Use of Sunscreen. A randomized trial in Queensland, Australia, showed that daily sun protective factor (SPF) 16 sunscreen application to the head and arms could prevent nonmelanoma skin cancers and invasive melanomas.[26,27] A prospective population-based cohort study of Norwegian women aged 40 to 75 years found that regularly using SPF ≥15 sunscreen was associated with a decreased melanoma risk compared to never using sunscreen and using SPF <15.[28] Case-control studies in the United States and Australia also showed that sunscreen use was associated with a decreased melanoma risk.[29,30]

Advise patients to use sunscreen with at least 30 SPF and broad-spectrum protection against both UVA and UVB radiation. U.S. Food and Drug Administration labeling guidelines make it easy to see these features on all bottles of sunscreen.[31] The AAD recommends using sunscreen to cover all exposed skin whenever going outside, even on cloudy days.[32] Sunscreen should be reapplied every 2 hours when outdoors and after being in the water.

Clinician Skin Cancer Screening

The USPSTF found insufficient evidence (I statement) regarding the benefits and harms of having clinicians performing visual skin examinations to screen for skin cancer, particularly melanoma.[33] Screening programs had been evaluated only in nonrandomized and ecologic studies. A national population-based screening program in Germany found no observable melanoma mortality benefit.[34]

The American Cancer Society (ACS) does not have a screening guideline for skin cancer but highlighted the importance of regular skin examinations for people at increased risk for skin cancer.[35]

Consider "*opportunistic screening*" as part of the complete PE for patients with significant sun exposure and patients age >50 years without a previous skin examination or who live alone.

Both new and changing nevi should be closely examined, as at least half of melanomas arise de novo from isolated melanocytes rather than pre-existing nevi. Detecting melanoma requires knowledge of how benign nevi change over time, often going from flat to raised or acquiring additional brown pigment.

Turn to Tables 12-4 through 12-6 on pp. 278–284 showing rough, pink, and brown nevi and their mimics.

Evaluating Moles for Melanoma: ABCDEs. Clinicians should apply the ABCDE method (see Box 12-5) when screening moles for melanoma (this does not apply for nonmelanocytic lesions like seborrheic keratoses). The sensitivity of the individual criterion for detecting melanomas when used by dermatologists ranges from 57% to 84%, and specificity ranges from 59% to 90%; using more than one criterion increases specificity but decreases sensitivity.[36] Pay close attention to nevi that have changed rapidly based on objective evidence and nevi

Review the ABCDE-EFG rule and photographs in Box 12-5, pp. 246–247. Also see Table 12-6, pp. 281–284, which provide additional helpful identifiers and comparisons of benign brown lesions with melanoma.

that appear markedly different than an individual's other nevi ("ugly duckling sign").[37] You should have a low threshold for referring a patient with a suspicious lesion to a dermatologist.

Skin Self-Examination

The USPSTF found insufficient evidence regarding counseling adults about skin self-examination (I statement).[24] The AAD recommended that individuals perform regular skin self-examinations and see a dermatologist for any new or suspicious spots and spots that are changing, itching, or bleeding.[32] The ACS also noted that many clinicians encourage patients to perform self-examinations.[35]

See Box 12-9, Patient Instructions for Skin Self-Examination, p. 258.

Approximately half of melanomas are initially detected by patients or their partners.

Instruct patients with risk factors for skin cancer and melanoma, especially those with a history of high sun exposure, prior or family history of melanoma, and ≥50 moles or >5 to 10 atypical moles, to perform regular skin self-examinations.

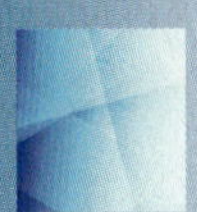

TABLE 12-1. Describing Primary Skin Lesions: Flat, Raised, and Fluid-Filled

Describe skin lesions accurately, including number, size, color, texture, shape, primary lesion, location, and configuration. *This table identifies common primary skin lesions and includes classic descriptions of each lesion with the diagnosis in italics.*

FLAT SPOTS

If you run your finger over the lesion but do not feel the lesion, the lesion is *flat*. If a flat spot is small (<1 cm), it is a *macule*. If a flat spot is larger (>1 cm), it is a ***patch***.

Macules (flat, small)

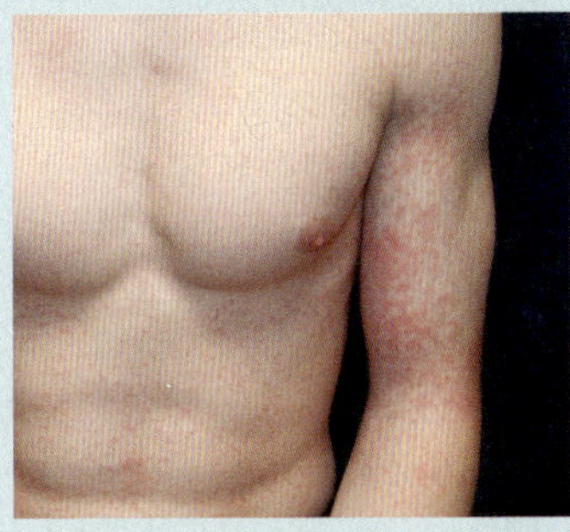

Multiple 3–8 mm erythematous confluent round macules on chest, back, and arms; *morbilliform drug eruption*

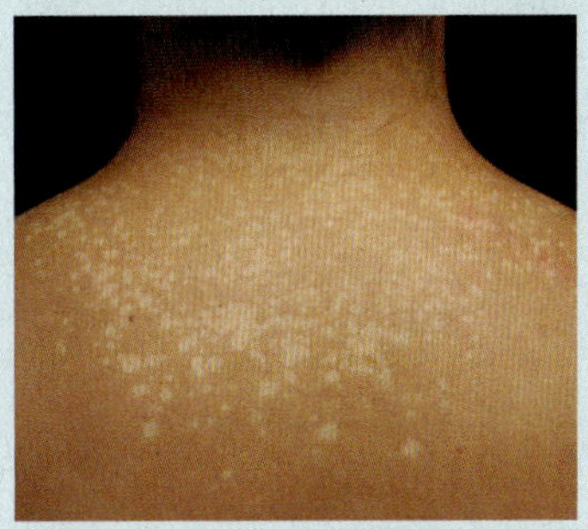

Multiple 2–5-mm hypopigmented, hyperpigmented, or tan round to oval macules on upper neck and back, upper chest, and arms with slight inducible scale on scraping (*tinea versicolor*)

Multiple scattered 2–4-mm round and oval brown macules, symmetrically pigmented, on back and chest with reticular pattern on dermoscopy; *benign melanocytic nevi*

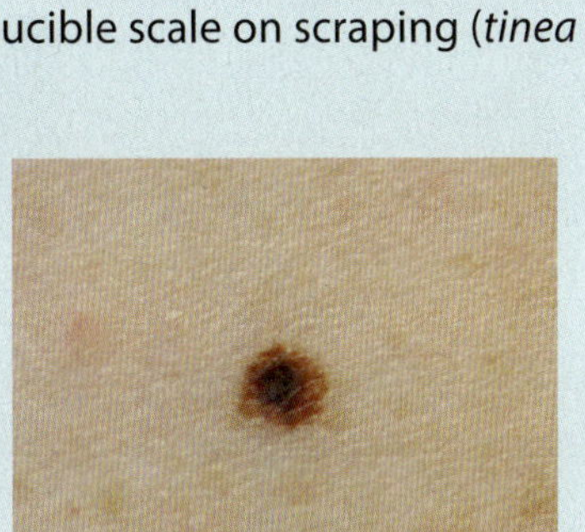

Solitary 6-mm dark brown round symmetric macule on upper back; *benign melanocytic nevus*

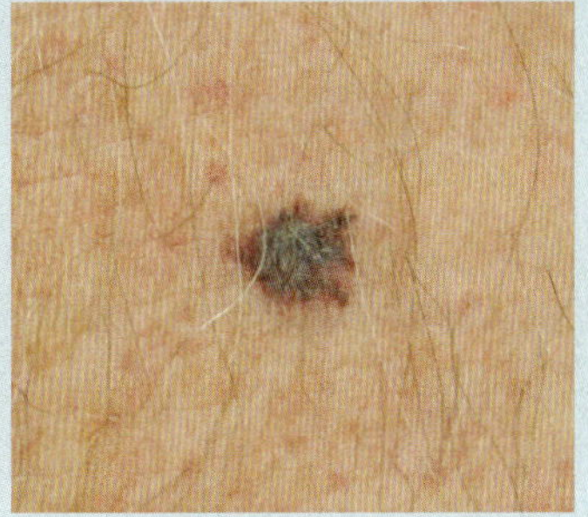

Solitary dark brown, blue-gray, and red 7-mm macule with irregular borders and fingerlike projections of pigment, on right forearm; *malignant melanoma*

(*continued*)

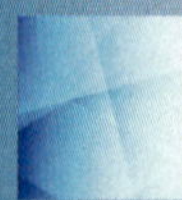

TABLE 12-1. Describing Primary Skin Lesions: Flat, Raised, and Fluid-Filled *(Continued)*

Patches (flat, large)

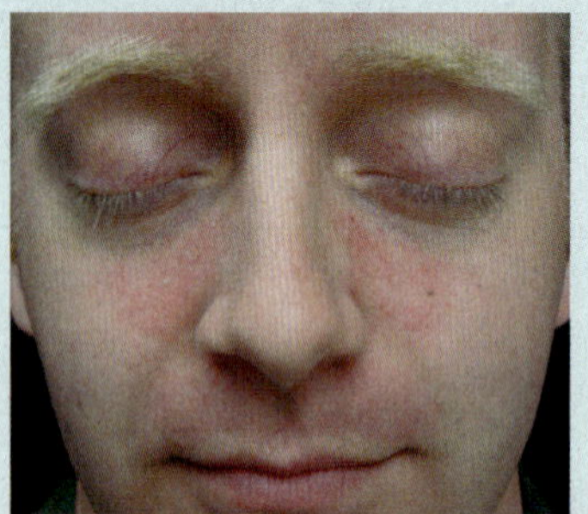

Bilaterally symmetric erythematous patches on central cheeks and eyebrows, some with overlying greasy scale; *seborrheic dermatitis*

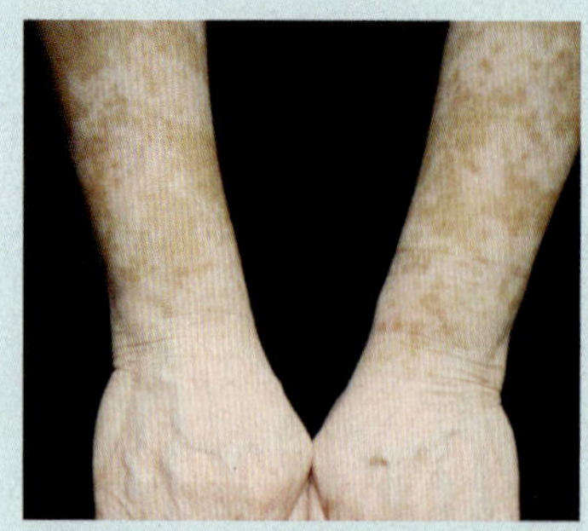

Large confluent completely depigmented patches on dorsal hands and distal forearms; *vitiligo*

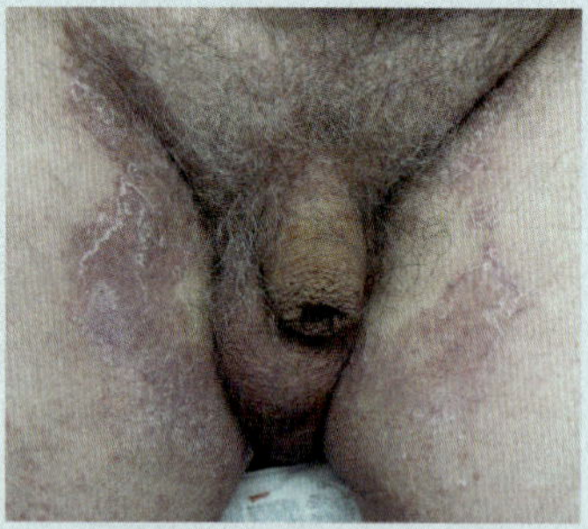

Bilateral erythematous, geographic patches with peripheral scaling, on inner thighs bilaterally, sparing the scrotum; *tinea cruris*

RAISED SPOTS

If you run your finger over the lesion and it is palpable above the skin, it is *raised.* If a raised spot is small (<1 cm), it is a *papule*. If a raised spot is larger (>1 cm), it is a *plaque*.

Papules (raised, small)

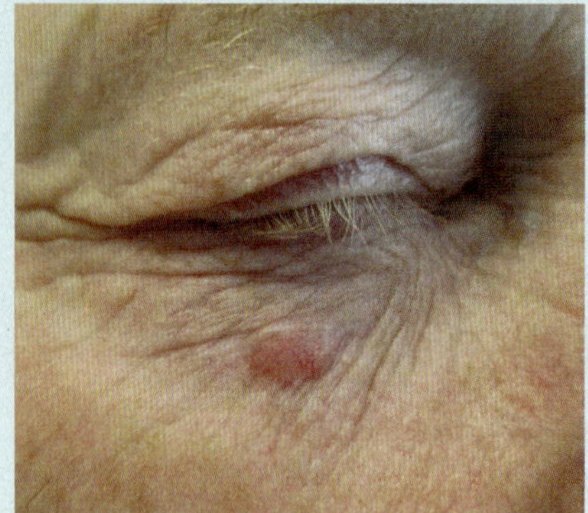

Solitary 7-mm oval pink pearly papule with overlying telangiectasias on right nasojugal fold; *basal cell carcinoma*

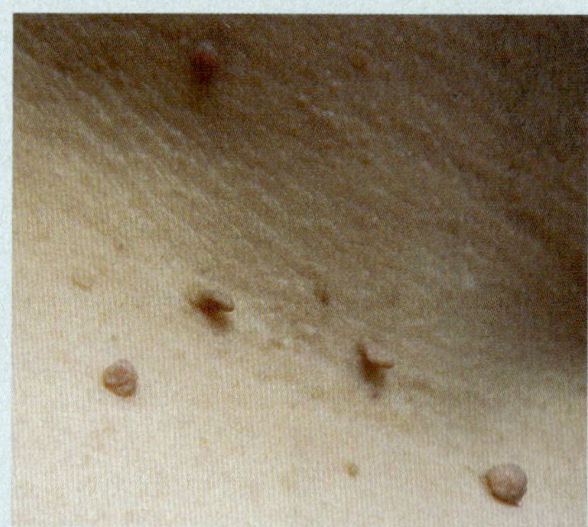

Multiple 2–4-mm soft, fleshy skin-colored to light brown papules on lateral neck and axillae in skin folds; *skin tags*

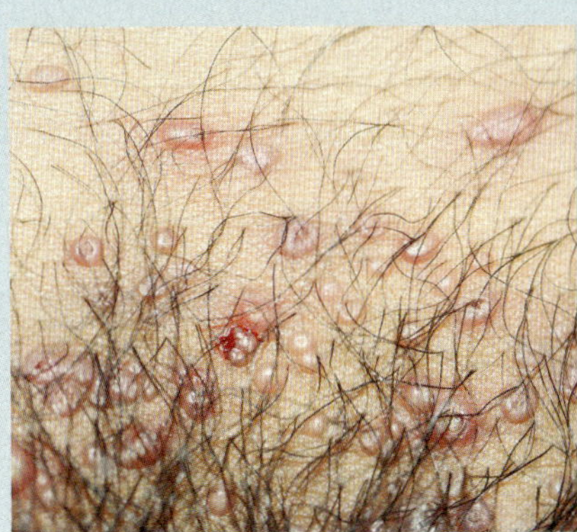

Multiple 3–5-mm pink firm smooth-domed papules with central umbilications, in mons pubis, and on penile shaft; *molluscum contagiosum*

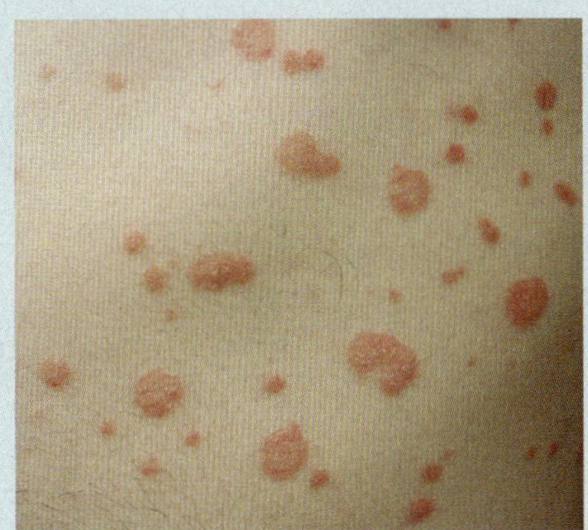

Scattered erythematous round drop-like, flat-topped well-circumscribed scaling papules and plaques on trunk; *guttate psoriasis*

Plaques (raised, large)

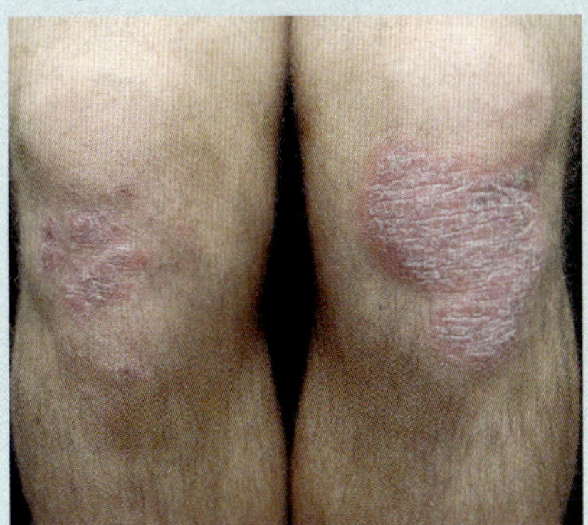

Scattered erythematous to bright pink well-circumscribed flat-topped plaques on extensor knees and elbows, with overlying silvery scale; *plaque psoriasis*

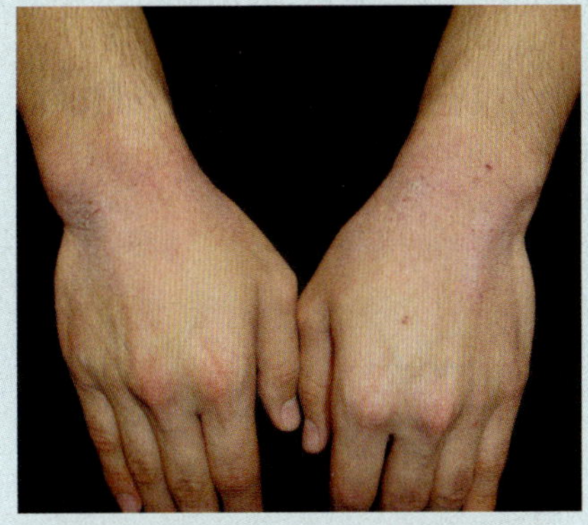

Bilateral erythematous, lichenified (thickened from rubbing) poorly circumscribed plaques on flexor wrists, antecubital fossae, and popliteal fossae; *atopic dermatitis*

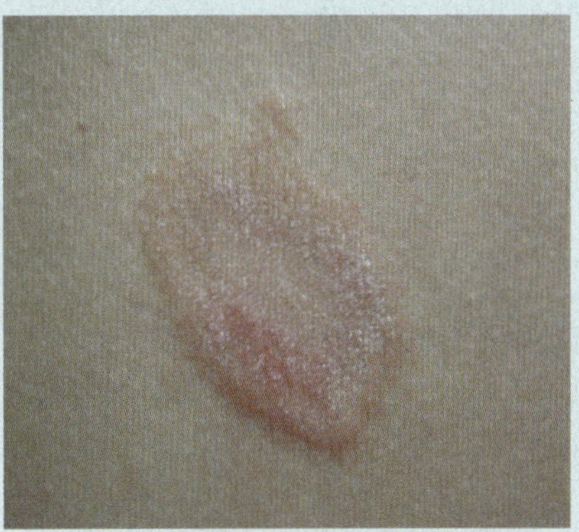

Single, oval, flat-topped superficial erythematous to skin-colored plaque on right abdomen; *herald patch of pityriasis rosea*

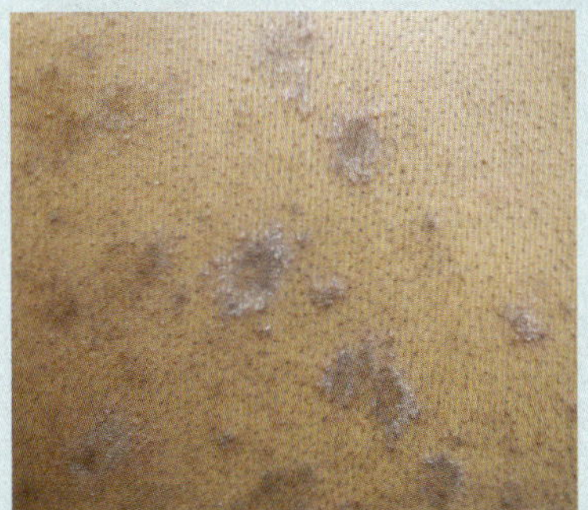

Multiple round to oval scaling violaceous plaques on abdomen and back; *pityriasis rosea*

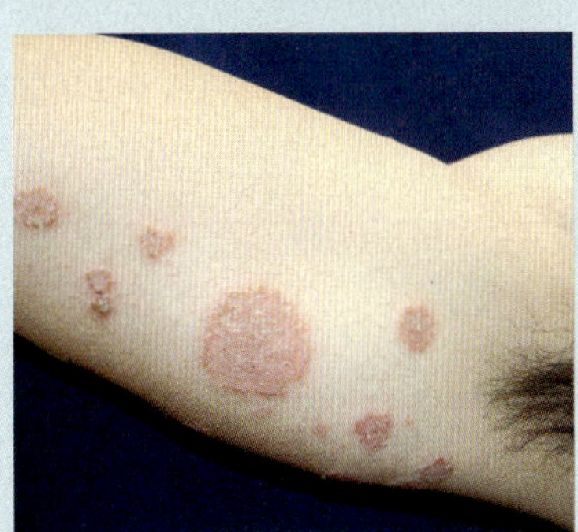

Multiple round coinlike eczematous plaques on arms, legs, and abdomen, with overlying dried transudate crust; *nummular dermatitis*

(continued)

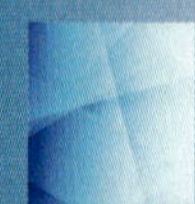

TABLE 12-1. Describing Primary Skin Lesions: Flat, Raised, and Fluid-Filled *(Continued)*

FLUID-FILLED LESIONS

If the lesion is raised, filled with fluid, and small (<1 cm), it is a *vesicle*. If a fluid-filled spot is larger (>1 cm), it is a *bulla*.

Vesicles (fluid-filled, small)

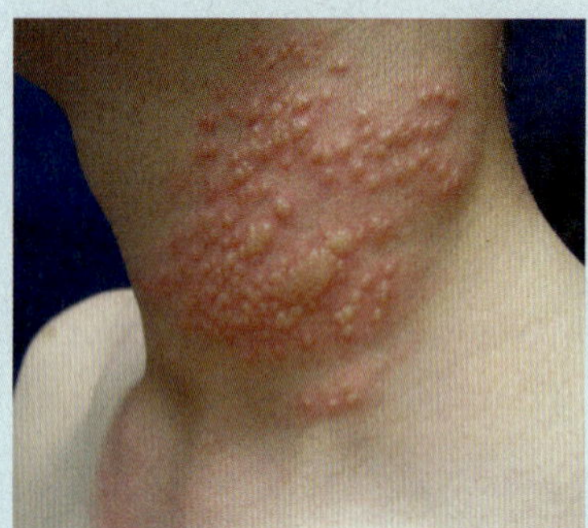

Multiple 2–4-mm vesicles and pustules on erythematous base, grouped together on left neck; *herpes simplex virus*

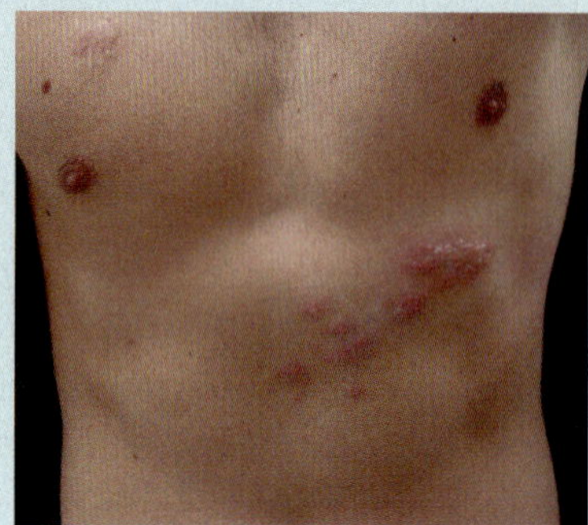

Grouped 2–5-mm vesicles on erythematous base on left upper abdomen and trunk in a dermatomal distribution that does not cross the midline; *herpes zoster, or* shingles

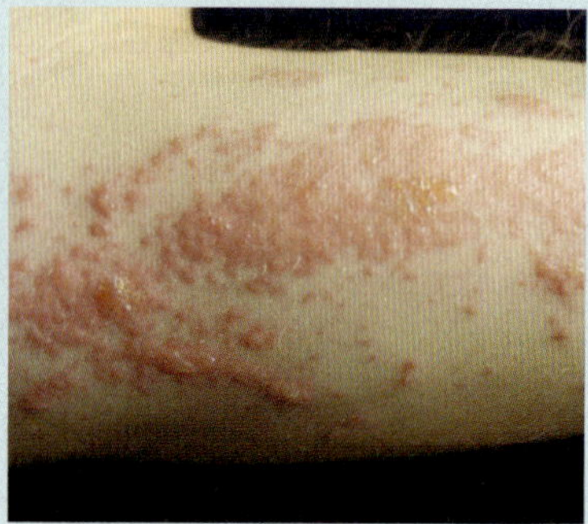

Scattered 2–5-mm erythematous papules and vesicles with transudate crust, some with linear arrays, on forearms, neck, and abdomen; *rhus dermatitis* or *allergic contact dermatitis* from poison ivy

Bullae (fluid-filled, large)

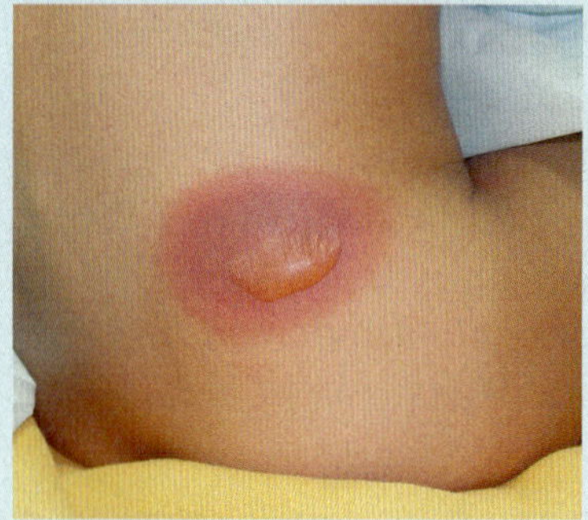

Solitary 8-cm dusky oval patch with smaller inner violaceous patch and central 3.5 cm tense bulla, on right posterior lower back; *bullous fixed drug eruption*

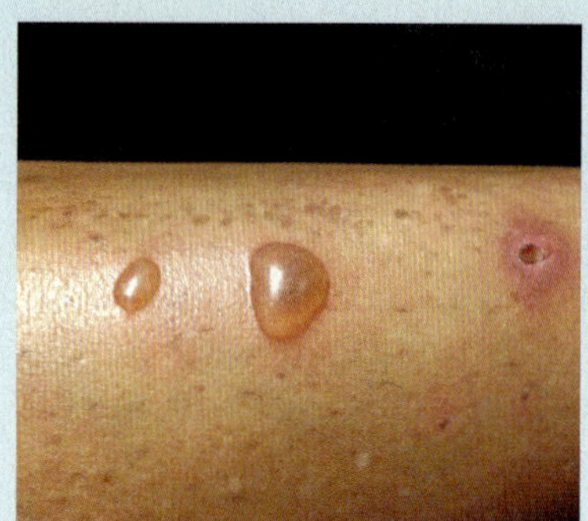

Several tense bullae on lower legs; *insect bites*

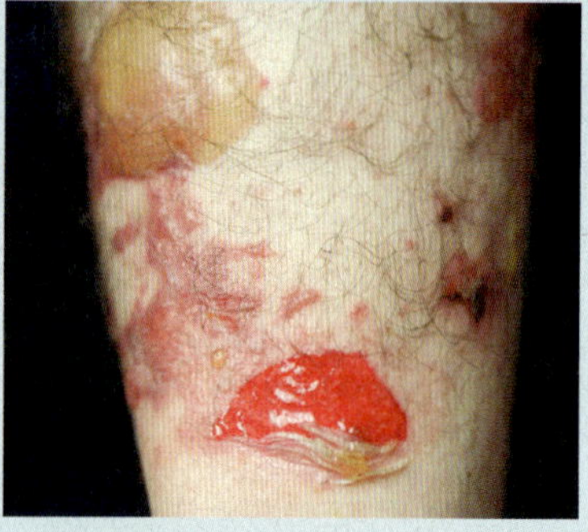

Many vesicles and tense bullae up to 4 cm, some having unroofed and left large (4 cm) erosions, on lower legs bilaterally up to the line of the top of combat boots; *an inherited skin fragility disorder*

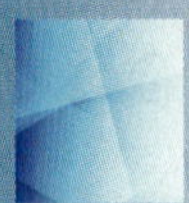

TABLE 12-2. Additional Primary Lesions: Pustules, Furuncles, Nodules, Cysts, Wheals, Burrows

Pustule: Small palpable collection of neutrophils or keratin that appears white

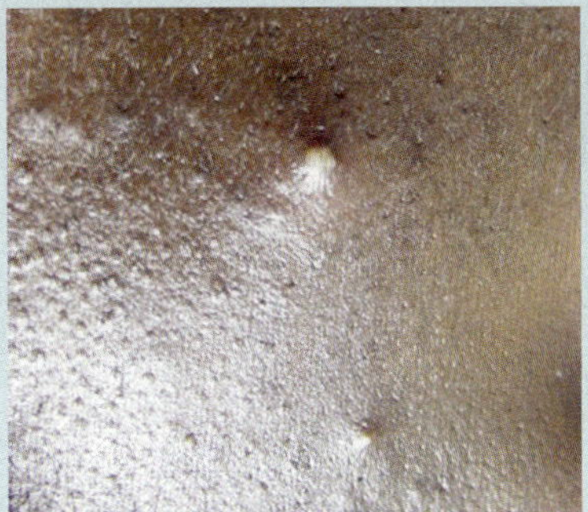

Around 15–20 pustules and acneiform papules on buccal and parotid cheeks bilaterally; *acne vulgaris*

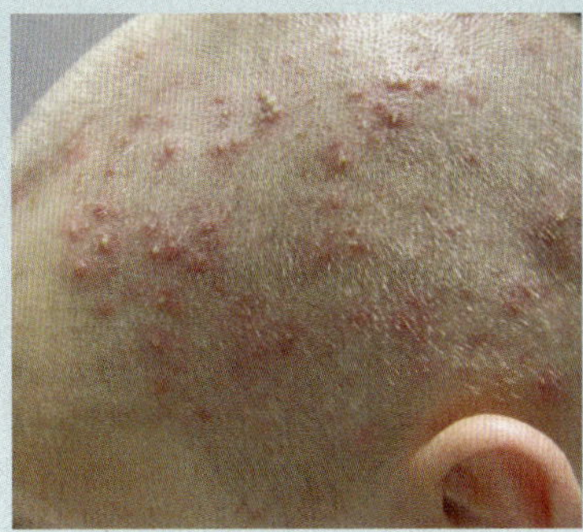

Around 30 2–5-mm erythematous papules and pustules on frontal, temporal, and parietal scalp; *bacterial folliculitis*

Furuncle: Inflamed hair follicle; multiple furuncles together form a *carbuncle*

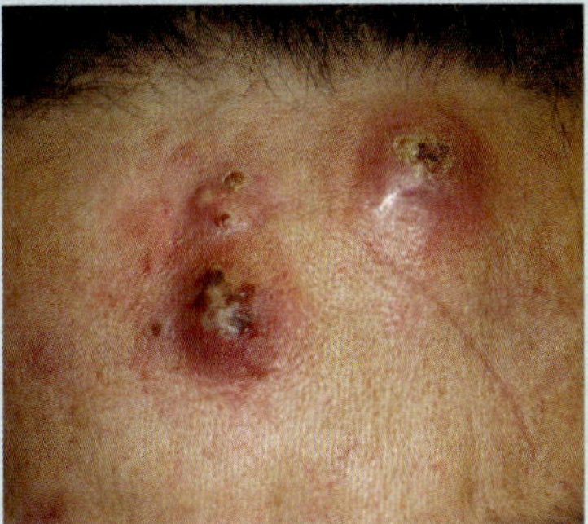

Two large (2-cm) furuncles on forehead, without fluctuance; *furunculosis* (Note: fluctuant deep infections are *abscesses*)

Nodule: Larger and deeper than a papule

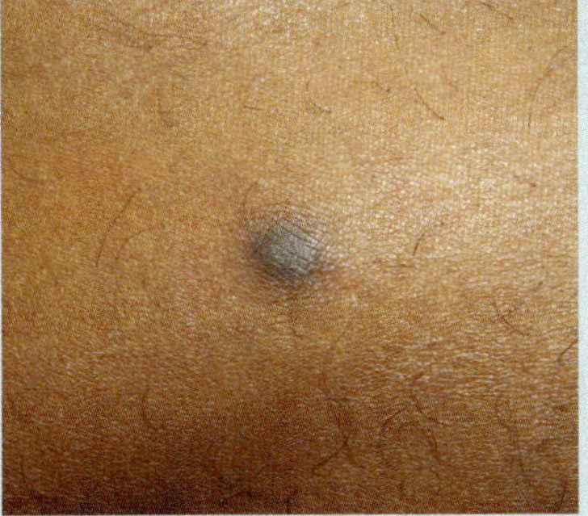

Solitary blue-brown 1.2-cm firm nodule with positive dimple sign and hyperpigmented rim on left lateral thigh; *dermatofibroma*

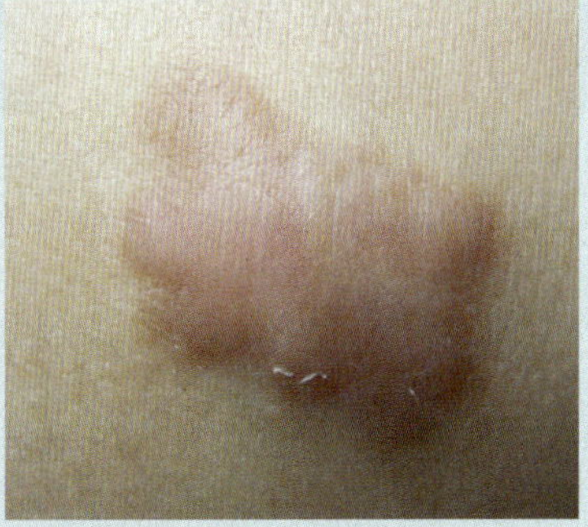

Solitary 4-cm pink and brown scarlike nodule on central chest at site of previous trauma; *keloid*

(*continued*)

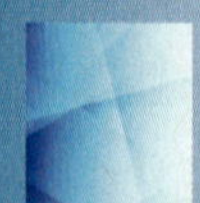

TABLE 12-2. Additional Primary Lesions: Pustules, Furuncles, Nodules, Cysts, Wheals, Burrows *(Continued)*

Subcutaneous Mass/Cyst: Whether mobile or fixed, cysts are encapsulated collections of fluid or semisolid

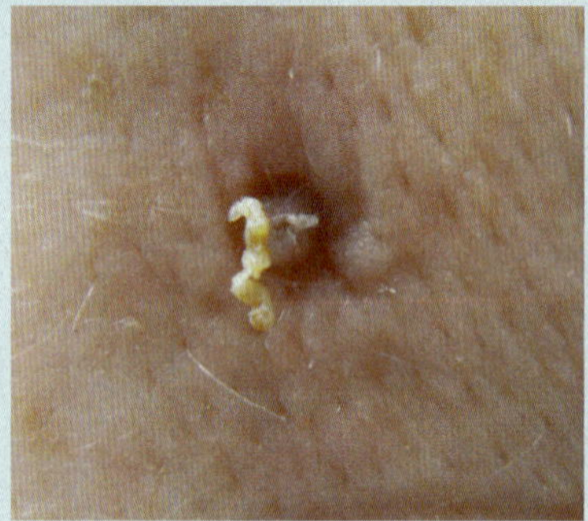

Solitary 2-cm tethered subcutaneous cyst with overlying punctum releasing caseous whitish yellow substance with foul odor; *epidermal inclusion cyst*

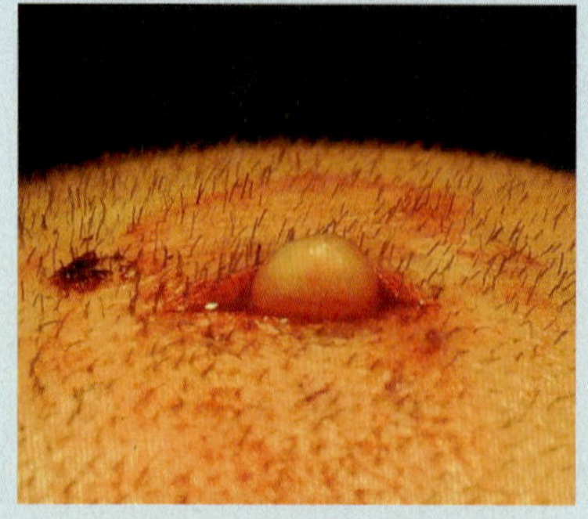

Three 6–8 mm mobile subcutaneous cysts on vertex scalp, that on excision reveal pearly white balls; *pilar cysts*

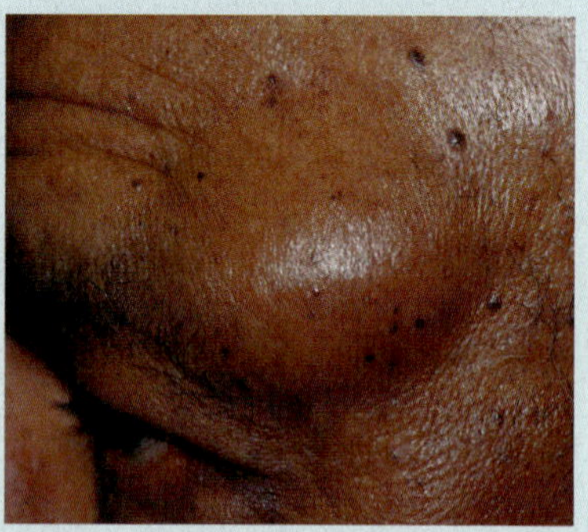

Solitary 9-cm mobile rubbery subcutaneous mass on left temple; *lipoma*

Wheal: Area of localized dermal edema that evanesces (comes and goes) within a period of 1–2 days; this is the essential primary lesion of *urticaria*

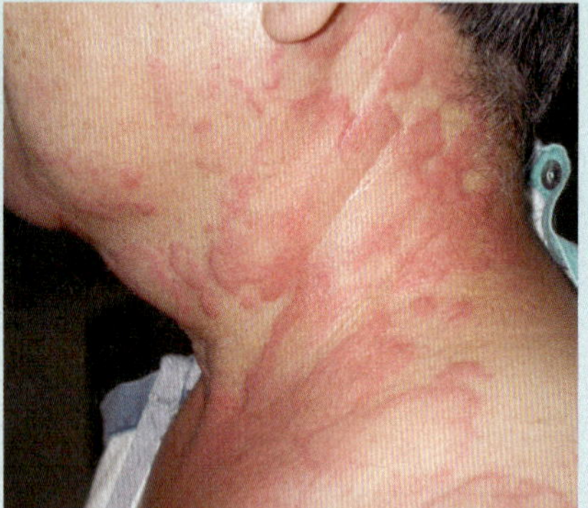

Many variably sized (1–10-cm) wheals on lateral neck, shoulders, abdomen, arms, and legs; *urticaria*

Burrow: Small linear or serpiginous pathways in the epidermis created by the scabies mite

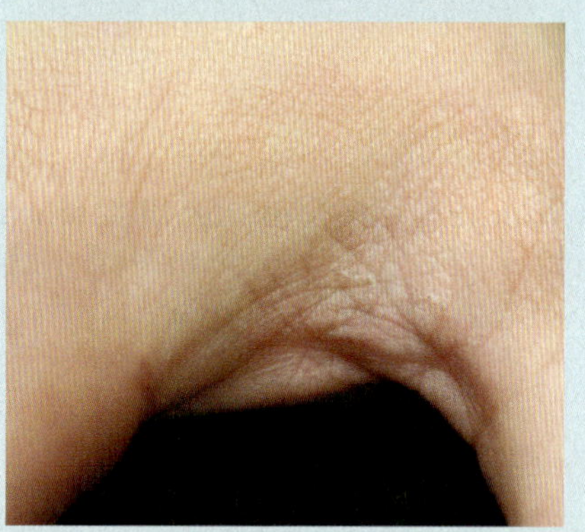

Multiple small (3–6-mm) erythematous papules on abdomen, buttocks, scrotum, and shaft and head of penis, with four *burrows* noted on interdigital web spaces; *scabies*

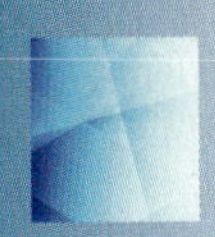

TABLE 12-3. Dermatology Safari: Benign Lesions

Practice makes perfect. Look for these common lesions during your clinical rotations. Perform a skin examination on as many patients as you can. If you are unsure about identifying the lesion, ask your instructors or supervising clinicians for help.

Cherry Angiomas

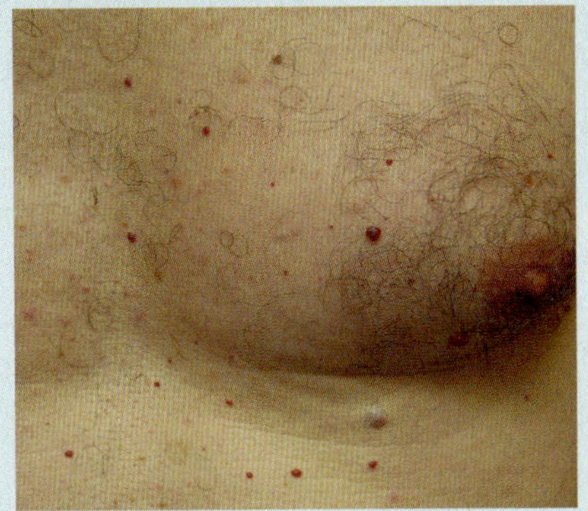

Seborrheic Keratosis

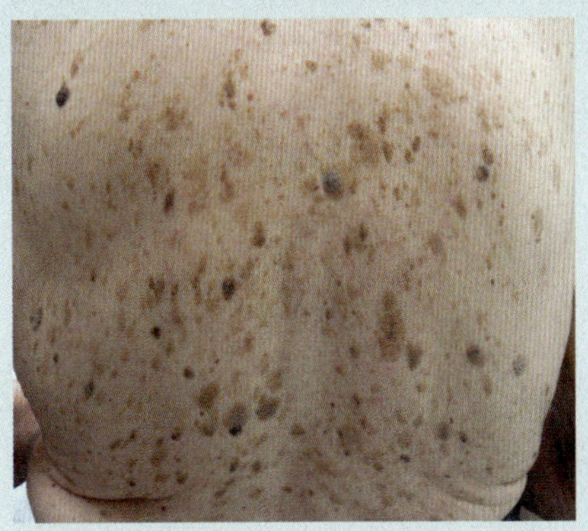

Solar Lentigines

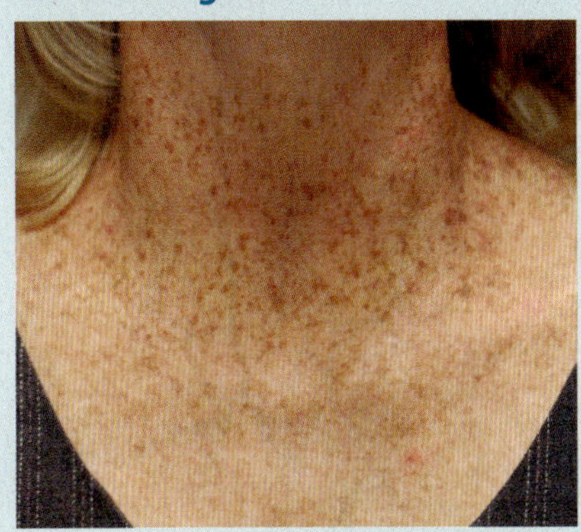

Benign Melanocytic Nevi

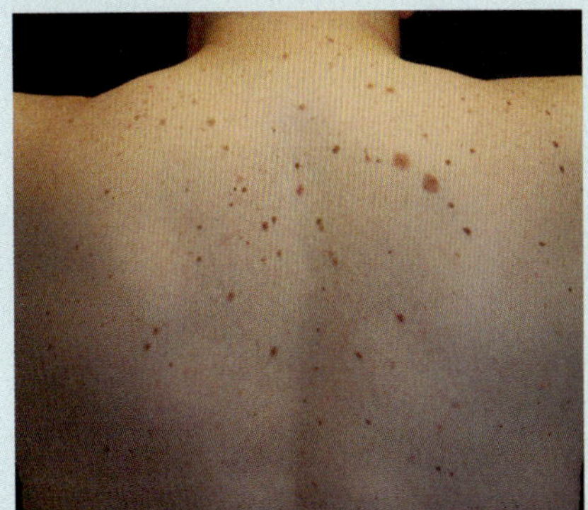

Dermatofibroma

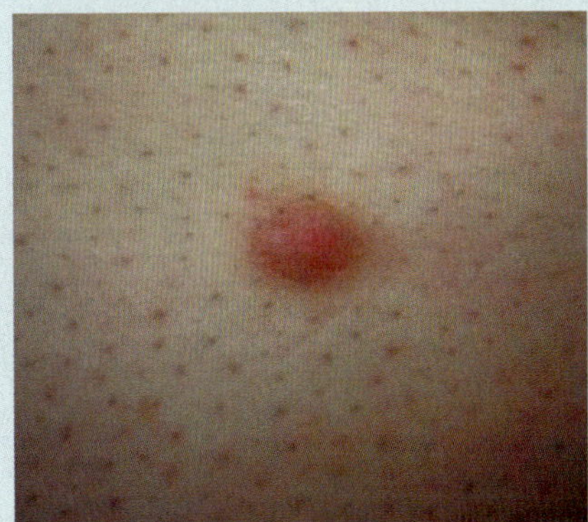

Keloids

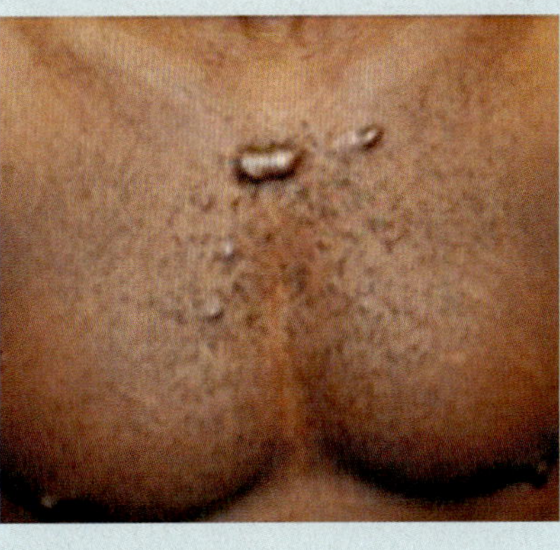

Epidermal Inclusion Cyst

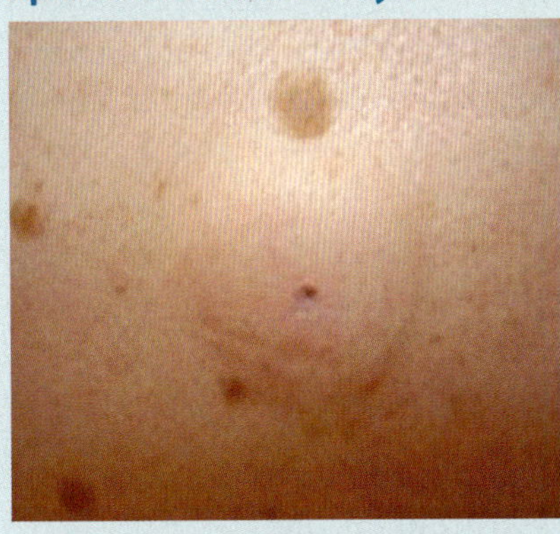

Pilar Cyst

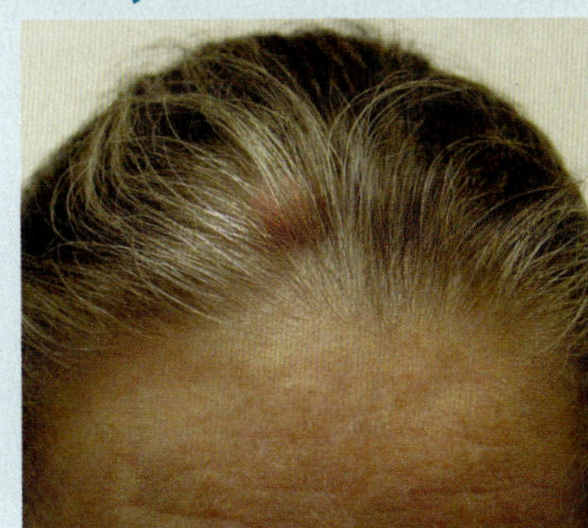

Lipoma

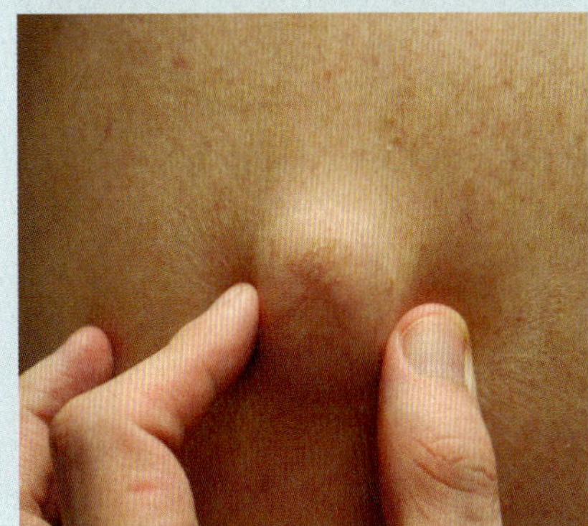

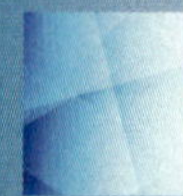

TABLE 12-4. Rough Lesions: Actinic Keratoses, Squamous Cell Carcinoma, and their Mimics

Patients commonly report feeling rough lesions. Many are benign, like seborrheic keratoses or warts, but squamous cell carcinoma (SCC) and its precursor actinic keratosis can also feel rough or keratotic. *SCC* most commonly arises on sun-damaged skin of the head, neck, and dorsal arms and hands and can metastasize if left untreated. It consists of more mature cells usually resembling the spinous layer of the epidermis and accounts for ~16% of skin cancers. If left untreated, *actinic keratoses* progress to SCC at a rate of about 1 in 1,000 per year. Counsel affected patients about sun avoidance and use of sunscreen and offer treatment to prevent progression to SCC.

ACTINIC KERATOSIS AND SQUAMOUS CELL CARCINOMA

Actinic Keratosis

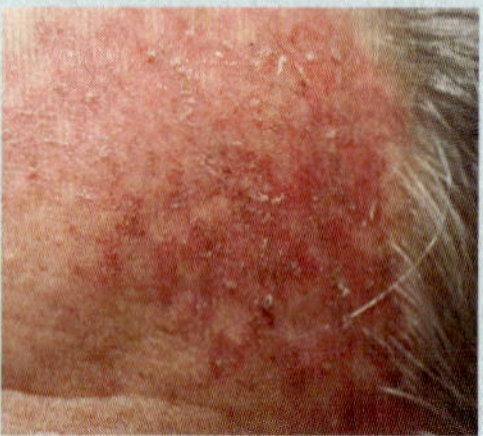
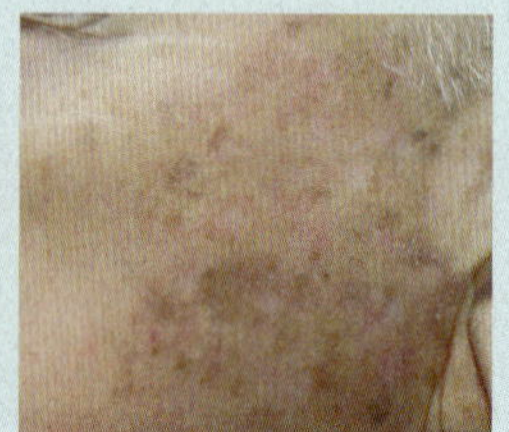

- Actinic keratosis after field therapy with 5-fluorouracil (left photo)
- Often easier to feel than to see
- Superficial keratotic papules "come and go" on sun-damaged skin

Cutaneous Horn/Keratotic Scale

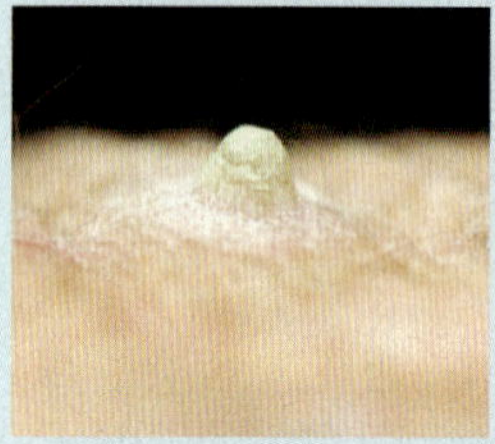
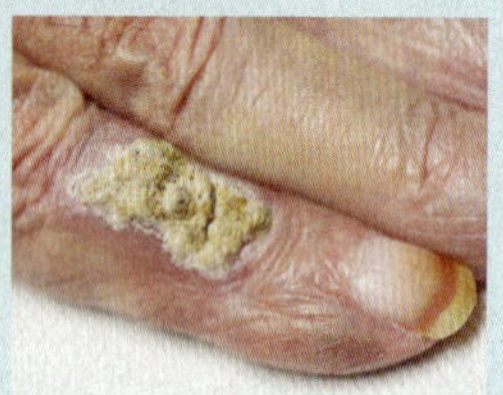

- The prototypic keratotic scale of actinic keratoses and SCC is formed by keratin and can result in a cutaneous horn
- Cutaneous horns should generally be biopsied to rule out SCC

Squamous Cell Carcinoma

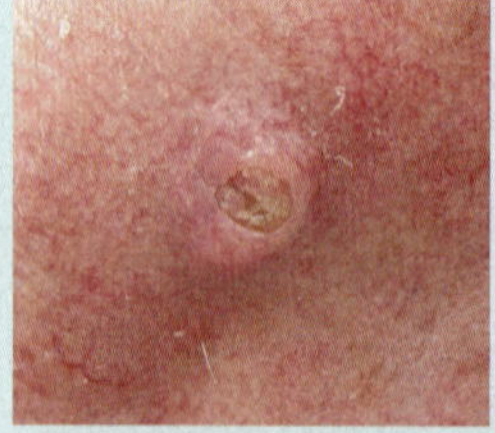
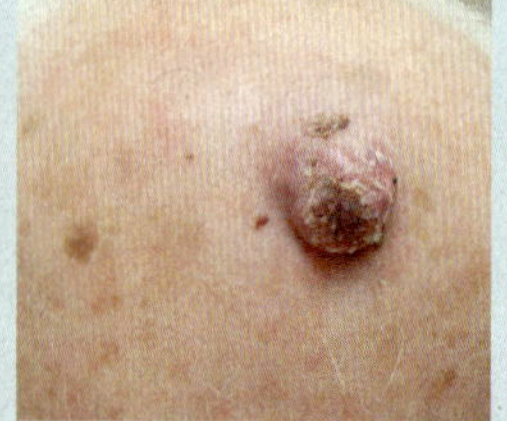

- Keratoacanthomas are SCCs that arise rapidly and have a crateriform center
- Often have a smooth but firm border
- SCCs can become quite large if left untreated (Note: highest sites of metastasis are the scalp, lips, and ears)

MIMICS

Superficial Xerosis or Seborrheic Dermatitis

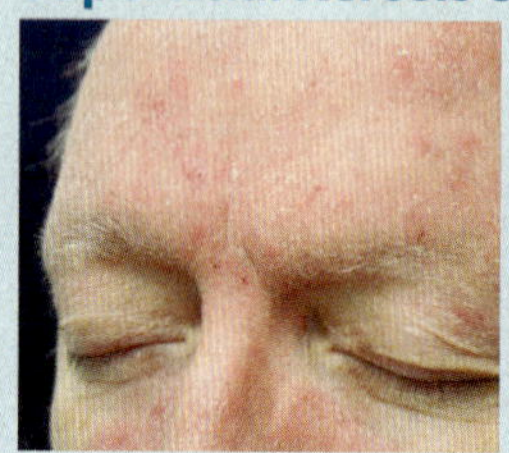

- May occur in same distribution on forehead, central face
- Scale is less keratotic and will improve with moisturizers, mild topical steroids

Warts

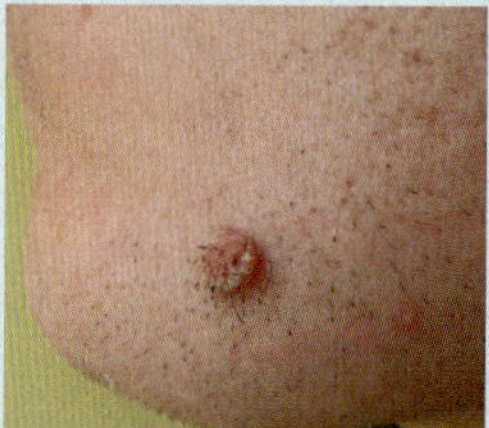
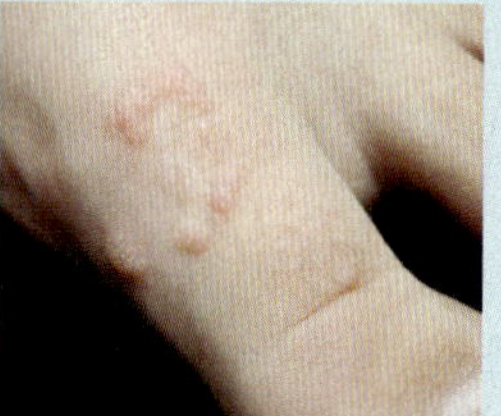

- Usually skin-colored to pink, texture more verrucous than keratotic
- May be filiform
- Often have hemorrhagic punctae that can be seen with a magnifying glass or dermoscope

Seborrheic Keratosis

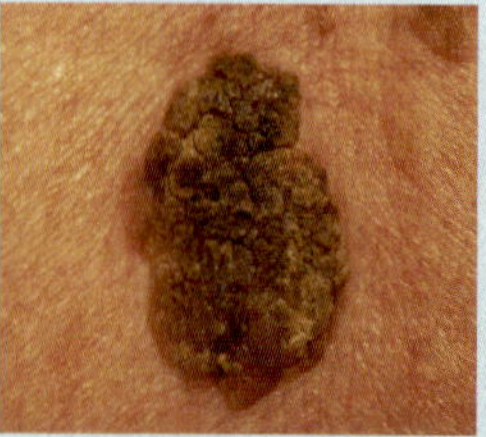
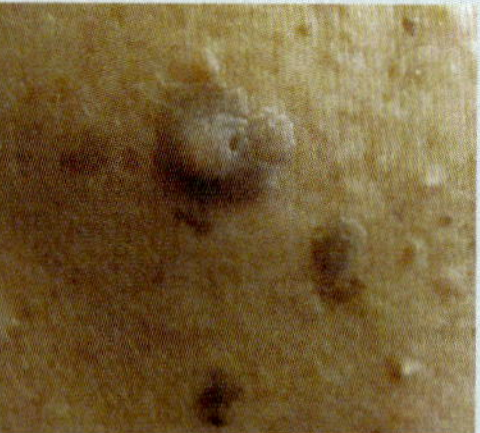

- Often have a verrucous texture
- Appear like a "stuck-on" or flattened ball of wax
- May crumble or bleed if picked
- Specific features on dermoscopy such as milia-like cysts or comedone-like openings are reassuring, if present
- May be erythematous, if inflamed

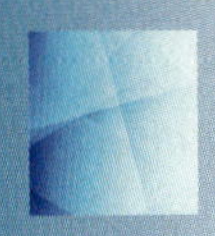

TABLE 12-5. Pink Lesions: Basal Cell Carcinoma and Its Mimics

Basal cell carcinoma (BCC) is the most common cancer in the world. Fortunately, it rarely spreads to other parts of the body. Nonetheless, it can invade and destroy local tissues, causing significant morbidity to the eye, nose, or brain. BCC consists of immature cells similar to those in the basal layer of the epidermis, and accounts for roughly 80% of all skin cancers. BCCs should be biopsied for confirmation before treatment. Review the BCC features below and how they contrast with mimics that are benign.

BASAL CELL CARCINOMAS

Superficial Basal Cell Carcinoma

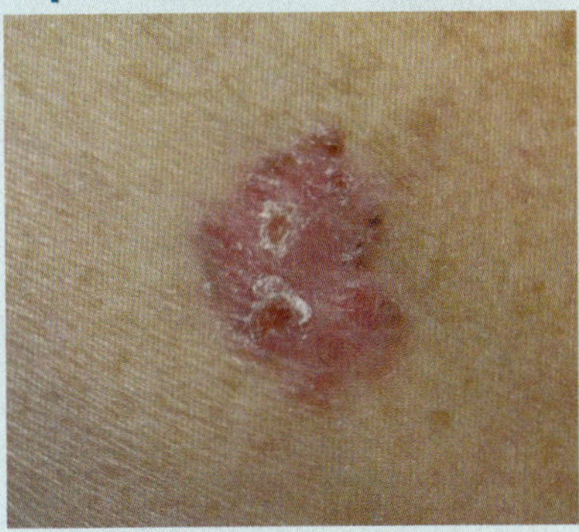

- Pink patch that does not heal
- May have focal scaling

Nodular Basal Cell Carcinoma

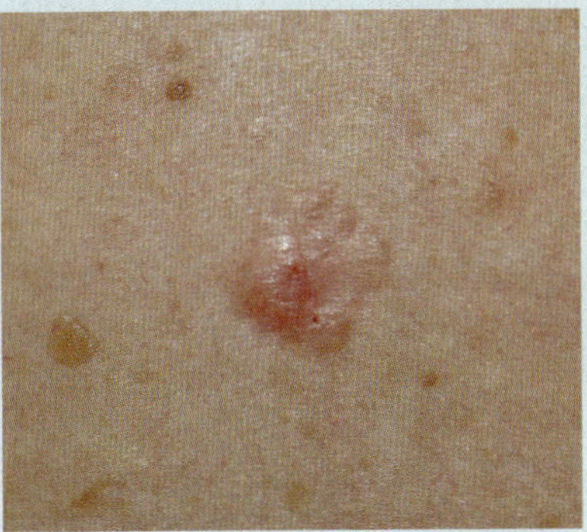

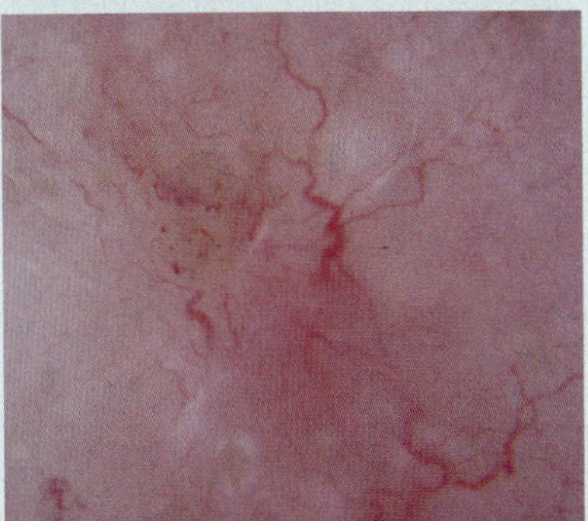

- Pink papule (top), often with translucent or pearly appearance and overlying telangiectasias
- May have focal pigmentation
- Dermoscopy (bottom) shows arborizing vessels, focal pigment globules, and other specific patterns

MIMICS

Actinic Keratosis and Squamous Cell Carcinoma In Situ

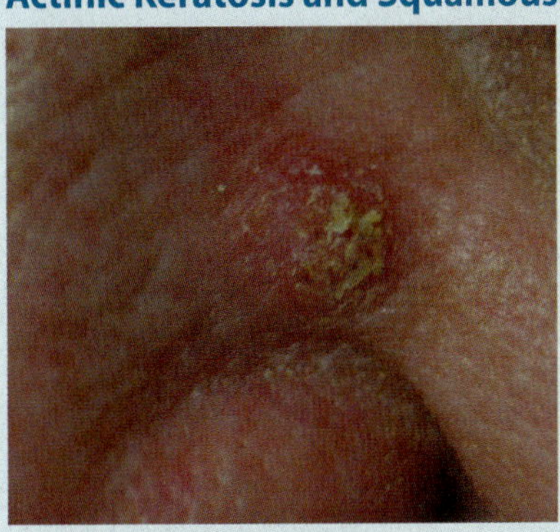

- Actinic keratosis or squamous cell carcinoma in situ usually has keratotic scaling

Sebaceous Hyperplasia

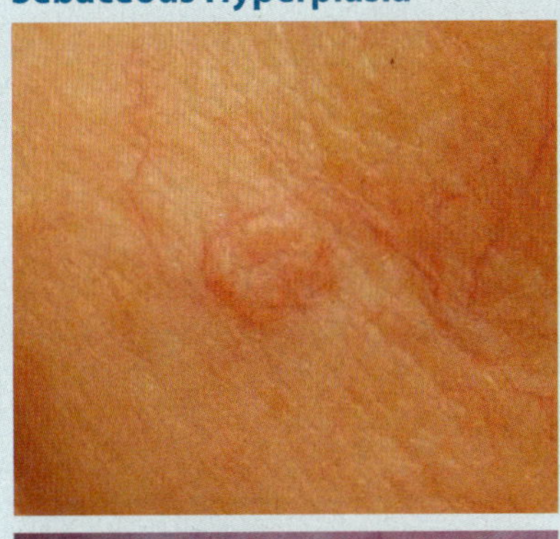

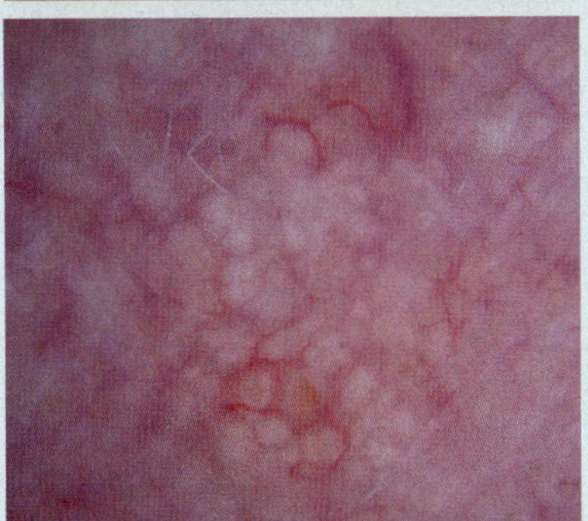

- Yellowish globular papules, often with central depression, on forehead and cheeks (top)
- Dermoscopy (bottom) shows telangiectasias that go around sebaceous glands rather than over them as in BCC

(continued)

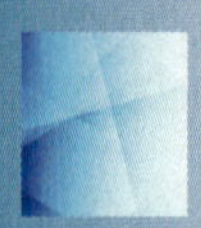

TABLE 12-5. Pink Lesions: Basal Cell Carcinoma and Its Mimics *(Continued)*

BASAL CELL CARCINOMAS

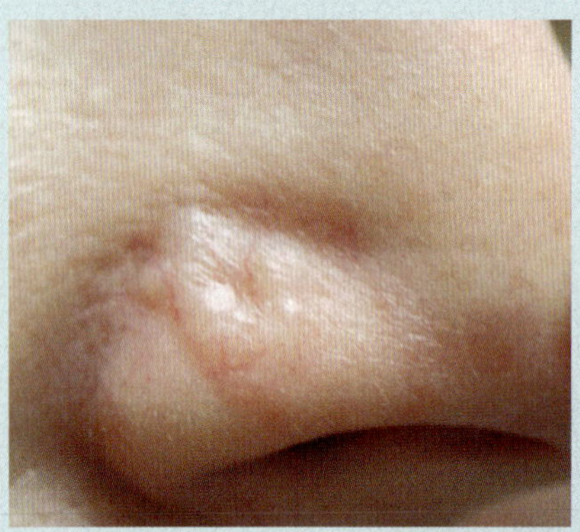

- 1 cm pearly pink plaque with central depression and overlying arborizing telangiectasias on nasal ala

Ulcerated Basal Cell Carcinoma

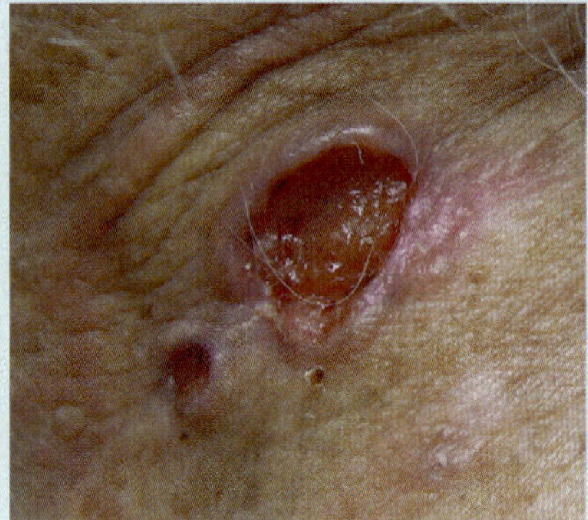

- Nonhealing ulcer, resulting in *"rolled border"*

MIMICS

Fibrous Papule

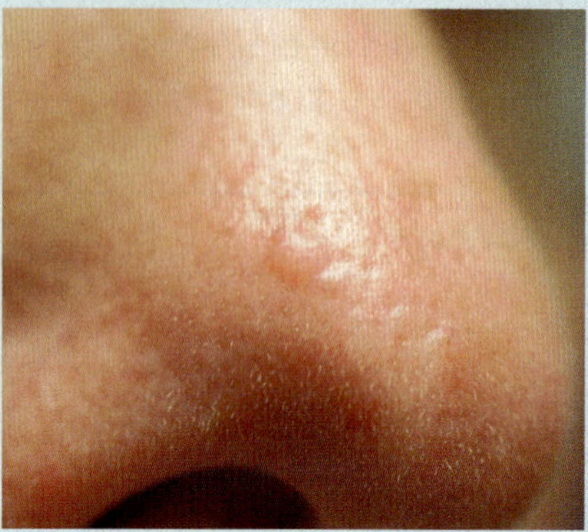

- Skin-colored to pink papule on the nose, without telangiectasias
- May become excoriated

Squamous Cell Carcinoma

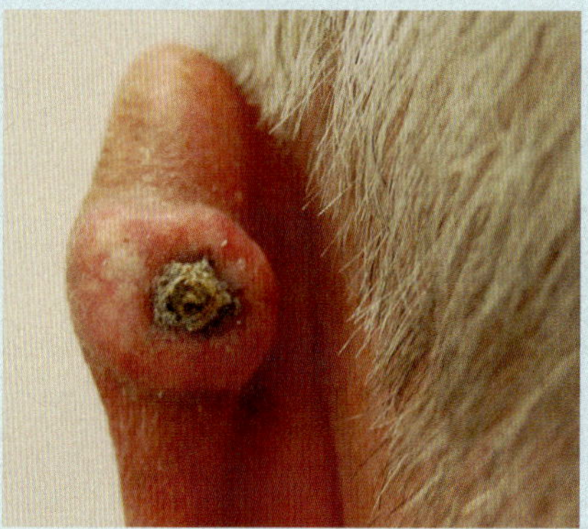

- May also be ulcerated
- Firmer at edges than BCC

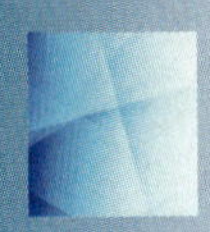

TABLE 12-6. Brown Lesions: Melanoma and Its Mimics

Most patients have brown spots on their body surface if you look thoroughly. Although these are usually freckles, benign nevi, solar lentigines, or seborrheic keratoses, you and the patient must look closely for any that stand out as a possible melanoma. The best way to detect a melanoma is to do numerous skin examinations so that you recognize brown lesions that are benign. With enough practice, when you see a melanoma, it will stick out as the "ugly duckling." Review the ABCDE rule and photographs on pp. 246–247, which provide additional helpful identifiers and comparisons.

MELANOMAS

Amelanotic Melanoma

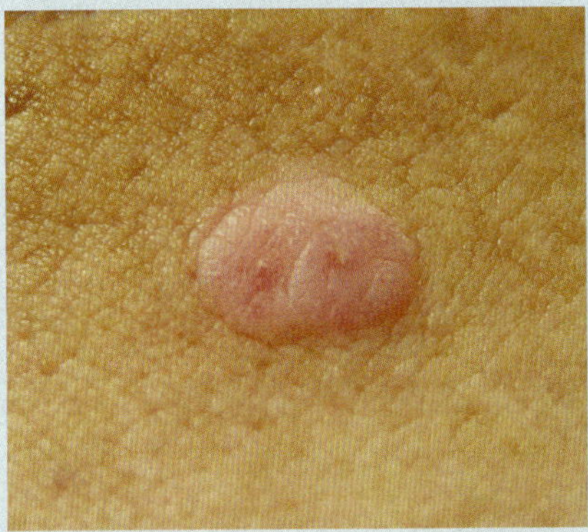

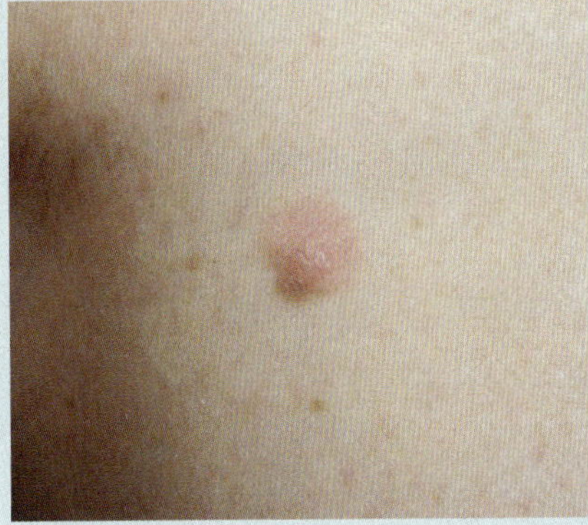

- Usually in very fair-skinned people
- *Evolution or rapid change* is the most important feature, because variegation or dark pigment is missing in this type

MIMICS

Skin Tags or Intradermal Nevi

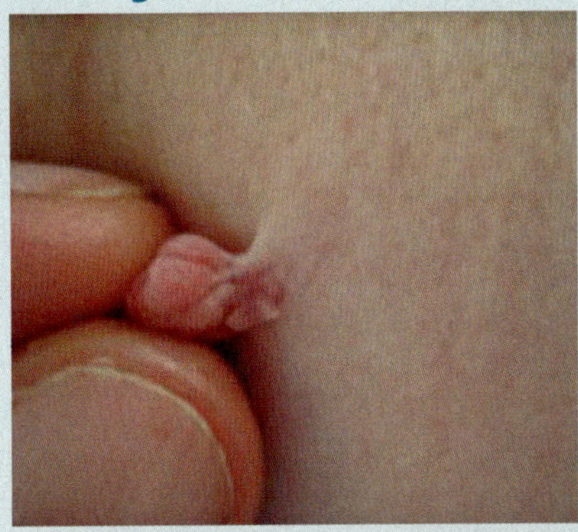

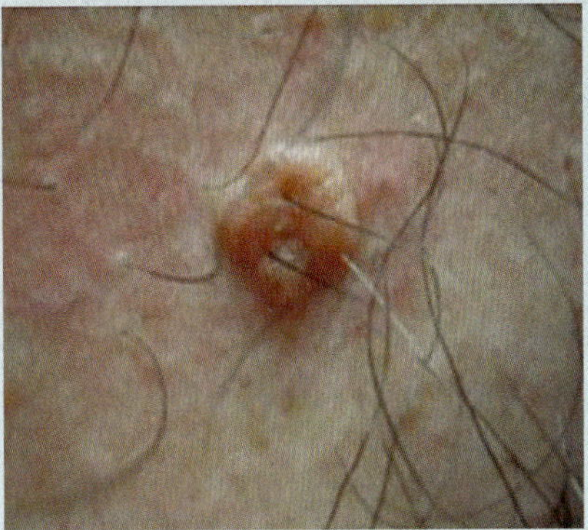

- Soft and fleshy
- Often around neck, axillae, or back
- Sessile nevi may have a hint of brown pigmentation

(*continued*)

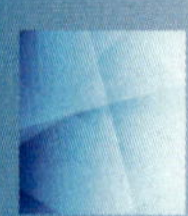

TABLE 12-6. Brown Lesions: Melanoma and Its Mimics *(Continued)*

MELANOMAS	MIMICS
Melanoma In Situ	**Solar Lentigo**
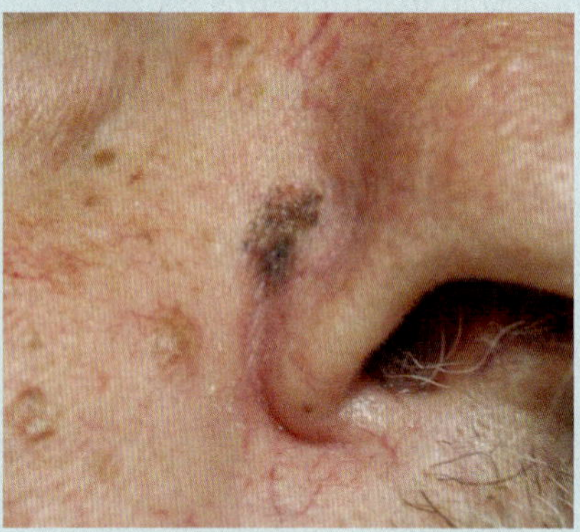	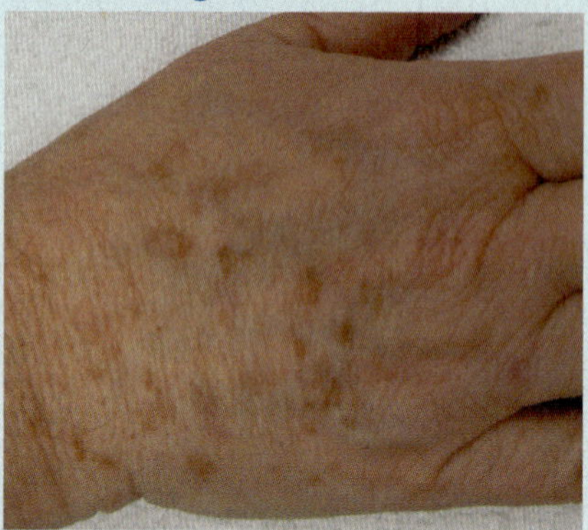
■ On sun-exposed or sun-protected skin ■ Look for ABCDE features	■ On sun-exposed skin ■ Light brown and uniform in color but may be asymmetric
Melanoma	**Dysplastic Nevus**
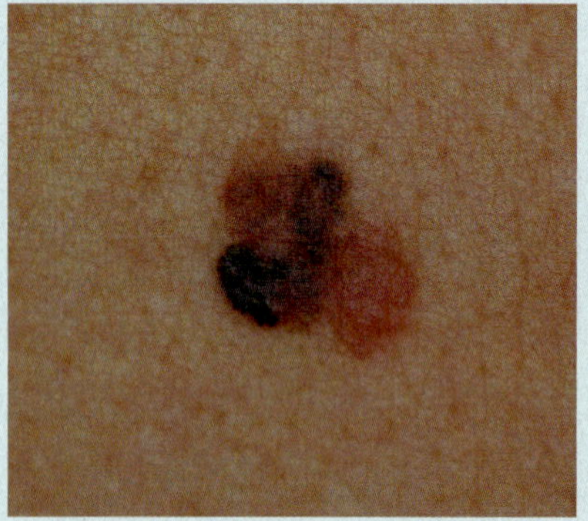	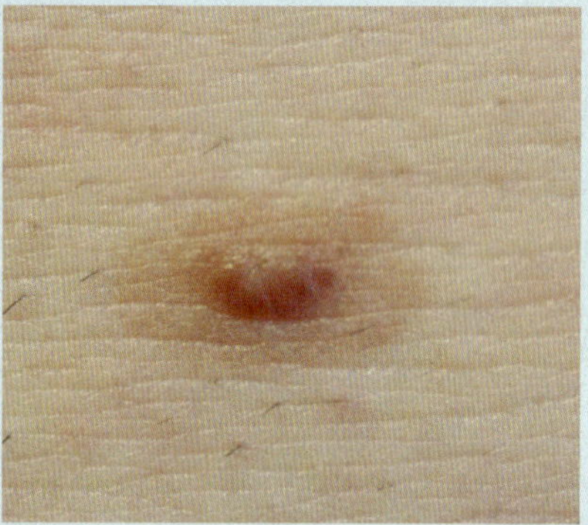
■ May arise de novo or in existing nevi and exhibits ABCDEs ■ Patients with many dysplastic nevi have increased risk of melanoma	■ May have macular base and papular central "fried egg" component ■ Compare to the patient's other nevi and monitor changes
Melanoma	**Inflamed Seborrheic Keratosis**
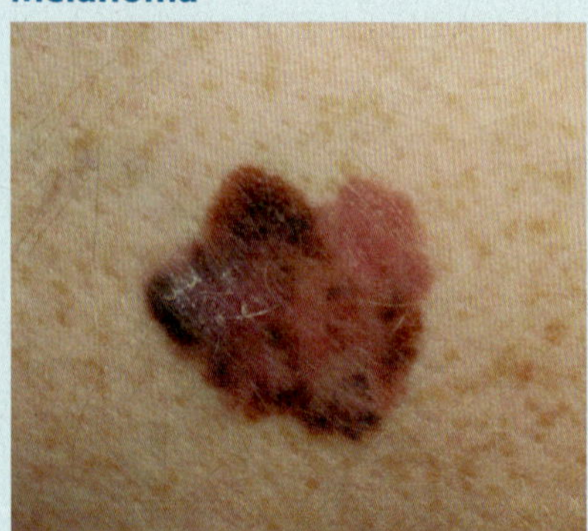	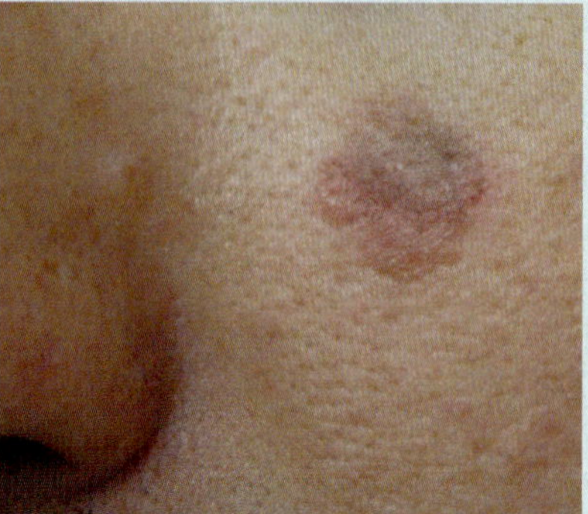
■ May have *variegated color* (browns, red) ■ Has melanocytic features on dermoscopy	■ Can sometimes mimic a melanoma if it has an erythematous base ■ Dermoscopy helps the trained eye distinguish these

MELANOMAS

Melanoma

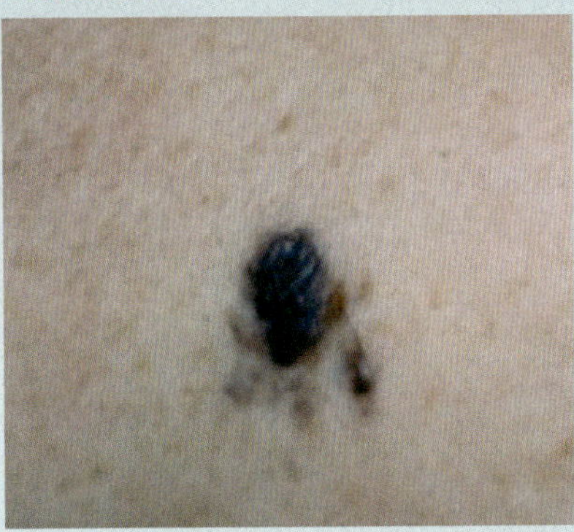

- May be uniform in color but *asymmetric;* key feature is *rapid change or evolution*

Acral Melanoma

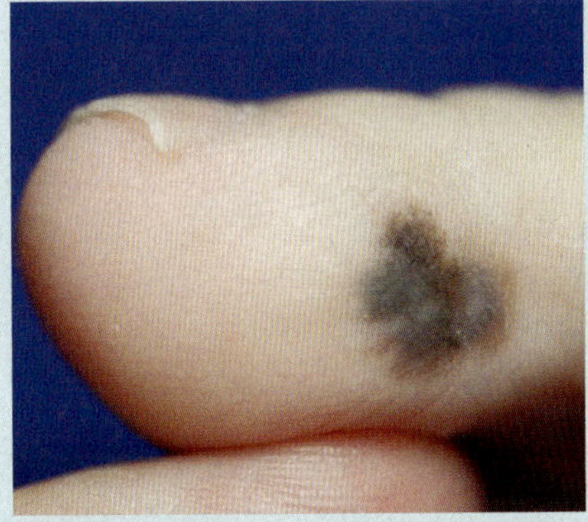

- Rapid change or evolution helps detect acral melanoma
- Consider biopsies if >7 mm, rapidly growing, or concerning features on dermoscopy

MIMICS

Seborrheic Keratosis

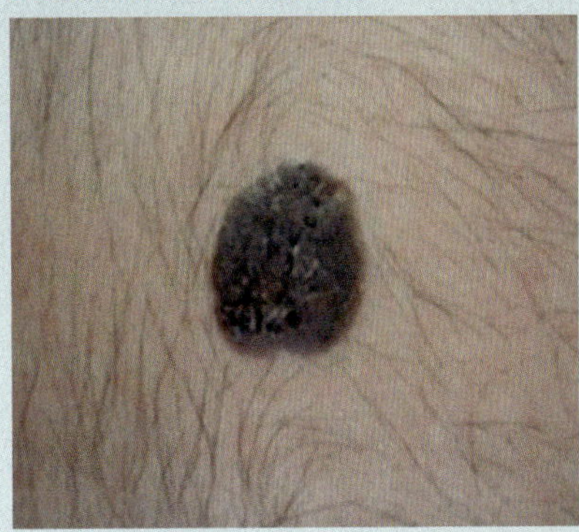

- Stuck-on and verrucous, may be darkly pigmented

Acral Nevus

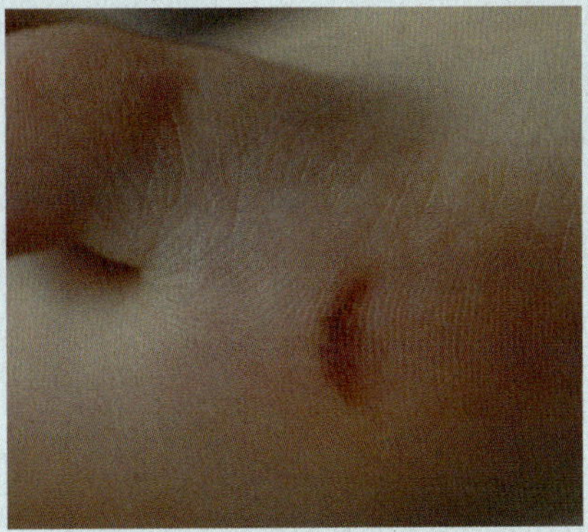

- Likely benign if <7 mm and has a reassurance pattern on dermoscopy, such as the parallel furrow or lattice patterns

(*continued*)

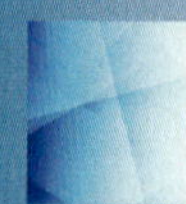

TABLE 12-6. Brown Lesions: Melanoma and Its Mimics *(Continued)*

MELANOMAS	MIMICS

Melanoma with Blue-Black Areas

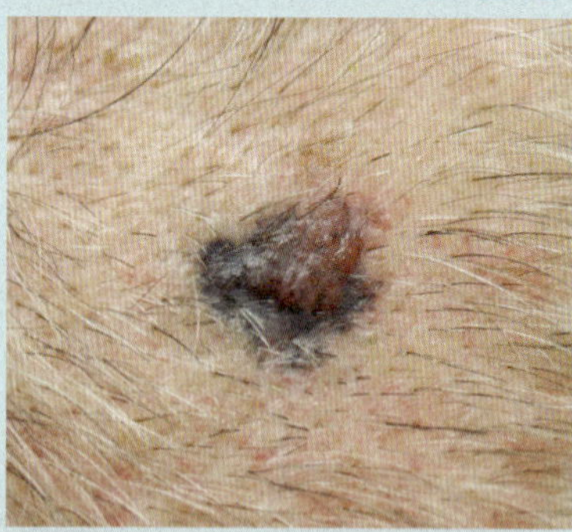

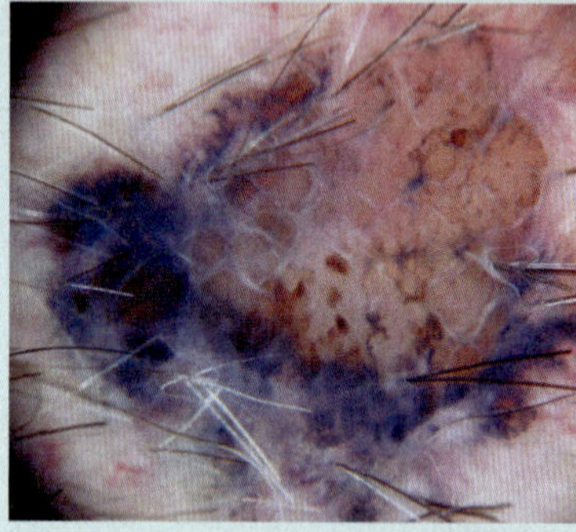

- Blue-black areas are concerning for melanoma, especially if they are asymmetric

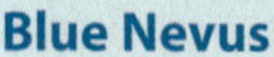

Blue Nevus

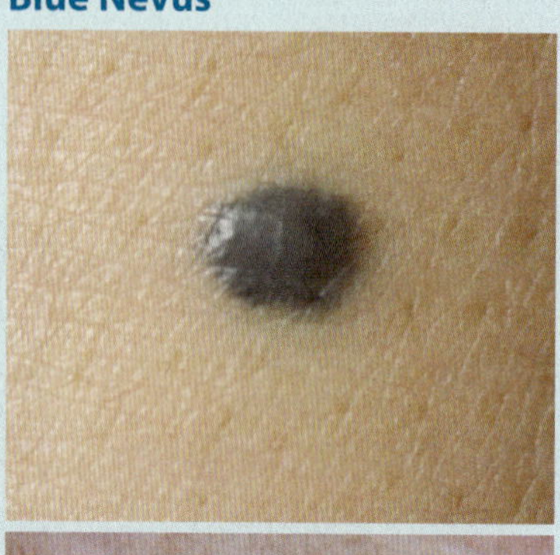

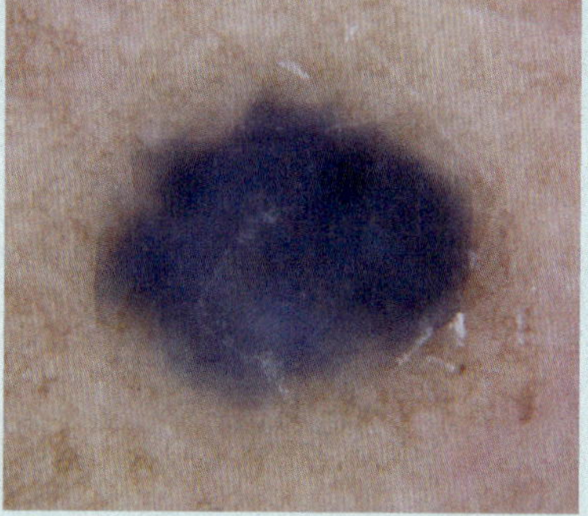

- Blue nevi have a homogeneous blue-gray appearance, clinically and on dermoscopy

Finding the Ugly Duckling: As you evaluate changing brown lesions in the context of the patient's other nevi and lentigines, the "ugly duckling" is the nevus that looks different from the patient's other nevi. A patient may make many atypical nevi with surrounding macular components and central acral components, but they all look the same. Find the patient's *signature nevus,* then search for the ugly duckling that looks different from the patient's typical "signature" nevi.

Most dermatologists now rely on a dermoscope to evaluate pigmented lesions, which allows them to detect melanomas when they are thinner. With training, dermoscopy can help distinguish nevi with reassuring patterns from possible early melanomas. Even without dermoscopy, however, a keen eye actively inspecting the skin for "ugly ducklings" is likely to detect melanomas when they arise.

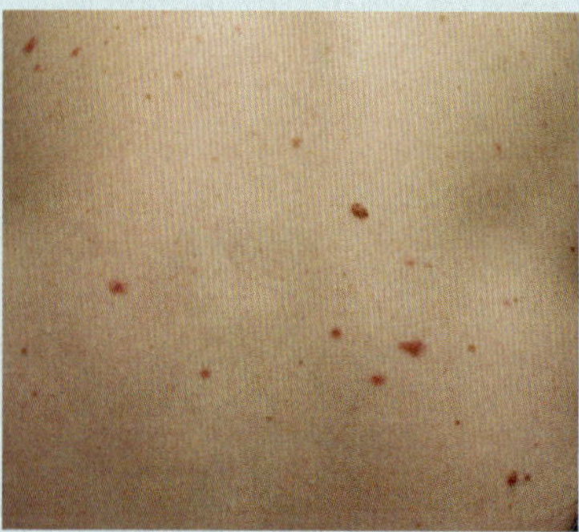

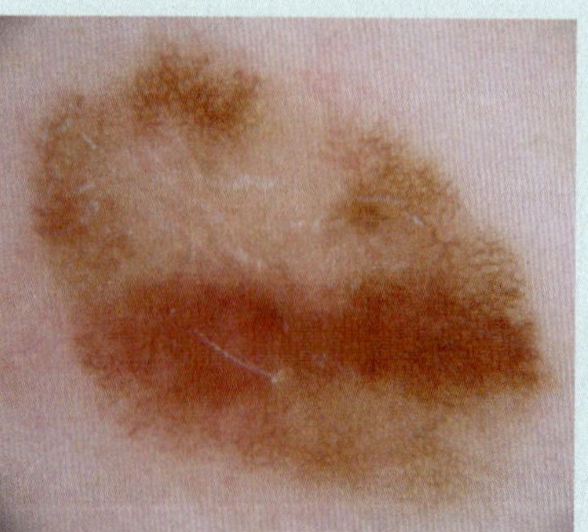

This patient has multiple atypical nevi on his back (left), but the one on his back just to the right of midline (enlarged right image) stands out as the "ugly duckling" because it has three colors; the white area showed melanoma in situ on biopsy.

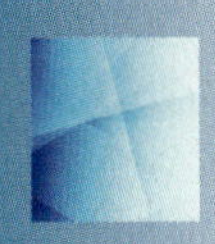

TABLE 12-7. Vascular and Purpuric Lesions of the Skin

	VASCULAR LESIONS		
	Spider Angioma[a]	Spider Vein[a]	Cherry Angioma
Color and Size	Fiery red; from very small to 2 cm	Bluish; size variable, from very small to several inches	Bright or ruby red; may become purplish with age; 1–3 mm
Shape	Central body, sometimes raised, surrounded by erythema and radiating legs	Variable; may resemble a spider or be linear, irregular, cascading	Round, flat, or sometimes raised; may be surrounded by a pale halo
Pulsatility and Effect of Pressure	Often seen in center of the spider when pressure with a glass slide is applied; pressure on the body causes blanching of the spider	Absent; pressure over the center does not cause blanching, but diffuse pressure blanches the veins	Absent; may show partial blanching, especially if pressure applied with edge of a pinpoint
Distribution	Face, neck, arms, and upper trunk; almost never below the waist	Most often on the legs, near veins; also on the anterior chest	Trunk; also extremities
Significance	Single spider angiomas are normal and are common on the face and chest; also seen in pregnancy and liver disease	Often accompanies increased pressure in the superficial veins, as in varicose veins	None; increases in size and numbers with aging

(continued)

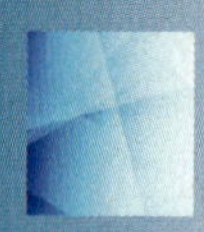

TABLE 12-7. Vascular and Purpuric Lesions of the Skin *(Continued)*

	PURPURIC LESIONS	
	Petechiae/Purpuras	**Ecchymosis**
Color and Size	Deep red or reddish purple, fading away over time; petechia, 1–3 mm; purpuras are larger	Purple or purplish blue, fading to green, yellow, and brown with time; variable size, larger than petechiae, >3 mm
Shape	Rounded, sometimes irregular; flat	Rounded, oval, or irregular; may have a central subcutaneous flat nodule (a hematoma)
Pulsatility and Effect of Pressure	Absent; no effect from pressure	Absent; no effect from pressure
Distribution	Variable	Variable
Significance	Blood outside the vessels; may suggest a bleeding disorder or, if petechiae, emboli to skin; palpable purpuras in *vasculitis*	Blood outside the vessels; often secondary to bruising or trauma; also seen in bleeding disorders

[a]These are telangiectasias, or dilated small vessels that look red or bluish.

Sources of photos: *Spider Angioma*—Marks R. *Skin Disease in Old Age*. JB Lippincott; 1987; *Petechia/Purpura*—Reprinted with permission from Kelley WN. *Textbook of Internal Medicine*. JB Lippincott; 1989.

TABLE 12-8. Hair Loss[4]

When taking a complete history of hair loss, include the duration, acuity of onset, cause from decreased hair density or increased shedding, the pattern (diffuse or localized), medication history, hair care practices, and associated medical conditions or stressors. *Decrease in hair density* is usually caused by male or female pattern hair loss, but less commonly by scarring alopecias. *Hair shedding from the roots* is often caused by *telogen effluvium, alopecia areata, anagen effluvium* (insults to the hair shaft from exposure to agents like chemotherapy) or less commonly, scarring alopecias. Perform a hair pull test to look for the percentage of telogen hairs. *Hair shedding from breakage at the hair shaft* is often caused by *tinea capitis,* improper hair care, and less commonly hair shaft disorders or *anagen effluvium.* Perform a tug test to look for hair fragility. See Figures 12-32 and 12-33 on p. 259 for examples of the hair pull test and tug test.

GENERALIZED OR DIFFUSE HAIR LOSS

Androgenetic alopecia affects over half of individuals assigned male at birth by their 50 years of age, and over half of those assigned female at birth by their 80 years of age. In those assigned male, look for frontal hairline regression and thinning on the posterior vertex; in those assigned female, look for thinning that spreads from the crown down without hairline regression. Severity is often described by standardized classifications such as the Norwood–Hamilton scale for those assigned male and the Ludwig scale for those assigned female. The *hair pull test* is normal or only pulls a few hairs.

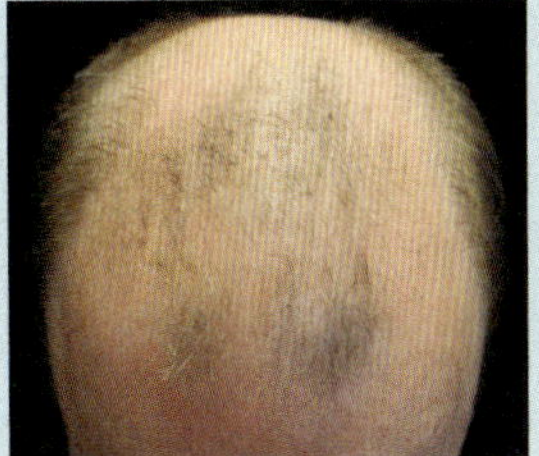

Male pattern hair loss (MPHL)

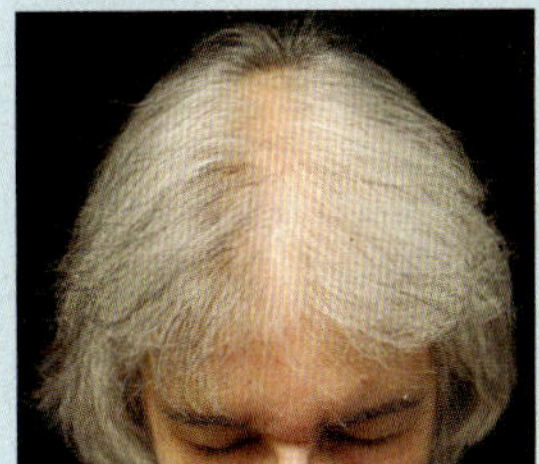

Female pattern hair loss (FPHL)

Telogen Effluvium and Anagen Effluvium

In *telogen effluvium,* overall, the patient's scalp and hair distribution appear normal, but a positive *hair pull test* reveals most hairs have telogen bulbs. In *anagen effluvium,* there is diffuse hair loss from the roots. The *hair pull test* shows few if any hairs with telogen bulbs.

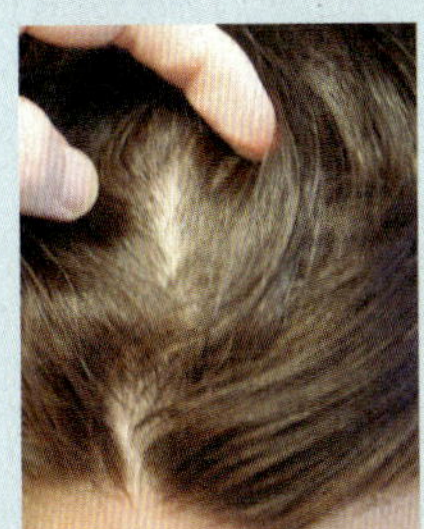

Normal hair part width in telogen effluvium

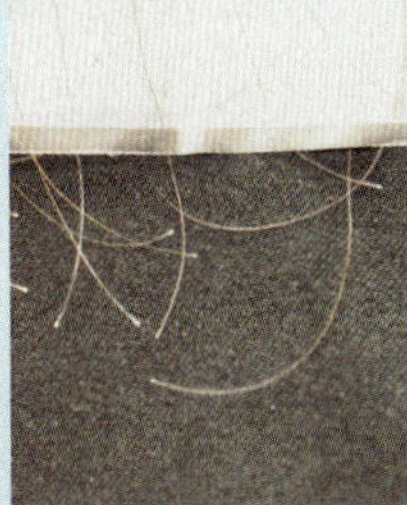

Positive hair pull test in telogen effluvium showing all hairs have telogen bulbs

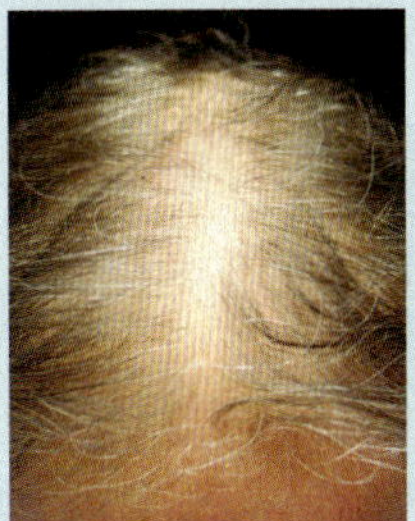

Anagen effluvium

(continued)

FOCAL HAIR LOSS

Alopecia Areata

There is sudden onset of clearly demarcated, usually localized, round or oval patches of hair loss leaving smooth skin without hairs, in children and young adults. There is no visible scaling or erythema.

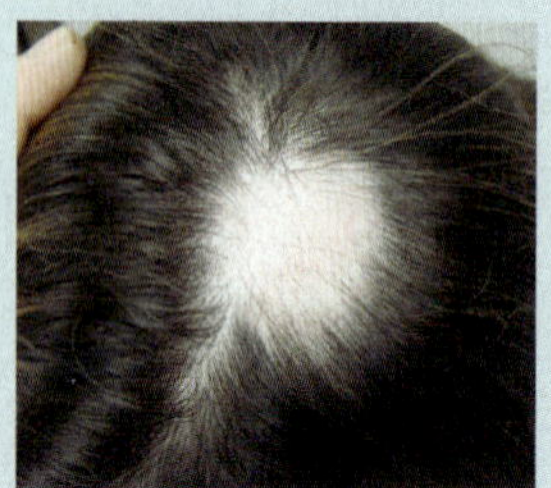

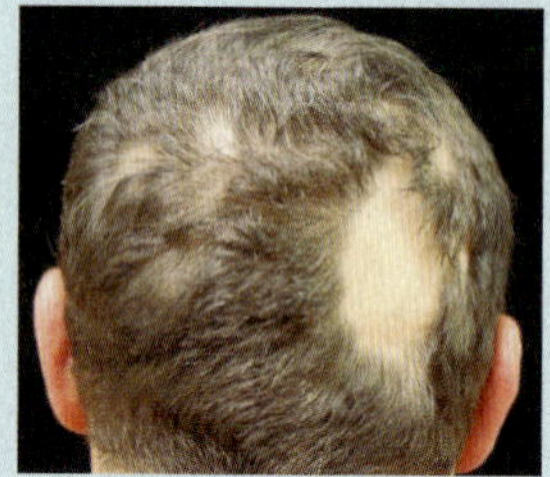

Tinea Capitis ("Ringworm")

Round scaling patches of alopecia are seen, mostly in children. There may be "black dots" of broken hairs and comma or corkscrew hairs on dermoscopy. Usually caused by *Trichophyton tonsurans* from humans, and less commonly, *Microsporum canis* from dogs or cats. Boggy plaques are called *kerions*.

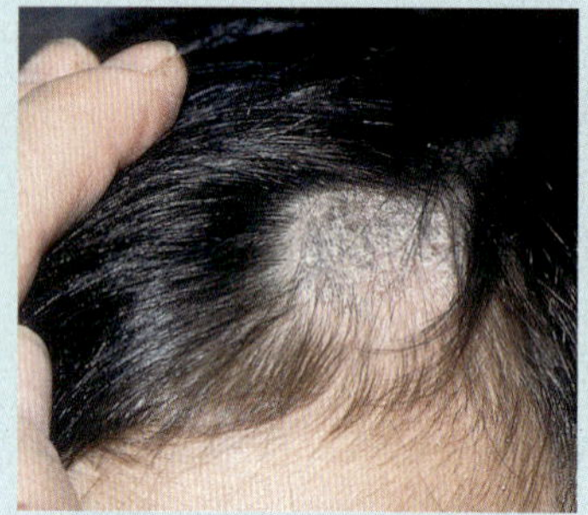

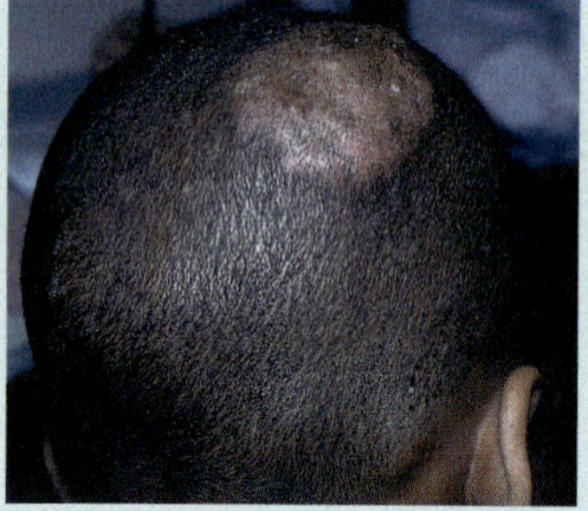

Scarring Alopecia

Scarring on the scalp is characterized by shiny skin, complete loss of hair follicles, and often, discoloration. Presence of any scarring should prompt referral to a dermatologist for possible scalp biopsy if the patient desires treatment. Examples of scarring alopecia include central centrifugal scarring alopecia and discoid lupus erythematosus, among others.

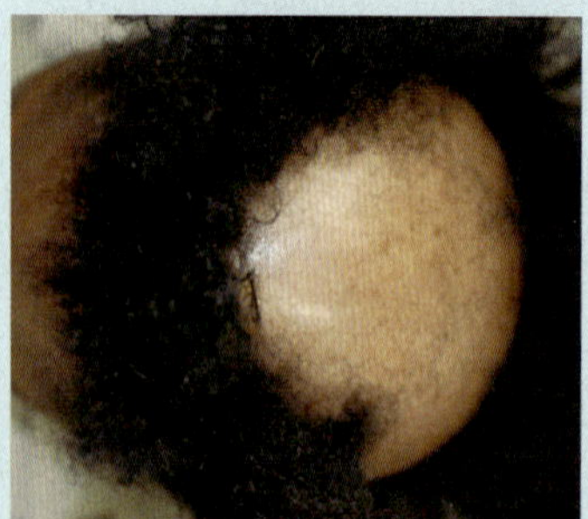

Central centrifugal scarring alopecia

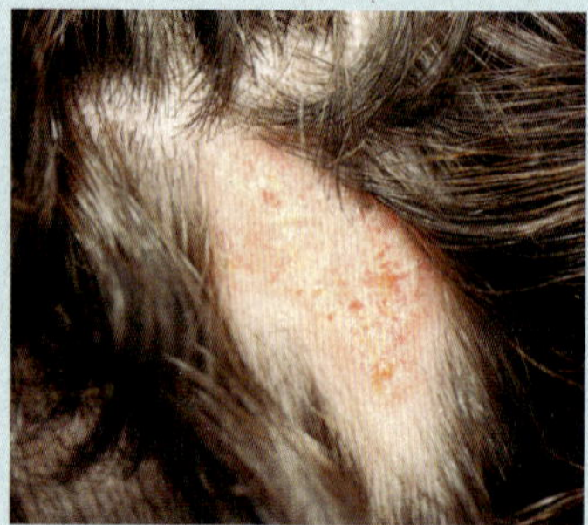

Discoid lupus scarring alopecia

Hair Shaft Disorders

Patients with abnormal hair from birth, as in this patient with a genetic condition called monilethrix, should be referred to dermatology.

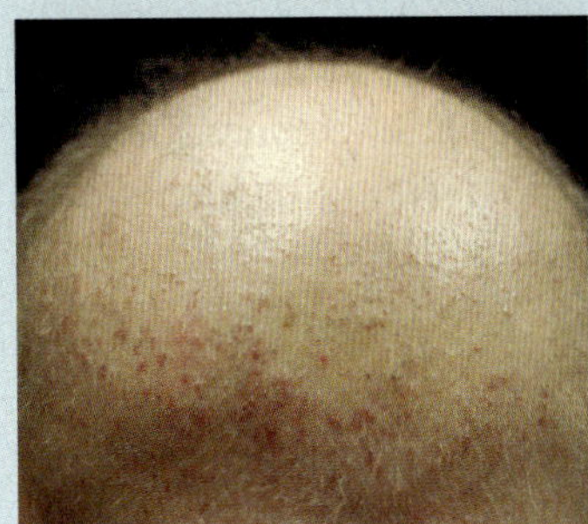

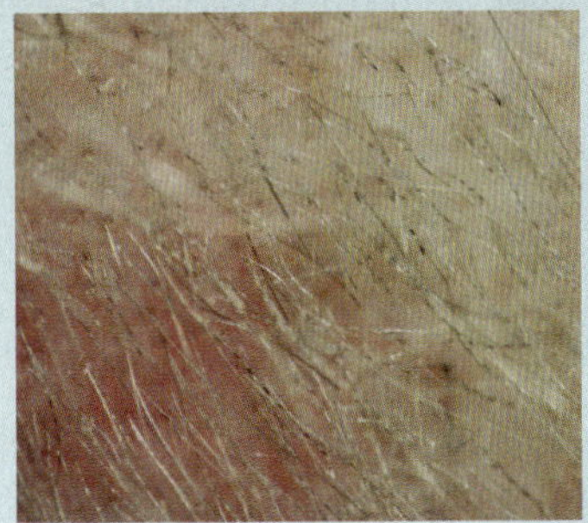

Hair shaft disorder with alternating bands

Source: Mubki T, Rudnicka L, Olszewska M, Shapiro J. Evaluation and diagnosis of the hair loss patient: part I. History and clinical examination. *J Am Acad Dermatol*. 2014;71(3):415.e1–415.e15.

Source of photo: *Alopecia Areata* [left]—Reprinted with permission from Goodheart HP, Gonzalez ME. *Goodheart's Photoguide to Common Pediatric and Adult Skin Disorders*. 4th ed. Wolters Kluwer; 2016. Appendix Figure 10.

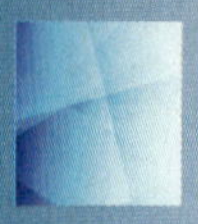

TABLE 12-9. Findings in or Near the Nails

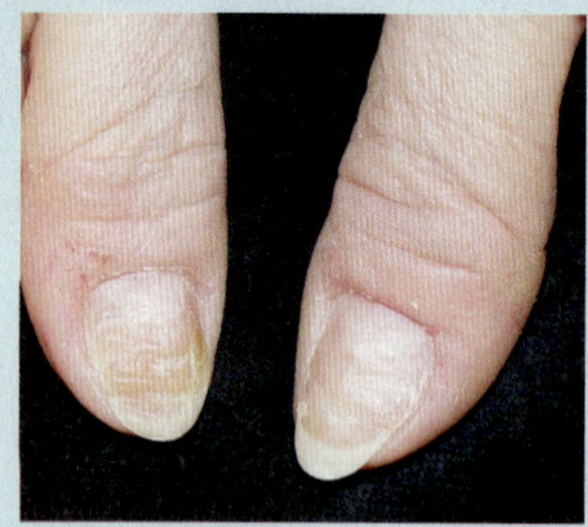

Paronychia

A superficial infection of the proximal and lateral nail folds adjacent to the nail plate. The nail folds are often red, swollen, and tender. Represents the most common infection of the hand, usually from *Staphylococcus aureus* or *Streptococcus* species, and may spread until it completely surrounds the nail plate. Creates a felon (closed-space infection) if it extends into the pulp space of the finger. Arises from local trauma due to nail biting, manicuring, or frequent hand immersion in water. Chronic infections may be related to *Candida.*

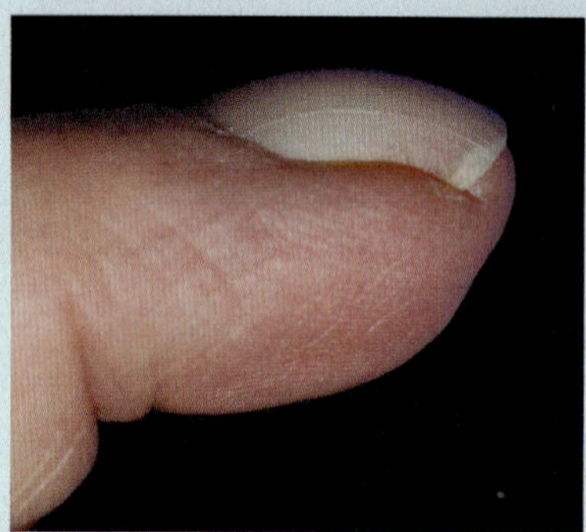

Clubbing of the Fingers

Clinically, a bulbous swelling of the soft tissue at the nail base, with loss of the normal angle between the nail and the proximal nail fold. The angle increases to 180 degrees or more, and the nail bed feels spongy or floating. The mechanism is still unknown but involves vasodilation with increased blood flow to the distal portion of the digits and changes in connective tissue, possibly from hypoxia, changes in innervation, genetics, or a platelet-derived growth factor from fragments of platelet clumps. Seen in congenital heart disease, interstitial lung disease and lung cancer, inflammatory bowel diseases, and malignancies.

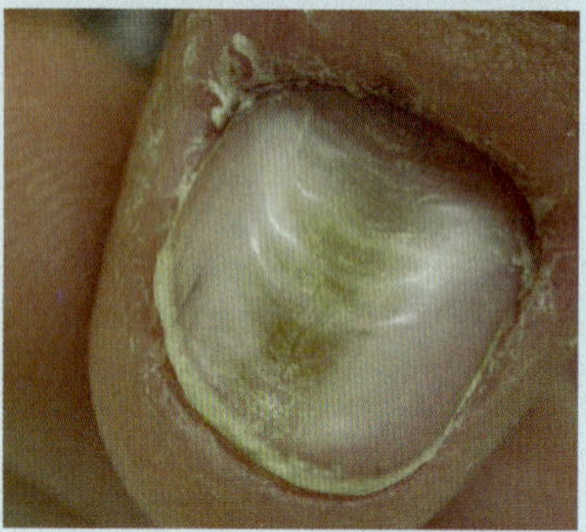

Habit Tic Deformity

There is depression of the central nail with a "Christmas tree" appearance from small horizontal depressions, resulting from repetitive trauma from rubbing the index finger over the thumb or vice versa. Pressure on the nail matrix causes the nail to grow out abnormally. Avoidance of the behavior leads to normal nail growth.

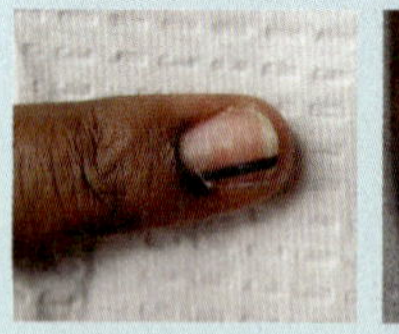

Melanonychia

Melanonychia is caused by increased pigmentation in the nail matrix, leading to a streak as the nail grows out. This may be a normal ethnic variation if found in multiple nails. A thin uniform streak may be caused by a nevus, but a wide streak, especially if growing or irregular, could represent a subungual melanoma.

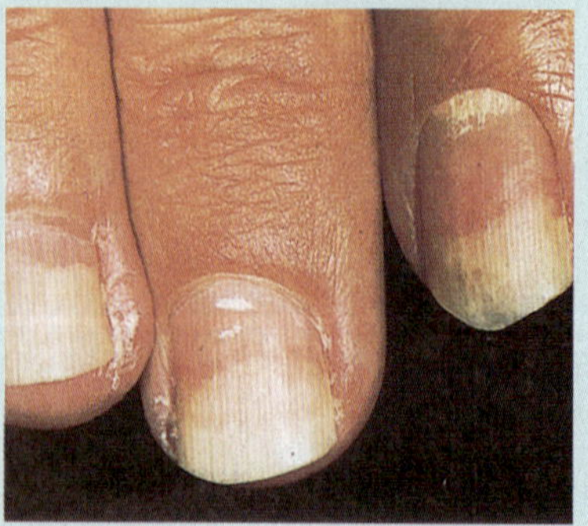

Onycholysis

A painless separation of the whitened opaque nail plate from the pinker translucent nail bed. Fingernails that extend past the fingertip are more likely to result in the traumatic shearing forces that produce onycholysis. Starts distally and progresses proximally, enlarging the free edge of the nail. Local causes include trauma from excess manicuring, psoriasis, fungal infection, and allergic reactions to nail cosmetics. Systemic causes include diabetes, anemia, photosensitive drug reactions, hyperthyroidism, peripheral ischemia, bronchiectasis, and syphilis.

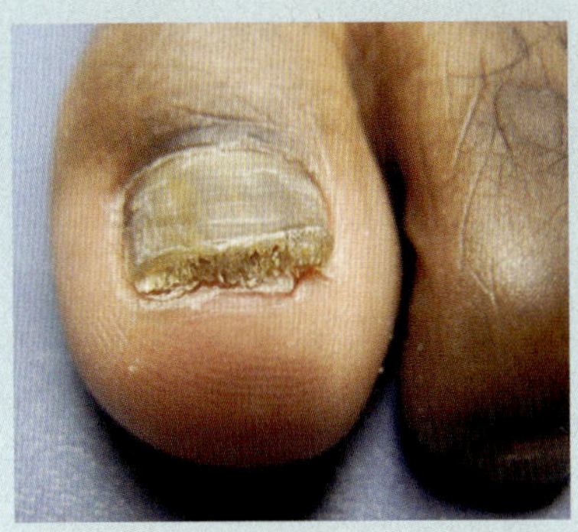

Onychomycosis

The most common cause of nail thickening and subungual debris is onychomycosis, most often from the dermatophyte *Trichophyton rubrum,* but also from other dermatophytes and some molds such as *Alternaria* and *Fusarium* species. Onychomycosis affects 1 in 5 over age 60. The best prevention is to treat and prevent tinea pedis. Only half of all nail dystrophies are caused by onychomycosis, so a positive fungal culture, potassium hydroxide examination, or pathologic evaluation of nail clippings is recommended before treating with oral antifungals.

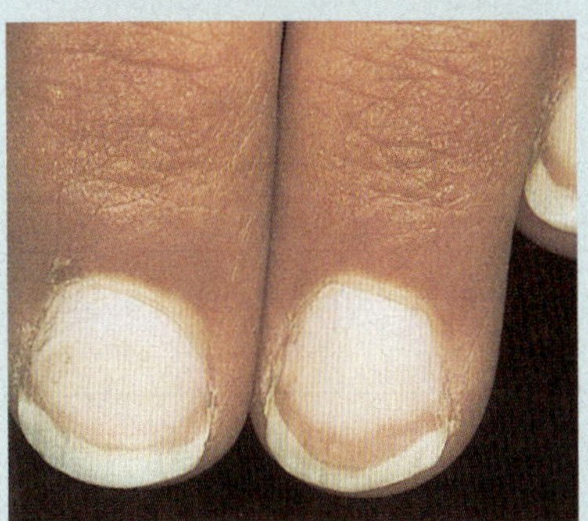

Terry Nails

Nail plate turns white with a ground-glass appearance, a distal band of reddish brown, and obliteration of the lunula. Commonly affects all fingers, although may appear in only one finger. Seen in liver disease, usually cirrhosis, heart failure, and diabetes. May arise from decreased vascularity and increased connective tissue in nail bed.

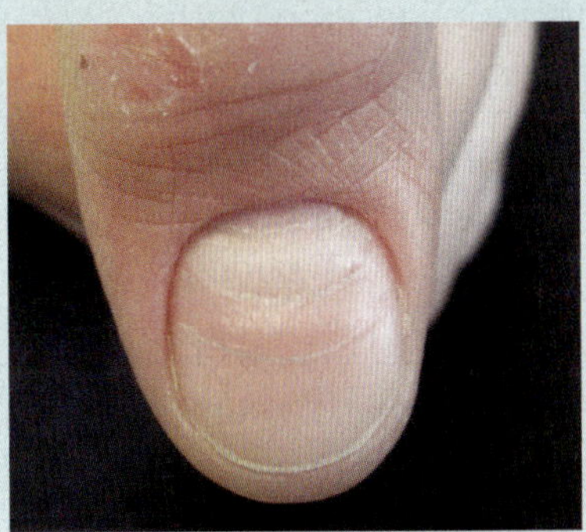

Transverse Linear Depressions (*Beau Lines*)

Transverse depressions of the nail plates, usually bilateral, resulting from temporary disruption of proximal nail growth from systemic illness. Timing of the illness may be estimated by measuring the distance from the line to the nail bed (nails grow approximately 1 mm every 6 to 10 days). Seen in severe illness, trauma, and cold exposure if Raynaud disease is present.

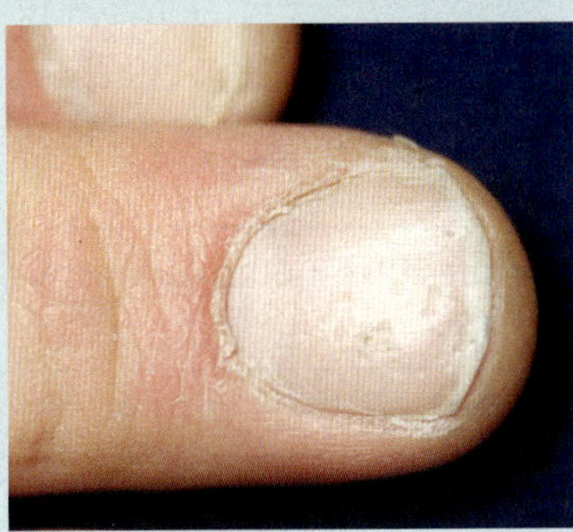

Pitting

Punctate depressions of the nail plate caused by defective layering of the superficial nail plate by the proximal nail matrix. Usually associated with psoriasis but also seen in reactive arthritis, sarcoidosis, alopecia areata, and localized atopic or chemical dermatitis.

Source of photos: *Onycholysis, Terry Nails*—Reprinted from Habif TP. *Clinical Dermatology: A Color Guide to Diagnosis and Therapy*. 2nd ed. CV Mosby; 1990.

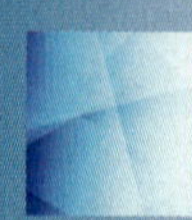

TABLE 12-10. Systemic Diseases and Associated Skin Findings

Systemic Disease	Associated Findings or Diagnoses
Addison disease	Hyperpigmentation of oral mucosa as well as sun-exposed skin, sites of trauma, and creases of palms and soles
Acquired immune deficiency syndrome	Human papillomavirus, herpes simplex virus, varicella zoster virus, cytomegalovirus, molluscum contagiosum, bacterial abscesses, mycobacterium (tuberculosis, leprae, avium) infections, candidiasis, deep fungal infections (cryptococcus, histoplasmosis), oral hairy leukoplakia, Kaposi sarcoma, oral and anal squamous cell carcinoma, acquired ichthyosis, severe psoriasis, severe seborrheic dermatitis, eosinophilic folliculitis
Chagas disease (American trypanosomiasis)	Unilateral conjunctivitis and lid edema associated with preauricular lymphadenopathy
Chronic renal disease	Pallor, xerosis, uremic frost, pruritus, "half and half" nails, calciphylaxis.
CREST syndrome	Calcinosis, Raynaud phenomenon, sclerodactyly, matted telangiectasias of face and hands (palms)
Crohn's disease	Erythema nodosum, pyoderma gangrenosum, enterocutaneous fistulas, aphthous ulcers
Cushing disease	Striae, atrophy, purpuras, ecchymoses, telangiectasias, acne, moon facies, buffalo hump, hypertrichosis
Dermatomyositis	Violaceous erythema as macules, patches, or papules in periocular region (heliotrope), on interphalangeal joints (Gottron sign), and on upper back and shoulders (shawl sign); poikiloderma in sun-exposed areas; periungual telangiectasia, ragged cuticles (Samitz sign)
Diabetes	Pruritus, diabetic dermopathy, acanthosis nigricans, candidiasis, neuropathic ulcers, necrobiosis lipoidica, eruptive xanthomas
Disseminated intravascular coagulation	Purpuras, petechiae, hemorrhagic bullae, induration, necrosis
Dyslipidemias	Xanthomas (tendon, eruptive, and tuberous), xanthelasma (may also occur in healthy people)
Gonococcemia	Purple to gray macules, papules or hemorrhagic pustules distributed over acral and periarticular surfaces
Hemochromatosis	Skin bronzing and hyperpigmentation
Hyperthyroidism	Warm, moist, soft, and velvety skin; thin and fine hair; alopecia; vitiligo; pretibial myxedema (in Graves disease); hyperpigmentation (local or generalized)
Hypothyroidism	Dry, rough, and pale skin; coarse and brittle hair; myxedema; alopecia (lateral third of the eyebrows to diffuse); skin cool to touch; thin and brittle nails
Infective endocarditis	Janeway lesions, Osler nodes, splinter hemorrhages, petechiae

Systemic Disease	Associated Findings or Diagnoses
Kawasaki disease	Mucosal erythema (lips, tongue, and pharynx), strawberry tongue, cherry red lips, polymorphous rash (primarily on trunk), erythema of palms and soles with later desquamation of fingertips
Leukemia/lymphoma	Pallor, exfoliative erythroderma, nodules, petechiae, ecchymoses, pruritus, vasculitis, pyoderma gangrenosum, bullous diseases
Leukocytoclastic vasculitis (postcapillary venules)	Palpable purpuras, purpuric wheals, hemorrhagic bullae in dependent areas
Liver disease	Jaundice, spider angiomas and other telangiectasias, palmar erythema, Terry nails, pruritus, purpuras, caput medusae
Lymphogranuloma venereum	Lymphadenopathy above and below Poupart ligament (groove sign)
Medium vessels vasculitides (e.g., polyarteritis nodosa, granulomatosis with polyangiitis, eosinophilic granulomatosis with polyangiitis, microscopic polyangiitis)	Livedo racemosa, purpuric nodules, ulcers
Meningococcemia	Angular or stellate purpuric patches and plaques with gunmetal gray center. Progresses to ecchymoses, bullae, necrosis
Neurofibromatosis 1 (von Recklinghausen syndrome)	Neurofibromas, café-au-lait spots, freckling in the axillae (Crowe sign), plexiform neurofibroma
Pancreatic carcinoma	Panniculitis, migratory thrombophlebitis (Trousseau sign)
Pancreatitis (hemorrhagic)	Bruising and induration over the costovertebral angle (Grey Turner sign), Cullen sign, panniculitis
Porphyria cutanea tarda	Photosensitivity with bullae and skin fragility on dorsal hands and forearms; bullae rupture and heal with scarring and milia; hypertrichosis of the face; bronzing of skin when associated with hemochromatosis
Pyoderma gangrenosum	Painful pustule quickly progressing to ragged ulcer with sharply marginated violaceous border and undermined edges
Rocky Mountain spotted fever	Pink or reddish papules progressing to purpuric papules; starts on wrists and ankles and spreads to palms and soles and then to trunk and face
Sarcoidosis	Red-brown plaques, often annular, typically involving the head and neck and especially the nose and ears; may show apple jelly color with dermoscopy
Systemic lupus erythematosus	Malar erythema (mid cheeks, spans bridge of nose), relative sparing of nasolabial folds, periungual erythema, interphalangeal erythema

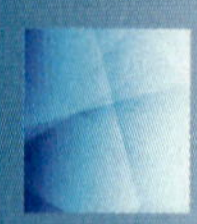

TABLE 12-11. Acne Vulgaris—Primary and Secondary Lesions

Acne vulgaris is the most common cutaneous disorder in the United States, affecting more than 85% of adolescents.[38] Acne is a disorder of the pilosebaceous unit that involves proliferation of the keratinocytes at the opening of the follicle; increased production of sebum, stimulated by androgens, which combines with keratinocytes to plug the follicular opening; growth of *Propionibacterium acnes,* an anaerobic diphtheroid normally found on the skin; and inflammation from bacterial activity and release of free fatty acids and enzymes from activated neutrophils. Cosmetics, humidity, heavy sweating, and stress are contributing factors. Most recommendations for treatment of acne are divided along its morphologic subdivisions: comedonal (mild), inflammatory (moderate), and nodulocystic (severe).

Lesions appear in areas with the greatest number of sebaceous glands, namely the face, neck, chest, upper back, and upper arms. They may be primary, secondary, or mixed.

Primary Lesions

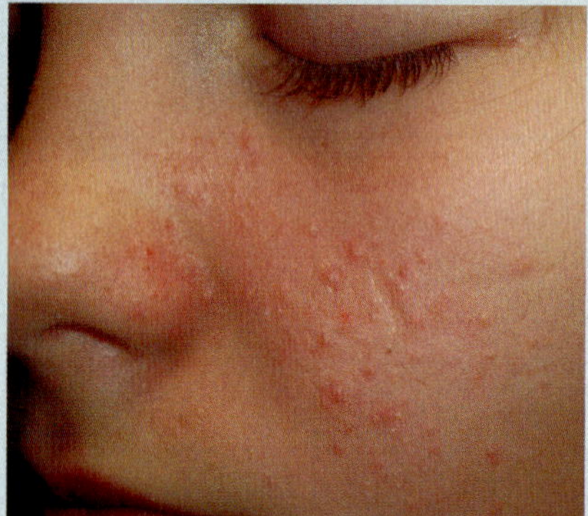

Mild Acne: Open and closed comedones, occasional papules

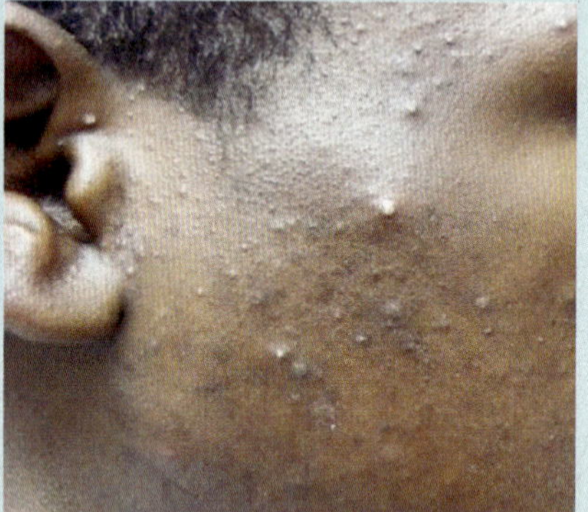

Moderate Acne: Comedones, papules, pustules

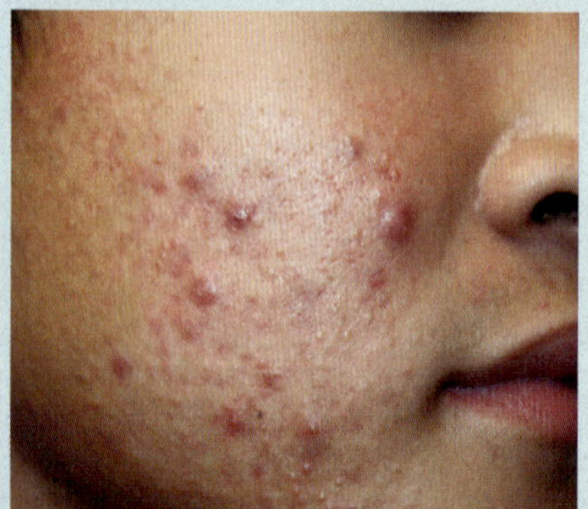

Severe Cystic Acne

Secondary Lesions

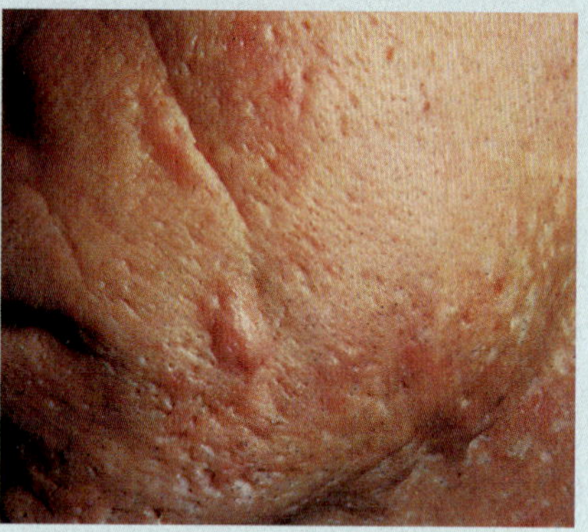

Acne with Pitting and Scars

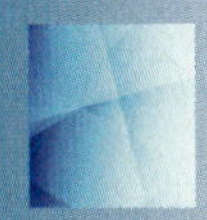

TABLE 12-12. Signs of Sun Damage

Sun damage is one of the most important clues that a patient is at risk of skin cancer. Study carefully the following indicators of sun damage accrued throughout life. These indicators should prompt close inspection for *pink lesions* that are possible basal cell carcinomas; rough or keratotic lesions that may be actinic keratoses or squamous cell carcinomas; or asymmetric, multicolored, or changing lesions that could be melanoma. Counsel affected patients about proper sun protection.

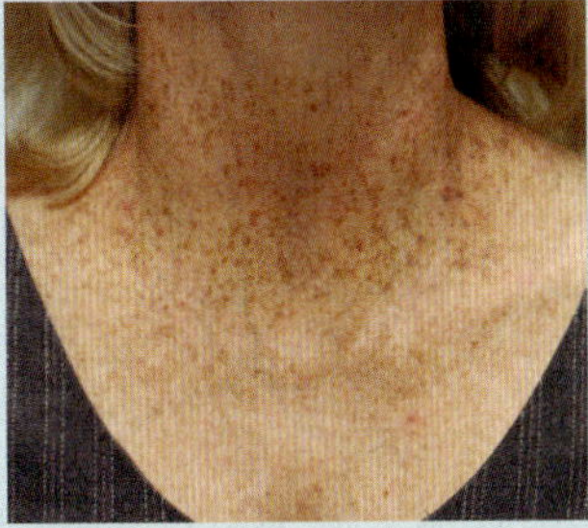

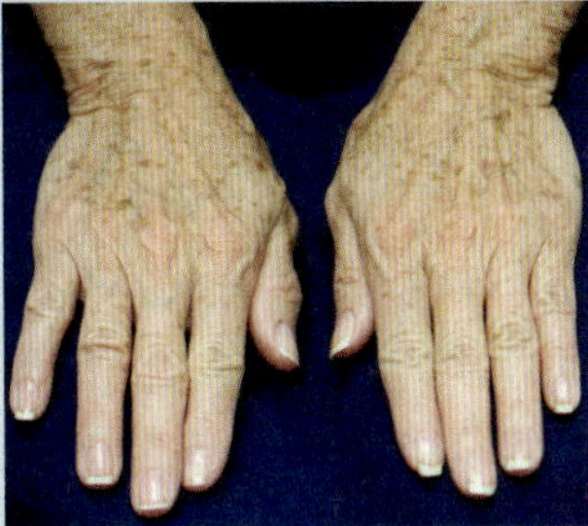

Solar Lentigo: Bilaterally symmetric brown macules located on sun-exposed skin, including the face, shoulders, and arms and hands

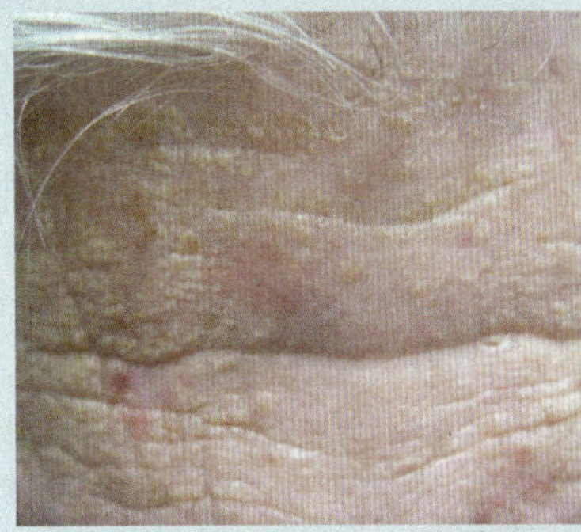

Solar Elastosis: Yellowish white macules or papules in sun-exposed skin, especially on the forehead

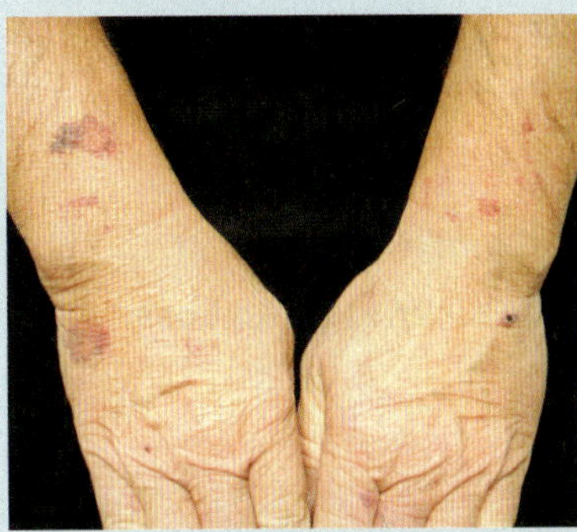

Actinic Purpura: Ecchymoses limited to the dorsal forearms and hands but not extending above the "shirt sleeve" line on the upper arm

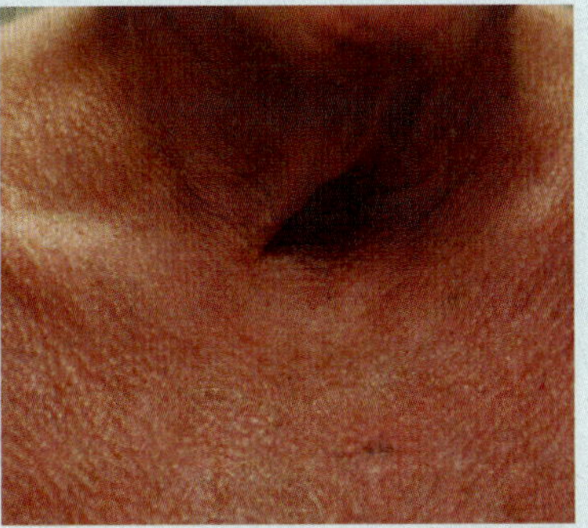

Poikiloderma: Red patches in sun-damaged areas, especially the V of the neck, and lateral neck (usually sparing the shadow inferior to the chin) with fine telangiectasias, and both hyper- and hypopigmentations

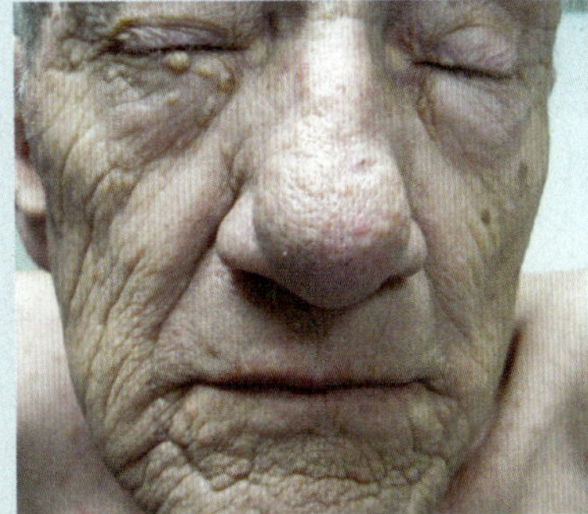

Wrinkles: Increased sun damage and tanning leads to deeper wrinkles at an earlier age

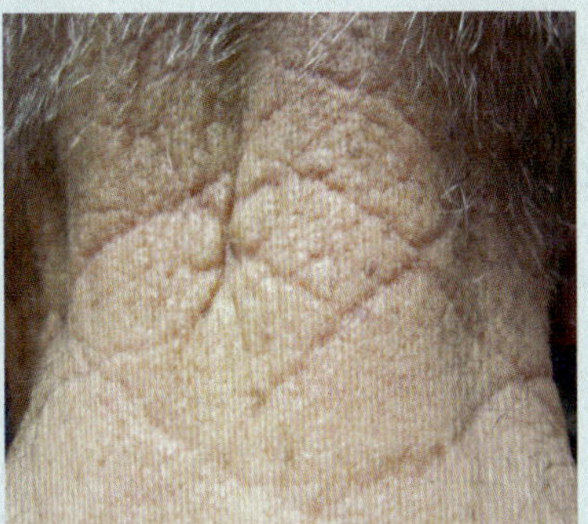

Cutis Rhomboidalis Nuchae: Deep wrinkles on the posterior neck that "crisscross"

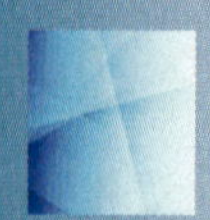

TABLE 12-13. Pressure Injuries

A pressure injury is localized damage to the skin and underlying soft tissue usually over a bony prominence or related to a medical or other device. The injury can present as intact skin or an open ulcer and may be painful. The injury occurs as a result of intense and/or prolonged pressure or pressure in combination with shear. The tolerance of soft tissue for pressure and shear may also be affected by microclimate, nutrition, perfusion, comorbidities, and condition of the soft tissue.

Pressure injuries or ulcers usually develop over bony prominences subject to unrelieved pressure, resulting in ischemic damage to underlying tissue. Prevention is important: inspect the skin thoroughly for early warning signs of erythema that still blanches with pressure, especially in patients with risk factors. Pressure injuries form most commonly over the sacrum, ischial tuberosities, greater trochanters, and heels.

A commonly applied staging system, based on depth of destroyed tissue, is illustrated below. Note that necrosis or eschar must be debrided before injuries can be staged. They may not progress sequentially through the four stages.

Address the patient's overall health, including comorbid conditions such as vascular disease, diabetes, immune deficiencies, collagen vascular disease, malignancy, psychosis, or depression; nutritional status; pain and level of analgesia; risk for recurrence; psychosocial factors such as learning ability, social supports, and lifestyle; and evidence of polypharmacy, overmedication, or abuse of alcohol, tobacco, or illicit drugs.[39]

RISK FACTORS FOR PRESSURE INJURIES

- Decreased mobility, especially if accompanied by increased pressure or movement causing friction or shear stress
- Decreased sensation, from brain or spinal cord lesions or peripheral nerve disease
- Decreased blood flow from hypotension or microvascular disease such as diabetes or atherosclerosis
- Fecal or urinary incontinence
- Presence of fracture
- Poor nutritional status or low albumin

Stage 1 Pressure Injury: Nonblanchable Erythema of Intact Skin

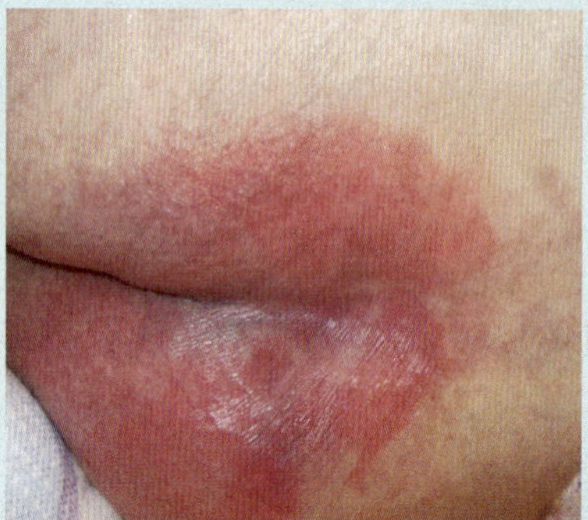

Intact skin with a localized area of nonblanchable erythema, which may appear differently in darkly pigmented skin. Presence of blanchable erythema or changes in sensation, temperature, or firmness may precede visual changes. Color changes do not include purple or maroon discoloration; these may indicate deep tissue pressure injury.

Stage 2 Pressure Injury: Partial-Thickness Skin Loss with Exposed Dermis

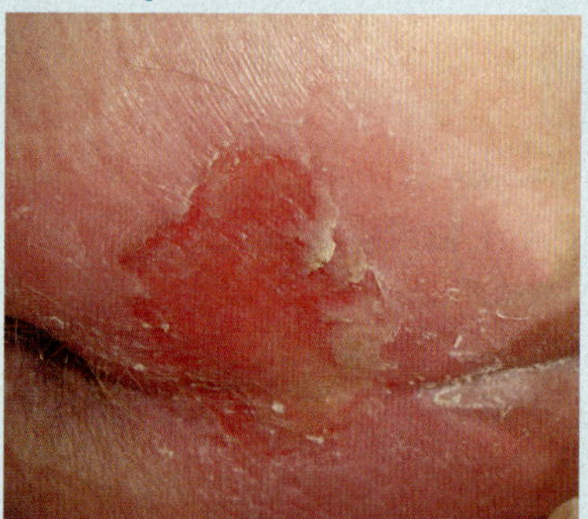

Partial-thickness loss of skin with exposed dermis. The wound bed is viable, pink or red, moist, and may also present as an intact or ruptured serum-filled blister. Adipose (fat) is not visible and deeper tissues are not visible. Granulation tissue, slough, and eschar are not present. These injuries commonly result from adverse microclimate and shear in the skin over the pelvis and shear in the heel. This stage should not be used to describe moisture-associated skin damage (MASD) including incontinence-associated dermatitis (IAD), intertriginous dermatitis (ITD), medical adhesive–related skin injury (MARSI), or traumatic wounds (skin tears, burns, abrasions).

RISK FACTORS FOR PRESSURE INJURIES

Stage 3 Pressure Injury: Full-Thickness Skin Loss

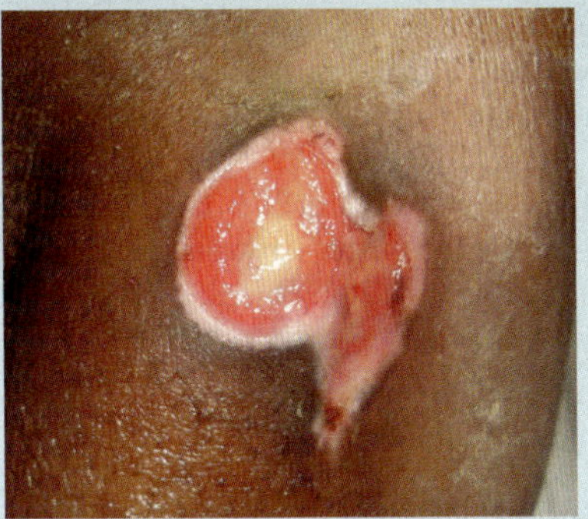

Full-thickness loss of skin, in which adipose (fat) is visible in the ulcer and granulation tissue and epibole (rolled wound edges) are often present. Slough and/or eschar may be visible. The depth of tissue damage varies by anatomical location; areas of significant adiposity can develop deep wounds. Undermining and tunneling may occur. Fascia, muscle, tendon, ligament, cartilage and/or bone are not exposed. If slough or eschar obscures the extent of tissue loss, this is an unstageable pressure injury.

Stage 4 Pressure Injury: Full-Thickness Skin and Tissue Loss

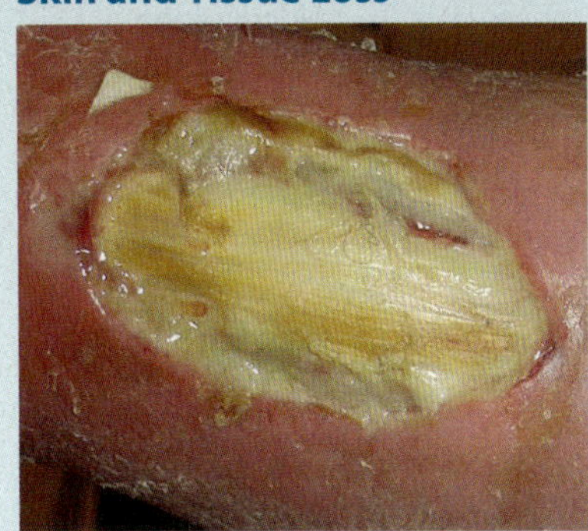

Full-thickness skin and tissue loss with exposed or directly palpable fascia, muscle, tendon, ligament, cartilage, or bone in the ulcer. Slough and/or eschar may be visible. Epibole (rolled edges), undermining and/or tunneling often occur. Depth varies by anatomical location. If slough or eschar obscures the extent of tissue loss, this is an unstageable pressure injury.

Unstageable Pressure Injury: Obscured Full-Thickness Skin and Tissue Loss

Full-thickness skin and tissue loss in which the extent of tissue damage within the ulcer cannot be confirmed because it is obscured by slough or eschar. If slough or eschar is removed, a stage 3 or stage 4 pressure injury will be revealed. Stable eschar (i.e., dry, adherent, intact without erythema or fluctuance) on the heel or ischemic limb should not be softened or removed.

Deep Tissue Pressure Injury: Persistent Nonblanchable Deep Red, Maroon, or Purple Discoloration

Intact or nonintact skin with localized area of persistent nonblanchable deep red, maroon, or purple discoloration or epidermal separation revealing a dark wound bed or blood-filled blister. Pain and temperature change often precede skin color changes. Discoloration may appear differently in darkly pigmented skin, often manifesting as deeper tones such as purple, blue, or a hue darker than the surrounding skin. This injury results from intense and/or prolonged pressure and shear forces at the bone–muscle interface. The wound may evolve rapidly to reveal the actual extent of tissue injury or may resolve without tissue loss. If necrotic tissue, subcutaneous tissue, granulation tissue, fascia, muscle, or other underlying structures are visible, this indicates a full-thickness pressure injury (unstageable, stage 3, or stage 4). Do not use DTPI to describe vascular, traumatic, neuropathic, or dermatologic conditions.

Source: Used with permission of National Pressure Injury Advisory Panel, Westford, MA.

REFERENCES

1. Coulson IH, Benton EC, Ogden S. Chapter 4: Diagnosis of skin disease. In: Griffiths CEM, Barker J, Bleiker TO, Chalmers R, Creamer D, eds. *Rook's Textbook of Dermatology*. 9th ed. Wiley-Blackwell; 2016.
2. Mayer JE, Swetter SM, Fu T, Geller AC. Screening, early detection, education, and trends for melanoma: current status (2007–2013) and future directions: part I. Epidemiology, high-risk groups, clinical strategies, and diagnostic technology. *J Am Acad Dermatol.* 2014;71(4):599.e1–599.e12.
3. Zalaudek I, Kittler H, Marghoob AA, et al. Time required for a complete skin examination with and without dermoscopy: a prospective, randomized multicenter study. *Arch Dermatol.* 2008;144(4):509–513.
4. Mubki T, Rudnicka L, Olszewska M, Shapiro J. Evaluation and diagnosis of the hair loss patient: part I. History and clinical examination. *J Am Acad Dermatol.* 2014;71(3):415.e1–415.e15.
5. Edsberg LE, Black JM, Goldberg M, McNichol L, Moore L, Sieggreen M. Revised national pressure ulcer advisory panel pressure injury staging system: revised pressure injury staging system. *J Wound Ostomy Continence Nurs.* 2016;43(6):585–597.
6. May L, Mullins P, Pines J. Demographic and treatment patterns for infections in ambulatory settings in the United States, 2006–2010. *Acad Emerg Med.* 2014;21(1):17–24.
7. Subramaniam S, Bober J, Chao J, Zehtabchi S. Point-of-care ultrasound for diagnosis of abscess in skin and soft tissue infections. *Acad Emerg Med.* 2016;23(11):1298–1306.
8. Adhikari S, Blaivas M. Sonography first for subcutaneous abscess and cellulitis evaluation. *J Ultrasound Med.* 2012;31(10):1509–1512.
9. Adams CM, Neuman MI, Levy JA. Point-of-care ultrasonography for the diagnosis of pediatric soft tissue infection. *J Pediatr.* 2016;169:122–7.e1.
10. Squire BT, Fox JC, Anderson C. ABSCESS: applied bedside sonography for convenient evaluation of superficial soft tissue infections. *Acad Emerg Med.* 2005;12(7):601–606.
11. Gottlieb M, Avila J, Chottiner M, Peksa GD. Point-of-care ultrasonography for the diagnosis of skin and soft tissue abscesses: a systematic review and meta-analysis. *Ann Emerg Med.* 2020;76(1):67–77.
12. Berger T, Garrido F, Green J, Lema PC, Gupta J. Bedside ultrasound performed by novices for the detection of abscess in ED patients with soft tissue infections. *Am J Emerg Med.* 2012;30(8):1569–1573.
13. Noble VE, Nelson BP. *Manual of Emergency and Critical Care Ultrasoun.* 2nd ed. Cambridge University Press; 2011.
14. Brian D, Euerle M, FACEP. Abscess Evaluation. Accessed October 27, 2023. https://www.acep.org/sonoguide/procedures/abscess-evaluation/
15. Euerle BD. Soft Tissue Ultrasound. Updated August 18, 2020. Accessed October 27, 2023. https://www.acep.org/sonoguide/basic/soft-tissue-ultrasound/
16. Stern RS. Prevalence of a history of skin cancer in 2007: results of an incidence-based model. *Arch Dermatol.* 2010;146(3):279–282.
17. American Cancer Society medical and editorial content team. *Key statistics for basal and squamous cell skin cancers.* American Cancer Society. Accessed August 1, 2023. https://www.cancer.org/cancer/types/basal-and-squamous-cell-skin-cancer/about/key-statistics.html
18. Siegel RL, Miller KD, Wagle NS, Jemal A. Cancer statistics, 2023. *CA Cancer J Clin.* 2023;73(1):17–48.
19. SEER*Explorer: an interactive website for SEER cancer statistics [Internet]. Surveillance Research Program, National Cancer Institute. Updated 2023, July 31. Accessed August 1, 2023. https://seer.cancer.gov/statistics-network/explorer/
20. American Cancer Society medical and editorial content team. *Key Statistics for Melanoma Skin Cancer.* American Cancer Society. Accessed August 1, 2023. https://www.cancer.org/cancer/types/melanoma-skin-cancer/about/key-statistics.html
21. PDQ® Screening and Prevention Editorial Board. PDQ Skin Cancer Prevention. National Cancer Instititute. Updated May 22, 2023. Accessed August 1, 2023. https://www.cancer.gov/types/skin/hp/skin-prevention-pdq
22. El Ghissassi F, Baan R, Straif K, et al. A review of human carcinogens–part D: radiation. *Lancet Oncol.* 2009;10(8):751–752.
23. Boniol M, Autier P, Boyle P, Gandini S. Cutaneous melanoma attributable to sunbed use: systematic review and meta-analysis. *BMJ.* 2012;345:e4757.
24. U. S. Preventive Services Task Force, Grossman DC, Curry SJ, et al. Behavioral counseling to prevent skin cancer: US Preventive Services Task Force Recommendation Statement. *JAMA.* 2018;319(11):1134–1142.
25. An S, Kim K, Moon S, et al. Indoor tanning and the risk of overall and early-onset melanoma and non-melanoma skin cancer: systematic review and meta-analysis. *Cancers (Basel).* 2021;13(23):5940.
26. Green A, Williams G, Neale R, et al. Daily sunscreen application and betacarotene supplementation in prevention of basal-cell and squamous-cell carcinomas of the skin: a randomised controlled trial. *Lancet.* 1999;354(9180):723–729.
27. Green AC, Williams GM, Logan V, Strutton GM. Reduced melanoma after regular sunscreen use: randomized trial follow-up. *J Clin Oncol.* 2011;29(3):257–263.
28. Ghiasvand R, Weiderpass E, Green AC, Lund E, Veierød MB. Sunscreen use and subsequent melanoma risk: a population-based cohort study. *J Clin Oncol.* 2016;34(33):3976–3983.
29. Lazovich D, Vogel RI, Berwick M, Weinstock MA, Warshaw EM, Anderson KE. Melanoma risk in relation to use of sunscreen or other sun protection methods. *Cancer Epidemiol Biomarkers Prev.* 2011;20(12):2583–2593.
30. Watts CG, Drummond M, Goumas C, et al. Sunscreen use and melanoma risk among young Australian adults. *JAMA Dermatol.* 2018;154(9):1001–1009.
31. Department of Health and Human Services. Labeling and effectiveness testing; sunscreen drug products for over-the-counter human use. Final rule. *Fed Regist.* 2011;76(117):35620–35665.
32. American Academy of Dermatology Association. How to prevent skin cancer. American Academy of Dermatology. Accessed August 2, 2023. https://www.aad.org/public/diseases/skin-cancer/prevent/how
33. U. S. Preventive Services Task Force, Mangione CM, Barry MJ, Nicholson WK, et al. Screening for skin cancer: US Preventive Services Task Force Recommendation Statement. *JAMA.* 2023;329(15):1290–1295.

REFERENCES

34. Henrikson NB, Ivlev I, Blasi PR, et al. Skin cancer screening: Updated Evidence Report and Systematic Review for the US Preventive Services Task Force. *JAMA*. 2023;329(15):1296–1307.
35. American Cancer Society medical and editorial content team. *How to Do a Skin Self-Exam*. American Cancer Society. Accessed August 1, 2023. https://www.cancer.org/cancer/risk-prevention/sun-and-uv/skin-exams.html
36. American Academy of Dermatology Ad Hoc Task Force for the ABCDEs of Melanoma, Tsao H, Olazagasti JM, Cordoro KM, et al. Early detection of melanoma: reviewing the ABCDEs. *J Am Acad Dermatol*. 2015;72(4):717–723.
37. Gaudy-Marqueste C, Wazaefi Y, Bruneu Y, et al. Ugly duckling sign as a major factor of efficiency in melanoma detection. *JAMA Dermatol*. 2017;153(4):279–284.
38. Kalkhoran S, Milne O, Zalaudek I, et al. Historical, clinical, and dermoscopic characteristics of thin nodular melanoma. *Arch Dermatol*. 2010;146(3):311–318.
39. Key statistics for melanoma skin cancer. American Cancer Society. Accessed November 12, 2018. http://www.cancer.org/cancer/skincancer-melanoma/detailedguide/melanoma-skin-cancer-key-statistics
40. Kalkhoran S, Milne O, Zalaudek I, et al. Historical, clinical, and dermoscopic characteristics of thin nodular melanoma. *Arch Dermatol*. 2010;146(3):311–318.
41. Benedetti J. Description of skin lesions. In: Falk S, ed. *Merck Manual: Professional Version*. Merck & Co, Inc. Accessed October 29, 2018. https://www.merckmanuals.com/professional/dermatologic-disorders/approach-to-the-dermatologic-patient/description-of-skin-lesions#v958357

CHAPTER 13

Head and Neck

This chapter introduces the organ systems and structures of the head and neck. Although the eyes, ears, nose, throat, and oral cavity are discussed in individual chapters, understand that they should be viewed as a unit. These structures are closely connected anatomically and can exhibit related symptoms. Physical examination (PE) of these structures should be performed sequentially to properly assess them.

ANATOMY AND PHYSIOLOGY

Head and Neck

Regions of the head take their names from the underlying facial skeleton. Knowing this anatomy helps to locate and describe physical findings (see Figs. 13-1 to 13-3).[1]

Two sets of salivary glands are located near the mandible: the *parotid gland*, visible and palpable when enlarged and located behind the mandible, and the *submandibular gland*, deep to the mandible. To locate the latter, press your tongue against your lower incisors and feel for its lobular surface against the tightened muscle. The oral cavity contains the openings of the *parotid duct* (*Stensen duct*) and *submandibular ducts.*

The *superficial temporal artery* passes in front of the ear and is easily palpable, with one of its branches often visible across the forehead, particularly in thin and elderly individuals.

To aid description, divide each side of the neck into two triangles by the *sternocleidomastoid (SCM) muscle* (Fig. 13-4):

- *Anterior cervical triangle:* mandible superiorly, SCM muscle laterally, and midline of the neck medially.
- *Posterior cervical triangle:* SCM muscle medially, trapezius laterally, and clavicle inferiorly. Note that the omohyoid muscle crosses the lower portion of this triangle, which can be mistaken for a lymph node or mass.

Great Vessels

Deep to the SCM muscles run the great vessels of the neck: the *carotid artery* and the *internal jugular vein* (Fig. 13-5). The *external jugular vein* passes diagonally over the surface of the SCM muscle and may be helpful when trying to identify the jugular venous pressure (see pp. 302–303).

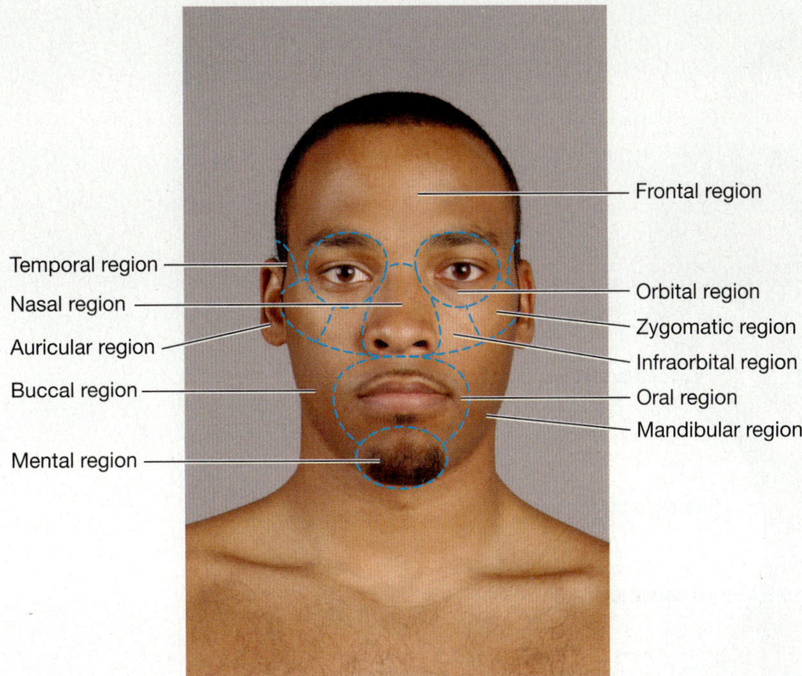

FIGURE 13-1. Surface anatomy of head, anterior view. (Reprinted with permission from Harrell KM, Dudek RW. *Lippincott® Illustrated Reviews: Anatomy.* Wolters Kluwer; 2019. Figure 8.23.)

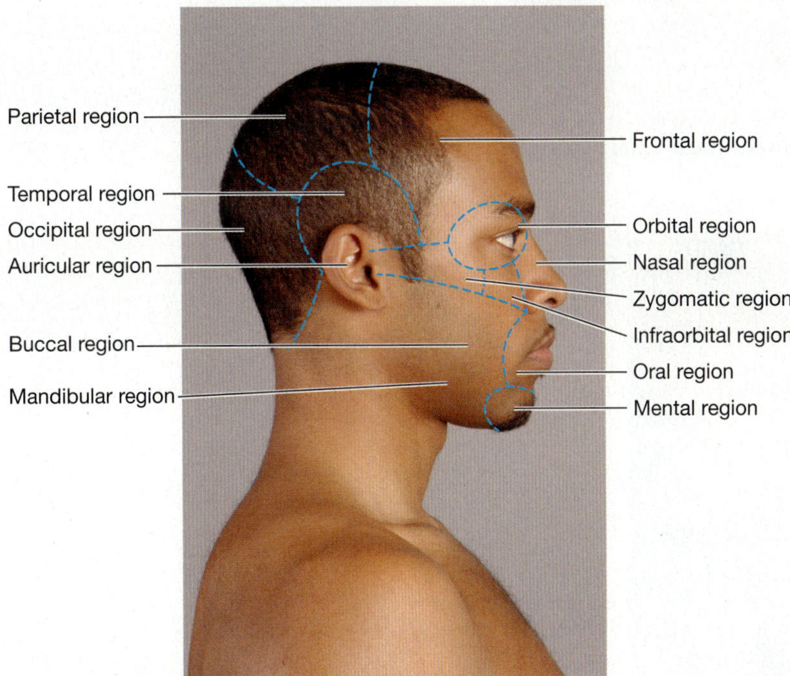

FIGURE 13-2. Surface anatomy of head, right lateral view. (Reprinted with permission from Harrell KM, Dudek RW. *Lippincott® Illustrated Reviews: Anatomy.* Wolters Kluwer; 2019. Figure 8.6.)

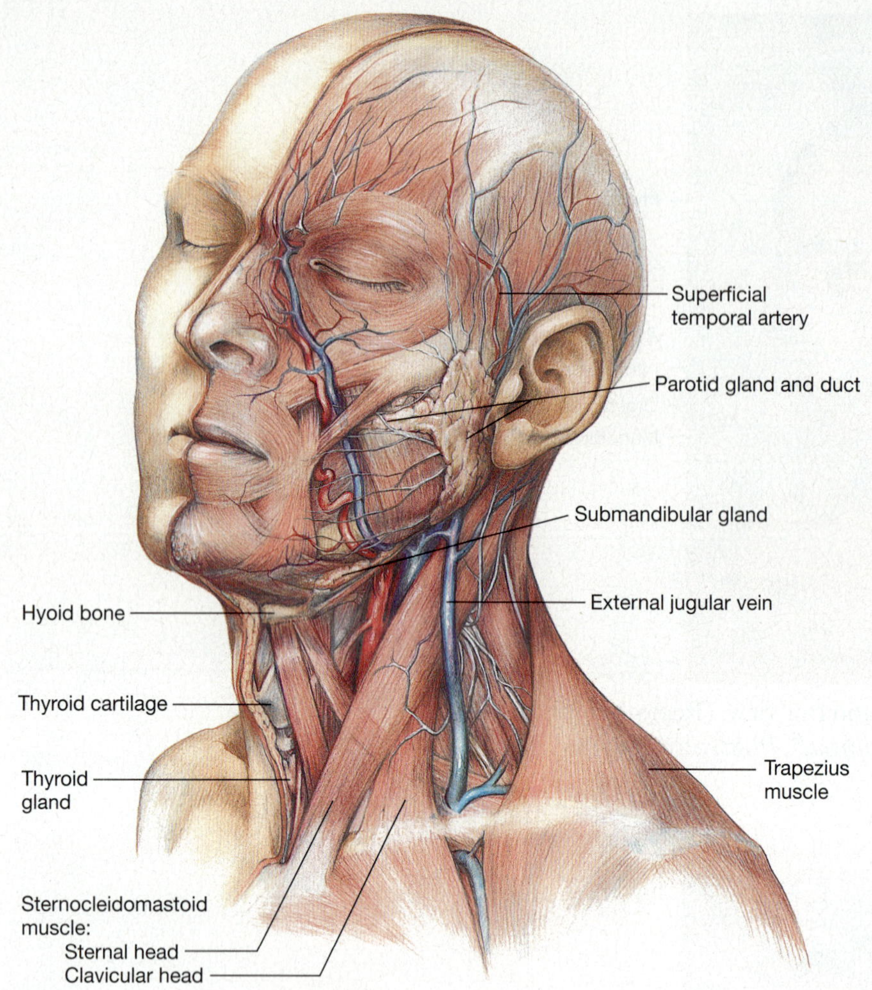

FIGURE 13-3. Anatomy of the head. (From Anatomical Chart Company: Head and Neck Anatomical Chart, 2000.)

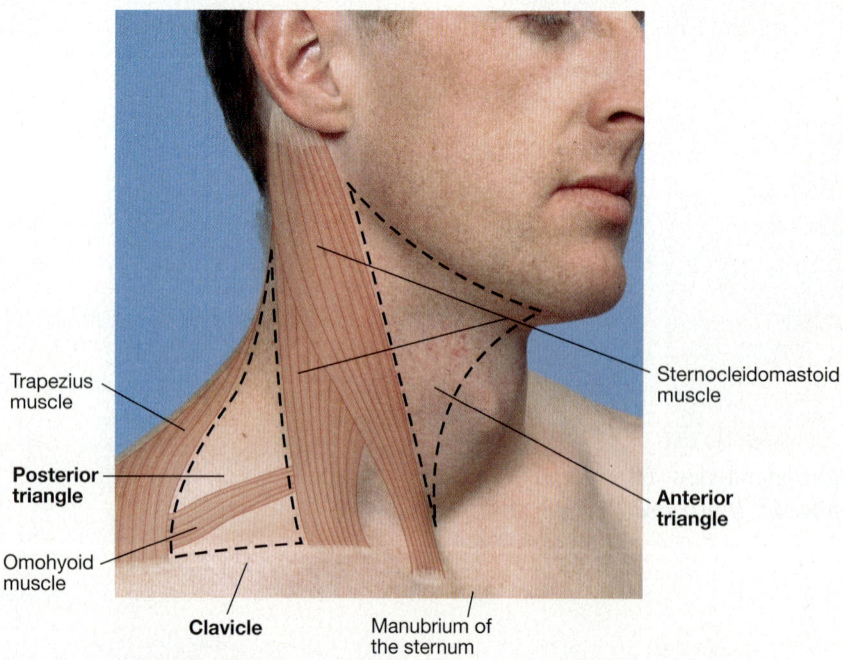

FIGURE 13-4. Anterior and posterior triangles of the neck.

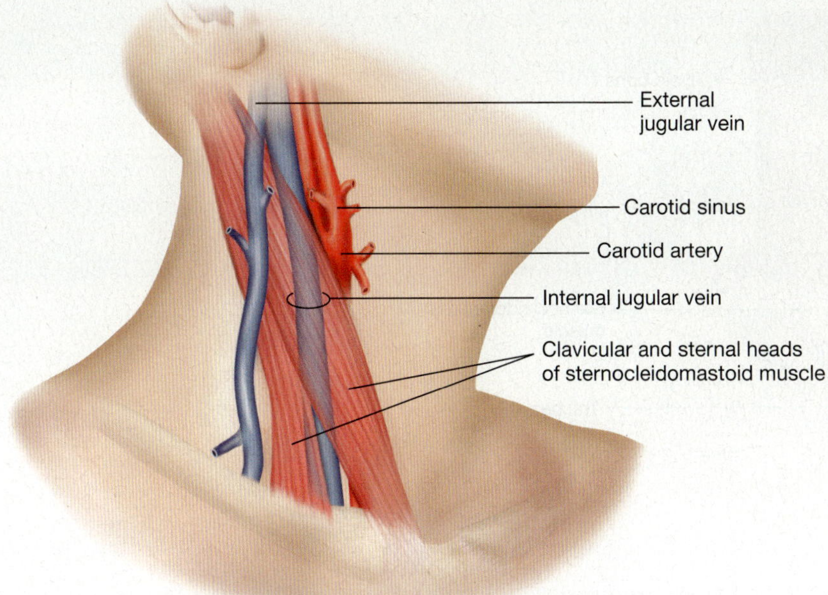

FIGURE 13-5. Great vessels of the neck.

Midline Structures and Thyroid Gland

Identify the following midline structures: the mobile hyoid bone located just below the mandible, the thyroid cartilage (which can be identified by the notch on its superior edge), cricoid cartilage, tracheal rings, and the thyroid gland (Figs. 13-6 and 13-7).

The *thyroid gland* is typically situated above the suprasternal notch, with the *thyroid isthmus* extending across the second to fourth tracheal rings just beneath the *cricoid cartilage*. Its lateral lobes curve posteriorly around the sides

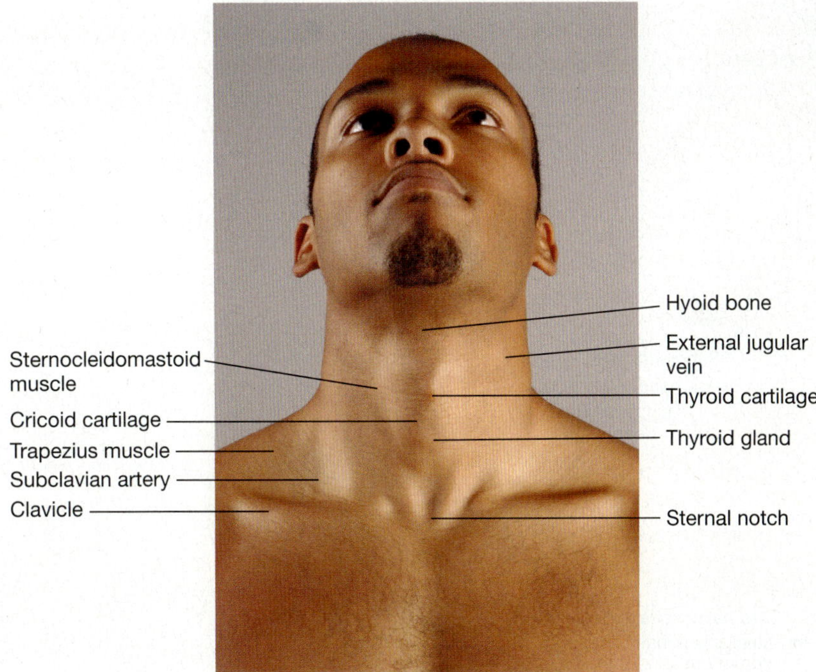

FIGURE 13-6. Surface anatomy of neck, anterior view.

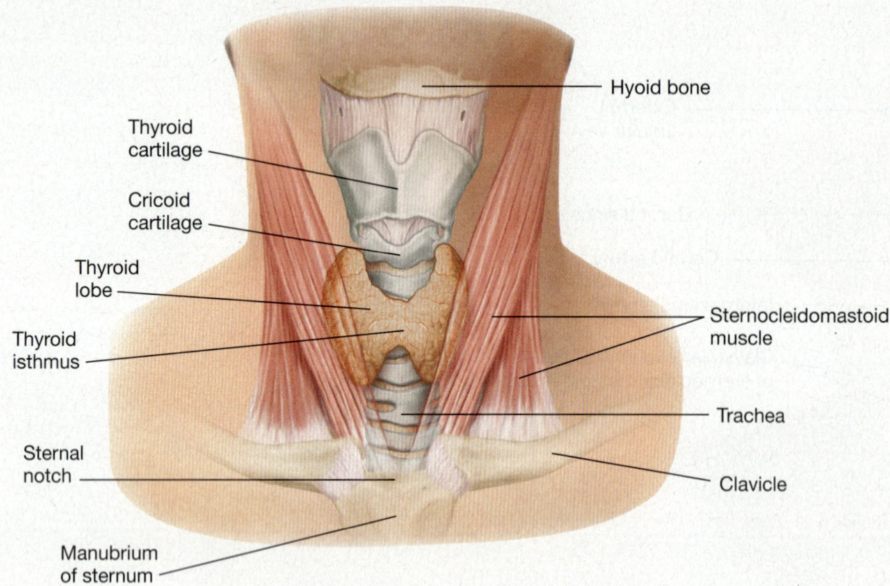

FIGURE 13-7. Midline structures of the neck.

of the trachea and the esophagus, measuring approximately 4 cm to 5 cm each. Except for the midline, the thyroid gland is covered by thin strap-like muscles that attach to the hyoid bone and more laterally by the visible SCM muscles.

Cervical Lymph Nodes

The lymph nodes of the head and neck are variably classified. One classification identifies nodes based on specific names of local anatomy as shown in Box 13-1 and Figure 13-8, together with the directions of lymphatic drainage.[2,3] Note

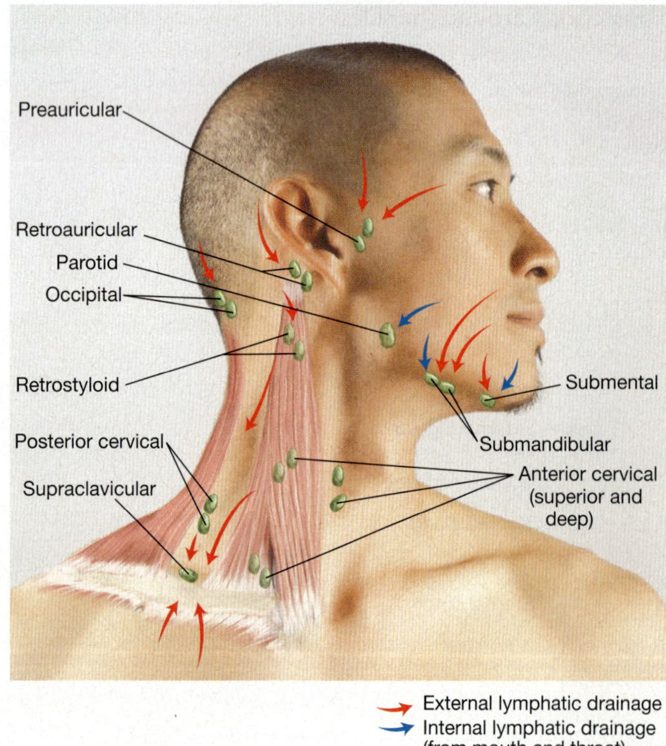

FIGURE 13-8. Lymph nodes of the neck.

Box 13-1. Cervical Lymph Node Groups

Lymph Node Group	Location
Submental lymph node group	Beneath the chin, in the midline of the anterior floor of the mouth.
Submandibular lymph node group	Below the lower jaw, along the underside of the mandible.
Jugular lymph node group	Along the jugular vein in the neck and are typically divided into superior, middle, and inferior groups.
Supraclavicular lymph node group	Located just above the clavicle. There are two main groups: the left-sided Virchow node and the right-sided lower deep cervical node.
Posterior triangle lymph node group	Found in the posterior triangle of the neck, which is bordered by the sternocleidomastoid muscle, the trapezius muscle, and the clavicle.
Anterior compartment group	Located in midline of neck extending between the hyoid and the manubrium.
Prevertebral compartment group	Located in front of the vertebrae, typically in the thoracic and abdominal regions and are not palpable on examination.
Retrostyloid node group	Situated posterior to the styloid process of the temporal bone, in the neck region.
Parotid lymph node group	Found around the parotid gland, situated in front of the ears and extending to the area beneath the earlobe.
Buccofacial lymph node group	Located in the facial and buccal (cheek) region.
Retroauricular and occipital lymph node groups	The retroauricular (also known as postauricular) lymph nodes are located behind the ears, while the occipital lymph nodes are found at the base of the skull, in the occipital region.

that this is a generalized location for these lymph nodes, and their exact position may slightly vary among individuals.

The jugular chain is mostly obscured by the SCM muscle, but palpable at its two extremes are the superior jugular nodes and supraclavicular nodes. Differentiate the submandibular nodes, which lie superficial to the submandibular gland. Normally, nodes are round or ovoid, smooth, and smaller than the submandibular gland, which has a larger, lobulated, slightly irregular surface (see p. 302).

Note that the jugular, submandibular, and submental nodes drain portions of the mouth, throat, and face. Assess lymphatic drainage patterns for possible malignancy or infection. Look for enlargement or tenderness of neighboring regional lymph nodes, and search for a source in its nearby drainage area.

HEALTH HISTORY: GENERAL APPROACH

Importantly, symptoms related to the head and neck may involve major structures such as sensory organs, cranial nerves (CNs), and major blood vessels originating in these areas. While many of these symptoms may represent benign processes, they can also indicate serious underlying conditions. As you engage with patients, be thorough in your interview and PE. Take note of features and findings that do not fit a typical benign pattern. This approach can help you differentiate between common head and neck conditions and potentially serious diseases.

Common or Concerning Symptoms

- Neck or thyroid mass or lump
- Neck pain (See Chapter 25, Musculoskeletal System: Neck, Shoulders, and Upper Extremities, p. 791.)
- Headache (See Chapter 27, Nervous System, pp. 909–911.)

Neck or Thyroid Mass or Lump

When encountering a patient with a thyroid mass or lump, a structured and comprehensive approach to the health history is essential.[4] This not only aids in the diagnostic process but also ensures that your patient's concerns are appropriately addressed. Box 13-2 lists key questions to consider when evaluating a neck or thyroid mass or lump.[5–7]

Box 13-2. Neck or Thyroid Mass or Lump: High-Yield Health History Questions

Domain	Questions	Rationale
Onset	*When did you first notice the neck mass or lump?*	This determines if the mass has a *sudden* or *gradual* onset, suggesting inflammatory/infectious processes or neoplastic/congenital etiologies, and helps assess progression and urgency.
Location	*Where exactly is the mass or lump located on your neck?*	*Midline* masses may indicate thyroglossal duct cysts, while *lateral* masses could suggest enlarged lymph nodes or branchial cleft cysts.
Size and consistency	*How would you describe the size and consistency of the mass (e.g., small, large, soft, firm, or hard)?*	This differentiates between causes based on size and consistency; *small firm masses* may indicate lymph nodes, *soft compressible masses* may suggest cysts, and *large hard masses* could point to neoplasms or abscesses.
Pain and tenderness	*Is the mass painful or tender when touched?*	A *painful or tender mass* suggests an infectious or inflammatory process, while a *nontender mass* may indicate a neoplastic or congenital etiology.
Associated symptoms	*Have you experienced any recent infections, weight loss, difficulty swallowing, or changes in your voice?*	Recent infections may point to reactive lymphadenopathy, while weight loss, difficulty swallowing, or voice changes might indicate a neoplastic process or compression of surrounding structures.
Medical history	*Do you have a history of head and neck cancer, radiation exposure, or a family history of thyroid disease or cancer?*	This can suggest potential causes or predisposing factors, such as recurrence, secondary malignancy, or thyroid-related issues.

Possible causes include **cervical lymphadenopathy** (enlarged lymph nodes due to infection, inflammation, or malignancy), **thyroglossal duct cyst** (remnant of thyroglossal duct that failed to regress during development, may become infected) and **head and neck cancer** (uncontrolled cell growth, often squamous cell carcinoma).

If the mass or lump is in the thyroid, possible causes include **thyroid nodule** (benign or malignant growth within thyroid gland), **thyroid cancer** (uncontrolled cell growth forming malignant tumors), and **goiter** (enlargement of the thyroid due to iodine deficiency, thyroid hormone dysfunction, or nodules).

See Table 13-1, Symptoms and Signs of Thyroid Dysfunction, p. 316.

PHYSICAL EXAMINATION: GENERAL APPROACH

An essential aspect of examining the head and neck is being familiar with your landmarks. You must know the surface anatomy and how deeper structures are positioned over the underlying skin. Proper examination requires adequate exposure of the head and neck up to the clavicles. You may need to ask patients to move or tilt their head in certain positions to examine the structures thoroughly.

Key Components of the Head and Neck Examination

- Examine the hair.
- Examine the scalp.
- Examine the skull.
- Inspect the skin on the head and face.
- Palpate the cervical lymph nodes.
- Examine the trachea.
- Inspect the thyroid gland.
- Palpate the thyroid gland: posterior approach.
- Palpate the thyroid gland: anterior approach.
- Examine the carotid arteries and jugular veins.

TECHNIQUES OF EXAMINATION

Examine the Hair

Observe hair quantity, distribution, texture, and any pattern of loss. Look for loose flakes of dandruff.

See Chapter 12, Skin, Hair, and Nails, Table 12-8, Hair Loss, pp. 287–289.

Examine the Scalp

Part the hair in several places and look for scaliness, lumps, nevi, and other lesions. To avoid missing abnormalities, inquire about any scalp issues the patient has noticed. Hairpieces and wigs should be removed to properly examine the scalp. For some individuals, wigs or hairpieces may be worn for cultural or religious reasons. In these cases, approach the issue with sensitivity and respect, and ensure the patient is comfortable and aware of their options. It may also be helpful to provide a private space for the patient to remove their wig or hairpiece, if needed.

Look for redness and scaling that may indicate seborrheic dermatitis or psoriasis, soft lumps that may be pilar cysts (wens), and pigmented nevi that raise concern of melanoma. See Table 12-6, Brown Lesions—Melanoma and Its Mimics, pp. 281–284.

Examine the Skull

Observe the general size and contour of the skull. Inspect for any deformities, depressions, lumps, or tenderness. Learn to recognize the irregularities in a normal skull, such as those near the suture lines between the parietal and occipital bones.

An enlarged skull may signify hydrocephalus or Paget disease of bone. Palpable tenderness or bony step-offs may be present after head trauma.

Inspect Facial Contours

Note the patient's facial contours. Inspect for asymmetry, involuntary movements, edema, and masses.

Inspect the Skin on the Head and Face

Inspect the skin on the face and head, noting its color, pigmentation, texture, thickness, hair distribution, and any lesions.

Acne is common in adolescents. *Hirsutism* (excessive facial hair) may appear in some individuals with polycystic ovary syndrome.

Palpate the Cervical Lymph Nodes

Gently palpate with the pads of your index and middle fingers in a rotary motion, moving the skin over underlying tissues in each area. The patient should be relaxed, with their neck slightly flexed forward and turned toward the side being examined if needed. Note that you can examine both sides at once, checking for lymph nodes and asymmetry. For submental nodes, feeling with one hand while bracing the top of the head with the other is helpful.

1. **Submental**—palpate in the midline a few centimeters behind the tip of the mandible.
2. **Submandibular**—midway between the angle and the tip of the mandible. These nodes are usually smaller and smoother than the lobulated submandibular gland against which they lie (Fig. 13-10).
3. **Parotid**—palpate in front of the ear (Fig. 13-9).
4. **Retroauricular**—palpate behind the ear and superficial to the mastoid process.
5. **Jugular**—deep in the SCM muscle and often inaccessible to examination. Hook your thumb and fingers around either side of the SCM muscle to find them.
6. **Occipital**—palpate at the base of the skull posteriorly.
7. **Anterior cervical**—palpate for these nodes in the midline between the SCM muscles and superior between the hyoid and manubrium.
8. **Posterior triangle**—palpate along the anterior edge of the trapezius by flexing the patient's neck slightly forward toward the side being examined (Fig. 13-10).
9. **Supraclavicular**—palpate deep in the angle formed by the clavicle and the SCM muscle (Fig. 13-11).

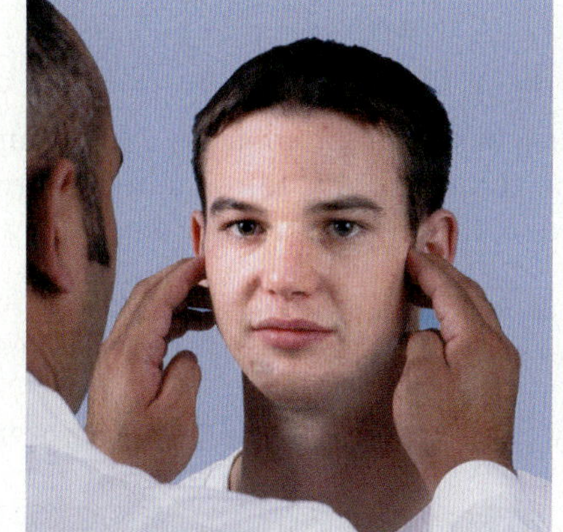

FIGURE 13-9. Palpating the parotid nodes.

A small hard tender superior jugular node, high and deep between the mandible and the SCM may be an elongated temporal styloid process or calcification of the stylohyoid ligament corresponding to Eagle's syndrome.

Enlargement of a supraclavicular node, especially on the left (**Virchow's node**), suggests possible metastasis from a thoracic or an abdominal malignancy.

Observe the size, shape, delimitation (discrete or matted together), mobility, consistency, and tenderness of the lymph nodes. Small, mobile, discrete, and nontender nodes, referred to as "*shotty*," are typically present in healthy individuals. To describe enlarged nodes, measure their maximal length and

Tender nodes suggest inflammation; hard or fixed nodes (fixed to underlying structures and not movable on palpation) suggest malignancy.

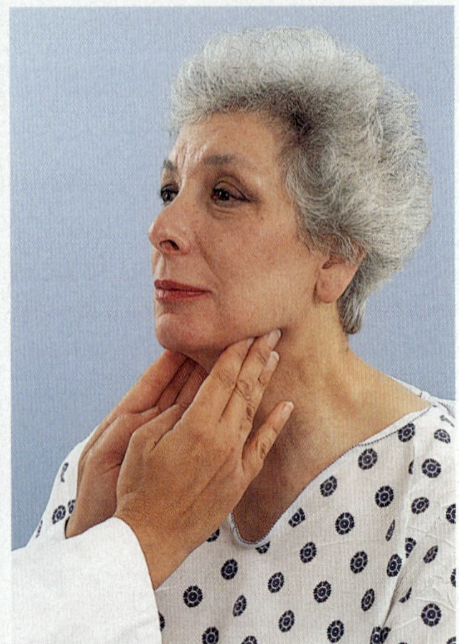

FIGURE 13-10. Palpating the submandibular nodes.

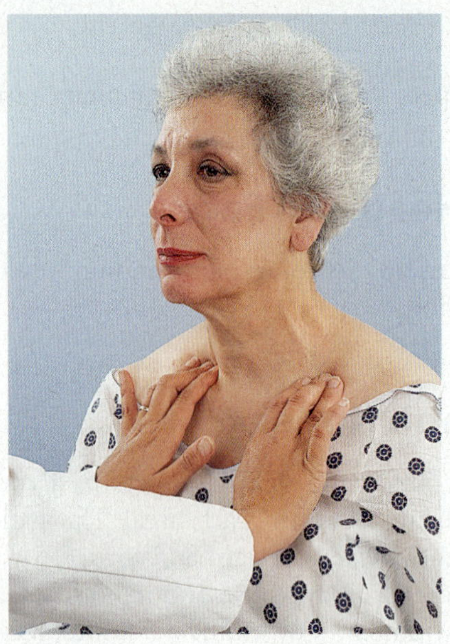

FIGURE 13-11. Palpating the supraclavicular nodes.

width in two dimensions, such as 1 cm × 2 cm. Also note any overlying skin changes like erythema, induration, drainage, or breakdown.

Enlarged or tender nodes, if unexplained, call for (1) re-examination of the regions they drain and (2) careful assessment of lymph nodes in other regions to identify regional from generalized lymphadenopathy.

Generalized lymphadenopathy is seen in multiple infectious, inflammatory, or malignant conditions such as HIV or AIDS, infectious mononucleosis, lymphoma, leukemia, and sarcoidosis.

Occasionally, you may mistake a band of muscle or an artery for a lymph node. Unlike a muscle or an artery, you should be able to roll a node in two directions: up and down and side to side. Neither a muscle nor an artery will pass this test.

Examine the Trachea

To orient yourself to the neck, identify the thyroid and cricoid cartilages and the trachea below them.

Inspect the trachea for any deviation from its usual midline position. Then palpate for any deviation. Place your finger along one side of the trachea and note the space between it and the SCM muscle (Fig. 13-12). Compare it with the other side. The spaces should be symmetric.

Masses in the neck may cause tracheal deviation to one side, raising suspicion for large thyroid masses, as well as conditions in the thorax such as a mediastinal mass, atelectasis, or a large pneumothorax.

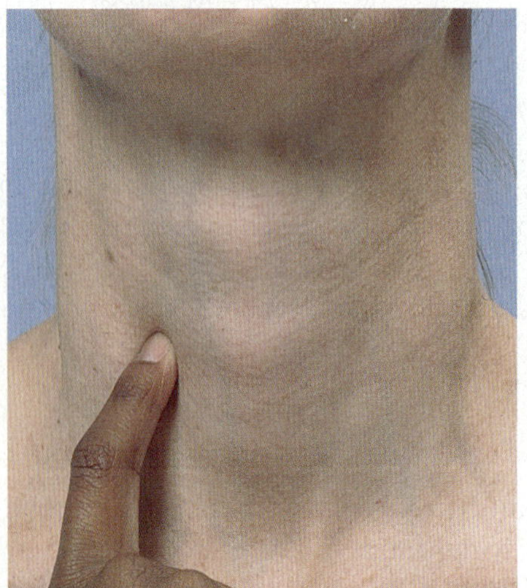

FIGURE 13-12. Palpating the trachea.

Auscultate breath sounds over the trachea. This allows subtle counting of the respiratory rate and establishes a point of reference when assessing upper versus lower airway causes of shortness of breath. When assessing shortness of breath, always remember to listen over the trachea for stridor for upper airway etiologies in addition to examining the lungs.

Stridor is an ominous, high-pitched musical sound from severe narrowing of the airway at the level of the supraglottis, the vocal cords, or the subglottis/trachea that signals a respiratory emergency. Causes include epiglottitis, tumors, foreign body, goiter, and stenosis from placement of an artificial airway.[12] See also Chapter 17, Thorax and Lungs, p. 467.

Inspect the Thyroid Gland

Inspect the thyroid gland. Tip the patient's head slightly back. Using tangential lighting directed downward from the tip of the patient's chin, inspect the region below the cricoid cartilage to identify the contours of the gland. The shadowed lower border of the thyroid glands shown in Figure 13-13 is outlined by arrows.

The patient in Figure 13-14 has a **goiter**, defined as enlargement of the thyroid gland to twice its normal size. Goiters may be simple, without nodules, or multinodular. See Table 13-2, Thyroid Enlargement and Function, p. 317.

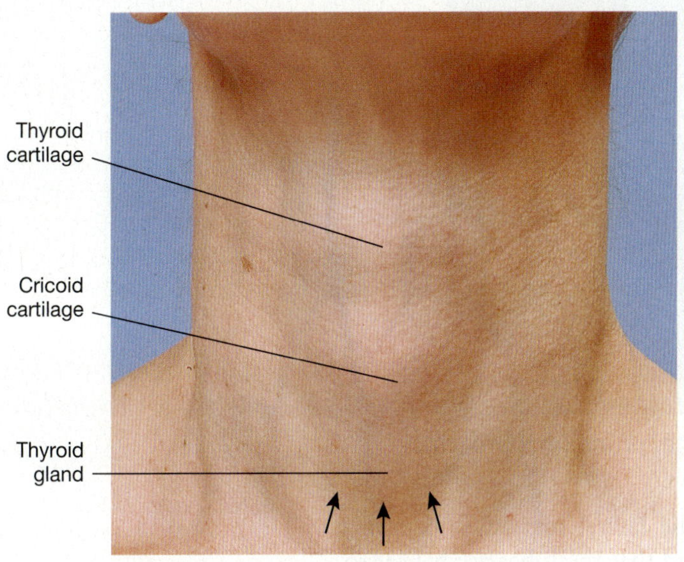

FIGURE 13-13. Thyroid gland position at rest.

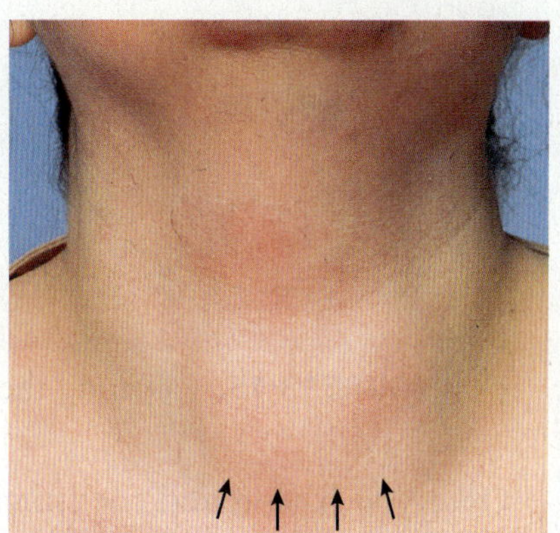

FIGURE 13-14. Thyroid gland with goiter.

Observe the patient swallowing. Ask them to sip some water and to extend the neck again and swallow. Watch for upward movement of the thyroid gland, noting its contour and symmetry. The thyroid cartilage, cricoid cartilage, and thyroid gland all rise with swallowing and then fall to their resting positions. With swallowing, the lower border of this large gland rises and looks less symmetric.

Confirm your visual observations by palpating the gland outlines as you stand facing the patient. This helps prepare you for the more systematic palpation to follow.

Palpate the Thyroid Gland: Posterior Approach

This may seem difficult at first. Use the cues from visual inspection. The thyroid gland is usually easier to palpate in a long slender neck. In shorter necks, hyperextension of the neck may be helpful. If the lower pole of the thyroid gland is not palpable, suspect a retrosternal location. If the thyroid gland is retrosternal, below the suprasternal notch, it is often not palpable.

Find your landmarks—the notched thyroid cartilage and the cricoid cartilage below it. Locate the thyroid isthmus, usually overlying the second, third, and fourth tracheal rings.

To begin the examination, position yourself behind the patient while they are seated or standing. Ask them to slightly flex their neck forward to relax the SCM muscles. Place the fingers of both hands gently on the patient's neck so that your index fingers rest just below the cricoid cartilage (Fig. 13-15). Have the patient sip and swallow water as before while you feel for the thyroid isthmus rising up under your finger pads. Although it is often palpable, it is not always so.

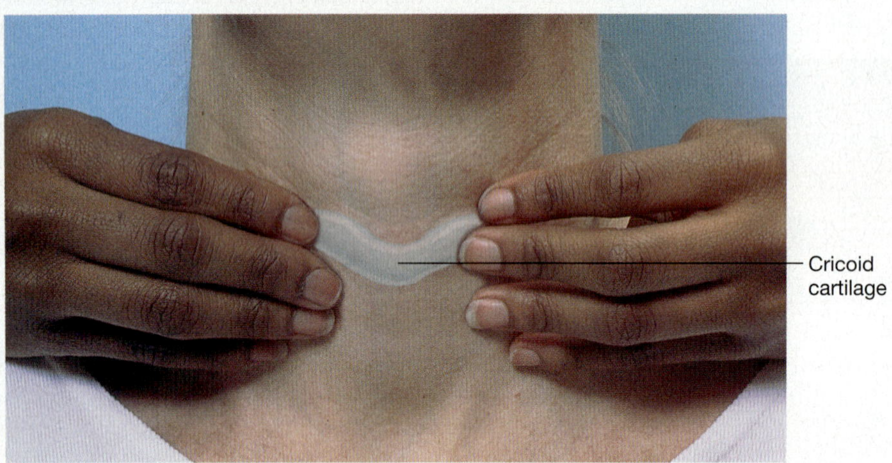

FIGURE 13-15. Palpating the thyroid gland, posterior approach.

Once you have found the isthmus, locate the lateral margin, and examine the left lobe in a similar fashion. Keep in mind that the lobes are harder to feel than the isthmus, so practice is necessary. The anterior surface of a lateral lobe is approximately the size of the distal phalanx of the thumb and feels somewhat rubbery.

To locate the right lobe of the thyroid, gently displace the trachea to the right using your left fingers, and then use the fingers of your right hand to palpate the area between the displaced trachea and the relaxed SCM muscle.

Retrosternal goiters can cause hoarseness, shortness of breath, stridor, or dysphagia from tracheal compression; neck hyperextension and arm elevation may cause flushing from compression of the thoracic inlet from the gland itself or from clavicular movement (**Pemberton's sign**). Approximately 17.5% to 32% of multinodular goiters harbor malignant thyroid cancers.[13–15]

Palpate the Thyroid Gland: Anterior Approach

During the examination, the patient should be seated or standing. To locate the thyroid isthmus, palpate the area between the cricoid cartilage and the suprasternal notch. Use one hand to gently retract the SCM muscle while using the other hand to palpate the thyroid gland. As you palpate, have the patient take a sip of water and swallow, and feel for the upward movement of the thyroid gland.

Observe the size, shape, and consistency of the thyroid gland and check for nodules or tenderness. Benign or colloid nodules tend to be uniform, ovoid structures, and are usually not fixed to surrounding tissue.

The thyroid is soft in Graves disease and may be nodular; it is firm in Hashimoto thyroiditis (though not always uniformly) and malignancy.[16]

The thyroid is tender in thyroiditis.

If the thyroid gland is enlarged, use a stethoscope to listen over the lateral lobes to detect a bruit, which is a sound similar to a cardiac murmur but is not of cardiac origin.

A localized systolic or continuous bruit may be heard in hyperthyroidism from Graves disease or toxic multinodular goiter.

Examine the Carotid Arteries and Jugular Veins

Detailed examination of the neck vessels should be deferred until the cardiovascular examination, when your patient is lying down in a supine position with their head elevated to 30°. If your patient has visible jugular venous distention in a sitting position, assess the heart and lungs promptly. In addition, be alert for unusually prominent arterial pulsations. For more information, refer to Chapter 18, Cardiovascular System, pages 492–497.

Jugular venous distention is a hallmark of heart failure.

RECORDING YOUR FINDINGS

At first, you might rely on full sentences to convey your observations; however, as you become more experienced, you will transition to using concise phrases. The following box provides phrasing styles suitable for most documentation.

Recording the Head, Eyes, Ears, Nose, and Throat (HEENT) Examination

HEENT:

Head—The skull is normocephalic/atraumatic (NC/AT). Hair with average texture.

Neck—Trachea midline. Neck supple; thyroid isthmus palpable, lobes not felt.

Lymph Nodes—No cervical adenopathy.

OR

HEENT:

Head—The skull is normocephalic/atraumatic. Frontal balding.

Neck—Trachea midline. Neck supple; thyroid isthmus midline, lobes palpable but not enlarged.

Lymph Nodes—Submandibular and anterior cervical lymph nodes tender, 1 cm × 1 cm, rubbery and mobile; no posterior cervical lymphadenopathy.

Dissecting PE documentation into comprehensive components illustrates the significant role of clinical observations in uncovering key diagnostic insights. The findings described in the PE examination note suggest a range of normal and mildly abnormal observations:

- *Head: normocephalic/atraumatic:* This indicates that the shape and size of the head are normal and without signs of recent or past injury.
- *Frontal balding:* This is a common finding and can be a normal part of aging, particularly in individuals assigned male at birth due to androgenetic alopecia (commonly known as male pattern baldness).
- *Neck: trachea midline, neck supple; thyroid isthmus midline, lobes palpable but not enlarged:* The midline position of the trachea is normal. A supple neck suggests no rigidity or muscle resistance, which is a good sign. The thyroid gland being palpable without enlargement indicates that it is detectable by touch but not abnormally large, which is generally a normal finding.
- *Lymph nodes: submandibular and anterior cervical lymph nodes tender, 1 cm × 1 cm, rubbery and mobile; no posterior cervical lymphadenopathy:* the presence of tender, rubbery, and mobile submandibular and anterior cervical lymph nodes that are about 1 cm in size can indicate a mild, likely reactive lymphadenopathy. This can be due to a variety of benign causes such as a recent infection (like a common cold or sore throat). The absence of posterior cervical lymphadenopathy is reassuring.

The patient's examination is largely normal, with the exception of mildly tender, small, and mobile lymph nodes in the submandibular and anterior cervical areas, which is most likely *benign reactive lymphadenopathy*, often seen in response to minor infections or inflammation in the region.

HEALTH PROMOTION AND COUNSELING: EVIDENCE AND RECOMMENDATIONS

Important Topics for Health Promotion and Counseling

- Screening for thyroid dysfunction
- Screening for thyroid cancer

In the following section, both traditional terms like "men," "women," "male," and "female" and inclusive terms such as "individuals assigned female at birth" and "individuals assigned male at birth" are used. This approach balances inclusivity with the need to accurately represent the original research.

Screening for Thyroid Dysfunction

Epidemiology. Thyroid dysfunction is characterized as either underactive (hypothyroidism) or overactive (hyperthyroidism) and can be either subclinical or overt. Dysfunction can be defined biochemically based on levels of thyroid-stimulating hormone (TSH) and thyroid hormones (thyroxine [T_4], triiodothyronine [T_3]). Subclinical hypothyroidism is associated with increased risk for cardiovascular disease, whereas subclinical hyperthyroidism is associated with cardiovascular mortality, atrial fibrillation, and decreased bone density.

The prevalence of subclinical hypothyroidism in the United States is estimated to be about 5% among individuals assigned female at birth and 3% among individuals assigned male at birth.[17,18] Only a small proportion is likely to progress to overt thyroid disease. The population prevalence of undiagnosed clinical hypothyroidism is estimated to be about 0.2%. The most common causes of hypothyroidism are chronic autoimmune thyroiditis and thyroid surgery. The population prevalence of subclinical hyperthyroidism is estimated to be about 2.3% in individuals assigned female at birth and 1.4% in individuals assigned male at birth; only 0.2% of the population have undiagnosed clinical hyperthyroidism. Graves disease, autoimmune thyroiditis, toxic nodules, toxic goiters, and high iodine intake can cause hyperthyroidism.

Screening. The U.S. Preventive Services Task Force (USPSTF) found no studies addressing the benefits and harms of screening with any thyroid tests for either subclinical or undiagnosed overt thyroid dysfunction.[17] They did find evidence that treating subclinical hypothyroidism was associated with a decreased risk for coronary disease events. However, they concluded that evidence was insufficient to recommend for or against screening asymptomatic nonpregnant adults (I statement).[19] The American Association of Clinical Endocrinologists/American Thyroid Association guideline advises an aggressive case-finding approach for patients with risk factors and nonspecific symptoms potentially suggesting thyroid dysfunction.[20]

Screening for Thyroid Cancer

Epidemiology. The incidence rate of thyroid cancer in the United States has nearly doubled over the past two decades, with over 43,000 cases expected to be diagnosed in 2023.[21,22] However, thyroid cancer mortality rates have remained relatively stable during this time, and only about 2,000 deaths were expected in 2023. The overall 5-year survival rate for thyroid cancer is 98.5%, ranging from 99.9% for early-stage (localized) cancers to 53.5% for distant-stage (metastatic) cancers.[22] About two-thirds of thyroid cancers are diagnosed at an early stage; only 3% are diagnosed at a distant stage. Risk factors for thyroid cancer include head and neck radiation exposure; having a first-degree relative diagnosed with thyroid cancer; and hereditary conditions such as familial medullary thyroid cancer, which may also be associated with multiple endocrine neoplasia syndrome type 2.[23] Individuals assigned female at birth are three times as likely to be diagnosed with thyroid cancer as those assigned male at birth.

Screening. The head and neck examination section describes palpating the thyroid gland to characterize glandular tissue and to identify nodules. Nodules are common findings and are usually benign; however, nodules that are ≥4 cm, firm, fixed to adjacent tissues, and associated with cervical lymphadenopathy or vocal cord paralysis are concerning for malignancy.[24] Ultrasound imaging is recommended to further evaluate thyroid nodules to determine whether biopsy is indicated. While neck palpation and ultrasound could potentially be used as thyroid cancer screening tests, the USPSTF has recommended against screening for thyroid cancer (grade D).[25] They found inadequate evidence that screening was beneficial but concluded that potential harms, related to overdiagnosis and overtreatment, were at least moderate.

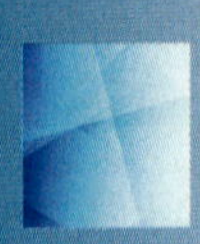

TABLE 13-1. Symptoms and Signs of Thyroid Dysfunction

	Hyperthyroidism	Hypothyroidism
Symptoms	Nervousness	Fatigue, lethargy
	Weight loss despite increased appetite	Modest weight gain with anorexia
	Excessive sweating and heat intolerance	Dry, coarse skin, and cold intolerance
	Palpitations	Swelling of face, hands, and legs
	Frequent bowel movements	Constipation
	Tremor and proximal muscle weakness	Weakness, muscle cramps, arthralgias, paresthesias, impaired memory, and hearing
Signs	Warm, smooth, moist skin	Dry, coarse, cool skin, sometimes yellowish from carotene, with nonpitting myxedema and loss of hair
	With Graves disease, eye signs such as stare, lid lag, and exophthalmos	Periorbital myxedema
	Increased systolic and decreased diastolic blood pressures	Low-pitched speech
	Tachycardia or atrial fibrillation	Decreased systolic and increased diastolic blood pressures
	Hyperdynamic cardiac pulsations with an accentuated S1	Bradycardia and, in late stages, hypothermia
	Tremor and proximal muscle weakness	Sometimes decreased intensity of heart sounds
		Prolonged relaxation phase during ankle reflex
		Impaired memory, mixed hearing loss, somnolence, peripheral neuropathy, carpal tunnel syndrome

Sources: Siminoski K. The rational clinical examination. Does this patient have a goiter? *JAMA*. 1995;273(10):813–817; McDermott MT. In the clinic. Hypothyroidism. *Ann Intern Med*. 2009;151(11):ITC61; McDermott MT. Hyperthyroidism. *Ann Intern Med*. 2012;157(1):ITC1–ITC16; Franklyn JA. Subclinical thyroid disorders–consequences and implications for treatment. *Ann Endocrinol (Paris)*. 2007;68(4):229–230.

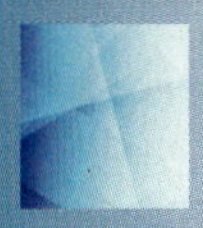

TABLE 13-2. Thyroid Enlargement and Function

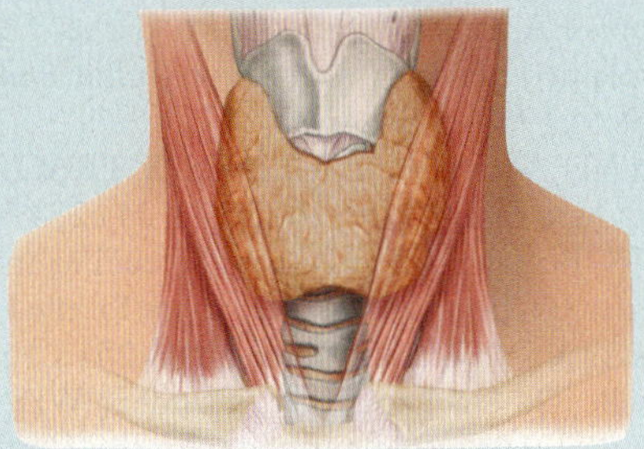

Diffuse Enlargement. Includes the isthmus and lateral lobes; there are no discretely palpable nodules. Causes include Graves disease, Hashimoto thyroiditis, and endemic goiter.

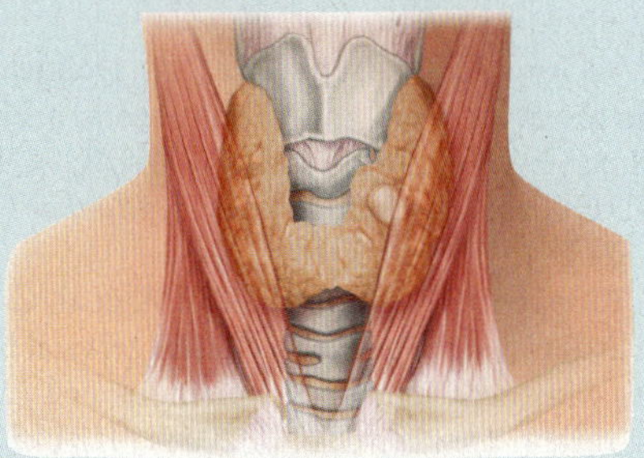

Single Nodule. May be a cyst, a benign tumor, or one nodule within a multinodular gland. It raises the question of malignancy. Risk factors are prior irradiation, hardness, rapid growth, fixation to surrounding tissues, enlarged cervical nodes, and occurrence in men.

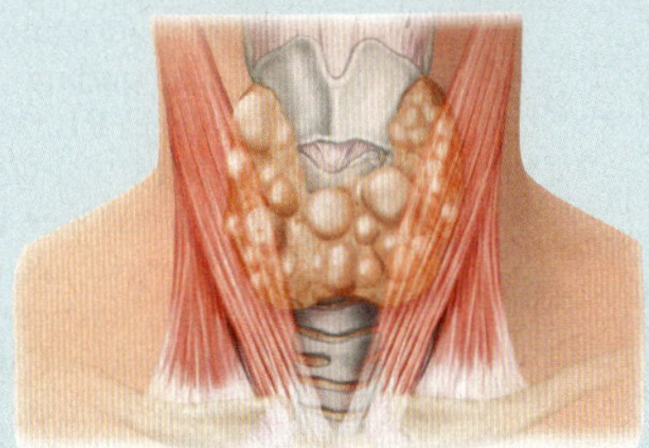

Multinodular Goiter. An enlarged thyroid gland with two or more nodules suggests a metabolic rather than a neoplastic process. Positive family history and continuing nodular enlargement are additional risk factors for malignancy.

REFERENCES

1. Norris CD, Anzai Y. Anatomy of neck muscles, spaces, and lymph nodes. *Neuroimaging Clin N Am*. © 2022 Elsevier Inc; 2022;32(4):831–849.
2. Grégoire V, Ang K, Budach W, et al. Delineation of the neck node levels for head and neck tumors: a 2013 update. DAHANCA, EORTC, HKNPCSG, NCIC CTG, NCRI, RTOG, TROG consensus guidelines. *Radiother Oncol*. 2014; 110(1):172–181.
3. Santer M, Kloppenburg M, Gottfried TM, et al. Current applications of artificial intelligence to classify cervical lymph nodes in patients with head and neck squamous cell carcinoma—a systematic review. *Cancers (Basel)*. 2022;14(21):5397.
4. Chorath K, Rajasekaran K. Evaluation and management of a neck mass. *Med Clin North Am*. © 2021 Elsevier Inc; 2021; 105(5):827–837.
5. Grani G, Sponziello M, Pecce V, Ramundo V, Durante C. Contemporary thyroid nodule evaluation and management. *J Clin Endocrinol Metab*. 2020;105(9):2869–2883.
6. Ospina NS, Papaleontiou M. Thyroid nodule evaluation and management in older adults: a review of practical considerations for clinical endocrinologists. *Endocr Pract*. 2021;27(3): 261–268.
7. Alexander EK, Cibas ES. Diagnosis of thyroid nodules. *Lancet Diabetes Endocrinol*. © 2022 Elsevier Ltd; 2022;10(7): 533–539.
8. Siminoski K. The rational clinical examination. Does this patient have a goiter? *JAMA*. 1995;273(10):813–817.
9. McDermott MT. In the clinic. Hypothyroidism. *Ann Intern Med*. 2009;151(11):ITC61.
10. McDermott MT. Hyperthyroidism. *Ann Intern Med*. 2012; 157(1):ITC1–ITC16.
11. Franklyn JA. Subclinical thyroid disorders–consequences and implications for treatment. *Ann Endocrinol (Paris)*. 2007; 68(4):229–230.
12. Pfleger A, Eber E. Assessment and causes of stridor. *Paediatr Respir Rev*. 2016;18:64–72.
13. Apostolou K, Zivaljevic V, Tausanovic K, et al. Prevalence and risk factors for thyroid cancer in patients with multinodular goitre. *BJS Open*. 2021;5(2).
14. Smith JJ, Chen X, Schneider DF, et al. Cancer after thyroidectomy: a multi-institutional experience with 1,523 patients. *J Am Coll Surg*. 2013;216(4):571–577; discussion 577–579.
15. De Filippis EA, Sabet A, Sun MRM, Garber JR. Pemberton's sign: explained nearly 70 years later. *J Clin Endocrinol Metab*. 2014;99(6):1949–1954.
16. Burman KD, Wartofsky L. CLINICAL PRACTICE. Thyroid nodules. *New Engl J Med*. 2015;373(24):2347–2356.
17. Rugge JB, Bougatsos C, Chou R. Screening and treatment of thyroid dysfunction: an evidence review for the U.S. Preventive Services Task Force. *Ann Intern Med*. 2015;162(1):35–45.
18. Hollowell JG, Staehling NW, Flanders WD, et al. Serum TSH, T(4), and thyroid antibodies in the United States population (1988 to 1994): National Health and Nutrition Examination Survey (NHANES III). *J Clin Endocrinol Metab*. 2002;87(2):489–499.
19. LeFevre ML; U. S. Preventive Services Task Force. Screening for thyroid dysfunction: U.S. Preventive Services Task Force recommendation statement. *Ann Intern Med*. 2015; 162(9):641–650.
20. Hennessey JV, Garber JR, Woeber KA, et al. American Association of Clinical Endocrinologists and American College of Endocrinology Position Statement on thyroid dysfunction case finding. *Endocr Pract*. 2016;22(2):262–270.
21. Siegel RL, Miller KD, Wagle NS, Jemal A. Cancer statistics, 2023. *CA Cancer J Clin*. 2023;73(1):17–48.
22. Surveillance E, and End Results Program. Cancer Stat Facts: Thyroid cancer. National Cancer Institute. https://seer.cancer.gov/statfacts/html/thyro.html
23. American Cancer Society. *Thyroid Cancer Risk Factors*. American Cancer Society. 2023. https://www.cancer.org/cancer/types/thyroid-cancer/causes-risks-prevention/risk-factors.html
24. Bomeli SR, LeBeau SO, Ferris RL. Evaluation of a thyroid nodule. *Otolaryngol Clin North Am*. 2010;43(2):229–238, vii.
25. Bibbins-Domingo K, Grossman DC, Curry SJ, et al. Screening for thyroid cancer: US Preventive Services Task Force Recommendation Statement. *JAMA*. 2017;317(18):1882–1887.

CHAPTER 14

Eyes

ANATOMY AND PHYSIOLOGY

Orbital Anatomy

The *eye* is positioned within a quadrilateral bony socket known as the *orbit*, which provides protection and support and optimizes the eye's functions. The *extraocular muscles (EOMs)* that stem from the orbit attach to the *sclera*, the tough white outer layer of the eyeball. Importantly, this external layer of the eye is continuous with the dura of the central nervous system.

Anterior Ocular Structures

The *iris*, a circular muscle, determines eye color and controls the amount of light entering the eye through the central aperture, the *pupil*. The *cornea*, a transparent external surface covering both the iris and the pupil, is continuous with the sclera (Figs. 14-1 and 14-2). Note that the upper eye-lid covers a portion of the iris but does not normally overlay the pupil. The opening between the eyelids is called the *palpebral fissure*.

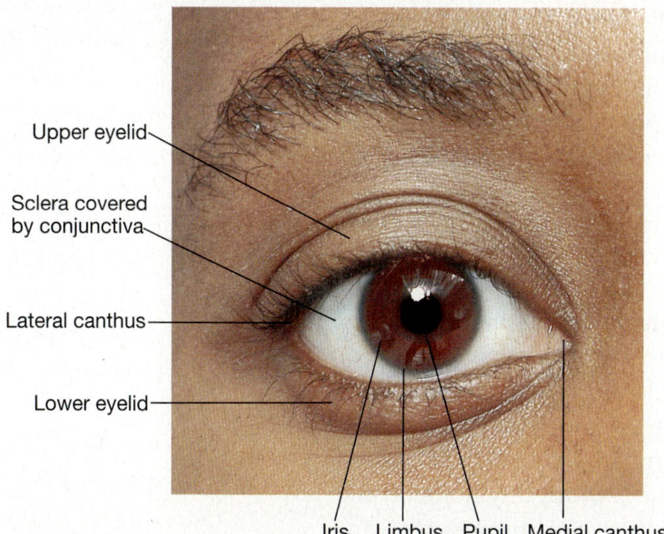

FIGURE 14-1. Surface anatomy of the eye and eyelids.

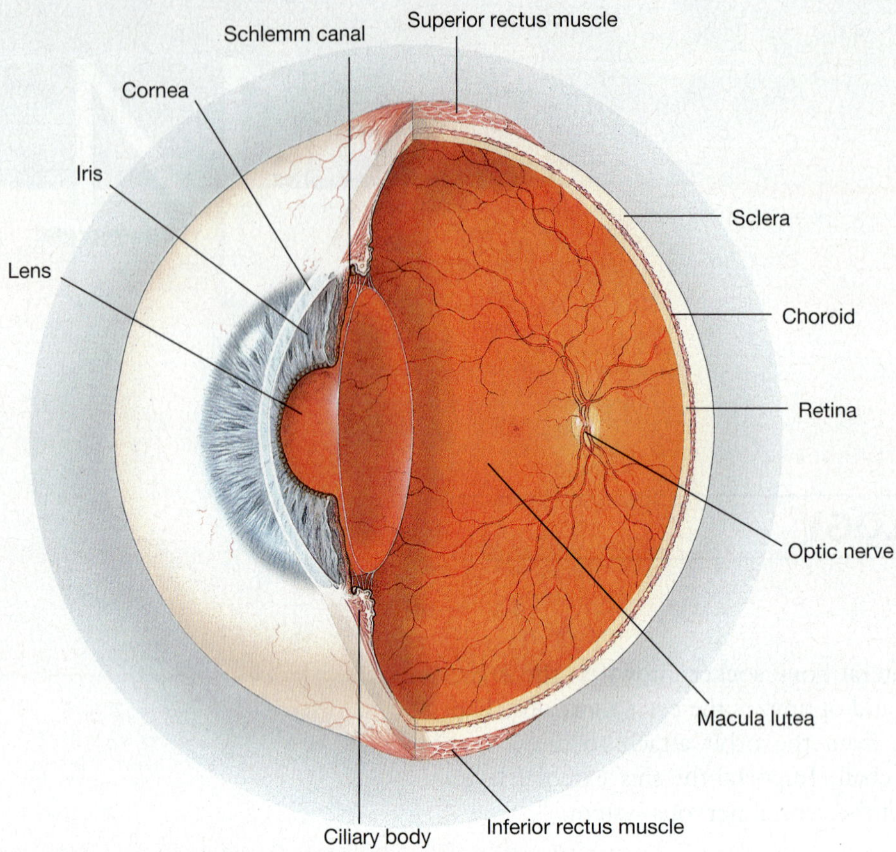

FIGURE 14-2. Normal eye, whole and cutaway views.

The *conjunctiva* is a clear, highly vascularized mucous membrane with two components: the *bulbar conjunctiva*, which covers most of the anterior eyeball and meets the cornea at the limbus, and the *palpebral conjunctiva* forms the inner lining of the eyelids. The two parts of the conjunctiva merge in a folded *fornix* that permits movement of the eyeball. The conjunctiva functions to lubricate and protect the eye.

The conjunctiva is usually transparent but can swell and become injected ("bloodshot") during times of infection, inflammation, or injury.

Tarsal plates, firm strips of connective tissue, lie along the eyelid margins and contain *meibomian glands* that provide oily lubrication to the ocular surface (Fig. 14-3). The *levator palpebrae superioris*, innervated by cranial nerve (CN) III, is the primary muscle that raises the upper eyelid, while the *Müller muscle*, innervated by the sympathetic nervous system, also contributes to lid elevation.

Lacrimal Apparatus

The *tear film* protects the conjunctiva and cornea from drying, inhibits microbial growth, and gives a smooth optical surface to the cornea. It consists of three layers: an *oily layer* from the meibomian glands, an *aqueous layer* from the lacrimal glands, and a *mucinous layer* from the conjunctival glands. The *lacrimal gland* is located in the superolateral orbit (Fig. 14-4). Tear fluid spreads across the eye and drains medially through *lacrimal puncta*, tiny holes on the superior and inferior medial eyelid margin. Tears then pass through the canaliculi into the *lacrimal sac* and on into the nose through the *nasolacrimal duct*.

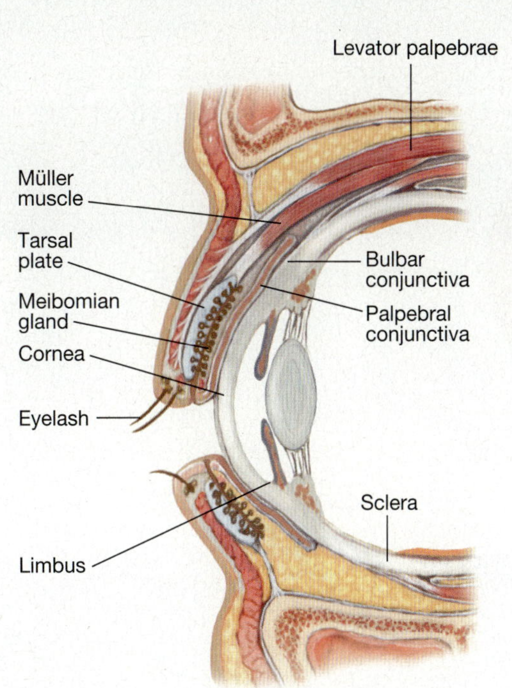

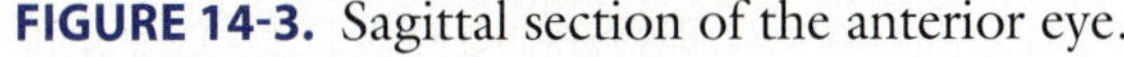

FIGURE 14-3. Sagittal section of the anterior eye.

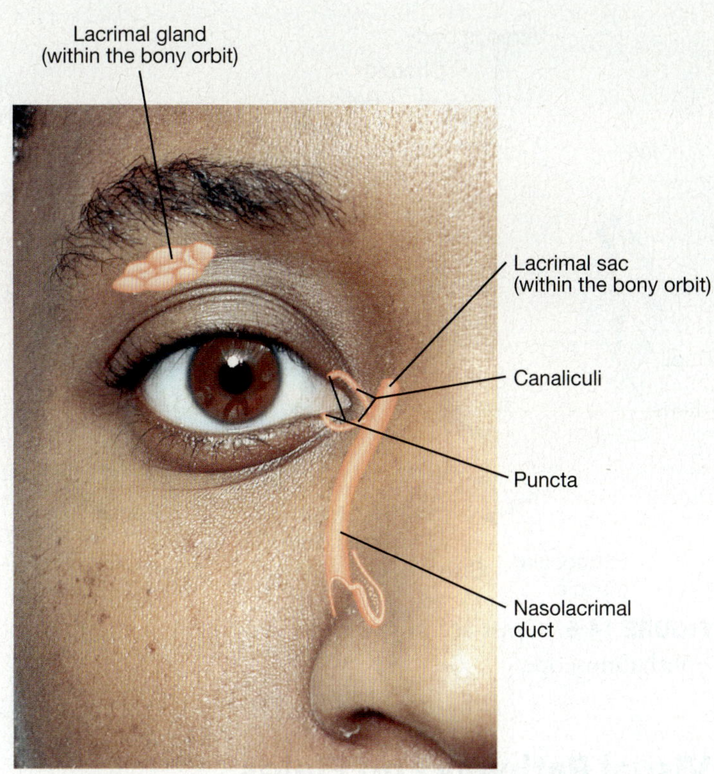

FIGURE 14-4. Lacrimal apparatus and drainage system.

Optical Structures

The *lens* is a transparent structure located behind the iris, suspended by fine ligaments called *zonule fibers*. These ligaments are controlled by muscles of the ciliary body to adjust the lens to focus on near or distant objects (*accommodation*) and project a clear image into the retina, the sensory part of the eye.

There are three fluid-filled chambers in the eye. The *anterior* and *posterior chambers*, between the cornea and iris, and between the iris and the lens, respectively, are filled with a clear liquid called the *aqueous humor*. The *vitreous chamber*, between the lens and the retina, is filled with a more viscous and gelatinous fluid, the *vitreous humor*, which helps maintain the shape of the eye. Aqueous humor is produced by the *ciliary body*, circulates from the posterior chamber through the pupil into the anterior chamber, and drains out through the *canal of Schlemm*, which helps control intraocular pressure (IOP) (Fig. 14-5).

Posterior Ocular Structures

The posterior portion of the eye visible through the ophthalmoscope is commonly called the *optic fundus* (Fig. 14-6). It includes the retina, choroid, vitreous, retinal vessels, macula, fovea, and optic disc. The *optic disc* denotes the entry point of the optic nerve and is visible with an ophthalmoscope. Lateral and slightly inferior to the disc is a small depression in the retinal surface marking the point of central vision. Around it is a darkened circular area called the *fovea*. The *macula* surrounds the fovea and lies within the flanking retinal vessels.

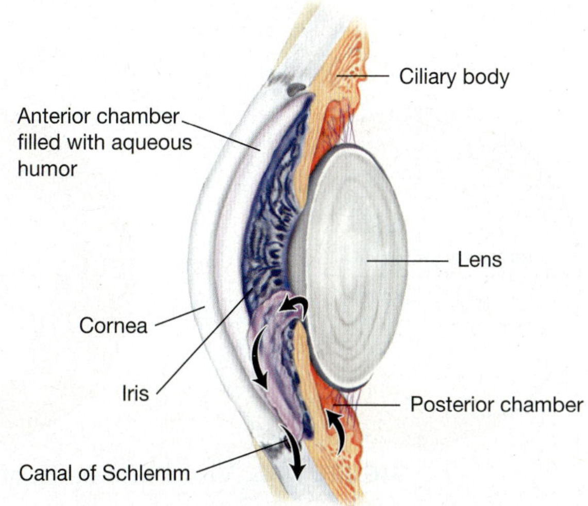

FIGURE 14-5. Circulation of aqueous humor.

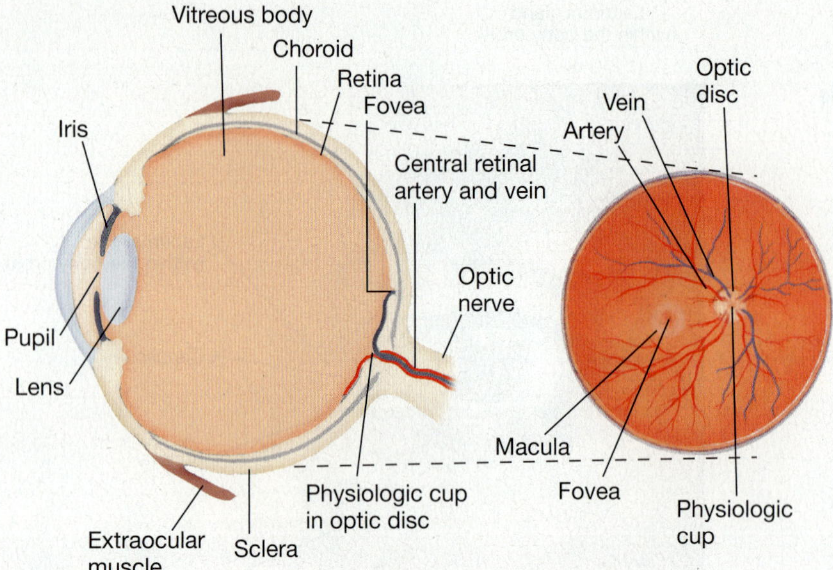

FIGURE 14-6. Cross-section of right eye showing the fundus as seen with an ophthalmoscope.

Visual Pathway and Fields

To see an image, light reflected from the target must pass through the pupil and be focused on *photoreceptors* in the retina. Nerve impulses, stimulated by light, are conducted from the retina through the *optic nerve* (CN II), *optic tract* on each side, and then on to a curving tract called the *optic radiation*. This ends in the *visual cortex*, a part of the occipital lobe.

A *visual field* is the entire area that an eye can see when focusing on a central point. To diagram visual fields, a cross is used to represent the focus of gaze, which can be divided into quadrants on a circle. The fields extend farthest on the temporal sides and are limited by the brows above, the cheeks below, and the nose medially. In the normal field of each eye, an oval blind spot is produced due to a lack of retinal receptors at the optic disc, which is located 15-degree temporal to the line of gaze. When using both eyes, the two visual fields overlap in an area of binocular vision, allowing for 3D depth perception (Fig. 14-7).

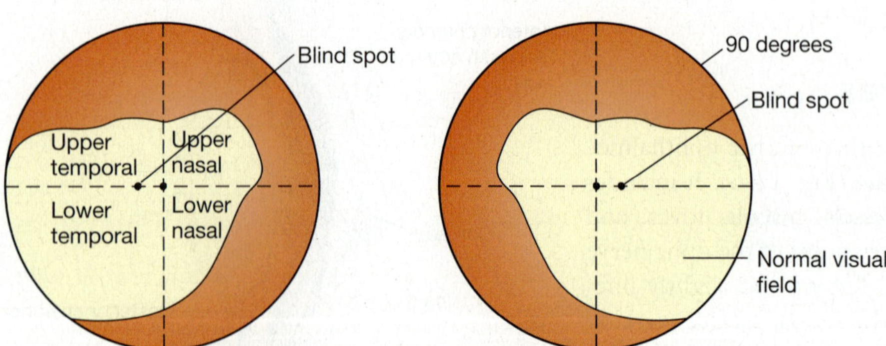

FIGURE 14-7. Visual field of left and right eyes.

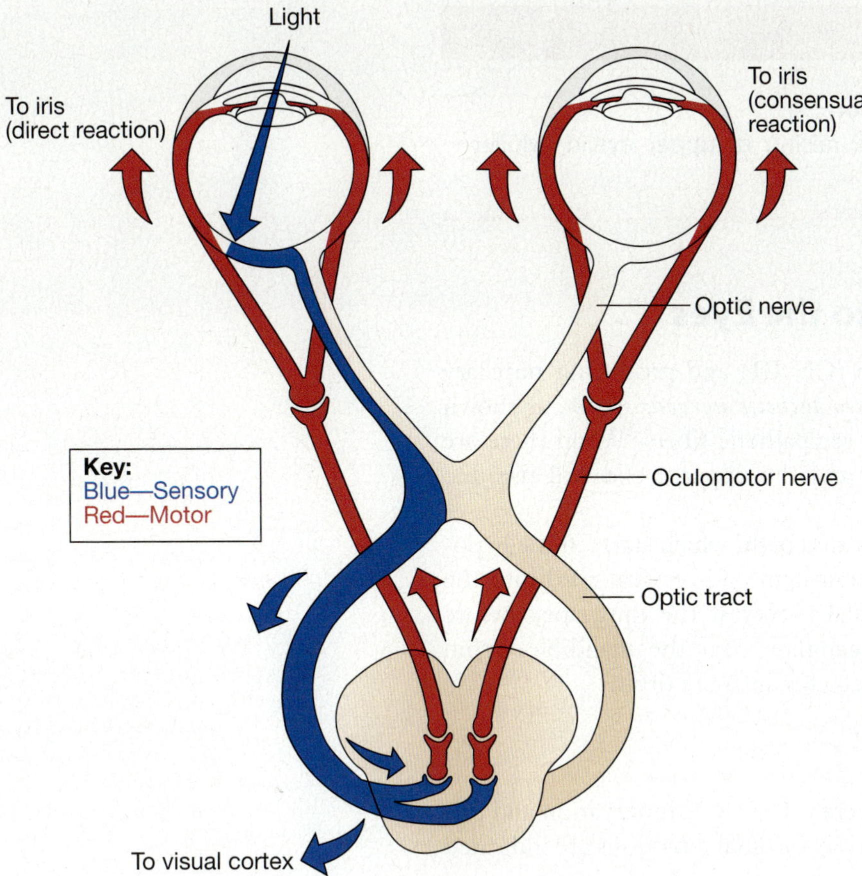

FIGURE 14-8. Pathways of the light reaction.

Visual Pathway: Pupillary Light Reaction. Pupillary size changes in response to light. A light beam shining onto one retina causes pupillary constriction in that eye, termed the *direct* reaction to light, and in the contralateral eye, the *consensual* reaction to light. The initial sensory pathways are similar to those described for vision: retina, optic nerve (CN II), and optic tract, which diverges in the midbrain. Motor impulses back to the constrictor muscles of the iris of each eye are transmitted through both oculomotor nerves (CN III) (Fig. 14-8).

Visual Pathway: Pupillary Near Reaction. Pupillary size also changes due to the effort of focusing on a near object. When a person shifts gaze from a far object to a near object, the pupils constrict (Fig. 14-9). This response, like the light reaction, is mediated by the oculomotor nerve (CN III). Coincident with this pupillary constriction, but not part of it, are (1) convergence of the eyes, a bilateral medial rectus movement; and (2) accommodation, an increased convexity of the lenses caused by contraction of the ciliary muscles. In accommodation, the change in shape of the lenses brings near objects into focus; physically, this takes place behind the iris and is not visible to the examiner.

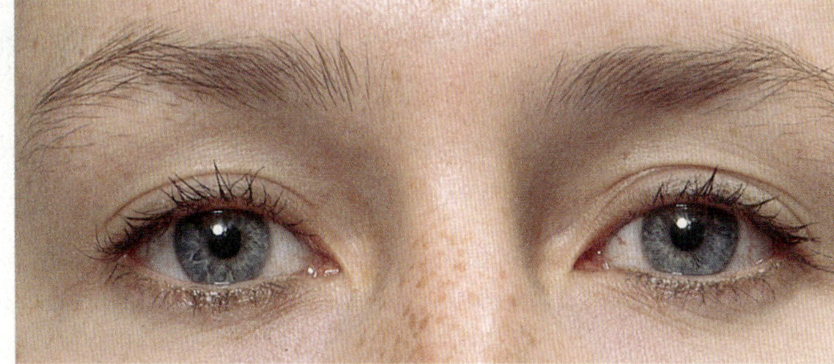

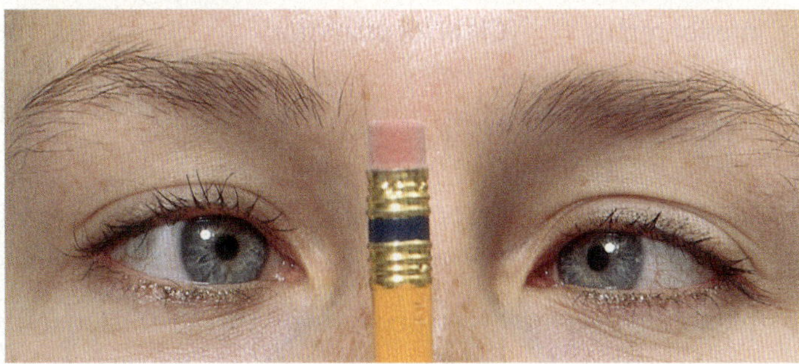

FIGURE 14-9. Pupils constrict when focus shifts to a close object.

Box 14-1. Autonomic Stimulation

- Parasympathetics: Pupillary constriction
- Sympathetics: Pupillary dilation and raising of upper eyelid (Müller muscle)

Autonomic Nerve Supply to the Eyes

Fibers traveling in the oculomotor nerve (CN III) and producing pupillary constriction (*miosis*) are part of the *parasympathetic nervous system*, as shown in Box 14-1. The iris is also supplied by sympathetic fibers. When these are stimulated, the pupil dilates (*mydriasis*), and the upper eyelid will rise due to stimulation of the Müller muscle.

The *sympathetic pathway* takes a complicated path, which starts in the hypothalamus and passes down through the brainstem and cervical cord into the neck. The neurons travel with the brachial plexus at the lung apex before returning back to the superior cervical ganglion near the mandible. From there, it follows the carotid artery or its branches into the orbit.

Extraocular Muscles

The EOMs are responsible for eye movements. Their CN innervation and primary actions are outlined in Box 14-2. The six cardinal directions are indicated by the lines in Figure 14-10.

Box 14-2. Extraocular Muscles, Innervation, and Primary Actions

Extraocular Muscle	Innervation	Primary Action
Medial rectus	Cranial nerve (CN) III (oculomotor nerve)	Adduction (inward movement)
Lateral rectus	CN VI (abducens nerve)	Abduction (outward movement)
Superior rectus	CN III (oculomotor nerve)	Elevation (upward movement) and intorsion (inward rotation), assists in adduction
Inferior rectus	CN III (oculomotor nerve)	Depression (downward movement), extorsion (outward rotation), assists in adduction
Superior oblique	CN IV (trochlear nerve)	Intorsion (inward rotation), depression and abduction
Inferior oblique	CN III (oculomotor nerve)	Extorsion (outward rotation), elevation and abduction

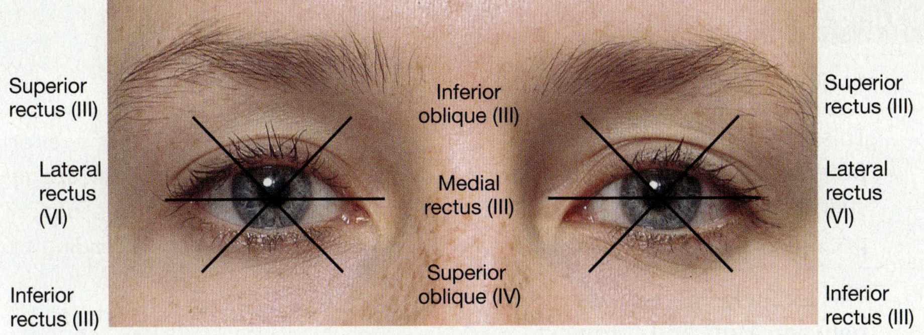

FIGURE 14-10. Cardinal directions of gaze, extraocular muscles, and their cranial nerve innervation.

In each position of gaze, a muscle of one eye is coupled (*yoked*) with a muscle of the other eye for conjugate gaze in a certain direction. If one of these muscles is paralyzed, the eye will deviate from its normal position in that direction of gaze, and the eyes will no longer appear conjugate, or parallel.

Nerve damage or injury to the muscle, due to head trauma, congenital causes, or central lesions, can cause aberrations in this yoked system and lead to *diplopia* (double vision).

HEALTH HISTORY: GENERAL APPROACH

Our visual system allows us to see and interact with the outside world, and changes in the eyes or vision can reflect our overall health. A thorough ophthalmologic history can provide important clues for generating a differential diagnosis and prompt further diagnostic work-up or a comprehensive neurologic examination. During the ophthalmologic history, start with general questions about vision and ocular function, then focus on specific areas of concern.

Common or Concerning Symptoms

- Blurred vision
- Eye redness or pain

Blurred Vision

Blurred vision refers to a loss of sharpness or clarity in vision, making objects appear hazy or out of focus. It can occur in one or both eyes and may be temporary or persistent. Box 14-3 guides you through high-yield questions for patients presenting with this condition.

Box 14-3. Blurred Vision: High-Yield Health History Questions

Domain	Questions	Rationale
Medical history	*Have you had any recent head injuries, infections, or surgeries?*	This can help narrow down potential causes of blurred vision, such as increased intraocular pressure or corneal damage.
Symptom onset	*When did your blurred vision begin, and was it sudden or gradual?*	This can help differentiate between acute and chronic conditions, such as retinal detachment (sudden) or cataracts (gradual).
Associated symptoms	*Are you experiencing any eye pain, redness, tearing, floaters, or light sensitivity?*	This can help identify potential causes, such as uveitis (eye pain and redness), retinal detachment (floaters), or corneal abrasion (sharp pain, tearing, and light sensitivity).
Medical conditions	*Do you have a history of diabetes, hypertension, or any autoimmune diseases?*	Certain medical conditions are known to affect vision, such as diabetic retinopathy (diabetes), hypertensive retinopathy (hypertension), or optic neuritis (autoimmune diseases like multiple sclerosis).
Medications	*Are you taking any medications, including over-the-counter or herbal remedies?*	Some medications can cause blurred vision as a side effect, such as corticosteroids or anticholinergic drugs.
Ocular history	*Have you had any previous eye problems or surgeries? Do you wear glasses or contact lenses?*	A history of ocular problems or surgeries may indicate a recurrence or complication, while the use of glasses or contact lenses may suggest refractive errors or poor lens hygiene as possible causes.

Possible causes include **dry eye** or **corneal issues**, **error of refraction** (mismatch between the eye's optical power and its axial length, leading to improperly focused images on the retina), **glaucoma** (increased intraocular pressure causing damage to the optic nerve), **macular degeneration** (age-related degeneration of the macula, the central part of the retina), **hypertensive retinopathy** (retinal damage due to chronic high blood pressure), **diabetic retinopathy** (retinal damage due to chronic high blood sugar levels), and **cataracts** (clouding of the lens in the eye, leading to impaired vision).

Common problems include **refractive errors** (like nearsightedness, farsightedness, and astigmatism, in which the eye does not focus light correctly), **age-related issues** (such as cataracts, which cloud the lens, and macular degeneration, affecting the central part of the retina), **diabetic retinopathy** (damages the retina's blood vessels leading to blurred vision), **glaucoma** (increase in eye pressure damaging the optic nerve), and **temporary conditions** like dry eyes or eye infections.

Eye Redness or Pain

Eye redness, also known as *conjunctival injection* or red eye, is a common condition in which the sclera (white part) of the eye appears red or pink due to dilation of the blood vessels on the surface of the eye. It is important to ask questions that can elicit the possible causes (Box 14-4).

Box 14-4. Eye Redness or Pain: High-Yield Health History Questions

Domain	Questions	Rationale
Onset and duration	*When did the eye redness or pain begin, and how long has it been going on?*	This can help narrow down the differential diagnosis, as certain conditions present with acute onset (e.g., conjunctivitis), while others develop more gradually (e.g., dry-eye syndrome).
Associated symptoms	*Are there any other symptoms accompanying the eye redness or pain, such as discharge, itching, or vision changes?*	Discharge may indicate infection, itching may suggest allergy, and chronic vision changes could signify a more serious condition like glaucoma or uveitis.
Exacerbating and relieving factors	*What factors, if any, worsen or improve the eye redness or pain?*	Worsening with light exposure may suggest uveitis, while relief with artificial tears could point toward dry-eye syndrome.
Medical history	*Do you have a history of any eye conditions or systemic diseases that may affect the eyes?*	Certain systemic diseases (e.g., diabetes, rheumatoid arthritis) and previous eye conditions can predispose individuals to eye redness or pain.
Environmental and lifestyle factors	*Have you been exposed to any new environments, allergens, or chemicals? Have you recently changed your contact lens habits or started using new eye products?*	Exposure to allergens or irritants, changes in contact lens habits, or new eye products may suggest a cause such as allergic conjunctivitis or contact–lens-related problems.
Trauma or infection	*Have you experienced any recent eye trauma or been exposed to someone with an eye infection?*	A history of eye trauma can lead to various conditions causing eye redness or pain, such as a corneal abrasion or hyphema; subconjunctival hemorrhage is common and painless; sick contacts raise the possibility of contagious causes like viral or bacterial conjunctivitis.

Possible causes include **conjunctivitis** (inflammation of the conjunctiva due to infection or allergy), **acute glaucoma** (increased intraocular pressure damaging optic nerve), **subconjunctival hemorrhage** (blood vessel rupture in conjunctiva, causing blood accumulation), and **corneal ulcers** (infection or inflammation causing corneal damage). Causes include **conjunctivitis** (inflammation of the eye's outer layer and eyelids) often leads to redness and irritation.

Allergic reactions (immune responses to allergens causing inflammation) typically cause redness, itching, and tearing, **dry-eye syndrome** (condition in which the eyes do not produce enough or good quality tears) results in redness and a gritty sensation, **uveitis** (inflammation within the eye), and **corneal abrasions** (scratches on the cornea, the eye's outer layer) are painful and cause redness. Redness and discomfort can also arise from **foreign objects** in the eye or **extended wear of contact lenses**.

See Table 14-1, Red Eyes, pp. 346–347.

PHYSICAL EXAMINATION: GENERAL APPROACH

When you are starting your ophthalmologic examination, remember that keen observation and a deep understanding of normal physiology are vital. The eyes can be windows into systemic health, and examining them can hint at underlying systemic diseases. Especially in nonverbal patients, an eye exam can shed light on aspects of the neurologic system, hidden intoxications, metabolic imbalances, and even life-threatening infections. There is a lot to cover in this exam, so approaching it systematically is key. As you progress in your studies, you will find that the most insightful ophthalmologic examinations come from meticulous observation and thorough documentation. Keep this in mind as you refine your skills.

Key Components of the Ophthalmologic Examination

- Test visual acuity
- Assess visual fields
- Test color vision and contrast sensitivity
- Assess eye position and alignment
- Inspect the eyebrows
- Inspect the eyelids and eyelashes
- Assess the lacrimal apparatus
- Inspect the conjunctivae and sclerae
- Inspect the cornea, iris, and lens
- Inspect the pupils
- Assess the pupillary light reactions
- Assess the pupillary near reaction
- Assess conjugate movements
- Test extraocular muscle movements
- Test for convergence
- Perform a funduscopic examination (direct ophthalmoscopy)

TECHNIQUES OF EXAMINATION

Test Visual Acuity

Test the acuity of central vision by using a *Snellen eye chart* in a well-lit area, if possible. Position your patient 20 ft from the chart and have them wear their glasses if they use them other than for reading. Ask your patient to cover one eye with a card to prevent peeking, and to read the smallest line of print possible. Encouraging them to attempt the next line may improve their performance. If your patient cannot read the largest letter, move them closer to the chart and note the intervening distance. Record the smallest line of print where your patient can identify more than half of the letters and the corresponding visual acuity, along with use of glasses, if any.

See Snellen eye chart in Chapter 4, Physical Examination, p. 69.

For patients who cannot identify the English alphabet, other options to test vision include *tumbling "E's,"* in which the patient points to the direction of the open face of the letter "E," and *Allen cards*, which display standardized pictures that can be recognized by children age >2 years.

Visual acuity is expressed as two numbers (e.g., 20/30): the first indicates the distance of the patient from the chart, and the second, the distance at which a normal eye can read the line of letters.[1] Vision of 20/200 means that, at 20 ft, the patient can read print that a person with normal vision could read at 200 ft. The larger the second number, the worse the vision. "20/40 corrected" means the patient could read the 20/40 line with glasses (a correction).

Myopia (near-sightedness) causes focusing problems for distance vision, whereas **hyperopia** (farsightedness) describes eyesight that is blurry for objects up close. **Astigmatism** is an imperfection of the cornea or lens causing distortion while looking at near and far objects (Fig. 14-11).

Testing near vision with a handheld card can help identify the need for reading glasses (*"readers," bifocals,* or *progressive lenses*) in patients older than age 45 years. You can also use this card to test visual acuity at the bedside. With proper correction and held 14 inches from the patient's eyes, the card simulates a Snellen chart.

Presbyopia causes focusing problems for near vision, found in middle-aged and older adults. A person with presbyopia often sees better when the card is farther away.

If you have no charts, screen visual acuity with any available print. If patients cannot read even the largest letters, test their ability to count your raised fingers, detect direction of hand motion, and distinguish light (such as a flashlight or penlight) from dark.

In the United States, an individual is typically deemed *legally blind* if their vision in the better eye, even with corrective glasses, is 20/200 or worse. Additionally, having a restricted field of vision, measuring 20 degrees or narrower in the better eye, can also qualify as legal blindness.

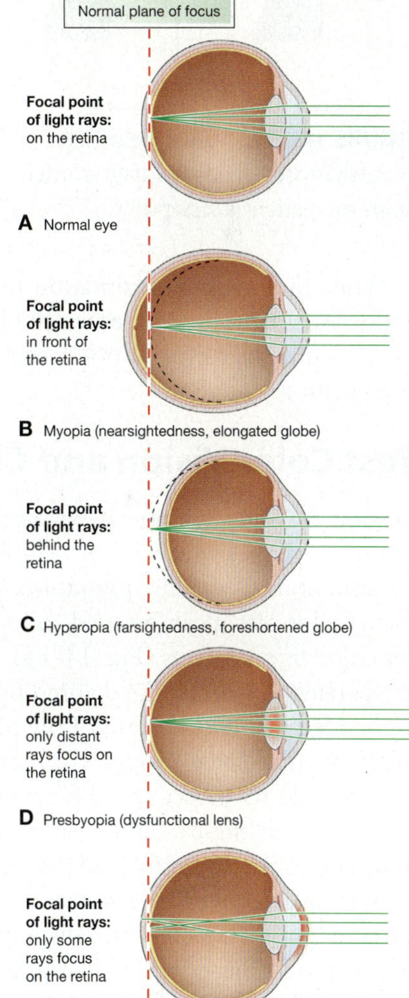

FIGURE 14-11. Refractive disorders. (Reprinted with permission from McConnell TH. *The Nature of Disease: Pathology for the Health Professions.* 2nd ed. Wolters Kluwer Health/ Lippincott Williams & Wilkins; 2014. Figure 20-6.)

Assess Visual Fields

Finger confrontation testing is a valuable screening technique for detection of lesions in the anterior and posterior visual pathway.

Position yourself in front of the patient and about an arm's length away. Close one of your eyes and have the patient cover the opposite eye while staring at your open eye. For example, when you close your left eye, you should have the patient cover their right eye to test the visual field of the patient's uncovered left eye. Place your hands about 2 ft apart out of the patient's view, roughly lateral to the patient's ears (Fig. 14-12).

While in this position, wiggle your fingers and slowly bring your moving fingers forward into the patient's center of view. Ask the patient to tell you as soon as they see your finger movement. Test each quadrant systematically. Test each eye individually and record the extent of visits in each area. Note any abnormal "*field cuts*" (Figs. 14-13A and 14-13B).

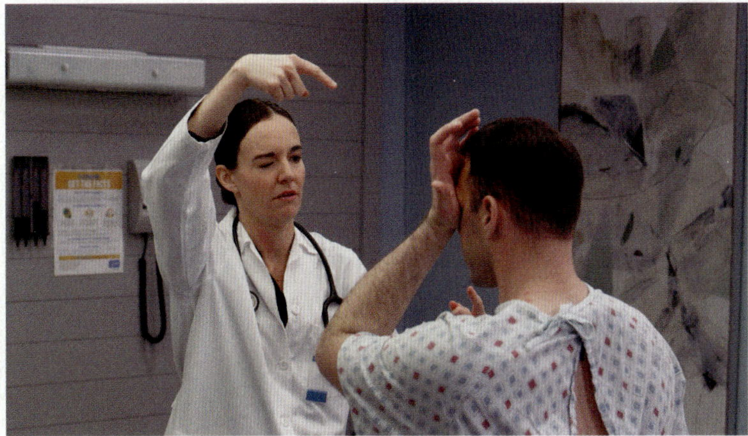

FIGURE 14-12. Testing the visual fields.

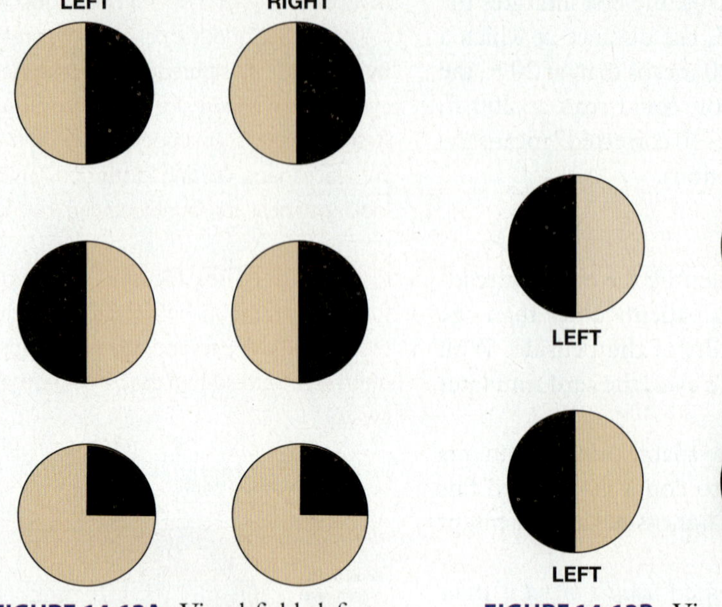

FIGURE 14-13A. Visual field defects. Note that visual fields are diagrammed from the patient's viewpoint.

FIGURE 14-13B. Visual field defects in a patient with left homonymous hemianopsia.

While the finger confrontation test can be useful for a quick assessment of gross visual field defects, especially in settings where more specialized equipment is unavailable, it is not a replacement for a comprehensive visual field examination.

Review these patterns in Table 14-2, Visual Field Defects, p. 348.

Test Color Vision and Contrast Sensitivity

Testing for *color vision* can be particularly helpful in ruling out damage to the optic nerve, which often exhibits red-green color deficits and red color desaturation. Generally, pseudoisochromatic color plates can be used to screen for color vision defects (Fig. 14-14). Ask the patient to identify the colored figure embedded in a background of the plate. With normal color vision, the patient will be able to detect the difference in hue between figure and background and, as a result, can easily read the figure.

Persons with defective color vision may fail to distinguish between figure and background colors in a pseudoisochromatic test and hence fail to read the figures.

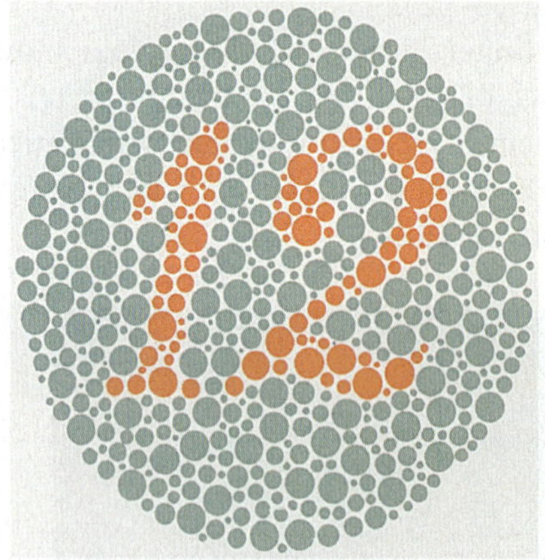

FIGURE 14-14. Pseudoisochromatic color plate for assessing color vision. (Reprinted with permission from Savino PJ, Danesh-Meyer HV. *Wills Eye Hospital Color Atlas & Synopsis of Clinical Ophthalmology: Neuro-Ophthalmology.* 3rd ed. Wolters Kluwer; 2019. Figure 1-3B.)

Testing for *contrast sensitivity* measures a person's ability to distinguish between an object and its background, based on the degree of contrast between them. This test is particularly important for detecting early changes in vision, especially in conditions like cataracts, glaucoma, and macular degeneration.

Though the most commonly recognized color vision abnormalities are sex-linked congenital red-green deficiencies, other color vision and contrast sensitivity anomalies can reflect acute or chronic optic nerve or retinal disease.

A method for testing contrast sensitivity is to have the patient observe a bright red object (e.g., a pen cap or a bottle cap). After alternating cover of the right and left eye, you can ask the patient if the color saturation is equal in both eyes. If the color is less saturated in one of the eyes, you can ask the patient to describe what percent brightness the less saturated color would be in comparison to the full-color saturation observed in the contralateral eye.

Assess Eye Position and Alignment

Stand in front of the patient and survey their eyes for position and alignment. If one or both eyes seems to protrude, have the patient look up and assess the axial projection of their eyes from below, looking up from the nostrils in a "worm's eye view" using other facial landmarks as a guide.

Abnormalities in eye movements include **esotropia** (inward deviation), **exotropia** (outward deviation), **hypertropia** (upward deviation), and **hypotropia** (downward deviation).

Hyper- or hypoglobus may refer to deviation in the globe position, which may result from congenital abnormalities, lacrimal gland enlargement, mucocele, fractures, or ocular tumors.

Abnormal protrusion or **proptosis** may be due to thyroid eye disease, congenital abnormalities, orbital infections, or ocular tumors.

Inspect the Eyebrows

Inspect the eyebrows, noting their fullness, hair distribution, tumors, and any underlying skin changes.

Scaliness occurs in seborrheic dermatitis, lateral sparseness in hypothyroidism.

Inspect the Eyelids and Eyelashes

Inspect the height of the *palpebral fissures*, or the opening between the eyelids, as well as any edema, or swelling, of the lids. The color of the lids should also be noted as well as any lesions or abnormalities that may be present. Another important aspect of eyelid examination is the condition and direction of the eyelashes. Any abnormalities or changes in the direction of the eyelashes could indicate an underlying problem. In addition, assess the adequacy of eyelid closure, especially if the eyes are unusually prominent or when there is facial paralysis.

See Table 14-3, Variations and Abnormalities of the Eyelids, p. 349.

Inspect the Lacrimal Apparatus

Briefly and gently inspect the regions of the lacrimal gland and lacrimal sac. First observe the height of the tear lake. Shine your light source toward the medial canthus of the eyelids. This will allow you to see where the lacrimal puncta are located. Observe the puncta for signs of swelling, inflammation, or discharge.

See Table 14-4, Lumps and Swellings in and Around the Eyes, p. 350.

Excessive tearing may be from increased production, caused by conjunctival inflammation or corneal irritation, or impaired drainage, caused by ectropion (p. 349) and/or obstruction of the nasolacrimal system. Dryness from impaired secretion is seen in Sjögren syndrome.

Inspect the Conjunctivae and Sclerae

Ask the patient to look up as you gently retract their lower lid with your thumbs, exposing the sclera and conjunctiva (Fig. 14-15). Inspect for color and the vascular pattern against the white scleral background. The slight vascularity of the sclera in Figure 14-15 is normal and present in most people. Look for any nodules or swelling (*chemosis*). If you need a fuller view of the eye, rest your thumb and finger on the bones of the cheek and brow, respectively, and spread the lids. Ask the patient to look to each side and down to examine the upper and lower conjunctival fornices. This technique gives you a good view of the sclera and bulbar conjunctiva but not of the palpebral conjunctiva of the upper lid. For this, you need to evert the lid (see pp. 340–341). Jaundice is shown in Figure 14-16.

See Table 14-1, Red Eyes, pp. 346–347.

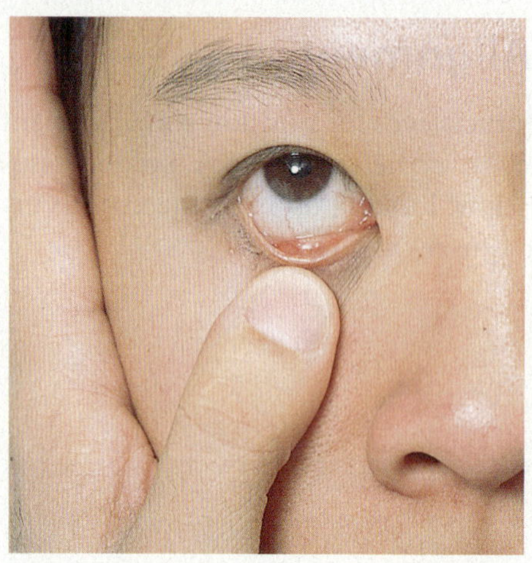

FIGURE 14-15. Inspecting the sclera and conjunctiva.

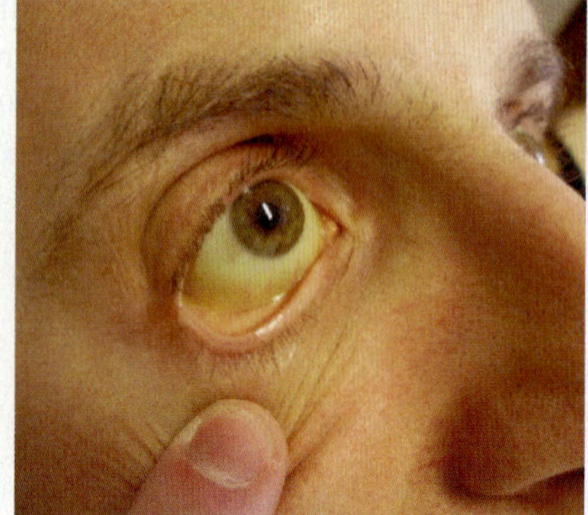

FIGURE 14-16. Yellowish discoloration of the sclera indicating jaundice. (Reprinted with permission from Weksler BB, Schechter GP, Ely S. *Wintrobe's Atlas of Clinical Hematology*. 2nd ed. Wolters Kluwer; 2018. Figure 3-61A.)

Inspect the Cornea, Iris, and Lens

With oblique lighting, inspect the cornea of each eye for opacities. It should appear clear, providing a clear view of the iris underneath. At the same time, inspect each iris, which is the colored ring of the eye underneath the cornea. The markings should be clearly defined.

Standing about 2 ft directly in front of the patient, shine a light into the patient's eyes and ask the patient to look at it. Inspect the light reflection in the corneas. Note any opacities in the lens that may be visible through the pupil.

See Table 14-5, Opacities of the Cornea and Lens, p. 351.

Inspect the Pupils

In dim light, inspect the size, shape, and symmetry of both pupils. Measure the pupils with a card showing black circles of varying sizes, and test the light reaction. Note if the pupils are large (>5 mm), small (<3 mm), or unequal (Fig. 14-17). *Miosis* refers to constriction of the pupils, *mydriasis* to dilation.

Simple *anisocoria*, or a difference in pupillary diameter ≥0.4 mm without a known pathologic cause, can be visible in approximately 20% of healthy people, although it rarely exceeds 1 mm.[2] Simple anisocoria is considered benign if it is equal in dim and bright light, and brisk pupillary constriction to light (the light reaction) occurs.

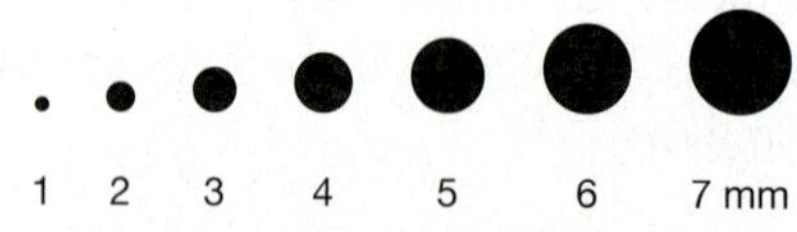

FIGURE 14-17. Pupillary sizes.

Compare benign anisocoria with Horner syndrome, oculomotor nerve paralysis, and tonic pupil. See Table 14-6, Pupillary Abnormalities, p. 352.

Assess the Pupillary Light Reactions

In dim light, test the pupillary reaction to light. Ask the patient to look into the distance, and shine a bright light obliquely into each pupil in turn.

Both the distant gaze and the oblique lighting help to prevent a near reaction. Look for:

- The *direct reaction* (pupillary constriction in the same eye)
- The *consensual reaction* (pupillary constriction in the opposite eye)

Always darken the room and use a bright light before deciding that a light reaction is abnormal or absent.

Assess the Pupillary Near Reaction

If the reaction to light is impaired or questionable, test the near reaction in both dim and normal light. Testing one eye at a time makes it easier to concentrate on pupillary responses, without the distraction of EOMs. Hold your finger or pencil about 10 cm from the patient's eye. Ask the patient to look alternately at it and into the distance directly behind it. Watch for pupillary constriction with near effort and convergence of the eyes. The third component of the near reaction, accommodation of the lens that brings the near object into focus, is not visible.

Testing the near reaction is helpful in diagnosing Argyll Robertson, tonic (Adie) pupils, and other neurologic syndromes (see p. 352).

See Table 14-6, Pupillary Abnormalities, p. 352.

Assess Conjugate Movements

The EOMs should be assessed for normal conjugate movements of the eyes in each direction. Any deviation from normal, such as *strabismus* or *dysconjugate* gaze, should be noted. *Nystagmus*, a fine rhythmic oscillation of the eyes, should also be checked. A few beats of nystagmus on extreme lateral gaze are normal, but, if this is observed, bring your finger into within the field of binocular vision and look again.

See Table 14-7, Dysconjugate Gaze, p. 353.

Sustained nystagmus within the binocular field of gaze is seen in congenital disorders, labyrinthitis, cerebellar disorders, and drug toxicity. See Table 27-10, Nystagmus, pp. 984–985.

Assess for *lid lag*. Ask the patient to follow your finger again as you move it slowly from up to down in the midline. The upper eyelid should overlap the iris slightly throughout this movement, as shown in Figure 14-18.

Note the rim of sclera from proptosis, an abnormal protrusion of the eyeballs in hyperthyroidism, leading to a characteristic "stare" on frontal gaze. If unilateral, consider Graves' disease, an orbital tumor, or retrobulbar hemorrhage from trauma.

In the lid lag of Graves disease, a rim of sclera is visible above the iris with downward gaze (Fig. 14-19).

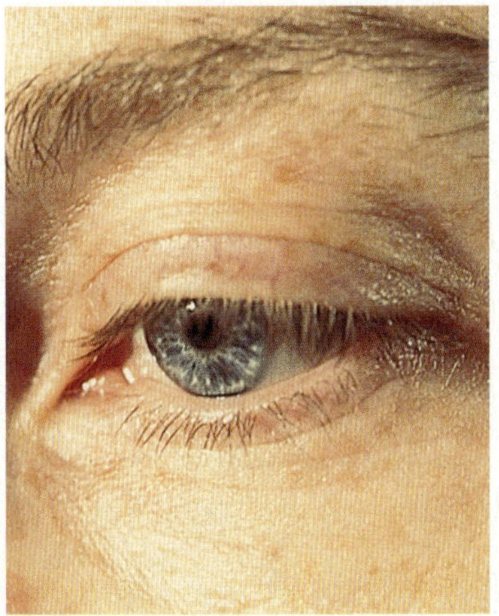

FIGURE 14-18. Normal upper lid overlap on downward gaze.

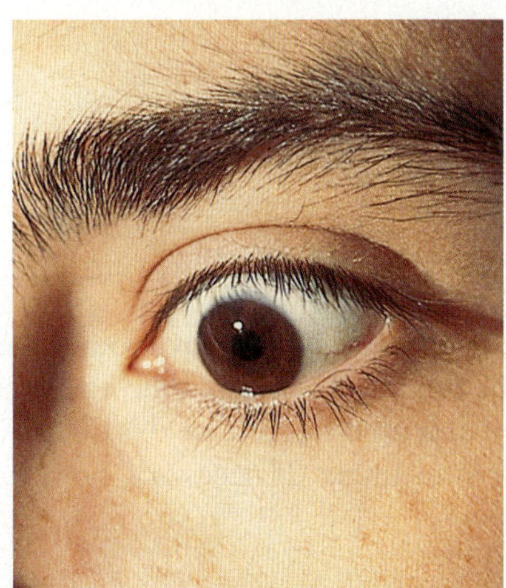

FIGURE 14-19. Lid lag. Note visible rim of sclera on downward gaze caused by proptosis.

Test Extraocular Muscle Movements

Ask the patient to follow your finger or pen as you sweep through the six cardinal directions of gaze. Making a wide "H" in the air, lead the patient's gaze (Fig. 14-20):

Review Box 14-2, Extraocular Muscles and Actions, p. 324.

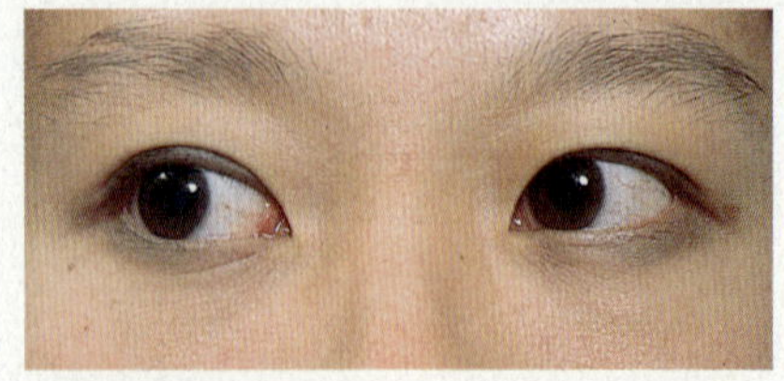

1. to the patient's extreme right,

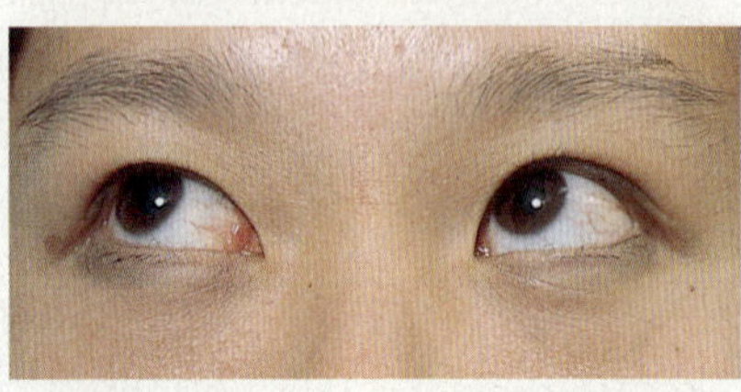

2. to the right and upward, and

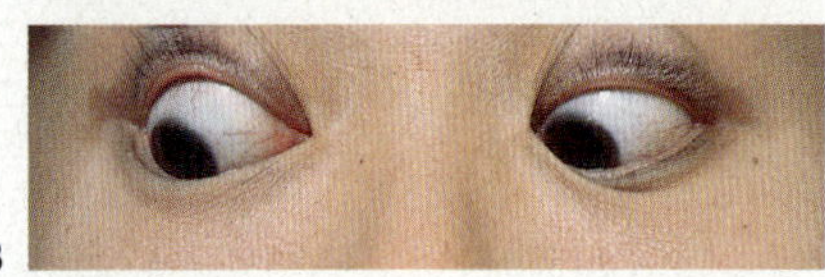

3. down on the right; then

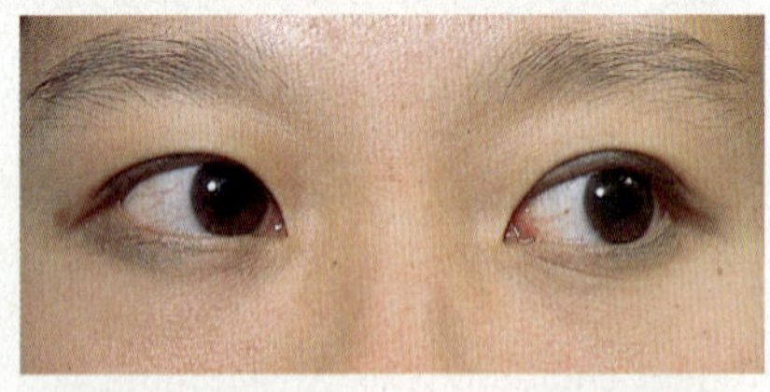

4. without pausing in the middle, to the extreme left,

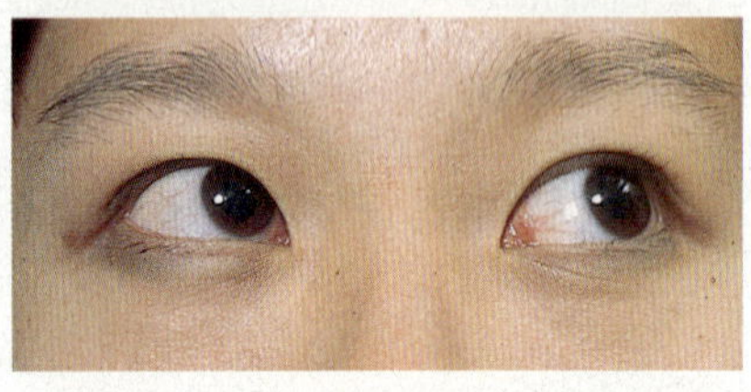

5. to the left and upward, and

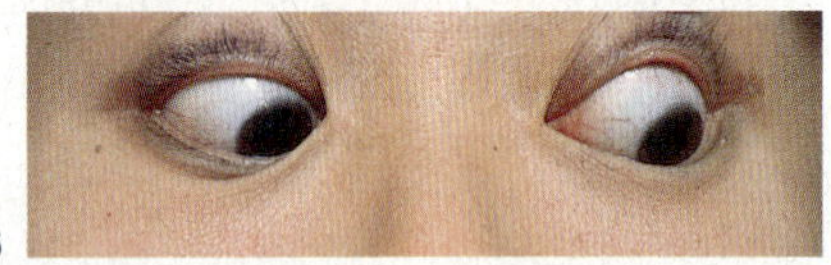

6. down on the left.

FIGURE 14-20. Test extraocular movements.

Pause during vertical and lateral gaze to detect *nystagmus.* Move your finger or pencil at a comfortable distance from the patient. Because middle-aged and older adults may have difficulty focusing on near objects, increase this distance. Some patients move their heads to follow your finger. If necessary, hold the head in the proper midline position.

Test for Convergence

Finally, if the near reaction has not already been tested, *test for convergence.* Ask the patient to follow your finger or pencil as you move it toward the bridge of

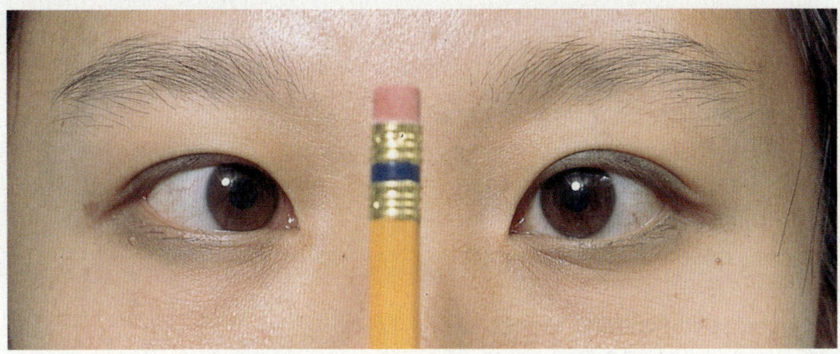

FIGURE 14-21. Testing for convergence.

their nose. The converging eyes normally follow the object to within 5 cm to 8 cm of the nose (Fig. 14-21).

Perform a Funduscopic Examination (Direct Ophthalmoscopy)

Most health care professionals will examine patients' eyes without dilating their pupils. Therefore, the view is limited to the optic nerve and a portion of the macula. To see more peripheral structures, to evaluate the macula closely, or to investigate unexplained visual loss, consider referral to ophthalmologists for pupillary dilation with mydriatic drops.

Contraindications for mydriatic drops include (1) recent head injury and coma, since continuing observations of pupillary reactions are essential, and (2) any suspicion of narrow-angle glaucoma. Pregnancy and breastfeeding are relative contraindications for administration of mydriatic drops.

This section reviews the technique for ophthalmoscopy for visualizing the fundus and optic nerve. Although some medical offices use the PanOptic ophthalmoscope, which provides a greater view of the fundus at an increased examination distance, the traditional direct ophthalmoscope is still widely used (Box 14-5). To use the ophthalmoscope effectively, remove your glasses (unless you have significant refractive error) and review the components of the ophthalmoscope (see Chapter 4, Physical Examination, p. 68). Proper technique and dedicated practice will allow the fundus, optic disc, and retinal vessels to come into focus. Over time, your examination skills will improve with commitment and repetition.

Box 14-5. Steps for Using the Ophthalmoscope

- Darken the room. Switch on the ophthalmoscope light and turn the light beam control with your finger until you see the large round beam of white light. Shine the light on the back of your hand to check the type of light, its desired brightness, and the power level of the ophthalmoscope.
- Turn the focusing wheel to the 0 diopter. (A *diopter* is a unit that measures the power of a lens to converge or diverge light.) At this diopter, the lens neither converges nor diverges light. Keep your finger on the edge of the lens disc so that you can turn the focusing wheel to focus the lens when you examine the fundus.

(*continued*)

Box 14-5. Steps for Using the Ophthalmoscope (*Continued*)

- Hold the ophthalmoscope in your right hand and *use your right eye to examine the patient's right eye*; hold it in your left hand and *use your left eye to examine the patient's left eye*. This keeps you from bumping the patient's nose and gives you more mobility and closer range for visualizing the fundus. With practice, you will become accustomed to using your nondominant eye.
- Hold the ophthalmoscope firmly braced against the medial aspect of your bony orbit, with the handle tilted laterally at about a 20-degree slant from the vertical. Check to make sure you can see clearly through the aperture. Instruct the patient to focus on a point slightly up and over your shoulder at a point directly ahead on the wall with their contralateral eye.
- Place yourself about 15 inches away from the patient at an angle of *15 degrees lateral to the patient's line of vision*. Shine the light beam on the pupil and look for the orange glow in the pupil—the *red reflex*. Note any opacities interrupting the red reflex. If you are nearsighted and have taken off your glasses, you may need to adjust the focusing wheel toward the minus/red diopters until the structures you see at a distance are in focus.

Absence of a red reflex through the pupil suggests an opacity of the lens (*cataract*) or, possibly, the vitreous (or even an artificial eye). Less commonly, a detached retina; mass; or; in children, a retinoblastoma may obscure this reflex.

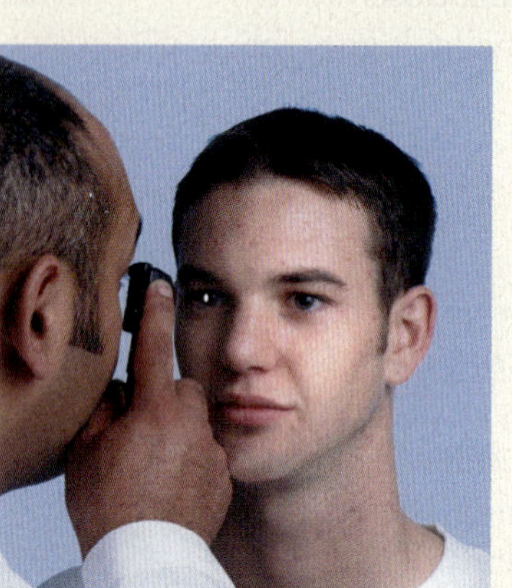

Examiner at 15-degree angle from patient's line of vision, eliciting red reflex.

- Now *place the thumb of your other hand across the patient's eyebrow* to stabilize your examining hand. Keep the light beam focused on the red reflex and move toward the patient pupil until you are almost touching the patient's eyelashes and the thumb of your examining hand.
- Try to keep both eyes open and relaxed, as if gazing into the distance, to help minimize any fluctuating blurriness as your eyes attempt to accommodate.
- You may need to lower the brightness of the light beam to make the examination more comfortable for the patient, avoid *hippus* (spasm of the pupil), and improve your view.

After familiarizing yourself with the ophthalmoscope, inspect the optic disc and retina. The optic disc is a circular structure with a yellow-orange to creamy-pink color, featuring a pink neuroretinal rim and central depression. Locating the optic disc can take practice, but with the ophthalmoscope's magnification of about 15 times the normal disc and retina, it becomes easier to observe.

The iris is also magnified about 4 times. Keep in mind that the optic disc measures around 1.5 mm in size. Refer to the steps provided in Box 14-6 to perform this important segment of the physical examination.

Box 14-6. Steps for Examining the Optic Disc and Retina

Optic Disc

- *First, locate the optic disc.* Look for the round yellowish-orange structure described above, or follow a blood vessel centrally until it enters the disc. The vessel size becomes progressively larger at each branch point as you approach the disc. Following each of the branch points back will lead you to the nerve.

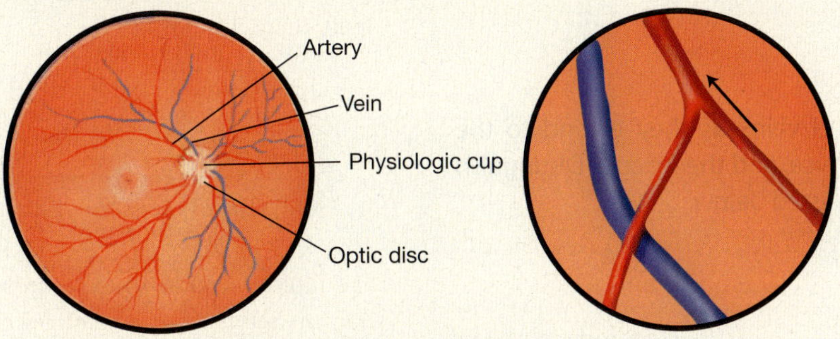

The optic disc and fundus.

- Now, bring the optic disc into sharp focus by adjusting the focusing wheel of your ophthalmoscope. If both you and the patient have no refractive errors, the retina should be in focus at 0 diopters.
- If structures are blurred, rotate the focusing wheel until you find the sharpest focus. For example, if the patient is myopic (nearsighted), rotate the focusing wheel counterclockwise to the minus/red diopters; in a hyperopic (farsighted) patient, move the focusing wheel clockwise to the plus/green diopters. You can correct your own refractive error in the same way.

In a *refractive error*, light rays from a distance do not focus on the retina. In *myopia*, they focus anterior to the retina, in *hyperopia*, posterior to it. Retinal structures in a myopic eye look larger than normal.

- *Inspect the optic disc.* Note the following features:
  - The sharpness or clarity of the disc outline.
  - The color of the disc, normally yellowish-orange to creamy-pink. White or pigmented crescents may ring the disc, a normal finding.
  - The size of the central physiologic *cup*, if present. It is usually yellowish-white. The horizontal diameter is usually less than half the horizontal diameter of the disc.
  - The comparative symmetry of the eyes and findings in the fundi.

See Table 14-8, Normal Variations of the Optic Disc, p. 354, and Table 14-9, Abnormalities of the Optic Disc, p. 355.

An enlarged cup may suggest glaucoma.

Importance of Detecting Papilledema

Swelling of the optic disc and anterior bulging of the physiologic cup suggest *papilledema* (Fig. 14-22), which is optic nerve head swelling associated with increased intracranial pressure. This pressure is transmitted to the optic nerve, causing stasis of axoplasmic flow, intra-axonal edema,

(*continued*)

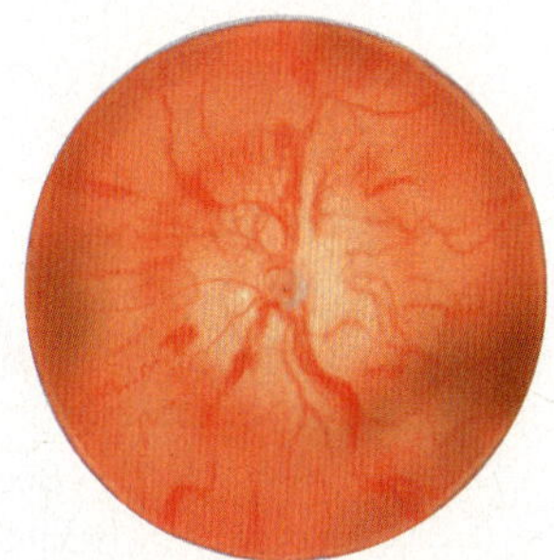

FIGURE 14-22. Papilledema.

Box 14-6. Steps for Examining the Optic Disc and Retina (*Continued*)

and swelling of the optic nerve head. Papilledema signals serious disorders of the brain, such as meningitis, subarachnoid hemorrhage, trauma, and mass lesions, so searching for this important disorder is a priority during all your funduscopic examinations (see technique as described on prior page).

Inspect the fundus for *spontaneous venous pulsations* (SVPs), rhythmic variations in the caliber of the retinal veins as they cross the fundus (narrower in systole; wider in diastole), present in 90% of healthy patients.

Loss of SVPs occurs with high intracranial pressures (>190 mm H_2O) that change the pressure gradient between cerebral spinal fluid pressure and intraocular pulse pressure in the optic disc. Other causes include glaucoma and retinal vein occlusion.[3,4]

Retina—Arteries, Veins, Fovea, and Macula

- *Inspect the retina,* including arteries and veins as they extend to the periphery, arteriovenous crossings, the fovea, and the macula. Distinguish arteries from veins based on the features listed below.

	Arteries	Veins
Color	Light red	Dark red
Size	Smaller (2/3 to 3/4 the diameter of veins)	Larger
Light reflex (*reflection*)	Bright	Inconspicuous or absent

See Tables 14-10 to 14-12 for information on retinal arteries and AV crossings, spots and streaks in the fundi, and light-colored spots in the fundi.

- Follow the vessels peripherally in each direction, noting their relative sizes and the character of the arteriovenous crossings.

Identify any lesions of the surrounding retina and note their size, shape, color, and distribution. As you search the retina, move your head and instrument as a unit, using the patient's pupil as an imaginary fulcrum. At first, you may lose your view of the retina because your light falls out of the pupil, but you will improve with practice. Lesions of the retina can be measured in terms of "disc diameters" from the optic disc.

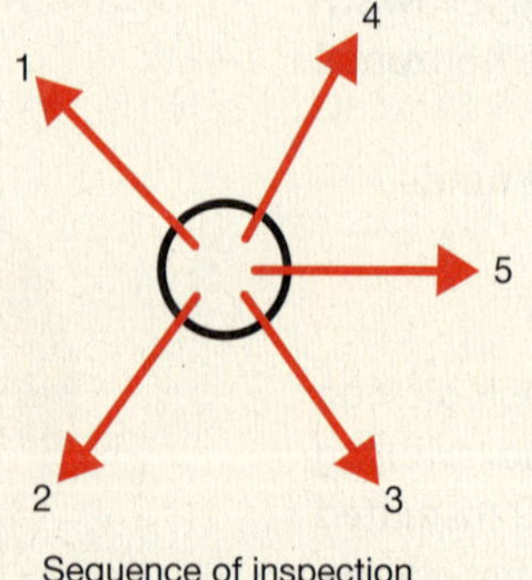

Sequence of inspection from disc to macula (left eye)

- *Inspect the fovea and surrounding macula.* Direct your light beam laterally or ask the patient to look directly into the light. In younger people, the tiny bright reflection at the center of the fovea helps to orient you; shimmering light reflections in the macular area are common.

Macular degeneration is an important cause of poor central vision in older adults. Types include *dry atrophic* (more common but typically progresses more slowly than the wet form) and *wet exudative, or neovascular.* Cellular debris, called *drusen,* maybe "hard" and sharply defined, as seen in Figure 14-23, or "soft" and confluent with altered pigmentation (see p. 358).

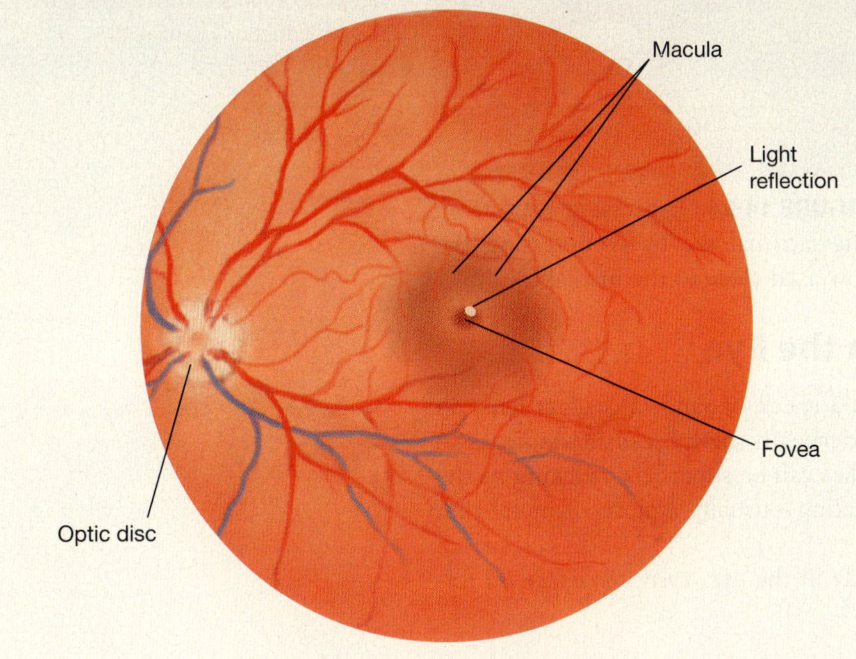

Structures of the left fundus.

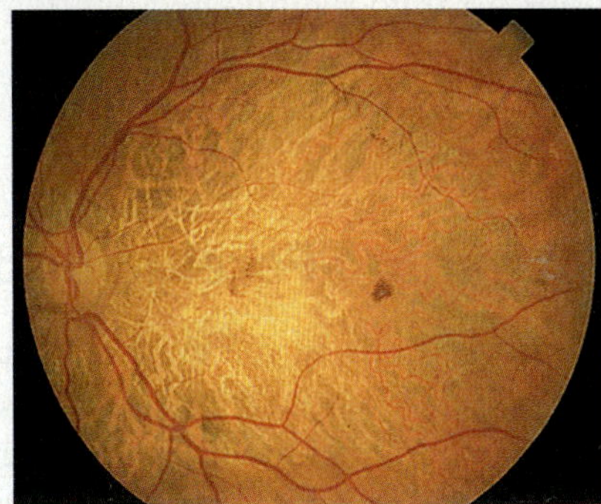

FIGURE 14-23. Hard drusen. (Reprinted with permission from Tasman W, Jaeger E, eds. *The Wills Eye Hospital Atlas of Clinical Ophthalmology.* 2nd ed. Lippincott Williams & Wilkins; 2001.)

- *Inspect the anterior structures.* Look for opacities in the vitreous or lens. Rotate the focusing wheel progressively to diopters of around +10 or +12, so you can focus on the more anterior structures in the eye.

Vitreous floaters are dark specks or strands seen between the fundus and the lens. *Cataracts* are densities in the lens (see p. 351).

SPECIAL TECHNIQUES AND MANEUVERS

Assessing Eye Protrusion (Proptosis or Exophthalmos)

For eyes with *exophthalmos* or increased axial projection, stand behind the seated patient and inspect from above. Draw their upper lids gently upward, then compare the protrusion of the eyes and the relationship of the corneas to the lower lids. For objective measurement, ophthalmologists use a Hertel exophthalmometer. This instrument measures the distance between the lateral angle of the orbit and an imaginary line across the most anterior point of the cornea. There is ethnographic variability, but upper limits of normal are 20 to 22 mm.[5–7] When protrusion is symptomatic and exceeds normal, further evaluation by computed tomography or magnetic resonance imaging often follows.[5]

Exophthalmos is a common finding in thyroid eye disease and is found in approximately 60% of patients with Graves disease. Other common symptoms of thyroid eye disease include eyelid retraction (91%), restricted ocular motility (43%), ocular pain (30%), lacrimation (23%), and dry eye (85%).[5–7] See also Table 13-1, Symptoms and Signs of Thyroid Disorders, p. 316.

Examining for Nasolacrimal Duct Obstruction

This test helps identify the cause of excessive tearing. Ask the patient to look up. Press on the lower lid close to the medial canthus, just inside the rim of the bony orbit; this compresses the lacrimal sac (Fig. 14-24). Look for fluid regurgitated out of the puncta into the eye. Avoid this test if the area is inflamed and tender.

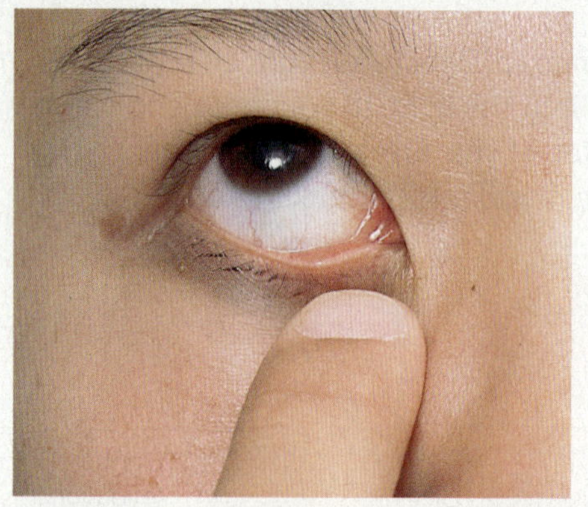

FIGURE 14-24. Expressing tears from the lacrimal sac by compressing the lower lid close to the medial canthus.

Discharge of mucopurulent fluid from the puncta suggests an obstructed nasolacrimal duct or a canaliculitis.

Managing Foreign Body in the Eye

A foreign body in the eye often involves a speck of sand, a contact lens, an insect, or a dislodged eyelash trapped underneath the lid, causing patients to sense something in their eye. Foreign bodies can be superficial, sticking to the eye surface or beneath the lid, or penetrating—usually a piece of metal that pierces the cornea or sclera.

To search thoroughly for a foreign body in the eye, *evert the upper lid* following the steps below.

- Wash your hands and ensure good lighting in the room. Ask the patient to sit down and explain the procedure to them. Make sure your patient understands what will happen and is comfortable with the procedure. While not always required, you can apply a topical anesthetic (like proparacaine) to the eye if you anticipate any patient discomfort. This can be especially useful if you plan to remove a foreign body.
- Gently stabilize the patient's forehead with your nondominant hand to prevent sudden movements. Ask the patient to look down and relax their eyes. Be reassuring and use gentle deliberate movements. With your dominant hand, obtain a clean cotton-tipped applicator or tongue depressor. Instruct the patient to keep looking downward throughout the procedure.
- With your nondominant hand, grasp the eyelashes of the upper lid between your thumb and index finger. While holding the lashes, gently pull the eyelashes outward (away from the eye) and upward (Fig. 14-25).
- Simultaneously, use the cotton-tipped applicator (or tongue depressor) to push downward on the upper tarsal plate (the firm part of the upper lid). This action will help evert the upper eyelid over the applicator (Fig. 14-26). This view allows

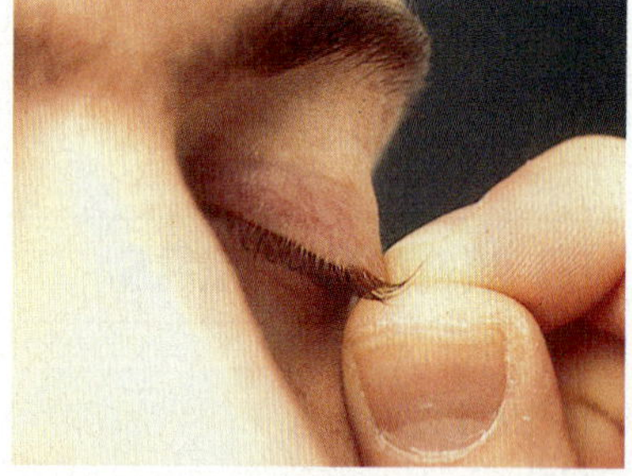

FIGURE 14-25. Start by pulling down on the upper eyelashes.

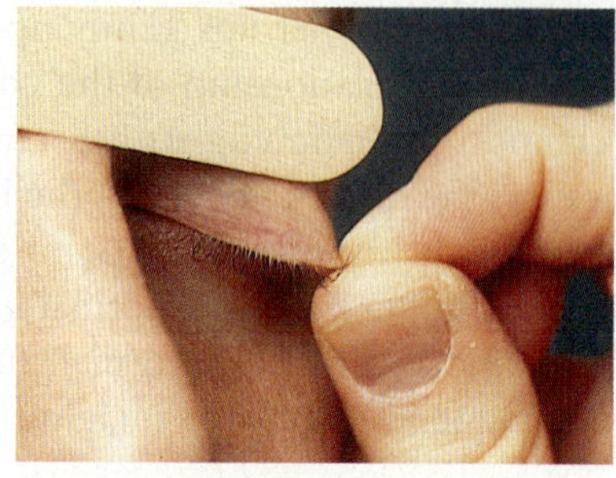

FIGURE 14-26. Everting the eyelid with the use of a tongue blade.

you to see the upper palpebral conjunctiva and look for a foreign body that might be lodged there.

- Secure the upper lashes against the eyebrow with your thumb and inspect the palpebral conjunctiva (Fig. 14-27). After your inspection, grasp the upper eyelashes and pull them gently forward. Ask the patient to look up. The eyelid will return to its normal position.

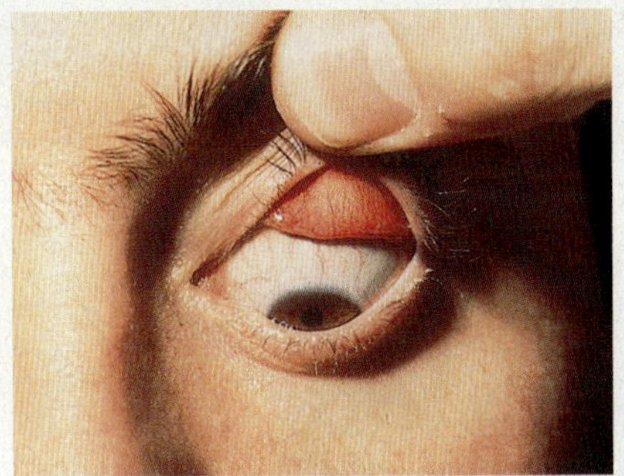

FIGURE 14-27. Securing the everted lid and inspecting the palpebral conjunctiva.

Testing for Functional Impairment of the Optic Nerves

The *swinging flashlight test* is a clinical test for functional impairment of the optic nerves (Fig. 14-28). In dim light, note the size of the pupils. After asking the patient to gaze into the distance, swing the beam of a penlight for 1 to 2 seconds first into one pupil, then into the other. Normally, each illuminated eye constricts promptly. The opposite eye should also constrict consensually.

In left-sided optic nerve damage, the pupils usually react as follows: When the light beam shines into the normal right eye, there is brisk constriction of both pupils (*direct response* on the right and *consensual response* on the left). When the light swings over to the abnormal left eye, partial dilation of both pupils will occur. The afferent stimulus on the left is reduced, so the efferent signals to both pupils are also reduced, and a net dilation occurs. This demonstrates an *afferent pupillary defect*, sometimes termed a **Marcus Gunn pupil**.

Modifications in Physical Examinations: Best Practices for Specialized Patient Populations

Prosthetic eyes provide not just a cosmetic solution but also play a role in socket health. Box 14-7 guides you through the unique examination considerations for these patients.

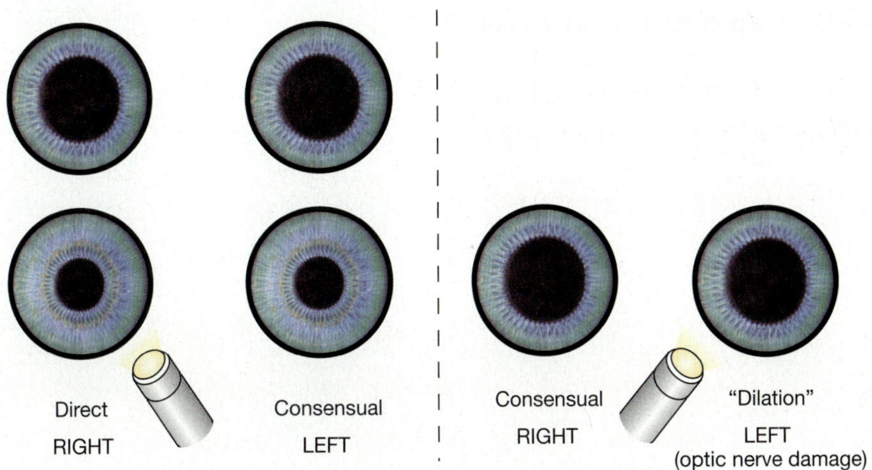

FIGURE 14-28. Swinging flashlight test.

Box 14-7. Eye Examination in the Presence of Medical Devices, Conditions, or Procedures

Patient with an Artificial Eye (Ocular Prosthesis)

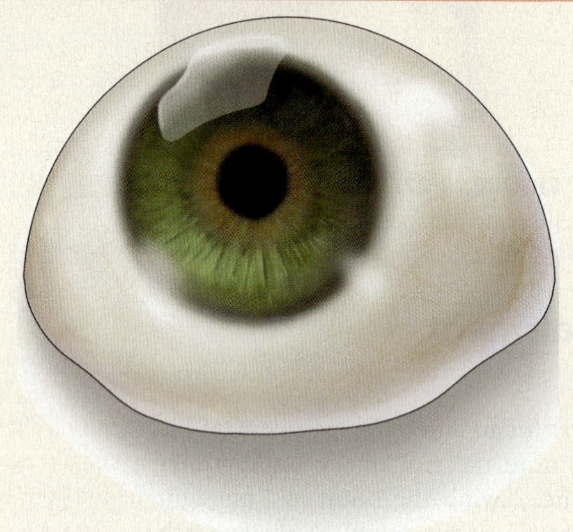

Device/condition	A prosthetic eye, often made of medical-grade acrylic or glass, designed to replace an absent natural eye.
General indication	Indicated for individuals who have lost an eye due to injury, disease, or other conditions, or were born with anophthalmia (absence of one or both eyes).
General location	Positioned within the eye socket (orbit), behind the eyelids.
Modification to the physical exam	1. Inspect the artificial eye for proper positioning, alignment with the other eye, and overall cosmetic appearance. 2. Check the surrounding eyelids and conjunctiva of the socket for any signs of irritation, infection, or inflammation. 3. Assess the movement of the prosthetic in relation to the natural eye when the patient looks in different directions. 4. Inquire about any discomfort, discharge, or changes in fit or appearance associated with the prosthetic eye.

RECORDING YOUR FINDINGS

Initially, your thorough sentence-based documentation of the PE is crucial for generating your diagnosis and hypothesis. As you gain experience, you will eventually shift to using brief, standard phrases for quicker and clearer documentation.

Recording the Head, Eyes, Ears, Nose, and Throat (HEENT) Examination

HEENT:

Eyes—Visual acuity 20/20 bilaterally. Lids and adnexa appear normal. Sclera white, conjunctiva quiet. Pupils are 5 mm constricting to 4 mm, equally round, and reactive to light. Disc margins sharp; no hemorrhages or exudates, no arteriolar narrowing.

OR

Eyes—Visual acuity 20/100 bilaterally. Eyelashes with scurf. Sclera white; conjunctiva injected. Pupils constrict 3 mm to 2 mm, equally round and reactive to light. Disc margins sharp; no hemorrhages or exudates. Arteriolar-to-venous ratio (AV ratio) 2:4; no AV nicking.

The detailed examination of PE documentation, breaking it down into individual elements, showcases the importance of clinical observations in guiding diagnosis. The findings described in the PE of the eyes suggest several potential concerns:

- *Visual acuity 20/100 bilaterally:* This indicates reduced visual acuity, which could be due to a variety of causes including refractive errors (like myopia or hyperopia), cataracts, macular degeneration, or other eye conditions affecting visual clarity.
- *Eyelashes with scurf:* Scurf on the eyelashes might suggest blepharitis, which is often associated with a bacterial infection or seborrheic dermatitis.
- *Sclera white; conjunctiva injected:* While the white sclera is normal, an injected conjunctiva suggests conjunctival irritation or inflammation, commonly seen in conjunctivitis, allergic reactions, or irritation from environmental factors.
- *Pupils constrict 3 mm to 2 mm, equally round and reactive to light:* This finding is typically normal, indicating that the pupils are functioning properly in response to light.
- *Disc margins sharp; no hemorrhages or exudates:* Sharp disc margins are normal. The absence of hemorrhages or exudates is a good sign.
- *Arteriolar-to-venous (AV) ratio 2:4; no AV nicking:* An AV ratio of 2:4 may suggest some narrowing of the retinal arterioles. Normally, the ratio is closer to 2:3. This could indicate chronic hypertension or other vascular conditions. The absence of AV nicking, in which arterioles compress the underlying veins, is a positive sign, as AV nicking is commonly associated with hypertension.

In summary, the findings of reduced visual acuity, eyelash scurf, conjunctival injection, and a slightly abnormal AV ratio suggest a combination of ocular conditions, possibly including *refractive errors, blepharitis, conjunctivitis,* and vascular changes indicating systemic issues like *hypertension.*

HEALTH PROMOTION AND COUNSELING: EVIDENCE AND RECOMMENDATIONS

Important Topics for Health Promotion and Counseling

- Visual impairment
- Screening for glaucoma
- UV-related eye injuries

Visual Impairment

Visual impairment is defined as having corrected visual acuity of only 20/40 or worse in the better eye, whereas legal blindness is having corrected visual acuity in the better eye of only 20/200 or worse.[8] More than 7 million Americans are estimated to be visually impaired, including more than 1 million who are legally blind.[9] The major causes of visual impairment are *cataracts* (affecting >30 million adults), *age-related macular degeneration* (affecting nearly 2 million adults), glaucoma (affecting >3 million adults), and *diabetic retinopathy* (affecting nearly 5 million adults).[8] Visual impairment is associated with decreased functional capacity, poor quality of life, loss of independent living, falls, cognitive decline, family stress, and increased risk for premature death and experiencing other medical comorbidities.[10] However, more than 80% of visually impaired Americans could achieve good visual acuity with correction.[11] Because onset can be gradual, those affected may not recognize their visual decline. The American Academy of Ophthalmology recommends a comprehensive screening medical eye examination, usually including testing visual acuity and visual fields, funduscopic examination, and IOP measurement, for all adults.[12] The recommended frequency for these examinations depends on age and risk factors.

Screening for Glaucoma

Primary open-angle glaucoma (POAG) is a leading cause of visual impairment and blindness in the United States, affecting nearly 3 million adults, including roughly 2% of adults older than age 40 years.[13] More than half are unaware of having the disease. In POAG, there is gradual loss of vision in the peripheral and/or central visual fields, resulting from optic nerve damage. Retinal examination may reveal optic nerve pallor and an increased optic nerve cup-to-disc ratio. Risk factors include older age, being African American or Latino/Hispanic, family history, diabetes, myopia, and ocular hypertension (intraocular pressure [IOP] ≥21 mm Hg).[14,15] Not all people with POAG have elevated IOP, and those with elevated IOP may not develop visual impairment. Glaucoma can be successfully treated with medical and surgical interventions. The U.S. Preventive Services Task Force concluded that available evidence was insufficient to support a recommendation for POAG screening.[15] However, the American Academy of Ophthalmology recommends periodic glaucoma testing, with a baseline examination starting at age 40 years and possibly earlier for at-risk patients with known family history.[12]

UV-Related Eye Injuries

Ultraviolet (UV) light can cause skin cancers on the eyelids, including basal cell carcinoma, squamous cell carcinoma, and melanoma.[16] Additionally, UV light is associated with developing cataracts, and directly staring at the sun can cause solar retinopathy.[17,18] Recommended preventive actions include using sunscreen on the face and eyelids and wearing eye protection against UV radiation.

See Regular Use of Sunscreen in Chapter 12, Skin, Hair, and Nails, pp. 268–269.

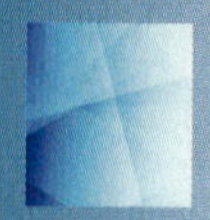

TABLE 14-1. Red Eyes

	Conjunctivitis	Subconjunctival Hemorrhage
	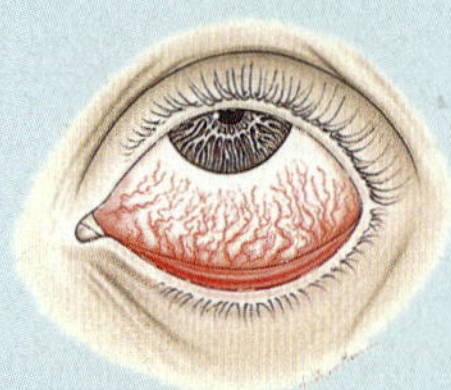	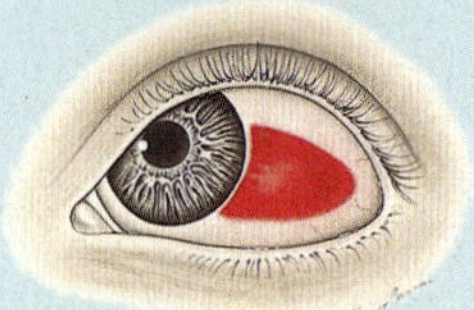
Pattern of Redness	Conjunctival injection: diffuse dilatation of conjunctival vessels with redness that tends to be maximal peripherally	Leakage of blood outside of the vessels, producing a homogeneous, sharply demarcated, red area that resolves over 2 wks
Pain	Mild discomfort rather than pain	Absent
Vision	Not affected except for temporary mild blurring due to discharge	Not affected
Ocular Discharge	Watery, mucoid, or mucopurulent	Absent
Pupil	Not affected	Not affected
Cornea	Clear	Clear
Significance	Bacterial, viral, and other infections; highly contagious; allergy; irritation	Often none. May result from trauma, bleeding disorders, or sudden increase in venous pressure, such as from cough

	Corneal Injury or Infection	Acute Iritis	Acute Angle Closure Glaucoma
	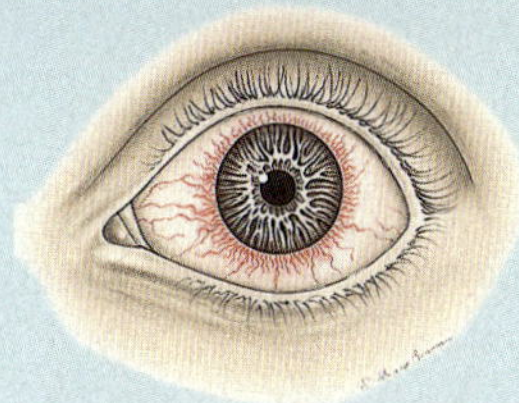	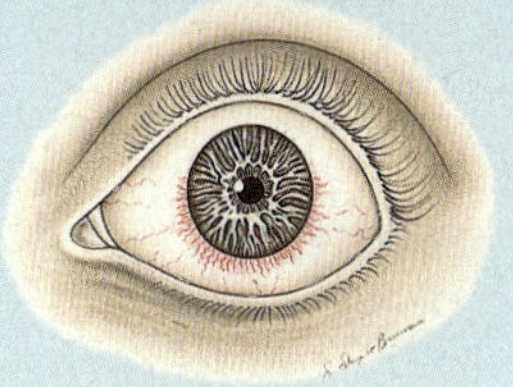	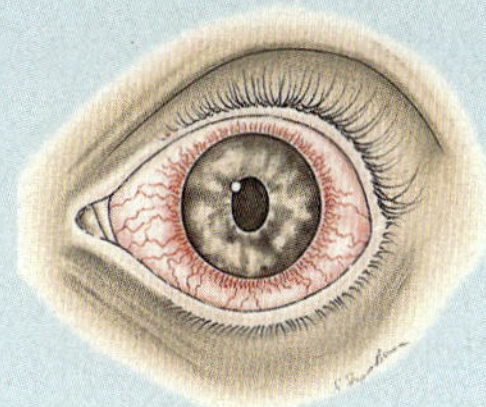
Pattern of Redness	Ciliary injection: Deeper vessels radiating from the limbus are dilated, creating a reddish-violet flush. The eye may also be diffusely red.	Ciliary injection: Redness more concentrated around the limbus, with deeper vessels involved.	Ciliary injection: Diffuse redness, often with a steamy cornea and marked circumcorneal flush.
Pain	Moderate to severe, superficial	Moderate, aching, deep, photophobia	Severe, aching, deep, severe photophobia
Vision	Usually decreased	Decreased	Decreased
Ocular Discharge	Watery or purulent	Absent	Absent
Pupil	Not affected unless iritis develops	Small and irregular	Dilated, fixed
Cornea	Changes depending on cause, often with epithelial defect. May have corneal opacity if infection involved.	Clear or slightly clouded; injection confined to corneal limbus	Steamy, cloudy
Significance	Abrasions, and other injuries; viral and bacterial infections	Associated with systemic infection, herpes zoster, tuberculosis, or autoimmune diseases; refer promptly	Acute increase in intraocular pressure constitutes an emergency

Source: Leibowitz HM. The red eye. *N Engl J Med*. 2000;343(5):345–351.

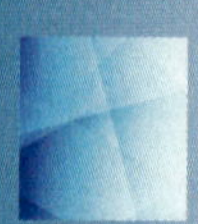

TABLE 14-2. Visual Field Defects

1. *Horizontal Defect* Occlusion of a branch of the central retinal artery may cause a horizontal (altitudinal) defect. Ischemia of the optic nerve can produce a similar defect.

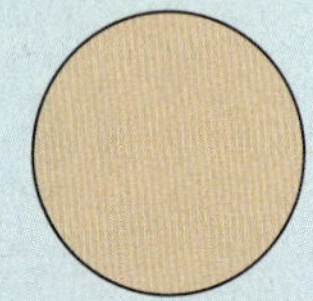
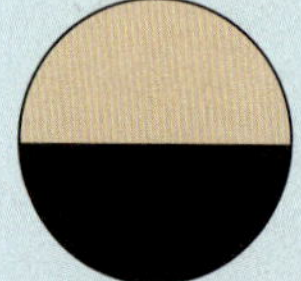

2. *Blind Right Eye (Right Optic Nerve)* A lesion of the optic nerve and, of course, of the eye itself, produces unilateral monocular blindness.

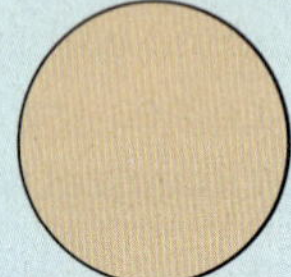

3. *Bitemporal Hemianopsia (Optic Chiasm)* A lesion at the optic chiasm (such as a pituitary tumor), may involve only fibers crossing over to the opposite side. Since these fibers originate in the nasal half of each retina, visual loss involves the temporal half of each field.

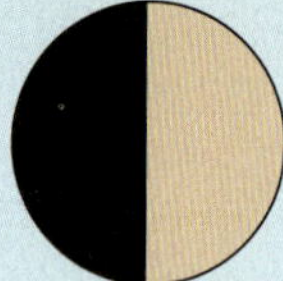
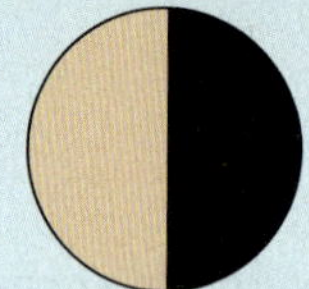

4. *Left Homonymous Hemianopsia (Right Optic Tract)* A lesion of the optic tract, interrupts fibers originating on the same side of both eyes. Visual loss in the eyes is, therefore, similar (homonymous) and involves half of each field (hemianopsia).

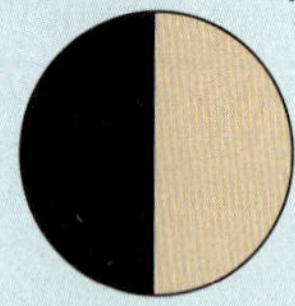
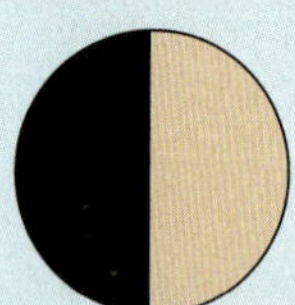

5. *Homonymous Left Superior Quadrantic Defect (Right Optic Radiation, Partial)* A partial lesion of the optic radiation in the temporal lobe, may involve only a portion of the nerve fibers, producing, for example, a homonymous quadrantic ("pie in the sky") defect.

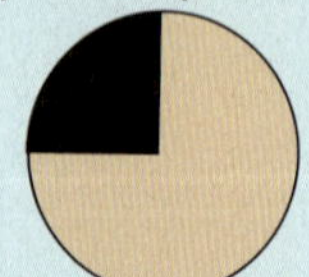
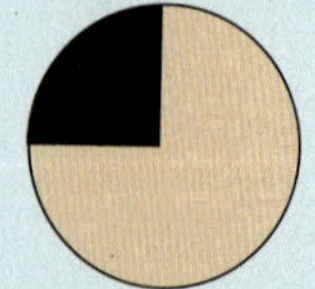

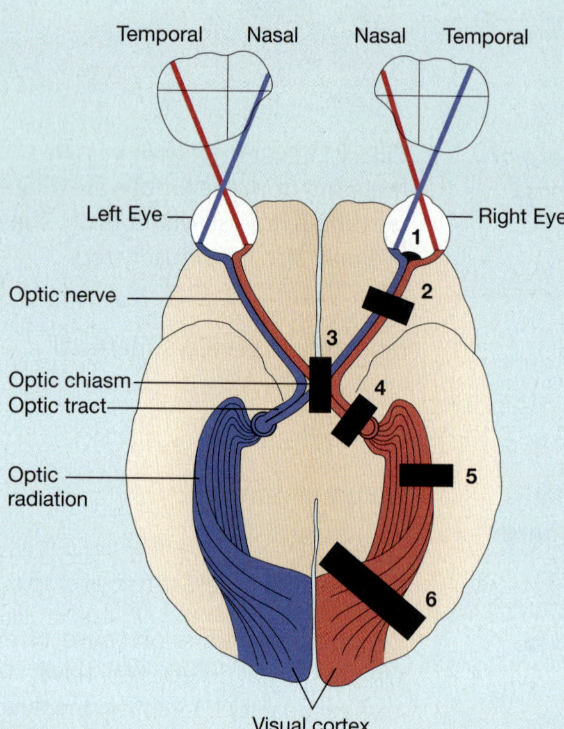

6. *Left Homonymous Hemianopsia (Right Optic Radiation)* A complete interruption of fibers in the optic radiation, produces a visual defect similar to that produced by a lesion of the optic tract.

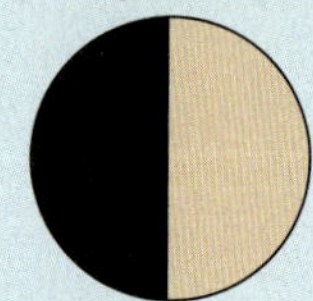
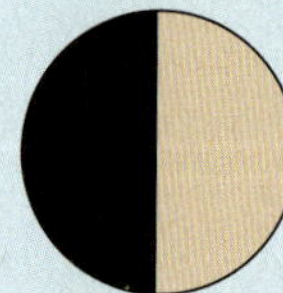

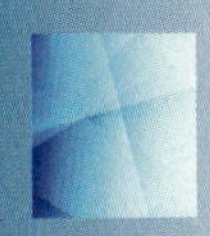

TABLE 14-3. Variations and Abnormalities of the Eyelids

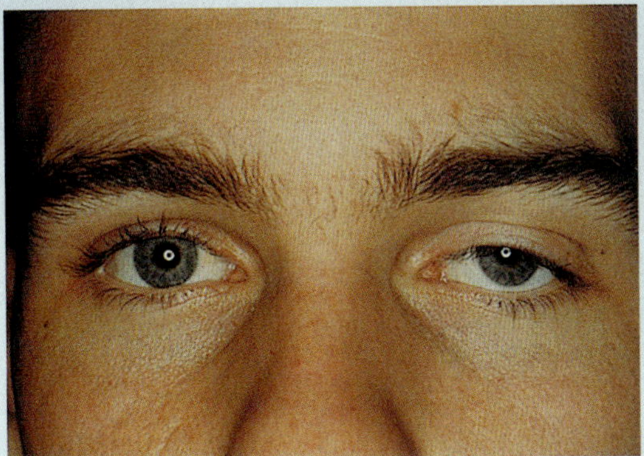

Ptosis

Ptosis is a drooping of the upper eyelid caused by involutional, myogenic, neurogenic, or mechanical etiologies. Senile ptosis often results from involutional changes, while congenital ptosis occurs due to myogenic factors.

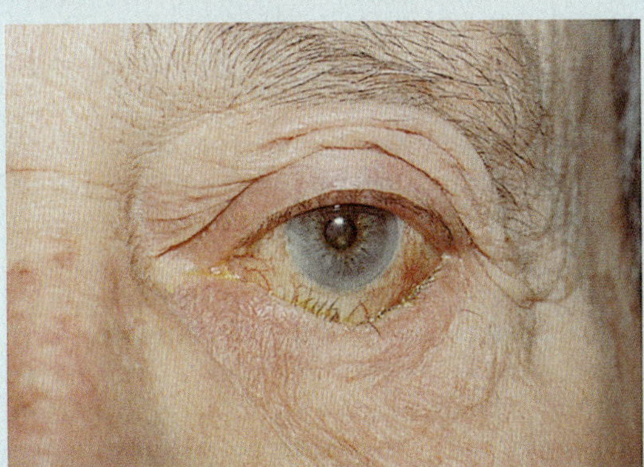

Entropion

In entropion, the lid margin turns inward, commonly seen in elderly patients. It can cause the lower lashes to irritate the conjunctiva and lower cornea. *Trichiasis*, by contrast, is inward growth of eyelashes. Squeezing the lids shut can reveal lower eyelid instability.

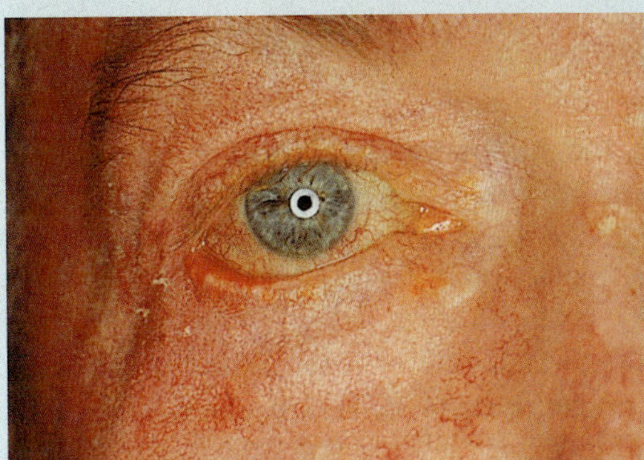

Ectropion

In ectropion, the lower eyelid margin turns outward, exposing the palpebral conjunctiva. This condition is more common in older adults with laxity of the lower eyelids. When the punctum of the lower eyelid turns outward, it can lead to poor eye drainage and tearing.

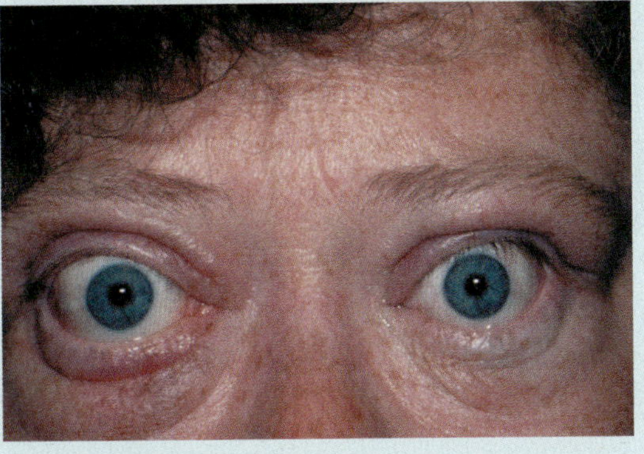

Lid Retraction and Exophthalmos

A wide-eyed stare can indicate retracted eyelids, which are characterized by a visible rim of sclera between the upper lid and the iris. This, along with "lid lag" when the eyes move from up to down, can be strong indicators of hyperthyroidism when accompanied by a fine tremor, moist skin, and heart rate of >90 beats per min.[19]

Exophthalmos is eye protrusion, commonly caused by thyroid eye disease due to autoreactive T-lymphocytes. Symptoms include retraction, lid lag, diplopia, dry eyes, pain, and tearing. Unilateral exophthalmos may be caused by thyroid eye disease, trauma, orbital tumors, sinus issues, and granulomatous disorders.[5]

Source of photos: *Ptosis, Ectropion, Entropion*—Reprinted with permission from Tasman W, Jaeger E, eds. *The Wills Eye Hospital Atlas of Clinical Ophthalmology*. 2nd ed. Lippincott Williams & Wilkins; 2001.

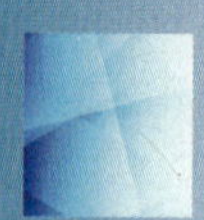

TABLE 14-4. Lumps and Swellings in and Around the Eyes

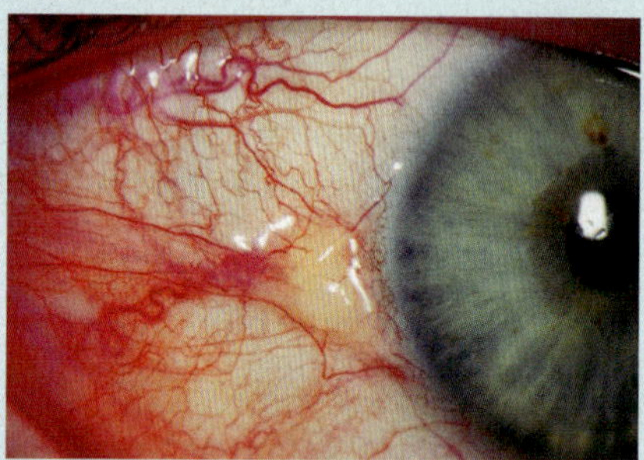

Pinguecula

Harmless yellowish triangular nodule in the bulbar conjunctiva on either side of the iris; appears frequently with aging, first on the nasal and then on the temporal side

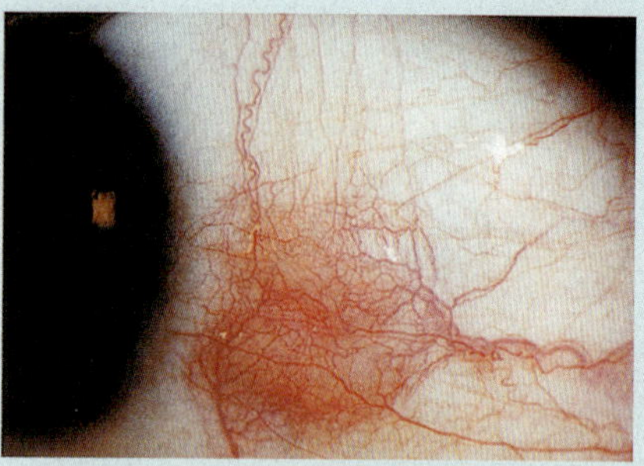

Episcleritis

Benign, usually painless localized ocular inflammation of the episcleral vessels; vessels appear movable over the scleral surface; may be nodular or show only redness and dilated vessels

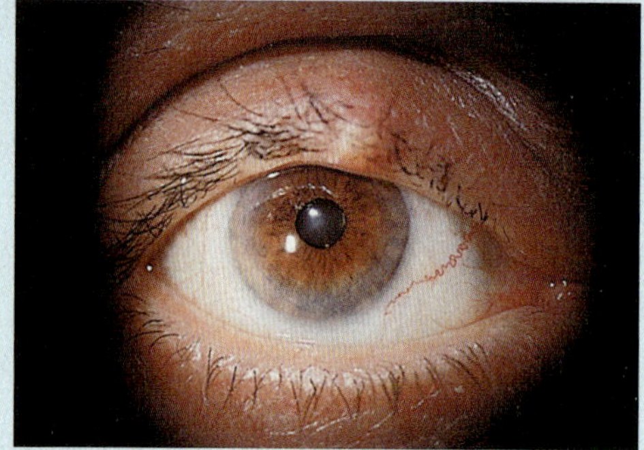

Stye (Hordeolum)

Painful, tender, red infection at the inner or outer margin of the eyelid, usually from *Staphylococcus aureus* (at the inner margin—from an obstructed meibomian gland; at the outer margin—from an obstructed eyelash follicle)

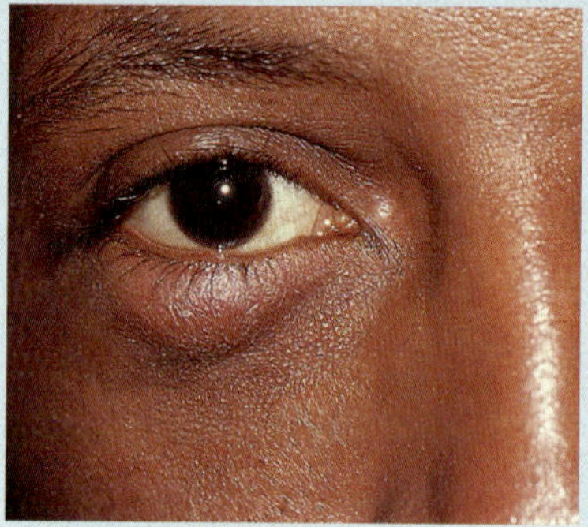

Chalazion

Subacute nontender, usually painless nodule caused by a blocked meibomian gland. may become acutely inflamed but, unlike a stye, usually points inside the lid rather than on the lid margin

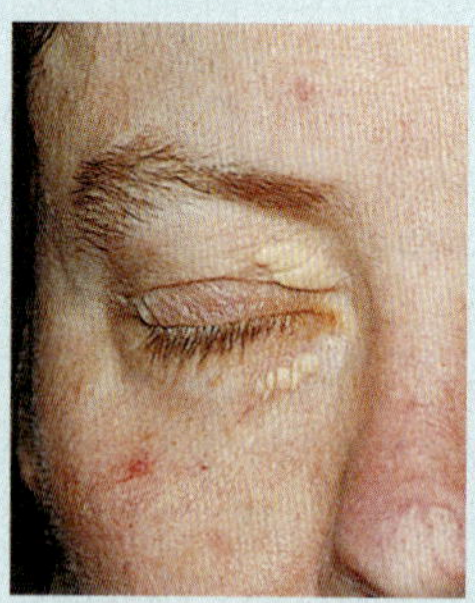

Xanthelasma

Slightly raised, yellowish, well-circumscribed cholesterol-filled plaques that appear along the upper or lower nasal portions of one or both eyelids; half of affected patients have hyperlipidemia; also common in primary biliary cirrhosis

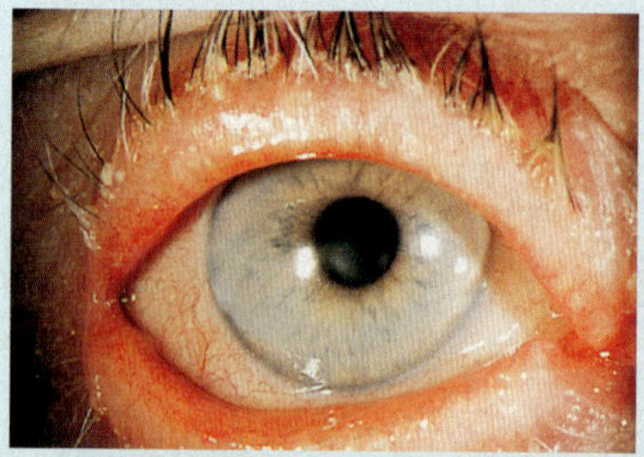

Blepharitis

Chronic inflammation of the eyelids at the base of the hair follicles, often from *S. aureus*; there is also a scaling seborrheic variant

TABLE 14-5. Opacities of the Cornea and Lens

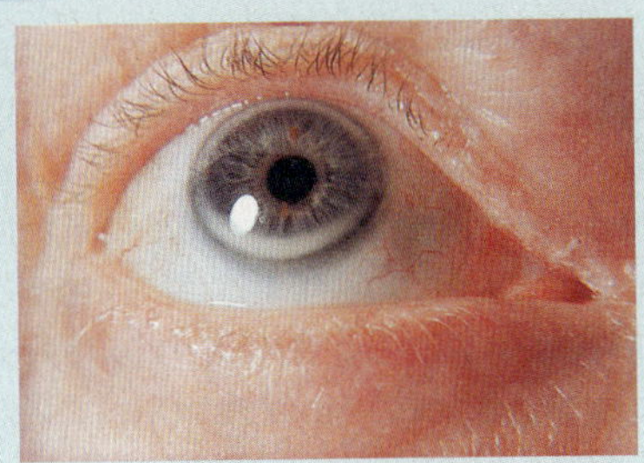

Corneal Arcus
Thin grayish-white arc or circle not quite at the edge of the cornea; accompanies normal aging but also seen in younger adults, especially African Americans; in young adults, suggests possible hyperlipoproteinemia; usually benign

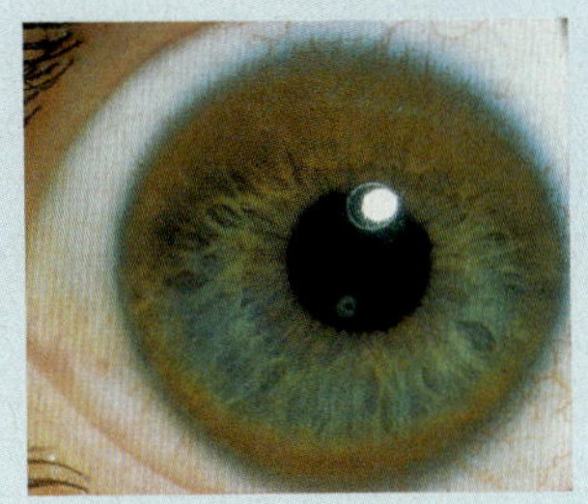

Kayser–Fleischer Ring
Golden to red-brown ring, sometimes shading to green or blue, from copper deposition in the periphery of the cornea found in Wilson disease; due to a rare autosomal recessive mutation of the *ATO7B* gene on chromosome 13 causing abnormal copper transport, reduced biliary copper excretion, and abnormal accumulation of copper in the liver and tissues throughout the body; patients present with liver disease, renal failure, and neurologic symptoms of tremor, dystonia, and a variety of psychiatric disorders[20]

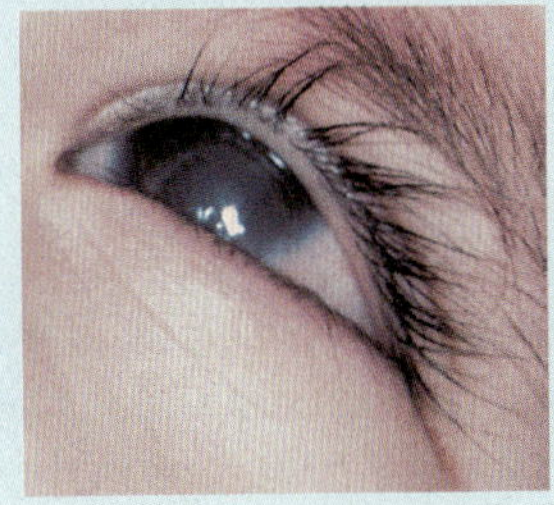

Corneal Scar
Superficial grayish-white opacity in the cornea, secondary to an old injury, infection, or inflammation; size and shape are variable; do not confuse with the opaque lens of a cataract, visible on a deeper plane and only through the pupil

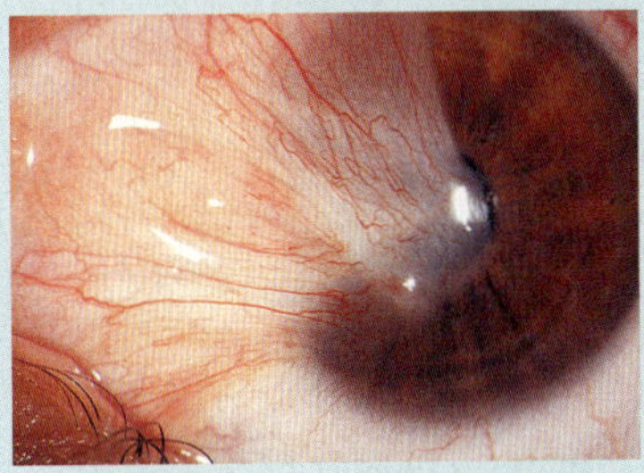

Pterygium
Triangular thickening of the bulbar conjunctiva that grows slowly across the outer surface of the cornea, usually from the nasal side, in response to excessive sun damage; reddening and irritation may occur, may interfere with vision as it encroaches on the pupil

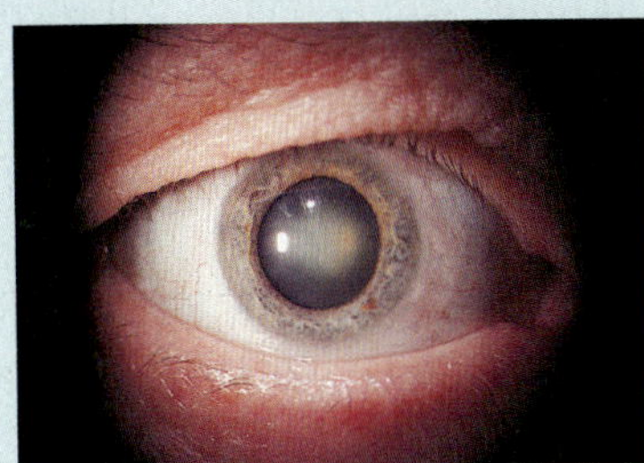

Cataracts
Opacity of the lenses visible through the pupil; risk factors are older age, smoking, trauma, diabetes, and corticosteroid use

Nuclear Cataract. Looks gray when seen by a flashlight; if the pupil is widely dilated, the gray opacity is surrounded by a black rim

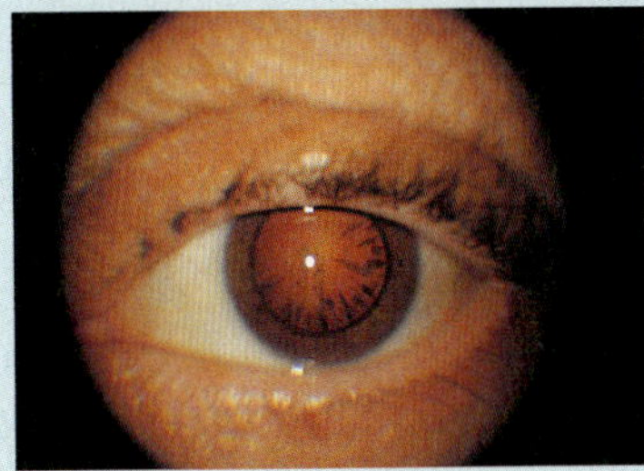

Peripheral Cataract. Produces spoke-like shadows that point—gray against black, as seen with a flashlight, or black against red with an ophthalmoscope; a dilated pupil, as shown here, facilitates this observation

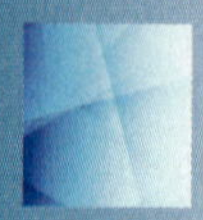

TABLE 14-6. Pupillary Abnormalities

Unequal Pupils (Anisocoria)—Anisocoria represents a defect in the constriction or dilatation of one pupil. Constriction to light and near effort is mediated by parasympathetic pathways, and pupillary dilatation by sympathetic pathways. The light reaction in bright and dim light identifies the abnormal pupil. When anisocoria is greater in bright light than in dim light, the larger pupil cannot constrict properly. Causes include blunt trauma to the eye, open-angle glaucoma (p. 347), and impaired parasympathetic innervation to the iris, as in tonic pupil and oculomotor nerve (cranial nerve [CN] III) paralysis. When anisocoria is greater in dim light, the smaller pupil cannot dilate properly, as in Horner syndrome, caused by an interruption of the sympathetic innervation. Assessing the near reaction is also important in determining the cause. See also Table 27-16, Pupils in Comatose Patients, p. 991.

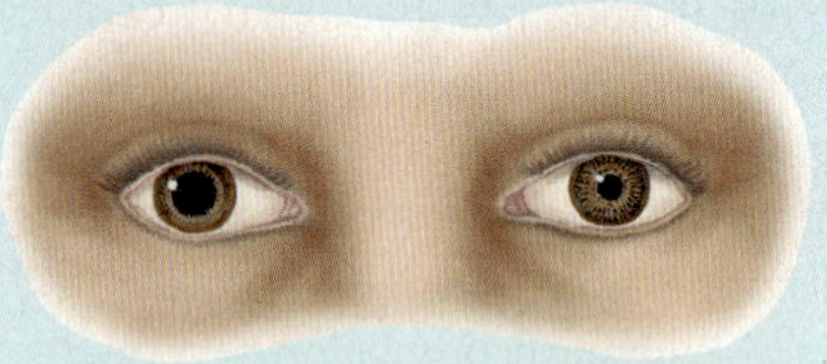

Tonic Pupil *(Adie Pupil)*. The pupil is unilaterally large (dilated), with slow or absent reaction to light, and slow tonic constriction during near vision due to parasympathetic denervation. Accommodation is slow, causing blurred vision.

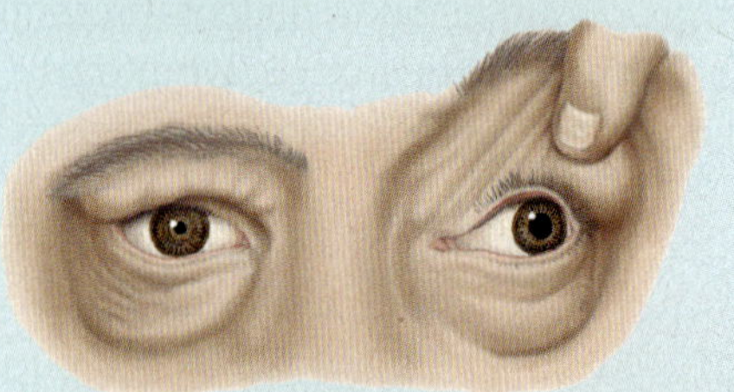

Oculomotor Nerve (CN III) Paralysis. The affected pupil is large and fixed, and there is ptosis of the upper eyelid and lateral deviation of the eye downward and outward due to impaired CN III innervation.

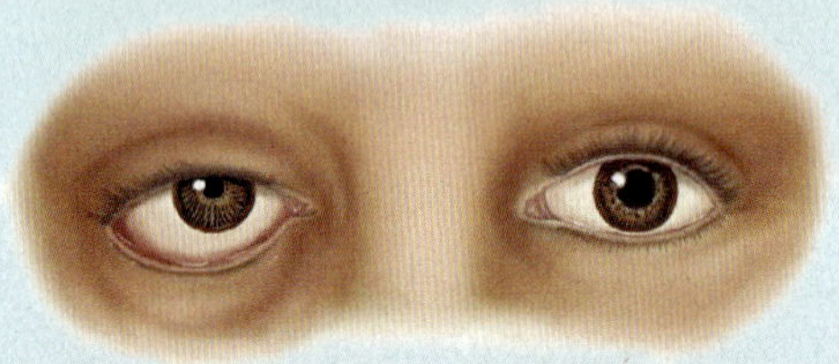

Horner Syndrome. Horner syndrome is characterized by a small, unilateral, slow-dilating pupil, ipsilateral ptosis, and ipsilateral anhidrosis. Anisocoria is >1 mm and may be caused by lesions in the sympathetic pathways, such as in the brainstem, neck and chest tumors, orbital trauma, or migraines. In congenital Horner syndrome, the iris on the affected side is lighter in color than the other side (heterochromia).[2]

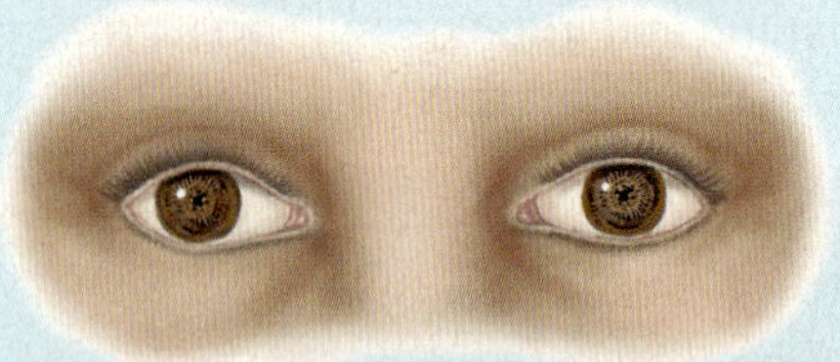

Small, Irregular Pupils (Argyll Robertson Pupils). The pupils are small and irregular, usually bilaterally. They constrict with near vision and dilate with far vision (a normal near reaction) but do not react to light. This is seen in neurosyphilis and rarely in diabetes.

Equal Pupils and One Blind Eye. Unilateral blindness does not cause anisocoria as long as the sympathetic and parasympathetic innervation to both irises is normal. A light directed into the seeing eye produces a direct reaction in that eye and a consensual reaction in the blind eye. A light directed into the blind eye, however, causes no response in either eye.

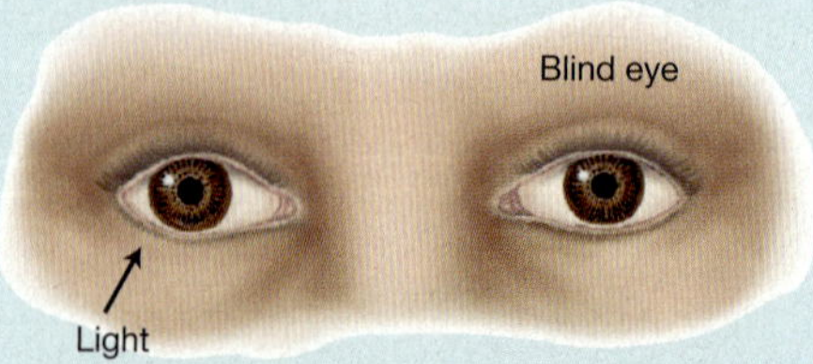

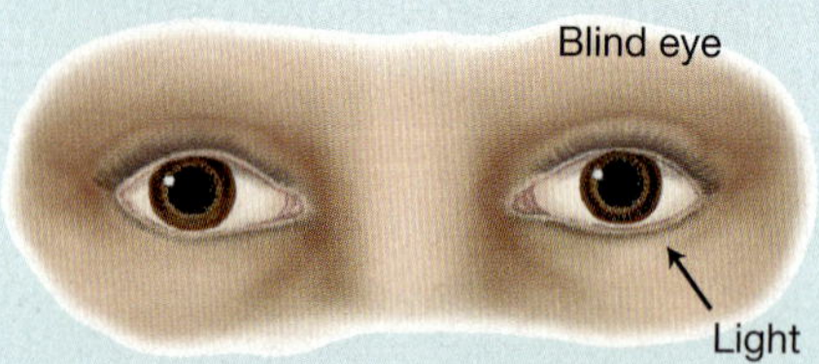

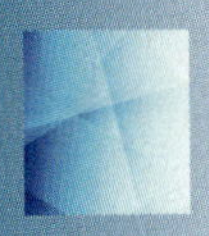

TABLE 14-7. Dysconjugate Gaze

A number of abnormal patterns of gaze are related to developmental disorders and cranial nerve (CN) abnormalities.

Developmental Disorders

Developmental dysconjugate gaze is caused by an imbalance in ocular muscle tone. This imbalance has many causes, may be hereditary, and usually appears in early childhood. These gaze deviations are classified according to direction:

Esotropia

Exotropia

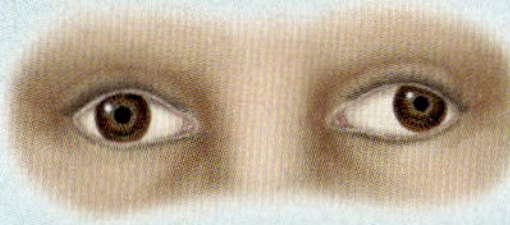

Disorders of Cranial Nerves

New onset of dysconjugate gaze in adults usually results from cranial nerve injuries, lesions, or abnormalities from causes such as trauma, multiple sclerosis, syphilis, and others.

Left CN VI Paralysis

LOOKING TO THE RIGHT

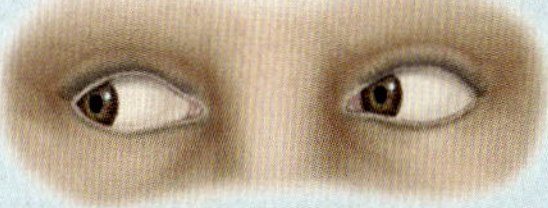

Eyes are conjugate.

Cover–Uncover Test

A cover–uncover test may be helpful. Here is what you would see in the right monocular esotropia illustrated above.

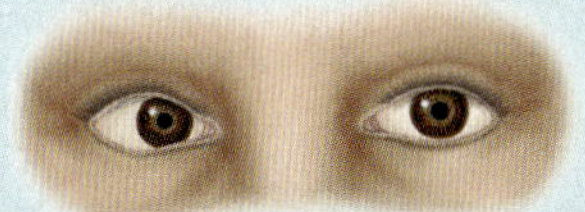

Corneal reflections are asymmetric.

COVER

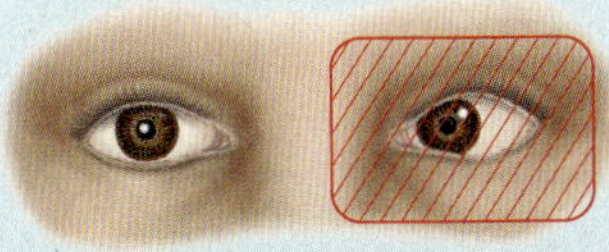

The right eye moves outward to fix on the light. (The left eye is not seen but moves inward to the same degree.)

UNCOVER

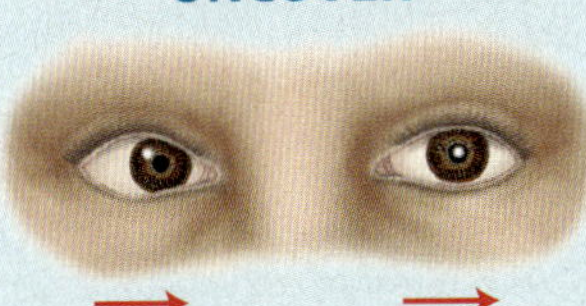

The left eye moves outward to fix on the light. The right eye deviates inward again.

LOOKING STRAIGHT AHEAD

Esotropia appears.

LOOKING TO THE RIGHT

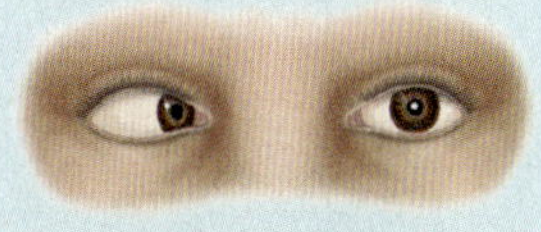

Esotropia is maximum.

Left CN IV Paralysis

LOOKING DOWN AND TO THE RIGHT

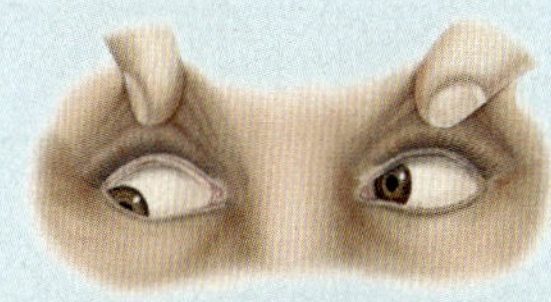

The left eye cannot look down when turned inward. Deviation is maximum in this direction.

Left CN III Paralysis

LOOKING STRAIGHT AHEAD

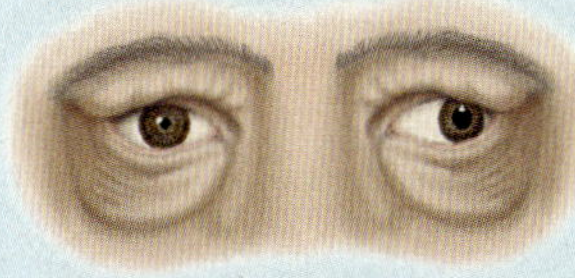

The eye is pulled outward by action of the CN VI. Upward, downward, and inward movements are impaired or lost. Ptosis and pupillary dilation may be associated.

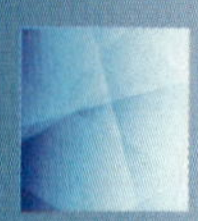

TABLE 14-8. Normal Variations of the Optic Disc

Physiologic Cupping

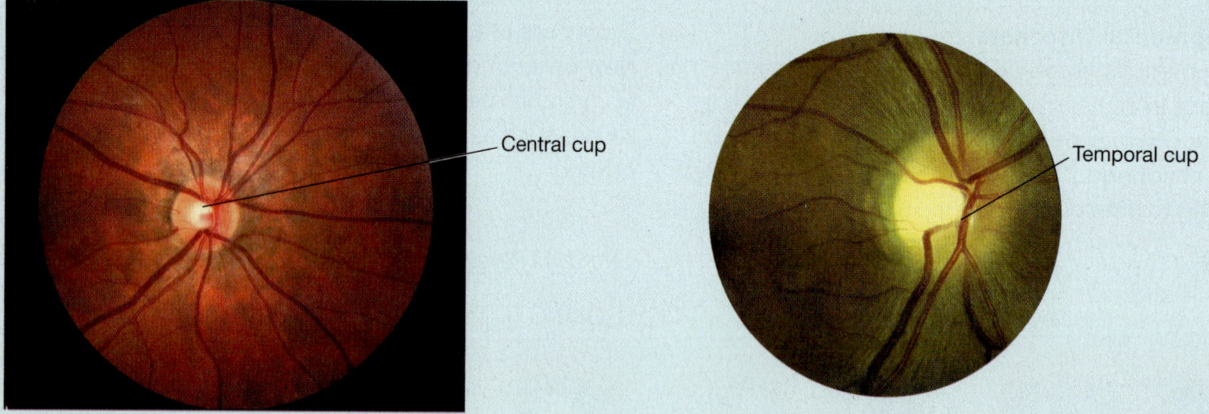

The physiologic cup is a small whitish depression in the optic disc, the entry point for the retinal vessels. Although sometimes absent, the cup is usually visible either centrally or toward the temporal side of the disc. Grayish spots are often seen at its base.

Medullated Nerve Fibers

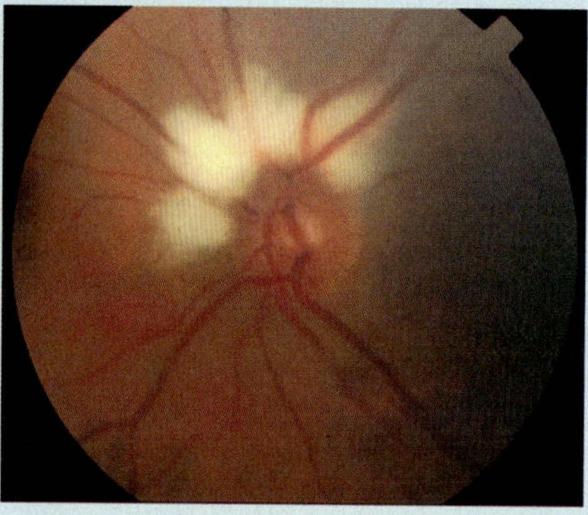

Medullated or myelinated nerve fibers are a less common but dramatic finding. Appearing as irregular white patches with feathered margins, they obscure the disc edge and retinal vessels. They have no pathologic significance.

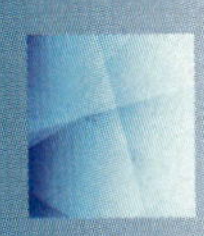

TABLE 14-9. Abnormalities of the Optic Disc

Normal

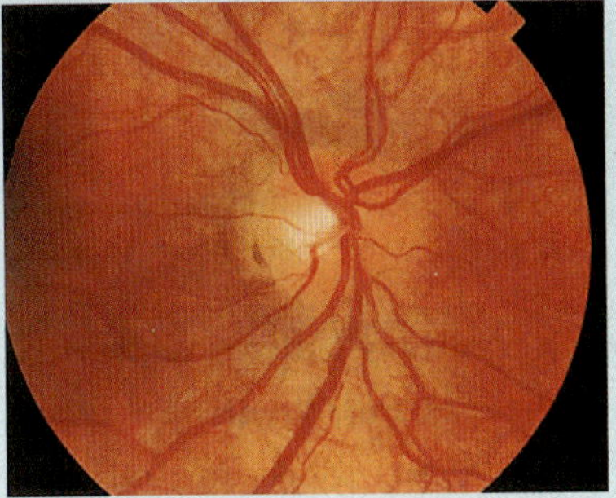

Process

Tiny disc vessels give normal color to the disc.

Appearance

Color yellowish-orange to creamy-pink
Disc vessels tiny
Disc margins sharp (except perhaps nasally)
The physiologic cup is located slightly temporally. Its diameter from side to side is usually less than half that of the disc.

Papilledema

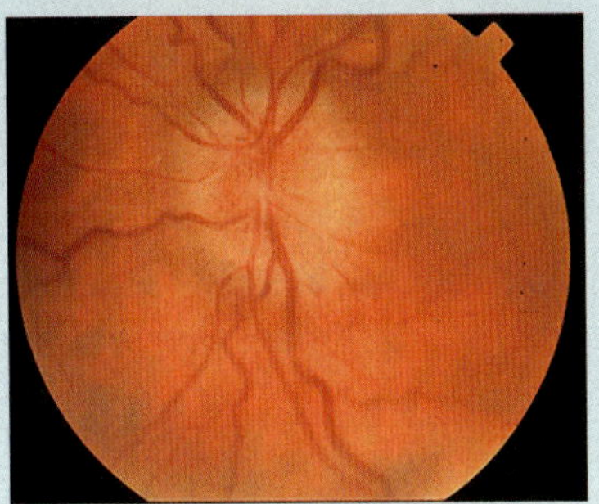

Process

Elevated intracranial pressure causes intra-axonal edema along the optic nerve, leading to engorgement and swelling of the optic disc.

Appearance

Color pink, hyperemic
Often with loss of venous pulsations
Disc vessels more visible, more numerous, curve over the borders of the disc
Disc swollen with margins blurred
Physiologic cup is not visible
Seen in intracranial mass, lesion, or hemorrhage, meningitis

Glaucomatous Cupping

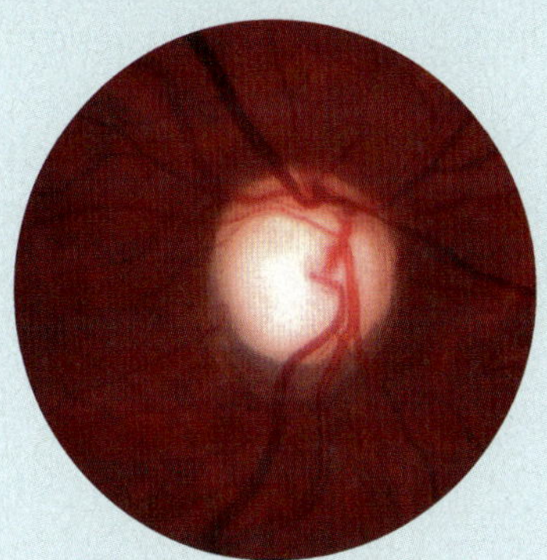

Process

Increased intraocular pressure within the eye leads to increased cupping (backward depression of the disc) and atrophy.

The base of the enlarged cup is pale.

Appearance

Death of optic nerve fibers leads to loss of the tiny disc vessels.

Optic Atrophy

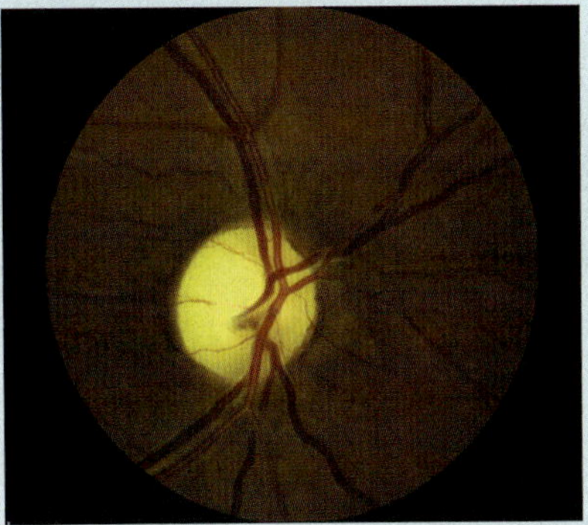

Process

The physiologic cup is enlarged, occupying more than half of the disc's diameter, at times extending to the edge of the disc. Retinal vessels sink in and under the cup, and may be displaced nasally.

Appearance

Color white
Tiny disc vessels absent
Seen in optic neuritis, multiple sclerosis, temporal arteritis

Sources of photos: *Normal*—Reprinted with permission from Tasman W, Jaeger E, eds. *The Wills Eye Hospital Atlas of Clinical Ophthalmology*. 2nd ed. Lippincott Williams & Wilkins; 2001; *Papilledema, Glaucomatous Cupping, Optic Atrophy*—Courtesy of Kenn Freedman, MD.

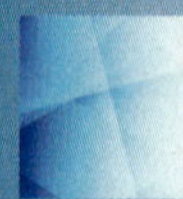

TABLE 14-10. Retinal Arteries and Arteriovenous Crossings: Normal and Hypertensive

Normal Retinal Artery and Arteriovenous (AV) Crossing

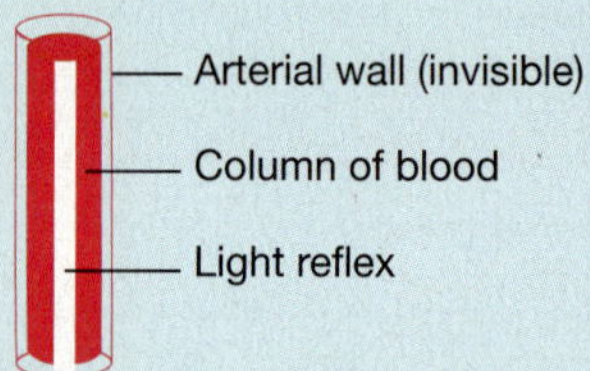

Normal artery wall is transparent with a narrow light reflex, about 1/4 of the diameter of the blood column. Vein crossing under the artery appears alongside the column of blood on both sides due to the transparent arterial wall.

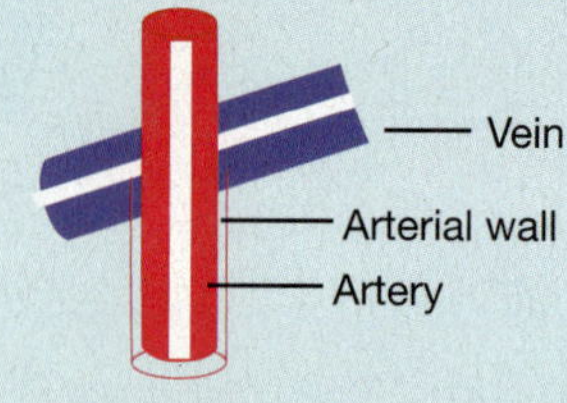

Retinal Arteries in Hypertension

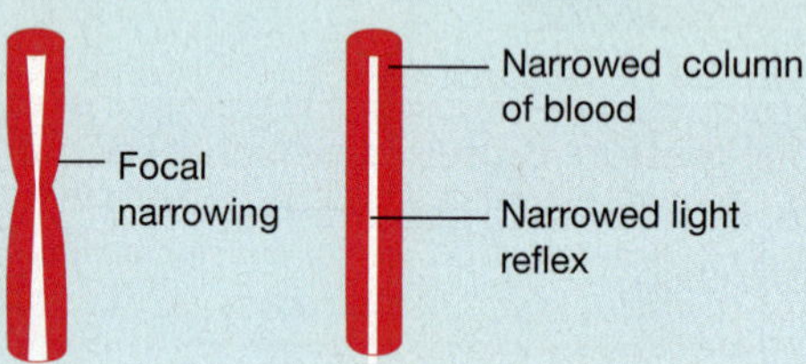

In hypertension, increased pressure damages the vascular endothelium, leading to deposition of plasma macromolecules and thickening of the arterial wall, causing focal or generalized narrowing of the lumen and the light reflex.

Copper Wiring

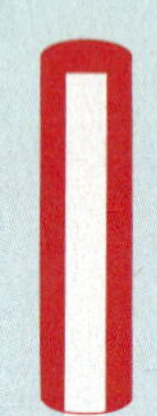

Sometimes the arteries, especially those close to the disc, become full and somewhat tortuous and develop an increased light reflex with a bright coppery luster, called copper wiring.

Silver Wiring

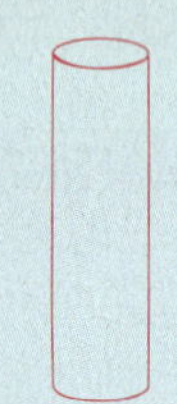

Occasionally the wall of a narrowed artery becomes opaque so there is no visible blood, called silver wiring.

AV Crossing

When the arterial walls lose their transparency, changes appear in the arteriovenous crossings. Decreased transparency of the retina probably also contributes to the first two changes shown below.

Concealment or AV Nicking. The vein appears to stop abruptly on either side of the artery.

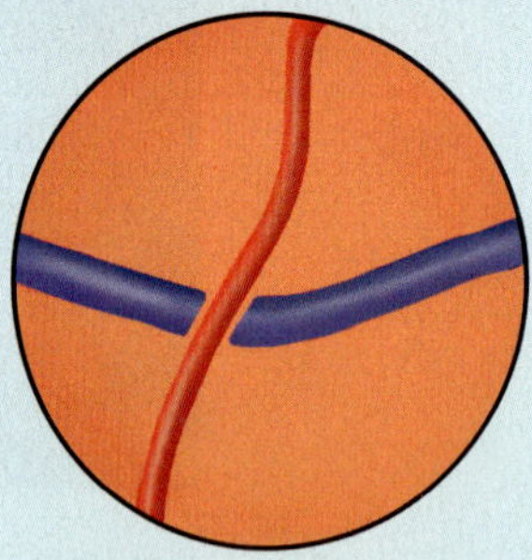

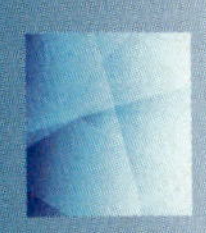

TABLE 14-11. Red Spots and Streaks in the Fundi

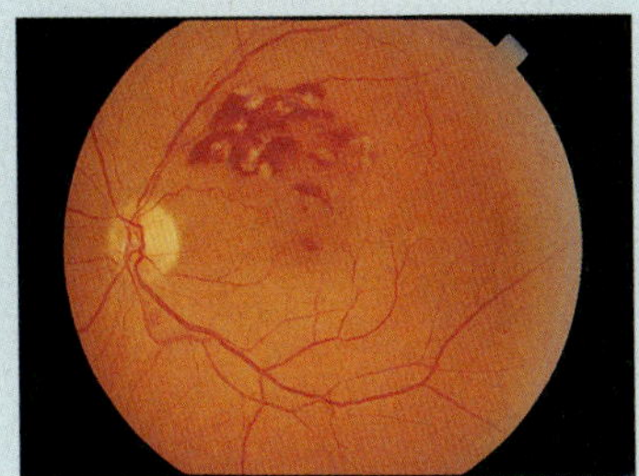

Superficial Retinal Hemorrhages

Small, linear, flame-shaped, red streaks in the fundi, shaped by the superficial bundles of nerve fibers that radiate from the optic disc in the pattern illustrated (O, optic disc; F, fovea). Sometimes the hemorrhages occur in clusters and look like a larger hemorrhage but can be identified by the linear streaking at the edges. These hemorrhages are seen in severe hypertension, papilledema, and occlusion of the retinal vein, among other conditions. An occasional superficial hemorrhage has a white center consisting of fibrin, which has many causes.

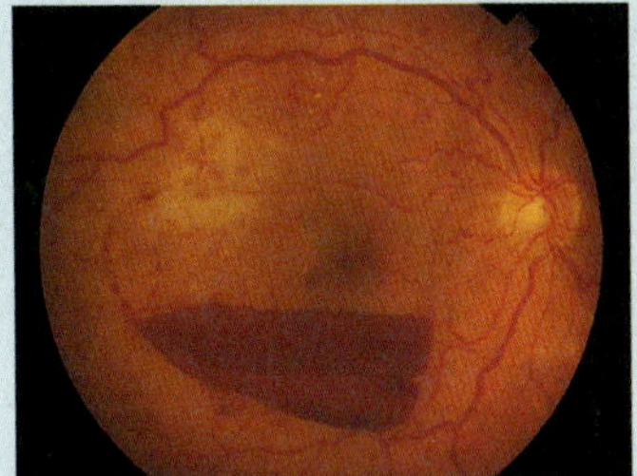

Preretinal Hemorrhage

Develops when blood escapes into the potential space between the retina and vitreous. This hemorrhage is typically larger than retinal hemorrhages. Because it is anterior to the retina, it obscures any underlying retinal vessels. Red blood cells settle with gravity, creating a horizontal line of demarcation between plasma above and cells below. Causes include a sudden increase in intracranial pressure.

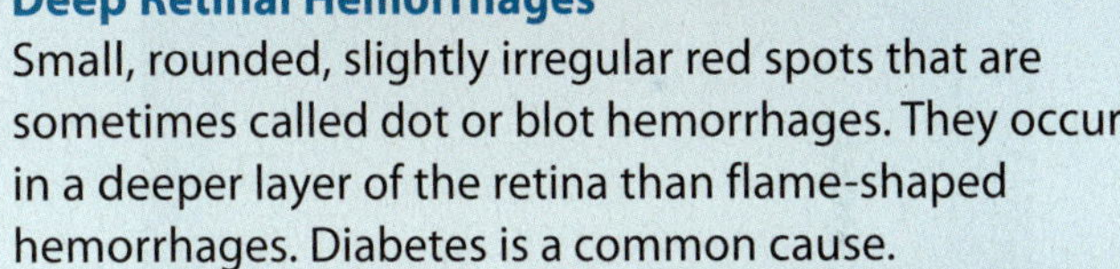

Deep Retinal Hemorrhages

Small, rounded, slightly irregular red spots that are sometimes called dot or blot hemorrhages. They occur in a deeper layer of the retina than flame-shaped hemorrhages. Diabetes is a common cause.

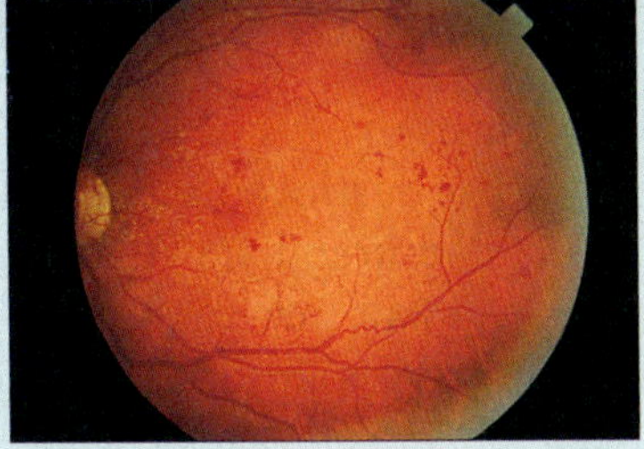

Microaneurysms

Tiny, round, red spots commonly seen in and around the macular area. They are minute dilatations of very small retinal vessels; the vascular connections are too small to be seen with an ophthalmoscope. A hallmark of diabetic retinopathy.

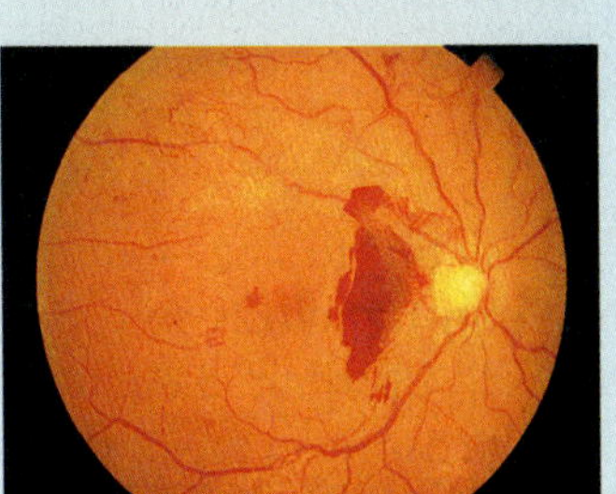

Neovascularization

Refers to the formation of new blood vessels. They are more numerous, more tortuous, and narrower than neighboring blood vessels in the area and form disorderly looking red arcades. A common feature of the proliferative stage of diabetic retinopathy. The vessels may grow into the vitreous, where retinal detachment or hemorrhage may cause loss of vision.

Source of photos: Reprinted with permission from Tasman W, Jaeger E, eds. *The Wills Eye Hospital Atlas of Clinical Ophthalmology*. 2nd ed. Lippincott Williams & Wilkins; 2001.

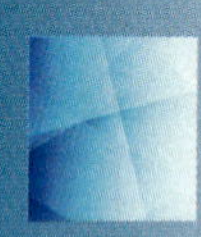

TABLE 14-12. Light-Colored Spots in the Fundi

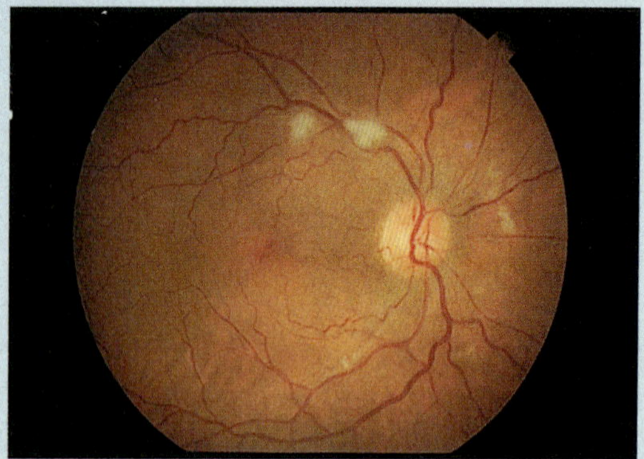

Soft Exudates: Cotton-Wool Spots

Cotton-wool spots are white or grayish, ovoid lesions caused by microinfarcts of the retinal nerve fiber layer. They have irregular "soft" borders and are moderate in size but usually smaller than the disc. Cotton-wool spots result from extruded axoplasm from retinal ganglion cells and are seen in conditions such as hypertension, diabetes, HIV, and other viruses.

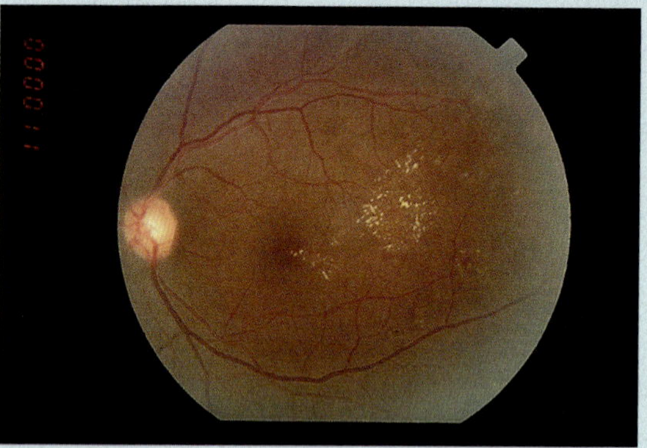

Hard Exudates

Hard exudates are lipid residues of serous leakage from damaged capillaries. They are creamy or yellowish, often bright, lesions with well-defined "hard" borders. These lesions are small and round, but they may coalesce into larger irregular spots. They can often be seen in clusters or in circular, linear, or star-shaped patterns. Hard exudates are commonly caused by diabetes and vascular dysplasias.

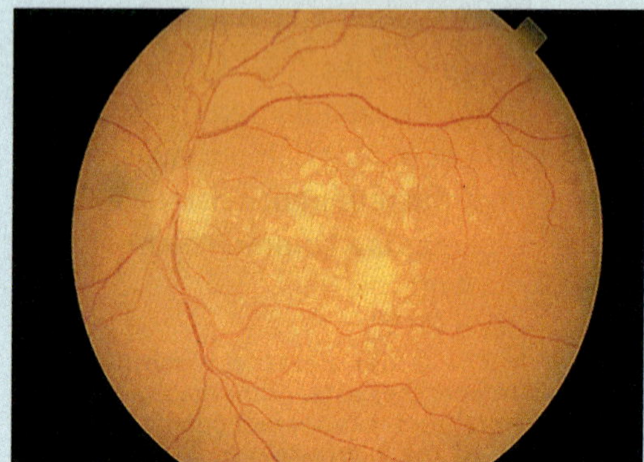

Drusen

Drusen are yellowish tiny to small round spots in the retina. The edges may be soft, as here, or hard (p. 339). They are haphazardly distributed but may concentrate at the posterior pole between the optic disc and the macula. Drusen consists of dead retinal pigment epithelial cells and is seen in normal aging and age-related macular degeneration.

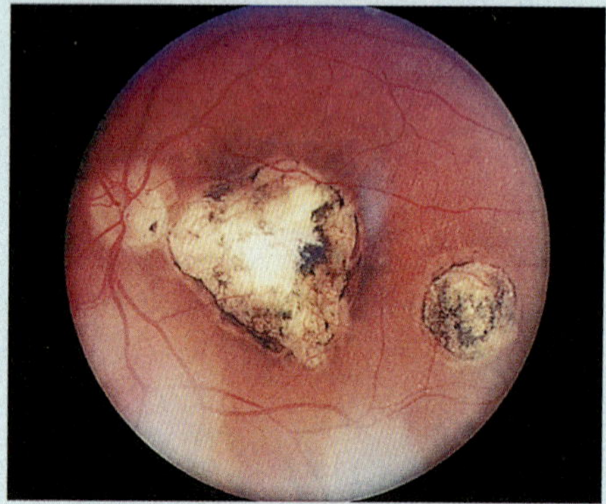

Healed Chorioretinitis

Here inflammation has destroyed the superficial tissues to reveal a well-defined, irregular patch of white sclera marked with dark pigment. Size varies from small to very large. Toxoplasmosis is illustrated. Multiple, small, somewhat similar-looking areas may be due to laser treatments. Here there is also a temporal scar near the macula.

Sources of photos: *Cotton-Wool Patches, Drusen, Healed Chorioretinitis*—Reprinted with permission from Tasman W, Jaeger E, eds. *The Wills Eye Hospital Atlas of Clinical Ophthalmology*. 2nd ed. Lippincott Williams & Wilkins; 2001; *Hard Exudates*—Courtesy of Kenn Freedman, MD, American Academy of Ophthalmology.

REFERENCES

1. Harper RA. *Basic Ophthalmology.* 9th ed. American Academy of Ophthalmology; 2010.
2. McGee SR. *Evidence-Based Physical Diagnosis.* 3rd ed. Elsevier/Saunders; 2012.
3. Morgan WH, Lind CR, Kain S, Fatehee N, Bala A, Yu DY. Retinal vein pulsation is in phase with intracranial pressure and not intraocular pressure. *Invest Ophthalmol Vis Sci.* 2012; 53(8):4676–4681.
4. Jacks AS, Miller NR. Spontaneous retinal venous pulsation: aetiology and significance. *J Neurol Neurosurg Psychiatry.* 2003; 74(1):7–9.
5. Bartalena L, Tanda ML. Clinical practice. Graves' ophthalmopathy. *N Engl J Med.* 2009;360(10):994–1001.
6. Bahn RS. Graves' ophthalmopathy. *N Engl J Med.* 2010; 362(8):726–738.
7. Phelps PO, Williams K. Thyroid eye disease for the primary care physician. *Dis Mon.* 2014;60(6):292–298.
8. Centers for Disease Control and Prevention. Common Eye Disorders and Diseases. Accessed July 7, 2023. https://www.cdc.gov/vision-health/about-eye-disorders/
9. Flaxman AD, Wittenborn JS, Robalik T, et al. Prevalence of visual acuity loss or blindness in the US: a Bayesian meta-analysis. *JAMA Ophthalmol.* 2021;139(7):717–723.
10. Rein DB, Wittenborn JS, Zhang P, et al. The economic burden of vision loss and blindness in the United States. *Ophthalmology.* 2022;129(4):369–378.
11. Chou CF, Frances Cotch M, Vitale S, et al. Age-related eye diseases and visual impairment among U.S. adults. *Am J Prev Med.* 2013;45(1):29–35.
12. Chuck RS, Dunn SP, Flaxel CJ, et al. Comprehensive adult medical eye evaluation preferred practice pattern(R). *Ophthalmology.* 2021;128(1):P1–P29.
13. Gupta P, Zhao D, Guallar E, Ko F, Boland MV, Friedman DS. Prevalence of glaucoma in the United States: the 2005–2008 National Health and Nutrition Examination Survey. *Invest Ophthalmol Vis Sci.* 2016;57(6):2905–2913.
14. Gedde SJ, Vinod K, Wright MM, et al. Primary open-angle glaucoma preferred practice pattern(R). *Ophthalmology.* 2021; 128(1):P71–P150.
15. Force USPST, Mangione CM, Barry MJ, et al. Screening for primary open-angle glaucoma: US Preventive Services Task Force recommendation statement. *JAMA.* 2022;327(20): 1992–1997.
16. Moran JM, Phelps PO. Periocular skin cancer: diagnosis and management. *Dis Mon.* 2020;66(10):101046.
17. Yam JC, Kwok AK. Ultraviolet light and ocular diseases. *Int Ophthalmol.* 2014;34(2):383–400.
18. Taylor J, Sousa DC. Solar retinopathy. *N Engl J Med.* 2023; 389(2):165.
19. Antonetti DA, Klein R, Gardner TW. Diabetic retinopathy. *N Engl J Med.* 2012;366(13):1227–1239.
20. Sullivan CA, Chopdar A, Shun-Shin GA. Dense Kayser-Fleischer ring in asymptomatic Wilson's disease (hepatolenticular degeneration). *Br J Ophthalmol.* 2002;86(1): 114.

CHAPTER 15

Ears and Nose

EAR: ANATOMY AND PHYSIOLOGY

The ear has three compartments: the external ear, the middle ear, and the inner ear.

External Ear

The *external ear* is comprised of the auricle and ear canal. The *auricle* is mainly made up of cartilage and is covered by skin, providing it with a firm, elastic consistency. The *helix*, a prominent curved outer ridge, is a defining feature of the auricle. Additionally, the *antihelix*, another curved prominence, is situated parallel and anterior to the helix. The *lobule*, a fleshy projection located inferiorly, forms the earlobe. The ear canal opens behind the *tragus*, which is a nodular protrusion that points backward over the entrance to the canal (refer to Fig. 15-1).

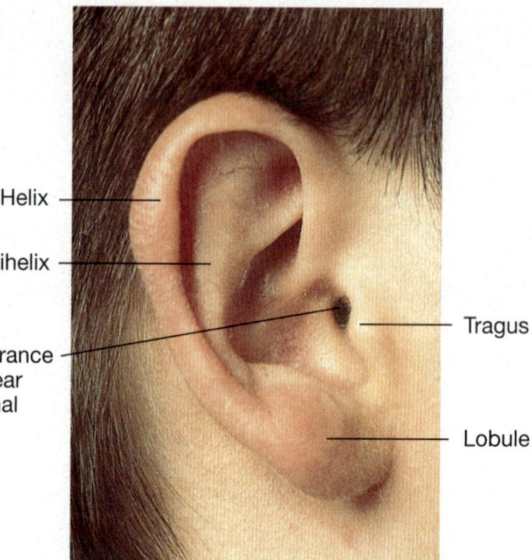

FIGURE 15-1. Anatomy of the external ear.

The *ear canal* is approximately 24 mm long, starting laterally at the external auditory meatus and extending inward to terminate at the eardrum. It has an S shape and travels anteriorly and inferiorly as it moves medially toward the eardrum. The outer one-third of the canal is encased in cartilage, covered by hair-bearing skin, and contains glands that produce *cerumen* (wax). In contrast, the inner two-thirds of the canal are surrounded by bone and lined by thin, hairless skin. Pressure on this inner two-thirds of the canal area causes pain—a point to remember during your examination. The lateral *tympanic membrane*, also known as the eardrum, marks the medial limit of the external ear at the end of the ear canal. The external ear functions by capturing sound waves and transmitting them into the middle and inner ear (Fig. 15-2).

Behind and below the ear canal is the mastoid portion of the temporal bone. The lowest portion of this bone, the *mastoid process*, is palpable behind the lobule.

Middle Ear

The middle ear, which is filled with air, contains three tiny bones called *ossicles*. These bones, namely the *malleus*, *incus*, and *stapes*, are responsible for transforming sound vibrations from the external ear into mechanical waves that

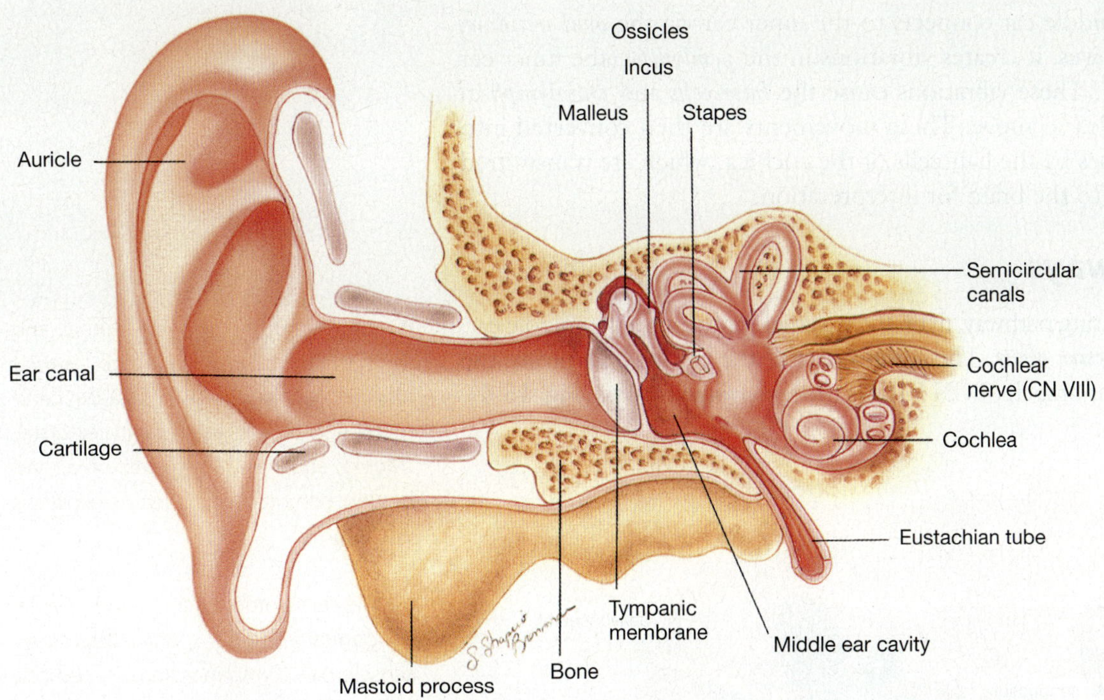

FIGURE 15-2. Anatomy of the external, middle, and inner ear.

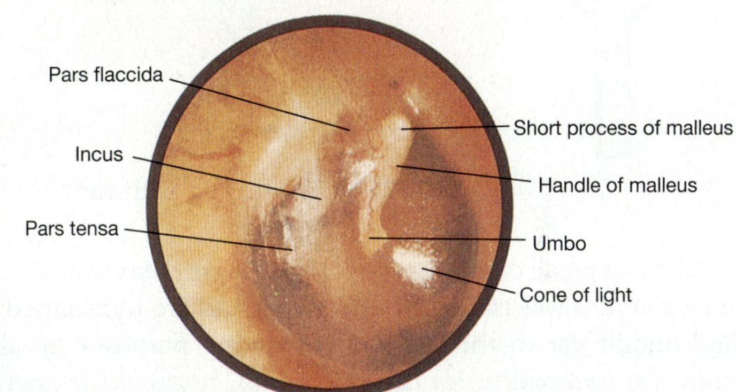

FIGURE 15-3. Right tympanic membrane.

then travel through the inner ear. The malleus and the incus, which are angled obliquely, are visible through the tympanic membrane. The malleus is attached to the center of the tympanic membrane, and its *handle* and *short process* are the two main landmarks. From the *umbo*, where the eardrum meets the tip of the malleus, a light reflection known as the *cone of light* fans downward and anteriorly. The *pars flaccida*, a small portion of the eardrum, lies above the short process, while the remainder of the eardrum is the *pars tensa*. The *anterior and posterior malleolar folds*, which extend obliquely upward from the short process of the malleus, separate the pars flaccida from the pars tensa, but they are usually invisible unless the eardrum is retracted. In some cases, the incus can also be seen through the drum in the posterior and superior area of the umbo (Fig. 15-3).

The middle ear connects to the nasopharynx via the proximal end of the *eustachian tube*, which ventilates the middle ear space and regulates pressure between the middle ear and surrounding environment. Additionally, it serves as a drainage pathway for mucus from the middle ear into the nasopharynx.

Inner Ear

The inner ear comprises the cochlea; semicircular canals; otolith organs located in the vestibule; and the *vestibulocochlear nerve*, also known as cranial nerve (CN) VIII. The cochlea is responsible for *hearing*, while the semicircular canals and otolith organs are dedicated to *balance*, collectively forming the *labyrinth*. Much of the middle ear and all of the inner ear is inaccessible to direct examination. You can assess their condition by testing auditory function.

The *stapes* in the middle ear connects to the inner ear via the *oval window*. As the stapes bone moves, it creates vibrations in the *perilymph* (the inner ear fluid) of the labyrinth. These vibrations cause the *hair cells* and *endolymph* in the ducts of the cochlea to move. These movements are then converted into electrical nerve impulses by the hair cells of the cochlea, which are transmitted by the auditory nerve to the brain for interpretation.

Hearing Pathways

The first part of the hearing pathway, from the external ear through the middle ear, is known as the *conductive phase*. The second part of the pathway, involving the cochlea and the cochlear branch of CN VIII, is the *sensorineural phase* (Fig. 15-4).

Hearing disorders of the external and middle ear cause *conductive hearing loss*. External ear causes include cerumen impaction, infection (otitis externa), trauma, squamous cell carcinoma, and benign bony growths such as exostosis or osteoma.

Middle ear disorders include otitis media, congenital conditions, cholesteatomas, otosclerosis, tympanosclerosis, tumors, and perforations of the tympanic membrane.

Disorders of the inner ear cause *sensorineural hearing loss* from congenital and hereditary conditions, presbycusis, viral infections such as rubella or cytomegalovirus, Ménière disease, noise exposure, ototoxic drug exposure, and acoustic neuromas.[1]

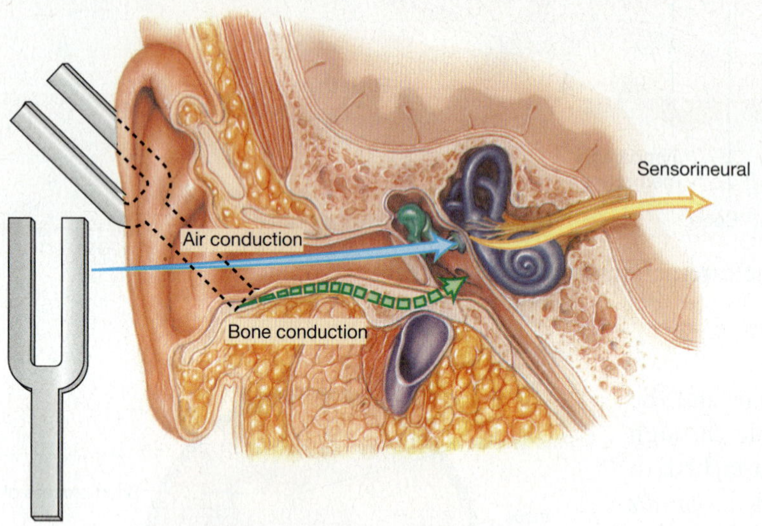

FIGURE 15-4. Hearing pathways.

The first phase of the hearing pathway is *air conduction (AC)*, which describes how sound waves travel through the air and are transmitted from the external and middle ear to the cochlea. For testing purposes, an alternative pathway known as *bone conduction (BC)* is used. BC bypasses the external and middle ear and directly stimulates the cochlea by setting the bone of the skull into vibration using a vibrating tuning fork placed on the head. In those with normal hearing, air conduction is *more sensitive* than bone conduction (AC > BC).

Vestibular System and Equilibrium

The vestibular system senses position and movements of the head contributing to our overall sense of balance and motion. The three semicircular canals in the inner ear sense *rotational movement*, whereas the otolith organs sense *linear movement*. Our visual and proprioceptive feedback also contribute to our overall sense of balance.

NOSE: ANATOMY AND PHYSIOLOGY

The nose consists of bone and cartilage, with approximately the upper third supported by bone and the lower two-thirds by cartilage (Fig. 15-5). Air enters

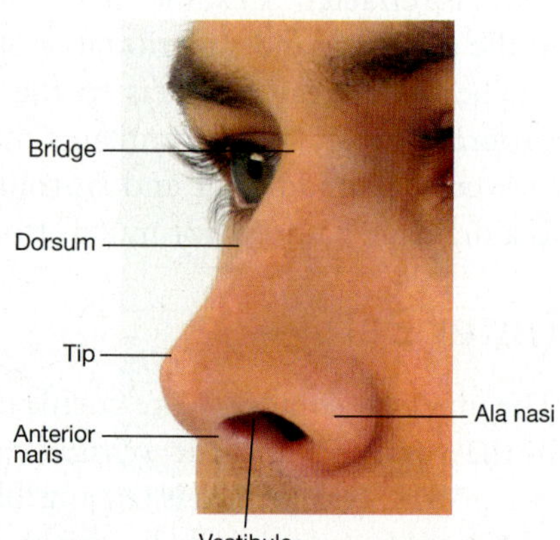

FIGURE 15-5. External anatomy of the nose.

the nasal cavity through the *anterior naris* on each side, then passes through the *vestibule*, a widened area, and on to the *nasopharynx* via the narrow nasal passage.

Nasal Septum

The *nasal septum* forms the medial wall of each nasal cavity, supported by both bone and cartilage, and is covered by a highly vascular *mucous membrane*. The vestibule, unlike the rest of the nasal cavity, is lined with hair-bearing skin instead of mucosa.

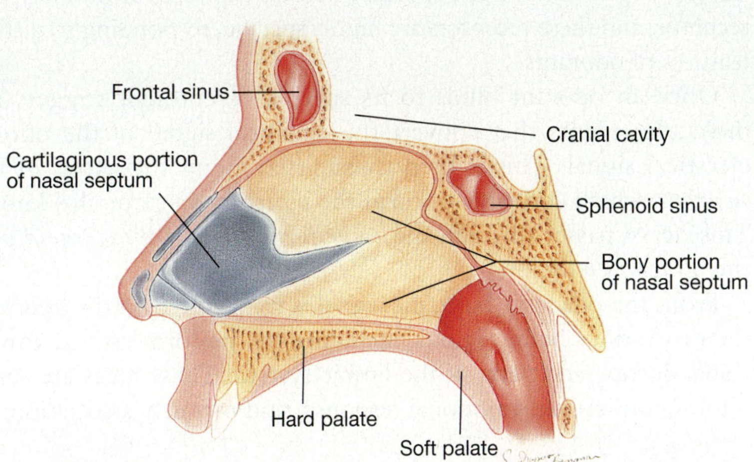

FIGURE 15-6. Medial wall—left nasal cavity (mucosa removed).

Turbinates and Meatuses

Laterally, the *turbinates*, bony structures covered by a highly vascular mucous membrane, curve and protrude into the nasal cavity. Each turbinate has a groove, or *meatus*, below it, named after the turbinate above it—*superior, middle*, and *inferior meatuses*. The inferior meatus drains the *nasolacrimal duct*, while most of the paranasal sinuses drain into the middle meatus (Figs. 15-6 and 15-7). Their openings are not usually visible. The turbinates and their overlying mucosa increase the surface area of the nasal cavities, aiding in the functions of cleansing, humidification, and temperature control of inspired air.

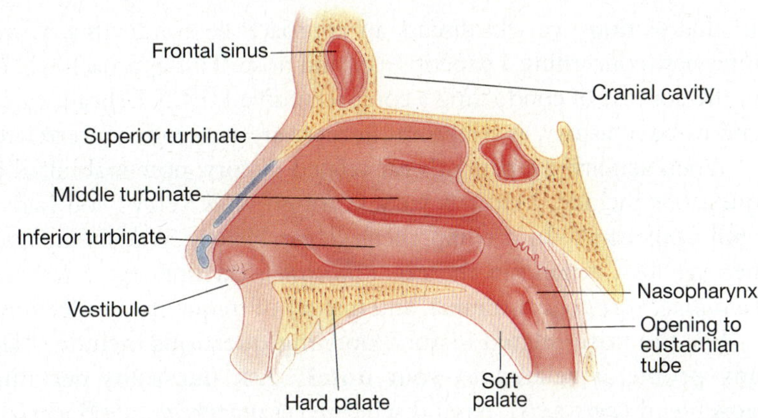

FIGURE 15-7. Lateral wall—right nasal cavity.

Paranasal Sinuses

The *paranasal sinuses* are four paired air-filled cavities located in the bones of the skull: the *maxillary, ethmoid, frontal, and sphenoid sinuses*. These cavities are lined with a mucous membrane and drain into the nasal cavities. The locations of all the sinuses are diagrammed in Figures 15-8 and 15-9. Only the frontal and maxillary sinuses are readily accessible on clinical examination

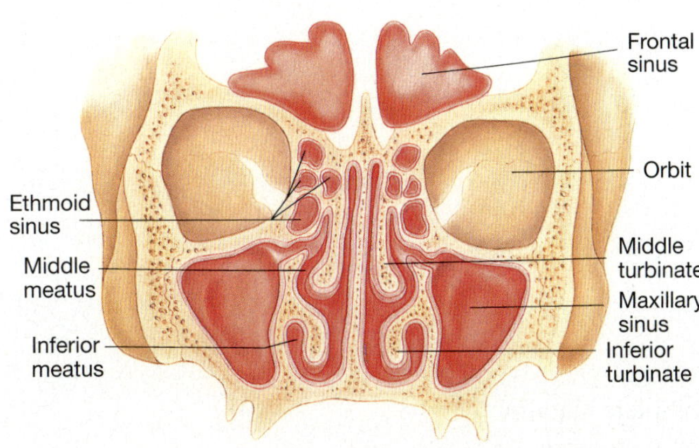

FIGURE 15-8. Cross-section of nasal cavity—anterior view.

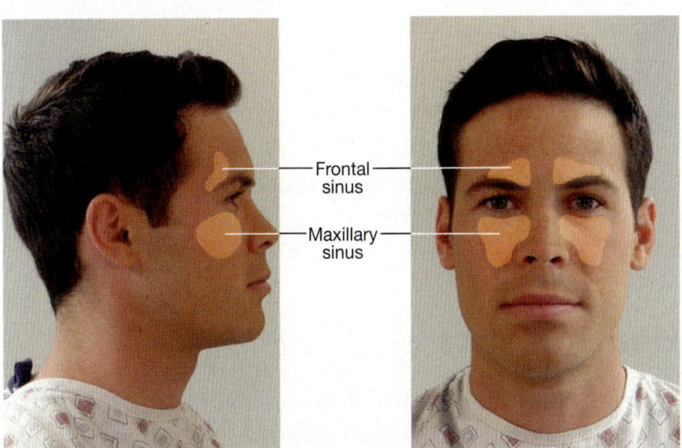

FIGURE 15-9. Frontal and maxillary sinuses.

Olfaction Pathway

The physiology of *olfaction*, or sense of smell, involves complex neurologic pathways. It begins when odorant molecules enter the nasal cavity and bind to olfactory receptors located on the cilia of olfactory sensory neurons within the olfactory epithelium. Each olfactory neuron expresses only one type of olfactory receptor, and these receptors are highly specific, responding to distinct chemical features of odorants.

Once an odorant binds to its specific receptor, it triggers a cascade of molecular events that convert the chemical signal of the odorant into an electrical signal. This is then transmitted along the axons of the *olfactory neurons*, which converge to form the *olfactory nerve* or also known as *CN I*. This nerve passes through the *cribriform plate of the ethmoid bone* to reach the *olfactory bulb*.

From the olfactory bulb, the signal is transmitted to the *olfactory tract* and then to various brain regions, including the piriform cortex, amygdala, entorhinal cortex, and parts of the limbic system. These areas are responsible for odor identification, emotional response, and memory association.

HEALTH HISTORY: GENERAL APPROACH

In this section, we will discuss an approach to conducting a health history interview concerning a patient's ears and nose. This approach will be beneficial in the context of conducting a comprehensive HEENT (head, ears, eyes, nose, and throat) history, as symptoms in these areas are often interrelated.

When acquiring a patient's ear-related history, potential initial open-ended questions include, "How is your hearing?" and "Have you had any trouble with your ears?" In a comprehensive ear history, you should inquire about hearing loss, ringing in the ears (*tinnitus*), ear drainage (*otorrhea*), ear pain (*otalgia*), vertigo, ear trauma, and history of frequent ear infections.

For the nose-related history, opening questions include, "Do you have any problems related to your nose?" Ask questions pertaining to any nosebleed (*epistaxis*), nasal discharge (*rhinorrhea*), nasal obstruction, and postnasal drip.

Common or Concerning Symptoms

- Hearing loss
- Earache and ear discharge
- Ringing in the ears (*tinnitus*)
- Dizziness and lightheadedness
- Nasal discharge (*rhinorrhea*) and nasal congestion
- Nosebleed (*epistaxis*)

Hearing Loss

Hearing loss, also known as *hearing impairment*, is a partial or complete inability to hear sounds in one or both ears. It can occur at any age and can be temporary or permanent, depending on the underlying cause. Sudden-onset hearing loss, particularly sensorineural hearing loss, without a known cause should be immediately referred to an otolaryngologist. These patients may benefit from urgent medical intervention. Pursue symptoms associated with hearing loss, such as earache or vertigo to help sort out likely causes. Ask about medications that might affect hearing and about sustained exposure to loud noise (Box 15-1).

Box 15-1. Hearing Loss: High-Yield Health History Questions

Domain	Questions	Rationale
Onset	*When did you first notice your hearing loss?*	*Sudden*: Sudden sensorineural hearing loss, acoustic trauma, barotrauma *Progressive*: Age-related hearing loss, noise-induced hearing loss, otosclerosis
Laterality	*Is your hearing loss in one ear or both ears?*	*Unilateral*: Acoustic neuroma, Ménière disease, sudden sensorineural hearing loss *Bilateral hearing loss*: Age-related hearing loss, noise-induced hearing loss, ototoxic medications
Severity	*How would you rate the severity of your hearing loss on a scale of 1–10?*	Severe hearing loss might suggest a more advanced or significant underlying condition
Associated symptoms	*Have you experienced any ringing in the ears (tinnitus), dizziness, or vertigo?*	*Tinnitus*: Age-related hearing loss, noise-induced hearing loss, Ménière disease, acoustic neuroma *Dizziness or vertigo*: Ménière disease, labyrinthitis, benign paroxysmal positional vertigo (BPPV)
Noise exposure	*Have you been exposed to loud noises or worked in a noisy environment?*	Can help identify noise-induced hearing loss, which can be gradual or sudden, depending on the intensity and duration of noise exposure
Medical history	*Do you have a history of ear infections, head or ear trauma, or family history of hearing loss?*	*Ear infections:* Recurrent otitis media, cholesteatoma *Head or ear trauma*: Tympanic membrane perforation, temporal bone fracture, disruption of the ossicular chain *Family history*: Genetic factors in sensorineural hearing loss, congenital hearing loss, syndromic or nonsyndromic hereditary hearing loss

Possible causes include **age-related hearing loss**, or **presbycusis** (degeneration of cochlea, loss of hair cells, neural changes); **noise-induced hearing loss** (damage to hair cells, cochlea from excessive noise); **ototoxic medication use** (damage to cochlea or vestibulocochlear nerve by ototoxic medications); and **trauma** (damage to ear structures, e.g., tympanic membrane, ossicles).

Earache and Ear Discharge

Earache, or pain in the ear, is especially common. Ask about discharge from the ear, especially if associated with earache or trauma. Cerumen (earwax) or debris in the ear is usually normal (Box 15-2).

Possible causes include **otitis externa** (inflammation of the external ear canal), **otitis media** (infection of the middle ear), and **temporomandibular joint (TMJ) disorder** (dysfunction of the jaw joint and muscles controlling jaw movement).

Box 15-2. Earache and Ear Discharge: High-Yield Health History Questions

Domain	Questions	Rationale
Onset	*When did the earache and ear discharge begin?*	Can help determine if the symptoms are *acute* (e.g., acute otitis media, external otitis) or *chronic* (e.g., chronic otitis media, cholesteatoma)
Laterality	*Are the earache and discharge in one ear or both ears?*	Helps differentiate between *unilateral* (e.g., external otitis, acute otitis media, cholesteatoma) and *bilateral* conditions (e.g., eustachian tube dysfunction, upper respiratory infection)
Characteristics	*Can you describe the ear discharge (e.g., color, consistency, odor)?*	*Pus-like, yellow-green:* Acute or chronic otitis media, cholesteatoma *Clear, watery:* Eustachian tube dysfunction, cerebrospinal fluid leak (rare) *Foul-smelling:* External otitis, cholesteatoma
Associated symptoms	*Have you experienced any fever, hearing loss, or dizziness?*	*Fever*: Acute otitis media, external otitis *Hearing loss*: Otitis media, cholesteatoma, eustachian tube dysfunction *Dizziness*: Labyrinthitis, inner ear involvement in middle ear infection
Medical history	*Do you have a history of ear infections, sinusitis, or upper respiratory infections?*	History of ear infections, sinusitis, or upper respiratory infections can provide valuable information on potential causes and predisposing factors for the current symptoms (e.g., recurrent acute otitis media, cholesteatoma, chronic otitis media, or eustachian tube dysfunction secondary to sinusitis or upper respiratory infections)

Domain	Questions	Rationale
Recent events	*Have you recently been swimming, had an upper respiratory infection, or used cotton swabs in your ears?*	*Swimming*: Otitis externa, also known as "swimmer's ear," can result from water exposure and bacterial or fungal infection *Upper respiratory infection*: Eustachian tube dysfunction or acute otitis media can develop following an upper respiratory infection *Cotton swab use*: Ear canal trauma, impacted cerumen, or tympanic membrane perforation can occur as a result of using cotton swabs in the ears

Ringing in the Ear (Tinnitus)

Tinnitus is a perceived sound that has no external stimulus—commonly, a musical ringing or a rushing or roaring noise in one or both ears. Tinnitus may accompany hearing loss and often remains unexplained (Box 15-3).

Box 15-3. Tinnitus: High-Yield Health History Questions

Domain	Questions	Rationale
Onset	*When did the tinnitus begin?*	Can help determine if the symptoms are *acute* (e.g., sudden sensorineural hearing loss) or *chronic* (e.g., age related hearing loss, chronic loud noise exposure)
Laterality	*Is the tinnitus in one ear or both ears?*	Helps differentiate between *unilateral* (e.g., vestibular schwannoma, vascular tumor, Ménière disease, asymmetric hearing loss) and *bilateral* conditions (e.g., age-related hearing loss, ototoxic medication exposure)
Characteristics	*Can you describe the tinnitus (e.g., pulsatile, objective)?*	*Pulsatile*: Vascular lesions, systemic cardiovascular illness, intracranial hypertension, patulous eustachian tube *Objective*: Palate myoclonus, vascular abnormalities

(continued)

Possible causes include **age-related hearing loss** (gradual deterioration of hair cells in the cochlea due to aging), **noise-induced hearing loss** (damage to hair cells in the cochlea due to exposure to loud noise), **ototoxic medications** (toxic effects on hair cells in the cochlea due to certain medications), **Ménière disease** (increased pressure in the cochlea due to excess fluid build-up), and **wax build-up in the ear canal** (blockage of the ear canal by earwax).

Box 15-3. Tinnitus: High-Yield Health History Questions (*Continued*)

Domain	Questions	Rationale
Associated symptoms	*Have you experienced any hearing loss, vertigo/imbalance?*	*Hearing loss*: Conductive hearing loss, sensorineural hearing loss; *Vertigo/imbalance*: Ménière disease, superior semicircular canal dehiscence, vestibular schwannoma
Medical history	*Do you have a history of cardiovascular or neurologic disease?*	History of *cardiovascular* (e.g., carotid stenosis, vascular aneurysm, heart murmur, hypertension) or *neurologic* conditions (e.g., intracranial arteriovenous malformations) can contribute to sources of pulsatile tinnitus
Medication history	*What medications do you currently take, or have you taken recently?*	Aspirin, nonsteroidal anti-inflammatory drugs, loop diuretics, and quinines can cause temporary tinnitus; aminoglycosides and some chemotherapeutic drugs (cisplatin) can cause permanent hearing loss/tinnitus

Dizziness and Lightheadedness

Dizziness and *lightheadedness* are challenging because these symptoms are often nonspecific and suggest a diverse set of conditions ranging from vertigo to presyncope, weakness, unsteadiness, and disequilibrium (Box 15-4). Clarify by asking the patient to describe how they are feeling without using the word "dizzy."

If there is true vertigo, distinguish peripheral from central neurologic causes (see Chapter 27, Nervous System, pp. 911–912).

See Table 15-1, Dizziness and Vertigo, p. 384 for distinguishing symptoms and time course.

Box 15-4. Dizziness: High-Yield Health History Questions

Domain	Questions	Rationale
Type	*How would you describe your dizziness (e.g., lightheadedness, spinning sensation, unsteadiness)?*	*Lightheadedness*: Vasovagal syncope, orthostatic hypotension, dehydration *Spinning sensation (vertigo):* Benign paroxysmal positional vertigo (BPPV), Ménière disease, vestibular neuritis *Unsteadiness*: Cerebellar dysfunction, peripheral neuropathy
Onset	*When did your dizziness begin?*	*Sudden:* BPPV, vestibular neuritis, stroke *Gradual:* Some cases of Ménière disease

Possible causes include **benign positional vertigo** (displacement of inner ear crystals [*otoconia*]), **acute labyrinthitis** (inflammation of the inner ear, often due to viral or bacterial infections, causing disturbance in the balance system), **vestibular neuritis** (inflammation of the vestibular nerve, typically caused by viral infections, leading to impaired balance and vertigo), and **Ménière disease** (disorder of the inner ear causing abnormal fluid accumulation, affecting the balance and hearing systems).

Domain	Questions	Rationale
Duration	*How long do your episodes of dizziness last?*	*Seconds to minutes*: BPPV, orthostatic hypotension *Hours to days*: Ménière disease, vestibular migraine *Days to weeks*: Vestibular neuritis, labyrinthitis *Persistent*: Central nervous system disorders, medication side effects
Triggers	*Are there any specific triggers for your dizziness (e.g., position changes, loud noises, certain situations)?*	*Position changes*: BPPV, orthostatic hypotension *Loud noises:* Perilymphatic fistula, superior semicircular canal dehiscence, Ménière disease *Certain situations*: Situational syncope (e.g., cough syncope, micturition syncope), anxiety or panic attacks
Associated symptoms	*Have you experienced any hearing loss, tinnitus, headache, or visual disturbances along with your dizziness?*	*Hearing loss or tinnitus*: Ménière disease, acoustic neuroma, labyrinthitis *Headache*: Migraine-associated vertigo, vestibular migraine, cerebrovascular event *Visual disturbances*: Migraine-associated vertigo, vestibular migraine, transient ischemic attack (TIA) or stroke
Medical history	*Do you have a history of heart disease, hypertension, diabetes, or neurologic disorders?*	*Heart disease:* Arrhythmias, valvular heart disease, or other cardiovascular causes of dizziness *Hypertension*: Orthostatic hypotension secondary to antihypertensive medications *Diabetes*: Peripheral neuropathy, autonomic neuropathy causing orthostatic hypotension *Neurologic disorders*: Multiple sclerosis, Parkinson disease, other central nervous system causes of dizziness

Nasal Discharge (Rhinorrhea) and Nasal Congestion

Rhinorrhea refers to drainage from the nose and is often associated with *nasal congestion*, a sense of stuffiness or obstruction. These symptoms are frequently accompanied by sneezing; watery eyes; throat discomfort; and itching in the eyes, nose, and throat (Box 15-5).[2]

Possible causes include **postnasal drip** (accumulation of mucus in the back of the throat), **sinusitis** (inflammation or infection of the paranasal sinuses), and **allergic rhinitis** (inflammation of the nasal mucous membranes caused by inhalation of an allergen).

Box 15-5. Rhinorrhea and Nasal Congestion: High-Yield Health History Questions

Domain	Questions	Rationale
Onset	*When did your rhinorrhea and nasal congestion begin?*	Can help determine if the symptoms are *acute* (e.g., viral upper respiratory infection, acute sinusitis) or *chronic* (e.g., allergic rhinitis, chronic sinusitis)
Characteristics	*Can you describe the characteristics of your nasal discharge (e.g., color, consistency)?*	*Clear, watery*: Viral upper respiratory infection, allergic rhinitis *Thick, yellow-green*: Bacterial sinusitis, chronic sinusitis *Bloody*: Nasal trauma, dry environment, septal perforation
Seasonality	*Do your symptoms occur seasonally or year-round?*	*Seasonal*: Allergic rhinitis related to specific allergens (e.g., grass, trees, pollen) *Year-round*: Nonallergic rhinitis, allergic rhinitis–related perennial allergen (dust, mold, dander), chronic sinusitis, vasomotor rhinitis
Triggers	*Are there any specific triggers for your rhinorrhea and nasal congestion (e.g., exposure to allergens, changes in weather, strong odors)?*	*Exposure to allergens*: Allergic rhinitis *Changes in weather or strong odors:* Vasomotor rhinitis *Upper respiratory infection*: Viral or bacterial sinusitis
Associated symptoms	*Have you experienced any fever, facial pain or pressure, or itchy/watery eyes along with your rhinorrhea and nasal congestion?*	*Fever*: Viral upper respiratory infection, bacterial sinusitis *Facial pain or pressure:* Sinusitis, either acute or chronic *Itchy/watery eyes*: Allergic rhinitis

Domain	Questions	Rationale
Medical history	*Do you have a history of allergies, asthma, or frequent sinus infections?*	*Allergies*: Allergic rhinitis, allergic sinusitis *Asthma*: Nasal symptoms related to allergic or nonallergic triggers, as both conditions may coexist *Frequent sinus infections*: Recurrent acute sinusitis, predisposition to developing chronic sinusitis

Nosebleed (Epistaxis)

Epistaxis or nosebleed is characterized by bleeding from the blood vessels inside the nose. It is a common condition that can range from a minor annoyance to a medical emergency, depending on the severity and duration of the bleeding (Box 15-6). Nosebleeds can occur in any age group but are more common in children and elderly patients.

Box 15-6. Epistaxis: High-Yield Health History Questions

Domain	Questions	Rationale
Onset	*When did the nosebleed begin?*	Spontaneous or related to an inciting event: trauma, nose-picking, use of nasal sprays
Laterality	*Is the bleeding from one nostril or both?*	*One nostril*: Localized causes (e.g., nasal septal irritation, foreign body) *Both nostrils*: Systemic causes (e.g., coagulopathy, hypertension)
Severity	*How would you rate the severity of the bleeding (e.g., slow drip, steady flow, gushing)?*	More severe bleeding might suggest a more significant underlying cause (e.g., arterial bleeding, coagulopathy)
Duration	*How long has the bleeding been occurring, and have you been able to stop it?*	Long-lasting, uncontrolled bleeding might suggest a more severe underlying cause or require more aggressive management

(continued)

Possible causes include **trauma** (injury to the blood vessels in the nose due to trauma), **dry air** (dry nasal lining can get irritated, leading to the formation of crusts or scabs that can bleed when disturbed), **nose picking** (injury to the blood vessels in the nose due to mechanical trauma), **infections** (inflammation and irritation of the nasal lining due to infections such as sinusitis or rhinitis), **high blood pressure** (damage to the blood vessels in the nose due to uncontrolled high blood pressure), and **blood-thinning medications** (interference with the clotting of blood, making it easier for nosebleeds to occur).

Box 15-6. Epistaxis: High-Yield Health History Questions (*Continued*)

Domain	Questions	Rationale
Precipitating factors	*Were there any factors that may have caused or contributed to the nosebleed (e.g., trauma, dry environment, use of blood-thinning medications, recent nasal surgery)?*	*Trauma*: Nasal fracture, foreign body, nose-picking *Dry environment*: Nasal mucosal dryness and irritation *Blood-thinning medications*: Anticoagulants, antiplatelet agents *Nasal surgery*: Postoperative epistaxis may be more difficult to control with conservative measures
Medical history	*Do you have a history of bleeding disorders, hypertension, or chronic sinusitis?*	*Bleeding disorders*: Coagulopathy, hemophilia, von Willebrand disease, hereditary hemorrhagic telangiectasia *Hypertension*: Increased risk of spontaneous nosebleeds due to high blood pressure *Chronic sinusitis*: Inflammation, irritation, or infections affecting the nasal passages and sinuses, which can predispose to bleeding

PHYSICAL EXAMINATION: GENERAL APPROACH

Both the ears and the nose require external and internal examinations. When you examine the ear, start externally by inspecting and palpating the auricle and the surrounding tissues. Then, delve deeper to explore the internal structures like the ear canal and eardrum using an otoscope. Similarly, for the nose, initiate your examination externally, and then progress to inspecting the anterior nasal cavity with an otoscope. This structured approach will serve you well in your clinical training.

EAR: TECHNIQUES OF EXAMINATION

Key Components of the Ear Examination

- Examine the auricle and surrounding tissue and palpate the tragus and mastoid.
- Examine the ear canals and tympanic membranes and malleus (otoscopy).
- Test auditory acuity (gross hearing).
- Test for conductive versus sensorineural hearing loss.

Examine the Auricle and Surrounding Tissue and Palpate the Tragus and Mastoid

Inspect the auricle and surrounding tissue for deformities, lumps, pits, or skin lesions.

See Table 15-2, Lumps on or Near the Ear, p. 385.

If ear pain, discharge, or inflammation is present, move the auricle up and down, press the tragus (*tug test*), and press firmly just behind the ear over the mastoid.

Movement of the auricle and tragus is painful in **acute otitis externa** (inflammation of the ear canal), but *not* in **otitis media** (inflammation of the middle ear).

Examine the Ear Canals and Tympanic Membranes (Otoscopy)

To examine the ear canal and tympanic membrane, use an otoscope with the largest ear speculum that can insert easily into the canal, as shown in Box 15-7.

Tenderness behind the ear occurs in otitis media and mastoiditis.

Otitis media can occasionally progress to acute mastoiditis, which presents with postauricular swelling, fluctuance, erythema, ear proptosis, and significant tenderness. *Bullous myringitis* is also a common sequela presenting with painful hemorrhagic vesicles on the tympanic membrane. Both of these conditions require urgent, often surgical, management by an otolaryngologist.

Box 15-7. Examining the Ears with the Otoscope

- Position the patient's head for optimal visibility through the otoscope.
- Use the fingers of your left hand to gently grasp the auricle and straighten the right ear canal by pulling it upward, backward, and slightly away from the head.
- Securely hold the otoscope handle between your thumb and fingers of your right hand, and brace your remaining fingers against the patient's face to allow for unexpected movements.

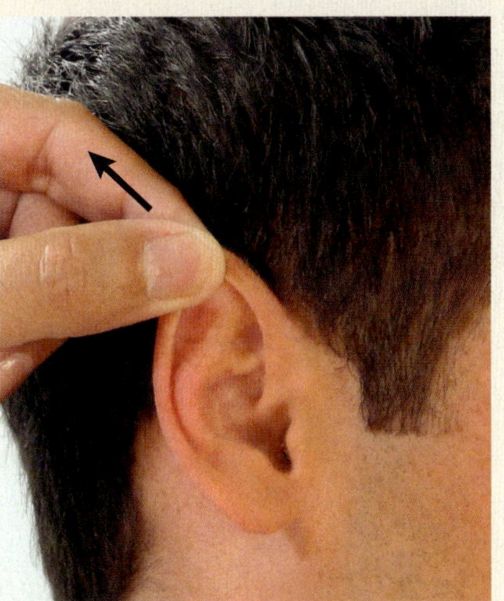

Straightening the ear canal to insert the otoscope speculum.

(*continued*)

Box 15-7. Examining the Ears with the Otoscope (*Continued*)

- Insert the speculum gently into the ear canal, directing it somewhat down and forward through any hairs present.
- When examining the left ear, switch hands by holding the otoscope with your left hand and straightening the ear canal with your right hand.
- If you find it uncomfortable to switch hands for examining the left ear, use your left hand to reach over the ear to pull it up and back, while holding the otoscope steady with your right hand to gently insert the speculum.

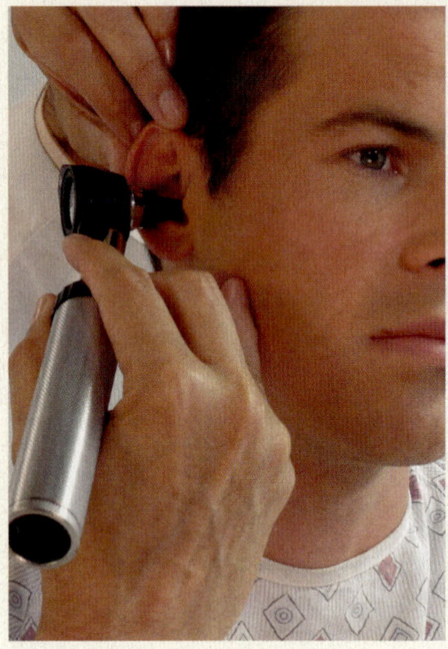

Bracing the otoscope with the right hand against the face and examining the right ear.

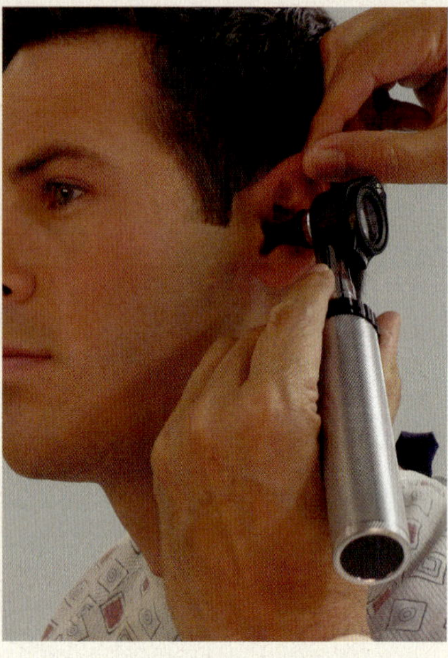

Bracing the otoscope with the left hand against the face and examining the left ear.

Nontender nodular swellings covered by normal skin deep in the ear canals suggest osteomas or exostoses (Fig. 15-10). These are nonmalignant overgrowths, which may obscure the tympanic membrane.

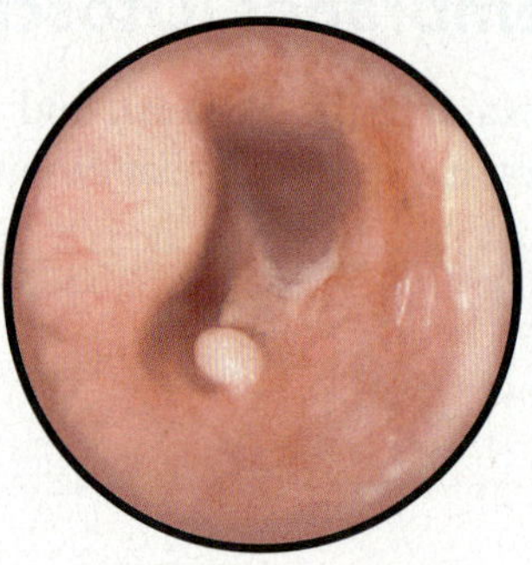

FIGURE 15-10. Exostosis.

Begin by inspecting the ear canal, noting any discharge, foreign bodies, redness of the skin, or swelling. Cerumen, which varies in color and consistency from yellow and flaky to brown and sticky, or even to dark and hard, may obstruct your view partially or completely.

In acute otitis externa, the canal is often swollen, narrowed, moist, erythematous or pale, and tender (Fig. 15-11).

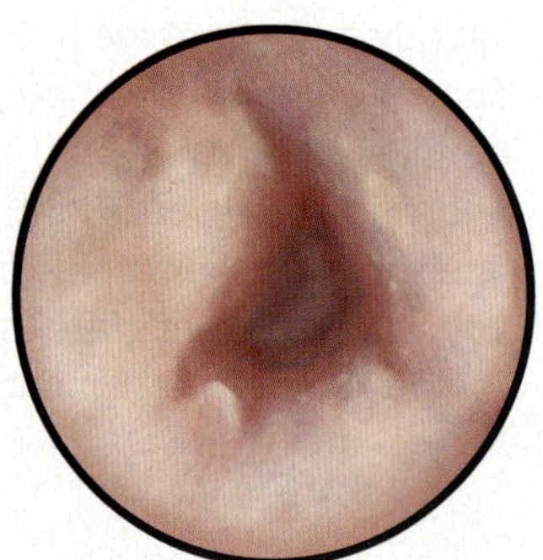

FIGURE 15-11. Acute otitis externa.

Inspect the tympanic membrane next, noting its color and contour (refer to Fig. 15-12). The cone of light, which is usually visible, can help orient you.

Look for the red, bulging tympanic membrane of acute purulent otitis media[3] and for the amber color of a serous effusion.

See Table 15-3, Abnormalities of the Tympanic Membrane, pp. 386–387 and Chapter 28, Children: Infancy Through Adolescence, Table 28-8, Abnormalities of the Eyes, Ears, and Mouth, p. 1109.

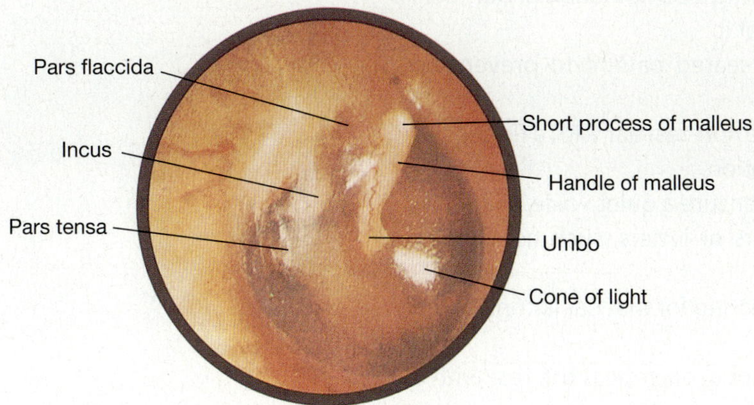

FIGURE 15-12. Anatomy of the right tympanic membrane.

Identify the handle of the malleus and inspect the short process of the malleus, noting its position.

An unusually prominent short process and a prominent handle that looks more horizontal suggest a retracted tympanic membrane.

Gently adjust the speculum to view as much of the tympanic membrane as possible, including the pars flaccida superiorly and the margins of the pars tensa. Check for any perforations. Note that the curving wall of the ear canal may obscure the anterior and inferior margins of the drum. To evaluate the mobility of the eardrum, use a *pneumatic otoscope* (refer to Chapter 28, Children: Infancy Through Adolescence, p. 1060).

A serous effusion, a thickened tympanic membrane, or purulent otitis media may decrease mobility. If there is a perforation, there will be no mobility.

Test Auditory Acuity (Gross Hearing)

To begin screening, ask the patient "Do you feel you have hearing loss or difficulty hearing?" Ask if the hearing loss or difficulty is more pronounced in one ear compared to the other.

Patients who answer "yes" are twice as likely to have a hearing deficit; for patients who report normal hearing, the likelihood of moderate to severe hearing impairment is only 0.13.[4]

If the patient reports hearing loss, proceed to the *whispered voice test* (Box 15-8). The whispered voice test is a reliable screening test for hearing loss if the examiner uses a standardized and consistent method of testing. Positive likelihood ratio (LR) is 2.3, and negative LR is 0.73.[4–7] This test is used to detect significant hearing loss greater than 30 dB, but a formal hearing test remains the reference standard.

Test for Conductive versus Sensorineural Hearing Loss

The *Weber* and *Rinne* fork tests may help determine if the hearing loss is conductive or sensorineural in origin for patients who fail the whispered voice test. However, questions have been raised about their precision, or test-retest reproducibility, and their accuracy when compared to air–bone gap reference standards.[6] Keep these factors in mind when interpreting the results of these tests.

Sensitivity of the Weber test is about 55%; specificity for sensorineural loss is about 79%, and for conductive loss, 92%. Sensitivity and specificity of the Rinne test are 60% to 90% and 95% to 98%.[8]

Box 15-8. Whispered Voice Test for Auditory Acuity

- Inform the patient that you will be whispering a combination of numbers and letters and then asking them to repeat it.
- Stand at arm's length (2 ft) behind the seated patient to prevent lip reading.
- Test each ear individually by occluding the non-test ear with a finger and gently rubbing the tragus in a circular motion.
- Exhale a full breath before whispering to ensure a quiet voice.
- Whisper a combination of three numbers or letters, such as 4-K-2 or 5-B-6.
  - If the patient responds correctly, the hearing for that ear is considered normal.
  - If the patient responds incorrectly or not at all, repeat the test with a different combination to exclude learning effects.
  - If the patient repeats at least three out of six letters or numbers correctly, they pass the screening test.
  - If the patient repeats less than three letters or numbers correctly, conduct further testing with audiometry.
- Repeat the same procedure for the other ear using a different number/letter combination.

Older adults with presbycusis, a type of sensorineural hearing loss related to age-related changes in the auditory system, may have difficulty hearing sibilant consonants due to their higher frequency. This type of hearing loss is usually gradual, progressive, and affects both ears.

To conduct the Weber and Rinne fork tests, ensure that the room is quiet and use a 512-Hz tuning fork. This frequency falls within the range of conversational speech, which is typically between 500 and 3,000 Hz and 45 to 60 dB.

Briskly stroke the prongs of a 512-Hz tuning fork between your thumb and index finger or tap them on your forearm just in front of your elbow to set the fork into light vibration.

Test for Lateralization (Weber Test). Firmly place the base of the vibrating tuning fork on top of the patient's head or on their midforehead (Fig. 15-13). Ask the patient where they hear the sound best: "On one side or both sides?" Normally, the vibration is heard in the midline or equally in both ears. If nothing is heard, try again while pressing the fork more firmly on the head. Restrict this test to patients with unilateral hearing loss because patients with normal hearing may lateralize, and patients with bilateral conductive or sensorineural deficits will not lateralize.

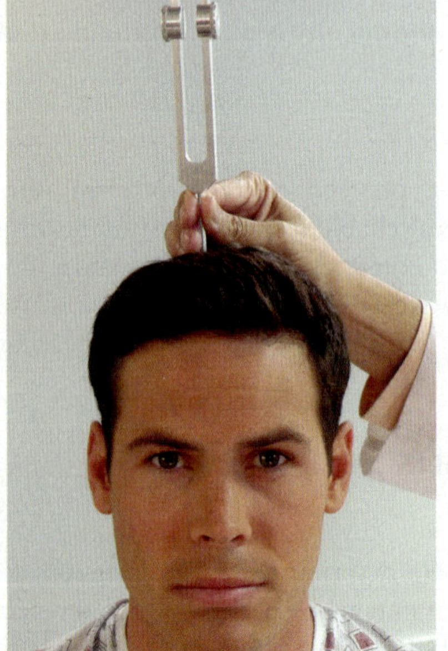

FIGURE 15-13. Lateralization (Weber) test.

In unilateral conductive hearing loss, sound is heard in (lateralized to) the impaired ear. Explanations include otosclerosis, otitis media, perforation of the eardrum, and cerumen. See Table 15-4, Patterns of Hearing Loss, p. 388.

In unilateral sensorineural hearing loss, sound is heard in the good ear.

Compare Air Conduction and Bone Conduction (Rinne Test). Place the base of a lightly vibrating tuning fork on the patient's mastoid bone, level with the ear canal (Fig. 15-14). Once the patient can no longer hear the sound, move the prongs of the fork close to their ear canal and ask if they detect any vibration (Fig. 15-15). Ensure that the prongs of the fork face forward to maximize sound transmission. Typically, sound is heard longer through air than through bone (AC > BC).

In conductive hearing loss, sound is heard through bone as long as or longer than it is through air (BC = AC or BC > AC). In sensorineural hearing loss, sound is heard longer through air (AC > BC) but may be reduced in absolute terms.

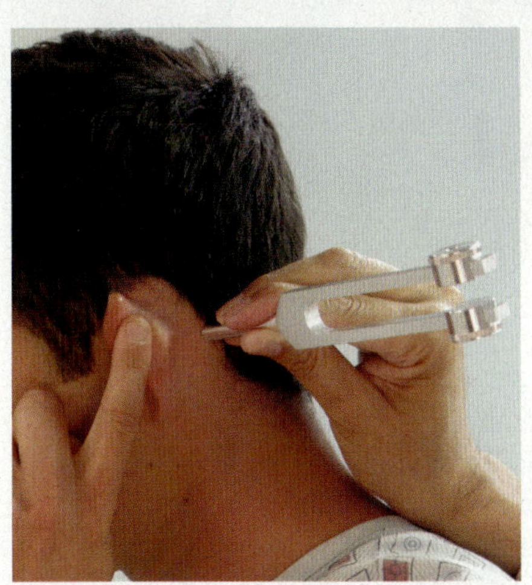

FIGURE 15-14. Rinne: Testing bone conduction.

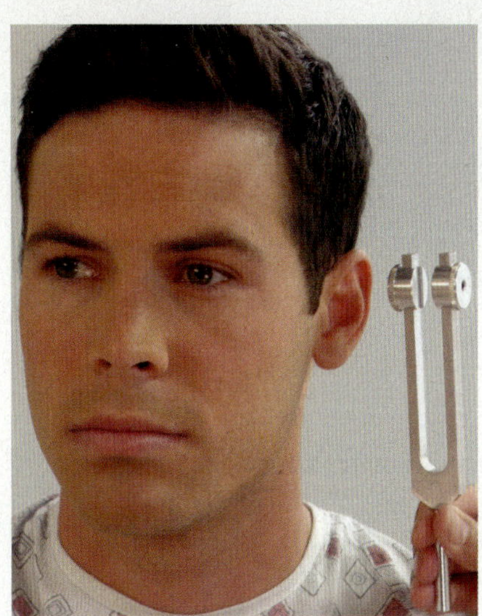

FIGURE 15-15. Rinne: Testing air conduction.

EAR: SPECIAL TECHNIQUES AND MANEUVERS

Modifications in Physical Examinations: Best Practices for Specialized Patient Populations

As you go through your training, you will increasingly encounter patients using hearing augmentation devices. Both hearing aids and cochlear implants present unique challenges during the assessment. Box 15-9 guides you through the ear examination in the presence of these devices to ensure thoroughness, patient comfort, and accuracy in assessment.

Box 15-9. Ear Examination in the Presence of Medical Devices, Conditions or Procedures

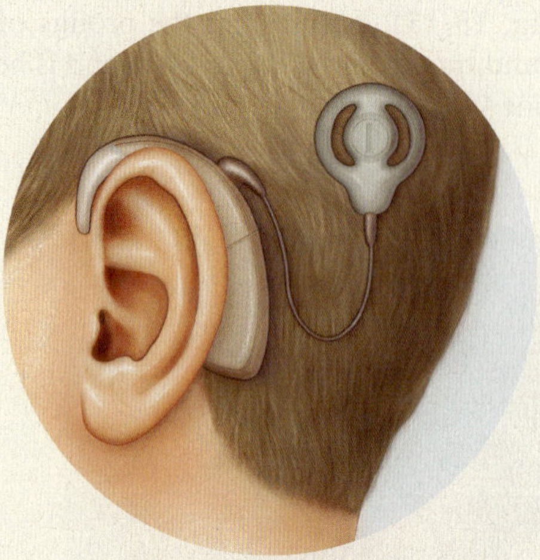

	Hearing Aid	Cochlear Implant
	Behind the ear; In the ear; In the canal	
Device/ condition	Electronic device that amplifies sound to assist individuals with hearing loss	Surgically implanted electronic device that bypasses damaged portions of the ear to directly stimulate the auditory nerve, allowing individuals with severe hearing loss to perceive sound
General indication	Used for individuals with mild to severe hearing loss when the auditory pathway is intact but sound amplification is needed	Used for individuals with moderate-to-profound sensorineural hearing loss who have had limited benefit from traditional hearing aids, particularly when the cochlea or auditory nerve is damaged
General location	Multiple designs are available: ■ External, behind the ear (BTE) ■ In the ear (ITE), fit in the outer ear bowl/concha ■ In the canal (ITC), fit in the auditory canal ■ Completely in canal (CIC), not visible externally	Comprises two parts: an external component that sits behind the ear and an internal component that is surgically implanted under the skin and inserted into the cochlea
Modification to the physical exam	1. Ask the patient to remove the device before examination. 2. Inspect the ear canal for any signs of irritation from the device. 3. Check for accumulation of cerumen (earwax) or other debris, which can clog the device and affect its functioning. 4. Be gentle with otoscopy to avoid dislodging any in-the-ear devices or causing discomfort.	1. Examine the external component gently, avoid tugging or pulling. 2. When examining the ear and scalp, be cautious near the area where the internal device is implanted to avoid pressure or manipulation. 3. Inspect for signs of skin irritation or breakdown around the site of the external component. 4. Avoid deep otoscopy if there's uncertainty about the position of the cochlear implant, to prevent damage or dislodgement.

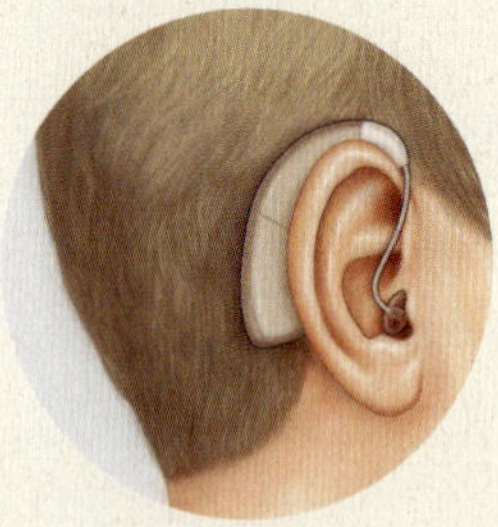

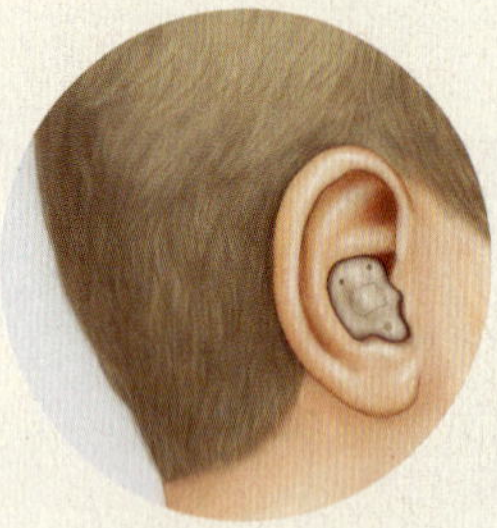

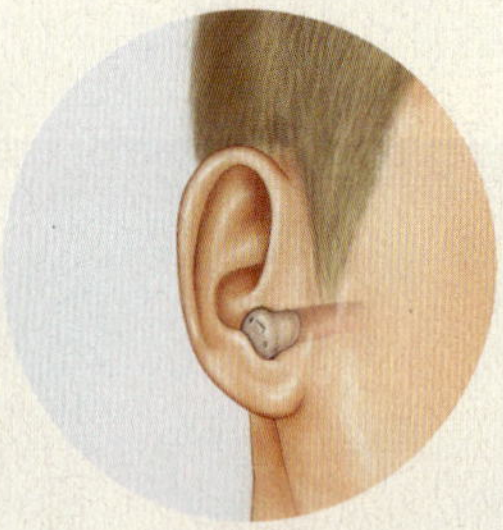

NOSE AND PARANASAL SINUS: TECHNIQUES OF EXAMINATION

Key Components of the Nose and Paranasal Sinus Examination

- Inspect the anterior and inferior surfaces of the nose.
- Test for nasal obstruction.
- Inspect the nasal cavity and mucosa.
- Inspect the nasal septum.
- Inspect the nasal turbinates and meatuses.
- Palpate the paranasal sinuses.

Ask your patient to sit upright and tilt their head slightly backward. This gives you a better view into the nasal cavity.

Inspect the Anterior and Inferior Surfaces of the Nose

Inspect the anterior and inferior surfaces of the nose by gently applying pressure on the tip of the nose with your thumb to widen the nostrils. Use a penlight or otoscope light to examine each nasal vestibule. Note any asymmetry or deformity of the nose. Use caution when examining a tender nasal tip, and manipulate the nose as little as possible.

Tenderness of the nasal tip or ala suggests local infection such as a furuncle, particularly if there is a small erythematous and swollen area.

Test for Nasal Obstruction

Test for nasal obstruction, if indicated, by pressing on each ala nasi in turn and asking the patient to breathe in.

Inspect the Nasal Cavity and Mucosa

To inspect the inside of the nostrils, use an otoscope and the largest available ear speculum. Tilt the patient's head back slightly and insert the speculum gently into the vestibule of each nostril, being careful to avoid the sensitive nasal septum (Fig. 15-16). Use one hand to hold the otoscope handle to the side and improve mobility. Direct the speculum posteriorly and then upward in small steps to visualize the inferior and middle turbinates, the nasal septum, and the narrow nasal passage between them (Fig. 15-17). Some asymmetry between the two sides is normal.

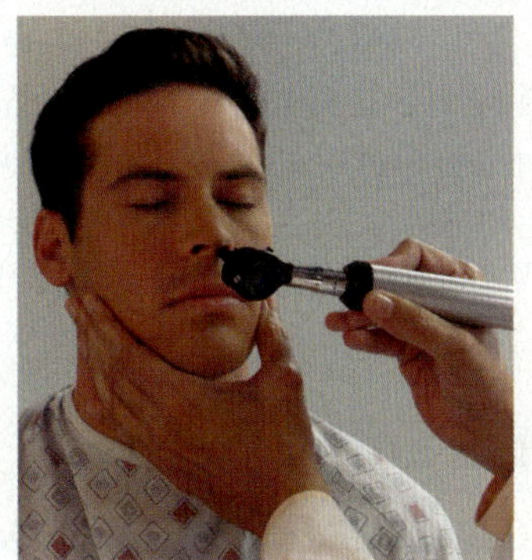

FIGURE 15-16. Inspecting inside the nares with an otoscope.

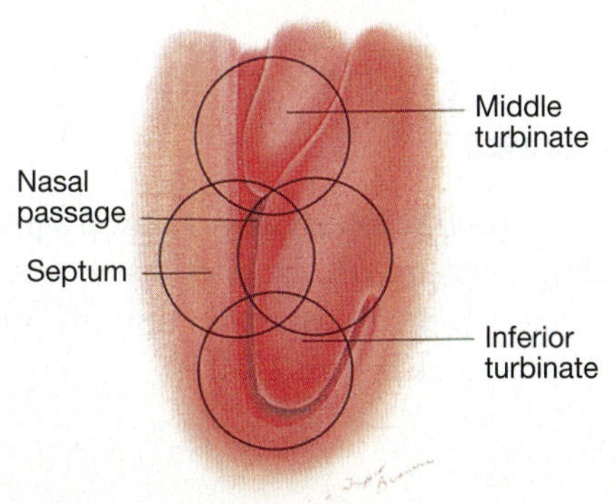

FIGURE 15-17. Inferior and middle turbinates.

Deviation of the lower septum is common and may be easily visible, as in Figure 15-18. Deviation seldom obstructs airflow.

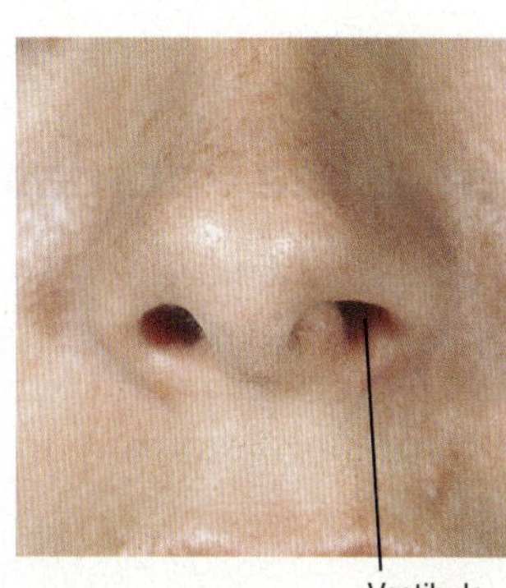

FIGURE 15-18. Deviation of the lower septum.

Inspect the nasal mucosa covering the septum and turbinates, noting its color and any signs of inflammation such as swelling, bleeding, or exudate. If present, identify the character of any exudate, such as clear, mucopurulent, or purulent. The nasal mucosa normally appears somewhat redder than the oral mucosa.

In viral rhinitis, the mucosa is reddened and swollen; in allergic rhinitis, it may be pale, bluish, or red.

Inspect the Nasal Septum

Note any deviation, inflammation, or perforation of the septum. The lower anterior portion of the septum (where the patient's finger can reach) is a common source of *epistaxis* (nosebleed). Inspect for any abnormalities such as ulcers or polyps (Fig. 15-19).

Fresh blood or crusting may be seen. Causes of septal perforation include trauma, surgery, rheumatologic diseases including granulomatosis with polyangiitis, and intranasal use of cocaine or amphetamines, which also cause septal ulceration.

Nasal polyps are pale saclike growths of inflamed mucosa that can obstruct the air passage or sinuses, seen in allergic rhinitis, aspirin sensitivity, asthma, chronic sinus infections, and cystic fibrosis.[9]

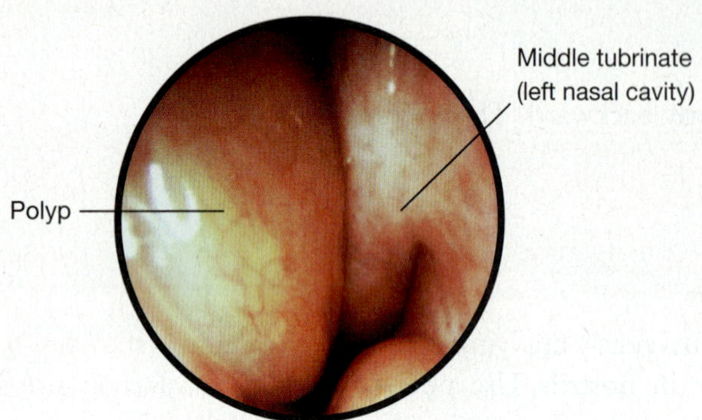

FIGURE 15-19. Nasal polyp.

Importantly, inspection of the nasal cavity through the anterior naris is limited to the vestibule, anterior portion of the septum, and lower and middle turbinates. To examine posterior abnormalities, a *nasopharyngeal mirror* is required, which is outside the scope of this book. You must discard or clean and disinfect all nasal and ear specula after use to prevent the spread of infection.

Inspect the Nasal Turbinates and Meatuses

Note the condition of the *inferior and middle turbinates.* They should appear pink and moist. Swelling, polyps, or other growths are abnormal. Examine the corresponding *meatuses* (spaces between the turbinates and the nasal septum). Look for discharge, inflammation, or foreign bodies. Repeat the process for the other nostril.

Palpate the Paranasal Sinuses

Palpate for sinus tenderness. To examine the *frontal sinuses*, apply upward pressure under the bony brows while avoiding pressure on the eyes, as shown in Figure 15-20. Similarly, to examine the *maxillary sinuses*, apply upward pressure beneath the zygomatic bones, as illustrated in Figure 15-21.

Local tenderness, together with symptoms such as facial pain, pressure or fullness, purulent nasal discharge, nasal obstruction, and smell disorder, especially when present for greater than 7 days, suggest acute bacterial rhinosinusitis involving the frontal or maxillary sinuses.[9–12]

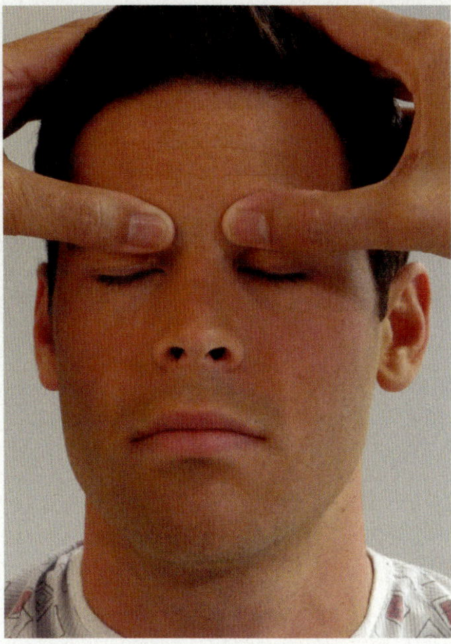

FIGURE 15-20. Palpating the frontal sinuses.

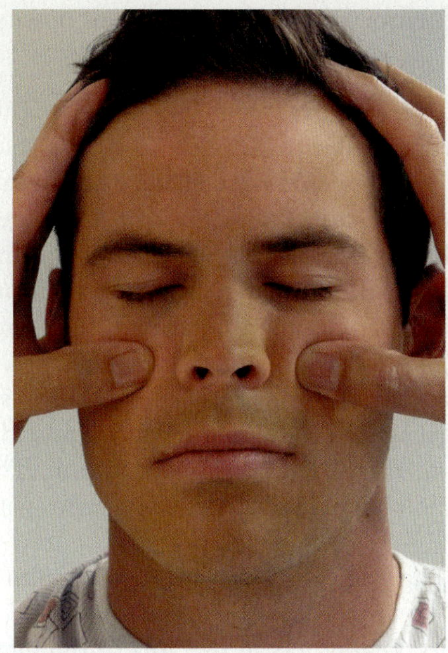

FIGURE 15-21. Palpating the maxillary sinuses.

RECORDING YOUR FINDINGS

The sample documentation provided is commonly adhered to in clinical settings. As you begin your training, you may rely on full sentences to detail findings comprehensively. However, with experience and familiarity, you will naturally transition to using concise phrases. These not only highlight the observed abnormalities but also efficiently denote what is absent or within normal limits.

Recording the Ears and Nose Examination

HEENT:

Ears—Acuity good to whispered voice. External auditory canals (EACs) intact bilaterally. Tympanic membranes (TMs) intact and mobile, with good cone of light. 512 Tuning Fork (TF): Weber midline. Rinne AC > BC bilaterally.

Nose—Nasal mucosa pink, septum midline; no sinus tenderness.

OR

Ears—Acuity diminished to whispered voice; intact to spoken voice. Bilateral external auditory canals and TMs clear.

Nose—Mucosa swollen with erythema and clear drainage. Septum midline. Tender over bilateral maxillary sinuses.

The approach of segmenting physical examination documentation into granular details exemplifies the profound impact clinical observations have on forming a diagnosis. The clinical findings described for the ears and nose in the second note suggest a combination of sensory changes and signs of possible inflammation or infection:

- *Ears: Acuity diminished to whispered voice; intact to spoken voice:* This indicates a reduction in hearing acuity, as the patient is able to hear normal spoken voice but has difficulty with softer sounds like a whispered voice. This could indicate mild hearing loss, which can have various causes including age-related changes, exposure to loud noises, earwax buildup, or an early stage of an ear infection.
- *Bilateral external auditory canals and TMs clear:* The external auditory canals and tympanic membranes appearing clear is a normal finding, suggesting no visible signs of infection, blockage, or damage in these areas.
- *Nose: Mucosa swollen with erythema and clear drainage:* Swollen nasal mucosa with erythema and clear drainage indicate inflammation, possibly due to an upper respiratory infection, allergies, or a sinus condition. The clear drainage suggests a bacterial infection, which often presents with yellow or green mucus, is less likely.
- *Septum midline:* This is a normal finding, indicating that the nasal septum is properly aligned and not deviated.
- *Tender over bilateral maxillary sinuses:* Tenderness in the area of the maxillary sinuses can be a sign of sinusitis. This is often accompanied by symptoms like a stuffy nose, pain in the face, and nasal discharge.

In summary, the ear findings suggest a possible *mild hearing impairment*, while the nasal findings point to inflammation or infection, likely *sinusitis,* or *allergic rhinitis.*

HEALTH PROMOTION AND COUNSELING: EVIDENCE AND RECOMMENDATIONS

Important Topic for Health Promotion and Counseling

- Screening for hearing loss

Screening for Hearing Loss

As of 2019, 20.3% of the world was estimated to have some degree of hearing loss.[13] In 2020, about 12% of adults in the United States 18 years and older reported some difficulty hearing; among those 65 years and older, nearly 30% reported difficulty hearing.[14] Hearing loss is commonly considered the inability to hear tones at frequencies between 250 and 8,000 Hz, the most important for speech processing.[15] This impairment, which can adversely affect social, psychological, and cognitive functioning, often goes undetected and untreated.[16] Unlike vision prerequisites for driving, there are no requirements for widespread hearing testing, and many adults avoid using hearing aids.

Hearing loss can be accurately and reliably detected by a number of screening tests, including single-item screening test (e.g., "Do you have difficulty with your hearing?"), multi-item questionnaires (such as the Hearing Handicap Inventory for the Elderly—Screening Version), handheld audiometers, the watch tick test, the whispered voice test (see pp. 375–376), the finger rub test, mobile apps, and smartphone- or tablet-based portable audiometers.[16]

The most common cause of hearing loss is *presbycusis*, age-related degeneration of hair cells in the ears, which leads to gradually progressive hearing loss, particularly for high-frequency sounds.[17] Exposure to hazardous noise levels, including from occupational and other environmental sources, is the next leading risk factor for hearing loss, particularly in younger adults.[18] Other risk factors for hearing loss in adults include family history of hearing loss, ototoxic drug exposures, tobacco use, and systemic illnesses such as diabetes mellitus. Risk factors for children include hereditary syndromes, perinatal infections, and craniofacial abnormalities.[16,19]

Removing impacted cerumen may substantially improve conductive hearing loss. Hearing-related function can be improved by using hearing aids for individuals with mild to moderate sensorineural hearing loss. Cochlear implants are a treatment option for those with severe sensorineural hearing loss.[16,17,19] Noise reduction and avoidance are strongly recommended strategies for preventing or delaying hearing loss.[16,19]

While screening trials can identify adults with hearing loss, the subsequent use of hearing aids is low, particularly among those without self-perceived hearing loss.[20,21] The U.S. Preventive Services Task Force found insufficient evidence evaluating the effect of screening on clinical outcomes to make a determination about screening adults ages 50 years and older for hearing loss (I statement).[17]

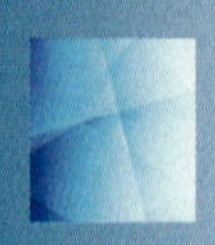

TABLE 15-1. Dizziness and Vertigo

"Dizziness" is a nonspecific term used by patients encompassing several disorders that clinicians must carefully sort out. A detailed history usually identifies the primary etiology. Learn the specific meanings of the following terms or conditions:

- *Vertigo*—a spinning sensation accompanied by nystagmus and ataxia; usually from peripheral vestibular dysfunction (~40% of "dizzy" patients), but may be from a central brainstem lesion (~10%; causes include atherosclerosis, multiple sclerosis, vertebrobasilar migraine, or transient ischemic attack)
- *Presyncope*—a near faint from "feeling faint or lightheaded"; causes include orthostatic hypotension, especially from medication, arrhythmias, and vasovagal attacks (~5%)
- *Dysequilibrium*—unsteadiness or imbalance when walking, especially in older patients; causes include fear of walking, visual loss, weakness from musculoskeletal problems, and peripheral neuropathy (up to 15%)
- *Psychiatric*—causes include anxiety, panic disorder, hyperventilation, depression, somatization disorder, alcohol, and substance abuse (~10%)
- *Multifactorial or unknown* (up to 20%)

Peripheral and Central Vertigo

	Onset	Duration and Course	Hearing	Tinnitus	Additional Features
Peripheral Vertigo					
Benign Positional Vertigo	Sudden, often when rolling onto the affected side or tilting up the head	Onset a few seconds to <1 min Lasts a few weeks, may recur	Not affected	Absent	Sometimes nausea, vomiting, nystagmus
Vestibular Neuronitis	Sudden	Onset hours to up to 2 wk May recur over 12–18 mo	Not affected	Absent	Nausea, vomiting, nystagmus
Acute Labyrinthitis	Sudden	Onset hours to up to 2 wk May recur over 12–18 mo	Sensorineural hearing loss—unilateral	May be present	Nausea, vomiting, nystagmus
Ménière Disease	Sudden	Onset several hours to ≥1 day Recurrent	Sensorineural hearing loss—fluctuating, recurs, eventually progresses	Present, fluctuating	Pressure or fullness in affected ear; nausea, vomiting, nystagmus
Drug Toxicity	Insidious or acute—linked to loop diuretics, aminoglycosides, salicylates, alcohol	May or may not be reversible Partial adaptation occurs	May be impaired	May be present	Nausea, vomiting
Acoustic Neuroma	Insidious from cranial nerve VIII compression, vestibular branch	Variable	Impaired, one side	Present	May involve cranial nerves V and VII
Central Vertigo	Often sudden (see causes above)	Variable but rarely continuous	Not affected	Absent	Usually with other brainstem deficits—dysarthria, ataxia, crossed motor and sensory deficits

Sources: Chan Y. Differential diagnosis of dizziness. *Curr Opin Otolaryngol Head Neck Surg.* 2009;17(3):200–203; Kroenke K, Lucas CA, Rosenberg ML, et al. Causes of persistent dizziness. A prospective study of 100 patients in ambulatory care. *Ann Intern Med.* 1992;117(11):898–904; Tusa RJ. Vertigo. *Neurol Clin.* 2001;19(1):23–55; Lockwood AH, Salvi RJ, Burkard RF. Tinnitus. *N Engl J Med.* 2002;347(12):904–910.

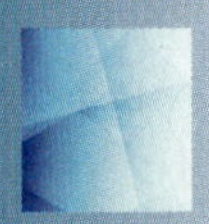

TABLE 15-2. Lumps on or Near the Ear

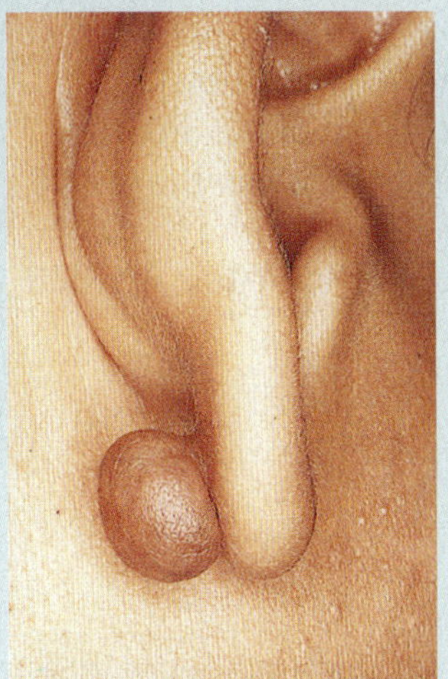

Keloid. A firm, nodular, hypertrophic mass of scar tissue extending beyond the area of injury.

It may develop in any scarred area but is most common on the shoulders and upper chest. A keloid on a pierced earlobe may have unwanted cosmetic effects.

Keloids are more common in people with darker skin and may recur following treatment.

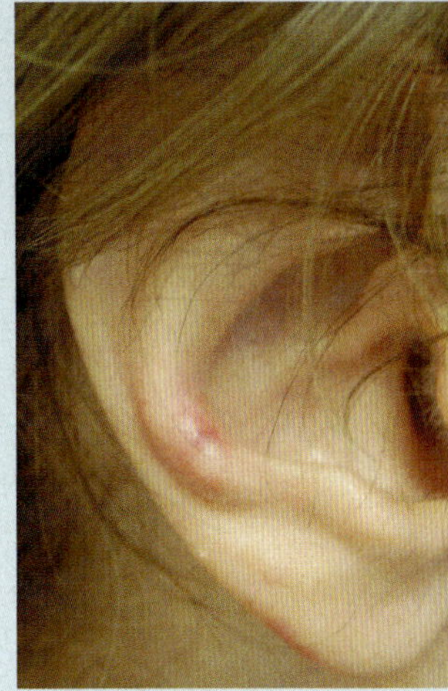

Chondrodermatitis helicis. This chronic inflammatory lesion starts as a painful, tender papule on the helix or antihelix. Reddening may occur. Biopsy is needed to rule out carcinoma.

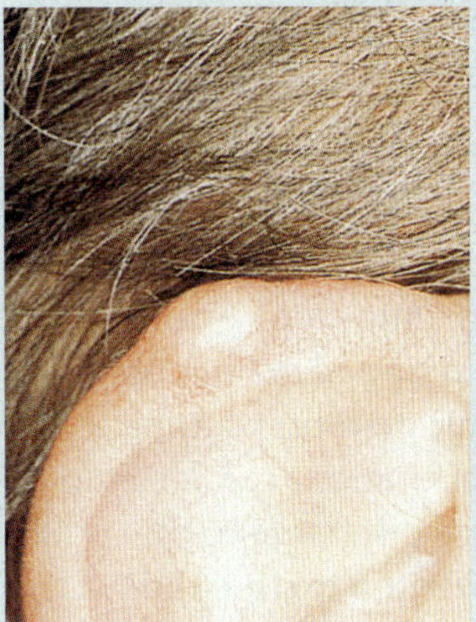

Tophi. A deposit of uric acid crystals characteristic of chronic tophaceous gout.

It appears as hard nodules in the helix or antihelix and may discharge chalky white crystals through the skin. It also may appear near the joints, hands, feet, and other areas. It usually develops after chronic sustained high blood levels of uric acid.

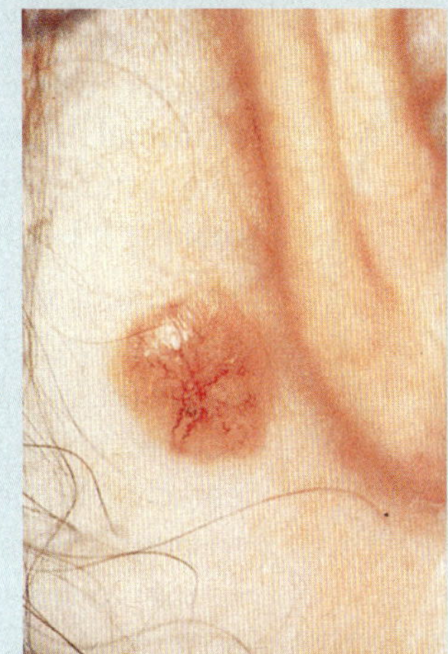

Basal cell carcinoma. This raised nodule shows the lustrous surface and telangiectatic vessels of basal cell carcinoma, a common slow-growing malignancy that rarely metastasizes. Growth and ulceration may occur.

These are more frequent in people with fair skin overexposed to sunlight.

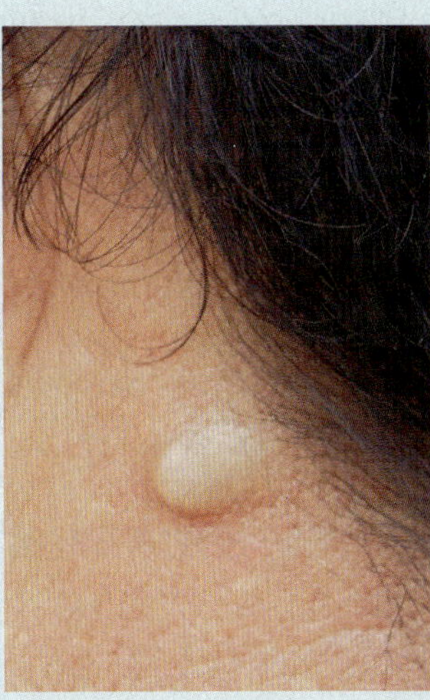

Cutaneous cyst. Also known as a sebaceous cyst, a dome-shaped lump in the dermis forms a benign closed firm sac attached to the epidermis.

A dark dot (blackhead) may be visible on its surface. Histologically, it is usually either (1) an epidermoid cyst, common on the face and neck, or (2) a pilar (trichilemmal) cyst, common in the scalp. Both may become inflamed.

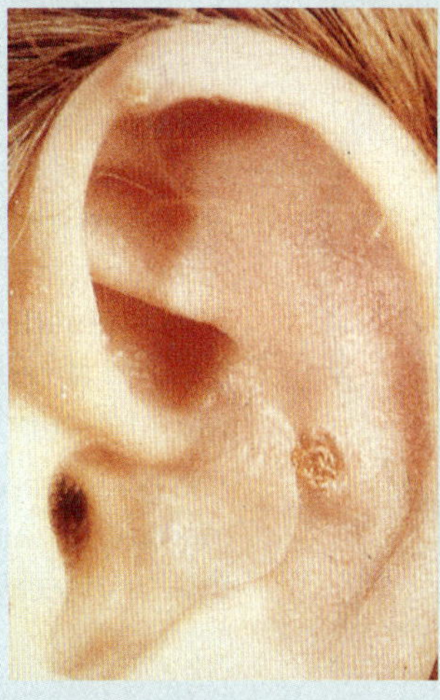

Rheumatoid nodules. In chronic rheumatoid arthritis, look for small lumps on the helix or antihelix and additional nodules elsewhere on the hands and along the surface of the ulna distal to the elbow, and on the knees and heels. Ulceration may result from repeated injuries. These nodules may antedate the arthritis.

Sources of photos: *Keloid*—Reprinted from Sams WM Jr, Lynch PJ, eds. *Principles and Practice of Dermatology*. Churchill Livingstone; 1990. Copyright © 1990 Elsevier. With permission; *Chondrodermatitis Helicis*—Image provided by Stedman's; *Tophi*—Reprinted with permission from Weber J, Kelley J. *Health Assessment in Nursing*. 2nd ed. Lippincott Williams & Wilkins; 2003. Figure 12-2; *Cutaneous Cyst*—Shutterstock photo by jaojormami; *Rheumatoid Nodules*—From Champion RH, Burton JL, Ebling FJG, eds. *Rook/Wilkinson/Ebling Textbook of Dermatology*. 5th ed. Blackwell Scientific; 1992. Copyright © 1992 by Blackwell Scientific Publications. Reprinted by permission of John Wiley & Sons, Inc.

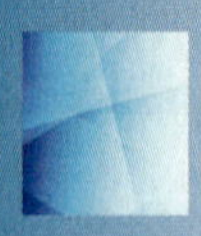

TABLE 15-3. Abnormalities of the Tympanic Membrane

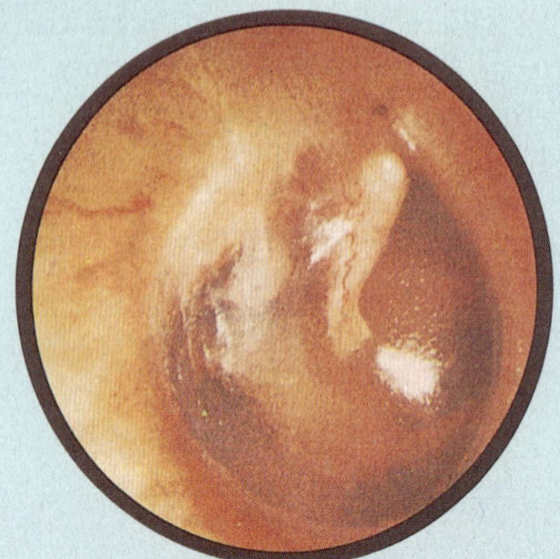

Normal Tympanic Membrane (Right)

This normal right eardrum has a pinkish-gray color with visible landmarks such as the malleus behind the upper part of the drum, the pars flaccida above the short process, and the pars tensa for the rest of the drum. A bright cone of light fans down and forward from the umbo, and part of the incus is visible behind the eardrum. Normal small blood vessels are present along the handle of the malleus.

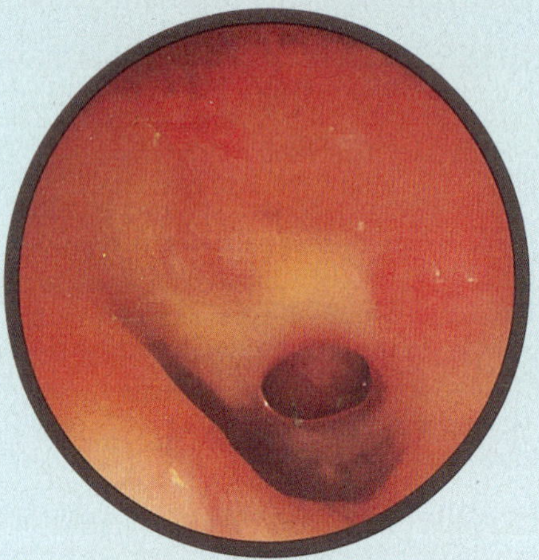

Perforation of the Tympanic Membrane

Perforations are holes in the eardrum caused by middle ear infections, which can result in earache and hearing loss. They can be central or marginal depending on whether the edge of the drum is involved. When they heal, the covering membrane may be thin and transparent, making it hard to distinguish from a true perforation.

This photo shows a common type of perforation known as a central perforation, which is surrounded by a reddened ring of granulation tissue indicating chronic infection. The tympanic membrane appears scarred, and no landmarks are visible. Large perforations can result in earache and hearing loss as infections can cause discharge to drain out through the perforated opening, which may eventually close during the healing process.

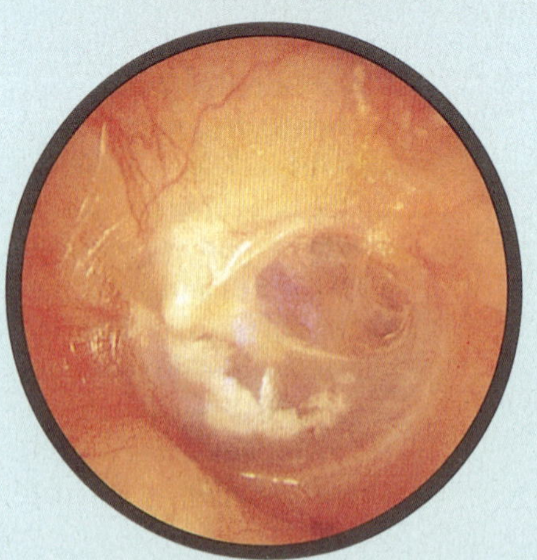

Tympanosclerosis

Tympanosclerosis is a scarring process in the middle ear due to otitis media, which can result in conductive hearing loss. It is characterized by deposition of hyaline, calcium, and phosphate crystals in the tympanic membrane and middle ear. In severe cases, it can entrap the ossicles. It is caused by the deposition of hyaline material within the layers of the tympanic membrane, often following a severe episode of otitis media. While generally not clinically significant and does not usually impair hearing, it can cause a large, irregularly margined, chalky white patch in the inferior portion of the tympanic membrane.

The photo also shows a healed perforation, signs of a retracted membrane, and a foreshortened, more horizontal handle of the malleus due to inward pull at the umbo.

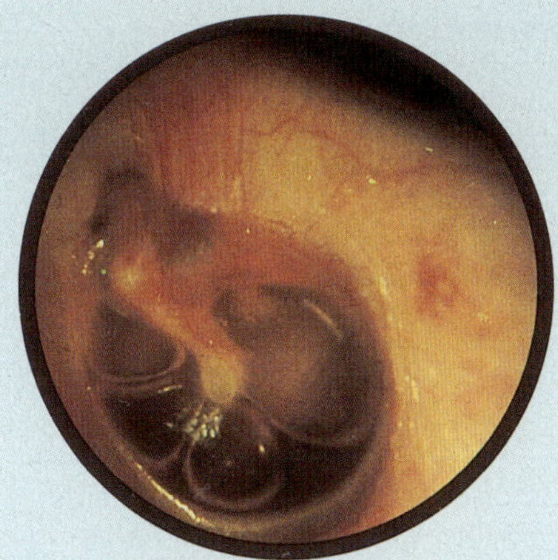

Serous Effusion

Serous effusions are usually caused by viral upper respiratory infections (otitis media with serous effusion) or by sudden changes in atmospheric pressure as from flying or diving (*otitic barotrauma*). The eustachian tube cannot equalize the air pressure in the middle ear and outside air. Air is absorbed from the middle ear into the bloodstream, and serous fluid accumulates in the middle ear instead. Symptoms include fullness and popping sensations in the ear, mild conduction hearing loss, and, sometimes, pain.

Amber fluid behind the eardrum is characteristic, as in this patient with otitic barotrauma. A fluid level, a line between air above and amber fluid below, can be seen on either side of the short process. Air bubbles (not always present) can be seen here within the amber fluid.

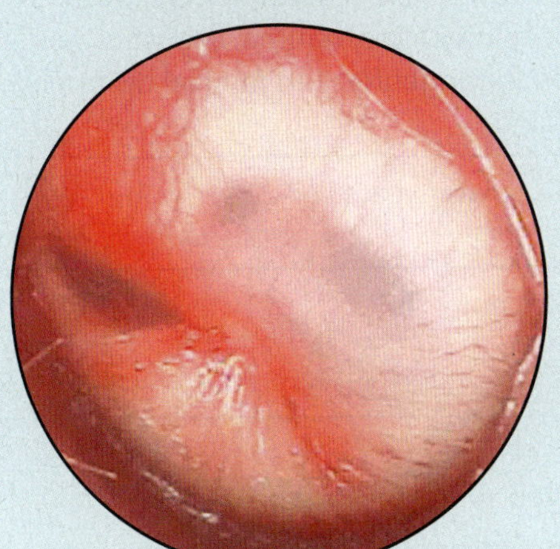

Acute Otitis Media With Purulent Effusion

Acute otitis media with purulent effusion is commonly caused by bacterial infection from *Streptococcus pneumoniae* or *Haemophilus influenzae*. Symptoms include earache, fever, and hearing loss. The tympanic membrane reddens, loses its landmarks, and bulges laterally, toward the examiner's eye.

Here the tympanic membrane appears bulging and erythematous, with a cloudy and opaque appearance. The normal landmarks, such as the light reflex, are obscured, indicating possible fluid buildup behind the eardrum. There is diffuse redness across the membrane. Spontaneous rupture of the tympanic membrane could occur, leading to the discharge of purulent material into the ear canal. Hearing loss in this case would be of the conductive type. Acute otitis media is more common in children, though it can occur in adults as well.

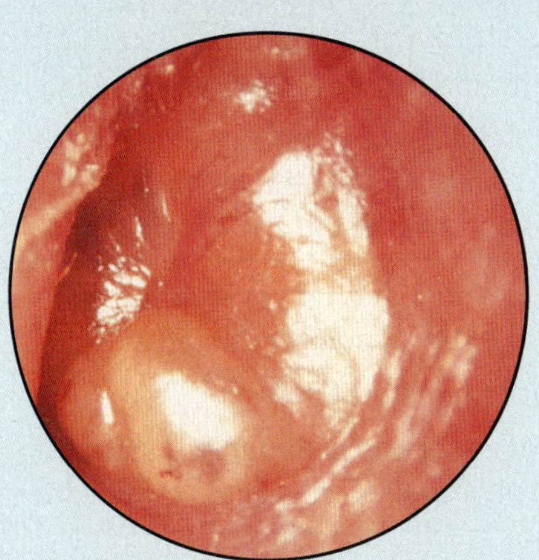

Bullous Myringitis

In bullous myringitis, painful hemorrhagic vesicles appear on the tympanic membrane, the ear canal, or both. Symptoms include earache, blood-tinged discharge from the ear, and conductive hearing loss.

In this image, a large vesicle (bulla) is discernible on the tympanic membrane. The eardrum is reddened, and its landmarks are obscured.

This condition is caused by *Mycoplasma*, viral, and bacterial otitis media.

Sources of photos: *Normal Eardrum*—Reprinted from Hawke M, Keene M, Alberti PW. *Clinical Otoscopy: A Text and Colour Atlas*. Churchill Livingstone; 1984. Copyright © 1984 Elsevier. With permission; *Perforation of the Tympanic membrane, Tympanosclerosis*—Courtesy of Michael Hawke, MD, Toronto, Canada; *Serous Effusion*—Reprinted from Hawke M, Keene M, Alberti PW. *Clinical Otoscopy: A Text and Colour Atlas*. Churchill Livingstone; 1984. Copyright © 1984 Elsevier. With permission; *Acute Otitis Media*—From Johnson JT, Rosen CA. *Bailey's Head and Neck Surgery*. 5th ed. Wolters Kluwer Health/Lippincott Williams & Wilkins; 2014. Figure 99-1. Courtesy of Alejandro Hoberman, MD, Children's Hospital of Pittsburgh of UPMC; *Bullous Myringitis*—Reprinted with permission from Jensen S. *Nursing Health Assessment: A Best Practice Approach*. 2nd ed. Wolters Kluwer Health/Lippincott Williams & Wilkins; 2011:370.

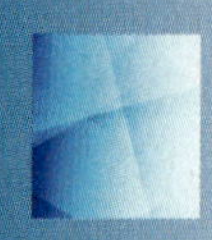

TABLE 15-4. Patterns of Hearing Loss

	Conductive Loss	Sensorineural Loss
	Tympanic membrane Middle ear Cochlear nerve	Tympanic membrane Middle ear Cochlear nerve
Pathophysiology	External or middle ear disorder impairs sound conduction to inner ear. Causes include foreign body, otitis media, perforated eardrum, and otosclerosis of ossicles.	Inner ear disorder involves cochlear nerve and neuronal impulse transmission to the brain. Causes include loud noise exposure, inner ear infections, trauma, acoustic neuroma, congenital and familial disorders, and aging.
Usual Age of Onset	Childhood and young adulthood, up to age 40 y	Middle or later years
Ear Canal and Tympanic Membrane	Abnormality usually visible, except in otosclerosis	Problem not visible
Effects	Little effect on sound Hearing seems to improve in noisy environment Voice remains soft because inner ear and cochlear nerve are intact	Higher registers are lost, so sound may be distorted Hearing worsens in noisy environment Voice may be loud because hearing is difficult
Weber Test (in Unilateral Hearing Loss)	Base of tuning fork at vertex Sound lateralizes to impaired ear—room noise not well heard, so detection of vibrations improves	Base of tuning fork at vertex Sound lateralizes to good ear—inner ear or cochlear nerve damage impairs transmission to affected ear
Rinne Test	Base of tuning fork on mastoid bone; then prongs at external auditory meatus Bone conduction (BC) longer than or equal to air conduction (AC) (BC ≥ AC) While air conduction through the external or middle ear is impaired, vibrations through bone bypass the problem to reach the cochlea.	Base of tuning fork on mastoid bone; then prongs at external auditory meatus AC longer than BC (AC > BC) The inner ear or cochlear nerve is less able to transmit impulses regardless of how the vibrations reach the cochlea. The normal pattern prevails.

REFERENCES

1. Lasak JM, Allen P, McVay T, Lewis D. Hearing loss: diagnosis and management. *Prim Care.* 2014;41(1):19–31.
2. Wheatley LM, Togias A. Clinical practice. Allergic rhinitis. *N Engl J Med.* 2015;372(5):456–463.
3. Siddiq S, Grainger J. The diagnosis and management of acute otitis media: American Academy of Pediatrics Guidelines 2013. *Arch Dis Child Educ Pract Ed.* 2015;100(4):193–197.
4. Bagai A, Thavendiranathan P, Detsky AS. Does this patient have hearing impairment? *JAMA.* 2006;295(4):416–428.
5. McShefferty D, Whitmer WM, Swan IR, Akeroyd MA. The effect of experience on the sensitivity and specificity of the whispered voice test: a diagnostic accuracy study. *BMJ Open.* 2013;3(4):e002394.
6. Pirozzo S, Papinczak T, Glasziou P. Whispered voice test for screening for hearing impairment in adults and children: systematic review. *BMJ.* 2003;327(7421):967.
7. Eekhof JA, de Bock GH, de Laat JA, Dap R, Schaapveld K, Springer MP. The whispered voice: the best test for screening for hearing impairment in general practice? *Br J Gen Pract.* 1996;46(409):473–474.
8. McGee SR. *Evidence-Based Physical Diagnosis.* 4th ed. Elsevier; 2018.
9. Seidman MD, Gurgel RK, Lin SY, et al. Clinical practice guideline: allergic rhinitis executive summary. *Otolaryngol Head Neck Surg.* 2015;152(2):197–206.
10. Foden N, Burgess C, Shepherd K, Almeyda R. A guide to the management of acute rhinosinusitis in primary care: management strategy based on best evidence and recent European guidelines. *Br J Gen Pract.* 2013;63(616):611–613.
11. Rosenfeld RM, Piccirillo JF, Chandrasekhar SS, et al. Clinical practice guideline (update): adult sinusitis executive summary. *Otolaryngol Head Neck Surg.* 2015;152(4):598–609.
12. Kaplan A. Canadian guidelines for acute bacterial rhinosinusitis: clinical summary. *Can Fam Physician.* 2014;60(3):227–234.
13. GBD Hearing Loss Collaborators. Hearing loss prevalence and years lived with disability, 1990–2019: findings from the Global Burden of Disease Study 2019. *Lancet.* 2021;397(10278):996–1009.
14. QuickStats: percentage* of adults aged >/= 18 years who have difficulty hearing even when using a hearing aid,† by age group—National Health Interview Survey, United States, 2020§. *MMWR Morb Mortal Wkly Rep.* 2022;71(12):475.
15. Feltner C, Wallace IF, Kistler CE, Coker-Schwimmer M, Jonas DE. Screening for hearing loss in older adults: updated evidence report and systematic review for the US Preventive Services Task Force. *JAMA.* 2021;325(12):1202–1215.
16. Nieman CL, Oh ES. Hearing Loss. *Ann Intern Med.* 2020;173(11):ITC81–ITC96.
17. U.S. Preventive Services Task Force; Krist AH, Davidson KW, Mangione CM, et al. Screening for hearing loss in older adults: US Preventive Services Task Force Recommendation Statement. *JAMA.* 2021;325(12):1196–1201.
18. Carroll YI, Eichwald J, Scinicariello F, et al. Vital signs: noise-induced hearing loss among adults—United States 2011–2012. *MMWR Morb Mortal Wkly Rep.* 2017;66(5):139–144.
19. Cunningham LL, Tucci DL. Hearing loss in adults. *N Engl J Med.* 2017;377(25):2465–2473.
20. Yueh B, Collins MP, Souza PE, et al. Long-term effectiveness of screening for hearing loss: the screening for auditory impairment–which hearing assessment test (SAI-WHAT) randomized trial. *J Am Geriatr Soc.* 2010;58(3):427–434.
21. Thodi C, Parazzini M, Kramer SE, et al. Adult hearing screening: follow-up and outcomes. *Am J Audiol.* 2013;22(1):183–185.

CHAPTER

16

Throat and Oral Cavity

ANATOMY AND PHYSIOLOGY

Mouth, Gingiva, and Teeth

The *lips* are muscular folds that encircle the mouth's entrance and, when opened, reveal the gums (*gingiva*) and *teeth* (Fig. 16-1). Note the scalloped shape of the gingival margins and pointed *interdental papillae*.

The *gingiva* is firmly attached to the teeth and jawbone, appearing pale pink or coral with a light stipple in people with lighter skin and diffusely or partly brown in people with darker skin (Fig. 16-2). A *labial frenulum*, a midline mucosal fold, connects each lip with the gingiva. The *gingival sulcus*, a shallow groove between the gum's margin and the tooth, is not visible but probed and measured by dental professionals. The *alveolar mucosa*, adjacent to the gingiva, blends with the lip's labial mucosa (see Fig. 16-2).

Each tooth has a *dentin* composition, with only its enamel-covered *crown* exposed above the bony socket. Small blood vessels and nerves enter the tooth through its apex and pass into the *pulp canal* and *pulp chamber* (Fig. 16-3).

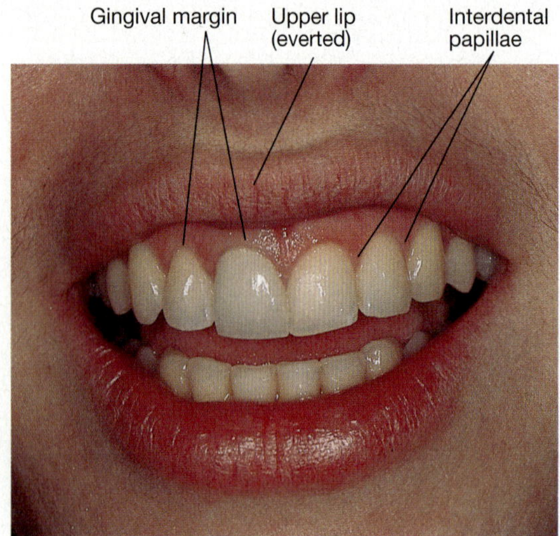

FIGURE 16-1. Mouth, gingiva, and teeth.

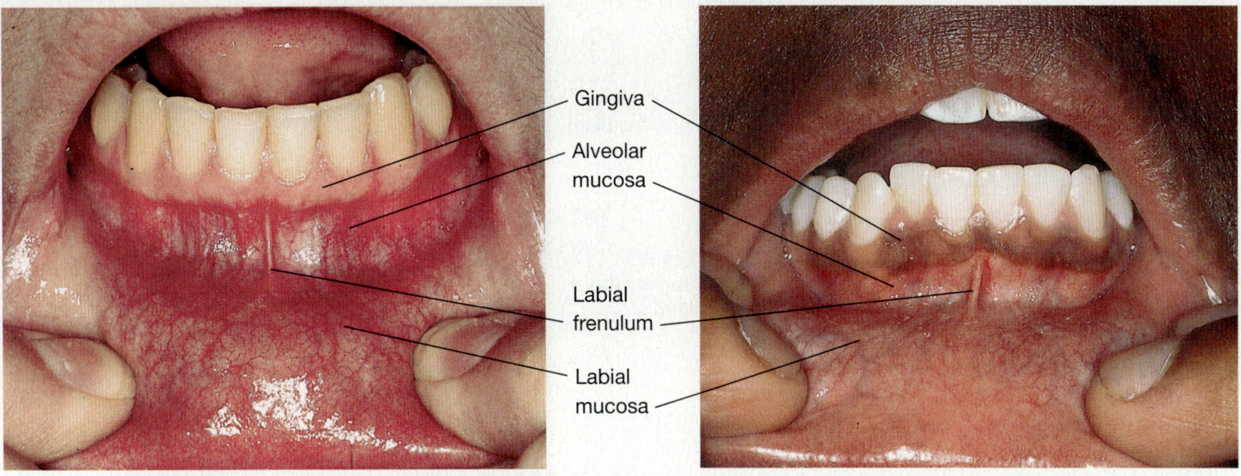

FIGURE 16-2. Alveolar and labial mucosa, labial frenulum.

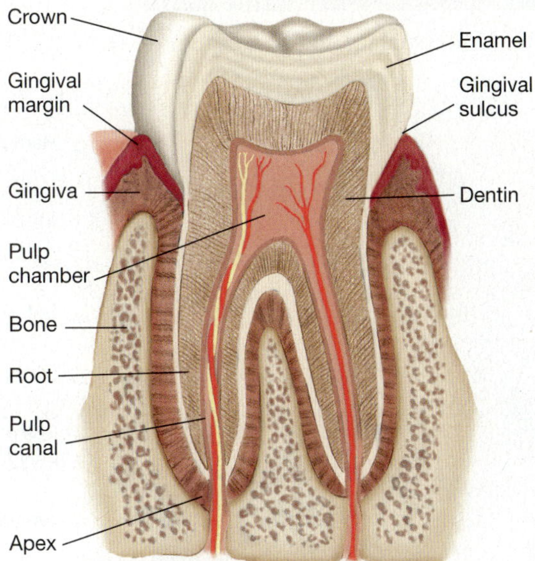

FIGURE 16-3. Anatomy of a tooth.

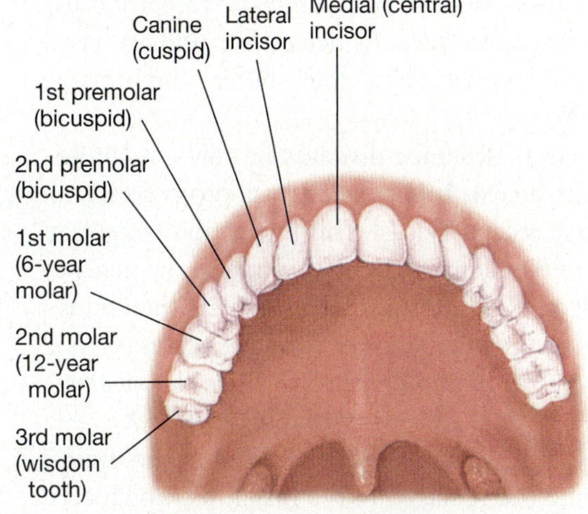

FIGURE 16-4. Adult teeth (upper jaw).

Adults have 32 teeth, numbered 1 to 16 on the upper jaw from right to left and 17 to 32 on the lower jaw from left to right (Fig. 16-4).

Tongue

The surface of the tongue is covered with papillae, giving it a rough texture. Some papillae appear as red dots that contrast with the thin white coating that often covers the tongue (Fig. 16-5).

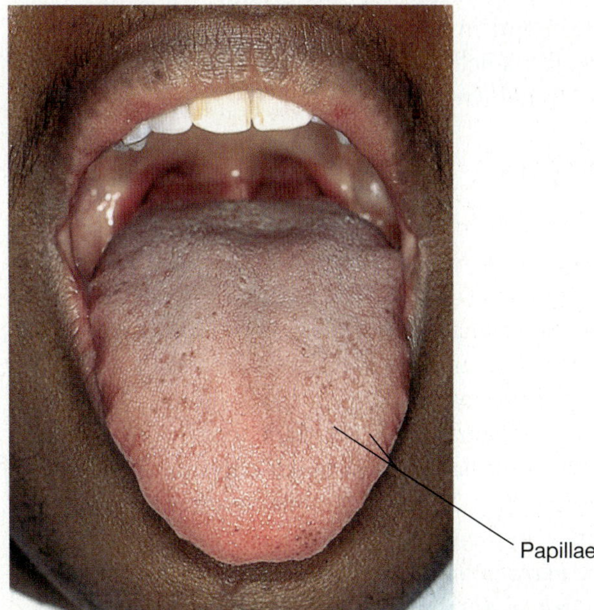

FIGURE 16-5. Dorsal papillae of the tongue.

The underside of the tongue has no papillae. Note the midline *lingual frenulum* that connects the tongue to the floor of the mouth and the ducts of the *submandibular gland (Wharton ducts)*, which pass forward and medially (Fig. 16-6). These ducts open on papillae located on each side of the lingual frenulum. The paired *sublingual salivary glands* are situated just under the mucosa of the floor of the mouth.

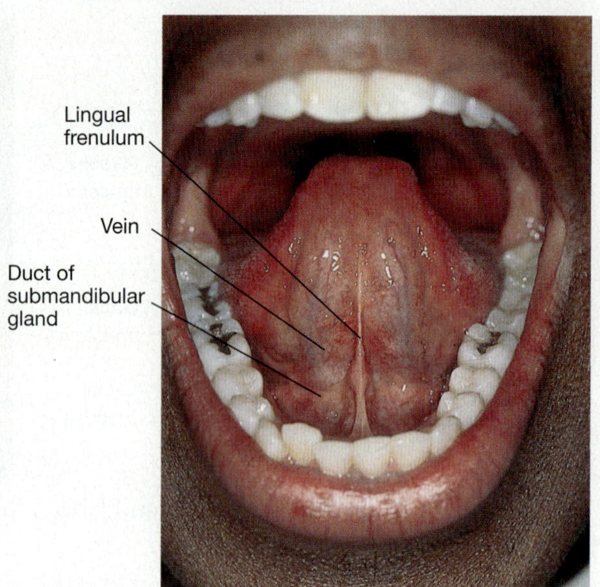

FIGURE 16-6. Undersurface of the tongue.

Gustation Pathway

Gustation, or the *sense of taste*, is a complex process that begins when food or other substances come into contact with taste buds on the tongue and other areas of the mouth and throat. *Taste buds* are small sensory organs containing taste receptor cells, which are specialized to detect five primary taste sensations: sweet, salty, sour, bitter, and umami (savory).

When a substance dissolves in saliva, its molecules interact with *microvilli* (small projections) on the taste receptor cells. This interaction triggers a chain of biochemical events, leading to the generation of an electrical signal. This signal is then transmitted to the brain via several cranial nerves (CNs), primarily the *facial nerve (CN VII), glossopharyngeal nerve (CN IX), and vagus nerve (CN X).*

The taste signal is first processed in the brainstem and then relayed to the thalamus, which acts as a relay station, forwarding the information to the *gustatory cortex* in the cerebral cortex. This cortex is responsible for interpreting the taste sensation and integrating it with other sensory inputs, like smell and texture, which contribute to the overall flavor perception.

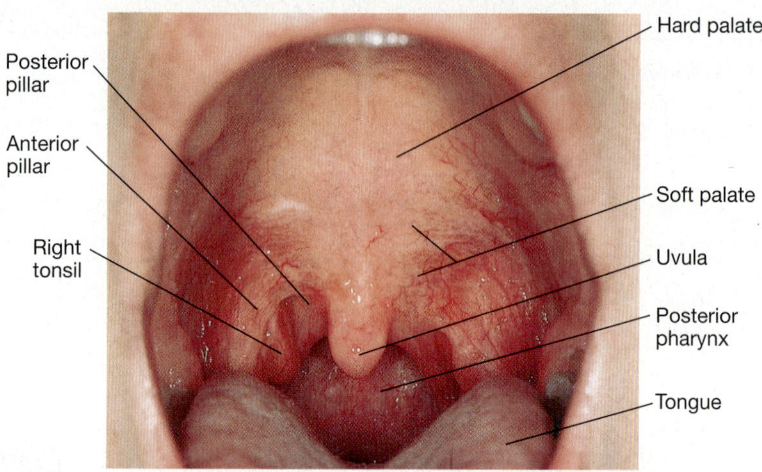

FIGURE 16-7. Anatomy of the posterior pharynx.

Pharynx

The arch formed by the anterior and posterior pillars, *soft palate*, and *uvula* rises above and behind the tongue (Fig. 16-7). The soft palate may have a meshwork of small blood vessels. The recess behind the soft palate and tongue allows for visualization of the *posterior pharynx.*

Note in Figure 16-7, the right tonsil protrudes from the tonsillar fossa between the anterior and posterior pillars. In adults, tonsils are often small or absent, as in the empty left tonsillar fossa.

The *buccal mucosa* lines the cheeks, and the *parotid duct (Stensen duct)* usually opens near the upper second molar and is marked by a small papilla (Fig. 16-8).

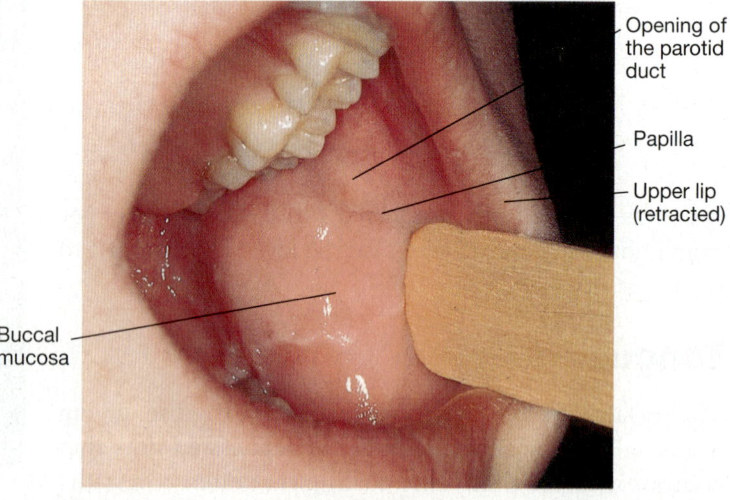

FIGURE 16-8. Buccal mucosa and opening of the parotid duct.

HEALTH HISTORY: GENERAL APPROACH

Throat and oral cavity symptoms can be indicative of either common or serious underlying conditions. Conducting a thorough medical interview and physical examination (PE) is essential in distinguishing between the two. As you delve deeper into the "HEENT" history, you will recognize the interconnectedness of head and neck symptoms, underscoring the importance of a holistic approach in your evaluations.

Common or Concerning Symptoms

- Sore throat
- Bleeding or swollen gums
- Hoarseness
- Malodorous breath (*halitosis*)

Sore Throat

In the clinical setting, a sore throat or *pharyngitis* is a frequent presentation. While a sore throat may seem like a straightforward symptom, recognizing the broad range of potential causes is essential. Conduct a comprehensive and structured assessment of the patient's health history. Box 16-1 offers a set of key questions to guide the evaluation of a patient with a sore throat. These questions probe into aspects such as the onset, duration, related symptoms, and factors that might worsen or alleviate the discomfort.

See Table 16-4, Findings in or under the Tongue, pp. 414–415.

Box 16-1. Sore Throat: High-Yield Health History Questions

Domain	Questions	Rationale
Onset	*When did your sore throat begin?*	Helps determine if the sore throat is acute or chronic, suggesting potential causes such as viral or bacterial infection, or underlying chronic conditions like allergies, gastroesophageal reflux disease (GERD), or postnasal drip
Severity	*How severe is your sore throat?*	Assesses the intensity of pain and discomfort, guiding further evaluation and management; a more severe sore throat may warrant additional investigations or interventions
Associated symptoms	*Are you experiencing fever, cough, or runny nose?*	Presence suggests a viral or bacterial infection; absence may indicate noninfectious causes like allergies, GERD, or postnasal drip

(*continued*)

Common causes to consider include **viral pharyngitis** (throat infection typically caused by viruses like the common cold), **bacterial pharyngitis** (infection due to bacteria, commonly known as "strep throat"), and **reflux-induced laryngopharyngitis** (throat irritation from acid reflux, also known as "heartburn"). Abnormalities may also include **aphthous ulcers** and **glossitis** (sore smooth tongue of nutritional deficiency).

Box 16-1. Sore Throat: High-Yield Health History Questions (*Continued*)

Domain	Questions	Rationale
Swallowing	*Is it painful to swallow, or does it feel like something is stuck in your throat?*	*Painful swallowing:* May indicate pharyngitis or tonsillitis *Sensation of something stuck in the throat:* Might suggest globus sensation or a foreign body
Exposures	*Have you been exposed to anyone with a similar illness or a known throat infection?*	Increases the likelihood of a contagious cause, such as viral or bacterial pharyngitis
Medical history	*Do you have a history of recurrent sore throats or any chronic medical conditions?*	*Recurrent:* May indicate an underlying condition (e.g., allergies, GERD) *Chronic:* Some conditions (e.g., diabetes, immunosuppression) may influence the risk and management of pharyngitis

Bleeding or Swollen Gums

When you encounter patients reporting symptoms like bleeding or swollen gums, remember that these can be more than isolated concerns. They might be signs of broader underlying health conditions or systemic issues. As a novice clinician, you must take a meticulous approach in evaluating the patient's oral health, while also thoroughly reviewing their general health history (Box 16-2).

See Table 16-3, Findings in the Gums and Teeth (pp. 412–413).

Box 16-2. Bleeding or Swollen Gums: High-Yield Health History Questions

Domain	Questions	Rationale
Onset	*When did you first notice bleeding or swollen gums?*	Determines if the issue is acute or chronic, suggesting potential causes such as acute gingival inflammation, trauma, or underlying chronic conditions like gingivitis or periodontitis
Triggers	*Do your gums bleed or swell during or after brushing, flossing, or eating certain foods?*	Can help determine if the issue is related to oral hygiene practices, dental devices, or specific food sensitivities

Common causes to consider include **gingivitis** (inflammation of the gums, commonly linked to poor oral hygiene), **periodontitis** (progressive gum disease), **medication-induced gingival enlargement** (swelling caused by certain medications such as antiseizure drugs, calcium-channel blockers, and immunosuppressants), and **systemic diseases** (conditions like diabetes, blood disorders, or hormonal fluctuations that may manifest orally).

Domain	Questions	Rationale
Dental hygiene	*How often do you brush and floss your teeth?*	Poor dental hygiene can lead to plaque buildup, resulting in gingivitis or periodontitis; maintaining good oral hygiene is important for gum health
Dental history	*When was your last dental checkup or cleaning?*	Regular dental checkups and cleanings can prevent and identify gum issues early; infrequent dental care may contribute to gum problems
Associated symptoms	*Are you experiencing tooth pain, sensitivity, or bad breath?*	*Tooth pain or sensitivity:* May indicate dental caries or periodontal disease *Bad breath* (*halitosis*): Can be a sign of poor oral hygiene, gingivitis, or periodontitis
Medical history	*Do you have a history of diabetes, smoking, or any medications that may affect your gums?*	*Diabetes* and *smoking:* Increase the risk of gum disease *Certain medications:* Antihypertensives and immunosuppressants can affect gum health and may cause gingival overgrowth or inflammation

Hoarseness

Hoarseness refers to a change in voice quality, often described as husky, rough, harsh, or lower pitched than usual. While a common presentation, it can be a signpost to numerous underlying conditions.[1–3] The key to distinguishing between these conditions lies in a diligent assessment of your patient's voice and medical history. Highlighted in Box 16-3 are high-yield questions tailored for the evaluation of hoarseness.

Box 16-3. Hoarseness: High-Yield Health History Questions

Domain	Questions	Rationale
Onset	*When did you first notice your hoarseness?*	Determines if the hoarseness is *acute* or *chronic*, which can suggest potential causes such as acute laryngitis, vocal cord nodules, or underlying chronic conditions like gastroesophageal reflux disease (GERD) or thyroid disease
Duration	*How long have you been experiencing hoarseness?*	Helps determine the severity and persistence of hoarseness; *persistent* hoarseness lasting >2 weeks may indicate an underlying chronic condition, while *acute* hoarseness may be related to an infection or injury
Voice changes	*Have you noticed any changes in your voice quality?*	Assessing changes in voice quality (e.g., breathiness, raspiness, pitch changes) can help identify the potential location and nature of the problem (e.g., vocal cords, larynx, or upper airway)
Associated symptoms	*Have you experienced any pain, difficulty swallowing, or breathing difficulties?*	*Pain with hoarseness:* May suggest an infectious or inflammatory process *Difficulty swallowing:* May indicate an obstruction *Breathing difficulties:* May indicate a more severe underlying condition (e.g., anaphylaxis, angioedema, tumors)
Triggers	*Does your hoarseness worsen with voice use or certain activities?*	*Hoarseness that worsens with voice use* may suggest vocal cord lesions, while *hoarseness that worsens with specific activities* (e.g., exercise, allergen exposure) may indicate asthma, laryngeal hypersensitivity, or upper airway obstruction
Medical history	*Do you have a history of smoking, GERD, or any recent upper respiratory infections?*	Smoking and GERD can cause *chronic hoarseness*; recent upper respiratory infections may cause *acute hoarseness* due to inflammation or vocal cord irritation; other medical conditions like allergies, asthma, or neurologic disorders can also contribute to hoarseness

Frequent causes include **laryngitis**, (inflammation of the larynx, usually due to viral infections, overuse of the voice, or irritation), **vocal cord abnormalities** (such as nodules or polyps, which can arise from prolonged voice strain), **gastroesophageal reflux disease** ([**GERD**] in which stomach acid irritates the throat and larynx), **systemic diseases** including thyroid disorders, and **throat cancer**, particularly in individuals with risk factors like smoking or heavy alcohol use.

Malodorous Breath (Halitosis)

Malodorous breath (*halitosis*) is an unpleasant or offensive odor emanating from the breath. Not all persons with malodorous breath are aware of it, and it can often be more than just an embarrassing concern. It sometimes serves as a clue to underlying health issues, both within the oral cavity and systemically. Evaluate your patient's oral hygiene practices, dietary habits, and medical history (Box 16-4).

Box 16-4. Halitosis: High-Yield Health History Questions

Domain	Questions	Rationale
Onset	*When did you first notice the malodorous breath?*	Determines if the malodor is acute or chronic, which can suggest potential causes such as recent oral hygiene issues, tonsillitis, or underlying chronic conditions like gastroesophageal reflux disease (GERD) or lung infections
Triggers	*Do certain foods or drinks trigger the malodor?*	Can help determine if the issue is related to diet, oral hygiene, or underlying medical conditions; certain foods like garlic, onions, or coffee can cause *transient* bad breath, while *persistent* bad breath may indicate dental or respiratory infections, GERD, or other systemic conditions
Dental hygiene	*How often do you brush and floss your teeth?*	Poor dental hygiene can lead to plaque buildup, which can cause bad breath and gum disease; maintaining good oral hygiene is important for breath freshness
Dental history	*When was your last dental checkup or cleaning?*	Regular dental checkups and cleanings can prevent and identify oral issues early; infrequent dental care may contribute to bad breath
Associated symptoms	*Have you noticed any other oral symptoms like gum bleeding, dry mouth, or a persistent cough?*	*Gum bleeding:* May indicate gingivitis or periodontitis, while dry mouth can lead to bacterial overgrowth and bad breath *Persistent cough:* May suggest respiratory infections, bronchitis, or chronic obstructive pulmonary disease (COPD)
Medical history	*Do you have a history of diabetes, liver or kidney disease, or acid reflux?*	Medical conditions like diabetes, liver or kidney disease, and GERD can lead to changes in breath odor: *a fruity breath odor* may indicate diabetic ketoacidosis, while a *fishy or musty breath odor* may suggest liver or kidney dysfunction; GERD can also cause bad breath due to stomach acid regurgitation

One thing to note is that even for a healthy mouth, there is often malodor upon waking from sleep, probably due to putrefaction of debris not cleared by low-level salivation during sleep.

Typical causes include **poor dental hygiene** (accumulation of food particles and bacterial growth leading to plaque formation), **mouth appliances** (such as retainers and dentures), **dental cavities** (holes or structural damage in the teeth caused by decay), **gum diseases** (such as gingivitis or periodontitis), **consumption of certain foods** (garlic, onions, and spices), and **systemic conditions** (GERD, hepatic cirrhosis, poorly controlled diabetes mellitus, impaired fat digestion, and inborn errors of metabolism such as trimethylaminuria).[4–8]

PHYSICAL EXAMINATION: GENERAL APPROACH

When examining the mouth and pharynx, the importance of meticulous observation cannot be overstated. Adequate lighting is pivotal for discerning subtle nuances, and a systematic visual inspection, paired with palpation, ensures a holistic assessment. Pay close attention to the oral mucosa, noting the condition of the lips, teeth, gums, palate, oral tongue, and the pharynx, especially the tonsils. This examination is an integral part of the overarching head and neck evaluation. If a patient has dentures, consider providing a paper towel and politely request their removal, allowing for a thorough inspection of the underlying mucosa.

Key Components of the Mouth and Pharynx Examination

- Inspect the lips and oral mucosa.
- Palpate the oral mucosa.
- Inspect the gingiva and teeth.
- Inspect the roof and floor of the mouth.
- Inspect the tongue.
- Test the hypoglossal nerve.
- Palpate the tongue.
- Inspect the soft palate, anterior and posterior pillars, uvula, tonsils, and pharynx.
- Test the vagus nerve.

TECHNIQUES OF EXAMINATION

Inspect the Lips and Oral Mucosa

Inspect the lips. Observe their color and moisture, and note any lumps, ulcers, cracking, or scaliness.

Watch for central cyanosis or pallor from anemia. See Table 16-1, Abnormalities of the Lips, pp. 406–407.

Inspect the oral mucosa. Look inside the patient's mouth with a good light source and the help of a tongue blade (Fig. 16-9). Inspect for discoloration, white patches, nodules, and ulcers (Fig. 16-10).

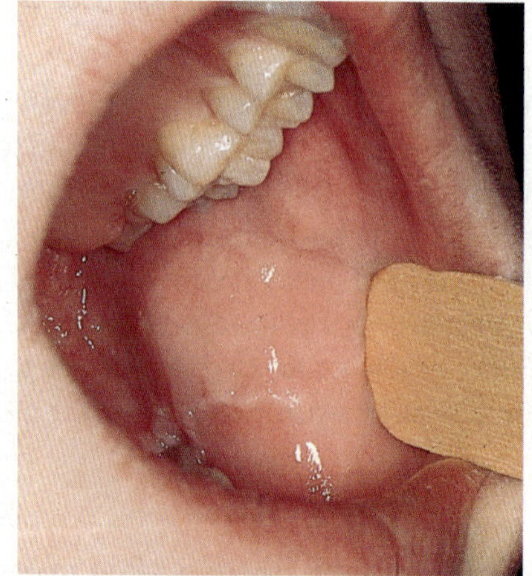

FIGURE 16-9. Inspecting the oral mucosa with a tongue blade.

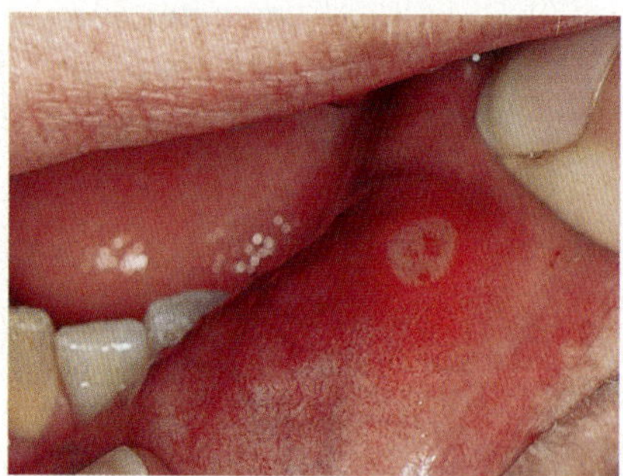

FIGURE 16-10. Aphthous ulcer on the labial mucosa of the lip.

Palpate the Oral Mucosa

If you notice any unusual sores or bumps in the mouth, put on gloves and palpate the area, taking note of any thickening or infiltration of tissues that could indicate a potential malignancy.

See Table 16-2, Findings in the Pharynx, Palate, and Oral Mucosa, pp. 408–411.

Bright red edematous mucosa underneath a denture suggests **denture stomatitis** (denture sore mouth). There may be ulcers or papillary granulation tissue.

Inspect the Gingiva and Teeth

Inspect the gingiva. Note the color of the gums, which are normally pink. Brown patches may be present, especially but not exclusively in dark-skinned individuals.

Redness of the gingiva suggests gingivitis; a black line might indicate lead poisoning.

Inspect the gum margins and the interdental papillae for swelling or ulceration.

The interdental papillae are swollen in gingivitis. See Table 16-3, Findings in the Gums and Teeth, pp. 412–413.

Inspect the teeth for any missing, discolored, misshapen, or abnormally positioned teeth. To assess tooth, jaw, or facial pain, gently palpate the teeth for looseness and the gums with a gloved thumb and index finger.[9,10]

Inspect the Roof and Floor of the Mouth

Inspect the *roof* of the mouth (hard palate). Note for any erythema, discoloration, nodules, ulcerations, or deformities.

Torus palatinus is a startling but benign midline lump (Fig. 16-11).

Inspect the *floor* of the mouth. Note any white or reddened areas, nodules, or ulcerations.

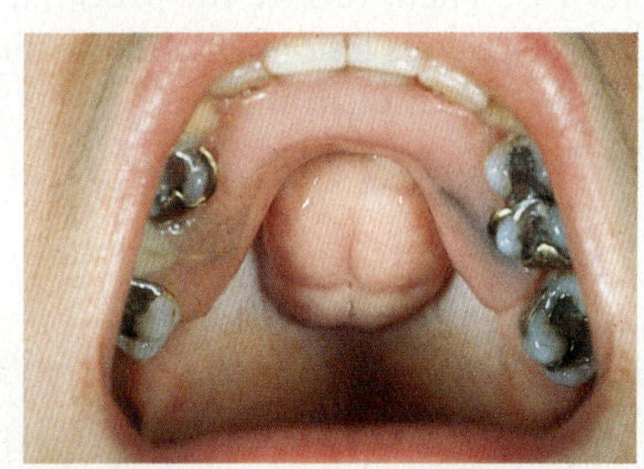

FIGURE 16-11. Torus palatinus. In this example, an upper denture has been fitted around the torus.

Inspect the Tongue

Look especially at the sides and undersurface of the tongue, areas where cancer often develops. Note the color and texture of the dorsum of the tongue.

Individuals aged >50 years who smoke or heavily use chewing tobacco and alcohol are at a higher risk for developing cancers of the tongue and oral cavity, usually in the form of squamous cell carcinomas on the side or base of the tongue. Be aware of any persistent nodules or ulcers, whether they appear red or white, as they may be signs of **erythroplakia** or **leukoplakia**, respectively, and should be biopsied, especially if they are indurated.

Test the Hypoglossal Nerve

The hypoglossal nerve (CN XII) is responsible for the motor function of the tongue. To test its integrity and function, start by asking the patient to open their mouth and protrude their tongue (Fig. 16-12). Ask them to move their tongue side to side inside the mouth to assess for any restrictions in range of motion. Also, inspect it for symmetry (Fig. 16-13).

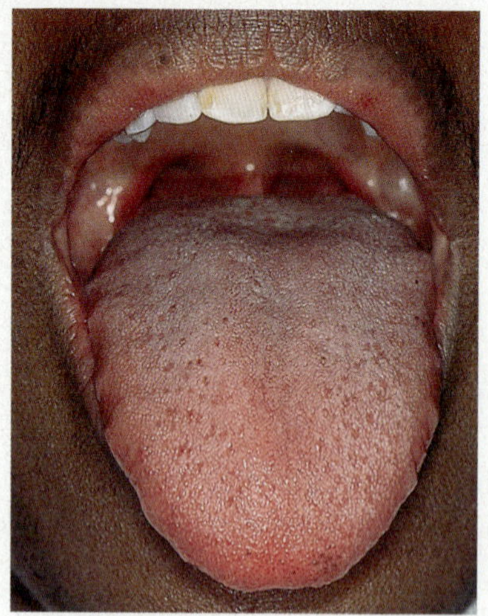

FIGURE 16-12. Inspecting the dorsum of the tongue.

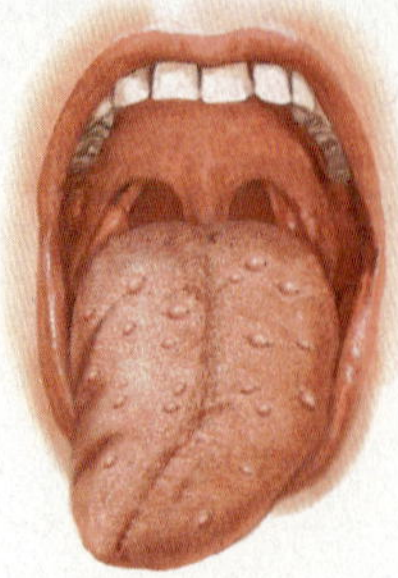

FIGURE 16-13. Asymmetric protrusion suggests a lesion of CN XII (tongue points toward the side of the lesion).

A unilateral weakness will result in the tongue deviating to the side of the lesion or injury when protruded ("points toward the lesion").

Palpate the Tongue

If indicated, to palpate the tongue, first ask the patient to protrude it. Using a gauze, grasp the tip of the tongue with your right hand and gently pull it toward the patient's left. Inspect the side of the tongue and palpate it with your gloved left hand, feeling for any lumps or bumps (Figs. 16-14 and 16-15). Then, reverse the procedure to examine the other side. If you detect any suspicious lesions or abnormalities, palpate them with your gloved hands for further evaluation.

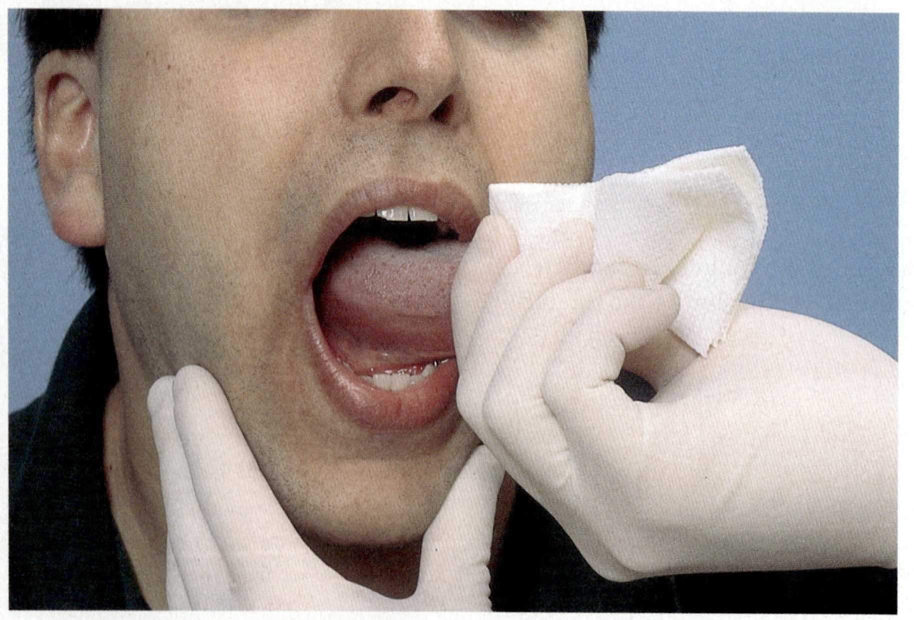

FIGURE 16-14. Grasping the tongue and inspecting its lateral margins.

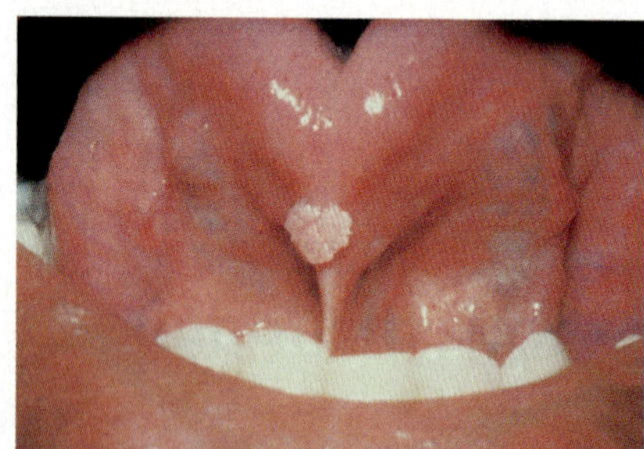

FIGURE 16-15. Carcinoma on the tongue. (Courtesy of the U.S. Department of Veteran's Affairs.)

Note the carcinoma on the left side of the tongue in Figure 16-15. Inspection and palpation remain the standard for detection of oral cancers.[11–13]

See Table 16-4, Findings in or under the Tongue, pp. 414–415.

Inspect the Soft Palate, Anterior and Posterior Pillars, Uvula, Tonsils, and Pharynx

Inspect the soft palate, anterior and posterior pillars, uvula, and tonsils by noting their color and symmetry and looking for any exudate, swelling, ulceration, or tonsillar enlargement.

To visualize the posterior pharynx, have the patient open their mouth without protruding the tongue and ask them to say "ahh." This action elevates the soft palate and uvula, allowing for a clearer view of the posterior pharynx. Look for any signs of redness, swelling, exudate (pus-like discharge), or lesions. Note the size and appearance of the tonsils. You should also note any asymmetry, growths, or discolorations.

Asymmetric tonsils, particularly when associated with other symptoms, may signify an underlying pathology such as lymphoma.

Tonsillar exudates with a beefy red uvula are common in streptococcal pharyngitis but warrant rapid antigen-detection testing or throat culture for diagnosis.[14]

In CN X paralysis, the soft palate fails to rise and the uvula deviates to the opposite side and "points away from the lesion" (Fig. 16-16).

Test the Vagus Nerve

To test the function of the vagus nerve (CN X), Ask the patient to open their mouth and say "ahh" or yawn. Observe the soft palate and uvula's elevation. Both should rise symmetrically.

To prevent the spread of infections, discard the tongue blade after use. Proper disposal practices are essential in clinical settings to maintain hygiene and patient safety.

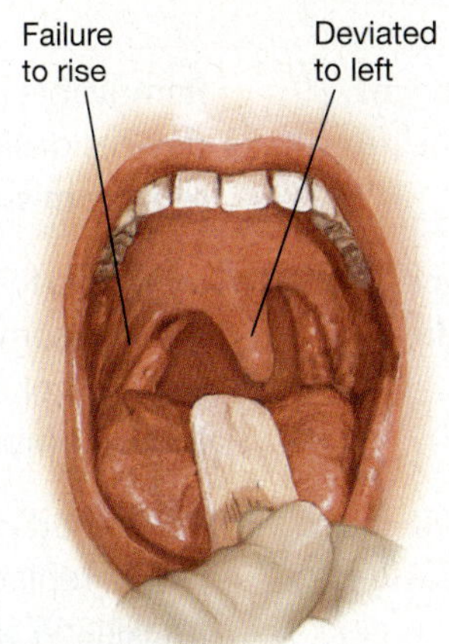

FIGURE 16-16. Cranial nerve X paralysis with the uvula pointing away from the lesion.

SPECIAL TECHNIQUES AND MANEUVERS

Modifications in Physical Examinations: Best Practices for Specialized Patient Populations

For many, dentures are a life-changing solution to tooth loss. As such, unique considerations are required during an oral examination. Box 16-5 delineates these special aspects.

RECORDING YOUR FINDINGS

For guiding your diagnosis and validating your hypotheses, a detailed PE documentation is essential. However, with your eventual exposure to various clinical experiences, your notetaking will evolve to include concise, universally accepted phrases for efficiency.

Box 16-5. Oral Cavity Examination in the Presence of Medical Devices, Conditions, or Procedures

	Patient with Dentures	Patient with Dental Implants
	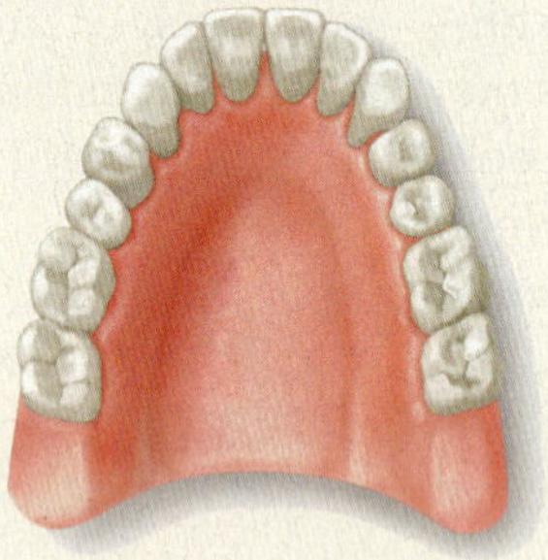	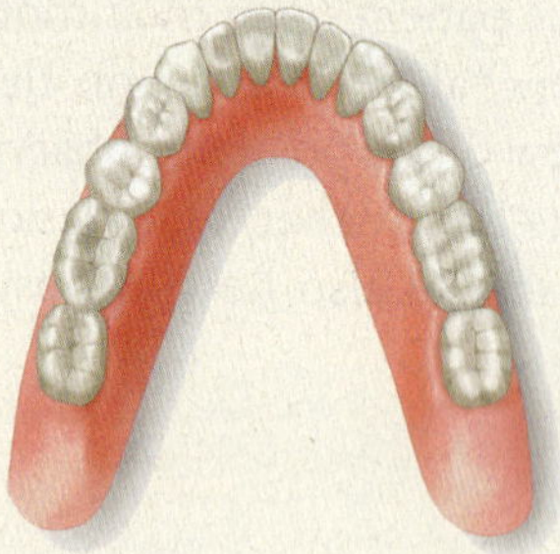
Device/ condition	Removable prosthetic devices designed to replace missing teeth	Fixed prosthetic devices anchored into the jawbone to replace missing teeth
General indication	Indicated for individuals missing some (partial denture) or all of their teeth (complete denture)	Indicated for individuals missing one or more teeth and seeking a permanent solution
General location	Positioned in the oral cavity, replacing upper (maxillary) and/or lower (mandibular) teeth	Implanted into the jawbone, replacing single or multiple missing teeth in either the upper (maxillary) or lower (mandibular) regions
Modification to the physical exam	1. Ask the patient if they can remove the dentures for a thorough oral examination. 2. Inspect the oral mucosa beneath the dentures for any signs of irritation, inflammation (*denture stomatitis*), ulceration, or tumors. 3. Examine the fit and condition of the dentures themselves. 4. Inquire about any discomfort, pain, or changes in fit or bite with the dentures. 5. Recommend daily cleaning and overnight soaking of dentures in an appropriate solution.	1. No removal is necessary as these are fixed prosthetics. 2. Inspect the surrounding gum tissue for signs of inflammation, infection, or recession, which could indicate *peri-implantitis*. 3. Check the stability and condition of the dental implant crown or bridge. 4. Inquire about any discomfort, pain, or changes in bite or fit with the implants. 5. Recommend regular oral hygiene practices to maintain the health of the surrounding gum tissue and to prevent plaque buildup around the implant.

Recording the Head, Eyes, Ears, Nose, and Throat (HEENT) Examination

HEENT:

Throat (or Mouth)—Oral mucosa pink, dentition good, tongue midline, tonsils absent bilaterally, pharynx without exudates or erythema.

OR

Throat—Oral mucosa pink, dental caries in lower molars, tongue midline, pharynx erythematous, bilateral tonsils enlarged, no exudates.

By dissecting PE documentation into its detailed parts, we see a clear example of how thorough clinical observations provide critical diagnostic clues. The clinical findings described for the throat area present a combination of normal and abnormal signs:

- *Oral mucosa pink:* This is a normal finding, indicating healthy oral mucosa without signs of inflammation or infection.
- *Dental caries in lower molars:* Their presence indicates a need for dental care to prevent further decay and potential complications such as toothache, infection, or tooth loss.
- *Tongue midline:* This is a normal finding, and there are no issues with CNs that would cause deviation.
- *Pharynx erythematous:* An erythematous pharynx indicates inflammation, which can be due to pharyngitis caused by a viral or bacterial infection, allergies, or irritants.
- *Bilateral tonsils enlarged, no exudates:* Enlarged tonsils without exudates can be a sign of a viral infection or a chronic condition. The absence of exudates makes a bacterial infection like streptococcal pharyngitis less likely.

Overall, these findings suggest possible *viral pharyngitis.*

HEALTH PROMOTION AND COUNSELING: EVIDENCE AND RECOMMENDATIONS

Important Topics for Health Promotion and Counseling

- Oral health
- Screening for oral and pharyngeal cancer

In the following section, both traditional terms like "men," "women," "male," and "female" and inclusive terms such as "individuals assigned female at birth" and "individuals assigned male at birth" are used. This approach balances inclusivity with the need to accurately represent the original research.

Oral Health

Clinicians should actively promote oral health because it is vital for an individual's overall health and well-being. Among adolescents aged 12 to 19 years and adults aged 20 years and older, 54% and 90% have had at least one cavity in a permanent tooth, respectively. One in four adults has an untreated cavity. Roughly 11% of those ages 65 years and older have no teeth at all (*edentulous*), and the prevalence increases with age.[15–18]

More than 40% of nonedentulous adults ages 30 years and older have some form of periodontal disease, including 7.8% with severe disease.[19] Periodontal disease is associated with low income, male sex at birth, smoking, diabetes, poor oral hygiene, and infrequent dental visits.

Counsel patients to adopt daily hygiene measures to improve oral health. Using fluoride-containing toothpastes reduce tooth decay, and brushing and flossing help prevent periodontal disease by removing dental plaques. Encourage patients to seek dental care at least annually to receive more specialized preventive care such as scaling, root planing, and applying topical fluorides.

Address diet and tobacco use. Children and adults should avoid excessive intake of foods high in starches and refined sugars such as sucrose, which enhance attachment and colonization of cariogenic bacteria. Urge patients to avoid using any tobacco products and to limit alcohol consumption to reduce risk of oral cancer.

Saliva cleanses and lubricates the mouth. Many medications reduce salivary flow, increasing risk for tooth decay, mucositis, and gum disease from xerostomia, especially for older adults.[20] If medications cannot be changed, recommend drinking higher amounts of water and chewing sugarless gum. For those wearing dentures, recommend removal and cleaning each night to reduce bacterial load and risk of bad breath.[21] Regular massage of the gums with a soft-bristled toothbrush or washcloth relieves soreness and pressure from dentures on the underlying soft tissue.

Screening for Oral and Pharyngeal Cancer

An estimated 50,000 Americans were diagnosed with cancer of the oral cavity and oropharynx in 2023, and more than 11,000 deaths were attributed to these cancers.[22] Individuals assigned male at birth are more than twice as likely as Individuals assigned female at birth to be diagnosed with and die from these cancers. Tobacco and alcohol account for about 75% of oral cavity cancers.[23] Sexually transmitted human papillomavirus (HPV) infection is an increasingly important cause of oropharyngeal cancers (lesions of the tonsils, oropharynx, and base of the tongue), accounting for about 70% of cases.[24] Risk for oropharyngeal HPV infection is associated with age (highest prevalence among those ages 35 to 39 years and 50 to 54 years), Individuals assigned male at birth, a higher number of lifetime sexual partners, sexual behaviors (oral sex), alcohol use in the previous year, and tobacco and marijuana smoking.[25]

The primary screening test for these cancers is a thorough examination of the oral cavity. However, in 2014, the U.S. Preventive Services Task Force (USPSTF) concluded that there was insufficient evidence to assess the balance of benefits and harms of routinely screening asymptomatic adults for oral cancer (I statement).[23] The USPSTF conducted another literature search in 2020 and found no new studies evaluating screening outcomes.[26] The American Dental Association does recommend that patients with a suspicious oral mucosal lesion be promptly referred to a specialist for biopsy evaluation.[27]

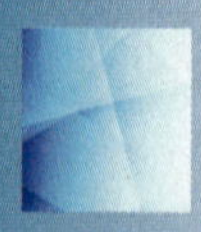

TABLE 16-1. Abnormalities of the Lips

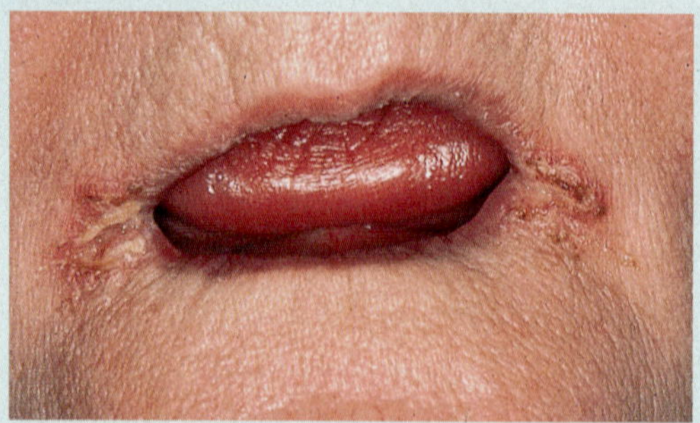

Angular Cheilitis

Angular cheilitis starts with softening of the skin at the angles of the mouth, followed by fissuring. It may be due to nutritional deficiency or, more commonly, overclosure of the mouth, seen in people with no teeth or with ill-fitting dentures. Saliva wets and macerates the infolded skin, often leading to secondary infection with *Candida,* as seen here.

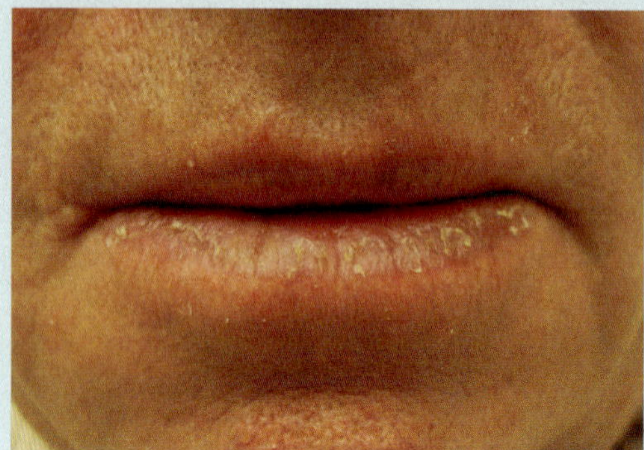

Actinic Cheilitis

Actinic cheilitis is a precancerous condition that results from excessive exposure to sunlight and affects primarily the lower lip. Fair-skinned individuals who work outdoors are most often affected. The lip loses its normal redness and may become scaly, somewhat thickened, and slightly everted. Solar damage predisposes to squamous cell carcinoma of the lip, so examine these skin lesions carefully.

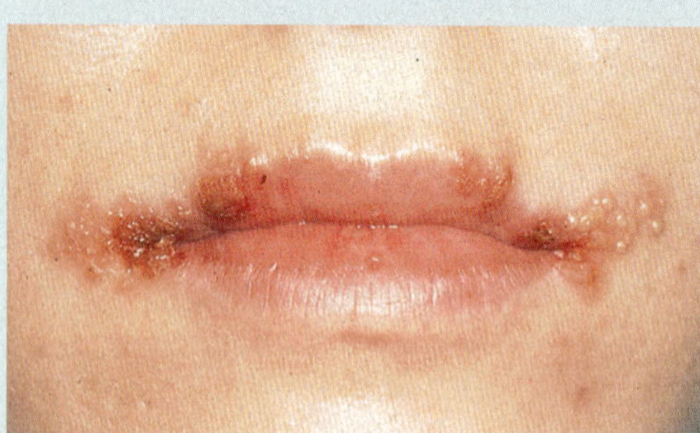

Herpes Simplex (*Cold Sore, Fever Blister*)

Herpes simplex virus (HSV) produces recurrent and painful vesicular eruptions of the lips and surrounding skin. A small cluster of vesicles first develops. As these break, yellow-brown crusts form. Healing takes 10–14 days. Both new and erupted vesicles are visible here.

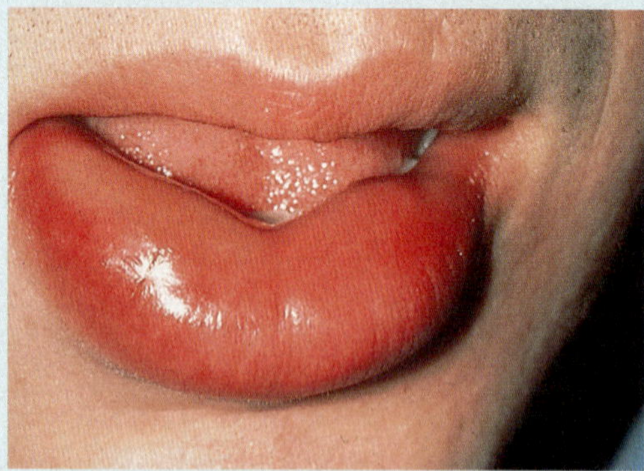

Angioedema

Angioedema is a localized subcutaneous or submucosal swelling caused by leakage of intravascular fluid into interstitial tissue. Two types are common. When vascular permeability is triggered by mast cells in allergic and nonsteroidal anti-inflammatory drug reactions, look for associated urticaria and pruritus. These are uncommon in angioedema from bradykinin and complement-derived mediators, the mechanism in angiotensin-converting enzyme inhibitor reactions. Angioedema is usually benign and resolves within 24–48 h. It can be life threatening when it involves the larynx, tongue, or upper airway or develops into anaphylaxis.

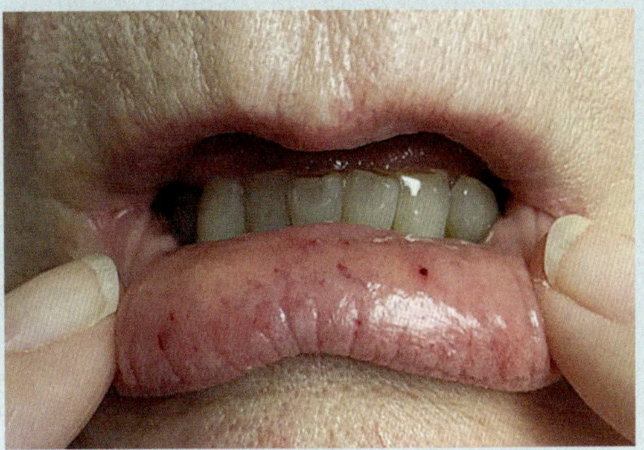

Hereditary Hemorrhagic Telangiectasia (Osler–Weber–Rendu Syndrome)

Multiple small red spots on the lips strongly suggest hereditary hemorrhagic telangiectasia, an autosomal dominant endothelial disorder causing vascular fragility and arteriovenous malformations (AVMs). Telangiectasias are also visible on the oral mucosa, nasal septal mucosa, and fingertips. Nosebleeds, gastrointestinal bleeding, and iron deficiency anemia are common. AVMs in the lungs and brain can cause life-threatening hemorrhage and embolic disease.

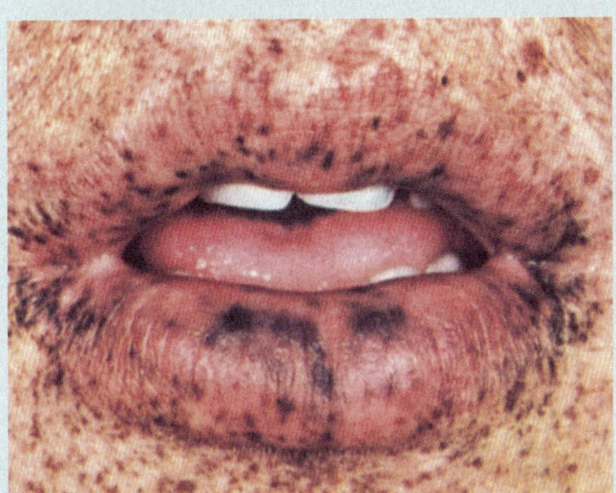

Peutz–Jeghers Syndrome

Look for prominent small brown pigmented spots in the dermal layer of the lips, buccal mucosa, and perioral area. These spots may also appear on the hands and feet. In this autosomal dominant syndrome, these characteristic skin changes accompany numerous intestinal polyps. The risk of gastrointestinal and other cancers ranges from 40% to 90%.

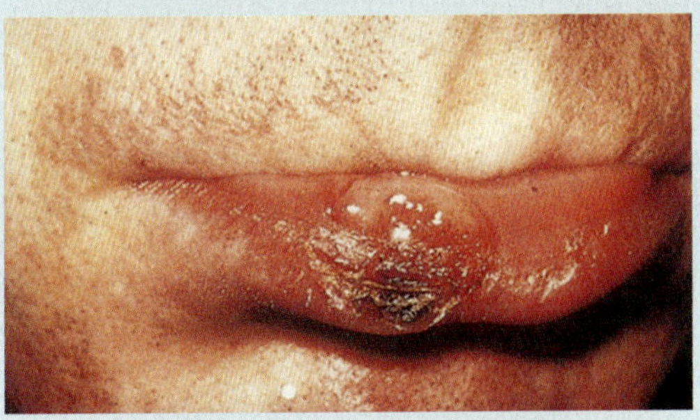

Chancre of Primary Syphilis

This ulcerated papule with an indurated edge usually appears after 3–6 wk of incubating infection from the spirochete *Treponema pallidum*. These lesions may resemble a carcinoma or crusted cold sore. Similar primary lesions are common in the pharynx, anus, and vagina but may escape detection since they are painless, nonsuppurative, and usually heal spontaneously in 3–6 wk. Wear gloves during palpation since these chancres are infectious.

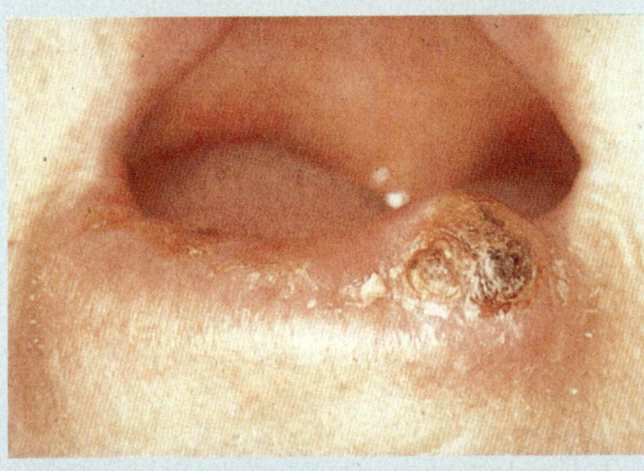

Carcinoma of the Lip

Like actinic cheilitis, squamous cell carcinoma usually affects the lower lip. It may appear as a scaly plaque, as an ulcer with or without a crust, or as a nodular lesion, as illustrated here. Fair skin and prolonged exposure to the sun are common risk factors.

Sources of photos: *Angular Cheilitis, Herpes Simplex, Angioedema*—Reprinted with permission from Neville BW. *Color Atlas of Clinical Oral Pathology*. Lea & Febiger; 1991; *Hereditary Hemorrhagic Telangiectasia*—Reprinted with permission from Mansoor N. *Frameworks for Internal Medicine*. Wolters Kluwer; 2019. Figure 40-2; *Peutz-Jeghers Syndrome*—Reprinted with permission from Robinson HBG, Miller AS. *Colby, Kerr, and Robinson's Color Atlas of Oral Pathology*. 5th ed. JB Lippincott; 1990; *Chancre of Syphilis*—Reprinted from Wisdom A. *A Colour Atlas of Sexually Transmitted Diseases*. 2nd ed. Wolfe Medical Publications; 1989. Copyright © 1989 Elsevier. With permission; *Carcinoma of the Lip*—Reprinted from Tyldesley WR. *A Colour Atlas of Orofacial Diseases*. 2nd ed. Wolfe Medical Publications; 1991. Copyright © 1991 Elsevier. With permission.

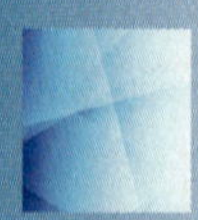

TABLE 16-2. Findings in the Pharynx, Palate, and Oral Mucosa

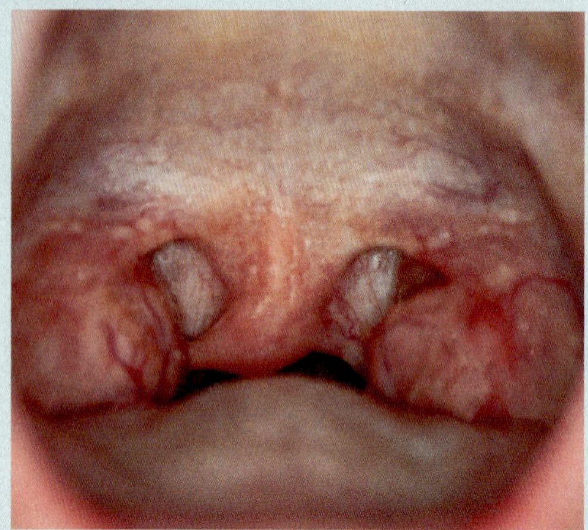

Large Normal Tonsils

Normal tonsils may be large without being infected, especially in children. They may protrude medially beyond the pillars and even to the midline. Here they slightly obscure the pharynx. Their color is pink.

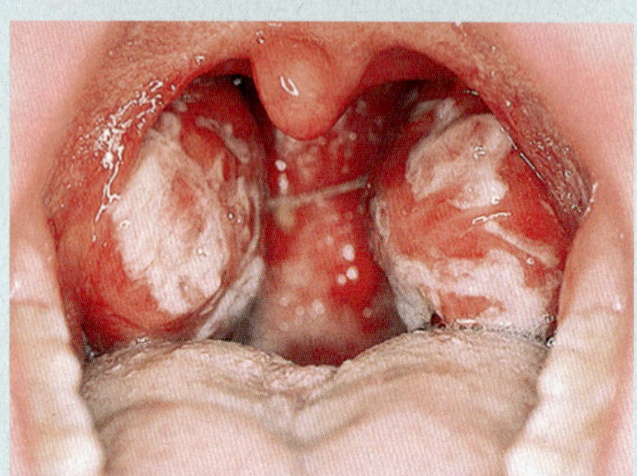

Exudative Tonsillitis

This red throat has thick white exudates on the tonsils. This, together with fever and enlarged cervical nodes, increases the probability of *group A streptococcal infection* or *infectious mononucleosis.* Anterior cervical lymph nodes are usually enlarged in the former, posterior nodes in the latter.

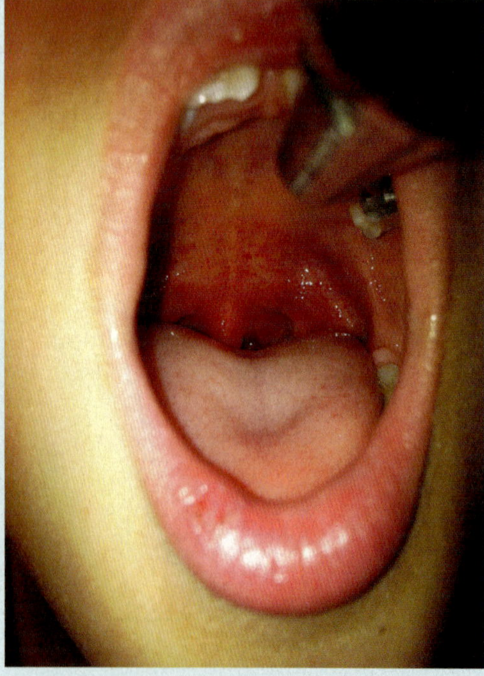

Pharyngitis

This photo shows a reddened throat without exudate. Redness and vascularity of the pillars and uvula are mild to moderate.

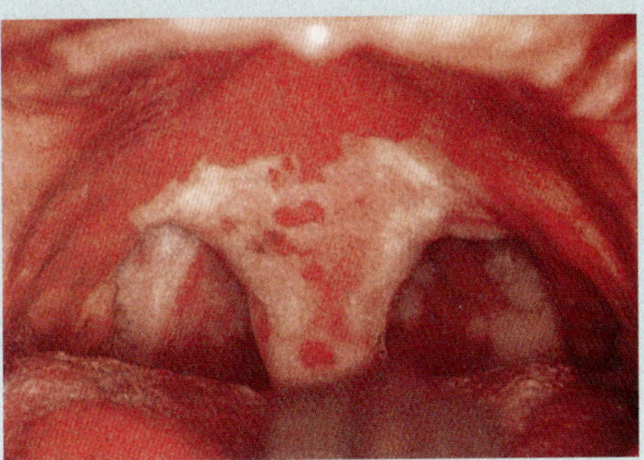

Diphtheria

Diphtheria, an acute infection caused by *Corynebacterium diphtheriae*, is now rare but still important. Prompt diagnosis may lead to life-saving treatment. The throat is dull red, and a gray exudate (*pseudomembrane*) is present on the uvula, pharynx, and tongue. The airway may become obstructed. Prompt diagnosis may lead to life-saving treatment.

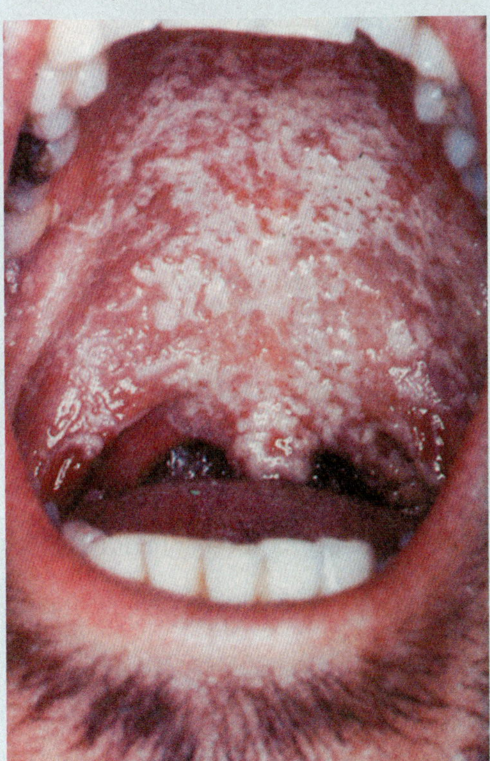

Thrush on the Palate (Candidiasis)

Thrush is a yeast infection from *Candida* species. Shown here on the palate, it may appear as cream-colored or bluish-white pseudomembranous patches on the tongue, mouth, or pharynx. Thick, white plaques are somewhat adherent to the underlying mucosa. Predisposing factors include prolonged treatment with antibiotics or corticosteroids and immunocompromised status.

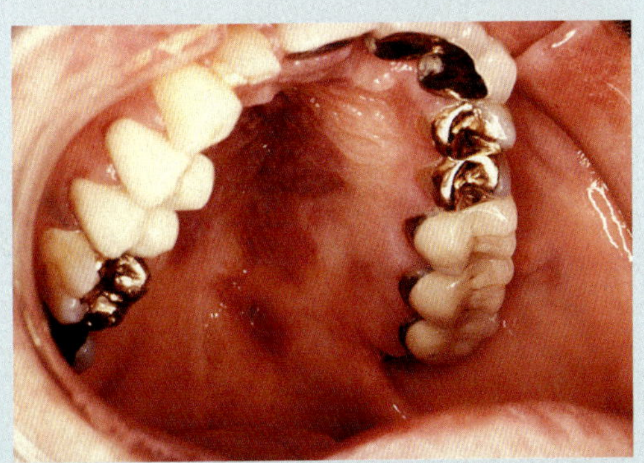

Kaposi Sarcoma in HIV/AIDS

The deep purple color of these lesions suggests Kaposi sarcoma (KS), a low-grade vascular tumor associated with human herpesvirus 8 (HHV-8). These nontender lesions may be raised or flat. About a third of patients with KS have lesions in the oral cavity; other affected sites are the gastrointestinal tract and the lungs.

(*continued*)

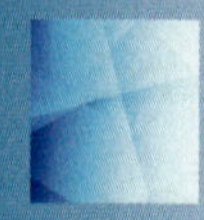

TABLE 16-2. Findings in the Pharynx, Palate, and Oral Mucosa *(Continued)*

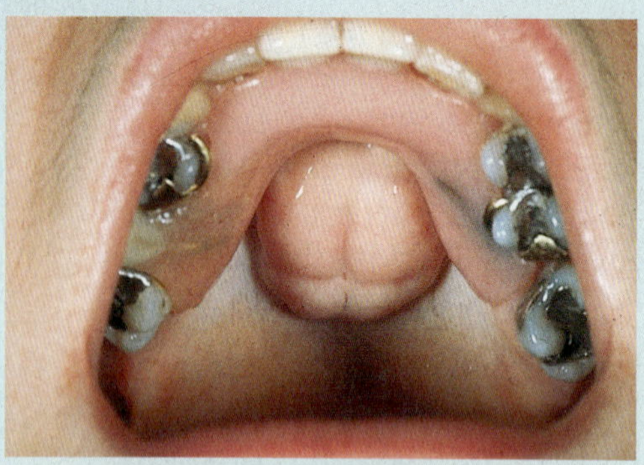

Torus Palatinus

A torus palatinus is a midline bony growth in the hard palate that is fairly common in adults. Its size and lobulation vary. Although alarming at first glance, it is harmless. In this example, an upper denture has been fitted around the torus.

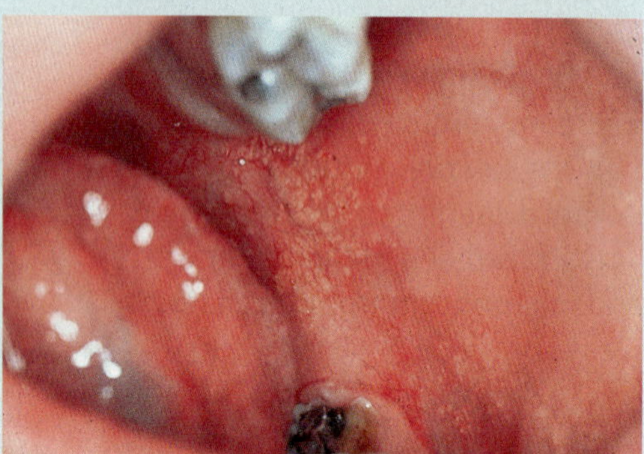

Fordyce Spots (Fordyce Granules)

Fordyce spots are normal sebaceous glands that appear as small yellowish spots in the buccal mucosa or on the lips. Here they are seen best anterior to the tongue and lower jaw. These spots are usually not numerous.

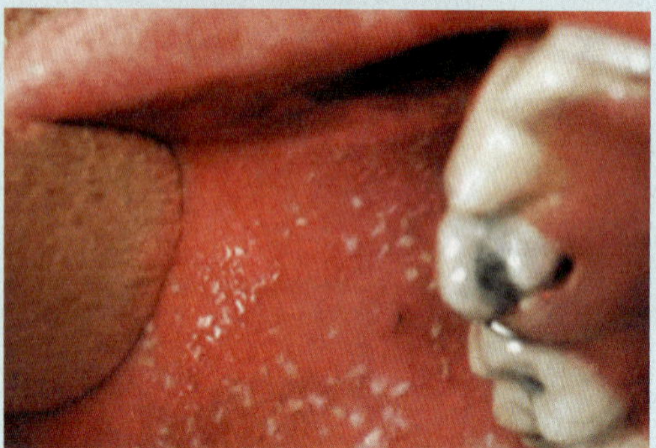

Koplik Spots

Koplik spots are an early sign of measles (*rubeola*). Search for small white specks that resemble grains of salt on a red background. They usually appear on the buccal mucosa near the first and second molars. In this photo, look also in the upper third of the mucosa. The rash of measles appears within a day.

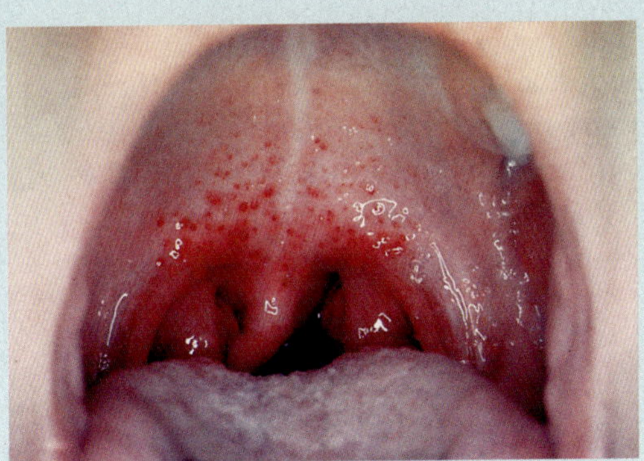

Petechiae

Petechiae are small red spots caused by blood that escapes from capillaries into the tissues. Petechiae in the buccal mucosa are often caused by accidentally biting the cheek. Oral petechiae may be due to infection or decreased platelets, and trauma.

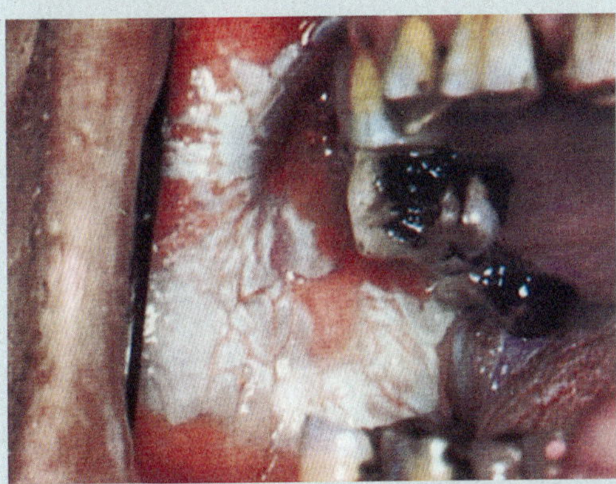

Leukoplakia

A thickened white patch (*leukoplakia*) may occur anywhere in the oral mucosa. The extensive example shown on this buccal mucosa resulted from frequent chewing of tobacco, a local irritant. This benign reactive process of the squamous epithelium may lead to cancer and should be biopsied. Another risk factor is human *papillomavirus* infection.

Sources of photos: *Large Normal Tonsils*—Reprinted with permission from Moore KL, Agur AMR, Dalley AF. *Essential Clinical Anatomy*. 5th ed. Wolters Kluwer; 2015. Figure 9-23A; *Exudative Tonsillitis*—Reprinted with permission from Hatfield NT, Kincheloe CA. *Introductory Maternity & Pediatric Nursing*. 4th ed. Wolters Kluwer; 2018. Figure 41-12; *Pharyngitis*—Courtesy of Naline Lai, MD; *Thrush on the Palate (Candidiasis)*—Reprinted with permission from Engleberg NC, DiRita V, Dermody TS. *Schaechter's Mechanisms of Microbial Disease*. 5th ed. Wolters Kluwer Health/Lippincott Williams & Wilkins; 2013. Figure 48-2; *Kaposi Sarcoma in AIDS*—From the Centers for Disease Control Public Health Image Library, photo credit Sol Silverman Jr, DDS; ID #6071; *Fordyce Spots*—Reprinted with permission from Neville BW. *Color Atlas of Clinical Oral Pathology*. Lea & Febiger; 1991; *Koplik Spots*—Reprinted with permission from Cornelissen CN, Fisher BD, Harvey RA. *Lippincott's Illustrated Reviews: Microbiology*. 3rd ed. Wolters Kluwer Health/Lippincott Williams & Wilkins; 2013:313; *Petechiae*—From the Centers for Disease Control Public Health Image Library, photo credit Heinz F. Eichenwald, MD; ID #3185; *Leukoplakia*—Reprinted with permission from Robinson HBG, Miller AS. *Colby, Kerr, and Robinson's Color Atlas of Oral Pathology*. 5th ed. JB Lippincott; 1990.

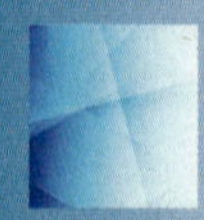

TABLE 16-3. Findings in the Gums and Teeth

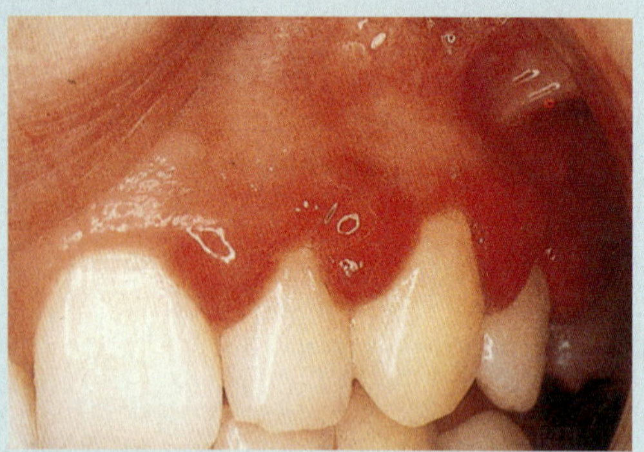

Marginal Gingivitis

Marginal gingivitis is common during adolescence, early adulthood, and pregnancy. The gingival margins are reddened and swollen, and the interdental papillae are blunted, swollen, and red. Brushing the teeth often makes the gums bleed. *Plaque*—the soft white film of salivary salts, protein, and bacteria that covers the teeth and leads to gingivitis—is not readily visible.

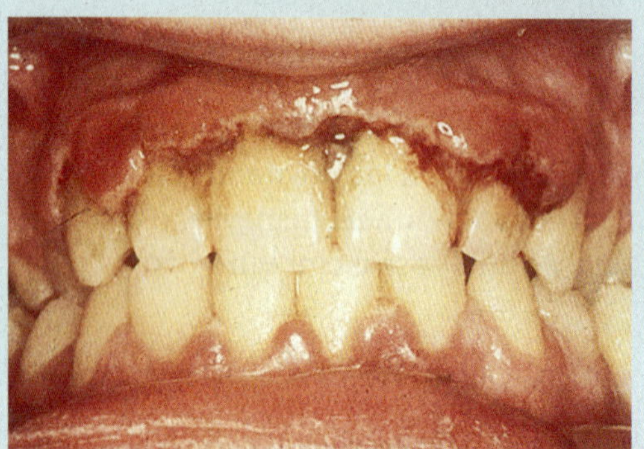

Acute Necrotizing Ulcerative Gingivitis

This uncommon form of gingivitis occurs suddenly in adolescents and young adults and is accompanied by fever, malaise, and enlarged lymph nodes. Ulcers develop in the interdental papillae. Then the destructive (necrotizing) process spreads along the gum margins, where a grayish pseudomembrane develops. The red, painful gums bleed easily; the breath is foul.

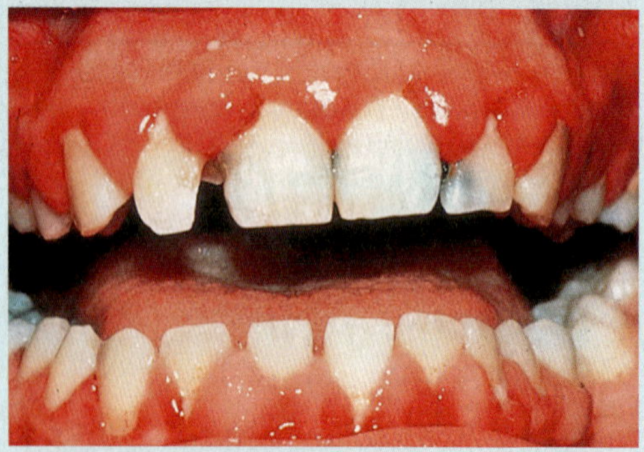

Gingival Hyperplasia

Gums enlarged by hyperplasia are swollen into heaped-up masses that may even cover the teeth. The redness of inflammation may coexist, as in this example. Causes include phenytoin therapy (as in this case), puberty, pregnancy, and leukemia.

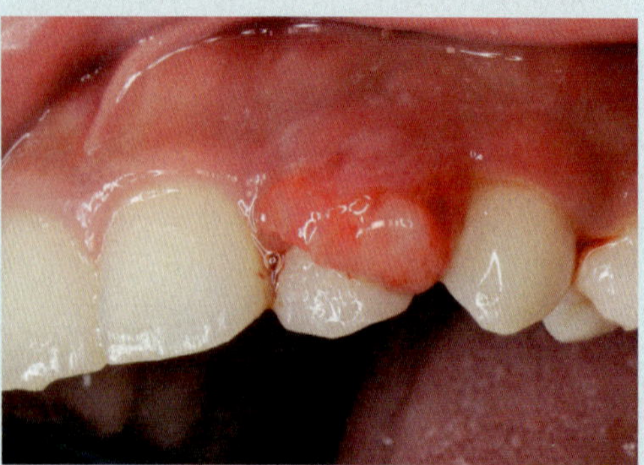

Pregnancy Tumor (Pregnancy Epulis or Pyogenic Granuloma)

Red purple papules of granulation tissue form in the gingival interdental papillae, in the nasal cavity, and sometimes on the fingers. They are red, soft, painless, and usually bleed easily. They occur in 1–5% of pregnancies and usually regress after delivery. Note the accompanying gingivitis.

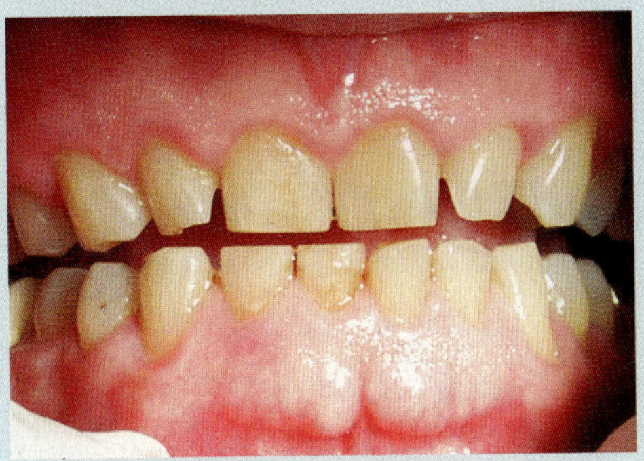

Tooth Attrition; Gum Recession

In many older adults, the chewing surfaces of the teeth are worn down by repetitive use so that the yellow-brown dentin becomes exposed—a process called *attrition. Recession of the gums,* which exposes the roots of the teeth may occur, giving a "long in the tooth" appearance.

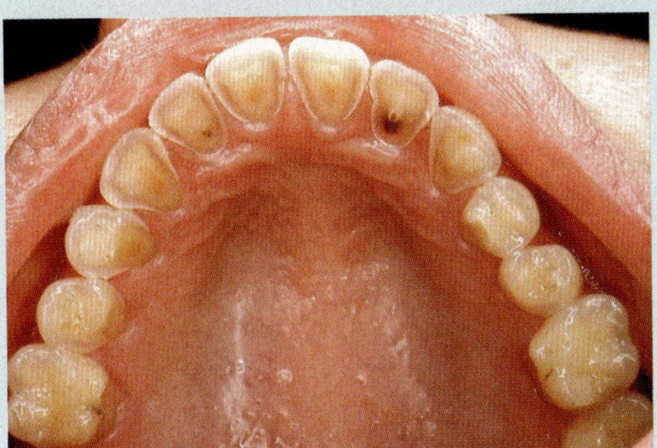

Tooth Erosion

Severe erosion is evident on the lingual surfaces of these maxillary teeth, especially the anterior teeth exposing the yellow-brown dentin. This pattern of tooth destruction typically results from recurrent regurgitation of stomach contents as in bulimia and in persons with severe acid reflux.

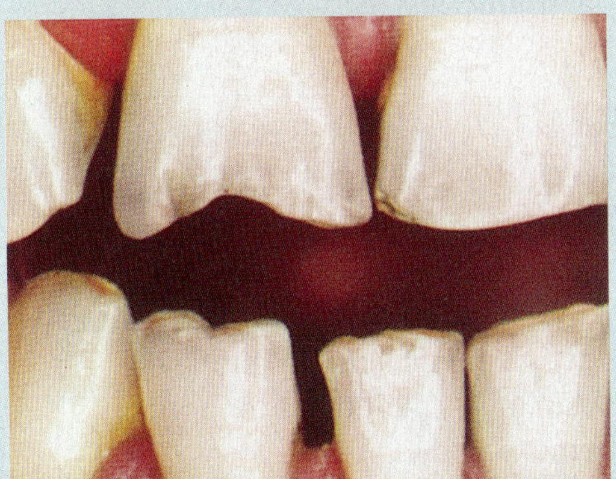

Tooth Abrasion with Notching

The biting surface of the teeth may become abraded or notched by recurrent trauma, such as holding nails or opening bobby pins between the teeth. Unlike Hutchinson teeth, the sides of these teeth show normal contours; size and spacing of the teeth are unaffected.

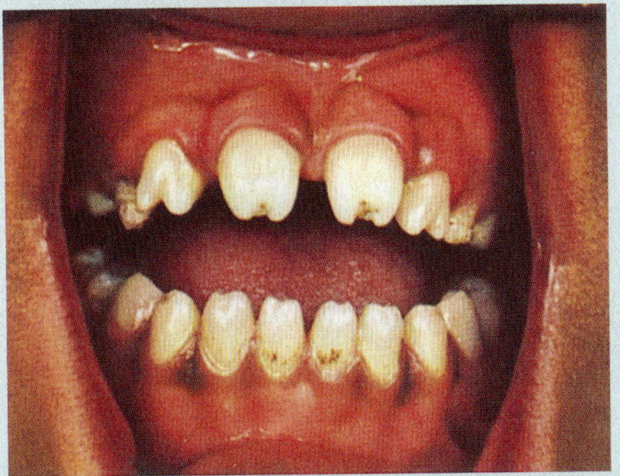

Hutchinson Teeth in Congenital Syphilis

Hutchinson teeth are smaller and more widely spaced than normal and are notched on their biting surfaces. The sides of the teeth taper toward the biting edges. The upper central incisors of the permanent (not the deciduous) teeth are most often affected. These teeth are a sign of congenital syphilis.

Sources of photos: *Marginal Gingivitis, Acute Necrotizing Ulcerative Gingivitis*—Reprinted from Tyldesley WR. *A Colour Atlas of Orofacial Diseases*. 2nd ed. Wolfe Medical Publications; 1991. Copyright © 1991 Elsevier. With permission; *Gingival Hyperplasia*—Courtesy of Dr. James Cottone; *Pregnancy Tumor*—Shutterstock photo by Kasama Kanpittaya; *Attrition of Teeth*—Reprinted with permission from DeLong L, Burkhart NW. *General and Oral Pathology for the Dental Hygienist*. 2nd ed. Wolters Kluwer Health/Lippincott Williams & Wilkins; 2013. Figure 21-1; *Erosion of Teeth*—Reprinted with permission from Timby BK, Smith NE. *Introductory Medical-Surgical Nursing*. 12th ed. Wolters Kluwer; 2018. Figure 70-2B; *Abrasion of Teeth, Hutchinson Teeth*—Reprinted with permission from Robinson HBG, Miller AS. *Colby, Kerr, and Robinson's Color Atlas of Oral Pathology*. 5th ed. JB Lippincott; 1990.

TABLE 16-4. Findings in or under the Tongue

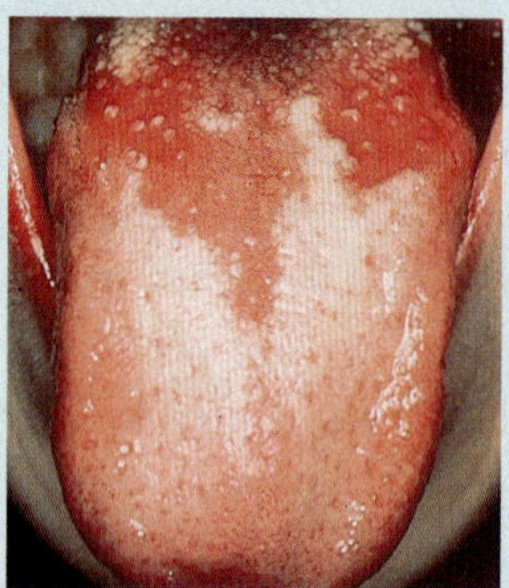

Geographic Tongue. In this benign condition, the dorsum shows scattered smooth red areas denuded of papillae. Together with the normal rough and coated areas, they give a map-like pattern that changes over time.

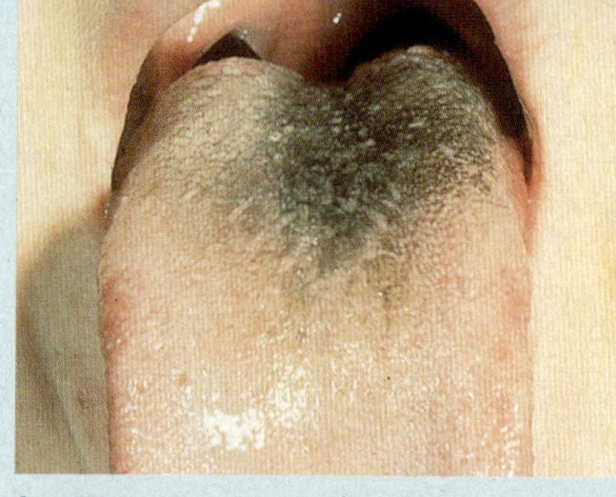

Black Hairy Tongue. Note the "hairy" yellowish to brown and black hypertrophied and elongated papillae on the tongue's dorsum. This benign condition is associated with *Candida* and bacterial overgrowth, antibiotic therapy, and poor dental hygiene. It also may occur spontaneously.

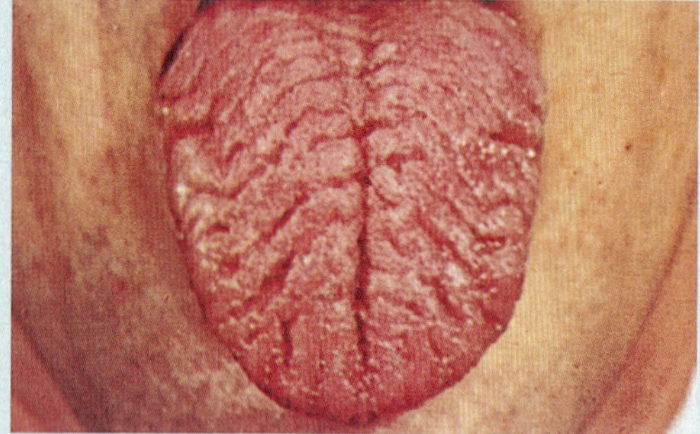

Fissured Tongue. Fissures appear with increasing age, sometimes termed *furrowed tongue.* Food debris may accumulate in the crevices and become irritating, but a fissured tongue is benign.

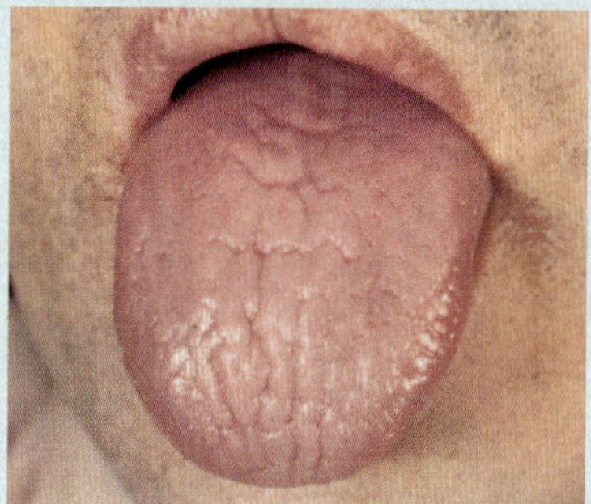

Smooth Tongue (*Atrophic Glossitis*). A smooth and often sore tongue that has lost its papillae, sometimes just in patches, suggests a deficiency in riboflavin, niacin, folic acid, vitamin B_{12}, pyridoxine, or iron, or treatment with chemotherapy.

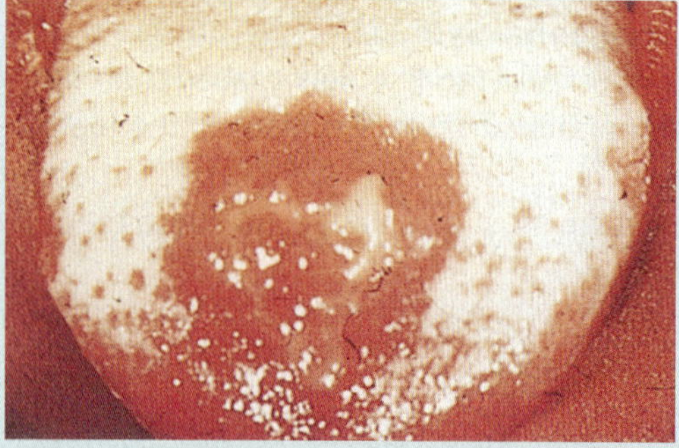

Candidiasis. Note the thick white coating from *Candida* infection. The raw red surface is where the coat was scraped off. Infection may also occur without the white coating. It is seen in immunosuppression from chemotherapy or prednisone therapy.

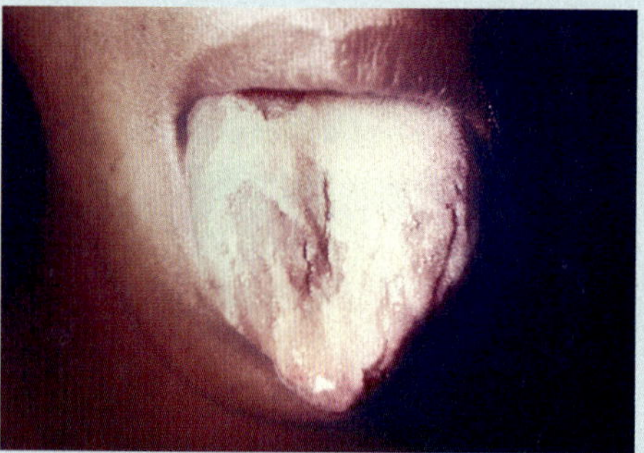

Oral Hairy Leukoplakia. These whitish raised asymptomatic plaques with a feathery or corrugated pattern occur most often on the sides of the tongue. Unlike candidiasis, these areas cannot be scraped off. This condition is caused by Epstein–Barr virus infection and is seen in HIV and AIDS infection.

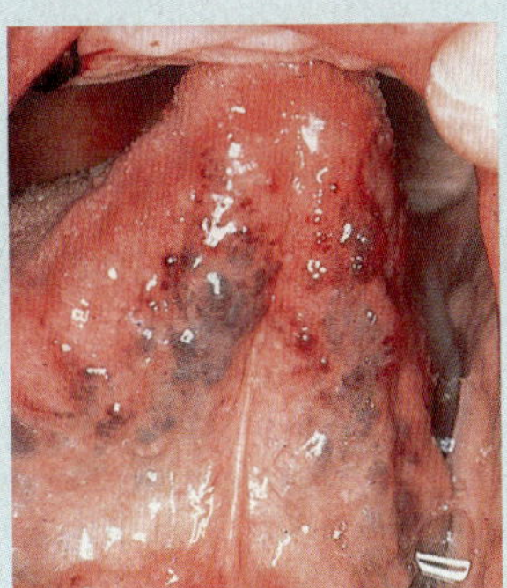

Varicose Veins. Small purplish or blue-black round swellings appear under the tongue with age. These dilatations of the lingual veins have no clinical significance.

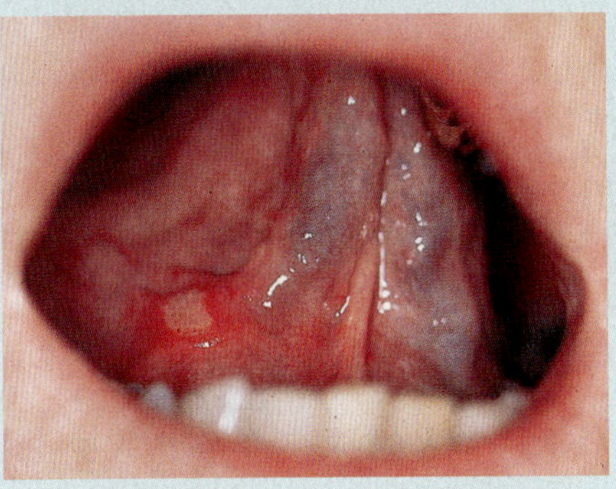

Aphthous Ulcer (*Canker Sore*). A painful, shallow whitish-gray oval ulceration surrounded by a halo of reddened mucosa. It may be single or multiple and may also occur on the gingiva and oral mucosa. It heals in 7–10 days, but may recur, as in Behçet disease.

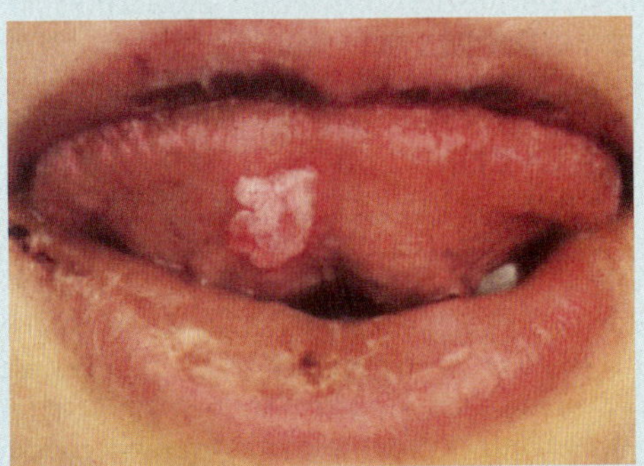

Mucous Patch of Syphilis. This painless lesion of secondary syphilis is highly infectious. It is slightly raised, oval, and covered by a grayish membrane. It may be multiple and occur elsewhere in the mouth.

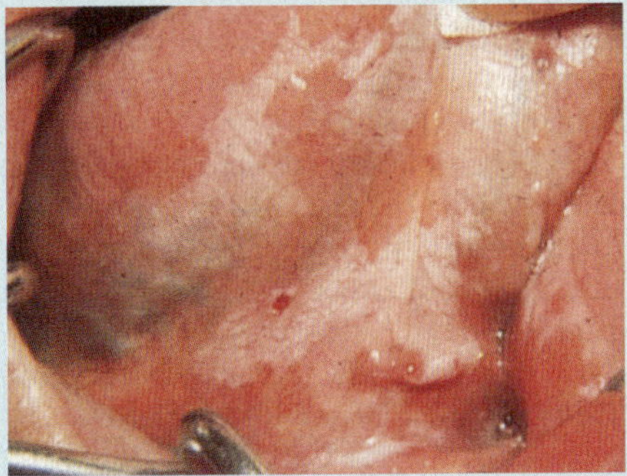

Leukoplakia. With this persisting painless white patch in the oral mucosa, the undersurface of the tongue appears painted white. Patches of any size raise the possibility of squamous cell carcinoma and require biopsy.

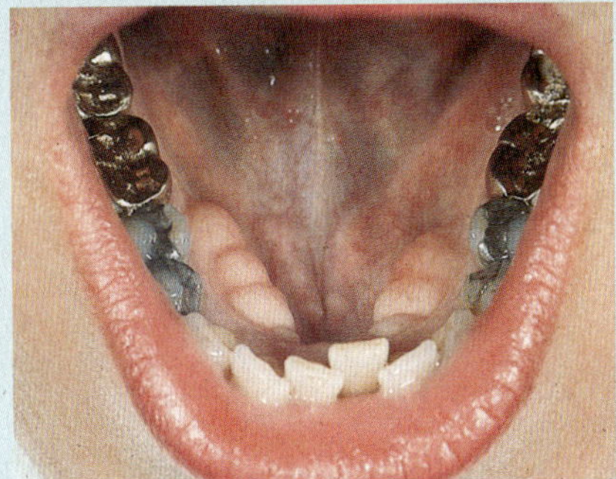

Tori Mandibularis. Rounded bony growths on the inner surfaces of the mandible are typically bilateral, asymptomatic, and harmless.

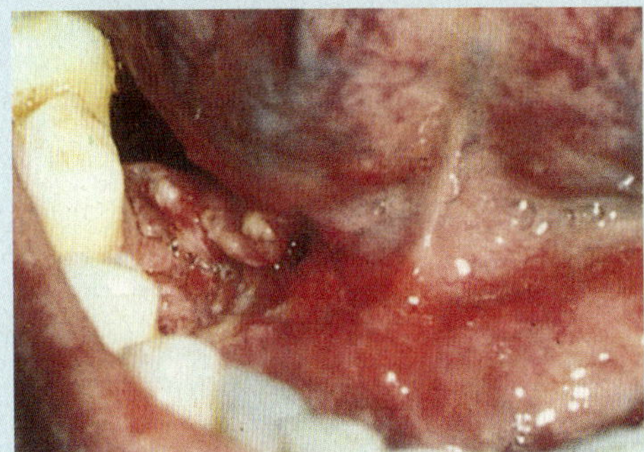

Carcinoma, Floor of the Mouth. This ulcerated lesion is in a common location for carcinoma. Medially, note the reddened area of mucosa, called *erythroplakia,* which is suspicious for malignancy and should be biopsied.

Sources of photos: *Fissured Tongue, Candidiasis, Mucous Patch, Leukoplakia, Carcinoma*—Reprinted with permission from Robinson HBG, Miller AS. *Colby, Kerr, and Robinson's Color Atlas of Oral Pathology*. 5th ed. JB Lippincott; 1990; *Smooth Tongue*—Reprinted with permission from Jensen S. *Nursing Health Assessment: A Best Practice Approach*. 3rd ed. Wolters Kluwer; 2019. Figure 15-25; *Geographic Tongue*—From the Centers for Disease Control Public Health Image Library; ID #16520; *Oral Hairy Leukoplakia*—From the Centers for Disease Control Public Health Image Library, photo credit Sol Silverman, Jr., DDS; ID #6061; *Varicose Veins*—Reprinted with permission from Neville BW. *Color Atlas of Clinical Oral Pathology*. Lea & Febiger; 1991.

REFERENCES

1. Cooper L, Quested RA. Hoarseness: an approach for the general practitioner. *Aust Fam Physician.* 2016;45(6):378–381.
2. Stachler RJ, Francis DO, Schwartz SR, et al. Clinical practice guideline: hoarseness (dysphonia) (update). *Otolaryngol Head Neck Surg.* 2018;158(1_suppl):S1–S42.
3. Born H, Rameau A. Hoarseness. *Med Clin North Am.* 2021; 105(5):917–938.
4. Kapoor U, Sharma G, Juneja M, Nagpal A. Halitosis: current concepts on etiology, diagnosis and management. *Eur J Dent.* 2016;10(2):292–300.
5. Özen ME, Aydin M. Subjective halitosis: definition and classification. *J N J Dent Assoc.* 2015;86(4):20–24.
6. Izidoro C, Botelho J, Machado V, et al. Revisiting standard and novel therapeutic approaches in halitosis: a review. *Int J Environ Res Public Health.* 2022;19(18):11303.
7. Scully C, el-Maaytah M, Porter SR, Greenman J. Breath odor: etiopathogenesis, assessment and management. *Eur J Oral Sci.* 1997;105(4):287–293.
8. Scully C. Halitosis. *BMJ Clin Evid.* 2014;2014:1305.
9. Lucas PW, van Casteren A. The wear and tear of teeth. *Med Princ Pract.* 2015;24(Suppl 1):3–13.
10. Brosnan MG, Natarajan AK, Campbell JM, Drummond BK. Management of the pulp in primary teeth–an update. *N Z Dent J.* 2014;110(4):119–123.
11. Messadi DV. Diagnostic aids for detection of oral precancerous conditions. *Int J Oral Sci.* 2013;5(2):59–65.
12. Hunter KD, Yeoman CM. An update on the clinical pathology of oral precancer and cancer. *Dent Update.* 2013;40(2): 120–122, 125–126.
13. Mangold AR, Torgerson RR, Rogers RS III. Diseases of the tongue. *Clin Dermatol.* 2016;34(4):458–469.
14. Weber R. Pharyngitis. *Prim Care.* 2014;41(1):91–98.
15. Fleming E, Afful J. Prevalence of Total and Untreated Dental Caries Among Youth: United States, 2015–2016. *NCHS Data Brief, no 307.* 2018. https://www.cdc.gov/nchs/data/databriefs/db307.pdf
16. Centers for Disease Control and Prevention. Oral Health Conditions. Accessed July 27, 2023. https://www.cdc.gov/oralhealth/conditions/index.html
17. Gupta N, Vujicic M, Yarbrough C, Harrison B. Disparities in untreated caries among children and adults in the U.S., 2011–2014. *BMC Oral Health.* 2018;18(1):30.
18. Parker ML, Thornton-Evans G, Wei L, Griffin SO. Prevalence of and changes in tooth loss among adults aged >/=50 years with selected chronic conditions—United States, 1999–2004 and 2011–2016. *MMWR Morb Mortal Wkly Rep.* 2020;69(21):641–646.
19. Eke PI, Thornton-Evans GO, Wei L, Borgnakke WS, Dye BA, Genco RJ. Periodontitis in US Adults: National Health and Nutrition Examination survey 2009–2014. *J Am Dent Assoc.* 2018;149(7):576–588.e6.
20. American Dental Association. Xerostomia. Accessed July 27, 2023. https://www.ada.org/en/resources/research/science-and-research-institute/oral-health-topics/xerostomia
21. American Dental Association. Denture care and maintenance. Accessed July 27, 2023. https://www.ada.org/resources/research/science-and-research-institute/oral-health-topics/dentures
22. Siegel RL, Miller KD, Wagle NS, Jemal A. Cancer statistics, 2023. *CA Cancer J Clin.* 2023;73(1):17–48.
23. Moyer VA, U.S. Preventive Services Task Force. Screening for oral cancer: U.S. Preventive Services Task Force recommendation statement. *Ann Intern Med.* 2014;160(1):55–60.
24. Centers for Disease Control and Prevention. HPV and Oropharyngeal Cancer. Accessed July 27, 2023. https://www.cdc.gov/cancer/hpv/basic_info/hpv_oropharyngeal.htm
25. Sonawane K, Suk R, Chiao EY, et al. Oral human papillomavirus infection: differences in prevalence between sexes and concordance with genital human papillomavirus infection, NHANES 2011 to 2014. *Ann Intern Med.* 2017;167(10): 714–724.
26. U.S. Preventive Services Task Force. Literature Surveillance Report. Oral Cancer: Screening. Accessed August 30, 2024. https://www.uspreventiveservicestaskforce.org/uspstf/document/literature-surveillance-report/oral-cancer-screening
27. Lingen MW, Abt E, Agrawal N, et al. Evidence-based clinical practice guideline for the evaluation of potentially malignant disorders in the oral cavity: a report of the American Dental Association. *J Am Dent Assoc.* 2017;148(10): 712–727.e10.

CHAPTER

17

Thorax and Lungs

ANATOMY AND PHYSIOLOGY

The *thorax* is a structure located in the chest region and is delimited anteriorly by the sternum and ribs, laterally by the ribs, and posteriorly by the thoracic spine and ribs. The clavicles and neck tissues form the superior boundary while the diaphragm forms the inferior boundary. Within the thorax lie important organs such as the lungs and heart, and the thorax plays a crucial role in the process of breathing. Study the anatomy of the chest wall and be able to identify the various structures illustrated in Figure 17-1.

Describe chest findings in two dimensions: along the vertical axis and around the circumference of the chest.

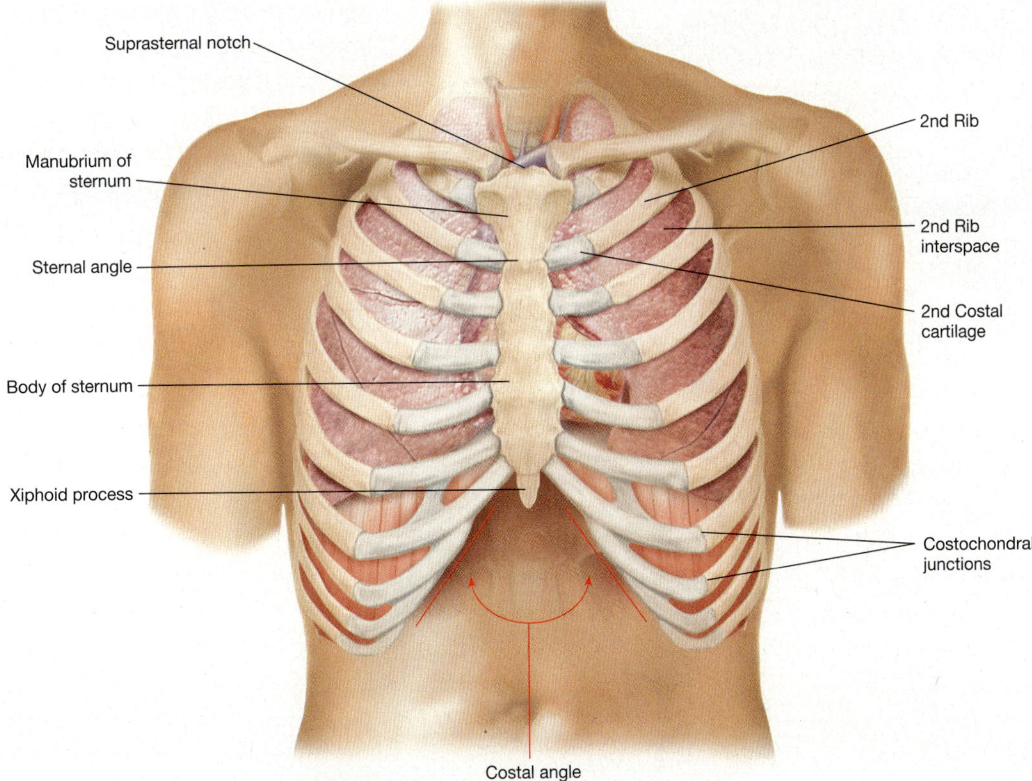

FIGURE 17-1. Chest wall anatomy.

Surface Anatomy: Vertical Axis

To locate findings in the thorax, *count the ribs* and *intercostal spaces* (Fig. 17-2). Start by placing your finger in the hollow curve of the *suprasternal notch,* and then move it down about 5 cm to the horizontal bony ridge where the manubrium joins the body of the sternum, also known as the *sternal angle* or the *angle of Louis.* The 2nd rib and its costal cartilage are located directly adjacent to the sternal angle. Using two fingers, "walk down" the interspaces on an oblique line, indicated by the red numbers in Figure 17-2.

Note that the ribs at the lower edge of the sternum may be too close together to count accurately. In patients with breasts, it may be necessary to displace them laterally by having them lie supine or palpate more medially, taking care not to press too hard on tender breast tissue. Note that the number of the intercostal space between two ribs is the same as the number of the rib above it, which can be a useful reference point during examination.

Note that the first 7 ribs articulate with the sternum via their costal cartilages, while the cartilages of the 8th, 9th, and 10th ribs connect to the cartilages above them. The 11th and 12th ribs, known as the "*floating ribs,*" have no anterior attachments. The cartilaginous tip of the 11th rib is usually palpable laterally, and the 12th rib can be felt posteriorly. Both costal cartilages and ribs feel identical when palpated.

Posteriorly, the 12th rib can serve as a starting point for counting ribs and intercostal spaces and provides an alternative to the anterior approach (Fig. 17-3). To do this, press in and up against the lower border of the 12th rib with one

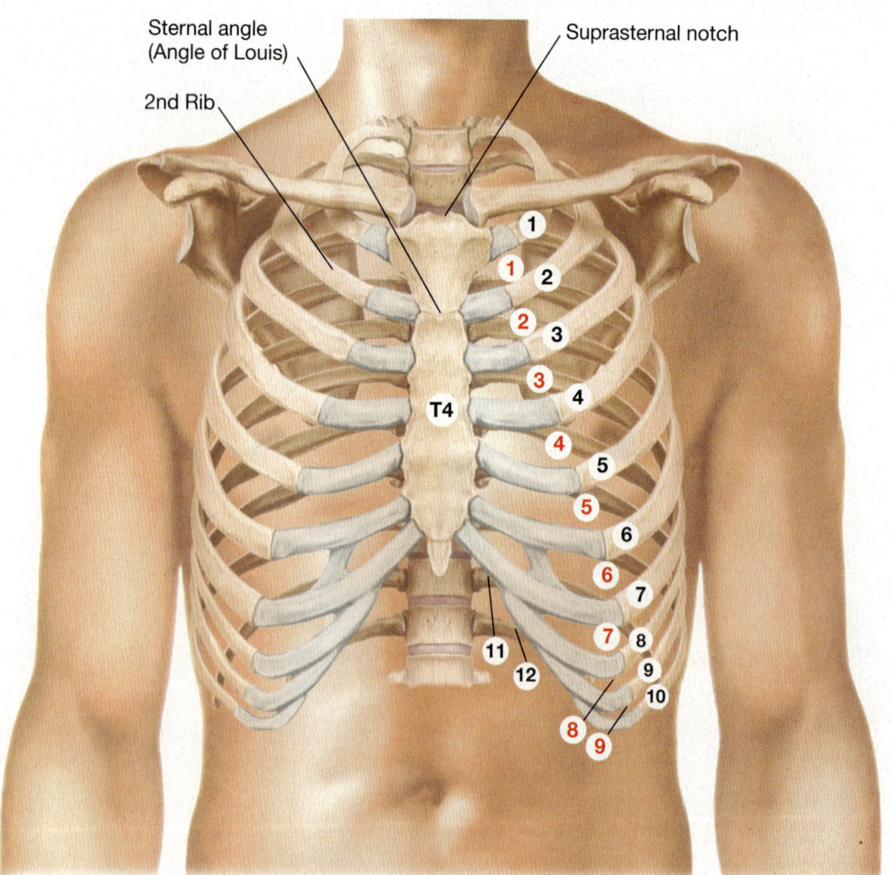

FIGURE 17-2. Anterior ribs (*black*) and intercostal spaces (*red*).

Note special landmarks:

- Second intercostal space for needle insertion for decompression of a tension pneumothorax
- Intercostal space between the 4th and 5th ribs for chest tube insertion
- Level of the 4th rib for the lower margin of a well-placed endotracheal tube on a chest x-ray.

Neurovascular structures run along the inferior margin of each rib, so needles and tubes should be placed just at the superior rib margins.

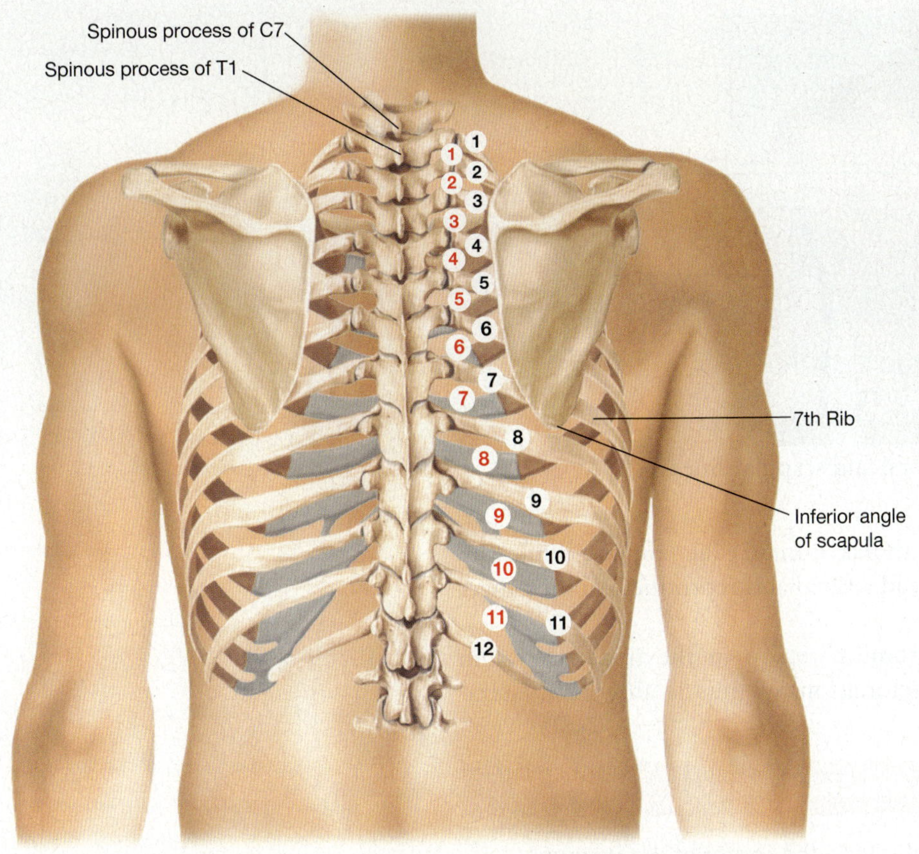

FIGURE 17-3. Posterior ribs (*black*) and intercostal spaces (*red*).

Note the intercostal space between the 7th and 8th ribs as a landmark for thoracentesis with needle insertion immediately superior to the 8th rib.

hand and then "walk up" the intercostal spaces, which are numbered in red in Figure 17-3. Alternatively, you can follow a more oblique line up and around to the front of the chest.

The inferior tip of the scapula is a helpful bony landmark that usually lies at the level of the 7th rib or intercostal space.

Surface Anatomy: Chest Circumference

To better visualize and locate structures in the thorax, use a series of vertical lines as demonstrated in Figures 17-4 through 17-6. Using these lines can help

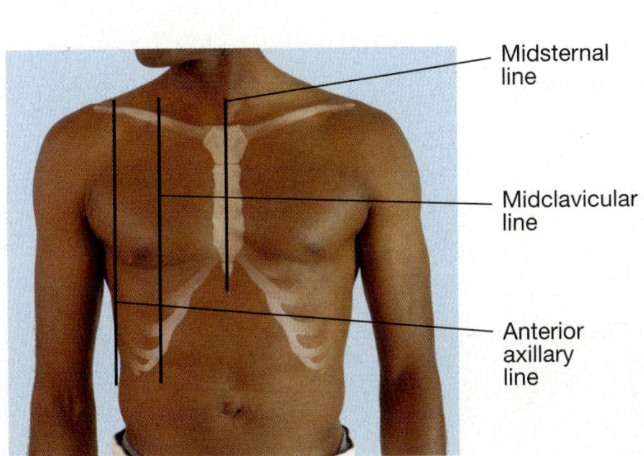

FIGURE 17-4. Midsternal and midclavicular lines.

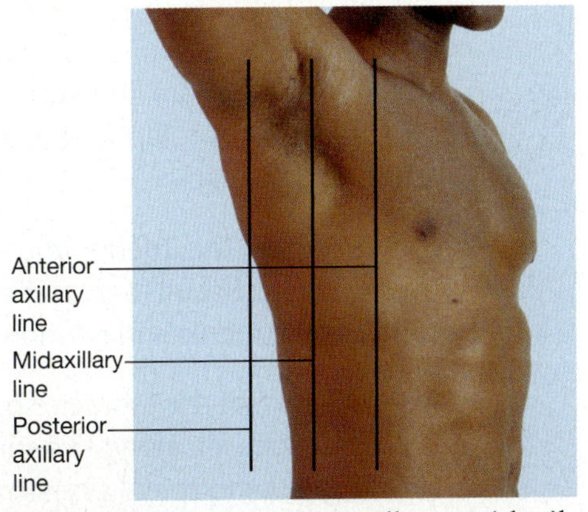

FIGURE 17-5. Anterior axillary, midaxillary, and posterior axillary lines.

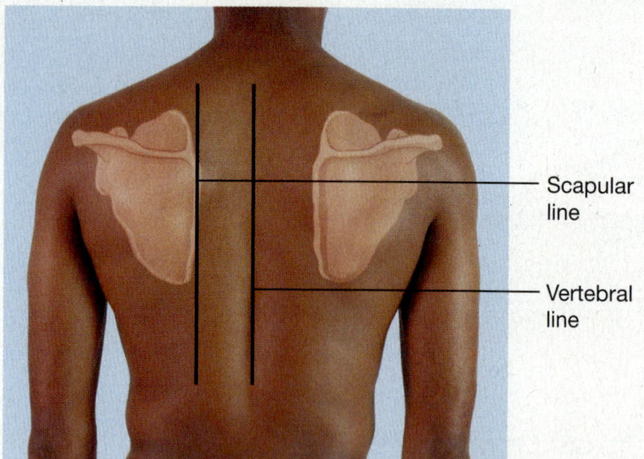

FIGURE 17-6. Vertebral and scapular lines.

in locating specific landmarks in the thorax during examination. While the midsternal and vertebral lines are easily identified and reproducible, the others may require visualization (Box 17-1).

The "*triangle of safety*" is an anatomical region in the midaxillary line formed by the lateral border of the pectoralis major muscle anteriorly, lateral

Box 17-1. Anatomical Lines in the Chest Wall

Midsternal line	Runs vertically along the center of the sternum (breastbone) and divides the chest into left and right halves
Midclavicular line	Runs vertically from the midpoint of the clavicle (collarbone) and is used as a reference point for clinical assessments of the chest and abdomen
Anterior axillary line	Runs vertically from the front (anterior) axillary fold, which is the junction between the chest and the upper arm; helps in identifying specific landmarks on the chest wall
Midaxillary line	Runs vertically from the apex of the axilla (armpit) and is used to locate structures in the middle of the axillary region
Posterior axillary line	Like the anterior axillary line, runs vertically from the posterior axillary fold, helping to identify specific landmarks on the back
Scapular line	Drops down from the inferior angle of the scapula (shoulder blade); useful for assessing back injuries or identifying structures in relation to the scapula
Vertebral line	Follows the path of the thoracic spinous processes (bony projections felt along the spine); used for reference during spinal assessments and procedures

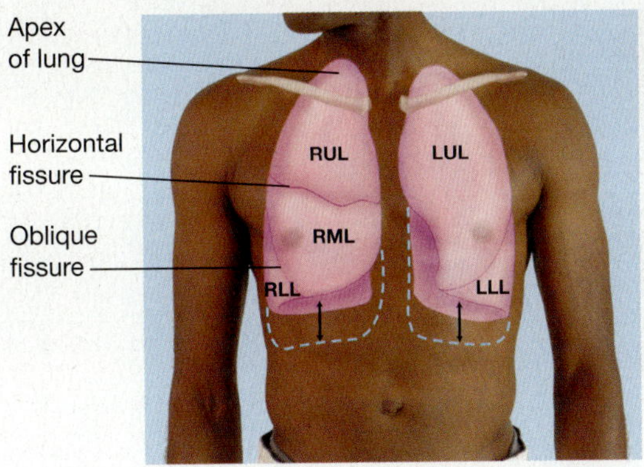

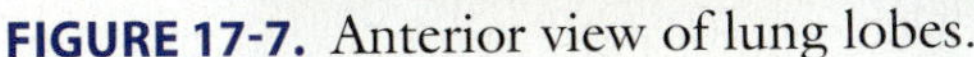

FIGURE 17-7. Anterior view of lung lobes.

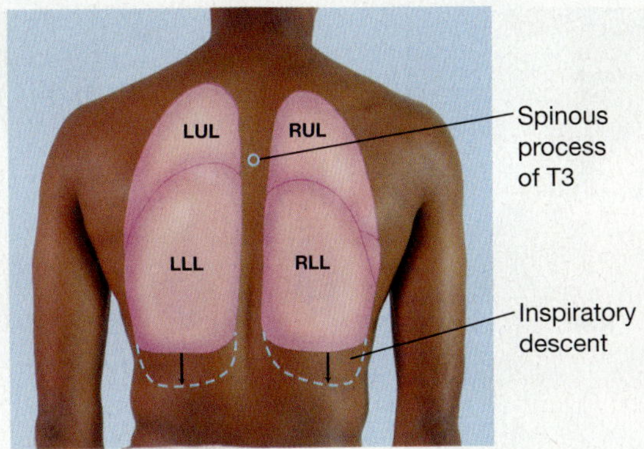

FIGURE 17-8. Posterior view of lung lobes.

border of the latissimus dorsi posteriorly, and the nipple line (4th or 5th intercostal space) inferiorly. This triangle represents a "safe position" for chest tube insertion.

Lungs, Fissures, and Lobes

Visualize the lungs and their lobes on the chest wall. Anteriorly, the apex of each lung rises approximately 2 to 4 cm above the inner third of the clavicle (Fig. 17-7). Moving inferiorly, the lower border of the lung crosses the 6th rib at the midclavicular line and the 8th rib at the midaxillary line. Posteriorly, the lower border of the lung lies at about the level of the T10 spinous process (Fig. 17-8). During inspiration, the lungs expand as the diaphragm contracts and descends, causing the lower border to descend in the chest cavity. To identify the right and left lungs on a chest x-ray, refer to Figure 17-9.

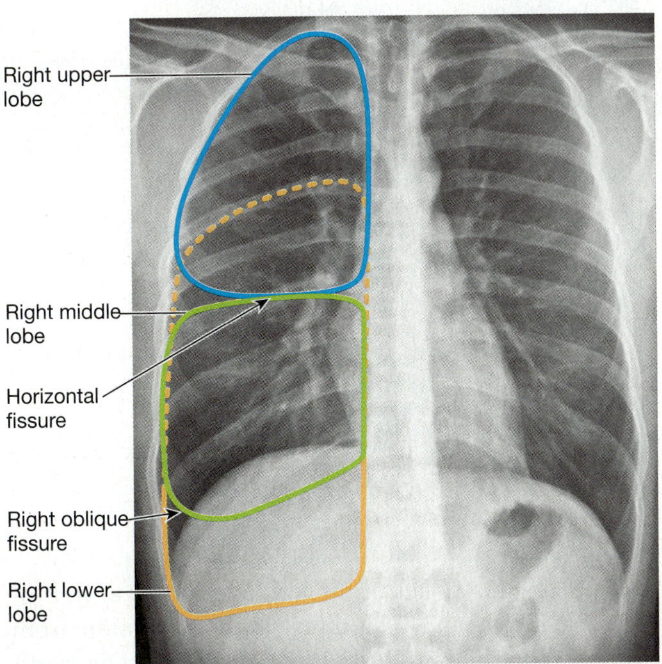

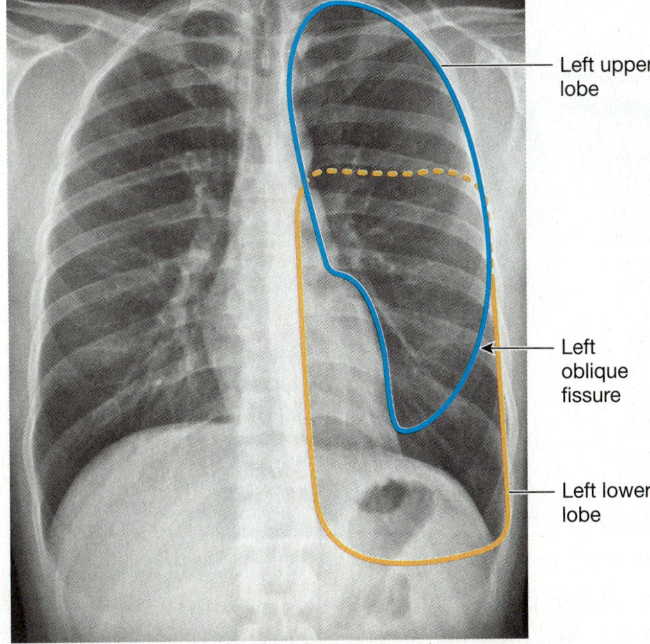

FIGURE 17-9. Right and left lungs in anterior view of a chest radiograph. (Reprinted with permission from Brant WE, Helms CA. *Fundamentals of Diagnostic Radiology*. 3rd ed. Lippincott Williams & Wilkins; 2007. Figure 1-5.)

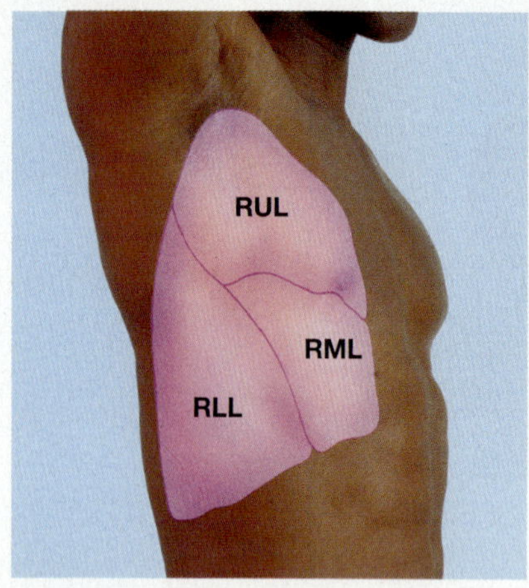

FIGURE 17-10. Right lung lobes and fissures.

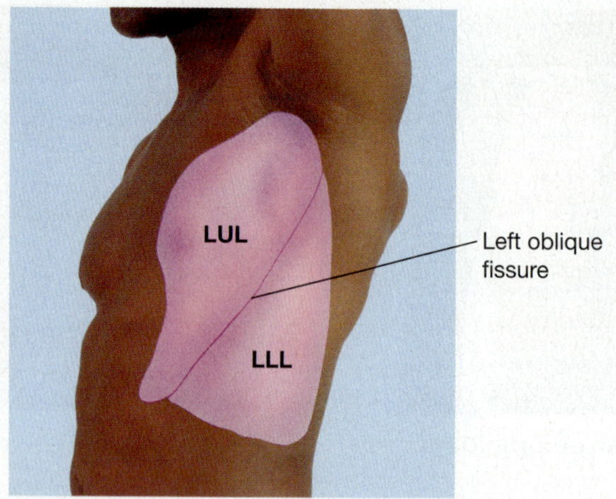

FIGURE 17-11. Left lung lobes and fissures.

Each lung is separated into two parts by an *oblique fissure* that roughly divides the lung in half. To locate this fissure, imagine a string running from the T3 spinous process obliquely down and around the chest to the 6th rib at the midclavicular line (Fig. 17-10). The right lung is further divided by the *horizontal (minor) fissure.* This fissure runs close to the 4th rib anteriorly and meets the oblique fissure in the midaxillary line near the 5th rib. As a result, the right lung is divided into upper, middle, and lower lobes (RUL, RML, and RLL), while the left lung has only two lobes, upper and lower (LUL, LLL), as shown in Figure 17-11. You can identify the lobes of the right and left lungs on chest x-rays in Figures 17-12 and 17-13.

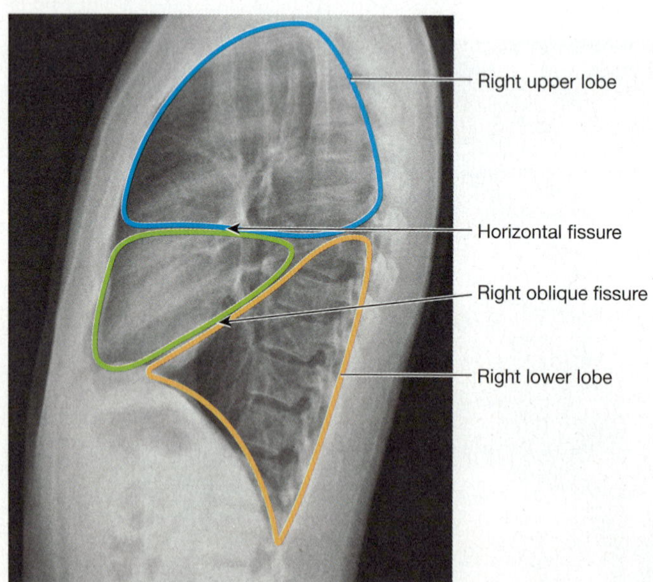

FIGURE 17-12. Lobes of the right lung in lateral view of a chest radiograph. (Modified with permission from Brant WE, Helms CA. *Fundamentals of Diagnostic Radiology.* 3rd ed. Lippincott Williams & Wilkins; 2007. Figure 21-2.)

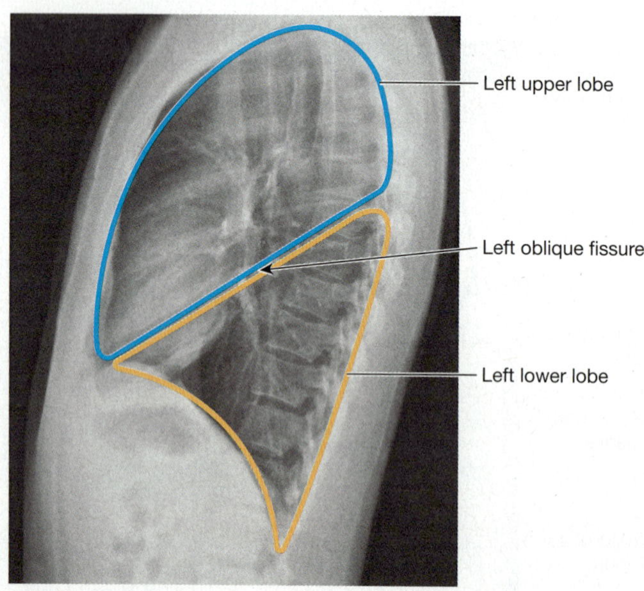

FIGURE 17-13. Lobes of the left lung in lateral view of a chest radiograph. (Modified with permission from Brant WE, Helms CA. *Fundamentals of Diagnostic Radiology.* 3rd ed. Lippincott Williams & Wilkins; 2007. Figure 21-2.)

Box 17-2. Anatomic Descriptors of the Chest

- Supraclavicular—above the clavicles
- Infraclavicular—below the clavicles
- Interscapular—between the scapulae
- Infrascapular—below the scapulae
- Apices of the lungs—uppermost portions of the lungs
- Bases of the lungs—lowermost portions of the lungs
- Upper, middle, and lower lung fields—describe the divisions of the lungs into different regions for clinical evaluation and auscultation

Learn the general anatomic terms used to locate chest findings during physical examination (PE) and when assessing lung sounds and conditions, as given in Box 17-2.

Consider the location of the PE findings as they typically correlate with the underlying lobes. For instance, signs identified in the right upper lung field are likely to originate from the right upper lobe, whereas signs found laterally in the right middle lung field may originate from any of the three different lobes.

Trachea and Major Bronchi (Tracheobronchial Tree)

Breath sounds produced over the trachea and bronchi are generally more intense and louder compared to those heard over the lung tissue. Therefore, familiarizing yourself with the locations of these structures is essential.

The *trachea* divides into its *mainstem bronchi* at the level of the sternal angle anteriorly and the T4 spinous process posteriorly, as illustrated in Figures 17-14 and 17-15. The *right main bronchus* is broader, shorter, and *more vertical* than the left main bronchus, entering the lung hilum directly.

Aspiration pneumonia is more common in the right middle and lower lobes because the right main bronchus is more vertical. For this same reason, if an endotracheal tube is advanced too far during intubation, it will more likely enter the right mainstem bronchus.

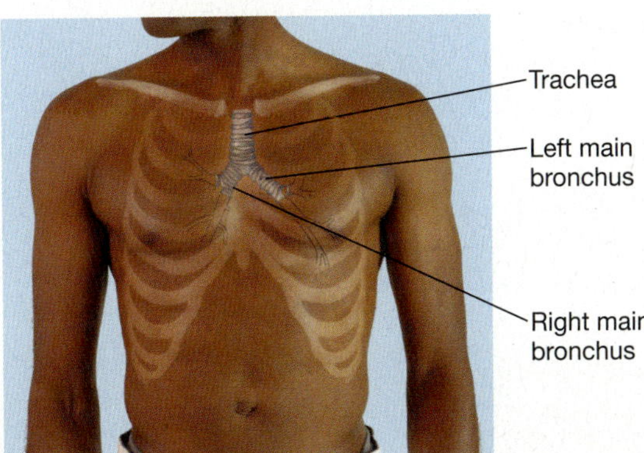

FIGURE 17-14. Trachea and mainstem bronchi, anterior view.

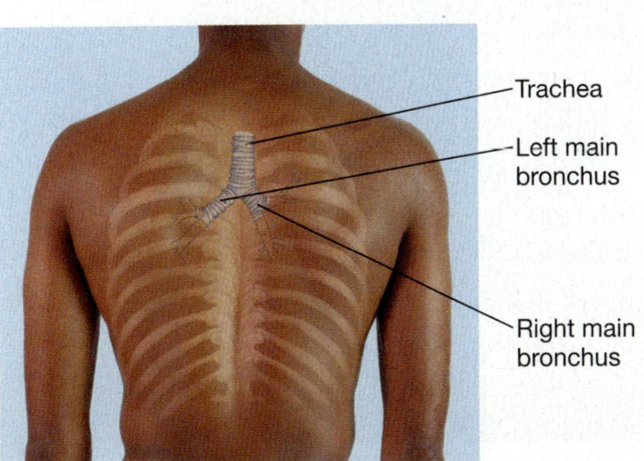

FIGURE 17-15. Trachea and mainstem bronchi, posterior view.

On the other hand, the *left main bronchus* extends inferolaterally from below the aortic arch and anterior to the esophagus and thoracic aorta before entering the lung hilum. Each main bronchus then divides into *lobar*, *segmental bronchi*, and *bronchioles* before terminating in the sac-like *alveoli*, where the crucial process of gas exchange occurs.

Pleurae

The lungs are separated from the chest wall by two continuous serous membranes known as *pleural surfaces*. The outer surface of the lungs is covered by the *visceral pleura*, while the *parietal pleura* lines the inner rib cage and the upper surface of the diaphragm. The space between these two layers, known as the *pleural space*, contains serous pleural fluid, which allows the lung to expand and contract during respiration. Although the visceral pleura lacks sensory nerves, the parietal pleura is richly innervated by the intercostal and phrenic nerves.

Accumulations of pleural fluid, or *pleural effusions*, may be *transudates*, seen in heart failure, cirrhosis, and nephrotic syndrome, or *exudates*, seen in numerous conditions including pneumonia, malignancy, pulmonary embolism, tuberculosis, and pancreatitis.

Irritation of the parietal pleura produces *pleuritic pain* with deep inspiration in viral pleurisy, pneumonia, pulmonary embolism, pericarditis, and collagen vascular diseases.

Mechanics and Physiology of Breathing

Breathing is primarily an automatic process controlled by *respiratory centers* in the brainstem that generate neuronal impulses for respiratory muscles. The *diaphragm* is the primary muscle responsible for inspiration, contracting, and descending in the chest to expand the thoracic cavity. Rib cage muscles, such as the *scalenes* and *parasternal intercostal muscles*, also help to expand the thorax. This expansion decreases intrathoracic pressure, allowing air to enter the lungs and fill the alveoli, while oxygen diffuses into pulmonary capillaries and carbon dioxide is exchanged out.

Expiration occurs passively as the chest and lungs recoil, and the diaphragm relaxes and rises. Abdominal muscles assist in expiration, and the chest and abdomen return to their resting positions.

Normal breathing is usually quiet and effortless, with minimal chest movement when a person is supine. However, during exercise and in certain diseases, extra effort is required to breathe, and *accessory muscles* such as the sternocleidomastoid (SCM) and scalenes may become visibly involved (Fig. 17-16).

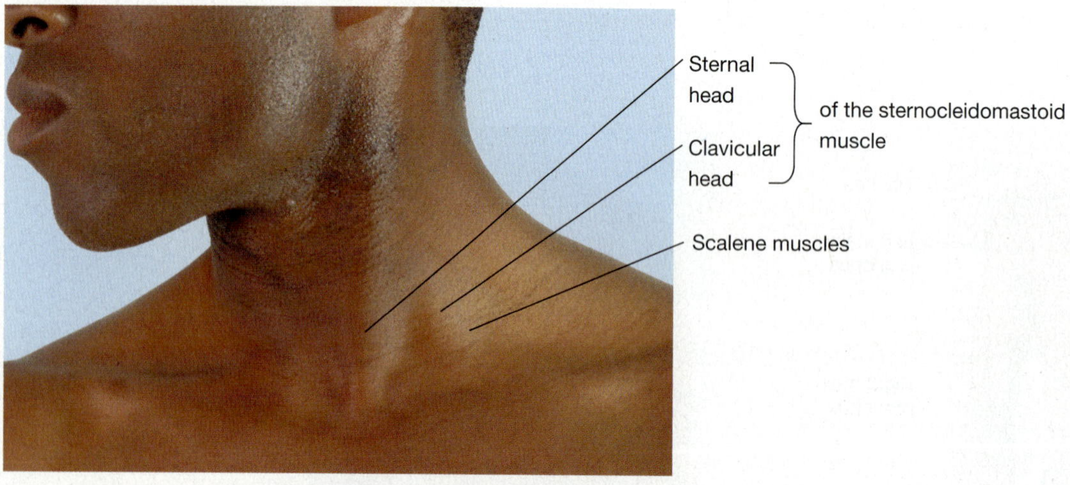

FIGURE 17-16. Accessory muscles in the neck.

Box 17-3. Characteristics of Breath Sounds[1–4]

	Duration of Sounds	Intensity of Expiratory Sound	Timing and Pattern	Locations Where Heard Normally
Vesicular[a]	Inspiratory sounds last longer than expiratory sounds.	Soft	Continuous through inspiration, fades 1/3 way through expiration	Throughout the lungs
Bronchovesicular	Inspiratory and expiratory sounds are almost equal.	Intermediate	At times separated by a silent interval; differences in pitch/intensity easier to detect during expiration	Often in the first and second interspaces anteriorly and between the scapulae
Bronchial	Expiratory sounds last longer than inspiratory ones.	Loud	Short silence between inspiratory and expiratory sounds; expiratory sounds last longer	Over the manubrium (larger proximal airways)
Tracheal	Inspiratory and expiratory sounds are almost equal.	Very loud	Continuous without pause	Over the trachea in the neck

[a]The thickness of the bars indicates intensity; the steeper their incline, the higher the pitch.

Breath Sounds (Lung Sounds)

Breath sounds, also known as lung sounds, are the noises produced by the respiratory system during the process of breathing. When you listen to the lungs, you are listening for these sounds to assess respiratory function and identify any abnormalities. Breath sounds provide valuable clues about the condition of the lungs and airways. The primary types of breath sounds are given in Box 17-3. You will learn to identify breath sounds by their intensity, their pitch, and the relative duration of their inspiratory and expiratory phases.

See Table 17-1, Normal and Altered Breath and Voice Sounds, p. 455.

HEALTH HISTORY: GENERAL APPROACH

Respiratory symptoms are a common cause for patients to seek medical attention, and identifying signs and symptoms that require prompt medical intervention by asking detailed questions to establish the cause and significance of their symptoms is crucial.

To obtain a comprehensive understanding of the patient's condition, you should allow them to describe their symptoms in their own words, with a particular focus on the effects of position and environmental exposures on their symptoms and the impact on their daily activities. As respiratory symptoms can also be a manifestation of other systemic disorders, such as cardiovascular and hematologic diseases, you should integrate the health history for other systems into the evaluation.

In addition to a thorough medical history and complete medication and allergy documentation, the social history is crucial in evaluating patients with known or suspected pulmonary diseases. Investigate tobacco and recreational drug use, occupational and environmental exposures, and travel history to gain a comprehensive understanding of the patient's condition.

Common or Concerning Symptoms

- Shortness of breath (*dyspnea*) and wheezing
- Cough
- Blood-streaked sputum (*hemoptysis*)
- Chest pain/discomfort (see also Chapter 18, Cardiovascular System)
- Daytime sleepiness, snoring, and disordered sleep

Shortness of Breath (Dyspnea) and Wheezing

Shortness of breath (SOB), or *dyspnea*, is a painless but uncomfortable awareness of breathing that is inappropriate to the level of exertion.[5] A thorough evaluation of dyspnea's pattern, onset, and triggers is crucial for determining its cause, particularly when focusing on lung-related conditions (Box 17-4). *Wheezes* are musical respiratory sounds that may be audible to the patient and to others.[6] Make every effort to determine its severity based on the patient's daily activities.

Box 17-4. Shortness of Breath (Dyspnea): High-Yield Health History Questions

Domain	Questions	Rationale
Onset	*When did you first notice the shortness of breath (SOB) or wheezing?*	*Acute:* May suggest an acute respiratory infection or asthma exacerbation *Chronic:* May suggest underlying conditions such as chronic obstructive pulmonary disease (COPD), interstitial lung disease (ILD), and heart failure
Triggers	*Do certain activities or environmental exposures trigger the symptoms?*	Exercise-induced SOB or wheezing may suggest asthma or cardiac dysfunction, while exposure to allergens or irritants may indicate allergic or occupational asthma
Severity	*How severe are your symptoms?*	Can guide the urgency and need for intervention, such as bronchodilators, oxygen therapy, or hospitalization

Common pulmonary sources include **asthma** (chronic inflammation of the airways causing wheezing, tightness, and difficulty in breathing), **chronic obstructive pulmonary disease** (**COPD**, long-term lung conditions, usually from smoking, that include emphysema and chronic bronchitis), **pneumonia** (infection in the lungs leading to inflammation and fluid accumulation), and **pulmonary embolism** (blood clot in the lung's arteries, which can impede blood flow and oxygenation).

See Table 17-2, Dyspnea, pp. 456–459.

Domain	Questions	Rationale
Associated symptoms	*Do you have cough, chest pain, or fever?*	*Cough:* May indicate bronchitis or pneumonia *Chest pain:* May suggest cardiac or pulmonary conditions *Fever:* May suggest an infectious etiology
Medical history	*Do you have a history of smoking, asthma, COPD, or heart disease?*	History of smoking or respiratory diseases increases the risk of respiratory issues; heart disease may cause shortness of breath or wheezing due to cardiac dysfunction
Medications	*Are you taking any medications that may affect your breathing?*	Certain medications like β-blockers and angiotensin-converting enzyme inhibitors may cause or exacerbate respiratory symptoms; conversely, bronchodilators or corticosteroids may help alleviate respiratory symptoms

Cough

Cough is a common symptom that ranges in significance from trivial to ominous.[7–18] Typically, cough is a reflex response to stimuli that irritate receptors in the larynx, trachea, or large bronchi. These stimuli include mucus, pus, and blood as well as external agents such as allergens, dust, foreign bodies, and even extremely hot or cold air. Cough may also be cardiovascular in origin. See Box 17-5. Establish the duration. Is the cough *acute*, lasting less than 3 weeks; *subacute*, lasting 3 to 8 weeks; or *chronic*, more than 8 weeks?

See Table 17-3, Cough and Hemoptysis, pp. 460–461.

Box 17-5. Cough: High-Yield Health History Questions

Domain	Questions	Rationale
Onset	*When did your cough begin?*	Determines if the cough is acute or chronic, suggesting potential causes such as acute respiratory infections, asthma, or underlying chronic conditions like chronic obstructive pulmonary disease (COPD), gastroesophageal reflux disease (GERD), and allergies
Duration	*How long have you been experiencing the cough?*	*Persistent:* Cough lasting more >2 weeks may indicate an underlying chronic condition *Acute:* May be related to an infection or allergy

(continued)

Common **pulmonary causes** are bronchitis, asthma, pneumonia, and COPD including emphysema and chronic bronchitis. Common **non-pulmonary causes** include **GERD**, **postnasal drip** (excess mucus from the nasal passages dripping down the back of the throat, often causing a persistent cough), **medications** (especially angiotensin-converting enzyme [ACE] inhibitors can induce coughing as a side effect), and **cardiac conditions** (congestive heart failure, for instance, can cause fluid accumulation in the lungs, resulting in a cough).

Box 17-5. Cough: High-Yield Health History Questions (*Continued*)

Domain	Questions	Rationale
Productivity	*Is the cough productive (produces phlegm) or nonproductive (dry)?*	*Productive:* May suggest an infection or chronic bronchitis *Nonproductive:* May indicate asthma or interstitial lung disease
Triggers	*Do certain activities or exposures trigger your cough?*	Cough that worsens with exposure to allergens or irritants may indicate allergic or occupational asthma, while cough that worsens with exercise may indicate exercise-induced asthma
Associated symptoms	*Do you have fever, sputum production, or chest pain?*	*Fever and sputum:* Suggest an infectious or inflammatory cause *Chest pain:* May indicate a more serious underlying condition such as pneumonia or pulmonary embolism
Medical history	*Do you have a history of smoking, asthma, COPD, or heart disease?*	History of smoking or respiratory diseases increases the risk of respiratory issues; asthma, COPD, or heart disease may cause or exacerbate cough
Medications	*Are you taking any medications that may affect your cough?*	Certain medications like angiotensin-converting enzyme inhibitors may cause or exacerbate cough; conversely, bronchodilators or corticosteroids may help alleviate cough

Blood-Streaked Sputum (Hemoptysis)

Hemoptysis refers to blood coughed up from the lower respiratory tract; it may vary from blood-streaked sputum to frank blood. Given its potential gravity, understanding the nature, volume, and associated factors of hemoptysis is of paramount importance (Box 17-6). Hemoptysis is rare in infants, children, and adolescents.

See Table 17-3, Cough and Hemoptysis, pp. 460–461. *Massive hemoptysis* (>500 mL over a 24-hour period or ≥100 mL/h) may be life-threatening.[19]

Box 17-6. Hemoptysis: High-Yield Health History Questions

Domain	Questions	Rationale
Onset	*When did you first notice the blood in your sputum?*	Determines if the hemoptysis is acute or chronic, which can suggest potential causes such as acute respiratory infections, bronchitis, or underlying chronic conditions like tuberculosis, lung cancer, or bronchiectasis
Amount	*How much blood have you coughed up?*	*Massive hemoptysis:* >600 mL/ 24 hours can be life-threatening and requires urgent intervention *Smaller amount:* May suggest a less severe underlying cause
Associated symptoms	*Do you have cough, chest pain, or shortness of breath (SOB)?*	*Cough and SOB:* Common symptoms associated with hemoptysis *Chest pain:* May suggest pulmonary embolism or pneumonia
Medical history	*Do you have a history of smoking, tuberculosis, lung disease, or cancer?*	Smoking and a history of tuberculosis or lung disease increase the risk of hemoptysis and may suggest a more severe underlying condition such as lung cancer or bronchiectasis
Medications	*Are you taking any medications that may affect your bleeding?*	Anticoagulants and antiplatelet agents may increase the risk of bleeding, including hemoptysis
Other symptoms	*Have you experienced weight loss or night sweats?*	Weight loss and night sweats may suggest an underlying infection or malignancy, particularly tuberculosis or lung cancer

Pulmonary causes include **bronchitis** (inflammation of the bronchial tubes, which can sometimes lead to blood in the sputum), **tuberculosis** (bacterial lung infection that may manifest with persistent coughing and blood in the sputum), **lung cancer** (malignant growth in the lungs in which hemoptysis may be one of the presenting symptoms), **pulmonary embolism** (blood clot in the lung's arteries can lead to hemoptysis alongside other symptoms like chest pain and shortness of breath), and **bronchiectasis** (chronic condition where the airways in the lungs become damaged and widened, leading to recurrent lung infections and hemoptysis).

Before using the term "hemoptysis," try to confirm the source of the bleeding. Blood or blood-streaked material may originate in the nose, mouth, pharynx, or gastrointestinal (GI) tract and is easily mislabeled. If vomited, it probably originates in the GI tract. Occasionally, however, blood from the nasopharynx or the GI tract is aspirated and then coughed out.

Chest Pain/Discomfort

Chest pain and chest discomfort raise concerns about the heart but often arise from other structures in the thorax and lungs. Sources of chest pain are listed in Box 17-7, 17-14, and 17-16. To assess this symptom, you must pursue a dual investigation of both thoracic and cardiac causes (Box 17-8). Distinguishing pulmonary sources of chest pain is fundamental to directing appropriate investigations and interventions. So, for this important symptom, you should keep all of these possibilities in mind.

See Table 17-4, Chest Pain, pp. 462–463.

Box 17-7. Sources of Chest Pain and Related Causes

Source	Possible Causes
Myocardium	Angina pectoris, myocardial infarction, myocarditis
Pericardium	Pericarditis
Aorta	Aortic dissection
Trachea and large bronchi	Bronchitis
Parietal pleura	Pericarditis, pneumonia, pneumothorax, pleural effusion, pulmonary embolus, connective tissue disease
Chest wall, including the skin, musculoskeletal, and neurologic systems	Costochondritis, herpes zoster
Esophagus	Gastroesophageal reflux disease, esophageal spasm, esophageal tear
Extrathoracic structures such as the neck, gallbladder, and stomach	Cervical arthritis, biliary colic, gastritis

Box 17-8. Chest Pain: High-Yield Health History Questions

Domain	Questions	Rationale
Onset	*When did your chest pain start?*	*Acute:* May suggest pulmonary embolism or pneumothorax *Chronic:* May suggest underlying lung conditions such as interstitial lung disease (ILD) or chronic obstructive pulmonary disease (COPD)
Location	*Where is the chest pain located?*	Pain in the chest area or *pleuritic* chest pain (pain that worsens with deep breaths or coughing) may suggest pulmonary causes such as pleurisy or pneumonia
Quality	*Can you describe the type of pain you're experiencing?*	Sharp, stabbing, or burning pain may suggest pulmonary causes such as pleurisy or pneumonia
Associated symptoms	*Do you have cough, shortness of breath (SOB), or fever?*	May suggest pulmonary causes of chest pain such as pneumonia or acute exacerbation of COPD.

Key pulmonary causes of chest pain include **pneumonia** (lung infection characterized by inflammation and fluid accumulation, often presenting with sharp or stabbing chest pain, especially during deep breaths), **pleurisy** (inflammation of the pleura, the lining of the lung and chest wall, leading to sharp chest pain that intensifies with breathing or coughing), **pulmonary embolism** (sudden blockage in a lung artery, usually due to a blood clot, can trigger sharp, sudden chest pain and difficulty breathing), and **pneumothorax** (collapsed lung, in which air leaks into the space between the lung and chest wall, resulting in sudden chest pain and shortness of breath).

Domain	Questions	Rationale
Medical history	*Do you have a history of smoking or lung disease?*	Increases the risk of pulmonary causes of chest pain such as COPD, ILD, and lung cancer
Medications	*Are you taking any medications that may affect your chest pain?*	Bronchodilators and corticosteroids may alleviate chest pain associated with pulmonary causes

This section focuses on *pulmonary problems.* For symptoms of exertional chest pain, palpitations, SOB when supine (*orthopnea*) or at night relieved by sitting upright (*paroxysmal nocturnal dyspnea*), and edema, see Chapter 18, Cardiovascular System (see pp. 485–489).

Daytime Sleepiness, Snoring, and Disordered Sleep

Navigating the intricate relationship between daytime sleepiness, snoring, and disordered sleep can be challenging as it often spans various medical domains. As you delve into this area, be mindful of how nighttime symptoms can infiltrate daytime activities, affecting your patient's overall well-being and functionality. When you engage with your patient, consider inquiring about issues such as snoring, witnessed *apneas* (periods where they stop breathing for ≥10 seconds), waking up with a choking sensation, and experiencing morning headaches (Box 17-9).

Box 17-9. Daytime Sleepiness, Snoring, and Disordered Sleep: High-Yield Health History Questions

Domain	Questions	Rationale
Daytime sleepiness	*Do you often feel excessively sleepy during the day?*	May suggest underlying sleep disorders such as obstructive sleep apnea (OSA), narcolepsy, and periodic limb movement disorder (PLMD)
Snoring	*Do you snore during sleep?*	*Loud, persistent:* Hallmark symptom of OSA *Intermittent/associated with other symptoms:* May suggest other sleep disorders such as upper airway resistance syndrome (UARS) or snoring-related sleep disturbance

(*continued*)

Prevalent causes related to these sleep disturbances include **obstructive sleep apnea** (**OSA**, condition in which breathing repeatedly stops and starts during sleep due to throat muscle relaxation, leading to loud snoring and profound daytime fatigue), **restless leg syndrome** (**RLS**) (neurologic condition causing an irresistible urge to move the legs, often interrupting sleep and resulting in daytime drowsiness), **narcolepsy** (chronic sleep disorder characterized by overwhelming daytime drowsiness and sudden sleep attacks, irrespective of having a full night's sleep), and **insomnia** (persistent difficulties in falling and/or staying asleep, which can lead to prolonged periods of wakefulness at night and consequent daytime sleepiness).

Box 17-9. Daytime Sleepiness, Snoring, and Disordered Sleep: High-Yield Health History Questions (*Continued*)

Domain	Questions	Rationale
Sleep patterns	*Do you have difficulty falling asleep or staying asleep?*	Can help identify potential sleep disorders such as insomnia, circadian rhythm disorders, and sleep-related movement disorders
Disordered sleep	*Do you experience pauses in breathing during sleep?*	Patients with OSA experience repeated episodes of upper airway obstruction during sleep, leading to disrupted sleep and symptoms such as daytime sleepiness and snoring
Associated symptoms	*Do you experience morning headaches or dry mouth?*	Can suggest underlying sleep-disordered breathing such as OSA
Medical history	*Do you have a history of obesity, hypertension, or heart disease?*	Associated with increased risk of OSA and other sleep-related breathing disorders
Medications	*Are you taking any medications that may affect your sleep?*	Sedatives and antidepressants may affect sleep patterns or exacerbate sleep disorders

PHYSICAL EXAMINATION: GENERAL APPROACH

When examining the thorax and lungs, the four classic techniques of inspection, palpation, percussion, and auscultation are used with observation beginning during the patient interview.

As you assess your patient, pay close attention to their speech patterns. This can offer invaluable insights, such as difficulty speaking in full sentences or signs of increased breathing effort. You must precisely measure vital signs, especially the respiratory rate and oxygen saturation levels during physical activity. Take note of indicators like hypoxemia, anemia, and other symptoms not directly related to the lungs during your general check. While examining the chest, look for symmetric movement and remember to perform percussion and auscultation. Inspect the posterior thorax and lungs with the patient seated and the anterior thorax and lungs while they are lying down.

A careful cardiac examination is necessary to identify signs of increased pressure on the right side of the heart, malfunctioning left ventricle, or valve disease. Examine the abdomen for paradoxical movement during inspiration, indicating diaphragmatic weakness.

TECHNIQUES OF EXAMINATION

Key Components of the Thorax and Lung Examination

- Survey the thorax and respiration
- Inspect the thorax
- Palpate the thorax
- Assess for thoracic expansion (lung excursion)
- Assess for tactile fremitus
- Percuss the thorax
- Identify extent of diaphragmatic excursion
- Auscultate the lungs for breath sounds
- Listen for adventitious (added) breath sounds
- Assess transmitted voice sounds

Survey the Thorax and Respiration

Even though the respiratory rate might already be recorded, again carefully observe the *rate, rhythm, depth*, and *effort of breathing*. A healthy resting adult breathes quietly and regularly about 12 to 18 times a minute. Note whether expiration lasts longer than usual.

See Table 17-5, Abnormalities in Rate and Rhythm of Breathing, p. 464, including bradypnea, tachypnea, hyperventilation, Cheyne–Stokes breathing, and ataxic breathing. Delayed expiration occurs in COPD.

Begin by observing the patient for signs of *respiratory distress*. Assess the respiratory rate for *tachypnea* (>25 breaths/min). Inspect the patient's color for *cyanosis* or *pallor*. Recall earlier relevant findings, such as the shape and color of the fingernails.

Observe for signs of accessory muscle use, such as contraction of the SCM and scalene muscles or supraclavicular retractions during inspiration. Also, note any contraction of the intercostal or abdominal oblique muscles during expiration.

Also observe the shape of the chest, which is normally wider than it is deep. The ratio of the anteroposterior (AP) diameter to the lateral chest diameter is usually 0.7 to 0.75 up to 0.9 and increases with aging.

Listen for audible sounds of breathing.

Inspect the Thorax

In the examination of the thorax and lungs, it is customary to begin with the posterior aspect before moving to the anterior chest. Although the techniques employed for the posterior and anterior thorax and lung examinations are essentially identical, adhering to this sequence for a systematic and comprehensive assessment is essential. For the purposes of this section, we will discuss the examination techniques for both regions together to avoid redundancy. However, you should be particularly mindful of the recommended sequence, starting with the posterior examination first, followed by the anterior thorax and lungs.

Posterior Thorax. To inspect the posterior thorax, have the patient sit with their hands resting comfortably on the sides.

Box 17-10. Chest Findings

Findings	Clinical Implications
Deformities or asymmetry in chest expansion	Suggestive of large pleural effusions
Abnormal muscle retraction of intercostal spaces during inspiration	Indicates conditions like severe asthma, chronic obstructive pulmonary disease (COPD), or upper airway obstruction
Impaired respiratory movement on one/both sides or unilateral lag	Associated with pleural disease (asbestosis, silicosis), phrenic nerve damage, or trauma
Cyanosis of the lips, tongue, and oral mucosa	Sign of hypoxia
Pallor and sweating (*diaphoresis*)	Commonly seen in acute coronary syndromes and heart failure
Nail clubbing	Present in conditions like bronchiectasis, congenital heart disease, pulmonary fibrosis, cystic fibrosis, lung abscess, and malignancy
Leaning forward posture with pursed lips	Characteristic of individuals with severe COPD
Use of accessory muscles	Suggestive of increased ventilatory needs from airways/parenchymal lung disease or respiratory muscle fatigue
Increased anteroposterior ratio (>0.9)	Indicative of COPD with a potential barrel-chest appearance[1,20,21] (evidence varies)
Audible high-pitched inspiratory whistling (*stridor*)	Warning sign of upper airway obstruction in larynx or trachea; urgent evaluation needed

Standing in a midline position behind the patient, visualize the underlying lobes and compare the right lung field with the left, noting any asymmetries. Observe the shape of the chest, such as a *barrel chest*, and how it moves. Note possible findings on inspection of the chest in Box 17-10.

Anterior Thorax. With the patient supine, inspect the anterior thorax and lungs. For patients with breasts, this position allows the breasts to be gently displaced. When examined in the supine position, the patient should lie comfortably with their arms somewhat abducted. If the patient is having difficulty breathing, raise the head of the examining table or the bed to increase respiratory excursion and ease of breathing.

Observe the shape of the patient's chest and the movement of the chest wall. Note deformities or asymmetry of the thorax, abnormal retraction of the lower intercostal spaces during inspiration, supraclavicular retraction, local lag, or impairment in respiratory movement.

See Table 17-6, Deformities of the Thorax, p. 465.

Palpate the Thorax

Posterior Thorax. Palpate the posterior chest and identify tender areas. Carefully palpate any area where the patient reports pain or has visible lesions or bruises. Note any palpable *crepitus*, defined as a crackling or grinding sound over bones, joints, or skin, with or without pain, due to air in the subcutaneous tissue. Assess any skin abnormalities such as masses or *sinus tracts* (blind, inflammatory, tube-like structures opening onto the skin).

Tenderness, bruising, and bony "step-offs" are common over a fractured rib. Crepitus may be palpable in overt fractures and arthritic joints; crepitus and chest wall edema are seen in mediastinitis.

Anterior Chest. Palpate the anterior chest wall and identify any tender areas. Assess for the presence of bruising, sinus tracts, or other skin changes.

Tender pectoral muscles or costal cartilages suggest, but do not prove, that chest pain has a localized musculoskeletal origin.

Assess for Thoracic Expansion (Lung Excursion)

Posterior Thorax. Assess chest expansion posteriorly. Place your thumbs at about the level of the 10th ribs posteriorly, with your fingers loosely grasping and parallel to the lateral rib cage (Fig. 17-17). As you position your hands, slide them medially to raise a loose fold of skin over the spine between your thumbs. Ask the patient to inhale deeply, and carefully observe the distance between your thumbs as they move apart during inspiration. Additionally, feel for the range and symmetry of the rib cage as it expands and contracts, which is sometimes referred to as *lung excursion*.

Anterior Chest. Assess chest expansion anteriorly. Place your thumbs along each costal margin, your hands along the lateral rib cage (Fig. 17-18). As you position your hands, slide them medially a bit to raise loose skin folds between your thumbs. Ask the patient to inhale deeply. Observe how far your thumbs diverge as the thorax expands and feel for the extent and symmetry of respiratory movement.

Unilateral decrease or delay in chest expansion occurs in chronic fibrosis of the underlying lung or pleura, pleural effusion, lobar pneumonia, pleural pain with associated splinting, unilateral bronchial obstruction, and paralysis of the hemidiaphragm.

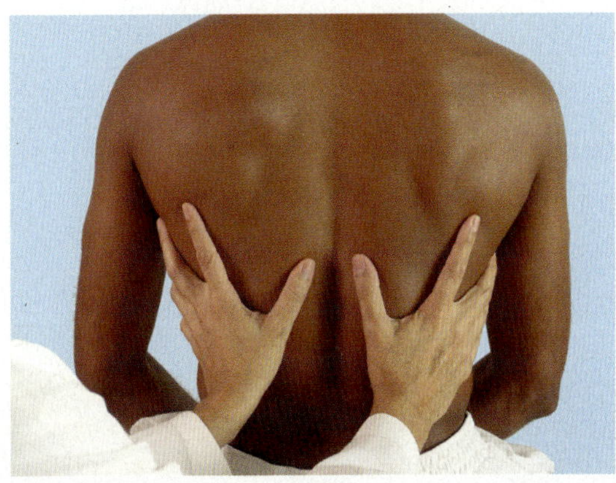

FIGURE 17-17. Assessing chest expansion posteriorly.

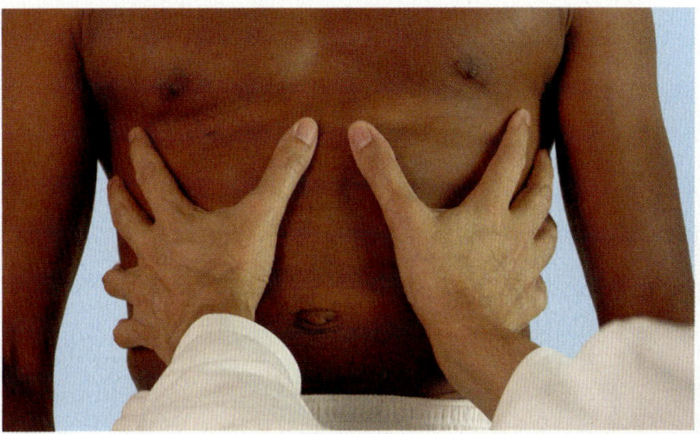

FIGURE 17-18. Assessing chest expansion anteriorly.

Box 17-11. Chest Tactile Fremitus[1,16,22]

Tactile Fremitus	Relative Intensity	Example of Location	Pathologic Examples
Decreased	Soft	Over a thickened chest wall	Pleural effusion, pneumothorax
Normal	Medium	Over healthy lung tissue	–
Increased	Loud	Over consolidated lung tissue	Lobar pneumonia, pulmonary edema
Absent	Very soft	Over areas with no airflow	Large pleural effusion, complete lung collapse

Assess for Tactile Fremitus

Tactile fremitus is the palpable vibration transmitted through the bronchopulmonary tree to the chest wall as the patient speaks. It is typically more prominent in the interscapular area than in the lower lung fields and easier to detect over the right lung than the left. It disappears below the diaphragm.

While tactile fremitus is not always precise, it can highlight asymmetries that require further investigation. To confirm any disparities, listen for underlying breath sounds, voice sounds, and whispered voice sounds (Box 17-11). These attributes should increase or decrease together.

Posterior Chest. Assess tactile fremitus posteriorly. Use the ball or ulnar surface of your hand to feel the transmitted vibrations as the patient repeats the words "*ninety-nine*" or "*one-one-one*" (Fig. 17-19). Palpate and compare symmetric areas of the lungs and identify any areas of increased, decreased, or absent fremitus. If fremitus is faint, ask the patient to speak more loudly or in a deeper voice.

Anterior Chest. If clinically indicated, assess tactile fremitus anteriorly. Compare both sides of the chest, using the ball or ulnar surface of your hand. Fremitus is usually decreased or absent over the precordium. When examining a female patient, gently displace the breasts as necessary (Fig. 17-20).

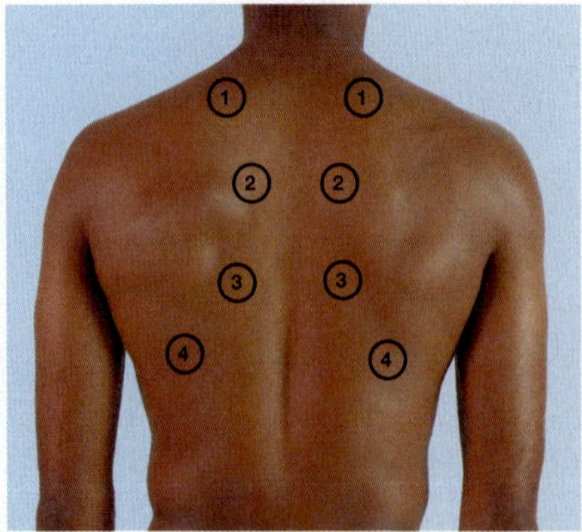

FIGURE 17-19. Locations for palpating fremitus.

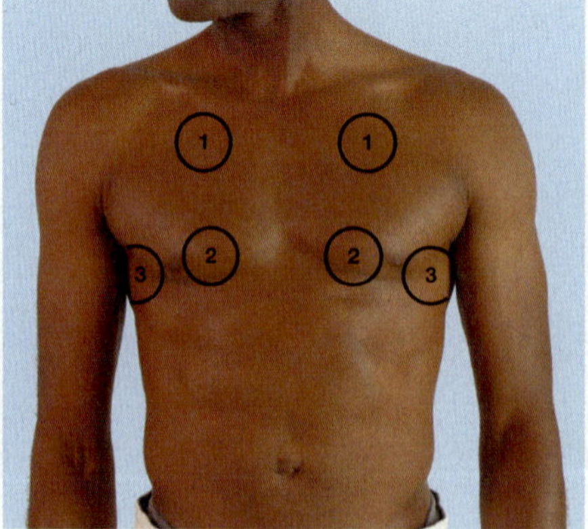

FIGURE 17-20. Locations for palpating tactile fremitus in the anterior chest.

Percuss the Thorax

Percussion is a key technique in chest examination, producing palpable vibrations and audible sounds. Percussion sets the chest wall and underlying tissues in motion, producing audible sound and palpable vibrations, and helps determine whether the underlying tissues are air-filled, fluid-filled, or consolidated. Percussion is practiced on any surface and is limited to a depth of 5 to 7 cm. As you practice, listen for changes in percussion notes over different types of materials or different parts of the body. The key points for good technique, described for a right-handed person, are detailed in Box 17-12. Healthy lungs produce a resonant percussion note.

Box 17-12. Chest Percussion Techniques

Step Description

- Hyperextend the middle finger of your left hand, known as the pleximeter finger (Fig. 17-21). Press its distal interphalangeal joint firmly on the lung surface intended for percussion. Ensure only this joint makes contact to avoid dampening of vibrations. Avoid letting the thumb and other fingers touch the chest wall.

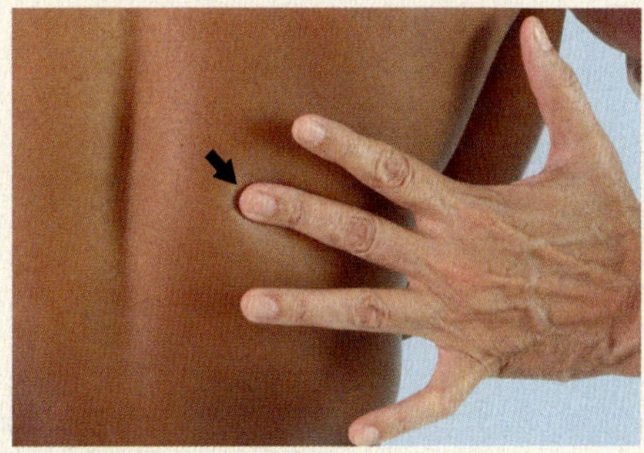

FIGURE 17-21. Pleximeter finger is placed firmly on the chest wall.

- With your right forearm close to the surface, cock your hand upward. The middle finger should be partially flexed, relaxed, and prepared to strike.

- Using a swift, sharp, yet relaxed wrist motion, strike the pleximeter finger with the right middle finger, termed the plexor finger (Fig. 17-22). Direct your aim at your distal interphalangeal joint to transmit vibrations through its bones to the chest wall below. Ensure consistent force and pleximeter pressure with each strike to maintain uniformity in the percussion note. The movement originates at the wrist, being directed, brisk, yet relaxed and slightly bouncy.

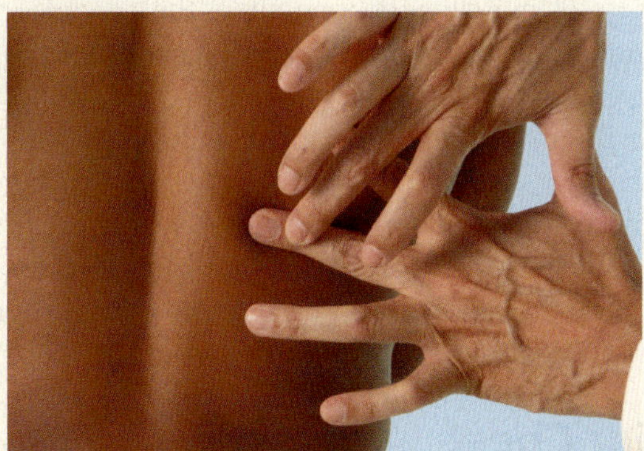

FIGURE 17-22. Striking the pleximeter finger with the right middle finger.

(*continued*)

Box 17-12. Chest Percussion Techniques (*Continued*)

Step Description

- Strike using the tip of the plexor finger, not the finger pad. The striking finger should be almost at right angles to the pleximeter. Consider keeping your fingernails short to avoid injuring your knuckle. Use the lightest percussion that produces a clear note. A thick chest wall requires a more forceful percussion blow than a thin one.

- Withdraw your striking finger quickly to avoid damping the vibrations you have created (Fig. 17-23).

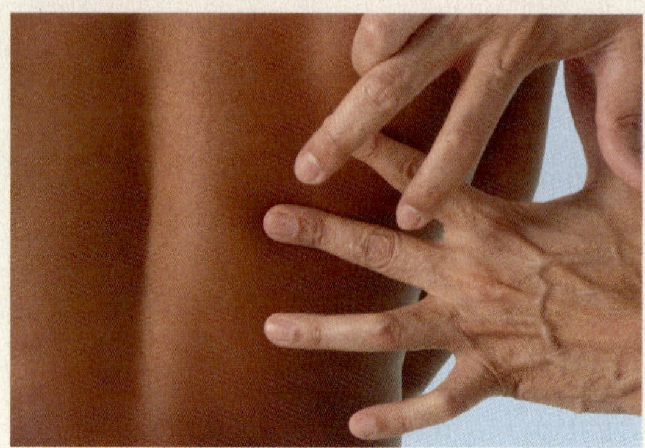

FIGURE 17-23. Withdraw the striking finger quickly.

Posterior Chest

Percuss the thorax posteriorly in symmetric locations on each side from the apex to the base. Percuss one side of the chest and then the other at each level in a *ladder-like pattern*, as shown in Figure 17-24. Omit the areas over the scapulae—the thickness of muscle and bone alters the percussion notes over the lungs. Identify and locate the area and quality of any abnormal percussion note.

When percussing the lower posterior chest, stand somewhat to the side rather than directly behind the patient. In this position, it is easier to place your pleximeter finger more firmly on the chest, making your plexor strike more effective by creating a better percussion note.

When comparing two areas, use the same percussion technique in both areas. Percuss or strike twice in each location and listen for differences in the percussion notes at the two locations.

Anterior Chest

If clinically indicated, percuss the anterior and lateral chest. Use the *ladder pattern* suggested for percussion, moving from one side to the other and comparing symmetric areas of the lungs (Fig. 17-25). The heart normally produces an area of dullness to the left of the sternum from the third to the fifth interspaces. In a female patient, to enhance percussion, gently displace the breast with your left hand while percussing with the right or ask the patient to move the breast for you. Identify and locate any area with an abnormal percussion note.

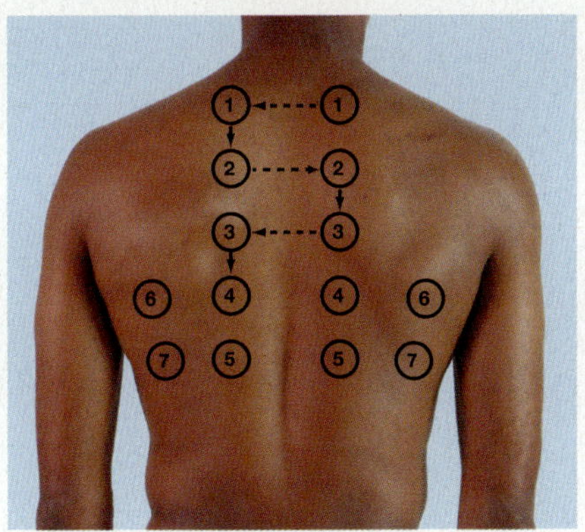

FIGURE 17-24. "Ladder" pattern for percussion and auscultation.

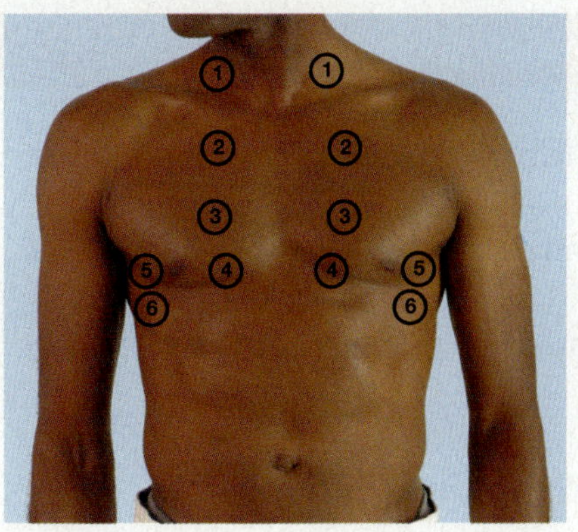

FIGURE 17-25. Ladder pattern for palpating and percussing the anterior chest.

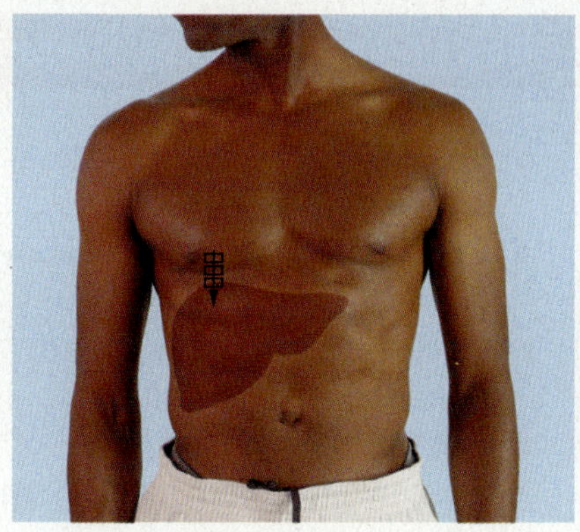

FIGURE 17-26. Percussing for liver dullness and gastric tympany.

When you percuss the anterior *left chest*, the typical lung resonance generally transitions to the *tympany* associated with the *gastric air bubble*. Conversely, as you percuss the anterior *right chest*, the familiar lung resonance usually shifts to the *dullness* characteristic of the *liver* (Fig. 17-26).

To develop proficiency in percussion, learn to identify the five percussion notes: *flat, dull, resonant, hyper-resonant,* and *tympanitic* (Box 17-13). These notes differ in their sound, intensity, pitch, and duration. Train your ear by focusing on one quality at a time, percussing in different locations.

Identify Extent of Diaphragmatic Excursion

Identify the descent of the diaphragm, or *diaphragmatic excursion* (Box 17-14).[1,24] This technique allows you to appreciate the range of movement and efficiency of

Box 17-13. Chest Percussion Notes

	Relative Intensity/Pitch	Relative Duration	Examples of Percussed Locations	Pathologic Examples
Flat	Soft/high	Short	Thigh	Large pleural effusion
Dull	Medium/medium	Medium	Liver	Lobar pneumonia due to alveoli filled with fluid and blood cells Pleural accumulations, such as serous fluid (*pleural effusion*), blood (*hemothorax*), pus (*empyema*), fibrous tissue, tumor[6,23]
Resonant	Loud/low	Long	Healthy lung	Simple chronic bronchitis
Hyper-resonant	Very loud/lower	Longer	Usually none	Chronic obstructive pulmonary disease, where it may obscure heart dullness Pneumothorax Asthma Large air-filled bulla
Tympanitic	Loud/high	Longer	Gastric air bubble or puffed-out cheek	Large pneumothorax

Box 17-14. Assessing Diaphragmatic Excursion

- Begin by determining the level of diaphragmatic dullness during quiet respiration.
- Hold the pleximeter finger above and parallel to the anticipated level of dullness.
- Percuss downward in progressive steps until you observe a clear shift from resonance to dullness.
- Confirm the identified level of change by percussing downward from adjacent areas both medially and laterally (Fig. 17-27).

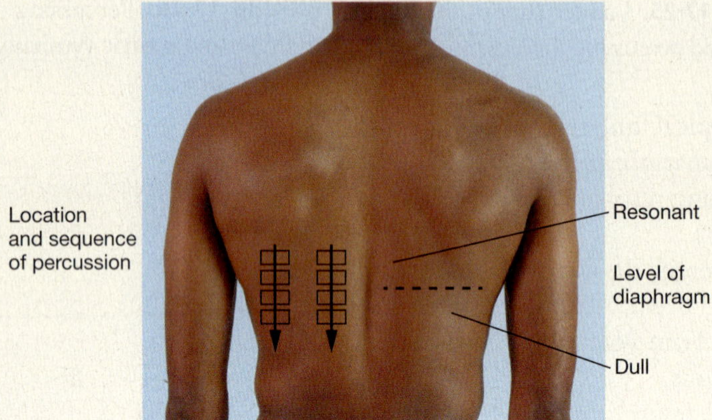

FIGURE 17-27. Identifying the extent of diaphragmatic excursion.

- Understand that with this technique, you are pinpointing the boundary between resonant lung tissue and the duller structures below the diaphragm. You are not directly percussing the diaphragm.
- Infer the probable position of the diaphragm based on the level of dullness identified. An abnormally high level suggests a pleural effusion or an elevated hemidiaphragm from atelectasis or phrenic nerve paralysis (Fig. 17-28).[12,25]

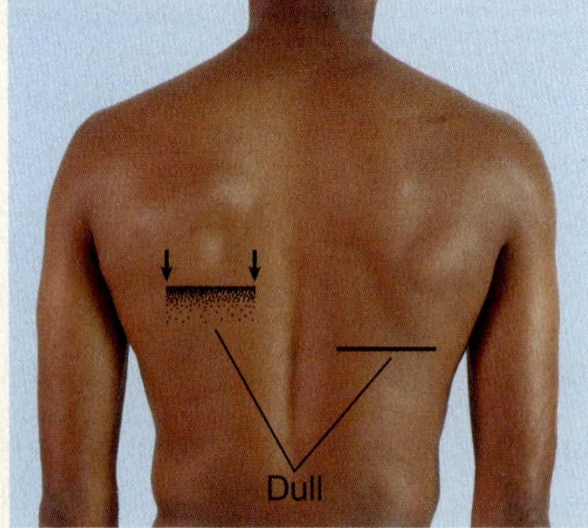

FIGURE 17-28. Absent descent of the diaphragm can indicate pleural effusion.

- To estimate diaphragmatic excursion, measure the distance between the dullness level on full expiration and the dullness level on full inspiration. This is typically between 3 and 5.5 cm.[23,26]

the diaphragm. Not only does it highlight potential diaphragmatic dysfunction, but it can also be indicative of underlying conditions that could restrict diaphragmatic movement, such as pleural effusion and tumors.

Auscultate the Lungs for Breath Sounds

Auscultation is the most important examination technique for assessing air flow through the tracheobronchial tree. Auscultation involves (1) listening to the sounds generated by breathing; (2) listening for any *adventitious* (added) sounds; and (3) if abnormalities are suspected, listening to the sounds of the patient's spoken or whispered voice as they are transmitted through the chest wall. Review the primary types of breath sounds in Box 17-3, p. 425.

Before beginning auscultation, ask the patient to cough once or twice to clear mild atelectasis or airway mucus that can produce unimportant added sounds. Bedclothes, paper gowns, and even chest hair can generate confusing crackling sounds that interfere with auscultation. For chest hair, press harder or moisten the hair.

See Considerations for Auscultating Through Clothing in Clinical Settings in Chapter 4, Physical Examination, pp. 66–67.

Posterior Chest. Listen to the breath sounds posteriorly with the *diaphragm* of your stethoscope after instructing the patient to breathe deeply through an open mouth. Always place the stethoscope directly on the skin. Clothing alters the characteristics of the breath sounds and can introduce friction and added sounds.

Like auscultating over clothing, air movement through a partially obstructed nose or nasopharynx can also introduce abnormal sounds.

Listen to at least one full breath—both inspiration and expiration—in each location. If you hear or suspect abnormal sounds, auscultate adjacent areas to assess the extent of any abnormality. If the patient becomes lightheaded from hyperventilation, allow the patient to take a few normal breaths.

Note the *intensity* of the breath sounds, which reflects the airflow rate at the mouth, and may vary from one area to another. Breath sounds are usually louder in the lower posterior lung fields. If the breath sounds seem faint, ask the patient to breathe more deeply. Both shallow breathing and a thick chest wall can alter breath sound intensity.

Breath sounds may be decreased when air flow is decreased (as in obstructive lung disease or respiratory muscle weakness) or when the transmission of sound is poor (as in pleural effusion, pneumothorax, or COPD).

Listen for the *pitch, intensity*, and *duration* of the *inspiratory and expiratory sounds*. Are *vesicular breath sounds* distributed normally over the chest wall? Are breath sounds diminished, or are there bronchovesicular or bronchial breath sounds in unexpected places? If so, in what distribution?

Anterior Chest. Listen to the chest anteriorly and laterally as the patient breathes with mouth open, and somewhat more deeply than normal. Compare symmetric areas of the lungs, using the pattern suggested for percussion and extending it to adjacent areas, if indicated.

Auscultate for Adventitious (Added) Sounds

Listen for any added, or *adventitious*, sounds that are superimposed on the usual breath sounds. Detection of adventitious sounds—*crackles* (sometimes called *rales*), *wheezes*, and *rhonchi*—is an important focus of your examination, often leading to diagnosis of cardiac and pulmonary conditions (Box 17-15). Many clinicians use the term *rhonchi* to describe sounds from secretions in large airways that may change with coughing.

For further discussion and other added sounds, see Table 17-7, Adventitious (Added) Lung Sounds: Causes and Qualities, pp. 466–467.

If you hear crackles, especially those that do not clear after coughing, listen carefully for the following characteristics[1,2,16,25,28,29] listed in Box 17-16. These are clues to the underlying condition.

Box 17-15. Adventitious or Added Breath Sounds[2,27]

	Crackles (or Rales)	Wheezes and Rhonchi
Sound Continuity	**Discontinuous**	**Continuous**
Description	Intermittent, nonmusical, and brief	Sinusoidal, musical, prolonged
Temporal Pattern	Like dots in time	Like dashes in time
	Fine crackles: soft, high-pitched (–650 Hz), very brief (5–10 ms)	*Wheezes:* high-pitched (≥400 Hz) with hissing/ shrill quality (>80 ms)
	• • • • •	
	Coarse crackles: louder, lower in pitch (–350 Hz), brief (15–30 ms)	*Rhonchi:* low-pitched (150–200 Hz) with snoring quality (>80 ms)
	• • • • •	
Clinical Implications	Crackles can arise from abnormalities of the lung parenchyma (pneumonia, interstitial lung disease, pulmonary fibrosis, atelectasis, heart failure) or of the airways (bronchitis, bronchiectasis).	Wheezes arise in the narrowed airways of asthma, chronic obstructive pulmonary disease, and bronchitis.

In some healthy people, crackles may be heard at the anterior lung bases after maximal expiration. Crackles in dependent portions of the lungs may also occur after prolonged recumbency.

If you hear wheezes or rhonchi, note their timing and location. Do they change with deep breathing or coughing? Beware of the silent chest, in which air movement is minimal. Note that tracheal sounds originating in the neck such as stridor and vocal cord dysfunction can be transmitted to the chest and mistaken for wheezing, leading to inappropriate or delayed treatment. Stridor and laryngeal sounds are loudest over the neck, whereas true wheezes and rhonchi are faint or absent over the neck.[1]

Note any *pleural friction rubs*, which are coarse, grating biphasic sounds heard primarily during expiration.

Pleural friction rubs may be heard in pleurisy, pneumonia, and pulmonary embolism.

See Table 17-7, Adventitious (Added) Lung Sounds: Causes and Qualities, pp. 466–467, and Table 17-8, Physical Findings in Selected Chest Disorders, pp. 468–469.

Box 17-16. Crackles

Characteristics	Details	Clinical Implications	Examples
Loudness, pitch, and duration	Fine or coarse crackles?	Fine late inspiratory crackles that persist suggest abnormal lung tissue.	*Fine:* interstitial pulmonary fibrosis, early congestive heart failure (CHF) *Coarse:* pulmonary edema, bronchitis
Number	Few or many?	Multiple crackles might indicate a more severe or widespread pulmonary condition.	*Few:* early stages of pneumonia, mild CHF *Many:* advanced pneumonia, severe CHF
Timing in the respiratory cycle	Inspiratory or expiratory?	Crackles during inspiration might indicate interstitial lung issues; during expiration, bronchial issues.	*Inspiratory:* pneumonia, pulmonary fibrosis *Expiratory:* chronic bronchitis, asthma
Location on the chest wall	Varies depending on the underlying condition	Crackles due to heart failure are best heard in the posterior inferior lung fields.	*Posterior:* CHF, lower-lobe pneumonia *Anterior:* upper-lobe pneumonia, tuberculosis
Persistence of their pattern from breath to breath	Consistent or variable?	Persistent patterns may indicate chronic conditions, while variable patterns can suggest acute issues or movement of secretions.	*Persistent:* pulmonary fibrosis, advanced CHF *Variable:* acute bronchitis resolving pneumonia
Any change after a cough or change in the patient's position	Changes or remains the same?	If crackles clear after coughing or changing position, it suggests inspissated secretions or atelectasis. If they persist, it could indicate fibrosis or other tissue abnormalities.	*Changes:* bronchiectasis, early CHF *Persists:* advanced pulmonary fibrosis, severe CHF

Box 17-17. Transmitted Voice Sounds in Pulmonary Examination

Test Name	Instructions to Patient	Normal Findings	Abnormal Findings	Typical Location of Abnormal Sounds
Egophony	Ask the patient to say "*Ee*."	You will normally hear a muffled long E sound	"*Ee*" sounds more like "*Aa*" (known as "E-to-A" change)	Detects a nasal or "bleating" quality; more distinct in conditions like pneumonia[1,24]
Bronchophony	Ask the patient to say "*ninety-nine*."	Normally, the sounds transmitted through the chest wall are muffled and indistinct	Louder voice sounds (bronchophony)	Focuses on clarity and volume of normal voice[1,24]; in conditions of consolidation, the voice becomes louder and clearer than normal
Whispered Pectoriloquy	Ask the patient to whisper "*ninety-nine*" or "*one-two-three*."	Whispered voice is normally heard faintly and indistinctly, if at all	Clearer whispered voice	Might be more sensitive in early or subtle consolidations than bronchophony[1,24]

Assess Transmitted Voice Sounds

If you hear abnormally located bronchovesicular or bronchial breath sounds, assess *transmitted voice sounds* using the three techniques listed in Box 17-17. With the diaphragm of your stethoscope, listen in symmetric areas over the chest wall for abnormal vocal resonances suspicious of pneumonia or pleural effusion.

Increased transmitted voice sounds suggest that embedded airways are blocked by inflammation or secretions. See Table 17-1, Normal and Altered Breath and Voice Sounds, p. 455.

SPECIAL TECHNIQUES AND MANEUVERS

Clinically Assess Pulmonary Function

Walk tests are practical, simple ways to assess cardiopulmonary function commonly used in rehabilitation and pre- and postoperative settings. The 2023 American Thoracic Society guidelines that standardize the 6-minute walk test continue to predict clinical outcomes in most patients with COPD.[6,16,30,31] The test is easy to administer and requires only a 100-foot hallway. It measures "the distance that a patient can quickly walk on a flat, hard surface in a period of 6 minutes" and provides a global evaluation of the pulmonary and cardiovascular systems, neuromuscular units, and muscle metabolism.[31]

Assess Forced Expiratory Time

This test assesses the expiratory phase of breathing, which is typically slowed in obstructive pulmonary disease. Ask the patient to take a deep breath in and then breathe out as quickly and completely as possible with their mouth open. Listen over the trachea with the diaphragm of a stethoscope and time the

Patients aged ≥60 years with a forced expiratory time of ≥9 seconds are four times more likely to have COPD.[32]

audible expiration. Try to get three consistent readings, allowing a short rest between efforts, if necessary.

Identify a Fractured Rib

Local pain and tenderness of one or more ribs raise the question of fracture. By compression of the chest in the AP plane, you can help to distinguish a fracture from a soft-tissue injury. With one hand on the sternum and the other on the thoracic spine, squeeze the chest. Ask "Is this painful, and where"?

An increase in the local pain (distant from your hands) suggests rib fracture rather than just soft-tissue injury.

Modifications in Physical Examinations: Best Practices for Specialized Patient Populations

Respiratory challenges often necessitate a variety of interventions and supports. From mechanical ventilation in critical care settings to home-based oxygen support, understanding each device's role is essential. Box 17-18 details the examination approach for patients benefiting from these vital respiratory tools.

Box 17-18. Thorax and Lung Examination with Medical Devices, Conditions, or Procedures Present

	Patient with a Tracheostomy Tube	Patient on a Mechanical Ventilator	Patient with a Chest Tube or Tube Thoracostomy
	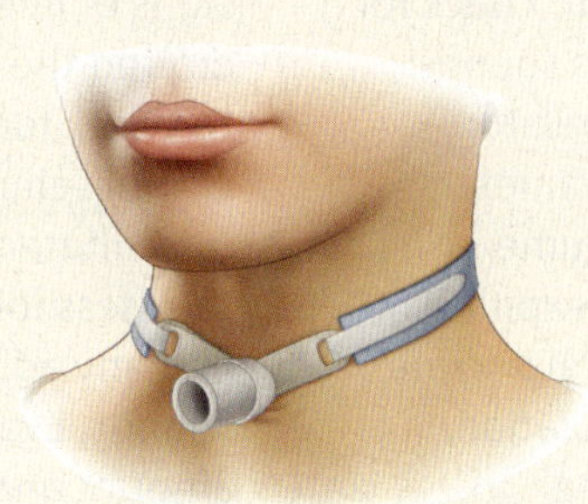	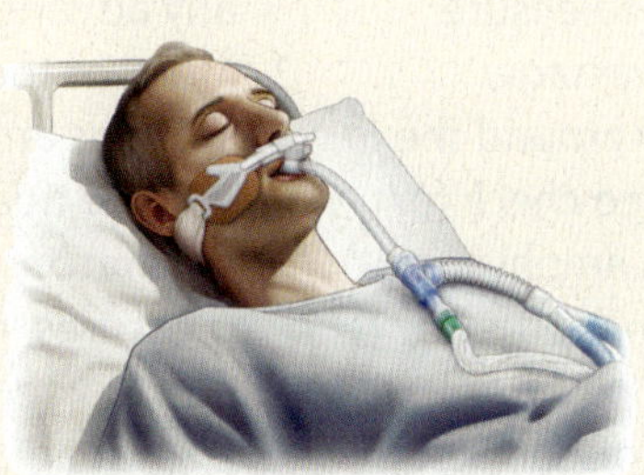	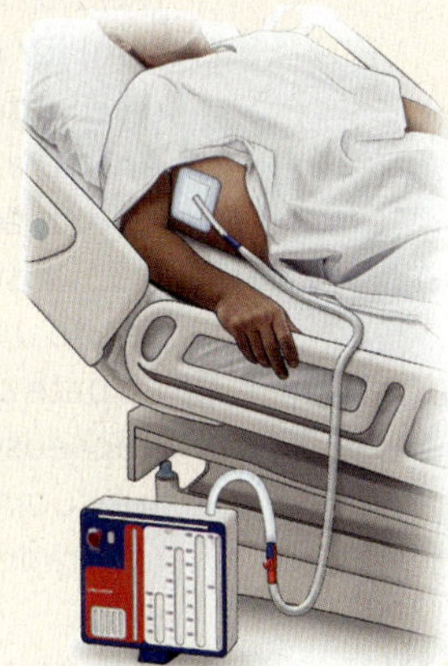
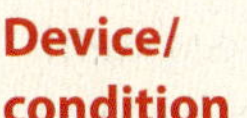 **Device/ condition**	Tube inserted into a surgically created direct airway, through an incision in the anterior neck and the trachea (windpipe)	Machine that provides artificial ventilation by moving breathable air into and out of the lungs	Flexible plastic tube inserted through the chest wall into the pleural space or mediastinum to remove pathologic air, fluid, blood, or pus; sutured in place on the chest wall and covered with dressing; usually connected to a three-chamber chest drainage system that may be attached to wall suction

(continued)

Box 17-18. Thorax and Lung Examination with Medical Devices, Conditions, or Procedures Present (*Continued*)

	Patient with a Tracheostomy Tube	Patient on a Mechanical Ventilator	Patient with a Chest Tube or Tube Thoracostomy
General indication	Indicated for long-term mechanical ventilation to bypass an upper airway obstruction or to facilitate clearance of secretions	Indicated for patients unable to breathe on their own due to respiratory failure, general anesthesia for surgery, or certain medical conditions (e.g., severe pneumonia or asthma)	Indicated to treat pneumothorax, hemothorax, empyema, and large pleural effusions
General location	Positioned in the anterior midline neck, entering directly into the trachea	Usually at the bedside in the intensive care unit or medical wards; tubes connect from the machine to the patient's endotracheal or tracheostomy tube	Typically inserted in the fifth intercostal space slightly anterior to the midaxillary line and directed toward the base or apex of the lung, depending on the condition being treated
Physical exam modification	1. Inspect the skin around the tracheostomy site for redness, swelling, and signs of infection. Assess the stoma (opening at the skin) for patency and any discharge. 2. Auscultate for breath sounds around the tracheostomy to ensure adequate air passage. 3. Palpate gently around the tracheostomy to check for subcutaneous emphysema (air trapped under the skin). 4. Inquire about discomfort, difficulty breathing, and any other changes associated with the tracheostomy. 5. Do not remove the tracheostomy tube without the assistance of an experienced provider.	1. Inspect the connections and position of the tubes. Ensure none of the tubes are being pulled or are at risk of being dislodged or disconnected. 2. Auscultate lung fields bilaterally to ensure even ventilation and to check for any adventitious sounds. 3. Monitor the ventilator settings and parameters, such as tidal volume, inspiratory and expiratory pressures, respiratory rate, and oxygen saturation. Do not adjust the ventilator settings without the assistance of an experienced provider. 4. Inquire about any evidence of discomfort, changes in respiratory status, and episodes of ventilator alarms.	1. Remove any kinks, loops, or obstructions in the tubing. Ensure the tubing is not under tension or at risk of being dislodged or disconnected. Inspect the chest wall insertion site for redness, swelling, and signs of infection. Palpate around the chest tube site to check for subcutaneous emphysema. 2. Auscultate all lung fields to assess for breath sounds and any adventitious sounds. Evaluate the amount and type of fluid being drained. Evaluate the chest drainage system for bubbling. Bubbling is normal during coughing or exhalation, but continuous bubbling is concerning for a system leak or air leak from the lung. 3. Do not manipulate the chest tube without the assistance of an experienced clinician.

RECORDING YOUR FINDINGS

For the novice clinician, the practice of documenting the PE with detailed sentences is key for initial diagnosis and hypothesis evaluation. With time and experience, you will often shift to a more streamlined approach, employing brief, universally accepted phrases in your notes.

Recording the Thorax and Lungs Examination

"Thorax is symmetric with good expansion. Lungs resonant. Breath sounds vesicular; no crackles, wheezes, or rhonchi. Diaphragms descend 4 cm bilaterally."

OR

"Thorax symmetric with moderate kyphosis and increased AP diameter, decreased expansion. Lungs are hyper-resonant. Breath sounds distant with delayed expiratory phase and scattered expiratory wheezes. Fremitus decreased; no bronchophony, egophony, or whispered pectoriloquy. Diaphragms descend 2 cm bilaterally."

The practice of splitting PE documentation into detailed segments underscores how specific clinical findings can offer vital clues for diagnosis. The findings from the thoracic examination described in the second note suggest a possible obstructive lung disease:

- *Thorax symmetric with moderate kyphosis and increased AP diameter, decreased expansion:* The symmetric thorax is normal, but moderate kyphosis and increased AP diameter are common in COPD. Decreased chest expansion indicates restricted lung movement, which is also typical in such conditions.
- *Lungs are hyper-resonant:* Hyper-resonance on percussion of the lungs indicates too much air in the lungs, as seen in conditions like emphysema, in which lung tissue is damaged and air gets trapped.
- *Breath sounds distant with delayed expiratory phase and scattered expiratory wheezes:* Distant breath sounds with a prolonged expiratory phase and wheezing are characteristic of obstructive lung diseases. These findings suggest narrowed airways and difficulty in air movement, typical in COPD or asthma.
- *Fremitus decreased:* Decreased fremitus is often found in hyperinflated lungs due to air trapping, as seen in emphysema.
- *No bronchophony, egophony, or whispered pectoriloquy:* The absence of these signs is typically normal. Their presence would suggest consolidation of the lung tissue, often seen in pneumonia, which does not seem to be the case here.
- *Diaphragms descend 2 cm bilaterally:* This finding suggests that the diaphragms are moving downward somewhat during inhalation, but the extent of movement might be limited. In chronic lung diseases, the diaphragm's ability to move effectively can be reduced due to lung hyperinflation.

These findings collectively point toward a *chronic obstructive pulmonary condition*, likely *emphysema* or *chronic bronchitis*, components of COPD. The presence of kyphosis and the increased AP diameter of the thorax suggests a long-standing condition.

POINT-OF-CARE ULTRASOUND EXAMINATION

The thoracic region, crucial for respiratory function, can present with subtle abnormalities. Point-of-care ultrasound (POCUS) examination can provide very useful and accurate information on the pleura, subpleural space, and thoracic cavity.[33,34] Ultrasound is exceedingly well-suited to detect the difference between air and fluid. Unlike many other ultrasound applications, which rely on visualizing the appearance or behavior of specific organs, many techniques in thoracic sonography use the appearance or behavior of artifacts. Thus, the artifacts that had long been considered a hindrance to ultrasound use in medicine are leveraged to make diagnoses. While we explore the added value of POCUS in thoracic assessments, it's important to note that our discussion will not delve into its step-by-step use and only highlight its diagnostic power.

Detecting Congestive Heart Failure, Pneumothorax, and Pleural Effusion

Physical Examination. Many PE techniques (auscultation, percussion, egophony, etc.) attempt to assess for the presence of fluid where there should be air for various conditions from pneumothorax to pleural effusions (Box 17-19). Each condition can present with nuanced variations in chest expansion, tactile fremitus, and other exam findings, leading to potential overlap or ambiguity. While conditions like pleural effusion might be noticeable when they are significant, others like congestive heart failure (CHF) and pneumothorax might be subtler in their presentation. Their exam findings can sometimes intertwine or be less pronounced, making it challenging to isolate just by traditional methods. POCUS should be considered when assessing a patient with heart failure, a potential pneumothorax, or pleural effusions.[35–38]

Box 17-19. Comparison of Physical Examination Findings: Heart Failure versus Pneumothorax versus Pleural Effusion

Physical Examination Finding	Heart Failure	Pneumothorax	Pleural Effusion
Respiratory Rate	Increased	Increased	May be increased
Chest Movement	Normal or reduced	Reduced on affected side	Reduced over effusion
Percussion Note	Dull if effusion	Hyper-resonant on side	Dull over effusion
Tactile Fremitus	Reduced	Reduced or absent on side	Reduced over effusion
Auscultation of Breath Sounds	Often diminished	Decreased or absent on side	Diminished over effusion

Ultrasound Technique

Basic Ultrasound Setup	
Patient positioning	Supine or sitting upright
Probe	Curvilinear probe for congestive heart failure or pleural effusion Curvilinear or linear probe for pneumothorax assessment
Ultrasound setting	"Lung" setting for assessment of pneumothorax or congestive heart failure; "abdomen" setting to assess for pleural effusion, B-mode for all applications, M-mode may be used for pneumothorax assessment

Evaluation of Congestive Heart Failure. POCUS evaluation of the thorax for CHF is typically performed with the patient in a supine or semirecumbent position, as illustrated in Figure 17-29.

Although many different schemas have been described to divide the lung into "zones" for scanning, one of the first and simplest divides the lung into three zones on each hemithorax.[36,37,39] As shown in Figure 17-30, *zone 1* includes the anterior chest, *zone 2* is the lateral chest wall, and *zone 3* is the posterolateral chest wall.

With the probe oriented toward the patient's head, carefully scan each zone. A normally aerated lung will present as shown in Figure 17-31, characterized by a bright pleural line and equally spaced reflections of this line—equivalent to the distance from the chest wall to the pleura.

"A-lines" represent normally aerated lungs and can be seen in conditions where the lung remains aerated, such as COPD or asthma. However, "wet" lungs or lungs with interstitial edema will demonstrate B-lines, characterized by bright echogenic reflections. These "laser-like" reflections arise from the pleura and negate any A-lines they cross (Fig. 17-32).

Assessment of Pneumothorax. For pneumothorax, the patient should lie flat during the POCUS evaluation. This is important because POCUS is used to assess for air in between the visceral and parietal pleura. In a patient with

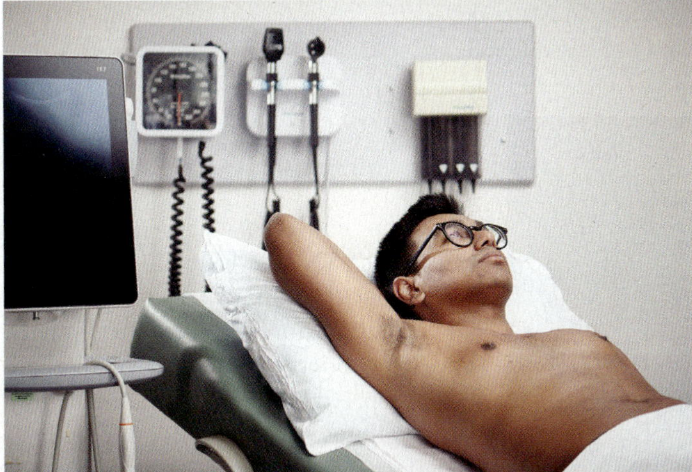

FIGURE 17-29. Patient positioning for thoracic ultrasound.

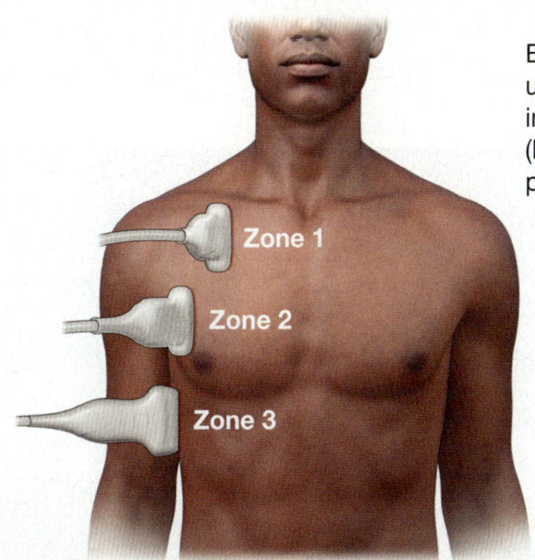

FIGURE 17-30. Lung zones for assessment of congestive heart failure.

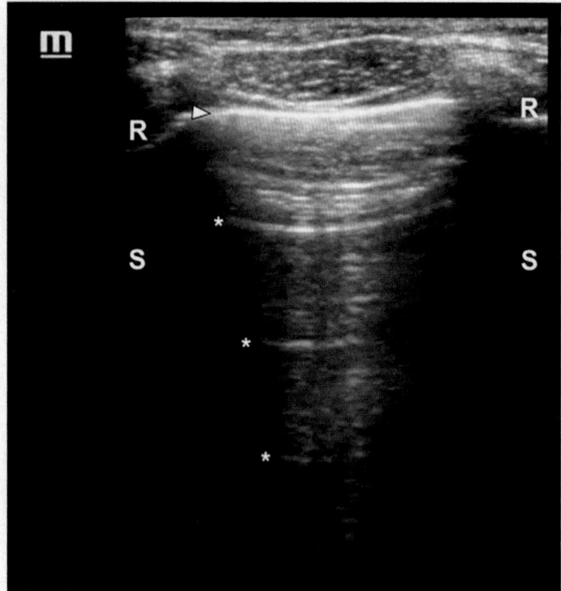

FIGURE 17-31. Normal lung appearance showing bright echogenic pleural line and A-lines. The probe marker is directed toward the patient's head. Note the ribs (*R*) and their shadows (*S*), the bright echogenic pleural line (*P*) (*arrowhead*), and A-lines (*), each occurring at multiples of the pleural depth.

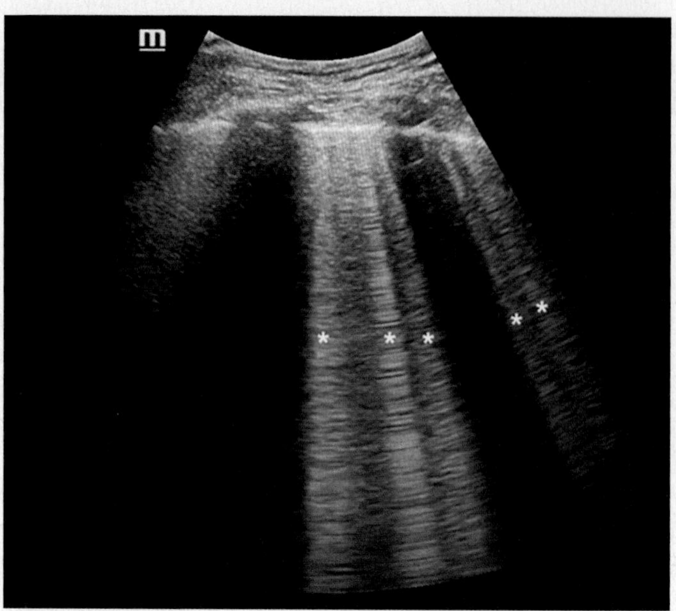

FIGURE 17-32. Note the B-lines (*) are as bright as the pleura and originate from the pleura.

pneumothorax but otherwise normal lung anatomy, air will rise to the most anterior part of the thoracic cavity, which is approximately at the level of the nipple. Thus, assessing both hemithoraces at the level of the nipple just above the diaphragm will give the most accurate assessment for pneumothorax. As Figure 17-33 indicates, scanning zone 1's caudal aspect yields optimal results.

In a healthy lung, the visceral and parietal pleura rub against each other with each respiratory cycle. The parietal pleura remains in a fixed position, but the visceral pleura slides up (cranial) and down (caudal) with each breath. In the setting of pneumothorax, air between the visceral and parietal pleura blocks the deeper visceral pleura from being visualized. Thus, only the immobile parietal pleura is visualized, and lung sliding is absent. *Lung sliding*, an essential indicator in pneumothorax detection, can be visualized using M-mode or motion mode. In M-mode, different motions are represented in distinct patterns, as depicted in Figure 17-33.

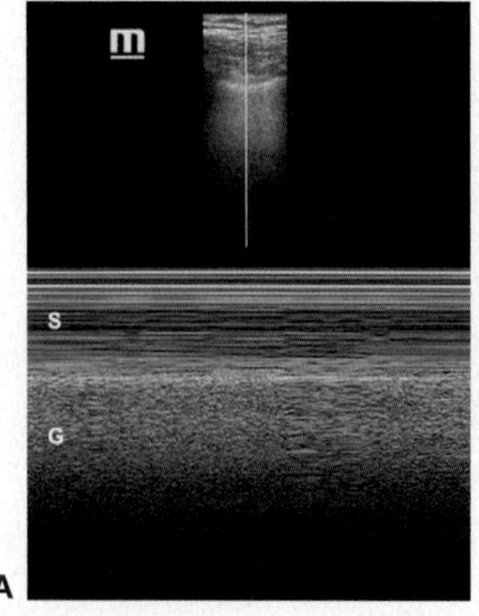

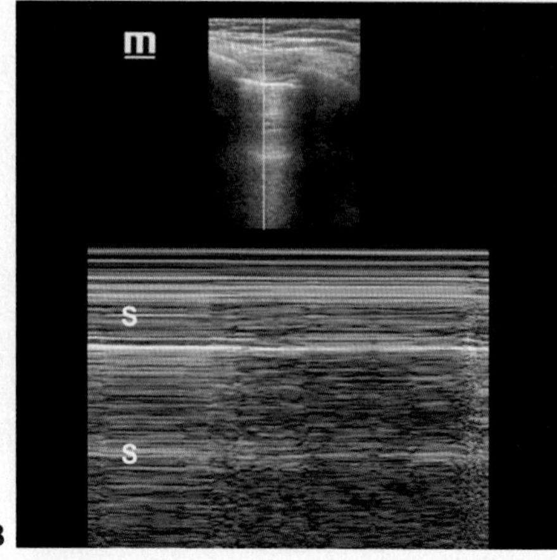

FIGURE 17-33. M-Mode in the evaluation of pneumothorax. (**A**) Normal lung, (**B**) Pneumothorax. Note the straight lines (*S*) above the pleura where there is no appreciable motion. Normal lung demonstrates motion, and grainy lines (*G*) deep to the pleura. With pneumothorax, there is no motion below the pleura and the lines are straight (*S*).

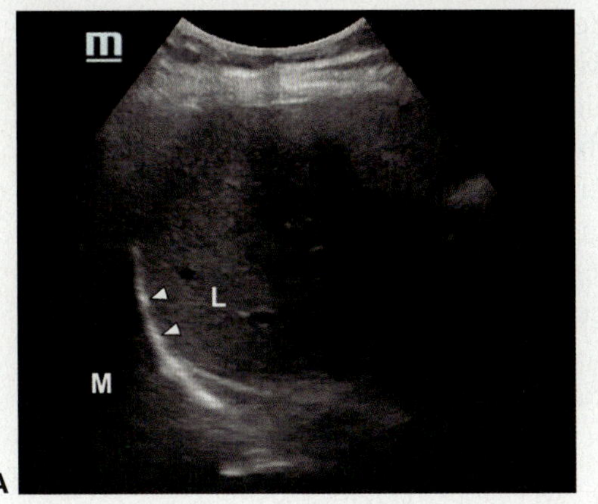

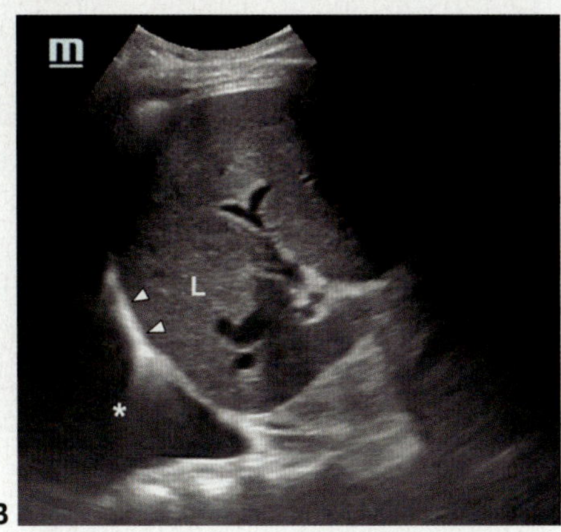

FIGURE 17-34. Normal costophrenic angles (**A**), and pleural effusion (**B**). Note the echogenic curve of the diaphragm (*arrowheads*), the medium echotexture of the liver (*L*), the mirror artifact in normal (*M*), and the anechoic/black echotexture of the pleural effusion (*).

Detection of Pleural Effusion. As with PE, the most sensitive area to examine for pleural effusion is the costophrenic angle. With the patient supine, position the probe with the marker directed toward the patient's head and scan near the posterior axillary line at the costal margin. On the left side of the screen, visualize the diaphragm and beneath it in a caudal direction the liver or spleen. Figure 17-34 shows a clear distinction between a normally aerated lung and one with pleural effusion. In a normally aerated lung with no effusion, the area cranial to the diaphragm will display a mirror image of the liver or spleen or will appear as indistinct gray. In the setting of pleural effusion, black fluid will fill the space just cranial to the diaphragm, highlighting the boundaries of the diaphragm below and the lung above.

HEALTH PROMOTION AND COUNSELING: EVIDENCE AND RECOMMENDATIONS

Important Topics for Health Promotion and Counseling

- Lung cancer
- Latent tuberculosis
- Obstructive sleep apnea
- Tobacco cessation (See Chapter 7, Health Maintenance and Screening, pp. 130–131)
- Immunizations—influenza and streptococcal pneumonia vaccines (See Chapter 7, Health Maintenance and Screening, pp. 132–133)

In the following section, both traditional terms like "men," "women," "male," and "female" and inclusive terms such as "individuals assigned female at birth" and "individuals assigned male at birth" are used. This approach balances inclusivity with the need to accurately represent the original research.

Lung Cancer

Epidemiology. Lung cancer is the third most frequently diagnosed cancer in the United States and the leading cause of cancer death.[40] More people die of lung cancer than of colon, breast, and prostate cancer combined. More than

238,000 new cases and nearly 130,000 deaths (accounting for 21% of all cancer deaths) were expected in 2023. However, incidence rates and death rates have been decreasing over the past few decades, concurrent with a decline in smoking rates.[41,42] Cigarette smoking is by far the leading risk factor for lung cancer and accounts for 80% to 90% of lung cancer deaths.[43] *Radon*, an invisible, odorless, radioactive gas released from soil and rocks in the ground, is the second leading cause of lung cancer in the United States. Other environmental and occupational exposures include second-hand smoke, asbestos, diesel exhaust, heavy metals, organic chemicals, ionizing radiation, and air pollution. Lung cancer also has a familial risk, especially if the relative was diagnosed at a younger age.

Prevention. Longer smoking histories and greater number of cigarettes smoked are associated with higher lung cancer risk. Tobacco cessation and prevention (see Chapter 7, Health Maintenance and Screening, pp. 130–131) have the greatest effect on reducing the burden of lung cancer.

Screening. Screening for lung cancer is an appealing strategy because cancers diagnosed at an early stage (confined to the lung) have a 62% 5-year relative survival compared to a dismal 7.8% relative survival for cancers diagnosed at a distant stage (metastatic).[41] Unfortunately, only 23% of lung cancers are diagnosed at an early stage. Numerous studies have shown that lung cancer screening with chest x-ray or sputum cytology is not effective.[44] However, in 2011, the National Lung Screening Trial (NLST) showed that 3 years of annual screening with low-dose computed tomography (LDCT) reduced the risk of dying from lung cancer compared to chest x-ray screening by 20% after nearly 7 years of follow-up.[45] In 2020, the NELSON trial, conducted in the Netherlands and Belgium, reported that four rounds of LDCT screening reduced the risk of dying from lung cancer compared to no screening by 24% in men and 33% in women after 10 years of follow-up.[46]

The U.S. Preventive Services Task Force (USPSTF) has given lung cancer screening with LDCT a B grade, meaning that there is a net benefit to offering screening.[47] Annual LDCT screening is recommended for those currently smoking (or those who have quit within the last 15 years) if they have smoked an average of one pack of cigarettes for 20 years and are aged 50 to 80 years. The USPSTF also recommended offering smoking cessation interventions to those who currently smoke. Screening with LDCT, though, can lead to harms, including false-positive results, unnecessary tests and invasive diagnostic procedures, overdiagnosis, radiation exposure, and incidental findings. Accordingly, clinicians were encouraged to discuss the potential benefits, limitations, and harms of screening and then order an LDCT for those expressing a preference for screening. Clinicians should also emphasize that screening is not a substitute for smoking cessation.

Latent Tuberculosis

Epidemiology. An estimated 10.6 million people worldwide developed active tuberculosis in 2021, and about 1.6 million tuberculosis-related deaths occurred.[48] Unlike patients with active tuberculosis, those with latent tuberculosis have no symptoms and are not contagious. However, they may develop active tuberculosis if they do not receive treatment. The estimated prevalence of latent tuberculosis in the United States is 5% for U.S.-born people and

15.9% for foreign-born people.[49] Immunocompetent patients with latent tuberculosis have a 5% to 10% lifetime risk of developing active tuberculosis.[50] The risk for latent tuberculosis is increased for those born in or previously residing in countries with high tuberculosis prevalence, those living in high-risk settings such as homeless shelters or correctional facilities, and those who are immunosuppressed.

Screening. Screening tests include interferon-gamma release assay (IGRA) blood tests and the tuberculin skin test (TST). IGRA requires a single venous blood sample and laboratory processing within 8 to 30 hours after collection. The TST requires intradermal placement of purified protein derivative and interpretation of response 48 to 72 hours later. The skin test reaction is measured in millimeters of *induration* (palpable, raised, hardened area or swelling). The interpretation of the TST depends upon the degree of induration and a person's clinical risk factors. An online tool can be used to estimate the likelihood (positive predictive value) that a person has latent tuberculosis and the annual risk of developing active disease based on the TST result and/or an IGRA result (http://www.tstin3d.com). The USPSTF issued a grade B recommendation favoring screening for latent tuberculosis in asymptomatic adults at increased risk for tuberculosis.[50] The USPSTF cited evidence that treating latent tuberculosis was moderately beneficial in preventing progression to active disease and that the harms from screening and treatment were small. The primary harm of treatment is hepatotoxicity.

Obstructive Sleep Apnea

Epidemiology. Obstructive sleep apnea (OSA) is a disorder characterized by repeated episodes of upper airway collapse, particularly during rapid eye movement (REM) sleep, leading to hypoxemia and disrupted sleep. OSA can cause excessive daytime sleepiness, which increases risk for vehicular and occupational accidents and is associated with higher risks for cognitive impairment, diabetes, cardiovascular morbidity, and all-cause mortality.[51,52] The estimated prevalence of moderate to severe OSA in adults ages 30 to 70 years is about 13% for men and 6% for women.[53] Risk factors for OSA include obesity, male sex, older age, treatment-resistant hypertension, CHF, atrial fibrillation, type 2 diabetes, stroke, polycystic ovary syndrome, craniofacial and upper airway abnormalities, and being postmenopausal.[51] Symptoms and signs suggesting OSA include excessive daytime sleepiness (which can be assessed with the Epworth sleepiness scale[54] shown in Box 17-20), witnessed apneic episodes, loud snoring, nocturnal awakenings, choking or gasping during sleep, and nonrestorative sleep.[51]

Screening. In 2022, the USPSTF concluded that the evidence was insufficient to assess the balance of benefits and harms of screening asymptomatic adults for OSA (I statement).[53] However, the American College of Physicians offered weak recommendations for ordering sleep studies in patients with unexplained daytime somnolence and in patients suspected to have OSA.[56] The American Academy of Sleep Medicine suggested that primary care physicians use standardized tools to annually screen high-risk patients for OSA and refer those with a positive screening for further evaluation.[57] A number of screening questionnaires and clinical prediction tools have been developed to assess whether patients are likely to have OSA, including the STOP-Bang Questionnaire

Box 17-20. Epworth Sleepiness Scale[55]

Consider how you have felt over the past week or two. How likely are you to doze off or fall asleep in the following situations?

0 = Never

1 = Slight chance

2 = Moderate chance

3 = High chance

Situation	Score
Sitting and reading	
Watching television	
Sitting inactive in a public space (e.g., theater or meeting)	
As a passenger in a car for an hour without a break	
Lying down in the afternoon when able	
Sitting quietly after lunch without alcohol	
In a car while stopped for a few minutes in traffic	
Total:	

Scores >10 are consistent with excessive daytime sleepiness.

Source: From Johns MW. A new method for measuring daytime sleepiness: the Epworth sleepiness scale. *Sleep*. 1991;14(6):540–545. Reproduced by permission from American Sleep Disorders Association and Sleep Research Society.

(Box 17-21).[58] In a sleep clinic population, positive responses to five or more items had a 58% positive predictive value for severe OSA.[59] However, the diagnostic performance of the screening questionnaires and tools has not been adequately evaluated in primary care settings.[53]

Box 17-21. STOP-Bang[58]

STOP

S: Do you *snore* loudly (louder than talking or loud enough to be heard through closed doors)?

T: Do you often feel *tired*, fatigued, or sleepy during the day?

O: Has anyone *observed* you stop breathing during the day?

P: Do you have or are you being treated for high blood *pressure*?

Bang

B: *Body* mass index >35 kg/m^2

A: *Age* >50 years?

N: *Neck* circumference >40 cm (16 inches)?

G: *Gender* male?

Patients receive 1 point for each "Yes." A total score is then calculated to assess the patient's risk level for OSA: **Score 0–2:** Low risk; **Score 3–4:** Intermediate risk; **Score 5–8:** High risk of OSA.

Adapted with permission from Dr. Frances Chung and University Health Network. www.stopbang.ca

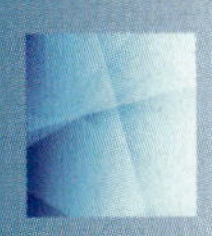

TABLE 17-1. Normal and Altered Breath and Voice Sounds[1,3,4,69]

The origins of breath sounds continue to be investigated.[1] Acoustic studies indicate that turbulent air flow in the pharynx, glottis, and subglottic region produces tracheal breath sounds, which are similar to bronchial sounds. The inspiratory component of vesicular breath sounds seems to arise in the lobar and segmental airways; the expiratory component arises in the more central larger airways. Normally, tracheal and bronchial sounds may be heard over the trachea and mainstem bronchi; vesicular breath sounds predominate throughout most of the lungs. When lung tissue loses airflow, there is increased transmission of high-pitched sounds. If the tracheobronchial tree is open, bronchial breath sounds may replace the normal vesicular sounds over airless areas of the lung. This change occurs in lobar pneumonia when the alveoli get filled with fluid and cellular debris—a process called *consolidation*. Other causes include pulmonary edema or, rarely, hemorrhage. Bronchial breath sounds usually correlate with an increase in tactile fremitus and transmitted voice sounds. These findings are summarized below.

	Normal Air-Filled Lung	Consolidated Airless Lung (Lobar Pneumonia)
	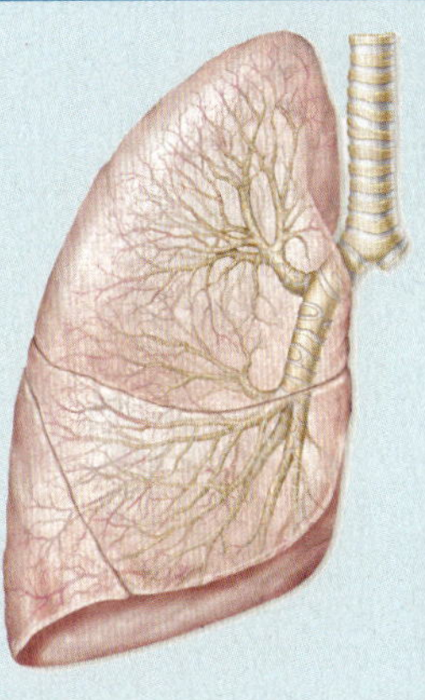 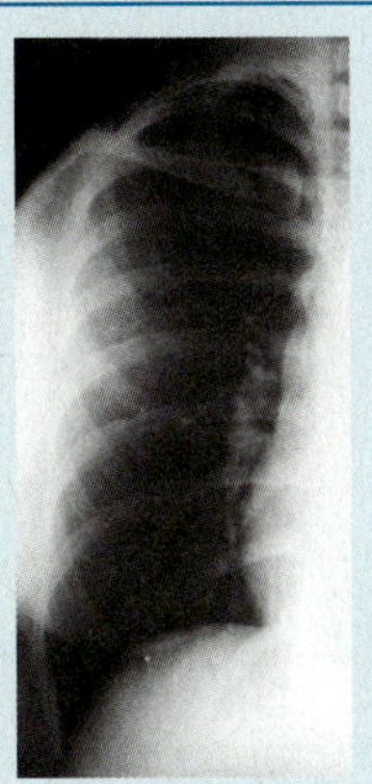	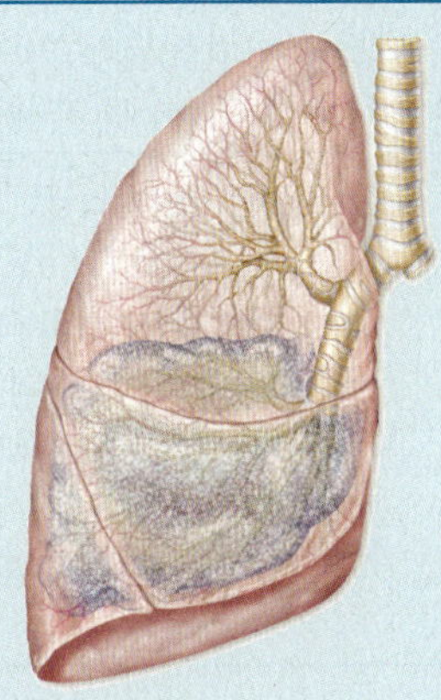 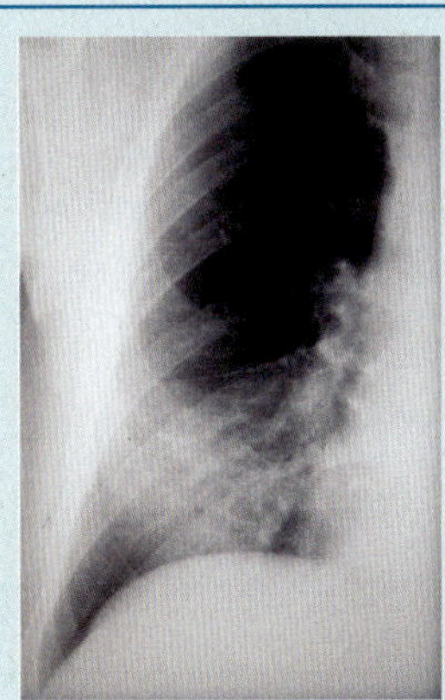
Breath Sounds	Predominantly vesicular	Bronchial or bronchovesicular over the involved area
Transmitted Voice Sounds	Spoken words muffled and indistinct Spoken "*ee*" heard as "*ee*" Whispered words faint and indistinct, if heard at all	Spoken "*ee*" heard as "*ay*" (*egophony*) Spoken words louder (*bronchophony*) Whispered words louder, clearer (*whispered pectoriloquy*)
Tactile Fremitus	Normal NOTE: In the hyperinflated lung of chronic obstructive pulmonary disease, breath sounds are decreased (muffled to distant) to absent, and transmitted voice sounds and fremitus are decreased.	Increased NOTE: In the dull lung of pleural effusion, breath sounds are decreased to absent (bronchial sounds possible at upper margin of effusion). Transmitted voice sounds are decreased to absent (but may be increased at upper margin of effusion). Fremitus is decreased.

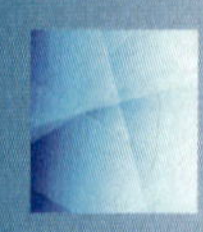

TABLE 17-2. Dyspnea

Problem	Process	Timing	Factors That Aggravate
Left-Sided Heart Failure (Left Ventricular Failure or Mitral Stenosis)	Elevated pressure in pulmonary capillary bed with transudation of fluid into interstitial spaces and alveoli, decreased compliance (increased stiffness) of the lungs, increased work of breathing	Dyspnea may progress slowly, or suddenly as in acute pulmonary edema	Exertion, lying down
Chronic Bronchitis	Excessive mucus production in bronchi, followed by chronic obstruction of airways	Chronic productive cough followed by slowly progressive dyspnea	Exertion, inhaled irritants, respiratory infections
Chronic Obstructive Pulmonary Disease (COPD)	Overdistention of air spaces distal to terminal bronchioles, with destruction of alveolar septa, alveolar enlargement, and limitation of expiratory air flow	Slowly progressive dyspnea; relatively mild cough later	Exertion
Asthma	Reversible bronchial hyper-responsiveness involving release of inflammatory mediators, increased airway secretions, and bronchoconstriction	Acute episodes, separated by symptom-free periods. Nocturnal episodes common	Variable, including allergens, irritants, respiratory infections, exercise, cold, and emotion
Diffuse Interstitial Lung Diseases (e.g., Sarcoidosis, Widespread Neoplasms, Idiopathic Pulmonary Fibrosis, and Asbestosis)	Abnormal and widespread infiltration of cells, fluid, and collagen into interstitial spaces between alveoli; many causes	Progressive dyspnea, which varies in its rate of development with the cause	Exertion
Pneumonia	Infection of lung parenchyma from the respiratory bronchioles to the alveoli	An acute illness, timing varies with the causative agent	Exertion, smoking

Factors That Relieve	Associated Symptoms	Setting
Rest, sitting up, though dyspnea may become persistent	Often cough, orthopnea, paroxysmal nocturnal dyspnea; sometimes wheezing	History of heart disease or its predisposing factors
Expectoration; rest, though dyspnea may become persistent	Chronic productive cough, recurrent respiratory infections; wheezing may develop	History of smoking, air pollutants, recurrent respiratory infections; often present with COPD
Rest, though dyspnea may become persistent	Cough, with scant mucoid sputum	History of smoking, air pollutants, sometimes a familial deficiency in α_1-antitrypsin
Separation from aggravating factors	Wheezing, cough, tightness in chest	Environmental conditions
Rest, though dyspnea may become persistent	Often weakness, fatigue; cough less common than in other lung diseases	Varied; exposure to trigger substances
Rest, though dyspnea may become persistent	Pleuritic pain, cough, sputum, fever, though not necessarily present	Varied

(*continued*)

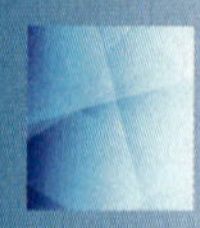

TABLE 17-2. Dyspnea *(Continued)*

Problem	Process	Timing	Factors That Aggravate
Spontaneous Pneumothorax	Leakage of air into pleural space through blebs on visceral pleura, with resulting partial or complete collapse of the lung	Sudden onset of dyspnea	
Acute Pulmonary Embolism	Sudden occlusion of part of pulmonary arterial tree by a blood clot that usually originates in deep veins of legs or pelvis	Sudden onset of tachypnea, dyspnea	Exertion
Anxiety with Hyperventilation	Overbreathing, with resultant respiratory alkalosis and fall in arterial partial pressure of carbon dioxide (pCO_2)	Episodic, often recurrent	Often occurs at rest; an upsetting event may not be evident

Factors That Relieve	Associated Symptoms	Setting
	Pleuritic pain, cough	Often a previously healthy young adult or adult with emphysema
Rest, though dyspnea may become persistent	Often none; retrosternal oppressive pain if massive occlusion; pleuritic pain, cough, syncope, hemoptysis, and/or unilateral leg swelling and pain from instigating deep vein thrombosis; anxiety (see below)	Postpartum or postoperative periods; prolonged bed rest; heart failure, chronic lung disease, and fractures of hip or leg; deep venous thrombosis (often not clinically apparent); also hypercoagulability, hereditary (i.e., protein C, S, factor V Leiden deficiency) or acquired (e.g., cancer, hormonal therapy)
Breathing in and out of a paper or plastic bag may help	Sighing, lightheadedness, numbness or tingling of the hands and feet, palpitations, chest pain	Other manifestations of anxiety may be present, such as chest pain diaphoresis, palpitations

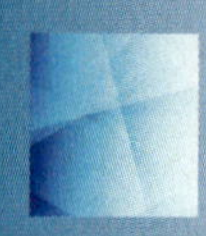

TABLE 17-3. Cough and Hemoptysis

Problem	Cough and Sputum	Associated Symptoms and Setting
Acute Inflammation		
Laryngitis	Dry cough, may become productive of variable amounts of sputum	Acute fairly minor illness with hoarseness. Often associated with viral rhinosinusitis
Acute Bronchitis	Cough, may be dry or productive	Acute, often viral, illness generally without fever or dyspnea; at times with burning retrosternal discomfort
Mycoplasma and Viral Pneumonias	Dry hacking cough, may become productive of mucoid sputum	Acute febrile illness, often with malaise, headache, and possibly dyspnea
Bacterial Pneumonias	Sputum is mucoid or purulent; may be blood-streaked, diffusely pinkish, or rusty	Acute illness with chills, often high fever, dyspnea, and chest pain. Commonly from *Streptococcus pneumoniae*; *Haemophilus influenzae*; *Moraxella catarrhalis*; *Klebsiella pneumoniae* in alcoholism, especially if underlying smoking, chronic bronchitis, and chronic obstructive pulmonary disease; cardiovascular disease; diabetes
Chronic Inflammation		
Postnasal Drip	Chronic cough; sputum mucoid or mucopurulent	Postnasal discharge may be seen in posterior pharynx. Associated with allergic rhinitis, with or without sinusitis
Chronic Bronchitis	Chronic cough; sputum mucoid to purulent, may be blood-streaked or even bloody	Often with recurrent wheezing and dyspnea, and prolonged history of tobacco abuse
Bronchiectasis	Chronic cough; sputum purulent, often copious and foul-smelling; may be blood-streaked or bloody	Recurrent bronchopulmonary infections common; sinusitis may coexist
Pulmonary Tuberculosis	Cough, dry or with mucoid or purulent sputum; may be blood-streaked or bloody	Early, no symptoms. Later, anorexia, weight loss, fatigue, fever, and night sweats
Lung Abscess	Sputum purulent and foul-smelling; may be bloody	Usually from aspiration pneumonia with fever and infection from oral anaerobes and poor dental hygiene; often with dysphagia or episode of impaired consciousness
Asthma	Cough, at times with thick mucoid sputum, especially near end of an attack	Episodic wheezing and dyspnea, but cough may occur alone. Often with a history of allergies
Gastroesophageal Reflux	Chronic cough, especially at night or early in the morning	Wheezing, especially at night (often mistaken for asthma), early morning hoarseness, and repeated attempts to clear the throat. Often with heartburn and regurgitation

Problem	Cough and Sputum	Associated Symptoms and Setting
Neoplasm		
Lung Cancer	Cough, dry to productive; sputum may be blood-streaked or bloody	Commonly with dyspnea, weight loss, and history of tobacco abuse
Cardiovascular Disorders		
Left Ventricular Failure or Mitral Stenosis	Often dry, especially on exertion or at night; may progress to the pink frothy sputum of pulmonary edema or to frank hemoptysis	Dyspnea, orthopnea, paroxysmal nocturnal dyspnea
Pulmonary Embolism	Dry cough, at times with hemoptysis	Tachypnea, chest or pleuritic pain, dyspnea, fever, syncope, anxiety; factors that predispose to deep venous thrombosis
Irritating Particles, Chemicals, or Gases	Variable. There may be a latent period between exposure and symptoms	Exposure to irritants. Eyes, nose, and throat may be affected

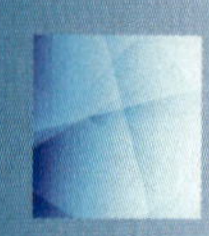

TABLE 17-4. Chest Pain[18,60–67]

Problem	Process	Location	Quality	Severity
Cardiovascular				
Angina Pectoris	Temporary myocardial ischemia, usually secondary to coronary atherosclerosis	Retrosternal or across the anterior chest, often radiates to the shoulders, arms, neck, lower jaw, or upper abdomen	Pressing, squeezing, tight, heavy, occasionally burning	Mild to moderate, sometimes perceived as discomfort rather than pain
Myocardial Infarction	Prolonged myocardial ischemia, resulting in irreversible muscle damage or necrosis	Same as in angina	Same as in angina	Often, but not always, a severe pain
Pericarditis	Irritation of parietal pleura adjacent to the pericardium	Retrosternal or left precordial, may radiate to the tip of left shoulder	Sharp, knifelike	Often severe
Aortic Dissection	A splitting within the layers of the aortic wall, allowing passage of blood to dissect a channel	Anterior or posterior chest, radiating to the neck, back, or abdomen	Ripping, tearing	Very severe
Pulmonary				
Pleuritic Pain	Inflammation of the parietal pleura, as in pleurisy, pneumonia, pulmonary infarction, or neoplasm; rarely, subdiaphragmatic abscess	Chest wall overlying the process	Sharp, knifelike	Often severe
Gastrointestinal and Other				
Gastrointestinal Reflux Disease	Irritation or inflammation of the esophageal mucosa due to reflux of gastric acid from lowered esophageal sphincter tone	Retrosternal, may radiate to the back	Burning, may be squeezing	Mild to severe
Diffuse Esophageal Spasm	Motor dysfunction of the esophageal muscle	Retrosternal, may radiate to the back, arms, and jaw	Usually squeezing	Mild to severe
Chest Wall Pain, Costochondritis	Variable, including trauma, inflammation of costal cartilage	Often below the left breast or along the costal cartilages	Stabbing, sticking, or dull, aching	Variable
Anxiety, Panic Disorder	Unclear	Precordial, below the left breast, or across the anterior chest	Stabbing, sticking, or dull, aching	Variable

Note: Chest pain may be referred from extrathoracic structures in the neck (*arthritis*) and abdomen (*biliary colic, acute cholecystitis*).

Problem	Timing	Factors That Aggravate	Factors That Relieve	Associated Symptoms
Cardiovascular				
Angina Pectoris	Usually 1–3 min but up to 10 min. Prolonged episodes up to 20 min	Often exertion, especially in the cold; meals; emotional stress. May occur at rest	Often, but not always, rest, nitroglycerin	Sometimes dyspnea, nausea, sweating
Myocardial Infarction	20 min to several hours	Not always triggered by exertion	Not relieved by rest	Dyspnea, nausea, vomiting, sweating, weakness
Pericarditis	Persistent	Breathing, changing position, coughing, lying down, sometimes swallowing	Sitting forward may relieve it	Seen in autoimmune disorders, postmyocardial infarction, viral infection, chest irradiation
Aortic Dissection	Abrupt onset, early peak, persistent for hours or more	Hypertension		If thoracic, hoarseness, dysphagia; also syncope, hemiplegia, paraplegia
Pulmonary				
Pleuritic Pain	Persistent	Deep inspiration, coughing, movements of the trunk		Of the underlying illness
Gastrointestinal and Other				
Gastrointestinal Reflux Disease	Variable	Large meal; bending over, lying down	Antacids, sometimes belching	Sometimes regurgitation, dysphagia; also cough, laryngitis, asthma
Diffuse Esophageal Spasm	Variable	Swallowing of food or cold liquid; emotional stress	Sometimes nitroglycerin	Dysphagia
Chest Wall Pain, Costochondritis	Fleeting to hours or days	Coughing; movement of chest, trunk, arms		Often local tenderness
Anxiety, Panic Disorder	Fleeting to hours or days	May follow effort, emotional stress		Breathlessness, palpitations, weakness, anxiety

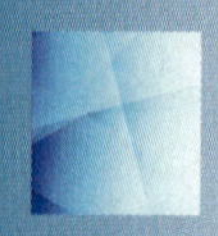

TABLE 17-5. Abnormalities in Rate and Rhythm of Breathing

When observing respiratory patterns, note the rate, depth, and regularity of the patient's breathing. Traditional terms, such as tachypnea, are given below so that you will understand them, but simple descriptions are recommended.

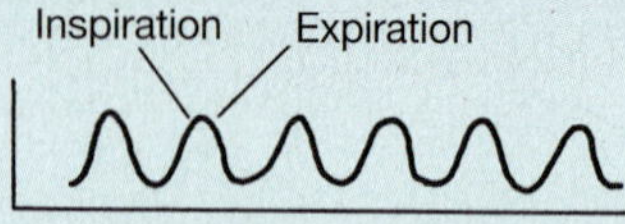

Normal

The respiratory rate is about 14–20/min in normal adults and up to 44/min in infants.

Slow Breathing (*Bradypnea*)

Slow breathing with or without an increase in tidal volume that maintains alveolar ventilation. Abnormal alveolar hypoventilation without increased tidal volume can arise from uremia, drug-induced respiratory depression, and increased intracranial pressure.

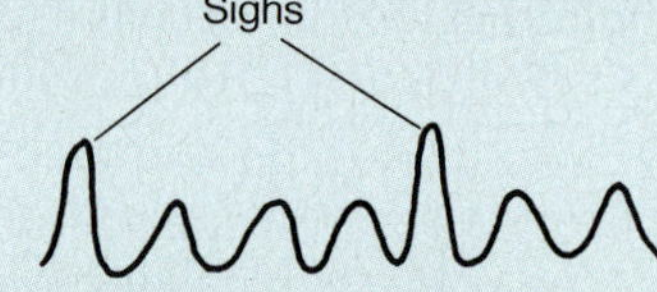

Sighing Respiration

Breathing punctuated by frequent sighs suggests *hyperventilation syndrome*—a common cause of dyspnea and dizziness. Occasional sighs are normal.

Rapid Shallow Breathing (*Tachypnea*)

Rapid shallow breathing has numerous causes, including salicylate intoxication, restrictive lung disease, pleuritic chest pain, and an elevated diaphragm.

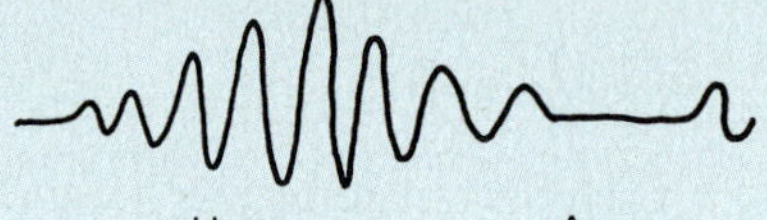

Cheyne–Stokes Breathing

Periods of deep breathing alternate with periods of *apnea* (no breathing). This pattern is normal in children and older adults during sleep. Causes include heart failure, uremia, drug-induced respiratory depression, and brain injury (typically bihemispheric).

Prolonged expiration

Obstructive Breathing

In obstructive lung disease, expiration is prolonged due to narrowed airways increase the resistance to air flow. Causes include asthma, chronic bronchitis, and chronic obstructive pulmonary disease.

Rapid Deep Breathing (*Hyperpnea, Hyperventilation*)

In *hyperpnea,* rapid deep breathing occurs in response to metabolic demand from causes such as exercise, high altitude, sepsis, and anemia. In *hyperventilation,* this pattern is independent of metabolic demand, except in respiratory acidosis. Lightheadedness and tingling may arise from decreased CO_2 concentration. In the comatose patient, consider hypoxia, or hypoglycemia affecting the midbrain or pons. *Kussmaul breathing* is compensatory overbreathing due to systemic acidosis. The breathing rate may be fast, normal, or slow.

Ataxic Breathing (*Biot Breathing*)

Breathing is irregular—periods of apnea alternate with regular deep breaths that stop suddenly for short intervals. Causes include meningitis, respiratory depression, and brain injury, typically at the medullary level.

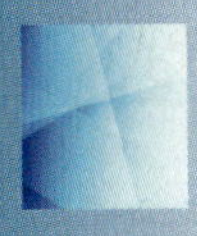

TABLE 17-6. Deformities of the Thorax

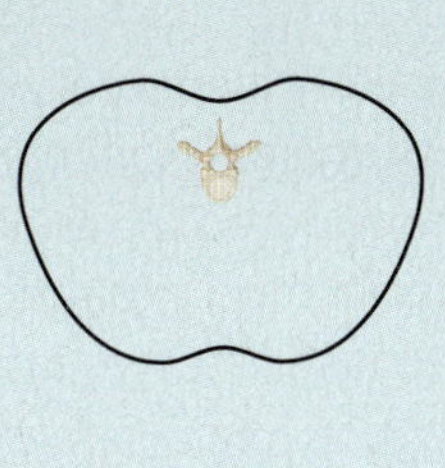

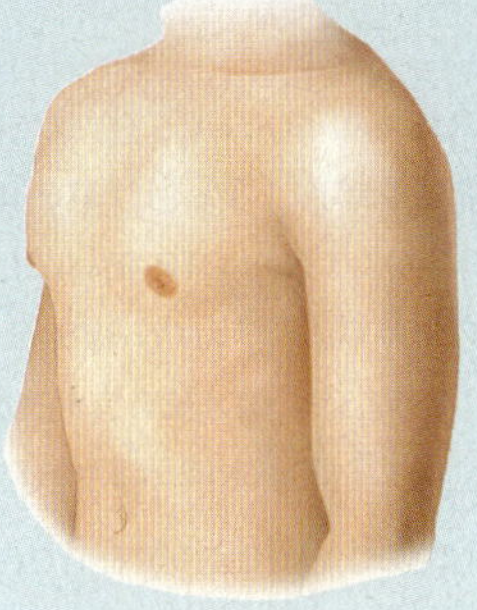

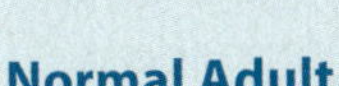

Normal Adult

The lateral diameter of the thorax in the normal adult is greater than its anteroposterior (AP) diameter. The ratio of its AP diameter to the lateral diameter is normally 0.7 up to 0.9 and increases with aging.[68]

Funnel Chest (*Pectus Excavatum*)

Note depression in the lower portion of the sternum. Compression of the heart and great vessels may cause murmurs.

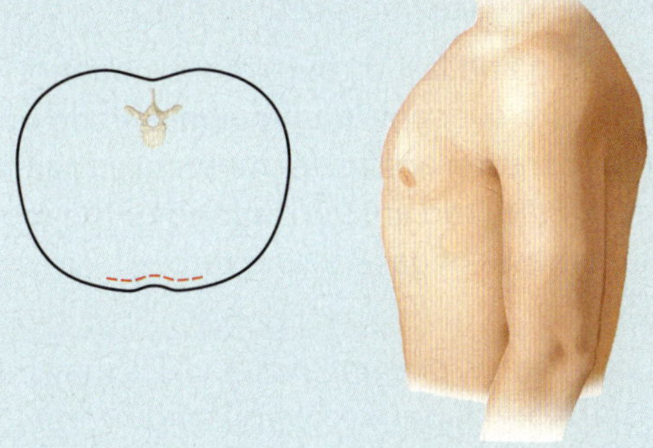

Barrel Chest

AP diameter is increased. This shape is normal during infancy, and often accompanies aging and chronic obstructive pulmonary disease.

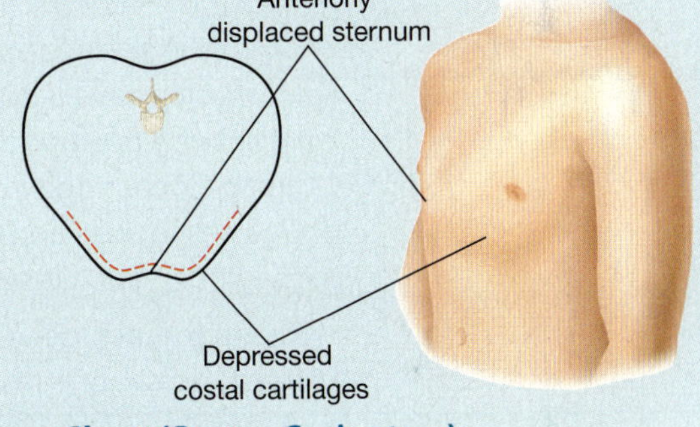

Pigeon Chest (*Pectus Carinatum*)

The sternum is displaced anteriorly, increasing the AP diameter. The costal cartilages adjacent to the protruding sternum are depressed.

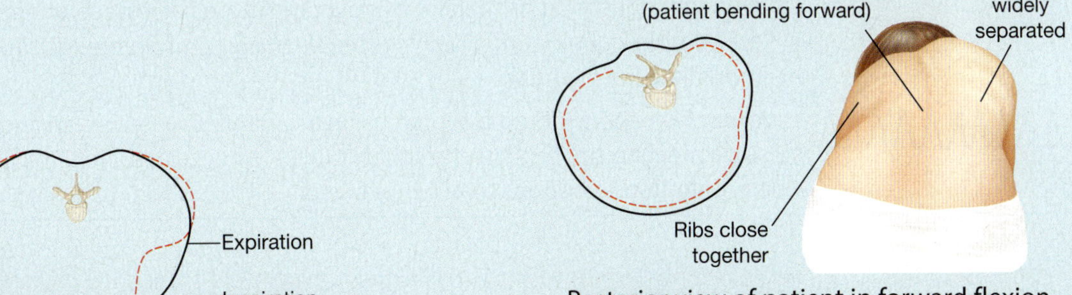

Traumatic Flail Chest

Multiple rib fractures may result in paradoxical movements of the thorax. As descent of the diaphragm decreases intrathoracic pressure, on inspiration, the injured area caves inward; on expiration, it moves outward.

Posterior view of patient in forward flexion.

Thoracic Kyphoscoliosis

Abnormal spinal curvatures and vertebral rotation deform the chest. Distortion of the underlying lungs may make interpretation of lung findings very difficult.

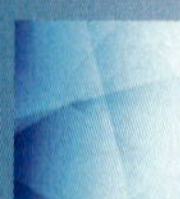

TABLE 17-7. Adventitious (Added) Lung Sounds: Causes and Qualities[1–4,69]

Sound	Causes and Qualities
Crackles	**Crackles** are discontinuous nonmusical sounds that can be early inspiratory (as in *chronic obstructive pulmonary disease [COPD]*), late inspiratory (as in *pulmonary fibrosis*), or biphasic (as in *pneumonia*). They are currently considered to result from a series of tiny explosions when small distal airways, deflated during expiration, pop open during inspiration. With few exceptions, recent acoustic studies indicate that the role of secretions as a cause of crackles is less likely.[1,32]
	Fine crackles are softer, higher pitched, and more frequent per breath than coarse crackles. They are heard from *mid to late inspiration*, especially in the dependent areas of the lung, and change according to body position. They have a shorter duration and higher frequency than coarse crackles. Fine crackles appear to be generated by the "sudden inspiratory opening of small airways held closed by surface forces during the previous expiration."[1] Examples include *pulmonary fibrosis* (known for "Velcro® rales") and interstitial lung diseases such as *interstitial fibrosis* and *interstitial pneumonitis*.
	Coarse crackles appear in early inspiration and last throughout expiration (*biphasic*), have a popping sound, are heard over any lung region, and do not vary with body position. They have a longer duration and lower frequency than fine crackles, change or disappear with coughing, and are transmitted to the mouth. Coarse crackles appear to result from "boluses of gas passing through airways as they open and close intermittently."[1] Examples include *COPD, asthma, bronchiectasis, pneumonia* (crackles may become finer and change from mid to late inspiratory during recovery), and *heart failure*.
Wheezes and Rhonchi	***Wheezes*** are continuous musical sounds that occur during rapid airflow when bronchial airways are narrowed almost to the point of closure. Wheezes can be inspiratory, expiratory, or biphasic. They may be localized, due to a foreign body, mucous plug, or tumor, or heard throughout the lung. Although wheezes are typical of asthma, they can occur in a number of pulmonary diseases. Recent studies suggest that as the airways become more narrowed, wheezes become less audible, culminating finally in "*the silent chest*" of severe asthma requiring immediate intervention.
	Rhonchi are considered by some to be a variant of wheezes, arising from the same mechanism, but lower in pitch. Unlike wheezes, rhonchi may disappear with coughing, so secretions may be involved.[1]

Sound	Causes and Qualities
Stridor	***Stridor*** is a continuous, high-frequency, high-pitched musical sound produced during airflow through a narrowing in the upper respiratory tract. Stridor is best heard over the neck during inspiration but can be biphasic. Causes of the underlying airway obstruction include tracheal stenosis from intubation, airway edema after device removal, epiglottitis, foreign body, and anaphylaxis. Immediate intervention is warranted.
Pleural Rub	A ***pleural rub*** is a discontinuous, low-frequency, grating sound that arises from inflammation and roughening of the visceral pleura as it slides against the parietal pleura. This nonmusical sound is biphasic, heard during inspiration and expiration, and often best heard in the axilla and base of the lungs.
Mediastinal Crunch (*Hamman Sign*)	A ***mediastinal crunch*** is a series of precordial crackles synchronous with the heartbeat, not with respiration. Best heard in the left lateral position, it arises from air entry into the mediastinum causing mediastinal emphysema (*pneumomediastinum*). It usually produces severe central chest pain and may be spontaneous. It has been reported in cases of tracheobronchial injury, blunt trauma, pulmonary disease, use of recreational drugs, childbirth, and rapid ascent from scuba diving.[1]

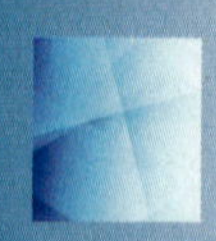

TABLE 17-8. Physical Findings in Selected Chest Disorders

The red boxes in this table provide a framework for the clinical assessment of common chest disorders. Start with the three boxes under percussion. Note resonant, dull, and hyper-resonant. Then move from each of these to other boxes that emphasize some of the key differences among various conditions. The changes described vary with the extent and severity of the disorder. Abnormalities deep in the chest usually produce fewer signs than superficial ones and may cause no signs at all. Use the table for the direction of typical changes, not for absolute distinctions.

Condition	Percussion Note	Trachea	Breath Sounds	Adventitious Sounds	Tactile Fremitus and Transmitted Voice Sounds
Normal Tracheobronchial tree and alveoli are open; pleurae are thin and close together; mobility of the chest wall is unimpaired	**Resonant**	Midline	Vesicular, except perhaps bronchovesicular and bronchial sounds over the large bronchi and trachea, respectively	None, except a few transient inspiratory crackles at the bases of the lungs	Normal
Left-Sided Heart Failure Increased pressure in the pulmonary veins causes congestion and interstitial edema (around the alveoli); bronchial mucosa may become edematous	**Resonant**	Midline	Vesicular (normal)	Late inspiratory crackles in the dependent portions of the lungs; possibly wheezes	Normal
Chronic Bronchitis Bronchi are chronically inflamed, and a productive cough is present. Airway obstruction may develop	**Resonant**	Midline	Vesicular (normal)	None; possible scattered coarse crackles in early inspiration and expiration; possible wheezes or rhonchi	Normal
Lobar Pneumonia (*Consolidation*) Alveoli fill with fluid, as in pneumonia	**Dull** over the airless area	Midline	Bronchial over the involved area	Late inspiratory crackles over the involved area	Increased over the involved area, with egophony, bronchophony, and whispered pectoriloquy

Condition	Percussion Note	Trachea	Breath Sounds	Adventitious Sounds	Tactile Fremitus and Transmitted Voice Sounds
Partial Lobar Obstruction (*Atelectasis*) When a plug (from mucus or a foreign object) obstructs bronchial air flow, affected alveoli collapse and become airless	**Dull** over the airless area	May be shifted toward involved side	Usually absent when bronchial plug persists; exceptions include right upper lobe atelectasis, where adjacent tracheal sounds may be transmitted	None	Usually absent when the bronchial plug persists; right upper lobe may be increased in atelectasis
Pleural Effusion Fluid accumulates in the pleural space and separates the air-filled lung from the chest wall, blocking the transmission of breath sounds	**Dull** to flat over the fluid	Shifted toward the unaffected side in a large effusion	Decreased to absent; bronchial breath sounds may be heard near top of large effusion	None, except a possible pleural rub	Decreased to absent, but may be increased toward the top of a large effusion
Pneumothorax When air leaks into the pleural space, usually unilaterally, the lung recoils away from the chest wall. Pleural air blocks sound transmission	**Hyper-resonant** or tympanitic over the pleural air	Shifted toward the unaffected side if tension pneumothorax	Decreased to absent over the pleural air	None, except a possible pleural rub	Decreased to absent over the pleural air
Chronic Obstructive Pulmonary Disease (COPD) Slowly progressive disorder in which the distal air spaces enlarge and lungs become hyperinflated. Chronic bronchitis may precede or follow the development of COPD	Diffusely **hyper-resonant**	Midline	Decreased to absent, with delayed expiration	None, or the crackles, wheezes, and rhonchi of associated chronic bronchitis	Decreased
Asthma Widespread, usually reversible, airflow obstruction with bronchial hyper-responsiveness and underlying inflammation. During attacks, as air flow decreases, the lungs hyperinflate	**Resonant** to diffusely **hyper-resonant**	Midline	Often obscured by wheezes	Wheezes, possibly crackles	Decreased

REFERENCES

1. Bohadana A, Izbicki G, Kraman SS. Fundamentals of lung auscultation. *N Engl J Med.* 2014;370(8):744–751.
2. Loudon R, Murphy RL Jr. Lung sounds. *Am Rev Respir Dis.* 1984;130(4):663–673.
3. Bohadana AB, Coimbra FT, Santiago JR. Detection of lung abnormalities by auscultatory percussion: a comparative study with conventional percussion. *Respiration.* 1986;50(3): 218–225.
4. Bohadana AB. Lung sounds in asthma and chronic obstructive pulmonary disease. *Monaldi Arch Chest Dis.* 2000;55(6): 484–487.
5. Parshall MB, Schwartzstein RM, Adams L, et al; American Thoracic Society Committee on Dyspnea. An official American Thoracic Society statement: update on the mechanisms, assessment, and management of dyspnea. *Am J Respir Crit Care Med.* 2012;185(4):435–452.
6. Agustí A, Anzueto A, Celli BR, Mortimer K, Salvi S, Vogelmeier CF; GOLD Scientific Committee. GOLD 2023 Executive Summary: responses from the GOLD Scientific Committee. *Eur Respir J.* 2023;61(6):2300616.
7. Smith JA, Woodcock A. Chronic cough. *N Engl J Med.* 2016; 375(16):1544–1551.
8. Wunderink RG, Waterer GW. Clinical practice. Community-acquired pneumonia. *N Engl J Med.* 2014;370(6):543–551.
9. Bel EH. Clinical practice. Mild asthma. *N Engl J Med.* 2013; 369(6):549–557.
10. Braman SS. Chronic cough due to acute bronchitis: ACCP evidence-based clinical practice guidelines. *Chest.* 2006; 129(1 Suppl):95S–103S.
11. Chung KF, McGarvey L, Song WJ, et al. Cough hypersensitivity and chronic cough. *Nat Rev Dis Primers.* 2022;8(1):45.
12. Gibson PG, McDonald VM, Marks GB. Asthma in older adults. *Lancet.* 2010;376(9743):803–813.
13. Morice AH, Millqvist E, Bieksiene K, et al. ERS guidelines on the diagnosis and treatment of chronic cough in adults and children. *Eur Respir J.* 2020;55(1):1901136.
14. Metlay JP, Waterer GW, Long AC, et al. Diagnosis and treatment of adults with community-acquired pneumonia. An official Clinical Practice Guideline of the American Thoracic Society and Infectious Diseases Society of America. *Am J Respir Crit Care Med.* 2019;200(7):e45–e67.
15. McCracken JL, Veeranki SP, Ameredes BT, Calhoun WJ. Diagnosis and management of asthma in adults: a review. *JAMA.* 2017;318(3):279–290.
16. Celli BR, Wedzicha JA. Update on clinical aspects of chronic obstructive pulmonary disease. *N Engl J Med.* 2019;381(13): 1257–1266.
17. Gibson P, Wang G, McGarvey L, Vertigan AE, Altman KW, Birring SS; CHEST Expert Cough Panel. Treatment of unexplained chronic cough: CHEST Guideline and Expert Panel Report. *Chest.* 2016;149(1):27–44.
18. Gulati M, Levy PD, Mukherjee D, et al. 2021 AHA/ACC/ASE/CHEST/SAEM/SCCT/SCMR guideline for the evaluation and diagnosis of chest pain: a report of the American College of Cardiology/American Heart Association Joint Committee on clinical practice guidelines. *J Am Coll Cardiol.* 2021;78(22):e187–e285.
19. Davidson K, Shojaee S. Managing massive hemoptysis. *Chest.* 2020;157(1):77–88.
20. McGee SR. Chapter 26: inspection of the chest. In: *Evidence-Based Physical Diagnosis.* 3rd ed. Elsevier/Saunders; 2012: 233–234.
21. Gottlieb DJ, Punjabi NM. Diagnosis and management of obstructive sleep apnea: a review. *JAMA.* 2020;323(14): 1389–1400.
22. McGee SR. Chapter 27: palpation and percussion of the chest. In: *Evidence-Based Physical Diagnosis.* 3rd ed. Elsevier/Saunders;2012:240.
23. Feller-Kopman D, Light R. Pleural disease. *N Engl J Med.* 2018;378(18):1754.
24. McGee SR. Chapter 27: palpation and percussion of the chest. In: *Evidence-Based Physical Diagnosis.* 3rd ed. Elsevier/Saunders; 2012:248.
25. Nath AR, Capel LH. Lung crackles in bronchiectasis. *Thorax.* 1980;35(9):694–699.
26. Wong CL, Holroyd-Leduc J, Straus SE. Does this patient have a pleural effusion? *JAMA.* 2009;301(3):309–317.
27. Bohadana A, Izbicki G, Kraman SS. Fundamentals of lung auscultation. *N Engl J Med.* 2014;370(21):2053.
28. Epler GR, Carrington CB, Gaensler EA. Crackles (rales) in the interstitial pulmonary diseases. *Chest.* 1978;73(3):333–339.
29. Nath AR, Capel LH. Inspiratory crackles and mechanical events of breathing. *Thorax.* 1974;29(6):695–698.
30. Qaseem A, Wilt TJ, Weinberger SE, et al; American College of Physicians; American College of Chest Physicians; American Thoracic Society; European Respiratory Society. Diagnosis and management of stable chronic obstructive pulmonary disease: a clinical practice guideline update from the American College of Physicians, American College of Chest Physicians, American Thoracic Society, and European Respiratory Society. *Ann Intern Med.* 2011;155(3):179–191.
31. Holland AE, Cox NS, Houchen-Wolloff L, et al. Defining modern pulmonary rehabilitation. An official American Thoracic Society Workshop report. *Ann Am Thorac Soc.* 2021; 18(5):e12–e29.
32. McGee SR. Chapter 30: pneumonia. In: *Evidence-Based Physical Diagnosis.* 3rd ed. Elsevier/Saunders; 2012:272.
33. Lichtenstein D. Lung ultrasound in the critically ill. *Curr Opin Crit Care.* 2014;20(3):315–322.
34. Demi L, Wolfram F, Klersy C, et al. New international guidelines and consensus on the use of lung ultrasound. *J Ultrasound Med.* 2023;42(2):309–344.
35. Pereira ROL, Convissar DL, Montgomery S, et al. Point-of-care lung ultrasound in adults: image acquisition. *J Vis Exp.* 2023;(193).
36. Chiu L, Jairam MP, Chow R, et al. Erratum to 'Meta-analysis of point-of-care lung ultrasonography versus chest radiography in adults with symptoms of acute decompensated heart failure' The American Journal of Cardiology Volume 174, 1 July 2022, Pages 89–95. *Am J Cardiol.* 2022;180:173.
37. Chiu L, Jairam MP, Chow R, et al. Meta-analysis of point-of-care lung ultrasonography versus chest radiography in adults with symptoms of acute decompensated heart failure. *Am J Cardiol.* 2022;174:89–95.
38. Noble VE, Nelson BP. *Manual of Emergency and Critical Care Ultrasound.* 2nd ed. Cambridge University Press; 2011.
39. Eckel RH, Jakicic JM, Ard JD, et al; American College of Cardiology/American Heart Association Task Force on Practice Guidelines. 2013 AHA/ACC guideline on lifestyle management to reduce cardiovascular risk: a report of the American College of Cardiology/American Heart Association

Task Force on Practice Guidelines. *Circulation*. 2014;129(25 Suppl 2):S76–S99.

40. Siegel RL, Miller KD, Wagle NS, Jemal A. Cancer statistics, 2023. *CA Cancer J Clin*. 2023;73(1):17–48.
41. Surveillance Research Program. SEER*Explorer: an interactive website for SEER cancer statistics. National Cancer Institute. Updated July 31, 2023. Accessed October 26, 2023. https://seer.cancer.gov/statistics-network/explorer/
42. Cornelius ME, Loretan CG, Wang TW, Jamal A, Homa DM. Tobacco product use among adults – United States, 2020. *MMWR Morb Mortal Wkly Rep*. 2022;71(11):397–405.
43. Centers for Disease Control and Prevention. What are the risk factors for lung cancer? Accessed October 28, 2023. https://www.cdc.gov/cancer/lung/basic_info/risk_factors.htm
44. Manser R, Lethaby A, Irving LB, et al. Screening for lung cancer. *Cochrane Database Syst Rev*. 2013;2013(6): CD001991.
45. National Lung Screening Trial Research Team; Aberle DR, Adams AM, Berg CD, et al. Reduced lung-cancer mortality with low-dose computed tomographic screening. *N Engl J Med*. 2011;365(5):395–409.
46. de Koning HJ, van der Aalst CM, de Jong PA, et al. Reduced lung-cancer mortality with volume CT screening in a randomized trial. *N Engl J Med*. 2020;382(6):503–513.
47. U. S. Preventive Services Task Force; Krist AH, Davidson KW, Mangione CM, et al. Screening for lung cancer: US Preventive Services Task Force recommendation statement. *JAMA*. 2021;325(10):962–970.
48. World Health Organization. Global Tuberculosis Report 2022. 2022. https://iris.who.int/bitstream/handle/10665/363752/9789240061729-eng.pdf?sequence=1
49. Jonas DE, Riley SR, Lee LC, et al. Screening for latent tuberculosis infection in adults: updated evidence report and systematic review for the US Preventive Services Task Force. *JAMA*. 2023;329(17):1495–1509.
50. U. S. Preventive Services Task Force, Mangione CM, Barry MJ, Nicholson WK, et al. Screening for latent tuberculosis infection in adults: US Preventive Services Task Force recommendation statement. *JAMA*. 2023;329(17):1487–1494.
51. Patel SR. Obstructive sleep apnea. *Ann Intern Med*. 2019; 171(11):ITC81–ITC96.
52. Dodds S, Williams LJ, Roguski A, et al. Mortality and morbidity in obstructive sleep apnoea-hypopnoea syndrome: results from a 30-year prospective cohort study. *ERJ Open Res*. 2020; 6(3):00057–2020.
53. U. S. Preventive Services Task Force; Mangione CM, Barry MJ, Cabana M, et al. Screening for obstructive sleep apnea in adults: US Preventive Services Task Force recommendation statement. *JAMA*. 2022;328(19):1945–1950.
54. Johns MW. A new method for measuring daytime sleepiness: the Epworth sleepiness scale. *Sleep*. 1991;14(6):540–545.
55. Johns MW. Polysomnography at a sleep disorders unit in Melbourne. *Med J Aust*. 1991;155(5):303–308.
56. Qaseem A, Dallas P, Owens DK, et al; Clinical Guidelines Committee of the American College of Physicians. Diagnosis of obstructive sleep apnea in adults: a clinical practice guideline from the American College of Physicians. *Ann Intern Med*. 2014;161(3):210–220.
57. Aurora RN, Quan SF. Quality measure for screening for adult obstructive sleep apnea by primary care physicians. *J Clin Sleep Med*. 2016;12(8):1185–1187.
58. Chung F, Subramanyam R, Liao P, Sasaki E, Shapiro C, Sun Y. High STOP-Bang score indicates a high probability of obstructive sleep apnoea. *Br J Anaesth*. 2012;108(5):768–775.
59. Nagappa M, Liao P, Wong J, et al. Validation of the STOP-Bang Questionnaire as a screening tool for obstructive sleep apnea among different populations: a systematic review and meta-analysis. *PLoS One*. 2015;10(12):e0143697.
60. Katerndahl DA. Chest pain and its importance in patients with panic disorder: an updated literature review. *Prim Care Companion J Clin Psychiatry*. 2008;10(5):376–383.
61. Hamel S, Denis I, Turcotte S, et al. Anxiety disorders in patients with noncardiac chest pain: association with health-related quality of life and chest pain severity. *Health Qual Life Outcomes*. 2022;20(1):7.
62. Abrams J. Clinical practice. Chronic stable angina. *N Engl J Med*. 2005;352(24):2524–2533.
63. Demiryoguran NS, Karcioglu O, Topacoglu H, et al. Anxiety disorder in patients with non-specific chest pain in the emergency setting. *Emerg Med J*. 2006;23(2):99–102.
64. Fletcher KC, Goutte M, Slaughter JC, Garrett CG, Vaezi MF. Significance and degree of reflux in patients with primary extraesophageal symptoms. *Laryngoscope*. 2011;121(12): 2561–2565.
65. Goldman L, Kirtane AJ. Triage of patients with acute chest pain and possible cardiac ischemia: the elusive search for diagnostic perfection. *Ann Intern Med*. 2003;139(12):987–995.
66. Huffman JC, Pollack MH, Stern TA. Panic disorder and chest pain: mechanisms, morbidity, and management. *Prim Care Companion J Clin Psychiatry*. 2002;4(2):54–62.
67. McConaghy JR, Oza RS. Outpatient diagnosis of acute chest pain in adults. *Am Fam Physician*. 2013;87(3):177–182.
68. Kahwati LC, Feltner C, Halpern M, et al. Primary care screening and treatment for latent tuberculosis infection in adults: evidence report and systematic review for the US Preventive Services Task Force. *JAMA*. 2016;316(9):970–983.
69. Bohadana AB, Kanga JF, Kraman SS. Does airway closure affect lung sound generation? *Clin Physiol*. 1988;8(4):341–349.

CHAPTER 18

Cardiovascular System

ANATOMY AND PHYSIOLOGY

Mediastinum, Heart, and Great Vessels

The *mediastinum* is a compartment located centrally in the thoracic cavity, bordered by the lungs on either side, the sternum anteriorly, and the thoracic vertebral bodies posteriorly. It houses several vital structures, including the heart and its great vessels, esophagus, trachea, thoracic duct, and lymph nodes.

To thoroughly understand the anterior chest and underlying cardiac structures, you must consider not only the exterior margins but also the internal anatomy of the heart. The *right ventricle* (*RV*) occupies the most anterior aspect of the heart and, in conjunction with the pulmonary artery, forms a structure that is wedge-shaped, sitting just behind and to the left of the sternum, as depicted in Figure 18-1.

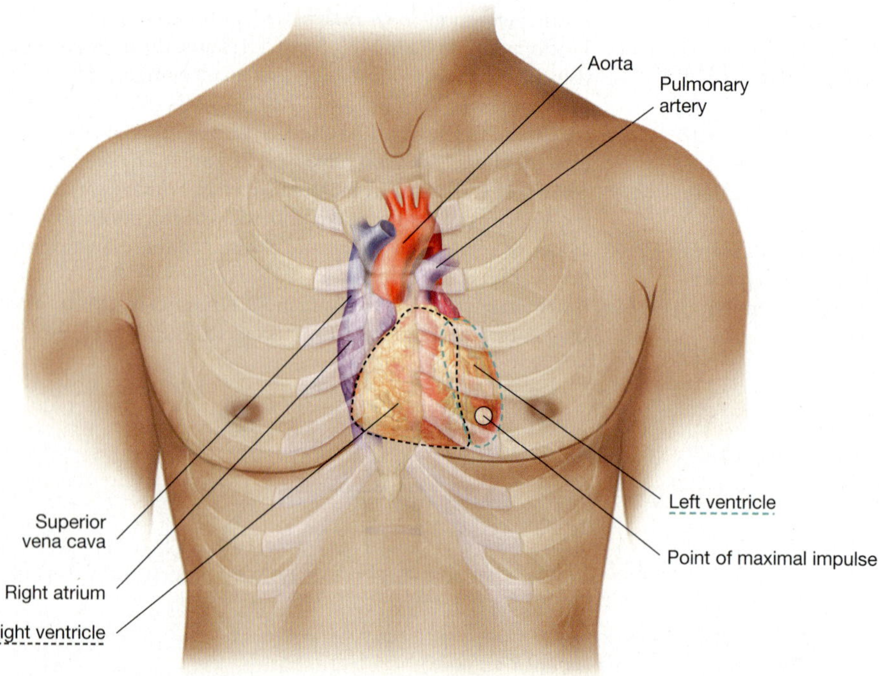

FIGURE 18-1. Major cardiac structures as visualized through the chest wall.

Internally, the heart's RV is separated from the left ventricle (LV) by the *interventricular septum*, a thick muscular wall (Fig. 18-2). The *tricuspid valve*, located between the right atrium (RA) and RV, manages blood flow between these chambers. Within the RV, the *papillary muscles* and *chordae tendineae* play critical roles in valve function during the cardiac cycle. The *pulmonic valve*, situated at the exit of the RV, controls blood flow into the pulmonary artery and lungs. The *LV*, nestled behind the RV and toward the left, establishes the heart's left lateral contour. Deep within the LV, the *mitral valve* regulates the flow from the left atrium, ensuring efficient passage into the ventricle. The intricate network of the LV's internal musculature contributes to its powerful contractions, propelling blood through the *aortic valve* into the systemic circulation. The *cardiac apex*, part of the LV, is crucial in clinical examinations for its role in generating the *apical impulse*.

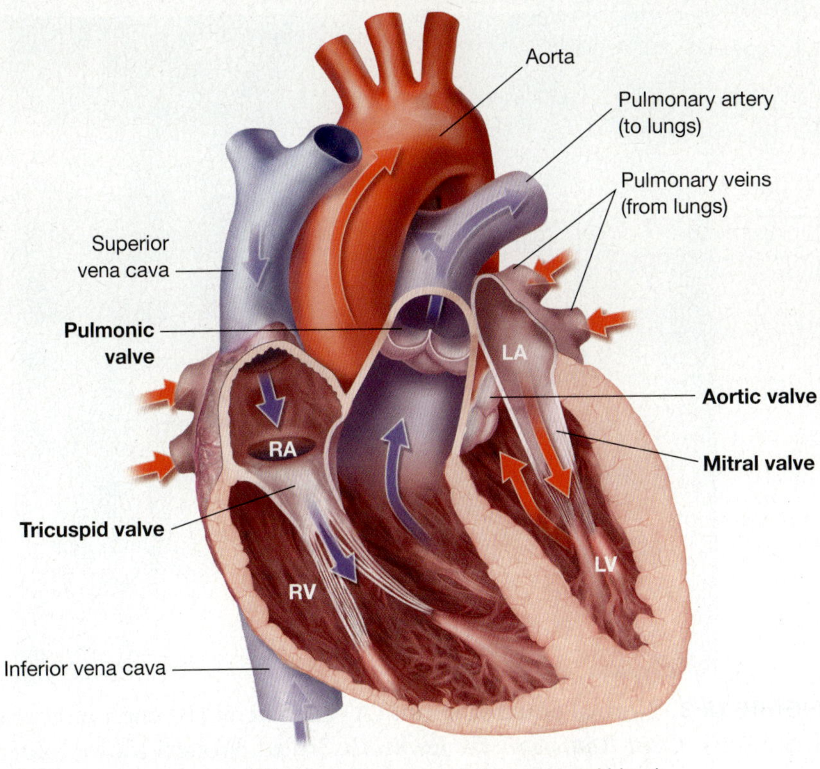

FIGURE 18-2. Cardiac chambers, valves, and circulation. RA, right atrium; LA, left atrium; RV, right ventricle; LV, left ventricle.

On palpation of the precordium, the apical impulse, felt at the *point of maximal impulse* (*PMI*), is normally detected in the fifth intercostal space, medially or just medial to the midclavicular line. The PMI delineates the left heart border and typically measures about 1 to 2.5 cm in diameter in supine patients.

The heart's internal structures, such as the atria located above the ventricles, contribute to the complete *cardiac silhouette*. The *left atrium* receives oxygenated blood from the *pulmonary veins* and serves as a reservoir before blood enters the LV. The *RA* receives deoxygenated blood from the systemic circulation and channels it into the RV.

The great vessels are located above the heart and mark the course of arterial outflow. The *pulmonary artery* quickly divides into its left and right branches transporting blood to the lungs. The *aorta* originates from the LV, arches upward to the level of the sternal angle, and then bends posteriorly to the left and downward. The *superior and inferior venae cavae* are located on the medial border and drain venous blood from the upper and lower parts of the body into the RA.

Additionally, familiarize yourself with the appearance of the heart and great vessels in a chest radiograph (Figs. 18-3 and 18-4), as this can aid in describing the location of any pathologic processes.

Conduction System

The contraction of the cardiac muscle is stimulated and coordinated by an electrical conduction system. Normally, this system starts with an electrical impulse from the *sinus node*, a group of specialized cells in the RA near the vena cava junction. The sinus node acts as the *pacemaker*, generating impulses that occur anywhere from 60 to 100 times a minute.

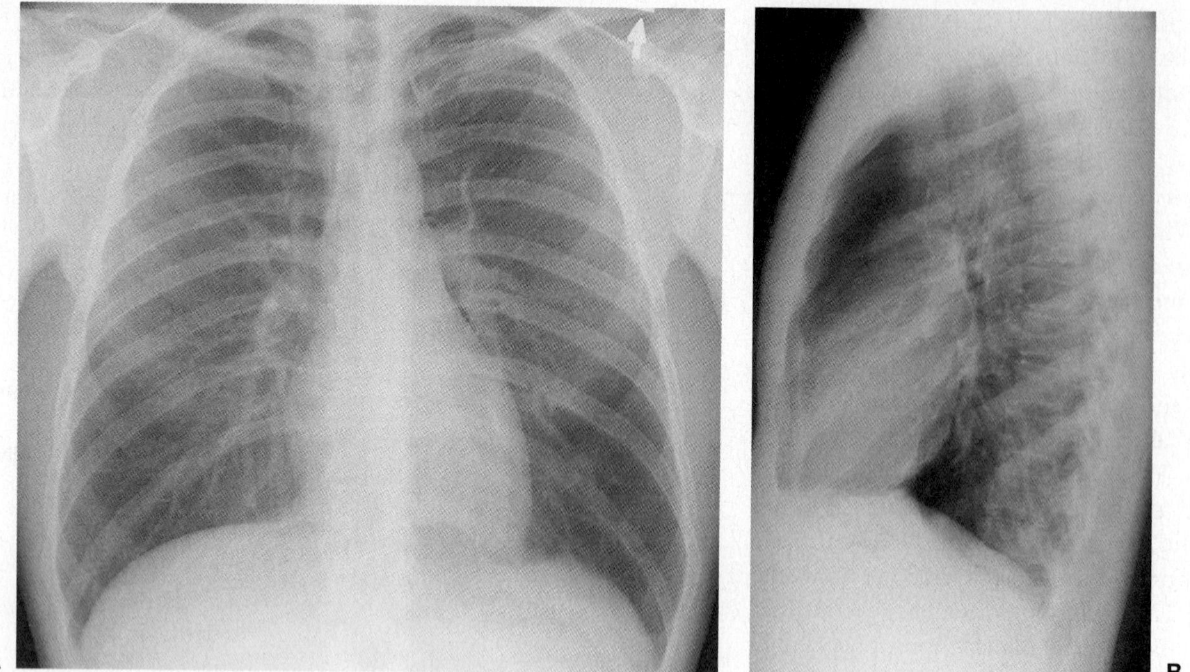

FIGURE 18-3. Normal posteroanterior (**A**) and lateral (**B**) chest radiographs. (Reprinted with permission from Collins J, Stern EJ. *Chest Radiology: The Essentials.* 3rd ed. Wolters Kluwer; 2015. Figure 1-2A-B.)

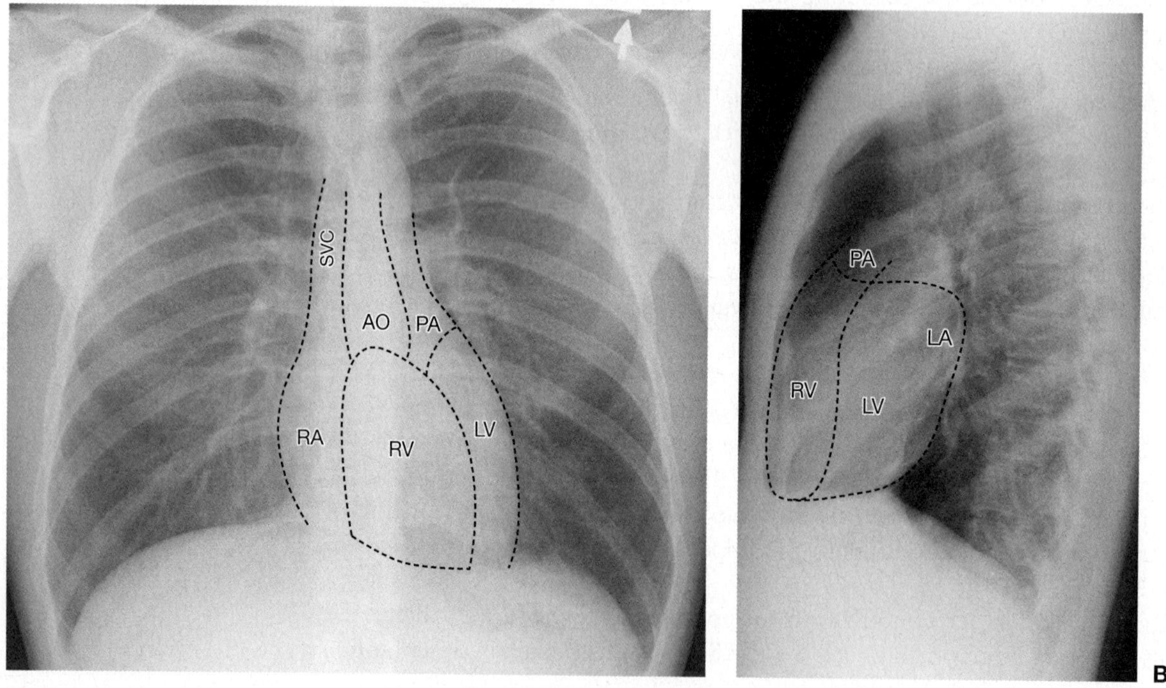

FIGURE 18-4. Normal posteroanterior (**A**) and lateral (**B**) chest radiographs with cardiac chambers and great vessels outlined. AO, aorta; LA, left atrium; LV, left ventricle; PA, pulmonary artery; RA, right atrium; RV, right ventricle; SVC, superior vena cava. (Modified with permission from Collins J, Stern EJ. *Chest Radiology: The Essentials.* 3rd ed. Wolters Kluwer; 2015. Figure 1-2A-B.)

From there, the impulse travels through both atria to the *atrioventricular* (*AV*) *node*, a group of cells located low in the atrial septum, where it is delayed before continuing down the bundle of His and its branches to the ventricular myocardium. The atria contract first, followed by the ventricles. Figure 18-5 depicts the normal conduction system in a simplified form. This electrical activity produces waves on an *electrocardiogram* (ECG). Note that interpreting ECG recordings from patients requires further instruction and considerable practice.

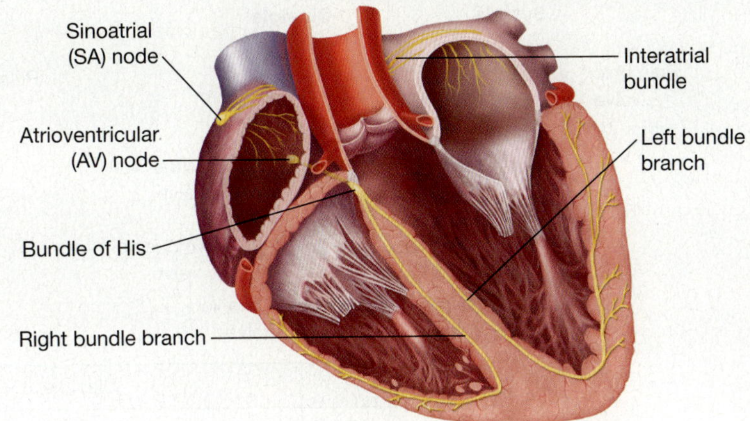

FIGURE 18-5. Cardiac conduction system.

Heart as a Pump

The LV and RV pump blood into the systemic and pulmonary arterial trees, respectively. *Cardiac output*, the volume of blood ejected from each ventricle in 1 minute, is the product of heart rate and stroke volume. *Stroke volume* is the volume of blood ejected with each heartbeat, and it is dependent on preload, myocardial contractility, and afterload. The *ejection fraction* (*EF*) is the percentage of ventricular volume ejected during each heartbeat and is normally 60%.

The heart's ability to function efficiently as a pump hinges on intricate interactions among various physiologic parameters. These dynamics—*preload*, *myocardial contractility*, and *afterload*—operate synchronously, dictating the heart's performance. Breaking down these components provides a comprehensive understanding of cardiac mechanics, their physiologic effects, and clinical implications (Box 18-1).

Box 18-1. Components Defining the Heart's Mechanical Efficiency

Feature	Definition	Influencing Factors	Physiologic Effects
Preload	Initial stretching of the cardiac muscle fibers prior to contraction	■ Venous return to the right heart ■ Inspiration increasing venous flow ■ Enhanced blood flow from exercising muscles ■ Conditions like heart failure affecting fluid volume	Influences end-diastolic volume and filling pressure in the ventricles
Myocardial Contractility	Cardiac muscle's intrinsic ability to contract forcefully at a given preload	■ Stimulation by the sympathetic nervous system ■ Adequacy of blood flow and oxygen delivery to the myocardium	Affects strength and velocity of myocardial fiber shortening during systole
Afterload	Resistance the ventricles face when ejecting blood during systole	■ Vascular tone in the aorta and peripheral arteries ■ Blood volume and pressure already present in the aorta	Dictates the pressure against which the heart must work to eject blood

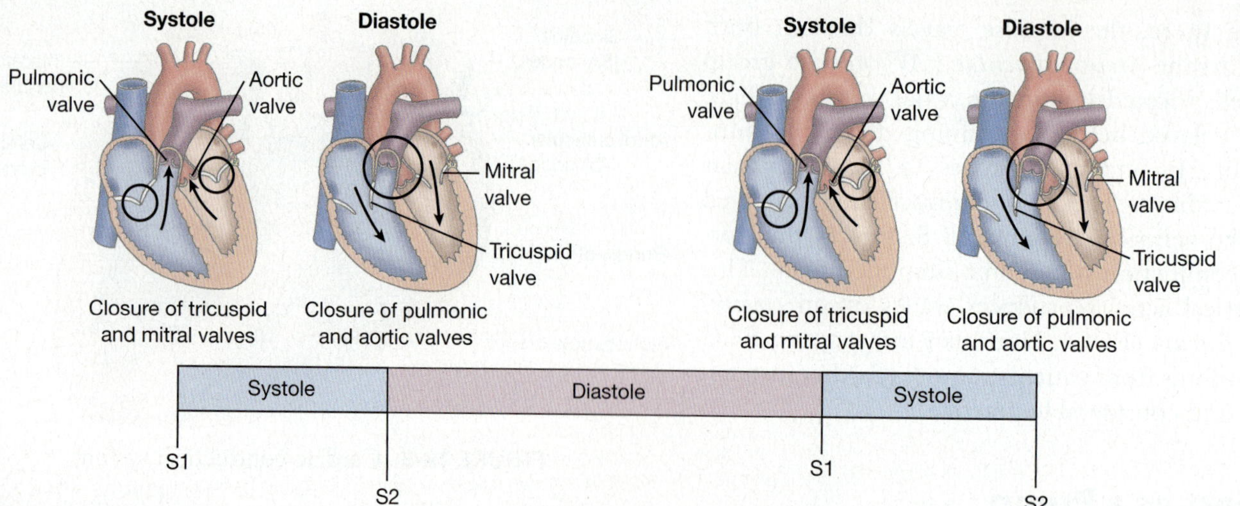

FIGURE 18-6. Cardiac cycle, direction of blood flow. (Modified with permission from Jensen S. *Nursing Health Assessment: A Best Practice Approach.* 3rd ed. Wolters Kluwer; 2019. Figure 17-8.)

Cardiac Circulation

Figure 18-6 depicts blood circulation through the heart, delineating the complex interplay between various cardiac structures. Pay particular attention to the orientation and function of the heart's chambers and valves, and the directionality of blood flow.

At the core of the heart's structure lie the *AV valves*: the *mitral valve* on the left side and the *tricuspid valve* on the right. These valves serve as critical conduits, regulating blood flow from the atria to the ventricles. Their unique design ensures that blood moves in a forward direction while preventing any backflow during ventricular contraction. The closure of these valves marks the generation of the first heart sound, S_1.

The *semilunar valves*, comprising the *aortic valve* and the *pulmonic valve* and named for their crescent-shaped cusps, are strategically positioned at the juncture where blood exits the heart. The aortic valve regulates the flow from the LV into the aorta, ushering oxygen-rich blood to the systemic circulation. Similarly, the pulmonic valve controls the passage of blood from the RV into the pulmonary arteries, directing oxygen-depleted blood to the lungs for oxygenation. These valves close at the end of ventricular contraction, and their closure is associated with the second heart sound, S_2.

Understanding the roles and locations of these valves is integral to grasping how the heart functions as an efficient pump, maintaining a unidirectional flow of blood (Box 18-2).

Box 18-2. Chest Wall Location and Origin of Valve Sounds and Murmurs

Typical Origin	Chest Wall Location
Aortic valve	Right second intercostal space
Pulmonic valve	Left second and third intercostal spaces close to the sternum
Tricuspid valve	Left fourth intercostal space at or near the lower left sternal border
Mitral valve	Left fifth intercostal space at the midclavicular line at and around the cardiac apex

Cardiac Cycle

The *cardiac cycle* is a complex process that involves the synchronized interaction of the heart's structural components and its electrical conduction system, resulting in the rhythmic contraction and relaxation of the myocardium: *systole* and *diastole*. *Systole* is the period of ventricular contraction; the heart muscle contracts and pumps blood from the chambers into the arteries. During systole, the LV ejects blood into the aorta, while the aortic valve is open, and the mitral valve is closed to prevent blood from regurgitating back into the left atrium.

As the ventricle ejects most of its blood into the aorta, the pressure levels off and starts to fall, and blood flows from the atrium to the ventricle. This period of ventricular relaxation is called diastole. In *diastole*, the heart muscle relaxes and allows the chambers to fill with blood, following the contraction phase. During this phase, the aortic valve is closed, preventing regurgitation of blood from the aorta back into the LV, and the mitral valve is open, allowing blood to flow from the left atrium into the relaxed LV. Late in diastole, ventricular pressure rises slightly during inflow of blood from atrial contraction.

In addition to the LV and aorta, the cardiac cycle also involves the RV and pulmonary artery. During systole, the pulmonic valve opens, and the tricuspid valve closes as blood is ejected from the RV into the pulmonary artery. During diastole, the pulmonic valve closes, and the tricuspid valve opens as blood flows into the relaxed RV. As the heart valves close, vibrations from the leaflets, adjacent cardiac structures, and the flow of blood create S_1 and S_2.

Although the cardiac cycle is a complex sequence of events, starting at the point in diastole when the heart is relaxed and the chambers are being filled with blood, right after the closure of the aortic and pulmonic valves, aids your ability to visualize and understand its dynamic phases. Box 18-3 provides a step-by-step overview.

Arterial Pulses and Blood Pressure

With every heartbeat, the LV propels a volume of blood into the aorta, initiating a pressure wave that travels rapidly through the arterial tree and can be detected as a pulse. While this pressure wave moves much faster than the actual blood flow, there is a noticeable lag between the contraction of the ventricle and the palpable pulse in peripheral limbs. This lag makes arm and leg pulses less reliable for precise timing of events within the cardiac cycle.

The difference between the highest arterial pressure during systole and the lowest pressure during diastole is known as the *pulse pressure*. This measurement reflects the force the heart generates each time it contracts and is directly influenced by stroke volume and arterial compliance. For example, if a blood pressure (BP) reading is 120/80 mm Hg, the pulse pressure is 40 mm Hg (120 – 80). A typical pulse pressure is usually between 30 and 40 mm Hg and can be influenced by a host of physiologic factors.

An elevated pulse pressure may indicate arterial stiffness and could be a risk factor for cardiovascular events. In contrast, a narrow pulse pressure might suggest a reduced stroke volume, as seen in heart failure or hypovolemia.

BP in the arterial system varies during the cardiac cycle, peaking in systole and falling to its lowest trough in diastole. These are the pressure levels that are measured with a BP monitor, or *sphygmomanometer*. These values are not

Box 18-3. Cardiac Cycle Phases and Corresponding Heart Sounds

Isovolumetric relaxation: The cycle often starts here, just after systole, when the left ventricle (LV) and right ventricle (RV) are relaxing, and both the aortic and pulmonary valves have just closed, leading to the **second heart sound (S_2)**. At this point, all four valves are closed, and there is no change in the volume of blood within the ventricles (isovolumetric).

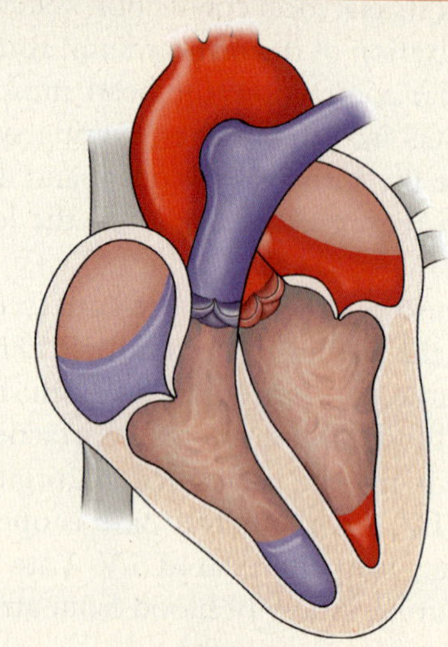

Early diastole: As the ventricles relax, the pressure within them drops. Once the LV pressure falls below that of the left atrium (LA), the mitral valve opens, allowing blood to flow passively into the LV from the LA.

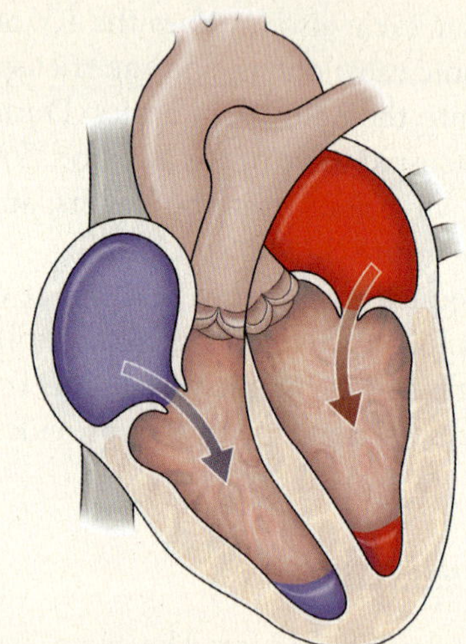

Rapid ventricular filling: Blood pours rapidly into the LV from the LA, and this phase may be accompanied by the **third heart sound (S_3)** in conditions of high cardiac output or heart failure.

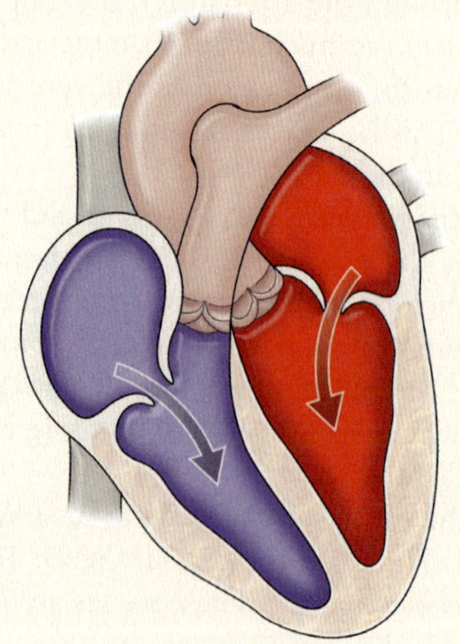

Atrial contraction: The atria contract, pushing the remaining blood into the ventricles. This "atrial kick" can contribute to the **fourth heart sound (S_4)**, especially in the setting of decreased ventricular compliance.

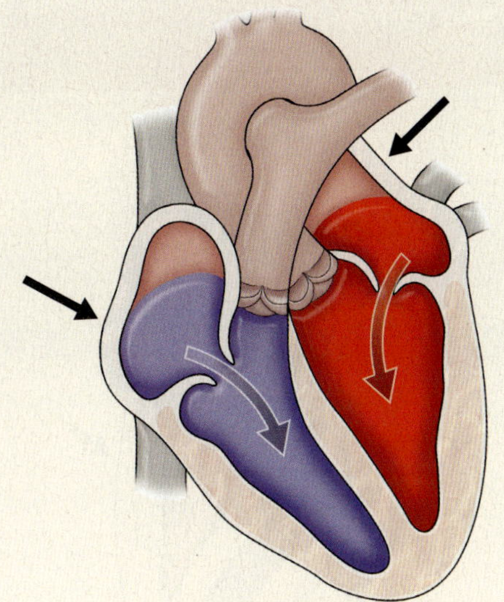

Systole begins: The ventricles start contracting. The pressure in the LV rises and exceeds that in the LA, causing the mitral valve to close and contributing to the **first heart sound (S_1)**.

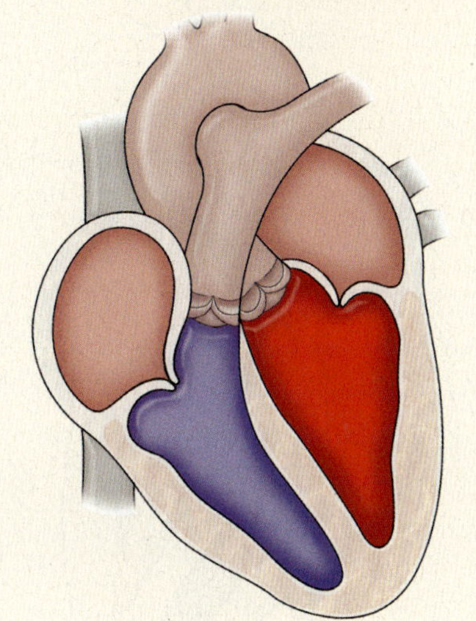

Isovolumetric contraction: All valves are closed. The LV pressure increases until it exceeds the pressure in the aorta, but no blood is ejected yet because the aortic valve is still closed.

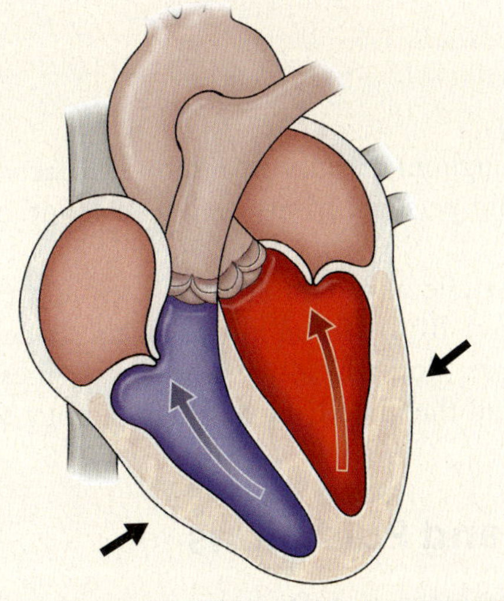

(*continued*)

Box 18-3. Cardiac Cycle Phases and Corresponding Heart Sounds (*Continued*)

Ventricular ejection: Following the isovolumetric contraction phase, the aortic valve opens, and the LV ejects blood into the aorta.

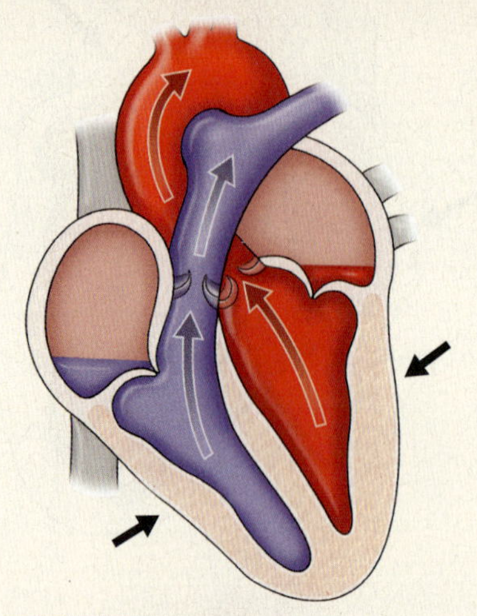

Isovolumetric relaxation: Once the ejection is complete, the LV pressure falls below the aortic pressure, causing the aortic valve to close, leading again to the **second heart sound (S_2)**, signaling the end of systole and the beginning of the next cardiac cycle.

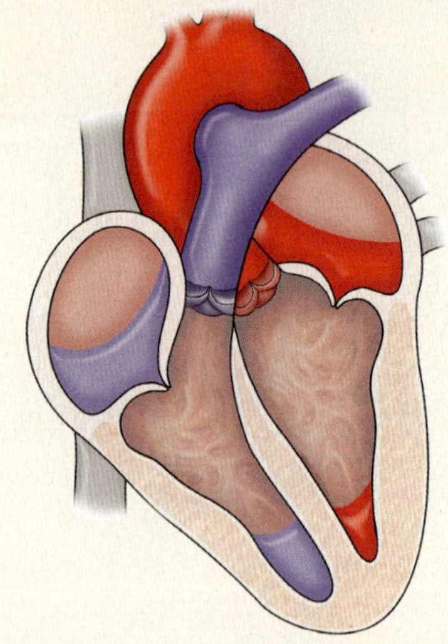

static; they are dynamic, changing throughout the day in response to activity, emotions, environmental factors, and personal habits such as caffeine or tobacco use.

Recognizing how the nuances of systolic and diastolic pressures as well as the significance of pulse pressure affect BP is critical in the diagnosis and management of cardiovascular conditions. You will learn to integrate these measurements with patient symptoms and the underlying pathophysiology to develop appropriate treatment strategies.

Jugular Venous Pressure and Pulsations

The jugular veins provide an important index of right heart pressures and cardiac function. Jugular venous pressure (JVP) reflects right atrial pressure, which, in turn, equals central venous pressure and right ventricular end-diastolic pressure. The JVP is best estimated from the right internal jugular vein, which has the most direct channel into the RA. Because the jugular veins

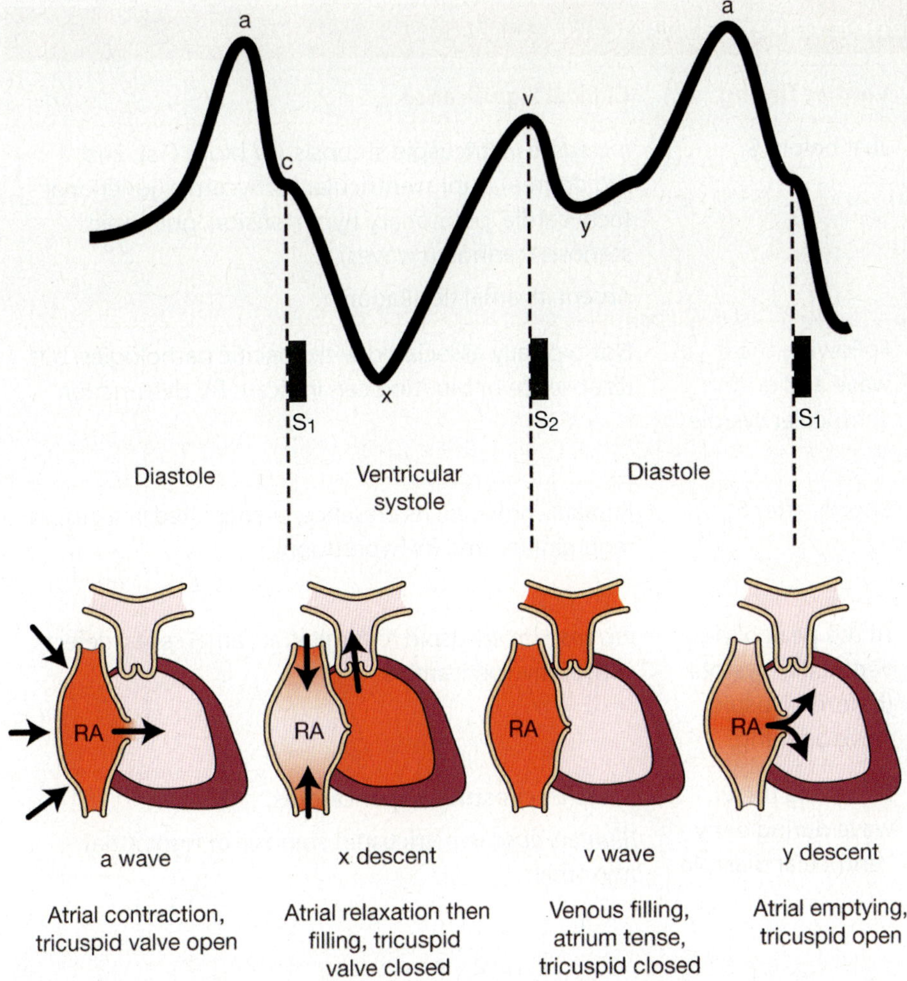

FIGURE 18-7. Jugular venous pulsations and corresponding wave patterns caused by changing pressures in the right atrium during diastole and systole.

lie deep to the sternocleidomastoid (SCM) muscles, learn to identify the pulsations they transmit to the surface of the neck, briefly described below, and measure their highest point of oscillation.

During the cardiac cycle, changing pressures in the RA lead to oscillations of filling and emptying in the jugular veins, which are known as *jugular venous pulsations* (as shown in Fig. 18-7 and Box 18-4). Atrial contraction causes an *a wave* in the jugular veins just before S_1, while systole is caused by retrograde blood flow into the neck veins. This is followed by the *x descent*, which occurs due to continued atrial relaxation. As the right atrial pressure begins to rise with inflow from the vena cava during RV systole, there is a second elevation known as the *v wave*. This is followed by the *y descent* as blood passively empties from the RA into the RV during early and mid-diastole.

See pp. 492–495 for more detailed discussion of the JVP and techniques for its examination.

Relation of Cardiac Findings to the Chest Wall

As you familiarize yourself with auscultatory findings, including heart sounds and murmurs, you must understand the chest wall locations where these sounds are best heard. This knowledge will assist you in pinpointing the specific valves or chambers from which they originate (see Box 18-2 and Figure 18-8).

Box 18-4. Jugular Venous Pulsation Waves and Descents

Wave	Associated Event	Cardiac Timing	Clinical Significance
***a* wave**	Atrial contraction	Just before S_1	*Increased in:* tricuspid stenosis, AV block (1st, 2nd, 3rd degree), supraventricular tachycardia, junctional tachycardia, pulmonary hypertension, pulmonic stenosis (cannon *a* waves) *Absent in:* atrial fibrillation
***x* descent**	Atrial relaxation and downward displacement of the tricuspid valve	Following the *a* wave and during ventricular systole	Not typically associated with specific pathologies, but its absence or blunting can indicate RV dysfunction
***c* wave**	Carotid transmission or closure of the tricuspid valve[1]	Shortly after S_1	Primarily noted for its presence; exaggerated in tricuspid regurgitation and RV hypertrophy
***v* wave**	Venous filling of the right atrium	At the peak of right ventricular systole (before tricuspid valve opening)	*Increased in:* tricuspid regurgitation, atrial septal defects, constrictive pericarditis
***y* descent**	Opening of the tricuspid valve and RV filling	Following the *v* wave during early ventricular diastole	*Sharp in:* constrictive pericarditis. *Blunted/absent in:* tricuspid stenosis or right atrial myxoma

Identify the anatomical location of cardiac findings in terms of intercostal spaces and the distance of the PMI from the midclavicular line. The midclavicular line correlates with LV pathology, as long as the midpoint between the acromioclavicular and sternoclavicular joints is carefully identified.[2]

The regions where heart sounds and murmurs can be auscultated often intersect, as depicted in Figure 18-8. Correlating the location of the sound or murmur with its occurrence during systole or diastole is a critical initial step in their accurate identification. This approach commonly results in precise bedside diagnoses, especially when combined with other cardiac examination findings.

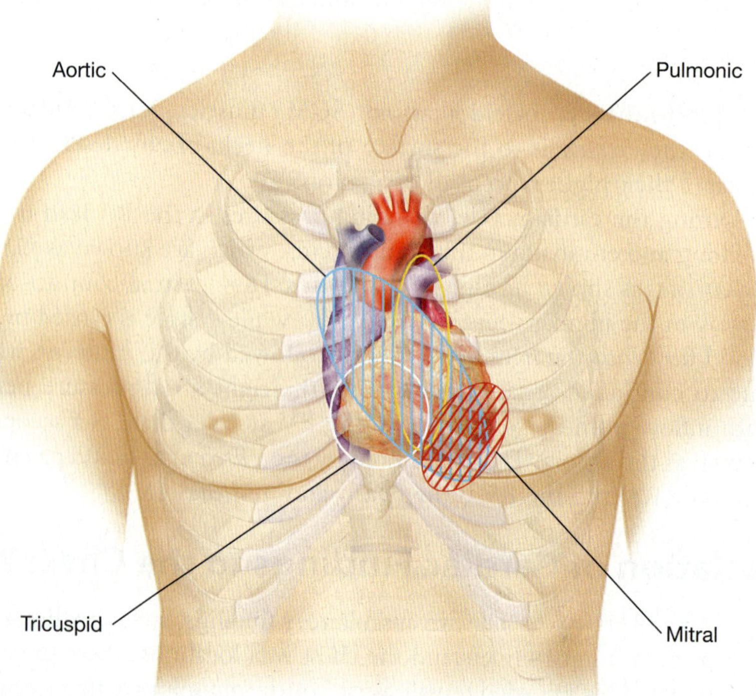

FIGURE 18-8. Precordial areas of cardiac auscultation.

Heart Sounds

The heart sounds of S_1 and S_2 emerge from the vibrations generated by the heart valves and the flow of blood, as they close during the

Box 18-5. Definitions and Locations of Cardiac Auscultation Sounds

	Definition	Timing	Best Auscultation Location
S_1	Associated with closure of atrioventricular valves (mitral and tricuspid) at the start of systole	Onset of systole	Apex of the heart, specifically the mitral area (fourth intercostal space at the midclavicular line)
S_2	Associated with closure of semilunar valves (aortic and pulmonic) at the end of systole Split S_2, with P_2 delayed after A_2, is best appreciated during inspiration	Onset of diastole	Base of the heart, aortic area (right second intercostal space at the right sternal border) for A_2 and the pulmonic area (left second intercostal space at the left sternal border) for P_2
S_3	Associated with rapid filling of the ventricles after the mitral valve opens	Early diastole	Apex of the heart, with the patient in the left lateral decubitus position to enhance detection
S_4	Associated with atrial contraction resulting in increased flow of blood into a ventricle with decreased compliance	Late diastole	Apex of the heart, near the mitral area, best heard with the patient in the left lateral decubitus position and at the end of expiration

S_3 is normal in young and pregnant individuals and suggests volume overload conditions such as heart failure in others ("**ventricular gallop**").[3,4]

S_4 is almost always pathologic in adults, indicating decreased ventricular compliance and referred to as "**atrial gallop**."[3,4]

cardiac cycle. You must understand the opening and closing of the AV and semilunar valves in correlation with cardiac events to enhance your diagnostic precision during auscultation (Box 18-5).

Timing. Identify the timing of heart sounds in relation to the cardiac cycle. Timing of sounds is often possible through auscultation alone but is aided by inspection and palpation. In most patients with normal or slow heart rates, it is easy to identify the paired heart sounds of S_1 and S_2 that mark the onset of systole and diastole. The relatively long diastolic interval after S_2 separates one pair from the next (Fig. 18-9).

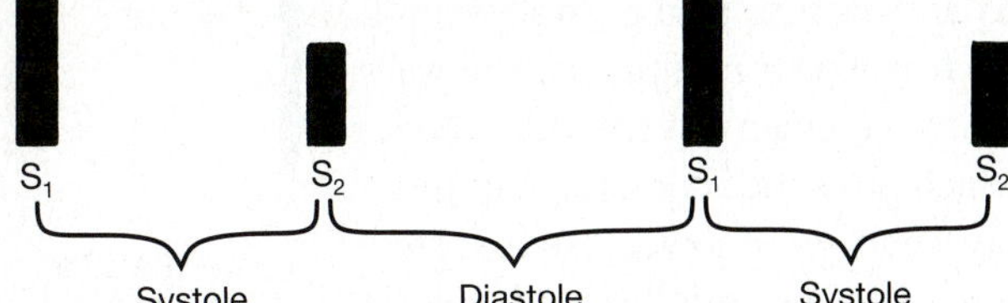

FIGURE 18-9. Diastole (S_2 to S_1) lasts longer than systole (S_1 to S_2).

Splitting of S_2. The left side involves the left atrium, mitral valve, LV, aortic valve, and aorta, and the right side involves the RA, tricuspid valve, RV, pulmonic valve, and pulmonary arteries. However, both sides generate the second heart sound (S_2), which has two components, A_2 and P_2, primarily caused by the closure of the aortic and pulmonic valves, respectively (Box 18-6). During inspiration, the right heart filling time is increased, leading to an extended right ventricular ejection period and P_2 delay, which splits S_2 into two audible components.

Box 18-6. Split Components of Heart Sounds S_1 and S_2

Heart Sound Component	Origin	Description	Best Auscultation Location
Mitral component of S_1	Mitral valve closure	Louder component of S_1, can sometimes mask the tricuspid component. Does not vary with respiration.	Apex of the heart
Tricuspid component of S_1	Tricuspid valve closure	Softer component of S_1, can be masked by the mitral component. Does not vary with respiration.	Lower left sternal border
Aortic component of S_2 (A_2)	Aortic valve closure	Louder component of S_2, reflecting the high pressure in the aorta during inspiration.	Throughout the precordium
Pulmonic component of S_2 (P_2)	Pulmonic valve closure	Softer and delayed component of S_2 during inspiration due to increased hangout time in the pulmonary vascular bed, leading to audible splitting.	Second and third left intercostal spaces close to the sternum

Conversely, during expiration, the RV ejection period is faster, and A_2 and P_2 fuse into a single sound, S_2. It is worth noting that the walls of veins contain less smooth muscle, which gives the venous system more capacitance and lower systemic pressure. The distensibility and impedance in the pulmonary vascular bed contribute to the "hangout time" that delays P_2 (Fig. 18-10).[5]

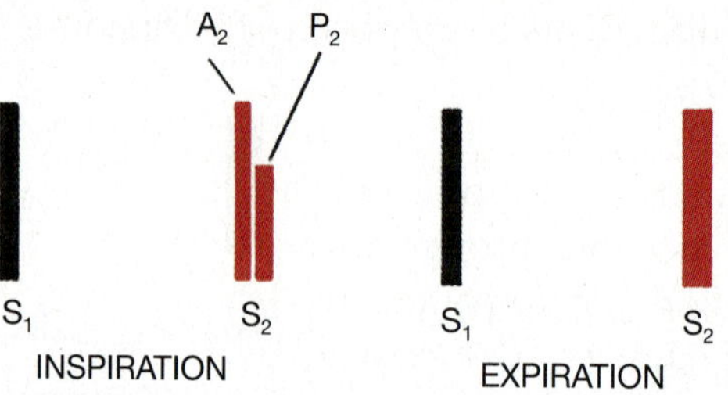

FIGURE 18-10. Splitting of S_2 during inspiration.

Splitting of S_1. S_1, heard at the beginning of systole, is also composed of two components: mitral and tricuspid sounds. The mitral component is audible throughout the precordium and is loudest at the apex of the heart. The tricuspid component is softer and is heard best at the lower left sternal border. Splitting of S_1, which is a normal finding, can be heard as the two components of S_1 are heard separately. Splitting of S_1 does not vary with respiration.

Heart Murmurs

Heart murmurs are abnormal heart sounds characterized by their pitch and longer duration. They are usually caused by turbulent blood flow and indicate valvular heart disease but can also be "innocent" flow murmurs in young adults. Narrowing of a valve orifice, such as in aortic stenosis, causes a characteristic murmur, while abnormal valve closure can result in regurgitation, allowing blood to leak backward, producing a regurgitant murmur.

To accurately identify murmurs, learn where they are best heard on the chest wall (see Box 18-2); their timing in systole or diastole; and their descriptive qualities, such as shape, maximal intensity, direction of radiation, grade of intensity, pitch, and quality. These factors can be integrated during examination to better understand and diagnose the underlying condition (see pp. 503–510).

HEALTH HISTORY: GENERAL APPROACH

Common or Concerning Symptoms

- Chest pain
- Palpitations
- Shortness of breath
- Swelling (*edema*)
- Fainting (*syncope*)

For chest symptoms, be systematic as you think through the range of possible cardiac and pulmonary etiologies as well as those outside the thoracic cavity. *This section approaches chest symptoms from a cardiac standpoint.*

For noncardiac causes of chest pain, review the Health History section of Chapter 17, Thorax and Lungs, pp. 429–431.

Chest Pain

Chest pain is one of the most serious of all patient symptoms and accounts for 1% of primary care outpatient visits.[6] It is the most common symptom of coronary heart disease (CHD), which affects more than 15 million Americans aged 20 years and older.[7] In 2009, approximately 683,000 patients were hospitalized with an acute coronary syndrome (ASD), and, at present, the 1-year mortality for patients who present with an ST-elevation ASD is an estimated 7% to 18%.[8] Classic exertional pain; pressure; or discomfort in the chest, shoulder, back, neck, or arm in angina pectoris is seen in 18% of patients with acute myocardial infarction (MI)[7]; atypical descriptors also are common, such as cramping; grinding; pricking; or, rarely, tooth or jaw pain.[9] To accurately diagnose and treat chest pain, asking the right questions is vital (Box 18-7).

Possible causes include **ACS** (reduced blood flow to the heart, leading to myocardial ischemia or infarction), **stable angina** (reduced blood flow to the heart due to partial blockage of coronary arteries), **aortic stenosis** (narrowing of the aortic valve, restricting blood flow from the heart to the body), **pericarditis** (inflammation of the pericardium, often due to infection or autoimmune disease), **gastroesophageal reflux disease** ([**GERD**] stomach acid refluxing into the esophagus, causing irritation and inflammation), and **pulmonary embolism (PE)** (blood clot in the pulmonary arteries, obstructing blood flow to the lungs).

Box 18-7. Chest Pain: High-Yield Health History Questions

Domain	Questions	Rationale
Onset	*When did your chest pain start?*	*Acute onset:* may suggest cardiovascular causes such as acute coronary syndrome (ACS) or aortic dissection *Chronic onset* may suggest underlying cardiovascular conditions such as angina or coronary artery disease (CAD)
Location	*Where is the chest pain located?*	Substernal and radiating to the left arm, neck, or jaw may suggest cardiac etiology
Quality	*How do you describe the type of pain you're experiencing?*	*Cardiac:* typically described as pressure, tightness, or squeezing *Noncardiac:* sharp, stabbing, or burning
Severity	*How severe is your chest pain?*	*Severe:* may suggest a more serious underlying condition such as ACS or aortic dissection *Mild or moderate:* may suggest stable angina or noncardiac causes.
Associated symptoms	*Do you have shortness of breath, nausea, or excessive sweating?*	Shortness of breath may indicate heart failure; nausea or diaphoresis may indicate ACS or other cardiovascular conditions
Medical history	*Do you have a history of high blood pressure, high cholesterol, or diabetes?*	These increase the risk of cardiovascular disease, including CAD and atherosclerosis

Palpitations

Palpitations involve an unpleasant awareness of the heartbeat. Patients use various terms to describe palpitations, such as skipping, racing, fluttering, pounding, and stopping of the heart. Palpitations may be irregular, rapidly slow down or accelerate, or arise from the increased forcefulness of cardiac contraction. Palpitations do not necessarily mean heart disease. Diagnosis of palpitations hinges on key questions (Box 18-8).

Possible causes include **arrhythmia** (abnormal heart rhythm due to issues with electrical conduction), **panic disorder** (sudden episodes of intense fear or anxiety), **generalized anxiety disorder** (persistent, excessive worry and fear about everyday situations), and **hyperthyroidism** (overproduction of thyroid hormones, leading to an increased metabolic rate).

See Table 18-1, Selected Heart Rates and Rhythms, and Table 18-2, Selected Irregular Rhythms (pp. 522–523).

Box 18-8. Palpitations: High-Yield Health History Questions

Domain	Questions	Rationale
Onset	*When did you first experience palpitations?*	*Acute onset:* may suggest arrhythmia or other underlying cardiovascular conditions such as pulmonary embolism or thyrotoxicosis *Chronic:* may suggest benign conditions such as anxiety or mitral valve prolapse
Frequency	*How often do you experience palpitations?*	*Intermittent:* may suggest arrhythmia *Persistent:* may suggest underlying conditions such as anxiety or hyperthyroidism
Duration	*How long do your palpitations last?*	More than a few seconds may suggest arrhythmia; brief palpitations may suggest benign conditions such as anxiety
Triggers	*Do certain activities or events trigger your palpitations?*	*Physical activity:* may suggest underlying cardiovascular conditions such as hypertrophic cardiomyopathy *Emotional stress:* may suggest anxiety or panic disorder
Associated symptoms	*Do you experience chest pain, dizziness, or syncope?*	Chest pain or pressure may suggest angina or MI; dizziness or syncope may suggest bradycardia, tachycardia, or other arrhythmias
Medical history	*Do you have a history of heart problems or issues with your thyroid?*	These increase the risk of arrhythmia and other underlying cardiovascular conditions

Shortness of Breath

Shortness of breath is a common patient concern that can represent dyspnea, orthopnea, or paroxysmal nocturnal dyspnea (PND). *Dyspnea* is an uncomfortable awareness of breathing that is inappropriate for a given level of exertion. This is common in patients with cardiac or pulmonary problems. *Orthopnea* is dyspnea that occurs when the patient is supine and improves when the patient sits up. Classically, it is quantified by the number of pillows the patient uses for sleeping, or by the fact that the patient needs to sleep sitting up. Nighttime episodes of sudden dyspnea that awakens the patient usually 1 or 2 hours after falling sleep is *paroxysmal nocturnal dyspnea (PND)*. See Box 18-9.

Possible cardiac causes include **congestive heart failure** (**[CHF]** inability of the heart to pump blood effectively, leading to fluid build-up), **coronary artery disease** (**[CAD]** narrowing or blockage of coronary arteries, reducing blood flow to the heart), **cardiomyopathy** (diseases of the heart muscle affecting structure and function), **valvular heart disease** (dysfunction of one or more heart valves), **atrial fibrillation** (rapid, irregular heartbeats due to disorganized atrial electrical activity), and **pulmonary hypertension** (high BP in the arteries supplying the lungs).

See Table 17-2, Dyspnea, pp. 456–459, in Chapter 17, Thorax and Lungs.

Box 18-9. Shortness of Breath: High-Yield Health History Questions

Domain	Questions	Rationale
Onset	*When did you first experience shortness of breath?*	*Acute onset:* may suggest underlying conditions such as acute heart failure or pulmonary embolism (PE) *Chronic:* may suggest underlying conditions such as chronic heart failure or valvular heart disease
Quality	*Can you describe the type of shortness of breath you have?*	Sudden, severe, and associated with chest pain or pressure may suggest underlying acute conditions such as acute coronary syndrome or PE
Triggers	*Do certain activities or events trigger your shortness of breath?*	*Physical activity:* may suggest underlying conditions such as chronic heart failure *Emotional stress:* may suggest anxiety or panic disorder
Associated symptoms	*Do you experience chest pain or pressure, palpitations, or edema?*	Chest pain or pressure may suggest underlying CAD; palpitations may suggest arrhythmia; edema may suggest heart failure or venous insufficiency
Medical history	*Do you have a history of heart problems or high blood pressure?*	These increase the risk of underlying cardiovascular conditions such as heart failure or CAD
Medications	*Are you taking any medications for your heart or blood pressure?*	Diuretics may be used to manage fluid overload in heart failure; others such as β-blockers may be used to manage hypertension or arrhythmias

Swelling (Edema)

Swelling, or *edema*, refers to the accumulation of excessive fluid in the extravascular interstitial space. Interstitial tissue can absorb up to 5 L of fluid, accommodating up to a 10% weight gain, before pitting edema appears.[10,11] Causes vary from systemic to local (Box 18-10). Consider asking patients who retain fluid to record daily morning weights because edema may not be obvious until several liters of extra fluid have accumulated; however, rapid weight gain (>1 to 2 lb/day) will occur prior to visible edema.

Possible cardiac causes include **left-sided heart failure** (impaired LV function, leading to fluid build-up in the lungs), **right-sided heart failure** (impaired RV function, causing fluid accumulation in peripheral tissues), **cor pulmonale** (right-sided heart enlargement and dysfunction from increased pressure in pulmonary arteries), **chronic obstructive pulmonary disease** ([**COPD**] chronic inflammatory lung disease causing airflow limitation), **hypoalbuminemia** (low blood albumin levels causing fluid leakage into tissues), and **dependent edema** (fluid accumulation in the lower extremities due to gravity and venous insufficiency).

Box 18-10. Swelling: High-Yield Health History Questions

Domain	Questions	Rationale
Onset	*When did you first notice the swelling or edema?*	*Acute onset:* may suggest underlying conditions such as acute heart failure or venous thromboembolism *Chronic:* may suggest underlying conditions such as chronic heart failure or venous insufficiency
Location	*Where is the swelling or edema located?*	*Bilateral and involving the lower extremities:* may suggest underlying cardiovascular conditions such as chronic heart failure or venous insufficiency *Unilateral:* can be related to cardiovascular issues though less common
Severity	*How severe is the swelling or edema?*	*Severe:* may suggest underlying conditions such as acute heart failure or deep vein thrombosis *Mild or moderate:* may suggest underlying chronic conditions such as chronic heart failure or venous insufficiency
Associated symptoms	*Do you experience shortness of breath, fatigue, or chest pain?*	Shortness of breath may suggest heart failure or pulmonary hypertension; fatigue may suggest anemia or heart failure; chest pain may suggest underlying CAD
Medical history	*Do you have a history of heart problems or high blood pressure?*	These increase the risk of underlying cardiovascular conditions such as heart failure or CAD
Medications	*Are you taking any medications for your heart or blood pressure?*	Diuretics may be used to manage fluid overload in heart failure; other medications such as calcium-channel blockers may be used to manage hypertension or peripheral edema

Fainting (Syncope)

Syncope, a temporary loss of consciousness, can arise from multiple etiologies, both cardiac and noncardiac. While often benign, fainting may signal serious cardiac issues, such as arrhythmias, structural heart defects, or vascular disorders that impair cerebral perfusion. Careful elicitation of the patient's health history through targeted questions can reveal the potential cardiac origins of syncope and guide further diagnostic evaluation and management (Box 18-11).

Cardiac-related causes include **arrhythmias** (abnormal heart rhythms, either too fast or too slow, which can compromise blood flow to the brain), **structural heart disease** (conditions such as hypertrophic cardiomyopathy or aortic stenosis, in which the heart's structure impedes normal blood flow), **cardiac ischemia** (reduced blood supply to the heart muscle, often due to CAD, which can lead to transient loss of consciousness), **valvular heart disease**, and **cardiac tamponade** (fluid accumulation around the heart, limiting its ability to pump efficiently).

See Chapter 27, Nervous System, pp. 915–916, and see Table 27-6, Syncope and Similar Disorders, pp. 976–977 for discussion of the symptoms and causes of cardiac and noncardiogenic syncope.

Box 18-11. Syncope: High-Yield Health History Questions

Domain	Questions	Rationale
Timing	*Can you describe what happened before, during, and after you passed out?*	Typically occurs without warning and is often preceded by symptoms such as palpitations, chest pain, or shortness of breath; the episode itself is often brief, with rapid recovery upon return to consciousness
Prodrome	*Did you experience anything unusual before you fainted, such as palpitations or lightheadedness?*	Prodromal symptoms may suggest underlying cardiovascular conditions such as arrhythmia or heart failure; palpitations or chest pain may suggest underlying coronary artery disease; lightheadedness or dizziness may suggest hypotension or arrhythmia
Past medical history	*Do you have a history of heart problems or a history of irregular heartbeats?*	These increase the risk of underlying cardiovascular causes of syncope
Family history	*Does anyone in your family have a history of heart problems or sudden death?*	Family history may suggest an inherited arrhythmia syndrome such as long QT syndrome
Medications	*Are you taking any medications that may affect your heart or blood pressure?*	β-blockers or antiarrhythmics may be used to manage underlying cardiovascular conditions; antipsychotics or tricyclic antidepressants may cause arrhythmia or hypotension
Physical exam	*Did your doctor find anything unusual when they checked your heart?*	Murmur or irregular rhythm may suggest underlying cardiovascular conditions such as valvular heart disease or arrhythmia

PHYSICAL EXAMINATION: GENERAL APPROACH

Listening to the heart is considered an essential aspect of physical examination for diagnosing cardiac issues. However, due to the evolving technology and time constraints of clinical practice,[12,13] physical examination skills are declining, particularly for the cardiovascular system.[14–16] Currently, cardiac point-of-care ultrasound (POCUS) is being used to enhance the physical examination and to teach cardiac anatomy and physiology.[17]

Although auscultation is the focus of the cardiovascular examination, other parts of the physical examination provide important information about whether the heart is adequately supplying blood to the rest of the body. These findings predict the presence or absence of cardiac disease, including their sensitivity, specificity, and likelihood ratios, which are provided when available. Excellent resources are available for students who need more detailed information.[18,19]

TECHNIQUES OF EXAMINATION

Key Components of the Cardiovascular Examination

- Measure blood pressure and heart rate.
- Identify jugular venous pressure.
- Auscultate for carotid bruits.
- Palpate the carotid arteries.
- Inspect the precordium.
- Palpate the precordium.
- Auscultate the precordium.
- Auscultate S_1 and S_2.
- Auscultate for splitting of heart sounds.
- Auscultate for heart murmurs.

When conducting a cardiac examination, you will typically stand on the patient's right side for the best access to the heart. However, if you are left-handed, standing on their left side may be more advantageous for using your dominant hand. Choose a position that allows for the most effective examination and ensures comfort for both you and the patient, highlighting the value of adaptability in clinical practice (Box 18-12).

Box 18-12. Sequence of Patient Positions in the Cardiac Examination

Patient Position	Examination	Accentuated Abnormal Findings
Supine, with the head elevated 30°	After examining the JVP and carotid pulse, inspect and palpate the precordium: the second right and left intercostal spaces; the RV; and the LV, including the apical impulse (diameter, location).	
Left lateral decubitus	Palpate the apical impulse to assess its diameter. Listen at the apex with the *bell* of the stethoscope.	Left lateral decubitus: low-pitched extra sounds such as an S_3, opening snap, diastolic rumble of *mitral stenosis*
Supine, with the head elevated 30°	Listen at the second right and left intercostal spaces, down the left sternal border to the fourth and fifth intercostal spaces, and across to the apex the six listening areas with the *diaphragm,* then the *bell* (see p. 501). As indicated, listen at the lower right sternal border for right-sided murmurs and sounds, often accentuated with inspiration, with the *diaphragm* and *bell.*	
Sitting, leaning forward, after full exhalation	Listen down the left sternal border and at the apex with the *diaphragm.*	Sitting, leaning forward: Soft decrescendo higher-pitched diastolic murmur of *aortic regurgitation*

Measure Blood Pressure and Heart Rate

Measure the BP and heart rate using optimal technique.[20,21] To take accurate BP and heart rate measurements, follow these steps.

First, ensure that the patient has been resting for at least 5 minutes in a quiet environment with their feet on the floor. Choose a cuff that fits correctly, and position the patient's unclothed arm at heart level, either on a table if seated, or supported at midchest level if standing or supine. The fourth intercostal space at the sternum is usually at heart level. At higher arm levels, the BP recordings will be lower; at lower levels, the BP recordings will be higher.

Make sure the bladder of the cuff is centered over the brachial artery, then inflate the cuff to around 30 mm Hg above the pressure at which the brachial or radial pulse disappears. As you deflate the cuff, listen for the Korotkoff sounds of at least two consecutive heartbeats to mark the *systolic pressure*, followed by the disappearance point of the heartbeats to mark the *diastolic pressure*.

To improve the accuracy and precision of BP measurements, obtain multiple averaged measurements, preferably through the use of automated home and ambulatory BP readings. These readings are more reliable, accurate, and have a better correlation with cardiovascular outcomes compared to clinic readings.[22,23]

For heart rate, either palpate the radial pulse using the pads of your index and middle fingers, or auscultate the apical pulse with your stethoscope.

Review Box 10-11, "ABC QUES" Mnemonic for Blood Pressure Measurement Positioning, p. 176, in Chapter 10, General Survey, Vital Signs, and Pain.

Identify Jugular Venous Pressure

The JVP closely parallels pressure in the RA, or central venous pressure, related primarily to volume in the venous system[24] and is best assessed from pulsations in the right internal jugular vein, which is directly in line with the superior vena cava and RA.[25–27]

The internal jugular veins lie deep into the SCM muscles in the neck and are not directly visible, so you must learn to identify the pulsations of the internal jugular vein transmitted to the surface of the neck (Fig. 18-11). Pulsations in the *right external jugular vein* can also be used,[28] but the route from the vena cava is more tortuous, and examination can be impaired by kinking and obstruction at the base of the neck and by obesity.[25,29] Note that the jugular veins and pulsations are difficult to see in children younger than age 12 years, so inspection is not useful in this age group.

See discussion of the double peak of the *a* and *v* waves and of the *x* and *y* descent on p. 482.

Although the JVP accurately predicts elevations in fluid volume in heart failure, its prognostic value for heart failure outcomes and mortality is unclear.[30]

Pressure changes from right atrial filling, contraction, and emptying cause fluctuations in the JVP and its waveforms that are visible to the examiner. The dominant movement of the JVP is inward, coinciding with the *x descent*.[25] In contrast, the dominant movement of the carotid pulse, often confused with the JVP, is outward. Careful observation of the fluctuations of the JVP yields clues about volume status, right and left ventricular function, patency of the tricuspid and pulmonary valves, pressures in the pericardium, and arrhythmias caused by junctional rhythms and AV blocks.

JVP falls with loss of blood or decreased venous vascular tone and increases with right or left heart failure, pulmonary hypertension, tricuspid stenosis, AV dissociation, increased venous vascular tone, and pericardial compression or tamponade.

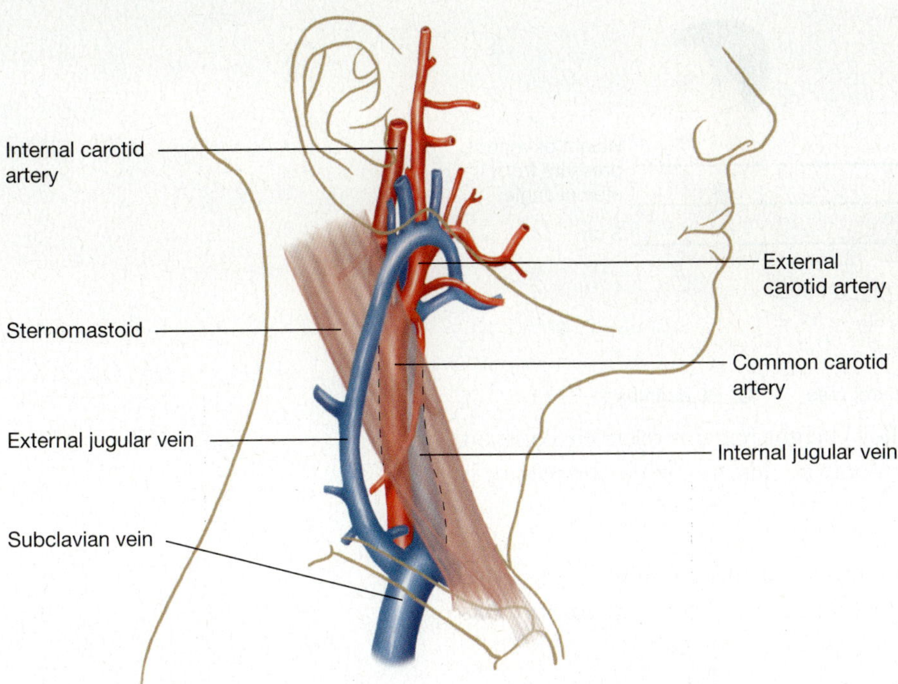

FIGURE 18-11. Internal and external jugular veins.

Estimate Jugular Venous Pressure. To estimate the level of the JVP, learn to find the *highest point of oscillation*, or *meniscus, in the internal jugular vein* or, alternatively, the point above which the external jugular vein appears collapsed.

The JVP is usually measured in vertical distance above the *sternal angle* (also called the *angle of Louis*), the bony ridge located around T4 adjacent to the second rib, where the manubrium joins the body of the sternum (Fig. 18-12).

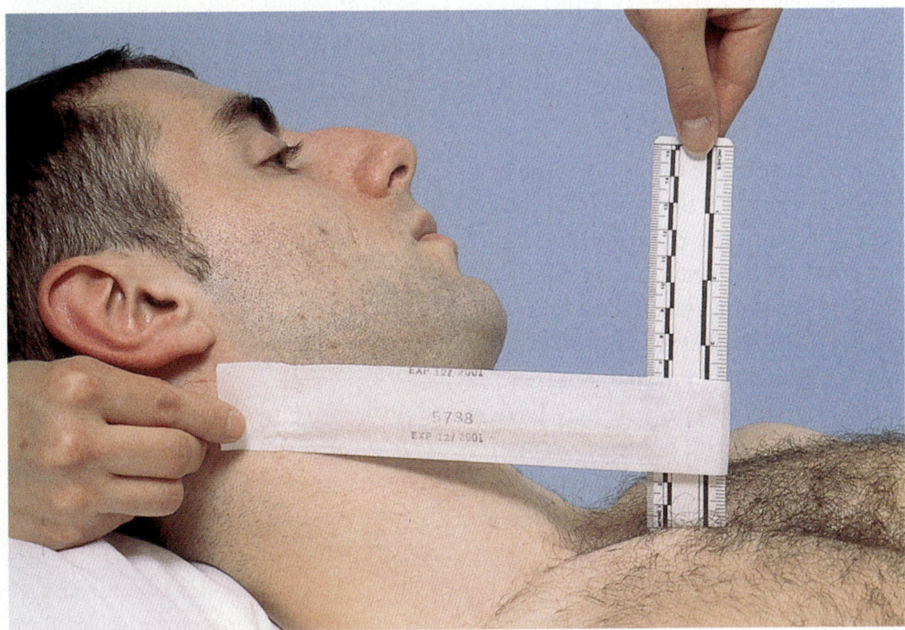

FIGURE 18-12. Measuring the jugular venous pressure with a horizontal card and vertical ruler.

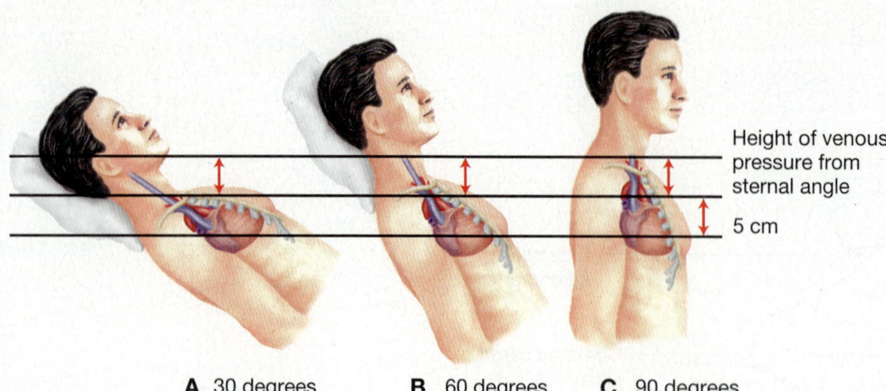

FIGURE 18-13. Jugular venous pressure (JVP) height remains relatively constant in three positions. Sometimes, the JVP can only be detected while the patient is recumbent or upright.

In Figure 18-13, note that the sternal angle remains roughly 5 cm above the right midatrium. In this patient, the pressure in the internal jugular vein is somewhat elevated.

- In Position A, the head of the bed is raised to the usual level, approximately 30°, but the JVP cannot be measured because the *level of oscillation* is above the jaw and, therefore, not visible.
- In Position B, the head of the bed is raised to 60°. The "top" of the internal jugular vein is now easily visible, so the vertical distance from the sternal angle or RA can now be measured.
- In Position C, the patient is upright, and the veins are barely discernible above the clavicle, making measurement untenable.

Note that the height of the venous pressure as measured from the sternal angle is *similar* in all three positions, but your ability to *measure* the height of the column of venous blood, or JVP, differs according to how you position the patient.

To help you learn the techniques for this challenging portion of the cardiac examination, steps for assessing the JVP are outlined in Box 18-13. The features listed in Box 18-14 also help distinguish jugular from carotid artery pulsations.

Jugular Venous Pressure and Volume Status. As you begin your assessment, consider the patient's volume status and whether you need to alter the elevation of the head of the bed or examining table. The usual starting position for the head of the bed or examining table when assessing the JVP is 30°.[31,32] Turn the patient's head lightly to the left, then the right, and identify the external jugular vein on each side. Then focus on the internal jugular venous pulsations on the right, transmitted from deep in the neck to the overlying soft tissues. The JVP is the highest oscillation point of the jugular venous pulsations that is usually evident in euvolemic patients.

In conditions in which you anticipate *the JVP will be low*, you may have to *lower the head of the bed*, sometimes even to 0°, to see the point of oscillation best. Likewise, if you suspect that *the JVP will be high*, you may have to *raise the head of the bed*. In some patients, the JVP will only be measurable when the patient is upright.

JVP measured at >3 cm above the sternal angle, or >8 cm in total distance above the RA, is considered *elevated* above normal. Such an elevation is strongly associated with both acute and chronic heart failure[25,33–37] and can also be observed in tricuspid stenosis, chronic pulmonary hypertension, superior vena cava obstruction, cardiac tamponade, and constrictive pericarditis.[38–40]

Box 18-13. Steps for Measuring the Jugular Venous Pressure

1. Make the patient comfortable. Raise the head slightly on a pillow to relax the sternocleidomastoid (SCM) muscles.
2. Raise the head of the bed or examining table to about 30°. Turn the patient's head slightly away from the side you are inspecting.
3. Use tangential lighting and examine both sides of the neck. Identify the external jugular vein on each side, then find the internal jugular venous pulsations.
4. If necessary, raise or lower the head of the bed until you can see the oscillation point or meniscus of the internal jugular venous pulsations in the lower half of the neck.
5. Focus on the right internal jugular vein. Look for pulsations in the suprasternal notch, between the attachments of the SCM muscle on the sternum and clavicle, or just posterior to the SCM. Distinguish the pulsations of the internal jugular vein from those of the carotid artery (see Box 18-14).
6. Identify the highest point of pulsation in the right jugular vein. Extend a long rectangular object or card horizontally from this point and a centimeter ruler vertically from the sternal angle, making an exact right angle. Measure the vertical distance in centimeters above the sternal angle where the horizontal object crosses the ruler and add to this distance 5 cm, the distance from the sternal angle to the center of the right atrium (see Fig. 18-20). The sum is the JVP.

Box 18-14. Distinguishing Internal Jugular and Carotid Pulsations

Internal Jugular Pulsations	Carotid Pulsations
■ Rarely palpable	■ Palpable
■ Soft biphasic undulating quality, usually with two elevations and *characteristic inward deflection* (x descent)	■ A more vigorous thrust with a *single outward component*
■ Pulsations eliminated by light pressure on the vein(s) just above the sternal end of the clavicle	■ Pulsations not eliminated by pressure on veins at sternal end of clavicle
■ Height of pulsations changes with position, normally dropping as the patient becomes more upright, and usually falls with inspiration	■ Height of pulsations unchanged by position
	■ Height of pulsations not affected by inspiration

Auscultate for Carotid Bruits

Next, auscultate both the carotid arteries to listen for a bruit. A *bruit* is a murmur-like sound arising from turbulent arterial blood flow. Ask the patient to stop breathing for ~10 seconds, then listen with the diaphragm of the stethoscope, which generally detects the higher-frequency sounds of arterial bruits better than the bell.[41]

Note that higher-grade stenoses may have lower-frequency or even absent sounds, more amenable to detection with the bell.

To best detect carotid bruits, place the diaphragm of the stethoscope near the upper end of the thyroid cartilage, below the angle of the jaw. This location overlies the bifurcation of the common carotid artery into the external and internal carotid arteries, reducing the likelihood of confusion with a transmitted murmur from the heart or subclavian or vertebral artery bruits. However, in some patients, carotid bruits may only be detected by auscultation over the mastoid process, which is located posterior to the ear.

Bruits are also caused by a tortuous carotid artery, external carotid arterial disease, aortic stenosis, hypervascularity of hyperthyroidism, and external compression from thoracic outlet syndrome. Bruits do not correlate with clinically significant underlying disease.[1,42,43]

Palpate the Carotid Arteries

As the presence of carotid atherosclerosis could potentially narrow the carotid arteries, it is important to auscultate the carotid arteries prior to palpating the carotid pulse. Palpate the carotid pulse, including the carotid upstroke, its amplitude and contour, and the presence or absence of *thrills*. The carotid pulse provides valuable information about cardiac function, especially aortic valve stenosis and regurgitation. Never palpate both carotid arteries at the same time. This may decrease blood flow to the brain and induce syncope.

The most feared complication of carotid artery palpation is the dislodgment of an atherosclerotic plaque, which could result in stroke.

To assess *amplitude* and *contour*, the patient should be supine with the head of the bed elevated to about 30°. First inspect the neck for carotid pulsations, often visible just medial to the SCM muscles. Then place your index and middle fingers or left thumb on the right carotid artery in the lower third of the neck and palpate for pulsations (Figs. 18-14 and 18-15).

A tortuous and kinked carotid artery may produce a unilateral pulsatile bulge.

Causes of decreased pulsations include decreased stroke volume from shock or MI and local atherosclerotic narrowing or occlusion.

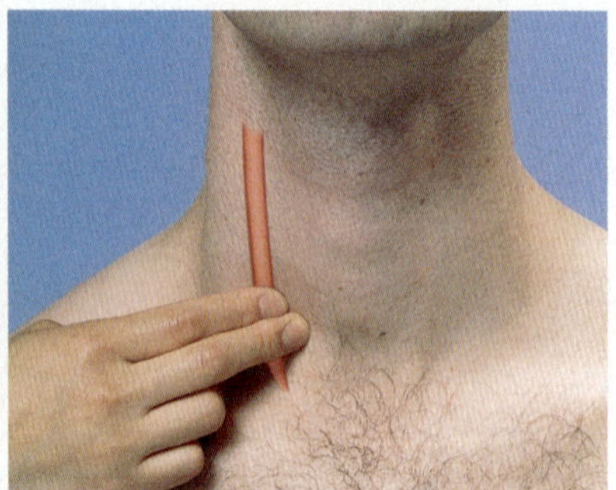

FIGURE 18-14. Palpating the carotid pulse with index and middle fingers.

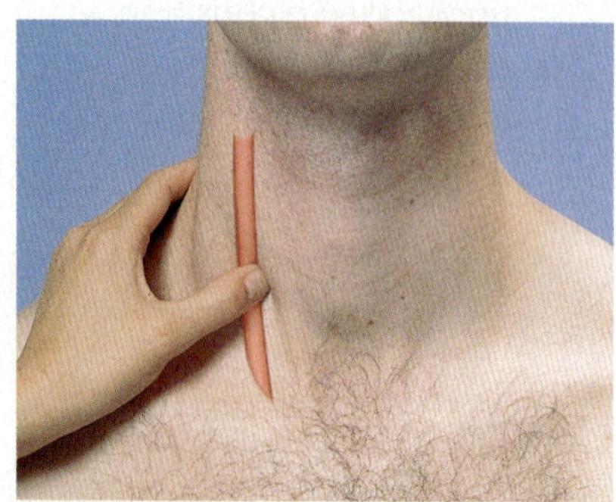

FIGURE 18-15. Palpating the carotid pulse with the thumb.

Box 18-15. Assessment Characteristics of the Carotid Pulse

- The *amplitude of the pulse.* This correlates reasonably well with the pulse pressure.

The carotid pulse is small, *thready* (barely detectable), or weak in cardiogenic shock; the pulse is bounding in aortic regurgitation.

- The *contour of the pulse wave,* namely the speed of the upstroke, the duration of its summit, and the speed of the downstroke. The normal upstroke is *brisk;* it is smooth, rapid, and follows S_1 almost immediately. The summit is smooth, rounded, and roughly midsystolic. The downstroke is less abrupt than the upstroke.

The carotid upstroke is delayed in aortic stenosis.

See Table 18-3, Abnormalities of the Arterial Pulse and Pressure Waves, p. 524.

- Any *variations in amplitude,* either from beat to beat or with respiration.
- *The timing of the carotid upstroke in relation to S_1 and S_2.* Note that the normal carotid upstroke follows S_1 and precedes S_2. This relationship is very helpful in correctly identifying S_1 and S_2, especially when the heart rate is increased and the duration of diastole, normally longer than systole, is shortened and approaches the duration of systole.

Press just inside the medial border of a relaxed SCM muscle, roughly *at the level of the cricoid cartilage.* Avoid pressing on the *carotid sinus,* which lies adjacent to the top of the thyroid cartilage. For the left carotid artery, use your right fingers or thumb. Slowly increase pressure until you feel a maximal pulsation, then slowly decrease pressure until you best sense the arterial pressure and contour. Assess the pulse characteristics as listed in Box 18-15.

Pressure on the carotid sinus may cause reflex bradycardia or drop in blood pressure.

As you palpate the carotid artery, you may detect *pulsus alternans, pulsus paradoxus (paradoxical pulse),* vibrations, or *thrills,* which are like the throat vibrations of a cat when it purrs (Box 18-16).

Thrills in aortic stenosis are transmitted to the carotid arteries from the suprasternal notch or second right intercostal space.

Inspect the Precordium

Carefully inspect the anterior chest and precordium, which may reveal the location of the *apical impulse* or *PMI,* or less commonly, the ventricular movements of a left-sided S_3 or S_4. Shine a tangential light across the chest wall over the cardiac apex to make these movements more visible. Plan to further characterize these movements as you proceed to palpation.

Palpate the Precordium

Palpate for various indicators such as heave or thrill, palpable S_1, S_2, S_3, or S_4, the apical impulse and PMI, the systolic impulse of the RV, the pulmonary artery area, and the aortic outflow area. Keep in mind the anatomic locations diagrammed in Figure 18-16.

Palpation is less useful in patients with a thickened chest wall (obesity) or increased anteroposterior (AP) diameter (obstructive lung disease).

Palpate for Heaves or Thrills. To palpate *heaves,* use your palm and/or hold your finger pads flat or obliquely against the chest. Heaves are sustained impulses that rhythmically lift your fingers, usually produced by an enlarged right or LV (depending on the location of the heave) and, occasionally, by ventricular aneurysms.

Box 18-16. Pulsus Alternans and Pulsus Paradoxus

Pulsus Alternans	Pulsus Paradoxus (Paradoxical Pulse)
Pulse rhythm is regular, but the force alternates due to varying ventricular contraction strength.	Systolic blood pressure abnormally decreases during inhalation.
Detect by palpating the pulse with light pressure on the radial or femoral arteries.	Detect by observing the pulse and blood pressure changes during the respiratory cycle, especially during inspiration.
Use a blood pressure cuff: Inflate the cuff, then slowly lower pressure to just below systolic level to hear the strong beats. Continue to lower the cuff to capture the alternating weaker beats, which will eventually disappear, causing the remaining Korotkoff sounds to appear to double.	Use a blood pressure cuff: Note the pressure at which Korotkoff sounds first appear during quiet respiration. Lower the cuff pressure slowly until sounds are heard throughout the respiratory cycle, then note this pressure level. The difference between these two pressures is the measure of the paradoxical pulse. The difference between these two levels is normally <3 or 4 mm Hg.
May indicate potential left ventricular dysfunction or heart failure.	May indicate conditions like cardiac tamponade, constrictive pericarditis, or severe asthma or chronic obstructive pulmonary disease, which can lead to changes in intrathoracic pressure during the respiratory cycle affecting cardiac output.

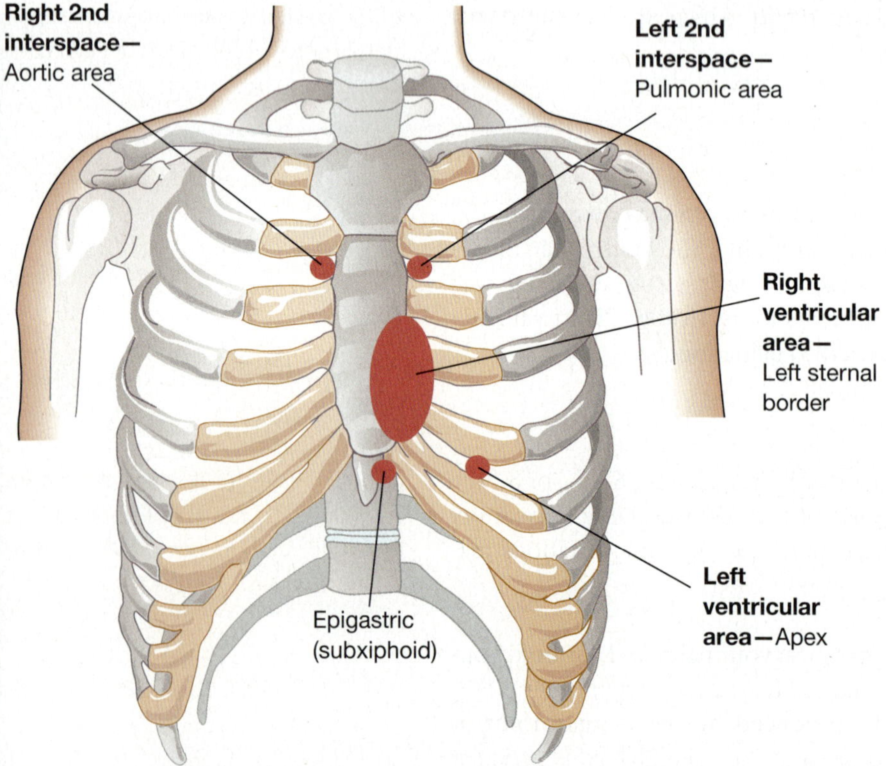

FIGURE 18-16. Palpation areas on the chest wall.

For *thrills*, press the ball of your hand (the padded area of your palm near the wrist) firmly on the chest to check for a buzzing or vibratory sensation caused by underlying turbulent flow. If present, auscultate the same area for murmurs. Conversely, once a murmur is detected, it is easier to palpate a thrill in the position that accentuates the murmur, such as the leaning forward position after detecting aortic regurgitation.

The presence of a thrill changes the grading of the murmur, as described on p. 508.

Palpate impulses from the *RV*, normally at the lower left sternal border and in the subxiphoid area (see p. 498).

Palpate for Apical Impulse and Point of Maximal Impulse. Next, identify the apical impulse and the PMI. The apical impulse represents the brief early pulsation of the LV as it moves anteriorly during systole and contacts the chest wall. In most examinations, the apical impulse is the PMI. If you cannot find the apical impulse, ask the patient to exhale fully and stop breathing for a few seconds. When examining a patient with breasts, it may be helpful to displace the left breast upward or laterally as necessary, or ask the patient to assist in doing this.

If you cannot identify the apical impulse with the patient supine, ask them to roll partly onto their left side in the *left lateral decubitus* position. Palpate again, using the palmar surfaces of several fingers (Fig. 18-17). The apex beat is palpable in 25% to 40% of adults in the supine position and 50% to 73% of adults in the left lateral decubitus position, especially those who are thin.[2]

Once you have found the apical impulse, make finer assessments with your fingertips, then with one finger to note the characteristics in Box 18-17. With experience, you will learn to palpate the apical impulse in most patients.

See Table 18-4, Variations and Abnormalities of the Ventricular Impulses, p. 525.

Auscultate the Precordium

Auscultation of heart sounds and murmurs using a stethoscope is a crucial skill that can lead to significant clinical diagnoses (Box 18-18).[44] Review the six auscultatory areas depicted in Figure 18-19. Heart sounds and murmurs originating from the four cardiac valves can spread across a broad area, which

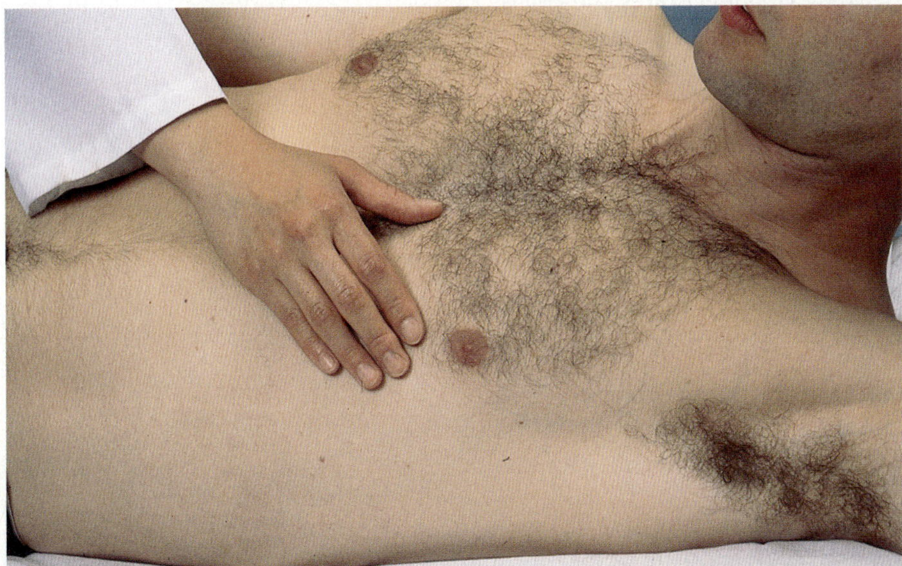

FIGURE 18-17. Palpating the apical impulse in the left lateral decubitus position.

Box 18-17. Characteristic Features of the Point of Maximal Impulse

Feature	Description	Condition
Vertical location	Usually in the fifth or possibly the fourth intercostal spaces	Rare conditions such as pregnancy or a high left diaphragm can shift the apical impulse upward and to the left. Dextrocardia may position the PMI on the right side of the chest.
Horizontal location	Measured in centimeters from the midclavicular line (or midsternal line; Fig. 18-18)	Lateral displacement of the PMI, either toward the anterior axillary line or lateral to the midclavicular line (or >10 cm from the midsternal line), may indicate ventricular dilatation, left ventricular hypertrophy, heart failure, cardiomyopathy, ischemic heart disease, thoracic deformities, or a mediastinal shift.
Diameter or area	Normally <2.5 cm in the supine patient, occupying one interspace	Diffuse PMI usually >3 cm indicates left ventricular enlargement from conditions like LVH, seen in hypertension or dilated cardiomyopathy.
Amplitude and duration	Typically brisk and nonsustained (a tap)	Sustained, forceful PMI can occur in hypermetabolic states or volume overload of the left ventricle from aortic regurgitation. In hyperkinetic states, the PMI is forceful and terminates quickly. In some patients, the most prominent impulse may be felt in the xiphoid or epigastric area which may indicate right ventricular hypertrophy, commonly seen in COPD.

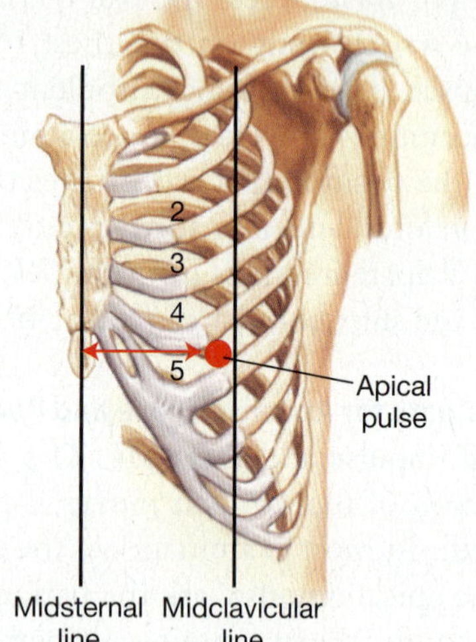

FIGURE 18-18. Describing the location of the point of maximal impulse in relation to the midsternal or midclavicular lines.

is clearly depicted in Figure 18-20. Therefore, it is important to describe auscultatory findings based on their anatomical location on the chest, rather than referring to the specific valve areas, to ensure accuracy in your clinical assessments.[7–9,45]

Throughout your examination, take your time at each of the six auscultatory areas. Concentrate on each of the events in the cardiac cycle, listening carefully to S_1, then S_2, other sounds and murmurs occurring in systole and diastole.

Box 18-18. Appropriate Use of the Stethoscope for the Cardiac Examination

It is important to understand the uses of both the diaphragm and the bell.

- *The diaphragm.* The diaphragm is better for picking up the relatively high-pitched sounds of S_1 and S_2, the murmurs of aortic and mitral regurgitation, and pericardial friction rubs. *Listen throughout the precordium* with the diaphragm, pressing it firmly against the chest.
- *The bell.* The bell is more sensitive to the low-pitched sounds of S_3 and S_4 and the murmur of mitral stenosis. Apply the bell lightly, with just enough pressure to produce an air seal with its full rim. *Use the bell at the apex, then move medially along the lower sternal border.* Resting the heel of your hand on the chest like a fulcrum may help you to maintain light pressure.

Firm pressure on the bell can stretch the underlying skin and make it function more like the diaphragm. Low-pitched sounds like S_3 and S_4 may then disappear—an observation that can help identify them. In contrast, high-pitched sounds such as a midsystolic click, an ejection sound, or an opening snap (OS) will persist or get louder.

See Tools of the Trade, pp. 68–71, in Chapter 4, Physical Examination.

Pattern of Auscultation. In a quiet room, auscultate the heart with your stethoscope with the patient's head and upper chest elevated to 30°. Start at either the base or apex, listening first with the diaphragm, then with the bell.

If starting at the base, gradually move your stethoscope inch by inch toward the apex. With your stethoscope in the right second intercostal space close to the sternum, move along the left sternal border in each intercostal space from the second through the fifth, and then toward the apex, making sure to auscultate in each of the six anatomic areas marked by the white circles in Figure 18-19.

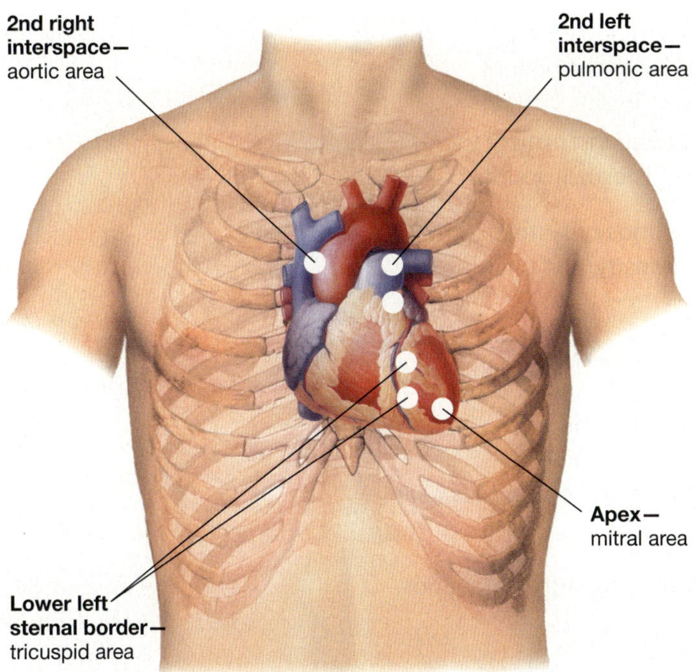

FIGURE 18-19. Auscultatory areas on the chest wall.

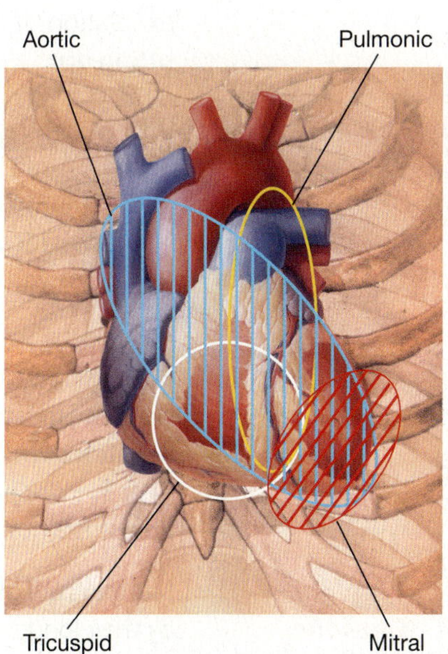

FIGURE 18-20. Radiation of heart sounds and murmurs.

Some recommend starting at the apex and moving toward the base. Move the stethoscope from the PMI medially to the left sternal border, superiorly to the second intercostal space, then across the sternum to the second intercostal space at the right sternal border. To clarify findings, move the stethoscope in smaller increments as needed (see p. 501). Review the guides to auscultation in Box 18-19 and learn the tips for identifying heart murmurs that follow in the next section.

Box 18-19. Auscultatory Sounds

Heart Sounds	Guides to Auscultation
S_1	▪ Note its intensity and any apparent splitting. ▪ S_1 splitting is a normal finding detectable along the lower left sternal border.
S_2	▪ Note its intensity.
Split S_2	▪ Listen for splitting of this sound in the second and third left intercostal spaces. Ask the patient to breathe quietly and then slightly more deeply than normal. ▪ Does S_2 split into its two components, as it normally does? If not, ask the patient to (1) breathe a little more deeply, or (2) sit up. Listen again. ▪ A thick chest wall may make the pulmonic component of S_2 inaudible. ▪ *Width of split.* How wide is the split? It is normally quite narrow. ▪ *Timing of split.* When in the respiratory cycle do you hear the split? It is normally heard late in inspiration. ▪ Does the split disappear as it should, during exhalation? If not, listen again with the patient sitting up. ▪ *Intensity of A_2 and P_2.* Compare the intensity of the two components, A_2 and P_2; A_2 is usually louder.
Extra Sounds in Systole	▪ These may include ejection sounds or systolic clicks. ▪ Note their location, timing, intensity, and pitch, and variations with respiration.
Extra Sounds in Diastole	▪ Such as S_3, S_4, or an opening snap[46] ▪ Note the location, timing, intensity, and pitch and variations with respiration. ▪ S_3 or S_4 in individuals with high levels of cardiovascular fitness is a normal finding.
Systolic and Diastolic Murmurs	▪ Murmurs are differentiated from S_1, S_2, and extra sounds by their longer duration.

See Table 18-5, Variations in the First Heart Sound—S_1, p. 526.

Note that S_1 is louder at more rapid heart rates, and PR intervals are shorter.

See Table 18-6, Variations in the Second Heart Sound—S_2, p. 527.

When either A_2 or P_2 is absent, as in aortic or pulmonic valve disease, S_2 is persistently single.

Expiratory splitting suggests a valvular abnormality (p. 503).

Persistent splitting results from delayed closure of the pulmonic valve or early closure of the aortic valve.

A loud P_2 points to pulmonary hypertension.

The systolic click of mitral valve prolapse (MVP) is the most common extra sound. See Table 18-7, Extra Heart Sounds in Systole, p. 528.

See Table 18-8, Extra Heart Sounds in Diastole, p. 529.

See Table 18-9, Midsystolic Murmurs, pp. 530–531; Table 18-10, Pansystolic (Holosystolic) Murmurs, p. 532; and Table 18-11, Diastolic Murmurs, p. 533.

Auscultate for S_1 and S_2

By carefully noting the intensities of S_1 and S_2, you will confirm each of these sounds and thereby correctly identify *systole*, the interval between S_1 and S_2, and *diastole*, the interval between S_2 and S_1. The correct timing of systole and diastole is the fundamental prerequisite for identifying events in the cardiac cycle.

To facilitate the correct identification of systole and diastole, as you auscultate the chest, palpate the right carotid artery in the lower third of the neck with your index and middle fingers—S_1 falls just before the carotid upstroke, and S_2 follows the carotid upstroke (See Figs. 18-14 and 18-15). Be sure to compare the intensities of S_1 and S_2 as you move your stethoscope through the listening areas. At the *base*, you will note that S_2 is louder than S_1 and may split with respiration. At the *apex*, S_1 is usually louder than S_2 unless the PR interval is prolonged.

Auscultate for Splitting of Heart Sounds

The second heart sound, S_2, and its two components, *A_2 and P_2*, are primarily caused by the closure of the aortic and pulmonic valves, respectively. During inspiration, right heart filling time is prolonged, resulting in increased RV stroke volume and duration of RV ejection, compared with the neighboring LV. This delay in the closure of the pulmonic valve, P_2, splits S_2 into its two audible components. Conversely, during expiration, the RV ejection period is faster, causing A_2 and P_2 to fuse into a single sound, S_2. Distensibility and impedance in the pulmonary vascular bed contribute to the "hangout time" that delays P_2.[5]

A_2, the component of S_2 reflecting the high pressure in the aorta, is normally louder and heard throughout the precordium. In contrast, P_2 is relatively soft and best auscultated near its anatomic location, the second and third left intercostal spaces close to the sternum, where you should search for the splitting of S_2.

Recall that S_1 also has two components. While it can be detected, the splitting of S_1 does not vary with respiration and is less frequently used in diagnostic evaluation.

Auscultate for Heart Murmurs

To correctly identify heart murmurs, a systematic approach is crucial. This requires a thorough understanding of cardiac anatomy and physiology as well as dedication to the practice and mastery of examination techniques. It can also be helpful to compare your findings with those of experienced clinicians to improve your skills.

To aid in the identification of heart murmurs, review the tips provided in Box 18-20. Additionally, carefully study the subsequent sections on the timing, shape, location, radiation, intensity, pitch, and quality of heart murmurs for more detailed information. Tables provided at the end of the chapter can also be a valuable resource for further expanding your skills.[73] To reinforce your learning, consider listening to heart sound recordings, as research has shown that this can improve accurate identification of heart murmurs and transfer to real-world patients.[7–9]

Murmur Timing. First decide if you are hearing a *systolic murmur*, falling between S_1 and S_2, or a *diastolic murmur*, falling between S_2 and S_1 (Boxes 18-21 and 18-22).

Diastolic murmurs usually represent valvular heart disease. Systolic murmurs point to valvular disease but can be physiologic flow murmurs arising from normal heart valves.

Box 18-20. Tips for Identifying Heart Murmurs

- *Time* the murmur—is it in systole or diastole? What is its duration?
- *Locate* where on the precordium the murmur is loudest—at the base, along the sternal border, at the apex? Does it radiate?
- Conduct any necessary *maneuvers,* such as having the patient lean forward and exhale or turn to the left lateral decubitus position to accentuate the murmurs.
  - Ask the patient to roll into the left lateral decubitus position, which brings the LV closer to the chest wall. Place the bell of your stethoscope lightly on the apical impulse (see Fig. 18-21).
  - Ask the patient to *sit up, lean forward, exhale completely, and briefly stop breathing after expiration.* Pressing the diaphragm of your stethoscope on the chest, listen along the left sternal border and at the apex, pausing periodically so the patient may breathe (see Fig. 18-22).
- Determine the *shape* of the murmur—for example, is it crescendo, decrescendo, or holosystolic?
- Grade the *intensity* of the murmur from 1 to 6 (systolic) or 1 to 4 (diastolic) and determine its *pitch* (high, medium, or low) and *quality* (blowing, harsh, rumbling, or musical).
- Identify *associated features* such as the quality of S_1 and S_2, the presence of extra sounds such as S_3, S_4, or an OS, the presence of additional murmurs, and the respiratory variation in murmur intensity.
- Be sure you are listening in a quiet room!

Right-sided heart murmurs generally increase with inspiration; left-sided murmurs generally increase with expiration.[44]

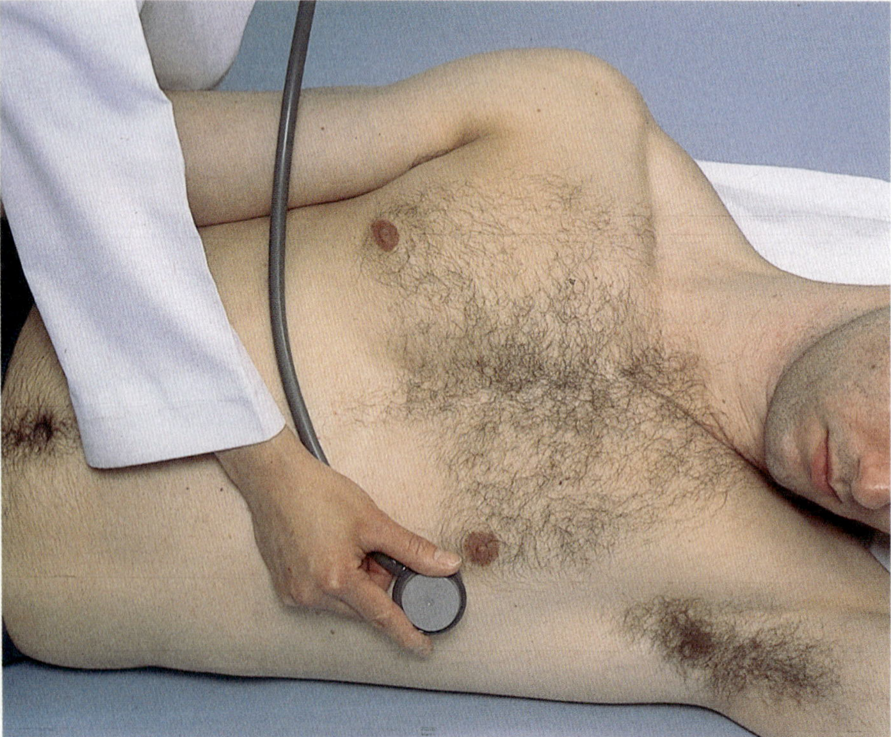

FIGURE 18-21. Auscultating for mitral stenosis in the left lateral decubitus position.

This position accentuates a left-sided S_3 and S_4 and mitral murmurs, especially mitral stenosis. Otherwise, you may miss these important findings.

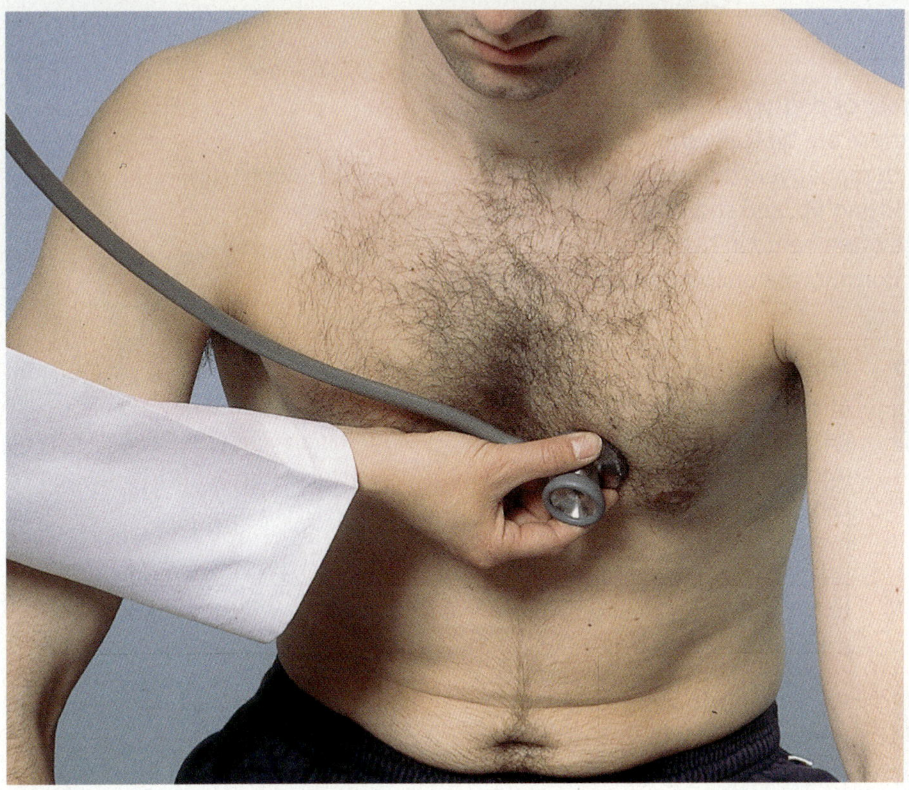

FIGURE 18-22. Auscultating for aortic regurgitation with the patient leaning forward.

You may easily miss the soft diastolic decrescendo murmur of aortic regurgitation unless you listen at this position.

Palpating the carotid pulse as you listen can help you with timing. Murmurs that coincide with the carotid upstroke are systolic.

Murmur Shapes. The shape of a heart murmur refers to its pattern of intensity over time. Murmurs can be *crescendo* (gradually getting louder), *decrescendo* (gradually getting softer), *crescendo–decrescendo* (gradually getting louder and then softer), or *plateau* (steady intensity throughout). The shape of a murmur can provide important diagnostic information, as certain murmurs are associated with specific underlying conditions. Box 18-23 shows continuous murmurs, and Box 18-24 shows murmur shapes.

Murmur Intensity and Grade. The intensity of a murmur refers to its loudness or softness and is graded on a scale from 1 to 6 and expressed as a fraction. The *numerator* describes the intensity of the murmur wherever it is loudest; the *denominator* indicates the scale you are using. Intensity is influenced by the thickness of the chest wall and the presence of intervening tissue.

An identical degree of turbulence would cause a louder murmur in a thin person than in a very muscular or obese person. Emphysematous lungs may diminish the intensity of murmurs.

Box 18-21. Systolic Murmurs

Systolic murmurs are typically *midsystolic* or *pansystolic.* Midsystolic murmurs can be *functional murmurs;* these are typically short midsystolic murmurs that decrease in intensity with maneuvers that reduce left ventricular volume, such as standing, sitting up, and straining during the Valsalva maneuver. These murmurs are often heard in healthy patients and are not pathologic. Early systolic murmurs are uncommon and are not depicted below.

Murmurs detected during pregnancy should be promptly evaluated for possible risk to the mother and fetus, especially those of aortic stenosis or pulmonary hypertension.[74]

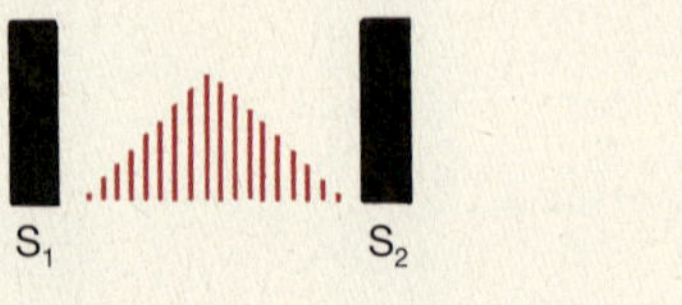

Midsystolic murmur: Begins after S_1 and stops before S_2. Brief gaps are audible between the murmur and the heart sounds. Listen carefully for the gap just before S_2, which is more readily detected and, if present, usually confirms the murmur as midsystolic, not pansystolic.

Midsystolic murmurs typically arise from blood flow across the semilunar (aortic and pulmonic) valves. See Table 18-10, Midsystolic Murmurs, p. 532.

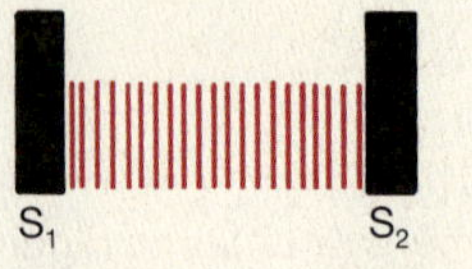

Pansystolic (holosystolic) murmur: Starts with S_1 and stops at S_2, without a gap between murmur and heart sounds.

Pansystolic murmurs often occur with regurgitant (backward) flow across the AV valves. See Table 18-10, Pansystolic (Holosystolic) Murmurs, p. 532.

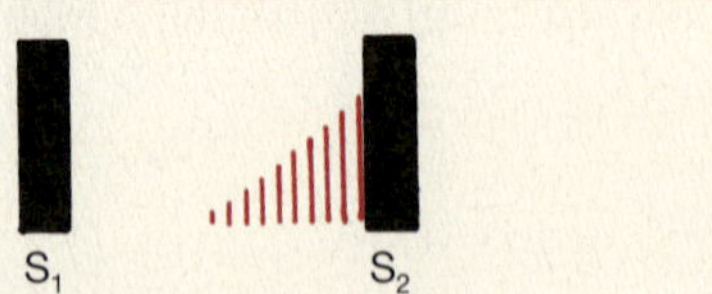

Late systolic murmur: Usually starts in mid- or late systole and persists up to S_2.

This is the murmur of mitral valve prolapse and is often, but not always, preceded by a systolic click (see p. 528); the murmur of mitral regurgitation may also be late systolic.

Box 18-22. Diastolic Murmurs

Diastolic murmurs may be early diastolic, mid-diastolic, or late diastolic.

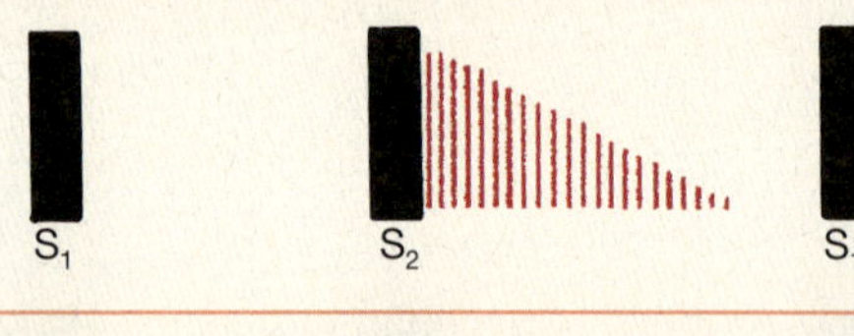

Early diastolic murmur: Starts immediately after S_2, without a discernible gap, then usually fades into silence before the next S_1.

Early diastolic murmurs typically reflect regurgitant flow across incompetent semilunar valves.

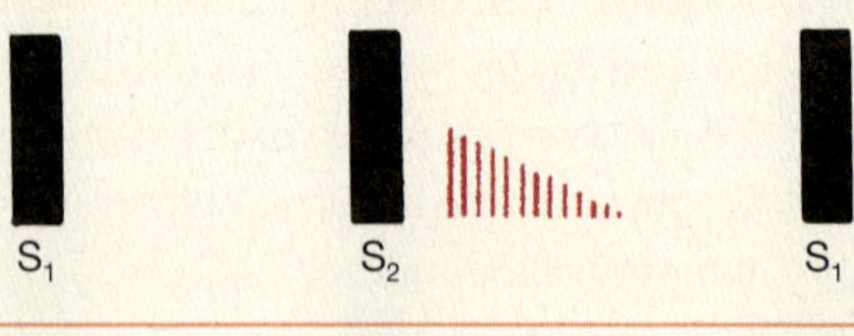

Mid-diastolic murmur: Starts a short time after S_2. It may fade away, as illustrated, or merge into a late diastolic murmur.

Middiastolic and presystolic murmurs reflect turbulent flow across the AV valves. See Table 18-11, Diastolic Murmurs, p. 533.

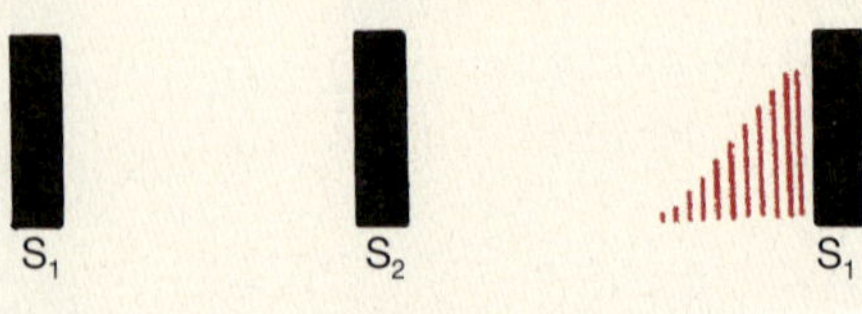

Late diastolic (presystolic) murmur: Starts late in diastole and typically continues up to S_1.

Box 18-23. Continuous Murmurs

Some congenital and clinical conditions produce continuous murmurs.

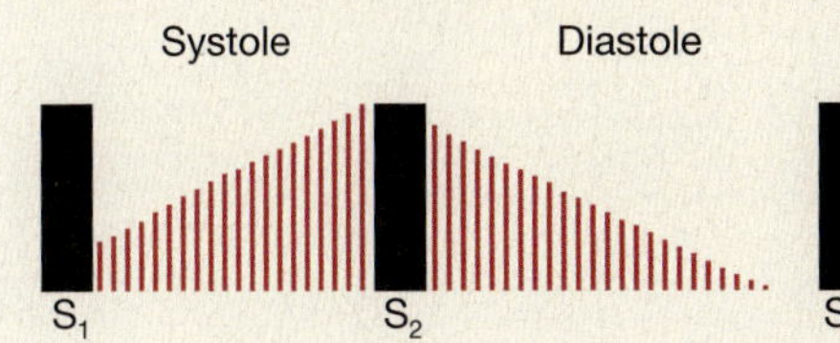

Continuous murmur: Begins in systole and extends into all or part of diastole (but is not necessarily uniform throughout).[73]

Congenital patent ductus arteriosus and AV fistulas, common in dialysis patients, produce continuous murmurs that are nonvalvular in origin. Venous hums and pericardial friction rubs also have both systolic and diastolic components. See Table 18-12, Cardiovascular Sounds with Both Systolic and Diastolic Components, p. 534.

Grade systolic murmurs using the 6-point scale in Box 18-25 (Levine grading system) based on the loudness or intensity of the murmur during systole.[76,77] Note that grades 4 through 6 require the added presence of a palpable thrill. Grade diastolic murmurs using the four-point scale in Box 18-26. This different scale is used by convention for diastolic murmurs as they are not commonly associated with a palpable thrill and is based on the duration of the murmur during diastole.[78,79]

Location of Maximal Intensity and Its Radiation/Transmission. This is determined by the site where the murmur originates. Find the location by exploring the area where you hear the murmur. Describe where you hear it best in terms of the intercostal space and its proximity to the sternum; apex; or its measured distance from the midclavicular, midsternal, or one of the axillary lines. For example, a murmur best heard in the second right intercostal space often

The murmur of aortic stenosis often radiates to the neck in the direction of arterial flow, especially on the right side. In mitral regurgitation, the murmur often radiates to the axilla, supporting transmission by bone conduction.[56,80]

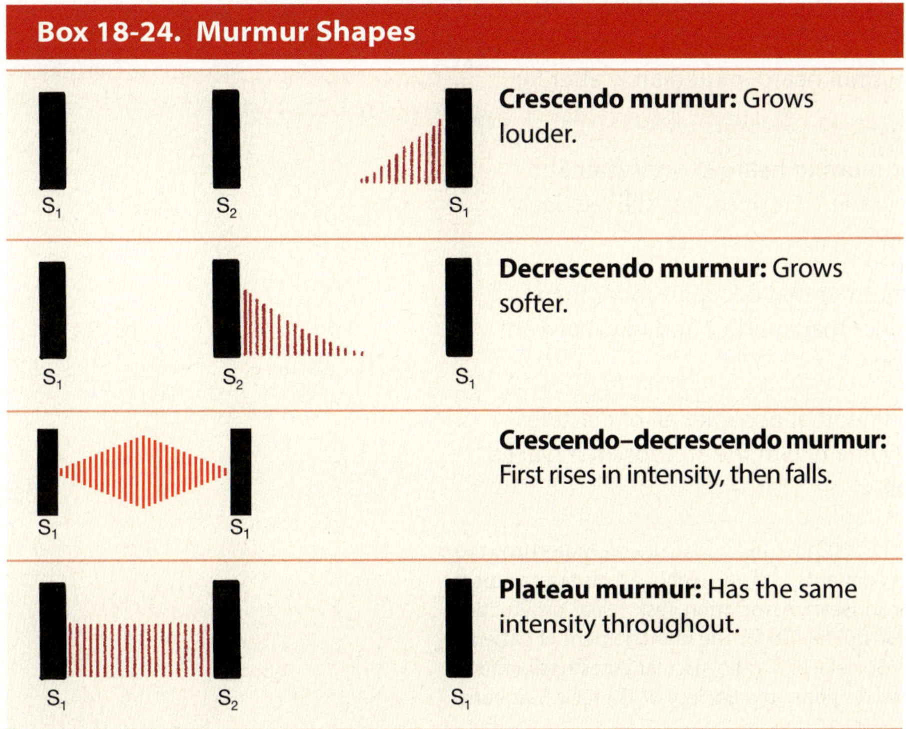

Note the presystolic murmur of mitral stenosis in normal sinus rhythm.

Note the early diastolic murmur of aortic regurgitation.

Listen for the midsystolic murmur of aortic stenosis and innocent flow murmurs.

Note the pansystolic murmur of mitral regurgitation.

Box 18-25. Grading System of Systolic Murmurs Based on the Loudness or Intensity of the Murmur During Systole

Grade	Description
Grade 1/6	Softer in volume than S_1 and S_2; very faint, heard only after listener has "tuned in"; may not be heard in all positions
Grade 2/6	Equal in volume to S_1 and S_2; quiet, but heard immediately upon placing the stethoscope on the chest
Grade 3/6	Louder in volume than S_1 and S_2, moderately loud
Grade 4/6	Loud with palpable thrill (vibration)
Grade 5/6	Very loud with thrill; may be heard when the stethoscope is partly off the chest
Grade 6/6	Loudest with thrill; may be heard with stethoscope entirely off the chest

originates at or near the aortic valve. This reflects not only the site of origin but also the intensity of the murmur, the direction of blood flow, and bone conduction in the thorax. Explore the area around a murmur and determine where else you can hear it.

Box 18-26. Grading System of Diastolic Murmurs Based on the Duration of the Murmur During Diastole[79]

Grade	Description
Grade 1/4	Short, early diastolic murmur heard immediately after S_2; often difficult to hear
Grade 2/4	Slightly longer diastolic murmur heard shortly after S_2; typically louder than a grade 1 murmur, but still relatively quiet and difficult to hear
Grade 3/4	Longer, mid-diastolic murmur that occupies more than half of diastole' typically louder than grade 2 and may have an associated opening snap
Grade 4/4	Long, pan-diastolic murmur that occupies all of diastole; typically loud and easily heard with the stethoscope placed lightly on the chest wall

Source: Bonow RO, Carabello BA, Chatterjee K, et al. 2008 focused update incorporated into the ACC/AHA 2006 guidelines for the management of patients with valvular heart disease: a report of the American College of Cardiology/American Heart Association Task Force on Practice Guidelines (Writing Committee to revise the 1998 guidelines for the management of patients with valvular heart disease). Endorsed by the Society of Cardiovascular Anesthesiologists, Society for Cardiovascular Angiography and Interventions, and Society of Thoracic Surgeons. *J Am Coll Cardiol.* 2008;52(13):e1–e142.

Murmur Pitch. The pitch of a murmur refers to the frequency of the sound it produces. A *high-pitched murmur* has a higher frequency and may be described as a whistling or blowing sound, while a *low-pitched murmur* has a lower frequency and may be described as a rumbling or humming sound. Pitch can provide important information about the underlying pathology causing the murmur.

A fully described murmur might be: a "medium-pitched, grade 2/4, blowing decrescendo diastolic murmur, best heard in the fourth left intercostal space, with radiation to the apex" (aortic regurgitation).

Murmur Quality. The quality of a murmur refers to its musical or vibratory characteristics. For example, it may be described as rough, harsh, blowing, or rumbling. Quality can provide important clues to the underlying cause of the murmur, as different conditions can produce murmurs with different qualities.

SPECIAL TECHNIQUES AND MANEUVERS

Bedside Maneuvers to Identify Murmurs and Heart Failure

Box 18-27 summarizes key bedside techniques to help you differentiate and identify various cardiac murmurs and signs of heart failure. Familiarize yourself with each maneuver, as mastering these can significantly enhance your clinical diagnostic skills in cardiology.

Box 18-27. Bedside Maneuvers to Identify Systolic Murmurs[57,58,81–84]

Maneuver	Mechanism	How to Perform
Standing and squatting	When a person is standing up, venous return to the heart decreases, as does peripheral vascular resistance. Arterial blood pressure, stroke volume, and the volume of blood in the LV all decline. With squatting, vascular and volume changes occur in the opposite direction.	Secure the patient's gown so that it will not interfere with your examination and prepare for prompt auscultation. Instruct the patient to squat next to the examining table and hold on to it for balance. Listen to the heart with the patient in the squatting position and again in the standing position. These maneuvers help (1) to identify a prolapsed mitral valve and (2) to distinguish hypertrophic cardiomyopathy from aortic stenosis.

(continued)

Box 18-27. Bedside Maneuvers to Identify Systolic Murmurs[57,58,81–84] (*Continued*)

Maneuver	Mechanism	How to Perform
Valsalva maneuver	Involves forcible exhalation against a closed glottis after full inspiration, causing increased intrathoracic pressure.	To distinguish the murmur of *hypertrophic cardiomyopathy*, ask the supine patient to *"bear down, like straining during a bowel movement."* Alternatively, place one hand on the patient's midabdomen and ask the patient to push against it. With your other hand, place your stethoscope on the patient's chest and listen at the lower left sternal border. To identify *heart failure* and *pulmonary hypertension*, place the blood pressure cuff on the upper arm, inflate it to 15 mm Hg above the systolic blood pressure, and ask the patient to perform the Valsalva maneuver for 10 s, then resume normal respiration. Keep the cuff pressure locked at 15 mm Hg above the baseline systolic pressure during the entire maneuver and for 30 s afterward. Listen for Korotkoff sounds over the brachial artery throughout.
Isometric handgrip	Increases the systolic murmurs of mitral regurgitation, pulmonic stenosis, and ventricular septal defect as well as the diastolic murmurs of aortic regurgitation and mitral stenosis.	To perform this maneuver, have the patient grip a hand dynamometer and squeeze it for at least 3 min. Listen to the heart during the maneuver and compare the intensity of any murmurs to that heard at baseline.
Transient arterial occlusion	Transient compression of both arms by bilateral blood pressure cuff inflation to 20 mm Hg greater than peak systolic blood pressure augments the murmurs of mitral regurgitation, aortic regurgitation, and ventricular septal defect.	To perform this maneuver, place a blood pressure cuff on each arm and inflate both to 20 mm Hg greater than the patient's peak systolic blood pressure and listen to the heart during the maneuver. Compare the intensity of any murmurs to that heard at baseline.

Modifications in Physical Examinations: Best Practices for Specialized Patient Populations

The presence of cardiac devices, including pacemakers and automatic implantable cardioverter defibrillators (AICDs), introduces unique considerations when conducting a cardiac physical examination. While these devices serve critical roles in rhythm management and life-saving interventions, they also necessitate specific adaptations in the traditional PE approach. Trainees must be aware of these modifications to ensure a comprehensive assessment while safeguarding the device's functionality. Box 18-28 provides guidance on tailoring the cardiac PE for patients with these devices.

Box 18-28. Cardiovascular Examination in the Presence of Medical Devices, Conditions, or Procedures

	Patient with a Pacemaker	Patient with an Automated Implantable Cardioverter-Defibrillator (AICD or ICD)
Device/condition	Implanted device that generates electrical impulses to maintain a normal heart rate in patients with abnormal heart rhythms, especially those that are too slow	Implanted device that monitors for and corrects life-threatening rapid heart rhythms, including ventricular tachycardia (VT) and ventricular fibrillation (VF), by delivering a defibrillation, or shock
General indications	Sinus node dysfunction, including symptomatic bradycardia and sick sinus syndrome; high-grade or symptomatic AV nodal dysfunction, including complete (third-degree) heart block and advanced second-degree heart block	Prevention of sudden cardiac death in patients with an increased risk of VT or VF (e.g., Brugada syndrome, heart failure with a severely reduced ejection fraction) Patients with prior life-threatening arrhythmias (sustained VT or VF)

(*continued*)

Box 18-28. Cardiovascular Examination in the Presence of Medical Devices, Conditions, or Procedures (*Continued*)

	Patient with a Pacemaker	Patient with an Automated Implantable Cardioverter-Defibrillator (AICD or ICD)
General location	Pulse generator is implanted on the anterior chest wall in the infraclavicular area. Transvenous electrodes, or leads, extend from the generator into the myocardium	Similar to a pacemaker, usually implanted on the anterior chest wall in the infraclavicular area, with leads extending into the myocardium
Modification to the physical exam	1. Begin with a visual inspection: Note the presence of any surgical scars, device protrusion, erythema, edema, or other skin changes over the device. 2. Palpate gently over the device to assess for warmth, tenderness, or local complications. Avoid pressing too hard. 3. With cardiac auscultation, be aware that you might hear a soft ticking sound related to the device's operation. 4. Document the presence of the pacemaker in the patient's medical record, including the model, date of implantation and the most recent battery change. 5. If indicated, obtain a 12-lead ECG to evaluate the functioning of the device. 6. If possible, obtain previous device interrogation reports for additional information on the device's functioning.	1. Visual inspection: Look for surgical scars, device protrusion, erythema, edema, or other skin changes. 2. Palpate gently, being cautious not to press hard over the device. 3. During auscultation, in addition to the heart's sounds, there might be soft electrical sounds related to the device's operation. 4. Always document the presence and type of device in the patient's record, including the date of implantation and the most recent battery change. 5. As with pacemakers, previous device interrogation reports can provide valuable insights on the device's performance and any arrhythmic episodes.

RECORDING YOUR FINDINGS

Initially, you will write thorough sentences of the PE which is crucial for diagnosis and hypothesis generation. As you gain experience, you will often shift to using brief, standard phrases for quicker and clearer documentation.

Recording the Cardiovascular Examination

"The JVP is 3 cm above the sternal angle with the head of bed elevated to 30°. Carotid upstrokes are brisk, without bruits. The PMI is tapping, 1 cm lateral to the midclavicular line in the fifth intercostal space. Crisp S_1 and S_2. At the base, S_2 is louder than S_1 with physiologic split of $A_2 > P_2$. At the apex, S_1 is louder than S_2. There are no murmurs or extra sounds."

OR

"The JVP is 5 cm above the sternal angle with the head of bed elevated to 50°. Carotid upstrokes are brisk; a bruit is heard over the left carotid artery. The PMI is diffuse, 3 cm in diameter, palpated at the anterior axillary line in the fifth and sixth intercostal spaces. S_1 and S_2 are soft. S_3 is present at the apex. High-pitched harsh 2/6 holosystolic murmur best heard at the apex, radiating to the axilla."

The practice of dissecting PE documentation into detailed components exemplifies how clinical observations can offer pivotal clues for diagnosis. This process highlights specific findings and nuances that might otherwise be overlooked, directly contributing to the accuracy and efficiency of the diagnostic process. The described findings in the patient's cardiovascular examination are indicative of several cardiac issues:

- *JVP 5 cm above the sternal angle at 50° elevation*: This elevated JVP suggests increased central venous pressure, commonly associated with right heart failure or fluid overload conditions like CHF.
- *Bruit over the left carotid artery:* A carotid bruit indicates turbulent blood flow, often due to stenosis of the carotid artery, which can be a marker of generalized atherosclerosis and increased risk of cerebrovascular events.
- *Diffuse, laterally displaced PMI:* This finding suggests ventricular hypertrophy or dilation, common in conditions like hypertensive heart disease or cardiomyopathy.
- *Soft S_1 and S_2, presence of S_3 at the apex:* A soft S_1 and S_2 can be due to various factors including low cardiac output. An S_3 heart sound is typically associated with heart failure or a volume-overloaded state.
- *High-pitched harsh 2/6 holosystolic murmur best heard at the apex, radiating to the axilla:* This description is characteristic of mitral regurgitation, a condition in which the mitral valve does not close properly during systole, causing blood to flow backward into the left atrium.

In summary, these findings are suggestive of *left-sided heart failure*, possibly secondary to mitral valve disease (mitral regurgitation), with evidence of increased cardiac workload (evidenced by LV hypertrophy/dilation) and systemic effects like fluid overload.[37,45,85,86]

POINT-OF-CARE ULTRASOUND EXAMINATION

POCUS can provide visual information to support clinical findings in the cardiovascular system PE.[16] Normal anatomy, physiology, and pathophysiology can be assessed rapidly and can support or change management of the patient. POCUS evaluation of the heart through the chest wall is also known as transthoracic echocardiography (TTE).

One common use of POCUS to augment the cardiovascular physical exam is to assess global left-ventricular systolic function (LVSF).[87] The 2014 International Evidence-Based Recommendations for Focused Cardiac Ultrasound concluded that not only can clinicians be adequately trained to assess global function, but that this improves diagnostic accuracy compared to the PE. Also clearly established is that visual estimation of LVSF in trained observers is comparable to formal estimates of function.[88,89] Visual estimation is most accurate when observers distinguish LVSF as "normal," "reduced," or "severely reduced."[89–91] POCUS evaluation of LVSF can be instrumental in guiding clinical decisions regarding administration of fluids or vasopressors in a hypotensive patient.[90–92]

Assessing Left Ventricular Systolic Function

Physical Examination. CHF is a complex syndrome characterized by the heart's inability to pump blood effectively. Physical signs of CHF, detailed in Box 18-29, can vary and may not be specific, making diagnosis based on PE alone difficult. For example, right-sided CHF may present with jugular venous distention and edema, while left-sided CHF often manifests with pulmonary symptoms. Furthermore, overlapping symptoms like dyspnea and swelling may also occur in renal, pulmonary, and liver diseases, complicating the diagnosis.

Box 18-29. Physical Examination Findings: Congestive Heart Failure

Physical Examination Finding	Maneuver/Technique	Possible Implication
Heart sounds (S_3)	Auscultation with a stethoscope over the cardiac apex	Suggestive of left ventricular dysfunction
Weak or thready pulse	Palpation of a peripheral artery (e.g., radial, or carotid artery)	Indicates decreased cardiac output
Jugular venous distention (JVD)	Inspection of the neck while the patient is at a 45° angle	Typically indicative of right-sided heart issues but can be seen in overall heart failure
Peripheral edema	Palpation and inspection of the lower extremities	Indicates heart failure
Pulmonary crackles	Auscultation of the lungs using a stethoscope	Suggestive of pulmonary edema due to left ventricular failure
Palpable apical impulse	Palpation of the chest wall in the midclavicular line, usually at the fifth or sixth intercostal space	Suggests cardiac enlargement if laterally displaced

Ultrasound Technique

Basic Ultrasound Setup	
Patient positioning	Supine or left lateral decubitus
Probe	Phased array probe (smaller footprint, easier to visualize cardiac structures between the ribs)
Ultrasound setting	"Cardiac" setting for the phased array probe, B-mode

POCUS can greatly aid in distinguishing CHF from other conditions by providing real-time visualization of cardiac function and fluid status. We discuss two methods of assessing LVSF in this chapter. For further details on other cardiac views, refer to *Essential Ultrasound Anatomy* by Loukas and Burns.[93]

POCUS evaluation for LVSF is performed with the patient in a supine or left lateral decubitus position. The study is performed with the phased array probe. The smaller footprint is useful for finding a good window for visualization of the cardiac motion between the ribs. The ultrasound machine is set to the "cardiac" preset, which will place the screen marker on the right side of the screen. This convention is only used for cardiac views to keep with classic echocardiography.

LVSF can be assessed by two methods in two views, the parasternal long (PSL) and the parasternal short (PSS) views (Box 18-30). In both views, visual estimation of LVSF is labeled as normal, reduced, or severely reduced.

The *parasternal long axis view* is obtained with the probe marker generally pointed toward the patient's right shoulder in approximately the fourth intercostal space. The probe should be oriented along the sagittal or "long" axis of the heart, and the location and angle of that long axis should be considered from a surface anatomy perspective as the operator is applying the probe (Fig. 18-23).

The *parasternal short axis view* is obtained by rotating the probe marker 90° clockwise from the PSL view (generally toward the patient's left shoulder). The probe should now be oriented in a transverse view through the ventricles with the focus on the LV in the middle of the screen (Fig. 18-24).

In general, remember that the best cardiac window may vary in each patient based on body habitus and prior cardiac disease (e.g., a patient with known heart failure with reduced EF may have a "boot-shaped" heart, and the cardiac window for the parasternal long may be in a more horizontal position across the chest wall).

Box 18-30. Echocardiographic Views and Their Evaluation Focus for Left Ventricular Function

View	Evaluation Focus
Parasternal long axis (PSL)	Evaluate if the anterior leaflet of the mitral valve is making contact with the ventricular septal wall during diastole
Parasternal short axis (PSS)	Best view for LVSF Evaluate the overall global function of the LV (i.e., are the walls coming together in a strong, symmetrical "squeeze"?)
Both views	Evaluate if the myocardium is thickening as it contracts

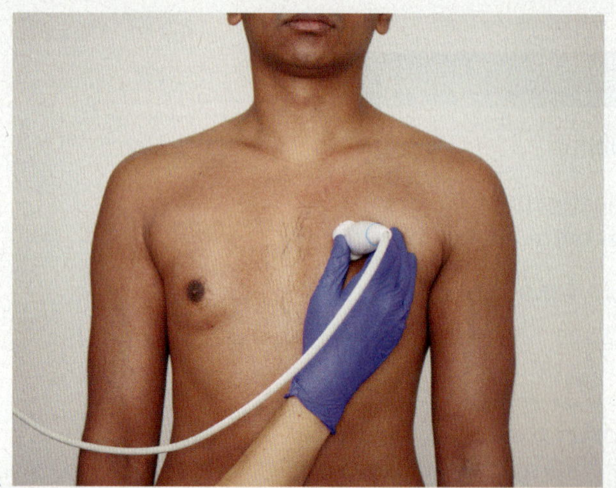

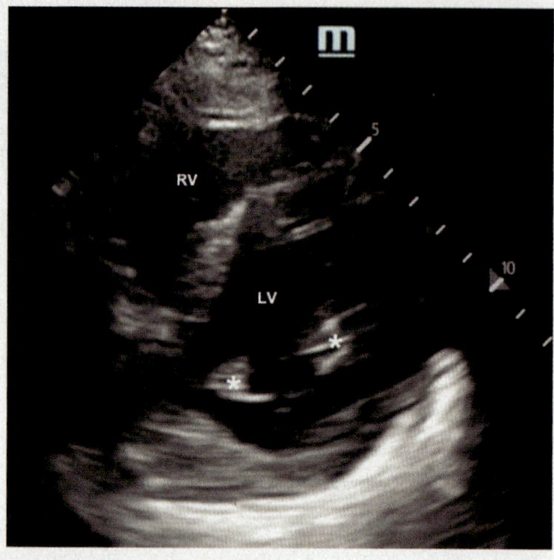

FIGURE 18-23. (**A**) Parasternal long axis (PSL) hand and probe positioning on the patient, with the probe marker oriented toward the patient's right shoulder; (**B**) PSL screen view showing labeled structures: LA (left atrium), LV (left ventricle), RV (right ventricle), Ao (aorta), DA (descending aorta), * (myocardium), arrowhead (anterior leaflet of the mitral valve).

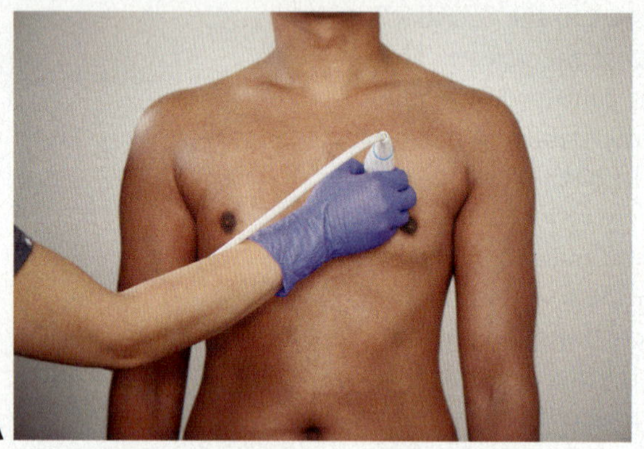

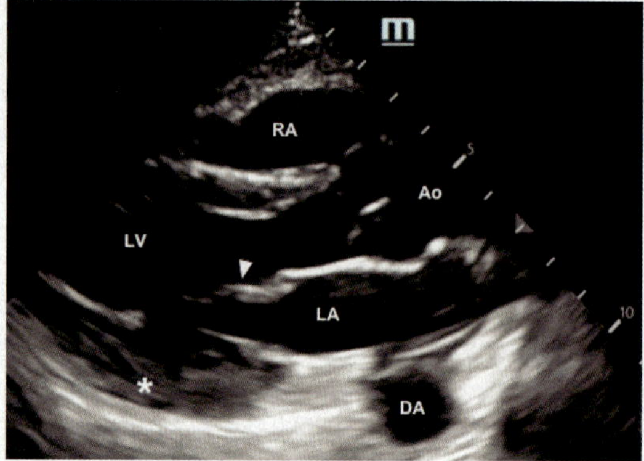

FIGURE 18-24. (**A**) Parasternal Short-Axis (PSS) hand and probe positioning on the patient, with the probe marker oriented toward the patient's left shoulder; (**B**) PSS screen view showing labeled structures: LV (left ventricle), RV (right ventricle), S (ventricular septal wall), * (papillary muscle).

As discussed in Chapter 9, Basic Principles and Techniques: Point-of-Care Ultrasound (POCUS), pp. 157–158, small adjustments will need to be made for each cardiac POCUS evaluation using rotation, sliding, and sweeping motions of the probe to obtain the ideal view of the heart. Adjustments to gain and depth will also be needed to optimize each view.

HEALTH PROMOTION AND COUNSELING: EVIDENCE AND RECOMMENDATIONS

Important Topics for Health Promotion and Counseling

- Screening for hypertension
- Initiating statin therapy for primary prevention
- Promoting lifestyle changes and risk factor modification
- Addressing excessive dietary sodium

In the following section, both traditional terms like "men," "women," "male," and "female" and inclusive terms such as "individuals assigned female at birth" and "individuals assigned male at birth" are used. This approach balances inclusivity with the need to accurately represent the original research.

Background

Cardiovascular disease (CVD), including hypertension (which accounts for the vast majority of diagnoses), CHD, heart failure, and stroke, is the leading global cause of mortality, with an estimated 19 million CVD deaths in 2021.[94] CVD is also the leading cause of death in the United States, accounting for more than a quarter of all deaths in 2020.[95,96] Modifiable risk factors, including hypertension, dyslipidemia, diabetes, tobacco use, overweight and obesity, unhealthy diet, and physical inactivity contribute to a substantial proportion of CVD events and mortality.[97,98] Health promotion strategies to prevent CVD include screening for hypertension, initiating statin therapy for primary prevention, and counseling to promote healthy lifestyles.

Screening for Hypertension

Epidemiology. Hypertension accounts for more atherosclerotic cardiovascular deaths than any other modifiable risk factor.[99] Nearly half of adults ages 20 years and older have *hypertension* (systolic blood pressure [SBP] ≥130 mm Hg or a diastolic blood pressure [DBP] ≥80 mm Hg), representing more than 120 million people (Box 18-31).[95] Individuals assigned male at birth (51%) have a higher prevalence of hypertension than those assigned female at birth (40%); prevalence markedly increases with age, ranging from 22% among adults ages 18 to 39 years, to 55% among adults ages 40 to 59 years, to 75% for adults

Box 18-31. Key Reports on Cardiovascular Health and Risk Assessment

- Heart Disease and Stroke Statistics—2018 Update: A Report From the American Heart Association (AHA)[102]; *updated annually*
- 2013 ACC/AHA Guideline on the Assessment of Cardiovascular Risk: A Report of the ACC/AHA Task Force on Practice Guidelines[103]
- Effectiveness-Based Guidelines for the Prevention of Cardiovascular Disease in Women—2011 Update: A Guideline From the AHA[104]
- Clinical Practice Guidelines for the Management of Hypertension in the Community: A Statement by the American Society of Hypertension and the International Society of Hypertension[105]
- Guidelines for the Primary Prevention of Stroke: A Guideline for Healthcare Professionals From the AHA/American Stroke Association (ASA), 2014.[106]
- Guidelines for the Prevention of Stroke in Women: A Statement for Healthcare Professionals From the AHA/ASA[107]
- Standards of Medical Care in Diabetes—2018: American Diabetes Association[108]; *updated annually*
- 2017 ACC/AHA/AAPA/ABC/ACPM/AGS/APhA/ASH/ASPC/NMA/PCNA Guideline for the Prevention, Detection, Evaluation, and Management of High Blood Pressure in Adults: Executive Summary: A Report of the ACC/AHA Task Force on Clinical Practice Guidelines[109]
- 2018 AHA/ACC/AACVPR/AAPA/ABC/ACPM/ADA/AGS/APhA/ASPC/NLA/PCNA Guideline on the Management of Blood Cholesterol: A Report of the ACC/AHA Task Force on Clinical Practice Guidelines[110]

ages 60 years and older. Non-Hispanic Black adults (57%) have the highest prevalence of hypertension in the United States, followed by White (44%) and Hispanic (44%) adults.[100] Data from the 2017 to 2020 National Health and Nutrition Examination Survey estimated that 62% of U.S. adults with hypertension were aware of their diagnosis, 53% were receiving treatment, but only 26% had their blood pressure under control.[95] Uncontrolled hypertension is a major risk factor for ischemic heart disease, cerebrovascular disease, CHF, and chronic kidney disease. In 2021, hypertension was a primary or contributing cause of more than 700,000 U.S. deaths.[101]

These differences in hypertension prevalence may be influenced by Social Determinants of Health (SDH), including access to healthcare, socioeconomic status, neighborhood environment, and experiences of chronic stress. These factors can impact health behaviors, stress levels, and healthcare access, contributing to disparities in hypertension across racial and ethnic groups.

- *Primary (essential) hypertension* is the most common cause of hypertension: risk factors include age, genetic predisposition, having a Black racial or ethnic background, obesity and weight gain, high salt intake, physical inactivity, and excessive alcohol consumption.
- *Secondary hypertension* accounts for <5% of hypertension cases. Causes include obstructive sleep apnea, chronic kidney disease, renovascular disease, medications, thyroid disease, parathyroid disease, Cushing syndrome, hyperaldosteronism, pheochromocytoma, and coarctation of the aorta.

Screening. The U.S. Preventive Services Task Force (USPSTF) has issued a grade A recommendation strongly encouraging annual BP screening of adults ages 40 years and older and those at increased risk for high BP.[111] Determinants of increased risk include having high-normal BPs (130–139/85–89 mm Hg), being overweight or obese, and having a Black racial or ethnic background. Average-risk adults ages 18 to 39 years can be screened every 3 to 5 years. The USPSTF has consistently found good-quality evidence that screening provides substantial benefits for reducing CVD events.[112] The most important potential harm of screening is overdiagnosis, leading to unnecessary medication.[113] However, the USPSTF guideline emphasizes the importance of generally not beginning pharmacologic treatment until confirming elevated office readings with ambulatory blood pressure monitoring (ABPM) or home blood pressure monitoring (HBPM). Immediate pharmacologic treatment is still recommended for patients with severe hypertension, particularly those with acute end-organ damage. In 2017, the American College of Cardiology (ACC) and American Heart Association (AHA) released a Guideline for the Prevention, Detection, Evaluation, and Management of High Blood Pressure in Adults.[109] They recommended obtaining automated BP measurements in the clinic and confirming hypertension with ABPM and HBPM. The ACC/AHA guideline defined hypertension as SBP higher than 130 mm Hg or DBP higher than 80 mm Hg. Adults with SBP between 120 and 129 mm Hg and DBP higher than 80 mm Hg were classified as having elevated BP. A 1-year reassessment was recommended for adults with normal BP, while those with elevated BP should be reassessed in 3 to 6 months.

These differences may be due to genetic factors, socioeconomic conditions, healthcare access, and chronic stress impacting certain groups more significantly.

Initiating Statin Therapy for Primary Prevention

Elevated blood cholesterol levels are associated with an increased risk for atherosclerotic CVD.[110] HMG-CoA reductase inhibitors (statins) can substantially lower levels of low-density lipoprotein (LDL) cholesterol levels and modestly increase levels of high-density lipoprotein (HDL) cholesterol. Statin therapy reduces the risk of overall mortality and CVD events in persons at increased CVD risk.[114] Determining whether to consider prescribing a statin begins with assessing CVD risk. Use the CVD risk calculators shown in Box 18-32 to

While CVD risk calculators are valuable, they may include race or ethnicity as variables, potentially reinforcing health disparities and oversimplifying social, economic, and environmental factors. Clinicians should use them cautiously, considering individual and broader social contexts.

Box 18-32. Selected Web-Based Cardiovascular Disease Risk Calculators

ASCVD Risk Estimator Plus (American College of Cardiology/American Heart Association)	https://tools.acc.org/ASCVD-Risk-Estimator-Plus/#!/calculate/estimate
QRISK3 (University of Nottingham/ClinRisk Ltd.)	https://qrisk.org/

establish 10-year and lifetime risk for patients aged 40 to 79 years. These risk estimates, which incorporate factors such as age, sex, smoking history, total cholesterol level, HDL level, systolic blood pressure (SBP), antihypertensive therapy, and diabetes, are derived from pooled data from population-based studies. However, there is insufficient data to reliably predict risk for individuals younger than 40 or older than 79 years. The primary purpose of these risk estimates is to facilitate crucial clinician–patient discussions about risk reduction strategies.

Treatment guidelines are based on the 10-year CVD risk. The USPSTF issued a grade B recommendation for initiating moderate-intensity statins for primary CVD prevention in asymptomatic adults ages 40 to 75 years who have one or more CVD risk factors (high cholesterol, diabetes, hypertension, or smoking) and a 10-year calculated CVD event risk 10% or higher.[115] Implementing this recommendation means periodically (every 5 years is considered a reasonable interval) measuring lipid levels in all adults ages 40 to 75 years who do not have existing CVD. The USPSTF further recommended that clinicians selectively consider offering a statin for those with a 10-year CVD risk of 7.5% to less than 10.0% (grade C). Evidence was insufficient (I statement) to make recommendations for prescribing a statin for adults ages 76 years and older.

An ACC/AHA Task Force also published a clinical practice guideline for managing cholesterol based on CVD risk (Fig. 18-25).[110] Clinicians were encouraged to engage patients in shared decision-making discussions, addressing the potential benefits and harms of prescribing statins and eliciting patient preferences before initiating therapy. Clinicians may consider obtaining a coronary artery calcium score for persons who remain uncertain after the treatment discussion.

Promoting Lifestyle Changes and Risk Factor Modification

The USPSTF has given a grade B recommendation to offer or refer adults with CVD risk factors to behavioral counseling interventions to promote a healthy diet and physical activity.[116] The target population is adults ages 18 years and older with hypertension or elevated BP, dyslipidemia, or mixed or multiple risk factors such as an estimated 10-year CVD risk 7.5% or higher or metabolic syndrome (Box 18-33).

Metabolic syndrome is diagnosed when any three of the following five risk factors are present: (1) elevated waist circumference, (2) elevated triglycerides, (3) reduced HDL cholesterol, (4) elevated BP, and (5) elevated fasting plasma glucose.[95] The USPSTF concluded that behavioral counseling interventions had a moderate net benefit in reducing CVD events and improving risk factor profiles. They considered the key elements of the interventions to include intensive and multiple sessions that address (1) dietary changes such as reducing saturated fats, sodium, and sugar and increasing consumption of fruits, vegetables, and whole grains and (2) achieving 90 to 180 minutes weekly of moderate to vigorous activity. Counseling can include strategies such as motivational interviewing

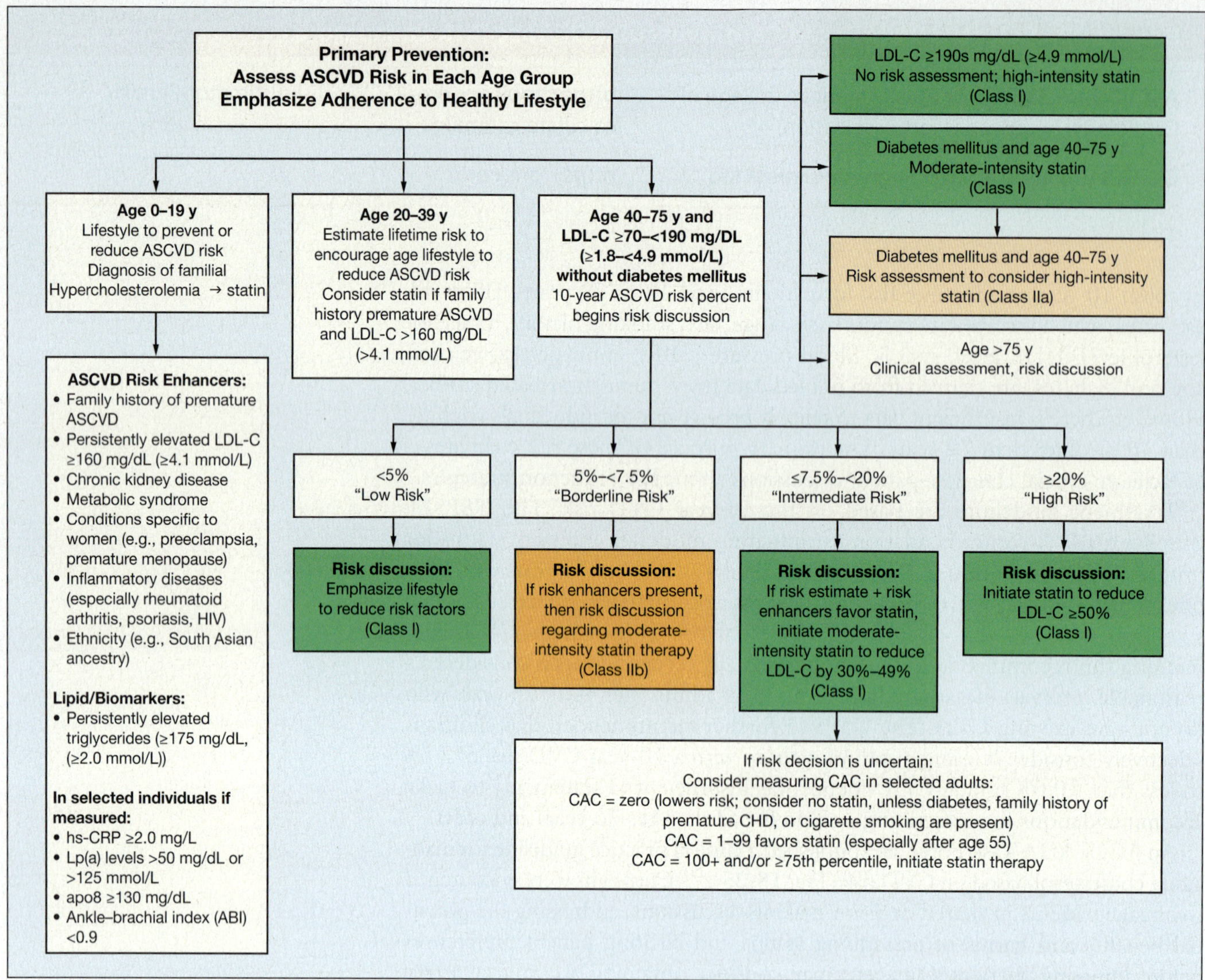

FIGURE 18-25. American College of Cardiology/American Heart Association cholesterol guideline, 2018. ASCVD, atherosclerotic cardiovascular disease; CAC, coronary artery calcium; CHD, coronary heart disease; HIV, human immunodeficiency syndrome; hs-CRP, high-sensitivity C-reactive protein; LDL-C, low-density lipoprotein cholesterol. (Reprinted with permission from Grundy SM, Stone NJ, Bailey AL, et al. 2018 AHA/ACC/AACVPR/AAPA/ABC/ACPM/ADA/AGS/APhA/ASPC/NLA/PCNA guideline on the management of blood cholesterol: a report of the American College of Cardiology/American Heart Association Task Force on clinical practice guidelines. *Circulation.* 2019;139(25):e1082–e1143. Copyright © 2018 American Heart Association, Inc., and the American College of Cardiology Foundation.)

and behavioral change techniques and be delivered by primary care clinicians or nonphysicians. The USPSTF recommended individualizing decisions about behavioral counseling intervention for those without CVD risk factors (grade C).[117] The ACC and AHA have issued an evidence-based summary of strategies for implementing primary prevention of CVD, highlighting the importance of a heart-healthy lifestyle and optimizing control of BP, cholesterol, and diabetes.[99]

In addition to the grade B recommendations to screen for hypertension[111] and initiate statins for high-risk adults,[115] the USPSTF has addressed other CVD risk factors. They recommended offering tobacco cessation interventions to persons currently smoking (grade A) (see Chapter 7, Health Maintenance and Screening, pp. 130–131),[126] offering behavioral weight loss interventions

Box 18-33. Screening for Major Cardiovascular Risk Factors

Risk Factor	Screening Recommendation	Goal
Family history of premature CVD[118]	Ask about family history	Estimate CVD risk
Cigarette smoking[119]	Ask about tobacco use	Cessation or continued abstinence
Unhealthy diet[120,121]	Ask about diet	Improved overall eating pattern
Physical inactivity[122,123]	Ask about physical activity.	30 min moderate-intensity exercise five times weekly
Obesity[10,45]	Estimate BMI and/or measure waist circumference.	BMI ≤25 kg/m^2; waist circumference: ≤40 in for individuals assigned male at birth, ≤35 in for individuals assigned female at birth
Hypertension[109]	Measure blood pressure.	<130/80 mm Hg for adults
Dyslipidemias[110,124]	Obtain baseline fasting lipids at age 21. Measure fasting lipids in average-risk adults every 5 y from ages 40 to 75.	Initiate statin therapy if meeting ACC/AHA guidelines
Diabetes[107]	Check hemoglobin A_{1c} or fasting glucose every 3 y (if normal) beginning at age 45 y; more frequently at any age if with risk factors.	Prevent/delay diabetes for those with HbA_{1c} of 5.7% to 6.4%
Atrial fibrillation[125]	Assess heart rhythm.	Identify and treat atrial fibrillation

to obese adults (grade B) (see Chapter 10, General Survey, Vital Signs, and Pain, pp. 192–194),[127] and screening for prediabetes and type 2 diabetes in adults ages 35 to 70 years who are overweight or obese (grade B).[128]

Addressing Excessive Dietary Sodium

In 2019, an estimated 1.9 million deaths worldwide were attributed to high sodium intake.[129] Although the AHA considers the ideal daily sodium intake to be less than 1,500 mg,[99] the National Academy of Medicine (NAM) has determined that a daily dietary intake of 2,300 mg of sodium is the acceptable upper intake level for adults.[130] While reducing sodium intake to 1,500 mg provides better BP control, the NAM found no evidence of benefit for overall health outcomes below the 2,300 mg level.[131] However, the average sodium intake among Americans is 3,468 mg/day, and nearly 90% of adults exceed the recommended upper intake level.[132]

Because more than 70% of consumed sodium comes from processed foods, the AHA and the NAM jointly recommended population-wide salt-reduction measures, including government standards for manufacturers, restaurants, and food service operators.[133,134] Advise patients to read the Nutrition Facts panel on food labels closely to help them adhere to the 2,300-mg/day guideline. Following eating plans such as the Dietary Approaches to Stop Hypertension (DASH) diet or the American Heart Association Healthy Diet, which limits foods high in sodium, saturated fats, sugar, and dairy and increase vegetable, fruit, and whole grain consumption, can reduce CVD risk.[99,116]

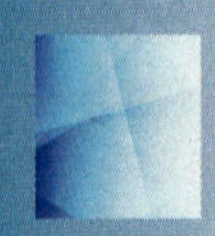

TABLE 18-1. Selected Heart Rates and Rhythms

Cardiac rhythms may be classified as regular or irregular. When rhythms are irregular, or rates are either fast or slow, obtain an ECG to identify the origin of the beats (sinus node, AV node, atrium, or ventricle) and the conduction pattern. The normal range for normal sinus rhythm is reported at 60–100 beats/min. Note that AV nodal rhythms, including AV block, may have a fast, normal, or slow ventricular rate.

IS THE RHYTHM REGULAR OR IRREGULAR?

REGULAR → WHAT IS THE RATE?

Rate	ECG Pattern	Usual Resting Rate
FAST (>100)	Sinus tachycardia	100–180
	Supraventricular (atrial or nodal) tachycardia	150–250
	Atrial flutter with a regular ventricular response	100–175
	Ventricular tachycardia	110–250
OR		
NORMAL (60–90)	Normal sinus rhythm	60–90
	Second-degree AV block	60–100
	Atrial flutter with a regular ventricular response	75–100
OR		
SLOW (<60)	Sinus bradycardia	<60
	Second-degree AV block	30–60
	Complete heart block	<40

IRREGULAR → WHAT IS THE PATTERN OF IRREGULARITY?

Pattern	ECG Pattern	Usual Resting Rate
SPORADIC	Premature or extra beats at random intervals, but normal underlying rhythm: e.g., atrial or ventricular premature contractions, sinus arrhythmia	See Table 18-2
OR		
REGULARLY IRREGULAR	Regular pattern of cadences: e.g., ventricular trigeminy	See Table 18-2
OR		
IRREGULARLY IRREGULAR	No discernible regularity: e.g., atrial fibrillation, atrial flutter	See Table 18-2

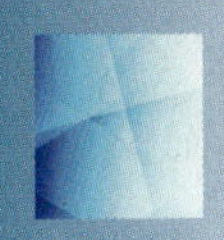

TABLE 18-2. Selected Irregular Rhythms

Type of Rhythm	ECG Waves and Heart Sounds	
SPORADIC Sinus Arrhythmia	S_1 S_2 S_1 S_2 S_1 S_2 S_1 S_2 S_1 S_2 INSPIRATION EXPIRATION	**Rhythm.** The heart varies cyclically, usually speeding up with inspiration and slowing down with expiration. **Heart Sounds.** Normal, although S_1 may vary with the heart rate.
Atrial or Nodal Premature Contractions (*Supraventricular*)	Aberrant P wave; Normal QRS and T QRS; P; T S_1 S_2 Early beat; Pause	**Rhythm.** A beat of atrial or nodal origin comes earlier than the next expected normal beat. A pause follows, and then the rhythm resumes. **Heart Sounds.** S_1 may differ in intensity from the S_1 of normal beats, and S_2 may be decreased.
SPORADIC Ventricular Premature Contractions (*Ventricular bigeminy or trigeminy*)	No P wave; Aberrant QRS and T S_1 S_2 Early beat with split sounds; Pause	**Rhythm.** A beat of ventricular origin comes earlier than the next expected normal beat. A pause follows, and the rhythm resumes. **Heart Sounds.** S_1 may differ in intensity from the S_1 of the normal beats, and S_2 may be decreased. Both sounds are likely to be split.
IRREGULARLY IRREGULAR Atrial Fibrillation and Atrial Flutter with Varying AV Block	No P waves; Fibrillation waves S_1 S_2 S_1 S_2 S_1 S_2 S_1 S_2	**Rhythm.** The ventricular rhythm is totally irregular, although short runs of the irregular ventricular rhythm may seem regular. **Heart Sounds.** S_1 varies in intensity.

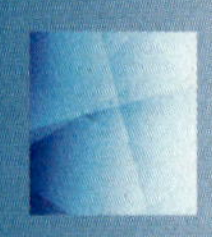

TABLE 18-3. Abnormalities of the Arterial Pulse and Pressure Waves

Normal

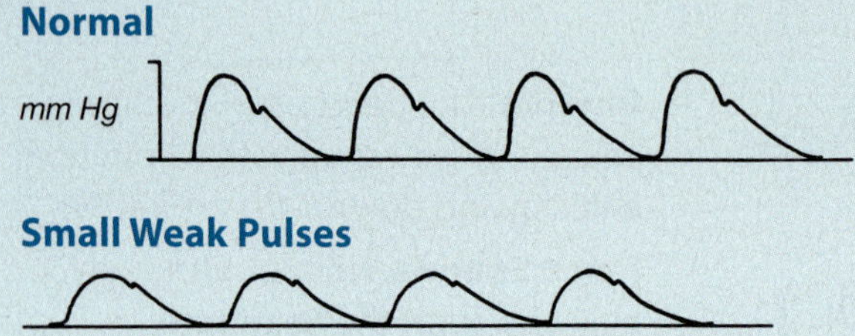

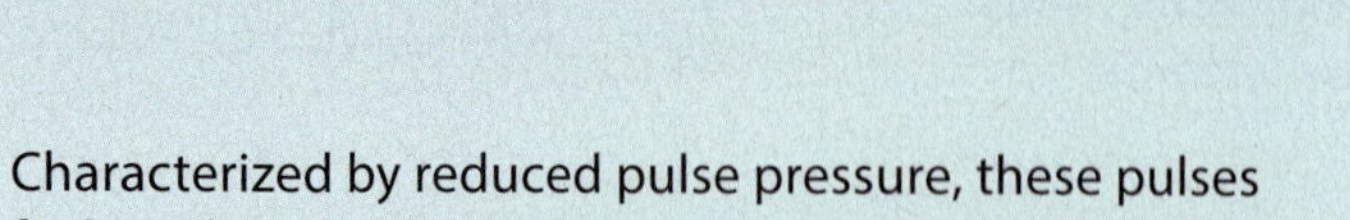

Pulse pressure ranges from 30 to 40 mm Hg with a smooth, rounded contour. The descending notch is impalpable.

Small Weak Pulses

Characterized by reduced pulse pressure, these pulses feel weak and indicate a slowed upstroke and elongated peak. Causes may include decreased stroke volume due to heart failure, hypovolemia, aortic stenosis, or increased peripheral resistance from cold exposure or severe heart failure.

Large Bounding Pulses

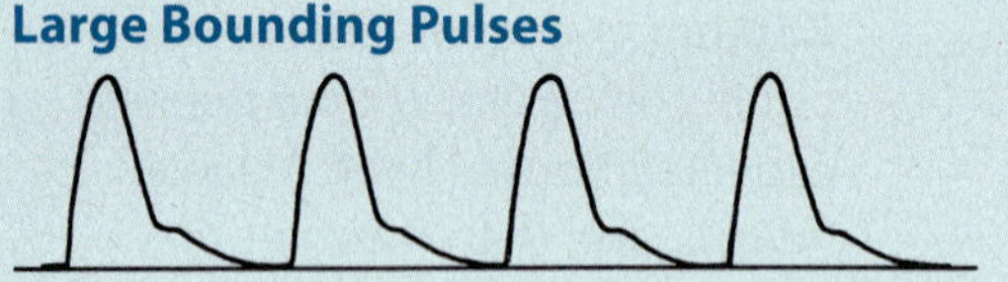

These are pulses with elevated pulse pressure, presenting as strong and bounding. They are often rapid in both ascent and descent with a short-lived peak. Possible etiologies include enhanced stroke volume, reduced peripheral resistance, or a combination thereof, as seen in conditions like fever, anemia, and various cardiovascular anomalies or from reduced aortic wall compliance due to aging or atherosclerosis.

Bisferiens Pulse

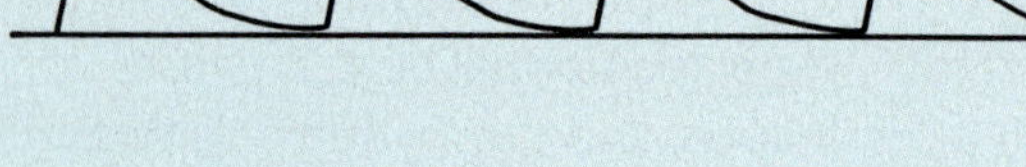

Characterized by an arterial pulse with a dual systolic peak, discernible with moderate arterial compression, this is typically associated with aortic regurgitation, combined aortic valve disease, or hypertrophic cardiomyopathy.

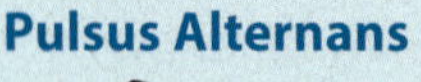

Pulsus Alternans

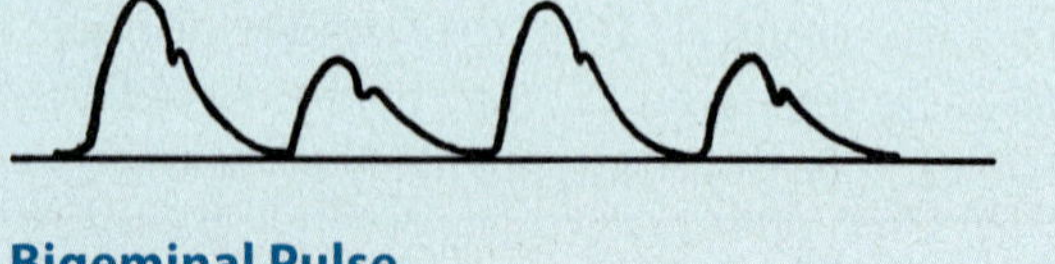

This regular pulse pattern alternates in amplitude between strong and weak beats and often signifies severe left ventricular dysfunction. Minor variations might necessitate a blood pressure cuff for detection (see p. 498).

Bigeminal Pulse

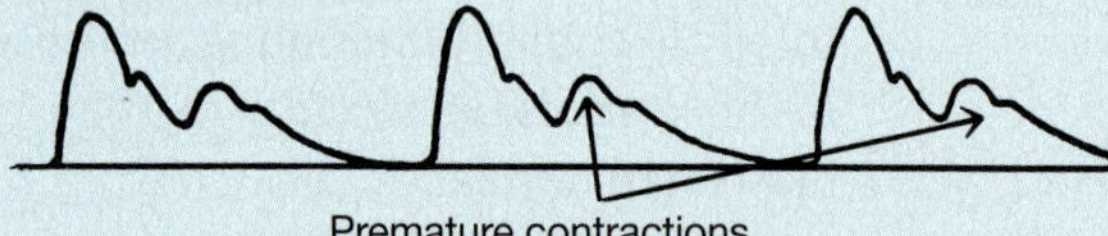

Similar to pulsus alternans, this involves a sequence of a normal beat followed by a premature contraction, resulting in alternating pulse amplitude correlated to the varying stroke volume.

Paradoxical Pulse

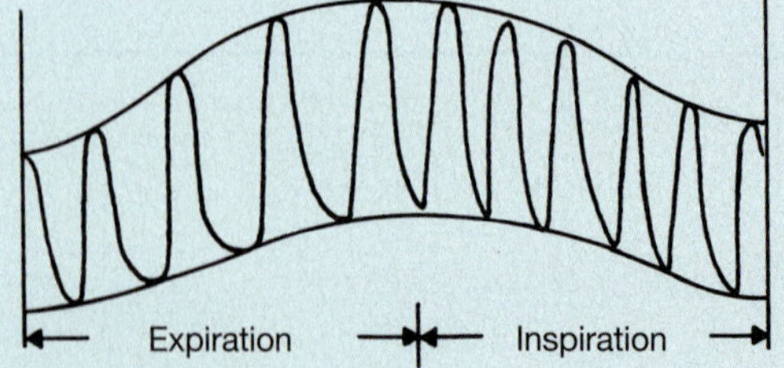

Identifiable by a detectable decrease in pulse amplitude during quiet inspiration and, in less obvious cases, by a drop in systolic pressure exceeding 10–12 mm Hg as measured with a cuff. It is commonly observed in pericardial tamponade, respiratory condition exacerbations, and constrictive pericarditis.

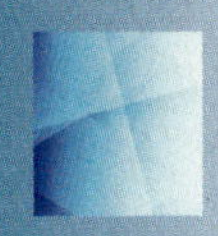

TABLE 18-4. Variations and Abnormalities of the Ventricular Impulses

In a healthy heart, the point of maximal impulse (PMI) is typically the *left ventricular impulse*, a fleeting sensation produced by the apex's contact with the chest wall during contraction. The *right ventricular impulse* is typically impalpable after infancy, with undefined characteristics. Familiarize yourself with the classic descriptors of the normal left ventricular PMI.

- *Location:* in the fourth or fifth left intercostal space, at the midclavicular line
- *Diameter:* discrete, or ≤2 cm
- *Amplitude:* brisk and tapping
- *Duration:* ≤2/3 of systole

A thorough assessment of the ventricular impulse can reveal critical insights into cardiovascular hemodynamics. The attributes of the ventricular impulse evolve in response to high-output conditions (such as anxiety, hyperthyroidism, and severe anemia) and pathologic states of chronic pressure or volume overload. Beyond the typical brisk tapping PMI, identify three other ventricular impulse types and their unique characteristics as detailed in the table below:

- *Hyperkinetic:* vigorous ventricular impulse due to a temporary increase in stroke volume, which is not necessarily a sign of heart disease
- *Sustained:* prolonged ventricular impulse resulting from ventricular hypertrophy due to a persistent pressure load, indicating *increased afterload*
- *Diffuse:* widespread ventricular impulse caused by ventricular dilation from chronic volume overload, reflecting *increased preload*

	Left Ventricular Impulse			Right Ventricular Impulse		
	Hyperkinetic	**Pressure Overload**	**Volume Overload**	**Hyperkinetic**	**Pressure Overload**	**Volume Overload**
Examples of Causes	Anxiety, hyperthyroidism, severe anemia	Aortic stenosis, hypertension	Aortic or mitral regurgitation; cardiomyopathy	Anxiety, hyperthyroidism, severe anemia	Pulmonic stenosis, pulmonary hypertension	Atrial septal defect
Location	Normal	Normal	Displaced to the left and possibly downward	Third, fourth, or fifth left intercostal spaces	Third, fourth, or fifth left intercostal spaces, subxiphoid area	Left sternal border, extending toward the left cardiac border, subxiphoid area
Diameter	–2 cm, though increased amplitude may make diameter feel larger	>2 cm	>2 cm	Not useful	Not useful	Not useful
Amplitude	More forceful tapping	More forceful tapping	*Diffuse*	Slightly more forceful	More forceful	Slightly to markedly more forceful
Duration	<2/3 systole	*Sustained* (up to S_2)	Often slightly sustained	Normal	*Sustained*	Normal to slightly sustained

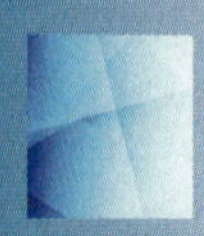

TABLE 18-5. Variations in the First Heart Sound—S_1

Normal Variations	S_1 S_2	S_1 is generally softer than S_2 at the *base* (right and left second intercostal spaces)
	S_1 S_2	S_1 is often but not always louder than S_2 at the apex
Accentuated S_1	S_1 S_2	Amplified during tachycardia, short PR interval rhythms, high cardiac output states (like during exercise, anemia, hyperthyroidism), and mitral stenosis
Diminished S_1	S_1 S_2	Decreased in first-degree heart block, left bundle-branch block, myocardial infarction, and premature mitral valve closure as seen in severe aortic regurgitation
Varying S_1	S_1 S_2 S_1 S_2	Intensity fluctuates in complete heart block, where atrial and ventricular beats are asynchronous, and in irregular rhythms such as atrial fibrillation, due to varying positions of the mitral valve at the time of ventricular contraction
Split S_1	S_1 S_2	Indicates delayed tricuspid valve closure; best heard along the lower left sternal border and more pronounced in right bundle-branch block Occasionally audible at the apex but should not be confused with S_4, an aortic ejection sound, or an early systolic click

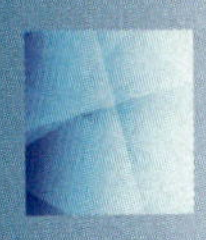

TABLE 18-6. Variations in the Second Heart Sound—S_2

	Inspiration	Expiration	
Physiologic Splitting	S_1 S_2 (A_2 P_2)	S_1 S_2	Splitting of S_2 should be assessed in the second or third left intercostal space. At the apex or aortic area, S_2 typically sounds singular, representing aortic valve closure since the pulmonic component is too soft to detect. Normal respiratory variation causes S_2 splitting to widen during inspiration, due to delayed P_2 following A_2, and to disappear upon expiration.
Pathologic Splitting	S_1 S_2	S_1 S_2	Wide physiologic splitting of S_2 persists throughout the respiratory cycle, indicating delayed pulmonic valve closure (as in pulmonic stenosis or right bundle branch block) or premature aortic valve closure (as in mitral regurgitation).
	S_1 S_2	S_1 S_2	Fixed splitting of S_2, not affected by breathing, usually indicates prolonged right ventricular systole, such as in atrial septal defect.
	S_1 S_2	S_1 S_2 (P_2 A_2)	Paradoxical or reversed splitting occurs when S_2 splits on expiration and merges on inspiration, often caused by a delayed aortic valve closure, as seen in left bundle branch block, where A_2 follows P_2 on expiration.

A_2 and P_2: Second Right Intercostal Space

A_2 with Increased Intensity (A_2 can usually be heard only in right second intercostal space): occurs in systemic hypertension because of the increased pressure load. Increased intensity also occurs when the aortic root is dilated, attributed to the increased proximity of the aortic valve to the chest wall.

A_2 Decreased or Absent: occurs in calcific aortic stenosis due to valve immobility. If A_2 is inaudible, no splitting is heard.

P_2 with Increased Intensity: When P_2 is equal to or louder than A_2, suspect pulmonary hypertension. Other causes include a dilated pulmonary artery and an atrial septal defect. When a split S_2 is heard widely, extending to the apex and the right base, P_2 is accentuated.

P_2 Decreased or Absent: This usually occurs from the increased AP diameter of the chest associated with aging. It can also result from pulmonic stenosis. If P_2 is inaudible, no splitting is heard.

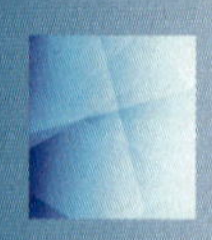

TABLE 18-7. Extra Heart Sounds in Systole

There are two kinds of extra heart sounds in systole: (1) early ejection sounds and (2) clicks, commonly heard in mid- and late systole.

Early Systolic Ejection Sounds

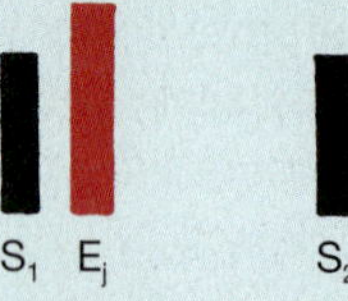

Early systolic ejection sounds are high-pitched, clicking noises occurring just after S_1, marking the abrupt stop of the aortic and pulmonic valves when they open in early systole.[47] Best heard with the diaphragm, these sounds suggest cardiovascular disease.

An *aortic ejection* sound can be detected at the base and apex of the heart, often louder at the apex and typically unaltered by respiration. It may indicate an enlarged aorta or aortic valve abnormalities, including congenital stenosis or a bicuspid aortic valve.[48,49]

A *pulmonic ejection* sound is most audible in the second and third left intercostal spaces and may be mistaken for a loud S_1. Its intensity usually *lessens upon inspiration* and can be a sign of pulmonary artery dilation, pulmonary hypertension, or pulmonic stenosis.

Systolic Clicks

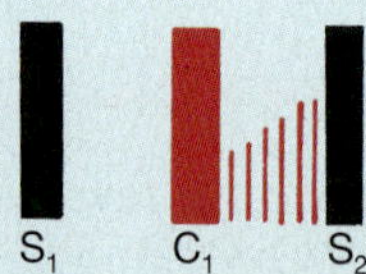

Systolic clicks are usually caused by *mitral valve prolapse (MVP)*—often mid-to-late systolic, are produced by the abnormal ballooning of the mitral valve into the left atrium due to leaflet redundancy and chordae tendineae elongation. MVP affects about 2–3% of the population without gender disparity.[50–52]

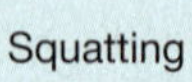

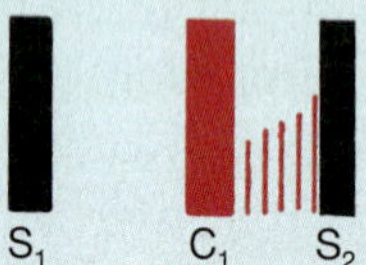

The click is typically high-pitched, heard best at or medial to the apex and the lower left sternal border, and may precede a late systolic murmur from mitral regurgitation. The presence and character of clicks and murmurs in MVP can vary significantly, with some patients presenting only a click, others only a murmur, and some both. These auscultatory findings can change between examinations and with different body positions.

Standing

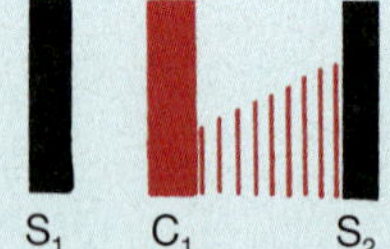

MVP auscultation findings are position-dependent, with squatting (and Valsalva release) delaying the click and murmur, and standing (and Valsalva strain) advancing them closer to S_1. Multiple positions, including supine, seated, squatting, and standing, are recommended for a thorough evaluation.

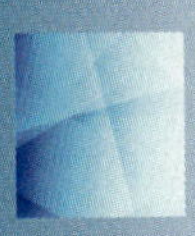

TABLE 18-8. Extra Heart Sounds in Diastole

Opening Snap (OS)

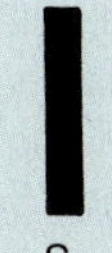

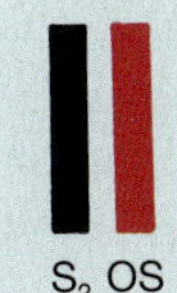

Early diastolic sound from the abrupt halting at the opening of a stenotic mitral valve, heard just medial to the apex and the lower left sternal border. Loud OS can radiate to the apex and pulmonic area, potentially mimicking the pulmonic component of split S_2. Its distinct high pitch and snapping quality differentiate it from S_2, though calcification of the valve leaflets can make it less audible, best heard with the diaphragm.

S_3

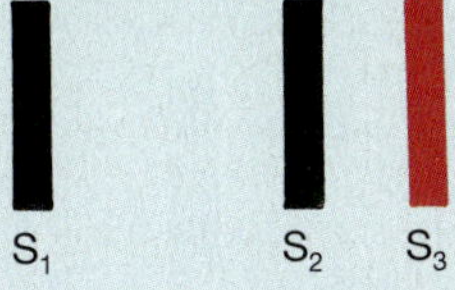

Physiologic S_3 is common in children, young adults up to 35 or 40 y, and often in the last pregnancy trimester. It occurs early in diastole during rapid ventricular filling, sounding later than an OS, and is dull and low pitched. Best detected at the apex in the left lateral decubitus position using the bell of the stethoscope with light pressure.

Pathologic S_3, or ventricular gallop, resembles a physiologic S_3 but is typically considered abnormal in adults over 40, indicating high left ventricular filling pressures and abrupt inflow deceleration across the mitral valve at diastole's rapid filling end. Common causes are reduced myocardial contractility, heart failure, ventricular volume overload from aortic or mitral regurgitation, and left-to-right shunts.[53,54]

For detection, a *left-sided S_3* is best heard at the apex in the left lateral decubitus position, while a *right-sided S_3* is audible along the lower left sternal border or below the xiphoid when the patient is supine, intensifying during inspiration. The term "gallop" describes the rhythm of three heart sounds, mimicking "Kentucky" at faster heart rates.

S_4 (atrial gallop)

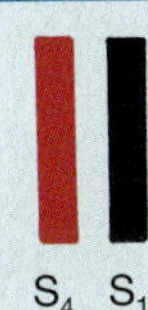

Precedes S_1 and is characterized by a dull, low pitch, optimally heard at the apex with the bell. A right ventricular S_4 may be detected at the lower left sternal border or subxiphoid area, especially in cases of obstructive lung disease. While an S_4 can be normal in athletes and the elderly, it often signifies ventricular hypertrophy or fibrosis, leading to stiffness and resistance (or decreased compliance) during filling after atrial contraction.[3,55]

Causes of a left-sided S_4 include hypertensive heart disease, aortic stenosis, ischemic, and hypertrophic cardiomyopathy.

Left-sided S_4 is optimally heard at the apex in the left lateral decubitus position, producing a "Tennessee" cadence. The rarer *right-sided S_4* can be detected along the lower left sternal border or below the xiphoid, often amplifying during inspiration, with causes like pulmonary hypertension and pulmonic stenosis.

An S_4 may result from delayed atrioventricular conduction, making the usually faint atrial sound distinguishable from the louder S_1. An S_4 cannot be present in the absence of atrial contractions, such as during atrial fibrillation.

In some cases, a patient exhibits both an S_3 and an S_4, creating a quadruple rhythm. When heart rates are high, these sounds may blend into a singular loud extra heart sound, known as a *summation gallop.*

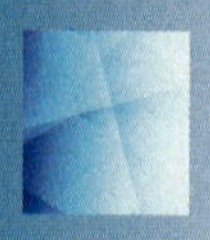

TABLE 18-9. Midsystolic Murmurs

Midsystolic ejection murmurs are the most common kind of heart murmur. They may be (1) *innocent*—without any detectable physiologic or structural abnormality; (2) *physiologic*—from physiologic changes in body metabolism; or (3) *pathologic*—arising from structural abnormalities in the heart or great vessels.[56–58] Midsystolic murmurs tend to peak near midsystole and usually stop before S_2. The crescendo–decrescendo or "diamond" shape is not always audible. The gap between the murmur and S_2 helps to distinguish midsystolic from pansystolic murmurs.

	Innocent Murmurs	Physiologic Murmurs
	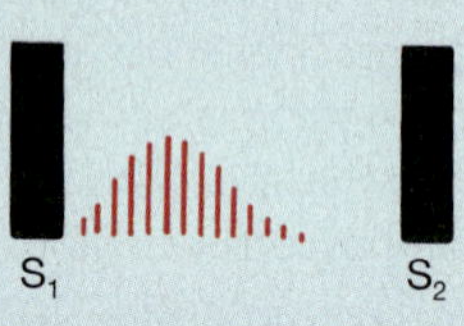	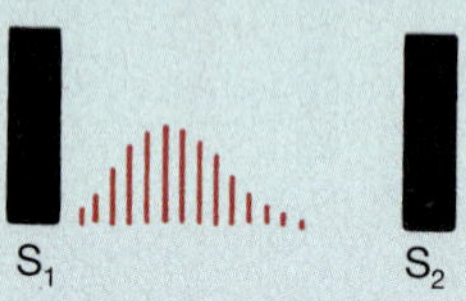
Murmur	*Location.* Left second to fourth intercostal spaces between the left sternal border and the apex *Radiation.* Minimal *Intensity.* Grades 1 to 2, possibly 3 *Pitch.* Soft to medium *Quality.* Variable *Maneuvers.* Usually decreases or disappears on sitting	Similar to innocent murmurs
Associated Findings	None: normal splitting, no ejection sounds, no diastolic murmurs, and no palpable evidence of ventricular enlargement. Occasionally, both an innocent murmur and pathologic murmur are present.	Signs of physiologic causes (see mechanisms below)
Mechanism	Turbulent blood flow, probably generated by ventricular ejection of blood into the aorta from the left and occasionally the right ventricle. Very common in children and young adults but may also be present in older adults. There is no underlying CVD.	Turbulence due to a temporary increase in blood flow in predisposing conditions such as anemia, pregnancy, fever, and hyperthyroidism.

Pathologic Murmurs

Aortic Stenosis[49,59,60]	Hypertrophic Cardiomyopathy[61]	Pulmonic Stenosis[62]
May be decreased S_1 S_2	S_1 S_1	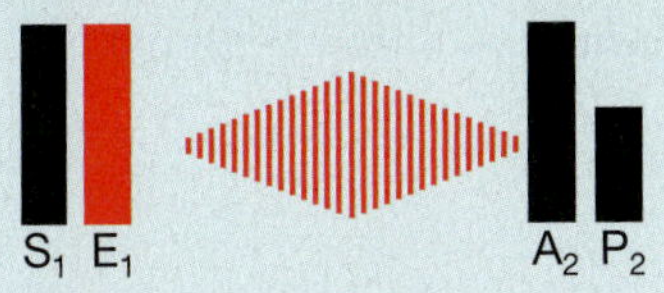
Location. Right second and third intercostal spaces *Radiation.* Often to the carotids, down the left sternal border, even to the apex. If severe, may radiate to left second and third intercostal spaces *Intensity.* Sometimes soft, but often loud, with a thrill *Pitch.* Medium, harsh; crescendo–decrescendo may be higher at the apex *Quality.* Often harsh; may be more musical at the apex *Maneuvers.* Heard best with the patient sitting and leaning forward	*Location.* Left third and fourth intercostal spaces *Radiation.* Down the left sternal border to the apex, possibly to the base, but not to the neck *Intensity.* Variable. See Maneuvers. *Pitch. Medium* *Quality.* Harsh *Maneuvers.* Intensity decreases with squatting and Valsalva release phase (increases venous return), *increases with standing and Valsalva strain phase* (decreases left ventricular volume) (see p. 510)	*Location.* Left second and third intercostal spaces *Radiation.* If loud, toward the left shoulder and neck *Intensity.* Soft to loud; if loud, associated with a thrill *Pitch.* Medium; crescendo–decrescendo *Quality.* Often harsh *Maneuvers:* No specific maneuvers noted beyond the typical auscultation guidelines.
As aortic stenosis worsens, the murmur peaks later in systole, and A_2 decreases in intensity. A_2 may be delayed and merged with $P_2 \rightarrow$ single S_2 on expiration or a paradoxical S_2 split. Carotid upstroke may be delayed, with a slow rise, small amplitude, and decreased volume. The hypertrophied left ventricle may produce a sustained apical impulse and an S_4 due to decreased compliance. After age 40 y there may be a dilated aorta and murmur of aortic regurgitation. Subendocardial ischemia due to poor coronary perfusion distal to the valve causes angina and syncope.	The carotid upstroke rises quickly, unlike aortic stenosis. The apical impulse is sustained. S_2 may be single. An S_4 is usually present at the apex (unlike mitral regurgitation). Usually benign, but progresses in 25% to syncope, ischemia, atrial fibrillation, dilated cardiomyopathy and heart failure, and stroke, with increased risk of sudden death.	The JVP is usually normal but may have prominent a wave. The right ventricular impulse is often sustained. An early pulmonic ejection sound is present in mild to moderate stenosis. In severe stenosis, S_2 is widely split and P_2 softens. May hear a right-sided S_4 over the left sternal border.
Significant stenosis causes turbulent blood flow across the valve and increases left ventricular afterload. The most common cause is valve calcification in older adults, at times progressing from nonobstructing sclerosis (present in 25%) to stenosis. The second most common cause is a congenital bicuspid aortic valve, often not recognized until adulthood.	Unexplained diffuse or focal ventricular hypertrophy with myocyte disarray and fibrosis associated with unusually rapid ejection of blood from the left ventricle during systole. Outflow tract obstruction of flow may coexist. Associated distortion of the mitral valve may cause mitral regurgitation.	Primarily a congenital disorder with valvular, supravalvular, or subvalvular stenosis. Stenosis impairs flow across the valve, increasing right ventricular afterload. In an atrial septal defect, increased flow across the pulmonic valve may mimic pulmonic stenosis.

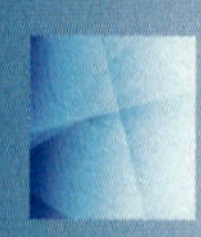

TABLE 18-10. Pansystolic (Holosystolic) Murmurs

Pansystolic (holosystolic) murmurs are pathologic, arising from blood flow from a chamber with high pressure to one of lower pressure, through a valve or other structure that should be closed. The murmur begins immediately with S_1 and continues up to S_2.

	Mitral Regurgitation[51,63–65]	Tricuspid Regurgitation[66–68]	Ventricular Septal Defect
	Decreased; S_1 S_2 S_3	S_1 S_2 S_3	S_1 S_2
Murmur	*Location.* Apex	*Location.* Lower left sternal border. If right ventricular pressure is high and the ventricle is enlarged, the murmur may be loudest at the apex and confused with mitral regurgitation	*Location.* Left third, fourth, and fifth intercostal spaces
	Radiation. To the left axilla, less often to the left sternal border	*Radiation.* To the right of the sternum, to the xiphoid area, and at times to the left midclavicular line, but not into the axilla	*Radiation.* Often wide, depending on the size of the defect
	Intensity. Soft to loud; if loud, associated with an apical thrill	*Intensity.* Variable	*Intensity.* Often very loud, with a thrill. Smaller defects have louder murmurs
	Pitch. Medium to high	*Pitch.* Medium	*Pitch.* High, holosystolic. Smaller defects have murmurs with a higher pitch
	Quality. Blowing, holosystolic	*Quality.* Blowing, holosystolic	*Quality.* Often harsh
	Maneuvers. The intensity of the murmur does not change with inspiration	*Maneuvers.* The intensity increases with inspiration, known as *Carvallo's sign.*	*Maneuvers:* Unlike tricuspid regurgitation, the intensity of the VSD murmur does not change with inspiration, but it does increase with inspiration, unlike mitral regurgitation.
Associated Findings	S_1 normal (75%), loud (12%), soft (12%) An apical S_3 reflects volume overload of the left ventricle. The apical impulse may be *diffuse* and laterally displaced. There may be a sustained lower left parasternal impulse from a dilated left atrium.	The right ventricular impulse is increased in amplitude and may be sustained. The JVP is often elevated in severe tricuspid regurgitation, with large *v* waves in the jugular veins, a pulsatile liver, ascites, and edema.	S_2 may be obscured by the loud murmur. Findings and associated findings vary with the size of the defect. Larger defects cause left-to-right shunts, pulmonary hypertension, and RV overload.
Mechanism	When the *mitral valve fails to close fully in systole,* blood regurgitates from left ventricle to left atrium, causing the murmur and increasing left ventricular preload, ultimately leading to left ventricular dilatation. Causes are structural, from mitral valve prolapse, infectious endocarditis, rheumatic heart disease, and collagen vascular disease; and functional, from ventricular dilatation and dilatation of the mitral valve annulus and from leaflet, papillary muscle, or chordae tendineae dysfunction.	When the *tricuspid valve fails to close fully in systole,* blood regurgitates from RV to right atrium, producing a murmur. The most common causes are RV failure and dilatation, with resulting enlargement of the tricuspid orifice, often induced by pulmonary hypertension or LV failure; and endocarditis—the RV and pulmonary artery pressures are low, so the murmur is early systolic.	A ventricular septal defect is a congenital abnormality classified according to one of four locations in the ventricular septum. The defect is a conduit for *blood flow from the relatively high-pressure left ventricle into the low-pressure right ventricle.* The defect may be accompanied by aortic regurgitation, tricuspid regurgitation, and aneurysms of the ventricular septum; an uncomplicated lesion is described here.

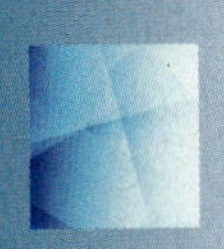

TABLE 18-11. Diastolic Murmurs

Diastolic murmurs are always pathologic. There are two basic types in adults. Early decrescendo diastolic murmurs signify regurgitant flow through an incompetent semilunar valve, usually the aortic. Rumbling diastolic murmurs in mid- or late diastole point to stenosis of an AV valve, usually the mitral. Diastolic murmurs are less common than systolic murmurs and more difficult to hear, requiring more meticulous examination.

	Aortic Regurgitation[69–72]	Mitral Stenosis[68,70]
	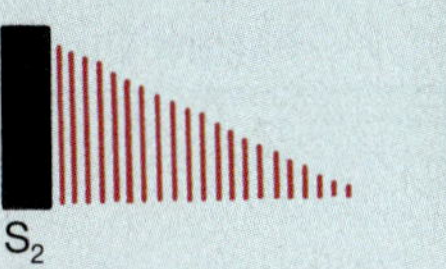	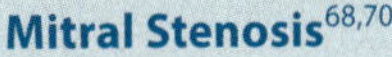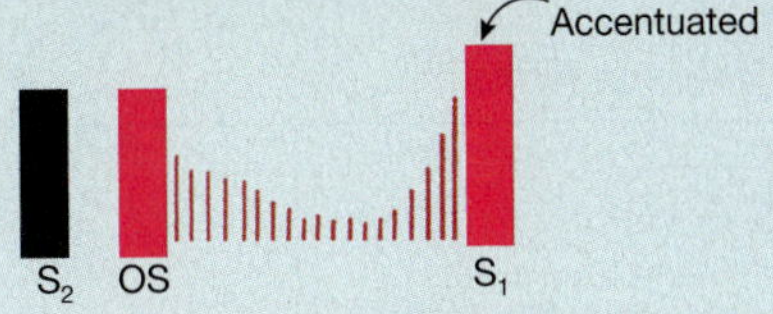
Murmur	*Location.* Left second to fourth intercostal spaces *Radiation.* If loud, to the apex, perhaps to the right sternal border *Intensity.* Grades 1–4 *Pitch.* High. *Use the diaphragm.* *Quality.* Blowing decrescendo; may be mistaken for breath sounds *Maneuvers.* The murmur is heard best with the *patient sitting, leaning forward,* with breath held after exhalation.	*Location.* Usually limited to the apex *Radiation.* Little or none *Intensity.* Grades 1–4 *Pitch.* Decrescendo low-pitched rumble with presystolic accentuation. *Use the bell.* *Maneuvers.* Placing the bell exactly on the apical impulse, turning the patient into *a left lateral position,* and mild exercise like handgrips make the murmur audible. It is heard better in exhalation.
Associated Findings	With advancing severity, the diastolic pressure drops to as low as 50 mm Hg; the pulse pressure can widen by >80 mm Hg. The apical impulse becomes *diffuse,* displaced laterally and downward, and increased in diameter, amplitude, and duration. A systolic ejection sound may be present; S_2 is increased in aortic root dilatation and decreased if leaflets are thickened and calcified; and an S_3 often reflects ventricular dysfunction from both volume and pressure overload. A midsystolic flow murmur or a mitral diastolic (*Austin Flint*) murmur, usually with mid-diastolic and presystolic components, reflect increased regurgitant flow. The arterial pulse wave collapses suddenly creating bounding arterial pulses with *pistol shot sounds* on light pressure of the diaphragm, especially with arm elevation (*Corrigan pulse*), a *to–fro murmur* over the brachial or femoral artery with firm pressure (*Duroziez sign*), and capillary pulsations with nail blanching (*Quincke pulses*).	S_1 is loud and may be palpable at the apex. An OS often follows S_2 and initiates the murmur. If pulmonary hypertension develops, P_2 is accentuated, the right ventricular parasternal impulse becomes palpable, and the *a* wave of the JVP is more prominent. The apical impulse is small and tapping. Atrial fibrillation occurs in about a third of symptomatic patients, with ensuing risks of thromboembolism.
Mechanism	The aortic valve leaflets fail to close completely during diastole, causing regurgitation from the aorta back into the left ventricle and left ventricular overload. The associated midsystolic flow murmur results from the ejection of this increased stroke volume across the aortic valve. The mitral diastolic (*Austin Flint*) murmur is seen in moderate to severe disease and attributed to diastolic impingement of the regurgitant flow on the anterior leaflet of the mitral valve. Causes include leaflet abnormalities, aortic pathology (Marfan syndrome), and subvalvular abnormalities such as subaortic stenosis or an atrial septal defect.	The stiffened mitral valve leaflets move into the left atrium in midsystole and narrow the valve opening, causing turbulence. The resulting murmur has two components: (1) mid-diastolic (during rapid ventricular filling) and (2) presystolic accentuation, possibly related to ventricular contraction. The most common cause worldwide is rheumatic fever, which causes fibrosis, calcification, and thickening of the leaflets and commissures, and chordal fusion.

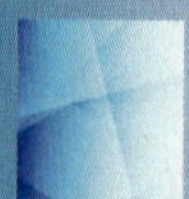

TABLE 18-12. Cardiovascular Sounds with Both Systolic and Diastolic Components

Some cardiovascular sounds extend beyond one phase of the cardiac cycle. Three examples, all nonvalvular in origin, are: (1) a *venous hum,* a benign sound produced by turbulence of blood in the jugular veins—common in children; (2) a *pericardial friction rub,* produced by inflammation of the pericardial sac; and (3) *patent ductus arteriosus,* a congenital anomaly that persists after birth causing a left-to-right shunt from the aorta to the pulmonary artery. *Continuous murmurs* begin in systole and extend through S_2 into all or part of diastole, as in *patent ductus arteriosus.* Arteriovenous fistulas, common in patients on hemodialysis, also produce continuous murmurs.

	Venous Hum	Pericardial Friction Rub[73,75]	Patent Ductus Arteriosus
	Systole, Diastole, S_1, S_2, S_1	Ventricular systole, Ventricular diastole, Atrial systole, S_1, S_2, S_1	Systole, Diastole, S_1, S_2, S_1
Timing	Continuous murmur without a silent interval. Loudest in diastole	Inflammation of the visceral and parietal pericardium from pericarditis produces a coarse grating sound with one, two, or three components (ventricular systole; ventricular filling and atrial contraction during diastole). Rubs are heard with and without pericardial effusions	Continuous murmur in both systole and diastole, often with a silent interval late in diastole. Loudest in late systole, obscures S_2, and fades in diastole
Location	Above the medial third of the clavicles, especially on the right, often when the head is turned in the opposite direction. Best heard when patient in sitting position; disappears when patient supine	Usually best heard in the left third intercostal space next to the sternum with the patient sitting and leaning forward with breath held after forced expiration. (In contrast, a pleural rub is heard only during inspiration.) May come and go spontaneously and require auscultation in several positions. Causes include myocardial infarction, uremia, connective tissue disease	Left second intercostal space
Radiation	Right or left first and second intercostal spaces	Minimal	Toward the left clavicle
Intensity	Soft to moderate. The hum is obliterated by pressure on the internal jugular vein.	Superficial sound of varying intensity that seems "close to the stethoscope"	Usually loud, sometimes associated with a thrill
Quality	Humming, roaring	Scratchy, scraping, grating	Harsh, machinery-like
Pitch	Low (heard better with the *bell*)	High (heard better with the *diaphragm*)	Medium

REFERENCES

1. Shorr RI, Johnson KC, Wan JY, et al. The prognostic significance of asymptomatic carotid bruits in the elderly. *J Gen Intern Med.* 1998;13(2):86–90.
2. McGee SR. Chapter 38: palpation of the heart. In: *Evidence-Based Physical Diagnosis.* 4th ed. Elsevier; 2018.
3. Shah SJ, Nakamura K, Marcus GM, et al. Association of the fourth heart sound with increased left ventricular end-diastolic stiffness. *J Card Fail.* 2008;14(5):431–436.
4. Minami Y, Kajimoto K, Sato N, et al. Third heart sound in hospitalised patients with acute heart failure: insights from the ATTEND study. *Int J Clin Pract.* 2015;69(8):820–828.
5. O'Gara PT, Loscalzo J. Chapter 267: physical examination of the cardiovascular system. In: Kasper DL, Fauci AS, Hauser SL, Longo DL, Jameson JL, Loscalzo J, eds. *Harrison's Principles of Internal Medicine.* 19th ed. McGraw-Hill Education; 2015.
6. McConaghy JR, Oza RS. Outpatient diagnosis of acute chest pain in adults. *Am Fam Physician.* 2013;87(3):177–182.
7. Writing Group Members; Mozaffarian D, Benjamin EJ, Go AS, et al; American Heart Association Statistics Committee; Stroke Statistics Subcommittee. Heart disease and stroke statistics-2016 update: a report from the American Heart Association. *Circulation.* 2016;133(4):e38–e360.
8. O'Gara PT, Kushner FG, Ascheim DD, et al. 2013 ACCF/AHA guideline for the management of ST-elevation myocardial infarction: a report of the American College of Cardiology Foundation/American Heart Association Task Force on Practice Guidelines. *J Am Coll Cardiol.* 2013;61(4):e78–e140.
9. Abrams J. Clinical practice. Chronic stable angina. *N Engl J Med.* 2005;352(24):2524–2533.
10. Cho S, Atwood JE. Peripheral edema. *Am J Med.* 2002; 113(7):580–586.
11. Clark AL, Cleland JG. Causes and treatment of oedema in patients with heart failure. *Nat Rev Cardiol.* 2013;10(3): 156–170.
12. Clark D 3rd, Ahmed MI, Dell'italia LJ, Fan P, McGiffin DC. An argument for reviving the disappearing skill of cardiac auscultation. *Cleve Clin J Med.* 2012;79(8):536–537, 544.
13. Markel H. The stethoscope and the art of listening. *N Engl J Med.* 2006;354(6):551–553.
14. Vukanovic-Criley JM, Hovanesyan A, Criley SR, et al. Confidential testing of cardiac examination competency in cardiology and noncardiology faculty and trainees: a multicenter study. *Clin Cardiol.* 2010;33(12):738–745.
15. Wayne DB, Butter J, Cohen ER, McGaghie WC. Setting defensible standards for cardiac auscultation skills in medical students. *Acad Med.* 2009;84(10 Suppl):S94–S96.
16. Marcus GM, Vessey J, Jordan MV, et al. Relationship between accurate auscultation of a clinically useful third heart sound and level of experience. *Arch Intern Med.* 2006; 166(6):617–622.
17. Johri AM, Durbin J, Newbigging J, et al. Cardiac point-of-care ultrasound: state-of-the-art in medical school education. *J Am Soc Echocardiogr.* 2018;31(7):749–760.
18. McGee SR. *Evidence-Based Physical Diagnosis.* 4th ed. Elsevier; 2018.
19. Simel DL, Rennie D, eds. *The Rational Clinical Examination: Evidence-Based Clinical Diagnosis.* McGraw-Hill Education; 2009. Accessed January 10, 2024. http://jamaevidence.mhmedical.com/book.aspx?bookID=845
20. Pickering TG, Hall JE, Appel LJ, et al. Recommendations for blood pressure measurement in humans and experimental animals: part 1: blood pressure measurement in humans: a statement for professionals from the Subcommittee of Professional and Public Education of the American Heart Association Council on High Blood Pressure Research. *Circulation.* 2005;111(5):697–716.
21. Powers BJ, Olsen MK, Smith VA, Woolson RF, Bosworth HB, Oddone EZ. Measuring blood pressure for decision making and quality reporting: where and how many measures? *Ann Intern Med.* 2011;154(12):781–788, W-289–W-290.
22. Appel LJ, Miller ER 3rd, Charleston J. Improving the measurement of blood pressure: is it time for regulated standards? *Ann Intern Med.* 2011;154(12):838–840.
23. Whelton PK, Carey RM, Aronow WS, et al. 2017 ACC/AHA/AAPA/ABC/ACPM/AGS/APhA/ASH/ASPC/NMA/PCNA guideline for the prevention, detection, evaluation, and management of high blood pressure in adults: a report of the American College of Cardiology/American Heart Association Task Force on Clinical Practice Guidelines. *Hypertension.* 2018;71(6):e13–e115.
24. Guarracino F, Ferro B, Forfori F, Bertini P, Magliacano L, Pinsky MR. Jugular vein distensibility predicts fluid responsiveness in septic patients. *Crit Care.* 2014;18(6):647.
25. Chua Chiaco JM, Parikh NI, Fergusson DJ. The jugular venous pressure revisited. *Cleve Clin J Med.* 2013;80(10): 638–644.
26. Cook DJ, Simel DL. The Rational Clinical Examination. Does this patient have abnormal central venous pressure? *JAMA.* 1996;275(8):630–634.
27. Davison R, Cannon R. Estimation of central venous pressure by examination of jugular veins. *Am Heart J.* 1974;87(3): 279–282.
28. Vinayak AG, Levitt J, Gehlbach B, Pohlman AS, Hall JB, Kress JP. Usefulness of the external jugular vein examination in detecting abnormal central venous pressure in critically ill patients. *Arch Intern Med.* 2006;166(19):2132–2137.
29. Constant J. Using internal jugular pulsations as a manometer for right atrial pressure measurements. *Cardiology.* 2000; 93(1–2):26–30.
30. Omar HR, Guglin M. Clinical and prognostic significance of positive hepatojugular reflux on discharge in acute heart failure: insights from the ESCAPE trial. *Biomed Res Int.* 2017;2017:5734749.
31. McGee SR. Chapter 36: inspection of the neck veins. In: *Evidence-Based Physical Diagnosis.* 4th ed. Elsevier; 2018.
32. Seth R, Magner P, Matzinger F, van Walraven C. How far is the sternal angle from the mid-right atrium? *J Gen Intern Med.* 2002;17(11):852–856.
33. Yancy CW, Jessup M, Bozkurt B, et al; American College of Cardiology Foundation; American Heart Association Task Force on Practice Guidelines. 2013 ACCF/AHA guideline for the management of heart failure: a report of the American College of Cardiology Foundation/American Heart Association Task Force on Practice Guidelines. *J Am Coll Cardiol.* 2013;62(16):e147–e239.
34. Rame JE, Dries DL, Drazner MH. The prognostic value of the physical examination in patients with chronic heart failure. *Congest Heart Fail.* 2003;9(3):170–175, 178.

35. Drazner MH, Rame JE, Stevenson LW, Dries DL. Prognostic importance of elevated jugular venous pressure and a third heart sound in patients with heart failure. *N Engl J Med.* 2001;345(8):574–581.
36. Badgett RG, Lucey CR, Mulrow CD. Can the clinical examination diagnose left-sided heart failure in adults? *JAMA.* 1997;277(21):1712–1719.
37. Meyer T, Shih J, Aurigemma G. In the clinic. Heart failure with preserved ejection fraction (diastolic dysfunction). *Ann Intern Med.* 2013;158(1): ITC5-1–ITC5-15; quiz ITC5-16.
38. Straka C, Ying J, Kong FM, Willey CD, Kaminski J, Kim DWN. Review of evolving etiologies, implications and treatment strategies for the superior vena cava syndrome. *Springerplus.* 2016;5:229.
39. Barst RJ, Ertel SI, Beghetti M, Ivy DD. Pulmonary arterial hypertension: a comparison between children and adults. *Eur Respir J.* 2011;37(3):665–677.
40. LeWinter MM. Clinical practice. Acute pericarditis. *N Engl J Med.* 2014;371(25):2410–2416.
41. Sandercock PAG, Kavvadia E. The carotid bruit. *Practic Neurol.* 2002;2(4):221.
42. Ratchford EV, Jin Z, Di Tullio MR, et al. Carotid bruit for detection of hemodynamically significant carotid stenosis: the Northern Manhattan Study. *Neurol Res.* 2009;31(7):748–752.
43. Sauvé JS, Laupacis A, Ostbye T, Feagan B, Sackett DL. Does this patient have a clinically important carotid bruit? *JAMA.* 1993;270(23):2843–2845.
44. Nishimura RA, Otto CM, Bonow RO, et al; American College of Cardiology/American Heart Association Task Force on Practice Guidelines. 2014 AHA/ACC guideline for the management of patients with valvular heart disease: a report of the American College of Cardiology/American Heart Association Task Force on Practice Guidelines. *J Am Coll Cardiol.* 2014;63(22):e57–e185.
45. Braverman AC. Aortic dissection: prompt diagnosis and emergency treatment are critical. *Cleve Clin J Med.* 2011;78(10): 685–696.
46. Michaels AD, Khan FU, Moyers B. Experienced clinicians improve detection of third and fourth heart sounds by viewing acoustic cardiography. *Clin Cardiol.* 2010;33(3):E36–E42.
47. McGee SR. Chapter 40: miscellaneous heart sounds. In: *Evidence-Based Physical Diagnosis.* 3rd ed. Elsevier/Saunders; 2012:345.
48. Kari FA, Beyersdorf F, Siepe M. Pathophysiological implications of different bicuspid aortic valve configurations. *Cardiol Res Pract.* 2012;2012:735829.
49. Siu SC, Silversides CK. Bicuspid aortic valve disease. *J Am Coll Cardiol.* 2010;55(25):2789–2800.
50. Topilsky Y, Michelena H, Bichara V, Maalouf J, Mahoney DW, Enriquez-Sarano M. Mitral valve prolapse with mid-late systolic mitral regurgitation: pitfalls of evaluation and clinical outcome compared with holosystolic regurgitation. *Circulation.* 2012;125(13):1643–1651.
51. Foster E. Clinical practice. Mitral regurgitation due to degenerative mitral-valve disease. *N Engl J Med.* 2010;363(2):156–165.
52. Hayek E, Gring CN, Griffin BP. Mitral valve prolapse. *Lancet.* 2005;365(9458):507–518.
53. Shah SJ, Marcus GM, Gerber IL, et al. Physiology of the third heart sound: novel insights from tissue Doppler imaging. *J Am Soc Echocardiogr.* 2008;21(4):394–400.
54. Shah SJ, Michaels AD. Hemodynamic correlates of the third heart sound and systolic time intervals. *Congest Heart Fail.* 2006;12(Suppl 1):8–13.
55. McGee SR. Chapter 39: the third and fourth heart sounds. In: *Evidence-Based Physical Diagnosis.* 3rd ed. Elsevier/Saunders; 2012:341.
56. McGee S. Etiology and diagnosis of systolic murmurs in adults. *Am J Med.* 2010;123(10):913–921.e1.
57. Lembo NJ, Dell'Italia LJ, Crawford MH, O'Rourke RA. Bedside diagnosis of systolic murmurs. *N Engl J Med.* 1988; 318(24):1572–1578.
58. Felker GM, Cuculich PS, Gheorghiade M. The Valsalva maneuver: a bedside "biomarker" for heart failure. *Am J Med.* 2006;119(2):117–122.
59. Otto CM, Prendergast B. Aortic-valve stenosis–from patients at risk to severe valve obstruction. *N Engl J Med.* 2014; 371(8):744–756.
60. Manning WJ. Asymptomatic aortic stenosis in the elderly: a clinical review. *JAMA.* 2013;310(14):1490–1497.
61. Ho CY. Hypertrophic cardiomyopathy in 2012. *Circulation.* 2012;125(11):1432–1438.
62. Fitzgerald KP, Lim MJ. The pulmonary valve. *Cardiol Clin.* 2011;29(2):223–227.
63. Asgar AW, Mack MJ, Stone GW. Secondary mitral regurgitation in heart failure: pathophysiology, prognosis, and therapeutic considerations. *J Am Coll Cardiol.* 2015;65(12):1231–1248.
64. Bonow RO. Chronic mitral regurgitation and aortic regurgitation: have indications for surgery changed? *J Am Coll Cardiol.* 2013;61(7):693–701.
65. Enriquez-Sarano M, Akins CW, Vahanian A. Mitral regurgitation. *Lancet.* 2009;373(9672):1382–1394.
66. Irwin RB, Luckie M, Khattar RS. Tricuspid regurgitation: contemporary management of a neglected valvular lesion. *Postgrad Med J.* 2010;86(1021):648–655.
67. Mutlak D, Aronson D, Lessick J, Reisner SA, Dabbah S, Agmon Y. Functional tricuspid regurgitation in patients with pulmonary hypertension: is pulmonary artery pressure the only determinant of regurgitation severity? *Chest.* 2009; 135(1):115–121.
68. McGee SR. Chapter 44: miscellaneous heart murmurs. In: *Evidence-Based Physical Diagnosis.* 3rd ed. Elsevier/Saunders; 2012:394.
69. McGee SR. Chapter 43: aortic regurgitation. In: *Evidence-Based Physical Diagnosis.* 3rd ed. Elsevier/Saunders; 2012:379.
70. Maganti K, Rigolin VH, Sarano ME, Bonow RO. Valvular heart disease: diagnosis and management. *Mayo Clin Proc.* 2010;85(5):483–500.
71. Enriquez-Sarano M, Tajik AJ. Clinical practice. Aortic regurgitation. *N Engl J Med.* 2004;351(15):1539–1546.
72. Babu AN, Kymes SM, Carpenter Fryer SM. Eponyms and the diagnosis of aortic regurgitation: what says the evidence? *Ann Intern Med.* 2003;138(9):736–742.
73. Chizner MA. Cardiac auscultation: rediscovering the lost art. *Curr Probl Cardiol.* 2008;33(7):326–408.
74. Pessel C, Bonanno C. Valve disease in pregnancy. *Semin Perinatol.* 2014;38(5):273–284.
75. McGee SR. Chapter 45: disorders of the pericardium. In: *Evidence-Based Physical Diagnosis.* 3rd ed. Elsevier/Saunders; 2012:400.
76. Levine SA. Notes on the gradation of the intensity of cardiac murmurs. *JAMA.* 1961;177:261.
77. Freeman AR, Levine SA. The clinical significance of the systolic murmur: a study of 1000 consecutive "non-cardiac" cases. *Ann Intern Med.* 1933;6:1371–1385.
78. Fischer DB, Lilly LS. Chapter 2: the cardiac cycle: mechanisms of heart sounds and murmurs. In: Lilly LS, ed. *Pathophysiology*

of Heart Disease: A Collaborative Project of Medical Students and Faculty. 6th ed. Lippincott Williams & Wilkins; 2016.
79. Bonow RO, Carabello BA, Chatterjee K, et al; American College of Cardiology/American Heart Association Task Force on Practice Guidelines. 2008 focused update incorporated into the ACC/AHA 2006 guidelines for the management of patients with valvular heart disease: a report of the American College of Cardiology/American Heart Association Task Force on Practice Guidelines (Writing Committee to revise the 1998 guidelines for the management of patients with valvular heart disease). Endorsed by the Society of Cardiovascular Anesthesiologists, Society for Cardiovascular Angiography and Interventions, and Society of Thoracic Surgeons. *J Am Coll Cardiol.* 2008;52(13):e1–142.
80. McGee SR. Chapter 43: heart murmurs: general principles. In: *Evidence-Based Physical Diagnosis.* 4th ed. Elsevier; 2018.
81. Zarzeczny R, Tomza C, Polak A, Nawrat-Szołtysik A. Blood pressure response to isometric handgrip testing and aerobic capacity and associations with sprint performance in middle-aged men following high-intensity interval training. *J Sports Med Phys Fitness.* 2018;58(4):525–533.
82. Porth CJ, Bamrah VS, Tristani FE, Smith JJ. The Valsalva maneuver: mechanisms and clinical implications. *Heart Lung.* 1984;13(5):507–518.
83. Zema MJ. Bedside assessment of cardiac hemodynamics: role of the simple Valsalva maneuver. *Am J Med.* 2012; 125(8):e13; author reply e15–e16.
84. Mar PL, Nwazue V, Black BK, et al. Valsalva maneuver in pulmonary arterial hypertension: susceptibility to syncope and autonomic dysfunction. *Chest.* 2016;149(5):1252–1260.
85. Cheng RK, Cox M, Neely ML, et al. Outcomes in patients with heart failure with preserved, borderline, and reduced ejection fraction in the Medicare population. *Am Heart J.* 2014;168(5):721–730.
86. Gheorghiade M, Vaduganathan M, Fonarow GC, Bonow RO. Rehospitalization for heart failure: problems and perspectives. *J Am Coll Cardiol.* 2013;61(4):391–403.
87. Ward RP, Mansour IN, Lemieux N, Gera N, Mehta R, Lang RM. Prospective evaluation of the clinical application of the American College of Cardiology Foundation/American Society of Echocardiography Appropriateness Criteria for transthoracic echocardiography. *JACC Cardiovasc Imaging.* 2008;1(5):663–671.
88. Via G, Hussain A, Wells M, et al; International Liaison Committee on Focused Cardiac UltraSound (ILC-FoCUS); International Conference on Focused Cardiac UltraSound (IC-FoCUS). International evidence-based recommendations for focused cardiac ultrasound. *J Am Soc Echocardiogr.* 2014;27(7):683.e1–683.e33.
89. Albaroudi B, Haddad M, Albaroudi O, Abdel-Rahman ME, Jarman R, Harris T. Assessing left ventricular systolic function by emergency physician using point of care echocardiography compared to expert: systematic review and meta-analysis. *Eur J Emerg Med.* 2022;29(1):18–32.
90. Labovitz AJ, Noble VE, Bierig M, et al. Focused cardiac ultrasound in the emergent setting: a consensus statement of the American Society of Echocardiography and American College of Emergency Physicians. *J Am Soc Echocardiogr.* 2010; 23(12):1225–1230.
91. Moore CL, Rose GA, Tayal VS, Sullivan DM, Arrowood JA, Kline JA. Determination of left ventricular function by emergency physician echocardiography of hypotensive patients. *Acad Emerg Med.* 2002;9(3):186–193.
92. Noble VE, Nelson BP. *Manual of Emergency and Critical Care Ultrasound.* Cambridge University Press; 2007.
93. Loukas M, Burns D. *Essential Ultrasound Anatomy.* Wolters Kluwer; 2020.
94. Vaduganathan M, Mensah GA, Turco JV, Fuster V, Roth GA. The global burden of cardiovascular diseases and risk: a compass for future health. *J Am Coll Cardiol.* 2022; 80(25):2361–2371.
95. Tsao CW, Aday AW, Almarzooq ZI, et al; American Heart Association Council on Epidemiology and Prevention Statistics Committee and Stroke Statistics Subcommittee. Heart Disease and Stroke Statistics-2023 update: a report from the American Heart Association. *Circulation.* 2023;147(8): e93–e621.
96. Ahmad FB, Cisewski JA, Xu J, Anderson RN. Provisional mortality data – United States, 2022. *MMWR Morb Mortal Wkly Rep.* 2023;72(18):488–492.
97. Global Cardiovascular Risk Consortium; Magnussen C, Ojeda FM, Leong DP, et al. Global effect of modifiable risk factors on cardiovascular disease and mortality. *N Engl J Med.* 2023;389(14):1273–1285.
98. Yusuf S, Joseph P, Rangarajan S, et al. Modifiable risk factors, cardiovascular disease, and mortality in 155 722 individuals from 21 high-income, middle-income, and low-income countries (PURE): a prospective cohort study. *Lancet.* 2020; 395(10226):795–808.
99. Arnett DK, Blumenthal RS, Albert MA, et al. 2019 ACC/AHA Guideline on the Primary Prevention of Cardiovascular Disease: a Report of the American College of Cardiology/American Heart Association Task Force on Clinical Practice Guidelines. *Circulation.* 2019;140(11):e596–e646.
100. Ostchega Y, Fryer CD, Nwankwo T, Nguyen DT. *Hypertension prevalence among adults aged 18 and over: United States, 2017–2018. NCHS Data Brief, no 364.* 2020. https://www.cdc.gov/nchs/products/databriefs/db364.htm
101. Centers for Disease Control and Prevention. Facts About Hypertension. Accessed January 29, 2024. https://www.cdc.gov/high-blood-pressure/data-research/facts-stats/
102. Benjamin EJ, Virani SS, Callaway CW, et al. Heart disease and stroke statistics-2018 update: a report from the American Heart Association. *Circulation.* 2018;137(12):e67–e492.
103. Goff DC Jr, Lloyd-Jones DM, Bennett G, et al. 2013 ACC/AHA guideline on the assessment of cardiovascular risk: a report of the American College of Cardiology/American Heart Association Task Force on Practice Guidelines. *J Am Coll Cardiol.* 2014;63(25 Pt B):2935–2959.
104. Mosca L, Benjamin EJ, Berra K, et al. Effectiveness-based guidelines for the prevention of cardiovascular disease in women–2011 update: a guideline from the American Heart Association. *Circulation.* 2011;123(11):1243–1262.
105. Weber MA, Schiffrin EL, White WB, et al. Clinical practice guidelines for the management of hypertension in the community: a statement by the American Society of Hypertension and the International Society of Hypertension. *J Clin Hypertens (Greenwich).* 2014;16(1):14–26.
106. Meschia JF, Bushnell C, Boden-Albala B, et al. Guidelines for the primary prevention of stroke: a statement for healthcare professionals from the American Heart Association/American Stroke Association. *Stroke.* 2014;45(12):3754–3832.
107. Bushnell C, McCullough LD, Awad IA, et al. Guidelines for the prevention of stroke in women: a statement for healthcare professionals from the American Heart Association/American Stroke Association. *Stroke.* 2014;45(5):1545–1588.

108. Professional Practice Committee: standards of medical care in diabetes-2018. *Diabetes Care.* 2018;41(Suppl 1):S3. Accessed January 10, 2024.
109. Whelton PK, Carey RM, Aronow WS, et al. 2017 ACC/AHA/AAPA/ABC/ACPM/AGS/APhA/ASH/ASPC/NMA/PCNA guideline for the prevention, detection, evaluation, and management of high blood pressure in adults: executive summary: a report of the American College of Cardiology/American Heart Association Task Force on Clinical Practice Guidelines. *Hypertension.* 2018;71(6):1269–1324.
110. Grundy SM, Stone NJ, Bailey AL, et al. 2018 AHA/ACC/AACVPR/AAPA/ABC/ACPM/ADA/AGS/APhA/ASPC/NLA/PCNA guideline on the management of blood cholesterol: a report of the American College of Cardiology/American Heart Association Task Force on Clinical Practice Guidelines. *Circulation.* 2019;139(25):e1082–e1143.
111. U. S. Preventive Services Task Force; Krist AH, Davidson KW, Mangione CM, et al. Screening for hypertension in adults: US Preventive Services Task Force reaffirmation recommendation statement. *JAMA.* 2021;325(16):1650–1656.
112. Guirguis-Blake JM, Evans CV, Webber EM, Coppola EL, Perdue LA, Weyrich MS. Screening for hypertension in adults: updated evidence report and systematic review for the US Preventive Services Task Force. *JAMA.* 2021;325(16):1657–1669.
113. Siu AL; U. S. Preventive Services Task Force. Screening for high blood pressure in adults: U.S. Preventive Services Task Force recommendation statement. *Ann Intern Med.* 2015; 163(10):778–786.
114. Chou R, Dana T, Blazina I, Daeges M, Jeanne TL. Statins for prevention of cardiovascular disease in adults: evidence report and systematic review for the US Preventive Services Task Force. *JAMA.* 2016;316(19):2008–2024.
115. U. S. Preventive Services Task Force; Mangione CM, Barry MJ, Nicholson WK, et al. Statin use for the primary prevention of cardiovascular disease in adults: US Preventive Services Task Force recommendation statement. *JAMA.* 2022;328(8):746–753.
116. U. S. Preventive Services Task Force, Krist AH, Davidson KW, Mangione CM, et al. Behavioral counseling interventions to promote a healthy diet and physical activity for cardiovascular disease prevention in adults with cardiovascular risk factors: US Preventive Services Task Force recommendation statement. *JAMA.* 2020;324(20):2069–2075.
117. U. S. Preventive Services Task Force; Mangione CM, Barry MJ, Nicholson WK, et al. Behavioral counseling interventions to promote a healthy diet and physical activity for cardiovascular disease prevention in adults without cardiovascular disease risk factors: US Preventive Services Task Force recommendation statement. *JAMA.* 2022;328(4):367–374.
118. Greenland P, Alpert JS, Beller GA, et al. 2010 ACCF/AHA guideline for assessment of cardiovascular risk in asymptomatic adults: executive summary: a report of the American College of Cardiology Foundation/American Heart Association Task Force on Practice Guidelines. *Circulation.* 2010;122(25):2748–2764.
119. Siu AL. Behavioral and pharmacotherapy interventions for tobacco smoking cessation in adults, including pregnant women: U.S. Preventive Services Task Force recommendation statement. *Ann Intern Med.* 2015;163(8):622–634.
120. Lloyd-Jones DM, Hong Y, Labarthe D, et al. Defining and setting national goals for cardiovascular health promotion and disease reduction: the American Heart Association's strategic Impact Goal through 2020 and beyond. *Circulation.* 2010;121(4):586–613.
121. Eckel RH, Jakicic JM, Ard JD, et al. 2013 AHA/ACC guideline on lifestyle management to reduce cardiovascular risk: a report of the American College of Cardiology/American Heart Association Task Force on Practice Guidelines. *Circulation.* 2014;129(25 Suppl 2):S76–S99.
122. Sallis RE, Matuszak JM, Baggish AL, et al. Call to action on making physical activity assessment and prescription a medical standard of care. *Curr Sports Med Rep.* 2016;15(3):207–214.
123. Obesity in Adults: Screening and Management. U.S. Preventive Services Task Force. Accessed January 10, 2024. https://www.uspreventiveservicestaskforce.org/uspstf/recommendation/obesity-in-adults-screening-and-management-2012
124. Jensen MD, Ryan DH, Apovian CM, et al; American College of Cardiology/American Heart Association Task Force on Practice Guidelines; Obesity Society. 2013 AHA/ACC/TOS guideline for the management of overweight and obesity in adults: a report of the American College of Cardiology/American Heart Association Task Force on Practice Guidelines and The Obesity Society. *J Am Coll Cardiol.* 2014;63(25 Pt B):2985–3023.
125. Goldstein LB, Bushnell CD, Adams RJ, et al; American Heart Association Stroke Council; Council on Cardiovascular Nursing; Council on Epidemiology and Prevention; Council for High Blood Pressure Research; Council on Peripheral Vascular Disease; and Interdisciplinary Council on Quality of Care and Outcomes Research. Guidelines for the primary prevention of stroke: a guideline for healthcare professionals from the American Heart Association/American Stroke Association. *Stroke.* 2011;42(2):517–584.
126. U. S. Preventive Services Task Force; Krist AH, Davidson KW, Mangione CM, et al. Interventions for tobacco smoking cessation in adults, including pregnant persons: US Preventive Services Task Force recommendation statement. *JAMA.* 2021;325(3):265–279.
127. U. S. Preventive Services Task Force, Curry SJ, Krist AH, Owens DK, et al. Behavioral weight loss interventions to prevent obesity-related morbidity and mortality in adults: US Preventive Services Task Force recommendation statement. *JAMA.* 2018;320(11):1163–1171.
128. U. S. Preventive Services Task Force; Davidson KW, Barry MJ, Mangione CM, et al. Screening for prediabetes and type 2 diabetes: US Preventive Services Task Force recommendation statement. *JAMA.* 2021;326(8):736–743.
129. GBD 2019 Risk Factors Collaborators. Global burden of 87 risk factors in 204 countries and territories, 1990–2019: a systematic analysis for the Global Burden of Disease Study 2019. *Lancet.* 2020;396(10258):1223–1249.
130. National Academies of Sciences, Engineering, and Medicine. *Dietary Reference Intakes for Sodium and Potassium.* 2019.
131. Institute of Medicine. *Sodium Intake in Populations. Assessment of Evidence.* 2013. https://nap.nationalacademies.org/catalog/18311/sodium-intake-in-populations-assessment-of-evidence
132. Clarke LS, Overwyk K, Bates M, Park S, Gillespie C, Cogswell ME. Temporal trends in dietary sodium intake among adults aged >/=19 years—United States, 2003–2016. *MMWR Morb Mortal Wkly Rep.* 2021;70(42):1478–1482.
133. Appel LJ, Frohlich ED, Hall JE, et al. The importance of population-wide sodium reduction as a means to prevent cardiovascular disease and stroke: a call to action from the American Heart Association. *Circulation.* 2011;123(10):1138–1143.
134. Institute of Medicine (IOM). *Strategies to Reduce Sodium Intake in the United States.* The National Academies Press; 2010.

CHAPTER

19

Peripheral Vascular System

ANATOMY AND PHYSIOLOGY

Arterial System

Arteries contain three concentric layers of tissue: the *intima*, *media*, and *adventitia* (Figs. 19-1 and 19-2). The internal elastic membrane borders the intima and the media; the external elastic membrane separates the media from the adventitia.

Atherosclerosis is a chronic inflammatory disease initiated by injury (i.e., smoking or hypertension) to vascular endothelial cells, provoking atheromatous plaque formation.

The innermost layer of all blood vessels is the *intima*, a single continuous lining of endothelial cells with remarkable metabolic properties.[1] Atherosclerotic plaque formation begins in the intima, where circulating cholesterol particles, especially low-density lipoproteins (LDLs), are exposed to proteoglycans from the extracellular matrix, undergo oxidative modification, and trigger a local inflammatory response that attracts mononuclear phagocytes (Box 19-1). Once in the intima, phagocytes mature into macrophages, ingest lipids, and become *foam cells* that develop into fatty streaks.

The *media* is composed of smooth muscle cells with elastic properties to accommodate blood pressure and flow. Its inner and outer boundaries consist

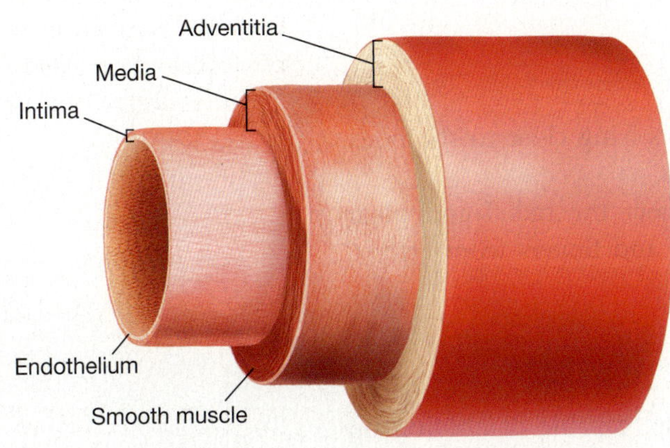

FIGURE 19-1. Artery anatomy.

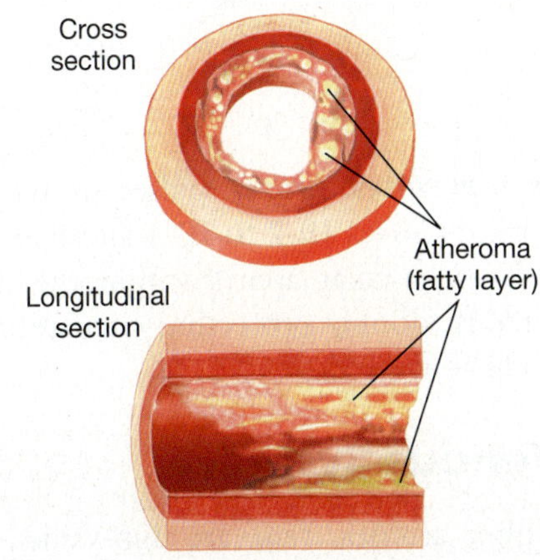

FIGURE 19-2. Atherosclerotic plaque.

Box 19-1. Atherosclerotic Plaque Formation

- In atherosclerotic plaques, there is a proliferation of smooth muscle cells and extracellular matrix that breaches the endothelial lining.
- Atherosclerotic plaques contain a fibrous cap of smooth muscle cells that overlies a necrotic lipid-rich core, vascular cells, and a wide range of immune cells and prothrombotic molecules.
- Inflammatory mediators that alter collagen repair and cap fibrosis are increasingly implicated in plaque rupture and plaque erosion, which expose thrombogenic factors in the plaque core to coagulation factors in the blood, resulting in overlying thrombus formation.
- If in the coronary arteries, these thrombi can result in acute myocardial infarction. If in the carotid arteries, the thrombi can dislodge and travel to the brain, resulting in stroke.

Plaque activation and instability, in addition to luminal stenosis, are well-recognized as critical factors contributing to ischemia and infarction.[2–4]

of elastic fibers, or elastin, and are called *internal* and *external elastic laminae*, or membranes. The media receives its blood supply from small blood vessels called the *vasa vasorum*.

The outer layer of the artery is the *adventitia*, the connective tissue containing nerve fibers and the vasa vasorum.

Arterial Branching. *Arteries* play a crucial role in accommodating the varying cardiac output during systole and diastole, and their anatomy and size vary based on their proximity to the heart. The *aorta* and its immediate branches, such as the *common carotid* and *iliac arteries*, are large and highly elastic. These arteries then transition into medium-sized muscular arteries, such as the *coronary* and *renal arteries*. The media of large and medium-sized arteries contributes to the propagation of blood flow and arterial pulsatile flow through a combination of elastic recoil and smooth muscle contraction and relaxation.

As the arteries continue to branch out, medium-sized arteries divide into smaller arteries and *arterioles*, with the latter having a diameter of 20 to 100 μm, making them known as the *"resistance vessels."* The tone of their smooth muscle is a significant determinant of *systemic vascular resistance*, a key component of blood pressure. Arterioles eventually lead to the vast network of *capillaries*, each only 7 to 8 μm across, which have an endothelial cell lining but no media, facilitating rapid diffusion of oxygen and carbon dioxide.

If an artery is obstructed, anastomoses between branching networks of smaller arteries can increase in size over time to form collateral circulation that perfuses structures distal to the occlusion.

Arterial Pulses. Arterial pulses are palpable in arteries lying close to the body surface (Boxes 19-2 to 19-4 and Figs. 19-3 to 19-5).

Two vascular arches within the hand interconnect the radial and ulnar arteries, doubly protecting circulation to the hand and fingers from arterial occlusion.

Venous System

Unlike arteries, *veins* are thin-walled and distensible, capable of holding up to two-thirds of the circulating blood flow. The venous intima consists of

Box 19-2. Arterial Pulses in the Arms and Hands

Arterial Pulses	Location for Palpation
Brachial artery	At the bend of the elbow just medial to the biceps tendon
Radial artery	On the lateral flexor surface of the wrist
Ulnar artery	On the medial flexor surface of the wrist, though it may be obscured by overlying tissues

Box 19-3. Arterial Pulses in the Abdomen

Arterial Pulses	Location for Palpation
Aorta	In the epigastrium
Celiac trunk	Not palpable; supplies the esophagus, stomach, proximal duodenum, liver, gallbladder, pancreas, spleen (foregut)
Superior mesenteric artery	Not palpable; supplies the small intestine (jejunum, ileum, cecum) and large intestine (ascending and transverse colon, right splenic flexure [midgut])
Inferior mesenteric artery	Not palpable; supplies the large intestine (descending and sigmoid colon and proximal rectum [hindgut])

Despite the rich collateral network that protects the three abdominal branches against hypoperfusion, occlusion of the mesenteric arteries can result in **acute mesenteric ischemia**, a potentially life-threatening condition.

Box 19-4. Arterial Pulses in the Legs

Arterial Pulses	Location for Palpation
Femoral artery	Just below the inguinal ligament, midway between the anterior superior iliac spine and the symphysis pubis
Popliteal artery	An extension of the femoral artery that passes medially behind the femur; palpable just behind but deep in the knee
Posterior tibial artery	Lies behind the medial malleolus of the ankle; an interconnecting arch between its two chief arterial branches protects circulation to the foot
Dorsalis pedis artery	On the dorsum of the foot just lateral to the extensor tendon of the big toe

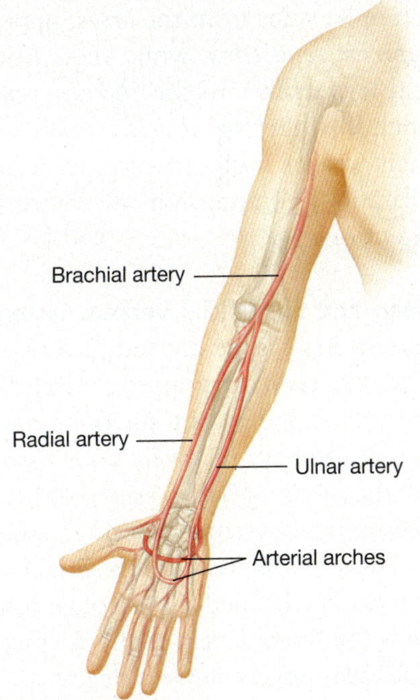

FIGURE 19-3. Arteries of the right upper extremity.

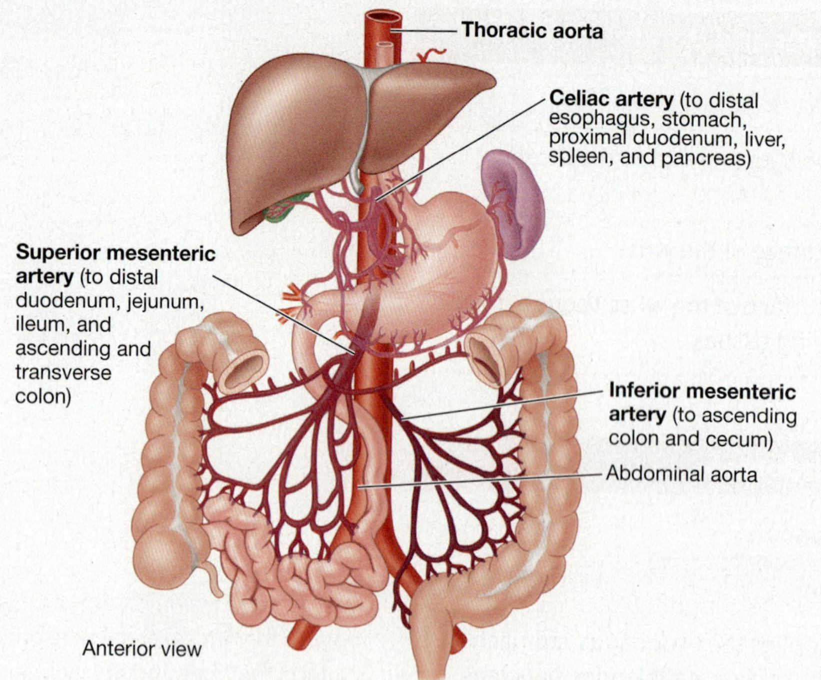

FIGURE 19-4. Abdominal aorta and its branches.

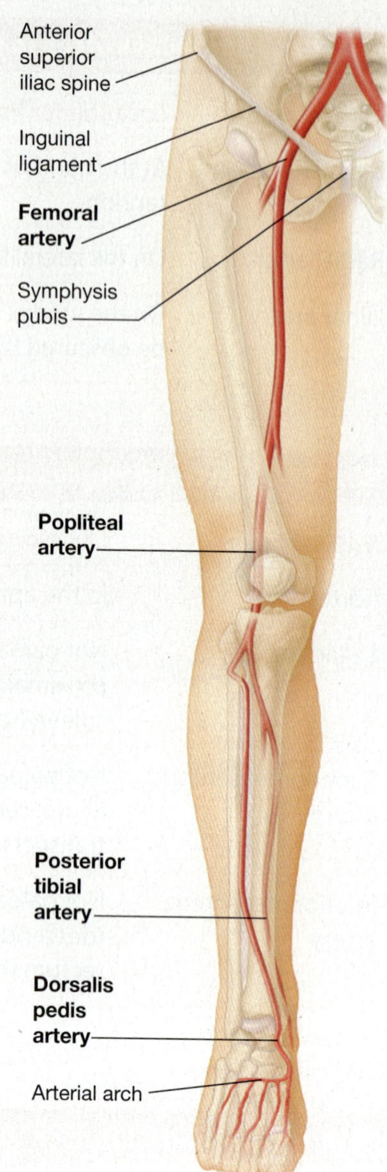

FIGURE 19-5. Arteries of the right lower extremity.

nonthrombogenic endothelium, and the media contains circumferential rings of elastic tissue and smooth muscle that regulate vein caliber in response to even minor changes in venous pressure. The smallest veins, or *venules*, drain capillary beds and form interconnecting *venous plexuses.*

Veins from different regions of the body drain into specific locations. For example, veins from the arms, upper trunk, and head and neck drain into the *superior vena cava*, while veins from the abdominal wall, liver, lower trunk, and legs drain into the *inferior vena cava*. Veins from the abdominal viscera drain into the *portal vein*, which supplies blood flow to the liver. Because of their weaker wall structure, leg veins are particularly susceptible to irregular dilatation, compression, ulceration, and tumor invasion and require special attention.

Deep and Superficial Venous Systems of the Legs. The veins of the lower extremities can be divided into two systems: deep veins and superficial veins. The *deep veins* carry approximately 90% of the venous return from the legs and are well supported by surrounding tissues. The *superficial veins* are subcutaneous and have relatively poor tissue support. The two main superficial veins are the *great saphenous vein* and the *small saphenous vein*, which connect to the deep venous system at specific points (Fig. 19-6).

The *great saphenous vein* originates on the dorsum of the foot, passes just anterior to the medial malleolus, continues up the medial aspect of the leg, and joins the femoral vein of the deep venous system below the inguinal ligament. The *small saphenous vein* begins on the lateral side of the foot, passes upward along the posterior calf, and joins the deep venous system in the popliteal fossa. Anastomotic veins connect the two saphenous veins and are readily visible when dilated.

In addition, *bridging* or *perforating veins* connect the superficial system with the deep system, allowing for the efficient return of blood to the heart

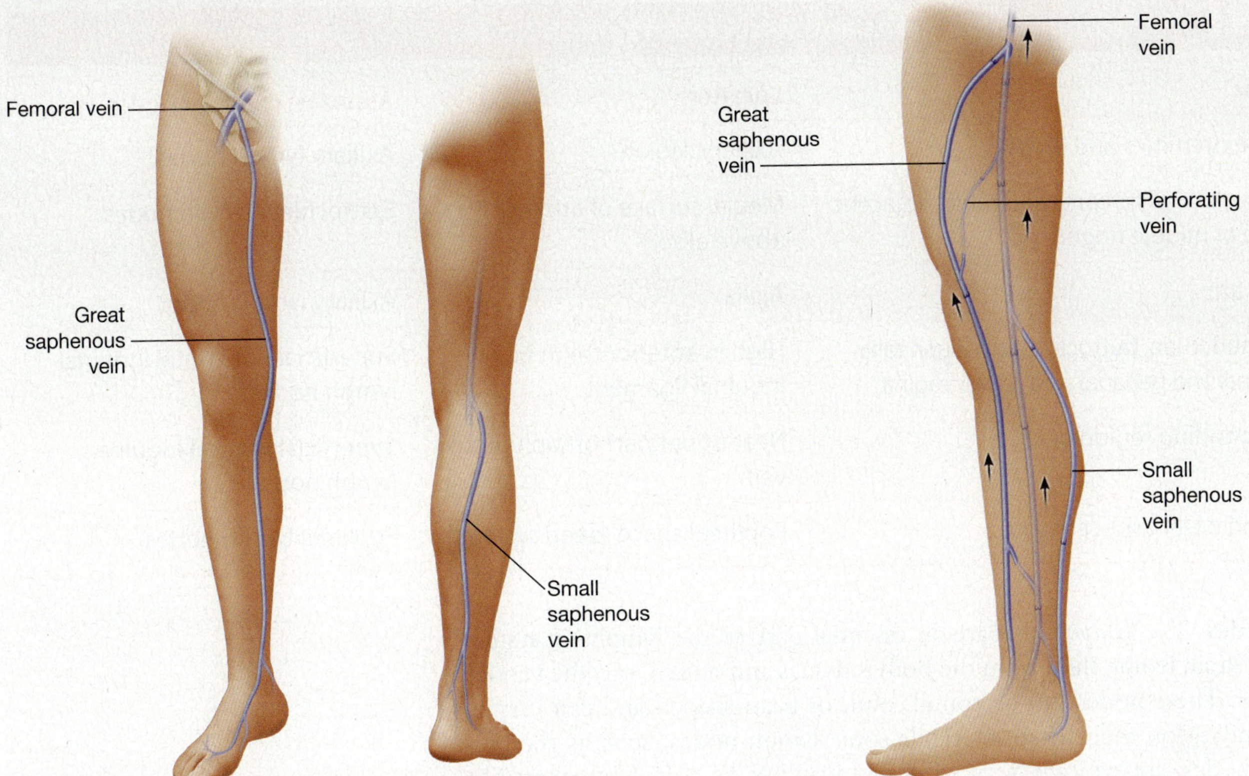

FIGURE 19-6. Superficial veins of the right lower extremity.

FIGURE 19-7. Deep, superficial, and perforating veins of the right lower extremity.

(Fig. 19-7). Pay special attention to the leg veins because of their weaker wall structure, which makes them susceptible to irregular dilatation, compression, ulceration, and invasion by tumors.

The *one-way valves* found in the deep, superficial, and perforating veins play a crucial role in the proper blood flow toward the heart. They prevent pooling, venous stasis, and backward flow by propelling the blood forward. The calf muscles also contribute to the venous return by contracting during walking, acting as a venous pump to move the blood upward against gravity.

Lymphatic System

The lymphatic system is a complex network of vessels responsible for draining *lymph fluid* from the body's tissues and returning it to the venous circulation. The *lymphatic plexuses*, which are networks of lymphatic capillaries, originate in the extracellular spaces and collect tissue fluid, plasma proteins, cells, and cellular debris via their porous endothelium. These capillaries then continue centrally as thin vascular channels and collecting ducts, eventually emptying into the major veins at the neck.

The *right lymphatic duct* drains fluid from the right side of the head, neck, thorax, and right upper limb and empties into the junction of the right internal jugular and the right subclavian veins. The *thoracic duct* collects lymph fluid from the rest of the body and empties into the junction of the left internal jugular and the left subclavian veins. Along these channels, lymph fluid is filtered through *lymph nodes*, which are interposed at regular intervals.

Box 19-5. Key Lymphatic Regions and Associated Lymph Nodes

Regions	Location	Associated Lymph Nodes
Upper extremities and breast	Axillary region	Axillary lymph nodes
Ulnar surface of forearm and hand, adjacent surface of middle finger	Medial surface of arm just above elbow	Epitrochlear lymph nodes
Rest of arm	Axilla	Axillary lymph nodes
Lower abdomen, buttock, external genitalia, anal canal and perianal area, lower vagina	High in anterior thigh below inguinal ligament	Superficial horizontal inguinal lymph nodes
Corresponding region of leg	Near upper part of saphenous vein	Superficial vertical inguinal lymph nodes
Heel and outer aspect of foot	Popliteal space (deep system)	Popliteal lymph nodes

Lymph Nodes. The *lymph nodes* are an essential part of the lymphatic system that helps drain lymph fluid from the body's tissues and return it to the venous circulation. These nodes can be round, oval, or bean-shaped and can vary in size depending on their location. While some lymph nodes, such as the preauricular nodes, are typically very small and may not be palpable, others like the inguinal nodes are relatively larger, usually measuring up to 1 to 2 cm in diameter in an adult.

Apart from its vascular functions, the lymphatic system plays a crucial role in the immune system by helping to engulf cellular debris and bacteria and produce antibodies. However, only the superficial lymph nodes are accessible for physical examination, including cervical nodes, axillary nodes, and nodes in the arms and legs (Box 19-5 and Figs. 19-8 and 19-9).

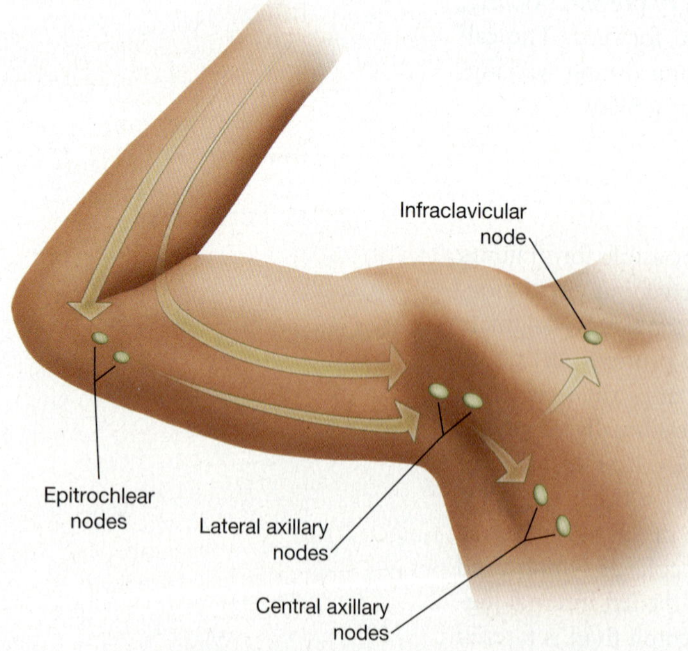

FIGURE 19-8. Lymph nodes of the arm.

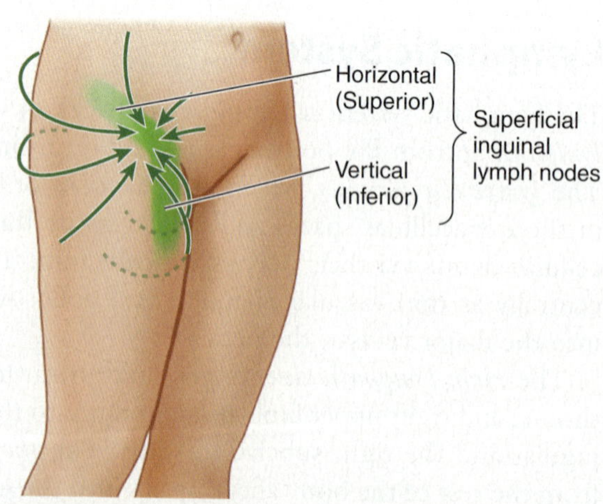

FIGURE 19-9. Superficial lymphatic drainage from gluteal region and thigh.

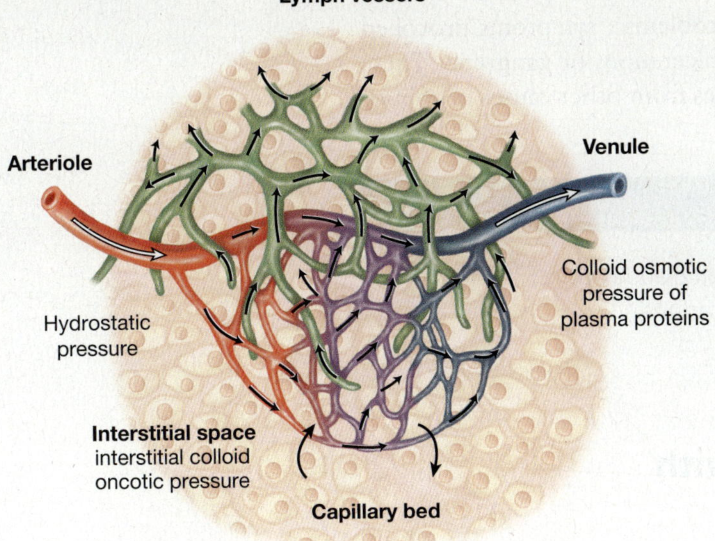

FIGURE 19-10. Capillary fluid exchange.

Transcapillary Fluid Exchange

Blood travels from arteries to veins through a network of capillaries, and most filtered fluid returns to the circulation as lymph (Fig. 19-10). The kidneys also help retain sodium and water when plasma volume decreases. However, abnormalities in venous capillary pressure, capillary osmotic pressure, or fluid balance can lead to *edema*, which presents as swelling, especially in the lower extremities.[5–7] *Pitting edema* is compressible and reduces in size with external pressure, while *lymphedema*, caused by blocked lymphatic drainage, is typically noncompressible.

Enlarged lymph nodes, known as *lymphadenopathy*, may or may not be accompanied by tenderness. It is important to differentiate between localized and generalized lymphadenopathy by identifying a causative lesion in the drainage area or enlarged nodes in at least two noncontiguous lymph node regions.

Mechanisms for the development of edema include increased plasma volume from sodium retention, altered capillary dynamics resulting in net filtration, inadequate removal of filtered lymph fluid, lymphatic or venous obstruction, and increased capillary permeability.[8,9] See Table 19-1, Types of Peripheral Edema, p. 569.

HEALTH HISTORY: GENERAL APPROACH

To approach a patient with signs and symptoms related to the peripheral vascular system, *assess the integrity of the system*, which includes the arteries, veins, and lymphatics.

To achieve this, you will need to ask targeted questions to differentiate nonspecific symptoms from those that may have a neurologic or musculoskeletal cause. Questions such as the onset and trigger of symptoms may be less helpful in this case. Instead, focus on determining the perfusion of the affected limb, as musculoskeletal and neurologic disorders should not affect blood supply. Symptoms related to the peripheral vascular system tend to worsen during exertion when oxygen consumption exceeds supply.

To assess perfusion, ask about skin color; throbbing or pulsatile quality; temperature; hair loss (especially for chronic problems); symptoms provoked by exertion; and the presence of any swelling, ulceration, or gangrene. These details can help distinguish specific vascular issues from other causes of pain or weakness.

Common or Concerning Symptoms

- Pain and/or swelling of legs with intermittent claudication
- Pain and/or swelling of legs without claudication
- Abdominal, flank, or back pain

Pain and/or Swelling of Legs with Intermittent Claudication

Swelling in legs or arms, known as *edema* or *peripheral edema*, is the accumulation of fluid in the soft tissues of the body. This can cause the affected area to become swollen, puffy, and sometimes painful. *Claudication* is a term derived from the Latin word "*claudicare*," which means "*to limp*." It describes a symptom characterized by muscle pain, cramping, or discomfort that occurs in the legs during exercise, such as walking or climbing stairs, and is relieved by rest.

Intermittent claudication is a more specific term that emphasizes the temporary nature of the pain. It refers to the same set of symptoms—pain, cramping, or discomfort in the legs during physical activity that subsides with rest. The term "intermittent" highlights that the pain comes and goes, typically occurring during exertion and resolving during rest. When dealing with leg pain and swelling, a detailed patient history can help identify the vascular problems involved (Box 19-6).

Causes include **peripheral artery disease** ([**PAD**] narrowing or blockage of leg arteries, leading to reduced blood flow and resulting in pain during exertion, especially walking), **deep vein thrombosis** ([**DVT**] formation of a blood clot in deep veins, typically in the leg, causing pain and swelling in the affected region), **chronic venous insufficiency** ([CVI] impaired return of blood from the legs to the heart, leading to leg swelling, pain, and varicose veins), **musculoskeletal conditions** (strains, sprains, or fractures can cause pain and swelling in the legs), and **neurogenic claudication** (leg pain due to spinal conditions like lumbar spinal stenosis, distinguished by pain worsening with prolonged standing or walking but relieved by forward bending or sitting).

Box 19-6. Pain and/or Swelling of Legs with Intermittent Claudication: High-Yield Health History Questions

Domain	Questions	Rationale
Location	*How do you describe the location of the pain or discomfort?*	*Calves:* may suggest peripheral artery disease (PAD) *Thighs or buttocks:* may suggest more proximal disease such as aortic stenosis or iliac artery disease
Timing	*When do you experience the pain or discomfort?*	*With exercise and improving with rest (intermittent claudication):* may suggest PAD *At rest and not relieved with rest:* may suggest more advanced disease or acute thrombosis

Domain	Questions	Rationale
Quality	*Can you describe the type of pain or discomfort?*	*Cramping or aching:* may suggest PAD *Sharp or stabbing:* may suggest underlying spinal stenosis
Duration	*How long does the pain or discomfort last?*	*Resolves within a few minutes of rest:* may suggest PAD *Persists:* may suggest more advanced disease or acute thrombosis
Swelling	*Do you have any swelling in your legs or ankles?*	May suggest underlying venous insufficiency or deep vein thrombosis
Risk factors	*Do you smoke or have a history of vascular disease?*	These increase the likelihood of underlying PAD

Pain and/or Swelling in Legs without Claudication

Unlike intermittent claudication, *leg pain without claudication* can persist irrespective of activity levels, making its diagnosis and treatment particularly challenging. A thorough patient history becomes indispensable, as it can illuminate the potential underlying conditions contributing to these symptoms (Box 19-7).

Possible causes of leg pain and/or swelling *without* claudication linked to the peripheral vascular system include **DVT**, **chronic venous insufficiency** ([**CVI**] veins in the legs cannot pump blood back to the heart effectively due to valve dysfunction or vein wall weakness), **varicose veins** (enlarged, twisted veins due to weak or damaged valves, leading to blood pooling and increased pressure in the veins), and **lymphedema** (swelling due to damage or blockage in the lymphatic system, leading to a buildup of lymphatic fluid).[11]

See Table 19-2, Painful Peripheral Vascular Disorders and Their Mimics, pp. 570–573.

Box 19-7. Pain and/or Swelling of Legs without Claudication: High-Yield Health History Questions

Domain	Questions	Rationale
Location	*Can you describe the location of the pain or swelling?*	*Unilateral:* may suggest underlying deep vein thrombosis (DVT) or venous insufficiency *Bilateral:* may suggest underlying systemic conditions such as heart failure or liver disease
Onset	*When did the pain or swelling start?*	*Acute onset:* may suggest underlying DVT or cellulitis *Chronic:* may suggest underlying venous insufficiency or lymphedema
Quality	*Can you describe the type of pain or discomfort?*	*Sharp or stabbing:* may suggest underlying nerve compression *Dull or aching:* may suggest underlying musculoskeletal conditions such as arthritis or myofascial pain syndrome

(continued)

Box 19-7. Pain and/or Swelling of Legs without Claudication: High-Yield Health History Questions (*Continued*)

Domain	Questions	Rationale
Swelling	*Can you describe the extent and characteristics of the swelling?*	*Unilateral, warm, tender, and associated with erythema:* may suggest underlying DVT or cellulitis *Bilateral pitting:* may suggest underlying systemic conditions such as heart failure or liver disease
Associated symptoms	*Do you have any associated symptoms such as fever or shortness of breath?*	These may suggest underlying systemic conditions such as infection or heart failure
Risk factors	*Do you have any underlying medical conditions or risk factors?*	These may suggest underlying venous or systemic conditions such as heart failure or liver disease

Abdominal, Flank, or Back Pain

Clarifying abdominal complaints related to the vasculature is difficult; however, they still relate to the perfusion of the organ systems. The acute onset of symptoms in the abdomen should raise the concern of arterial thrombosis, and a thorough determination of relevant health history is essential (Box 19-8). Symptoms here can also be related to oxygen supply–demand mismatch. For example, if the symptoms are provoked when the patient is eating (and thus, the abdominal viscera needs a greater oxygen supply), the symptoms likely result from arterial pathology. This can evoke fear of eating (*food fear*) or progress to anorexia.

Possible vascular causes include **abdominal aortic aneurysm** ([**AAA**] enlarged area in the lower part of the aorta), **renal artery stenosis** (blood vessels become narrowed, potentially leading to flank pain and hypertension), **mesenteric ischemia** (decreased blood flow to the intestines, often due to a blockage, can manifest as abdominal pain, especially after eating), **dissecting aortic aneurysm** (inner layer of the aorta tears, causing the inner and middle layers to separate/dissect; pain usually manifests in the chest or back), **pelvic congestion syndrome** (varicose veins develop around the ovaries, leading to chronic pain in the lower abdomen and back), and **nutcracker syndrome** (compression of the left renal vein between the abdominal aorta and the superior mesenteric artery, leading to left flank pain and possible blood in the urine).

Box 19-8. Abdominal, Flank, or Back Pain: High-Yield Health History Questions

Domain	Questions	Rationale
Location	*Can you describe the location of the pain or discomfort?*	*Midepigastric or left upper quadrant abdominal or flank pain:* may suggest underlying cardiac conditions such as ischemic heart disease or aortic dissection. *Back pain in the thoracic or lumbar spine:* may suggest underlying aortic aneurysm or spinal stenosis

Domain	Questions	Rationale
Timing	*When do you experience the pain or discomfort?*	*Exertional or worsens with exertion:* may suggest underlying cardiac conditions such as ischemic heart disease or aortic stenosis *Constant or worsens with standing:* may suggest underlying venous insufficiency or peripheral artery disease (PAD)
Quality	*Can you describe the type of pain or discomfort?*	*Sharp or stabbing:* may suggest underlying aortic dissection or renal colic *Dull or aching:* may suggest underlying ischemic heart disease or musculoskeletal conditions
Radiation	*Does the pain or discomfort radiate to other areas of the body?*	*Radiates to the jaw or left arm:* may suggest underlying ischemic heart disease *Radiates to the back:* may suggest underlying aortic dissection
Associated Symptoms	*Do you have any associated symptoms such as shortness of breath or leg swelling?*	These may suggest underlying cardiac or peripheral vascular conditions such as heart failure or venous insufficiency
Risk Factors	*Do you have any underlying medical conditions or risk factors?*	These risk factors, such as high blood pressure, diabetes, smoking, and high cholesterol, may increase the likelihood of underlying cardiac or peripheral vascular conditions

PHYSICAL EXAMINATION: GENERAL APPROACH

As with your clinical interview, examine the integrity of the arterial, venous, and lymphatic systems of the extremities and abdomen. Ensure that pulses are equal throughout the extremities and that the perfusion is intact. Progress through the examination in a top-down fashion: start with the carotid arteries, then move to the upper extremities, followed by the abdomen, and finally the lower extremities. In doing so, compare and contrast the (1) quality of pulses, (2) size of the arteries, (3) temperature of the extremities, (4) hair patterns on the extremities, and (5) presence or absence of edema from side to side. When examining the abdomen, remember to palpate the abdominal aorta. Should you discover a pulsatile mass, you might have identified an AAA, a condition that can be life threatening. As you deepen your understanding of the peripheral vascular system, remember that PAD is frequently asymptomatic and often goes underdiagnosed, which can lead to significant morbidity and mortality.

TECHNIQUES OF EXAMINATION

Key Components of the Peripheral Vascular System Examination

- Inspect the upper extremities.
- Palpate the radial pulse.
- Palpate the brachial pulse.
- Palpate for epitrochlear nodes.
- Examine the abdominal aorta.
- Palpate the superficial inguinal lymph nodes.
- Inspect the lower extremities.
- Assess the temperature of the feet and legs.
- Palpate the femoral pulse.
- Palpate the popliteal pulse.
- Palpate the posterior tibial (PT) pulse.
- Palpate the dorsalis pedis (DP) pulse.
- Palpate for pitting edema.
- Palpate for venous tenderness or cords.

In addition, review the techniques for assessing blood pressure, the carotid artery, the aorta, and the renal and femoral arteries on the pages indicated below.

- Measure the blood pressure in both arms (see Chapter 10, General Survey, Vital Signs, and Pain, p. 173).
- Palpate the carotid upstroke, auscultate for bruits (see Chapter 18, Cardiovascular System, pp. 496–497).
- Palpate the aorta and assess its maximal diameter (see Chapter 21, Abdomen, p. 637).

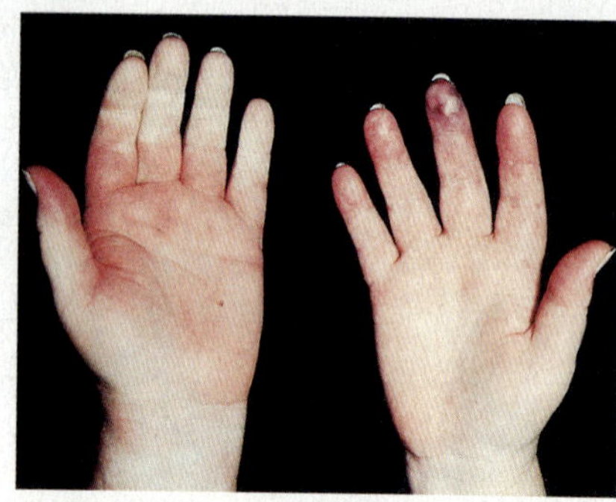

FIGURE 19-11. Raynaud disease.

Inspect the Upper Extremities

Inspect both arms from the fingertips to the shoulders and take note of the size, symmetry, any swelling, venous pattern, color of the skin and nail beds, and the texture of the skin.

Swelling from lymphedema of the arm and hand may follow axillary node dissection and radiation therapy.

In Raynaud disease, wrist pulses are typically normal, but spasm of more distal arteries causes episodes of sharply demarcated pallor of the fingers, as shown in Figure 19-11.

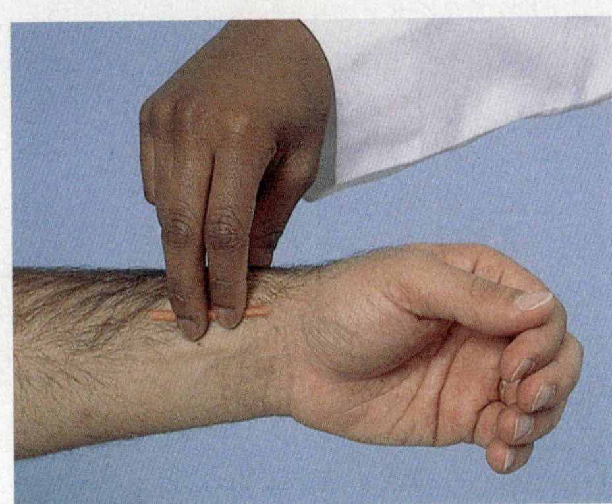

FIGURE 19-12. Palpating the radial pulse.

Bounding carotid, radial, and femoral pulses are present in aortic regurgitation.

Pulsus parvus refers to weak pulses, usually seen with atherosclerotic PVD, while **pulsus tardus** refers to sluggish pulses, usually occurring in the setting of aortic stenosis or low cardiac output.

Capillary refill time in the digits of >5 seconds has low sensitivity and specificity and is not considered diagnostically helpful.[10]

Palpate the Radial Pulse

Palpate the radial pulse with the pads of your fingers on the flexor surface of the lateral wrist (Fig. 19-12). Partially flexing the patient's wrist may help you feel this pulse. Compare the pulses in both arms. Assess the amplitude using a recommended scale (Box 19-9).

Palpate the Brachial Pulse

Flex the patient's elbow slightly and palpate the artery just medial to the biceps tendon at the antecubital crease (Fig. 19-13). The brachial pulse can also be palpated higher in the arm in the groove between the biceps and triceps muscles.

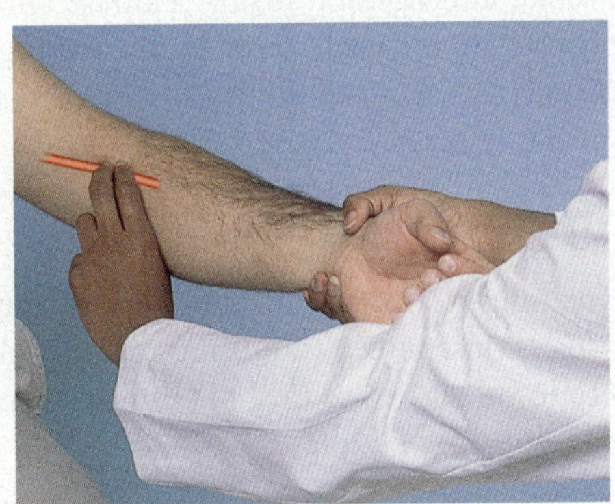

FIGURE 19-13. Palpating the brachial pulse.

Box 19-9. Recommended Grading of Pulses

There are several recommended systems for grading the amplitude of arterial pulses. One system proposed in the 2016 American College of Cardiology (ACC)/American Heart Association (AHA) guidelines uses a scale of 0 to 3.[13]

Scale	Description
+3	Bounding
+2	Brisk, expected (normal)
+1	Diminished, weaker than expected
0	Absent, unable to palpate

Palpate for Epitrochlear Nodes

With the patient's elbow flexed to about 90° and the forearm supported by your hand, reach around behind their arm and feel in the groove between their biceps and triceps muscles, about 3 cm above the medial epicondyle (Fig. 19-14). If a node is present, note its size, consistency, and tenderness. Epitrochlear nodes are usually not palpable in healthy individuals.

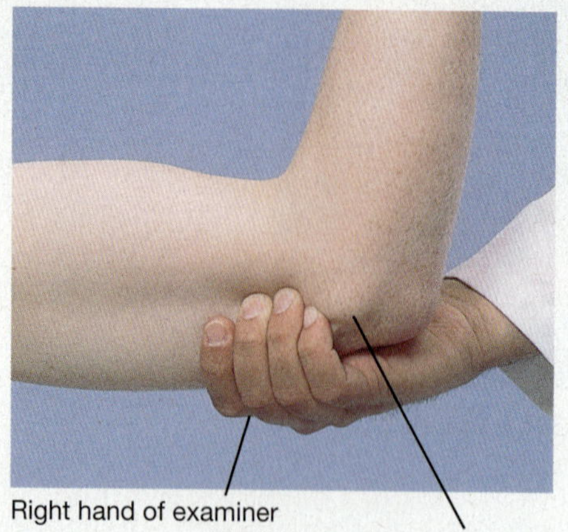

FIGURE 19-14. Palpating the epitrochlear of the left arm.

An enlarged epitrochlear node suggests local or distal infection or may be associated with lymphadenopathy from lymphoma or HIV.

Examine the Abdominal Aorta

For techniques of examination of the abdominal aorta, see Chapter 21, Abdomen, p. 637. In brief, listen for aortic, renal, and femoral bruits. Palpate and estimate the width of the abdominal aorta in the epigastric area by measuring the aortic width between two fingers, especially in older adults and smokers due to higher risk of AAA. Assess for a pulsatile mass.[14]

Palpate the Superficial Inguinal Nodes

Palpate the superficial inguinal nodes, including both the horizontal and the vertical groups (Fig. 19-15). Note their size, consistency, and discreteness, and note any tenderness. Nontender, discrete inguinal nodes up to 1 cm or even 2 cm in diameter are commonly palpable in healthy people.

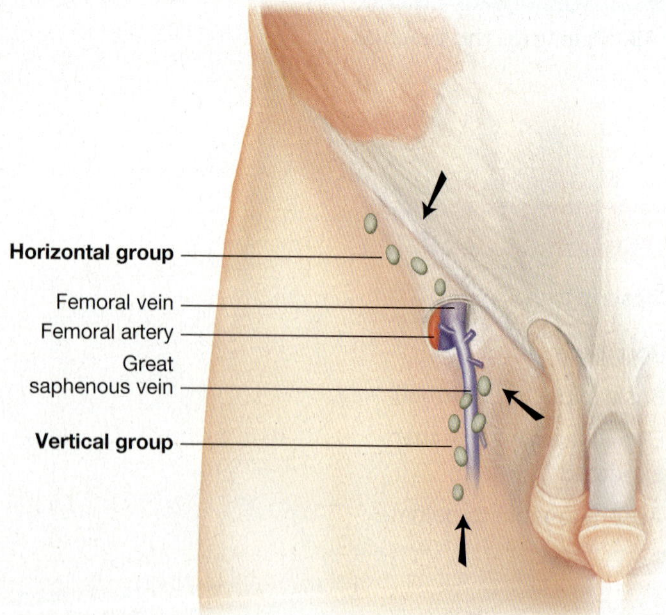

FIGURE 19-15. Superficial inguinal lymph nodes. (Reprinted with permission from Moore KL, Dalley AF II, Agur AMR. *Clinically Oriented Anatomy*. 8th ed. Wolters Kluwer; 2018. Figure 7-46.)

Box 19-10. Common Findings on Inspection of the Extremities

Aspect	Inspection Criteria	Potential Findings/Notes
Size and symmetry	Compare thighs, calves, and ankles for asymmetry using a tape ruler. Normally, the difference in calf circumference is <3 cm.	Calf asymmetry >3 cm increases the likelihood ratio (LR) for deep vein thrombosis (DVT) to >2.8.[10] Also consider a muscle tear, Baker cyst, or muscular atrophy.
Swelling or edema	Check if it is unilateral or bilateral and note the extent. Figure 19-16 illustrates a non-edematous ankle and foot. For comparison, Figure 19-17 depicts pretibial edema affecting the ankle and foot.	Local swelling, and redness, may suggest superficial thrombophlebitis, an emerging risk factor for DVT.[15] *Asymmetric* redness over calf indicate cellulitis. *Unilateral* swelling may suggest venous thromboembolism (VTE) from DVT, chronic venous insufficiency (CVI), or lymphedema. *Bilateral edema* is seen in heart failure, cirrhosis, and nephrotic syndrome. *Venous distention* indicates a venous cause for edema.
Saphenous system	Inspect for varicosities, especially when patient is standing.	Varicose veins are dilated, tortuous, which may also present with visible thickening (Fig. 19-18).
Skin and nails	Inspect for pigmentation, rashes, scars, ulcers, and observe the color and texture of skin and nail beds.	Foot ulcers raise the likelihood of peripheral vascular disease to 7.[10] Brownish discoloration or ulcers just above the malleolus indicate CVI. Visibly brawny skin suggests lymphedema and advanced venous insufficiency.
Hair distribution	Observe hair on lower legs, feet, and toes.	Specific patterns may suggest circulatory issues.

Inspect the Lower Extremities

Inspect both legs thoroughly, starting from the groin and buttocks down to the feet. Ensure the patient is in a supine position and is appropriately draped to maintain their dignity by covering their external genitalia while having their legs fully exposed. Always ask the patient to remove any stockings, leggings, or socks to facilitate a comprehensive examination.

Systematically evaluate various criteria to identify potential underlying conditions. Box 19-10 gives a summary of common findings to look for.

See also Table 19-3, Chronic Insufficiency of Arteries and Veins, p. 574 and Table 19-4, Common Ulcers of the Ankles and Feet, p. 575.

Assess the Temperature of the Feet and Legs

Assess the temperature of the feet and legs with the backs of your fingers. Compare one side with the other.

Poikilothermia is the relative hypothermia of one extremity as compared with another. Asymmetric coolness of the feet has a positive likelihood ratio (LR) of 5.9 for PAD.[10,16]

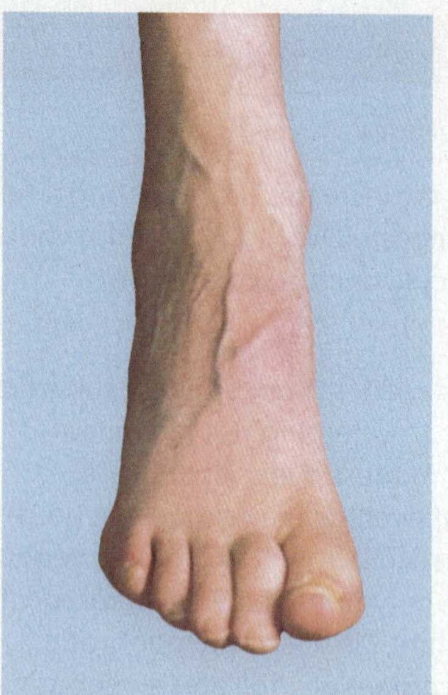

FIGURE 19-16. Non-edematous right ankle and foot. Note the prominent veins.

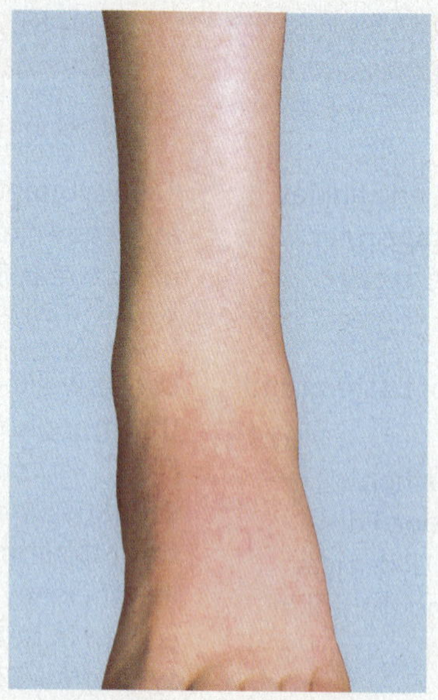

FIGURE 19-17. Pretibial edema of left ankle and foot. Note loss of vein prominence due to swelling.

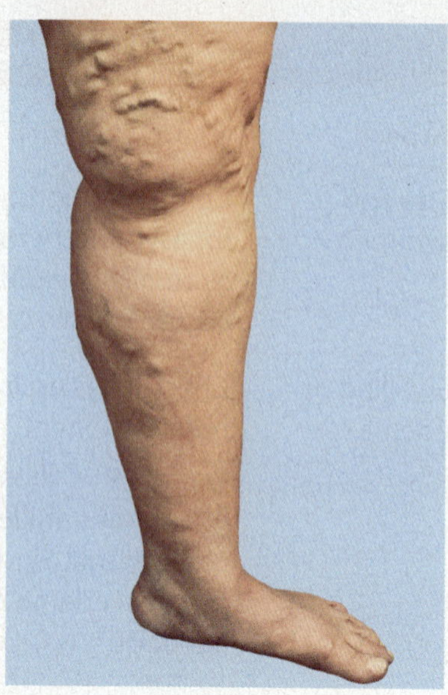

FIGURE 19-18. Varicose veins.

Palpate the Femoral Pulse

Press deeply below the inguinal ligament and about midway between the anterior superior iliac spine and the symphysis pubis (Fig. 19-19). As in deep abdominal palpation, the use of two hands, one on top of the other, may be helpful, especially in patients with a larger body size, in whom it can be particularly challenging to palpate the femoral pulse.

If the femoral pulse is absent, the LR of PAD is 4.7.[10,16] If the occlusion is at the aortic or iliac level, all pulses distal to the occlusion are typically affected and may cause postural color changes.

An exaggerated, widened femoral pulse suggests the pathologic dilatation of a femoral aneurysm.

FIGURE 19-19. Palpating the right femoral pulse.

Palpate the Popliteal Pulse

The patient's knee should be somewhat flexed, with the leg relaxed. Place the fingertips of both hands so that they just meet in the midline behind the knee and press them deeply into the popliteal fossa (Fig. 19-20). The popliteal pulse is more difficult to find than other pulses. It is deeper and feels more diffuse.

If you cannot palpate the popliteal pulse with this approach, try with the patient prone. Flex the patient's knee to about 90°, let the lower leg relax against your shoulder or upper arm, and press your two thumbs deeply into the popliteal fossa (Fig. 19-21).

An exaggerated, widened popliteal pulse suggests a popliteal artery aneurysm.

Popliteal and femoral aneurysms are uncommon. They are usually from atherosclerosis and occur primarily in individuals assigned male at birth aged ≥50 years.

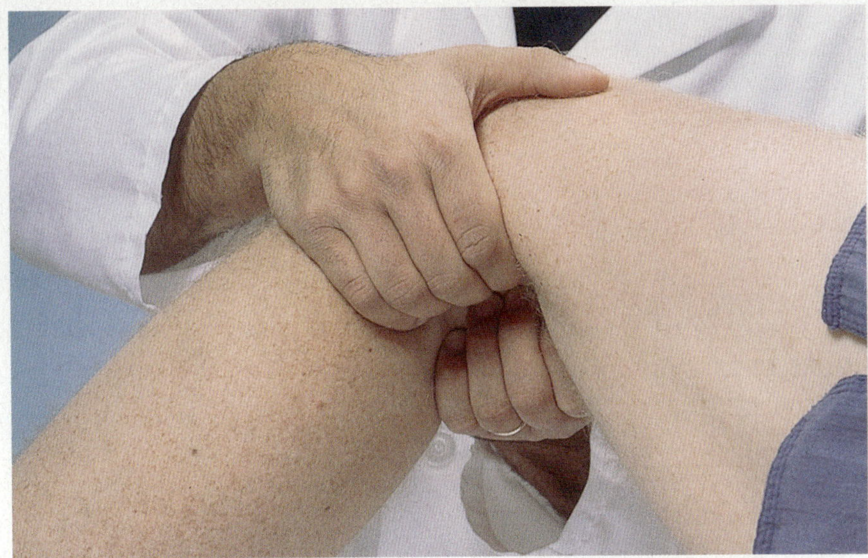

FIGURE 19-20. Palpating the popliteal in popliteal fossa, supine position.

FIGURE 19-21. Deeply palpating the popliteal pulse in popliteal fossa, prone position.

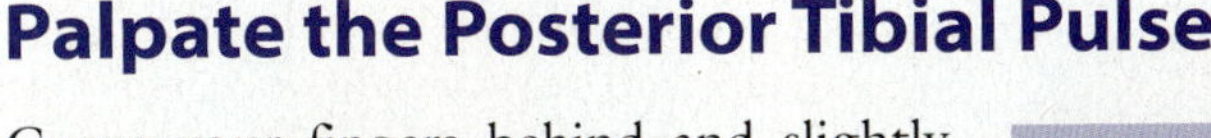

Palpate the Posterior Tibial Pulse

Curve your fingers behind and slightly below the medial malleolus of the ankle (Fig. 19-22). This pulse may be hard to feel in a swollen or a thick ankle due to surrounding fat (Box 19-11).

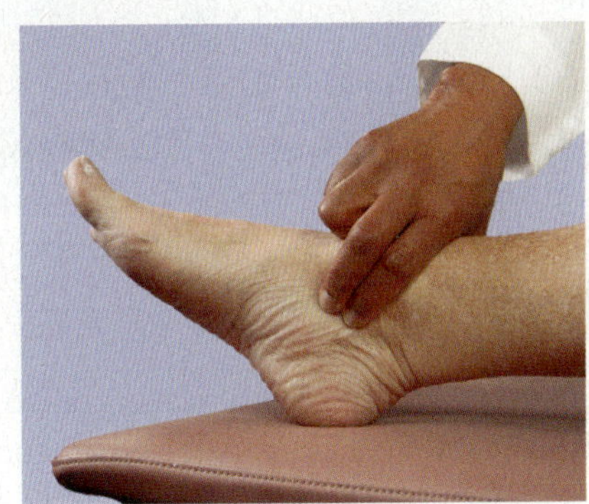

FIGURE 19-22. Palpating the posterior tibial pulse.

Acute arterial occlusion from embolism or thrombosis causes pain and numbness or tingling. The limb distal to the occlusion becomes cold, pale, and pulseless. Pursue emergency treatment.

Box 19-11. Tips for Palpating Difficult Peripheral Pulses

1. Position your body and examining hand comfortably; awkward positions decrease tactile sensitivity.
2. Once your hand is positioned properly, linger, varying the pressure of your fingers to pick up a weak pulsation. If unsuccessful, explore the area gently but more deliberately.
3. Think of the position and depth of the pulse. A pulse may require several fingers or may require two hands to properly palpate.
4. Do not mistake the patient's pulse with your own pulsating fingertips. If needed, count your own heart rate, and compare it to the patient's. The rates are usually different. Your carotid pulse is convenient for this comparison.
5. In some cases, it is helpful to compare the pulse you are trying to palpate with the patient's carotid or radial pulse simultaneously.

Palpate the Dorsalis Pedis Pulse

Palpate the dorsum of the foot (not the ankle) just lateral to the extensor tendon of the great toe (Fig. 19-23). The DP artery may be congenitally absent or branch higher in the ankle. If you cannot feel a pulse, explore the dorsum of the foot more laterally.

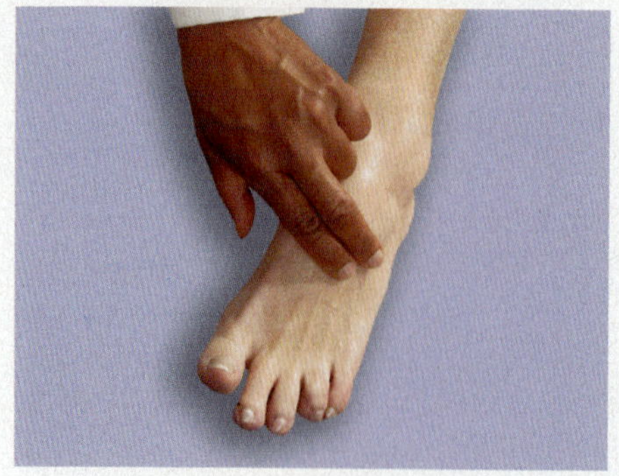

FIGURE 19-23. Palpating the dorsalis pedis pulse.

Absent pedal pulses with normal femoral and popliteal pulses raise the LR of PAD to >14.[10]

Palpate for Pitting Edema

If swelling or edema is present, palpate for pitting edema. Press firmly but gently with your thumb for at least 2 seconds over the dorsum of each foot, behind each medial malleolus, and over the shins (Fig. 19-24). Look for *pitting*—a depression caused by pressure from your thumb. Normally there is none.

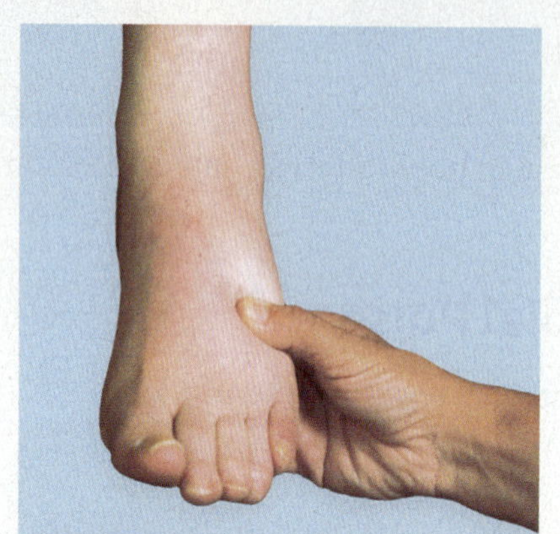

FIGURE 19-24. Palpating for pitting edema.

FIGURE 19-25. 3+ pitting edema.

The severity of edema is graded on a subjective four-point scale graded by the depth and duration of the indentation (Box 19-12). Figure 19-25 shows 3+ pitting edema.

See Table 19-1, Types of Peripheral Edema, p. 569.

Palpate for Venous Tenderness or Cords

Palpate the inguinal area just medial to the femoral pulse for tenderness of the femoral vein.

A painful, pale, swollen leg, together with tenderness in the groin over the femoral vein, suggests *iliofemoral deep vein thrombosis.* Risk of pulmonary embolism (PE) in proximal vein thrombosis range from 10% to 50%.[17]

Next, with the patient's leg flexed at the knee and relaxed, palpate the calf. With your fingerpads, gently compress the calf muscles against the tibia and search for any tenderness or cords.

Only half of patients with DVT in the calf have tenderness or venous cords, and absence of calf tenderness does not rule out thrombosis.

Box 19-12. Pitting Edema Scale

1+	Barely detectable impression when finger is pressed into skin
2+	Moderate pitting, indentation subsides rapidly
3+	Deep pitting, indentation remains for a short time
4+	Very deep pitting, indentation lasts a long time

SPECIAL TECHNIQUES AND MANEUVERS

Assess for Peripheral Arterial Disease Using the Ankle–Brachial Index

If the patient presents with history and examination findings suspicious of peripheral vascular disease, such as pain, claudication, numbness, weakness, weak-to-absent DP and PT pulses, or pallor of distal extremities (see Box 19-4), measuring the *ankle–brachial index* (*ABI*) is an important diagnostic technique. The ABI is the ratio of blood pressure measurements in the foot and arm. This noninvasive method is simple, reproducible, and accurate at detecting the decreased blood pressure distal to an arterial stenosis.[18] It is often used to assess PAD.

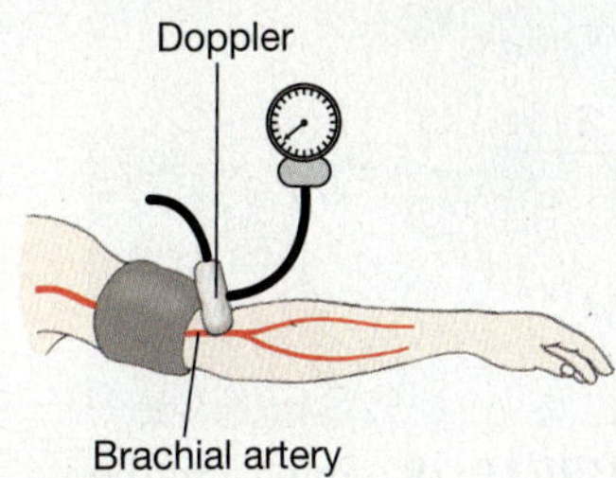

FIGURE 19-26. Measuring the brachial pressure.

Step 1: Measure the Brachial Pressure. After the patient has been resting in the supine position for 10 minutes, place a blood pressure cuff on the arm (Fig. 19-26). Apply ultrasound gel over the brachial pulse. Using the transducer of a handheld vascular Doppler, locate the brachial pulse. Inflate the cuff to 20 mm Hg above the last audible pulse. Deflate the cuff slowly (~1 mm Hg/sec) and record the pressure at which the pulse becomes audible again. Obtain two measures in each arm and record the average as the brachial pressure in that arm.

Step 2: Measure the Ankle Pressures. Now place the blood pressure cuff on the ankle proximal to the malleoli (Fig. 19-27). Apply ultrasound gel over the DP artery. Using the transducer of a handheld vascular Doppler, locate the DP pulse. Inflate the cuff to 20 mm Hg above the last audible pulse. Deflate the cuff slowly (~1 mm Hg/sec) and record the pressure at which the pulse becomes audible again. Repeat the previous steps for the PT artery. Then repeat both measurements on the opposite leg.

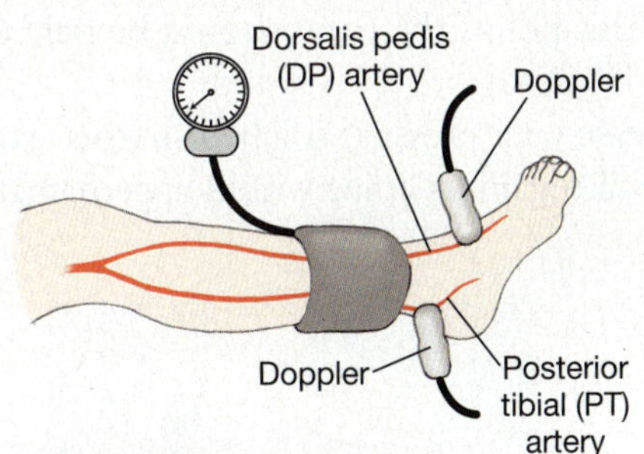

FIGURE 19-27. Measuring the ankle pressure.

In older adult patients or those with diabetes, the limb vessels may be fibrotic or calcified. In this case, the vessel may be resistant to collapse by the blood pressure cuff, and a signal may be heard at high cuff pressures. The persistence of a signal at a high pressure in these individuals results in an artifactually elevated blood pressure value.[19]

Step 3: Calculate the Ankle–Brachial Index. An ABI is calculated for each leg. The ABI value is determined by taking the higher pressure of the two arteries at the ankle, divided by the brachial arterial systolic pressure. Calculated ABI values should be recorded to two decimal places.[19]

$$\text{Right ABI} = \frac{\text{Highest Pressure in Right Foot}}{\text{Highest Pressure in Both Arms}}$$

$$\text{Left ABI} = \frac{\text{Highest Pressure in Left Foot}}{\text{Highest Pressure in Both Arms}}$$

Step 4: Interpret the Ankle–Brachial Index. Normal ABI ranges from 0.90 to 1.40 because the pressure is normally higher in the ankle than the arm.

Values >1.40 suggest a noncompressible calcified vessel. A value <0.90 is considered diagnostic of PAD; values <0.5 suggest severe PAD.

Evaluate Arterial Perfusion of the Hand Using the Allen Test

The *Allen test* evaluates the patency of both the ulnar and radial arteries (Fig. 19-28). It becomes especially significant before undertaking procedures such as drawing blood from the radial artery.

Begin by having the patient rest their hands on their lap with palms facing upward. Instruct them to make a tight fist with one hand. With your thumbs and fingers, compress both the radial and ulnar arteries of the selected hand (Fig. 19-29).

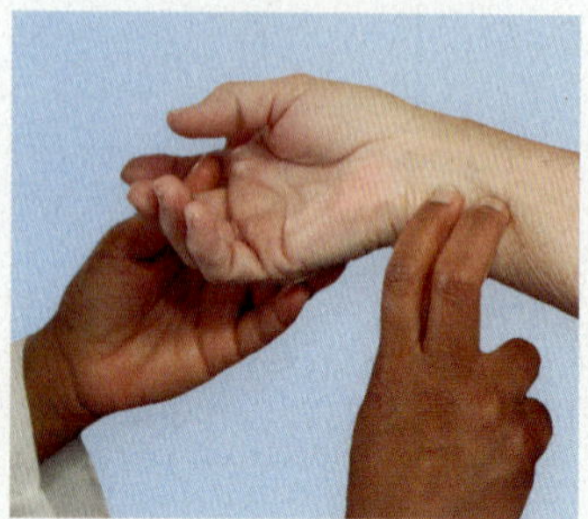

FIGURE 19-28. Palpating the ulnar pulse.

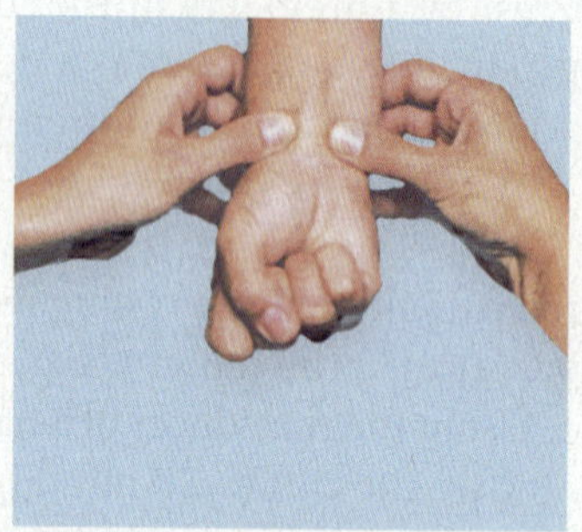

FIGURE 19-29. Compressing both the radial and ulnar arteries.

On your request, the patient should then open their hand, ensuring it remains relaxed and slightly flexed. At this point, the palm should be pale due to the obstruction of blood flow (Fig. 19-30).

Fully extending the hand can induce pallor, potentially leading to a falsely positive result.

To test the *ulnar artery's patency*, release your pressure solely from this artery. If the ulnar artery is patent, the palm will regain its color within approximately 3 to 5 seconds (Fig. 19-31).

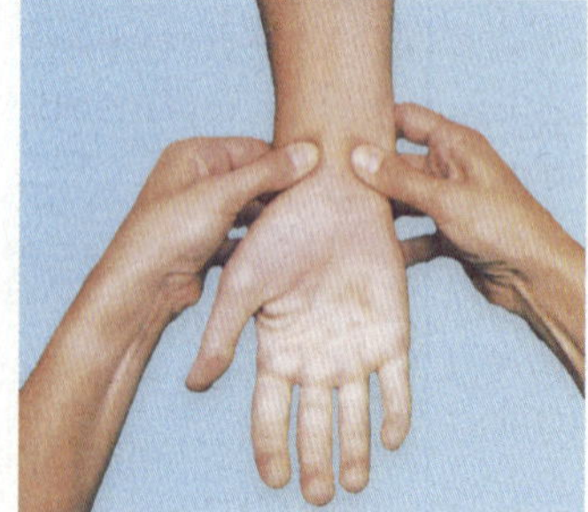

FIGURE 19-30. Pallor with relaxed hand.

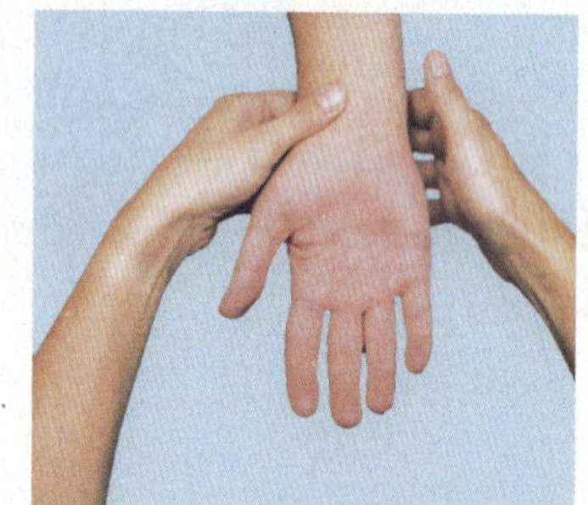

FIGURE 19-31. Palmar flushing—Allen test showing patent arterial circulation.

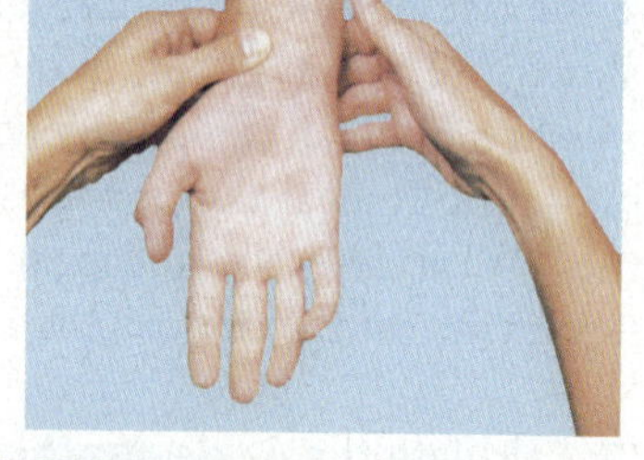

FIGURE 19-32. Palmar pallor—Allen test showing possible occlusive disease.

Then, to evaluate the *radial artery's patency*, maintain your compression on the ulnar artery and release pressure from the radial artery. If the radial artery is patent, the palm will once again regain its color.

If pallor persists, it suggests occlusion of the ulnar artery or its distal branches (see Fig. 19-32).

Modifications in Physical Examinations: Best Practices for Specialized Patient Populations

For patients requiring regular vascular access, such as those on dialysis or long-term intravenous (IV) therapy, devices like arteriovenous (AV) fistulas and access ports are paramount. Box 19-13 explores their characteristics and implications for the physical examination.

Box 19-13. Peripheral Vascular Examination in the Presence of Medical Devices, Conditions or Procedures

	Patient with an Arteriovenous (AV) Fistula or Graft	Patient with a Central Venous Access Port	Patient with a Tunneled Hemodialysis Catheter	Patient with a Peripherally Inserted Central Catheter (PICC) or Midline Catheter
	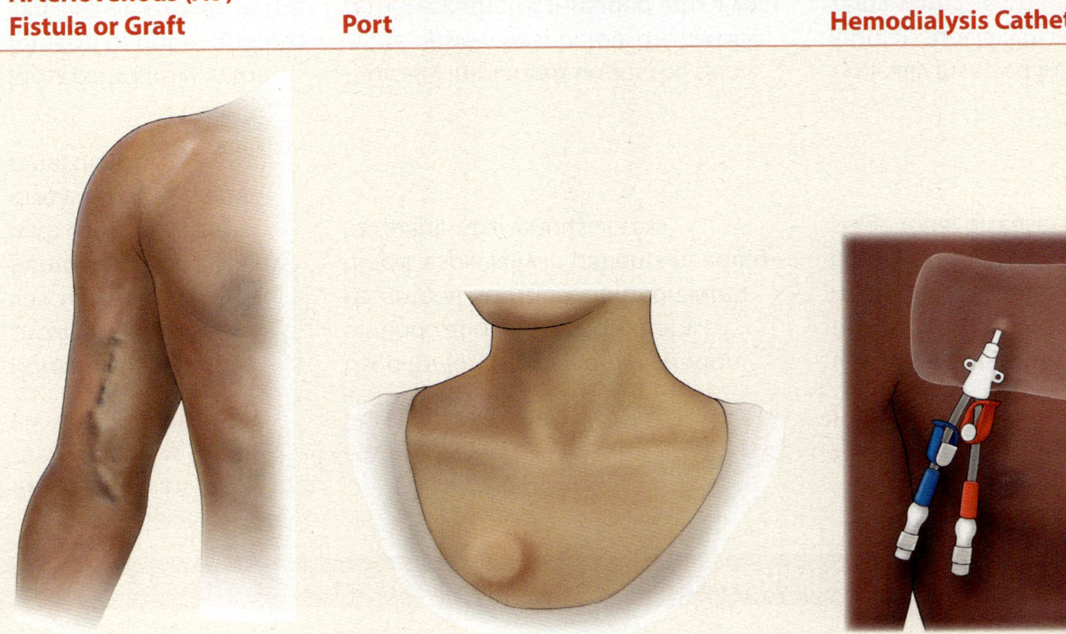			
Device/ condition	Permanent vascular access established surgically by either a side-by-side connection made between an artery and a vein, or a graft connecting an artery and vein, typically in the arm	Implanted venous access device with a reservoir that can be accessed externally with a special needle	Catheter specifically designed for hemodialysis, a blood exchange procedure to remove excess fluid and waste products when the kidneys fail	Catheter inserted in a peripheral vein and designed for prolonged vascular access

(continued)

Box 19-13. Peripheral Vascular Examination in the Presence of Medical Devices, Conditions or Procedures (*Continued*)

	Patient with an Arteriovenous (AV) Fistula or Graft	Patient with a Central Venous Access Port	Patient with a Tunneled Hemodialysis Catheter	Patient with a Peripherally Inserted Central Catheter (PICC) or Midline Catheter
General indication	Primarily used for providing long-term vascular access for hemodialysis in patients with chronic kidney disease or end-stage renal disease	Used for long-term administration of medications, chemotherapy, parenteral nutrition, or for drawing blood, especially in patients needing frequent intravenous access	Used as a temporary or permanent access for hemodialysis in patients with chronic kidney disease or end-stage renal disease	Used for short- and intermediate-term administration of medications, particularly prolonged courses of antibiotics that may be several weeks in duration
General location	Most commonly in the forearm or upper arm but can also be created in the leg	Typically implanted under the skin, in the upper chest below the clavicle, with the catheter threaded into a vein and terminating in the superior vena cava or right atrium.	Typically inserted in the internal jugular, subclavian or femoral veins, with the tip residing in the right atrium or superior vena cava.	Typically inserted at a peripheral venous site, typically the cubital vein or brachial vein in the upper arm, with its tip terminating in the superior vena cava. A midline is shorter, with the tip terminating in a vein near the shoulder.

Modification to the physical exam	1. Inspect the site for signs of infection, inflammation, or aneurysmal changes. 2. Use the palm of the hand to palpate for the characteristic "thrill," a palpable vibration or "buzz" over the fistula, indicating blood flow. Absence indicates a problem. 3. Auscultate for a bruit (low-pitched, soft, machinery-like, or whooshing sound) over the fistula, indicating blood flow; absence indicates a problem. 4. Examine the color, pulses, and capillary refill of the hand to evaluate for distal ischemia. 5. Be gentle and avoid using the limb with the AV fistula or graft for blood pressure measurements or venipuncture.	1. Inspect the skin overlying the port for signs of infection or inflammation, including erythema, edema, warmth, or skin erosion. 2. Palpate gently around the port to ensure it is flat against the chest and to check for tenderness. 3. Auscultate (if relevant based on the clinical scenario) over the port for any unusual sounds or if there is a suspicion of vascular complications. 4. Avoid accessing the port unless specially trained. Always ensure clean and aseptic technique when the port is accessed.	1. Inspect the catheter site for signs of infection or inflammation, including erythema, edema, warmth, or purulent discharge. 2. Palpate around the site to check for tenderness or induration. 3. Auscultate over the catheter insertion site if there is a suspicion of vascular complications. 4. Be cautious when accessing the catheter, always ensuring clean and aseptic technique. 5. Avoid using the area near the catheter for other venous accesses.	1. Inspect the catheter site for signs of infection or inflammation, including erythema, edema, warmth, or purulent discharge. 2. Palpate around the site to check for tenderness or induration. 3. Be cautious when accessing the catheter, always ensuring clean and aseptic technique. 4. Avoid using an area proximal to the catheter for other venous accesses.

RECORDING YOUR FINDINGS

The example documentation given is standard in clinical environments. As you commence your training, you might find yourself using complete sentences to thoroughly describe observations. As you gain experience and become more accustomed to the process, you will gravitate toward succinct phrases. These phrases quickly emphasize any irregularities and also indicate what is considered normal or missing.

Recording the Peripheral Vascular System Examination

"Extremities are warm and without edema. No varicosities or stasis changes. Calves are supple and nontender. No femoral or abdominal bruits. Brachial, radial, femoral, popliteal, DP, and PT pulses are 2+ and symmetric."

OR

"Extremities are pale below the midcalf, with notable hair loss. Erythema noted when legs dependent but no edema or ulceration. Bilateral femoral bruits; no abdominal bruits heard. Brachial and radial pulses 2+; femoral, popliteal, DP, and PT pulses 1+."

It is more helpful and less time consuming to record pulses in a table format:

	Radial	Brachial	Femoral	Popliteal	Posterior Tibial	Dorsalis Pedis
RT	2+	2+	1+	1+	1+	1+
LT	2+	2+	1+	1+	1+	1+

The meticulous analysis of physical examination findings in the extremities and vascular system is crucial, as it can uncover critical signs pointing to vascular pathologies.

- *Pale extremities below the midcalf with hair loss:* this finding typically indicates compromised blood flow to the lower extremities, often a sign of PAD, which can be associated with atherosclerosis or other vascular conditions.
- *Erythema upon dependency without edema or ulceration:* dependent erythema can signal arterial insufficiency, while the absence of edema and ulceration suggests that the condition might not yet have progressed to severe chronic arterial or venous insufficiency.
- *Bilateral femoral bruits without abdominal bruits:* bruits over the femoral arteries are indicative of turbulent flow, often due to narrowing or stenosis. The absence of abdominal bruits may help localize the vascular compromise to the peripheral arteries rather than the abdominal aorta or renal arteries.
- *Brachial and radial pulses 2+; diminished femoral, popliteal, DP, and PT pulses 1+:* the discrepancy in pulse strength between the upper and lower extremities further supports the presence of peripheral arterial disease, with a possible reduction in arterial caliber or blockage-reducing blood flow to the lower limbs.

These findings are suggestive of *peripheral arterial disease*, likely due to atherosclerotic changes, with notable compensation mechanisms such as hair loss from reduced nutrient supply and erythema due to vascular insufficiency. The presence of femoral bruits and diminished pulses in the lower extremities, compared to normal upper extremity pulses, reinforces this diagnosis.

POINT-OF-CARE ULTRASOUND EXAMINATION

The peripheral vascular system is complex and sometimes necessitates more than a manual assessment. Point-of-care ultrasound (POCUS) offers clarity in visualizing conditions like DVT or arterial anomalies. In this section, we will highlight the interpretive value of POCUS in vascular evaluations, while detailed procedural guidance on its use will not be covered.

Detecting Nonpalpable Pulses

Physical Examination. Patients with PAD can sometimes exhibit nontraditional symptoms, making clinical diagnosis a challenge. Traditional physical examination leans heavily on palpation, visual inspection, and auscultation (Box 19-14).[13,20] When faced with undetectable arterial pulses, using ultrasound to verify arterial blood flow becomes a pivotal step, especially if the extremity in question appears cold, discolored, or painful.

While the ABI remains the gold standard for gauging PAD, its accuracy may falter in cases involving fibrotic or calcified arteries. Therefore, integrating it with continuous Doppler ultrasound offers a more comprehensive diagnostic perspective. The typical approach involves a handheld continuous wave

Box 19-14. Physical Examination Findings: Peripheral Arterial Disease

Skin appearance	■ Pallor or blanching upon elevation ■ Dependent rubor (reddish-blue discoloration) ■ Atrophic skin changes ■ Hair loss on legs and feet ■ Thin, brittle nails ■ Skin ulcerations, particularly on toes ■ Gangrene
Pulse palpation	■ Absent or diminished pulses (e.g., dorsalis pedis, posterior tibial) ■ Decreased pulse amplitude
Temperature	■ Cool to touch in affected limb
Auscultation	■ Bruits over major arteries (indicative of turbulent blood flow)
Pain assessment	■ Claudication (pain with walking) ■ Rest pain (pain in limb even when at rest) ■ Pain relief upon hanging leg off bed (due to gravity-enhanced blood flow)

Doppler to detect an audible pulse, especially when it is not palpable.[21] This method relies on surface anatomy and key landmarks without offering direct visualization of the artery. Not only does POCUS provide a direct view of the artery in question, but its color Doppler and pulsed-wave Doppler features also grant us an in-depth look at arterial flow.

See Assess for Peripheral Arterial Disease Using the Ankle-Brachial Index, p. 557.

Ultrasound Technique

Basic Ultrasound Setup	
Patient Positioning	Supine or sitting upright
Probe	Linear probe
Ultrasound Setting	"Vascular" setting for the linear probe, B-mode, color Doppler, pulsed-wave Doppler

POCUS evaluation for PAD is performed with the patient in a supine or seated position. The probe can be placed in a transverse view over the appropriate anatomic area to evaluate the vessel of interest. Most commonly the vessel is identified in B-mode and then color Doppler or pulsed-wave Doppler is used to identify flow or lack of flow. At the bedside in the setting of a nonpalpable pulse, the simple yes or no clinical question, "*Is there flow*"? is critical in determining the next best steps (Box 19-15).[20]

Box 19-15. Comparative Evaluation of Peripheral Flow Characteristics and Corresponding POCUS Findings

Evaluation of Flow	Characteristics
Normal flow	■ Usually palpable ■ Normal is seen as pulsed-wave Doppler triphasic flow (Fig. 19-33).
Decreased flow	■ Usually nonpalpable with clinical findings as listed above ■ Color flow may be difficult to appreciate. ■ Severely decreased is seen as pulsed-wave Doppler monophasic flow (Fig. 19-34).

Detecting Deep Venous Thrombosis

Physical Examination. Patients with suspected lower extremity DVT can be rapidly and accurately assessed using POCUS.[22,23] The technique relies on visualization of the vein in question (e.g., femoral and popliteal veins), compression of the vein to ensure there is no thrombus within, and application of Doppler flow to ensure flow can be visualized within the vessel lumen. Clinical exam findings for lower extremity DVT are shown in Box 19-16.

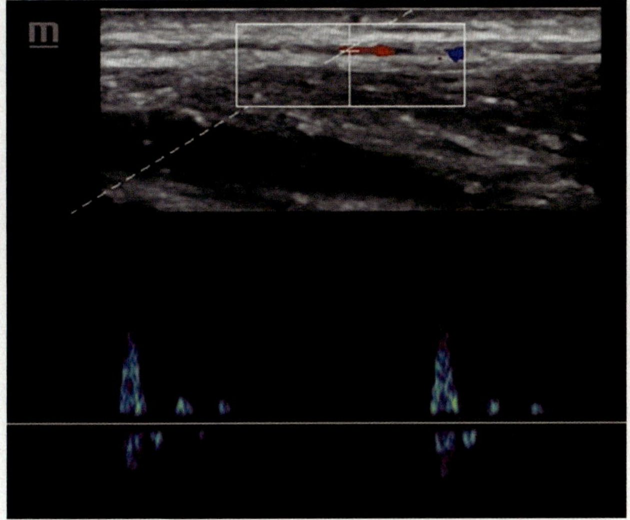

FIGURE 19-33. Normal Triphasic Blood Flow Pattern. The lower panel displays a triphasic Doppler waveform, featuring a strong systolic peak, brief reverse flow, and a secondary forward flow, indicating normal arterial function.

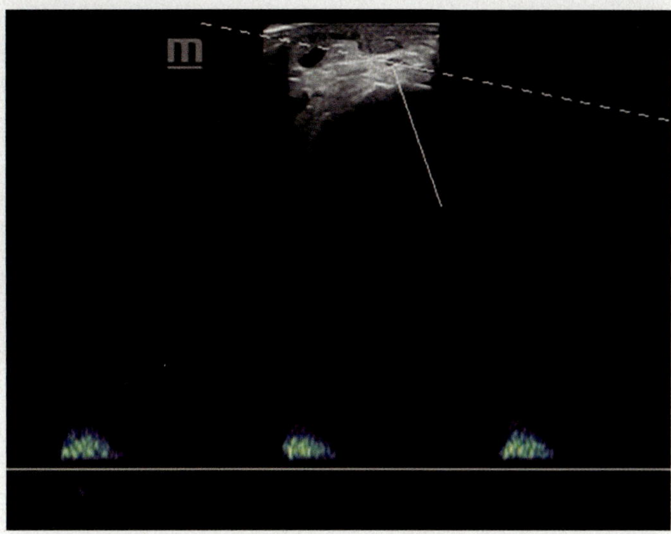

FIGURE 19-34. Monophasic Flow Pattern. The lower panel displays a monophasic spectral Doppler waveform, indicative of reduced or abnormal blood flow, often associated with downstream vascular obstruction or disease.

Ultrasound Technique

Basic Ultrasound Setup	
Patient Positioning	Supine with frog-leg (out-turned) positioning of lower extremity
Probe	Linear probe
Ultrasound Setting	"Vascular" or "Lower extremity" setting for the linear probe, B-mode, color Doppler

Box 19-16. Physical Examination Findings: Deep Venous Thrombosis	
Leg swelling (edema)	One leg may appear more swollen than the other, especially around the calf.
Pain or Tenderness	Pain often starts in the calf and can feel like cramping or soreness.
Warmth	Skin of the affected leg may feel warmer to touch than the other leg.
Discoloration	Skin on the affected leg may turn reddish or bluish.
Palpable Cord	Firm or tender area that can be felt beneath the skin of the affected leg, representing a thrombosed vein.
Distended Superficial Veins	Superficial veins may appear more prominent or engorged.

POCUS evaluation for DVT is performed with the patient in a supine with frog-leg (out-turned) positioning of lower extremity or seated position. The probe can be placed in a transverse view over the appropriate anatomical area to evaluate the vessel of interest. Most commonly, the vessel is identified in B-mode, and compressibility is assessed by placing pressure on the vessel as it is visualized (Box 19-17). Thrombus within the vessel can sometimes be seen in B-mode. Color Doppler can be used to identify flow or lack of flow.[24]

Box 19-17. Comparative Evaluation of Peripheral Flow Characteristics and Corresponding POCUS Findings

Evaluation of Flow	Characteristics
Normal vein	■ Fully compressible (anterior and posterior walls should touch); Figure 19-35 ■ Nonpulsatile
Deep vein thrombosis (DVT)	■ Partially or noncompressible ■ Visible thrombus ■ Limited color Doppler flow; Figure 19-36

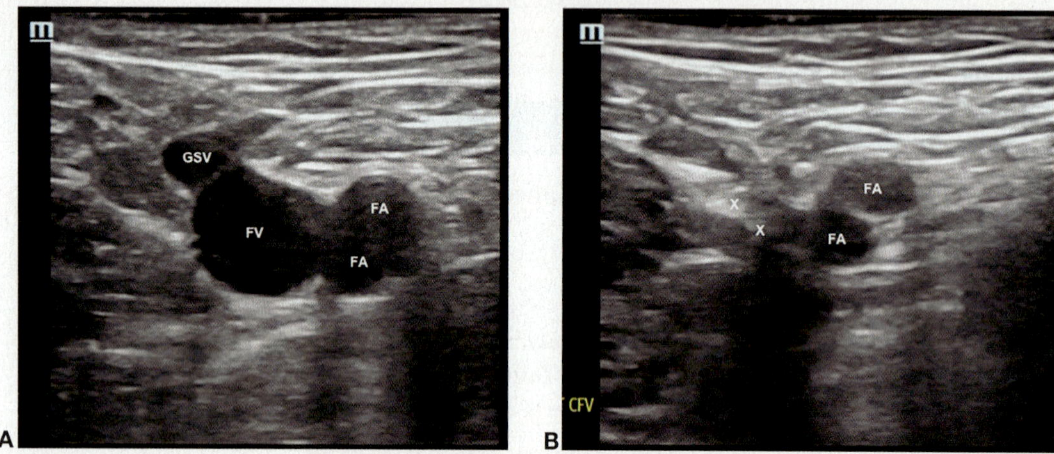

FIGURE 19-35. (A) Normal vein anatomy with labeled structures: FA (femoral artery), FV (femoral vein), and GSV (greater saphenous vein); (B) Compression applied to the vein, demonstrating vein collapse marked by "X" to indicate compression effectiveness.

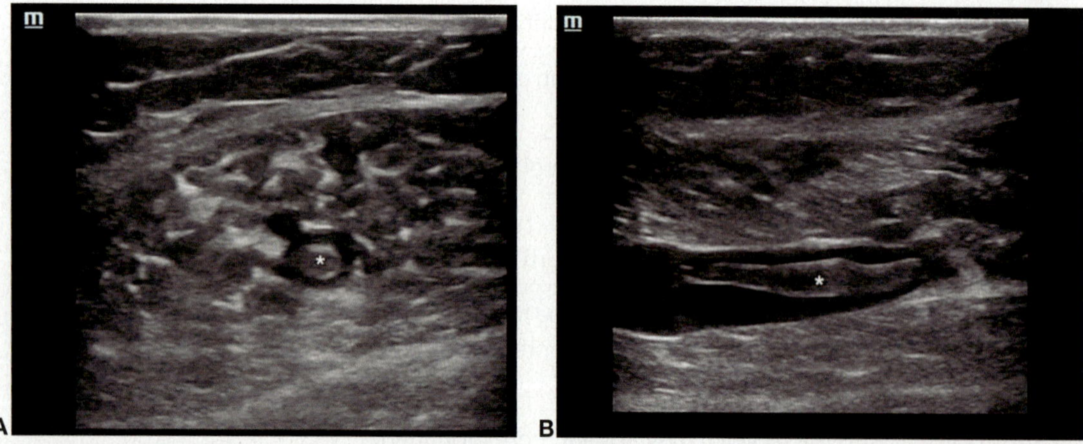

FIGURE 19-36. (A) Transverse view showing a thrombus within the vessel, marked by an asterisk (*); (B) Sagittal view of the same thrombus (*), demonstrating its longitudinal extent within the vessel.

HEALTH PROMOTION AND COUNSELING: EVIDENCE AND RECOMMENDATIONS

Important Topics for Health Promotion and Counseling

- Screening for lower extremity PAD
- Screening for AAA

In the following section, both traditional terms like "men," "women," "male," and "female" and inclusive terms such as "individuals assigned female at birth" and "individuals assigned male at birth" are used. This approach balances inclusivity with the need to accurately represent the original research.

Screening for Lower Extremity Peripheral Artery Disease

Epidemiology. An estimated 236 million people globally have atherosclerotic lower extremity PAD, although only a minority has classic claudication (exertional calf pain).[25,26] Prevalence increases with age and is higher in high-income countries than in low- and middle-income countries. Risk factors for PAD include age 65 years and older, risk factors for atherosclerosis (diabetes, tobacco use, hyperlipidemia, hypertension), and known atherosclerotic disease in another vascular area (coronary, carotid, subclavian, renal, or mesenteric artery or AAA).[27]

Screening. Detecting PAD is important because it is both a marker for cardiovascular morbidity and mortality and a harbinger of functional decline. Risk of death from myocardial infarction and stroke triples in adults with PAD. PAD can be detected noninvasively using the ABI (see p. 557). Values less than 0.90 are considered abnormal. The ABI is reliable, reproducible, and easy to perform in the office. Although the sensitivity of an abnormal ABI is low (15% to 20%), the specificity is 99%, and the test has high positive and negative predictive values (both >80%).[28] The U.S. Preventive Services Task Force (USPSTF) does not advocate PAD screening because it found the available evidence insufficient to estimate the relative benefits and harms of ABI testing (I statement).[29] However, the AHA suggests that using the ABI to screen for PAD in patients with risk factors is reasonable.[26,27]

Screening for Abdominal Aortic Aneurysm

Epidemiology. AAA is an infrarenal aortic diameter of at least 3 cm. The population prevalence of AAA increases with age and is higher in individuals assigned male at birth compared to those assigned female at birth.[30] The dreaded consequence of AAA is rupture, which is often fatal—most patients die before reaching a hospital. The chances of rupture and mortality markedly increase when the aortic diameter is 5.5 cm or larger.[31] The strongest risk factors for AAA are older age, being assigned male at birth, smoking, and family history; other risk factors include history of other vascular aneurysms, taller height, atherosclerotic cardiovascular disease, hypertension, and hyperlipidemia.

Screening. AAAs are detectable with abdominal ultrasound, which is a noninvasive, inexpensive, and accurate (sensitivity 94% to 100%; specificity 98% to 100%) screening test.[32] Palpation is not sensitive enough to be recommended for screening. Because symptoms are uncommon, and screening can reduce AAA-related mortality by about 50% over 13 to 15 years, the USPSTF makes a grade B recommendation for one-time abdominal ultrasound screening of men ages 65 to 75 years who have smoked more than 100 cigarettes in a lifetime.[31] Clinicians can selectively offer screening to men in this age range who have never smoked (grade C); evidence is insufficient regarding screening women in this age range who have ever smoked or have a family history of AAA (I statement). However, the USPSTF recommends against screening individuals assigned female at birth who have never smoked and have no family history of AAA (grade D).

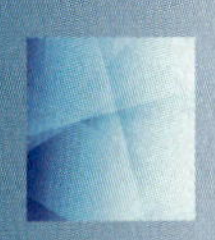

TABLE 19-1. Types of Peripheral Edema

Approximately one-third of body water is extracellular fluid, with 25% being plasma and the remainder being interstitial fluid. Edema is the accumulation of interstitial fluid due to disrupted forces, with pitting characteristics reflecting protein concentration. Pitting and recovery occur within seconds in low protein concentration, while high protein levels result in nonpitting, as in lymphedema. *Capillary leak syndrome*, where protein leaks into the interstitial space, can also cause edema.[9,10]

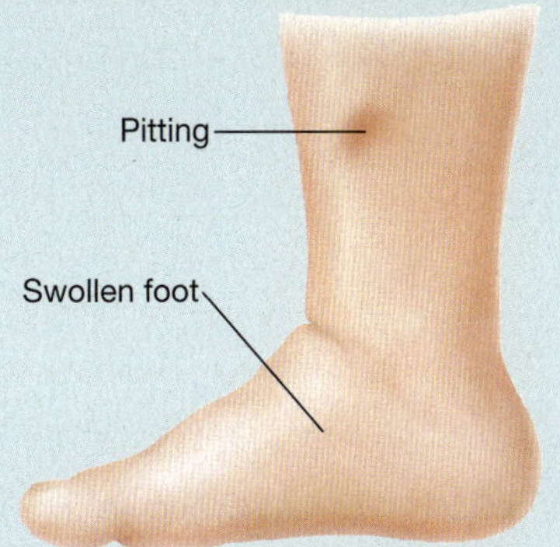

Pitting Edema

Edema is bilateral swelling from increased fluid and salt retention, shown by pitting after thumb pressure on the feet. It can result from prolonged standing/sitting, heart failure, nephrotic syndrome, cirrhosis, malnutrition, and some medications.

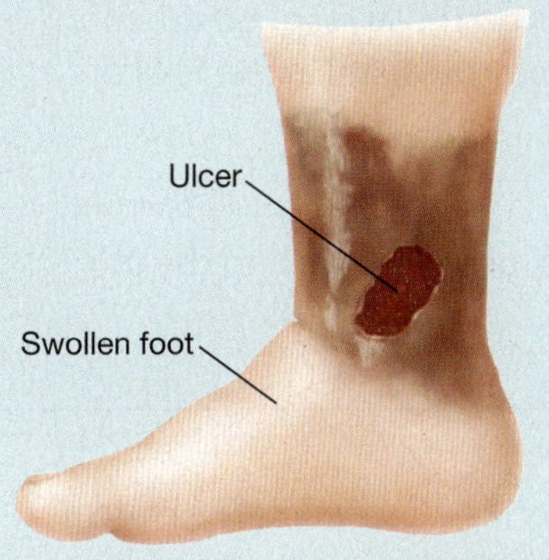

Chronic Venous Insufficiency

Edema is soft and may be bilateral, with pitting on pressure. Check for skin thickening and brawny changes, particularly near the ankle. Foot edema, brownish pigmentation, and ulceration are common. It results from deep venous system obstruction and incompetent valves. (See Table 19-2, Painful Peripheral Vascular Disorders and Their Mimics, pp. 570–573.)

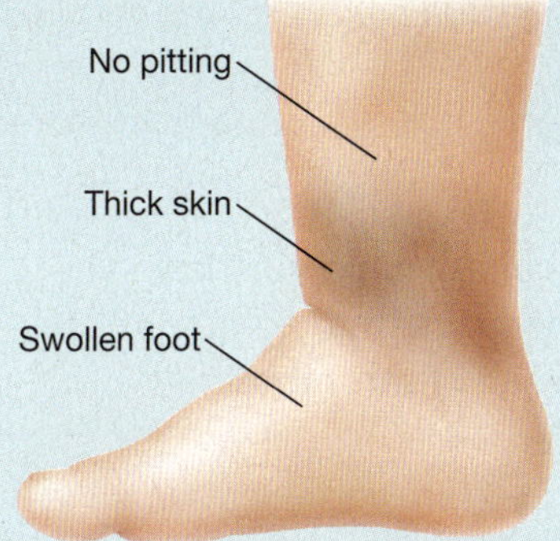

Lymphedema

Lymphedema causes initially soft and pitting edema that becomes indurated, hard, and nonpitting, with markedly thickened skin and rare ulceration. Bilateral edema in the feet and toes is common, with no pigmentation. It arises from protein-rich fluid accumulation due to obstruction or infiltration of lymph channels, fibrosis, inflammation, axillary node dissection, and/or radiation.

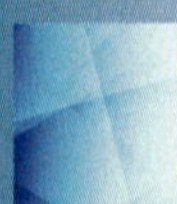

TABLE 19-2. Painful Peripheral Vascular Disorders and Their Mimics

Problem	Process	Location of Pain
Arterial Disorders		
Raynaud phenomenon: primary and secondary[12]	*Raynaud phenomenon, primary:* Episodic reversible vasoconstriction in the fingers and toes, usually triggered by cold temperatures (capillaries are normal); no definable cause *Raynaud phenomenon, secondary:* symptoms/signs related to autoimmune diseases—scleroderma, systemic lupus erythematosus, mixed connective tissue disease; cryoglobulinemia; also, to occupational vascular injury; drugs	Distal portions of one or more fingers Pain is usually not prominent unless fingertip ulcers develop; numbness and tingling are common
Peripheral Arterial Disease	Atherosclerotic disease leading to obstruction of peripheral arteries causing exertional claudication (muscle pain relieved by rest) and atypical leg pain; may progress to ischemic pain at rest	Usually calf muscles, but also occurs in the buttock, hip, thigh, or foot, depending on the level of obstruction; rest pain may be distal in the toes or forefoot
Acute Arterial Occlusion	Embolism or thrombosis	Distal pain, usually involving the foot and leg
Venous Disorders *(Lower Extremity)*		
Superficial Phlebitis and Superficial Vein Thrombosis	Involves inflammation of a superficial vein (*superficial phlebitis*), at times with venous thrombosis (*superficial vein thrombosis* when clot confirmed by imaging)	Pain and tenderness along the course of a superficial vein, most often in the saphenous system
Deep Venous Thrombosis (DVT)	DVT and PE are disorders of venous thromboembolic disease (VTE); DVTs are distal, limited to the deep calf veins, or proximal, in the popliteal, femoral, or iliac veins	Classically, painful or painless calf swelling with erythema; signs correlate poorly with site of thrombosis
Chronic Venous Insufficiency (Deep)	More severe form of chronic venous disease, with chronic venous engorgement from venous occlusion or incompetent venous valves	Diffuse aching of the leg(s), skin erythema which slowly progresses to brownish discoloration

Timing	Factors That Aggravate	Factors That Relieve	Associated Manifestations
Relatively brief (min), but recurrent	Exposure to cold, emotional upset	Warm environment	*Primary:* Distinct digital color changes of pallor, cyanosis, and hyperemia (redness); no necrosis *Secondary:* More severe, with ischemia, necrosis, and loss of digits; capillary loops are distorted
May be brief if relieved by rest; if there is *rest pain,* may be persistent and worse at night	Exercise such as walking; if *rest pain,* leg elevation, and bedrest	Rest usually stops the pain in 1–3 min; *rest pain* may be relieved by walking (increases perfusion), sitting with legs dependent	Local fatigue, numbness, progressing to cool dry hairless skin, trophic nail changes, diminished to absent pulses, pallor with elevation, ulceration, gangrene (see pp. 574–575)
Sudden onset; associated symptoms may occur without pain			Coldness, numbness, weakness, absent distal pulses
An acute episode lasting days or longer	Immobility, venous stasis, and chronic venous disease, venous procedure (such as IV cannula placement), obesity	Supportive care, walking; measures prompted by further testing	Local induration, erythema; if palpable nodules or cords, consider superficial or deep vein thrombosis, both associated with significant risk of DVT and PE
Often hard to determine due to lack of symptoms; one-third of untreated calf DVTs extend proximally	Immobilization or recent surgery, lower extremity trauma, pregnancy or postpartum state, hypercoagulable state (e.g., nephrotic syndrome, malignancy)	Antithrombotic and thrombolytic therapy	Asymmetric calf diameters more diagnostic than palpable cord or tenderness over femoral triangle; high risk of PE (50% with proximal DVT)
Chronic, increasing as the day wears on	Prolonged standing, sitting with legs dependent	Limb elevation, walking	Chronic edema, pigmentation, swelling, and possibly ulceration, especially if advanced age, pregnancy, increased weight, prior history, or trauma (see pp. 574–575)

(*continued*)

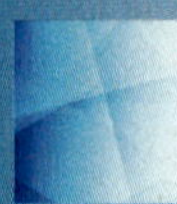

TABLE 19-2. Painful Peripheral Vascular Disorders and Their Mimics *(Continued)*

Problem	Process	Location of Pain
Thromboangiitis Obliterans *(Buerger Disease)*	Inflammatory nonatherosclerotic occlusive disease of small- to medium-sized arteries and veins, especially in smokers; occluding thrombus spares the blood vessel wall	Often digit or toe pain progressing to ischemic ulcerations
Compartment Syndrome	Pressure builds from trauma or bleeding into one of the four major muscle compartments between the knee and ankle; each compartment is enclosed by fascia that limits expansion to accommodate increasing pressure	Tight, bursting pain in calf muscles, usually in the anterior tibial compartment, sometimes with overlying dusky red skin
Acute Lymphangitis	Acute infection, usually from *Streptococcus pyogenes* or *Staphylococcus aureus,* spreading up the lymphatic channels from distal portal of entry such as skin abrasion, ulcer, or dog bite	An arm or a leg
Mimics *(Primarily of Acute Superficial Thrombophlebitis)*		
Acute Cellulitis	Acute bacterial infection of the skin and subcutaneous tissues, most commonly from beta-hemolytic streptococci (*erysipelas*) and *S. aureus*	In the arms, legs, or elsewhere
Erythema Nodosum	Painful raised, bilateral erythematous lesions from inflammation of subcutaneous fat tissue, seen in systemic conditions such as pregnancy, sarcoidosis, tuberculosis, streptococcal infections, inflammatory bowel disease, medications (oral contraceptives)	Anterior pretibial surfaces of both lower legs; can also appear on extensor arms, buttocks, and thighs

Timing	Factors That Aggravate	Factors That Relieve	Associated Manifestations
Ranges from brief recurrent to chronic persistent pain	Exercise	Rest; smoking cessation	May progress to gangrene at tips of digits; can move proximally, with migratory phlebitis and tender nodules along blood vessels; usually involves at least two limbs
Several hours if acute (pressure must be relieved to avert necrosis); during exercise if chronic	*Acute:* Anabolic steroids; surgical complication; crush injury *Chronic:* Occurs with exercise	*Acute:* Surgical incision to relieve pressure *Chronic:* Avoiding exercise; ice, elevation	Tingling, burning sensations in calf; muscles may feel tight, full; numbness, paralysis if unrelieved
An acute episode lasting day or longer			Red streak(s) on the skin, with tenderness, enlarged, tender lymph nodes, and fever
An acute episode lasting days or longer			Erythema, edema, and warmth *Erysipelas:* Lesion raised and demarcated from skin; involves upper dermis, lymphatics *Cellulitis:* Involves deeper dermis, adipose tissue; may include enlarged, tender lymph nodes and fever
Pain associated with a series of lesions over 2–8 wk			2–5-cm lesions, initially elevated, bright red then fade to violet or red-brown; do not ulcerate; often with polyarthralgia, fever, malaise

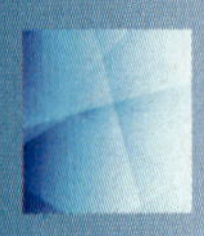

TABLE 19-3. Chronic Insufficiency of Arteries and Veins

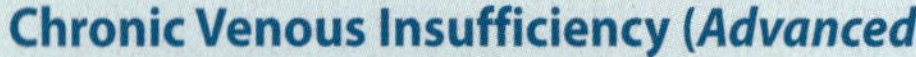

	Chronic Arterial Insufficiency (*Advanced*)	Chronic Venous Insufficiency (*Advanced*)
	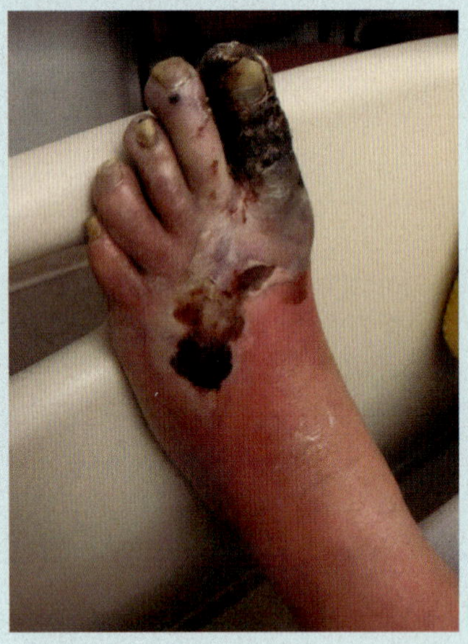	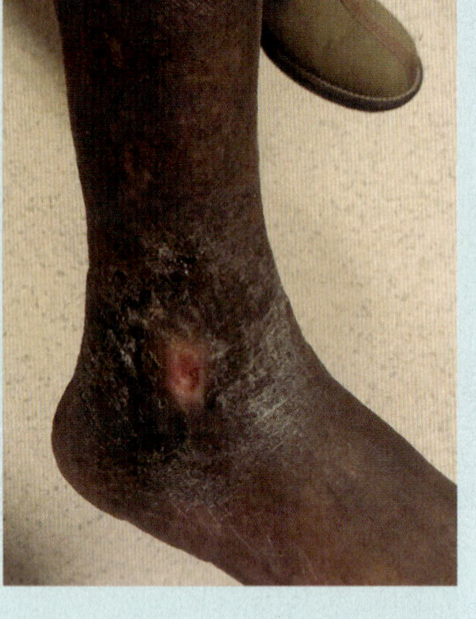
Pain	Intermittent claudication, progressing to pain at rest	Often painful
Mechanism	Tissue ischemia	Venous stasis and hypertension
Pulses	Decreased or absent	Normal, though may be difficult to feel through edema
Color	Pale, especially on elevation; dusky red on dependency	Normal, or cyanotic on dependency; petechiae and then brown pigmentation appear with chronicity
Temperature	Cool	Normal
Edema	Absent or mild; may develop as the patient tries to relieve rest pain by lowering the leg	Present, often marked
Skin Changes	Trophic changes: thin, shiny, atrophic skin; loss of hair over the foot and toes; nails thickened and ridged	Often brown pigmentation around the ankle, stasis dermatitis, and possible thickening of the skin and narrowing of the leg as scarring develops
Ulceration	If present, involves toes or points of trauma on feet	If present, develops at sides of ankle, especially medially
Gangrene	May develop	Does not develop

Source of photos: Courtesy of Daniel K. Han, Vascular Surgery, Icahn School of Medicine at Mount Sinai.

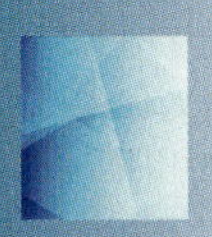

TABLE 19-4. Common Ulcers of the Ankles and Feet

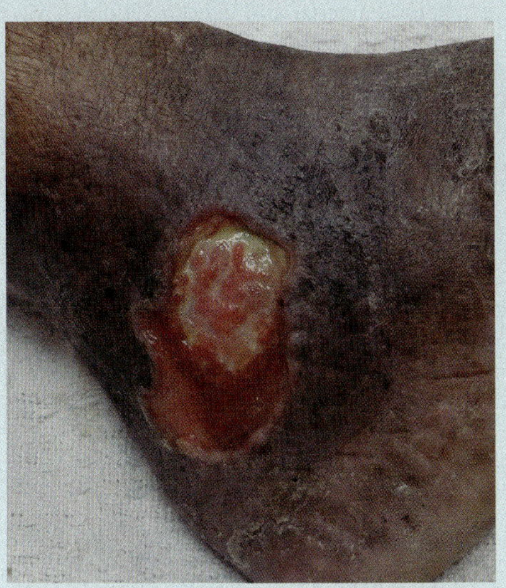

Chronic Venous Insufficiency

This condition usually appears over the medial and sometimes the lateral malleolus. The ulcer contains small, painful granulation tissue and fibrin; necrosis or exposed tendons are rare. Borders are irregular, flat, or slightly steep. Pain affects quality of life in 75% of patients. Associated findings include edema, reddish pigmentation and purpura, venous varicosities, the eczematous changes of stasis dermatitis (redness, scaling, and pruritus), and at times cyanosis of the foot when dependent. Gangrene is rare.

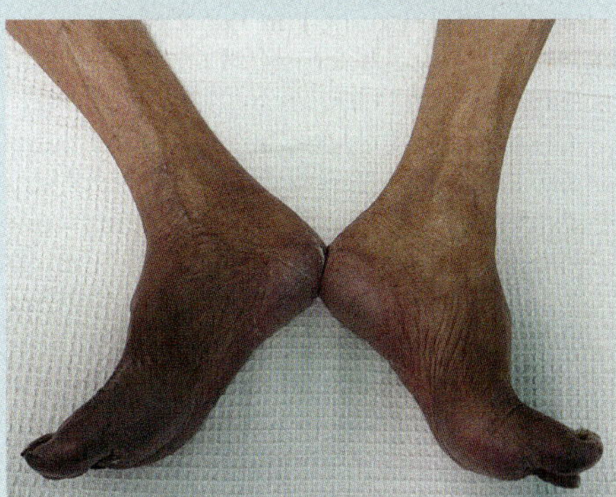

Arterial Insufficiency

This condition occurs in the toes, feet, or possibly areas of trauma (e.g., the shins). Surrounding skin shows no callus or excess pigment, although it may be atrophic. Pain often is severe unless masked by neuropathy. May be accompanied by gangrene, along with decreased pulses, trophic changes, foot pallor on elevation, and dusky rubor on dependency.

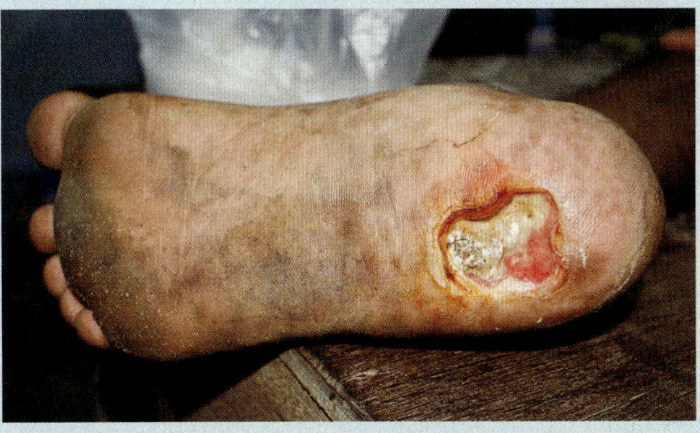

Neuropathic Ulcer

This condition develops in pressure points of areas with diminished sensation; seen in diabetic neuropathy, neurologic disorders, and Hansen disease. The surrounding skin is calloused. There is no pain, so the ulcer may go unnoticed. In uncomplicated cases, there is no gangrene. Associated signs include decreased sensation and absent ankle jerks.

Sources of photos: *Chronic Venous Insufficiency*—Shutterstock photo by Casa nayafana; *Arterial Insufficiency*—Shutterstock photo by Alan Nissa; *Neuropathic Ulcer*—Shutterstock photo by Zay Nyi Nyi.

REFERENCES

1. Mitchell RN, Halushka MK. Chapter 11: blood vessels. In: Kumar V, Abbas AK, Aster JC, eds. *Robbins and Cotran Pathologic Basis of Disease*. 9th ed. Elsevier; 2015.
2. Libby P. Mechanisms of acute coronary syndromes and their implications for therapy. *N Engl J Med*. 2013;368(21): 2004–2013.
3. Libby P. Chapter 291e: the pathogenesis, prevention, and treatment of atherosclerosis. In: Kasper DL, Fauci AS, Hauser SL, Longo DL, Jameson JL, Loscalzo J, eds. *Harrison's Principles of Internal Medicine*. 19th ed. McGraw-Hill Education; 2015.
4. Ketelhuth DF, Hansson GK. Modulation of autoimmunity and atherosclerosis–common targets and promising translational approaches against disease. *Circ J*. 2015;79(5):924–933.
5. Levick JR, Michel CC. Microvascular fluid exchange and the revised Starling principle. *Cardiovasc Res*. 2010;87(2):198–210.
6. Woodcock TE, Woodcock TM. Revised Starling equation and the glycocalyx model of transvascular fluid exchange: an improved paradigm for prescribing intravenous fluid therapy. *Br J Anaesth*. 2012;108(3):384–394.
7. Reed RK, Rubin K. Transcapillary exchange: role and importance of the interstitial fluid pressure and the extracellular matrix. *Cardiovasc Res*. 2010;87(2):211–217.
8. Braunwald E, Loscalzo J. Chapter 50: edema. In: Kasper DL, Fauci AS, Hauser SL, Longo DL, Jameson JL, Loscalzo J, eds. *Harrison's Principles of Internal Medicine*. 19th ed. McGraw-Hill Education; 2015.
9. Grada AA, Phillips TJ. Lymphedema: diagnostic workup and management. *J Am Acad Dermatol*. 2017;77(6):995–1006.
10. McGee SR. Chapter 52: peripheral vascular disease; Chapter 54: edema and deep vein thrombosis. In: *Evidence-Based Physical Diagnosis*. 3rd ed. Elsevier/Saunders; 2012:459–465, 470–476.
11. Kucher N. Clinical practice. Deep-vein thrombosis of the upper extremities. *N Engl J Med*. 2011;364(9):861–869.
12. Gerhard-Herman MD, Gornik HL, Barrett C, et al. 2016 AHA/ACC guideline on the management of patients with lower extremity peripheral artery disease: executive summary: a report of the American College of Cardiology/American Heart Association Task Force on Clinical Practice Guidelines. *J Am Coll Cardiol*. 2017;69(11):1465–1508.
13. Gerhard-Herman MD, Gornik HL, Barrett C, et al. 2016 AHA/ACC guideline on the management of patients with lower extremity peripheral artery disease: a report of the American College of Cardiology/American Heart Association Task Force on Clinical Practice Guidelines. *J Am Coll Cardiol*. 2017;69(11):e71–e126.
14. Kent KC. Clinical practice. Abdominal aortic aneurysms. *N Engl J Med*. 2014;371(22):2101–2108.
15. Decousus H, Frappé P, Accassat S, et al. Epidemiology, diagnosis, treatment and management of superficial-vein thrombosis of the legs. *Best Pract Res Clin Haematol*. 2012;25(3):275–284.
16. Khan NA, Rahim SA, Anand SS, Simel DL, Panju A. Does the clinical examination predict lower extremity peripheral arterial disease? *JAMA*. 2006;295(5):536–546.
17. Spandorfer J, Galanis T. In the clinic. Deep venous thrombosis. *Ann Intern Med*. 2015;162(9):ITC1–ITC16.
18. Klein S, Hage JJ. Measurement, calculation, and normal range of the ankle-arm index: a bibliometric analysis and recommendation for standardization. *Ann Vasc Surg*. 2006; 20(2):282–292.
19. Measuring and understanding the ankle brachial index (ABI). Stanford Medicine 25. Accessed February 25, 2024. https://stanfordmedicine25.stanford.edu/the25/ankle-brachial-index.html
20. Kim ES, Sharma AM, Scissons R, et al. Interpretation of peripheral arterial and venous Doppler waveforms: a consensus statement from the Society for Vascular Medicine and Society for Vascular Ultrasound. *Vasc Med*. 2020;25(5):484–506.
21. Cao P, Eckstein HH, De Rango P, et al. Chapter II: diagnostic methods. *Eur J Vasc Endovasc Surg*. 2011;42(Suppl 2):S13–S32.
22. Pomero F, Dentali F, Borretta V, et al. Accuracy of emergency physician-performed ultrasonography in the diagnosis of deep-vein thrombosis: a systematic review and meta-analysis. *Thromb Haemost*. 2013;109(1):137–145.
23. Fischer EA, Kinnear B, Sall D, et al. Hospitalist-operated compression ultrasonography: a point-of-care ultrasound study (HOCUS-POCUS). *J Gen Intern Med*. 2019;34(10):2062–2067.
24. Noble VE, Nelson B. *Manual of Emergency and Critical Care Ultrasound*. 2nd ed. Cambridge University Press; 2011.
25. Song P, Rudan D, Zhu Y, et al. Global, regional, and national prevalence and risk factors for peripheral artery disease in 2015: an updated systematic review and analysis. *Lancet Glob Health*. 2019;7(8):e1020–e1030.
26. Criqui MH, Matsushita K, Aboyans V, et al; American Heart Association Council on Epidemiology and Prevention; Council on Arteriosclerosis, Thrombosis and Vascular Biology; Council on Cardiovascular Radiology and Intervention; Council on Lifestyle and Cardiometabolic Health; Council on Peripheral Vascular Disease; and Stroke Council. Lower extremity peripheral artery disease: contemporary epidemiology, management gaps, and future directions: a scientific statement from the American Heart Association. *Circulation*. 2021;144(9):e171–e191.
27. Gerhard-Herman MD, Gornik HL, Barrett C, et al. 2016 AHA/ACC guideline on the management of patients with lower extremity peripheral artery disease: a report of the American College of Cardiology/American Heart Association Task Force on Clinical Practice Guidelines. *Circulation*. 2017;135(12):e726–e779.
28. Guirguis-Blake JM, Evans CV, Redmond N, Lin JS. Screening for peripheral artery disease using the Ankle-Brachial index: updated evidence report and systematic review for the US Preventive Services Task Force. *JAMA*. 2018;320(2):184–196.
29. U. S. Preventive Services Task Force, Curry SJ, Krist AH, Owens DK, et al. Screening for peripheral artery disease and cardiovascular disease risk assessment with the ankle-brachial index: US Preventive Services Task Force recommendation statement. *JAMA*. 2018;320(2):177–183.
30. Tsao CW, Aday AW, Almarzooq ZI, et al; American Heart Association Council on Epidemiology and Prevention Statistics Committee and Stroke Statistics Subcommittee. Heart disease and stroke statistics-2023 update: a report from the American Heart Association. *Circulation*. 2023;147(8):e93–e621.
31. U. S. Preventive Services Task Force; Owens DK, Davidson KW, Krist AH, et al. Screening for abdominal aortic aneurysm: US Preventive Services Task Force recommendation statement. *JAMA*. 2019;322(22):2211–2218.
32. Guirguis-Blake JM, Beil TL, Senger CA, Coppola EL. Primary care screening for abdominal aortic aneurysm: a systematic evidence review for the US Preventive Services Task Force. 2019. U.S. Preventive Services Task Force Evidence Syntheses, formerly Systematic Evidence Reviews.

CHAPTER 20

Breasts and Axillae

ANATOMY AND PHYSIOLOGY

Breast

The *breast* of a person assigned female at birth is positioned on the anterior thoracic wall, extending from the clavicle and second rib to the sixth rib, and from the sternum to the midaxillary line. Breast tissue may also extend into the axilla as the *axillary tail of the breast (Spence)*. The breast lies over the *pectoralis major* and *serratus anterior muscles* (Fig. 20-1).

The axillary tail of Spence is an important area to examine for breast health, as breast cancer can develop here just like in any other part of the breast.

The glandular tissue comprises 15 to 20 *lobes* that form *lactiferous ducts* and *sinuses*, opening onto the *nipple* and *areola*. Each duct drains a lobe containing 20 to 40 smaller lobules with milk-secreting *tubuloalveolar glands*. Adipose tissue primarily surrounds the breast in intraglandular, superficial, and peripheral areas.

The areola's surface has small, rounded elevations from Areolar (Montgomery) glands, sweat glands, and accessory areolar glands (Fig. 20-2). A few hairs may also be present. The breast has two fascial layers: the *superficial fascia* beneath the dermis and the *deep fascia* in front of the pectoralis major muscle. *Suspensory (Cooper) ligaments* attach the breast to the skin (Fig. 20-3).[1]

Supernumerary nipples can occasionally be found along the "milk line" (Fig. 20-4). Typically, only a small nipple and areola are present, which can

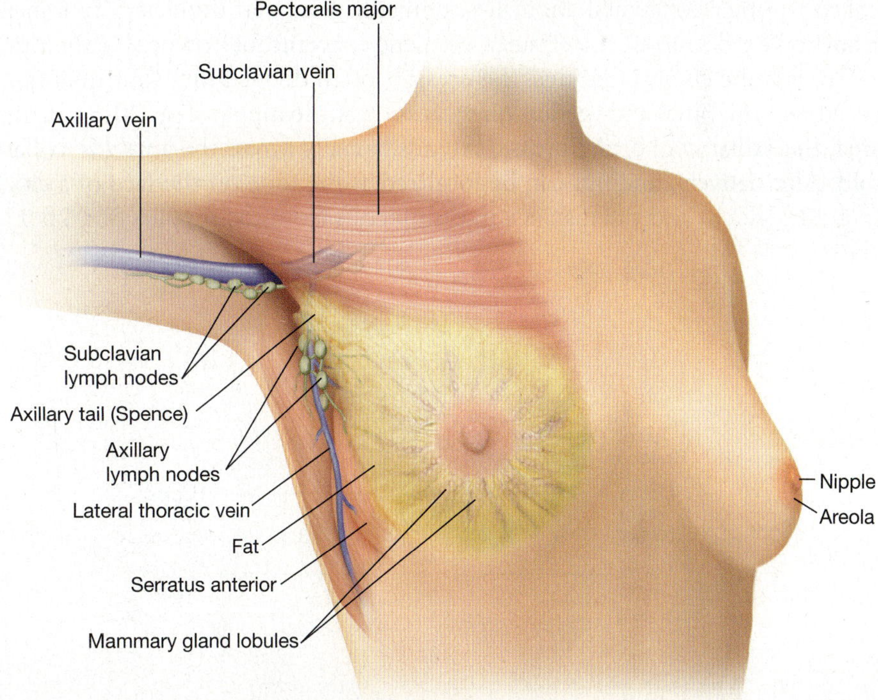

FIGURE 20-1. Breast anatomy.

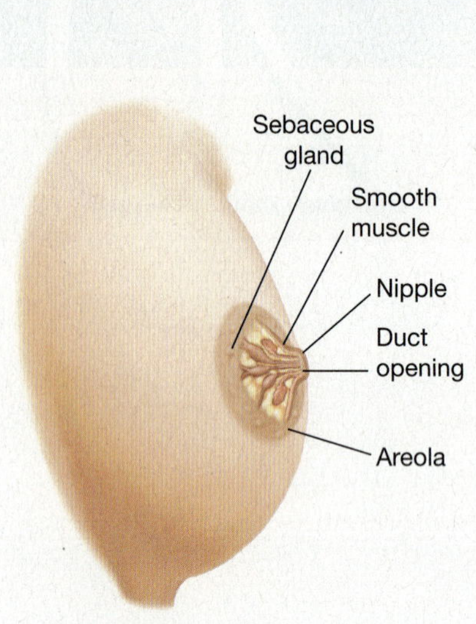

FIGURE 20-2. Nipple and areola.

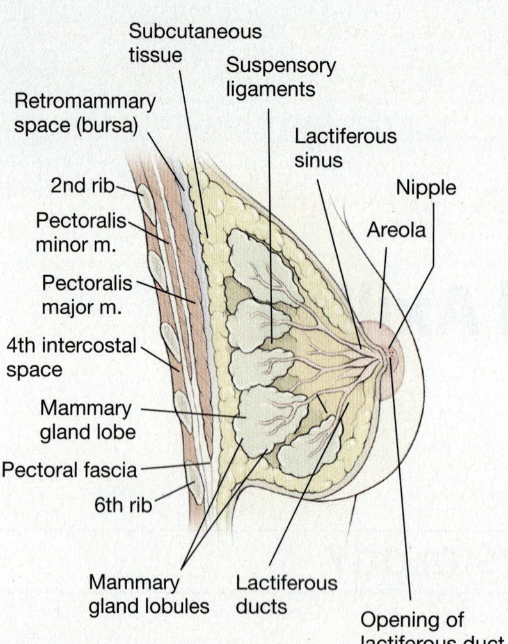

FIGURE 20-3. Sagittal section of breast. (Reprinted with permission from Tank PW. *Grant's Dissector*. 15th ed. Wolters Kluwer Health/Lippincott Williams & Wilkins; 2013. Figure 2-6.)

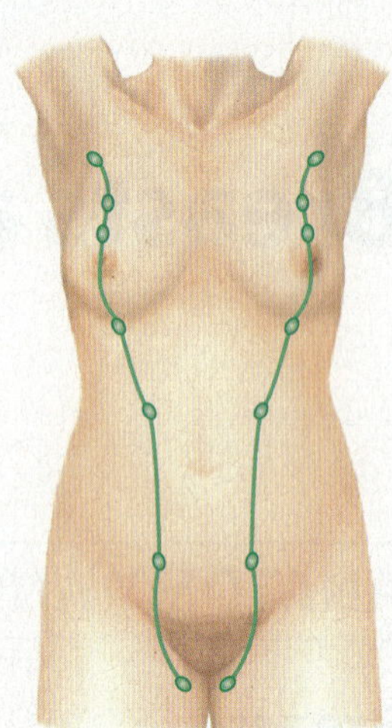

FIGURE 20-4. Milk lines.

be mistaken for a common mole. They may be familial and, without associated glandular tissue, show little association with other congenital anomalies. Glandular tissue-containing supernumerary nipples may exhibit pigmentation, swelling, tenderness, or lactation during puberty, menstruation, or pregnancy and can be linked to other congenital anomalies, primarily renal and thoracic.[2] Treatment is advised for diagnostic uncertainty, cosmetic concerns, or potential pathology.[3]

To describe clinical findings, the breast is often divided into four quadrants based on horizontal and vertical lines crossing at the nipple (Fig. 20-5). A fifth area, the axillary tail of the breast, extends laterally across the anterior axillary fold. Alternatively, findings can be localized as the time on the face of a clock (e.g., 3 o'clock) and the distance in centimeters from the nipple (Box 20-1).

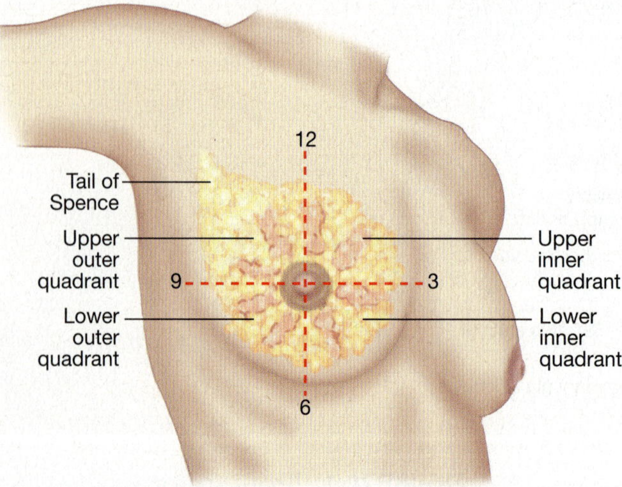

FIGURE 20-5. Breast quadrants and tail of Spence.

Box 20-1. Breast Quadrants: Location Descriptions and Clinical Significance

Quadrant/Area	Location Description	Clinical Significance
Upper outer quadrant (UOQ)	Above the horizontal line and outside the vertical line passing through the nipple, extending into the axillary area.	Most common site for breast cancer; includes the axillary tail of the breast.
Upper inner quadrant (UIQ)	Above the horizontal line and inside the vertical line.	Pathologies here are closer to the sternum.
Lower outer quadrant (LOQ)	Below the horizontal line and outside the vertical line.	Abnormalities may be more difficult to detect due to looser breast tissue structure.
Lower inner quadrant (LIQ)	Below the horizontal line and inside the vertical line.	Like the UIQ, closer to the sternum and important for lesion detection.

Breasts are hormonally sensitive tissues and respond to changes in hormonal cycles and aging. In individuals of various gender identities, adult breasts may be soft but often feel granular, nodular, or lumpy due to normal physiologic nodularity. This uneven texture is commonly bilateral and can occur throughout the breast or in specific areas. Nodularity may increase before hormonal fluctuations, a time when breasts often enlarge and become tender or even painful.

Furthermore, the composition of breasts varies with factors such as age, nutritional status, pregnancy, hormone use, and others. After certain life stages or hormone-related events, there may be atrophy of glandular tissue and a notable decrease in the number of lobules.

For breast changes during adolescence, see Chapter 28, Children: Infancy Through Adolescence, p. 1094 and in pregnancy in Chapter 29, Pregnant Persons, pp. 1123–1124.

Both the nipple and areola of breasts are supplied with smooth muscle that contracts to express milk from the ductal system during nursing. Rich sensory innervation, especially in the nipple, triggers *milk letdown* following neurohormonal stimulation from infant sucking. Tactile stimulation of the area, including breast examination, makes the nipple smaller, firmer, and more erect and causes the areola to pucker and wrinkle. These smooth muscle reflexes are normal and should not be mistaken for signs of breast disease.

Axilla

The *axilla* is a pyramid-shaped structure bordered by the axillary vein at the top, the *latissimus dorsi* muscle on the lateral side, and the *serratus anterior* muscle on the medial side.[4] Three significant nerves run through the axilla: the *thoracodorsal nerve*, *long thoracic nerve*, and the *intercostobrachial nerve*. The thoracodorsal nerve provides innervation to the latissimus dorsi muscle, while the long thoracic nerve supplies the serratus anterior muscle. The intercostobrachial nerve, a sensory nerve, innervates the skin of the axilla and the upper medial arm.[5]

The axillary lymph nodes are organized into six groups (Fig. 20-6 and Box 20-2).[5] They are positioned along the chest wall, typically high in the axilla and halfway between the anterior and posterior axillary folds. Among these groups, the central nodes are the most likely to be palpable during a physical examination (PE).

The lymphatic drainage of the breast is of great importance in the spread of carcinoma, and about 75% is to the axillary nodes.

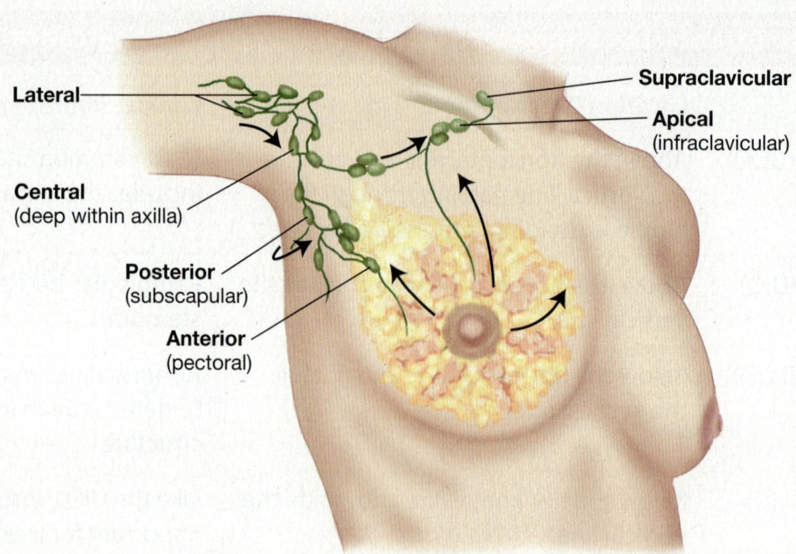

FIGURE 20-6. Direction of lymph flow.

Box 20-2. Axillary Lymph Node Groups: Locations and Associated Lymphatic Drainage

Group Name	Location	Lymph Vessels Received
Anterior (pectoral) group	Along the lower border of the pectoralis minor behind the pectoralis major	Lymph vessels from the lateral quadrants of the breast and superficial vessels from the anterolateral abdominal wall above the level of the umbilicus
Posterior (subscapular) group	In front of the subscapularis muscle	Superficial lymph vessels from the back, down as far as the level of the iliac crests
Lateral (humeral or deep) group	Along the medial side of the axillary vein	Most of the lymph vessels of the upper limb (except those superficial vessels draining the lateral side)
Central group	In the center of the axilla in the axillary fat	Lymph from the above three groups; nodes also located between the pectoralis minor and pectoralis major muscles in an area called the Rotter space (*Rotter nodes*)
Apical (terminal) group	At the apex of the axilla at the lateral border of the first rib	Efferent lymph vessels from all the other axillary nodes; the final common pathway for all of the axillary lymph nodes
Infraclavicular (deltopectoral) group	In the groove between the deltoid and pectoralis major muscles (outside the axilla)	Superficial lymph vessels from the lateral side of the hand, forearm, and arm

The apical nodes are the final common pathway for all of the axillary lymph nodes.

Breast tissue in individuals assigned male at birth predominantly consists of a small nipple and areola situated above a thin disc of undeveloped breast tissue, which is mainly composed of ducts. Without estrogen and progesterone stimulation, ductal branching and lobule development are minimal, making it challenging to differentiate this breast tissue from the pectoralis muscle on the chest wall.[6]

In some individuals assigned male at birth, benign breast enlargement can occur due to *gynecomastia*, a proliferation of palpable glandular tissue generally defined as >2 cm, or *pseudogynecomastia*, an accumulation of subareolar fat. Causes of gynecomastia include increased estrogen levels, decreased testosterone levels, and medication side effects.[7]

HEALTH HISTORY: GENERAL APPROACH

During the history or PE, inquire about any concerns related to the breasts. Ask the patient if they have experienced lumps, pain, or nipple discharge in their breasts, as these are the most common breast-related problems. If a patient presents with a breast concern, it is crucial to understand the nature and duration of the issue. When a patient reports a lump or pain, inquire about the location within the breast to focus your examination on that area. Always ask if the problem occurs or worsens at specific times during the menstrual cycle, as many benign breast symptoms are associated with hormonal changes. This conversation may also serve as an opportunity to increase the patient's awareness of screening guidelines.

Common or Concerning Symptoms

- Breast lump or mass
- Breast discomfort or pain
- Nipple discharge

Breast Lump or Mass

Palpable lumps or nodularity and premenstrual enlargement and tenderness are common.[8] Obtaining a thorough and accurate medical history through precise questions is essential for reaching an accurate diagnosis (Box 20-3).

Most likely causes include **fibrocystic changes** (benign changes in breast tissue; lumps, cysts, or thickening areas), **simple cysts** (fluid-filled sacs in breast tissue), **fibroadenomas** (noncancerous solid breast lumps), **intraductal papillomas** (small, benign, wart-like growths in milk ducts), **fat necrosis** (fatty breast tissue damage, forming a mass), and **breast cancer** (malignant growth in breast tissue).[9]

See Table 20-1, Common Breast Masses, p. 600 and Table 20-2, Visible Signs of Breast Cancer, p. 601.

Box 20-3. Breast Lump or Mass: High-Yield Health History Questions

Domain	Questions	Rationale
Characteristics	*How does the lump or mass feel? Is it big or small, round or not, and can you move it around?*	*Fibrocystic changes:* tend to be irregular and lumpy *Simple cysts:* smooth, round, and mobile *Fibroadenomas:* firm, round, smooth, and mobile *Fat necrosis* tends to be irregular, hard, and possibly painful *Breast cancer:* often hard, irregularly shaped, and immobile
Skin changes	*Have you seen any changes in the skin or nipple, like redness, pulling in, or any fluids coming out?*	*Intraductal papillomas:* commonly present with nipple discharge *Fat necrosis and breast cancer:* may cause skin or nipple retraction *Mastitis or breast abscess:* would show redness and warmth in the area
Medical and surgical history	*Have you had any recent injuries, surgeries, or radiation treatment on your breast?*	Can point to fat necrosis as the cause of the breast mass or lump
Relation to menstrual cycle	*Does the lump or mass change in size, hurt, or look different during your menstrual period?*	Fibrocystic changes and simple cysts are often related to hormonal fluctuations during the menstrual cycle; if the mass or lump changes in size or tenderness, it may suggest a benign cause such as fibrocystic changes or simple cysts
Personal and family history of breast cancer	*Do you or your family have any history of breast problems, including cancer?*	Can increase the risk of breast cancer or inform the likelihood of benign breast conditions
Nipple discharge	*Have you seen any fluid coming out of your nipple, especially if it is bloody?*	Can be one of the first signs of a pathologic process; unilateral serous, sanguinous, or serosanguinous discharge can indicate cancer, infection, or other benign processes
Medications	*What medications are you taking?*	Hormone-based medications may increase the risk of breast cancer

Breast Discomfort or Pain

Breast pain alone (*mastodynia* or *mastalgia*) is not typically a sign of breast cancer. Determine if the pain is *diffuse* (defined as involving >25% of the breast) or *focal* (involving <25% of the breast).[10] For a confident and accurate diagnosis, you must focus on obtaining a complete and precise medical history through accurate questioning (Box 20-4).

Most likely causes include **cyclical mastalgia** (hormonal fluctuations), **noncyclical mastalgia**, **fibrocystic changes** (benign breast tissue changes), **mastitis/breast abscess** (inflammation/infection), and **medication-related** (side effect of medications).[8]

Box 20-4. Breast Discomfort or Pain: High-Yield Health History Questions

Domain	Questions	Rationale
Association with menstrual cycle	*Does the breast pain or discomfort come and go with your monthly period?*	Helps distinguish between cyclical (related to the menstrual cycle) and noncyclical or other causes, which are not related to hormonal fluctuations
Skin characteristics	*Have you seen any changes in the skin or nipple, like redness, warmth, or fluids?*	*Mastitis/breast abscess:* typically presents with redness, warmth, and swelling in the affected area *Fibrocystic changes:* may be associated with breast lumps or cysts *Nipple discharge:* can suggest an alternative cause, such as intraductal papilloma
Medication history	*Have you started any new medications or made changes to your existing ones lately?*	Oral contraceptives, hormone-replacement therapy, selective serotonin-reuptake inhibitors, diuretics, and certain antipsychotics, can cause breast pain as a side effect
Breast lumps or masses	*Do you feel any lumps, bumps, or thicker parts in your breasts?*	Fibrocystic changes, which are often associated with lumps, cysts, or thickened areas, and other causes of breast pain or discomfort do not typically present with a mass or lump
Associated symptoms	*Are you experiencing any fever, chills, or flu-like symptoms?*	May suggest an infectious process, such as mastitis or a breast abscess, which typically causes localized pain, redness, and warmth in the affected breast

Nipple Discharge

Ask about any discharge from the nipples and when it occurs. It is important to differentiate *physiologic* from *pathologic discharge*. Physiologic hypersecretion is seen in pregnancy, lactation, chest wall stimulation, sleep, and stress (Box 20-5).

Most likely pathologic causes include **duct ectasia** (dilated milk ducts), **intraductal papilloma** (benign growth in duct), **fibrocystic changes**, **galactorrhea**[11,12] (discharge of milk-containing fluid unrelated to pregnancy or lactation), **mastitis**, and **breast cancer**.[6]

Box 20-5. Nipple Discharge: High-Yield Health History Questions

Domain	Questions	Rationale
Color and consistency of discharge	*What color and texture is the fluid coming from the nipple?*	*Thick, sticky:* may suggest duct ectasia *Bloody/sanguineous or blood tinged/serosanguinous:* may suggest intraductal papilloma or breast cancer *Green or brown:* may suggest fibrocystic changes *Milky or clear:* may suggest galactorrhea *Purulent:* may suggest mastitis/breast abscess
Laterality of discharge	*Is the fluid coming from one nipple or both?*	*Unilateral:* more concerning for breast cancer, intraductal papilloma, and fibrocystic changes, mastitis/breast abscess *Bilateral:* more commonly associated with galactorrhea
Breast lump or mass	*Do you feel any lumps in your breast when you have nipple discharge?*	More commonly seen with intraductal papilloma, fibrocystic changes, mastitis/breast abscess, and breast cancer
Breast pain	*Does your breast or nipple hurt or feel tender?*	More commonly associated with fibrocystic changes, mastitis/breast abscess, and intraductal papilloma; breast cancer can also cause pain
Medications	*Are you currently on any medications?*	Hormonal contraceptives and antidepressants can cause nipple discharge

PHYSICAL EXAMINATION: GENERAL APPROACH

When conducting a breast examination, prioritize the patient's comfort and privacy. Before beginning the examination, ask for their permission and ensure they feel comfortable with the process. Throughout the examination, maintain privacy by covering the opposite breast and ensuring that the patient feels comfortable and respected.

Communicate with the patient and explain the process to help them feel more comfortable and in control. Patients should be informed that an adequate breast examination initially requires full exposure of both breasts; later, one breast may be covered while the other is examined. Let the patient know that various positions will be required to properly examine specific areas of the entire breast, including the tail, periphery, and axilla. By doing so, you will be able to educate them on breast awareness at the same time.[13–15]

The best time for breast examination in a patient who is still menstruating is 5 to 7 days *after* the onset of menstruation because breasts tend to swell and become more nodular before menses from increasing estrogen stimulation. Nodules appearing during the premenstrual phase should be re-evaluated after the onset of menstruation. For individuals who have gone through menopause and those assigned male at birth, any time is appropriate for breast examination.

TECHNIQUES OF EXAMINATION

Key Components of the Breasts and Axillae Examination

- Inspect the breasts of individuals assigned female at birth in four views.
- Palpate the breasts (consistency, tenderness, nodules - presence, characteristics, mobility).
- Inspect the axillae (rash, irritation, infection, pigmentation).
- Palpate the axillary nodes.
- Inspect the breasts of individuals assigned male at birth.

Inspect the Breasts of Individuals Assigned Female at Birth in Four Views

Inspect the breasts and nipples with the patient in the sitting position and disrobed to the waist. A thorough examination of the breasts includes careful inspection for skin changes, symmetry, contours, and retraction in four views—arms at sides, arms over head, arms pressed against hips, and leaning forward (Boxes 20-6 and 20-7).

Box 20-6. Breast Examination: Key Inspection and Observation Components

Examination Component to Inspect	What to Inspect For	Abnormal Findings and Implications
Skin appearance	Color, thickness, and prominence of pores	Redness indicates possible infection or inflammatory carcinoma; thickening and prominent pores (*peau d'orange* or orange peel) suggest breast cancer.
Breast size/symmetry	Differences in size and symmetry	Significant asymmetry could point to breast cancer or other conditions.
Breast contour	Masses, dimpling, flattening	Breast flattening suggests cancer; asymmetrical nipple direction change indicates potential cancer.
Nipple characteristics	Size, shape, direction, rashes, discharge	Eczematous nipple changes, like rash, scaling, or ulceration, signal Paget disease with possible ductal or lobular carcinoma. Inward-pulled nipples, possibly retracted due to cancer, might appear depressed, flat, broad, or thickened.

Box 20-7. Breast Inspection: Four Views

Position	Position Purpose	Examination Procedure	Observations
Arms at sides (Fig. 20-7)	Provides a baseline view for initial assessment; most natural and relaxed position to observe the breasts in their usual state. Ideal for initial symmetry and standard anomaly detection.	Instruct the patient to stand upright with their arms relaxed at their sides. Begin your visual inspection of the breasts in this position.	Look for overall symmetry, skin texture and color. Note any visible lumps, nipple inversion, or skin changes like dimpling.
Arms over head (Fig. 20-8)	Elevating the arms stretches the breast tissue and skin, making it easier to detect subtle changes or irregularities in contour, especially those not visible in a relaxed posture.	Ask the patient to slowly raise their arms above their head.	Carefully observe any changes in the breasts' shape or skin during this movement. Check for contour changes, dimpling, or puckering of skin. Assess nipple alignment and note any unusual bulges.
Arms pressed against hips (Fig. 20-9)	Engages the pectoral muscles, which can highlight any asymmetry or distortions not evident in a relaxed stance. Useful for observing changes in breast shape and skin tension.	Have the patient place their hands on their hips and press down firmly to contract the pectoral muscles.	Watch for any alterations in the shape or surface of the breasts. Look for asymmetry, distortions, or changes in breast shape. Dimpling or retraction can be more apparent in this position.
Leaning forward (Fig. 20-10)	Utilizes gravity to separate the breasts from the chest wall, allowing for better visualization of the lower contours and sides of the breasts, particularly beneficial for examining larger breasts.	Instruct the patient to lean forward from the waist, allowing the breasts to hang downward. Observe the breasts from this angle.	Examine how breasts fall and their shape. Look for any skin changes or abnormalities, especially in larger breasts.

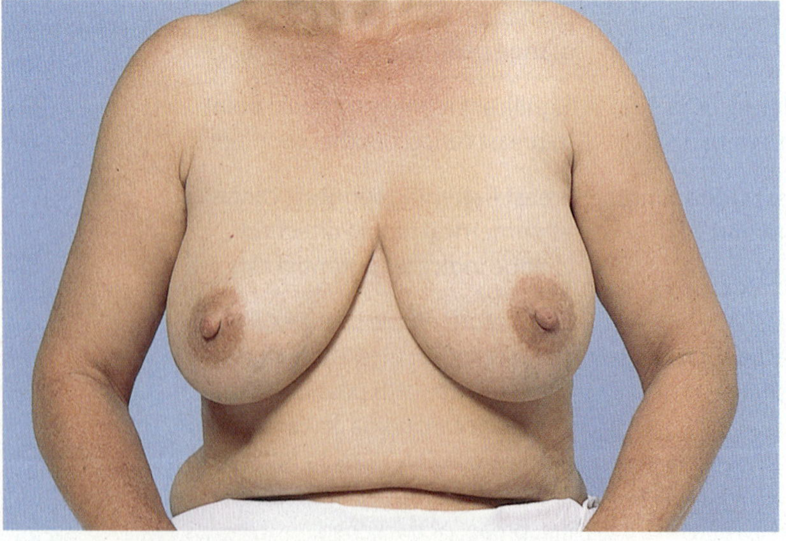

FIGURE 20-7. Inspection with arms at sides.

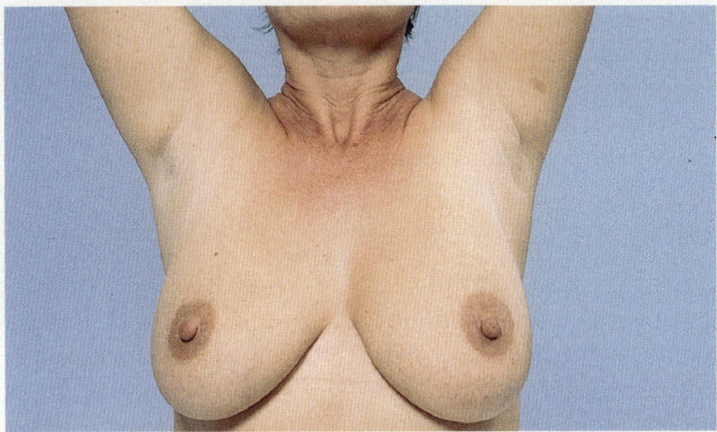

FIGURE 20-8. Inspection with arms overhead.

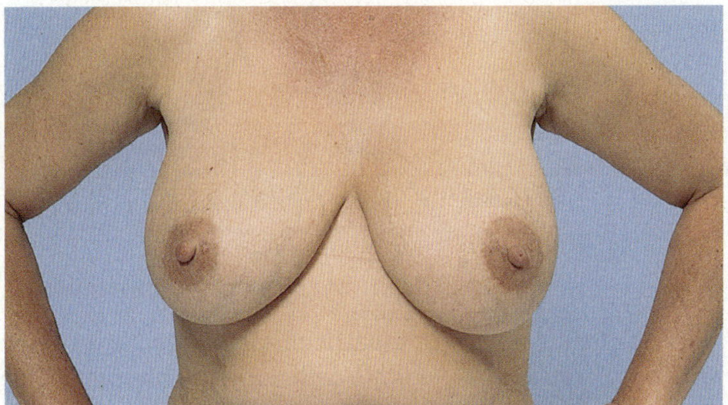

FIGURE 20-9. Inspection with hands pressed against hips.

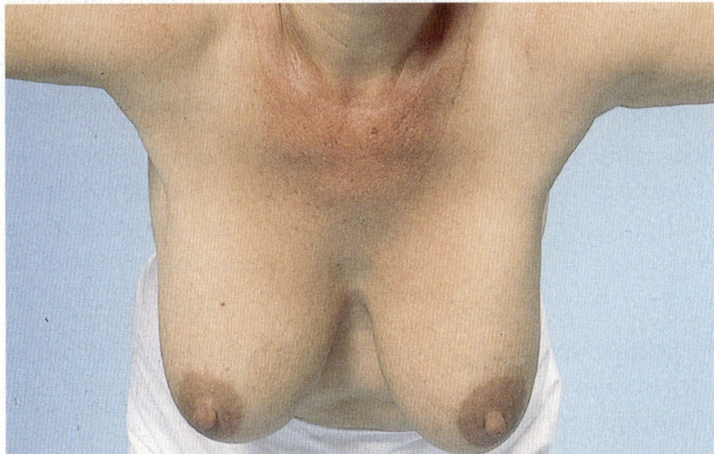

FIGURE 20-10. Inspection while leaning forward.

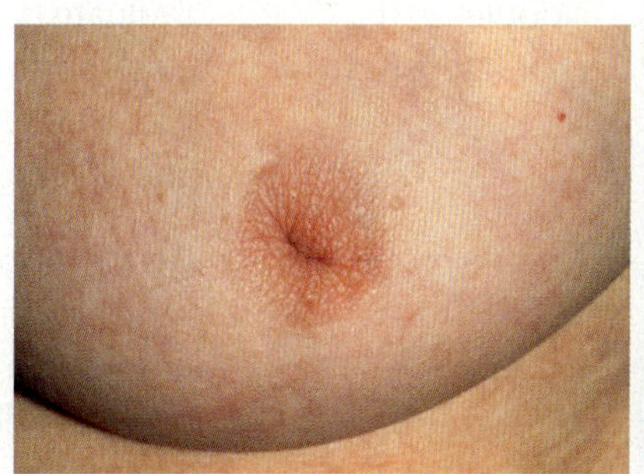

FIGURE 20-11. Inverted nipple.

Occasionally, the nipple is *inverted*, or points inward, depressed below the areolar surface. It may be enveloped by folds of areolar skin, as shown in Figure 20-11 but can be moved out from its sulcus. It is usually a normal variant of no clinical consequence, except for possible difficulty when breastfeeding or chestfeeding.

When performing a breast examination on adolescents, assess their breast development according to the Tanner sex maturity ratings. These ratings provide a standardized approach to evaluate breast development and range from stage 1, indicating prepubertal breast tissue, to stage 5, indicating mature breast tissue (see Chapter 28, Children: Infancy Through Adolescence, p. 1094).

Palpate the Breasts

Palpation is most effectively performed with the patient in a supine position, which helps to flatten the breast tissue for a more thorough examination. Start palpating the rectangular area that extends from the clavicle down to the inframammary fold or bra line, and from the midsternal line to the posterior axillary line, extending well into the axilla. This ensures a comprehensive examination, including the tail of the breast.

Tender subareolar cords suggest mammary duct ectasia, a benign but sometimes painful condition of dilated ducts with surrounding inflammation and, at times, with associated masses.

See Table 20-1, Common Breast Masses, p. 600.

Examine the breast tissue carefully for the examination components described in Box 20-8.

Box 20-8. Breast Examination: Key Palpation Components

Examination Component to Palpate	What to Palpate For	Abnormal Findings and Implications
Consistency of the tissues	Check consistency, considering glandular and fat tissue balance. Note nodularity and the inframammary ridge.	Unusual hardness or irregular texture may indicate pathology; misinterpretation of inframammary ridge could lead to false tumor concerns.
Tenderness	Assess for premenstrual tenderness.	Persistent or localized breast tenderness, especially when not linked to menstrual cycles, can be a sign of various breast conditions, including cysts, inflamed areas, or potentially more serious issues like cancer.
Presence of nodules	Palpate for lumps or masses differing from normal tissue, termed as *dominant mass*.	Persistent or growing dominant masses should be evaluated further for potential pathology. Nodules in the tail of Spence are sometimes mistaken for enlarged axillary lymph nodes.
Nodule characteristics	Evaluate nodule location (by quadrant or clock position and distance from the nipple), size, shape, consistency (soft, firm, or hard), and delimitation (well-circumscribed or not).	Irregular, hard, poorly circumscribed, or changing nodules could suggest malignancy or other serious conditions.
Nodule mobility	Gently move the breast near the mass and watch for dimpling. Next, try to move the nodule or mass with the patient's arm relaxed along the side of their body and then again while hands are pressed against the hip.	A mobile mass that becomes fixed when the arm relaxes is attached to the ribs and intercostal muscles; if fixed when the hand is pressed against the hip, it is attached to the pectoral fascia.

Use the pads of your second, third, and fourth fingers, kept slightly flexed for optimal sensitivity, and ensure to follow a systematic approach. The vertical strip pattern is the best validated technique currently known for detecting breast masses.[16]

During palpation, apply light, medium, and deep pressure with small, concentric circles at each point of examination (Box 20-9). For larger breasts, apply firmer pressure to assess the deeper tissues. Make sure to examine the entire breast, including its periphery, tail, and axilla.

When pressing deeply on the breast, a normal rib can be mistaken for a hard breast mass.

Box 20-9. Breast Palpation: Areas of the Breast

Breast Area	Examination Procedure	Findings and Clinical Implications
Lateral breast: assesses tissue that may be obscured in a standard position.	Ask the patient to roll onto their opposite hip, place their hand on her forehead, and keep their shoulders against the bed to flatten the lateral breast tissue. Begin palpation in the axilla, moving down to the bra line, then medially up to the clavicle in vertical overlapping strips, reaching the nipple (Fig. 20-12).	Changes or abnormalities in the lateral breast tissue may indicate conditions like cysts, masses, or other irregularities that require further medical evaluation.
Medial breast: targets tissue closer to the chest wall and midsternum	Instruct the patient to lie with their shoulders flat on the table and slide their flexed elbow to shoulder level (Fig. 20-13). Palpate from the nipple down to the bra line and back to the clavicle in vertical overlapping strips to the midsternum.	Irregularities or abnormalities in the medial breast tissue can be indicative of various conditions, and any unusual findings should be assessed.
Nipples: detects changes in elasticity and any discharge	Palpate each nipple, assessing its elasticity (Fig. 20-14). If nipple discharge is reported, compress the areola in radial positions around the nipple to determine the discharge's origin, observing the color, consistency, and quantity (Fig. 20-15).	Elasticity changes or discharge from nipples can be signs of underlying conditions, including infections or malignancies. The characteristics of any discharge should be noted.

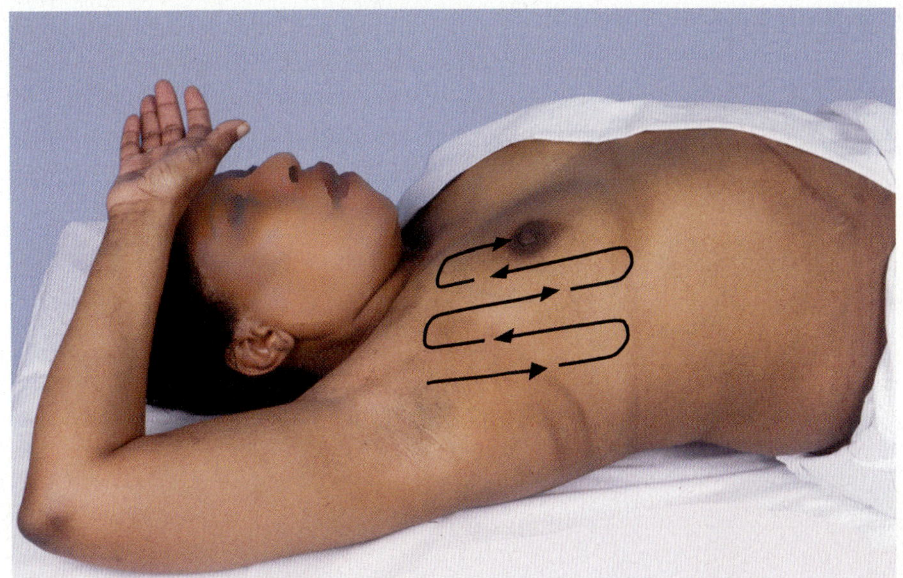

FIGURE 20-12. Vertical strip pattern, lateral breast.

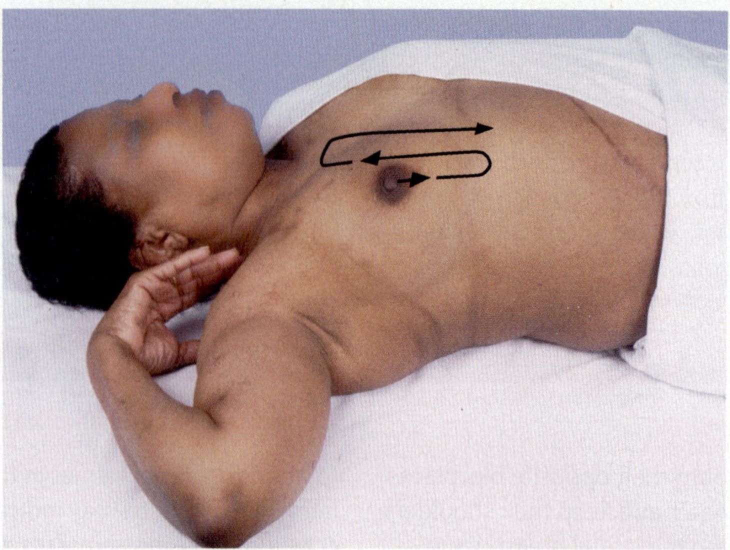

FIGURE 20-13. Vertical strip pattern, medial breast.

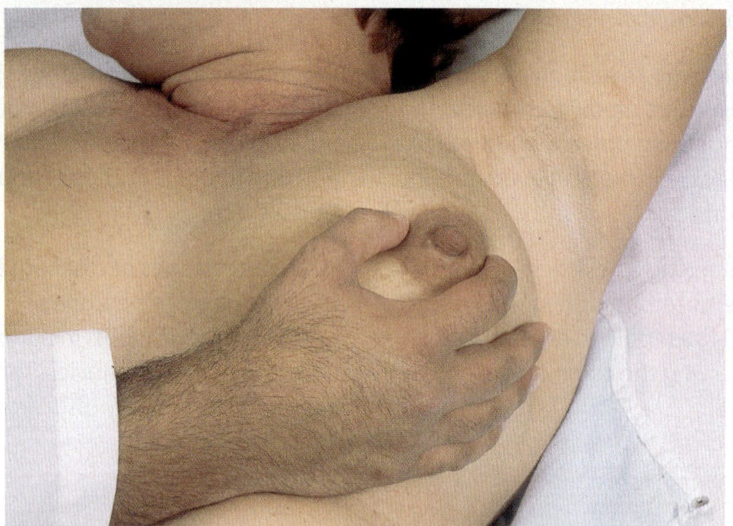

FIGURE 20-14. Palpating the nipple.

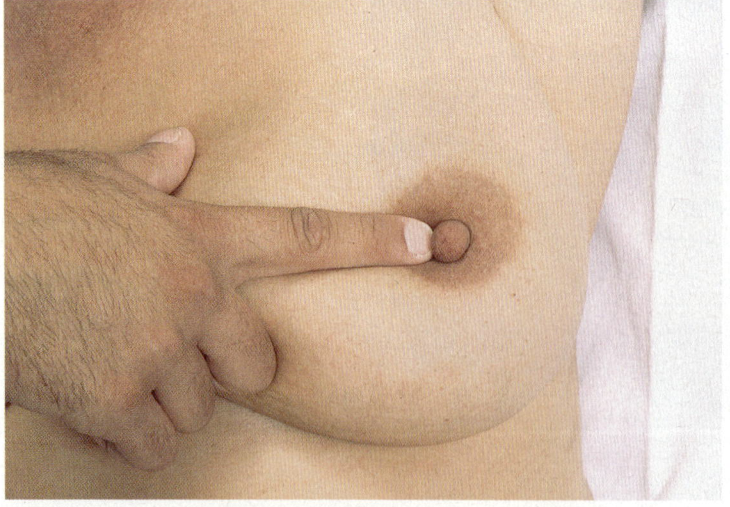

FIGURE 20-15. Compressing the areola for nipple discharge.

Milky discharge unrelated to a prior pregnancy and lactation is nonpuerperal **galactorrhea**. Causes include hyperthyroidism, pituitary prolactinoma, and dopamine antagonists, including psychotropics and phenothiazines.

Spontaneous unilateral bloody discharge from one or two ducts warrants further evaluation for intraductal papilloma, shown in Figure 20-16, ductal carcinoma in situ, or Paget disease of the breast. Clear, serous, green, black, or nonbloody discharges that are multiductal are usually benign.[8,17,18]

See Table 20-2, Visible Signs of Breast Cancer, p. 601.

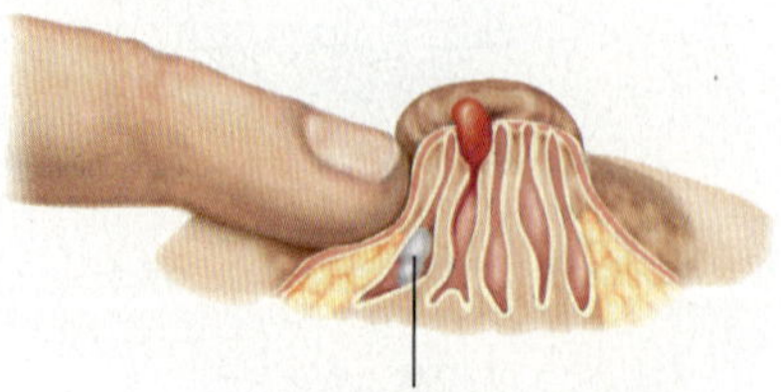

FIGURE 20-16. Intraductal papilloma.

Inspect the Axillae

Although the axillae may be examined with the patient lying down, a sitting position is preferable. Inspect the skin of each axilla, noting evidence of:

- Rash
- Irritation
- Infection
- Unusual pigmentation

Sweat gland infection from follicular occlusion (*hidradenitis suppurativa*) may be present.

Deeply pigmented velvety axillary skin suggests **acanthosis nigricans**—associated with diabetes; obesity; polycystic ovary syndrome; and, rarely, malignant paraneoplastic disorders.

Palpate the Axillary Lymph Nodes

The *central axillary nodes* are typically the most palpable among the axillary nodes. It is common to find one or more soft, small (<1 cm), and nontender nodes.

To examine the left axilla, use your right hand; for the right axilla, use your left hand. Encourage the patient to relax their arm on the side being examined and inform them that the procedure might cause some discomfort. Support the patient's wrist or hand (on the side being examined) with your other hand. Cup your examining hand's fingers and extend them toward the apex of the axilla, reaching as high as possible (as illustrated in Fig. 20-17). Position your fingers directly behind the pectoral muscles, aiming toward the midclavicle. Gently press your fingers toward the chest wall and slide them down, aiming to feel the central axillary nodes against the chest wall. Observe and record the size, shape, boundaries, mobility, consistency, and any tenderness of the nodes you palpate.

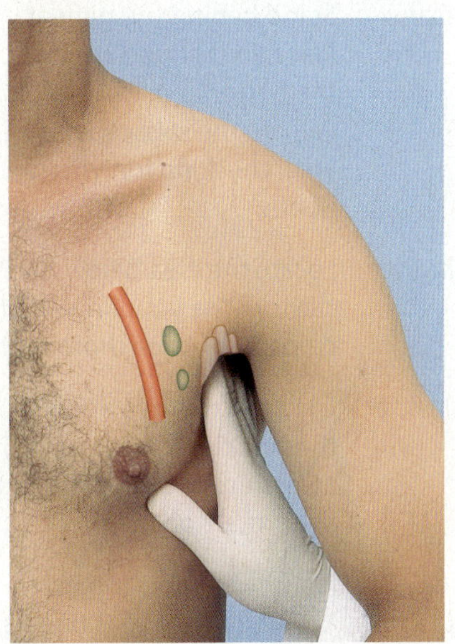

FIGURE 20-17. Palpating the left axilla.

If the central nodes feel large, hard, or tender, or if there is a suspicious lesion in the drainage areas for the axillary nodes, palpate for the other groups of axillary lymph nodes (Box 20-10).

For all lymph node groups, palpate for nodes that are large (≥1 to 2 cm), firm, hard, matted together, or fixed to the skin or underlying tissues, as these characteristics may suggest malignancy.

Enlarged axillary nodes may result from infection of the hand or arm, recent immunizations or skin tests, or generalized lymphadenopathy.

Box 20-10. Clinical Examination Techniques for Axillary and Related Lymph Node Groups

Axillary Lymph Node Group	Location	Palpation Technique
Anterior (pectoral) nodes	Anterior axillary fold	Grasp the anterior axillary fold between your thumb and fingers. Palpate inside the border of the pectoral muscle.
Lateral (humeral) nodes	High in the axilla, along the upper humerus	Position your hand high in the axilla. Gently palpate along the upper humerus, feeling for lymph nodes.
Posterior (subscapular) nodes	Posterior axillary fold	Stand behind the patient. Place your fingers inside the posterior axillary fold. Palpate the subscapular area, checking for lymph nodes.
Infraclavicular nodes	Below the clavicle	Locate the area below the clavicle. Use your fingers to palpate this area thoroughly.
Supraclavicular nodes	Above the clavicle	Focus on the area above the clavicle. Palpate gently, assessing for any enlarged or abnormal nodes.
Epitrochlear nodes	Medial to the elbow	Identify the area medial to the elbow. Use your fingers to palpate the epitrochlear region. This examination is particularly important if there are enlarged axillary nodes or signs of upper limb infection or malignancy.

Inspect the Breasts of Individuals Assigned Male at Birth

Although brief, the examination of the breast in individuals assigned male at birth is crucial. Start by inspecting the nipple and areola for any signs of nodules, swelling, or ulceration. Proceed to palpate the areola and surrounding breast tissue to check for nodules. If the breast appears enlarged (>2 cm), differentiate between *pseudogynecomastia*, characterized by soft fatty enlargement typically due to obesity, and *gynecomastia*, which presents as a benign firm disc of glandular enlargement. Note that breast tissue in gynecomastia is often tender.

Gynecomastia, typically caused by hormonal imbalances or medications, does not imply a risk for male breast cancer.

Most cases of breast cancer in individuals assigned male at birth present as painless breast masses, often with nipple involvement. Similar to breast cancer in individuals assigned female at birth, advanced cases also have palpable axillary lymph nodes.[6,19,20]

SPECIAL TECHNIQUES AND MANEUVERS

Modifications in Physical Examinations: Best Practices for Specialized Patient Populations

Patients who have undergone breast surgeries, whether it be breast augmentation, reduction, or mastectomy, require modified approaches during the PE. These procedures, each with its unique indications and outcomes, significantly alter the breast's natural anatomy, potentially masking or mimicking pathologic changes. Box 20-11 provides a detailed guide on the key distinctions and necessary modifications for the breast exam based on the specific surgical intervention.

Box 20-11. Breast Examination in the Presence of Medical Devices, Conditions, or Procedures

	Breast Augmentation or Reconstruction Surgery	Breast Reduction Surgery	Mastectomy
Device/condition	Surgery involving the insertion of breast implants (silicone gel, saline, etc.) under breast tissue or chest muscles	Surgery that involves removing excess breast tissue, fat, and skin	Surgical removal of one or both breasts, partially or completely
General indication	Desire for larger breasts, postmastectomy reconstruction, or addressing asymmetrical breasts	Addressing physical discomfort due to large breasts or for aesthetic reasons	Treatment of breast cancer, as a preventative measure in individuals at high risk for breast cancer, and as part of gender-affirming surgery.
General location	Implants positioned either behind breast tissue and above the pectoral muscle, or beneath the pectoral muscle.	Surgical incisions can vary but commonly are around the areola, vertically down from the areola to the breast crease, or horizontally along the breast crease.	Entire breast tissue is removed, often including the nipple and areola. Some patients may opt for reconstruction post-mastectomy, while others might choose different modifications to align more closely with their gender identity.

(continued)

Box 20-11. Breast Examination in the Presence of Medical Devices, Conditions, or Procedures (*Continued*)

	Breast Augmentation or Reconstruction Surgery	Breast Reduction Surgery	Mastectomy
Modification to the physical exam	1. Begin with visual inspection for asymmetry, skin changes, rippling, or signs of implant complications. 2. Gently but firmly palpate to distinguish between implant and natural tissue, feeling for implant edges. 3. Carefully assess tissue above and around the implant, feeling for any new masses. 4. If the implant is submuscular, palpate separately, asking the patient to flex the chest muscles. 5. Check for signs of implant rupture, such as asymmetry or changes in shape. 6. Use the pads of the first three fingers, and always ask about pain or discomfort during the exam. 7. Examine axillary lymph nodes to check for any enlargement that may suggest silicone migration	1. Start with a visual inspection for surgical scars, skin changes, or changes in nipple position. 2. Palpate gently using a circular motion, being mindful of areas that might be tender postsurgery. Check for lumpiness, tissue irregularities, or any thickening around surgical sites. 3. Assess nipple sensation, vascular supply, and whether there is any nipple discharge. 4. Examine both the inframammary fold and axillary region for any new masses or lymphadenopathy.	1. Begin by visually inspecting for surgical scars, skin changes, or contour irregularities. 2. Carefully palpate the chest wall, feeling for any new masses, chest wall irregularities, or tethering of the skin. 3. Check range of motion of the ipsilateral arm and examine for signs of lymphedema. 4. In reconstructed breasts, adapt and follow guidelines from the breast augmentation section. 5. Thoroughly examine the axillary and supraclavicular regions for any lymphadenopathy or masses.

RECORDING YOUR FINDINGS

For guiding your diagnosis and validating your hypotheses, detailed PE documentation is essential. However, with your eventual growth in clinical experience, your note-taking will evolve to include concise, universally accepted phrases for efficiency.

Recording the Breasts and Axillae Examination

Breasts:

"Breasts symmetric and smooth without nodules or masses. Nipples without discharge."

OR

"Breasts pendulous with diffuse fibrocystic changes. Single firm 1 × 1 cm mass, mobile, and nontender, with overlying peau d'orange appearance in right breast, upper outer quadrant at 11 o'clock, 2 cm from the nipple."

Axillary adenopathy usually included after Neck in section on Lymph Nodes; see pp. 309–310.

The technique of partitioning PE documentation into elaborate details demonstrates the essential role of clinical observations in pinpointing diagnostic clues. The findings described in the breast examination example are suspicious of several potential concerns:

- *Pendulous breasts:* Pendulous or drooping breasts are a natural result of aging and the effects of gravity on breast tissue. However, they can also be associated with factors such as genetics, pregnancy, and breastfeeding, chestfeeding or nursing.
- *Diffuse fibrocystic changes:* Fibrocystic changes in the breasts are common and can cause breast tissue to feel lumpy or have areas of increased density. These changes are often benign but can sometimes cause discomfort.
- *Single firm 1 × 1 cm mass:* The presence of a firm mass in the breast raises concerns about the possibility of a breast lump or tumor.
- *Mobile and nontender:* The fact that the mass is mobile and nontender can be both reassuring and concerning. It suggests that it may be more likely to be benign, but further evaluation is necessary.
- *Overlying peau d'orange appearance:* Dimpling or pitting of the skin (like an orange peel), is concerning as it can be associated with inflammatory breast cancer.

In summary, the findings are suspicious of a breast mass, which could be benign or potentially indicative of *breast cancer* especially given the overlying peau d'orange appearance.

HEALTH PROMOTION AND COUNSELING: EVIDENCE AND RECOMMENDATIONS

Important Topics for Health Promotion and Counseling

- Breast cancer in individuals assigned female at birth
- Breast cancer in individuals assigned male at birth

In the following section, both traditional terms like "men," "women," "male," and "female" and inclusive terms such as "individuals assigned female at birth" and "individuals assigned male at birth" are used. This approach balances inclusivity with the need to accurately represent the original research.

Breast Cancer in Individuals Assigned Female at Birth

Epidemiology. Breast cancer is the most commonly diagnosed cancer in the world and the leading cause of cancer death among individuals assigned female at birth.[21] In 2015, 2.4 million persons were diagnosed with breast cancer worldwide, and more than 500,000 deaths were attributed to this disease. Among individuals assigned female at birth in the United States, breast cancer is the most commonly diagnosed cancer and second only to lung cancer as a cause of cancer death.[22] A person born now in the United States has about a 12%, or 1 in 8, lifetime risk of developing invasive breast cancer and a 2.6%, or 1 in 38, lifetime risk of eventually dying from breast cancer.[23] About 80% of new breast cancer diagnoses occur after age 50, with a median age at diagnosis of 62.[17] The probability of being diagnosed with breast cancer increases with age (Box 20-12). Breast cancer mortality rates in the United States have been markedly declining since the early 1990s.

The American Cancer Society (ACS) reports that Black women continue to experience disproportionately higher mortality rates compared to other racial and ethnic groups. This increased likelihood of mortality is influenced by a range of factors, including delayed diagnosis, limited access to quality healthcare, differences in treatment options, and the impact of structural racism. These systemic inequities contribute to the persistent disparity in outcomes, underscoring the need for targeted efforts to address these challenges.

The strongest risk factors for breast cancer are increasing age, first-degree family members diagnosed with breast cancer (especially two or more diagnosed

Box 20-12. Probability of Developing Invasive Female Breast Cancer by Age Intervals[a,17]

Current Age (years)	10-Year Probability (%)
20	0.1 (1 in 1,567)
30	0.5 (1 in 220)
40	1.5 (1 in 68)
50	2.3 (1 in 43)
60	3.4 (1 in 29)
70	3.9 (1 in 25)
Lifetime Risk	12.4 (1 in 8)

[a]Probability is for women who are breast cancer free at the beginning of the age interval.

Source: American Cancer Society. *Breast Cancer Facts & Figures 2022–2024.* American Cancer Society, Inc.; 2022. Accessed January 1, 2024. https://www.cancer.org/research/cancer-facts-statistics/breast-cancer-facts-figures.html

Box 20-13. Calculators for Assessing Risk of Breast Cancer

- Gail model: http://www.cancer.gov/bcrisktool/
- Centers for Disease Control and Prevention Division of Cancer Prevention and Control—Know *BRCA* Tool: https://www.knowbrca.org/

at an early age), inherited genetic mutations, personal history of breast cancer or ductal or lobular carcinoma in situ, biopsy-confirmed precancerous lesions, relatively denser breasts on mammography, high-dose radiation to the chest at a young age, and high levels of endogenous hormones.[17]

A number of breast cancer risk assessment tools can be used to help determine personal risks of developing breast cancer (Box 20-13). This information can be used to guide decisions about when to start screening for breast cancer, how often to screen, which screening tests to perform, and whether to consider preventive interventions. One of the most commonly used tools is the National Cancer Institute's Breast Cancer Risk Assessment Tool (also known as the Gail model), which incorporates age, race/ethnicity, personal history of breast cancer or ductal or lobular carcinoma in situ, chest radiation, genetic mutations, first-degree relatives with breast cancer, previous breast biopsy results, age at menarche, and age at first delivery.[24]

Prevention. Healthy behaviors that may reduce breast cancer risk include physical activity, consuming diets high in fruits and vegetables, and limiting alcohol.[25] The U.S. Preventive Services Task Force (USPSTF) issued a grade B recommendation for using a risk tool to screen women for *BRCA* gene mutations if they have a family history of breast, ovarian, tubal, or peritoneal cancers.[26] *BRCA* gene mutations account for up to 10% of all breast cancers. Persons who screen positive should be referred to genetic counselors and considered for *BRCA* testing. Those with *BRCA* mutations can consider more intensive screening strategies (see Screening) and prophylactic bilateral mastectomy or chemoprophylaxis to prevent breast cancer. An evidence review found that bilateral mastectomy was associated with between an 80% and 100% reduction in breast cancer incidence and mortality.[27] Persons at high risk for breast cancer can also take *selective estrogen-receptor modulators (SERMs)*, such as tamoxifen and raloxifene, which are used to treat breast cancers, to reduce their risk of developing invasive breast cancer. However, taking SERMs also increases the risks of thromboembolic events and endometrial cancer. *Aromatase inhibitors* are another class of breast cancer treatment medications that have been shown effective for preventing breast cancer in high-risk postmenopausal women, but their use is not currently approved by the U.S. Food and Drug Administration for this indication.[25] The USPSTF issued a grade B recommendation encouraging clinicians to offer chemoprevention with either SERMs or aromatase inhibitors to women at increased risk for breast cancer who are also at low risk for medication complications.[28] National Health Interview Survey data suggest that the prevalence of chemoprevention use among eligible U.S. individuals is exceptionally low, perhaps due to clinician and patient concerns about side effects.[29]

Screening. Recommendations for breast cancer screening vary based on a person's age and risk for breast cancer. Mammography is the primary screening modality for breast cancer. Concerning findings on mammography may

Box 20-14. Benefits and Harms of Screening Mammography by Age Ranges, Average-Risk Individuals Assigned Female at Birth

Age Group (Years)	Breast Cancer Mortality: Relative Risk (95% CI)	Deaths Prevented over 10 Years (95% CI)[a]	False-Positive Test Results (n)[a]	Breast Biopsies (n)[a]
40–49	0.92 (0.75–1.02)	3 (0–9)	1,212	164
50–59	0.86 (0.68–0.97)	8 (2–17)	932	159
60–69	0.67 (0.51–1.28)	21 (11–32)	808	165
70–74	0.80 (0.51–1.28)	13 (0–32)	696	175
50–69	0.78 (0.68–0.95)	13 (6–20)	—	—

[a]Per 10,000 women screened for 10 years.

Sources: Adapted from Nelson HD, Fu R, Cantor A, Pappas M, Daeges M, Humphrey L. Effectiveness of breast cancer screening: systematic review and meta-analysis to update the 2009 U.S. Preventive Services Task Force Recommendation. *Ann Intern Med.* 2016;164(4):244–255; Nelson HD, Pappas M, Cantor A, Griffin J, Daeges M, Humphrey L. Harms of breast cancer screening: systematic review to update the 2009 U.S. Preventive Services Task Force Recommendation. *Ann Intern Med.* 2016;164(4):256–267.

be further evaluated with special mammographic views, breast ultrasound, magnetic resonance imaging (MRI), or digital breast tomosynthesis (DBT). The USPSTF has summarized results of studies evaluating the potential benefits and harms of screening mammography for average-risk women (no previous breast cancer or high-risk lesion, no genetic mutation, and no history of chest radiation at a young age).[30,31] Box 20-14 shows that the greatest mortality benefits are for individuals in their 60s, while those in their 40s are most likely to have false-positive results. Randomized trials also reported that screening was associated with overdiagnosis rates (finding cancers that would not otherwise be clinically detected during a person's lifetime) of 11% to 22%.

Based on these data, the USPSTF has issued a grade C recommendation for biennial mammography screening of women ages 40 to 74 years and an I statement (insufficient evidence) for women ages 75 and older.[32] Box 20-15 shows the breast cancer screening recommendations for mammography, clinical breast examination, and breast self-examination issued by the USPSTF,[32] the American Cancer Society,[33] and the American College of Obstetricians and Gynecologists.[34] Providers may want to perform clinical breast examinations or instruct women on performing breast self-exams when they are at very high risk for breast cancer. Breast self-examination, in combination with education efforts to address breast cancer, may also be advisable for women in limited-resource settings.

Evidence guiding screening practices for higher-risk persons is limited. Experts suggest that those with moderately increased risk due to increased breast density or a family history of one or two relatives with breast cancer could reasonably consider beginning screening at an earlier age, screening annually, and screening with DBT.[25] Those at very high risk due to genetic mutations are recommended to undergo annual screening beginning 10 years before the youngest family member was diagnosed (though not before age 30) using mammography and MRI.[35] Individuals who received thoracic radiation

Box 20-15. Recommendations for Breast Cancer Screening in Average-Risk Individuals Assigned Female at Birth

Organization	Mammography	Clinical Breast Examination	Breast Self-Examination
U.S. Preventive Services Task Force	50–74 y—biennially <50 y—individualize screening based on patient specific factors ≥75 y—insufficient evidence to assess the balance of benefits and harms	Insufficient evidence to assess the additional benefits and harms beyond screening mammography	Recommends against teaching breast self-examination, supports breast self-awareness
American Cancer Society—(2015)	40–45 y—optional annual screening 45–54 y—annual screening ≥55 y—biennial screening with option to continue annual screens Continue screening if good health and life expectancy ≥10 y	Not recommended	Not recommended; encourages breast self-awareness
American College of Obstetricians and Gynecologists	Offer screening starting at age 40 y Screening should be every 1 or 2 y based on a shared decision-making process Continue screening until at least age 75	May be offered in context of a shared decision-making process every 1–3 y for women aged 25–39 y and annually for women 40 y and older	Not recommended, but individuals should be counseled about breast self-awareness

Sources: Siu AL; U.S. Preventive Services Task Force. Screening for breast cancer: U.S. Preventive Services Task Force Recommendation Statement. *Ann Intern Med.* 2016;164(4):279–296; Oeffinger KC, Fontham ET, Etzioni R, et al. Breast cancer screening for women at average risk: 2015 guideline update from the American Cancer Society. *JAMA.* 2015;314(15):1599–1614; Practice bulletin no. 179 summary: breast cancer risk assessment and screening in average-risk women. *Obstet Gynecol.* 2017;130(1):241–243.

are advised to begin annual screening with mammography and MRI 10 years after completing radiation, but not before age 30.

Breast Cancer in Individuals Assigned Male at Birth

Breast cancer in individuals assigned male at birth accounts for less than 1% of breast cancer cases in the United States; an estimated 2,550 new cases were expected in 2018 with only 480 deaths attributed to this disease.[22] These individuals are more likely to present at an advanced stage because the diagnosis is often not suspected, and screening is not typically recommended for those assigned male at birth. Risk factors include increasing age, radiation exposure, *BRCA* gene mutations, Klinefelter syndrome, testicular disorders, alcohol use, liver disease, diabetes, and obesity.

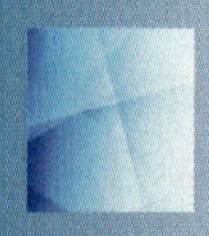

TABLE 20-1. Common Breast Masses

The three most common breast masses are *fibroadenoma* (a benign tumor), *cysts,* and *breast cancer.* The clinical characteristics of these masses are listed below. However, any breast mass should be carefully evaluated and usually warrants further investigation by ultrasound, aspiration, mammography, or biopsy.

The masses depicted below are large for purposes of illustration. *Fibrocystic changes,* not illustrated, are also commonly palpable as nodular, rope-like densities in women aged 25–50 y. They may be tender or painful. They are considered benign and not a risk factor for breast cancer.

	Fibroadenoma	Cysts	Cancer
Usual Age (in Years)	15–25 y, usually puberty and young adulthood, but up to age 55 y	30–50 y, regress after menopause except with estrogen therapy	30–90 y, most common over age 50 y
Number	Usually single, may be multiple	Single or multiple	Usually single, although may coexist with other nodules
Shape	Round, disc-like, or lobular; typically small (1–2 cm)	Round	Irregular or stellate
Consistency	May be soft, usually firm	Soft to firm, usually elastic	Firm or hard
Delimitation	Well delineated	Well delineated	Not clearly delineated from surrounding tissues
Mobility	Very mobile	Mobile	May be fixed to skin or underlying tissues
Tenderness	Usually nontender	Often tender	Usually nontender
Retraction Signs	Absent	Absent	May be present

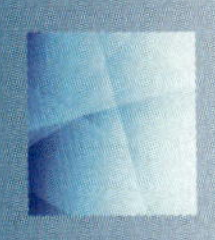

TABLE 20-2. Visible Signs of Breast Cancer

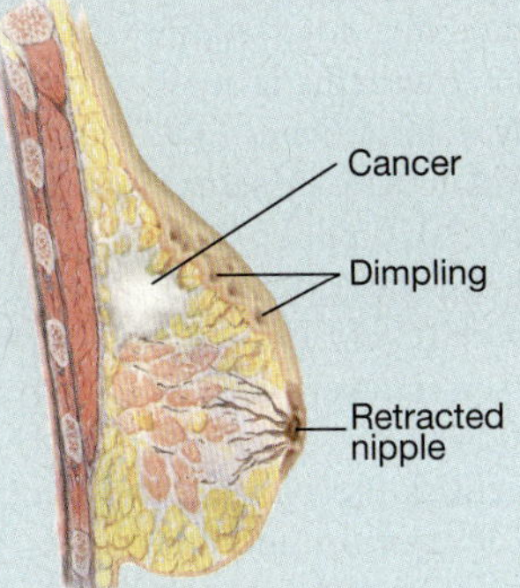

Retraction Signs

As breast cancer advances, it causes fibrosis (scar tissue). Shortening of this tissue produces *dimpling, changes in contour,* and *retraction or deviation of the nipple*. Other causes of retraction include fat necrosis and mammary duct ectasia.

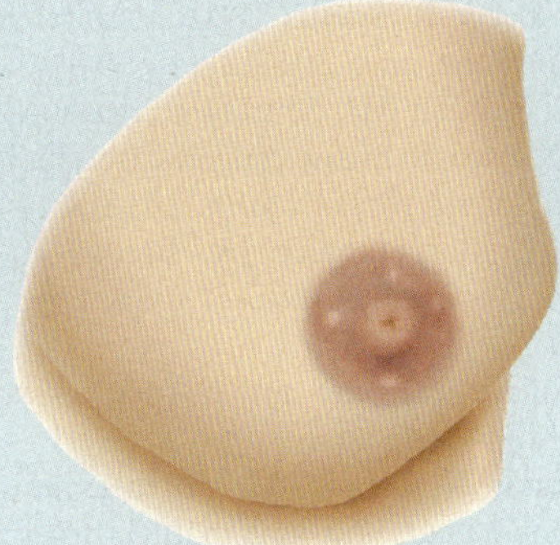

Abnormal Contours

Look for any variation in the normal convexity of each breast and compare one side with the other. Special positioning may again be useful. Shown here is marked flattening of the lower outer quadrant of the left breast.

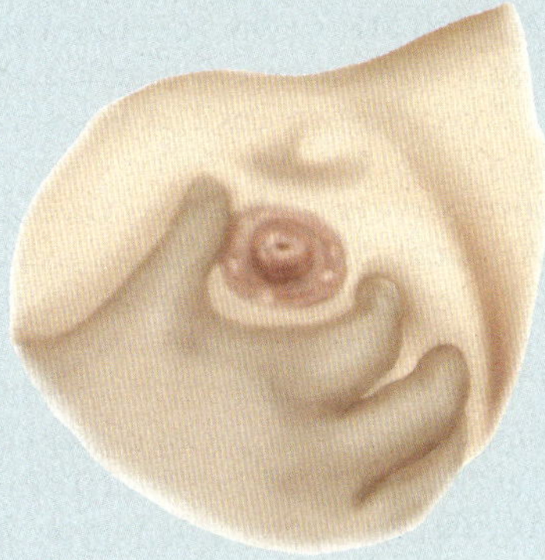

Skin Dimpling

Look for this sign with the patient's arm at rest, during special positioning, and on moving or compressing the breast, as illustrated here.

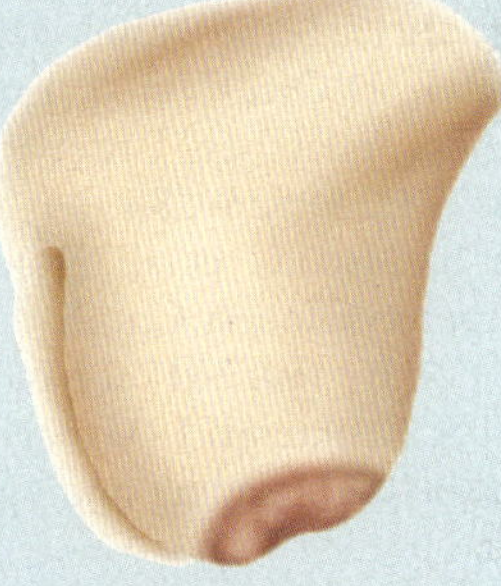

Nipple Retraction and Deviation

A retracted nipple is flattened or pulled inward, as illustrated here. It may also be broadened and feels thickened. When involvement is radially asymmetric, the nipple may deviate or point in a different direction from its normal counterpart, typically toward the underlying cancer.

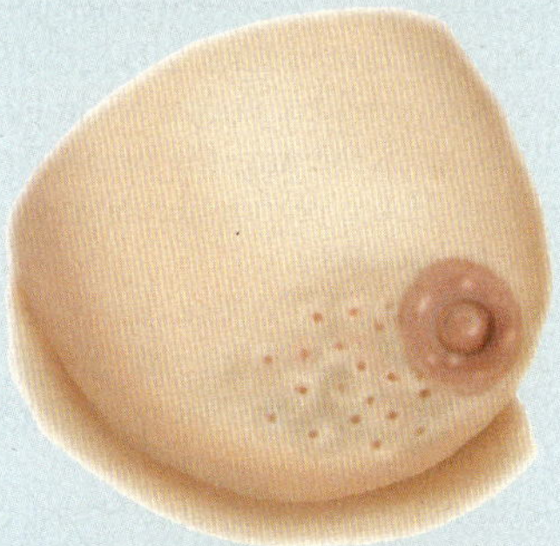

Edema of the Skin

Edema of the skin is produced by lymphatic blockade. It appears as thickened skin with enlarged pores—the so-called *peau d'orange* (orange peel) *sign*. It is often seen first in the lower portion of the breast or areola.

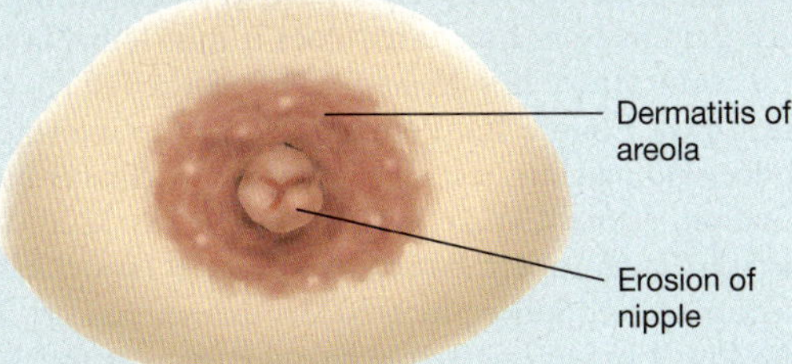

Paget Disease of the Nipple

This uncommon form of breast cancer usually starts as a scaly, eczema-like lesion on the nipple that may weep, crust, or erode. A breast mass may be present. Suspect Paget disease in any persisting dermatitis of the nipple and areola. Often (>60%) presents with an underlying in situ or invasive ductal or lobular carcinoma.

REFERENCES

1. Pandya S, Moore RG. Breast development and anatomy. *Clin Obstet Gynecol.* 2011;54(1):91–95.
2. Caouette-Laberge L, Borsuk D. Congenital anomalies of the breast. *Semin Plast Surg.* 2013;27(1):36–41.
3. Francone E, Nathan MJ, Murelli F, Bruno MS, Traverso E, Friedman D. Ectopic breast cancer: case report and review of the literature. *Aesthetic Plast Surg.* 2013;37(4):746–749.
4. Fayanju OM, Margenthaler JA. Breast. In: Klingensmith ME, ed. *The Washington Manual of Surgery.* 7th ed. Wolters Kluwer; 2016.
5. Wai CJ. Axillary anatomy and history. *Curr Probl Cancer.* 2012;36(5):234–244.
6. Chau A, Jafarian N, Rosa M. Male breast: clinical and imaging evaluations of benign and malignant entities with histologic correlation. *Am J Med.* 2016;129(8):776–791.
7. Johnson RE, Murad MH. Gynecomastia: pathophysiology, evaluation, and management. *Mayo Clin Proc.* 2009;84(11):1010–1015.
8. Salzman B, Fleegle S, Tully AS. Common breast problems. *Am Fam Physician.* 2012;86(4):343–349.
9. Expert Panel on Breast Imaging; Moy L, Heller SL, Bailey L, et al. ACR Appropriateness Criteria® palpable breast masses. *J Am Coll Radiol.* 2017;14(5S):S203–S224.
10. Jokich PM, Bailey L, D'Orsi C, et al; Expert panel on breast imaging. ACR Appropriateness Criteria® breast pain. *J Am Coll Radiol.* 2017;14(5S):S25–S33.
11. Lee S-J, Trikha S, Moy L, et al; Expert panel on breast imaging. ACR Appropriateness Criteria® evaluation of nipple discharge. *J Am Coll Radiol.* 2017;14(5S):S138–S153.
12. Patel BK, Falcon S, Drukteinis J. Management of nipple discharge and the associated imaging findings. *Am J Med.* 2015;128(4):353–360.
13. Rossouw JE, Anderson GL, Prentice RL, et al; Writing Group for the Women's Health Initiative Investigators. Risks and benefits of estrogen plus progestin in healthy postmenopausal women: principal results from the Women's Health Initiative randomized controlled trial. *JAMA.* 2002;288(3):321–333.
14. Breast cancer—patient version. National Cancer Institute. Accessed April 25, 2018. http://www.cancer.gov/cancertopics/types/breast
15. Fenton JJ, Barton MB, Geiger AM, et al. Screening clinical breast examination: how often does it miss lethal breast cancer? *J Natl Cancer Inst Monogr.* 2005;(35):67–71.
16. Barton MB, Elmore JG. Pointing the way to informed medical decision making: test characteristics of clinical breast examination. *J Natl Cancer Inst.* 2009;101(18):1223–1225.
17. American Cancer Society. *Breast Cancer Facts & Figures 2022–2024.* American Cancer Society, Inc.; 2022. Accessed January 1, 2024. https://www.cancer.org/research/cancer-facts-statistics/breast-cancer-facts-figures.html
18. Genetics of breast and gynecologic cancers (PDQ®)–health professional version. National Cancer Institute. Accessed January 1, 2024. http://www.cancer.gov/cancertopics/pdq/genetics/breast-and-ovarian/HealthProfessional
19. Key TJ. Endogenous oestrogens and breast cancer risk in premenopausal and postmenopausal women. *Steroids.* 2011;76(8):812–815.
20. Zeleniuch-Jacquotte A, Afanasyeva Y, Kaaks R, et al. Premenopausal serum androgens and breast cancer risk: a nested case-control study. *Breast Cancer Res.* 2012;14(1):R32.
21. Global Burden of Disease Cancer Collaboration; Allen C, Barber RM, Barregard L. Global, regional, and national cancer incidence, mortality, years of life lost, years lived with disability, and disability-adjusted life-years for 32 cancer groups, 1990 to 2015: a systematic analysis for the Global Burden of Disease study. *JAMA Oncol.* 2017;3(4):524–548.
22. Siegel RL, Miller KD, Jemal A. Cancer statistics, 2018. *CA Cancer J Clin.* 2018;68(1):7–30.
23. Howlader N, Noone A, Krapcho M, et al., eds. *SEER Cancer Statistics Review (CSR) 1975–2014.* National Cancer Institute; 2018. Accessed January 1, 2024. https://seer.cancer.gov/csr/1975_2014/
24. Breast Cancer Risk Assessment Tool: Online Calculator (The Gail Model). National Cancer Institute. Accessed January 1, 2024. https://www.cancer.gov/bcrisktool
25. Nattinger AB, Mitchell JL. Breast cancer screening and prevention. *Ann Intern Med.* 2016;164(11):ITC81–ITC96.
26. US Preventive Services Task Force; Owens DK, Davidson KW, Krist AH, et al. Risk assessment, genetic counseling, and genetic testing for BRCA-related cancer: US Preventive Services Task Force recommendation statement. *JAMA.* 2019;322(7):652–665.
27. Nelson HD, Smith ME, Griffin JC, Fu R. Use of medications to reduce risk for primary breast cancer: a systematic review for the U.S. Preventive Services Task Force. *Ann Intern Med.* 2013;158(8):604–614.
28. US Preventive Services Task Force; Owens DK, Davidson KW, Krist AH, et al. Medication use to reduce risk of breast cancer: US Preventive Services Task Force recommendation statement. *JAMA.* 2019;322(9):857–867.
29. Waters EA, McNeel TS, Stevens WM, Freedman AN. Use of tamoxifen and raloxifene for breast cancer chemoprevention in 2010. *Breast Cancer Res Treat.* 2012;134(2):875–880.
30. Nelson HD, Fu R, Cantor A, Pappas M, Daeges M, Humphrey L. Effectiveness of breast cancer screening: systematic review and meta-analysis to update the 2009 U.S. Preventive Services Task Force recommendation. *Ann Intern Med.* 2016;164(4):244–255.
31. Nelson HD, Pappas M, Cantor A, Griffin J, Daeges M, Humphrey L. Harms of breast cancer screening: systematic review to update the 2009 U.S. Preventive Services Task Force recommendation. *Ann Intern Med.* 2016;164(4):256–267.
32. US Preventive Services Task Force; Nicholson WK, Silverstein M, Wong JB, et al. Screening for breast cancer: US Preventive Services Task Force recommendation statement. *JAMA.* 2024;331(22):1918–1930.
33. Oeffinger KC, Fontham ET, Etzioni R, et al. Breast cancer screening for women at average risk: 2015 guideline update from the American Cancer Society. *JAMA.* 2015;314(15):1599–1614.
34. Practice bulletin no. 179 summary: breast cancer risk assessment and screening in average-risk women. *Obstet Gynecol.* 2017;130(1):241–243.
35. Bevers TB, Helvie M, Bonaccio E, et al. Breast Cancer Screening and Diagnosis, Version 3.2018, NCCN Clinical Practice Guidelines in Oncology. *J Natl Compr Canc Netw.* 2018;16(11):1362–1389.

CHAPTER 21

Abdomen

ANATOMY AND PHYSIOLOGY

The *abdomen* lies between the thorax and pelvis and is bordered superiorly by the inferior surface of the dome of the diaphragm (at about the fifth anterior intercostal space); posteriorly by the *lumbar vertebrae*; anterolaterally by flexible multilayered wall of muscles and sheet-like tendons (*rectus abdominis*, *transversus abdominis*, *internal* and *external obliques*); and inferiorly by the pelvic brim, which consists of the *iliac crest*, *anterior superior iliac spine*, *inguinal ligament pubic tubercle*, and *symphysis pubis*. Try to visualize these anatomic landmarks as shown in Figure 21-1.

The *abdominopelvic cavity* lies between the thoracic diaphragm and the pelvic diaphragm and contains two continuous cavities, the *abdominal cavity*, and the *pelvic cavity*. This extended cavity houses most of the digestive organs, the spleen, and parts of the urogenital system (Fig. 21-2). Several organs are often palpable except for the stomach and much of the liver and spleen, which lie high in the abdominal cavity close to the diaphragm, where they are protected by the thoracic ribs. Lining this cavity and folding over viscera are the *parietal* and *visceral* peritoneum.

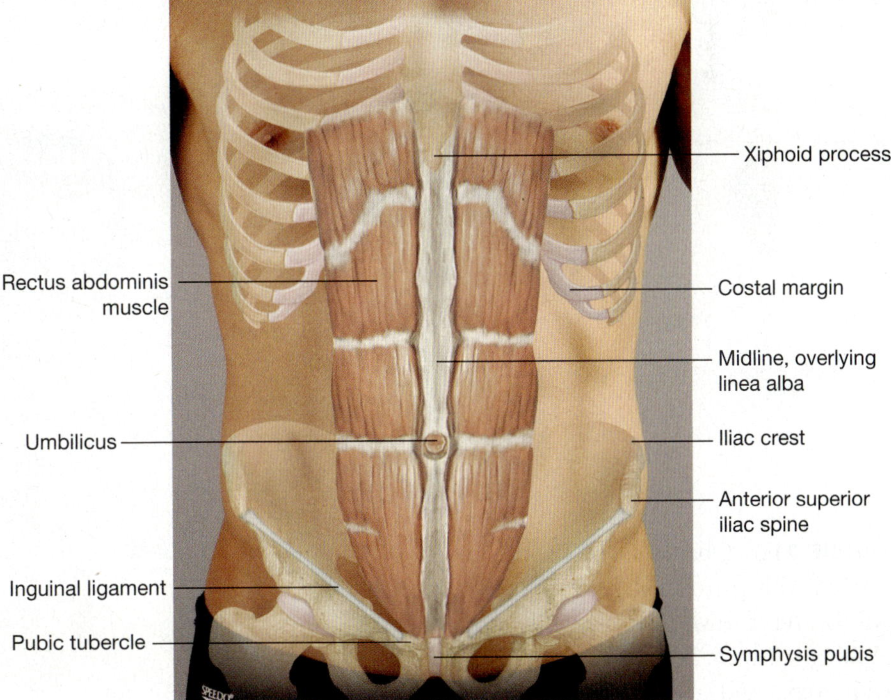

FIGURE 21-1. Landmarks of the abdomen.

Abdominal Division Methods and Contents

Quadrant Method. For descriptive purposes, the abdomen is often divided by imaginary horizontal and vertical lines crossing at the umbilicus, forming the right upper, right lower, left upper, and left lower quadrants (Fig. 21-3). Box 21-1 provides the anatomic structures located within each quadrant as pictured in Figure 21-4.

In the *right upper quadrant* (*RUQ*), the soft consistency of the *liver* makes it difficult to palpate through the abdominal wall. The lower margin of the liver, the liver edge, can be palpable at the right costal margin. The *gallbladder*, which rests against the inferior surface of the liver, and the more deeply lying *duodenum* are generally not palpable unless pathologic. Moving medially, the examiner encounters the rib cage with its *xiphoid process*, which protects the *stomach*. The *abdominal aorta* can have visible pulsations and may be palpable in the upper abdomen, or epigastrium in thin patients. At a deeper level, the lower pole of the right kidney and the tip of the 12th floating rib may be palpable, especially in children and thin individuals with relaxed abdominal muscles.

FIGURE 21-2. Abdominal viscera in situ.

In the *left upper quadrant* (*LUQ*), the *spleen* is lateral to and behind the stomach, just above the left kidney in the left midaxillary line. Its upper margin rests against the dome of the diaphragm. Ribs 9 through 11 protect most of the spleen. The tip of the spleen may be palpable below the left costal margin in a small percentage of adults (in contrast to readily palpable splenic enlargement, or *splenomegaly*). In healthy people, the *pancreas* cannot be detected.

The *left lower quadrant* (*LLQ*) contains the *sigmoid colon*. Portions of the distal colon (descending and sigmoid) may be palpable, especially if stool is present. In the lower midline are the *urinary bladder*, which can often be palpated when distended, and, in individuals with a *uterus and ovaries*, these organs may also be present and sometimes palpable.

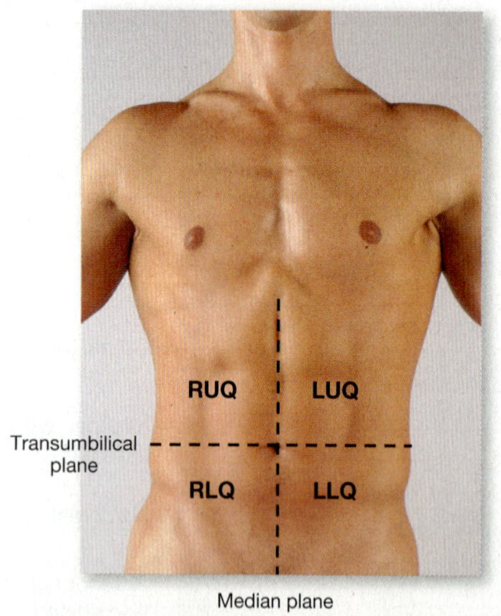

FIGURE 21-3. Quadrants of the abdomen. (Reprinted with permission. Base photo from Dalley AF II, Agur AMR. *Moore's Clinically Oriented Anatomy.* 9th ed. Wolters Kluwer; 2023. Modified with overlay and labels for Harrell KM, Dudek RW. *Lippincott® Illustrated Reviews: Anatomy.* Wolters Kluwer; 2019. Figure 4-2B.)

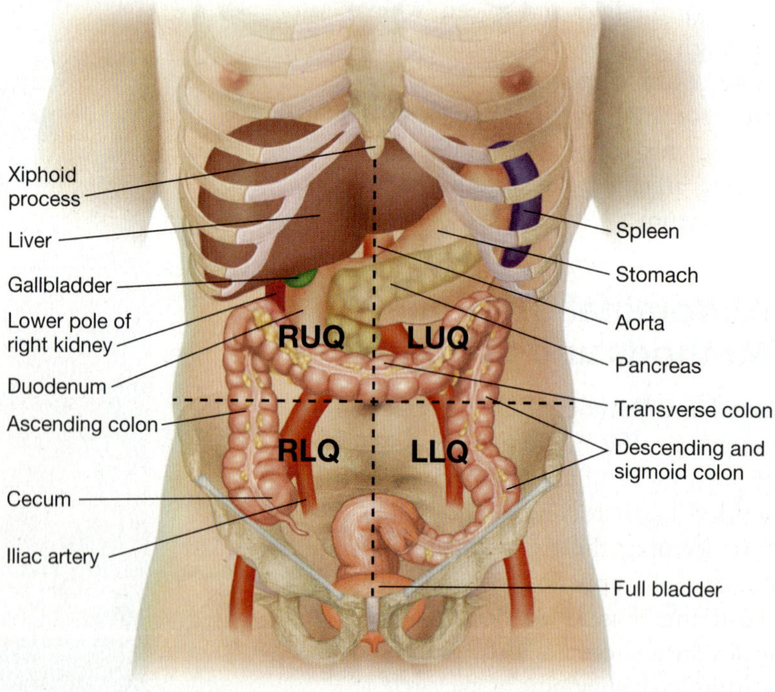

FIGURE 21-4. Abdominal quadrants and underlying structures.

Box 21-1. Abdominal Structures by Quadrant and by Region

Method	Location	Organs/Structures
By quadrant		
Right upper quadrant (RUQ)	Right of midline and above an imaginary horizontal line drawn across level of umbilicus	Liver (major part), gallbladder, part of the pancreas, part of the small and large intestines, right kidney (upper portion), and adrenal gland (right side)
Left upper quadrant (LUQ)	Left of midline and above level of umbilicus	Stomach, spleen, left lobe of the liver, body of the pancreas, left kidney (upper portion), adrenal gland (left side), and part of the small and large intestines
Left lower quadrant (LLQ)	Left of midline and below the level of the umbilicus	Part of the small intestines, descending colon, sigmoid colon, parts of the reproductive organs (left ovary and fallopian tube, left seminal vesicle and vas deferens), left ureter
Right lower quadrant (RLQ)	Right of midline and below the level of the umbilicus	Cecum, appendix, ascending colon, terminal ileum, parts of the reproductive organs (right ovary and fallopian tube, right seminal vesicle, and vas deferens), right ureter
By region		
Right hypochondriac	Under ribs, right side	Parts of the liver and gallbladder
Epigastric	Above umbilical region	Most of the stomach
Left hypochondriac	Under ribs, left side	Tail of the pancreas and part of the stomach
Right lumbar (or flank)	Right side of umbilical region	Parts of the intestines and the right kidney
Umbilical	Around umbilicus (navel)	Parts of the small intestine and transverse colon
Left lumbar (or flank)	Left side of umbilical region	Parts of the intestines and the left kidney
Right iliac (or inguinal)	Lower right part of abdomen	Appendix and parts of the small intestines
Hypogastric (or suprapubic)	Below umbilical region	Parts of the small intestine, bladder, uterus, and ovaries
Left iliac (or inguinal)	Lower left part of abdomen	Parts of the descending colon and small intestine

The *appendix* is located in the *right lower quadrant* (*RLQ*) at the base of the *cecum*, the first part of the large intestine, where the *terminal ileum* enters the large intestine at the *ileocecal valve*. In healthy people, these are not palpable.

The *kidneys* lie posteriorly in the abdominal cavity behind the peritoneum (*retroperitoneal*). The ribs protect their upper poles (Fig. 21-5). The *costovertebral angle* (*CVA*), formed by the lower border of the 12th rib and the transverse processes of the upper lumbar vertebrae, defines where to elicit kidney tenderness, called *CVA tenderness*.

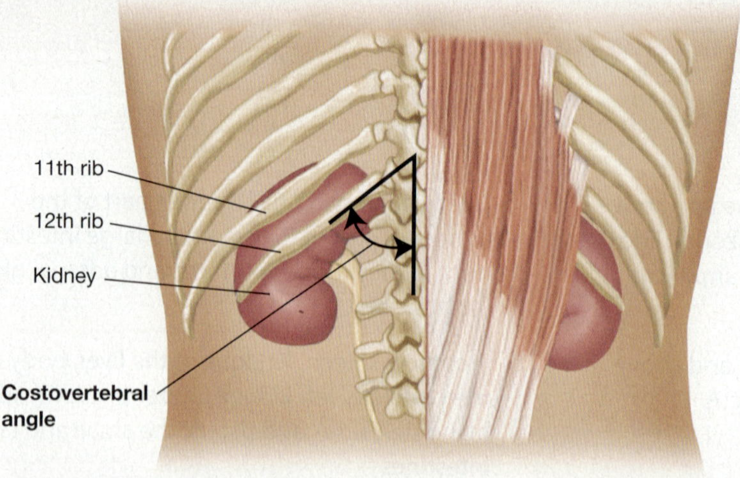

FIGURE 21-5. Posterior view of kidneys and costovertebral angles.

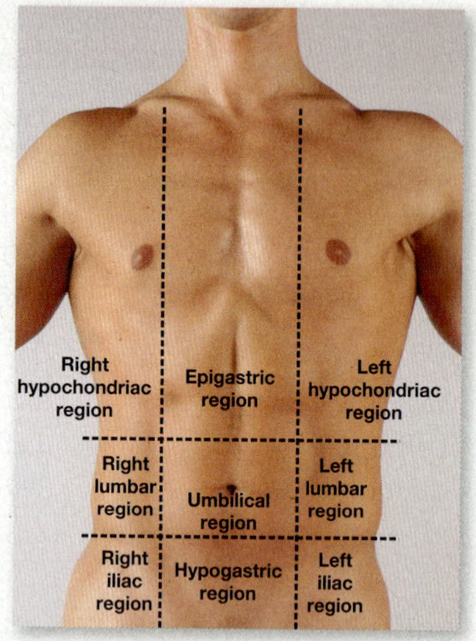

FIGURE 21-6. Regions of the abdomen. (Reprinted with permission. Base photo from Dalley AF II, Agur AMR. *Moore's Clinically Oriented Anatomy.* 9th ed. Wolters Kluwer; 2023. Modified with overlay and labels for Harrell KM, Dudek RW. *Lippincott® Illustrated Reviews: Anatomy.* Wolters Kluwer; 2019. Figure 4-2A.)

Nine-Region Method. Another system divides the abdomen into nine regions using a framework of two horizontal and two vertical imaginary lines (Fig. 21-6). The horizontal lines play a critical role in this division. The *upper horizontal line*, also known as the *transpyloric plane*, is situated midway between the top of the iliac crest and the bottom of the sternum. This line is significant as it often corresponds to the level of L1 in the spine. The *lower horizontal line*, known as the *intertubercular plane*, runs across the top of the hip bones. This line is generally aligned with L5, providing a clear lower boundary for the upper abdominal regions.

Complementing the horizontal lines are the vertical lines. The *right lateral line* runs vertically downward from the midpoint of the right clavicle. This line helps to define the right boundary of the central abdominal regions. Similarly, the *left lateral line* runs vertically downward from the midpoint of the left clavicle. It marks the left boundary of the central abdominal regions.

In clinical practice, the use of abdominal quadrants is often more prevalent than the nine-region division for its simplicity and speed in localizing symptoms, ease of communication, adequacy for initial assessments, and foundational role in education and training. However, the nine-region method is still valuable, particularly for more detailed diagnostic processes. It is often used in situations in which a more precise localization of symptoms is necessary. Most commonly referred to regions are *epigastric, umbilical, and hypogastric* (or *suprapubic*).

Physiology of the Abdominal Organs

Within the abdominal cavity, each organ contributes to a specific physiologic function:

- *Digestion:* The stomach and intestines chemically and mechanically break down food. Digestive enzymes from the pancreas and bile from the liver further aid in this process. Bile, crucial for fat digestion, is produced by the liver and stored in the gallbladder, being released into the duodenum during digestion.
- *Absorption:* The small intestine is the primary site for the absorption of nutrients into the bloodstream, facilitated by its extensive surface area. Here, the nutrients processed by the liver and enzymes from the pancreas are absorbed.
- *Metabolism:* The liver is central to metabolic processes, including glycogen storage, gluconeogenesis, protein synthesis, and detoxification. It processes

nutrients from the intestines, manages carbohydrate metabolism, and synthesizes vital proteins like albumin and clotting factors.

- *Excretion:* The large intestine concentrates waste into feces for excretion. The kidneys filter blood to remove waste products, which are excreted as urine. The liver also plays a role in excretion, as it conjugates bilirubin with bile salts for elimination via bile.
- *Endocrine Function:* The pancreas releases insulin and glucagon to regulate blood glucose levels. The adrenal glands, located atop the kidneys, secrete hormones that regulate metabolism and stress responses.
- *Immune Function:* The spleen filters blood, removes old red blood cells, and mounts an immune response to blood-borne pathogens.

Understanding these physiologic roles is fundamental for students as they learn to correlate abdominal anatomy with clinical conditions.

HEALTH HISTORY: GENERAL APPROACH

Gastrointestinal (GI) problems rank high among reasons for office and emergency room visits. You will encounter a wide variety of GI symptoms, including abdominal pain, reflux, nausea and vomiting with or without blood, difficulty or pain with swallowing, loss of appetite, and jaundice. Numerous symptoms also originate in the genitourinary (GU) tract and often accompany GI symptoms such as abdominal pain, nausea, and vomiting.

See Chapter 23, Pelvis and Genitourinary System: Penis, Scrotum, and Prostate, pp. 693–700 and Chapter 24, Pelvis and Genitourinary System: Vulva, Vagina, Uterus, and Adnexa, pp. 736–744.

In recent years, consensus statements from expert societies have clarified the definitions and classification of numerous abdominal symptoms, particularly the 2016 Rome IV criteria for functional GI disorders.[1]

See Table 21-1, Classification and Diagnosis of Selected Functional Gastrointestinal Disorders, p. 655.

When interviewing patients with abdominal symptoms, approach history taking systematically. Align your questions with the structures within the abdominopelvic cavity and its layers, keeping the anatomic placement of these structures in mind.

Clarifying questions are essential to understand the exact meaning of each symptom. For instance, the term *"heartburn"* may refer to pain from reflux or angina, while *"spitting up blood"* may indicate bleeding from the GI tract or upper airways.

As you gain experience, you can modify your approach to ask fewer but more focused questions that are relevant to the presenting concern. Remember that developing these skills takes time, but they are critical for sound clinical reasoning and an accurate differential diagnosis.

Common or Concerning Symptoms

- Abdominal pain (general)
- Regional pain:
  - Epigastric pain
  - Right upper quadrant abdominal pain

- Left upper quadrant abdominal pain
- Right lower quadrant abdominal pain
- Left lower quadrant abdominal pain
- Hypogastric (suprapubic) pain
- Nausea and vomiting
- Hematemesis (vomiting blood)
- Hematochezia (bright red blood in stool) and melena (black, tarry stool)
- Dysphagia (difficulty swallowing) and/or odynophagia (painful swallowing)
- Diarrhea
- Constipation
- Jaundice

Also see Chapter 23, Pelvis and Genitourinary System: Penis, Scrotum, and Prostate, pp. 693–700 and Chapter 24, Pelvis and Genitourinary System: Vulva, Vagina, Uterus, and Adnexa, pp. 736–744.

Abdominal Pain

In 2021, ~12.5 million ambulatory care visits for stomach and abdominal pain, cramps, and spasms occurred in the United States.[2,3] Attempt to clarify the presenting symptoms carefully and obtain clues from accompanying symptoms.[4] A careful history alone can lead to the correct diagnosis in 76% of cases.[3]

See Table 21-2, Abdominal Pain, pp. 656–659.

Before exploring common causes, review the mechanisms and clinical patterns of abdominal pain (Box 21-2).

Box 21-2. Types of Abdominal Pain and Their Clinical Features

Type of Pain	Description
Visceral	■ Typically originates from abdominal organs, whether hollow or solid, and can occur due to forceful contractions, distention, or stretching ■ Often nonspecific and challenging to localize, usually felt near the midline; precise location varies depending on involved structure ■ Can be triggered by ischemia (reduction in blood flow to the organ) ■ Often described as gnawing, cramping, or aching ■ May be accompanied by sweating, pallor, nausea, vomiting, and restlessness ■ Visceral periumbilical pain may indicate early stages of acute appendicitis; often evolves to sharper parietal pain in the right lower quadrant as inflammation extends to adjacent parietal peritoneum (Fig. 21-7)
Parietal (somatic)	■ Originates from inflammation of the parietal peritoneum (peritonitis) ■ Typically, steady and aching; usually more severe and precisely localized than visceral counterpart ■ Aggravated by movement or coughing, leading to significant discomfort; patients therefore often prefer to lie still ■ If symptoms are disproportionately intense compared to physical findings, consider intestinal mesenteric ischemia

Type of Pain	Description
Referred	■ Experienced in distant sites innervated at similar spinal levels as disordered structures ■ Discomfort originating from duodenum or pancreas may be referred to the back, while biliary tree issues could manifest as discomfort in the right scapular region or right posterior thorax; pleurisy or inferior wall myocardial infarction discomfort may present in epigastric area ■ Often develops as the initial discomfort intensifies and appears to radiate or travel from original site ■ Palpation at site of referred discomfort typically does not elicit tenderness

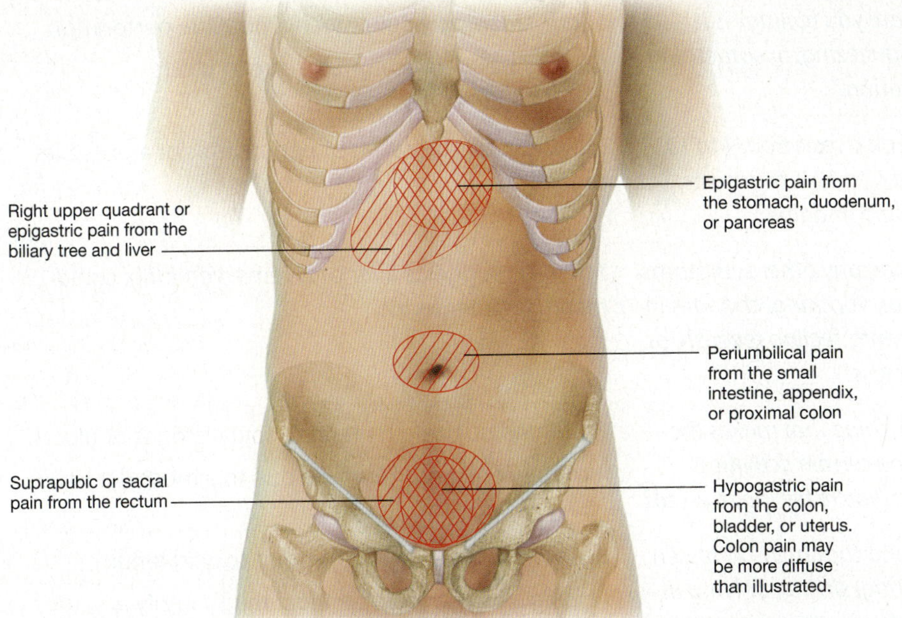

FIGURE 21-7. Areas of manifestation of visceral pain from abdominal viscera.

A key strategy in diagnosing abdominal pain is to consider the anatomic structures located in the area where the pain is experienced. Each quadrant or region of the abdomen—epigastric region, RUQ, LUQ, RLQ, LLQ, and hypogastric or suprapubic region—houses specific organs. Asking the patient to point to the pain and characterize all its features, combined with findings on the physical examination, is key to identifying possible causes.

By identifying the pain's location, you can narrow down the list of potential causes, as different regions correlate with different organs and possible conditions. Causes range from benign to life threatening, so take the time to conduct a careful interview by using high-yield health history questions (Box 21-3).

Box 21-3. General Health History Questions for Abdominal Pain

Domain	Questions	Rationale
Onset and duration	*When did you first notice the pain in your belly area, and how long has it lasted?*	*Sudden:* might point to appendicitis *Chronic:* suggests a condition like irritable bowel syndrome (IBS)

(continued)

Box 21-3. General Health History Questions for Abdominal Pain (*Continued*)

Domain	Questions	Rationale
Location	*Can you show or tell me exactly where it hurts in your belly?*	*RUQ:* could relate to the gallbladder *RLQ:* might involve the appendix
Radiation	*Does the pain you're feeling radiate or spread to any other part of your body?*	*Radiating to the back:* may be associated with pancreatic issues *Radiating to the shoulder:* could suggest gallbladder or liver problems
Characteristics	*What kind of pain are you feeling? Is it stabbing, aching, squeezing, or something like a burning sensation?*	*Sharp, stabbing:* could mean a possible perforation *Burning sensation:* might be due to ulcers
Severity	*How bad is the pain on a scale from 1 to 10, where 1 is very mild and 10 is the most intense pain you could imagine?*	*Intense:* could be a sign of pancreatitis or a possible organ rupture
Associated symptoms	*Have you been feeling any other symptoms like feeling nauseous, vomiting, changes in your bowel movements, feeling feverish, or unexpected weight loss?*	*Jaundice:* suggests liver problems. *Vomiting:* could mean gastroenteritis
Aggravating factors	*Can you think of anything that makes the pain worse, like doing certain activities, after eating, or when you're feeling stressed?*	*Postprandial:* could be related to gallstones or ulcers *Movement related:* might be due to a muscular issue
Alleviating factors	*What have you found that helps to lessen the pain? Does resting, sitting, or lying in a certain way, or any over-the-counter medications or common remedies help?*	*Relief from antacids:* might point to acid reflux *Finding a comfortable position:* might imply a musculoskeletal issue
Past medical history	*Have you ever had problems with digestion or with going to the bathroom?*	History of digestive problems may indicate a recurrence or ongoing issue such as Crohn's disease
Medication history	*Are you taking any medicine, vitamins, or herbal supplements that might be affecting how your belly feels?*	Certain medications can cause side effects or interact with others, affecting symptoms (e.g., NSAIDs are known to cause stomach issues, including ulcers)
Family history	*Do any of your family members have a history of belly or digestive issues, or any similar conditions?*	Can reveal a predisposition to conditions such as celiac disease or colorectal cancer, influencing the direction of the investigation

Epigastric Pain

Epigastric pain refers to discomfort or pain located in the upper central region of the abdomen (*epigastrium*), just below the ribcage and above the umbilicus. This region includes several important organs and structures, such as the stomach, the lower part of the esophagus, the upper part of the small intestine (duodenum), the pancreas, and the liver.

Dyspepsia is defined as chronic or recurrent discomfort or pain centered in the upper abdomen, characterized by epigastric pain or burning (or both) and postprandial fullness or early satiety (or both).[1,19] *Heartburn* is a rising retrosternal burning pain or discomfort occurring weekly or more often. It is typically aggravated by foods such as alcohol, chocolate, citrus fruits, coffee, onions, and peppermint and positions like bending over, exercising, lifting, and lying supine.

Possible common causes include **gastritis** (inflammation of gastric mucosa), **gastroesophageal reflux disease** ([**GERD**] reflux of stomach acid into the esophagus), **pancreatitis** (inflammation of the pancreas), **peptic ulcer disease** ([**PUD**] break in the lining of the stomach or duodenum), and **nonalcoholic fatty liver disease** ([**NALFD**] fat build-up in liver cells).

For key questions to ask during a health history and the reasons they help identify different diagnoses, see Box 21-4.

Box 21-4. Epigastric Abdominal Pain: High-Yield Health History Questions

Questions	Rationale
Have you felt a sudden, sharp pain in the middle of your upper abdomen, maybe spreading upwards toward your chest?	Could indicate peptic ulcer disease (PUD); location and radiation of the pain can help distinguish it from other causes like heartburn or pancreatitis
How often do you drink alcohol, and how much do you typically consume?	Frequent or heavy alcohol use can lead to gastritis or contribute to the development of PUD
Have you had any fever or chills recently, or noticed a yellowish tint to your skin or eyes?	*Fever and chills:* could suggest an inflammatory process like gastritis *Jaundice:* might indicate a problem with the liver or pancreas
Do you have conditions like excess body weight, diabetes, high blood pressure, or high cholesterol?	Can increase the risk of nonalcoholic fatty liver disease or pancreatitis
Have you experienced any changes in your hunger, unexpected weight loss, or noticed your stools turning very light in color?	*Appetite changes and weight loss:* could signal conditions such as gastritis or PUD *Pale stools:* may indicate a problem with the pancreas or liver

Right Upper Quadrant Abdominal Pain

RUQ abdominal pain refers to discomfort or pain in the upper right portion of the abdomen. This region contains several important organs and structures, including the liver; gallbladder; right kidney; part of the pancreas; and small and large intestines. RUQ pain can have various causes, and the nature and severity of the pain can differ based on the underlying condition (Box 21-5).

Possible common causes include **gallstones** (**cholelithiasis**, hardened deposits of bile that form in the gallbladder), **cholecystitis** (inflammation of the gallbladder), **hepatitis** (inflammation of the liver), and **NALFD**.

Box 21-5. Right Upper Quadrant Abdominal Pain: High-Yield Health History Questions

Questions	Rationale
Have you suddenly felt a severe pain on the upper right side of your abdomen that also reaches your back or shoulder?	*Gallstones:* typically cause sudden, sharp, and severe pain when obstructing the bile ducts *Cholecystitis:* may present with similar pain but is often steady and longer lasting *Hepatitis and nonalcoholic fatty liver disease (NALFD):* less likely to cause intense pain
Do you drink alcohol frequently or in large amounts?	*Heavy alcohol consumption:* more likely to cause alcoholic hepatitis or liver disease *Little to no alcohol intake:* NAFLD more likely
Have you had a fever or felt chills, or have you noticed your skin or the whites of your eyes turning yellow?	*Fever and chills:* may indicate an infectious or inflammatory process, such as hepatitis or cholecystitis *Jaundice:* more commonly associated with hepatitis, as it indicates impaired liver function or bile flow obstruction *Gallstones or NAFLD:* less likely unless there is a bile duct obstruction
Do you have any ongoing health conditions like excess weight, high blood sugar, elevated blood pressure, or raised cholesterol levels?	Could be related to NAFLD; these risk factors are less specific for gallstones, cholecystitis, or hepatitis, although they may still contribute to the development of these conditions
Have you noticed any recent changes in your appetite, weight loss, or a difference in the color of your bowel movements, such as them being light-colored or gray?	*Change in appetite or unexplained weight loss:* may be associated with hepatitis or NAFLD *Pale or clay-colored stools:* can indicate bile flow obstruction, which may occur with gallstones or cholecystitis

Left Upper Quadrant Abdominal Pain

The LUQ contains several organs and structures that could be the source of pain, including the stomach, spleen, part of the pancreas and colon (splenic flexure), and the left kidney. Box 21-6 contains relevant health history questions.

Possible common causes include **gastritis**, **GERD**, **pancreatitis**, and **PUD**. Additional common causes include **constipation** (infrequent bowel movements, leading to hard and difficult-to-pass stools) and **kidney stones** (formation of stones in the urinary tract, often due to dehydration or dietary factors). Although less common, **splenic disorders** such as **splenomegaly** (enlarged spleen) or **splenic infarction** can cause LUQ pain.

Box 21-6. Left Upper Quadrant Abdominal Pain: High-Yield Health History Questions

Questions	Rationale
Could you walk me through when you first noticed the pain, the duration of each episode, and whether the pain has been changing over time?	*Gradual, episodic (and can be chronic):* could be constipation *Sudden, severe pain that can come in waves:* could be kidney stones *Acute onset:* may be splenic trauma or infarction *Gradual and chronic:* can be splenomegaly (depending on the underlying cause)
Have you had any injuries or accidents lately that could be related to this pain?	*Blunt abdominal trauma (e.g., car accident or sports injury):* could be splenic injury *Less likely to be associated with recent trauma:* constipation, kidney stones, splenic infarction, and splenomegaly
Have there been any changes in your bowel movements recently?	Constipation is characterized by infrequent, hard stools or difficulty passing stools
Do you feel the pain moving towards your back or groin area?	*Radiates to the lower back or groin:* may be kidney stones *Referred to the left shoulder (Kehr sign), but typically not to the back or groin:* could be splenic disorders *Localized to the abdomen:* could be constipation *Localized to the LUQ:* could be splenomegaly
Have you had any symptoms of an infection, such as fever or chills?	Can indicate an underlying infection or inflammation Splenic infarction or embolic event: can be caused by a bacterial infection *Kidney stones:* may be associated with fever if infection is present *Splenic trauma:* less likely to present with fever unless a secondary infection develops *Splenomegaly:* can be associated with fever if caused by underlying infection or inflammatory condition

Right Lower Quadrant Abdominal Pain

RLQ region primarily includes the appendix, right ureter, right ovary and fallopian tube, part of the ascending colon, and the cecum. Pain in this area can have various causes, such as appendicitis, ovarian cysts, kidney stones, and inflammatory bowel diseases like Crohn's disease. The nature and severity of the pain can vary based on the underlying condition (Box 21-7).

For GU causes of RLQ pain, see Chapter 23, Pelvis and Genitourinary System: Penis, Scrotum, and Prostate, pp. 693–700 and Chapter 24, Pelvis and Genitourinary System: Vulva, Vagina, Uterus, and Adnexa, pp. 736–744.

Possible common causes include **appendicitis** (inflammation of the appendix), **gynecologic disorders** including **ovarian cyst/torsion** (ovarian cyst rupture or ovarian torsion)**, pelvic inflammatory disease** ([**PID**] infection of the reproductive tract), **ectopic pregnancy**, **inflammatory bowel disease** ([**IBD**] chronic inflammation of the gastrointestinal tract), and **kidney stones**.

Box 21-7. Right Lower Quadrant Abdominal Pain: High-Yield Health History Questions

Questions	Rationale
Could you tell me when the pain started, where you feel it, and what it feels like (sharp, dull, throbbing, others)?	*Vague pain around the umbilicus, later localizing to the RLQ:* could be appendicitis *Sudden, severe, unilateral:* could be ovarian cyst/torsion or ectopic pregnancy *Gradual, persistent, bilateral lower abdominal pain:* could be pelvic inflammatory disease (PID) *Crampy, episodic:* could be inflammatory bowel disease (IBD) *Severe, colicky (possibly radiating to groin):* could be kidney stones
Have you experienced any new or unusual changes with your bowel movements or when you urinate?	*Diarrhea, blood in stools, urgency:* could be IBD *Hematuria, dysuria, urinary frequency:* could be kidney stones *No changes:* Ovarian cyst/torsion, PID, ectopic pregnancy, appendicitis (although appendicitis sometimes causes mild constipation or diarrhea)
Have you had any changes in your vaginal health, such as new bleeding, discharge, or changes in your menstrual cycle?	*Vaginal bleeding and missed period:* can be ectopic pregnancy *Abnormal vaginal discharge, menstrual irregularities:* can be PID *No gynecologic symptoms:* can be appendicitis, IBD, kidney stones, ovarian cyst/torsion (ruptured cyst may cause bleeding)
Have you been experiencing any fever, unexpected weight loss, or sweating during the night?	*Fever:* may be appendicitis or PID *Weight loss, fever, night sweats:* may be IBD *No systemic symptoms:* can be ovarian cyst/torsion, ectopic pregnancy, kidney stones (although kidney stone can cause fever if associated infection)
Is this type of pain familiar to you, or do you have any existing health conditions we should be aware of?	*History of similar pain episodes:* suggests recurrent conditions such as IBD or kidney stones *History of previous gynecologic issues:* increases likelihood of ovarian cyst/torsion, PID, or ectopic pregnancy *Past abdominal surgeries or sexually transmitted infection:* can help guide the diagnostic process

Left Lower Quadrant Abdominal Pain

LLQ pain refers to pain or discomfort felt in the lower left side of the abdomen, below the navel, and above the left hip bone. The LLQ contains several important organs, including the descending colon, left ovary and fallopian tube, left ureter, and left part of the bladder, among others. In Box 21-8, you will find important questions to include in a health history and their rationales that are instrumental in distinguishing potential diagnoses.

For GU causes of LLQ pain, see Chapter 23, Pelvis and Genitourinary System: Penis, Scrotum, and Prostate, pp. 693–700 and Chapter 24, Pelvis and Genitourinary System: Vulva, Vagina, Uterus, and Adnexa, pp. 736–744.

Possible common causes include **diverticulitis** (inflammation or infection of the diverticula), **colitis** (inflammation of the colon, autoimmune or infectious), **ovarian cyst/torsion**, **kidney stones**, and **hernia** (weakness in the abdominal wall allowing protrusion).

Box 21-8. Left Lower Quadrant Abdominal Pain: High-Yield Health History Questions

Questions	Rationale
Could you describe where exactly you're feeling the pain, how long it typically lasts, and how severe it is, using a scale from 1 to 10 where 1 is very mild and 10 is the most severe?	*LLQ pain with tenderness:* could be diverticulitis or colitis *Sudden, severe, unilateral:* could be ovarian cysts/torsion *Severe, colicky pain in back or lower abdomen:* could be kidney stones *Pain and bulging in lower abdomen or groin area:* could be hernia
Have there been any changes in your bowel habits lately, such as experiencing diarrhea or becoming constipated?	*Diarrhea or constipation:* could be diverticulitis or colitis *No changes:* could be ovarian cysts/torsion, kidney stones, hernia
Have you been having fevers or chills, or have you noticed any other symptoms that might suggest an infection?	*Fever, chills:* could be diverticulitis or colitis; kidney stones if they lead to infection or obstruction *No systemic signs:* could be ovarian cysts/torsion, hernia
Did the pain start suddenly or have you had any injuries to that area recently?	*Acute, severe:* could be ovarian cysts/torsion, hernia *Gradual onset:* could be diverticulitis or colitis *Sudden onset, severe:* kidney stones may be lodged in the urinary tract
Have you noticed any unusual vaginal bleeding or discharge beyond your regular menstrual cycle?	Can help identify gynecologic causes of LLQ pain, such as ovarian cysts/torsion or pelvic inflammatory disease

Hypogastric (Suprapubic) Pain

Hypogastric pain is often used interchangeably with *suprapubic pain* and refers to pain or discomfort felt in the lower central region of the abdomen, below the umbilicus, and above the pubic bone. The lower central area of the abdomen contains several important organs, including the bladder, uterus, ovaries, prostate gland, and rectum, among others. Box 21-9 provides health history questions and the reasons behind them to separate potential diagnoses.

For GU causes of hypogastric or suprapubic pain, see Chapter 23, Pelvis and Genitourinary System: Penis, Scrotum, and Prostate, pp. 693–700 and Chapter 24, Pelvis and Genitourinary System: Vulva, Vagina, Uterus, and Adnexa, pp. 736–744.

Possible common causes include **urinary tract infection** (**UTI**), **bladder disorders** such as interstitial cystitis or bladder cancer, **gynecologic issues** (e.g., endometriosis, ovarian cysts, or PID), and **GI problems** (e.g., constipation, IBS, and IBD).[20]

Box 21-9. Hypogastric/Suprapubic Abdominal Pain: High-Yield Health History Questions

Questions	Rationale
Could you tell me exactly where your pain is, how long it lasts each time, and how intense it is on a scale from 1 to 10 where 1 is very mild and 10 is the most severe?	*Burning sensation or discomfort during urination:* could be urinary tract infection (UTI) *Chronic pelvic pain that may worsen with a full bladder:* can be interstitial cystitis or bladder cancer *Cyclic or intermittent pain that worsens during menstruation or sexual activity:* can be endometriosis, ovarian cysts, or pelvic inflammatory disease (PID) *Diffuse or crampy pain that may be associated with bowel movements:* can be constipation, irritable bowel syndrome (IBS), or inflammatory bowel disease (IBD)
Have you noticed any changes in how often you need to urinate, or is there a sudden need to go that wasn't there before?	*Increased frequency or urgency:* can be UTIs and bladder disorders *Painful or difficult urination:* can be gynecologic conditions *No changes in urinary habits:* can be gastrointestinal (GI) conditions
Are you experiencing any unusual bleeding or discharge that is different from your normal menstrual cycle?	*Abnormal bleeding or discharge:* can be endometriosis or ovarian cysts *Foul-smelling discharge or bleeding after sexual activity:* can be PID *No vaginal symptoms:* can be bladder or GI conditions
Have there been any recent changes in your bowel movements, like new cases of constipation or diarrhea?	*Changes in bowel habits or passage of mucus with stools:* can be constipation, IBS, or IBD may cause *No bowel changes:* can be bladder or gynecologic conditions
Do you have a history of any medical issues or procedures involving your pelvic region that we should be aware of?	*Previous UTI or bladder disorders:* may suggest a recurrent or chronic condition *Previous endometriosis or ovarian cysts:* increases the likelihood of these conditions *History of IBS or IBD:* suggests these conditions as the cause

Nausea and Vomiting

Nausea, often described as "having a queasy sensation in the stomach," may progress to retching and vomiting. *Retching* describes involuntary spasm of the stomach, diaphragm, and esophagus that precedes and culminates in *vomiting*, the forceful expulsion of gastric contents out of the mouth. Some patients may not actually vomit but raise esophageal or gastric contents without nausea or retching, called *regurgitation*. See Box 21-10 for targeted health history questions to help pinpoint potential diagnoses.

Gastroenteritis (inflammation of the stomach and intestines caused by viral or bacterial infection) is one of the most common disorders that present with vomiting as a prominent symptom followed by **food poisoning** and **medication side effects**. Vomiting and nausea with constipation or *obstipation* (severe constipation with inability to pass both stool and gas) are indicative of a bowel obstruction and warrant further workup.

Box 21-10. Nausea and Vomiting: High-Yield Health History Questions

Domain	Questions	Rationale
Onset and duration	*Can you share when you first began feeling nauseous and when the vomiting started? How long have these symptoms been present?*	*Acute onset:* suggests an infection or food poisoning *Chronic symptoms:* could indicate a more serious underlying condition, (e.g., gastroparesis or gastrointestinal [GI] obstruction)
Frequency and timing	*How frequently are you experiencing nausea and vomiting? Do you notice it happening at certain times of the day or after specific activities or events?*	More frequent in the morning or after eating could suggest gastroparesis or an ulcer
Associated symptoms	*Along with nausea and vomiting, are there other issues you're dealing with, like stomach pain, fever, diarrhea, or headaches?*	*Abdominal pain:* could suggest obstruction or inflammatory condition *Fever:* could indicate infection *Diarrhea:* could suggest a viral or bacterial infection *Headache:* could indicate migraine or other neurologic condition
Precipitating factors	*Have you noticed anything that tends to make your nausea and vomiting worse, like certain foods, smells, or types of movement? Is there anything that seems to alleviate these symptoms?*	*Worsening after eating certain foods or smelling certain odors:* could suggest a food intolerance or sensitivity *Worse with movement:* could indicate vertigo or other balance disorders
Medication history	*Are you taking any medications or supplements, even those that are over-the-counter? It would be helpful to know if any of these might be related to your symptoms.*	*Chemotherapy drugs, opioids, and antibiotics:* can cause nausea and vomiting as a side effect *Over-the-counter medications and supplements (e.g., aspirin or iron supplements):* can also cause GI irritation and lead to nausea and vomiting

Hematemesis

Clinical presentation of *hematemesis* (vomiting blood) can range from slight blood traces to copious bright red bleeding, often indicative of upper GI tract issues. The appearance of the vomit (e.g., bright red or coffee ground) along with symptoms like abdominal pain or lightheadedness, helps identify the severity and source of bleeding (Box 21-11).

PUD (sores in the lining of the stomach or small intestine caused by *Helicobacter pylori* infection or long-term use of nonsteroidal anti-inflammatory drugs [NSAIDs]), and **esophageal varices** (swollen veins in the lining of the esophagus, often caused by chronic liver disease such as cirrhosis) are two of the most common causes of hematemesis. Less common causes include **Mallory–Weiss tear** (tear in the lining of the esophagus caused by severe vomiting or retching), **gastritis** (inflammation of the stomach lining, often caused by alcohol use, NSAID use, or infection), **gastric cancer**, and certain **medications** (e.g., **blood thinners**).

Box 21-11. Hematemesis: High-Yield Health History Questions

Domain	Questions	Rationale
Onset and duration	*Could you tell me when you first noticed vomiting blood, and how long this has been going on?*	*Acute onset:* may suggest a bleeding ulcer *Chronic cases:* could indicate a more serious underlying condition (e.g., cirrhosis or esophageal varices)
Characteristics	*What does the blood you vomited look like in terms of color and amount?*	*Bright red:* could suggest active bleeding in the upper gastrointestinal (GI) tract *Darker or coffee-ground–like:* could indicate a slower, chronic bleed
Associated symptoms	*Besides vomiting blood, are you feeling any other symptoms like stomach pain, feeling dizzy, or lightheaded?*	*Abdominal pain:* could suggest peptic ulcer disease (PUD) *Dizziness or lightheadedness:* could indicate hypovolemia or shock from significant blood loss
Precipitating factors	*Have you identified anything in particular that seems to cause these episodes of vomiting blood, like eating certain foods, coughing, or physical exertion?*	*Postprandial:* could suggest PUD or esophagitis *Occurs with coughing:* could indicate bleeding from the respiratory system
Medical history	*Do you have any previous medical conditions related to your digestive system or liver, such as gastritis, cirrhosis, or inflammatory bowel disease?*	*GI conditions (e.g., gastritis or PUD):* can lead to upper GI tract bleeding *Liver conditions (e.g., cirrhosis):* can cause bleeding from esophageal varices

Hematochezia and Melena

Patients may report the presence of blood in their stool (*hematochezia*) or black, tarry stools (*melena*). Hematochezia often results from bleeding in the lower GI tract and may present as bright red blood, suggesting a more acute or active source of bleeding. On the other hand, melena, characterized by black and tarry stools, usually indicates bleeding in the upper GI tract, where blood has had time to be digested and altered during its passage through the intestines. The distinct presentations of hematochezia and melena can suggest different underlying causes, ranging from benign to potentially serious conditions (Box 21-12 and Table 21-6).

Common causes of hematochezia include **hemorrhoids** (swollen veins in the lowest part of the rectum and anus), **diverticulosis** (small bulges or pockets in the lining of the digestive system), and **IBD** like Crohn's disease and ulcerative colitis. **Anal fissures** (small tears in the lining of the anus) and **colorectal cancer** are also notable causes. For melena, common causes include **PUD**, **gastritis**, and **esophageal varices** (typically due to liver cirrhosis). Less common causes can include **gastric cancer** and certain **medications** like blood thinners.

Box 21-12. Hematochezia and Melena: High-Yield Health History Questions

Domain	Questions	Rationale
Onset and duration	*Could you tell me when you first noticed blood in your stool or black, tarry stools, and how long this has been going on?*	*Acute-onset hematochezia:* may suggest a lower gastrointestinal (GI) source (e.g., diverticulosis or hemorrhoids) *Melena:* often indicates an upper GI source (e.g., ulcer)

Domain	Questions	Rationale
Characteristics	*What does the blood or stool look like? Are there any changes in the consistency or color?*	*Bright red blood in stool (hematochezia):* typically indicates a lower GI source *Black, tarry stools (melena):* suggest upper GI source and slower bleeding
Associated symptoms	*Besides changes in your stool, are you experiencing any abdominal pain, weight loss, or changes in appetite?*	*Abdominal pain or weight loss:* could suggest inflammatory bowel disease (IBD), malignancies, or other serious conditions
Precipitating factors	*Have you identified anything that seems to trigger these symptoms, like certain foods, medications, or physical activities?*	*Certain foods, medications (e.g., nonsteroidal anti-inflammatory drugs [NSAIDs]), or activities:* can exacerbate gastrointestinal (GI) bleeding
Medical history	*Do you have any previous medical conditions related to your digestive system, liver, or blood disorders?*	*Diverticulosis, IBD, or coagulopathies:* can lead to hematochezia or melena *Liver diseases:* could be associated with upper GI bleeding
Medication and lifestyle	*Are you currently taking any medications, especially pain relievers or blood thinners? Do you consume alcohol or smoke?*	*NSAIDs, anticoagulants, and other medications:* increase risk of GI bleeding *Alcohol and smoking:* risk factors for GI disorders that can lead to hematochezia or melena

Dysphagia and/or Odynophagia

Patients may report difficulty swallowing from impaired passage of solid foods or liquids from the mouth to the stomach, or *dysphagia*. Food seems to stick or *"not go down right,"* suggesting motility disorders or structural anomalies. The sensation of a lump or foreign body in the throat at rest that improves or disappears with swallowing, called a *globus sensation*, is not true dysphagia. See Box 21-13 for high-yield health history questions to assist in distinguishing among possible diagnoses.

Common causes include **GERD** (reflux of stomach acid into the esophagus due to weakened lower esophageal sphincter), **esophagitis** (often due to GERD, infection, or medication), **hiatal hernia** (protrusion of a portion of the stomach into the chest through a hole in the diaphragm), **eosinophilic esophagitis** (caused by build-up of eosinophil white blood cells in the esophagus), and **pharyngitis** (often caused by a viral or bacterial infection).

A less common cause is **stricture** (narrowing of the esophagus due to scar tissue, often due to GERD or radiation therapy). Rare causes are **achalasia** (failure of the muscles in the lower esophageal sphincter to relax properly, causing difficulty swallowing) and **Zenker diverticulum** (pouch that develops in the esophagus, which can collect food and cause difficulty swallowing and discomfort).

For types of dysphagia, see Table 21-3, Dysphagia, p. 660.

Box 21-13. Dysphagia and Odynophagia: High-Yield Health History Questions

Domain	Questions	Rationale
Onset and duration	*Could you tell me when you first noticed you were having trouble swallowing and how long this has been going on?*	*Acute onset:* may suggest an obstruction or foreign body in the throat *Chronic cases:* could indicate a more serious underlying condition (e.g., esophageal cancer or neurologic disorders)
Type	*Is it harder for you to swallow solids, liquids, or are both equally difficult?*	*Difficulty swallowing solids:* could suggest esophageal obstruction *Difficulty swallowing liquids:* could indicate a motility disorder or neurologic condition
Associated symptoms	*Have you been experiencing any other related symptoms, like unexpected weight loss, food coming back up, or a burning sensation in your chest?*	*Weight loss:* could suggest underlying malignancy *Regurgitation or heartburn:* could indicate gastroesophageal reflux disease (GERD) or hiatal hernia
Location	*Can you pinpoint where the swallowing difficulty seems to start? Is it in your throat, chest, or down toward your stomach?*	*Throat or upper chest:* could suggest a problem with the esophagus or upper airway *Lower chest or abdomen:* could indicate an issue with the lower esophageal sphincter or stomach
Precipitating factors	*Have you noticed if certain types of food or body positions make it more difficult to swallow?*	*Occurs with certain foods or after eating:* could suggest mechanical obstruction or motility disorder *Occurs with certain positions or activities:* could indicate a muscular or neurologic problem
Medical history	*Do you have any existing neurologic or digestive conditions, like a history of stroke, Parkinson disease, or acid reflux?*	*Neurologic conditions:* can affect muscles involved in swallowing *Gastrointestinal conditions (e.g., GERD or hiatal hernia):* can cause reflux and irritation of the esophagus

Diarrhea

Diarrhea is defined as painless loose or watery stools during at least 75% of defecations for the prior 3 months, with symptom onset at least 6 months prior to diagnosis.[21,22] Stool volume may increase to more than 200 g in 24 hours. *Acute diarrhea* is diarrhea that lasts less than 14 days, *persistent diarrhea* lasts 14 to 30 days, and *chronic diarrhea* lasts more than 30 days. See Box 21-14 for high-yield health history questions to ask in a patient presenting with this symptom.

Common causes include **viral gastroenteritis**, **bacterial gastroenteritis** (Infection, inflammation, and toxin production), **food intolerance** (enzyme deficiency, malabsorption, or sensitivity to specific foods), **IBS**, **IBD**, **celiac disease** (autoimmune reaction to gluten, causing damage to the small intestine), **medication side effects** (e.g., antibiotics, antacids, laxatives), and **parasitic infections**.[23]

See Table 21-4, Diarrhea, pp. 661–663.

Box 21-14. Diarrhea: High-Yield Health History Questions

Domain	Questions	Rationale
Onset and duration	*When did the diarrhea begin, and how long has it been occurring?*	*Acute onset:* may suggest infection or food poisoning *Chronic symptoms:* could indicate a more serious underlying condition (e.g., inflammatory bowel disease [IBD] or irritable bowel syndrome [IBS])
Characteristics	*Can you tell me how often you have bowel movements, and what the amount and consistency usually look like?*	*Watery stools:* could suggest a viral or bacterial infection *Greasy or fatty stools:* could indicate malabsorption or pancreatic insufficiency
Associated symptoms	*Along with diarrhea, are you feeling any abdominal pain, fever, nausea, or have you been vomiting?*	*Abdominal pain:* could suggest inflammatory or infectious cause *Fever:* could indicate infection *Nausea and vomiting:* could suggest viral or bacterial infection *Bloody stools:* could indicate IBD or infection
Precipitating factors	*Have you noticed if certain foods, stress, or activities seem to trigger episodes of diarrhea?*	*Occurs after eating certain foods:* could suggest a food intolerance or sensitivity *Occurs during times of stress:* could indicate IBS
Medication history	*Are you currently taking any medications or supplements that may be affecting your bowel movements?*	Certain antibiotics and laxatives can disrupt the normal gut microbiota and lead to diarrhea as a side effect
Travel history	*Have you traveled abroad recently, and, if so, where to?*	Certain countries or regions have a higher risk for specific infections, such as cholera in areas with poor sanitation or *Giardia* in areas with contaminated water

Constipation

According to the Rome IV criteria, constipation must have been present for the past three months, with symptoms beginning at least six months before diagnosis and at least two of the following conditions must be met: less than three bowel movements per week, 25% or more defecations with either straining or sensation of incomplete evacuation, lumpy or hard stools, or the need for manual facilitation during defecation.[21,22] See Box 21-15 for high-yield health history questions to ask in a patient presenting with this symptom.

Lifestyle-related causes include inadequate fiber intake or a low-fiber diet, insufficient fluid intake or dehydration, and a sedentary lifestyle or lack of physical activity. **Medical causes** encompass IBS with predominant constipation (IBS-C), functional constipation[26,27] or chronic idiopathic constipation, slow transit constipation or *colonic inertia*, pelvic floor dysfunction or dyssynergic defecation, neurologic disorders such as Parkinson disease and multiple sclerosis, and metabolic and endocrine disorders like hypothyroidism and diabetes. **Medication-induced causes** involve the use of opioids, anticholinergics, calcium-channel blockers, and iron supplements.

See Table 21-5, Constipation, p. 664.

Box 21-15. Constipation: High-Yield Health History Questions

Domain	Questions	Rationale
Onset and duration	*When did the constipation begin, and for how long has it been a concern?*	*Acute onset:* may suggest a recent change in diet or medication *Chronic symptoms:* could indicate an underlying medical condition (e.g., hypothyroidism or irritable bowel syndrome)
Characteristics	*Can you tell me how often you go to the bathroom, and what the amount and consistency usually look like?*	*Infrequent or small bowel movements:* could suggest a lack of fiber or hydration *Hard, lumpy stools:* could indicate a more severe case
Associated symptoms	*Along with the constipation, are you experiencing any other discomforts, like stomach pain, feeling full, or feeling queasy?*	*Abdominal pain or bloating:* could indicate an obstruction or other gastrointestinal issue *Nausea or vomiting:* could suggest a more severe case
Lifestyle factors	*How would you describe your activity level and how much fiber you usually eat?*	*Sedentary lifestyle and low-fiber diet:* can increase risk
Medication history	*Are you taking any medications or supplements, even those available over the counter, that could be affecting your digestion?*	Opioids and certain anticholinergics can cause constipation as a side effect
Medical history	*Do you have any medical issues like an underactive thyroid, diabetes, or multiple sclerosis?*	*Neurologic conditions (e.g., multiple sclerosis):* can affect the muscles involved in bowel movements *Endocrine disorders (e.g., hypothyroidism or diabetes):* can alter the balance of hormones and lead to constipation

Jaundice

Jaundice (*icterus*) is a yellowish discoloration of the skin and sclerae from increased levels of *bilirubin*, a bile pigment derived chiefly from the breakdown of hemoglobin. Jaundice is usually apparent when plasma bilirubin is more than 3 mg/dL. The yellow color may have a greenish tinge in patients with longstanding jaundice, due to oxidation of bilirubin to biliverdin.[28]

Carotenemia, the presence of the orange pigment *carotene* in the blood due to ingestion of carrots, presents as a yellow discoloration of the skin, especially palms and soles, but not the sclerae or mucous membranes.[28]

Mechanisms of jaundice are listed in Box 21-16. Pay attention to patients with risk factors for liver disease and those on certain medications that can potentially cause liver damage (Boxes 21-17 and 21-18).

Box 21-16. Mechanisms of Jaundice

- Increased production of bilirubin
- Decreased uptake of bilirubin by hepatocytes
- Decreased ability by liver to conjugate bilirubin
- Decreased excretion of bilirubin into bile, resulting in absorption of conjugated bilirubin back into blood

Box 21-17. Risk Factors for Liver Disease

- *Infectious hepatitis:* travel or meals in areas of poor sanitation, ingestion of contaminated water or foodstuffs (*hepatitis A*); parenteral or mucous membrane exposure to infectious body fluids such as blood, serum, semen, and saliva, especially through sexual contact with an infected partner or use of shared needles for injection drug use (*hepatitis B*); illicit injection drug use or blood transfusion (*hepatitis C*). Hepatitis B is also endemic in certain regions of the world and can present in patients with no risk factors.
- *Nonalcoholic steatohepatitis:* in patients with metabolic syndrome
- *Alcoholic hepatitis* or *alcoholic cirrhosis*: screen patients carefully about alcohol use
- *Toxic liver damage:* from medications, industrial solvents, environmental toxins, or some anesthetic agents
- *Gallbladder disease* or *prior surgery:* may result in extrahepatic biliary obstruction
- *Hereditary disorders:* such as family history of hemolytic anemia or liver disease (e.g., hemochromatosis, α-1-antitrypsin deficiency, Wilson disease)

Box 21-18. Medications and Supplements Associated with Liver Damage and Jaundice

- Acetaminophen
- Amiodarone (an antiarrhythmic drug)
- Anabolic steroids and oral contraceptives
- Antibiotics (e.g., penicillins, sulfonamides, tetracyclines)
- Antiepileptic drugs (e.g., valproate, phenytoin)
- Antifungal medications (e.g., ketoconazole, fluconazole)
- Antipsychotic medications (e.g., chlorpromazine, haloperidol)
- Antithyroid medications (e.g., propylthiouracil, methimazole)
- Antitubercular medications (e.g., isoniazid, rifampin, pyrazinamide)
- Antiviral drugs for HIV and hepatitis C
- Chemotherapy drugs and other cancer medications
- Herbal and dietary supplements (e.g., kava [*Piper methysticum*], black cohosh [*Actaea racemosa* or *Cimicifuga racemosa*])
- Immunosuppressants (e.g., methotrexate, azathioprine)
- Nonsteroidal anti-inflammatory drugs (NSAIDs)
- Statins (cholesterol-lowering drugs)

For high-yield health history questions to ask in a patient presenting with this symptom, see Box 21-19.

The most common causes in adults are **gallstones or biliary obstruction**, **alcoholic liver disease** (liver damage from chronic alcohol use), **NAFLD**, **viral hepatitis** (liver inflammation and damage from viral infection), and **medications or drug-induced liver injury**.

Box 21-19. Jaundice: High-Yield Health History Questions

Domain	Questions	Rationale
Onset and duration	*When did you first notice the yellowing of your skin or eyes, and how long has this been apparent?*	*Acute onset:* may suggest obstruction or infection *Chronic symptoms:* could indicate a more serious underlying condition (e.g., liver disease or pancreatic cancer)
Associated symptoms	*Besides the change in color, are you feeling any stomach pain, fever, or an itch that won't go away?*	*Abdominal pain:* could suggest blockage or inflammation in the bile ducts or liver *Fever:* could indicate infection *Itching:* can occur due to the accumulation of bilirubin in the skin
Medical history	*Do you have any past liver or gallbladder issues like hepatitis, cirrhosis, or gallstones?*	Liver or gallbladder conditions (e.g., hepatitis or cirrhosis) can impair liver function and lead to the buildup of bilirubin in the blood, causing jaundice; ask about risk factors for liver diseases (Box 21-17)
Medication history	*Are you taking any medications or supplements, even nonprescription ones, that could be affecting your liver?*	Certain medications or supplements can cause liver damage and lead to jaundice; see Box 21-18
Alcohol use	*Could you tell me about your alcohol consumption habits, including any recent heavy drinking sessions?*	Heavy or chronic alcohol consumption can cause liver damage and lead to jaundice as well as other complications such as cirrhosis or liver cancer
Travel history	*Have you been on any trips abroad lately; if so, where did you go?*	Certain countries or regions have a higher risk for specific infections, such as hepatitis A in areas with poor sanitation
Family history	*Is there a history of liver conditions or jaundice-related illnesses in your family?*	Certain liver conditions (e.g., hereditary hemochromatosis or Wilson disease) can run in families and increase risk of liver damage and jaundice

PHYSICAL EXAMINATION: GENERAL APPROACH

Once you have carefully interviewed the patient, gathering more information through the physical examination (PE) helps narrow the possible causes to specific areas and/or organ systems. A complete PE includes a review of patients' vital signs and an inspection of other body areas outside of the GI system, particularly the GU system, cardiopulmonary system, and skin.

To begin, explain the steps for examining the abdomen to the patient and ensure you have good lighting. The patient should have an empty bladder. Pay special attention when draping to expose the abdomen, as pictured throughout, and detailed in Box 21-20.

Box 21-20. Tips for Examining the Abdomen

- Make the patient comfortable in the supine position, with a pillow under their head (and optionally under their knees).
- Ask the patient to keep their arms at their sides. When arms are above the head, the abdominal wall stretches and tightens, which hinders palpation.
- *Draping the patient.* Place the drape or sheet at the level of the patient's symphysis pubis, then expose their abdomen by raising their gown to just below the nipple line above the xiphoid process. The groin should be visible, but the genitalia should remain covered. The abdominal muscles should be relaxed to enhance all aspects of the examination, especially palpation.
- Before you begin, ask the patient to point to any areas of pain so you can examine these areas last.
- Warm your hands by rubbing them together or placing them under lukewarm water.
- Approach the patient calmly and avoid quick, unexpected movements.
- Avoid having long fingernails that can scratch or scrape their skin.
- Position yourself at the patient's *right side* and proceed in a systematic fashion with inspection, percussion, and palpation.
- Mentally visualize each organ in the region you are examining.
- *Watch the patient's face for any signs of pain or discomfort.*
- If necessary, distract the patient with conversation or questions. If they are frightened or ticklish, begin palpation with their hand under yours. After a few moments, slip your hand underneath to palpate directly.

TECHNIQUES OF EXAMINATION

Key Components of the Abdominal Examination

- Inspect the abdomen.
- Auscultate for bowel sounds.
- Auscultate for abdominal bruits.
- Percuss the abdomen.
- Palpate lightly in all four quadrants.
- Palpate deeply in all four quadrants.
- Estimate liver size by percussion.
- Palpate the liver edge.
- Percuss for splenic enlargement.
- Palpate for the splenic edge.
- Palpate for aortic pulsations.

Inspect the Abdomen

From the right side of the bed, inspect the surface, contours, and movements of the abdomen. Note for the abdominal features highlighted in Box 21-21. Watch for bulges or peristalsis. Try to also lower your viewing plane by bending over or stooping down so that you can observe the abdomen tangentially (Fig. 21-8).

See Table 21-7, Localized Bulges in the Abdominal Wall, p. 666 and Table 21-8, Protuberant Abdomens, p. 667.

Auscultate for Bowel Sounds

Auscultate the abdomen before performing percussion or palpation, maneuvers that may alter the characteristics of the bowel sounds. Place the diaphragm of your stethoscope gently on the abdomen for a maximum of 5 minutes (Fig. 21-9). Because bowel sounds are widely transmitted through the abdomen, listening

See Table 21-9, Sounds in the Abdomen, p. 668.

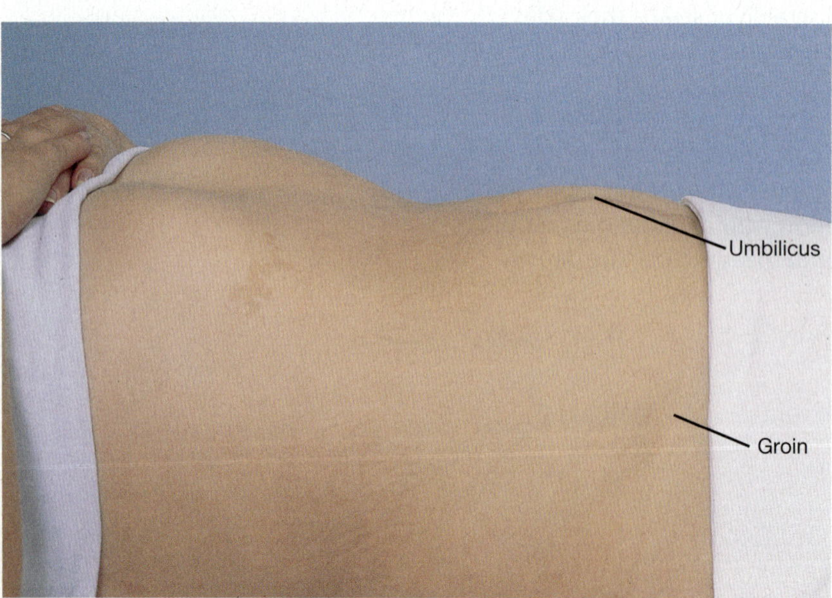

FIGURE 21-8. Inspecting the contours of the abdomen.

Box 21-21. Clinical Observations and Implications in Abdominal Examination

Abdominal Feature	Observations and Clinical Implications
Skin assessment	
■ Temperature	Warm is normal; cool and clammy may indicate circulatory problems.
■ Color	Check for bruises, erythema, or jaundice.
Integumentary changes	
■ Scars	Describe or diagram location; may indicate previous surgeries or trauma.
■ Striae	Old silver striae are normal; pink–purple striae may suggest Cushing syndrome.
Vascular indicators	
■ Dilated veins	Some small veins are normal; extensive dilatation may suggest portal hypertension (*caput medusae*) or inferior vena cava obstruction.
Skin lesions	
■ Rashes or ecchymoses	Absence is normal; ecchymosis may signify intraperitoneal or retroperitoneal hemorrhage.
Abdominal wall features	
■ Umbilicus	Normal contour; inflammation or bulges may suggest hernia.
■ Contour	Flat, rounded, protuberant, or scaphoid; protuberance may indicate conditions (see Table 21-8).
■ Bulges	No significant bulges should be present; bulging flanks suggest ascites and other bulges may indicate hernias or masses.
■ Symmetry	Symmetric is normal; asymmetry may suggest hernia, enlarged organ, or mass.
Organ enlargement	
■ Visible organs/ masses	None are typically visible; enlarged liver or spleen may descend below the rib cage; lower abdominal masses or hernias may be present.
Pulsations	
■ Aortic pulsation	Normal pulsation may be visible; increased pulsations may indicate abdominal aortic aneurysm or increased pulse pressure.

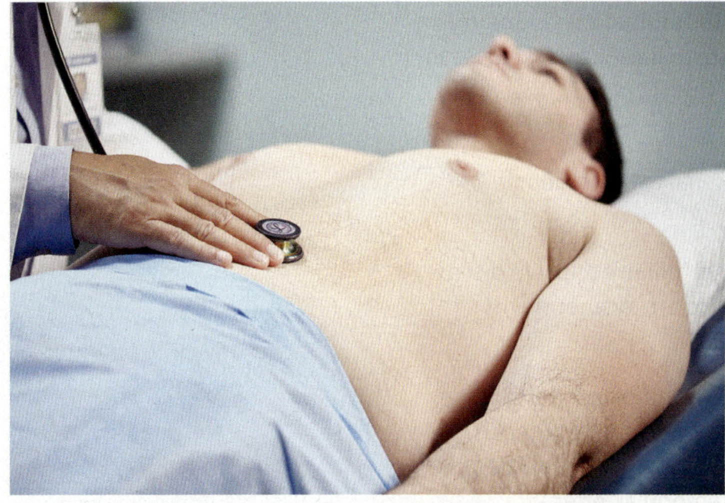

FIGURE 21-9. Auscultating the abdomen.

Box 21-22. Clinical Interpretation of Abdominal Auscultation Findings

Abdominal Auscultation Features	Observations and Clinical Significance
Bowel sounds	
■ Normoactive	Clicks and gurgles occurring 5 to 34 times per minute are considered normal.
■ Hypoactive	Frequency of fewer than 5 sounds per minute suggests hypoactivity.
■ Hyperactive	Frequency of more than 34 sounds per minute indicate hyperactivity, often referred to as *borborygmi* or more commonly as "stomach growling."
Abdominal bruits	Turbulent flow (bruits) over a pulsatile abdominal mass may suggest abdominal aortic aneurysm; 4% to 20% of healthy individuals have abdominal bruits (see Fig. 21-11).[29]
Friction rubs	Rare but can occur over the liver, spleen, or abdominal mass; associated with hepatoma, gonococcal infection around the liver, splenic infarction, and pancreatic carcinoma.

in one area, such as the RLQ, is usually sufficient. Listen for the auscultation features in Box 21-22.

Although auscultation of the abdomen is common, it might be of limited use. Changes in bowel sounds heard on auscultation are typically nonspecific and nondiagnostic.[30,31]

Auscultate for Abdominal Bruits

Abdominal bruits are characterized as distinctive whooshing or swishing sounds that are auscultated over the abdomen using a stethoscope. These auditory phenomena indicate turbulent blood flow within the abdominal vasculature. Common areas are highlighted in Box 21-23 and in Fig. 21-10.

Common causes include stenosis, aneurysms, or (occasionally) an increase in blood flow due to certain conditions such as portal hypertension or arteriovenous malformations.

Box 21-23. Auscultation Sites for Detecting Abdominal Bruits

Artery	Area of Auscultation	Possible Indications of Bruits
Aorta	Midline of the abdomen, may be slightly left of center in certain individuals	Abdominal aortic aneurysm, aortoiliac occlusive disease
Renal arteries	Above and lateral to umbilicus on both sides	Renal artery stenosis
Iliac arteries	Lower abdomen, along common iliac arteries course	Aortoiliac occlusive disease, iliac artery aneurysms
Femoral arteries	Groin area, midway between hip and pubic bones	Peripheral arterial disease, femoral artery stenosis, other vascular abnormalities in femoral arteries

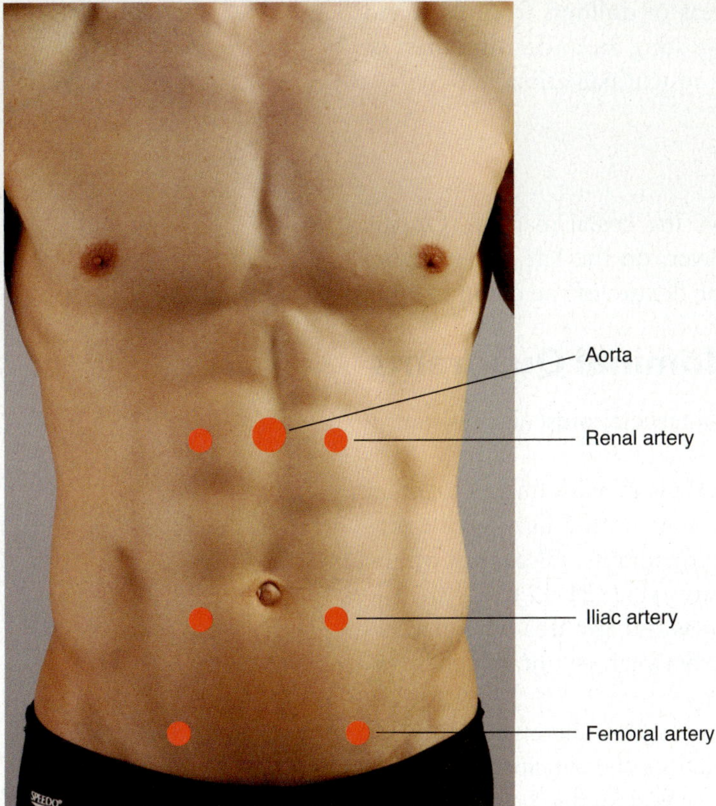

FIGURE 21-10. Abdominal auscultatory areas for bruits.

While sometimes normal in healthy individuals, abdominal bruits more commonly indicate underlying vascular pathologies. Their presence usually warrants further clinical evaluation and management to identify and address potential vascular issues.

Percuss the Abdomen

Percussion helps you assess the amount and distribution of gas in the abdomen, viscera, and masses that are solid or fluid-filled, and the size of the liver and spleen.

Percuss the abdomen lightly in all four quadrants to determine the distribution of *tympany* and *dullness* (Fig. 21-11). Tympany usually predominates

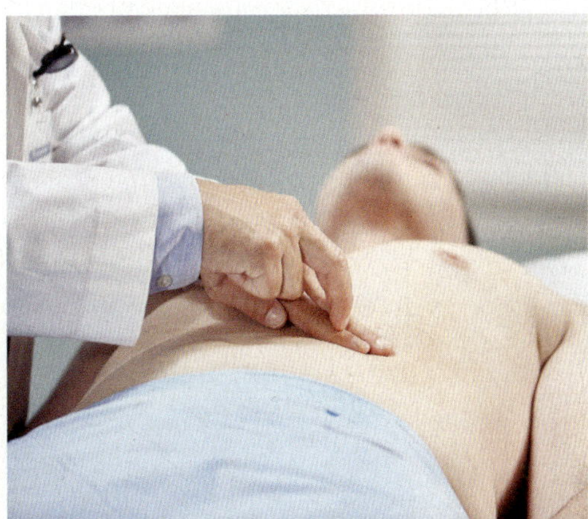

FIGURE 21-11. Percussing the abdomen.

because of gas in the GI tract, but scattered areas of dullness from fluid and feces are also common. Note any dull areas suggesting an underlying mass or enlarged organ. This observation will guide subsequent palpation.

A protuberant abdomen that is tympanitic throughout suggests intestinal obstruction or paralytic ileus. See Table 21-8, Protuberant Abdomens, p. 667.

Briefly percuss the lower anterior chest above the costal margins. On the right, you will usually find the dullness of the liver, on the left, the tympany that overlies the gastric air bubble and the splenic flexure of the colon.

Palpate Lightly in All Four Abdominal Quadrants

Gentle palpation aids detection of abdominal tenderness, muscular resistance, and some superficial organs and masses.

Keeping your hand and forearm on a horizontal plane, with fingers together and flat on the abdominal wall, palpate the abdomen with a light gentle dipping motion. As you move your hand to different quadrants, raise it just off the skin. Gliding smoothly, palpate in all four quadrants (Fig. 21-12).

Identify any superficial organs, masses, or hernias and any area of tenderness or increased resistance to palpation. Differentiate between voluntary and involuntary guarding of the abdominal muscles.

Voluntary guarding occurs when a patient consciously or subconsciously tenses the abdominal muscles, often as a reaction to anxiety or the anticipation of pain. This type of guarding can usually be reduced with techniques that help the patient relax:

- Ask them to bend their lower extremities at the hip to make the abdominal muscles less tense.
- Ask them to mouth-breathe with their jaws wide open.
- Palpate after asking them to exhale, which usually relaxes the abdominal muscles.

In contrast, *involuntary guarding* is an automatic, reflexive contraction of the abdominal muscles that the patient cannot consciously control. It often indicates peritoneal irritation (peritonitis) or underlying inflammation within the abdomen. Unlike voluntary guarding, involuntary guarding does not diminish with relaxation techniques.

See Table 21-10. Tender Abdomens, pp. 669–670.

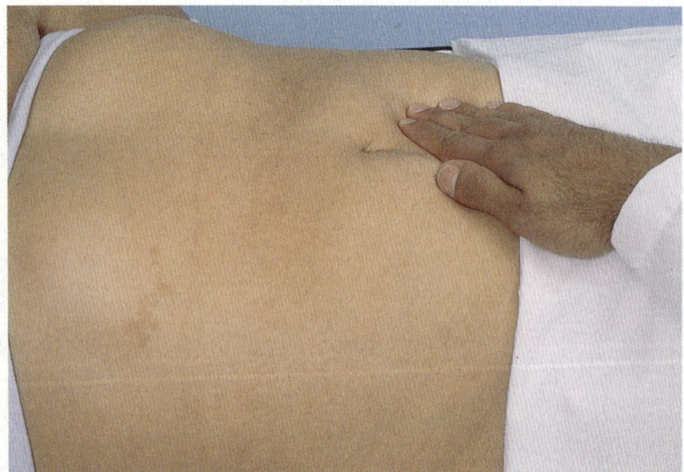

FIGURE 21-12. Using one hand to lightly palpate the abdomen in all four quadrants to assess for tenderness, surface masses, or rigidity.

Palpate Deeply in All Four Abdominal Quadrants

Deep palpation is usually required to delineate the liver edge, kidneys, and abdominal masses. Use one hand over the other to perform this technique. Again, using the palmar surfaces of your fingers, press down in all four quadrants (Fig. 21-13). Identify any masses; note their location, size, shape, surface, consistency, tenderness, and pulsations, and any mobility with respiration or pressure from the examining hand (Box 21-24). Correlate your findings from palpation with your percussion notes.

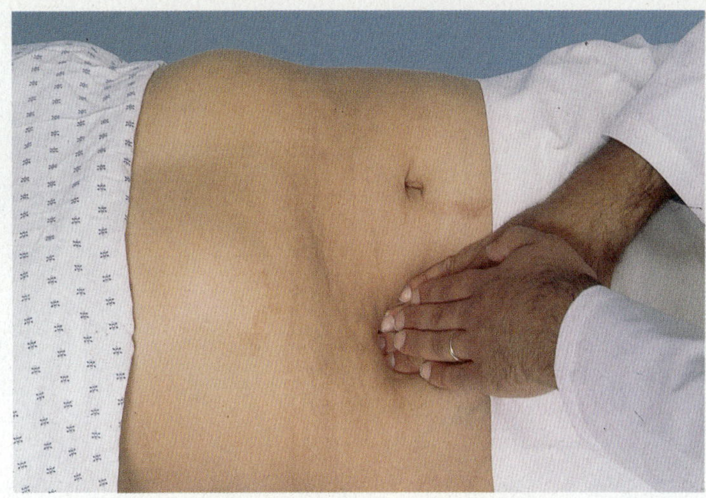

FIGURE 21-13. Using two hands to deeply palpate the abdomen in all four quadrants to assess for masses, organ enlargement, or deep tenderness.

Box 21-24. Characterization of Palpable Abdominal Masses: Key Features and Considerations

Feature	Description	Characteristics/Examples
Origin	Organic	Arising from an organ (e.g., hepatomegaly, splenomegaly)
	Neoplastic	Benign or malignant tumors (e.g., lipoma, carcinoma)
	Functional	Physiologic changes (e.g., pregnancy, full bladder)
Consistency	Soft	Cystic or fluid-filled (e.g., ovarian cyst, abscess)
	Firm	Solid organs or fibrous tumors (e.g., fibroma, enlarged kidney)
	Hard	Malignancy or calcifications (e.g., hardened lymph nodes)
Location	Epigastric	Near the stomach (e.g., pancreatic mass)
	Periumbilical	Around the umbilicus (e.g., mesenteric lymphadenopathy)
	Hypogastric	Lower abdomen (e.g., bladder distention)
	Flank	Side of the abdomen (e.g., renal mass)
Mobility	Mobile	Moves with palpation (e.g., floating kidney)
	Fixed	Does not move, attached to structures (e.g., invasive carcinoma)
Reproducibility	Reproducible	Felt consistently on examinations (e.g., enlarged liver)
	Nonreproducible	Intermittent conditions (e.g., bowel obstruction)
Pulsations	Pulsatile	Vascular origin (e.g., aortic aneurysm)
	Nonpulsatile	Solid or cystic mass without vascular component
Associated symptoms	Asymptomatic	Discovered incidentally, no symptoms
	Symptomatic	Accompanied by symptoms like pain, weight loss

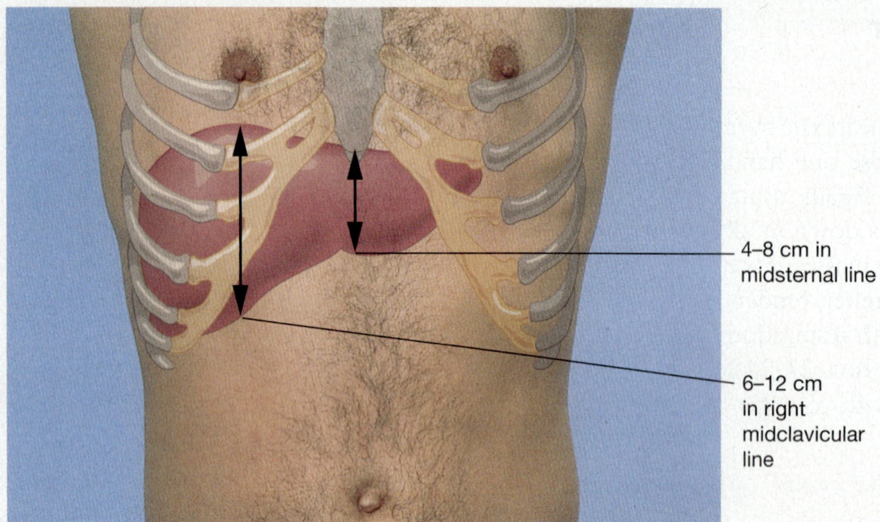

FIGURE 21-14. Area of percussion for estimating liver size along the right midclavicular line.

Estimate Liver Size by Percussion

Because the rib cage shelters most of the liver, direct assessment is limited. Liver size and shape can be estimated by palpation and percussion. Pressure from your palpating hand helps you evaluate the surface, consistency, and tenderness of the liver. Percussion helps you approximate liver size.

In chronic liver disease, finding an enlarged palpable liver edge below the ribs is suggestive of an enlarged liver and cirrhosis.[29]

Estimate the size of the liver by percussion. Measure the vertical span of liver dullness in the right midclavicular line after carefully locating the midclavicular line to improve accurate measurement (Fig. 21-14). Use a light to moderate percussion strike, because a heavier strike can lead to underestimation of liver size.[34]

Starting at a level well below the umbilicus in the RLQ (in an area of tympany, not dullness), percuss upward toward the liver. Identify the lower border of dullness in the midclavicular line (Fig. 21-15).

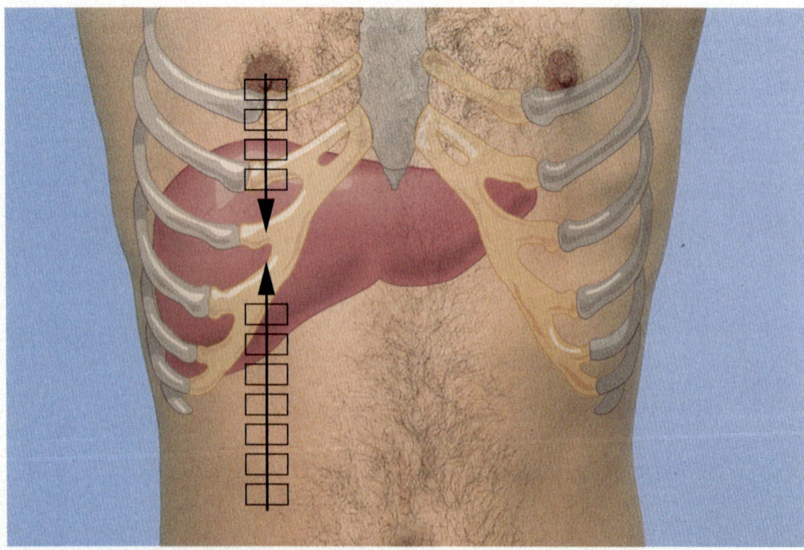

FIGURE 21-15. Percussing along the right midclavicular line to determine the upper and lower borders of liver dullness.

Next, identify the upper border of liver dullness. Start your examination at the nipple line and percuss downward along the midclavicular line. You are listening for a change from lung resonance to liver dullness. It may be necessary to gently displace the patient's breast to ensure that you start in a resonant area (Fig. 21-15). Once you detect the change in sound, mark this point. Next, identify the lower border of liver dullness at the same midclavicular line. The distance between these two points represents the vertical span of liver dullness, which should be measured in centimeters.

In adults, the normal liver span typically ranges from 6 to 12 cm in the midclavicular line. Estimates of liver span by percussion have a 60% to 70% correlation with actual span.

Palpate the Liver Edge

Palpate for the liver edge below the right costal margin. Place your right hand on the patient's right abdomen lateral to the rectus muscle, making light contact with your fingertips (Fig. 21-16). This is done to prevent mistaking the rectus muscle for the underlying and adjacent liver. Also place your hand well below where you would expect the lower border of the liver, which you previously percussed. Starting palpation too close to the right costal margin risks missing the lower edge of an enlarged liver that extends into the RLQ. Some examiners point their fingers up toward the patient's head, whereas others prefer a somewhat more oblique position. In either case, press gently in and up.

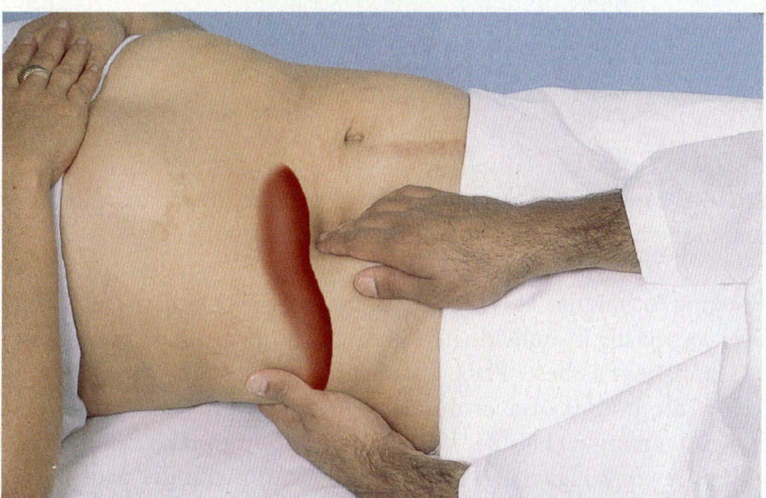

FIGURE 21-16. Palpating for the liver edge.

Ask the patient to take a deep breath. Try to feel the liver edge as the air-filled lungs and the diaphragm push the liver down to meet your fingertips. When palpable, the normal liver edge is soft, distinct in outline, and with a smooth surface. If you feel the edge, slightly lighten the pressure of your palpating hand so that the liver can slip under your fingerpads and you can feel its anterior surface. Note any tenderness (the normal liver may be slightly tender).

On inspiration, the liver is palpable about 3 cm below the right costal margin in the midclavicular line. Some patients breathe more with the chest than with the diaphragm. It may be helpful to ask such patients to *"breathe with the abdomen,"* which brings the liver, as well as the spleen and kidneys, into a palpable position during inspiration.

To palpate the liver edge, you may have to adapt your examining pressure to the thickness and resistance of the abdominal wall. If you cannot feel the edge, move your palpating hand closer to the costal margin and try again. A palpable liver edge does not reliably indicate hepatomegaly. Nevertheless, its examination is integral to your comprehensive physical assessment, as it helps you in identifying potential liver anomalies, establishing a baseline for future evaluations, and gathering information about the liver's overall health and the condition of surrounding structures.

See Table 21-11, Liver Enlargement: Apparent and Real, p. 671.

Trace the liver edge both laterally and medially. Palpation through the rectus muscles is especially difficult. Describe the liver edge and measure its distance from the right costal margin in the midclavicular line.

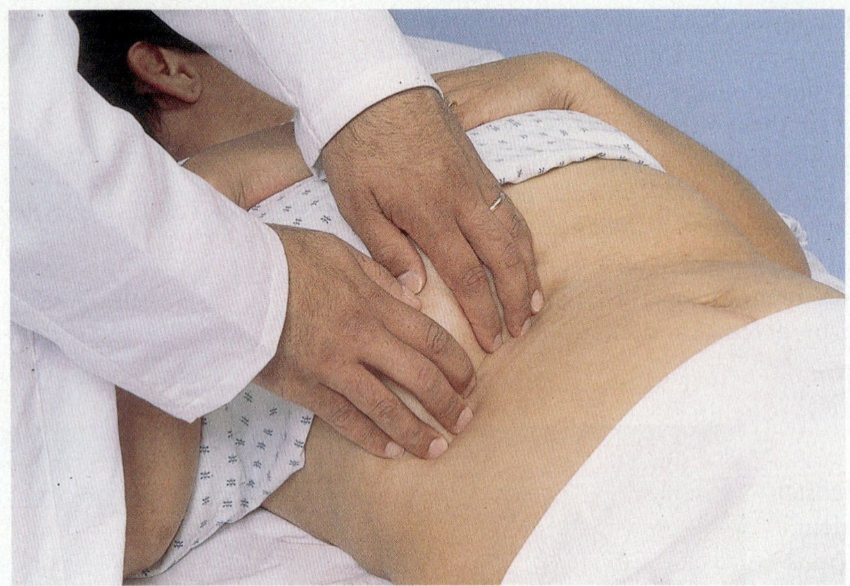

FIGURE 21-17. Positioning fingers along the costal margin in the hooking technique to prepare for palpating the liver edge.

FIGURE 21-18. Using the finger pads of both hands to palpate the liver edge during deep inspiration in the hooking technique.

Hooking Technique. This technique can be particularly useful for examining the liver, especially in individuals with a larger abdominal area. Stand to the right of the patient's chest. Place both hands, side by side, on their right abdomen below the border of liver dullness. Press in with your fingers and up toward the costal margin (Fig. 21-17). Ask the patient to take a deep breath. The liver edge shown in Figure 21-18 is palpable with the finger pads of both hands.

Percuss for Splenic Enlargement

When a spleen enlarges, it expands anteriorly, downward, and medially, often replacing the tympany of stomach and colon with the dullness of a solid organ. It then becomes palpable below the costal margin. Dullness to percussion suggests splenic enlargement but may be absent when an enlarged spleen lies above the costal margin. Continue to examine the patient from their right side.

The following two techniques may help you to detect *splenomegaly*.

Percussion is moderately accurate in detecting splenomegaly (sensitivity, 60% to 80%; specificity, 72% to 94%).[35]

Check for Splenic Enlargement along Traube's Space. Percuss the left lower anterior chest wall roughly from the border of cardiac dullness at rib 6 to the anterior axillary line and down to the costal margin, an area termed *Traube*, or *semilunar*, *space*. As you percuss along the routes marked by the arrows in Figures 21-19 and 21-20, you should note tympany. If tympany is prominent, especially laterally, splenomegaly is unlikely. Note that fluid or solids in the stomach or colon may cause dullness in the Traube space.

Check for a Splenic Percussion (Castell's Sign). Percuss the lowest interspace in the left anterior axillary line (Fig. 21-21). This area is usually tympanitic. Then ask the patient to take a deep breath to let their air-filled lungs and diaphragm push the spleen, and percuss again. When spleen size is normal, the percussion note usually remains tympanitic despite this downward displacement by the diaphragm.

A change in percussion note from tympany to dullness on inspiration is a *positive splenic percussion sign,* but this sign is only moderately useful for detecting splenomegaly (Fig. 21-22).

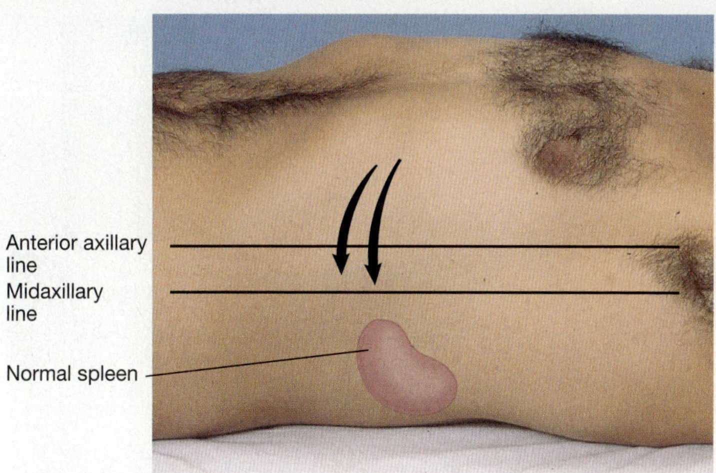

FIGURE 21-19. Percussion in Traube's space producing resonance, indicating a normal spleen size (negative finding for splenic enlargement).

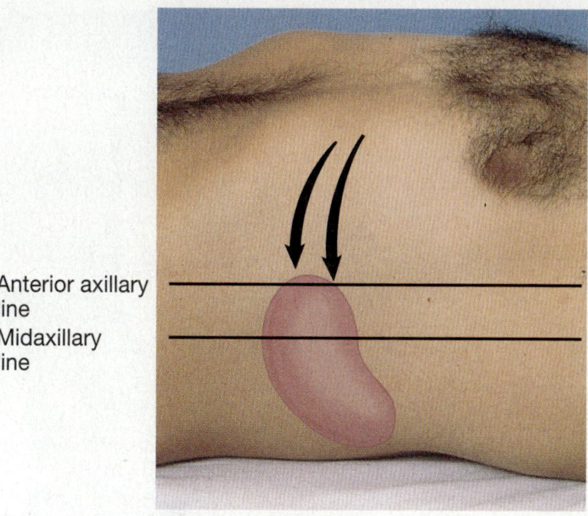

FIGURE 21-20. Percussion in Traube's space producing dullness, suggesting splenic enlargement (positive finding for splenic enlargement).

If either or both of these tests are positive, pay extra attention to palpation of the spleen.

Palpate for the Splenic Edge

To enhance relaxation of the abdominal wall, the patient should keep arms at their sides and, if needed, flex their hips and legs. With your left hand, reach over and around the patient to support and press forward their lower left rib cage and adjacent soft tissue. With your right hand below the left costal margin, press in toward the spleen. Begin palpation low enough so that you can detect an enlarged spleen. If your hand is too close to the costal margin, you will not be able to reach up under the rib cage. You may miss an enlarged spleen by starting palpation too high in the abdomen.

Splenomegaly is eight times more likely when the spleen is palpable.[29] Causes include portal hypertension, hematologic malignancies, HIV infection, infiltrative diseases like amyloidosis, and splenic infarct or hematoma.

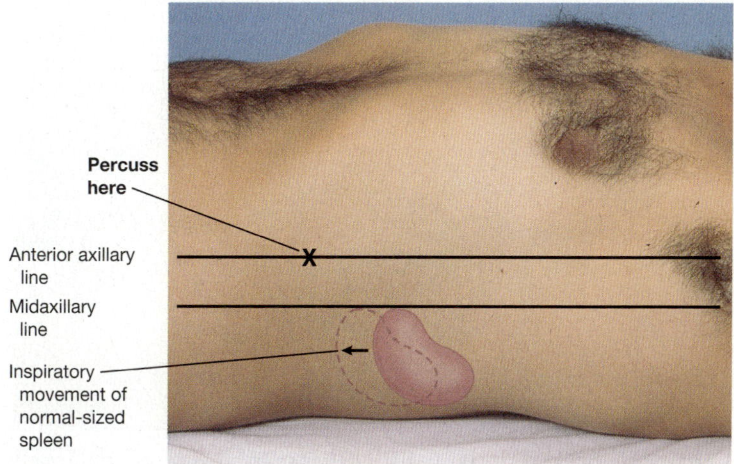

FIGURE 21-21. Percussion in the most inferior interspace along the left anterior axillary line on deep inspiration producing tympany, indicating a negative splenic percussion sign (normal spleen size).

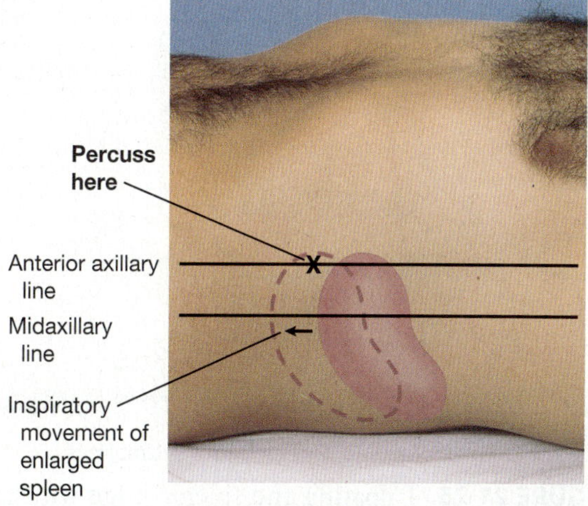

FIGURE 21-22. Percussion in the most inferior interspace along the left anterior axillary line on deep inspiration producing dullness, indicating a positive splenic percussion sign (suggesting splenomegaly).

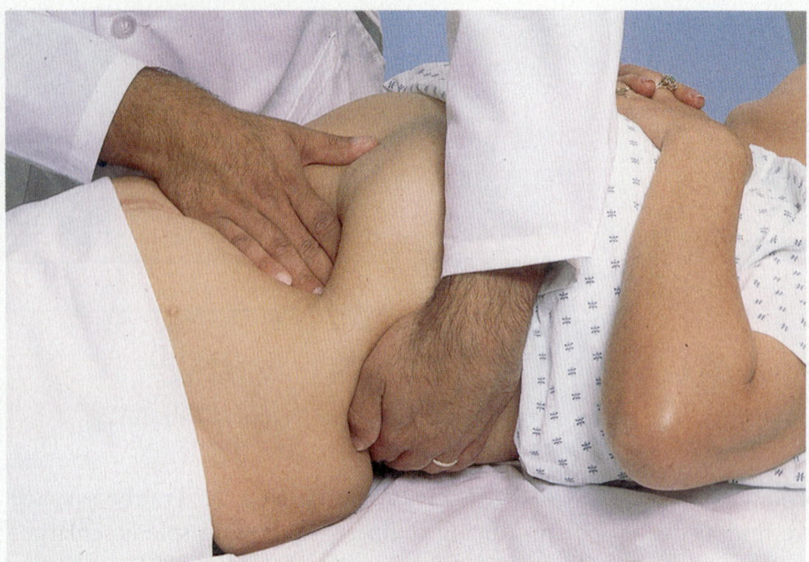

FIGURE 21-23. Examiner palpating for the splenic edge by placing hands under the left costal margin during deep inspiration.

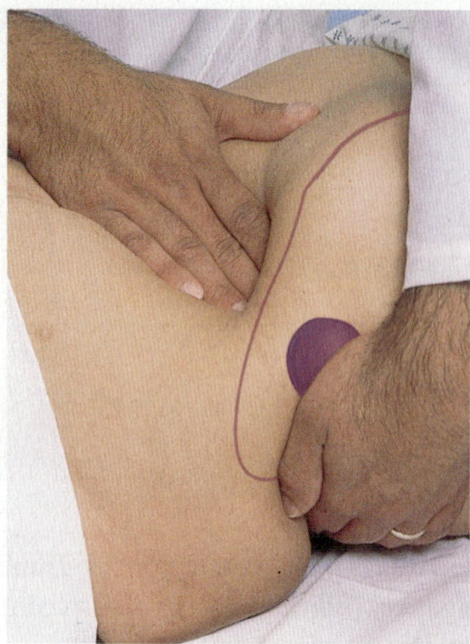

FIGURE 21-24. Palpable spleen tip (shown in purple) below the costal margin, indicating an enlarged spleen (splenomegaly).

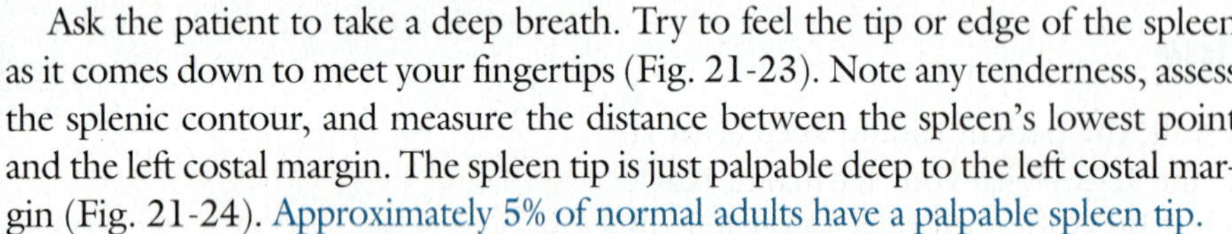

Ask the patient to take a deep breath. Try to feel the tip or edge of the spleen as it comes down to meet your fingertips (Fig. 21-23). Note any tenderness, assess the splenic contour, and measure the distance between the spleen's lowest point and the left costal margin. The spleen tip is just palpable deep to the left costal margin (Fig. 21-24). Approximately 5% of normal adults have a palpable spleen tip.

Repeat with the patient lying on their right side with their hips and knees partially flexed (Fig. 21-25). In this position, gravity may bring the spleen forward and to the right into a palpable location (Fig. 21-26).

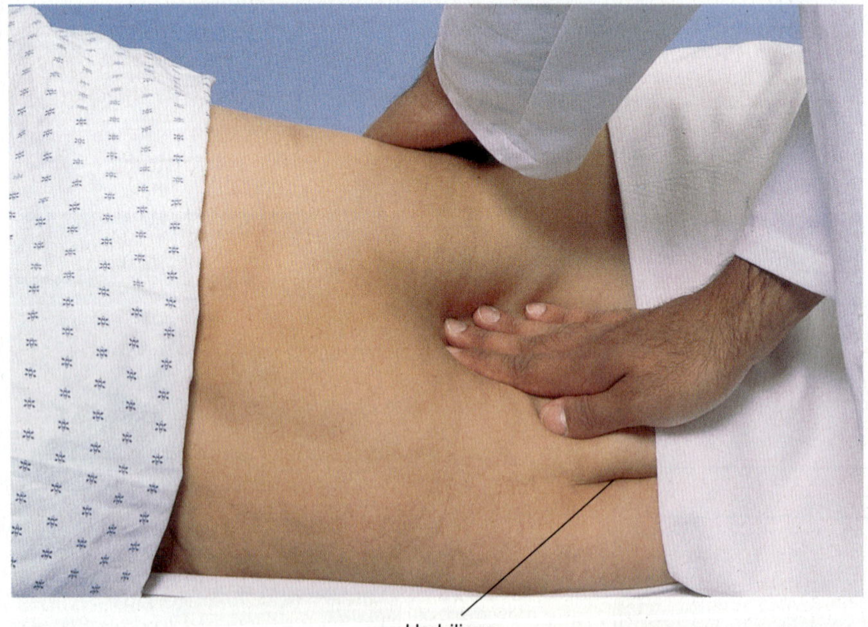

FIGURE 21-25. Palpating the splenic edge with the patient lying on the right side, which moves the spleen closer to the abdominal wall for better detection of splenomegaly.

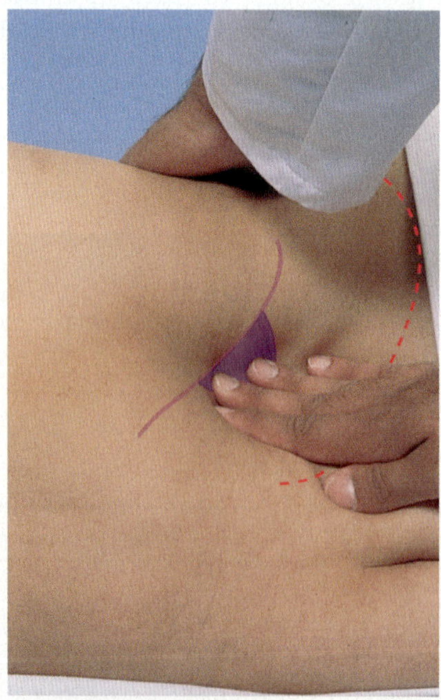

FIGURE 21-26. Edge of enlarged spleen palpable about 2 cm below the left costal margin on deep inspiration, suggesting splenomegaly.

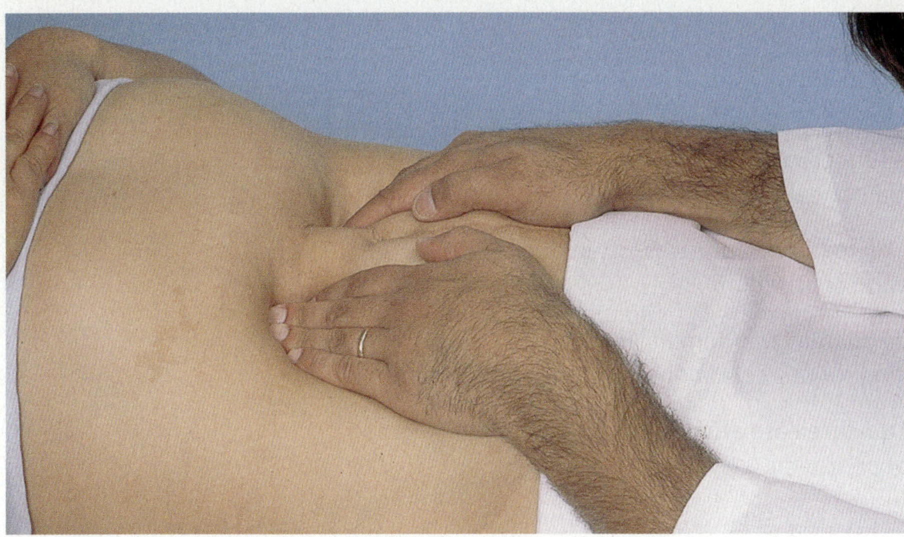

FIGURE 21-27. Palpating the periumbilical region on both sides of the aorta to assess for abnormal pulsations, which may indicate an abdominal aortic aneurysm.

Palpate for Aortic Pulsations

Press firmly deep in the epigastrium, slightly to the left of the midline, and identify the aortic pulsations. In adults older than age 50 years, those who smoke, and those with a history of hypertension or vascular disease, assess the width of the aorta by pressing deeply in the upper abdomen with one hand on each side of the aorta (Figs. 21-27 to 21-29). In this age group, a normal aorta is not more than 3 cm wide (average, 2.5 cm, excluding the thickness of the skin and abdominal wall).

A periumbilical or upper abdominal mass with expansile pulsations that is ≥3 cm in diameter suggests an abdominal aortic aneurysm (AAA). Its sensitivity varies with the size of the AAA. Larger aneurysms (≥5 cm) are more likely to be detected, with sensitivity increasing as the size of the aneurysm increases. While palpation is a valuable clinical tool, imaging techniques such as ultrasound or CT scans are more reliable for the precise diagnosis of AAAs, especially smaller ones.[36,37]

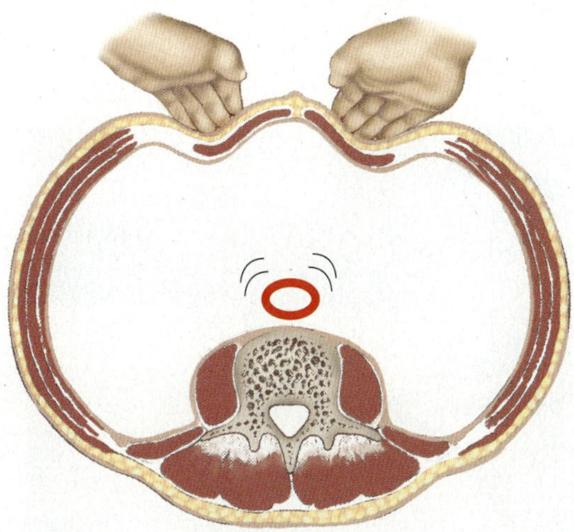

FIGURE 21-28. Detecting normal aortic pulsations by applying firm pressure on epigastrium, cross-section.

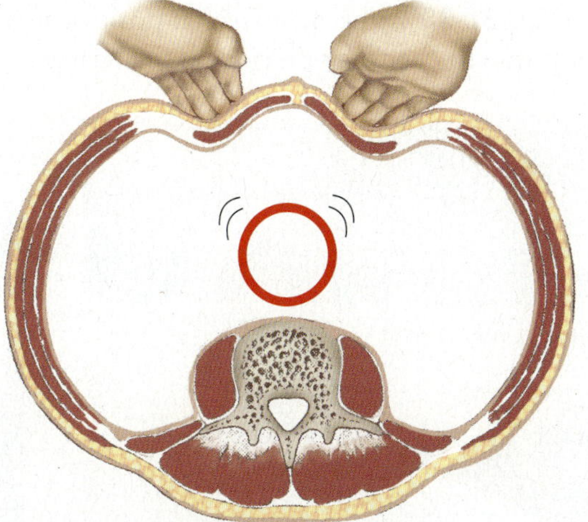

FIGURE 21-29. Identifying expanded aortic width on pressure on firm application of pressure on epigastrium, cross-section.

Box 21-25. Clinical Signs in Peritonitis

Clinical Sign	Description
Positive cough test	Pain in a specific area triggered or worsened by coughing, indicating potential peritoneal irritation
Involuntary guarding	Unconscious tensing of abdominal muscles, often due to abdominal inflammation or irritation
Rigidity	Severe form of muscle guarding; abdominal muscles are stiff and hard, indicating serious conditions like peritonitis
Rebound tenderness	Increased pain upon quick release after deep abdominal pressure, indicative of peritonitis

When positive, these signs roughly double the likelihood of peritonitis; rigidity makes peritonitis almost four times more likely.[32] Causes include any inflammatory, infectious, or ischemic intra-abdominal process, such as appendicitis, diverticulitis, cholecystitis, and bowel ischemia or perforation.

See also Table 21-10, Tender Abdomens, pp. 669–670.

SPECIAL TECHNIQUES AND MANEUVERS

Assessment techniques exist for possible peritonitis, ascites, abdominal wall mass, appendicitis, acute cholecystitis, ventral hernia, renal colic or pyelonephritis, and urinary bladder distention.

Assessing Possible Peritonitis

Inflammation of the parietal peritoneum, or *peritonitis*, signals an acute intra-abdominal inflammatory process requiring further urgent evaluation and workup.[29] Signs of peritonitis include a *positive cough test*, *involuntary guarding*, *rigidity*, *rebound tenderness*, and *percussion tenderness* (Box 21-25).

Even before palpation, ask the patient to cough and identify where the cough produces pain. Then palpate gently, starting with one finger and then with your hand, to localize the area of pain. As you palpate, check for peritoneal signs of guarding, rigidity, and rebound tenderness.

To assess rebound tenderness, ask the patient, *"Which hurts more, when I press or let go"*? Press down with your fingers firmly and slowly, then withdraw your hand quickly (Fig. 21-30). The maneuver is positive if withdrawal produces pain. Percuss gently to check for percussion tenderness.

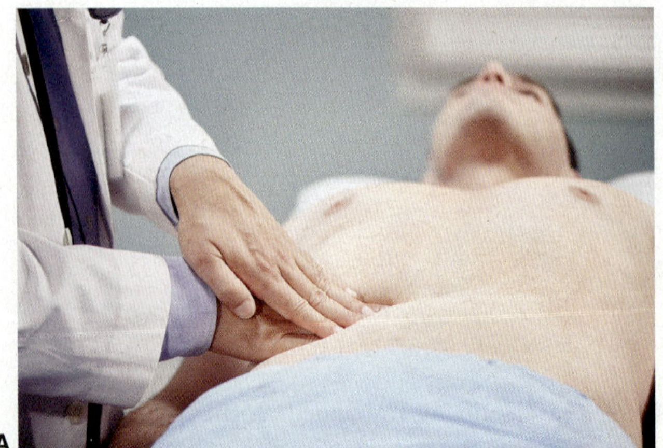

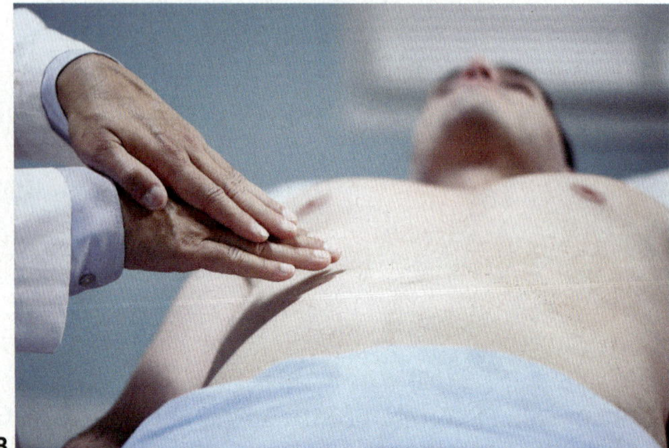

FIGURE 21-30. Detecting for rebound tenderness: (**A**) applying gentle pressure to the abdomen and (**B**) quickly releasing it.

Assessing Possible Ascites

A protuberant abdomen with bulging flanks is suspicious for *ascites,* the most common complication of cirrhosis.[38] Because ascitic fluid characteristically sinks with gravity, whereas gas-filled loops of bowel rise, dullness appears in the dependent areas of the abdomen. There are two techniques for comparative percussion for detecting ascites.

Percuss from Area of Central Tympany to Area of Dullness. Start with the patient lying supine. Percuss from the central area of the abdomen, which usually produces a tympanic or drum-like sound, and gradually move outward in various directions toward areas producing a dull sound. This mapping of the border between tympany and dullness helps identify fluid, which typically produces a dull sound (Fig. 21-31).

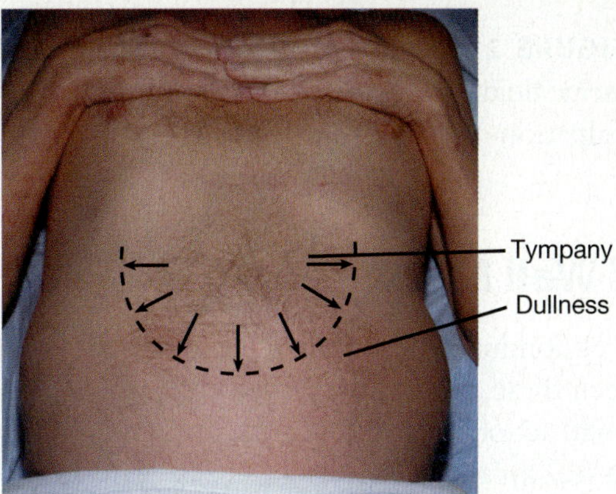

FIGURE 21-31. Mapping the area and direction of percussion dullness from the tympanic center outward, indicating the presence of ascites.

Test for Shifting Dullness. Percuss and mark the border between tympany and dullness with the patient's supine. Then ask them to roll onto one side and percuss and mark the borders again in this new position. In a person without ascites, the border between tympany and dullness remains relatively constant (Fig. 21-32).

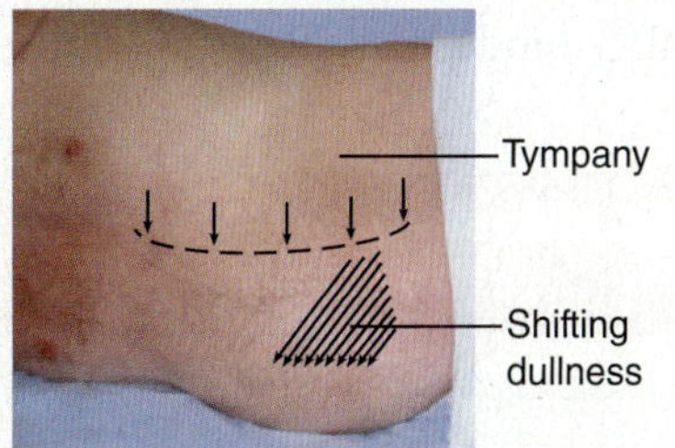

FIGURE 21-32. Mapping the boundary between tympany (top) and shifting dullness (bottom) in the abdomen, indicated by the dashed line (boundary) and arrows (direction of percussion), to detect ascitic fluid.

In ascites, dullness shifts to the more dependent side, whereas tympany shifts to the top. Sensitivity of this test is 83% with a specificity of 56%.[38]

The *fluid wave test,* once popular for detecting ascitic fluid by transmitting an impulse across the abdomen, is limited in usefulness. It frequently gives false negatives until ascites is advanced and can occasionally yield false positives.

Identifying Abdominal Organs and Masses in the Presence of Ascites

To perform the *ballottement technique* for examining an organ or mass, such as an enlarged liver as shown in Figure 21-33, follow these steps: Align and stiffen the fingers of one hand together, then place them on the abdominal surface over the area of the anticipated structure. Make a quick, jabbing movement directly toward the structure. This motion often displaces any intervening fluid, allowing your fingertips to briefly come into contact with the surface of the structure through the abdominal wall (Fig. 21-34).

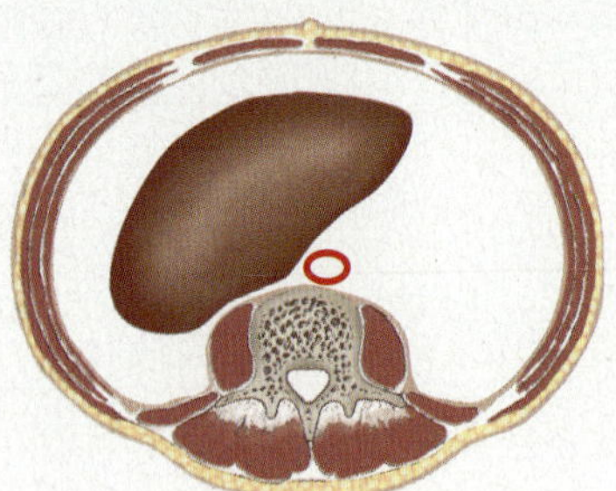

FIGURE 21-33. Note enlarged liver surrounded by ascitic fluid, cross-section.

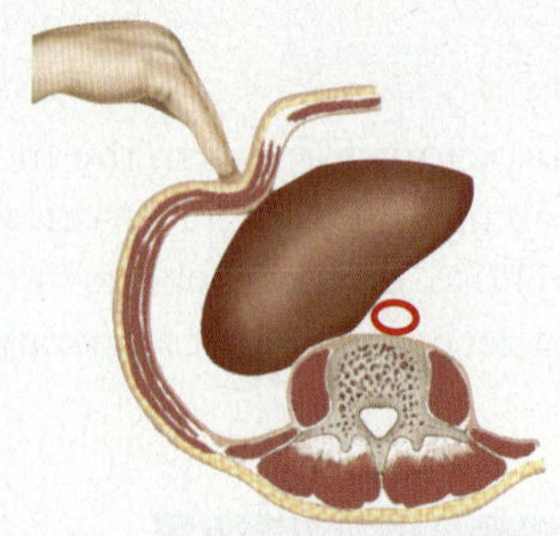

FIGURE 21-34. Displacement of ascitic fluid by ballottement allowing palpation of liver, cross-section.

Assessing for Abdominal Wall Mass

Occasionally, masses are located in the abdominal wall rather than inside the abdominal cavity. To differentiate between these, ask the patient to either raise their head and shoulders or to strain down, actions that tighten the abdominal muscles. Then, palpate the area again to feel for the mass.

A mass in the abdominal wall remains palpable; an intra-abdominal mass is obscured by muscular contraction.

Assessing Possible Appendicitis

Appendicitis is a common cause of acute abdominal pain, especially in the RLQ. Assess for signs of McBurney point tenderness, Rovsing sign (indirect tenderness), the psoas sign, and the obturator sign (Box 21-26). Appendicitis is twice as likely in the presence of RLQ tenderness, Rovsing sign (indirect

Box 21-26. Clinical Examination Maneuvers for Suspected Appendicitis

Maneuver	Description	Examples of Abnormalities
McBurney point tenderness	Palpate carefully for an area of local tenderness in the right lower quadrant (RLQ), particularly at the McBurney point. Assess for guarding, rigidity, and rebound tenderness. Classically, *McBurney point* lies 2 inches from the anterior superior iliac spine on a line drawn from that process to the umbilicus (Fig. 21-35).	Localized tenderness in the RLQ suggests appendicitis. Early voluntary guarding may be replaced by involuntary rigidity and signs of peritoneal inflammation. RLQ pain on quick withdrawal suggests appendicitis.
Rovsing sign	Press deeply in the left lower quadrant (LLQ), then quickly withdraw your fingers (Fig. 21-36).	Pain in the RLQ during left-sided pressure (indirect tenderness) indicates a positive Rovsing sign, suggesting appendicitis.
Psoas sign	With the patient supine, ask them to raise their right thigh against your hand placed above their knee, or, alternatively, turn them onto their left side and extend their right thigh at the hip. Flexion of the thigh at the hip makes the psoas muscle contract; extension stretches it (Fig. 21-37).	Increased abdominal pain with these movements suggests a positive psoas sign, indicating irritation of the right psoas muscle by an inflamed retrocecal appendix.
Obturator sign	Flex the patient's right thigh at the hip with their knee bent, and rotate their leg internally at the hip. This maneuver stretches the internal obturator muscle (Fig. 21-38).	Right hypogastric pain during this maneuver is a positive obturator sign, possibly indicating an inflamed appendix in the pelvis. The sensitivity of this sign is low.

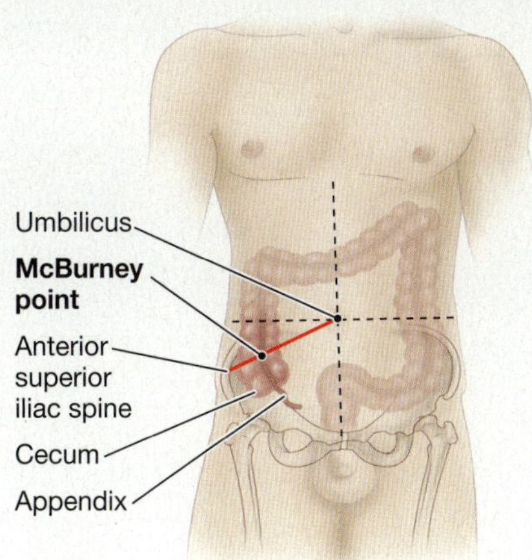

FIGURE 21-35. Surface projection of pelvis, cecum, and appendix showing McBurney point. (Reprinted with permission from Honan L. *Focus on Adult Health: Medical-Surgical Nursing*. 2nd ed. Wolters Kluwer; 2019. Figure 24-2.)

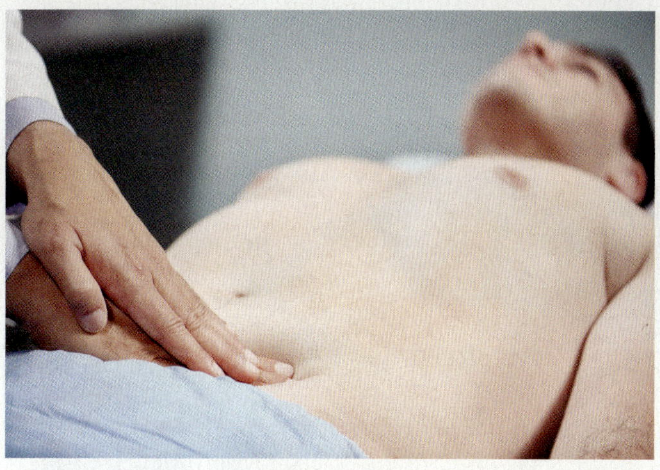

FIGURE 21-36. Assessing for Rovsing sign by applying pressure to the left lower quadrant. Pain in the right lower quadrant indicates a positive sign, suggesting possible appendicitis.

tenderness), and the psoas sign; it is three times more likely with McBurney point tenderness (McBurney sign).[32]

Perform a rectal examination and, when indicated, a pelvic examination. These maneuvers have low sensitivity and specificity, but they may identify an inflamed appendix atypically located within the pelvic cavity or other causes of the abdominal pain.

Right-sided rectal tenderness suggests appendicitis but may also be caused by an inflamed adnexa or seminal vesicle.

Assessing Possible Acute Cholecystitis

When a patient presents with RUQ pain suspicious of acute cholecystitis but does not have any tenderness on palpation in the RUQ, test for the *Murphy sign*. Deeply palpate the RUQ at the location of the pain. Ask the patient to take a deep breath, which forces the liver and gallbladder down toward the examining fingers (Fig. 21-39).

A sharp halting in inspiratory effort due to pain from palpation of the gallbladder on examination is a *positive Murphy sign*. When positive, the Murphy sign triples the likelihood of acute cholecystitis.[32]

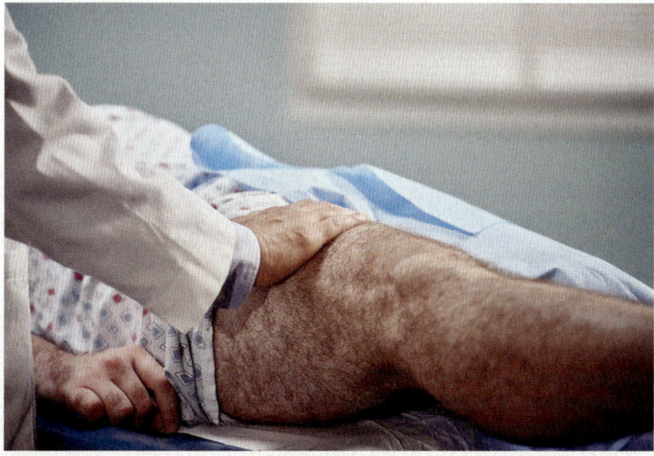

FIGURE 21-37. Performing the Psoas sign test by asking the patient to raise their right leg against resistance.

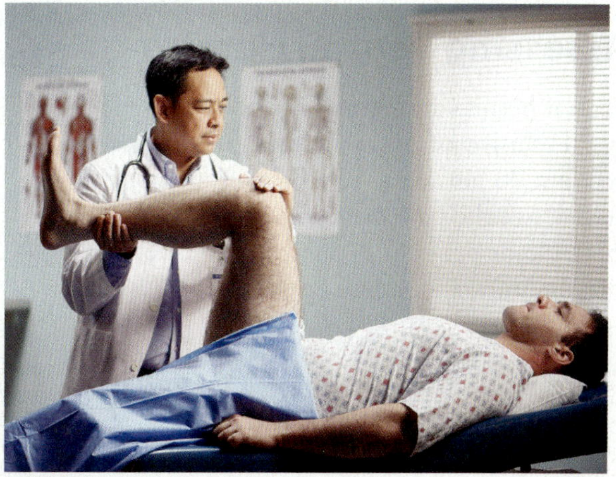

FIGURE 21-38. Assessing for the Obturator sign by flexing and internally rotating the patient's right hip.

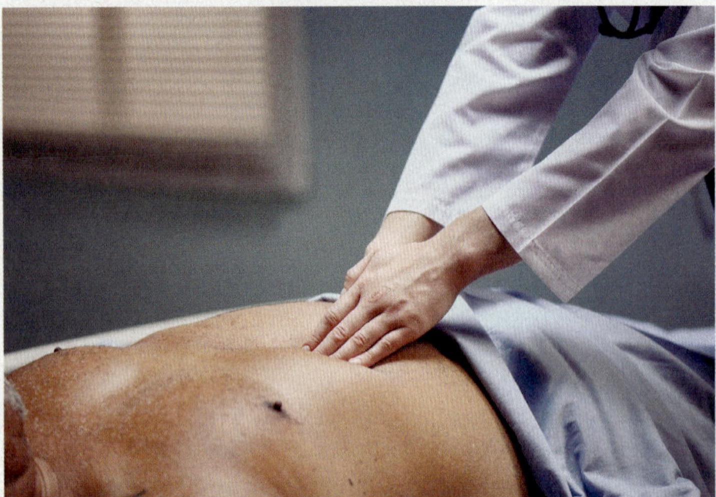

FIGURE 21-39. Performing Murphy's sign by palpating under the right costal margin while the patient inhales deeply.

Assessing Possible Renal Colic or Pyelonephritis

The kidneys are retroperitoneal and usually not palpable unless markedly enlarged. In patients suspected to have renal colic or pyelonephritis, *CVA tenderness* can be elicited due to inflammation of the renal capsule.

Start by explaining the maneuver to the patient. Place the palm of one hand along the CVA area. Then make a fist with the other hand and strike the hand already on the CVA with the ulnar surface of your fist (Fig. 21-40). Use enough force to cause a perceptible but painless jar or thud on the area. To save the patient from repositioning, integrate this assessment into your examination of the posterior thorax, lungs, or back.

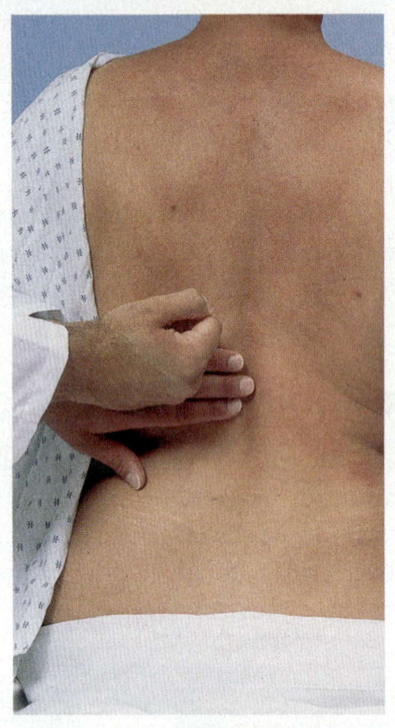

FIGURE 21-40. Fist percussion to detect costovertebral angle (CVA) tenderness.

Pain with pressure or fist percussion supports pyelonephritis if associated with fever and dysuria but may also be musculoskeletal.

Assessing Ventral Hernias

Ventral hernias are hernias in the abdominal wall exclusive of groin hernias. If you suspect but do not see an umbilical or incisional hernia, ask the patient to raise both legs off the table or perform a Valsalva maneuver to increase intra-abdominal pressure.

The bulge of a hernia will usually appear with this action, but should not be confused with *diastasis recti,* which is a benign 2- to 3-cm gap in the rectus muscles often seen in patients who are obese or postpartum.

Inguinal and femoral hernias are discussed in Chapter 23, Pelvis and Genitourinary System: Penis, Scrotum, and Prostate, pp. 704–706, and Chapter 24, Pelvis and Genitourinary System: Vulva, Vagina, Uterus, and Adnexa, pp. 754–755.

Assessing for Urinary Bladder Distention

Normally, the urinary bladder is not palpable unless it is distended above the symphysis pubis. Percuss for dullness and the height of the urinary bladder above the symphysis pubis. Bladder volume must be 400 to 600 mL before dullness appears.[29] On palpation, the dome of the distended bladder feels smooth and round. Check for tenderness.

Causes of bladder distention are outlet obstruction from a urethral stricture or prostatic hyperplasia; medication side effects; and neurologic disorders, such as stroke and multiple sclerosis.

See point-of-care ultrasound estimation of urinary bladder volume in Chapter 24, Pelvis and Genitourinary System: Vulva, Vagina, Uterus, and Adnexa, pp. 757–758.

Modifications in Physical Examinations: Best Practices for Specialized Patient Populations

Abdominal and pelvic interventions can drastically alter the landscape of PEs. Box 21-27 sheds light on the essential considerations when examining patients with percutaneous endoscopic gastrostomy (PEG) or jejunostomy (PEJ) tubes, peritoneal dialysis catheters, or ostomy bags.

Box 21-27. Abdominal Examination in the Presence of Medical Devices, Conditions or Procedures

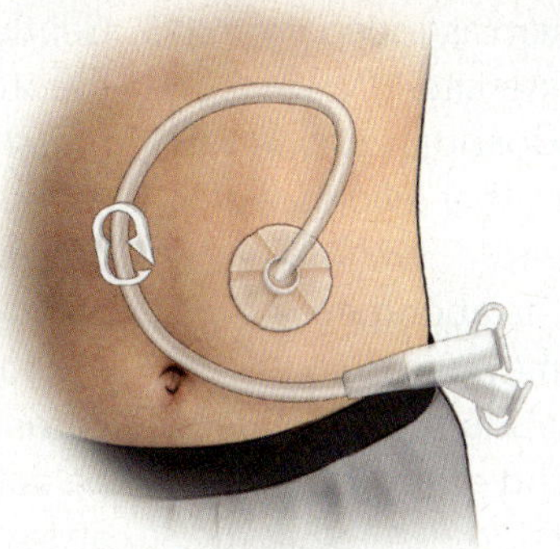

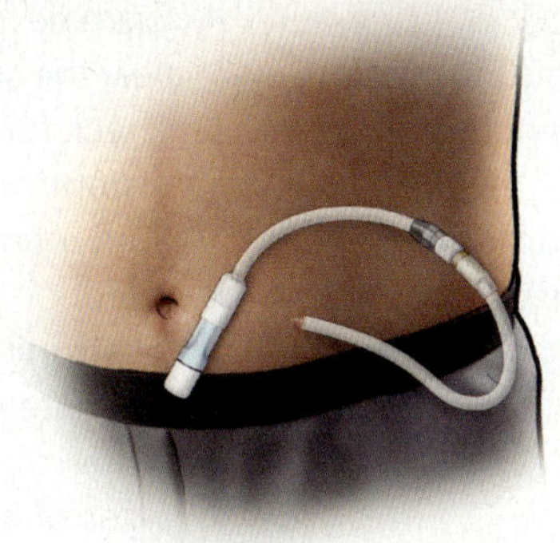

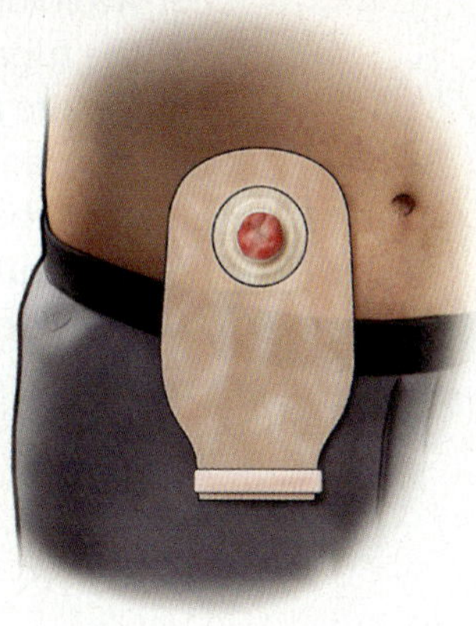

	Patient with a Percutaneous Endoscopic Gastrostomy (PEG) or Jejunostomy (PEJ) Tube	Patient with a Peritoneal Dialysis Catheter	Patient with an Ostomy
Device/ condition	Flexible tube inserted through the abdominal wall into the stomach (PEG) or jejunum (PEJ) for enteral nutrition.	Permanent catheter placed in the abdomen allowing dialysis solution to be filled and then drained from the peritoneal cavity, using the peritoneum as the membrane through which fluid, electrolytes, and waste products are exchanged with the blood.	Pouching system used to collect waste from a surgically diverted biologic system (e.g., ileostomy or colostomy). The pouch adheres to the skin surrounding a stoma, an artificial opening that channels feces or urine outside the body.

(*continued*)

Box 21-27. Abdominal Examination in the Presence of Medical Devices, Conditions or Procedures (*Continued*)

	Patient with a Percutaneous Endoscopic Gastrostomy (PEG) or Jejunostomy (PEJ) Tube	Patient with a Peritoneal Dialysis Catheter	Patient with an Ostomy
General indication	Nutritional support for patients with inadequate oral intake but a functioning gastrointestinal system	Treatment of end-stage renal disease or kidney failure; removing waste products and excess fluids	To bypass an injured or diseased part of the colon or to allow stool to leave the body after parts of the colon or rectum are removed.
General location	Typically, in the left upper quadrant of the abdomen	Typically inserted through the lower abdominal wall and into the peritoneal cavity	Depends on ostomy type but often on the lower abdomen.
Modification to the physical exam	1. Begin with visual inspection for signs of infection, skin irritation, or leakage. 2. Gently palpate around the tube site to check for tenderness, swelling, or discharge. 3. Avoid direct pressure over the tube site. 4. Inquire about discomfort, pain, and functioning of the tube. 5. Note tube dislodgement or evidence of blockage.	1. Inspect catheter site for signs of skin irritation or infection, including erythema, edema, or discharge. 2. Gently palpate around the catheter for warmth or tenderness 3. Don't tug or pull on the catheter. 4. Examine for hernias, especially near the catheter site. 5. Check for abdominal distention or other evidence of fluid retention 6. Infection of the abdomen (peritonitis) may occur, so evaluate for abdominal tenderness and other signs of infection.	1. Inspect the skin around the stoma for signs of irritation or infection, including erythema, warmth, and skin breakdown. 2. Check stoma color; it should be moist and pink/red. 3. Gently palpate around the stoma without pressing directly on it. 4. Assess ostomy bag output consistency, color, and quantity. 5. Ask for patient consent before inspecting or palpating and inquire about discomfort or changes in output.

RECORDING YOUR FINDINGS

The practice of documenting the PE with detailed sentences is key for initial diagnosis and hypothesis evaluation. With time and experience, you will shift to a more streamlined approach, employing brief, universally accepted phrases in your notes.

Recording the Abdominal Examination

"Abdomen is protuberant, soft and nontender; no palpable masses or hepatosplenomegaly. Liver span is 7 cm in the right midclavicular line;

edge is smooth and palpable 1 cm below the right costal margin. Spleen and kidneys not felt. No costovertebral angle (CVA) tenderness."

OR

"Abdomen is flat. No bowel sounds heard. It is firm and board like, with increased tenderness, guarding, and rebound in the right lower quadrant. Liver percusses to 7 cm in the midclavicular line; edge not felt. Spleen and kidneys not felt. No palpable masses. No CVA tenderness. Psoas sign positive."

The detailed examination of PE documentation, breaking it down into individual elements, showcases the importance of clinical observations in guiding diagnosis. The abdominal findings described are suggestive of several important clinical considerations:

- *Flat abdomen with absence of bowel sounds:* This can indicate a lack of intestinal activity, which might be seen in conditions like ileus (temporary cessation of bowel motility) or bowel obstruction.
- *Firm and board-like abdomen with increased tenderness, guarding, and rebound tenderness in the RLQ:* These are classic signs of peritonitis. This often indicates a serious intra-abdominal issue like appendicitis, especially when localized to the RLQ.
- *Positive psoas sign:* This suggests irritation of the psoas muscle, often associated with appendicitis or other inflammatory processes affecting the structures adjacent to the psoas muscle, such as an inflamed appendix.
- *Liver percussion to 7 cm in the midclavicular line; edge not felt:* This suggests a normal liver size. The inability to feel the liver edge might be due to the patient's body habitus or the liver's position within the abdomen.
- *Spleen and kidneys not felt:* This is generally a normal finding, as the spleen and kidneys are often not palpable in the absence of enlargement or disease.
- *No palpable masses or CVA tenderness:* The absence of these findings helps rule out certain conditions like masses in the abdominal cavity or kidney pathology.

Overall, the most concerning findings are those suggesting *peritonitis* and *potential appendicitis*, especially given the RLQ symptoms and positive psoas sign.

POINT-OF-CARE ULTRASOUND EXAMINATION

Point-of-care ultrasound (POCUS) enhances clinical assessments of the abdominal system by providing visual insights that complement findings from the PE. Conducting accurate abdominal exams can be complex due to patient body habitus variations. POCUS offers a swift method to examine the abdomen for different causes of pain, aiding in refining or altering patient management strategies. This section delves into using POCUS for identifying intraperitoneal free fluid (FF) and investigating the origins of RUQ and flank pain.

Estimation of urinary bladder volume can be found in Chapter 24, Pelvis and Genitourinary System: Vulva, Vagina, Uterus, and Adnexa, pp. 757–758.

The approach to abdominal POCUS is consistent across all evaluations, focusing on specific regions with the ultrasound probe to discern normal from pathologic findings. Typically conducted with the patient lying supine, the examination uses a curvilinear probe for its broad applicability. However, a phased array probe may be used for deeper anatomic investigations if necessary. The ultrasound settings are generally adjusted to either "FAST" or "Abdomen" mode to optimize the assessment. In the following subsections, we will detail the areas of interest for the probe and highlight key findings associated with each anatomic area.

Ultrasound Technique

Basic Ultrasound Setup	
Patient positioning	Supine
Probe	Curvilinear probe
Ultrasound setting	"FAST" or "Abdomen" setting, B-mode

Assessing the Liver Size

Physical Examination. When a patient presents with RUQ pain and elevated liver enzymes, POCUS can be instrumental in evaluating the liver for signs of hepatomegaly. Since the liver's edge may not always be palpable, especially due to its positioning beneath the ribcage, ultrasound becomes an invaluable tool for accurately determining liver size (see pp. 632–633). Hepatomegaly can arise from a variety of conditions, including acute or chronic hepatitis, fatty liver disease, congestive heart failure (CHF), and primary or metastatic cancer.[39] Liver size can vary based on several factors, such as body mass index (BMI), height, gender, and age.[40,41]

Ultrasound Technique. POCUS evaluation for liver size is done with the patient in the supine position. The probe should be placed with the probe marker toward the patient's head in the midaxillary line just distal to the diaphragm, often around the 10th to 11th intercostal space (Fig. 21-41). This probe positioning ensures that you are measuring the caudocranial dimension. If needed, rotate the probe to align between the intercostal spaces or slide the probe cranially to visualize the largest area of the liver. At maximal inspiration, identify an image that contains the liver, diaphragm, and kidney, then freeze the image and measure the liver from the diaphragm to the inferior liver edge (Fig. 21-42).

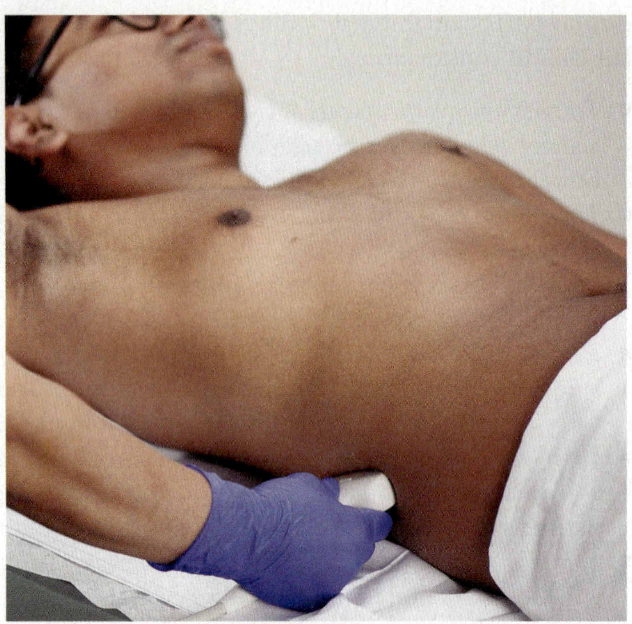

FIGURE 21-41. Probe positioning on a patient for liver evaluation.

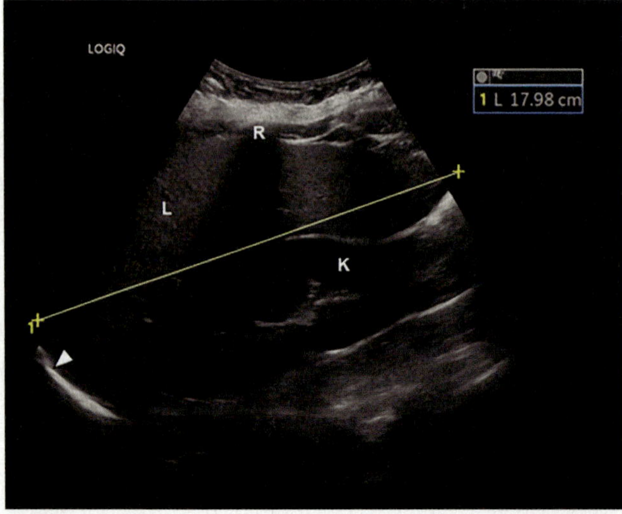

FIGURE 21-42. Measurement of liver size, noted to be abnormal. L, liver; K, kidney; R, rib shadow; arrowhead, diaphragm.

Evaluating the Gallbladder

Physical Examination. In cases involving gallbladder pathologies, patients often report pain in the RUQ, typically manifesting after eating (postprandial). This discomfort is frequently associated with additional symptoms, including nausea, vomiting, or fever.

Cholecystitis produces steady, constant pain. This pain is usually felt in the RUQ or epigastric region but is distinguished by a *positive Murphy sign*, signifying increased pain on palpation of the gallbladder area, which may also radiate to the right shoulder (see p. 641). In contrast, biliary colic, often caused by gallstones (*cholelithiasis*), typically

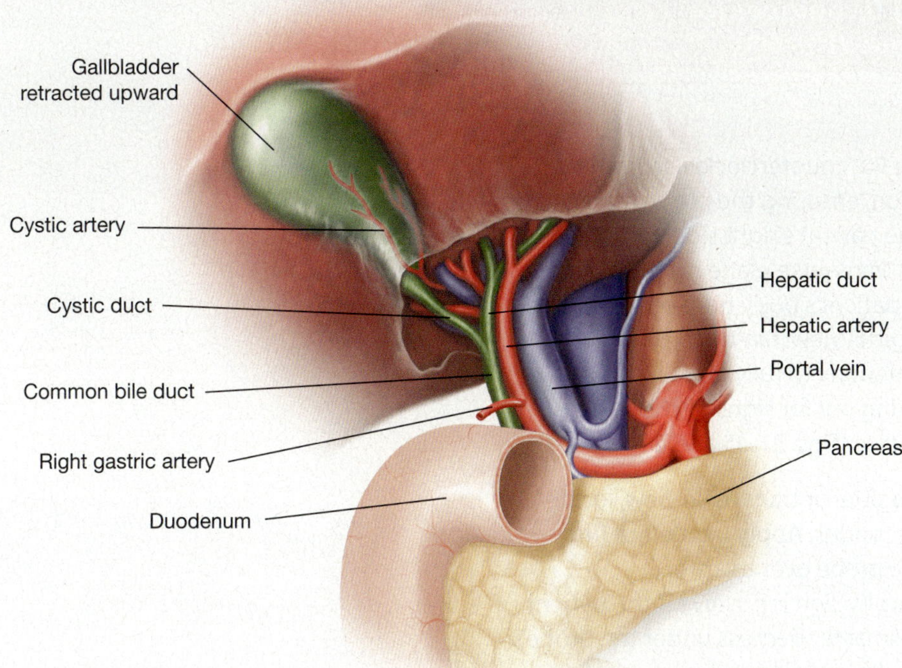

FIGURE 21-43. Biliary anatomy.

manifests as intermittent pain. This discomfort localizes in the epigastric area or the RUQ, without eliciting a Murphy sign.

Ultrasound Technique. The patient may start supine but may need to roll into a left lateral decubitus position since the gallbladder is a mobile organ (Box 21-28). The gallbladder neck is fixed in relation to the main lobar fissure (MLF) and the portal vein, so visualization of the MLF may help to identify the portal vein and the portal triad [portal vein, hepatic artery, common bile duct (CBD)].[42] Basic biliary anatomy is illustrated in Figure 21-43.

Box 21-28. Ultrasound Imaging Techniques for Gallbladder Assessment

Technique	Procedure
Sagittal View Technique	■ Begin by positioning the probe at the right anterior abdominal wall's costal margin, with the probe marker pointing towards the patient's head (Fig. 21-44). ■ Gently sweep the probe laterally along the costal margin until the gallbladder comes into view. ■ To align with the gallbladder's long axis (which might not perfectly match the patient's sagittal plane), rotate the probe, usually clockwise. This helps to elongate the gallbladder for a better examination. ■ Fan the probe both superiorly and inferiorly to comprehensively visualize the gallbladder, checking for gallstones or any other abnormalities.

(continued)

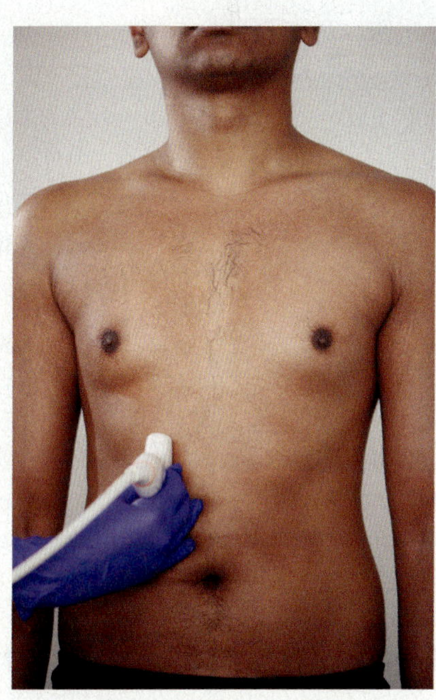

FIGURE 21-44. Sweeping the probe laterally along the costal margin to visualize the gallbladder.

Box 21-28. Ultrasound Imaging Techniques for Gallbladder Assessment (*Continued*)

Technique	Procedure
Transverse View Technique	■ Rotate the probe 90° counterclockwise from the sagittal orientation, ensuring the probe marker points toward the patient's right side. Note that the gallbladder's transverse plane may not align exactly with the patient's body transverse plane. ■ Similar to the sagittal view, fan the probe superiorly and inferiorly to fully visualize the gallbladder, looking out for signs of cholelithiasis or other pathologies (Figs. 21-45 and 21-46).
Sonographic Murphy sign	■ While in either sagittal or transverse view, locate the gallbladder's fundus. Apply gentle but firm pressure with the probe over this area. ■ Sonographic Murphy sign is positive if the patient experiences maximal tenderness under the probe's pressure at the gallbladder's fundus, suggesting acute cholecystitis. ■ Ensure the probe is positioned below the costal margin for this evaluation, avoiding intercostal spaces to prevent discomfort and achieve accurate results.

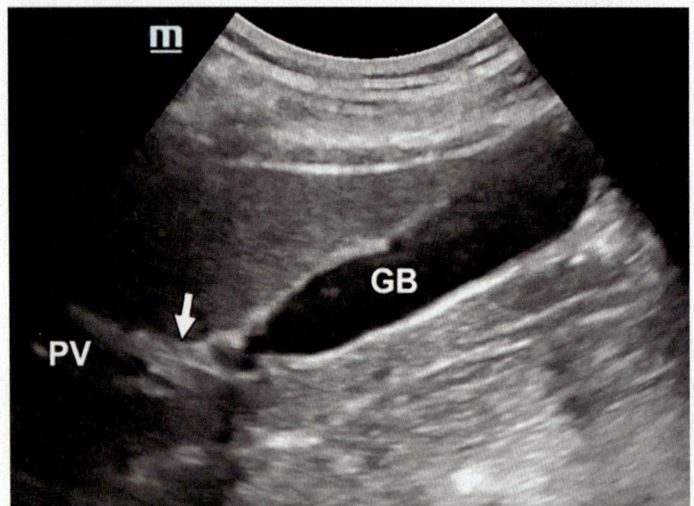

FIGURE 21-45. Normal gallbladder anatomy with clear delineation of wall layers. GB, body of gallbladder; arrow, main lobar fissure; PV, portal vein.

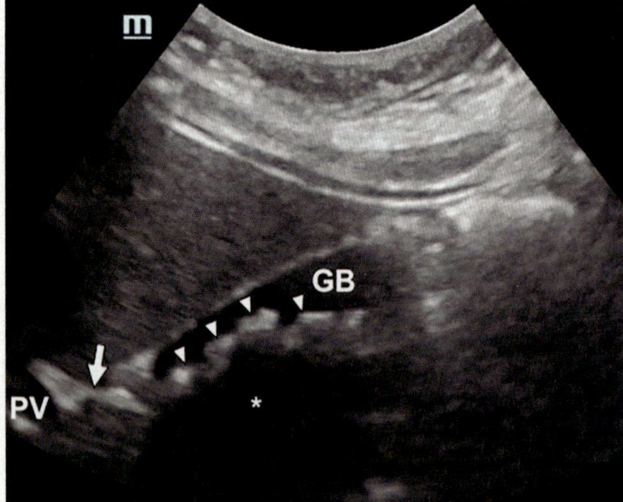

FIGURE 21-46. Cholelithiasis. GB, body of the gallbladder; arrow, main lobar fissure; PV, portal vein; arrowheads, stones; asterisk, shadowing from stones.

Evaluating for Intraperitoneal Free Fluid (FF)

Physical Examination. The assessment of intraperitoneal FF is a crucial aspect of diagnosing and managing patients with abdominal problems. Findings include a protuberant abdomen, tenderness, and bulging flanks, which are indicative of

Box 21-29. Physical Examination Findings Associated With Intraperitoneal Free Fluid[29,38]

Physical Examination Finding	Sensitivity	Specificity
Protuberant abdomen	Not available*	Not available*
Tenderness present	Not available*	Not available*
Bulging flanks	73–93%	44–70%
Flank dullness	80–94%	29–69%
Shifting dullness	60–87%	56–90%
Fluid wave	50–80%	82–92%

*Values not available as these findings are nonspecific and lack validated diagnostic data.

fluid accumulation, as shown in Box 21-29, which also presents the diagnostic sensitivity and specificity of various signs such as flank dullness, shifting dullness, and the fluid wave test.[43] These measures offer insights into the likelihood that these signs accurately identify the presence of intraperitoneal FF.

Ultrasound Technique. In patients experiencing abdominal pain and distention, POCUS is a valuable tool for detecting the presence of intraperitoneal FF. Since the 1970s, ultrasonography has proven to be highly sensitive in identifying as little as 100 mL of FF.[44] Various conditions can lead to its accumulation, including cirrhosis, malignancy, CHF, portal vein thrombosis, nephrotic syndrome, and malnutrition, with cirrhosis being the most prevalent cause of ascites. Box 21-30 outlines the essential POCUS imaging techniques for detecting intraperitoneal FF, especially in emergency settings where rapid assessment can significantly impact patient care.

Box 21-30. Ultrasound Techniques for Detecting Intraperitoneal Free Fluid

Technique	Procedure
Initial positioning	■ Position the patient in the supine posture to facilitate intraperitoneal free fluid detection, particularly in emergency trauma assessments.
Right upper quadrant visualization	■ Place the ultrasound probe in the midaxillary line just below the diaphragm, around the 10th or 11th intercostal space (Fig. 21-47), with the marker toward the patient's head. This approach targets the *Morison pouch (hepatorenal recess)*, the most common site for free fluid (Figs. 21-48 and 21-49). ■ The Morison pouch, when viewed on ultrasound, appears as a potential space between the liver and the right kidney. In the absence of fluid, it may not be distinctly visible because the liver and kidney are in close contact. However, when fluid accumulates, the Morison pouch becomes more apparent as an anechoic (dark or black) area on the ultrasound image, indicating the presence of free fluid.
Probe adjustment	■ Rotate or slide the probe cranially for optimal alignment and to enhance visualization of the space between the liver and the right kidney, ensuring a thorough assessment of free fluid.

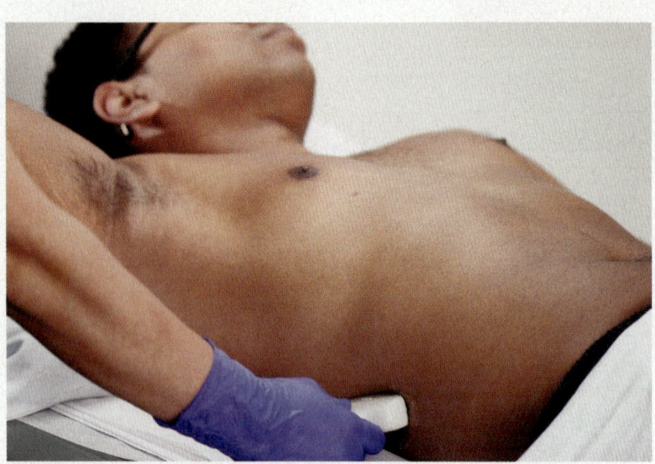

FIGURE 21-47. Probe positioning on a patient for right upper quadrant assessment.

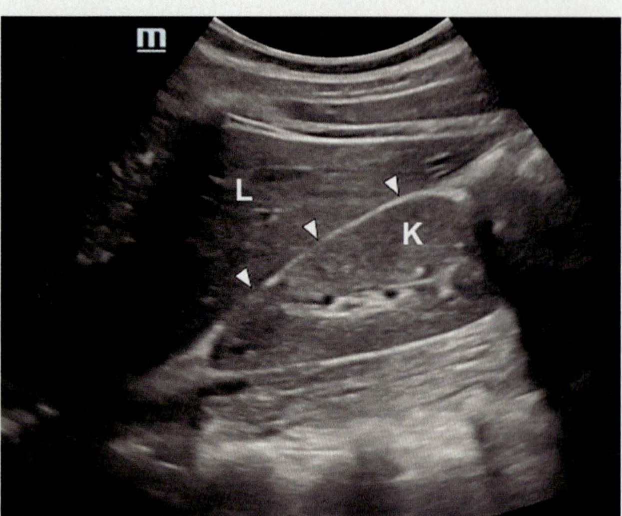

FIGURE 21-48. Normal right upper quadrant (RUQ). RUQ without free fluid. L, liver; K, kidney; arrowheads, Morison pouch.

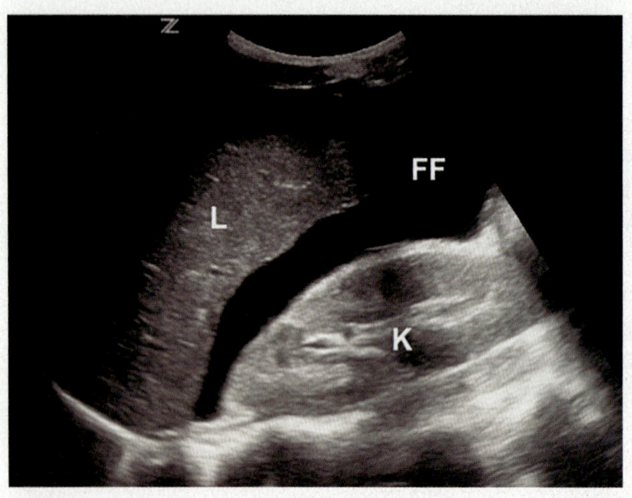

FIGURE 21-49. Right upper quadrant with anechoic free fluid (FF) noted in the Morison pouch between the liver (L) and kidney (K), indicating potential fluid accumulation.

HEALTH PROMOTION AND COUNSELING: EVIDENCE AND RECOMMENDATIONS

Important Topics for Health Promotion and Counseling

- Viral hepatitis A
- Viral hepatitis B
- Viral hepatitis C
- Colorectal cancer

In the following section, both traditional terms like "men," "women," "male," and "female" and inclusive terms such as "individuals assigned female at birth" and "individuals assigned male at birth" are used. This approach balances inclusivity with the need to accurately represent the original research.

Viral Hepatitis A

Epidemiology. An estimated 4,000 new cases of hepatitis A virus (HAV) occurred in 2016.[45] HAV infection is rarely fatal; it does not cause chronic hepatitis, and deaths usually occur only in those with other liver diseases. Viral transmission is primarily person to person through the fecal–oral route and can be reduced by handwashing with soap and water after using the bathroom or changing diapers and before preparing or eating food.[46]

Hepatitis A vaccination, initially recommended in 1996, has been associated with a more than 90% decrease in the annual number of reported HAV cases in the United States. The Advisory Committee on Immunization Practices (ACIP) recommends hepatitis A vaccination for all children at age 1 year, for persons with chronic liver disease, and for groups at increased risk of acquiring HAV—persons traveling to or working in countries with high endemic rates of infection, men who have sex with men (MSM), users of injection and illicit drugs, persons with occupational risk for infection, and persons who have clotting-factor disorders.[47] During a widespread outbreak, healthy individuals who have not been vaccinated may be considered for vaccination.

While the term 'men who have sex with men (MSM)' is widely used and appropriate in public health for clarity and precision, it may be seen as stigmatizing as it labels individuals based on behavior. Nevertheless, we retain its use in this section for consistency and to align with established public health terminology.

Prevention. Postexposure prophylaxis among previously unvaccinated individuals is a single dose of immune globulin administered as soon as possible, ideally within 2 weeks. Recommendations for immune globulin apply to close personal contacts of persons with confirmed HAV; coworkers of infected food handlers; and staff and attendees (and their household members) of childcare centers where HAV has been diagnosed in children, staff, or households of attendees. Hepatitis A vaccine is additionally recommended if the person also has an indication for vaccination. The vaccine alone may be administered at any time before traveling to endemic areas.

Viral Hepatitis B

Epidemiology. Hepatitis B virus (HBV) infection is a more serious health threat than HAV; the fatality rate for acute infection can be up to 1.5%, and HBV infection can become chronic.[45,48] HBV is spread by the blood, semen, or other bodily fluids of an infected person; sexual contact, injection drug use, and perinatal transmission are the most common pathways. Most infections in healthy adults are self-limited, with elimination of the virus and development of immunity. The U.S. Centers for Disease Control and Prevention (CDC) estimated that about 21,000 new cases of HBV occurred in the United States in 2016. Risk of chronic HBV infection is highest when the immune system is immature; chronic infection occurs in up to 90% of infected infants and 30% of children infected before the age of 6 years. Chronic HBV infection also develops more often in persons who are immunosuppressed or have diabetes. About 15% to 25% of those with chronic HBV infection die from cirrhosis or liver cancer, accounting for nearly 2,000 deaths each year in the United States. Most persons with chronic infection are asymptomatic until the onset of advanced liver disease.

Prevention. HBV infection is preventable. The HBV vaccine, first recommended in the early 1980s, has led to a 90% decline in the annual incidence of newly reported cases. The ACIP recommends universal vaccination for all infants beginning at birth as well as for previously unvaccinated children younger than age 19 years.[48]

Box 21-31. Recommendations for Hepatitis B Vaccination: High-Risk Groups and Settings

- *Sexual contacts*, including sex partners of hepatitis B surface antigen–positive persons, people with more than one sex partner in the prior 6 months, people seeking evaluation and treatment for sexually transmitted infections, and men who have sex with men
- *Persons with percutaneous or mucosal exposure to blood*, including injection drug users, household contacts of antigen-positive persons, residents and staff of facilities for the developmentally disabled, health care workers, persons with diabetes, and dialysis patients
- *Others*, including travelers to endemic areas, people with chronic liver disease and HIV infection, and people seeking protection from hepatitis B infection who do not acknowledge a specific risk factor
- *All adults in high-risk settings*, such as sexually transmitted infection clinics, HIV testing and treatment programs, drug-abuse treatment programs and programs for injection drug users, correctional facilities, programs for men having sex with men, chronic hemodialysis facilities and end-stage renal disease programs, and facilities for people with developmental disabilities

Source: Schillie S, Harris A, Link-Gelles R, Romero J, Ward J, Nelson N. Recommendations of the Advisory Committee on Immunization Practices for use of a Hepatitis B vaccine with a novel adjuvant. *MMWR Morb Mortal Wkly Rep*. 2018;67(15):455–458.

For adults, vaccine recommendations target high-risk groups (Box 21-31). HBV infection is also treatable. The U.S. Preventive Services Task Force (USPSTF) concluded that antiviral treatment in patients with chronic HBV could improve health outcomes and recommended screening for HBV in persons at high risk for infection (grade B), including those born in countries with a high endemic prevalence of HBV infection, unvaccinated US-born persons whose parents were from countries with a high endemic prevalence of HBV infection, persons with HIV, injection drug users, MSM, and household contacts or sexual partners of HBV-infected persons.[49] The CDC also recommends screening persons on hemodialysis or who are receiving immunosuppressive therapy.[50] The USPSTF (grade A) and ACIP recommend screening all pregnant women.[48,51]

Viral Hepatitis C

Epidemiology. Hepatitis C virus (HCV) is the most prevalent chronic bloodborne pathogen in the United States. Anti-HCV antibody is detectable in just under 2% of the population, although prevalence is markedly increased in high-risk groups.[52] In 2016, the CDC estimated that just over 40,000 cases of acute HCV infection occurred in the United States with over 18,000 HCV-related deaths.[45] HCV is mainly transmitted by percutaneous exposures, particularly from injection drug use, health care workers with needlestick injury or mucosal exposure to HCV-positive blood, blood transfusion or organ transplantation before 1992, and transfusion with clotting factors before 1987. Other causes include long-term hemodialysis, getting an unregulated tattoo, and birth from an HCV-positive mother; sexual transmission is uncommon, although it occurs among HIV-positive persons, particularly among MSM. Hepatitis C becomes a chronic illness in more than 75% of those who are infected and is a major risk factor for subsequently developing cirrhosis and hepatocellular carcinoma and for undergoing transplantation for end-stage liver disease. However, the majority of persons with chronic HCV are unaware of being infected.

Screening. Screening tests for HCV are very sensitive. Antiviral treatment regimens can achieve high rates of sustained virologic response (aviremia

≥24 weeks after completing treatment) and improve clinical outcomes. Consequently, the USPSTF concluded that screening for hepatitis C infection is of moderate benefit for persons at high risk for infection as well as those born between 1945 and 1965 (grade B).[52]

Colorectal Cancer

Epidemiology. Colorectal cancer is the third most frequently diagnosed cancer (>140,000 total new cases annually) and the third leading cause of cancer death (~50,000 deaths) in the United States.[53] Overall, about 80% of new cases and nearly 90% of deaths occur after age 55; the median age at diagnosis is 67 years; and the median age at death is 73 years.[54] The lifetime risk for being diagnosed with colorectal cancer is about 4%, while the lifetime risk for dying from colorectal cancer is just under 2%.[55]

Colorectal cancer incidence and mortality rates have been gradually but steadily declining in the United States over the past three decades.[55] These trends are attributed to changes in risk factor prevalence, such as decreased tobacco use; increased uptake of screening, which both prevents cancers and increases detection of early-stage curable cancers; and improved treatments.[56] The strongest risk factors for colorectal cancer are *increasing age; personal history of colorectal cancer, adenomatous polyps, or longstanding IBD; and family history of colorectal neoplasia*, particularly with diagnoses in multiple first-degree relatives, a single first-degree relative diagnosed before age 60, or a hereditary colorectal cancer syndrome.[57] While the lifetime risk of colorectal cancer is extremely high in patients with hereditary syndromes, about 75% of colorectal cancers arise in people without any obvious hereditary risk or family history.[58]

Prevention. The most effective prevention strategy is to screen for and remove precancerous adenomatous polyps. Screening programs using fecal blood testing or flexible sigmoidoscopy have been shown in randomized trials to reduce the risk of developing colorectal cancer by about 5% to 25%.[59,60] Physical activity, aspirin, other NSAIDs, and postmenopausal combined hormone replacement therapy (estrogen and progestin) also protect against colorectal cancer.[57]

The USPSTF recommends low-dose aspirin for preventing cardiovascular disease and colorectal cancer in select adults ages 50 to 59 years with an increased 10-year cardiovascular disease risk (grade B).[54] In contrast, it recommends individualized decision-making for adults ages 60 to 69 years (grade C). Hormone therapy for cancer chemoprevention is not advised; women receiving combined therapy were actually more likely to present with advanced-stage colorectal cancers, and they had a nonsignificantly higher risk than women receiving placebo for colorectal cancer mortality.[61] Furthermore, hormone therapy is associated with increased risks for breast cancer, cardiovascular events, and venous thromboembolism.[62–64] There is no convincing evidence that dietary changes or taking supplements can prevent colorectal cancer.[57]

Screening. Screening tests include stool tests that detect occult fecal blood, such as fecal immunochemical tests and high-sensitivity guaiac-based tests, and those that detect abnormal DNA in the stool. Endoscopic tests are also used for screening, including colonoscopy, which visualizes the entire colon and can remove polyps, and flexible sigmoidoscopy, which visualizes the distal 60 cm of the bowel. CT colonography is used to image the colon. Any abnormal finding on a stool test, imaging study, or flexible sigmoidoscopy warrants further evaluation with colonoscopy. Screening programs using fecal blood testing or flexible sigmoidoscopy have been shown in randomized trials to reduce the risk of colorectal cancer death by about 15% to 30%.[65]

Although colonoscopy is the gold standard diagnostic test for screening, there is no direct evidence from randomized trials that screening with colonoscopy reduces colorectal cancer incidence or mortality. Additionally, no randomized trials have evaluated the efficacy of screening with CT colonography or fecal DNA tests (which are now combined with fecal immunochemical tests).

Much of the evidence supporting colonoscopy's effectiveness in reducing cancer incidence and mortality comes from observational studies and extrapolated data from trials of other screening methods, such as fecal occult blood tests (FOBT) and sigmoidoscopy.

Guidelines. The USPSTF, the American Cancer Society, and the U.S. Multi-Society Task Force on Colorectal Cancer all published guidelines strongly endorsing colorectal cancer screening.[66–68] The USPSTF, which gives a grade A recommendation for colorectal screening in average-risk adults ages 45 to 50 years, suggests multiple screening options (Box 21-32). Performing digital rectal examination to test for fecal occult blood is *not recommended* for colorectal cancer screening.

Although screening reduces colorectal cancer incidence and mortality, only about two-thirds of the adult US population is current with recommended screening, while more than a quarter has never been screened.[69] Colonoscopy is the most commonly used test, although people may prefer other tests, such as fecal occult blood tests because they are safer and easier to perform.

Higher-risk persons, based on personal history of colorectal neoplasia or longstanding IBD, or a family history of colorectal neoplasia, are advised to begin screening at a younger age, usually with colonoscopy, and get tested more frequently than average-risk adults.[68]

Box 21-32. Screening Recommendations—U.S. Preventive Services Task Force 2021

- **Adults ages 45 to 49 years (Grade B recommendation) and Adults ages 50 to 75 years (Grade A recommendation)**—screening options:
  - Stool-based tests
    - Fecal immunochemical test (FIT) annually
    - High-sensitivity guaiac-based fecal occult blood test (HSgFOBT) annually
    - Stool DNA-FIT (sDNA-FIT) testing every 1 to 3 years
  - Direct visualization tests
    - Colonoscopy every 10 years
    - Flexible sigmoidoscopy every 5 years
    - Flexible sigmoidoscopy every 10 years plus FIT annual FIT
    - CT colonography every 5 years
- **Adults ages 76 to 85 years—individualized decision making (grade C recommendation),** decisions should take into consideration life expectancy and previous screening history. Previously unscreened adults might benefit from screening, if they are in good health and have a life expectancy sufficient to benefit from detection and treatment.
- **Adults older than age 85 years—do not screen (grade D recommendation)**, because "competing causes of mortality preclude a mortality benefit that would outweigh the harms"

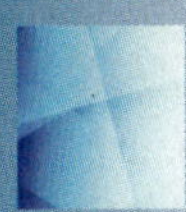

TABLE 21-1. Classification and Diagnosis of Selected Functional Gastrointestinal Disorders[1]

Disorder	Rome IV Criteria Definition
Cyclic vomiting syndrome	Intense vomiting episodes lasting hours or days with symptom-free intervals
Functional abdominal bloating/ distention	Recurrent episodes of bloating or distention, not fitting other functional disorder criteria
Functional anorectal pain	Conditions like proctalgia fugax (brief, intense rectal pain) and chronic proctalgia (ongoing or recurrent rectal pain)
Functional constipation	Presence of ≥2 of the following: straining in >25% of defecations, hard stools in >25% of defecations, incomplete evacuation sensation in >25% of defecations, anorectal obstruction sensation in >25% of defecations, need for manual maneuvers in >25% of defecations, <3 spontaneous bowel movements per week
Functional diarrhea	Loose or watery stools without pain, occurring in >25% of bowel movements
Functional dyspepsia	Characterized by ≥1 symptoms: postprandial fullness, early satiation, epigastric pain, epigastric burning, without evidence of structural disease
Functional gallbladder disorder	Chronic right upper quadrant pain without evidence of gallstones or other explanatory gallbladder pathology
Functional heartburn	Burning sensation in the retrosternal area, not due to gastroesophageal reflux disease, confirmed by normal acid exposure on reflux monitoring and no esophagitis
Functional nausea and vomiting disorders	Chronic nausea and vomiting without an underlying organic cause
Globus	Sensation of a lump or foreign body in the throat, unrelated to swallowing, pain, or heartburn
Irritable bowel syndrome (IBS)	Recurrent abdominal pain, at least once per week in the last 3 mo, associated with ≥2 of the following: related to defecation, change in stool frequency, change in stool form
Pelvic floor dysfunction	Disorders such as dyssynergic defecation, involving paradoxical contraction or inadequate relaxation of pelvic floor muscles during defecation
Rumination syndrome	Effortless regurgitation of recently ingested food, followed by rechewing, reswallowing, or spitting

Source: Drossman DA, Hasler WL. Rome IV-functional GI disorders: disorders of gut-brain interaction. *Gastroenterology*. 2016;150(6):1257–1261.

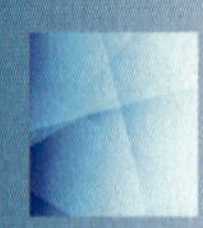

TABLE 21-2. Abdominal Pain

Problem[5]	Process	Location	Quality
Gastroesophageal reflux disease (GERD)[6,7]	Prolonged exposure of esophagus to gastric acid due to impaired esophageal motility or excess relaxations of the lower esophageal sphincter; *Helicobacter pylori* may be present	Chest or epigastric	Heartburn, regurgitation
Peptic ulcer and dyspepsia[8,9]	Mucosal ulcer in stomach or duodenum >5 mm, covered with fibrin, extending through the muscularis mucosa; *H. pylori* infection present in 90% of peptic ulcers	Epigastric, may radiate straight to the back	Variable: epigastric gnawing or burning (dyspepsia); may also be boring, aching, or hunger like No symptoms in up to 20%
Gastric cancer	Adenocarcinoma in 90–95%, either intestinal (older adults) or diffuse (younger adults, worse prognosis)	Increasingly in "cardia" and GE junction; also in distal stomach	Variable
Acute appendicitis[10,11]	Acute inflammation of the appendix with distention or obstruction	Poorly localized periumbilical pain, usually migrates to the right lower quadrant	Mild but increasing, possibly cramping Steady and more severe
Acute cholecystitis[12]	Inflammation of the gallbladder, from persistent obstruction of the cystic duct by gallstone in 90%	Right upper quadrant or epigastrium; may radiate to right shoulder or interscapular area	Steady, persistent, aching
Biliary colic	Intermittent obstruction of the cystic duct by a gallstone	Epigastric or right upper quadrant; may radiate to the right scapula and shoulder	Intermittent pain that resolves
Acute pancreatitis[4,13]	Intrapancreatic trypsinogen activation to trypsin and other enzymes, resulting in autodigestion and inflammation of the pancreas	Epigastric, may radiate straight to the back or other areas of the abdomen; 20% with severe sequelae of organ failure	Usually steady, progressive, severe

Timing	Aggravating Factors	Relieving Factors	Associated Symptoms and Setting
After meals, especially spicy foods	Lying down, bending over; physical activity; diseases such as scleroderma, gastroparesis; drugs like nicotine that relax the lower esophageal sphincter	Antacids, proton pump inhibitors; avoiding alcohol, smoking, fatty meals, chocolate, selected drugs such as theophylline, calcium channel blockers	Wheezing, chronic cough, shortness of breath, hoarseness, choking sensation, dysphagia, regurgitation, halitosis, sore throat; increases risk of Barrett esophagus and esophageal cancer
Intermittent; duodenal ulcer is more likely than gastric ulcer or dyspepsia to cause pain that (1) wakes the patient at night, and (2) occurs intermittently over a few weeks, disappears for months, then recurs	Variable	Food and antacids may bring relief (less likely in gastric ulcers)	Nausea, vomiting, belching, bloating; heartburn (more common in duodenal ulcer); weight loss (more common in gastric ulcer); dyspepsia is more common in the young (20–29 y), gastric ulcer in those over 50 y, and duodenal ulcer in those 30–60 y
Pain is persistent, slowly progressive; duration of pain is typically shorter than in peptic ulcer	Often food; *H. pylori* infection	Not relieved by food or antacids	Anorexia, nausea, early satiety, weight loss, and sometimes bleeding; most common in ages 50–70 y
Continues to worsen until intervention/treatment	Movement or cough	If it subsides temporarily, suspect perforation of the appendix.	Anorexia, nausea, possibly vomiting, which typically follow the onset of pain; low fever
Gradual onset; course longer than in biliary colic	Prior history of biliary colic symptoms		Anorexia, nausea, vomiting, fever; no jaundice
Rapid onset over a few minutes, lasts one to several hours, and subsides gradually; often recurrent	Large fatty meals		Anorexia, nausea, vomiting
Acute onset, persistent pain	Movement	Hydration, bowel rest	Nausea, vomiting, abdominal distention, 80% with history of alcohol abuse or gallstones

(*continued*)

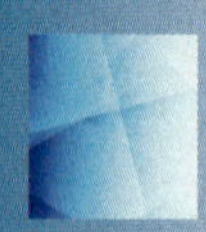

TABLE 21-2. Abdominal Pain *(Continued)*

Problem[5]	Process	Location	Quality
Chronic pancreatitis	Irreversible destruction of the pancreatic parenchyma from recurrent inflammation	Epigastric, radiating to the back	Longstanding persistent pain
Pancreatic cancer[14,15]	Predominantly adenocarcinoma (95%); 5% 5-y survival	If cancer in body or tail, epigastric, in either upper quadrant, often radiates to the back	Steady, deep, nonspecific
Acute diverticulitis[16]	Acute inflammation of colonic diverticula, outpouchings, usually in sigmoid or descending colon	Left lower quadrant, pelvic	May be cramping at first, then steady
Acute bowel obstruction	Obstruction of the bowel lumen, most commonly caused by (1) adhesions or hernias (small bowel), or (2) cancer or strictures (colon)	Generalized abdominal pain, nonspecific, result of distention	Cramping, colicky
Mesenteric ischemia[17,18]	Occlusion of blood flow to small bowel, from arterial or venous thrombosis, cardiac embolus, or hypoperfusion	Vague nonspecific	Pain out of proportion to examination is hallmark of mesenteric ischemia

Timing	Aggravating Factors	Relieving Factors	Associated Symptoms and Setting
Chronic or recurrent course	Alcohol, medication, frequent attacks of acute pancreatitis	None	Pancreatic enzyme insufficiency, diarrhea with fatty stools (*steatorrhea*), and diabetes mellitus
Persistent pain; relentlessly progressive illness	Smoking, chronic pancreatitis	Often intractable	Painless jaundice, anorexia, weight loss; glucose intolerance, depression
Often gradual onset		Analgesia, bowel rest, antibiotics	Fever, diarrhea, urinary symptoms, anorexia
Progressive, intermittent	Ingestion of food or liquids	Bowel rest, hydration	No passage of flatus or bowel movement, nausea, vomiting, progressive abdominal distention
Usually abrupt in onset, then persistent	Underlying thromboembolic disease, low flow states, hypercoagulable conditions	Volume resuscitation	Vomiting, bloody stool, soft distended abdomen, systemic shock

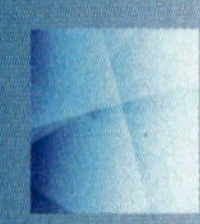

TABLE 21-3. Dysphagia

Process and Problem	Timing	Factors That Aggravate	Factors That Relieve	Associated Symptoms and Conditions
Oropharyngeal dysphagia	Acute or gradual onset and a variable course, depending on the underlying disorder	Attempts to start the swallowing process		Aspiration into the lungs or regurgitation into the nose with attempts to swallow; from motor disorders affecting the pharyngeal muscles such as stroke, bulbar palsy, or other neuromuscular conditions
Esophageal dysphagia				
Mechanical narrowing				
Mucosal rings and webs	Intermittent	Solid foods	Regurgitation of the bolus of food	Usually none
Esophageal stricture	Intermittent; may become slowly progressive	Solid foods	Regurgitation of the bolus of food	A long history of heartburn and regurgitation
Esophageal cancer	May be intermittent at first; progressive over months	Solid foods, with progression to liquids	Regurgitation of the bolus of food	Pain in the chest and back and weight loss, especially late in the course of illness
Motor disorders				
Diffuse esophageal spasm	Intermittent	Solids or liquids	Maneuvers described below; sometimes nitroglycerin	Chest pain that mimics angina pectoris or myocardial infarction and lasts minutes to hours; possibly heartburn
Scleroderma	Intermittent; may progress slowly	Solids or liquids	Repeated swallowing; movements such as straightening the back, raising the arms, or a Valsalva maneuver (straining down against a closed glottis)	Heartburn; other manifestations of scleroderma
Achalasia	Intermittent; may progress	Solids or liquids	Repeated swallowing; movements such as straightening the back, raising the arms, or a Valsalva maneuver (straining down against a closed glottis)	Regurgitation, often at night when lying down, with nocturnal cough; possibly chest pain precipitated by eating

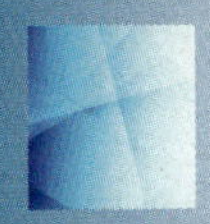

TABLE 21-4. Diarrhea

Problem	Process	Characteristics of Stool	Timing	Associated Symptoms	Setting, Persons at Risk
Acute Diarrhea[24] (≤14 days)					
■ *Secretory infection (noninflammatory)*	Infection by viruses, preformed bacterial toxins (e.g., *Staphylococcus aureus*, *Bacillus cereus*, *Clostridium perfringens*, toxigenic *Escherichia coli*, *Vibrio cholerae*), cryptosporidium, *Giardia lamblia*, rotavirus	Watery, without blood, pus, or mucus	Duration of a few days, possibly longer; lactase deficiency may lead to a longer course	Nausea, vomiting, periumbilical cramping pain; temperature normal or slightly elevated	Often travel, a common food source, or an epidemic
■ *Inflammatory infection*	Colonization or invasion of intestinal mucosa (nontyphoid *Salmonella*, *Shigella*, *Yersinia*, *Campylobacter*, enteropathic *E. coli*, *Entamoeba histolytica*, *Clostridioides difficile*)	Loose to watery, often with blood, pus, or mucus	Acute illness of varying duration	Lower abdominal cramping pain and often rectal urgency, tenesmus; fever	Travel, contaminated food or water; frequent anal intercourse
Drug-induced diarrhea	Action of many drugs, such as magnesium-containing antacids, antibiotics, antineoplastic agents, and laxatives	Loose to watery	Acute, recurrent, or chronic	Possibly nausea; usually little if any pain	Prescribed or over-the-counter medications
Chronic diarrhea (≥30 days)					
■ *Diarrheal syndrome*					
Irritable bowel syndrome[25]	Altered motility or secretion from luminal and mucosal irritants that change mucosal permeability, immune activation, and colonic transit, including maldigested carbohydrates, fats, excess bile acids, gluten intolerance, enteroendocrine signaling, and changes in microbiomes	Loose; ~50% with mucus; small to moderate volume Small, hard stools with constipation May be mixed pattern	Worse in the morning; rarely at night.	Crampy lower abdominal pain, abdominal distention, flatulence, nausea; urgency, pain relieved with defecation	Young and middle-aged adults, especially individuals assigned female at birth

(continued)

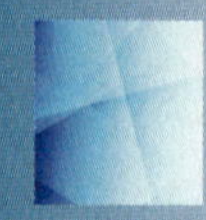

TABLE 21-4. Diarrhea *(Continued)*

Problem	Process	Characteristics of Stool	Timing	Associated Symptoms	Setting, Persons at Risk
Fecal impaction/ motility disorders	Partial obstruction by impacted stool only allowing passage of loose feces	Loose, small volume	Variable	Crampy abdominal pain, incomplete evacuation	Older adults immobilized and institutionalized patients; ensues from selected medications
Cancer of the sigmoid colon	Partial obstruction by a malignant neoplasm	May be blood-streaked	Variable	Change in usual bowel habits, crampy lower abdominal pain, constipation	Middle-age and older adults, especially >55 y
■ *Inflammatory bowel disease*					
Ulcerative colitis	Mucosal inflammation typically extending proximally from the rectum (*proctitis*) to varying lengths of the colon (*colitis to pancolitis*), with microulcerations and, if chronic, inflammatory polyps	Frequent, watery, bloody	Onset typically abrupt; often recurrent, persisting, and may awaken at night	Cramping, with urgency, tenesmus; fever, fatigue, weakness; abdominal pain if complicated by toxic megacolon; may include episcleritis, uveitis, arthritis, erythema nodosum	Often young adults, Ashkenazi Jewish descendants; linked to altered CD4+ T-cell Th2 response; increases risk of colon cancer
Crohn's disease of the small bowel (*regional enteritis*) or colon (*granulomatous colitis*)	Chronic transmural inflammation of the bowel wall, with skip pattern involving the terminal ileum and/or proximal colon (and rectal sparing); may cause strictures	Small, soft to loose or watery, with bleeding if colitis, obstructive symptoms, if enteritis	More insidious onset; chronic or recurrent	Crampy periumbilical, right lower quadrant (*enteritis*) or diffuse (*colitis*) pain, with anorexia, fever, and/or weight loss; perianal or perirectal abscesses and fistulas; may cause small or large bowel obstruction	Often teens or young adults, but also adults of middle age; more common in Ashkenazi Jewish descendants; linked to altered CD4+ T-cell helper (Th1 and 17) response; increases risk of colon cancer

Problem	Process	Characteristics of Stool	Timing	Associated Symptoms	Setting, Persons at Risk
■ *Voluminous diarrhea*					
Malabsorption syndrome	Defective membrane transport or absorption of intestinal epithelium (Crohn's and celiac diseases, surgical resection); impaired luminal digestion (pancreatic insufficiency); epithelial defects at brush border (lactose intolerance)	Typically, bulky, soft, light yellow to gray, mushy, greasy or oily, and sometimes frothy; particularly foul-smelling; usually floats in toilet (*steatorrhea*)	Onset of illness typically insidious	Anorexia, weight loss, fatigue, abdominal distention, often crampy lower abdominal pain. Symptoms of nutritional deficiencies such as bleeding (vitamin K), bone pain and fractures (vitamin D), glossitis (vitamin B), and edema (protein)	Variable, depending on cause
Osmotic diarrhea					
■ *Lactose intolerance*	Intestinal lactase deficiency	Watery diarrhea of large volume	Follows the ingestion of milk and milk products; relieved by fasting	Crampy abdominal pain, abdominal distention, flatulence	In >50% of African Americans, Asians, Native Americans, Hispanics; in 5–20% of Caucasians
■ *Abuse of osmotic purgatives*	Laxative habit, often surreptitious	Watery diarrhea of large volume	Variable	Often none	Persons with anorexia nervosa or bulimia nervosa
■ *Secretory diarrhea*	Variable: bacterial infection, secreting villous adenoma, fat or bile salt malabsorption, hormone-mediated conditions (gastrin in *Zollinger–Ellison syndrome,* vasoactive intestinal peptide)	Watery diarrhea of large volume	Variable	Weight loss, dehydration, nausea, vomiting, and cramping abdominal pain	Variable depending on cause

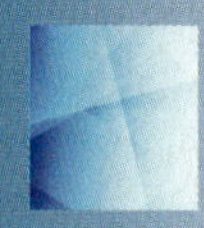

TABLE 21-5. Constipation

Problem	Process	Associated Symptoms and Setting
Life activities and habits		
Inadequate time or setting for the defecation reflex	Ignoring the sensation of a full rectum inhibits the defecation reflex	Hectic schedules, unfamiliar surroundings, bed rest
False expectations of bowel habits	Expectations of "regularity" or more frequent stools than a person's norm	Beliefs, treatments, and advertisements that promote the use of laxatives
Diet deficient in fiber	Decreased fecal bulk	Other factors such as debilitation and constipating drugs may contribute
Irritable bowel syndrome[25]	Functional change in frequency or form of bowel movement without known pathology; possibly from change in intestinal bacteria.	Three patterns: diarrhea—predominant, constipation—predominant, or mixed. Symptoms present ≥6 mo and abdominal pain for ≥3 mo plus at least two to three features (improvement with defecation; onset with change in stool frequency; onset with change in stool form and appearance)
Mechanical Obstruction		
Cancer of the rectum or sigmoid colon	Progressive narrowing of the bowel lumen from adenocarcinoma	Change in bowel habits; often diarrhea, abdominal pain, bleeding, occult blood in stool; in rectal cancer, tenesmus, and pencil-shaped stools; weight loss
Fecal impaction	A large, firm, immovable fecal mass, most often in the rectum	Rectal fullness, abdominal pain, and diarrhea around the impaction; common in debilitated, bedridden, and often older adults and institutionalized patients
Other obstructing lesions (e.g., diverticulitis, volvulus, intussusception, or hernia)	Narrowing or complete obstruction of the bowel	Colicky abdominal pain, abdominal distention, and in intussusception, often "currant jelly" stools (red blood and mucus)
Painful anal lesions	Pain may cause spasm of the external sphincter and voluntary inhibition of the defecation reflex.	Anal fissures, painful hemorrhoids, perirectal abscesses
Drugs	Variety of mechanisms	Opiates, anticholinergics, antacids containing calcium or aluminum, and many others
Depression	Mood disorder	Fatigue, anhedonia, sleep disturbance, weight loss
Neurologic disorders	Interference with the autonomic innervation of the bowel	Spinal cord injuries, multiple sclerosis, Hirschsprung disease, and other conditions
Metabolic conditions	Interference with bowel motility	Pregnancy, hypothyroidism, hypercalcemia

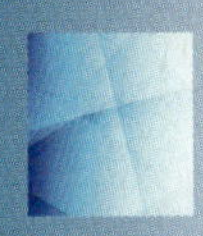

TABLE 21-6. Black and Bloody Stool

Problem	Selected Causes	Associated Symptoms and Setting
Melena		
■ Refers to passage of black tarry stool ■ Fecal blood tests are positive ■ Involves loss ≥60 mL of blood into the gastrointestinal (GI) tract (less in children), usually from the esophagus, stomach, or duodenum with transit time of 7–14 h ■ Less commonly, if slow transit, blood loss originates in the jejunum, ileum, or ascending colon ■ In infants, melena may result from swallowing blood during the birth	■ Gastritis, gastroesophageal reflux disease, peptic ulcer (gastric or duodenal) ■ Gastritis or stress ulcers ■ Esophageal or gastric varices ■ Reflux esophagitis, Mallory–Weiss tear in esophageal mucosa due to retching and vomiting	■ Usually epigastric discomfort from heartburn, dysmotility; if peptic ulcer, pain after meals (delay of 2–3 h if duodenal ulcer; may be asymptomatic) ■ Recent ingestion of alcohol, aspirin, or other anti-inflammatory drugs; recent bodily trauma, severe burns, surgery, or increased intracranial pressure ■ Cirrhosis of the liver or other causes of portal hypertension ■ Retching, vomiting, often recent ingestion of alcohol
Black stool		
■ Black stool from other causes with negative fecal blood tests; stool change has no pathologic significance	■ Ingestion of iron, bismuth salts, licorice, or even chocolate cookies	■ Asymptomatic
Stool with red blood (*hematochezia*)		
■ Usually originates in the colon, rectum, or anus; much less frequently from the jejunum or ileum	■ Colon cancer ■ Hyperplasia or adenomatous polyps	■ Often a change in bowel habits, weight loss
■ Upper GI hemorrhage may also cause red stool, usually with large blood loss ≥1 L	■ Diverticula of the colon	■ Often no other symptoms ■ Often no symptoms unless inflammation causes diverticulitis
■ Rapid transit leaves insufficient time for the blood to turn black from oxidation of iron in hemoglobin	■ Inflammatory conditions of the colon and rectum	
	■ Ulcerative colitis, Crohn's disease	■ See Table 21-4, Diarrhea, pp. 661–663
	■ Infectious diarrhea	■ See Table 21-4, Diarrhea, pp. 661–663
	■ Proctitis (various causes including anal intercourse)	■ Rectal urgency, tenesmus (see Table 21-4, Diarrhea, pp. 661–663)
	■ Ischemic colitis	■ Lower abdominal pain sometimes fever or shock in older adults; abdomen typically soft to palpation
	■ Hemorrhoids	■ Blood on the toilet paper, on the surface of the stool, or dripping into the toilet, typically painless
	■ Anal fissure	■ Blood on the toilet paper or on the surface of the stool; anal pain with defecation
Reddish but nonbloody stool	■ Ingestion of beets	■ Pink urine, which usually precedes the reddish stool; from poor metabolism of betacyanin

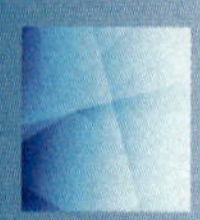

TABLE 21-7. Localized Bulges in the Abdominal Wall

Localized bulges in the abdominal wall include *ventral hernias* (defects in the wall through which tissue protrudes) and subcutaneous tumors such as *lipomas*. The more common ventral hernias are umbilical, incisional, and epigastric. Hernias and diastasis recti usually become more evident when the patient is supine and raises the head and shoulders.

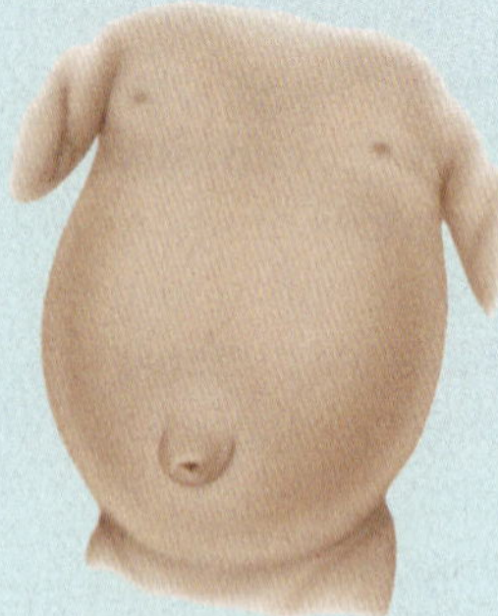

Umbilical hernia

A protrusion through a defective umbilical ring. When present in infants, it usually closes spontaneously within 1–2 y.

Diastasis recti

Separation of the two rectus abdominis muscles, through which abdominal contents form a midline ridge typically extending from the xiphoid to the umbilicus and seen only when the patient raises the head and shoulders. Often present in patients with repeated pregnancies, obesity, and chronic lung disease. It is clinically benign.

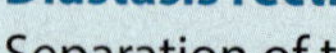

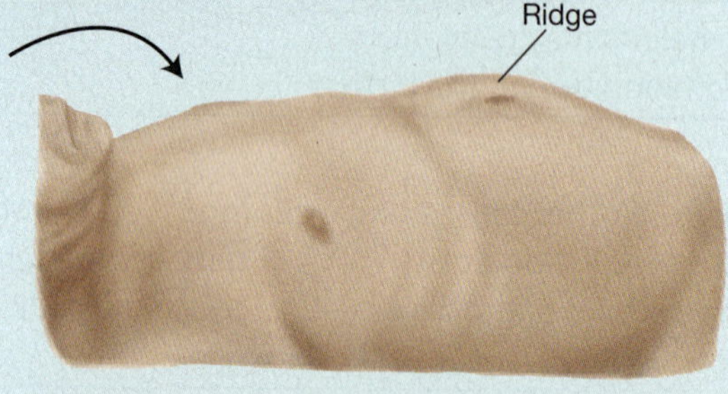

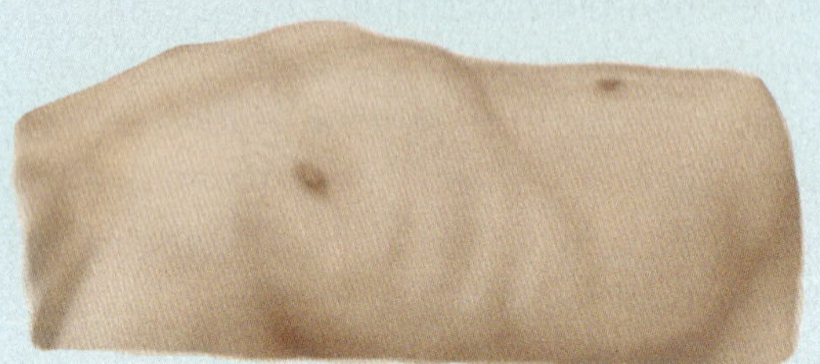

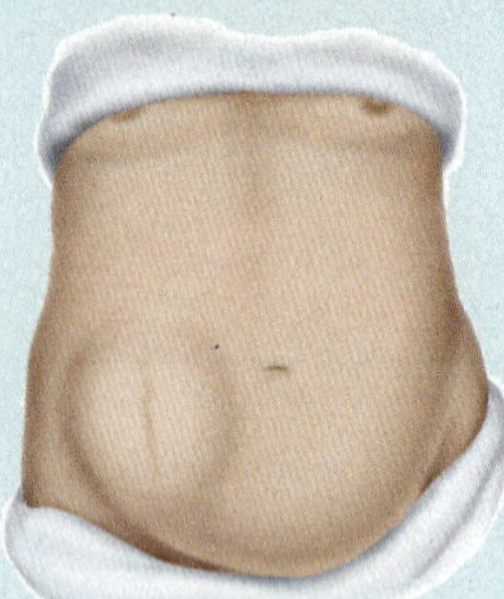

Incisional hernia

This is a protrusion through an operative scar. Palpate to detect the length and width of the defect in the abdominal wall. A small defect, through which a large hernia has passed, has a greater risk for complications than a large defect.

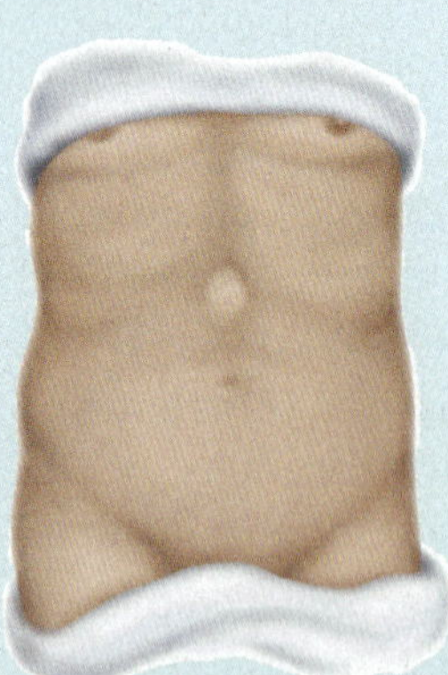

Epigastric hernia

A small midline protrusion through a defect in the linea alba occurs between the xiphoid process and the umbilicus. With the patient coughing or performing a Valsalva maneuver, palpate by running your finger pad down the linea alba.

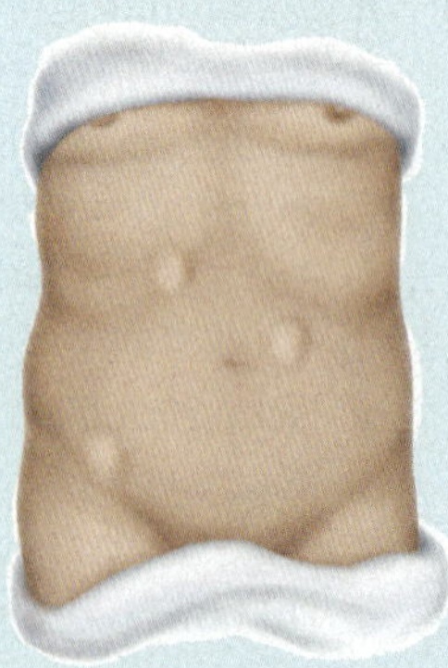

Lipoma

Common, benign, fatty tumors usually in the subcutaneous tissues almost anywhere in the body, including the abdominal wall. Small or large, they are usually soft and often lobulated. Press your finger down on the edge of a lipoma. The tumor typically slips out from under your finger and is well demarcated, nonreducible, and usually nontender.

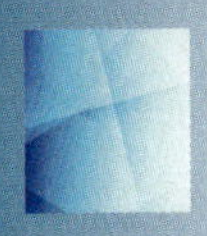

TABLE 21-8. Protuberant Abdomens

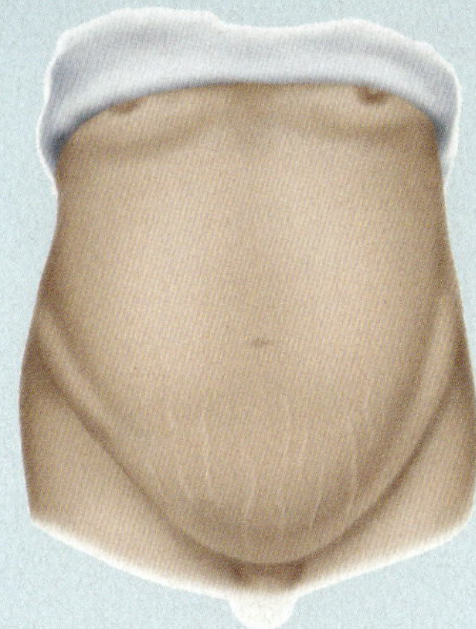

Fat

Fat is the most common cause of a protuberant abdomen. Fat thickens the abdominal wall, the mesentery, and omentum. The umbilicus may appear sunken. A *pannus,* or apron of fatty tissue, may extend below the inguinal ligaments. Lift it to look for inflammation in the skin folds or even for a hidden hernia.

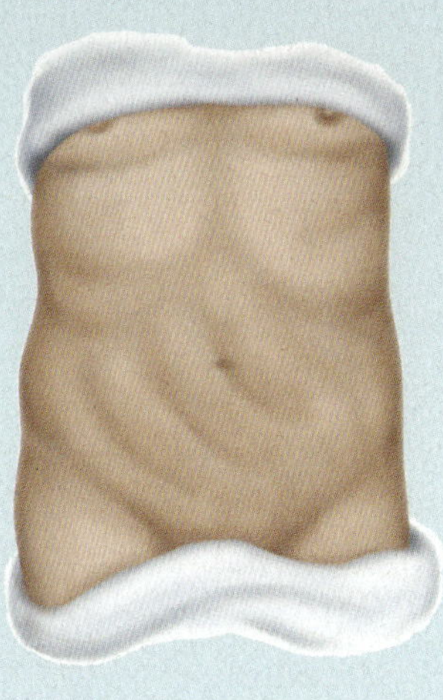

Gas

Gaseous distention may be localized or generalized. It causes a tympanitic percussion note. Selected foods may cause mild distention from increased intestinal gas production. More serious causes are intestinal obstruction and adynamic (paralytic) ileus. Note the location of the distention. Distention is more marked in obstruction in the colon than in the small bowel.

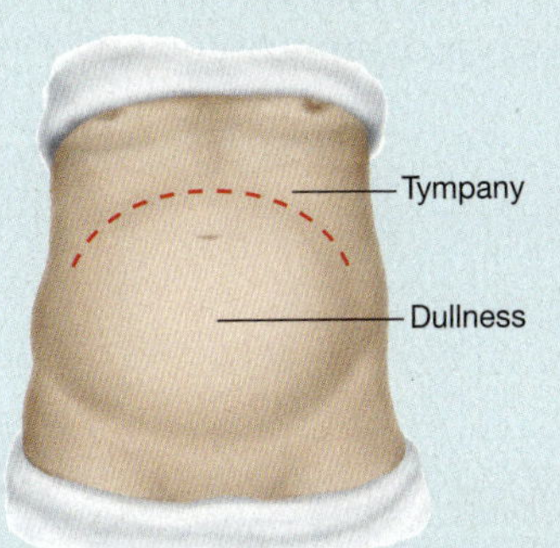

Tumor

A large solid tumor, usually rising out of the pelvis, is dull to percussion. Air-filled bowel is displaced to the periphery. Causes include ovarian tumors and uterine fibroids. Occasionally, a markedly distended bladder is mistaken for such a tumor.

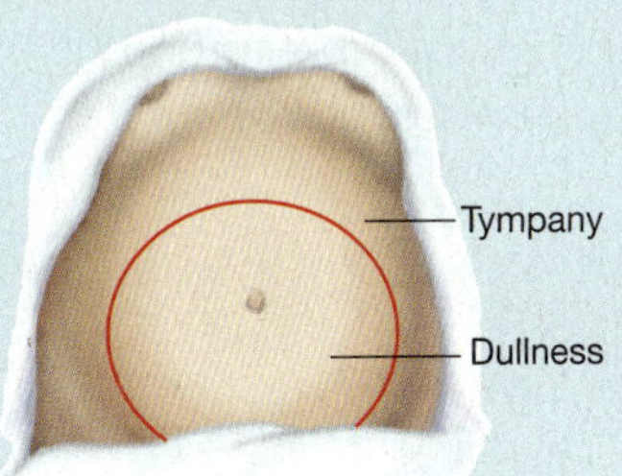

Fetal heart sounds present

Pregnancy

Pregnancy is a common pelvic "mass." Listen for the fetal heart (see p. 1134).

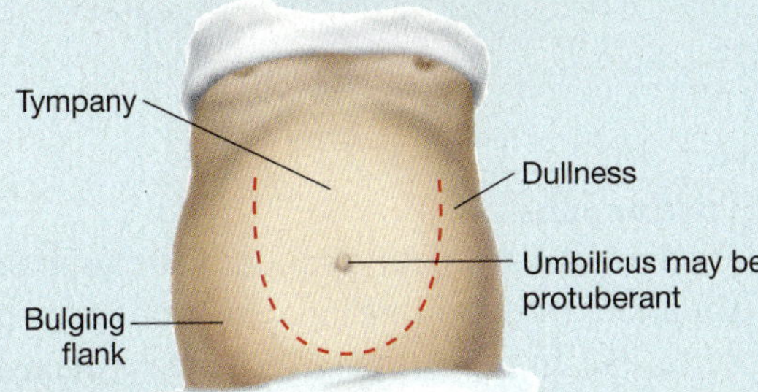

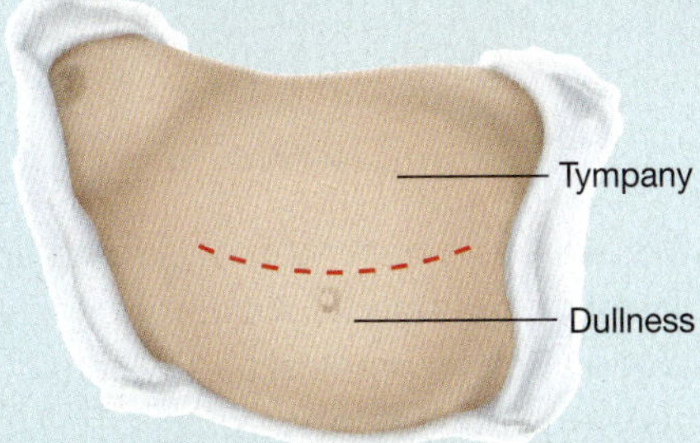

Ascitic fluid

Ascitic fluid seeks the lowest point in the abdomen, producing bulging flanks that are dull to percussion. The umbilicus may protrude. Turn the patient onto one side to detect the shift in position of the fluid level (shifting dullness). (See p. 639 for assessment of ascites.)

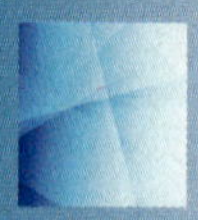

TABLE 21-9. Sounds in the Abdomen

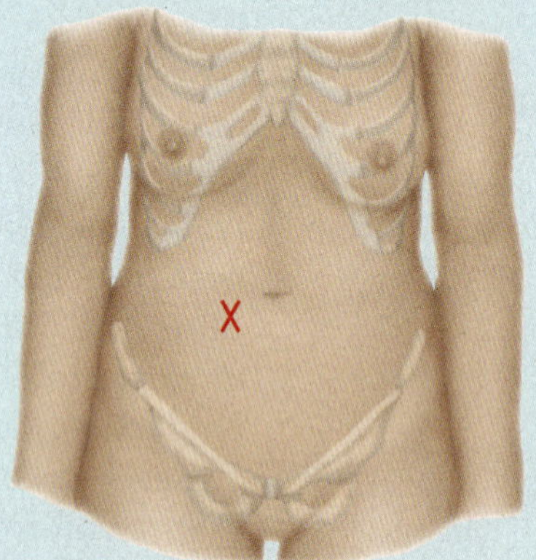

Bowel sounds

Bowel sounds may be:

- *Increased,* as in diarrhea or early intestinal obstruction
- *Decreased,* then absent, as in *adynamic ileus* and *peritonitis.* Before deciding that bowel sounds are absent, sit down and listen where shown for ≥2 min.

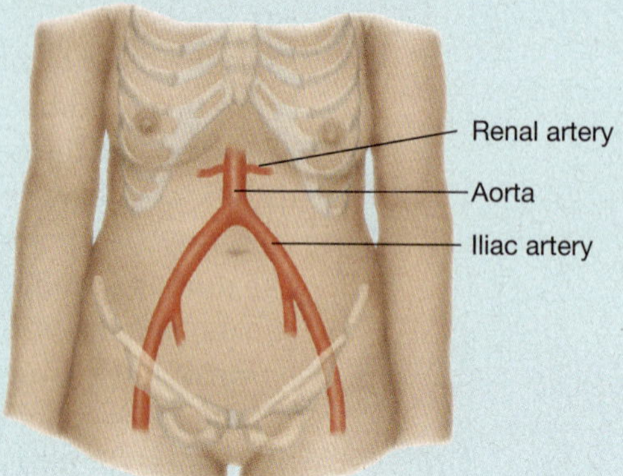

Bruits

A *hepatic bruit* suggests carcinoma of the liver or cirrhosis. *Arterial bruits* with both systolic and diastolic components suggest partial occlusion of the aorta or large arteries. Such bruits in the epigastrium are suspicious for renal artery stenosis or renovascular hypertension.

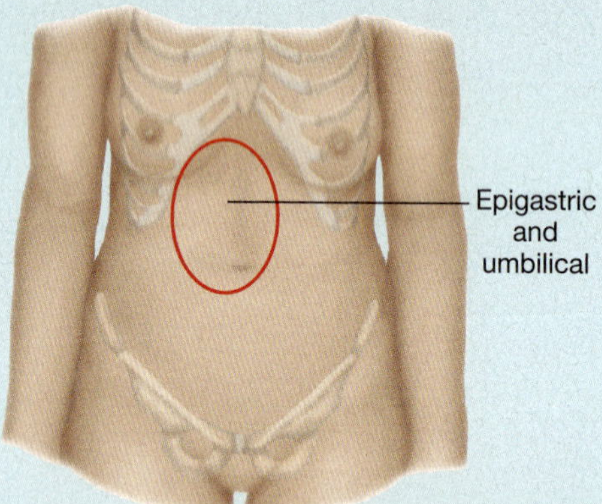

Venous hum

A venous hum is a rare soft humming noise with both systolic and diastolic components. It points to increased collateral circulation between portal and systemic venous systems, as in hepatic cirrhosis.

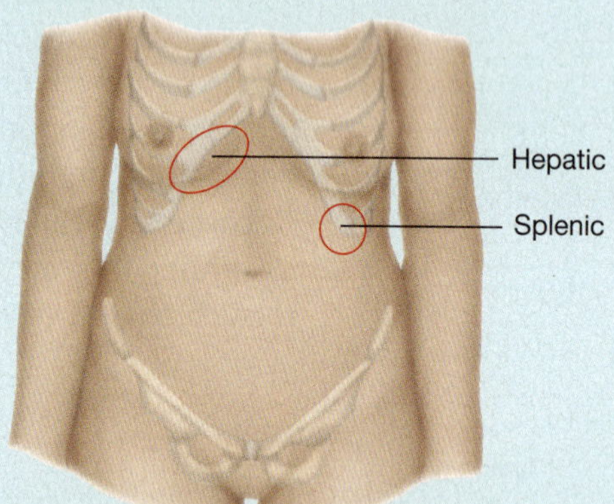

Friction rubs

Friction rubs are grating sounds with respiratory variation. They indicate inflammation of the peritoneal surface of an organ, as in liver cancer, chlamydial or gonococcal perihepatitis, recent liver biopsy, or splenic infarct. When a systolic bruit accompanies a hepatic friction rub, suspect carcinoma of the liver.

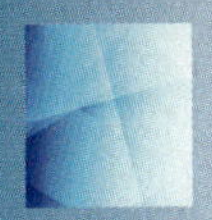

TABLE 21-10. Tender Abdomens

Abdominal wall tenderness

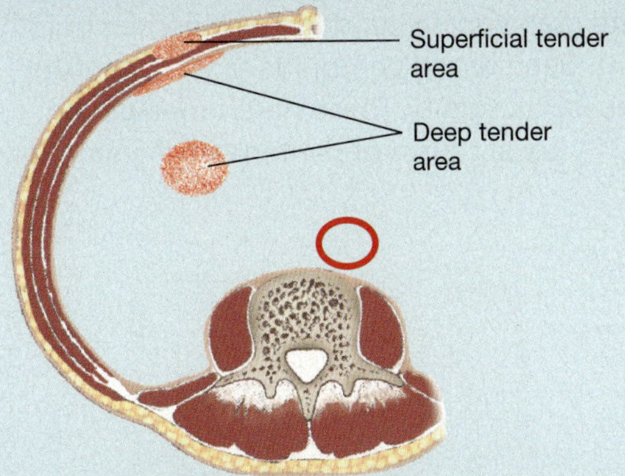

Tenderness may originate in the abdominal wall. When the patient raises the head and shoulders, this tenderness persists, whereas tenderness from a deeper lesion (protected by the tightened muscles) decreases.

Visceral tenderness

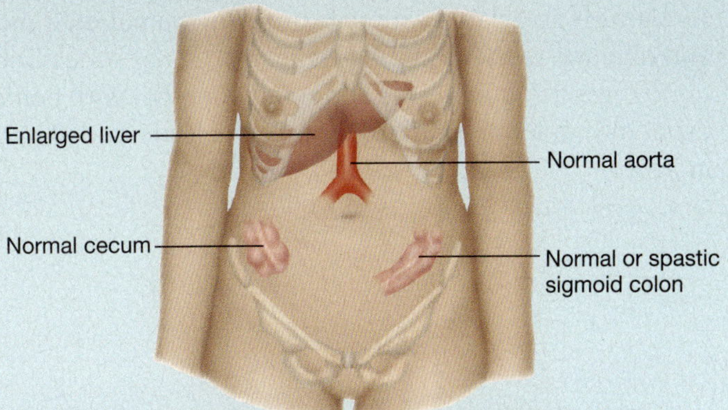

The structures shown may be tender to deep palpation. Usually, the discomfort is dull with no muscular rigidity or rebound tenderness. A reassuring explanation to the patient may prove helpful.

Tenderness from disease in the chest and pelvis

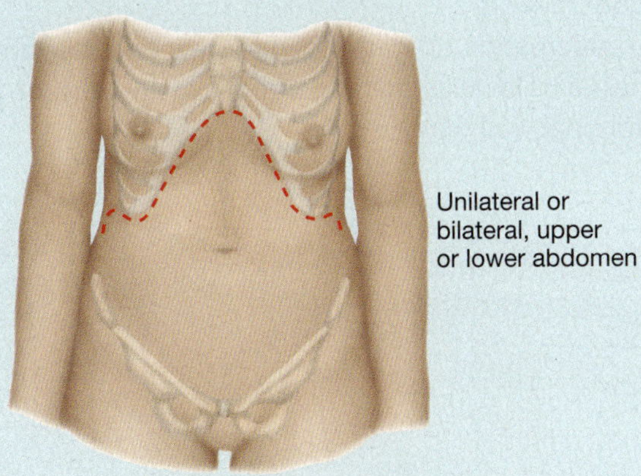

Acute pleurisy

Abdominal pain and tenderness may result from acute pleural inflammation. When unilateral, it can mimic acute cholecystitis or appendicitis. Rebound tenderness and rigidity are less common; chest signs are usually present.

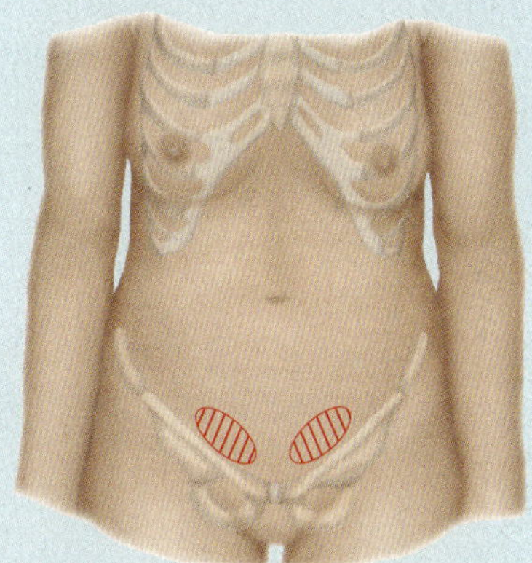

Acute salpingitis

Frequently bilateral, the tenderness of acute salpingitis (inflammation of the fallopian tubes) is usually maximal just above the inguinal ligaments. Rebound tenderness and rigidity may be present. On pelvic examination, motion of the cervix and uterus causes pain.

(*continued*)

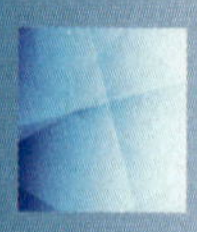

TABLE 21-10. Tender Abdomens *(Continued)*

Tenderness of peritoneal inflammation

Tenderness associated with peritoneal inflammation is more severe than visceral tenderness. Muscular rigidity and rebound tenderness are frequently but not necessarily present. Generalized peritonitis causes exquisite tenderness throughout the abdomen, together with board-like muscular rigidity. These signs on palpation, especially abdominal rigidity, double the likelihood of peritonitis.[32,33] Local causes of peritoneal inflammation include:

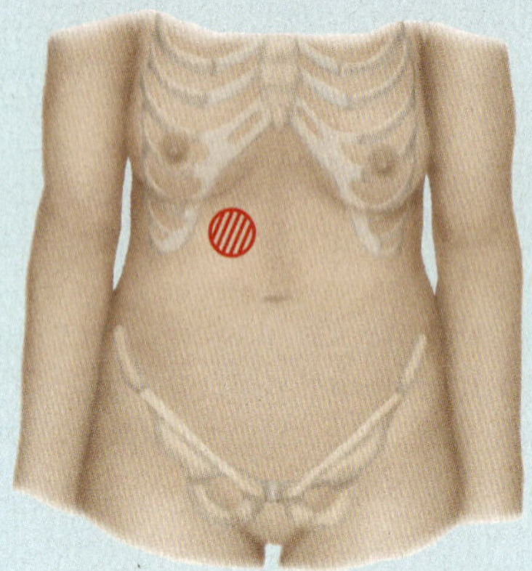

Acute cholecystitis[12]

Signs are maximal in the right upper quadrant. Check for Murphy sign (see pp. 641–642).

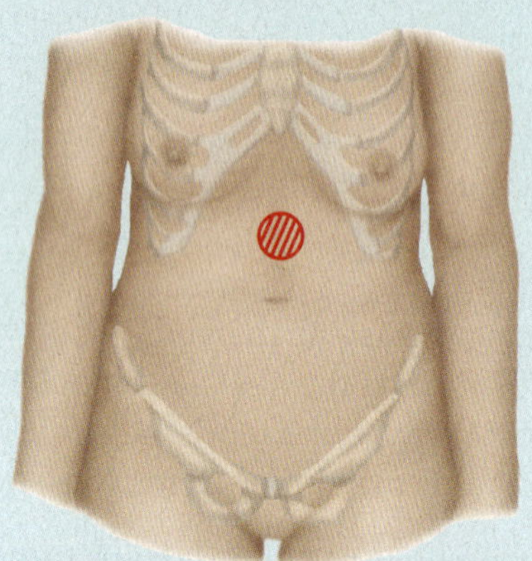

Acute pancreatitis

In acute pancreatitis, epigastric tenderness and rebound tenderness and localized guarding are usually present, but the abdominal wall may be soft.

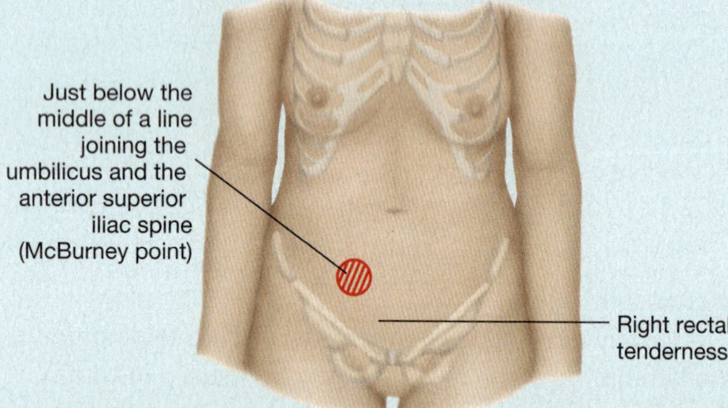

Acute appendicitis[10,11]

Right lower quadrant signs are typical of acute appendicitis but may be absent early in the course. The typical area of tenderness, McBurney point, is illustrated. Examine other areas of the right lower quadrant as well as the right flank.

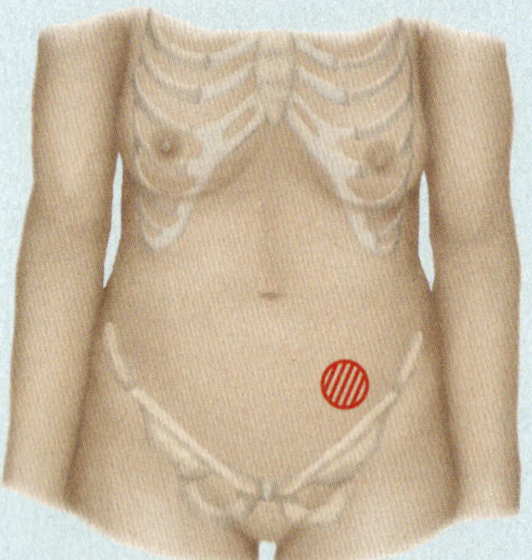

Acute diverticulitis

Acute diverticulitis is a confined inflammatory process, usually in the left lower quadrant, that involves the sigmoid colon. If the sigmoid colon is redundant there may be suprapubic or right-sided pain. Look for localized peritoneal signs and a tender underlying mass. Microperforation, abscess, and obstruction may ensue.

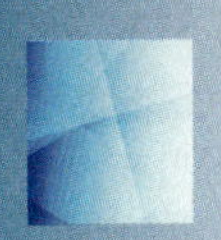

TABLE 21-11. Liver Enlargement: Apparent and Real

A palpable liver does not necessarily indicate hepatomegaly (an enlarged liver), but more often results from a change in consistency—from the normal softness to an abnormal firmness or hardness, as in cirrhosis. Clinical estimates of liver size should be based on both percussion and palpation, although even these techniques are imperfect compared to ultrasound.

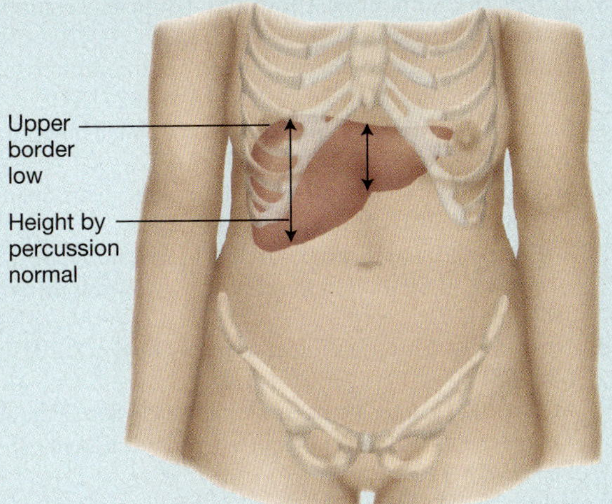

Downward displacement of the liver by a low diaphragm

This finding is common when the diaphragm is flattened and low, as in COPD. The liver edge may be palpable well below the costal margin. Percussion, however, reveals a low upper edge, and the vertical span of the liver is normal.

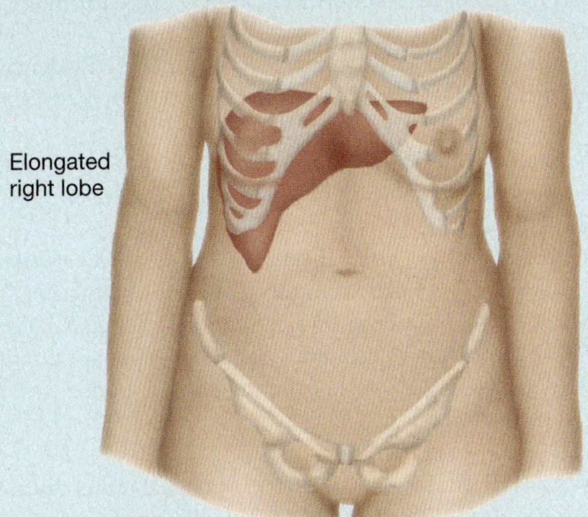

Normal variations in liver shape

In some individuals, the right lobe of the liver may be elongated and easily palpable as it projects downward toward the iliac crest. Such an elongation, sometimes called *Riedel lobe,* represents a variation in shape, not an increase in liver volume or size.

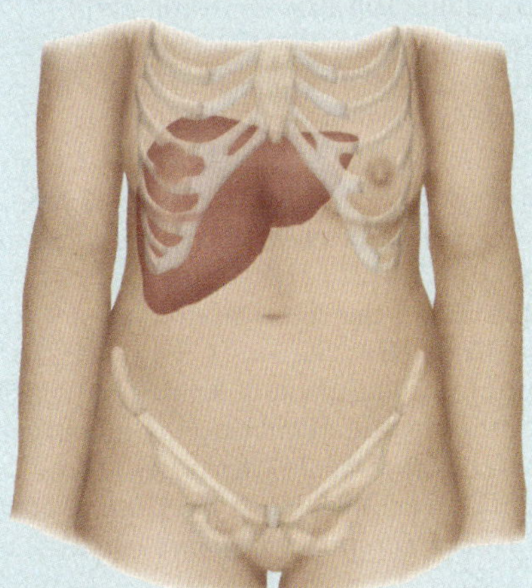

Smooth large liver

Cirrhosis may produce an enlarged liver with a firm, *nontender* edge. The cirrhotic liver may also be scarred and contracted. Many other diseases may produce similar findings such as hemochromatosis, amyloidosis, and lymphoma. An enlarged liver with a smooth, *tender* edge suggests inflammation, as in hepatitis, or venous congestion, seen in right-sided heart failure.

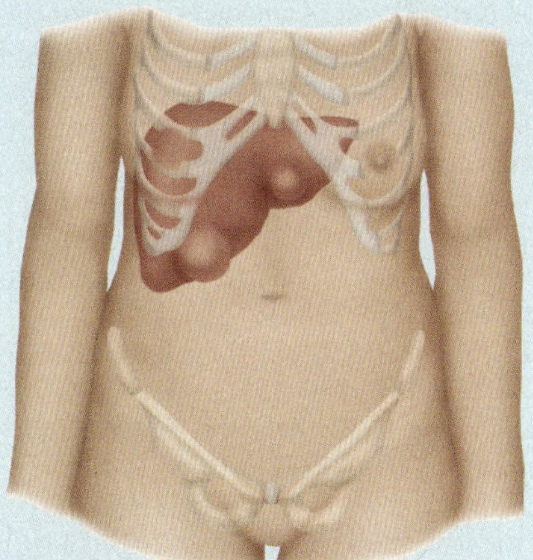

Irregular large liver

An enlarged liver that is firm or hard with an irregular edge or surface suggests *hepatocellular carcinoma*. There may be one or more nodules. The liver may or may not be tender.

REFERENCES

1. Drossman DA, Hasler WL. Rome IV-functional GI disorders: disorders of gut-brain interaction. *Gastroenterology.* 2016; 150(6):1257–1261.
2. National Center for Health Statistics. *National Hospital Ambulatory Medical Care Survey: 2021 Emergency Department Summary Tables.* Centers for Disease Control and Prevention, 2021. Accessed January 7, 2024. https://www.cdc.gov/nchs/data/nhamcs/web_tables/2021-nhamcs-ed-web-tables-508.pdf
3. Natesan S, Lee J, Volkamer H, Thoureen T. Evidence-based medicine approach to abdominal pain. *Emerg Med Clin North Am.* 2016;34(2):165–190.
4. Schneider L, Büchler MW, Werner J. Acute pancreatitis with an emphasis on infection. *Infect Dis Clin North Am.* 2010; 24(4):921–941.
5. *Gastroenterology and Hepatology–Medical Knowledge Self-Assessment Program.* American College of Physicians; 2013.
6. Shaheen NJ, Weinberg DS, Denberg TD, Chou R, Qaseem A, Shekelle P. Upper endoscopy for gastroesophageal reflux disease: best practice advice from the clinical guidelines committee of the American College of Physicians. *Ann Intern Med.* 2012;157(11):808–816.
7. Wilson JF. In the clinic. Gastroesophageal reflux disease. *Ann Intern Med.* 2008;149(3):ITC2-1–ITC2-16.
8. Talley NJ, Vakil NB, Moayyedi P. American Gastroenterological Association technical review on the evaluation of dyspepsia. *Gastroenterology.* 2005;129(5):1756–1780.
9. Tack J, Talley NJ. Functional dyspepsia–symptoms, definitions and validity of the Rome III criteria. *Nat Rev Gastroenterol Hepatol.* 2013;10(3):134–141.
10. Howell JM, Eddy OL, Lukens TW, Thiessen ME, Weingart SD, Decker WW. Clinical policy: critical issues in the evaluation and management of emergency department patients with suspected appendicitis. *Ann Emerg Med.* 2010;55(1):71–116.
11. Andersson RE. The natural history and traditional management of appendicitis revisited: spontaneous resolution and predominance of prehospital perforations imply that a correct diagnosis is more important than an early diagnosis. *World J Surg.* 2007;31(1):86–92.
12. Strasberg SM. Clinical practice. Acute calculous cholecystitis. *N Engl J Med.* 2008;358(26):2804–2811.
13. Fogel EL, Sherman S. ERCP for gallstone pancreatitis. *N Engl J Med.* 2014;370(2):150–157.
14. Ryan DP, Hong TS, Bardeesy N. Pancreatic adenocarcinoma. *N Engl J Med.* 2014;371(11):1039–1049.
15. Yadav D, Lowenfels AB. The epidemiology of pancreatitis and pancreatic cancer. *Gastroenterology.* 2013;144(6):1252–1261.
16. Katz LH, Guy DD, Lahat A, Gafter-Gvili A, Bar-Meir S. Diverticulitis in the young is not more aggressive than in the elderly, but it tends to recur more often: systematic review and meta-analysis. *J Gastroenterol Hepatol.* 2013;28(8): 1274–1281.
17. Acosta S. Mesenteric ischemia. *Curr Opin Crit Care.* 2015; 21(2):171–178.
18. Sise MJ. Acute mesenteric ischemia. *Surg Clin North Am.* 2014;94(1):165–181.
19. Peterson MC, Holbrook JH, Von Hales D, Smith NL, Staker LV. Contributions of the history, physical examination, and laboratory investigation in making medical diagnoses. *West J Med.* 1992;156(2):163–165.
20. Lacy BE, Patel NK. Rome criteria and a diagnostic approach to irritable bowel syndrome. *J Clin Med.* 2017;6(11):99.
21. Schmulson MJ, Drossman DA. What is new in Rome IV. *J Neurogastroenterol Motil.* 2017;23(2):151–163.
22. Longstreth GF, Thompson WG, Chey WD, Houghton LA, Mearin F, Spiller RC. Functional bowel disorders. *Gastroenterology.* 2006;130(5):1480–1491.
23. Leffler DA, Lamont JT. Clostridium difficile infection. *N Engl J Med.* 2015;372(16):1539–1548.
24. DuPont HL. Acute infectious diarrhea in immunocompetent adults. *N Engl J Med.* 2014;370(16):1532–1540.
25. Camilleri M. Peripheral mechanisms in irritable bowel syndrome. *N Engl J Med.* 2012;367(17):1626–1635.
26. Shah BJ, Rughwani N, Rose S. In the clinic. Constipation. *Ann Intern Med.* 2015;162(7):ITC1–ITC17.
27. Gallegos-Orozco JF, Foxx-Orenstein AE, Sterler SM, Stoa JM. Chronic constipation in the elderly. *Am J Gastroenterol.* 2012; 107(1):18–25.
28. Novo C, Welsh F. Jaundice. *Surgery (Oxford).* 2017;35(12): 675–681.
29. McGee SR. Chapter 49: palpation and percussion of the abdomen. *Evidence-Based Physical Diagnosis.* 3rd ed. Elsevier/Saunders; 2012:428–440.
30. Felder S, Margel D, Murrell Z, Fleshner P. Usefulness of bowel sound auscultation: a prospective evaluation. *J Surg Educ.* 2014;71(5):768–773.
31. Cope Z. *The Early Diagnosis of the Acute Abdomen.* Oxford University Press; 1972.
32. McGee SR. Chapter 50: abdominal pain and tenderness. *Evidence-Based Physical Diagnosis.* 3rd ed. Elsevier/Saunders; 2012:441–452.
33. Cartwright SL, Knudson MP. Evaluation of acute abdominal pain in adults. *Am Fam Physician.* 2008;77(7):971–978.
34. de Bruyn G, Graviss EA. A systematic review of the diagnostic accuracy of physical examination for the detection of cirrhosis. *BMC Med Inform Decis Mak.* 2001;1:6.
35. Grover SA, Barkun AN, Sackett DL. Does this patient have splenomegaly? *JAMA.* 1993;270(18):2218–2221.
36. Kent KC. Clinical practice. Abdominal aortic aneurysms. *N Engl J Med.* 2014;371(22):2101–2108.
37. Lederle FA. In the clinic. Abdominal aortic aneurysm. *Ann Intern Med.* 2009;150(9):ITC5-1–ITC5-16.
38. Cattau EL Jr, Benjamin SB, Knuff TE, Castell DO. The accuracy of the physical examination in the diagnosis of suspected ascites. *JAMA.* 1982;247(8):1164–1166.
39. Walker HK, Hall WD, Hurst JW. *Clinical Methods: The History, Physical, and Laboratory Examinations.* 3rd ed. Butterworths; 1990:1087.
40. Kratzer W, Fritz V, Mason RA, Haenle MM, Kaechele V, Group RS. Factors affecting liver size: a sonographic survey of 2080 subjects. *J Ultrasound Med.* 2003;22(11):1155–1161.
41. Patzak M, Porzner M, Oeztuerk S, et al. Assessment of liver size by ultrasonography. *J Clin Ultrasound.* 2014;42(7): 399–404.
42. Noble VE, Nelson B. *Manual of Emergency and Critical Care Ultrasound.* 2nd ed. Cambridge Medicine. Cambridge University Press; 2011:346.

43. Cattau EL Jr, Benjamin SB, Knuff TE, Castell DO. The accuracy of the physical examination in the diagnosis of suspected ascites. *JAMA.* 1982;247(8):1164–1166.
44. Goldberg BB, Goodman GA, Clearfield HR. Evaluation of ascites by ultrasound. *Radiology.* 1970;96(1):15–22.
45. Centers for Disease Control and Prevention. *Viral Hepatitis Surveillance—United States, 2016.* 2018, Accessed January 17, 2024. https://stacks.cdc.gov/view/cdc/53558
46. Centers for Disease Control and Prevention. "Hepatitis A." *Centers for Disease Control and Prevention.* 2023, Accessed January 17, 2024. https://www.cdc.gov/hepatitis-a/index.html
47. Fiore AE, Wasley A, Bell BP. Prevention of hepatitis A through active or passive immunization: recommendations of the Advisory Committee on Immunization Practices (ACIP). *MMWR Recomm Rep.* 2006;55(RR-07):1–23.
48. Schillie S, Harris A, Link-Gelles R, Romero J, Ward J, Nelson N. Recommendations of the Advisory Committee on Immunization Practices for use of a hepatitis B vaccine with a novel adjuvant. *MMWR Morb Mortal Wkly Rep.* 2018;67(15):455–458.
49. LeFevre ML. Screening for hepatitis B virus infection in nonpregnant adolescents and adults: U.S. Preventive Services Task Force recommendation statement. *Ann Intern Med.* 2014; 161(1):58–66.
50. Weinbaum CM, Williams I, Mast EE, et al. Recommendations for identification and public health management of persons with chronic hepatitis B virus infection. *MMWR Recomm Rep.* 2008;57(RR-08):1–20.
51. US Preventive Services Task Force (USPSTF). Screening for hepatitis B virus infection in pregnant women: US Preventive Services Task Force reaffirmation recommendation statement. *JAMA.* 2019;322(4):349–354.
52. Moyer VA. Screening for hepatitis C virus infection in adults: U.S. Preventive Services Task Force recommendation statement. *Ann Intern Med.* 2013;159(5):349–357.
53. Siegel RL, Miller KD, Jemal A. Cancer statistics, 2018. *CA Cancer J Clin.* 2018;68(1):7–30.
54. National Cancer Institute. *Cancer stat facts: colorectal cancer.* Accessed January 17, 2024. https://seer.cancer.gov/statfacts/html/colorect.html
55. National Cancer Institute. *SEER Cancer Statistics Review, 1975–2014.* Accessed January 17, 2024. https://seer.cancer.gov/csr/1975_2014/
56. Edwards BK, Ward E, Kohler BA, et al. Annual report to the nation on the status of cancer, 1975–2006, featuring colorectal cancer trends and impact of interventions (risk factors, screening, and treatment) to reduce future rates. *Cancer.* 2010;116(3):544–573.
57. National Cancer Institute. *Colorectal cancer prevention (PDQ®)–health professional version.* Accessed January 17, 2024. https://www.cancer.gov/types/colorectal/hp/colorectal-prevention-pdq
58. National Cancer Institute. *Genetics of colorectal cancer (PDQ®)–health professional version.* Accessed January 17, 2024. https://www.cancer.gov/types/colorectal/hp/colorectal-genetics-pdq#section/_1
59. Holme Ø, Schoen RE, Senore C, et al. Effectiveness of flexible sigmoidoscopy screening in men and women and different age groups: pooled analysis of randomised trials. *BMJ.* 2017;356:i6673.
60. Holme Ø, Bretthauer M, Fretheim A, Odgaard-Jensen J, Hoff G. Flexible sigmoidoscopy versus faecal occult blood testing for colorectal cancer screening in asymptomatic individuals. *Cochrane Database Syst Rev.* 2013;2013(9):CD009259.
61. Simon MS, Chlebowski RT, Wactawski-Wende J, et al. Estrogen plus progestin and colorectal cancer incidence and mortality. *J Clin Oncol.* 2012;30(32):3983–3990.
62. Chlebowski RT, Hendrix SL, Langer RD, et al. Influence of estrogen plus progestin on breast cancer and mammography in healthy postmenopausal women: the Women's Health Initiative randomized trial. *JAMA.* 2003;289(24):3243–3253.
63. Manson JE, Hsia J, Johnson KC, et al. Estrogen plus progestin and the risk of coronary heart disease. *N Engl J Med.* 2003;349(6):523–534.
64. Cushman M, Kuller LH, Prentice R, et al. Estrogen plus progestin and risk of venous thrombosis. *JAMA.* 2004;292(13): 1573–1580.
65. Lin JS, Piper MA, Perdue LA, et al. Screening for colorectal cancer: updated evidence report and systematic review for the US Preventive Services Task Force. *JAMA.* 2016;315(23): 2576–2594.
66. Davidson KW, Barry MJ, Mangione CM, et al. Screening for colorectal cancer: US Preventive Services Task Force recommendation statement. *JAMA.* 2021;325(19):1965–1977.
67. Wolf AMD, Fontham ETH, Church TR, et al. Colorectal cancer screening for average-risk adults: 2018 guideline update from the American Cancer Society. *CA Cancer J Clin.* 2018; 68(4):250–281.
68. Shaukat A, Kahi CJ, Burke CA, et al. ACG Clinical Guidelines: colorectal cancer screening 2021. *Am J Gastroenterol.* 2021;116(3):458–479.
69. Centers for Disease Control and Prevention. "Quick Facts: Colorectal Cancer Screening in U.S. Behavioral Risk Factor Surveillance System—2016." *Centers for Disease Control and Prevention.* Accessed January 17, 2024. https://www.cdc.gov/brfss/annual_data/annual_2016.html

CHAPTER

22

Anus and Rectum

ANATOMY AND PHYSIOLOGY

The *sigmoid colon* concludes at the *rectum*, the furthest section of the lower gastrointestinal (GI) tract. The rectum stretches from the rectosigmoid junction near the sacral promontory to the anorectal junction, just in front of the S3 vertebra. Following the rectum is the brief portion known as the *anal canal* (see Fig. 22-1).

The anus begins at the *anorectal ring* and extends to the *anal verge*, which is where hair-bearing skin transitions to hairless skin at the external anus. Beyond the anal verge lies the perianal skin, also known as the *anal margin*. The *external anal sphincter* consists of voluntary skeletal muscle, while the *internal anal sphincter*, an extension of the rectum's outer smooth muscle layer, is involuntary. The anorectal ring can be felt above the external anal sphincter.[1,2]

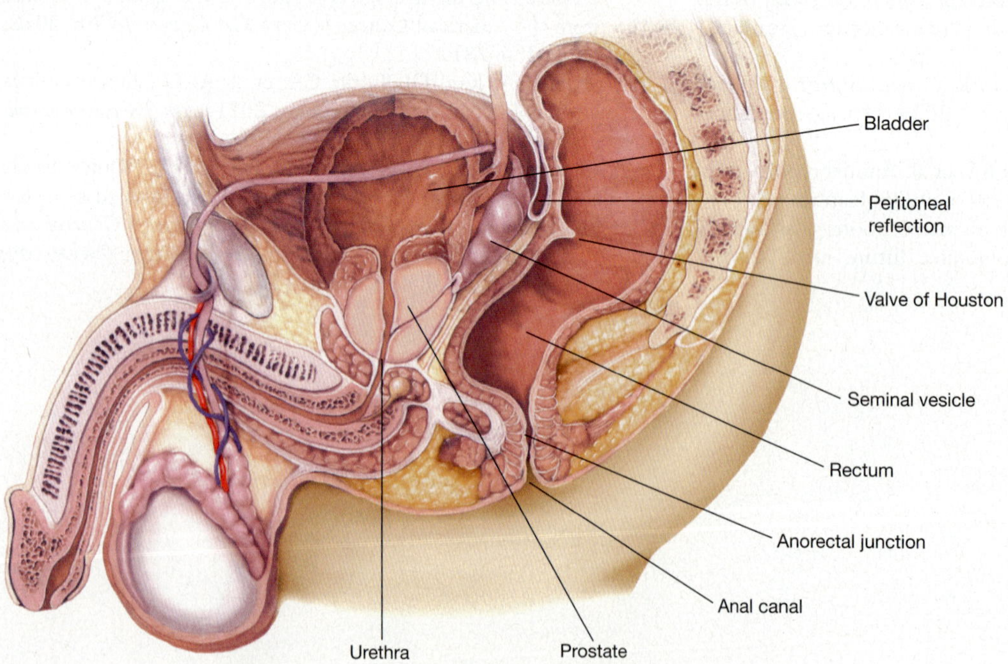

FIGURE 22-1. Anus, rectum, and prostate, sagittal view.

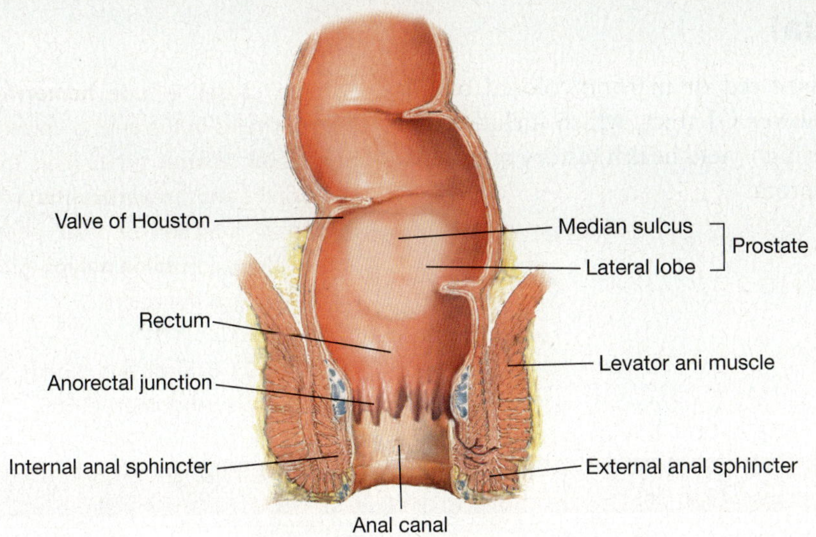

FIGURE 22-2. Anus and rectum, coronal view showing the anterior wall.

Take note of the anal canal's angle, which aligns approximately between the anus and umbilicus. Unlike the rectum, the canal has an abundant supply of somatic sensory nerves, so an improperly directed examining finger or instrument may cause pain.

The anal canal is distinguished from the rectum by a serrated line that marks the transition from skin to mucous membrane (Fig. 22-2). This anorectal junction, commonly known as the *pectinate* or *dentate line*, also separates somatic and visceral nerve supplies. Here, transitional columnar epithelium is found next to the distal squamous epithelium.[2] The junction is readily visible during anoscopic or endoscopic examinations but cannot be felt.

The uterine cervix usually is palpable through the anterior wall of the rectum.

Within the rectal wall are three inward folds, known as the *valves of Houston*. The lowest valve can sometimes be detected, typically on the patient's left side. Most of the rectum accessible during digital examination lacks a peritoneal surface, except for the anterior rectum, which may be reachable with the tip of your examining finger.

Peritoneal inflammation or nodularity from peritoneal metastases may cause tenderness.

HEALTH HISTORY: GENERAL APPROACH

When addressing the rectosigmoid and anal regions in patients presenting with GI tract symptoms, keep in mind the possible diagnoses related to these symptoms. Be aware that some answers may not be easily disclosed by patients due to the sensitive nature of certain causes, particularly those linked to sexual health and practices.

Common or Concerning Symptoms

- Bloody stool (hematochezia); also see Chapter 21, Abdomen, pp. 618–619
- Pain on defecation
- Anal and perianal lesions

Bloody Stool (Hematochezia)

Hematochezia refers to the passage of bright red or maroon-colored blood in the stool.[3] The blood comes from the lower GI tract, which includes the rectum, colon, and anus. Box 22-1 provides high-yield health history questions to ask in a patient presenting with this symptom.

Possible causes include **hemorrhoids** (swollen veins in the anus or lower rectum), **anal fissures** (small tears in the lining of the anus), **diverticulitis** (inflammation or infection of small pouches in the colon), and **colon polyps** (growth on the lining of the colon).

See Table 21-6, Black and Bloody Stool in Chapter 21, Abdomen, p. 665.

Box 22-1. Bloody Stool (Hematochezia): High-Yield Health History Questions

Domain	Questions	Rationale
Onset and duration	*When did you start noticing blood in your stool, and how long have you been experiencing it?*	Helps differentiate acute from chronic hematochezia and provides clues to potential causes *Acute onset:* may suggest infection or ischemia *Chronic:* could indicate inflammatory bowel disease (IBD) or colorectal cancer
Amount and appearance	*How do you describe the amount and appearance of the blood in your stool (e.g., bright red, dark red, or mixed with stool)?*	Provides insight into the source and severity of bleeding *Bright red:* may suggest a lower GI source *Darker:* could indicate bleeding higher up in the GI tract
Associated symptoms	*Are you experiencing any other symptoms, such as abdominal pain, diarrhea, weight loss, or fever?*	*Fever and diarrhea:* could suggest infection *Weight loss and abdominal pain:* might indicate IBD or cancer
Past medical history	*Do you have a history of any digestive system or blood disorders?*	Identifies potential underlying medical conditions that could contribute to hematochezia, such as IBD, diverticular disease, or bleeding disorders
Medication history	*Are you taking any medicines, including those you can buy without a prescription and any supplements, that could be causing blood in your stool?*	Helps identify potential medication-induced hematochezia (e.g., anticoagulants, nonsteroidal anti-inflammatory drugs)
Family history	*Does your family have a history of digestive system or blood disorders?*	Provides insight into potential genetic or hereditary factors such as a family history of colorectal cancer or inherited bleeding disorders
Bowel movement habits	*Have there been any recent changes in how often you go to the bathroom, the texture of your stool, or difficulty during bowel movements?*	Helps identify potential causes related to bowel habits, such as hemorrhoids or anal fissures caused by straining, or changes associated with infections or IBD
Dietary habits	*Have you recently eaten any red or dark-colored foods, or taken iron supplements that could look like blood in your stool?*	Rules out potential false alarms due to diet or supplements, which can sometimes mimic the appearance of blood in the stool

Pain on Defecation

Pain on defecation can range from mild to severe and can be described in various ways, such as sharp, burning, throbbing, or aching.[4] Box 22-2 provides high-yield health history questions to ask in a patient presenting with this symptom.

The most common causes of pain on defecation are **hemorrhoids** affecting approximately 50% of the population by age 50 and **anal fissures** affecting up to 10% of the general population. Additional common causes include **irritable bowel syndrome** ([**IBS**] swollen veins in the anus or lower rectum), **inflammatory bowel disease** ([**IBD**] small tears in the lining of the anus), and **proctitis** (growth on the lining of the colon).

Box 22-2. Pain on Defecation: High-Yield Health History Questions

Domain	Questions	Rationale
Onset and duration	*When did you first start feeling pain when passing stool, and how long has this been going on?*	*Acute onset:* may suggest infection or trauma *Chronic:* could indicate hemorrhoids or an anal fissure
Location	*Can you show where it hurts when you pass stool, or describe where the pain is?*	Helps localize the source of pain (e.g., anal pain could suggest hemorrhoids or an anal fissure)
Characteristics	*How would you describe the pain (e.g., sharp, burning, throbbing, or aching)?*	*Sharp pain:* might indicate an anal fissure *Throbbing pain:* could suggest a perianal abscess
Severity	*How severe is the pain on a scale of 1 to 10, with 10 being the worst pain imaginable?*	Assesses the intensity of the pain, which can help guide further evaluation and management
Associated symptoms	*Are you experiencing any other symptoms, such as bleeding, swelling, itching, or discharge?*	Helps identify additional symptoms that may provide clues about the underlying cause (e.g., itching and swelling could suggest hemorrhoids or an allergic reaction)
Aggravating factors	*What makes the pain worse, such as certain foods, straining, or sitting?*	Identifies potential triggers or causes of pain with defecation (e.g., straining could worsen pain from hemorrhoids or an anal fissure)
Alleviating factors	*What makes the pain better, such as rest, warm sitz baths, or over-the-counter medications?*	Provides insight into the nature of the pain and potential treatments or management strategies
Past medical history	*Do you have a history of any digestive, rectal, or related health issues?*	Identifies potential underlying medical conditions that could contribute to pain
Medication history	*Are you taking any medicines, including those you can buy without a prescription and any supplements, that could be causing pain when you pass stool?*	Helps identify potential medication-induced pain and guides further evaluation and management
Bowel movement habits	*Have there been any recent changes in how often you go to the bathroom, the texture of your stool, or difficulty during bowel movements?*	Helps identify potential causes of pain related to bowel habits, such as constipation leading to straining, or changes associated with infections or inflammatory bowel disease

Anal and Perianal Lesions

Anal and perianal lesions refer to any abnormal growths or marks around the anus or on the skin of the perianal area.[5] These lesions can present with a variety of symptoms, such as itching, pain, and bleeding, or without any discomfort at all. They can have a range of appearances from bumps and ulcers to skin tags.[6] Box 22-3 provides high-yield health history questions to assist in the evaluation of a patient presenting with anal or perianal lesions.

Common anal and perianal lesions include **hemorrhoids**[7] and **anal fissures.**[5] Other conditions are **anal warts**, often associated with HPV infection, and **perianal abscesses** (infected cavities filled with pus). Less common but serious considerations include **malignancies** such as anal carcinoma.[8]

Box 22-3. Anal and Perianal Lesions: High-Yield Health History Questions

Domain	Questions	Rationale
Onset and duration	*When did you first notice the lesion? How long has it been present?*	*Acute lesions:* might suggest an infection or recent trauma *Chronic:* might be due to persistent conditions like warts or malignancies
Location	*Where is the lesion located? Is it inside the anal canal, on the edge, or outside around the anus?*	*Internal:* may be hemorrhoids or polyps *External:* might be warts or skin tags
Appearance	*What does the lesion look like (e.g., color, size, shape)? Is there more than one lesion?*	Can offer important diagnostic clues (e.g., warts have a distinct look compared to skin tags or abscesses)
Symptoms	*Are you experiencing any symptoms associated with the lesion, such as pain, bleeding, itching, or discharge?*	*Abscess:* may be painful and discharge pus *Warts:* may be painless but itchy
Aggravating factors	*Do certain activities or factors seem to worsen the lesion or symptoms, like bowel movements, physical activity, or sitting?*	Identifies potential irritants or activities that exacerbate the condition, which can be helpful in management and treatment
Alleviating factors	*Have you found anything that relieves the symptoms or appears to reduce the size of the lesions?*	*Sitz bath:* may soothe hemorrhoids *Topical treatments:* may reduce wart size
Past medical history	*Do you have a history of any conditions that could be associated with these lesions, such as HPV or gastrointestinal disorders?*	*Human papillomavirus (HPV):* can predispose to warts *Inflammatory bowel disease:* can lead to various anal lesions
Sexual and bowel history	*Have you had any sexual practices that might have contributed to the lesions? What are your bowel movement habits?*	Certain sexual practices can increase the risk of anal lesions like warts or fissures. Bowel habits can contribute to lesions; for example, chronic diarrhea or constipation can lead to hemorrhoids or fissures.
Medication and treatment history	*Are you using any treatments or medications for the lesions? Have you had similar issues treated in the past?*	Can help track the progress of the condition and guide future management decisions

PHYSICAL EXAMINATION: GENERAL APPROACH

Before beginning the examination, let the patient know that you will be examining the anorectal area, as this examination can be very sensitive. Although the rectal examination may cause discomfort, it is rarely painful. Thus, the approach to this section of the examination requires effective and constant communication on what is about to happen as well as the expected outcomes of the examination. Be sure to warn the patient about what they may feel—including pressure; wetness from the lubricant; possible discomfort; and the slow, gentle movement of your examining finger.

TECHNIQUES OF EXAMINATION

Key Components of the Anorectal Examination

- Properly position the patient.
- Inspect the sacrococcygeal and perianal areas.
- Inspect the anus.
- Perform a digital rectal examination (DRE).

Properly Position the Patient

Choose one of several suitable patient positions for conducting the examination, with input from the patient when needed. Usually, the side-lying position with the hips and knees partially flexed is satisfactory and allows good visualization of the perianal and sacrococcygeal areas (Fig. 22-3). Some clinicians ask the patient to stand and lean forward with their upper body resting across the examining table and hips flexed, although this approach might be perceived as less dignified by some patients. In either position, your examining finger cannot reach the full length of the rectum.

Ask the patient to lie on their left side with their buttocks close to the edge of the examining table near you. Partially flexing the patient's hips and knees,

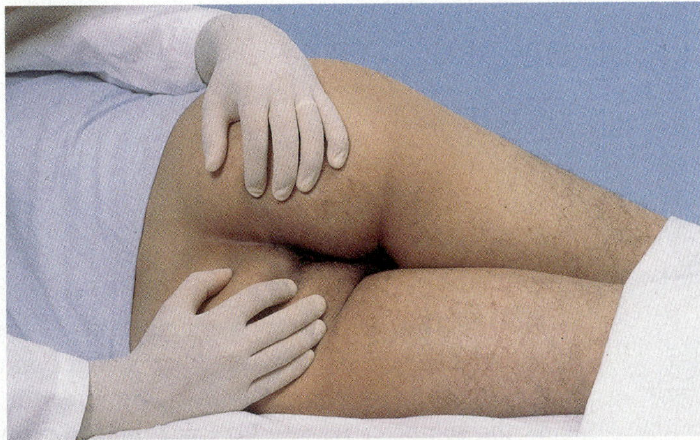

FIGURE 22-3. Positioning the patient on the left side for the anorectal examination.

especially in the upper leg, stabilizes their position and improves visibility. Drape the patient appropriately and adjust the light to ensure good visualization of the perirectal and anal area. Glove your hands and spread the buttocks apart.

If only a rectal examination is needed, the lateral position is satisfactory and affords a better view of the perianal and sacrococcygeal areas. Note that the cervix is readily palpated through the anterior rectal wall. Sometimes, a retroverted uterus is also palpable. Do not mistake either of these or a tampon in the vagina, for a suspicious mass.

Inspect the Sacrococcygeal and Perianal Areas

Inspect for lesions, ulcers, inflammation, rashes, and excoriations. Adult perianal skin is normally more pigmented and somewhat coarser than the skin over the buttocks. Palpate any abnormal areas, noting masses or tenderness.

Inspect the Anus

Inspect the anus noting any external lesions, masses, or areas of skin breakdown.

Perform a Digital Rectal Examination

Lubricate your gloved index finger and explain to the patient that you are going to perform a DRE. The patient will feel some pressure but should not feel pain. Place the pad of your gloved and lubricated finger over the anus (Fig. 22-4A).

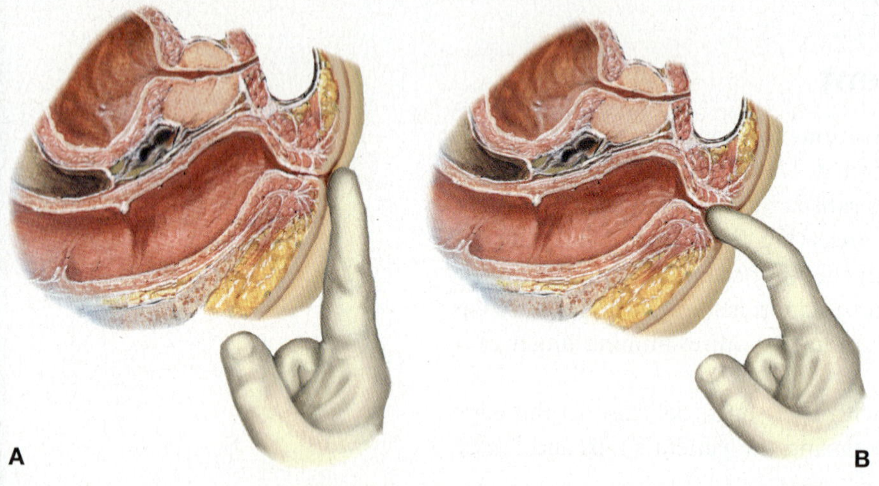

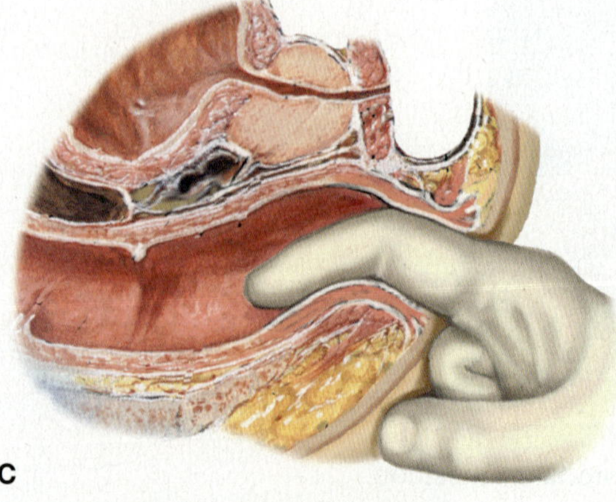

FIGURE 22-4. Digital rectal examination. **A.** Placing the pad of a gloved and lubricated index finger on the anus. **B.** Gradually inserting the examining finger in the anus as the sphincter relaxes. **C.** Palpating the rectal surface (sagittal view).

The sphincter will initially tighten, and, as it gradually relaxes, gently insert your fingertip into the anal canal (Fig. 22-4B). Occasionally, severe tenderness prevents entry and internal examination. Do not apply force. Instead, place your fingers on both sides of the anus, gently spread the orifice, and ask the patient to bear down. Proceed in the general direction of the umbilicus.

Palpate the Rectum. Palpate circumferentially noting any masses, areas of tenderness, or breaks in the mucosa.

A tender fluctuant mass with overlying redness and induration is suggestive of a perirectal or perianal abscess.[9] These patients may or may not have accompanying systemic signs of infection such as fever or chills. Chronic abscesses with persistent drainage from an external opening on the skin surface represent a perirectal fistula. Fistulas may ooze blood, pus, or feculent mucus.

Ask the Patient to Squeeze the External Anal Sphincter. To assess muscular tone, ask the patient to squeeze their external anal sphincter. Normally, the muscles of the anal sphincter close snugly around your examining finger. Initial resting tone reflects the integrity of the internal anal sphincter.

Sphincter tightness may occur with anxiety, inflammation, or scarring.[10] Sphincter laxity occurs in neurologic diseases, such as S2–S4 cord lesions, and signals possible changes in the urinary sphincter and detrusor muscle. Consider testing perianal sensation.

Palpate the Rectal Surface. Insert your examining finger into the rectum as far as possible. Rotate your hand clockwise to palpate as much of the rectal surface as possible on the patient's right side, then counterclockwise to palpate the surface posteriorly on their left side (see Fig. 22-4C). Note any masses with irregular borders suspicious of rectal cancer, nodules, irregularities, or induration (Fig. 22-5). To bring a possible lesion into reach, take your finger off the rectal surface, ask the patient to bear down, and palpate again.

See Table 22-1, Abnormalities of the Anus, Surrounding Skin, and Rectum, pp. 684–685.

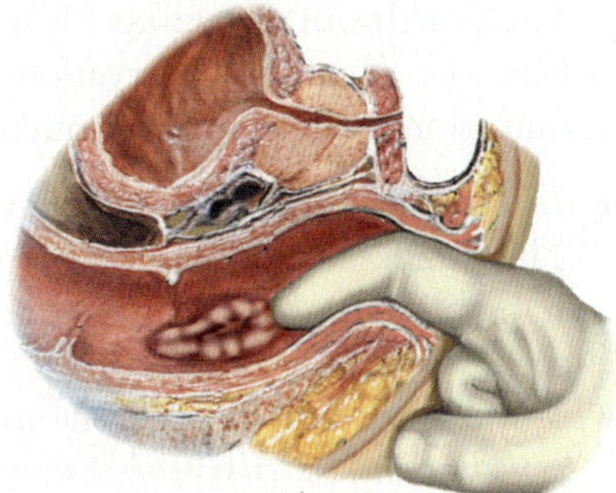

FIGURE 22-5. Palpable rectal cancer.

Gently Withdraw the Examining Finger. Gently withdraw your finger and wipe the anal area or give the patient a disposable absorbent paper. Note the appearance of any fecal matter on your glove. Test the fecal matter for occult blood when indicated.

SPECIAL TECHNIQUES AND MANEUVERS

Perform a Prostatic Examination (When Indicated)

A prostatic examination is a crucial component of the genitourinary assessment. It involves evaluating the prostate gland for size, texture, and any irregularities that may indicate conditions such as benign prostatic hyperplasia or prostate cancer. For detailed steps on conducting a prostatic examination and its clinical significance, refer to Chapter 23, Pelvis and Genitourinary System: Penis, Scrotum, and Prostate, p. 710.

Perform a Rectovaginal Examination (When Indicated)

You may also examine the rectum after internal examination of the vagina and surrounding structures while the patient is in the lithotomy position. This position allows you to conduct the examination, delineate a possible adnexal or pelvic mass, and test the integrity of the rectovaginal wall; it may also help you to palpate a cancer high in the rectum. For the indications and technique of the rectovaginal examination, see Chapter 24, Pelvis and Genitourinary System: Vulva, Vagina, Uterus, and Adnexa, p. 753.

RECORDING YOUR FINDINGS

In clinical notes, your initial detailed documentation of the PE is key for diagnosis and hypothesis testing. Once you gain experience, you will gradually adopt brief, widely recognized phrases for efficiency and clarity.

Recording the Anus and Rectum Examination

"No perirectal lesions or fissures. External sphincter tone intact. Rectal vault without masses. (Or, uterine cervix nontender.) Stool brown; no fecal blood."

OR

"Perirectal area inflamed; no ulcerations, warts, or discharge. Unable to examine external sphincter, rectal vault, or prostate because of spasm of external sphincter and marked inflammation and tenderness of anal canal."

The practice of dissecting PE findings into precise details underscores the critical role of clinical observations in formulating a diagnosis. The perirectal examination findings for this patient reveal:

- *Inflammation in the perirectal area without ulcerations, warts, or discharge:* This suggests an inflammatory condition that is not currently exhibiting signs of common infectious causes known to produce specific lesions or secretions.
- *Spasm of the external sphincter and marked tenderness of the anal canal, preventing examination of the external sphincter, rectal vault, or prostate:* These findings indicate significant irritation or inflammation, which could be associated with a variety of anorectal conditions, such as abscesses, acute proctitis, or severe hemorrhoidal disease.
- *Absence of ulcerations:* This decreases the likelihood of certain infectious etiologies, such as herpes simplex virus or syphilis.
- *Lack of warts:* Suggests that HPV infection is not present.

- *No discharge:* Generally rules out bacterial or parasitic infections characterized by rectal discharge.
- The *spasm and inflammation* may reflect a protective physiologic reaction to minimize further injury or irritation from clinical examination.

The most likely working diagnosis could be an *anorectal abscess* or *acute proctitis.* The absence of ulcerations, warts, and discharge makes infectious etiologies like STIs less likely, although they cannot be completely ruled out without further testing.

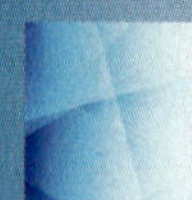

TABLE 22-1. Abnormalities of the Anus, Surrounding Skin, and Rectum

Pilonidal Cyst and Sinus

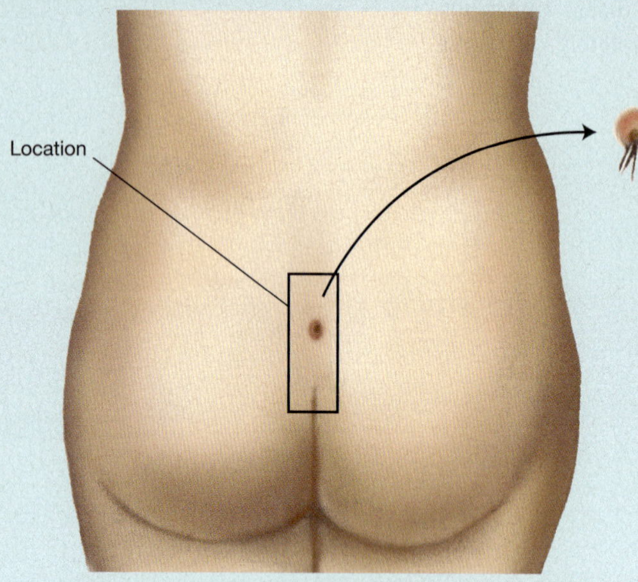

Pilonidal cysts are fairly common, probably congenital, abnormalities located in the midline natal cleft. Look for the opening of a sinus tract, sometimes with a small tuft of hair surrounded by a halo of erythema. These cysts are generally asymptomatic, except for slight drainage, but abscess formation and secondary sinus tracts may occur.[11]

External Hemorrhoids (*Thrombosed*)

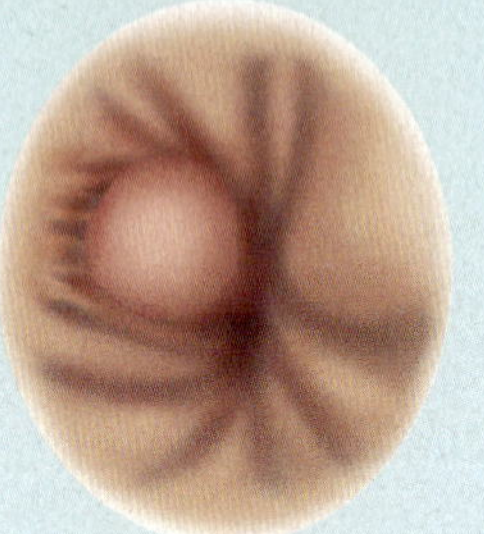

External hemorrhoids are dilated hemorrhoidal veins that originate below the pectinate line that are covered with skin. They seldom produce symptoms unless thrombosis occurs. Thrombosis causes acute local pain that increases with defecation and sitting. A tender, swollen, bluish, ovoid mass is visible at the anal margin.[12,13]

Internal Hemorrhoids (*Prolapsed*)

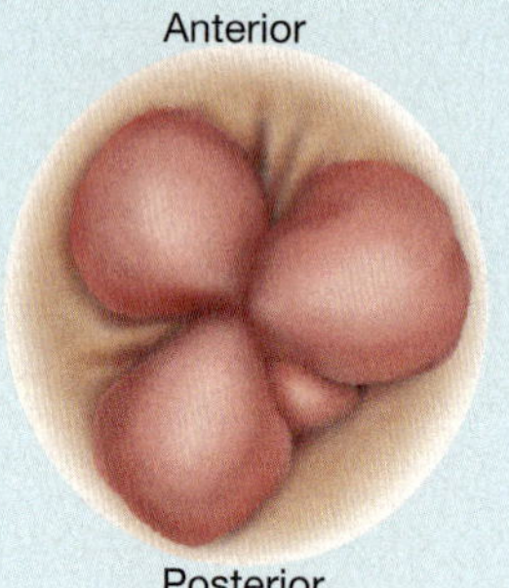

Internal hemorrhoids are enlargements of the normal vascular cushions located above the pectinate line, usually not palpable.[7] Internal hemorrhoids may cause bright red bleeding, especially during defecation. They may also prolapse through the anal canal and appear as reddish, moist, protruding masses, typically located in one or more of the positions illustrated.

Prolapse of the Rectum

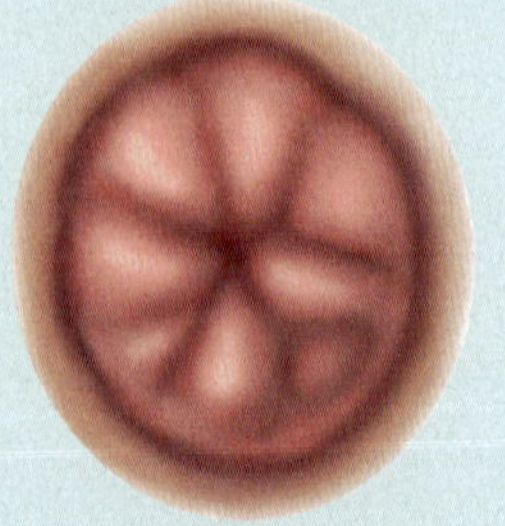

On straining for a bowel movement, the rectal mucosa, with or without its muscular wall, may prolapse through the anus, telescoping through the anal verge. A prolapse involving only mucosa is relatively small and shows radiating folds, as illustrated. When the entire bowel wall is involved, the prolapse is larger and covered by concentrically circular folds.

Anal Fissure

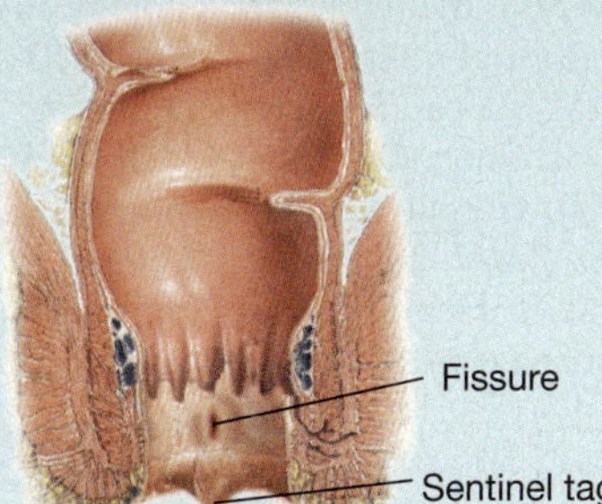

An anal fissure is a very painful tear/ulceration of the anoderm, found most commonly in the midline posteriorly, less commonly in the midline anteriorly. Its long axis lies longitudinally. There may be a swollen "sentinel" skin tag just below it. Gentle separation of the anal margins may reveal the lower edge of the fissure.[5] The sphincter is spastic; the examination is painful. An examination under anesthesia may be necessary to fully characterize the lesion.

Anorectal Fistula

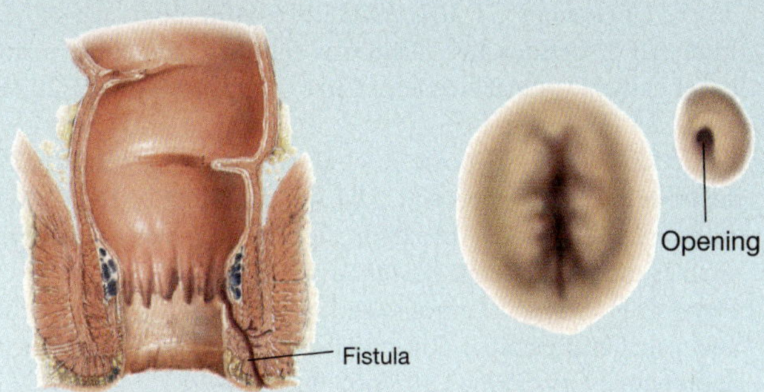

An anorectal fistula is an abnormal connective tract that originates from anal glands to an external opening on the skin (as shown here). Fistulas are the result of previous anorectal abscess/infections.[9] Look for the fistulous opening or openings anywhere in the skin around the anus.

Rectal Polyps

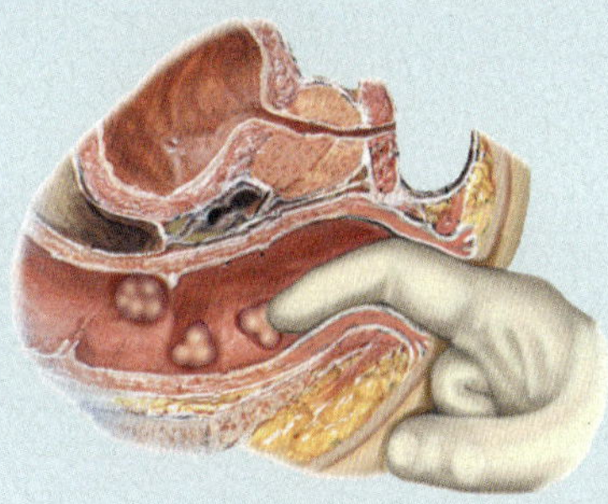

Polyps of the rectum are fairly common.[14] Variable in size and number, they can develop on a stalk (pedunculated) or lie on the mucosal surface (sessile). They are soft and may be difficult or impossible to feel even when in reach of the examining finger. Endoscopy and biopsy are needed for differentiation of benign from malignant lesions.

Rectal Cancer

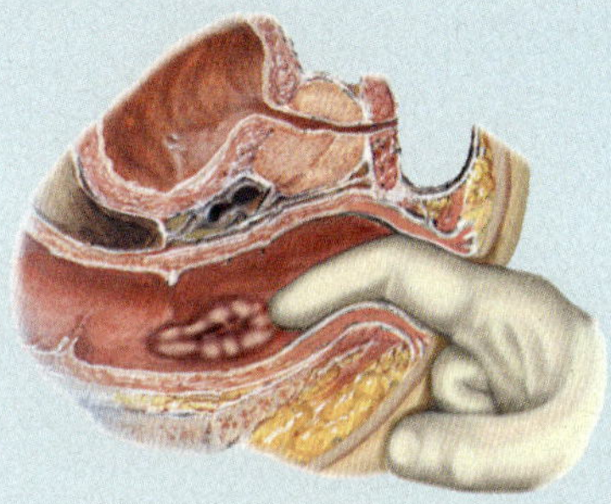

Illustrated here is the firm, nodular, rolled edge of an ulcerated cancer.[8]

Rectal Shelf

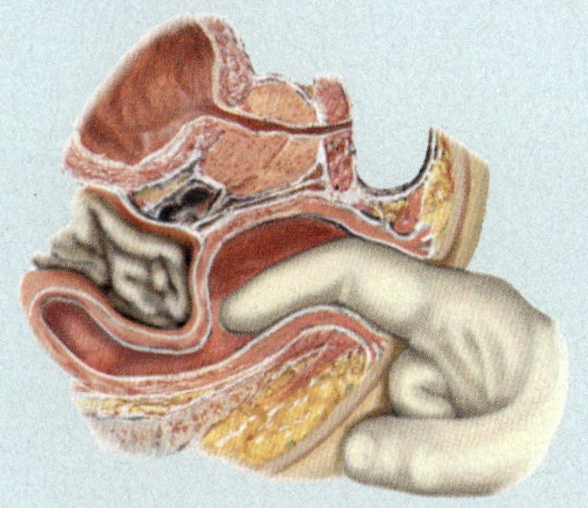

Widespread peritoneal metastases from any source may develop in the area of the peritoneal reflection anterior to the rectum. A firm-to-hard nodular rectal "shelf" may be just palpable with the tip of the examining finger. In female patients, this shelf of metastatic tissue develops in the rectouterine pouch, behind the cervix and the uterus.

REFERENCES

1. Jorge JM, Wexner SD. Anatomy and physiology of the rectum and anus. *Eur J Surg*. 1997;163(10):723–731.
2. Bennett AE. Correlative anatomy of the anus and rectum. *Semin Ultrasound CT MR*. 2008;29(6):400–408.
3. Elimeleh Y, Gralnek IM. Diagnosis and management of acute lower gastrointestinal bleeding. *Curr Opin Gastroenterol*. 2024; 40(1):34–42.
4. Lukic S, Mijac D, Filipovic B, et al. Chronic abdominal pain: gastroenterologist approach. *Dig Dis*. 2022;40(2):181–186.
5. Abbass MA, Valente MA. Premalignant and malignant perianal lesions. *Clin Colon Rectal Surg*. 2019;32(5):386–393.
6. Dawson H, Serra S. Tumours and inflammatory lesions of the anal canal and perianal skin revisited: an update and practical approach. *J Clin Pathol*. 2015;68(12):971–981.
7. Sandler RS, Peery AF. Rethinking what we know about hemorrhoids. *Clin Gastroenterol Hepatol*. 2019;17(1):8–15.
8. Wilkinson N. Management of rectal cancer. *Surg Clin North Am*. 2020;100(3):615–628.
9. Seidman MD, Gurgel RK, Lin SY, et al. Clinical practice guideline: allergic rhinitis executive summary. *Otolaryngol Head Neck Surg*. 2015;152(2):197–206.
10. Spiesman MG, Malow L. The etiology and surgical management of anal tightness. *Surg Forum*. 1951:129–131.
11. Kober MM, Alapati U, Khachemoune A. Treatment options for pilonidal sinus. *Cutis*. 2018;102(4):E23–E29.
12. Cengiz TB, Gorgun E. Hemorrhoids: a range of treatments. *Cleve Clin J Med*. 2019;86(9):612–620.
13. Lohsiriwat V. Hemorrhoids: from basic pathophysiology to clinical management. *World J Gastroenterol*. 2012;18(17): 2009–2017.
14. Cowan ML, Silviera ML. Management of rectal polyps. *Clin Colon Rectal Surg*. 2016;29(4):315–320.

CHAPTER 23

Pelvis and Genitourinary System: Penis, Scrotum, and Prostate

ANATOMY AND PHYSIOLOGY

Pelvis

The pelvis is a complex structure that supports various organs, offers attachment points for muscles and ligaments, and houses pelvic organs (Figs. 23-1 and 23-2). It comprises the hip bones (ilium, ischium, and pubis), sacrum, and coccyx. The *ilium* forms the uppermost part of the hip bone; the *ischium*, the lower and posterior part; and the *pubis*, the anterior and medial part. The *sacrum* is a triangular bone made from five fused sacral vertebrae, articulating with the ilium at the sacroiliac joints. The *coccyx* is a small triangular bone at the base of the sacrum.

The centrally located *urinary bladder* is a muscular sac situated at the base of the pelvis, responsible for storing urine. Anterior to the bladder is the *prostate gland*, a walnut-sized organ integral to the reproductive system, encircling part of the urethra and contributing to semen production. The *urethra*, running through the prostate, serves as a conduit for urine and semen to exit the body. Behind the bladder lies the *rectum*, the terminal part of the large intestine, leading to the *anus*. Lying on either side of the bladder are the seminal vesicles and vas deferens. The *seminal vesicles* produce a fluid that forms part of the semen, while the *vas deferens*, extending from the epididymis, transport sperm. In addition, the pelvis contains various blood vessels; nerves; and muscles, including the *pelvic floor muscles*, which support these organs and assist in functions like urination, defecation, and sexual activity.

Urogenital System

Examine the urogenital system in Figure 23-3. The *kidneys*, located in the abdominal cavity, filter waste and excess substances from the blood to form *urine*. Urine flows through the *ureters*, connecting the kidneys to the *bladder*, which stores urine until it is expelled. The *urethra* transports urine outside the body.

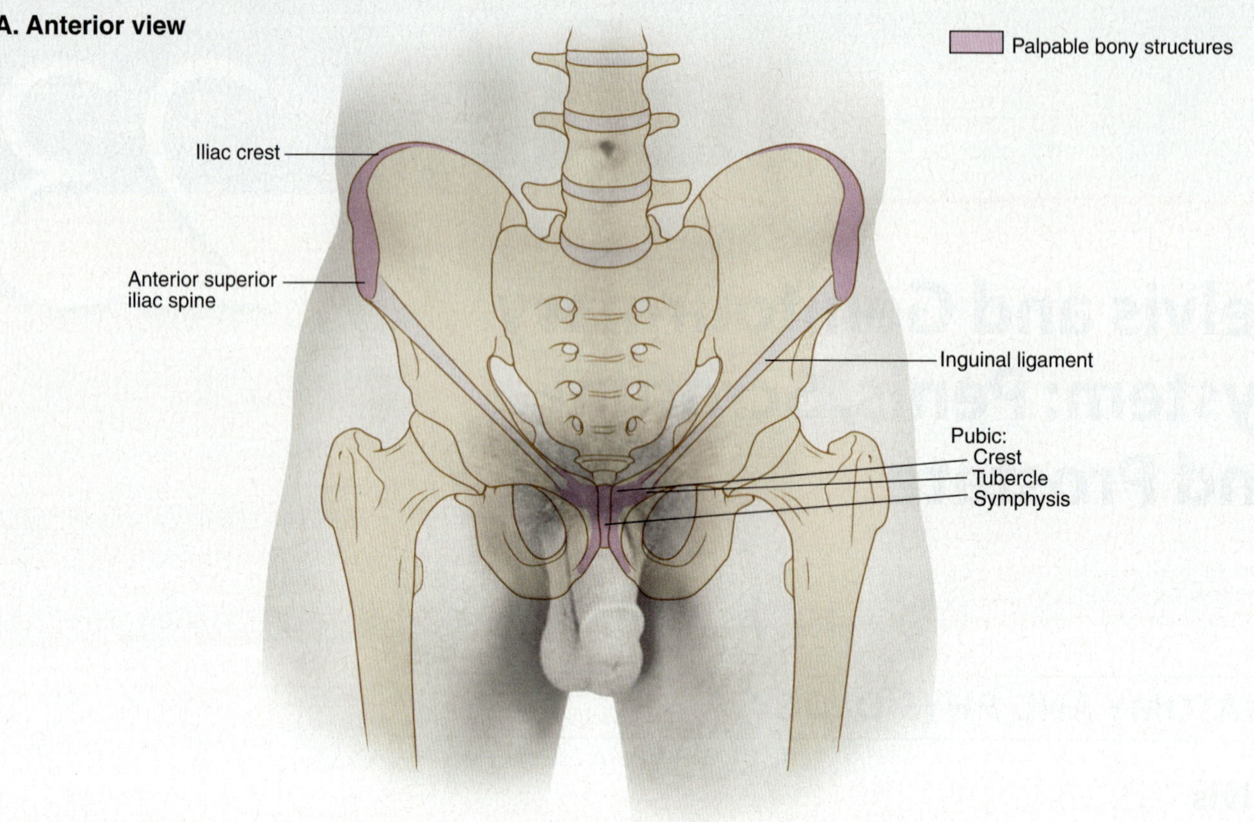

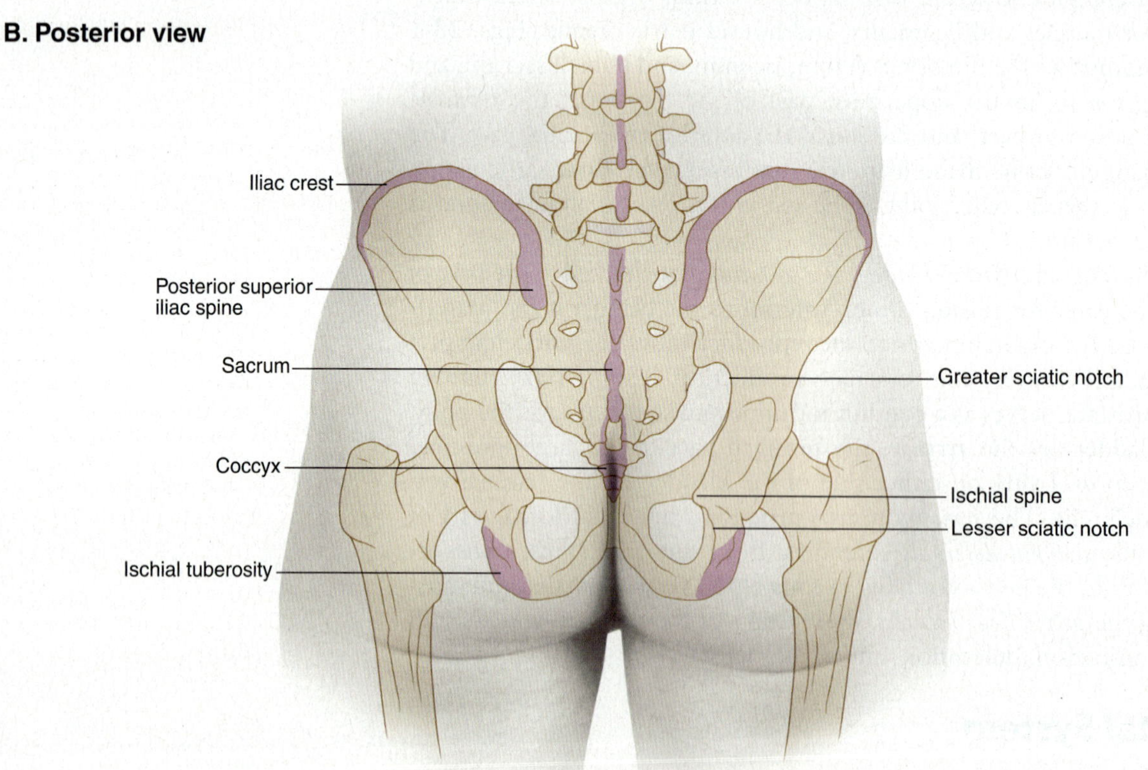

FIGURE 23-1. Surface anatomy of the pelvis and perineum. (Reprinted with permission from Gest TR. *Lippincott® Atlas of Anatomy*. 2nd ed. Wolters Kluwer; 2020. Plate 6-2.)

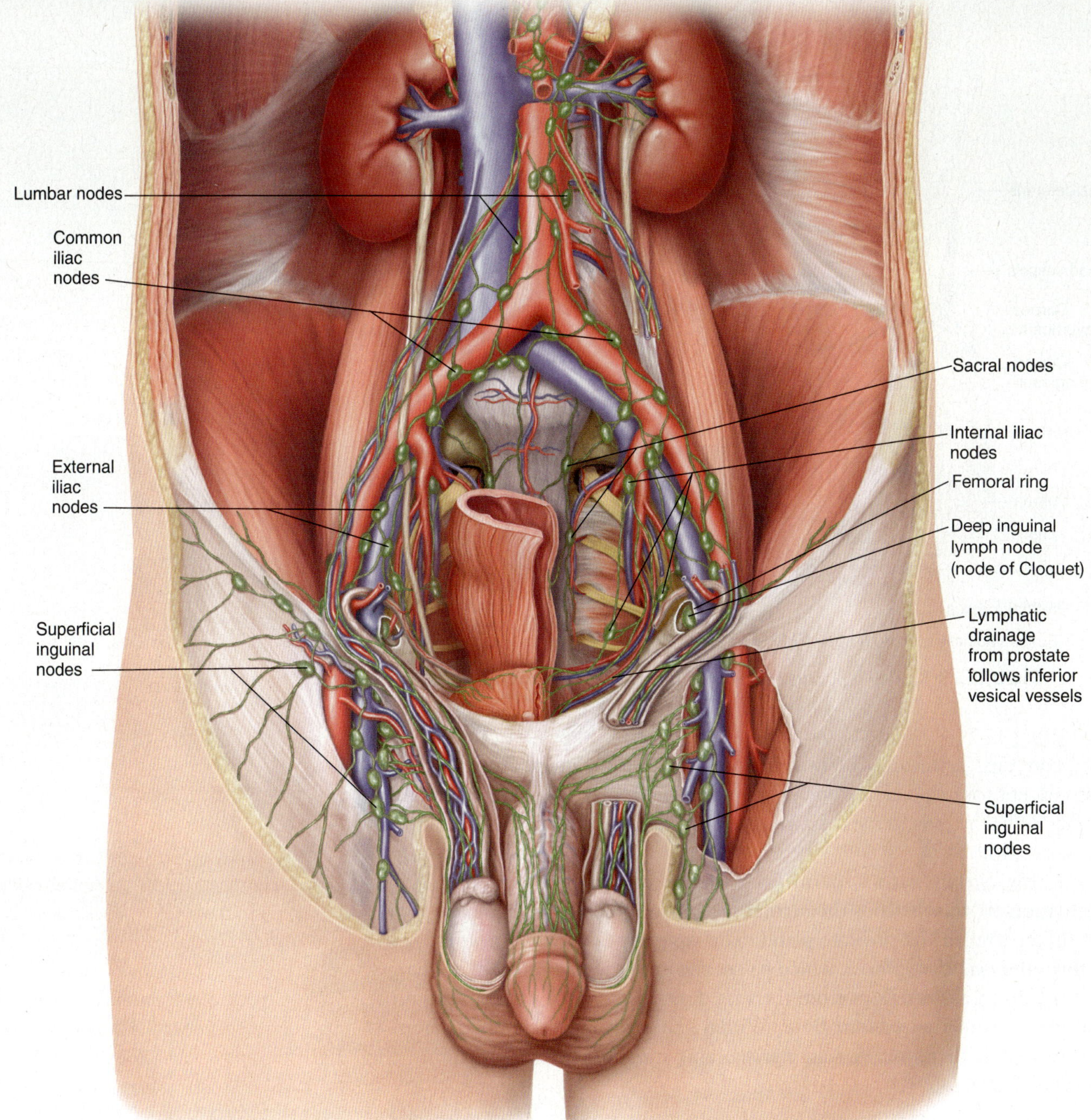

FIGURE 23-2. Lower abdomen, pelvis, and their contents. (Reprinted with permission from Gest TR. *Lippincott® Atlas of Anatomy*. 2nd ed. Wolters Kluwer; 2020. Plate 6-37.)

The *penile shaft* has three columns of erectile tissue: the *corpus spongiosum*, housing the urethra, and two *corpora cavernosa*. The corpus spongiosum extends to the glans, featuring a widened base called the *corona*. The *glans* of an uncircumcised penis is covered by the *prepuce* (*foreskin*), which can accumulate *smegma*, a substance consisting of secretions from the glans. The urethra runs along the penile shaft's ventral midline and terminates at the *urethral meatus* on the glans tip.

The *testes* are oval-shaped glands consisting of seminiferous tubules and interstitial tissue, enclosed by the *tunica albuginea*. The *scrotum*, a pouch of

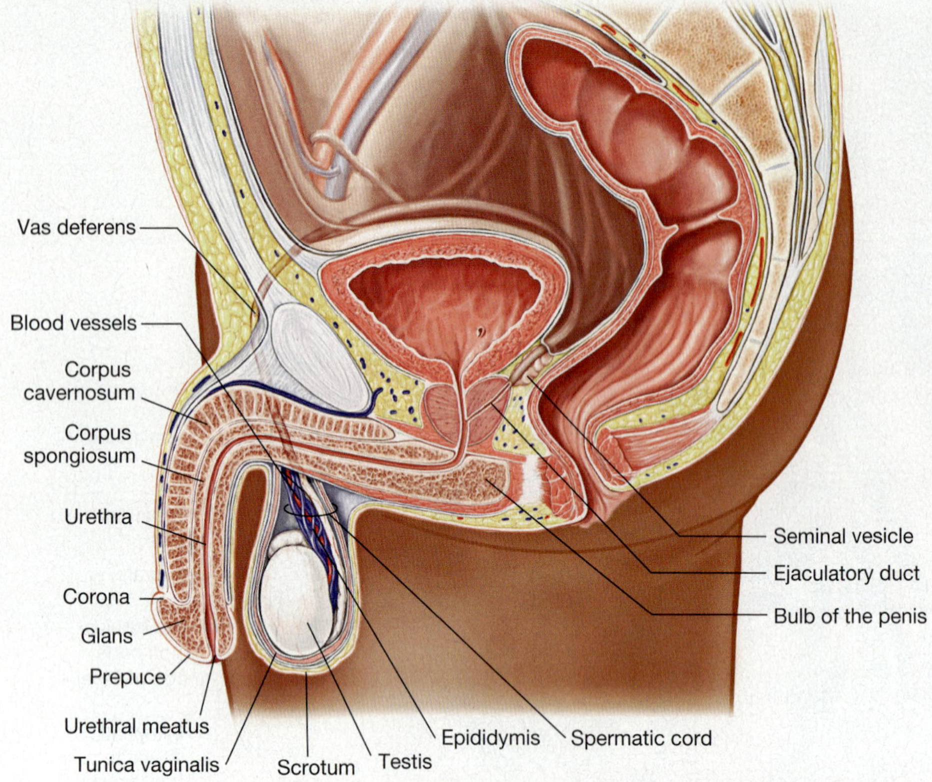

FIGURE 23-3. Pelvis, penis, scrotum and prostate, sagittal view.

skin, contains the testes. The *tunica vaginalis*, a serous membrane, covers the testis except for its posterior side. The *epididymis*, located on the posterolateral surface of each testis, serves as a reservoir for sperm storage, maturation, and transportation.

The *vas deferens* carries sperm from the epididymis to the urethra during ejaculation. It travels from the scrotal sac into the pelvic cavity, arching over the ureter toward the prostate gland. The vas merges with the *seminal vesicle* to form the *ejaculatory duct*, which passes through the prostate and discharges into the urethra. Secretions from the vasa deferens, seminal vesicles, and prostate gland form the *seminal fluid*. Within the scrotum, each vas deferens is intertwined with blood vessels, nerves, and muscle fibers, constituting the spermatic cord.

If the peritoneal lining remains an open channel to the scrotum, it can give rise to an *indirect inguinal hernia.*

The parietal and visceral layers form a potential space for the abnormal fluid accumulation of a *hydrocele.*

Prostate

The *prostate gland* surrounds the urethra and lies next to the bladder outlet (see Fig. 23-3). It is small during childhood, but, between puberty and approximately age 20 years, it increases roughly fivefold in size (to about the size of a chestnut). Prostate volume further expands as the gland becomes hyperplastic with age (see p. 710). The *base of the prostate gland* is the broad top and is directed upward near the inferior surface of the bladder. The greater part of this surface is directly continuous with the bladder wall (normally palpable during examination). The *apex of the prostate* is the pointed bottom of the gland and is in contact with the superior fascia of the urogenital diaphragm.

The prostate is divided into several lobes. The main mass of the prostate, the *right and left lateral lobes,* lie against the anterior rectal wall, where they

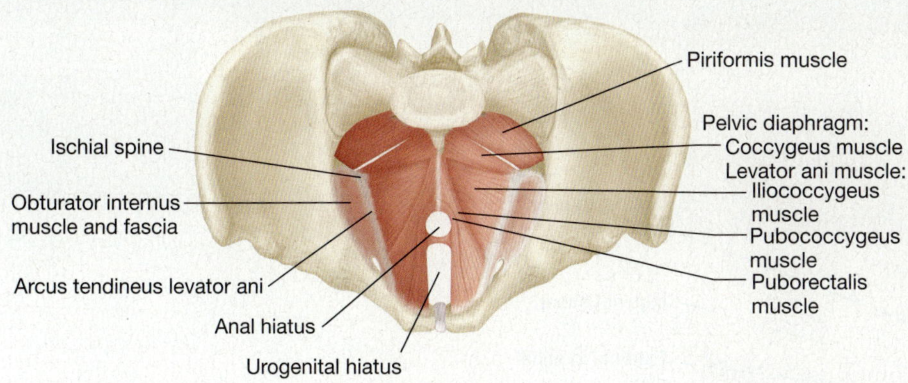

FIGURE 23-4. Pelvic diaphragm, superior view. (Reprinted with permission from Pansky B, Gest TR. *Lippincott's Concise Illustrated Anatomy: Thorax, Abdomen & Pelvis.* Wolters Kluwer Health/Lippincott Williams & Wilkins; 2012. Figure 3.12F.)

are palpable as a rounded, heart-shaped structure approximately 2.5 cm long. They are separated by a shallow *median sulcus* or *groove*, also palpable. The posteromedial part of the lateral lobes that can be palpated through the rectum during an examination is often referred to as the *posterior lobe.* Note that the *anterior* and *median* lobes of the prostate cannot be examined, as they are not in contact with the rectal wall. The seminal vesicles, shaped like rabbit ears above the prostate, are also not normally palpable.

Pelvic Floor Muscles

Pelvic floor muscles, like the *levator ani* and *coccygeus*, provide support to pelvic organs and maintain continence (Fig. 23-4). Other muscles, including the *obturator internus* and *piriformis*, contribute to hip movement and stability. The *sacrospinous*, *sacrotuberous*, and *inguinal ligaments* provide support and stability to the pelvic organs and bony pelvis.

Groin or Inguinal Area

The *groin*, or *inguinal area*, is at the junction between the lower abdomen and thigh on either side of the pubic bone. Key landmarks include the *anterior superior iliac spine*, the *pubic tubercle*, and the connecting *inguinal ligament* (Fig. 23-5).

The *inguinal canal*, medial and parallel to the inguinal ligament, serves as a passageway for the vas deferens through the abdominal muscles. The internal opening, the *internal inguinal ring*, is about 1 cm above the midpoint of the ligament. The external opening, the *external inguinal ring*, is a triangular, slit-like structure palpable just above and lateral to the pubic tubercle.

Indirect inguinal hernias form at the internal inguinal ring, where the spermatic cord leaves the abdomen. *Direct inguinal hernias* occur more medially due to weakness in the inguinal canal floor and are associated with straining and heavy lifting. See Table 23-7, Course, Presentation, and Differentiation of Hernias in the Groin, p. 722.

The *femoral canal* is beneath the inguinal ligament. To approximate its location, place your right index finger on the right femoral artery from below, middle finger on the femoral vein, and third finger on the femoral canal.

Femoral hernias protrude at this location and are more likely to present as emergencies with bowel incarceration or strangulation.

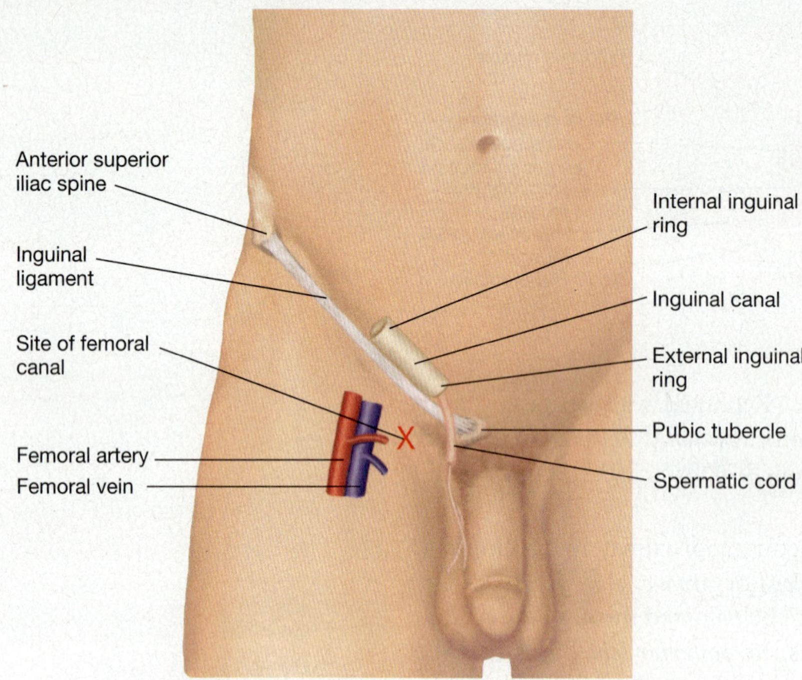

FIGURE 23-5. Anatomic landmarks of the right groin.

The femoral artery enters the thigh from behind the inguinal ligament as the *common femoral artery.* The femoral vein, draining blood from the lower extremity, terminates at the lower edge of the inguinal ligament, becoming the *external iliac vein.* The femoral vein runs alongside and medial to the femoral artery within the femoral sheath, just behind the inguinal ligament.

Blood, Lymphatic, and Nerve Supplies

Blood supply to the pelvis comes primarily from the *internal iliac arteries*, which branch into smaller arteries. Blood is drained by the *internal iliac veins* and other smaller veins.

Lymph drainage from the penis and nearby structures passes primarily to the deep inguinal and external inguinal nodes. Lymph vessels from the scrotum drain into the superficial inguinal lymph nodes. Lymphatic drainage from the testes parallels their venous drainage: the left testicular vein empties into the left renal vein, and the right testicular vein empties into the inferior vena cava. The connecting lumbar and preaortic lymph nodes in the abdomen are clinically undetectable.

When you find an inflammatory or suspect a possible malignant lesion on the penis, scrotum, or testis, assess the inguinal nodes carefully for enlargement or tenderness. See Chapter 19, Peripheral Vascular System, p. 552 for further discussion of the inguinal nodes.

The *nervous system* in the pelvis includes the *sacral plexus*, giving rise to nerves that innervate the pelvic organs, muscles, and skin. Notable nerves include the *pudendal nerve*, which innervates external genitalia and perineum, and the *pelvic splanchnic nerves*, providing parasympathetic innervation to the pelvic organs.

Micturition Cycle

The *micturition* or *urination cycle* is a process involving the coordinated interaction between the urinary bladder, urethra, and nervous system and consists of four stages:

- *Filling:* Urine produced by the kidneys flows through the ureters into the bladder. The detrusor muscle stays relaxed, while the internal and external urethral sphincters contract to prevent leakage.
- *Storage:* As the bladder fills, its walls stretch and pressure increases. The detrusor muscle remains relaxed, allowing the bladder to expand. The internal and external urethral sphincters stay contracted to maintain continence.
- *Voiding:* When the bladder is full, stretch receptors initiate the micturition reflex. The detrusor muscle contracts, and both urethral sphincters relax, forcing urine out through the urethra.
- *Postvoiding:* After emptying, the detrusor muscle relaxes, and the urethral sphincters contract, returning to their resting states. The bladder begins the filling phase again, repeating the cycle.

The urethra coordinates its urinary function with the reproductive system to prevent simultaneous passage of urine and semen. This is achieved by closing the bladder neck during ejaculation, ensuring semen only exits through the urethra.

Sexual Development and Function

The hypothalamus releases *gonadotropin-releasing hormone* (*GnRH*), which stimulates the pituitary gland to secrete *luteinizing hormone* (*LH*) and *follicle-stimulating hormone* (*FSH*). LH activates interstitial *Leydig cells* to produce *testosterone*, which is converted to *5α-dihydrotestosterone* (*5α-DHT*) in target tissues. This hormone triggers genitalia growth, secondary sexual characteristics, and sperm production, regulated by FSH in the seminiferous tubules.

See the Tanner stages of sexual maturity in Chapter 28, Children: Infancy Through Adolescence, pp. 1091–1097.

Sexual function in individuals assigned male at birth relies on adequate testosterone levels, arterial blood flow, and neural innervation through α-adrenergic and cholinergic pathways. Erection occurs due to venous engorgement of the corpora cavernosa and two types of stimuli. Higher brain centers respond to visual, auditory, and erotic cues, while tactile stimulation activates sensory impulses from the genitalia. Both stimuli increase nitric oxide and cyclic guanosine monophosphate levels, leading to local vasodilation.

HEALTH HISTORY: GENERAL APPROACH

Discussing a patient's sexual and genital health history can be challenging. Although clinicians and educators understand the importance of thorough sexual health education, training, and expertise may be limited.[1–5] To encourage patients to openly discuss their history and symptoms, approach your questions respectfully, directly, nonjudgmentally, and sensitively. Incorporating inclusive language is a cornerstone of this approach. By using language respectful of diverse gender identities and experiences, you create a welcoming space for individuals to share their unique perspectives and concerns. Your confidence and skill will improve with practice, so be patient and develop your own style for addressing sexual health topics. This aspect of the patient interview is vital, transcending factors such as age, sexual orientation, gender identity, comorbidities, socioeconomic factors, and disabilities.

Common or Concerning Symptoms

- Lower urinary tract storage symptoms
- Lower urinary tract voiding symptoms
- Lower urinary tract postmicturition symptoms
- Urinary incontinence (See also Chapter 24, Pelvis and Genitourinary System: Vulva, Vagina, Uterus, and Adnexa, pp. 743–744.)
- Penile discharge or lesions
- Scrotal or testicular pain, swelling, or lesions
- Erectile dysfunction (ED)

Lower urinary tract symptoms (LUTS) refer to a group of symptoms related to the dysfunction of the bladder, urethra, and surrounding muscles and nerves[6–8] are typically divided into three main categories: storage symptoms, voiding symptoms, and postmicturition symptoms.

For hypogastrium or suprapubic pain, see Chapter 21, Abdomen, pp. 615–616 and Chapter 24, Pelvis and Genitourinary System: Vulva, Vagina, Uterus, and Adnexa, pp. 741–742.

Lower Urinary Tract Storage Symptoms

Lower urinary tract *storage* symptoms involve difficulty storing urine in the bladder, leading to increased *urinary frequency* (needing to urinate more often than usual during the day), *urgency* (an unusually intense and immediate desire to void), and *nocturia* (waking up to urinate during the night). Box 23-1 provides high-yield health history questions for these symptoms.

Possible causes include **benign prostatic hyperplasia** ([**BPH**] enlarged prostate compressing the urethra), **overactive bladder** ([**OAB**] involuntary bladder contractions), **prostatitis** (inflammation or infection of the prostate), **urinary tract infection** (**UTI**), and **neurogenic bladder** (disruption of nerve signals to the bladder due to neurologic conditions).

See Table 23-1, Urinary Frequency, Nocturia, and Polyuria, pp. 714–715.

Box 23-1. Lower Urinary Tract Storage Symptoms: High-Yield Health History Questions

Domain	Questions	Rationale
Medical history	*Have you ever had bladder infections, any infections passed through sexual contact, or problems with your prostate?*	History of urinary tract infections (UTIs), sexually transmitted infections (STIs), or prostate issues may indicate a predisposition to recurrent infections or other complications, which can cause urinary frequency, urgency, and nocturia
Current symptoms	*Other than needing to go to the bathroom often, feeling a sudden need to urinate, or waking up at night to urinate, are you feeling any pain, seeing blood when you urinate, or have a fever?*	Additional symptoms like pain, hematuria, or fever may suggest an infection, such as a UTI or prostatitis, or other conditions like urinary stones or bladder cancer

Domain	Questions	Rationale
Fluid intake	*Can you tell me about what you drink every day? How much and what kinds of drinks?*	High fluid intake, particularly of diuretic beverages such as coffee, tea, or alcohol, can contribute to urinary frequency, urgency, and nocturia
Medications	*Are you taking any medicines or health supplements that might be affecting how often you need to go to the bathroom?*	Diuretics, anticholinergics, α-blockers, and calcium-channel blockers can cause or exacerbate urinary frequency, urgency, and nocturia
Bowel habits	*Have you noticed any changes in how often you go to the toilet for a bowel movement, or have you been constipated lately?*	Constipation and changes in bowel habits can cause increased pressure on the bladder, leading to urinary frequency, urgency, and nocturia

Lower Urinary Tract Voiding Symptoms

Voiding symptoms are related to difficulties in emptying the bladder completely or comfortably. They can include *weak* or *intermittent urine stream* (reduced urine flow or one that stops and starts), *hesitancy* (difficulty starting the urine flow), and *straining to urinate*. Box 23-2 provides high-yield health history questions for these symptoms.

Common causes include **BPH**, **prostatitis**, **UTI**, and **neurogenic bladder**. Other possible causes include **urethral stricture** (narrowing of the urethra due to scar tissue or inflammation), **bladder outlet obstruction**, and **medication side effects**.

See Table 23-9, Abnormalities of the Prostate, p. 724.

Box 23-2. Lower Urinary Tract Voiding Symptoms: High-Yield Health History Questions

Domain	Questions	Rationale
Medical history	*Have you ever had any problems with your bladder or kidneys, like infections or kidney stones, or needed surgery for them?*	May be relevant to the presenting symptoms and help guide further evaluation and management
Symptoms and duration	*When did you first start noticing these symptoms? Do they come and go or are they constant?*	*Acute onset:* may suggest an infection or obstruction *Chronic or progressive course:* might indicate an underlying structural issue, such as benign prostatic hyperplasia (BPH) or a stricture
Associated symptoms	*Are you feeling any pain or fever, getting the shivers, or noticing any unusual fluid coming out?*	May suggest an infection, such as a urinary tract infection (UTI) or prostatitis
Voiding pattern	*Have you noticed any changes in how often you need to urinate, like going more often, suddenly needing to go, or getting up at night to go?*	*Increased frequency or urgency:* may point to an overactive bladder, infection, or inflammation *Nocturia:* can be associated with BPH or other conditions that impair bladder emptying

(*continued*)

Box 23-2. Lower Urinary Tract Voiding Symptoms: High-Yield Health History Questions (*Continued*)

Domain	Questions	Rationale
Medications and allergies	*Are you taking any medicines or health supplements right now? Do you have allergies to any medications?*	Anticholinergics or α-blockers can cause or exacerbate urinary symptoms by affecting bladder function or urethral tone
Social and lifestyle factors	*Do you smoke, drink alcohol, or use any recreational drugs? Are there any parts of your lifestyle that might be affecting how you're feeling?*	*Smoking:* associated with bladder cancer and can exacerbate urinary symptoms *Alcohol and some recreational drugs:* can affect bladder function and urethral tone

Lower Urinary Tract Postmicturition Symptoms

Postmicturition symptoms include *sensation of incomplete bladder emptying* (sensation of residual urine in the bladder) and *postmicturition dribbling* (leakage of a small amount of urine after the main urinary stream has finished). These symptoms can be bothersome and affect daily life, pointing to issues with how the bladder empties or the muscles involved in urination. Box 23-3 outlines key health history questions for these symptoms.

Common causes include **weakened bladder** or **pelvic floor muscles** and **neurologic conditions** such as spinal cord injuries or neurodegenerative diseases. **Aging** and certain **medications that affect bladder muscle tone** may further contribute to these symptoms.

Box 23-3. Lower Urinary Tract Postmicturition Symptoms: High-Yield Health History Questions

Domain	Questions	Rationale
Symptoms and duration	*Do you feel like you haven't completely emptied your bladder after urinating?*	Sensation of incomplete emptying can indicate issues such as a weak bladder, bladder outlet obstruction, or neurogenic bladder (nerves controlling bladder function are impaired)
Associated symptoms	*Do you experience any dribbling or leakage of urine after you finish urinating?*	Often occurs due to residual urine in the urethra, especially in individuals with prostate enlargement or those with weakened pelvic floor muscles; could also indicate incomplete bladder emptying
Voiding pattern	*How often do these symptoms occur and do they seem to be getting worse?*	Regular occurrence and progression can signal worsening of an underlying condition, such as chronic bladder obstruction or deteriorating bladder muscle function
Medications and allergies	*Are you on any new medications that might affect bladder function?*	Certain medications can influence the bladder's ability to contract or relax properly, affecting posturination symptoms (e.g., drugs affecting the nervous system might impact bladder emptying)
Lifestyle factors	*Have there been any recent changes in your diet or fluid intake?*	Dietary habits and fluid intake can directly affect bladder function (e.g., high caffeine or alcohol intake can lead to increased urine production and subsequently affect postmicturition symptoms)

Urinary Incontinence

Up to 30% of older adults are concerned about *urinary incontinence*, involuntary loss of urine that can be socially restricting and cause problems with hygiene.[9–11] Bladder control involves complex neuroregulatory and motor mechanisms (see p. 693). Several central or peripheral nerve lesions affecting S2 to S4 spinal nerves can affect normal voiding. Box 23-4 provides a list of health history questions designed to help differentiate between possible causes.

Possible causes include **overflow incontinence** (incomplete bladder emptying often due to an obstruction or weak bladder muscle), **functional incontinence** (physical or cognitive impairments that hinder timely toilet access), **stress incontinence** (involuntary leakage occurs during activities that increase abdominal pressure), **urge incontinence** (sudden, intense urge to urinate followed by involuntary leakage), **mixed incontinence** (combination of stress and urge symptoms), and **neurogenic incontinence** (neurologic disorders or damage affecting bladder control). Also see Table 23-2, Urinary Incontinence in Individuals Assigned Male at Birth, pp. 716–717.

Box 23-4. Urinary Incontinence in Individuals Assigned Male at Birth: High-Yield Health History Questions

Domain	Questions	Rationale
Onset and pattern	*When did you first notice you were losing control of your bladder? What seems to trigger it, or is there a pattern to it?*	Helps differentiate between stress, urge, overflow, and functional incontinence
Severity and impact	*How often do you lose control of your bladder? How is this affecting your daily life and how you feel emotionally?*	Helps prioritize interventions and determine the urgency of addressing the issue
Voiding habits	*Can you tell me about your usual bathroom habits and any recent changes you've noticed?*	Can reveal factors contributing to urinary incontinence, such as excessive fluid intake, caffeine or alcohol consumption, or infrequent voiding
Urologic history	*Have you ever had any surgery, been pregnant, or had any serious injuries to your lower abdomen and pelvic area?*	Can indicate structural or functional changes contributing to urinary incontinence
Neurologic status	*Lately, have you noticed any changes in how you feel physically, like any numbness, a tingling feeling, or weakness in your body?*	Neurologic changes can signal central or peripheral nervous system issues that may contribute to urinary incontinence, such as spinal cord injuries or neurodegenerative diseases
Medical history	*Do you have any other health problems, and are you taking any medicines for them?*	Can help determine if the incontinence is related to an underlying condition (e.g., diabetes or multiple sclerosis) or a side effect of medications (e.g., diuretics or α-blockers).

Penile Discharge or Lesions

Review any previous genital symptoms or past history of infection from herpes, gonorrhea, or syphilis.[12–16] Ask about any discharge from the penis, dripping, or staining of underwear. If penile discharge is present, clarify the amount; color; and any fever, chills, rash, or associated symptoms (Box 23-5).

Possible causes include **sexually transmitted infections (STIs)**, **nongonococcal urethritis** ([**NGU**] inflammatory response to various pathogens, often noninfectious), **balanitis** (inflammation of the glans penis and foreskin), **herpes simplex virus** ([**HSV**] viral infection affecting skin and mucous membranes), and **human papillomavirus** ([**HPV**], viral infection causing warts and, rarely, malignancy).

See Table 23-4, Abnormalities of the Penis and Scrotum, p. 719, and Table 23-5, Abnormalities of the Testis, p. 720.

Box 23-5. Penile Discharge or Lesions: High-Yield Health History Questions

Domain	Questions	Rationale
Onset and duration	*When did you first notice any discharge or sores on your penis, and have they gotten better or worse over time?*	*Sexually transmitted infections (STIs):* often present with acute purulent discharge (e.g., gonorrhea) Chronic dermatologic conditions: might present with progressive whitish lesions over months or years (e.g., lichen sclerosis) *Evolution (e.g., from vesicles to ulcers):* may suggest herpes infection *Painless, nonprogressing ulcers:* could indicate syphilis
Sexual history	*Have you recently started a sexual relationship with someone new, or had sex without protection?*	Recent unprotected sex or new partners increases the likelihood of STI as a cause of penile discharge or lesions
Associated symptoms	*Are you feeling any pain, itching, or burning either around your genitals or when you urinate?*	Can help narrow down the potential causes, as some conditions (e.g., herpes) are more likely to cause these symptoms than others
Medical history	*Do you have any other health issues or a history of infections in your genital area?*	*Diabetes:* can predispose an individual to infections *History of genital infections:* may indicate a recurrent issue
Medication use	*Are you currently on any medications, or have you recently started or stopped taking any?*	*Antibiotics:* can cause changes in the genital area or predispose an individual to infections *Others:* may cause a hypersensitivity reaction
Hygiene practices	*How would you describe your personal hygiene practices, particularly in the genital area?*	*Poor personal hygiene:* can contribute to the development of infections or irritations *Aggressive cleaning:* may cause trauma or irritation to the genital area

Scrotal or Testicular Pain, Swelling, or Lesions

Evaluating scrotal or testicular pain, swelling, or lesions is critical, as these symptoms could indicate serious health issues. Direct and detailed questioning about the symptoms' onset, duration, and characteristics is essential for accurate diagnosis and effective treatment (Box 23-6).

Possible causes include **epididymitis** (infection of epididymis), **orchitis** (inflammation of testicle), **varicocele** (dilated veins in pampiniform plexus), **hydrocele** (fluid collection around testicle), **inguinal hernia** (protrusion of bowel or fat), **spermatocele** (cyst within epididymis), **testicular torsion** (twisting of spermatic cord), and **testicular cancer** (malignant testicular tumor).

Box 23-6. Scrotal or Testicular Pain, Swelling, or Lesions: High-Yield Health History Questions

Domain	Questions	Rationale
Symptoms	*When did you first start feeling pain, swelling, or notice a sore? Is this feeling constant, or does it come and go?*	*Sharp and sudden:* might mean testicular torsion, which is a medical emergency If *Mild and persistent:* could be a long-term issue like a hydrocele or varicocele *Intermittent:* might be epididymitis *Constant, especially with a lump:* might mean something serious like testicular cancer
Pain characteristics	*How do you describe what the pain feels like? Is it sharp, dull, or throbbing? Does it spread to other areas like your groin or lower stomach?*	*Quick, severe:* could be torsion or a tear *Constant, dull:* might be from an infection, inflammation, or varicocele *Unilateral:* might be torsion or a varicocele *Spreading to the groin or lower abdomen:* could be epididymitis or orchitis
Swelling characteristics	*Where is the swelling, and how big it is? Does it hurt or feel tender when you touch it?*	*Small, specific:* might be a cyst or abscess *Larger:* could be a hydrocele or varicocele *Sore or painful:* could be an infection like epididymitis or orchitis *Painless:* could be a long-term condition like a hydrocele or varicocele
Aggravating and relieving factors	*What makes the pain worse or better?*	*Not relieved by elevation of the testicle (negative* Prehn sign*):* might be testicular torsion *Relieved by elevation:* might be epididymitis *Aggravated by physical activity:* may suggest trauma or strain
Associated symptoms	*Are you experiencing any other symptoms like fever, problems with urinating, or any fluid coming out?*	*Fever and urinary symptoms:* may suggest infection, such as epididymitis or orchitis *Penile discharge:* could indicate a sexually transmitted infection (STI) *Absence of associated symptoms:* may point to noninfectious causes, such as torsion or varicocele
Medical and surgical history	*Have you ever had surgery or an injury to your scrotum or testicles? Do you have any health conditions that might be causing these symptoms?*	*History of inguinal hernia repair:* may predispose to recurrent hernias or postsurgical complications *History of STIs:* could suggest epididymitis or orchitis

Erectile Dysfunction

ED is a common condition that affects up to 30 million individuals assigned male at birth in the United States alone.[17,18] Proper questioning aids in identifying the underlying causes, which may range from physical issues like cardiovascular disease to psychological factors (Box 23-7).

Possible causes include **cardiovascular disease** affecting blood flow, **diabetes** affecting blood flow and nerve function, **low testosterone**, **neurologic disorders** (e.g., spinal cord injuries, multiple sclerosis, and Parkinson disease), **psychological factors** (such as stress, anxiety, or depression), **lifestyle choices** (smoking, excessive alcohol use, and lack of exercise), **certain medications** (blood pressure drugs, antidepressants), and **pelvic or genital injuries**.

Box 23-7. Erectile Dysfunction: High-Yield Health History Questions

Domain	Questions	Rationale
Medical history	*Do you have any health conditions like diabetes, high blood pressure, or heart problems? Have you had any surgeries or treatments that could affect your ability to be sexually active?*	*Diabetes, high blood pressure, or heart disease:* can cause or contribute to erectile dysfunction (ED) *Surgeries or treatments that affect the pelvic region or nerves (e.g., prostate surgery or radiation therapy):* can also affect sexual function
Medication history	*Are you taking any medicines, including things you can buy without a prescription or natural supplements? What are they, and how long have you been taking them?*	*Antidepressants, blood pressure medications, and antihistamines:* can cause or contribute to ED *Herbal supplements (e.g., yohimbe):* can also affect sexual function
Psychosocial history	*Are you going through any major stress or changes in your life, like issues at work or in your relationships? Have you been feeling anxious or down lately?*	Stress, anxiety, and depression can contribute to ED
Lifestyle factors	*Do you smoke? How much alcohol do you drink, and how often do you exercise?*	Smoking, excessive alcohol consumption, and sedentary behavior can contribute to ED
Sexual history	*Are you currently sexually active? Do you have any trouble getting an erection, either when you masturbate or when you're asleep?*	Patients who are unable to achieve an erection during any sexual activity may have a more severe form of ED

PHYSICAL EXAMINATION: GENERAL APPROACH

Many students beginning their training might feel apprehensive about examining the genitalia due to concerns about patient reactions, cooperation, or potential erections during the examination. To alleviate these concerns, thoroughly explain the examination process to the patient, ensuring they feel reassured and informed. If necessary, have an assistant accompany you. In the event of an erection, calmly explain that it is a normal response, complete the examination, and maintain a composed demeanor. If a patient refuses the examination, discuss their reasons for refusal.

During the examination, ensure the patient's comfort by exposing only the areas being examined at any given time, whether the patient is standing or sitting. For example, when the patient is supine, use a gown to cover their chest and abdomen, and place a drape at the midthigh. Expose the genitalia and inguinal areas as needed, and always wear gloves. When examining younger patients, review their sexual maturity rating to accurately document your findings.

TECHNIQUES OF EXAMINATION

Key Components of the Examination of the Penis and Scrotum

- Inspect the penile skin, prepuce, and glans.
- Inspect the urethral meatus.
- Palpate the shaft of the penis.
- Inspect the scrotum.
- Assess for groin hernias.
- Palpate each testis.
- Palpate the epididymis.
- Examine the spermatic cords.

Inspect the Penile Skin, Prepuce, and Glans

Inspect the skin on the ventral and dorsal surfaces and the base of the penis for excoriations or inflammation. If you encounter any such abnormalities, gently lift the penis when necessary to ensure a complete assessment.

Pubic or genital excoriations suggest *pediculosis pubis* (lice or crabs) or sometimes scabies in the pubic hair.

See Table 23-4, Abnormalities of the Penis and Scrotum, p. 719.

Inspect the prepuce or foreskin, which covers the glans. Retract the prepuce or ask the patient to retract it. Retraction of the prepuce is especially important for the detection of chancres and carcinomas, which may not be visible otherwise. After inspection, carefully return the foreskin to its original position. During this step, also note that *smegma*, a cheesy, whitish material, may accumulate normally under the foreskin. This accumulation is a typical finding and should not be a cause for concern.

Phimosis is a tight prepuce that cannot be retracted over the glans. **Paraphimosis** is a tight prepuce that, once retracted, cannot be returned and edema ensues.

Inspect the glans. Pay close attention to its color and texture. A healthy glans typically appears pink or a shade consistent with the patient's skin tone. Any significant changes in color, such as redness or pallor, should be noted. Also inspect for any ulcers, scars, nodules, or signs of inflammation.

Inspect the Urethral Meatus

Inspect the location of the urethral meatus. Compress the glans gently between your index finger above and your thumb below (Fig. 23-6). This maneuver should open the urethral meatus and allow you to inspect it for spontaneous discharge. Normally, there is none.

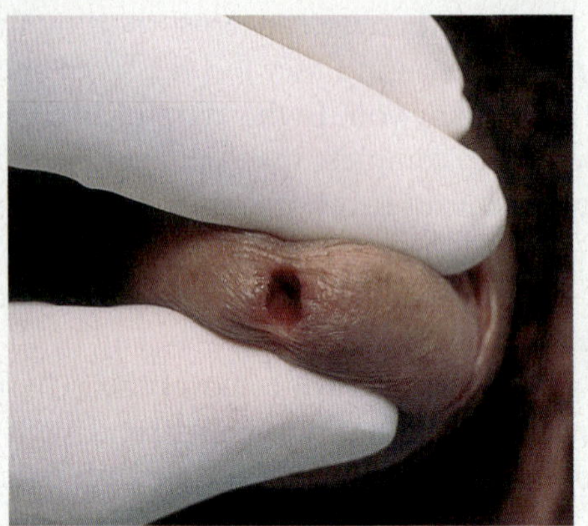

FIGURE 23-6. Gently compressing the glans to inspect the urethral meatus.

Hypospadias is a congenital ventral displacement of the meatus on the penis, while **epispadias** is a congenital dorsal displacement.

If the patient has reported urethral discharge that you are unable to see, instruct them to "strip" or "milk" the shaft of the penis from its base to the glans. Alternatively, you may perform this maneuver yourself. This technique may help expel some discharge from the urethral meatus for appropriate examination. Have culture swabs and appropriate materials ready to collect and test the discharged material.

Palpate the Shaft of the Penis

Palpate the shaft between your thumb and first two fingers, noting any induration. Palpate any abnormality of the penis, noting any induration or tenderness.

On the dorsal side of the penis, plaques of Peyronie disease can sometimes be palpated under the skin on the right or left aspect of the shaft in the corpora cavernosa.

Urethral strictures most commonly occur in the proximal urethra, but induration or firmness along the ventral surface of the penis suggests a urethral stricture or possibly a carcinoma.

Inspect the Scrotum

Inspect the scrotum. Begin by lifting the scrotum gently to access and inspect its posterior surface. Observe the skin closely for any irregularities, including lesions, scars, or other noticeable marks. Evaluate the distribution of pubic hair around the scrotal area. Note any abnormal patterns or hair loss.

Inspection may reveal scrotal nevi, hemangiomas, or telangiectasias as well as STIs including condyloma or ulcers from herpes and chancroid (painful) and syphilis and lymphogranuloma venereum (painless), with associated inguinal lymphadenopathy.[19]

Carefully examine scrotal contours for any signs of swelling, lumps, or unusual protrusions. Look for the presence of varicose veins or any bulging masses that may indicate underlying health issues.

Assess the symmetry of the left and right hemiscrotum. You should note any noticeable asymmetry.

A poorly developed scrotum on one or both sides suggests **cryptorchidism** (undescended testicle).

See Table 23-4, Abnormalities of the Penis and Scrotum, p. 719.

Now move to the inguinal areas, located on either side of the lower abdomen, just above the scrotum. Note any erythema, excoriation, or visible adenopathy. Observe for any visible bulges that may indicate an inguinal hernia or other conditions. Check both the left and right inguinal areas for consistency and symmetry.

Erythema and mild excoriation point to fungal infection, not uncommon in this moist area.

Epidermoid cysts are dome-shaped white or yellow papules or nodules formed by occluded follicles filled with keratin debris of desquamated follicular epithelium. They are common, frequently multiple, and benign (Fig. 23-7).

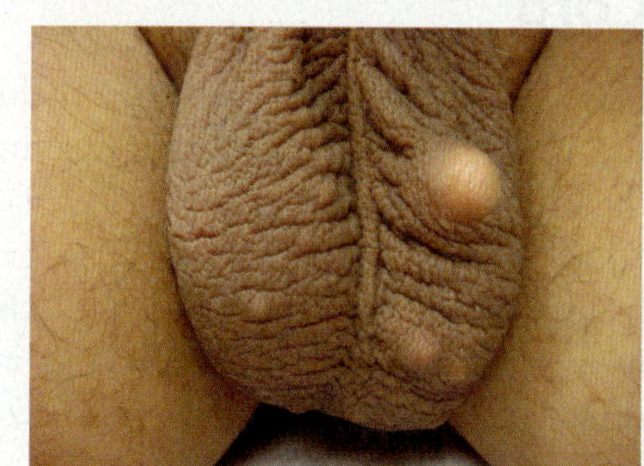

FIGURE 23-7. Benign scrotal epidermoid cysts. (Reprinted with permission from Goodheart HP, Gonzalez ME. *Goodheart's Photoguide to Common Pediatric and Adult Skin Disorders.* 4th ed. Wolters Kluwer; 2016. Figure 30-28.)

Assess for Groin Hernias

With the patient standing and you seated in front, begin by visually inspecting the inguinal regions and genitalia for any bulging areas or asymmetry, which might suggest a groin hernia. Note that groin hernias in individuals assigned female at birth often do not show a visible bulge, making them harder to detect visually. This difference underscores the importance of a thorough and careful examination in all patients, regardless of gender.[20]

After the initial inspection, proceed with palpation. Gently palpate the inguinal region, feeling for any lumps or protrusions. Ask the patient to cough or perform the Valsalva maneuver. Observe any changes in the inguinal area during these maneuvers. Note any bulges that appear or become more pronounced, as these indicate herniation.

If a hernia is suspected from your initial assessment, proceed with the further examination techniques outlined on pages 704–706. In addition, diagnostic measures like an ultrasound may be necessary for a more comprehensive evaluation.

See Table 23-7, Course, Presentation, and Differentiation of Hernias in the Groin, p. 722.

Palpate Each Testis

If using a one-handed technique, palpate each testis and epididymis between your thumb and first two fingers (Fig. 23-8). If using two hands, cradle the testis at both poles in the thumb and fingertips of both hands. Palpate the scrotal contents as you gently slide them back and forth from the fingertips of one hand to the other, without changing the position of your hands as they cup the scrotum. This technique is comfortable for the patient and allows accurate examination.

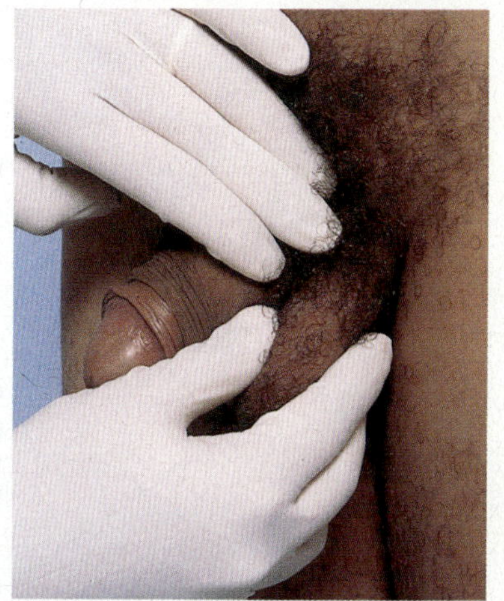

FIGURE 23-8. Palpating the testis and epididymis using one-handed technique.

See Table 23-5, Abnormalities of the Testis, p. 720, and Table 23-6, Abnormalities of the Epididymis and Spermatic Cord, p. 721.

For each testis, assess size, shape, consistency, and tenderness; feel for any nodules. The testes should be firm but not hard, descended, symmetric, or nontender, and

Any painless nodule on the testis raises the possibility of testicular cancer, a potentially curable cancer with a peak incidence ages 15–34 years.

they should also be without masses.[19] Pressure on the testis normally produces a deep visceral pain.

Palpate the Epididymis

Palpate the epididymis on the posterior surface of each testicle without applying excess pressure, which can cause discomfort. Assess for tenderness; the epididymis should not be tender under normal conditions. The epididymis feels nodular and cord-like and should not be confused with an abnormal lump.

Examine the Spermatic Cord

Palpate each spermatic cord, including the vas deferens, from the epididymis to the external inguinal ring (Fig. 23-9). Use your thumb and fingers for palpation, feeling along the cord. The vas deferens feels slightly stiff and tubular and is distinct from the accompanying vessels of the spermatic cord.

The vas deferens, if chronically infected, may feel thickened or beaded. A cystic structure in the spermatic cord suggests a hydrocele of the cord.

With the patient standing, palpate the spermatic cord about 2 cm above the testis. Have the patient hold their breath and "bear down" against a closed glottis for about 4 seconds (Valsalva maneuver).

During this maneuver, a temporary increase in the diameter of the spermatic cord indicates filling of abnormally dilated spermatic veins draining the testis, suggesting a **varicocele**.

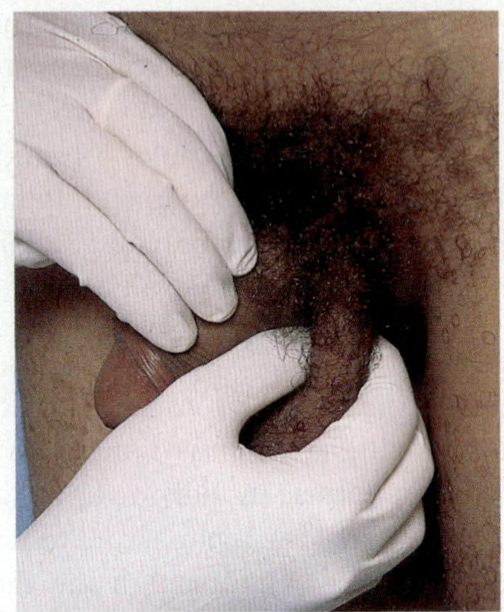

FIGURE 23-9. Palpating the spermatic cord.

SPECIAL TECHNIQUES AND MANEUVERS

The lifetime risk of developing a *groin hernia*, *inguinal* or *femoral hernia*, is approximately 25% in individuals assigned male at birth but less than 5% in individuals assigned female at birth. Approximately 96% of groin hernias are inguinal and 4% are femoral (Fig. 23-10). However, femoral hernias, which

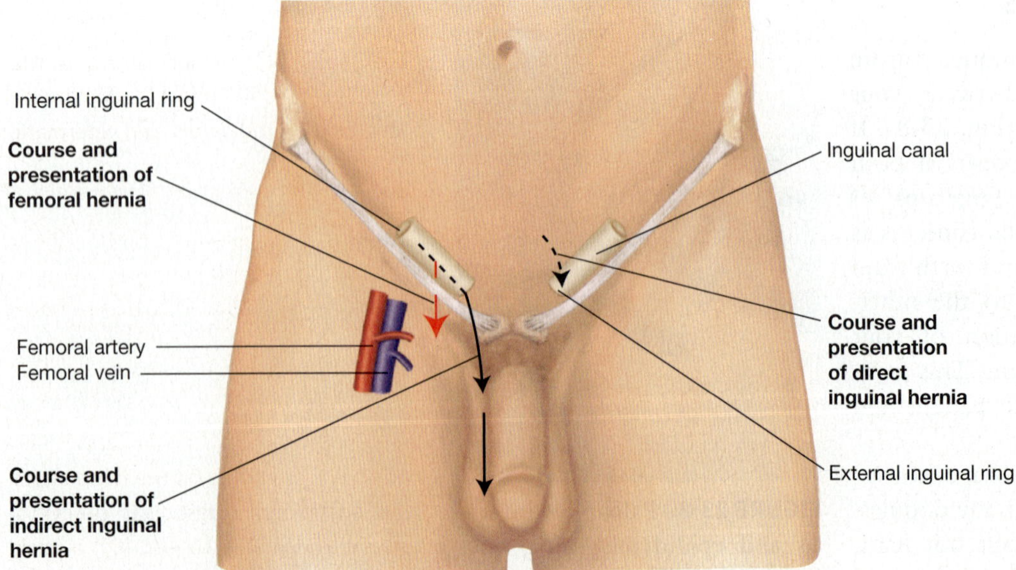

FIGURE 23-10. Course and presentation of groin hernias.

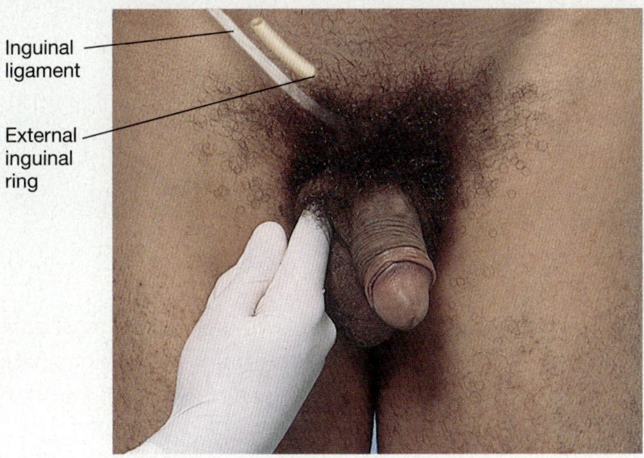

FIGURE 23-11. Invaginating redundant scrotal skin toward external inguinal ring to detect a right inguinal hernia.

occur more often in older individuals assigned female at birth (median age of presentation is 60 to 79 years), lead to a higher proportion of emergency operations due to the higher risk of the hernia contents being trapped within the hernia sac (*incarceration*) and causing ischemia and necrosis (*strangulation*).[20,21] Chance of incarceration is low, however, estimated at 0.3% to 3% per year, and is 10 times more common with indirect hernias.[22,23]

See Table 23-7, Course, Presentation, and Differentiation of Hernias in the Groin, p. 722.

Evaluating a Suspected Inguinal Hernia

To examine for an inguinal hernia on either side, place the tip of your dominant index finger at the anterior inferior margin of the scrotum, staying superficial to the testes (Fig. 23-11). Gently move your finger and hand upward toward the external inguinal ring, invaginating the redundant scrotal skin beneath the peripubic fat pad next to the base of the penis.

Follow the spermatic cord upward to the inguinal ligament. Identify the triangular slit-like opening of the *external inguinal ring* just above and lateral to the pubic tubercle. Palpate the external inguinal ring and its floor.

Ask the patient to cough, and feel for a distinct bulge or mass that moves against your stationary finger during the cough.

A bulge near the external inguinal ring suggests a *direct* inguinal hernia. A bulge near the internal inguinal ring suggests an *indirect* inguinal hernia.[22]

Gently palpate obliquely along the inguinal canal toward the *internal inguinal ring*. Again, ask the patient to cough, and check for a bulge that slides down the inguinal canal and taps against your fingertip. Use the same techniques with the same dominant finger to examine both sides.

If a hernia is suspected but does not return to the abdomen when the patient lies down, attempt gentle reduction with sustained finger pressure. Do not attempt this maneuver if the mass is tender or the patient reports nausea and vomiting.

Suspect strangulation in the presence of tenderness, nausea, and vomiting, and consider surgical intervention.[24]

To assess a possible inguinal hernia presenting as a mass in the scrotum, ask the patient to lie down. If the mass disappears by returning to the abdomen by itself (*reducible*), it is likely to be an *indirect* inguinal hernia. The patient can often tell you what happens to their swelling when lying down and may be able to demonstrate how they reduce it themselves.

Evaluating a Suspected Femoral Hernia

Ensure the patient is in a comfortable and appropriate position, either standing or lying down with their legs slightly parted. This position provides better access to the femoral region. Position yourself in front of the patient, with easy access to their anterior thigh and inguinal region.

Start by locating the femoral pulse in the upper portion of the thigh. Once it is located, move your fingers medially toward the inner thigh and slightly upward, approaching the area of the pubic tubercle. The femoral canal is located in this region.

Femoral hernias most commonly present inferior to the inguinal ligament and medial to the femoral artery.[20]

Place your fingers gently but firmly in the region medial to the femoral canal. Ask the patient to cough or bear down (Valsalva maneuver), which increases intra-abdominal pressure, and carefully observe and feel for any bulge or swelling that appears during the strain. This could indicate the presence of a femoral hernia.

Note any tenderness in the area on palpation. Assess the consistency of any swelling detected. Compare the findings with the other side to check for asymmetry.

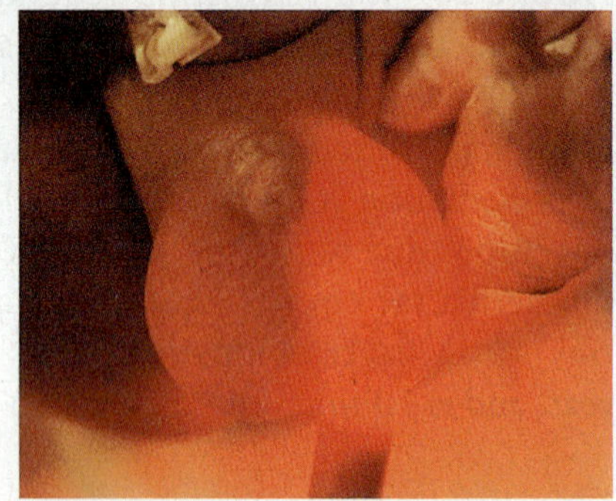

FIGURE 23-12. Transillumination of a hydrocoele. (Reprinted with permission from Fletcher MA. *Physical Diagnosis in Neonatology*. Lippincott-Raven; 1998.)

Assessing for Scrotal Contents by Transillumination

Transillumination is a simple, noninvasive technique that can provide valuable information about the nature of scrotal masses and swellings. After darkening the room, hold a strong light source behind the scrotum. Instruct the patient to hold or support their scrotum if needed, or you can do it with your free hand, ensuring the scrotum is slightly stretched for a clear view.

Position the light source directly behind the scrotum, shining the light through the scrotal skin and contents. Look for the way light passes through it. If the mass inside the scrotum is cystic, like a hydrocele, the light will pass through it, creating a red or pinkish glow (Fig. 23-12). If the mass is solid, such as a tumor or most types of hernias, the light will not pass through, and the mass will appear as a dark shadow.

Transillumination of the scrotal mass may help distinguish a *hydrocele* from an intestine-containing hernia. Those containing blood or tissue, such as a normal testis, a tumor, or most hernias, do not transilluminate.

Performing a Testicular Self-Examination

Testicular cancer, while not a common disease, affects about 1 in every 250 individuals assigned male at birth at some point in their lives.[25] The U.S. Preventive Services Task Force (USPSTF) recommends against routine screening for testicular cancer in asymptomatic adolescent and adult individuals, classifying it with a grade D recommendation. This is due to the low prevalence of the disease and the balance between the potential benefits and harms of screening.[26] The American Cancer Society (ACS), while not endorsing routine testicular self-examinations (TSEs) for screening purposes, emphasizes the importance of being aware of the signs and symptoms of testicular cancer. They advise seeking medical attention promptly if any changes, such as a lump in the testicle, are noticed.

Box 23-8. Patient Instructions for Testicular Self-Examination

This examination is best performed after a warm bath or shower.[27,40] This way, the scrotal skin is warm and relaxed. It is best to do the test while standing.

- Standing in front of a mirror, check for any swelling on the skin of the scrotum.
- With the penis out of the way, gently feel your scrotal sac to locate a testicle. Examine each testicle separately.
- Use one hand to stabilize the testicle. Using the fingers and thumb of your other hand, firmly but gently feel or roll the testicle between your fingers. Feel the entire surface. Find the epididymis. This is a soft, tube-like structure at the back of the testicle that collects and carries sperm and is not an abnormal lump. Check the other testicle and epididymis the same way.
- If you find a hard lump, an absent or enlarged testicle, a painful swollen scrotum, or any other differences that do not seem normal, do not wait. See your health care provider right away.

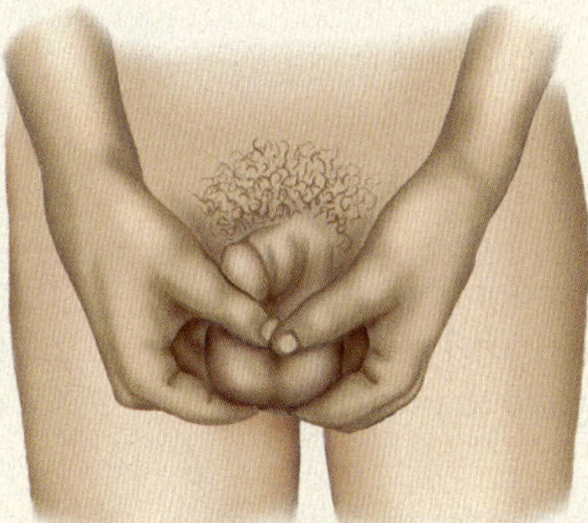

As noted by the ACS, "It's normal for one testicle to be slightly larger than the other, and for one to hang lower than the other. You should also know that each normal testicle has a small, coiled tube (epididymis) that can feel like a small bump on the upper or middle outer side of the testicle. Normal testicles also have blood vessels, supporting tissues, and tubes that carry sperm. Some individuals may confuse these with abnormal lumps at first. If you have any concerns, ask your doctor or clinician."

Although routine TSE is not universally recommended, it can be a valuable tool for increasing health awareness and self-care, particularly for individuals at higher risk of testicular cancer. Such risk factors include a family history of the disease, previous cancer in one testicle, or other relevant medical histories. You may consider teaching TSE to patients, especially those in high-risk categories, as a way of empowering them to monitor their own health (Box 23-8). This approach aligns with the concept of patient-centered care, enabling individuals to recognize normal conditions for their bodies and identify any concerning changes.[27]

For high-risk patients, review the risk factors for testicular carcinoma: cryptorchidism, which confers a high risk for testicular carcinoma in the undescended testicle; history of carcinoma in the contralateral testicle; mumps orchitis; inguinal hernia; hydrocele in childhood; and positive family history.

Modifications in Physical Examinations: Best Practices for Specialized Patient Populations

Box 23-9 provides guidance on how to adapt the genitalia examination based on various devices and surgical procedures.

Box 23-9. Genitalia Examination in the Presence of Medical Devices, Conditions, or Procedures

	Patient with an Indwelling Urinary Catheter (Foley Catheter)	Patient with a Suprapubic Catheter (Suprapubic Cystostomy)
	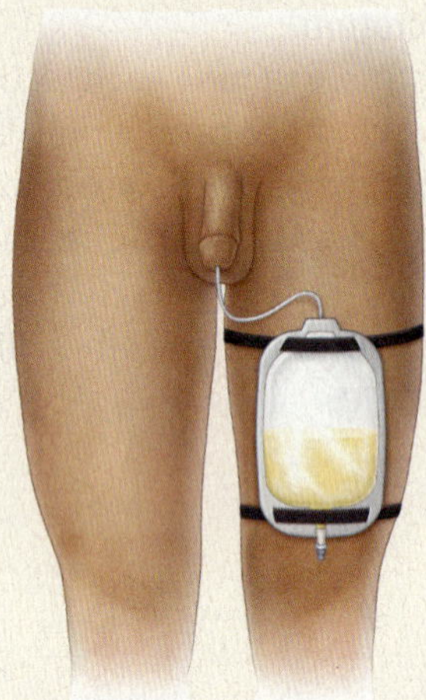	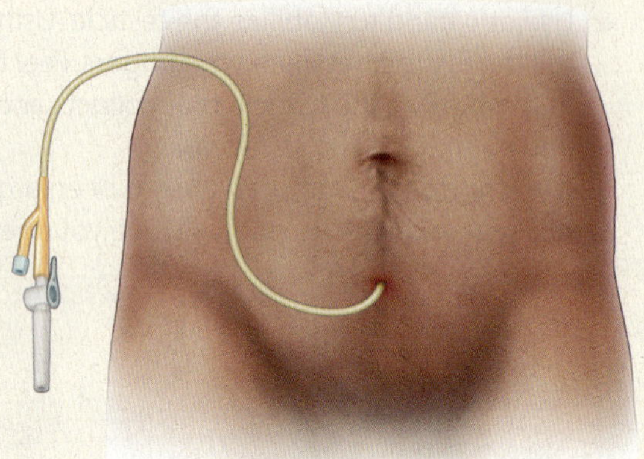
Device/ condition	Flexible tube inserted through the urethra and into the bladder to drain urine Typically has a saline-filled balloon at its tip to prevent it from slipping out Most have two channels, one for draining urine and one for inflating and deflating the balloon	Tube surgically inserted directly into the bladder through the abdominal wall to allow for urinary drainage
General indication	Drainage of urine to treat urinary retention, during surgery, or to monitor urine output	Direct drainage of urine; alternative to urethral catheterization
General location	Catheter passes through the urethra, with the tip in the bladder; external tubing is secured to the patient's thigh with adhesive to prevent inadvertent pulling or tension Urine drainage bag is either attached to the patient's thigh or hangs from the patient's stretcher	Catheter passes through the abdominal wall, with the tip terminating in the bladder
Modification to the physical exam	1. Ask permission and explain each step of the exam to ensure patient comfort. 2. Evaluate the urethral meatus for signs of irritation, urine leakage, or skin breakdown. Avoid retracting the foreskin, if present, to prevent catheter displacement. 3. Palpate and inspect the penis and scrotum carefully, avoiding any tension on the catheter. 4. Be aware of the balloon's location inside the bladder—do not exert pressure in this area. 5. Ask the patient about any discomfort, quantity and appearance of urine output, concerns for catheter obstruction, and any urine leakage around the catheter.	1. Ask permission and explain each step of the exam to ensure patient comfort. 2. Inspect the suprapubic area and genitalia, noting any redness, discharge, swelling, or urine leakage at the catheter insertion site. 3. Palpate the suprapubic area without applying direct pressure on the insertion site, which may be sensitive or painful. Avoid applying tension on the tubing. 4. Ask the patient about any discomfort, quantity and appearance of urine output, concerns for catheter obstruction, and any urine leakage around the catheter.

Patient with a Penile Implant (Prosthesis)	**Patient with a Phalloplasty**
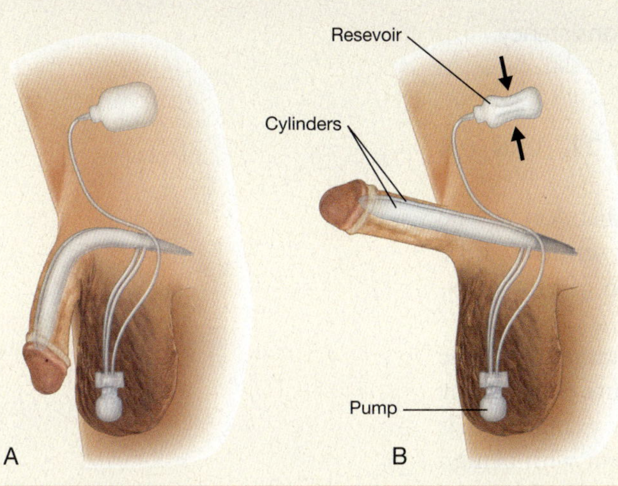	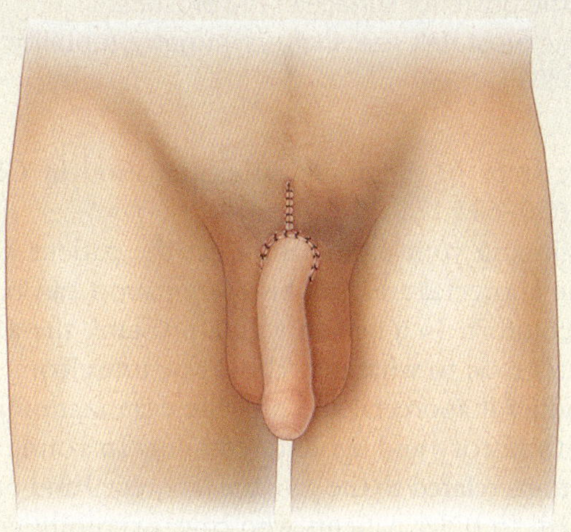
Inflatable cylinders or malleable rods implanted into the penis to allow patients with erectile dysfunction (ED) to achieve an erection	Neophallus (new penis) is constructed using tissue grafts typically from the patient's forearm, thigh, or back
Treatment of ED refractory to other treatments; treatment of penile injury or deformity	Gender confirmation surgery to align physical appearance with gender identity; reconstruction for congenital anomalies or after penile trauma
Devices are located in the corpora cavernosa of the penis; if inflatable, a saline reservoir is located in the lower abdomen or abdominal wall with an inflating pump in the scrotum	Depending on the surgery (e.g., phalloplasty creates a neophallus using tissue from other areas of the body)
1. Ask permission and explain each step of the exam to ensure patient comfort. 2. Prior to the examination, ask the patient about the type of implant (inflatable or malleable) and any special considerations. 3. Inquire about device function, issues with sexual activity, or issues with urination. 4. Inspect for signs of infection or inflammation including erythema, edema, or skin breakdown. 5. Palpate the penis gently, being cautious not to manipulate an inflatable device unintentionally. Evaluate for pain or discomfort during palpation. 6. Check for signs of device malfunction, such as asymmetry or firm nodules.	1. Approach with sensitivity, acknowledging the patient's surgical history. Always ask permission and explain each step of the exam to ensure patient comfort. 2. Begin by inquiring about any issues with sexual function ability to pass urine, or any other concerns. 3. Visually inspect the neophallus, noting surgical scars, skin grafts, general appearance, and patency of the urethral opening. 4. Inspect for signs of infection or inflammation, including erythema, edema, skin breakdown, or discharge from the urethral opening. 5. Gently palpate the neophallus, being mindful of the patient's sensitivity.

Key Components of the Prostate Examination

- Properly position the patient. (See Chapter 22, Anus and Rectum, pp. 680–681.)
- Palpate the posterior surface of the prostate.
- Assess the prostate's size, shape, symmetry, mobility, and consistency.

Review the steps of the anorectal examination in Chapter 22, Anus and Rectum, pp. 680–681.

Before beginning your examination, let the patient know that you will be examining the anorectal area, as this examination can be very sensitive and a source of discomfort. In a person with a prostate, the addition of this assessment adds extra time to what may already be unwelcome.

When deciding if anorectal and prostate examination is warranted, take the patient's health history and age into account. In young patients without any urinary symptoms related to the prostate, anorectal and prostate examination is rarely indicated. In older patients who have symptoms consistent with benign prostatic hyperplasia (BPH), a prostate examination should be part of the normal physical examination.

See Table 23-8. BPH Symptom Score: American Urological Association, p. 723.

Palpate the Posterior Surface of the Prostate Gland

Once in the rectum, rotate your hand further counterclockwise so that your finger can examine the posterior surface of the prostate gland (see Figs. 22-3 and 22-4). By turning your body slightly away from the patient, you can feel this area more easily. Tell the patient that examining their prostate gland may prompt an urge to urinate. Sweep your finger carefully over the prostate gland, identifying its lateral lobes and the groove of the *median sulcus* between them.

Assess the Prostate's Size, Shape, Symmetry, Mobility, and Consistency

Note the size, shape, mobility, and consistency of the prostate, and identify any nodules or tenderness. The normal prostate is rubbery and nontender, with no evidence of fixation to the surrounding tissues.

Take note of any asymmetry, such as a difference in firmness or size between each lobe. If possible, extend your finger above the prostate to the region of the seminal vesicles and the peritoneal cavity and sweep the anterior wall. Note any nodules or tenderness. This can be difficult in patients with an enlarged prostate.

Findings include a rectal "shelf" of peritoneal metastases (see p. 685) or the tenderness of peritoneal inflammation.

See Table 23-9, Abnormalities of the Prostate, p. 724.

Gently withdraw your finger and wipe the anal area or give the patient a disposable absorbent paper. Note the appearance of any fecal matter on your glove. Test the fecal matter for occult blood when indicated.

RECORDING YOUR FINDINGS

The documentation of your physical examination (PE) findings in your clinical notes is essential as it directly guides diagnosis and aids in hypothesis generation and validation. With increasing clinical experience, you will transition from detailed sentences to concise, universally accepted phrases, reflecting a deeper understanding and efficiency in clinical documentation.

Recording the Genitalia and Prostate Examination

"Circumcised penis. No penile discharge or lesions. No scrotal swelling or discoloration. Testes descended bilaterally, smooth, without masses. Epididymis is nontender. No inguinal or femoral hernias. Prostate smooth, symmetric and nontender with palpable median sulcus."

OR

"Uncircumcised penis; prepuce easily retractable. No penile discharge or lesions. No scrotal swelling or discoloration. Testes descended bilaterally; right testicle smooth; 1 × 1 cm firm nodule on left lateral testicle. It is fixed and nontender. Epididymis nontender. No inguinal or femoral hernias. Left lateral prostate lobe with 1 × 1 cm firm, hard nodule near the apex; right lateral lobe smooth; median sulcus obscured."

The breakdown of PE documentation into finer details serves as a prime example of how your clinical observations can yield crucial diagnostic clues. The findings described in the examination note raise several clinical suspicions:

- *Firm nodule on left lateral testicle:* The presence of a 1 × 1 cm firm, fixed, and nontender nodule on the left testicle is suspicious for testicular cancer, especially if the nodule is hard and does not move independently of the testicle. Testicular cancer often presents as a painless mass or nodule in the testicle.
- *Nodule on left lateral prostate lobe:* The 1 × 1 cm firm, hard nodule near the apex of the left lateral prostate lobe, combined with an obscured median sulcus, is concerning for prostate cancer. Prostate cancer typically presents as a hard, irregular nodule that can be palpated on digital rectal examination (DRE). The obscuration of the median sulcus is also concerning, as it may indicate an abnormal growth pattern.
- *Absence of other common genital pathologies:* The lack of penile discharge or lesions, absence of scrotal swelling or discoloration, and the normal condition of the right testicle and epididymis help to rule out other common conditions like infections, hydroceles, or varicoceles.
- *No inguinal or femoral hernias:* The absence of hernias is noted, but it does not contribute to the suspicion of malignancy. It is, however, part of a comprehensive genital examination.

In summary, the clinical findings of a firm nodule on the left testicle and a hard nodule on the left prostate lobe are suspicious for *testicular* and *prostate cancer*, respectively.

HEALTH PROMOTION AND COUNSELING: EVIDENCE AND RECOMMENDATIONS

Important Topics for Health Promotion and Counseling

- Prostate cancer

In the following section, both traditional terms like "men," "women," "male," and "female" and inclusive terms such as "individuals assigned female at birth" and "individuals assigned male at birth" are used. This approach balances inclusivity with the need to accurately represent the original research.

Prostate Cancer

Epidemiology. Prostate cancer is the most frequently diagnosed cancer (other than nonmelanoma skin cancers) among individuals in the U.S. and the second leading cause of cancer death.[28] The ACS estimated 288,300 new prostate cancer diagnoses in 2023 and 34,700 prostate cancer deaths. The overall lifetime risk of being diagnosed with prostate cancer is about 1 in 8, while the risk of dying from prostate cancer is about 1 in 43.[29] Age, ethnicity, and family history are the strongest risk factors for prostate cancer. Prostate cancer is rare before age 40 years; however, incidence rates begin increasing rapidly after age 45 years, and the median age at diagnosis is 67 years. Individuals of African American descent have the highest incidence and mortality rates from prostate cancer in the United States and, compared to individuals of European descent, are more likely to present before age 50 and with advanced-stage cancers. Family history of prostate cancer is associated with increased cancer risk, particularly when multiple first-degree relatives have been diagnosed and/or the relative's cancer was early onset (age ≤55 years).[30] Prostate cancer risk has also been associated with a family history of breast cancer, particularly due to the *BRCA2* mutation, and of colorectal cancer due to Lynch syndrome. Although the evidence is less convincing, other potential risk factors include Agent Orange (dioxin) exposure among Vietnam veterans, diets high in animal fat, and cadmium exposure.[31] However, BPH, a common finding in older individuals, is not a risk factor for prostate cancer.

Screening. The *prostate-specific antigen* (*PSA*) blood test is the primary prostate cancer screening test. The European Randomized Study of Screening for Prostate Cancer found that PSA screening every 2 to 4 years reduced the relative risk of dying from prostate cancer by 20% compared to no screening after 16 years of follow-up.[32] This corresponded to an absolute risk reduction of 1.8 prostate cancer deaths per 1,000 individuals screened. An American study, the Prostate, Lung Colorectal, and Ovarian Cancer Screening Trial (PLCO) found no prostate-cancer mortality benefit for prostate cancer screening with PSA and DRE compared to no screening.[33] However, the validity of the PLCO results have been questioned because many participants in the control group were actually screened, and a substantial fraction of individuals with abnormal PSA tests did not undergo biopsy.[34] Screening has been associated with harms, including false positive results, biopsy complications, overdiagnosis, overtreatment, and treatment complications.[34]

The USPSTF concluded that screening offered a small potential benefit for reducing the risk of dying from prostate cancer for some men, although many more men would experience harms. They issued a grade C recommendation that men ages 55 to 69 years make an individualized decision after discussing the potential benefits and harms of screening with their clinicians.[35] PSA testing should be offered only to those expressing a preference for screening. The USPSTF recommended against screening men ages 70 years and older (grade D). The American Urological Association recommended screening with PSA testing in combination with shared decision making.[36,37] Clinicians were advised to regularly offer PSA screening every 2 to 4 years to average-risk people ages 50 to 69 years; screening should be offered beginning at ages 40 to 45 years to people at increased risk for prostate cancer.

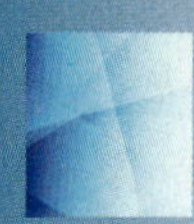

TABLE 23-1. Urinary Frequency, Nocturia, and Polyuria

Problem	Mechanisms	Selected Causes	Associated Symptoms
Frequency	Decreased bladder capacity		
	Increased bladder sensitivity to stretch because of inflammation	Infection, stones, tumor, or foreign body in the bladder	Burning on urination, urinary urgency, sometimes gross hematuria
	Decreased elasticity of the bladder wall	Infiltration by scar tissue or tumor	Symptoms of associated inflammation (see above) are common
	Decreased cortical inhibition of bladder contractions	Motor disorders of the central nervous system, such as a stroke	Urinary urgency; neurologic symptoms such as weakness and paralysis
	Impaired bladder emptying with residual urine in the bladder		
	Partial mechanical obstruction of the bladder neck or proximal urethra	Most commonly, benign prostatic hyperplasia; also urethral stricture and other obstructive lesions of the bladder or prostate	Prior obstructive symptoms: hesitancy in starting the urinary stream, straining to void, reduced size and force of the stream, and dribbling during or at the end of urination
	Loss of S2–S4 innervation to the bladder	Neurologic disease affecting the sacral nerves or nerve roots (e.g., diabetic neuropathy)	Weakness or sensory defects
Nocturia			
With High Volumes	Most types of polyuria		
	Decreased concentrating ability of the kidney with loss of the normal drop in nocturnal urine output	Chronic renal insufficiency due to a number of diseases	Possibly other symptoms of renal insufficiency
	Excessive fluid intake before bedtime	Habit, especially involving alcohol and coffee	
	Fluid-retaining, edematous states. Daytime accumulation of dependent edema that is excreted at night when the patient is supine	Heart failure, nephrotic syndrome, hepatic cirrhosis with ascites, chronic venous insufficiency	Edema and other symptoms of the underlying disorder; urinary output during the day may be reduced as fluid accumulates in the body tissues (see Table 19-1, Peripheral Causes of Edema, p. 569)

Problem	Mechanisms	Selected Causes	Associated Symptoms
With Low Volumes	Urinary frequency		
	Voiding while up at night without a real urge, a "pseudofrequency"	Insomnia	Variable
Polyuria	Deficiency of antidiuretic hormone (diabetes insipidus)	A disorder of the posterior pituitary and hypothalamus	Thirst and polydipsia, often severe and persistent; nocturia
	Renal unresponsiveness to antidiuretic hormone (nephrogenic diabetes insipidus)	A number of kidney diseases, including hypercalcemic and hypokalemic nephropathy; drug toxicity (e.g., from lithium)	Thirst and polydipsia, often severe and persistent; nocturia
	Solute diuresis		
	Electrolytes, such as sodium salts	Large saline infusions, potent diuretics, certain kidney diseases	Variable
	Nonelectrolytes, such as glucose	Uncontrolled diabetes mellitus	Thirst, polydipsia, and nocturia
	Excessive water intake	Primary polydipsia	Polydipsia tends to be episodic; thirst may not be present; nocturia is usually absent

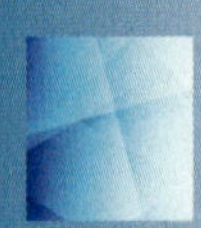

TABLE 23-2. Urinary Incontinence in Individuals Assigned Male at Birth

Problem	Mechanisms	Symptoms	Physical Signs
Stress Incontinence			
Urethral sphincter is weakened so that transient increases in intraabdominal pressure raise the bladder pressure to levels that exceed urethral resistance.	Often follows prostate surgery due to weakened urethral sphincter	Leakage of small amounts of urine with coughing, laughing, sneezing; urine loss is unrelated to the urge to urinate	May be demonstrable, especially if examined before voiding and in a standing position
Urge Incontinence			
Detrusor contractions are stronger than normal and overcome the normal urethral resistance. The bladder is typically small.	Detrusor contractions are stronger than normal and overcome normal urethral resistance. Causes include decreased cortical inhibition from neurologic conditions and hyperexcitability of sensory pathways.	Involuntary urine loss preceded by an urge to void; volume tends to be moderate	Small bladder not detectable on abdominal examination; signs of central nervous system disease, local pelvic problems, or fecal impaction may be present
	Hyperexcitability of sensory pathways, as in bladder infections, tumors, and fecal impaction	Urgency, frequency, and nocturia with small to moderate volumes; if acute inflammation is present, pain on urination	When cortical inhibition is decreased, mental deficits or motor signs of central nervous system disease are often present.
	Deconditioning of voiding reflexes, as in frequent voluntary voiding at low bladder volumes	Possibly "pseudo-stress incontinence"—voiding 10–20 s after stresses such as a change of position, going up- or downstairs, and possibly coughing, laughing, or sneezing.	When sensory pathways are hyperexcitable, signs of local pelvic problems or a fecal impaction may be present.

Problem	Mechanisms	Symptoms	Physical Signs
Overflow Incontinence			
Detrusor contractions are insufficient to overcome urethral resistance, causing urinary retention. The bladder is typically flaccid and large, even after an effort to void.	Can result from obstruction of the bladder outlet (e.g., benign prostatic hyperplasia) or weakness of the detrusor muscle	Dripping or dribbling incontinence; decreased force of the urinary stream	Enlarged, sometimes tender bladder; signs include prostatic enlargement, motor signs of peripheral nerve disease, decreased sensation, and diminished reflexes
Functional Incontinence			
Patient is functionally unable to reach the toilet in time because of impaired health or environmental conditions.	Due to impaired mobility (weakness, arthritis, poor vision) or environmental factors (unfamiliar setting, distant bathrooms)	Incontinence on the way to the toilet or in the early morning	Bladder undetectable on examination; physical or environmental clues point to likely causes
Incontinence Secondary to Medications			
Drugs may contribute to any type of incontinence listed.	Drugs affecting bladder control include sedatives, antipsychotics, anticholinergics, sympathetic blockers, and diuretics	Variable, depending on the medication	Variable, requiring a careful history and chart review

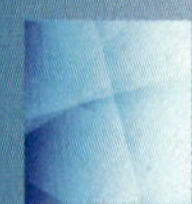

TABLE 23-3. Sexually Transmitted Infection–Associated Changes in Genital Anatomy

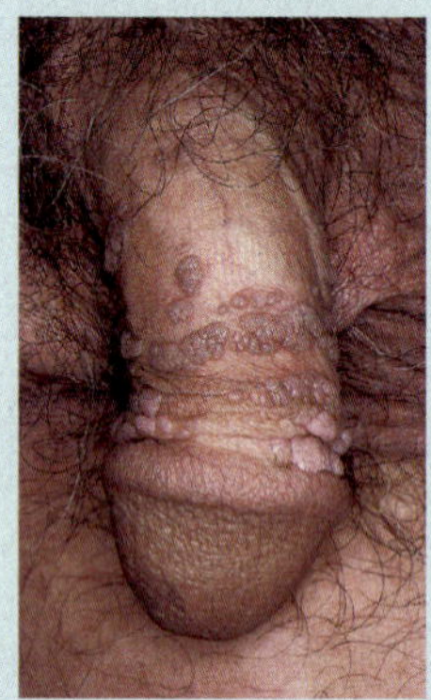

Genital Warts (Condylomata Acuminata)

- *Appearance:* Single or multiple papules or plaques of variable shapes; may be round, acuminate (pointed), or thin and slender. May be raised, flat, or cauliflower-like (verrucous).
- *Causative organism:* Human papillomavirus, usually subtypes 6, 11; carcinogenic subtypes rare, approximately 5–10% of all anogenital warts. *Incubation:* weeks to months; infected contact may have no visible warts.
- Can arise on penis, scrotum, groin, thighs, anus; usually asymptomatic, occasionally cause itching and pain.
- May disappear without treatment.

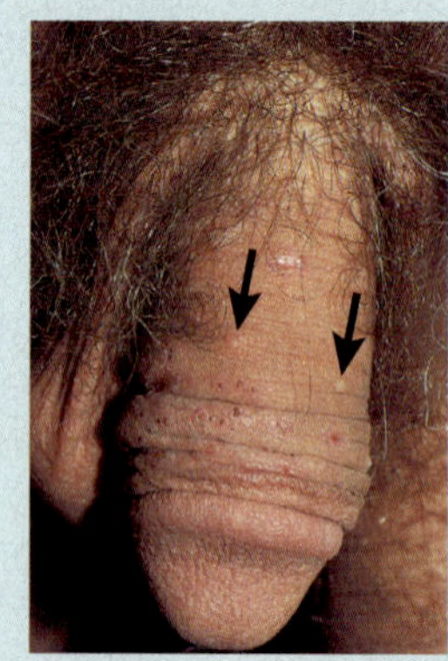

Genital Herpes Simplex

- *Appearance:* Small scattered or grouped vesicles, 1–3 mm in size, on glans or shaft of penis. Appear as erosions if vesicular membrane breaks.
- *Causative organism:* Usually *Herpes simplex virus* 2 (90%), a double-stranded DNA virus. *Incubation:* 2–7 days after exposure.
- Primary episode may be asymptomatic; recurrence usually less painful, of shorter duration.
- Associated with fever, malaise, headache, arthralgias; local pain and edema, lymphadenopathy.
- Need to distinguish from genital herpes zoster (usually in older patients with dermatomal distribution) and candidiasis.

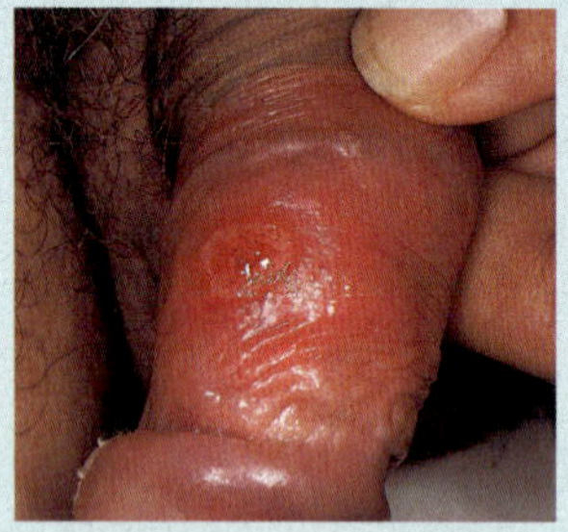

Primary Syphilis

- *Appearance:* Small red papule that becomes a chancre, painless erosion up to 2 cm in diameter. Base of chancre is clean, red, smooth, and glistening; borders are raised and indurated. Chancre heals within 3–8 wk.
- *Causative organism: Treponema pallidum*, a spirochete. *Incubation:* 9–90 days after exposure.
- May develop inguinal lymphadenopathy within 7 days; lymph nodes are rubbery, nontender, mobile.
- 20–30% of patients develop secondary syphilis while chancre still present (suggests coinfection with HIV).
- Distinguish from: genital herpes simplex; chancroid; granuloma inguinale from *Klebsiella granulomatis* (rare in the United States; four variants, so difficult to identify).

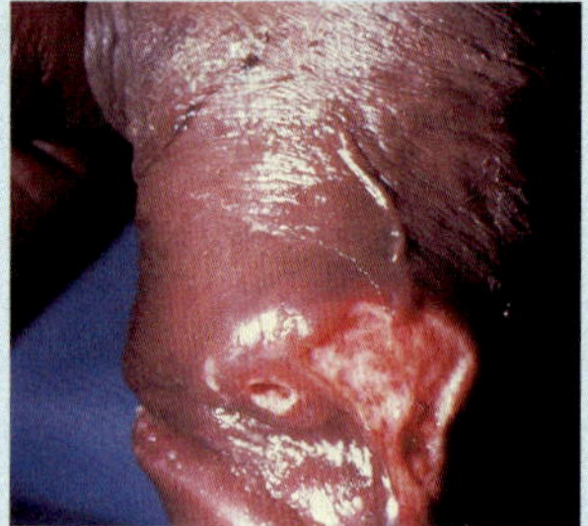

Chancroid

- *Appearance:* Red papule or pustule initially, then forms a painful deep ulcer with ragged nonindurated margins; contains necrotic exudate, has a friable base.
- *Causative organism: Haemophilus ducreyi*, an anaerobic bacillus. *Incubation:* 3–7 days after exposure.
- Painful inguinal adenopathy; suppurative buboes in 25% of patients.
- Need to distinguish from: primary syphilis; genital herpes simplex; lymphogranuloma venereum, granuloma inguinale from *K. granulomatis* (both rare in the United States).

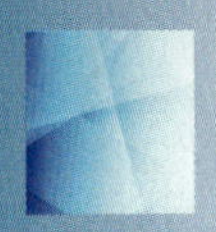

TABLE 23-4. Abnormalities of the Penis and Scrotum

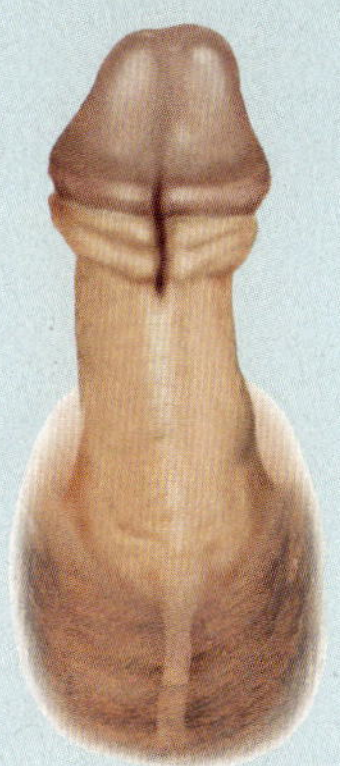

Hypospadias

A congenital displacement of the urethral meatus to the inferior surface of the penis. The meatus may be subcoronal, midshaft, or at the junction of the penis and scrotum (penoscrotal).

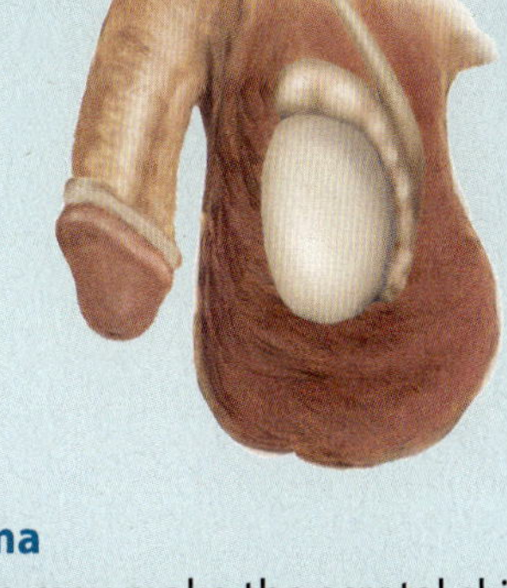

Scrotal Edema

Pitting edema may make the scrotal skin taut; seen in heart failure, liver failure, or nephrotic syndrome.

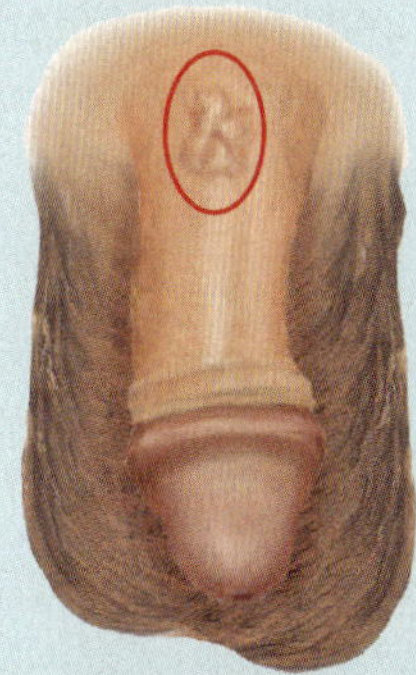

Peyronie Disease

Palpable, nontender, hard plaques are found just beneath the skin, usually along the dorsum of the penis. The patient complains of curved, painful erections.

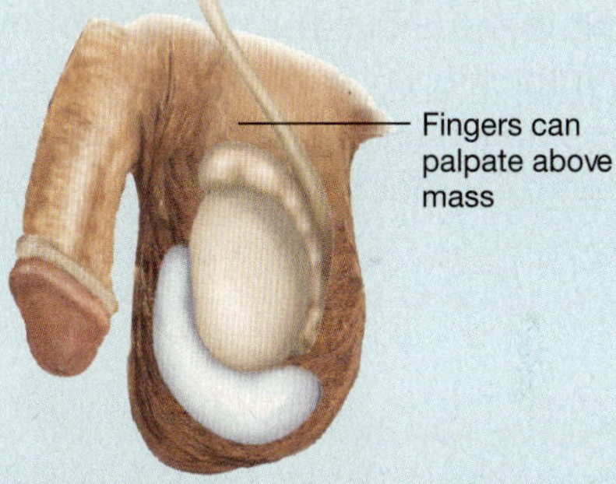

Hydrocele

A nontender, fluid-filled mass within the tunica vaginalis. It transilluminates, and the examining fingers can palpate above the mass within the scrotum.

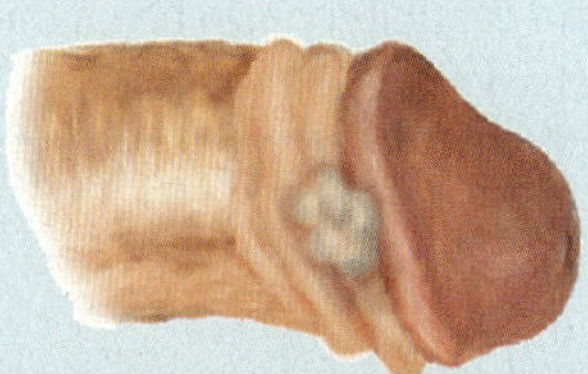

Carcinoma of the Penis

An indurated nodule or ulcer that is usually nontender. Limited almost completely to individuals who are not circumcised, it may be masked by the prepuce. Any persistent penile sore is suspicious.

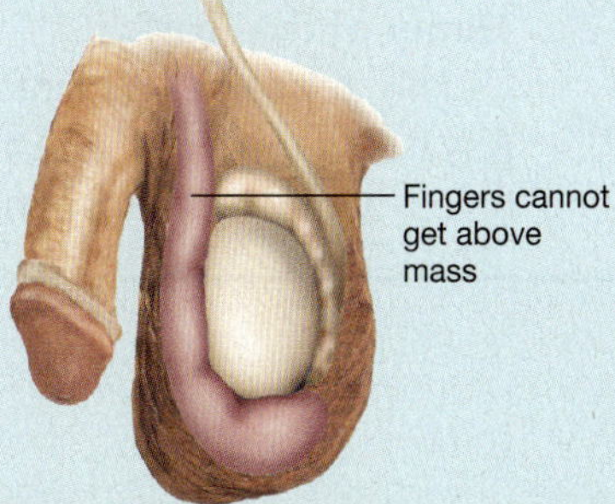

Scrotal Hernia

Usually an indirect inguinal hernia that comes through the external inguinal ring, so the examining fingers cannot get above it within the scrotum.

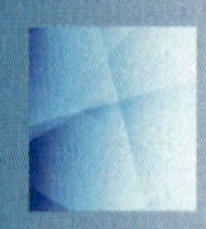

TABLE 23-5. Abnormalities of the Testis

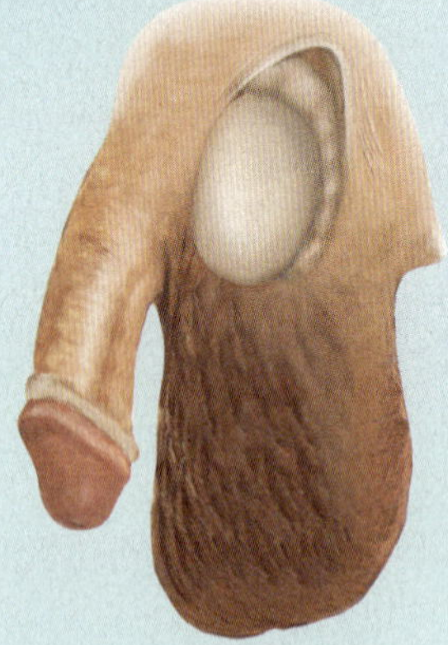

Cryptorchidism

The testis is atrophied and lies outside the scrotum in the inguinal canal, abdomen, or near the pubic tubercle; it may also be congenitally absent. There is no palpable testis or epididymis in the unfilled scrotum. Cryptorchidism, even with surgical correction, markedly raises the risk of testicular cancer.[38]

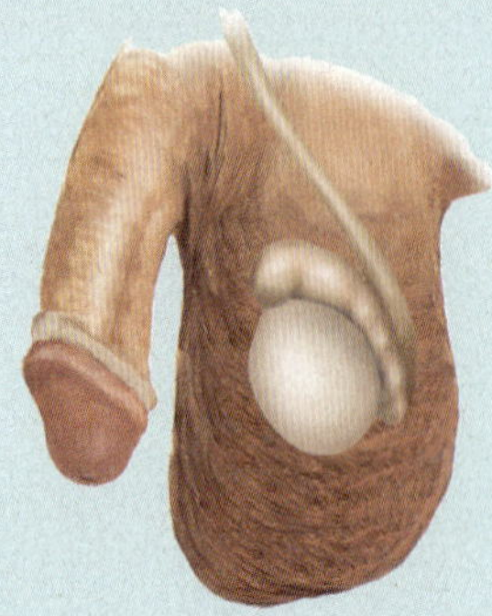

Small Testis

In adults, testicular length is usually ≤3.5 cm. Small firm testes usually ≤2 cm suggest Klinefelter syndrome. Small soft testes suggesting atrophy are seen in cirrhosis, myotonic dystrophy, use of estrogens, and hypopituitarism; may also follow severe orchitis.

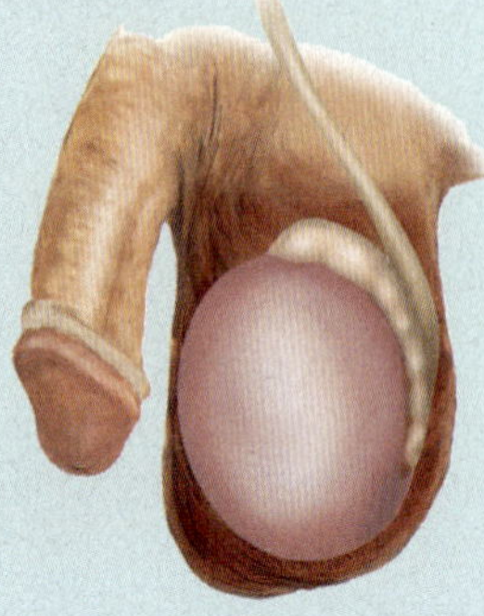

Acute Orchitis

The testis is acutely inflamed, painful, tender, and swollen. It may be difficult to distinguish from the epididymis. The scrotum may be reddened. Seen in mumps and other viral infections; usually unilateral.

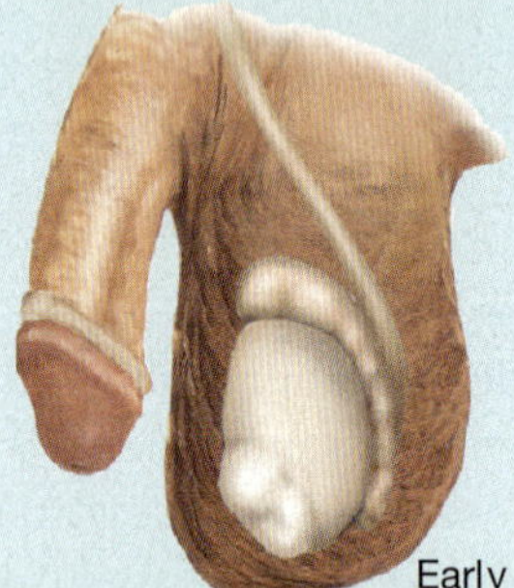

Tumor of the Testis

Usually appears as a painless nodule. Any nodule within the testis warrants investigation for malignancy.

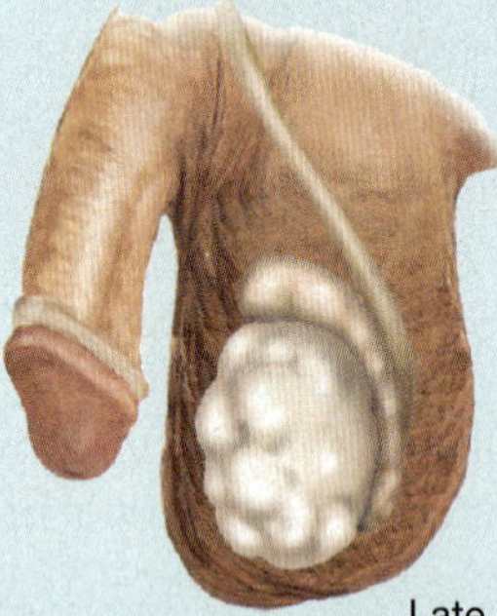

As a testicular neoplasm grows and spreads, it may seem to replace the entire organ. The testicle characteristically feels heavier than normal.

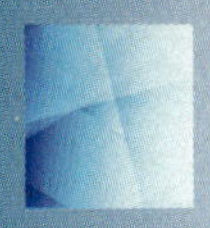

TABLE 23-6. Abnormalities of the Epididymis and Spermatic Cord

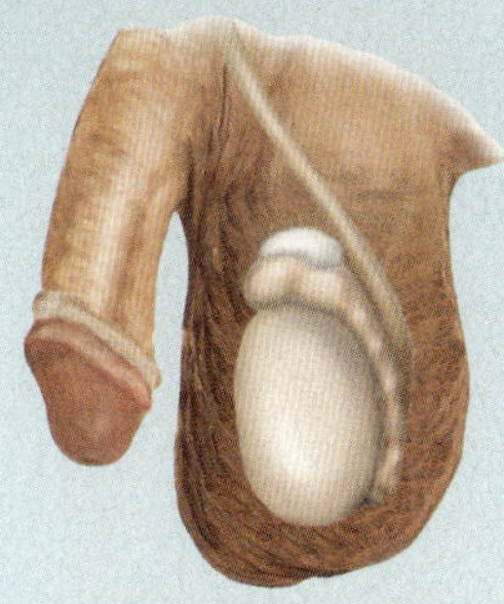

Spermatocele and Cyst of the Epididymis

A painless, movable cystic mass just above the testis suggests a spermatocele or an epididymal cyst. Both transilluminate. The former contains sperm, and the latter does not, but they are clinically indistinguishable.

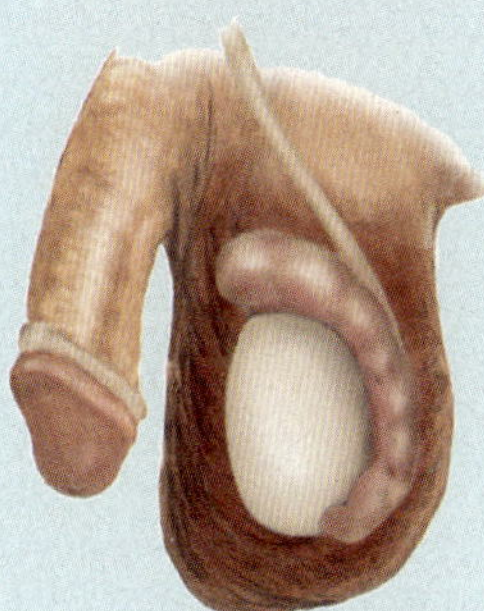

Acute Epididymitis

An acutely inflamed epididymis is indurated, swollen, and notably tender, making it difficult to distinguish from the testis. The scrotum may be reddened and the vas deferens inflamed. Causes include infection from *Neisseria gonorrhoeae, Chlamydia trachomatis* (younger adults), *Escherichia coli*, and *Pseudomonas* (older adults); trauma; and autoimmune disease. Barring urinary symptoms, urinalysis is often negative.

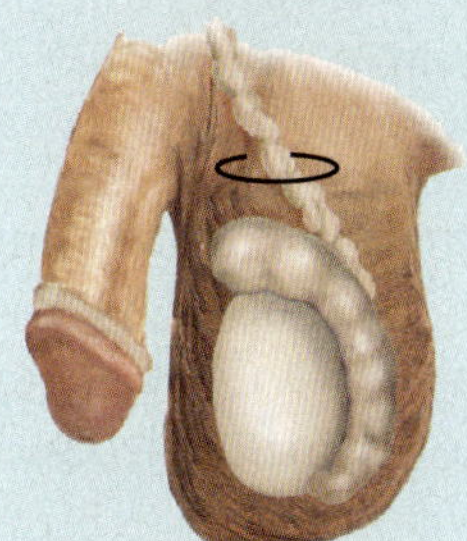

Tuberculous Epididymitis

The chronic inflammation of tuberculosis produces a firm enlargement of the epididymis, which is sometimes tender, with thickening or beading of the vas deferens.

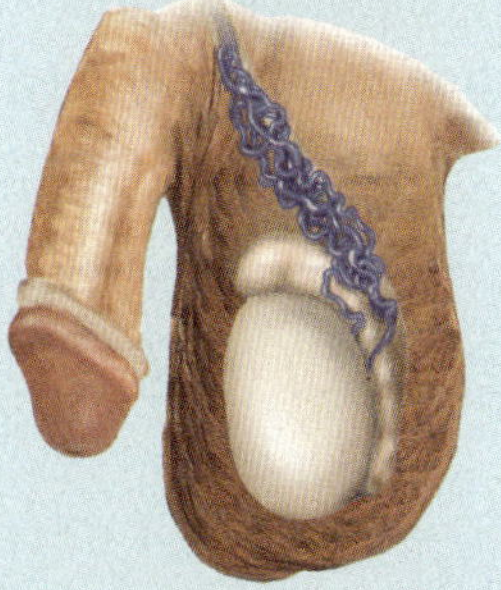

Varicocele of the Spermatic Cord

Varicocele refers to gravity-mediated varicose veins of the spermatic cord, usually found on the left. It feels like a soft "bag of worms" in the spermatic cord above the testis, and if prominent, appears to distort the contours of the scrotal skin. A varicocele collapses in the supine position, so examination should be both supine and standing. If the varicocele does not collapse when the patient is supine, suspect a left spermatic vein obstruction within the abdomen.

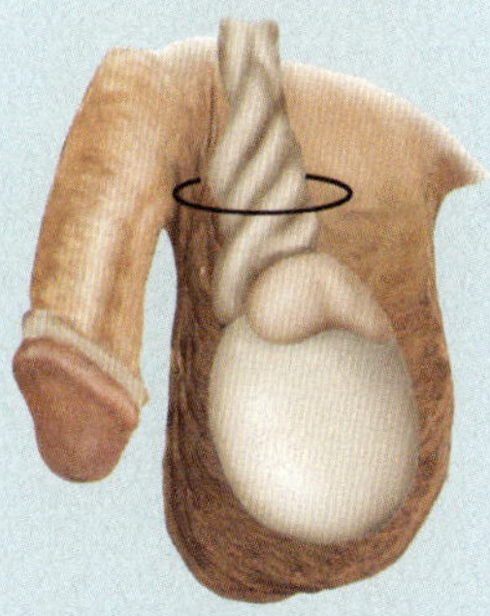

Testicular Torsion

Torsion, or twisting, of the testicle on its spermatic cord produces an acutely painful, tender, and swollen organ that is often retracted upward in the scrotum. The cremasteric reflex is nearly always absent on the affected side in individauls with testicular torsion, though this can be difficult to assess during acute pain episodes. If the presentation is delayed, the scrotum becomes red and edematous. There is no associated urinary infection. Torsion is most common in neonates and adolescents but can occur at any age. It is a surgical emergency because of obstructed circulation and requires urgent surgical consultation.

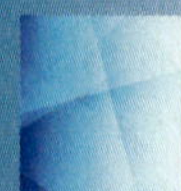

TABLE 23-7. Course, Presentation, and Differentiation of Hernias in the Groin

See Figure 23-10.

	Groin Hernias		
	Indirect	**Direct**	**Femoral Hernias**
Frequency, Age, and Sex	Most common, all ages and sexes. Often in children; may occur in adults.	Less common. Usually in individuals assigned male at birth older than 40 y; rare in individuals assigned female at birth.	Least common. More common in individuals assigned female at birth than in individuals assigned male at birth.
Point of Origin	Above inguinal ligament, near its midpoint (the internal inguinal ring).	Above inguinal ligament, close to the pubic tubercle (near the external inguinal ring).	Below the inguinal ligament; appears more lateral than an inguinal hernia. Can be hard to differentiate from lymph nodes.
Course *(Examining finger in inguinal canal during coughing or straining)*	Often into the scrotum. The hernia comes down the inguinal canal and touches the fingertip.	Rarely into the scrotum. The hernia bulges anteriorly and pushes the side of the finger forward.	Never into the scrotum. The inguinal canal is empty.

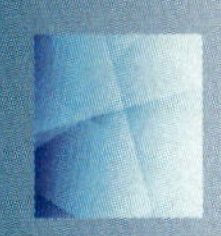

TABLE 23-8. BPH Symptom Score: American Urological Association

Score or ask the patient to score each of the questions below. Higher scores (maximum 35) indicate more severe symptoms; scores ≤7 are considered mild and generally do not warrant treatment.[39]

PART A	**Not at All**	**Less Than 1 Time in 5**	**Less Than Half the Time**	**About Half the Time**	**More Than Half the Time**	**Almost Always**	**Total Points for Each Row**
1. Incomplete emptying: Over the past month, how often have you had a sensation of not emptying your bladder completely after you finished urinating?	0	1	2	3	4	5	
2. Frequency: Over the past month, how often have you had to urinate again <2 h after you finished urinating?	0	1	2	3	4	5	
3. Intermittency: Over the past month, how often have you stopped and started again several times when you urinated?	0	1	2	3	4	5	
4. Urgency: Over the past month, how often have you found it difficult to postpone urination?	0	1	2	3	4	5	
5. Weak stream: Over the past month, how often have you had a weak urinary stream?	0	1	2	3	4	5	
6. Straining: Over the past month, how often have you had to push or strain to begin urination?	0	1	2	3	4	5	
PART B	**None**	**1 Time**	**2 Times**	**3 Times**	**4 Times**	**5 Times**	**Points for Part B**
7. Nocturia: Over the past month, how many times did you most typically get up to urinate from the time you went to bed at night until the time you got up in the morning?	0	1	2	3	4	5	

TOTAL PARTS A and B (maximum 35)________

Source: Adapted from Madsen FA, Bruskewitz RC. Clinical manifestations of benign prostatic hyperplasia. *Urol Clin North Am*. 1995;22(2):291–298. Copyright © 1995 Elsevier. With permission.

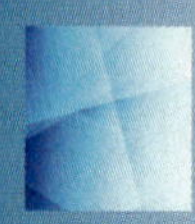

TABLE 23-9. Abnormalities of the Prostate

Normal Prostate Gland

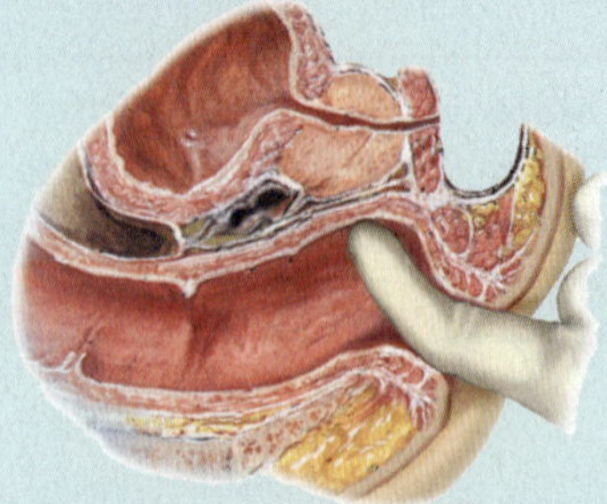

The normal prostate, felt through the anterior rectal wall, is rounded and heart-shaped, about 2.5 cm in length, with a palpable median sulcus between the lobes; only its posterior surface is accessible by examination.

Prostatitis

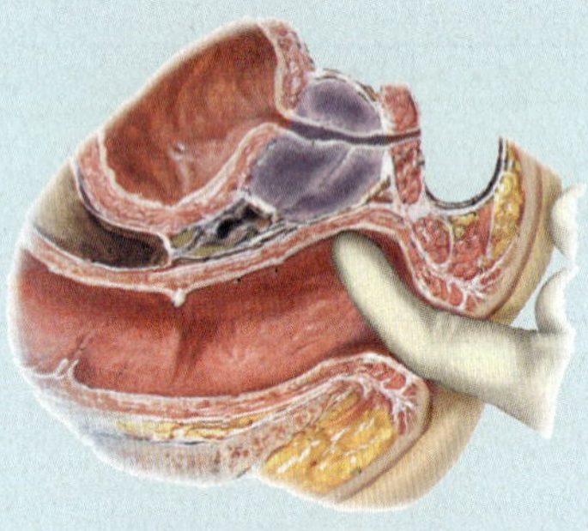

Acute bacterial prostatitis features fever, urinary discomfort, and a tender, swollen, warm prostate. Caused primarily by gram-negative aerobes like *E. coli*, and in younger men, sexually transmitted pathogens like *N. gonorrhea* and *C. trachomatis*.

Chronic bacterial prostatitis, often marked by recurrent urinary infections and sometimes asymptomatic, presents with a prostate that may feel normal on examination, with *E. coli* commonly isolated from prostatic fluid cultures.

Differentiating these from chronic pelvic pain syndrome, which lacks infection evidence but presents with urinary symptoms, requires physical examination to check for prostate irregularities, indicative of other acute conditions, BPH, or cancer.

Benign Prostatic Hyperplasia

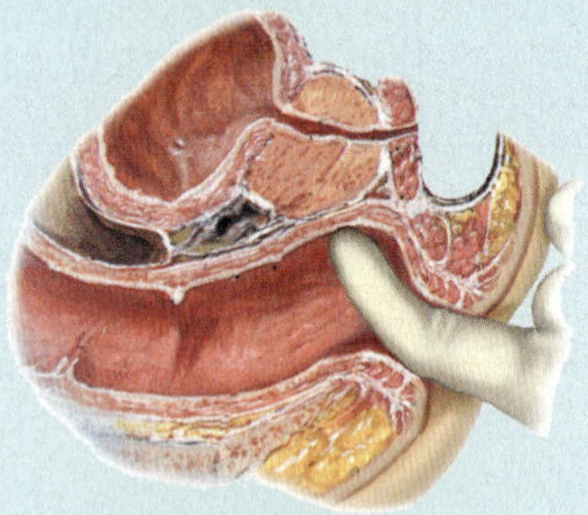

BPH, a benign prostate enlargement common with aging, can cause irritative and obstructive urinary symptoms. The prostate may feel symmetrically enlarged, smooth, and firm with a less distinct median sulcus.

Prostate Cancer

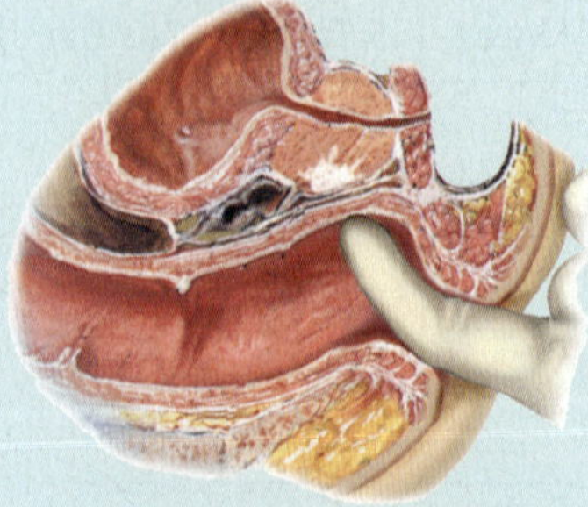

Prostate cancer may manifest as a hard nodule or firmness in the gland, often irregular in shape and potentially extending beyond the gland. Not all hard areas indicate cancer; they could also stem from stones, chronic inflammation, or other nonmalignant issues.

REFERENCES

1. Turner D, Driemeyer W, Nieder TO, Scherbaum N, Briken P. [“How much sex do medical studies need?”—A survey of the knowledge and interest in sexual medicine of medical students.] *Psychother Psychosom Med Psychol.* 2014;64(12):452–457. “Wie viel Sex braucht das Studium der Medizin?”—Eine Erhebung des Wissens und Interesses Medizinstudierender zum Thema Sexualmedizin.
2. Lapinski J, Sexton P. Still in the closet: the invisible minority in medical education. *BMC Med Educ.* 2014;14:171.
3. Moll J, Krieger P, Moreno-Walton L, et al. The prevalence of lesbian, gay, bisexual, and transgender health education and training in emergency medicine residency programs: what do we know? *Acad Emerg Med.* 2014;21(5):608–611.
4. Sack S, Drabant B, Perrin E. Communicating about sexuality: an initiative across the core clerkships. *Acad Med.* 2002; 77(11):1159–1160.
5. Rutherford K, McIntyre J, Daley A, Ross LE. Development of expertise in mental health service provision for lesbian, gay, bisexual and transgender communities. *Med Educ.* 2012; 46(9):903–913.
6. Sarma AV, Wei JT. Clinical practice. Benign prostatic hyperplasia and lower urinary tract symptoms. *N Engl J Med.* 2012; 367(3):248–257.
7. Hooton TM. Clinical practice. Uncomplicated urinary tract infection. *N Engl J Med.* 2012;366(11):1028–1037.
8. Gupta K, Trautner B. In the clinic. Urinary tract infection. *Ann Intern Med.* 2012;156(5):ITC3-1–ITC3-16.
9. Bettez M, Tu LM, Carlson K, et al. 2012 update: guidelines for adult urinary incontinence collaborative consensus document for the Canadian Urological Association. *Can Urol Assoc J.* 2012;6(5):354–363.
10. Markland AD, Vaughan CP, Johnson TM 2nd, Burgio KL, Goode PS. Incontinence. *Med Clin North Am.* 2011;95(3): 539–554.
11. Holroyd-Leduc JM, Tannenbaum C, Thorpe KE, Straus SE. What type of urinary incontinence does this woman have? *JAMA.* 2008;299(12):1446–1456.
12. Sexually transmitted infections treatment guidelines. Division of STD Prevention; National Center for HIV, Viral Hepatitis, STD, and TB Prevention; Centers for Disease Control and Prevention. Accessed January 1, 2024. https://www.cdc.gov/std/treatment-guidelines/default.htm
13. Final recommendation statement: chlamydia and gonorrhea: screening. U.S. Preventive Services Task Force. Accessed January 1, 2024. https://www.uspreventiveservicestaskforce.org/Page/Document/RecommendationStatementFinal/chlamydia-and-gonorrhea-screening
14. Final recommendation statement: Human Immunodeficiency Virus (HIV) infection: screening. U.S. Preventive Services Task Force. Accessed January 1, 2024. https://www.uspreventiveservicestaskforce.org/Page/Document/UpdateSummaryFinal/human-immunodeficiency-virus-hiv-infection-screening
15. Skarbinski J, Rosenberg E, Paz-Bailey G, et al. Human immunodeficiency virus transmission at each step of the care continuum in the United States. *JAMA Intern Med.* 2015; 175(4):588–596.
16. Meanley S, Gale A, Harmell C, Jadwin-Cakmak L, Pingel E, Bauermeister JA. The role of provider interactions on comprehensive sexual healthcare among young men who have sex with men. *AIDS Educ Prev.* 2015;27(1):15–26.
17. Liu RJ, Li SY, Xu ZP, et al. Dietary metal intake and the prevalence of erectile dysfunction in US men: Results from National Health and Nutrition Examination Survey 2001–2004. *Front Nutr.* 2022;9:974443.
18. Pellegrino F, Sjoberg DD, Tin AL, et al. Relationship between age, comorbidity, and the prevalence of erectile dysfunction. *Eur Urol Focus.* 2023;9(1):162–167.
19. Montgomery JS, Bloom DA. The diagnosis and management of scrotal masses. *Med Clin North Am.* 2011;95(1):235–244.
20. McIntosh A, Hutchinson A, Roberts A, Withers H. Evidence-based management of groin hernia in primary care–a systematic review. *Fam Pract.* 2000;17(5):442–447.
21. Miserez M, Peeters E, Aufenacker T, et al. Update with level 1 studies of the European Hernia Society guidelines on the treatment of inguinal hernia in adult patients. *Hernia.* 2014;18(2):151–163.
22. van den Berg JC, de Valois JC, Go PM, Rosenbusch G. Detection of groin hernia with physical examination, ultrasound, and MRI compared with laparoscopic findings. *Invest Radiol.* 1999;34(12):739–743.
23. Siegel RL, Miller KD, Jemal A. Cancer statistics, 2018. *CA Cancer J Clin.* 2018;68(1):7–30.
24. Simons MP, Aufenacker T, Bay-Nielsen M, et al. European Hernia Society guidelines on the treatment of inguinal hernia in adult patients. *Hernia.* 2009;13(4):343–403.
25. U.S. Preventive Services Task Force. Screening for testicular cancer: U.S. Preventive Services Task Force reaffirmation recommendation statement. *Ann Intern Med.* 2011;154(7): 483–486.
26. SEER Cancer Statistics Review (CSR) 1975–2015. National Cancer Institute. Accessed February 26, 2024. https://seer.cancer.gov/csr/1975_2015/
27. Testicular self-exam. National Library of Medicine. Accessed February 26, 2024. http://www.nlm.nih.gov/medlineplus/ency/article/003909.htm
28. Siegel RL, Miller KD, Wagle NS, Jemal A. Cancer statistics, 2023. *CA Cancer J Clin.* 2023;73(1):17–48.
29. Surveillance Research Program. SEER*Explorer: An interactive website for SEER cancer statistics. National Cancer Institute. Updated November 16, 2023. Accessed February 26, 2024. https://seer.cancer.gov/statistics-network/explorer/overview.html
30. National Cancer Institute. Genetics of Prostate Cancer (PDQ®). Updated March 17, 2023. Accessed February 26, 2024. https://www.cancer.gov/types/prostate/hp/prostate-genetics-pdq
31. National Cancer Institute. Prostate Cancer Prevention (PDQ®). Updated October 26, 2023. Accessed February 26, 2024. https://www.cancer.gov/types/prostate/hp/prostate-prevention-pdq#section/_17
32. Hugosson J, Roobol MJ, Mansson M, et al. A 16-yr Follow-up of the European Randomized study of Screening for Prostate Cancer. *Eur Urol.* 2019;76(1):43–51.
33. Pinsky PF, Prorok PC, Yu K, et al. Extended mortality results for prostate cancer screening in the PLCO trial with median follow-up of 15 years. *Cancer.* 2017;123(4):592–599.
34. Fenton JJ, Weyrich MS, Durbin S, Liu Y, Bang H, Melnikow J. Prostate-specific antigen-based screening for prostate cancer: evidence report and systematic review for the US Preventive Services Task Force. *JAMA.* 2018;319(18):1914–1931.

35. U. S. Preventive Services Task Force; Grossman DC, Curry SJ, et al. Screening for prostate cancer: US Preventive Services Task Force Recommendation Statement. *JAMA*. 2018; 319(18):1901–1913.
36. Wei JT, Barocas D, Carlsson S, et al. Early detection of prostate cancer: AUA/SUO guideline part I: prostate cancer screening. *The Journal of urology*. 2023;210(1):46–53.
37. U. S. Preventive Services Task Force; Davidson KW, Mangione CM, et al. Collaboration and shared decision-making between patients and clinicians in Preventive Health Care Decisions and US Preventive Services Task Force Recommendations. *JAMA*. 2022;327(12):1171–1176.
38. Kolon TF, Herndon CD, Baker LA, et al. Evaluation and treatment of cryptorchidism: AUA guideline. *J Urol*. 2014; 192(2):337–345.
39. Madsen FA, Bruskewitz RC. Clinical manifestations of benign prostatic hyperplasia. *Urol Clin North Am*. 1995;22(2):291–298.
40. Key statistics for testicular cancer. American Cancer Society. Accessed February 26, 2024. https://www.cancer.org/cancer/testicular-cancer/about/key-statistics.html

CHAPTER 24

Pelvis and Genitourinary System: Vulva, Vagina, Uterus, and Adnexa

ANATOMY AND PHYSIOLOGY

Pelvis

Pelvic anatomy varies widely among individuals, with certain trends observed in those assigned females at birth, often related to reproductive functions. Pelvises typically associated with these individuals tend to be lighter and broader, featuring a shallower and more spacious cavity. This design, generally seen in people with reproductive systems that include a *uterus*, *fallopian tubes*, and *ovaries*, facilitates the accommodation of a growing fetus and the process of childbirth (Fig. 24-1).

A notable variation in pelvic structure is observed in the shape of the pelvic inlet: it tends to be *oval or round* in individuals with these reproductive systems, contrasting with the more heart-shaped inlet often found in individuals with a reproductive system that includes testes. The pubic arch in pelvises associated with childbirth-capable reproductive systems is also typically wider, with an angle of about 90° to 100°, compared to the narrower angle of around 50° to 60° often observed in pelvises not associated with childbirth.

While housing reproductive organs, the *urinary bladder*, *urethra*, and *rectum*, the *musculature* and *ligament structures* in these pelvises resemble those in others. However, the pelvic floor muscles in individuals who have experienced pregnancy and childbirth may be more susceptible to weakness and injury. These muscles play a vital role in supporting pelvic organs and maintaining continence.

Despite variations in the fundamental aspects of pelvic anatomy, the arterial distribution, venous return, nerve innervation, and lymphatic drainage tend to follow similar patterns (Fig. 24-2). The *internal iliac arteries* supply blood to the pelvic organs, muscles, and bones, and the internal iliac veins and other smaller veins drain blood from the pelvis. The *sacral plexus* gives rise to nerves that innervate the pelvic organs, muscles, and skin, including the *pudendal nerve* and the *pelvic splanchnic nerves.*

Lymph from the external genital region and lower part of the vagina drains into lymph nodes located in the groin area. Meanwhile, lymph from the internal genital organs, including the upper vagina, uterus, fallopian tubes, and ovaries,

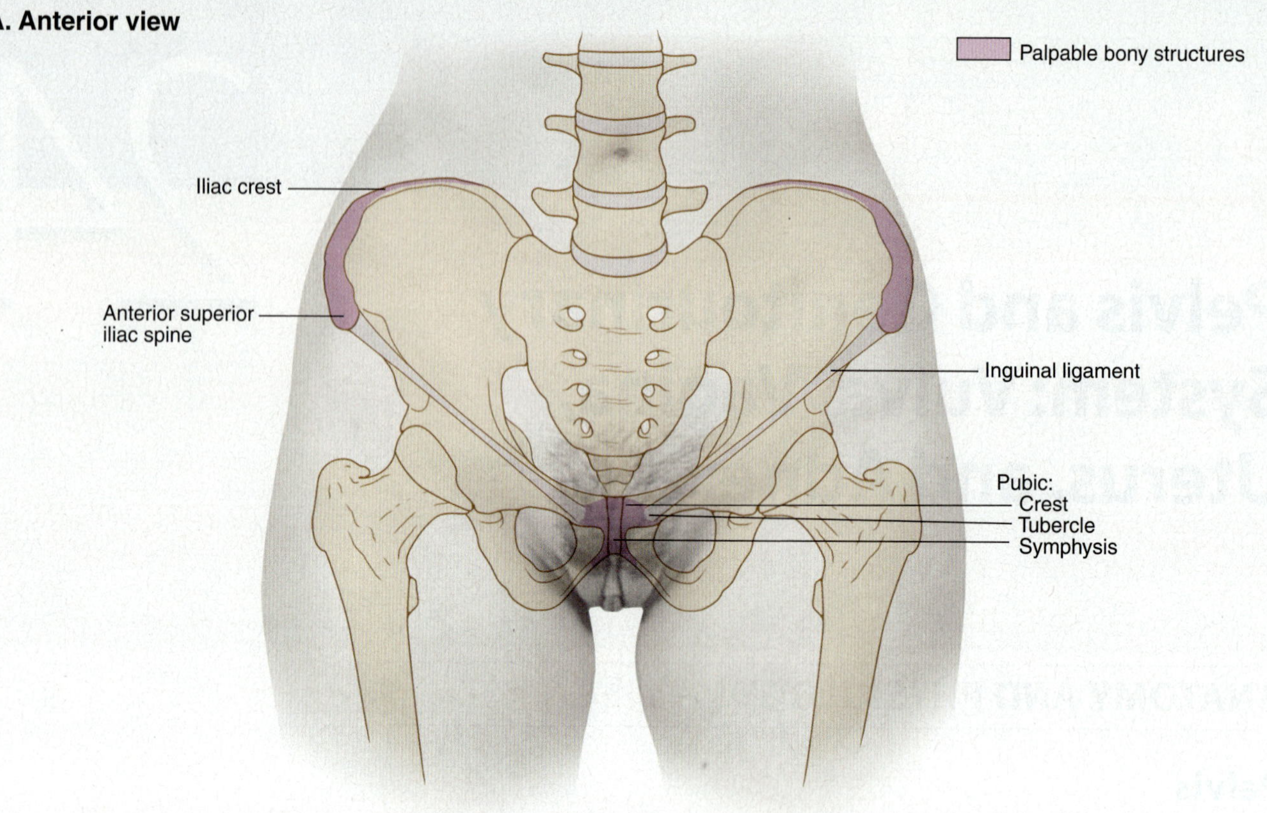

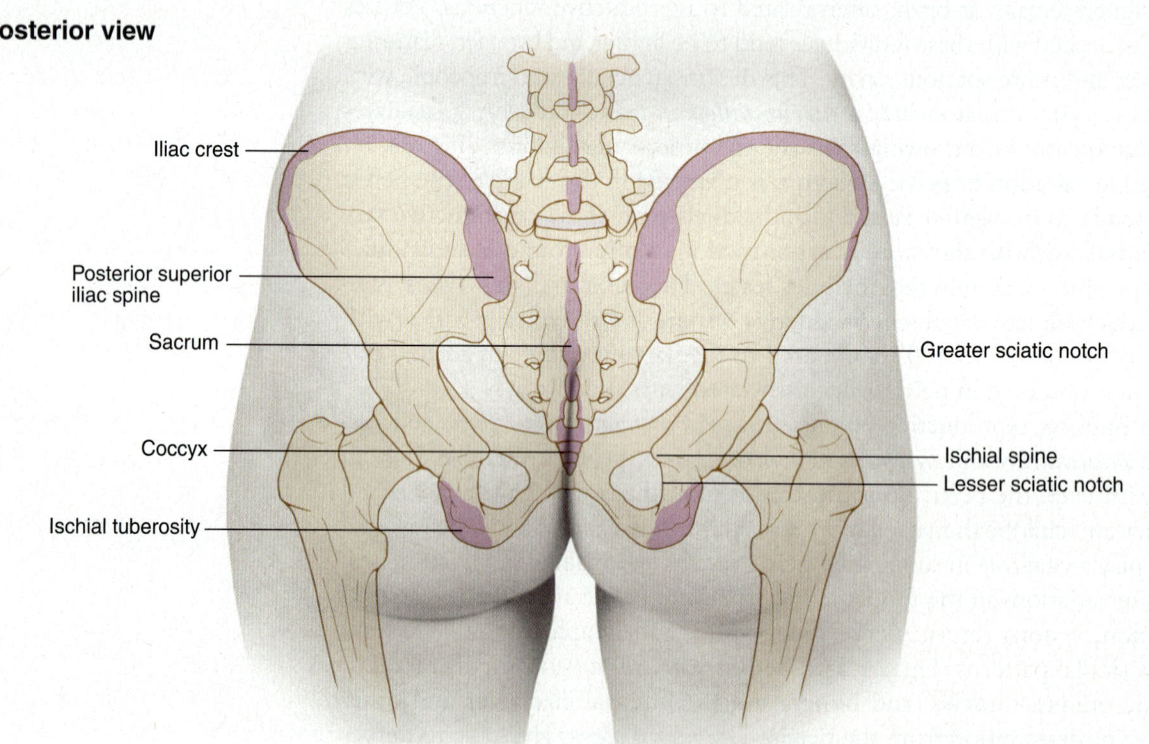

FIGURE 24-1. Surface anatomy of the pelvis and perineum. (Reprinted with permission from Gest TR. *Lippincott® Atlas of Anatomy.* 2nd ed. Wolters Kluwer; 2020. Plate 6-1.)

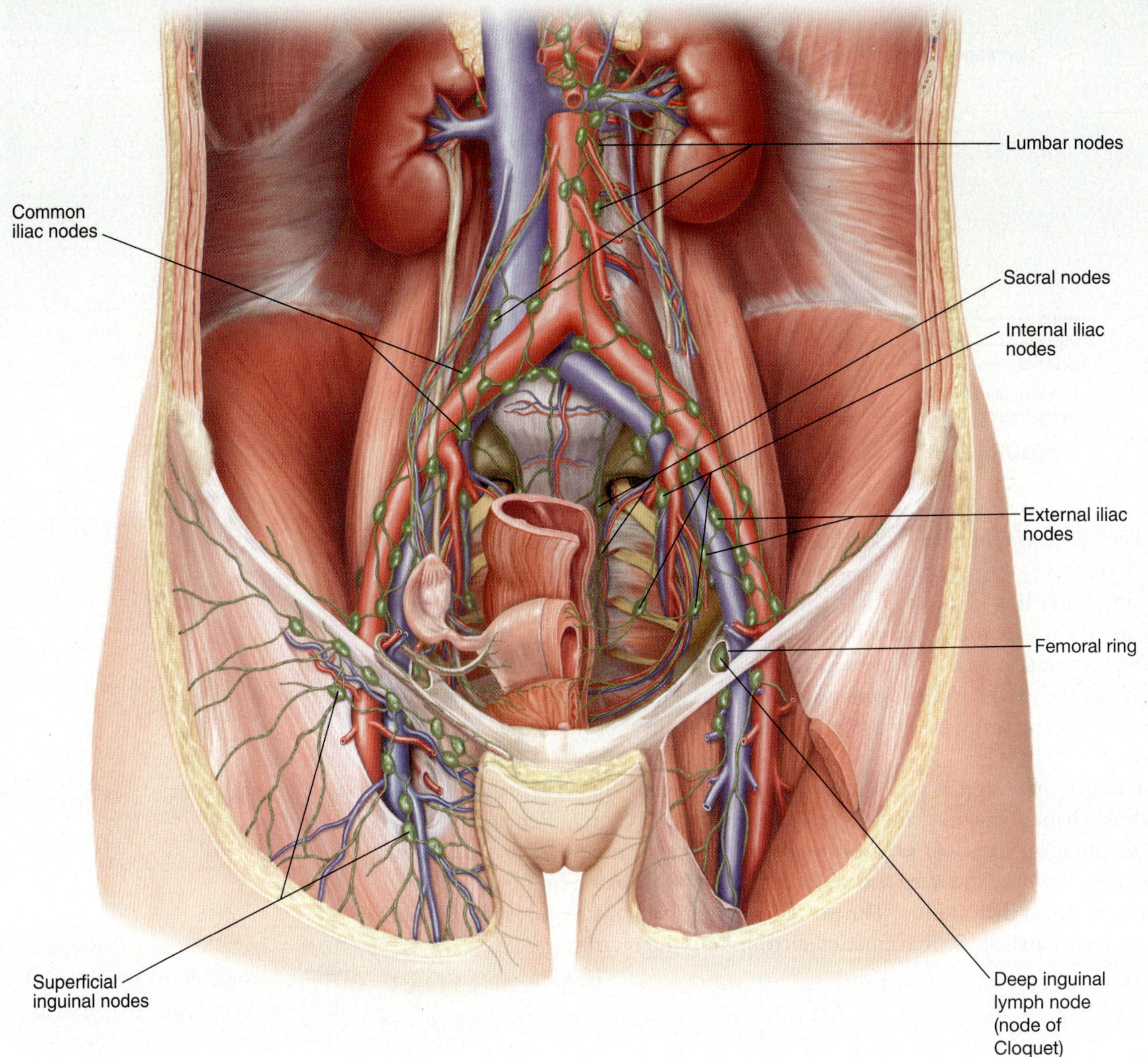

FIGURE 24-2. Lower abdomen, pelvis, and their contents. (Reprinted with permission from Gest TR. *Lippincott® Atlas of Anatomy.* 2nd ed. Wolters Kluwer; 2020. Plate 6-36.)

flows into deeper lymph nodes within the pelvic and abdominal regions. These nodes, situated deeper in the body, are typically not palpable.

Pelvic Floor

The pelvic organs are supported by a sling of tissues composed of muscle, ligaments, and endopelvic fascia called the *pelvic floor,* which helps support the pelvic organs above the outlet of the lesser pelvis (Fig. 24-3). Pelvic floor muscles also aid in sexual function (*orgasm*), urinary and fecal continence, and stabilization of connecting joints. The pelvic floor consists of the *pelvic diaphragm* and the *perineal membrane.*

Weakness of the pelvic floor muscles may cause prolapse of the pelvic organs that can produce a ***cystocele*** (prolapse of the bladder into the vagina), ***rectocele*** (prolapse of the rectum into the vagina), or ***enterocele*** (prolapse of the bowel into the vagina).

See Table 24-1, Bulges and Swelling of the Vulva, Vagina, and Urethra, p. 764.

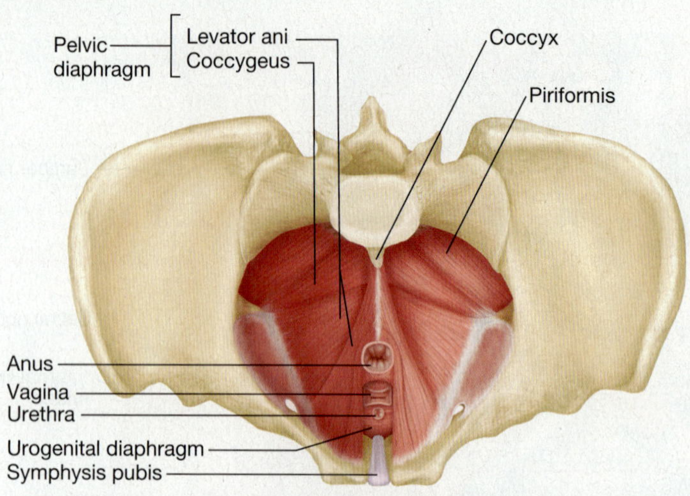

FIGURE 24-3. Pelvis and the pelvic floor, superior view.

The *pelvic diaphragm*, separating the pelvic cavity and perineum, consists of the *levator ani* and *coccygeal muscles* connected to the lesser pelvis. The levator ani comprises three muscles: *puborectalis, pubococcygeus, and iliococcygeus.* Below lies the *perineal membrane*, a triangular fibromuscular sheet housing *bulbocavernosus and ischiocavernosus muscles*, the *superficial transverse perineal body*, and the *external anal sphincter*. This membrane stretches across the anterior triangle, securing the urethra, vagina, and perineal body to the ischiopubic rami.

The urethra, vagina, and anorectum pass through the *urogenital hiatus*, a keyhole-shaped opening in the pelvic diaphragm's center. Beneath the pelvic diaphragm, the *deep urogenital diaphragm* contains the *external urethral sphincter, urethra,* and *deep transverse perineal muscle,* extending from the inferior ischium to the midline. The posterior triangle mainly features the external and internal anal sphincter muscles surrounding the rectum.

Loss of urethral support contributes to stress incontinence. Weakness of the perineal body from childbirth predisposes to rectoceles and enteroceles.

Regarding innervation, the pelvic diaphragm receives input from *sacral nerve roots S3 to S5,* while the perineal membrane and urogenital diaphragm are innervated by the *pudendal nerve*.

Vulva

Vulva is the collective term for the external part of the genitalia (Fig. 24-4). It consists of the *mons pubis,* a hair-covered fat pad overlying the symphysis pubis; *labia majora,* rounded folds of adipose tissue forming the outer lips of the vagina; *labia minora,* thinner pinkish red folds or inner lips that extend anteriorly to form the *prepuce*; and the *clitoris*. It also includes the *vestibule*, the boat-shaped fossa between the labia minora that surrounds the opening of the urethra, the *urethral meatus* anteriorly, and the vaginal opening, the *introitus*, posteriorly. The vaginal opening may be partially occluded by a membrane, the *hymen*. The term *perineum* refers to the tissue between the introitus and the anus.

The two major vulvar glands are the *greater vestibular (Bartholin) glands* and the *paraurethral (Skene) glands*. The openings of the greater vestibular glands are

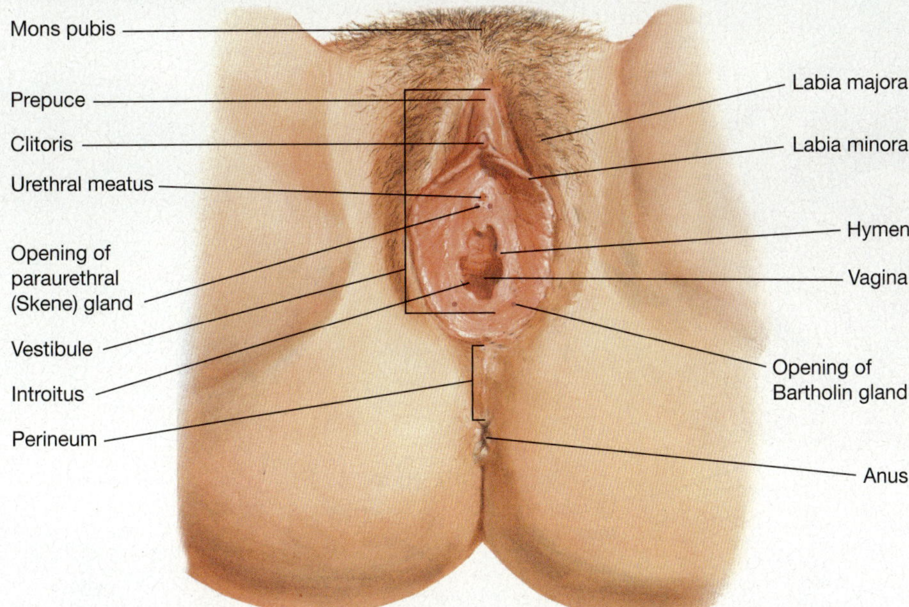

FIGURE 24-4. Vulva and perineum, patient in the lithotomy position.

located posteriorly on both sides of the vaginal opening but are not usually visible (Fig. 24-5). The glands themselves are situated more deeply. The greater vestibular glands' main function is to secrete mucus to lubricate the vagina and vulva. Just posterior and adjacent to the urethral meatus on either side lie the openings of the paraurethral (Skene) glands. These glands secrete transudate that lubricates the urethral opening and release fluid during intercourse.

See Table 24-2, Lesions of the Vulva, p. 765.

Vagina

The *vagina* is a musculomembranous tube extending upward and posteriorly between the urinary bladder and urethra and the rectum. Its upper third lies at a horizontal plane and terminates in the cup-shaped *fornix*. The vaginal mucosa lies in transverse folds, or *rugae*.

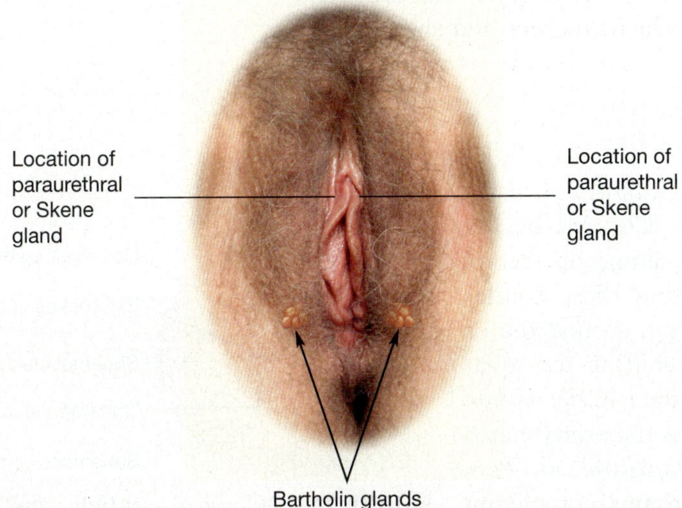

FIGURE 24-5. Paraurethral (Skene) and greater vestibular (Bartholin) glands.

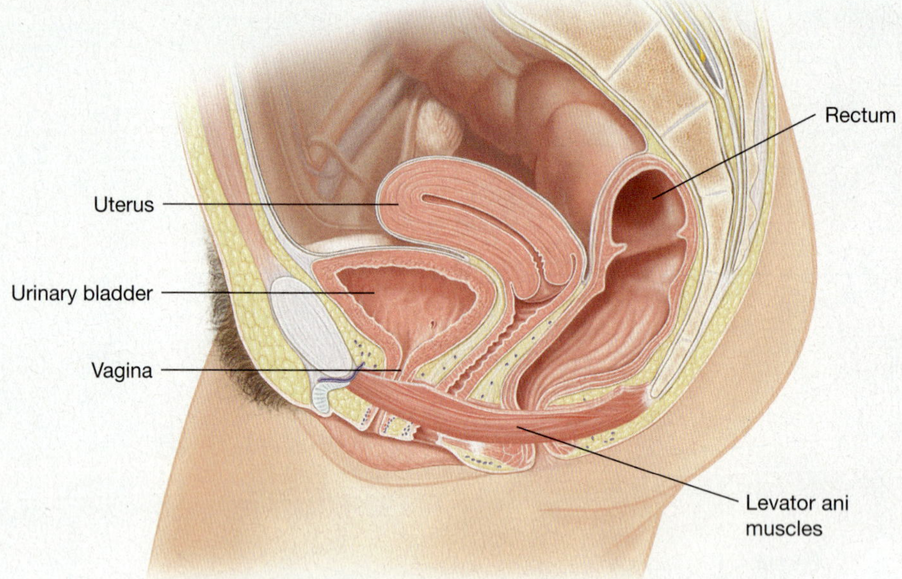

FIGURE 24-6. Pelvic anatomy, sagittal view.

The vaginal fornix lies at almost a right angle to the *cervix*, a firm, collagenous cylindrical organ with a central slit or depression, that is connected to the *uterus*, a thick-walled fibromuscular structure shaped like an inverted pear (Fig. 24-6). The cervix protrudes into the vagina, dividing the upper vagina into three recesses, the *anterior*, *posterior*, and *lateral fornices*.

Uterus

The *uterus*, a dynamic organ located centrally in the pelvic cavity between the bladder and rectum, primarily functions to house and nourish a developing fetus during pregnancy. Resembling an inverted pear, the uterus consists of the *body* (or *corpus*) and the *cervix*. The *fundus*, the superior broad portion, arches forward and upward, with its position varying based on bladder fullness. The body narrows into the *isthmus*, leading to the cervix. Internally, the uterine cavity is small in a nonpregnant state but expands significantly during pregnancy. The uterine walls feature three layers: the outer *perimetrium*; muscular *myometrium*; and the inner *endometrium*, which thickens and sheds in response to menstrual cycle hormonal changes.

Cervix

The *cervix*, visible with a speculum, features an *external os* marking the *endocervical canal* entrance (Fig. 24-7). Covered by red columnar epithelium and pink squamous epithelium, the cervix includes the *squamocolumnar junction*, delineating these epithelial types. During puberty, the columnar epithelium around the os (*ectropion*) is replaced by squamous epithelium, shifting the squamocolumnar junction toward the os and forming the *transformation zone*. This zone is crucial for cervical health, as it is the primary area of concern for dysplasia, typically sampled in *Papanicolaou* (*Pap*) *smears*. The cervix connects to the uterus at the isthmus, completing the link to the uterine cavity lined by the endometrium.

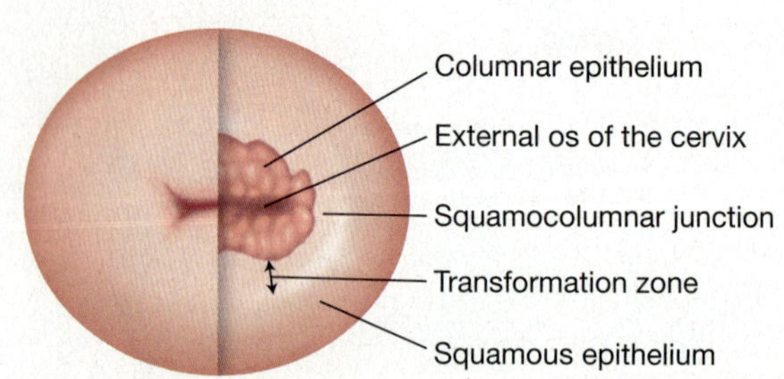

FIGURE 24-7. Cervical epithelia and transformation zone.

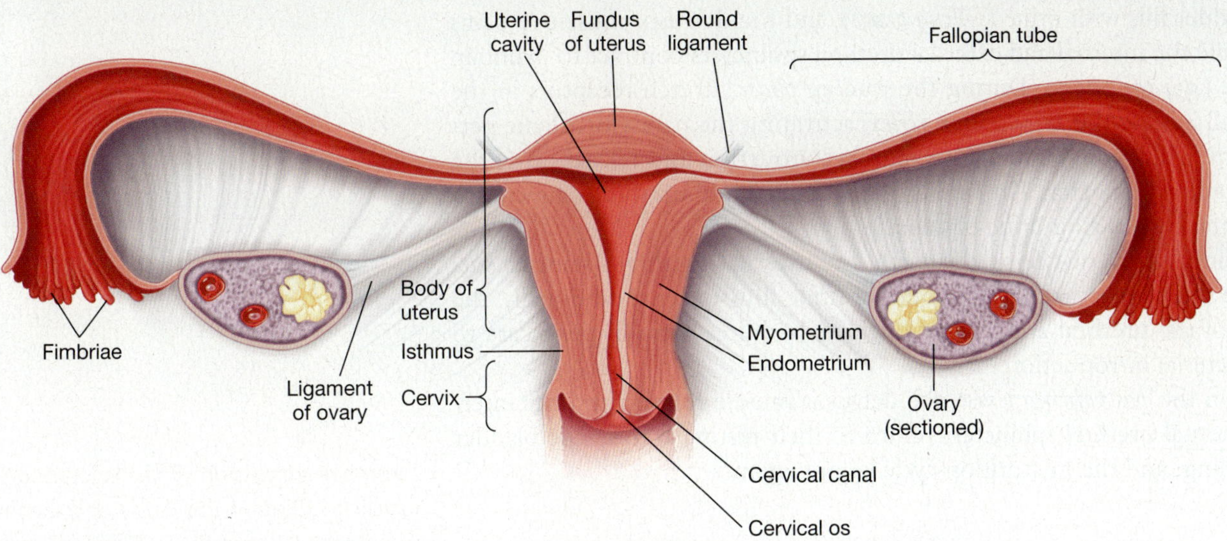

FIGURE 24-8. Uterus and adnexa, anterior cross-sectional view.

Adnexa

The term *adnexa* originates from the Latin verb "*adnectere*," which means "to bind together." It specifically refers to the anatomical structures that are adjunct or accessory to a primary organ. In gynecology, adnexa denotes the collective group of structures closely associated with the uterus, primarily including the *ovaries*, *fallopian tubes*, and the *supporting connective tissues* and *ligaments*. The two bilateral *fallopian tubes* insert into the uterine fundus. The fallopian tube has a fanlike tip, the *fimbria*, that extends to the *ovary* to each side of the uterus and collects the *oocyte* from the periovarian peritoneal cavity and conducts it to the uterine cavity (Fig. 24-8).

The two *ovaries* are almond-shaped glands that vary considerably in size but average approximately 3.5 × 2 × 1.5 cm from adulthood through menopause. The ovaries are palpable on pelvic examination in roughly half of patients during the reproductive years. Normally, the fallopian tubes are not palpable.

The ovaries have two primary functions: production of oocytes and secretion of hormones, including *estrogen*, *progesterone*, and *testosterone*. Increased hormonal secretion during puberty stimulates the growth of the uterus and its endometrial lining; enlargement of the vagina; thickening of the vaginal epithelium; and the development of *secondary sex characteristics*, including the breasts and pubic hair.

See the Tanner stages of sexual maturity in Chapter 28, Children: Infancy Through Adolescence, pp. 1091–1097.

The area behind the uterus is in the shape of a cul-de-sac called the *rectouterine pouch* (*pouch of Douglas*). You can palpate this area on rectovaginal examination.

Micturition Cycle

The *micturition* or *urination cycle* ensures efficient urine storage and elimination. In individuals assigned female at birth, the urethra is shorter and straighter, leading to a higher risk of urinary tract infections (UTIs) due to easier bacterial access. The urethra in these individuals is also not involved in the reproductive system, eliminating the need for coordination with ejaculation.

The bladder fills with urine (*filling phase*), and the detrusor muscle remains relaxed while the internal and external urethral sphincters contract to maintain continence (*storage phase*). During the *voiding phase*, stretch receptors in the bladder wall initiate the *micturition reflex*, activating the parasympathetic nervous system. This results in detrusor muscle contraction and relaxation of the internal urethral sphincter. The brain signals the external urethral sphincter to relax voluntarily, allowing urine passage.

In individuals assigned female at birth, the external urethral sphincter surrounds the shorter urethra, causing quicker urine flow onset. Additionally, the proximity of the urethral and vaginal openings requires extra hygiene care to prevent bacterial introduction.

Finally, in the *postvoiding phase*, the detrusor muscle relaxes, and the internal and external urethral sphincters return to their resting states. The bladder resumes filling, and the micturition cycle begins again.

Also see discussion of the micturition cycle in Chapter 23, Pelvis and Genitourinary System: Penis, Scrotum, and Prostate, p. 693.

Menstrual Cycle

The *menstrual cycle* is a complex hormonal process that occurs in the reproductive system, preparing the body for potential pregnancy. The average cycle lasts about 28 days but can vary between individuals, ranging from 21 to 35 days. It consists of several phases, including the *menstrual*, *follicular*, *ovulation*, and *luteal* phases (Box 24-1).

Throughout the menstrual cycle, hormonal interactions between the hypothalamus, pituitary gland, and ovaries regulate the growth and release of eggs as well as the preparation and maintenance of the endometrium for potential pregnancy.

Box 24-1. Phases of the Menstrual Cycle

Phase	Duration	Description
Menstrual	3–7 days	Endometrial lining of the uterus is shed, resulting in menstrual bleeding; estrogen and progesterone levels are low; marks the beginning of the menstrual cycle.
Follicular	Overlaps	Follows the menstrual phase; pituitary gland releases follicle-stimulating hormone, stimulating growth of ovarian follicles in the ovaries; follicles produce estrogen, leading to the thickening of the endometrial lining, preparing it for potential implantation of a fertilized egg; overlaps with the menstrual phase for a few days.
Ovulation	Around day 14	Mature egg is released from the dominant ovarian follicle in response to a surge of luteinizing hormone; egg travels down the fallopian tube, where it can be fertilized by sperm if sexual intercourse occurs during this time; occurs around day 14 of a 28-day cycle.
Luteal	After ovulation	Ruptured follicle transforms into the corpus luteum, which secretes progesterone and estrogen; hormones maintain the thickened endometrial lining in case of successful fertilization and implantation; if fertilization does not occur, corpus luteum breaks down, leading to a decline in progesterone and estrogen levels, triggering menstruation and a new cycle.

Menarche and Menses

Despite variations worldwide and within the US population, median age at menarche has remained relatively stable—between 12 and 13 years—across well-nourished populations in high-income countries.[1,2] Adolescents in the United States usually begin menstruation between ages 9 and 16 years, and it often takes at least 1 year for *menstrual cycles* to settle into a regular pattern. Environmental factors, including socioeconomic conditions, nutrition, and access to preventive health care, may influence the timing and progression of puberty.[3]

The *menstrual history* is an essential component of the health history, providing insight into the patient's reproductive health. The term *menarche* denotes the onset of menstruation in an individual's life. It is important to ascertain the date of the *last menstrual period* (*LMP*), which represents the commencement of the most recent menstrual cycle. Additionally, for a more comprehensive overview, some also refer to the *prior menstrual period* (*PMP*), marking the cycle immediately preceding the LMP.

The dates of previous menstrual periods provide clues to possible pregnancy or menstrual irregularities.

The *regularity* of the menstrual cycle is characterized by the *interval*, defined as the time elapsed from the start of one period to the beginning of the next. The interval between periods ranges roughly from 24 to 38 days; menstrual flow lasts from 3 to 7 days. An understanding of the flow is equally important. *Flow* can vary from light to heavy and can be approximated by the number of sanitary products used daily. However, there is subjective variability in the individual's interpretation of flow intensity.

In addition, any *intermenstrual bleeding* or *"spotting"* outside the expected menstrual dates should be assessed. *Postcoital bleeding*, denoting any bleeding episode following sexual intercourse, is another critical point to ask your patient about, given its implications for potential underlying pathologies.

Premenstrual Syndrome. *Premenstrual syndrome (PMS)* includes emotional and physical symptoms that interfere with normal daily life. These symptoms may include depression, anxiety, irritability, sleep disturbance, headache, appetite changes, abdominal pain, and social withdrawal.[4] Criteria for diagnosis are symptoms and signs in the 5 days prior to menses for at least three consecutive cycles, cessation of symptoms and signs within 4 days after onset of menses, and interference with daily activities.

Menopause

Menopause is characterized by the cessation of menstruation (*amenorrhea*) for 12 consecutive months, occurring without any other evident pathologic or physiologic cause. Typically manifesting between ages 48 and 55 years, with the median age being 51, it is preceded by *perimenopause*, the transitional period before menopause marked by irregular cycles of bleeding and vasomotor symptoms such as hot flashes, flushing, and sweating.

As the ovaries cease the production of estradiol and progesterone, *estrogen* levels significantly decline. Concurrently, a decrease in the negative feedback on the hypothalamus leads to increased secretion of *gonadotropin-releasing hormone* (*GnRH*), which, in turn, causes elevated levels of *luteinizing hormone* (*LH*) and *follicle-stimulating hormone* (*FSH*). Accompanying *menopausal symptoms* may include mood shifts, hot flashes, accelerated bone loss, increased cholesterol levels, and vulvovaginal atrophy, which can result in vaginal drying, painful urination (*dysuria*), and painful sexual intercourse (*dyspareunia*). Urinary symptoms may also manifest due to atrophy of the urethra and the urinary trigone.

HEALTH HISTORY: GENERAL APPROACH

When obtaining the patient's obstetrical and gynecologic history, always adopt a systematic approach. Inclusivity plays a pivotal role in establishing an environment that respects the diverse range of gender identities and experiences. Addressing these topics can be emotionally challenging for some patients. Ensure that the setting is relaxed and private, fostering an atmosphere of trust and comfort. Ideally, take the history with the patient fully clothed, especially during your first meeting. This approach helps alleviate any potential discomfort and aligns with the principles of patient-centered care.

Respecting the patient's autonomy and privacy is fundamental in this context. Whenever possible, you should interview the patient alone, unless they explicitly request the presence of a caregiver, friend, or family member for support. Exceptions can be made for children, adolescents, and patients with cognitive impairments, but, even in these cases, providing an opportunity for private conversation is important.

To enhance the patient's comfort and foster open communication, frame your questions in an open-ended and nonjudgmental manner. Embracing inclusive language not only ensures that the patient's identity and experiences are validated but also reinforces the principles of compassionate and patient-centered care.

Common or Concerning Symptoms

- Painful menstruation (dysmenorrhea)
- Absence of menses (amenorrhea)
- Abnormal uterine bleeding
- Pelvic pain (See also hypogastrium or suprapubic abdominal pain in Chapter 21, Abdomen, pp. 615–616 and Chapter 23, Pelvis and Genitourinary System: Penis, Scrotum, and Prostate, pp. 694–695.)
- Vulvovaginal symptoms
- Urinary incontinence (See also Chapter 23, Pelvis and Genitourinary System: Penis, Scrotum, and Prostate, p. 697.)

Questions about menarche, PMS, and menopause are essential as they pertain to the natural phases of the individual's menstrual lifecycle. These phases are generally considered "normative" or inherent to the reproductive journey of individuals assigned female at birth. Explore the patient's concerns and attitude about their body in relation to these stages and learn to describe patterns related to menstrual irregularities (Boxes 24-2 and 24-3).

Box 24-2. Menstrual Lifecycle: Health History Questions

Menstrual Lifecycle	Health History Questions
Menarche: onset of menses	■ *At what age did you have your first menstrual period?* ■ *Did you experience any discomfort or pain during your first period?* ■ *How did your menstrual cycles evolve over the first year after your first period?* ■ *Were there any noticeable changes in your body or mood leading up to your first period?* ■ *How did you feel about starting your period, and did you have anyone to talk to about it?*
Premenstrual syndrome (PMS): cluster of emotional, behavioral, and physical symptoms occurring 5 days before menses for three consecutive cycles	■ *Can you describe the specific symptoms you experience before your period?* ■ *How do these symptoms impact your daily life or routine?* ■ *Have you noticed any triggers that might worsen or alleviate your symptoms?* ■ *Have you tried any treatments or interventions to manage your PMS symptoms?* ■ *Do you track your menstrual cycle, and if so, have you noticed any patterns related to the onset of these symptoms?*
Menopause: absence of menses for 12 consecutive months, usually occurring between ages 48 and 55 years	■ *At what age did you notice your periods becoming less frequent or stopping altogether?* ■ *Have you experienced any hot flashes, night sweats, or other common menopausal symptoms?* ■ *Have there been any changes in your mood, sleep, or libido since you started noticing these changes in your cycle?* ■ *Are you currently on any hormone replacement therapy or other treatments for menopause symptoms?* ■ *How has menopause impacted your overall well-being and quality of life?*

Box 24-3. Glossary of Terms Related to Menstrual Irregularities

Abnormal uterine bleeding—bleeding between menses; includes infrequent, excessive, prolonged, or postmenopausal bleeding

Amenorrhea—absence of menses

Dysmenorrhea—pain with menses, often with bearing down, aching, or cramping sensation in the lower abdomen or pelvis

Menorrhagia—excessive menstrual flow or prolonged menstrual periods

Metrorrhagia—bleeding between menstrual periods

Oligomenorrhea—infrequent menstrual bleeding

Polymenorrhea—menstrual cycles with intervals of 21 days or fewer

Postmenopausal bleeding—bleeding occurring 6 months or more after cessation of menses

Postcoital bleeding—vaginal bleeding after sexual intercourse

Painful Menstruation (Dysmenorrhea)

Dysmenorrhea is reported by almost half of patients. It may be *primary* (menstrual pain that occurs without an underlying medical condition) or *secondary* (menstrual pain due to an underlying medical condition). To help determine the possible causes, see the health history questions listed in Box 24-4.

Possible secondary causes include **endometriosis** (endometrial tissue grows outside the uterus, leading to inflammation and scarring), **uterine fibroids** (benign, smooth muscle tumors grow in the uterus), **pelvic inflammatory disease** ([**PID**] infection of the upper reproductive tract), **adenomyosis** (endometrial tissue invading the uterine muscular wall [myometrium]), and **ectopic pregnancy** (fertilized egg implanted outside the uterus, typically in the fallopian tube).

Box 24-4. Painful Menstruation (Dysmenorrhea): High-Yield Health History Questions

Domain	Questions	Rationale
Timing and duration	*When does the pain start in relation to your period, and how long does it last?*	*Primary dysmenorrhea:* typically occurs within the first 1–2 days of menstruation and lasts 1–2 days *Secondary dysmenorrhea:* can occur throughout the menstrual cycle and may last longer
Pain characteristics	*How would you describe the pain, and where is it located?*	*Primary dysmenorrhea:* involves crampy lower abdomen or pelvic pain *Secondary dysmenorrhea:* pain varies with its cause; endometriosis pain is often sharp in the lower back or pelvis, and adenomyosis pain tends to be deep and widespread
Associated symptoms	*Are you experiencing any other symptoms, such as nausea, vomiting, or diarrhea?*	Could suggest a more severe case of primary dysmenorrhea or secondary dysmenorrhea due to endometriosis or adenomyosis
Medical history	*Do you have a history of any gynecologic conditions, such as endometriosis or adenomyosis?*	Endometriosis and adenomyosis are two common conditions associated with dysmenorrhea; others include fibroids, ovarian cysts, and pelvic inflammatory disease
Medication history	*Have you tried any over-the-counter (OTC) pain relievers, such as ibuprofen or acetaminophen, and do they help with the pain?*	Identifies potential treatment options for dysmenorrhea, which may include OTC pain relievers or hormonal contraceptives
Lifestyle factors	*Do any lifestyle factors seem to exacerbate or alleviate your symptoms, such as exercise or stress?*	Regular exercise and stress management techniques, such as meditation or yoga, may help alleviate symptoms of dysmenorrhea

Absence of Menses (Amenorrhea)

Primary amenorrhea is the absence of menstruation by age 15 years, and *secondary amenorrhea* is the absence of menstruation for 3 months or longer in patients who have previously had regular menstrual cycles. Pregnancy, lactation, and menopause are physiologic causes of secondary amenorrhea. The health history questions in Box 24-5 are tailored to help you identify possible causes.

Possible causes include **polycystic ovary syndrome** ([**PCOS**] hormonal imbalances lead to irregular ovulation and menstruation, with increased androgen production), **hypothalamic amenorrhea** (disruption in hypothalamic production of GnRH, LH, and FSH due to stress, low body weight, excessive exercise), **thyroid disorders** (hypothyroidism or hyperthyroidism), **hyperprolactinemia** (suppression of GnRH, LH, and FSH production, disrupting ovulation and menstruation), and **significant weight loss** (severe energy deficiency leads to decreased production of GnRH, LH, and FSH).

Box 24-5. Absence of Menses (Amenorrrhea): High-Yield Health History Questions

Domain	Questions	Rationale
Timing and duration	*How long have you gone without a period, and when was your last one?*	Helps differentiate primary amenorrhea from secondary amenorrhea
Associated symptoms	*Are you experiencing any other symptoms, such as hot flashes, night sweats, or vaginal dryness?*	Hot flashes, night sweats, and vaginal dryness could suggest menopause or premature ovarian failure
Medical history	*Do you have a history of any gynecologic conditions?*	Polycystic ovarian syndrome, premature ovarian failure, thyroid disorders, and pituitary gland disorders are common conditions that can cause amenorrhea
Medication history	*Are you currently taking any medications or supplements, including hormonal contraceptives, that might be contributing to your amenorrhea?*	Hormonal contraceptives and some antidepressants can cause menstrual irregularities and amenorrhea
Pregnancy history	*Are you sexually active, and have you taken a pregnancy test?*	Rule out pregnancy as a potential cause before pursuing further evaluation and management
Family history	*Do you have a family history of any medical conditions associated with amenorrhea, such as premature ovarian failure or thyroid disorders?*	Premature ovarian failure and thyroid disorders can run in families and increase the risk of amenorrhea

Abnormal Uterine Bleeding

The term *abnormal uterine bleeding* (*AUB*) encompasses several patterns. Asking targeted questions about the pattern, frequency, and severity of bleeding can uncover important clues about hormonal imbalances, uterine abnormalities, or systemic health issues (Box 24-6).

The **PALM-COEIN system** was developed to standardize the nomenclature and classification of AUB in the reproductive years (Box 24-7).[5]

Box 24-6. Abnormal Uterine Bleeding: High-Yield Health History Questions

Domain	Questions	Rationale
Timing and duration	*When did the abnormal bleeding start, and how long does it last?*	Timing, duration, and frequency of bleeding provide clues to potential causes and can help decide the type of testing the patient will need
Bleeding characteristics	*How heavy is your bleeding, and are you passing clots?*	*Heavy bleeding with clots:* may suggest structural causes such as fibroids or adenomyosis *Lighter bleeding:* may suggest hormonal imbalances
Associated symptoms	*Are you experiencing any pain or discomfort? Do you have any symptoms of anemia, like feeling tired or weak?*	*Pain or discomfort:* may suggest structural causes such as fibroids or endometriosis *Symptoms of anemia:* may suggest heavy bleeding
Medical history	*Do you have a history of any gynecologic conditions?*	*Structural:* fibroids, adenomyosis, and endometriosis *Hormonal imbalance:* polycystic ovarian syndrome and thyroid disorders
Medication history	*Are you taking any medications or supplements, such as hormonal contraceptives, that might affect your menstrual cycle?*	Hormonal contraceptives and anticoagulants can cause menstrual irregularities
Pregnancy history	*Are you sexually active, and have you recently taken a pregnancy test?*	Rule out pregnancy as a potential cause before pursuing further evaluation and management
Family history	*Does anyone in your family have any medical conditions associated with abnormal uterine bleeding, such as bleeding disorders or certain types of cancer?*	Bleeding disorders and certain types of cancer can run in families and increase the risk of AUB

Box 24-7. Major Causes of Abnormal Uterine Bleeding: PALM-COEIN Classification

PALM	
Polyp	Abnormal growths that extend from the surface of the endometrium, or the inner lining of the uterus; often benign but can cause irregular bleeding
Adenomyosis	Tissue that normally lines the inside of the uterus starts to grow within its muscular walls, often causing pain and heavy periods
Leiomyoma (fibroids)	Benign tumors of the uterus, often referred to as fibroids; can vary in size and location and may lead to heavy or prolonged menstrual periods
Malignancy and hyperplasia	Refers to cancerous growths and abnormal thickening of the endometrium, respectively; both can result in irregular or heavy bleeding; endometrial hyperplasia may increase the risk of developing uterine cancer

COEIN	
Coagulopathy	Conditions that affect the blood's ability to clot, like von Willebrand disease, can result in prolonged or excessive menstrual bleeding
Ovulatory dysfunction	Refers to irregularities in ovulation; AUB-O indicates ovulatory cycles, while AUB-A indicates anovulatory cycles; both can cause irregular bleeding patterns
Endometrial	Pertains to problems with the endometrial lining itself that are not due to any of the other listed causes
Iatrogenic	Bleeding issues that arise due to medical treatments or surgical procedures, such as the use of certain medications or interventions
Not yet classified	Causes of abnormal bleeding that do not fit into the other specific classifications

Pelvic Pain

Acute pelvic pain is of sudden onset and typically lasts for a short period (days to weeks). *Chronic pelvic pain* refers to pain that lasts for more than 6 months and does not respond to treatment.[6] It accounts for approximately 10% of ambulatory referrals to gynecologists and 20% of hysterectomies.[7–9] Acute pelvic pain in menstruating adolescents and adults warrants immediate attention. Box 24-8 provides health history questions to assist you in differentiating possible causes.

Possible causes include **PID**,[10] **endometriosis**, and **ectopic pregnancy**.[11,12] Additional causes include **sexually transmitted infections (STIs), ovarian cyst rupture or torsion, UTI or interstitial cystitis, and kidney stones** (crystals forming in kidneys).

Box 24-8. Pelvic Pain: High-Yield Health History Questions

Domain	Questions	Rationale
Location	*Where is it located? Can you describe the location of your pain?*	Helps narrow down potential causes by associating pain location with specific conditions (e.g., lower abdominal pain with ovarian cyst, pain near pubic bone with bladder infection, lower back pain with endometriosis)
Timing and duration	*When did the pain start? Is it constant or intermittent? How long does it last?*	Onset, constancy, and duration of pain can indicate specific conditions, such as chronic or acute issues
Pattern	*Is the pain constant or intermittent?*	*Constant:* can indicate infection, inflammation, or a mass (e.g., pelvic inflammatory disease [PID], interstitial cystitis, tumors) *Intermittent:* may suggest inflammatory bowel syndrome (IBS), kidney stones, or dysmenorrhea
Aggravating or relieving factors	*Do any factors worsen or improve the pain? How is your menstrual cycle? Do you experience pain during menstruation?*	*Worsens during menstruation:* suggests endometriosis or fibroids *Improves with bowel movements:* indicates IBS

(*continued*)

Box 24-8. Pelvic Pain: High-Yield Health History Questions (*Continued*)

Domain	Questions	Rationale
Associated symptoms	*Do you experience other symptoms, like nausea, fever, or vaginal discharge?*	Changes in bowel or urinary habits can help identify underlying issues, such as constipation, diarrhea, or urinary incontinence, which could contribute to pelvic pain; conditions like IBS, interstitial cystitis, or prostatitis may be associated
Past medical and surgical history	*Do you have a history of pelvic or abdominal surgery? Any chronic medical conditions?*	Recent infections or surgeries can cause inflammation, adhesions, or direct trauma to the pelvic structures, potentially leading to pain (e.g., PID after a sexually transmitted infection or adhesions following a gynecologic surgery)
Sexual and reproductive history	*Are you sexually active? Have you had any pregnancies, miscarriages, or abortions?*	*Pregnancy:* may lead to pelvic pains like round ligament pain, symphysis pubis dysfunction, and complications such as ectopic pregnancy or miscarriage *Past pregnancy:* can be significant for conditions like pelvic organ prolapse or pelvic floor dysfunction

Vulvovaginal Symptoms

Vulvovaginal symptoms experienced in the external genitalia or the vagina include burning sensation, discomfort or tenderness swelling, visible redness or rash, abnormal discharge, and odor. Box 24-9 contains specific health history questions useful for distinguishing between various causes.

Possible causes include **bacterial vaginosis** ([**BV**] overgrowth of certain bacteria, leading to an imbalance in vaginal flora), **candidiasis** (yeast infection), **trichomoniasis** (infection by *Trichomonas vaginalis*), **genital herpes**, and **atrophic vaginitis** (decreased estrogen levels, causing thinning and inflammation of vaginal walls).

See Table 24-3, Vaginal Discharge, p. 766.

Box 24-9. Vulvovaginal Symptoms: High-Yield Health History Questions

Domain	Questions	Rationale
Symptom description	*How do you describe the specific symptoms you are experiencing (e.g., itching, burning, discharge, pain)?*	Aids in identifying causes like infections (yeast, bacterial vaginosis, trichomoniasis), dermatologic conditions (lichen sclerosis, contact dermatitis), or other issues (atrophic vaginitis, vulvodynia)
Onset	*When did the symptoms begin?*	Can help differentiate between *acute* (e.g., infection, allergic reaction) and *chronic* conditions (e.g., lichen sclerosis, vulvodynia)

Domain	Questions	Rationale
Pattern	*Are the symptoms constant or intermittent?*	*Constant:* may suggest a persistent underlying cause (e.g., dermatologic conditions, atrophic vaginitis) *Intermittent:* can point to triggers or irritants (e.g., contact dermatitis, recurrent infections)
Severity	*How would you rate the severity of your symptoms on a scale of 1–10?*	Severe symptoms might suggest an acute infection or a significant dermatologic issue
Aggravating or relieving factors	*Do any factors worsen or improve the symptoms (e.g., menstrual cycle, sexual activity, hygiene practices)?*	*Worsen during menstruation:* might suggest a hormonal influence *Improve with hygiene changes:* may point to irritants or infections
Discharge characteristics	*Have you noticed any changes in vaginal discharge (e.g., color, consistency, odor)?*	*Thick, white:* yeast infection *Thin, grayish with a fishy odor:* bacterial vaginosis *Frothy, yellow-green:* trichomoniasis or other conditions like atrophic vaginitis
Sexual and reproductive history	*Have you had any new or multiple sexual partners recently?*	New or multiple sexual partners may increase the risk of sexually transmitted infections (e.g., trichomoniasis, chlamydia, gonorrhea)
Hygiene practices	*What type of personal hygiene products (e.g., soap, menstrual products, lubricants) do you use?*	May cause irritation or allergic reactions, leading to vulvovaginal symptoms

Urinary Incontinence

Up to 50% of individuals assigned female at birth experience *urinary incontinence*, which can disrupt daily life and hygiene.[13–15] Bladder control depends on the detrusor muscle, urethral sphincter, and pelvic floor, regulated by neural pathways (see pp. 733–734). Hormonal changes, pregnancy, childbirth, and aging can weaken pelvic support or sphincter function, leading to stress, urge, or mixed incontinence. Box 24-10 provides key health history questions to help identify causes and guide evaluation.

Possible causes include **overflow incontinence** (incomplete bladder emptying often due to an obstruction or weak bladder muscle), **functional incontinence** (caused by physical or cognitive impairments that hinder timely toilet access), **stress incontinence** (involuntary leakage during activities that increase abdominal pressure), **urge incontinence** (sudden, intense urge to urinate followed by involuntary leakage), **mixed incontinence** (combination of stress and urge symptoms), and **neurogenic incontinence** (neurologic disorders or damage affecting bladder control).

See Table 24-4, Urinary Incontinence in Individuals Assigned Female at Birth, p. 767.

Box 24-10. Urinary Incontinence in Individuals Assigned Female at Birth: High-Yield Health History Questions

Domain	Questions	Rationale
Onset and pattern	*When did you first notice you were losing control of your bladder? What seems to trigger it, or is there a pattern to it?*	Helps differentiate between stress, urge, overflow, or functional incontinence
Severity and impact	*How often do you lose control of your bladder? How is this affecting your daily life and how you feel emotionally?*	Helps prioritize interventions and determine the urgency of addressing the issue
Voiding habits	*Can you tell me about your usual bathroom habits and any recent changes you've noticed?*	Can reveal factors contributing to urinary incontinence, such as changes related to childbirth, menopause, excessive fluid intake, or urinary frequency and urgency
Pelvic and reproductive history	*Have you ever had any surgery, been pregnant, or had any serious injuries to your lower abdomen and pelvic area?*	History of childbirth, pregnancy, or pelvic surgeries can indicate structural or functional changes contributing to urinary incontinence, such as weakened pelvic floor muscles or changes in bladder position and function
Neurologic status	*Lately, have you noticed any changes in how you feel physically, like any numbness, a tingling feeling, or weakness in your body?*	Can signal central or peripheral nervous system issues that may contribute to urinary incontinence, such as spinal cord injuries or neurodegenerative diseases
Medical history	*Do you have any other health problems, and are you taking any medicines for them?*	Can help determine if the incontinence is related to an underlying condition (like diabetes or multiple sclerosis) or a side effect of medications (like diuretics or α-blockers)

PHYSICAL EXAMINATION: GENERAL APPROACH

To enhance the comfort and understanding of patients during pelvic examinations, foster an environment of trust and respect (Box 24-11). Begin by seeking the patient's explicit consent and maintaining open communication throughout the process. Clearly explain each step before proceeding, using phrases like, *"I will first examine the external area for any irregularities, and then gently insert a speculum to check the internal area and cervix,"* and *"Now, I'll collect samples for the Pap test and screenings for gonorrhea and chlamydia."* Encourage the patient to express any discomfort or concerns, and ensure they are as relaxed as possible. Always use gloves to maintain hygiene, and have all necessary tools readily accessible. It is also recommended to have a chaperone

Box 24-11. Tips for a Successful Genitalia Examination in Individuals Assigned Female at Birth

Patient Responsibilities	Examiner Responsibilities
Pre-examination preparations: ■ Refrain from intercourse, douching, or vaginal suppositories for 24–48 h. ■ Empty bladder before examination. **During the examination:** ■ Lie supine with head and shoulders elevated. ■ Place arms at sides or folded across chest to facilitate eye contact and reduce muscle tightening.	**Before the examination:** ■ Obtain permission and select a chaperone if needed. ■ Explain each examination step in advance. **Examination technique:** ■ Properly drape the patient for comfort and eye contact. ■ Avoid sudden movements. ■ Choose and warm the correct size speculum. ■ Monitor patient comfort by watching facial expressions and obtaining feedback. ■ Use gentle techniques, especially when inserting the speculum.

present for added reassurance and support. This approach helps create a more positive and less stressful experience for the patient. For patients younger than age 21 years, pelvic examinations should only be performed when indicated by the medical history.

Positioning

Drape the patient appropriately and then assist them into the lithotomy position. Place one heel, then the other into the foot holders. The patient may be more comfortable in socks or shoes than bare feet. Then ask the patient to slide all the way down the examining table until their buttocks extend slightly beyond the edge. Their thighs should be flexed, abducted, and externally rotated at the hips. Make sure their head is supported with a pillow.

Prepare the Equipment

Assemble equipment and review the supplies and procedures of your own facility before taking cultures and other samples. You will need the materials described in Box 24-12.

Vaginal specula are traditionally made of metal, but disposable plastic versions are also available and frequently used. The two primary shapes of specula are the *Pedersen* and *Graves* (Fig. 24-9). Both are available in small, medium, and large sizes. The medium Pedersen speculum is usually most comfortable for patients who are sexually active. The narrow-bladed Pedersen speculum is best for the patient with a small introitus, such as individuals who are sexually inexperienced and older adults. The Graves specula are best for parous patients with vaginal prolapse.

Box 24-12. Essential Equipment for Pelvic Examinations and Their Uses

Equipment and Description	Purpose/Usage
Movable light source	Ensures a clear visualization of the vaginal walls and cervix during the examination
Vaginal speculum	Opens the vaginal walls, allowing for a clear view of the cervix; selection of the appropriate size is crucial for ensuring patient comfort
Water-soluble lubricant	Aids in the comfortable insertion of the speculum; use sparingly, especially during Pap smears, to prevent interference with the test results
Pap smear equipment	Used to screen for conditions such as cervical dysplasia and cancer
Bacteriologic culture materials	Identifies bacterial infections, including bacterial vaginosis or group B streptococcus, through the collection of appropriate samples
DNA probes	Detect specific infections, such as human papillomavirus, which is crucial for patient diagnosis and treatment planning
Diagnostic testing materials (e.g., potassium hydroxide and normal saline)	Used for preparing and evaluating wet mounts, which are essential in diagnosing vaginal infections like yeast or trichomoniasis
Additional supplies	Gloves are a must for maintaining hygiene during internal exams; cotton swabs and brushes are used for collecting samples, and cytology fixative spray or solution helps preserve Pap smear samples before their analysis in the lab

Before using a speculum, practice opening and closing its blades, locking the blades in an open position, and releasing them again. Plastic specula might have a different locking mechanism than metal ones. Familiarize yourself with the particular design you are using.

The instructions in this chapter apply to a metal speculum; you can easily adapt them to a plastic speculum by handling it before use. When using a plastic speculum, warn the patient that it typically makes a loud click when locked or released.

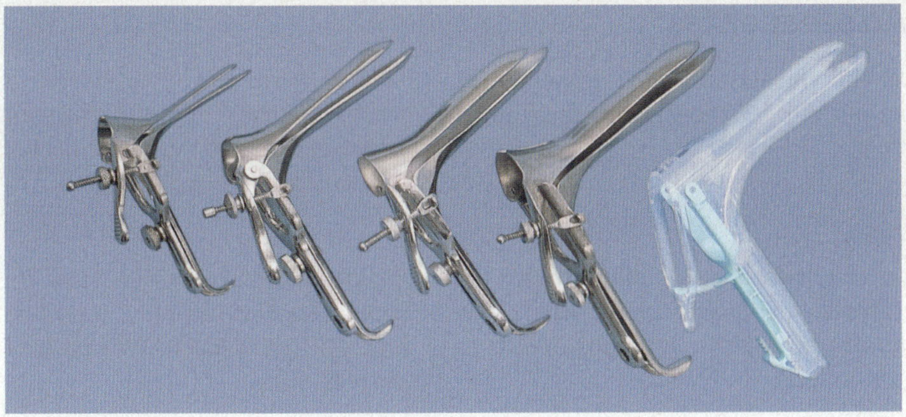

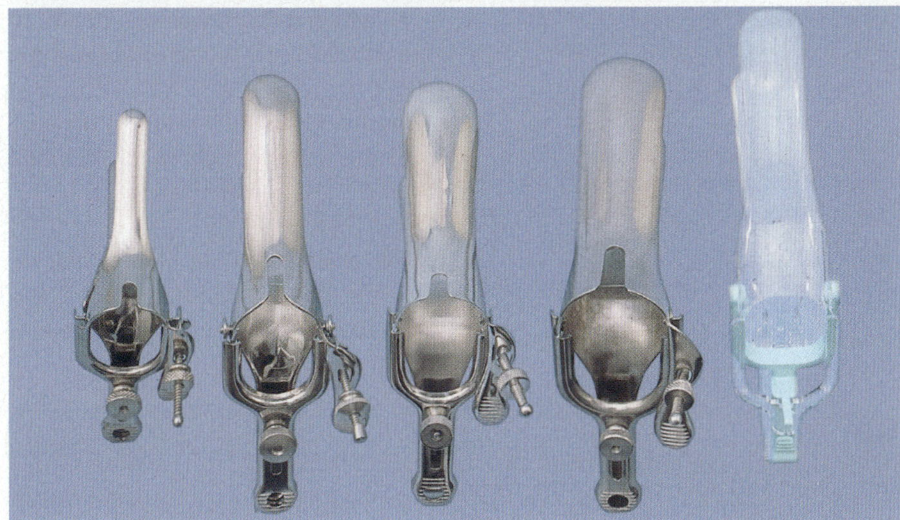

FIGURE 24-9. Specula, from left to right: small metal Pedersen, medium metal Pedersen, medium metal Graves, large metal Graves, and large plastic Pedersen.

TECHNIQUES OF EXAMINATION

Key Components of the Examination of the Vulva, Vagina, Uterus, and Adnexa

- Assess sexual maturity (adolescents)
- Inspect the vulva
- Insert the vaginal speculum
- Inspect the cervix
- Inspect the vagina
- Obtain specimens for cervical cytology (Pap smears)
- Perform a bimanual examination
- Assess the pelvic floor muscles for strength and tenderness
- Perform a rectovaginal examination (if indicated)

Assess Sexual Maturity (Adolescents)

You can assess pubic hair during either the abdominal or the pelvic examination. Note its characteristics and distribution, and rate it according to the Tanner stages, described on pp. 1091–1097.

Delayed puberty is often familial or related to chronic illness. It may also reflect disorders of the hypothalamus, anterior pituitary gland, or ovaries.

Inspect the Vulva

Visually inspect the *mons pubis*, *labia*, and *perineum*. Carefully separate the labia to examine the more delicate structures like the *labia minora*, *clitoris*, *urethral meatus*, and *vaginal opening* or *introitus*. Check for any signs of inflammation, ulceration, discharge, swelling, or nodules.

Excoriations or itchy, small, red maculopapules suggest *pediculosis pubis* (lice or "crabs"), often found at the bases of the pubic hairs.

An enlarged clitoris is seen in conditions associated with elevated androgen levels.

Inspect for urethral caruncle, prolapse of the urethral mucosa (p. 764), and tenderness in interstitial cystitis.

For descriptions of herpes simplex, Behçet disease, syphilitic chancre, and epidermoid cyst, see Table 24-2, Lesions of the Vulva, p. 765.

Insert the Vaginal Speculum

Select a speculum of appropriate size and shape and moisten it with warm water. Lubricants and gels may interfere with cytologic studies and bacterial or viral cultures, so use them sparingly. Let the patient know you are about to insert the speculum and will be applying downward pressure.

Gently separate the labia minora and introduce the closed speculum at approximately 30° downward toward the cervix (Fig. 24-10). You may carefully

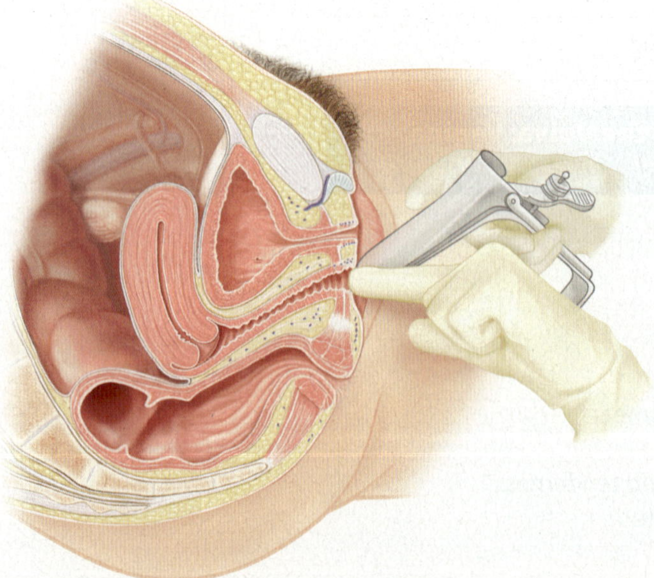

FIGURE 24-10. Gently inserting the vaginal speculum.

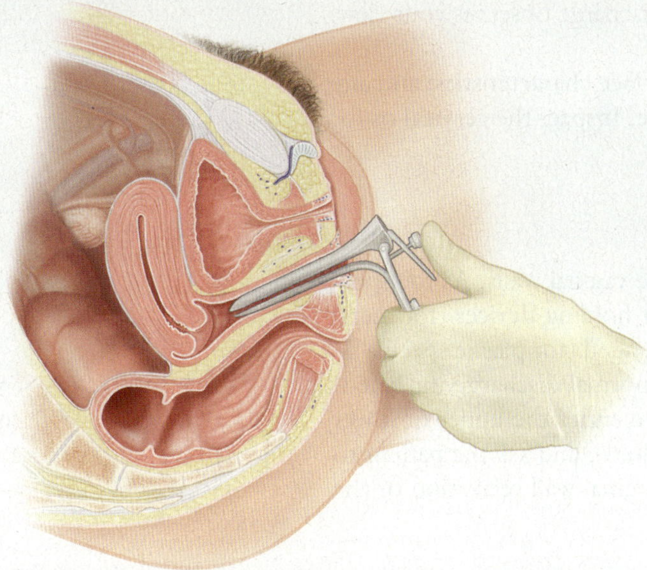

FIGURE 24-11. Inserting the speculum to its full length.

enlarge the vaginal introitus by lubricating one finger with water and applying downward pressure at its lower margin, then palpate the location of the cervix in order to angle the speculum more accurately.

Inspect the Cervix

After placing the speculum in the vagina, remove the fingers of your other hand from the introitus. Rotate the speculum into a horizontal position, maintaining pressure posteriorly, and insert it to its full length (Fig. 24-11). Then slowly open the speculum to visualize the cervix. Do not open the blades of the speculum prematurely. Rotate and adjust the speculum until it cups the cervix and brings it into full view (Fig. 24-12). Fix the speculum in its open position by tightening the thumbscrew. Position the light until you can see the cervix well. When the uterus is retroverted, the cervix points more anteriorly than illustrated. If you have difficulty finding the cervix, withdraw the speculum

See Table 24-5, Variations in the Cervical Surface, p. 768; Table 24-6, Shapes of the Cervical Os, p. 769; and Table 24-7, Abnormalities of the Cervix, p. 769.

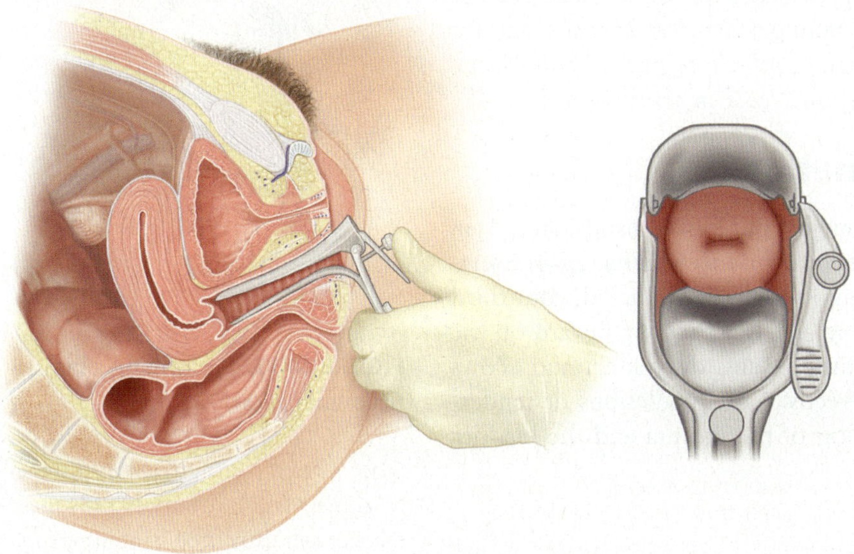

FIGURE 24-12. Visualizing the cervix.

slightly and reposition it on a different slope. If a discharge obscures your view, wipe it away gently with a large cotton swab.

Note the color of the cervix; its position and surface characteristics; and any ulcerations, nodules, masses, bleeding, or discharge. Inspect the cervical os for discharge.

Inspect the Vagina

Withdraw the speculum slowly while observing the vaginal walls. As the speculum clears the cervix, release any thumbscrews or holding devices (for metal specula) or ensure any locking mechanism is disengaged (for plastic specula).

Inspect the vaginal walls for masses, lesions, abnormal discharge, or bleeding. Check for bulging in the vaginal wall. Remove either the upper or lower blade of the speculum (or use a single-blade speculum), and ask the patient to bear down so that you can assess the location of vaginal wall relaxation or the degree of bladder, rectal, and uterine prolapse.

Look for lateral displacement or immobility of the cervix along with palpable nodularity in the posterior fornix in endometriosis involving the uterosacral ligaments.

See Table 24-3, Vaginal Discharge, p. 766.

Vaginal cancer is rare; diethylstilbestrol (DES) exposure in utero and HPV infection are risk factors.[16,17]

After inspection is completed, the speculum is gently closed and removed.

See Table 24-1, Bulges and Swelling of the Vulva, Vagina, and Urethra, p. 764.

Obtain Specimens for Cervical Cytology (Pap Smears)

Obtain one specimen from the endocervix and another from the ectocervix or a combination specimen using the cervical brush ("broom"); see Box 24-13. For best results, the patient should not be menstruating.

The patient should avoid intercourse and use of douches, tampons, contraceptive foams or creams, and vaginal suppositories for 48 hours before the examination. For sexually active individuals younger than age 25 years, and for other asymptomatic patients at increased risk of infection, plan to culture the cervix routinely for *Chlamydia trachomatis* and *Neisseria gonorrhoeae*.[18]

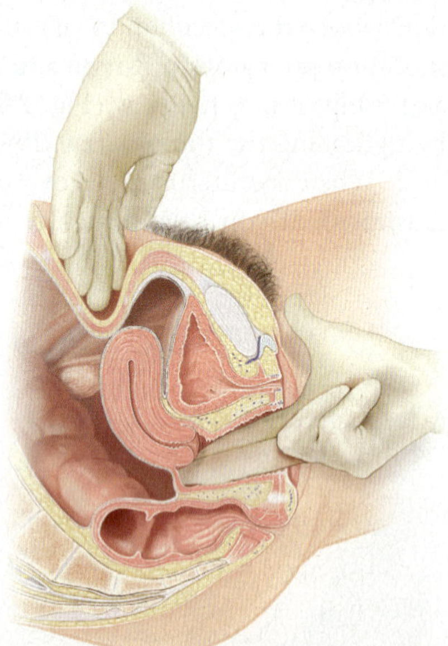

FIGURE 24-13. Performing a bimanual examination.

Perform a Bimanual Examination

Lubricate the index and middle fingers of one of your gloved hands, and, *from a standing position, insert your lubricated fingers into the vagina*, again exerting pressure primarily posteriorly. Your thumb should be abducted, your third and fourth fingers flexed into your palm (Fig. 24-13). Pressing inward on the perineum with your flexed fingers causes little, if any, discomfort and allows you to position your palpating fingers correctly. Note any lesions or tenderness in the vaginal wall, including the region of the urethra and the bladder anteriorly.

Stool in the rectum may simulate a rectovaginal mass, but, unlike a malignant mass, it can usually be dented by digital pressure. Rectovaginal examination confirms the distinction.

Box 24-13. Obtaining the Pap Smear: Options for Specimen Collection

Cervical Broom Method	Liquid-Based Cytology Handling	Traditional Slide Method Handling
Use a plastic brush with a broom-like tip. Rotate in the cervical os in a full clockwise direction.	Place the sample directly into a preservative.	Stroke each side of the brush on a glass slide, then fix promptly.
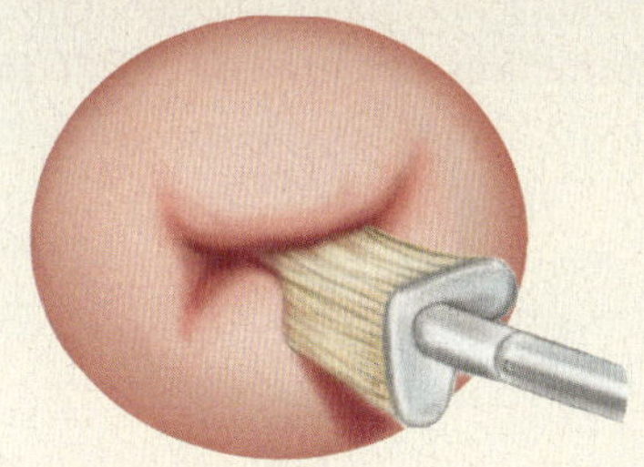		
Cervical Scrape	**Liquid-Based Cytology Handling**	**Traditional Slide Method Handling**
Use the longer end of the scraper in the cervical os. Press, turn, and scrape in a full circle, focusing on the transformation zone and squamocolumnar junction.	Place the scraped material directly into a preservative.	Smear the specimen on a glass slide, then place in a safe spot.
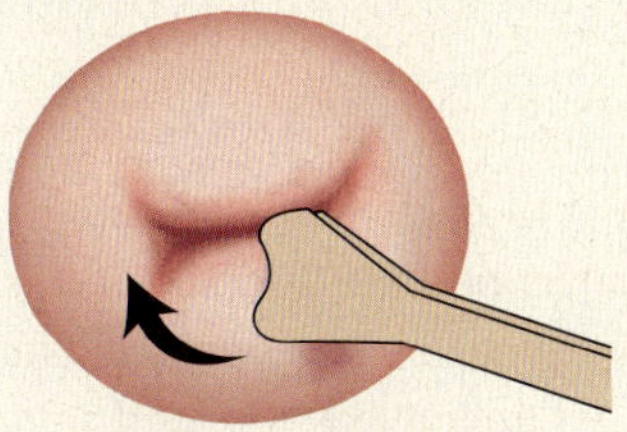		
Endocervical Brush	**Liquid-Based Cytology Handling**	**Traditional Slide Method Handling**
Insert the endocervical brush into the cervical os. Roll it between the thumb and index finger, both clockwise and counterclockwise.	Place the collected material into a preservative.	Gently smear the slide with the collected material, then fix promptly.
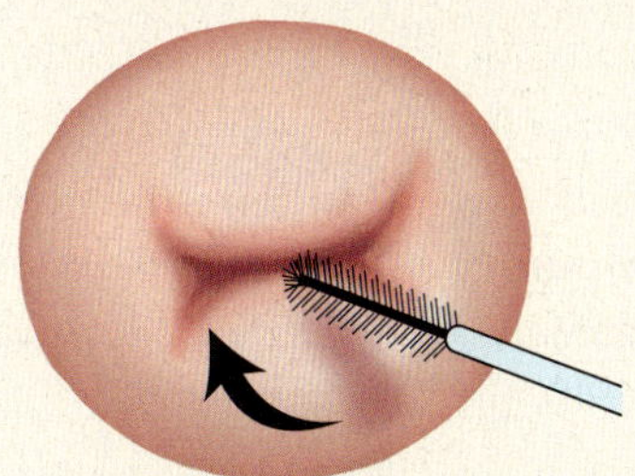		

For pregnant individuals, use a cotton-tipped applicator moistened with saline in place of the endocervical brush, especially for the traditional slide method to minimize discomfort and risk.

Palpate the Cervix. Note its position, shape, consistency, regularity, mobility, and tenderness. Normally, the cervix can be moved somewhat without pain. Feel the fornices around the cervix and note any nodularity, immobility, and tenderness in this area.

Cervical motion tenderness and/or adnexal tenderness are hallmarks of PID, ectopic pregnancy, and appendicitis.

Nodularity, immobility, and tenderness in the fornices may result from endometriosis.

Palpate the Uterus. Place your other hand on the lower abdomen just above the symphysis pubis. While you elevate the cervix and uterus with your pelvic hand, press your abdominal hand in and down, trying to grasp the uterus between your two hands (see Fig. 24-13). Note its size, shape, consistency, and mobility, and identify any tenderness or masses.

See Table 24-8, Positions of the Uterus, p. 770, and Table 24-9, Abnormalities of the Uterus, p. 771.

If you cannot feel the uterus with either of these maneuvers, it may be tipped posteriorly. Slide your pelvic fingers into the posterior fornix and feel for the uterus butting against your fingertips. In a patient who is obese or who has a poorly relaxed abdominal wall, you may not be able to feel the uterus even when it is located anteriorly.

See retroversion and retroflexion of the uterus (p. 770).

Palpate Each Ovary. Place your abdominal hand on the right lower quadrant, and your pelvic hand in the right lateral fornix (Fig. 24-14). Press your abdominal hand in and down, trying to push the adnexal structures toward your pelvic hand. Try to identify the right ovary or any adjacent adnexal masses. By moving your hands slightly, slide the adnexal structures between your fingers, if possible, and note their size, shape, consistency, mobility, and tenderness. Repeat the procedure on the left side.

Normal ovaries may be somewhat tender. They are usually palpable in slender, relaxed patients but are difficult or impossible to feel in patients who are obese or tense.

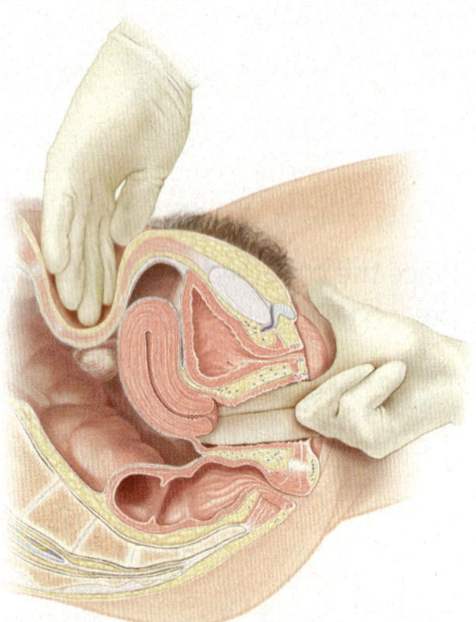

FIGURE 24-14. Palpating the ovaries.

Within 3 to 5 years after menopause, the ovaries become atrophic and usually nonpalpable. Pelvic pain, bloating, increased abdominal size, and urinary tract symptoms are more common in patients with ovarian cancer.[19]

Adnexal masses can also arise from a tubo-ovarian abscess, salpingitis, or inflammation of the fallopian tubes from PID, or ectopic pregnancy.

See Table 24-10, Adnexal Masses, p. 771.

Assess the Pelvic Floor Muscles for Strength and Tenderness

Ask the patient to squeeze around your fingers as long and as hard as they can. Snug compression of your fingers that lasts 3 or more seconds is full strength. Then, with your fingers still placed against the vaginal walls inferiorly, ask the patient to cough several times or to bear down (*Valsalva maneuver*). Look for

Muscle weakness arises from aging, vaginal deliveries, and neurologic conditions and contributes to the urine leakage of stress incontinence during increased abdominal pressure.

any urinary leakage during increased abdominal pressure. Watch for abdominal muscle over-recruitment or tightening of the adductor or gluteal muscles.

In patients with pelvic pain or vaginal wall tenderness, palpate the external pelvic floor muscles in a clockwise rotation to identify trigger points.

Trigger point tenderness in these muscles accompanies pelvic floor spasm and pelvic floor dysfunction from trauma, interstitial cystitis, and fibromyalgia. Pelvic floor disorders, present in ~25% of all individuals assigned female at birth and ≥30% of older patients, include urinary and fecal incontinence, pelvic organ prolapse, and other sensory and emptying abnormalities of the lower urinary and gastrointestinal tracts.[20]

Perform a Rectovaginal Examination (if Indicated)

The rectovaginal examination has the following primary purposes: to palpate a retroverted uterus, the uterosacral ligaments, cul-de-sac, and adnexa, and to assess pelvic pathology (Fig. 24-15).

Nodularity and thickening of the uterosacral ligaments occur in endometriosis as does pain with uterine movement.

After withdrawing your fingers from the bimanual examination, change your gloves and lubricate your fingers as needed. Slowly reintroduce your index finger into the vagina and your middle finger into the rectum. Ask the patient to strain down as you do this to relax the anal sphincter. Mention that this may stimulate an urge to move the bowels, but this will not occur. Apply pressure against the anterior and lateral walls with the examining fingers and downward pressure with the hand on the abdomen.

Check the *rectal vault* for masses. If fecal blood testing is planned, change gloves to avoid contaminating fecal material with any blood provoked by collecting the Pap smear. After the examination, wipe off the external genitalia and rectum, or offer wipes to the patient to do so.

See Chapter 22, Anus and Rectum, p. 682.

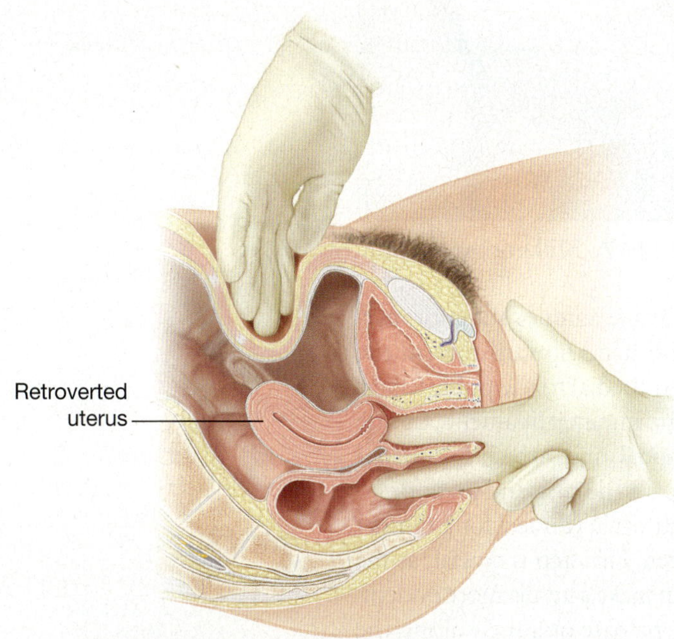

FIGURE 24-15. Examining the rectovaginal area.

SPECIAL TECHNIQUES AND MANEUVERS

Assessing Labial Swelling

If your patient reports labial swelling, a focused assessment of the greater vestibular (Bartholin) glands is necessary (Fig. 24-16). Gently insert your gloved index finger into the vagina near the posterior introitus and place your thumb on the outside of the posterior part of the labium majus. Examine each side, typically around the 4 o'clock and 8 o'clock positions, by palpating between your finger and thumb. Carefully assess for any swelling, tenderness, or discharge from the duct opening of the gland. If discharge is present, obtain a sample for culture to identify any underlying infection.

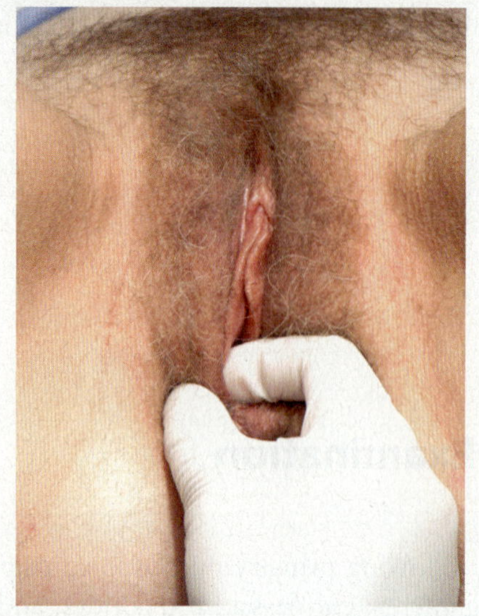

FIGURE 24-16. Palpating the greater vestibular (Bartholin) gland.

A greater vestibular gland may become acutely or chronically infected, resulting in swelling. See Table 24-1, Bulges and Swelling of the Vulva, Vagina, and Urethra, p. 764.

Assessing for Urethritis

To evaluate possible urethritis or inflammation of the paraurethral glands, insert your index finger into the vagina and milk the urethra gently outward from the inside (Fig. 24-17). Note any discharge from or about the urethral meatus. If present, culture it.

Causes of urethritis include infection from *C. trachomatis* and *N. gonorrhoeae.*

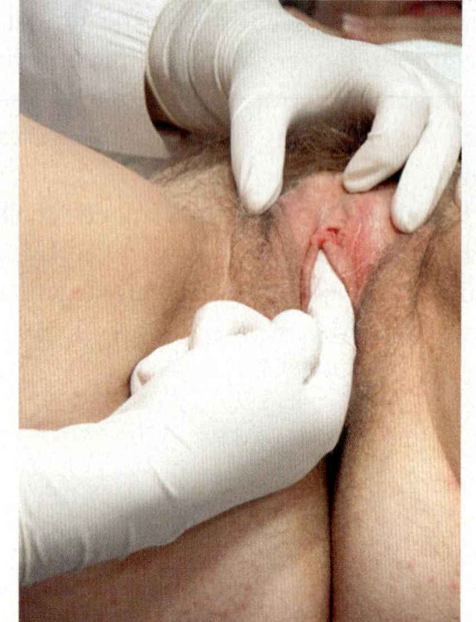

FIGURE 24-17. Milking the urethra.

Assessing for Suspected Inguinal Hernia

Have the patient first lie down and then stand, as some hernias may only be visible or palpable when standing. Look for any bulges or asymmetry, which could indicate a hernia, paying particular attention to the areas around the inguinal ligament and the femoral canal.

Then place the tip of your dominant index finger at the anterior superior margin of the labia majora. Gently move your finger and hand upward toward the external inguinal ring, ensuring your movement is just medial to the pubic tubercle. To identify the inguinal ring, follow the line of the inguinal ligament. Locate the triangular, slit-like opening of the external inguinal ring, which is situated just above and lateral to the pubic tubercle, and palpate the ring and its floor.

Next, conduct a *cough test.* Ask the patient to cough while you feel for a distinct bulge or mass that moves against your stationary finger. This step is crucial, as the increased intra-abdominal pressure during coughing can make a hernia more evident.

Continue by palpating the inguinal canal. Gently palpate obliquely along the canal, moving toward the internal inguinal ring. Ask the patient to cough again and check for any bulge that slides down the inguinal canal and taps against your fingertip.

Finally, ensure to examine both sides, using the same techniques and your dominant finger, to assess both the left and right inguinal areas thoroughly.

Assessing for Suspected Femoral Hernia

Femoral hernias occur when tissue pushes through a weak spot in the muscle wall near the femoral vein in the upper thigh. While these are less common overall compared to inguinal hernias, they are relatively common in individuals who are assigned female at birth due to their wider pelvis.

In examining the patient for a femoral hernia, the procedure is largely similar to that used for an inguinal hernia, with one notable difference in the approach: the focus on locating the femoral pulse in the upper thigh. After finding the femoral pulse, move your fingers medially toward the inner thigh, aiming toward the area around the pubic tubercle, which is where the femoral canal is situated.

See further discussion of assessing groin hernias in Chapter 23, Pelvis and Genitourinary System: Penis, Scrotum, and Prostate, pp. 704–706.

Modifications in Physical Examinations: Best Practices for Specialized Patient Populations

In the evolving landscape of reproductive and gender-affirming health care, you are increasingly likely to encounter patients with gender-confirmation surgery or intrauterine devices (IUDs). While the foundational principles of the genitalia examination remain consistent, the presence of these interventions demands specific modifications to ensure both diagnostic accuracy and patient comfort (Box 24-14).

RECORDING YOUR FINDINGS

While detailed sentences in physical examination (PE) documentation are crucial in developing your initial diagnostic and hypothesis-generation skills, as you gain experience, you will eventually condense your notes into universally recognized, succinct phrases.

Recording the Examination of the Vulva, Vagina, Uterus, and Adnexa

"No inguinal adenopathy. External genitalia without erythema, lesions, or masses. Vaginal mucosa pink. Cervix parous, pink, and without discharge. Uterus anterior, midline, smooth, and not enlarged. No adnexal tenderness. Pap smear obtained. Rectovaginal wall intact. Rectal vault without masses. Stool brown and negative for fecal blood."

OR

"Bilateral shotty inguinal adenopathy. External genitalia without erythema or lesions. Vaginal mucosa and cervix coated with thin white homogeneous discharge with a mild fish-like odor. After swabbing cervix, no discharge visible in the cervical os. Uterus midline; no adnexal masses. Rectal vault without masses. Stool brown and negative for fecal blood."

Box 24-14. Genitalia Examination in the Presence of Medical Devices, Conditions, or Procedures

	Patient with an Intrauterine Device (IUD)	Patient with a Vaginoplasty
	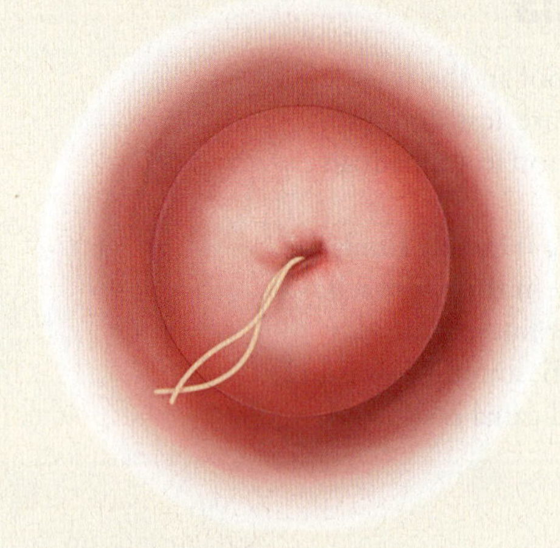	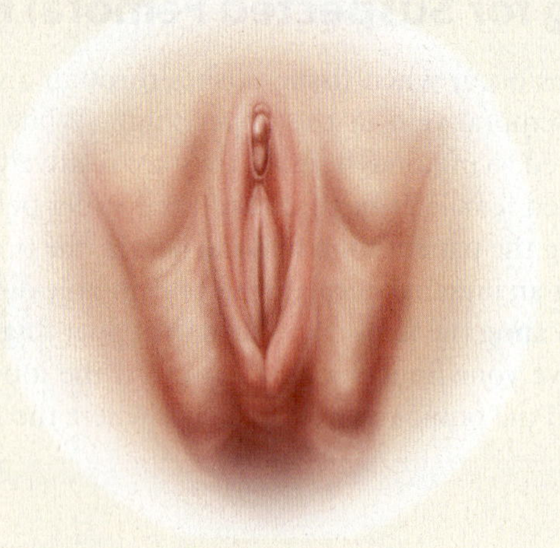
Device/ condition	Small T-shaped device inserted into the uterus to prevent pregnancy	Surgical procedure to construct or reconstruct the vagina
General indication	Long-term reversible contraception	Gender confirmation surgery to align physical appearance with gender identity; reconstruction for congenital anomalies; following surgery or trauma to restore normal appearance and function
General location	Within the uterine cavity, with strings extending through the cervix into the vagina	In the anatomic location of the vagina
Modification to the physical exam	1. Begin by explaining the examination steps to the patient, ensuring the patient understands the process and reason for the exam. 2. Visually inspect the cervix, noting the presence of the IUD strings protruding from the os. Avoid tugging or pulling these strings as it can displace the IUD. 3. During the bimanual exam, palpate gently, being cautious not to exert pressure that might inadvertently displace the IUD. 4. If unable to locate the IUD strings, consider further evaluation with ultrasound to confirm its location. 5. Advise the patient to regularly check for the presence of the IUD strings and to seek medical evaluation if they cannot be felt or if they feel unusually long or short.	1. Approach with sensitivity, acknowledging the patient's surgical history. Always ask permission and explain each step of the exam to ensure patient comfort. 2. Begin with a thorough history-taking, understanding the extent and type of surgery and any associated complications or concerns. 3. Be gentle and use adequate lubrication, recognizing that the neovagina might not have the same elasticity as native tissue. 4. When inspecting the external genitalia, note any scars, erythema, edema, discoloration, or signs of trauma. 5. For the internal exam, proceed gently, and ensure familiarity with the depth and angle of the neovagina, which can differ from nonsurgical anatomy. 6. On internal exam, note any strictures or narrowing of the vaginal orifice, bleeding, or discharge. 7. When palpating, note any masses or tender areas, and always inquire about the patient's comfort. 8. Understand that some individuals may have retained prostate tissue; be sensitive when discussing or assessing this.

The method of deconstructing PE documentation into specific details exemplifies the vital contribution of clinical observations to the diagnostic possibilities. The described findings suggest a potential infection or inflammatory condition:

- *Bilateral shotty inguinal adenopathy:* The presence of small, firm ("shotty") lymph nodes in the inguinal area can indicate a reaction to infection or inflammation in the genital or lower urinary tract.
- *Vaginal discharge:* Thin, white, homogeneous discharge with a mild **fish-like** odor is characteristic of bacterial vaginosis (BV).
- *Cervical findings:* The absence of discharge in the cervical os after swabbing, along with the absence of erythema or lesions on the external genitalia, might reduce the likelihood of an STI like chlamydia or gonorrhea, but does not rule it out.
- *Uterine and adnexal examination:* The uterus being midline and the absence of adnexal masses are normal findings and do not contribute to a specific diagnosis in this context.
- *Rectal exam and stool test:* The rectal vault without masses and stool negative for fecal blood are noncontributory to the primary concern but are important for a comprehensive pelvic examination.

In summary, these findings are most suggestive of *BV*, given the characteristic nature of the vaginal discharge.

POINT-OF-CARE ULTRASOUND EXAMINATION

Assessing bladder volume is essential for precise evaluation across all patients, and the anatomy of the genitourinary system often requires specific attention to detail. The evaluation of anuria or oliguria involves understanding whether there is a difficulty in urine production (in which case the bladder should be underfilled) or urine retention (when the bladder cannot empty normally). Detection of urinary retention can also help in the assessment of spinal cord compromise (which inhibits the innervation of the bladder and release of urine) or other structural causes of urinary retention caused by masses blocking the urethra (such as a prostate) or malfunction of a urinary catheter.

This section highlights the diagnostic utility of point-of-care ultrasound (POCUS) in accurately determining bladder volume.[21] While PE maneuvers can offer insights, POCUS provides a more direct and quantifiable evaluation. However, the hands-on procedural nuances of POCUS remain outside this book's purview.

Estimating Bladder Volume

Physical Examination. The bladder may be palpated when it exceeds 400 to 600 mL. Dullness to percussion over the lower abdomen indicates a filled or distended bladder, and the fundal height of the bladder can often be palpated above the pubic symphysis. A distended bladder is typically tender to palpation (Box 24-15).

Box 24-15. Physical Examination Findings: Urinary Bladder Volume

Examination Technique	Associated Finding
Inspection of the lower abdomen	Suprapubic fullness may suggest a distended bladder.
Palpation of the suprapubic area	A palpable bladder can indicate significant retention.
Percussion over the suprapubic region	Dullness can suggest bladder distension.
Asking the patient to attempt voiding	Absence of urinary stream can indicate significant retention or obstruction.

Ultrasound Technique

Basic Ultrasound Setup	
Patient positioning	Supine
Probe	Curvilinear probe
Ultrasound setting	"abdomen" setting

Begin just cranial to the pubic symphysis in the midline. Scan in both a transverse plane (with the probe marker facing toward the patient's right-hand side) and in a sagittal plane (with the probe marker facing the patient's head).

In a transverse plane, fan the probe angle cranially and caudally to find the largest bladder area visible. Freeze the image and measure the bladder diameter in two orthogonal planes: from anterior to posterior and from left to right (width). Next, obtain the largest diameter of the bladder in the sagittal plane, and measure the largest distance from cranial to caudal (Fig. 24-18).

Taking those three measurements, multiply them all together and then by 0.75 (i.e., length × width × height × 0.75) to obtain a noninvasive estimate of bladder volume.[22] Some machines have a built-in automated volume calculation (Fig. 24-18).

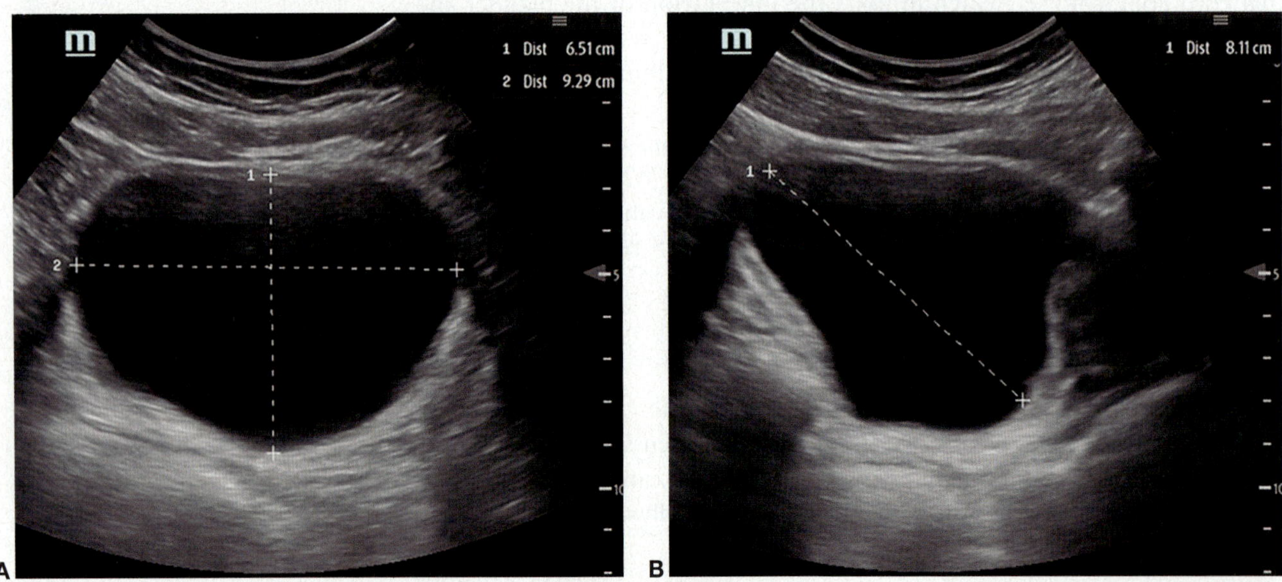

FIGURE 24-18. Bladder volume measurements in transverse (**A**) and sagittal (**B**) planes.

HEALTH PROMOTION AND COUNSELING: EVIDENCE AND RECOMMENDATIONS

Important Topics for Health Promotion and Counseling

- Cervical cancer
- Menopause and hormone replacement therapy
- Urinary incontinence

In the following section, both traditional terms like "men," "women," "male," and "female" and inclusive terms such as "individuals assigned female at birth" and "individuals assigned male at birth" are used. This approach balances inclusivity with the need to accurately represent the original research.

Cervical Cancer

Epidemiology. Worldwide, cervical cancer is the fourth most frequently diagnosed cancer among women and the fourth leading cause of cancer death in this group.[23] However, cancer incidence and mortality are much lower in high-income countries. In the United States, cervical cancers are not among either the top 10 most frequently diagnosed cancers or the top 10 leading causes of cancer death.[24] The lifetime risk for being diagnosed with cervical cancer in the United States is about 1 in 140, while the lifetime risk for dying from cervical cancer is about 1 in 500.[25] HPV, particularly genotypes 16 and 18, is found in virtually all cervical cancers. HPV is sexually transmitted, and having multiple sexual partners and an earlier age of sexual activity are risk factors for developing cervical cancer.[26] Other important risk factors include inadequate screening and treatment for precancers, immunosuppression, long-term use of oral contraception, coinfection with *C. trachomatis,* previous cervical cancer or high-grade precancerous lesion, tobacco smoking or exposure to second-hand smoke, in utero exposure to DES, and having three or more full-term pregnancies.

Cervical Cancer Prevention. HPV vaccination offers the opportunity to prevent cervical cancer and precancers. In the United States, the only available HPV vaccine is the 9-valent vaccine, which targets HPV genotypes that can cause cervical, vulvar, vaginal, anal, penile, and oropharyngeal cancers as well as most anogenital warts.

HPV Vaccine Recommendations. The U.S. Advisory Committee on Immunization Practices (ACIP) recommends routine vaccination for individuals beginning at age 11 or 12 years, although vaccinations can be first given at age 9.[27] For those being vaccinated before age 15, the recommendation is two doses of HPV vaccine within 6 to 12 months. For those first being vaccinated at ages 15 through 26 and immunocompromised persons ages 9 through 26, the recommendation is for three doses of HPV vaccine (0, 1 to 2, and 6 months). Catch-up vaccination is recommended for all people through age 26 who were not previously adequately vaccinated. The ACIP also recommends that clinicians consider discussing HPV vaccination for adults ages 27 through 45 years who were not adequately vaccinated and who are at risk for acquiring new HPV infections.

Box 24-16. Current Cervical Cancer Screening Guidelines for Individuals Assigned Female at Birth at Average Risk: U.S. Preventive Services Task Force, American Cancer Society, and American College of Obstetrics and Gynecology[31,44,45]

Variables	Recommendation
Age at which to begin screening	21 years[a]
Screening method and interval	Ages 21–29 years: cytology alone every 3 years Ages 30–65 years: screen every 3 years with cytology alone every 3 years; high-risk human papillomavirus (hrHPV) testing alone every 5 years; cotesting (hrHPV and cytology) every 5 years
Age at which to end screening	Age >65 years, assuming three consecutive negative results on cytology, two consecutive negative cotesting results, or two consecutive negative hrHPV testing within 10 years before cessation of screening, with the most recent test performed within 5 years
Screening after hysterectomy with removal of the cervix	Not recommended

[a]The American Cancer Society recommends that screening begin at age 25 years.

Vaccinated females should still get cervical cancer screening (Box 24-16) and recognize that using condoms does not eliminate the risk of cervical HPV infection.

Cervical Cancer Screening. Widespread organized cervical screening with the Pap smear has contributed to significant declines in cervical cancer incidence and mortality since the 1960s. Pap smears can identify high-risk precancerous changes or early cancers that can be further evaluated and treated by gynecologists.[28] However, the introduction of high-risk HPV (hrHPV) tests, which are more sensitive than Pap smears in identifying precancerous high-grade cervical intraepithelial neoplasia (CIN), has expanded options for screening. The U.S. Preventive Services Task Force (USPSTF) has issued guidelines on cervical cancer screening for average-risk women (see Box 24-16).[29] The guidelines defined average risk as having no history of a high-grade, precancerous cervical lesion or cervical cancer; not being immunocompromised; and having no in utero exposure to DES. The USPSTF gave a grade A recommendation for screening individuals ages 21 to 65 with a cervix. Those ages 21 to 29 years should be screened every 3 years with cytology alone. Individuals ages 30 to 65 years can be screened every 3 years with cytology alone, every 5 years with hrHPV testing alone, or every 5 years with both tests together (cotesting). They recommended against screening for individuals younger than age 21, those older than 65 with adequate previous screening, and individuals who had undergone hysterectomy with removal of the cervix (grade D).

Menopause and Hormone Replacement Therapy

Menopause may bring psychological and physiologic changes ranging from mood shifts to hot flashes to vaginal drying and bone loss. For many years, hormone-replacement therapy (HRT) with oral estrogen ± progestin was recommended to treat menopausal symptoms and protect against bone loss and cardiovascular disease events. However, the Women's Health Initiative, a large randomized, controlled trial investigating the use of postmenopausal HRT found that receiving hormones increased risks for cardiovascular disease events and breast cancer.[30] The USPSTF recommends against the use of either estrogen alone (for individuals who have had a hysterectomy) or combined use of estrogen and progestin for preventing chronic conditions in postmenopausal individuals (grade D).[31] However, the USPSTF recommendation did not address using HRT to treat menopausal symptoms. The North American Menopause Society advises individualized decision making regarding HRT for relieving menopausal symptoms based on a person's symptom severity and risk–benefit ratio.[32] Doses should be low, prescribed early in menopause, and for the shortest acceptable duration.

Urinary Incontinence

Epidemiology. Urinary incontinence is classified as urge, stress, mixed, and overflow.[33,34] Urge incontinence occurs with urgency to void, stress incontinence occurs with effort or physical exertion that increases intra-abdominal pressure, mixed is a combination of urge and stress symptoms, and overflow presents with continuous urinary leakage. An estimated 9.6 million US women ages 50 years and older reported bothersome incontinence on the 2001 to 2014 National Health and Nutrition Examination Surveys.[35] Urinary incontinence adversely impacts quality of life by interfering with physical, psychological, and social functioning. Urinary incontinence is also associated with perineal infections, falls, and fractures. Risk factors for urinary incontinence include increasing age, vaginal births, menopause, genitourinary surgery, cognitive and functional impairment, and chronic medical comorbidities (e.g., diabetes, neurologic disorders, and cardiovascular disease). Other contributing factors, which are potentially modifiable, include obesity and weight gain, constipation, vaginal atrophy, medications, tobacco use, and excessive caffeine intake. Although incontinence can be effectively treated with behavioral, nonpharmacologic, pharmacologic, and surgical interventions, studies suggest that clinicians are often unaware of the symptoms because patients are reluctant to discuss them.

Screening. Given the high prevalence and substantial impact of symptoms, the Women's Preventive Services Initiative (WPSI) issued a weak-level recommendation to annually screen women for urinary incontinence beginning in adolescence.[33] The WPSI identified numerous reasonably accurate screening instruments that assess whether women are experiencing urinary incontinence and whether the symptom is affecting their quality of life and activities. Examples of screening instruments include the *3 Incontinence Question (3IQ)*, which can distinguish between stress and urge incontinence,[36] and the *Bladder Control Self-Assessment Questionnaire (B-SAQ)*,[37] which assesses degree of symptom bothersomeness (Figs. 24-19 and 24-20). Results from the screening instruments can be used to guide decisions about further evaluation and treatment.

1. During the last three months, have you leaked urine (even a small amount)?

☐ Yes ☐ No → Questionnaire completed

2. During the last three months, did you leak urine:
(Check all that apply)

☐ a. When you were performing some physical activity, such as coughing, sneezing, lifting, or exercise?
☐ b. When you had the urge or the feeling that you needed to empty your bladder, but you could not get to the toilet fast enough?
☐ c. Without physical activity and without a sense of urgency?

3. During the last three months, did you leak urine *most often*:
(Check only one)

☐ a. When you were performing some physical activity, such as coughing, sneezing, lifting, or exercise?
☐ b. When you had the urge or the feeling that you needed to empty your bladder, but you could not get to the toilet fast enough?
☐ c. Without physical activity and without a sense of urgency?
☐ d. About equally as often with physical activity as with a sense of urgency?

Definitions of type of urinary incontinence are based on responses to question 3:

Response to question 3	Type of incontinence
a. Most often with physical activity	Stress only or stress predominant
b. Most often with the urge to empty the bladder	Urge only or urge predominant
c. Without physical activity or sense of urgency	Other cause only or other cause predominant
d. About equally with physical activity and sense of urgency	Mixed

Brown JS, Bradley CS, Subak LL, et al. The sensitivity and specificity of a simple test to distinguis between urge and stress urinary incontinence. Ann Intern Med. 2006;144:715–723.

Graphic 72319 Version 17.0

FIGURE 24-19. 3IQ to assess urinary incontinence.[36] (Source: Brown JS, Bradley CS, Subak LL, et al. The sensitivity and specificity of a simple test to distinguish between urge and stress urinary incontinence. *Ann Intern Med.* 2006;144(10):715–723. Copyright © 2006 American College of Physicians. All Rights Reserved. Reprinted with the permission of American College of Physicians, Inc.)

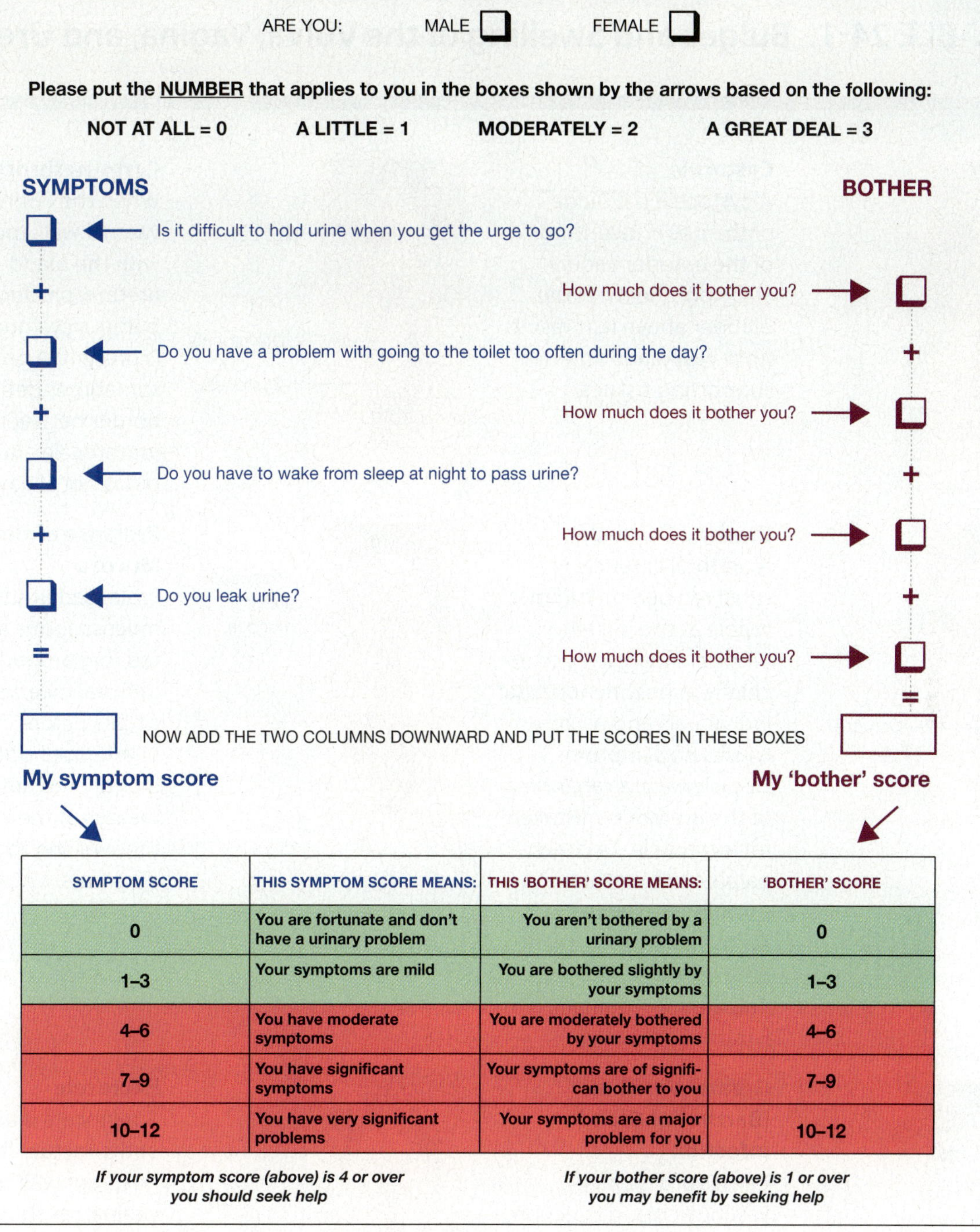

ARE YOU: MALE ☐ FEMALE ☐

Please put the NUMBER that applies to you in the boxes shown by the arrows based on the following:

NOT AT ALL = 0   A LITTLE = 1   MODERATELY = 2   A GREAT DEAL = 3

SYMPTOMS | **BOTHER**

☐ ← Is it difficult to hold urine when you get the urge to go?

+ How much does it bother you? → ☐

☐ ← Do you have a problem with going to the toilet too often during the day?

+ How much does it bother you? → ☐ +

☐ ← Do you have to wake from sleep at night to pass urine?

+ How much does it bother you? → ☐ +

☐ ← Do you leak urine?

= How much does it bother you? → ☐ +

=

☐ NOW ADD THE TWO COLUMNS DOWNWARD AND PUT THE SCORES IN THESE BOXES ☐

My symptom score | **My 'bother' score**

SYMPTOM SCORE	THIS SYMPTOM SCORE MEANS:	THIS 'BOTHER' SCORE MEANS:	'BOTHER' SCORE
0	You are fortunate and don't have a urinary problem	You aren't bothered by a urinary problem	0
1–3	Your symptoms are mild	You are bothered slightly by your symptoms	1–3
4–6	You have moderate symptoms	You are moderately bothered by your symptoms	4–6
7–9	You have significant symptoms	Your symptoms are of significan bother to you	7–9
10–12	You have very significant problems	Your symptoms are a major problem for you	10–12

If your symptom score (above) is 4 or over you should seek help

If your bother score (above) is 1 or over you may benefit by seeking help

IMPORTANT — if you have blood in your urine, have difficulty passing urine, or pain on passing urine, you MUST talk to your doctor about it.

FIGURE 24-20. Bladder Control Self-Assessment Questionnaire.[37] (Source: Basra RK, Cortes E, Khullar V, Kelleher C. A comparison study of two lower urinary tract symptoms screening tools in clinical practice: the B-SAQ and OAB-V8 questionnaires. *J Obstet Gynaecol.* 2012;32(7):666–671. Reprinted by permission of Taylor & Francis Ltd. http://www.tandfonline.com)

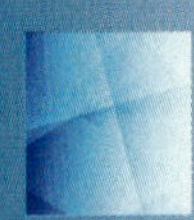

TABLE 24-1. Bulges and Swelling of the Vulva, Vagina, and Urethra

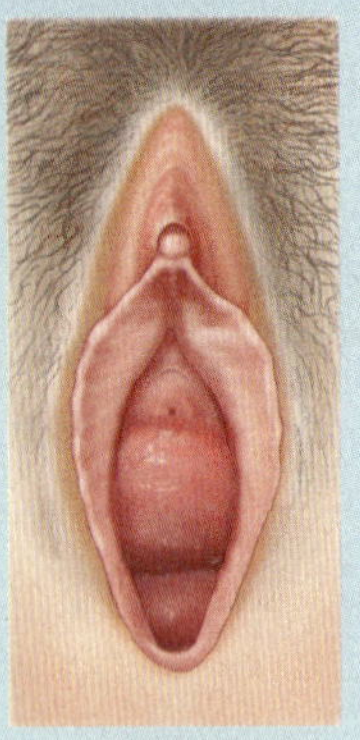

Cystocele

A cystocele is a bulge of the upper two-thirds of the anterior vaginal wall, together with the bladder above it. It results from weakened anterior supporting tissues.

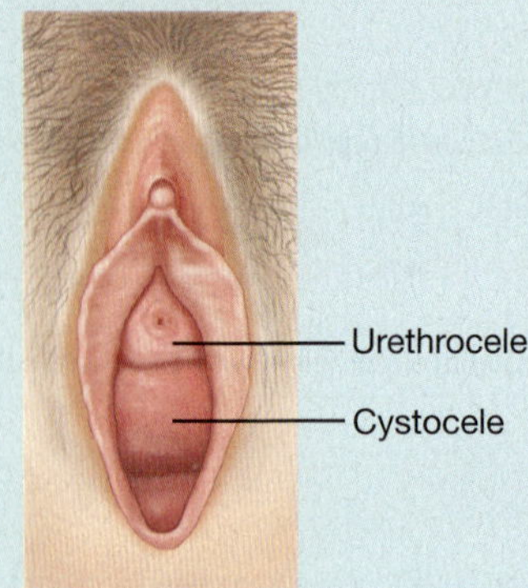

Cystourethrocele

When the entire anterior vaginal wall, together with the bladder and urethra, produces the bulge, a cystourethrocele is present. A groove sometimes defines the border between the urethrocele and cystocele, but is not always present.

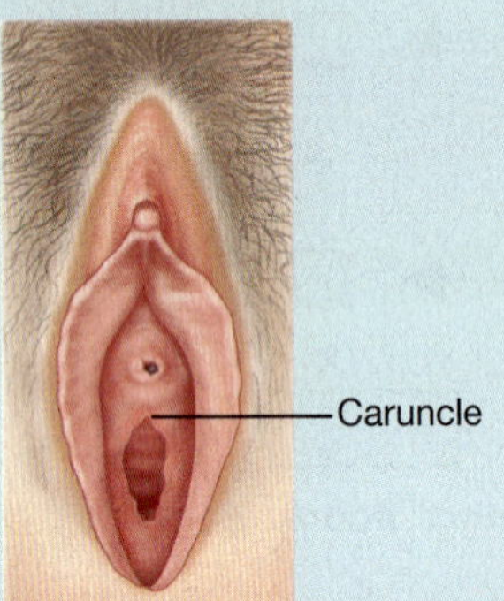

Urethral Caruncle

A urethral caruncle is a small red benign tumor visible at the posterior urethral meatus. It occurs chiefly in postmenopausal individuals and usually causes no symptoms. Occasionally, a carcinoma of the urethra is mistaken for a caruncle. To check, palpate the urethra through the vagina for thickening, nodularity, or tenderness, and palpate for inguinal lymphadenopathy.

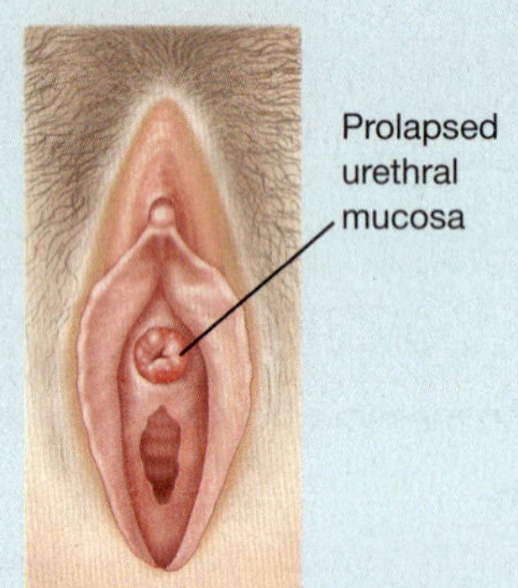

Prolapse of the Urethral Mucosa

Prolapsed urethral mucosa forms a swollen red ring around the urethral meatus. It usually occurs before menarche or after menopause. Identify the urethral meatus at the center of the swelling to make this diagnosis.

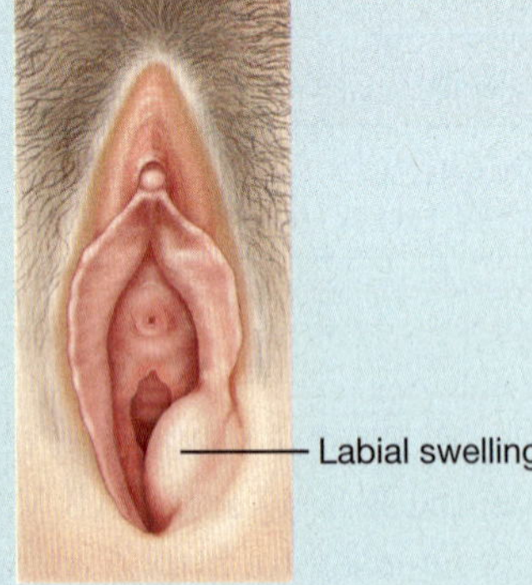

Greater Vestibular (Bartholin) Gland Infection

Causes of a greater vestibular gland infection include trauma, gonococci, anaerobes like bacteroides and peptostreptococci, and *C. trachomatis.* Acutely, the gland appears as a tense, hot, very tender abscess. Look for pus emerging from the duct or erythema around the duct opening. Chronically, a nontender cyst is felt that may be large or small.

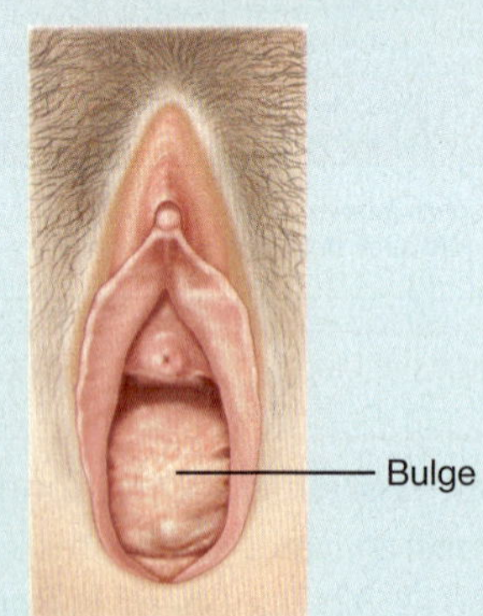

Rectocele

A rectocele is a herniation of the rectum into the posterior wall of the vagina, resulting from a weakness or defect in the endopelvic fascia.

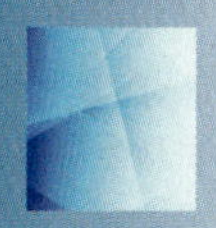

TABLE 24-2. Lesions of the Vulva

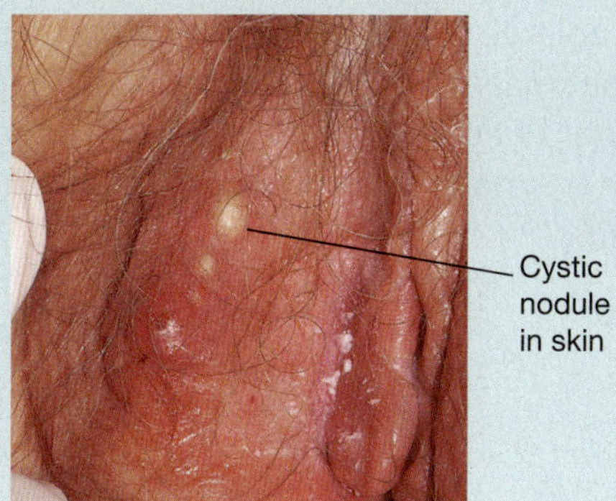

Epidermoid Cyst

A small firm round cystic nodule in the labia suggests an epidermoid cyst. These are yellowish in color. Look for the dark punctum marking the blocked opening of the gland.

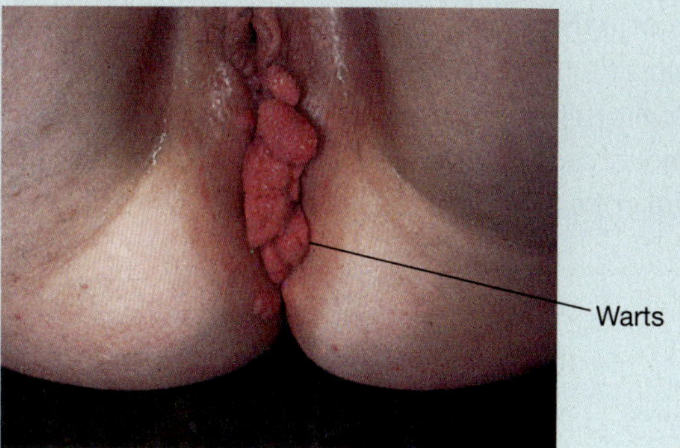

Venereal Wart (*Condyloma Acuminatum*)

Warty lesions on the labia and within the vestibule are often condyloma acuminata from infection with *human papillomavirus.*

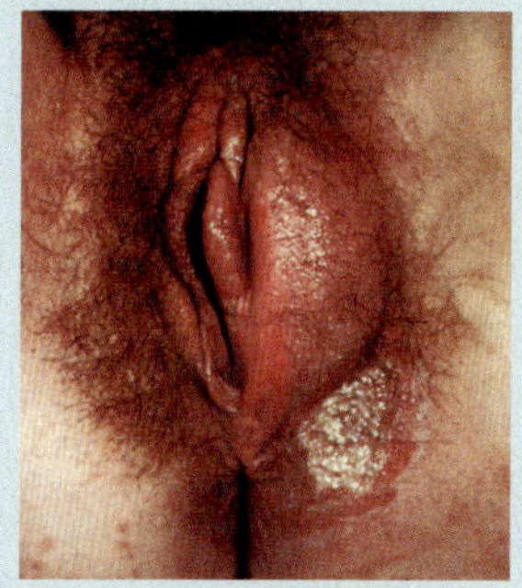

Syphilitic Chancre

This firm painless ulcer from primary syphilis forms—21 d after exposure to *Treponema pallidum.* It may remain hidden and undetected in the vagina and heals regardless of treatment in 3–6 wk.

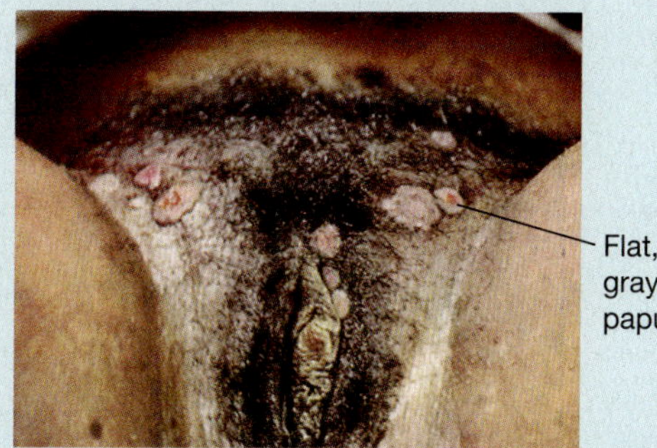

Secondary Syphilis (*Condyloma Latum*)

Large raised, round or oval, flat-topped gray or white lesions point to condylomata lata. These are contagious and, along with rash and mucous membrane sores in the mouth, vagina, or anus, are manifestations of secondary syphilis.

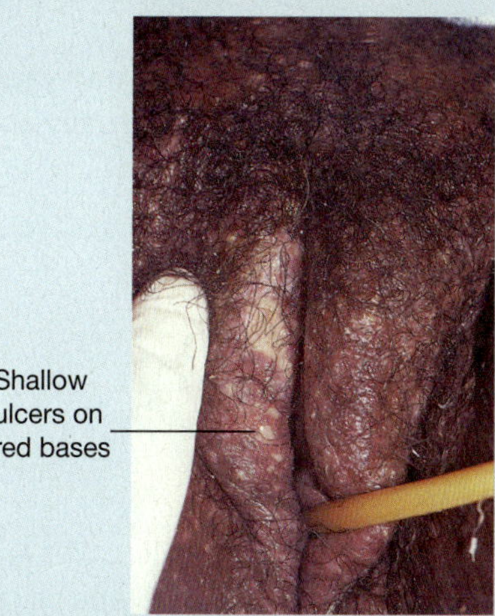

Genital Herpes

Shallow small painful ulcers on red bases are suspicious for infection from genital herpes simplex virus 1 or 2. Ulcers may take 2–4 wk to heal. Recurrent outbreaks of localized vesicles, then ulcers are common.

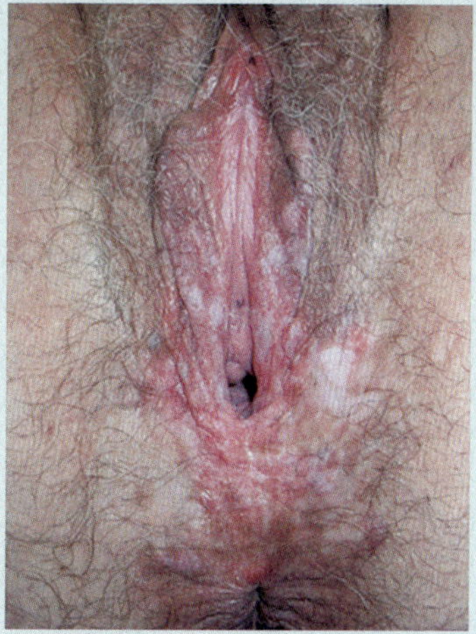

Carcinoma of the Vulva

An ulcerated or raised red vulvar lesion in an elderly patient may be a vulvar carcinoma, usually a squamous cell carcinoma arising on the labia.

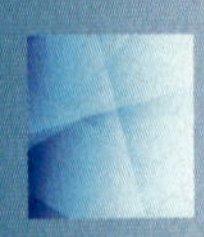

TABLE 24-3. Vaginal Discharge

Discharge from a vaginal infection must be distinguished from a physiologic discharge. A physiologic discharge is clear or white, may contain white clumps of epithelial cells, and is not malodorous. To distinguish vaginal from cervical discharges, use a large cotton swab to wipe off the cervix. If no cervical discharge is present in the os, suspect a vaginal origin and consider the causes below. Note that the diagnosis of cervicitis or vaginitis hinges on careful collection and analysis of the appropriate laboratory specimens.[16,17]

	Trichomonal Vaginitis	Candidal Vaginitis	Bacterial Vaginosis
	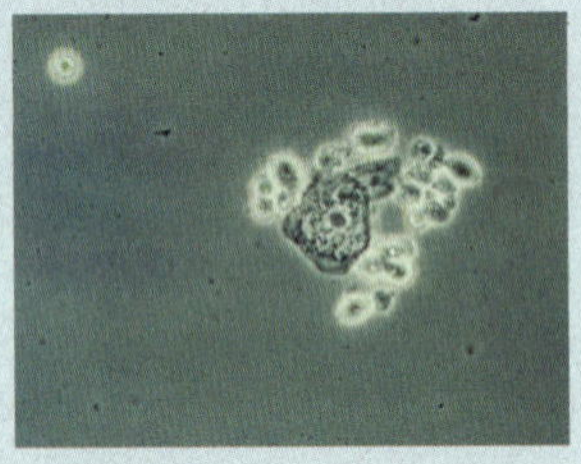	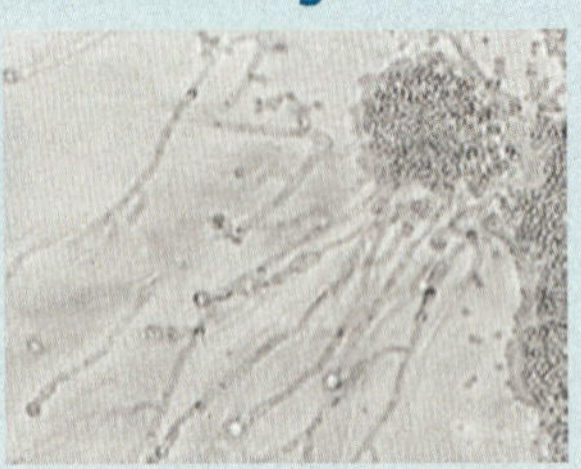	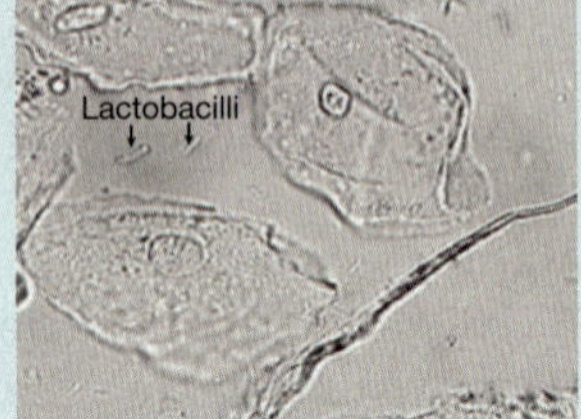
Cause	*Trichomonas vaginalis,* a protozoan; often but not always acquired sexually	*Candida albicans,* a yeast (normal overgrowth of vaginal flora); many factors predispose, including antibiotic therapy	Bacterial overgrowth probably from anaerobic bacteria; often transmitted sexually
Discharge	Yellowish green or gray, possibly frothy; often profuse and pooled in the vaginal fornix; may be malodorous	White and curdy; may be thin but typically thick; not as profuse as in trichomonal infection; not malodorous	Gray or white, thin, homogeneous, malodorous; coats the vaginal walls; usually not profuse, may be minimal
Other Symptoms	Pruritus (though not usually as severe as with *Candida* infection); pain on urination (from skin inflammation or possibly urethritis); dyspareunia	Pruritus; vaginal soreness; pain on urination (from skin inflammation); dyspareunia	Unpleasant strong, fish-like or musty quality genital odor; reported to occur after intercourse
Vulva and Vaginal Mucosa	Vestibule and labia minora may be erythematous; the vaginal mucosa may be diffusely reddened, with small red granular spots or petechiae in the posterior fornix; in mild cases, the mucosa looks normal	The vulva and even the surrounding skin are often inflamed and sometimes swollen to a variable extent; the vaginal mucosa is often reddened, with white tenacious patches of discharge; the mucosa may bleed when these patches are scraped off; in mild cases, the mucosa looks normal	The vulva and vaginal mucosa usually appear normal
Laboratory Evaluation	Scan saline wet mount for trichomonads	Scan potassium hydroxide (KOH) preparation for the branching hyphae of *Candida*	Scan saline wet mount for *clue cells* (epithelial cells with stippled borders); sniff for fish-like odor after applying KOH ("whiff test"); test the vaginal secretions for pH >4.5

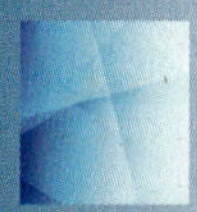

TABLE 24-4. Urinary Incontinence in Individuals Assigned Female at Birth

Problem	Mechanisms	Symptoms	Physical Signs
Stress Incontinence			
Urethral sphincter is weakened so that transient increases in intra-abdominal pressure raise the bladder pressure to levels that exceed urethral resistance.	Weakness of pelvic floor and inadequate support of the bladder neck and proximal urethra may be caused by childbirth, surgery, atrophy of the mucosa, and urethral infection.	Momentary leakage of small amounts of urine with coughing, laughing, sneezing; unrelated to the urge to urinate	Demonstrable stress incontinence, especially in a standing position; atrophic vaginitis may be evident; no bladder distention
Urge Incontinence			
Detrusor contractions are stronger than normal and overcome the normal urethral resistance; bladder is typically small	Detrusor contractions overcome normal urethral resistance; causes include decreased cortical inhibition from neurologic conditions or hyperexcitability of sensory pathways (bladder infections, tumors, fecal impaction)	Involuntary urine loss preceded by an urge to void, with urgency, frequency, nocturia, and (possibly) pain on urination	Small bladder not detectable on abdominal examination; signs of central nervous system disease, local pelvic problems, or fecal impaction may be present
Overflow Incontinence			
Detrusor contractions are insufficient to overcome urethral resistance, causing urinary retention; bladder is typically flaccid and large, even after an effort to void	Due to detrusor contractions insufficient to overcome urethral resistance, causing urinary retention	Continuous dripping or dribbling incontinence, decreased urinary stream force	Enlarged, sometimes tender bladder; other signs may include peripheral nerve disease symptoms, decreased sensation, and reflexes
Functional Incontinence			
Patient is functionally unable to reach the toilet in time because of impaired health or environmental conditions	Related to problems in mobility or environmental factors	Incontinence on the way to the toilet or only in the early morning	Bladder undetectable on examination; look for physical or environmental clues that point to the likely cause
Incontinence Secondary to Medications			
Drugs may contribute to any type of incontinence listed	Drugs contributing to incontinence include sedatives, antipsychotics, anticholinergics, sympathetic blockers, and potent diuretics.	Variable, depending on the medication	Variable, necessitating a careful history and chart review

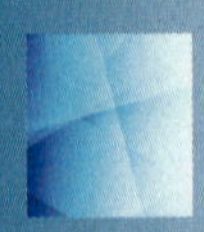

TABLE 24-5. Variations in the Cervical Surface

Two kinds of epithelia cover the cervix: (1) shiny pink *squamous epithelium,* which resembles the vaginal epithelium, and (2) deep red, plushy *columnar epithelium,* which is continuous with the endocervical lining. These meet at the *squamocolumnar junction.* When this junction is at or inside the cervical os, only squamous epithelium is seen. A ring of columnar epithelium is often visible to a varying extent around the os—the result of a normal process that accompanies fetal development, menarche, and the first pregnancy.[a]

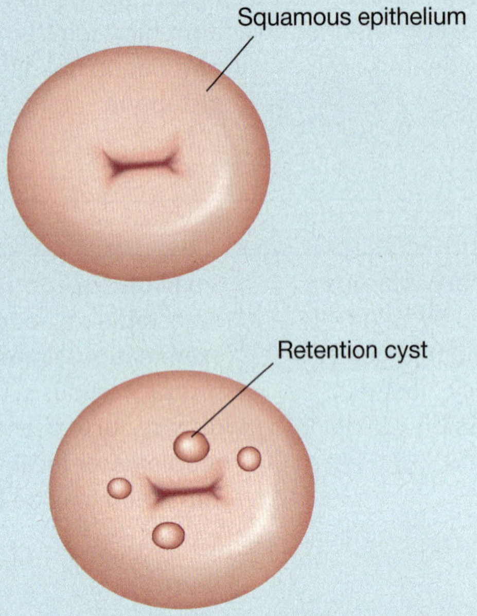

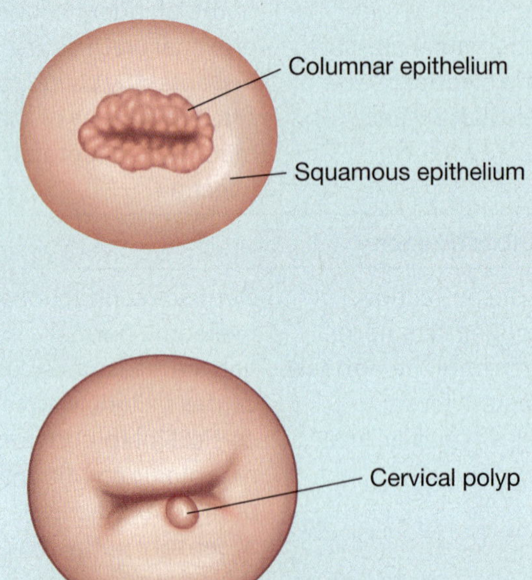

As estrogen stimulation increases during adolescence, all or part of this columnar epithelium is transformed into squamous epithelium by a process termed *metaplasia.* This change may block the secretions of columnar epithelium and cause *retention cysts,* also called *nabothian cysts.* These appear as translucent nodules on the cervical surface and have no pathologic significance.

A cervical polyp usually arises from the endocervical canal, becoming visible when it protrudes through the cervical os. It is bright red, soft, and rather fragile. When only the tip is seen, it cannot be differentiated clinically from a polyp originating in the endometrium. Polyps are benign but may bleed.

[a]Other terms for the columnar epithelium visible on the ectocervix are *ectropion, ectopy,* and *eversion.*

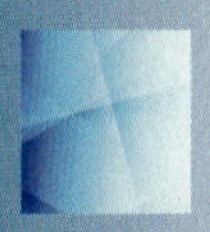

TABLE 24-6. Shapes of the Cervical Os

The table illustrates the different shapes of the cervical os, including both normal anatomical variations and changes that may occur from childbirth.

In individuals without a history of vaginal delivery, the cervical os typically appears as either an **oval** or **slit-like** opening. However, childbirth can lead to various types of **cervical lacerations**, which alter its appearance.

Common forms of delivery-related lacerations include the **bilateral transverse laceration**, characterized by a horizontal shape on both sides of the cervix; the **stellate laceration**, with multiple lacerations radiating outward in a star-like pattern; and the **unilateral transverse laceration**, marked by a single horizontal tear on one side. These variations are **normal findings** during gynecologic exams and provide insights into an individual's obstetric history.

Normal

Types of Lacerations from Delivery

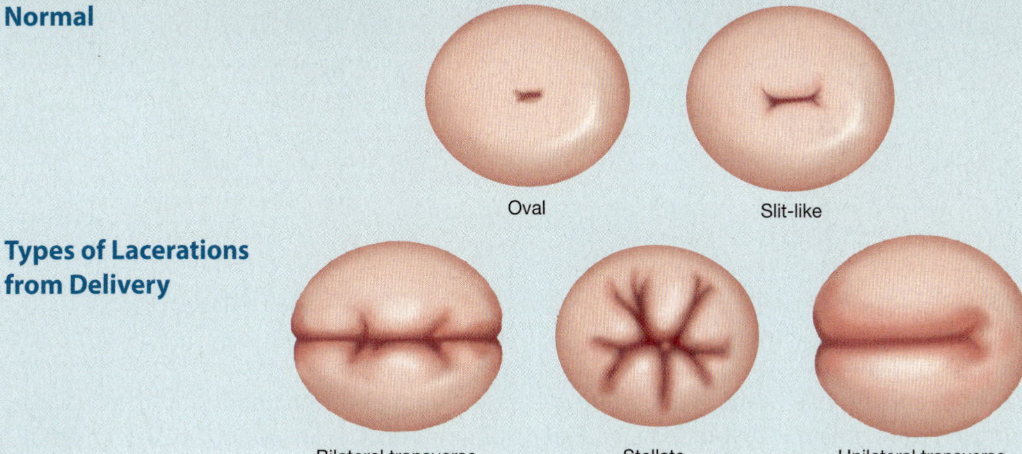

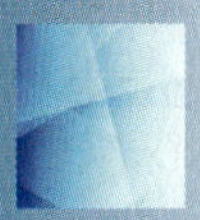

TABLE 24-7. Abnormalities of the Cervix

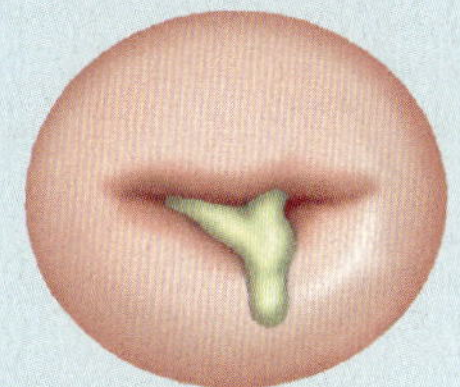

Mucopurulent Cervicitis

Mucopurulent cervicitis produces purulent yellow drainage from the cervical os, usually from *C. trachomatis, N. gonorrhoeae,* or herpes infection. These infections are sexually transmitted and may occur without symptoms or signs.

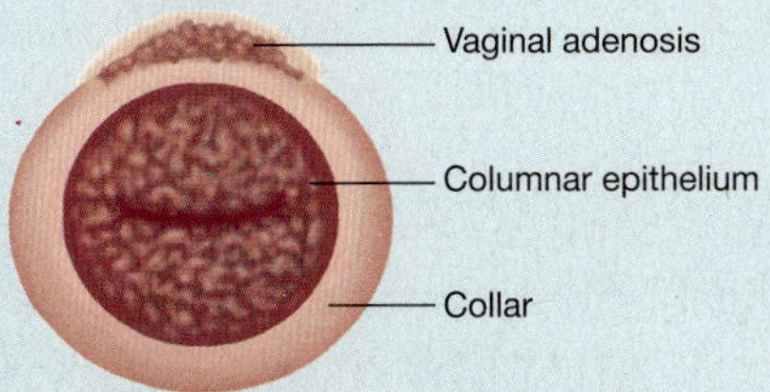

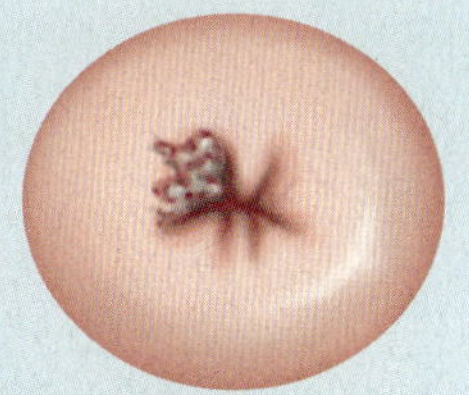

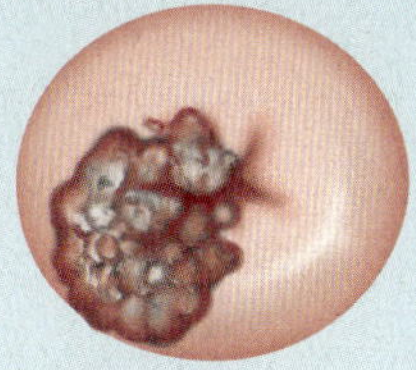

Carcinoma of the Cervix

Carcinoma of the cervix begins in an area of metaplasia. In its earliest stages, it cannot be distinguished from a normal cervix. In later stages, an extensive, irregular, cauliflower-like growth may develop. Early frequent intercourse, multiple partners, smoking, and infection with human papillomavirus increase the risk for cervical cancer.

Fetal Exposure to Diethylstilbestrol (DES)

Individuals exposed to DES in utero are at greatly increased risk for several abnormalities, including (1) columnar epithelium that covers most or all of the cervix, (2) vaginal adenosis (i.e., extension of this epithelium to the vaginal wall), and (3) a circular collar or ridge of tissue, of varying shapes, between the cervix and vagina. Much less common is an otherwise rare carcinoma of the upper vagina.

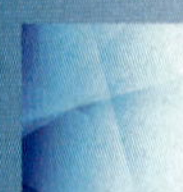

TABLE 24-8. Positions of the Uterus Retroversion and Retroflexion Are Usually Normal Variants

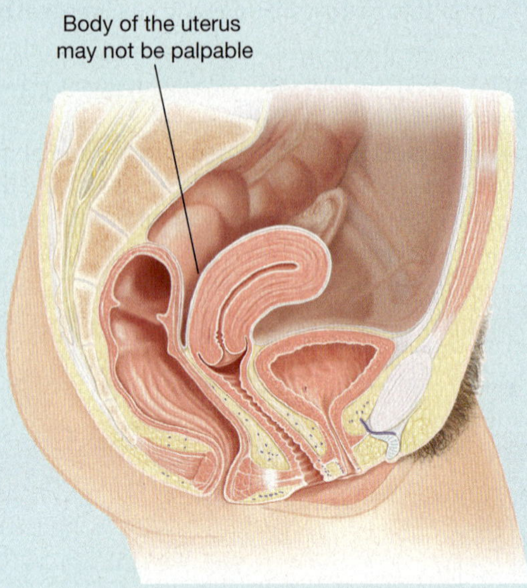

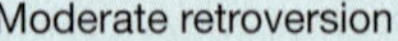
Moderate retroversion

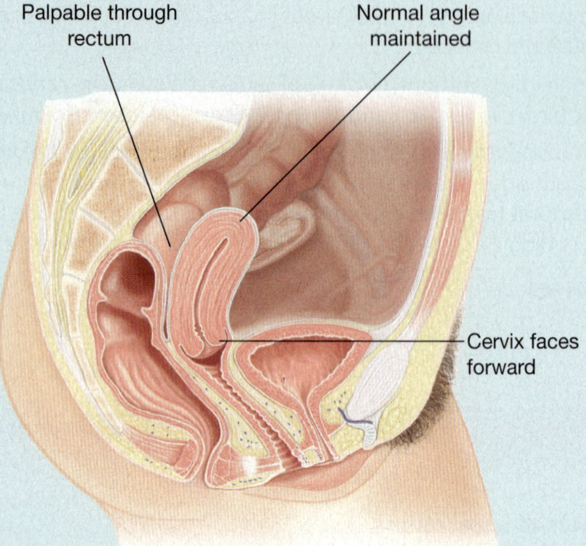

Marked retroversion

Retroversion of the Uterus

Retroversion of the uterus refers to a tilting backward of the entire uterus, including both the body and the cervix. It is a common variant occurring in approximately 20% of females. Early clues on pelvic examination are a cervix that faces forward and a uterine body that cannot be felt by the abdominal hand. In ***moderate retroversion,*** the body may not be palpable with either hand. In ***marked retroversion,*** the body can be felt posteriorly, either through the posterior fornix or through the rectum. A retroverted uterus is usually both mobile and asymptomatic. Occasionally, such a uterus is fixed and immobile, held in place by conditions such as endometriosis or PID.

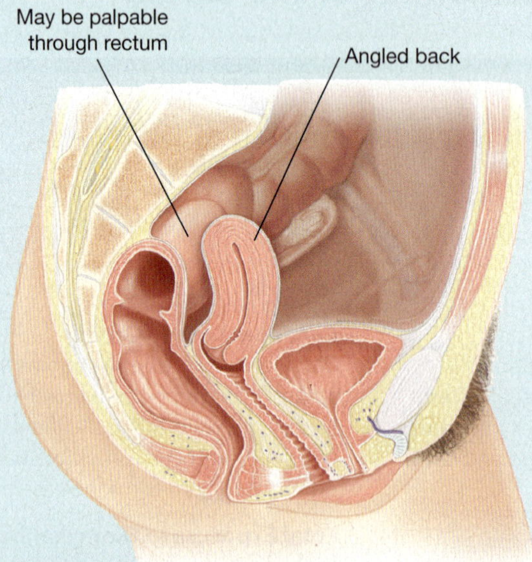

Retroflexion of the Uterus

Retroflexion of the uterus refers to a backward angulation of the body of the uterus in relation to the cervix. The cervix maintains its usual position. The body of the uterus is often palpable through the posterior fornix or through the rectum.

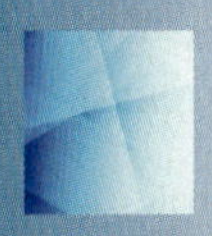

TABLE 24-9. Abnormalities of the Uterus

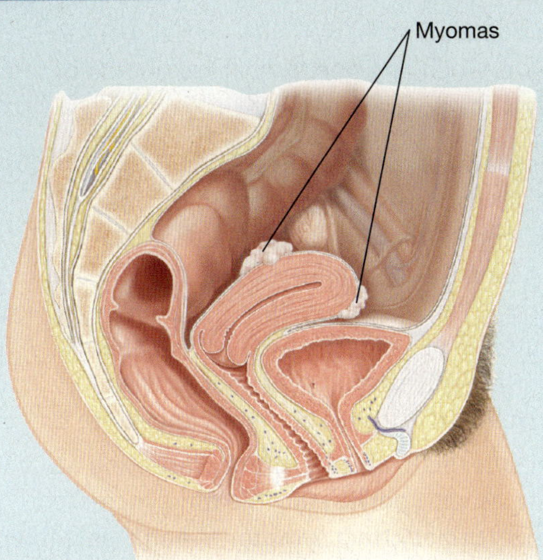

Myomas of the Uterus (Fibroids)

Myomas are very common benign uterine tumors. They may be single or multiple and vary greatly in size, occasionally reaching large proportions. They feel like firm irregular nodules that are continuous with the uterine surface. Occasionally, a myoma projecting laterally is confused with an ovarian mass; a nodule projecting posteriorly can be mistaken for a retroflexed uterus. Submucosal myomas project toward the endometrial cavity and are not palpable, although they may be suspected because of an enlarged uterus.

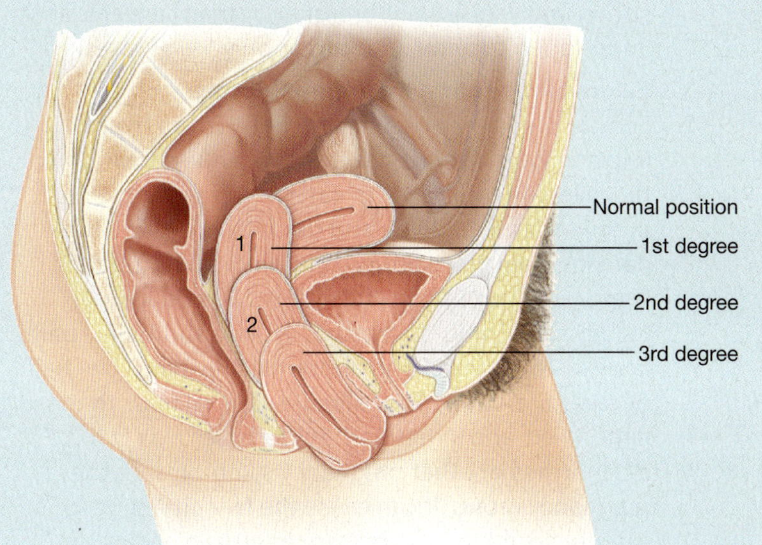

Prolapse of the Uterus

Prolapse of the uterus results from weakness of the supporting structures of the pelvic floor and is often associated with a cystocele and rectocele. In progressive stages, the uterus becomes retroverted and descends down the vaginal canal to the outside:

- In *first-degree prolapse*, the cervix is still well within the vagina.
- In *second-degree prolapse,* it is at the introitus.
- In *third-degree prolapse (procidentia)*, the cervix and vagina are outside the introitus.

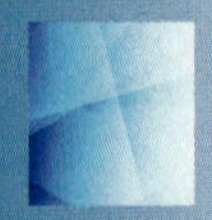

TABLE 24-10. Adnexal Masses

Adnexal masses typically result from disorders of the fallopian tubes or ovaries. Three examples—often hard to differentiate—are described. Note that inflammatory disease of the bowel (such as diverticulitis), carcinoma of the colon, and a pedunculated myoma of the uterus may simulate an adnexal mass.

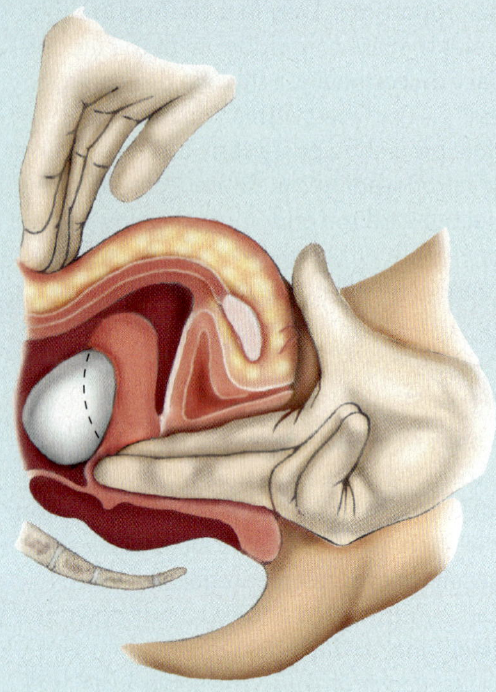

Ovarian Cysts and Ovarian Cancer

Ovarian cysts and tumors may cause adnexal masses, which can extend beyond the pelvis (see figure). Many benign simple and complex ovarian cysts resolve spontaneously. At times these cysts may rupture resulting in severe, acute pain. Enlarged ovaries with numerous follicles are commonly seen in polycystic ovarian syndrome which results from a hormonal imbalance.[38,39]

Ovarian cancer is relatively rare, often presenting at advanced stages with pelvic pain, bloating, increased abdominal size, urinary tract symptoms, and a palpable mass. Reliable screening tests are lacking, and while a strong family history of breast or ovarian cancer is an important risk factor, it occurs in only 5% of cases.[19]

Ectopic Pregnancy, Including Rupture

Ectopic pregnancy occurs when a fertilized ovum implants outside the endometrial cavity, primarily in the fallopian tube (90% of cases).[6,7] It affects 1–2% of pregnancies worldwide and risk factors include tubal damage from PID, prior ectopic pregnancy, tubal surgery, IUD presence, and assisted reproductive techniques. Common features include abdominal pain, adnexal tenderness, and abnormal bleeding. Over half of cases present with a palpable adnexal mass that is large, fixed, and ill-defined. Milder cases may involve amenorrhea or other pregnancy symptoms. As the pregnancy grows, it can cause the fallopian tube to rupture resulting in significant internal bleeding and shock. These severe cases can be life threatening and require emergency surgery.

Pelvic Inflammatory Disease

PID is due to "spontaneous ascension of microbes from the cervix or vagina to the endometrium, fallopian tubes, and adjacent structures."[40] STIs, primarily *N. gonorrhoeae* and *C. trachomatis,* are the main causes of PID. Hallmarks of acute disease are adnexal, cervical, and uterine tenderness. If not treated, serious reproductive sequelae such as tubo-ovarian abscesses and or infertility may ensue. Therefore, even though the clinical diagnosis of PID is imprecise, empiric treatment with antibiotics should be initiated without delay in order to protect the patients' reproductive future.

REFERENCES

1. Chumlea WC, Schubert CM, Roche AF, et al. Age at menarche and racial comparisons in US girls. *Pediatrics.* 2003;111(1):110–113.
2. Finer LB, Philbin JM. Trends in ages at key reproductive transitions in the United States, 1951–2010. *Women's Health Issues.* 2014;24(3):e271–e279.
3. Kaplowitz P. Pubertal development in girls: secular trends. *Curr Opin Obstet Gynecol.* 2006;18(5):487–491.
4. Freeman EW, Sammel MD, Lin H, Rickels K, Sondheimer SJ. Clinical subtypes of premenstrual syndrome and responses to sertraline treatment. *Obstet Gynecol.* 2011;118(6):1293–1300.
5. Munro MG, Critchley HO, Broder MS, Fraser IS, Disorders FWGoM. FIGO classification system (PALM-COEIN) for causes of abnormal uterine bleeding in nongravid women of reproductive age. *Int J Gynaecol Obstet.* 2011;113(1):3–13.
6. Orazulike NC, Konje JC. Diagnosis and management of ectopic pregnancy. *Women's Health (Lond).* 2013;9(4):373–385.
7. Barnhart KT. Clinical practice. Ectopic pregnancy. *N Engl J Med.* 2009;361(4):379–387.
8. Chronic Pelvic Pain (CPP). International Pelvic Pain Society. Accessed October 14, 2024. https://www.pelvicpain.org/images/pdf/Patient%20Info%20Handouts%202023/Chronic%20Pelvic%20Pain%20CPP%202023.pdf
9. Chapter 26: anatomy of the female pelvis. In: Johnson CT, Hallock JL, Bienstock JL, Fox HE, Wallach EE, eds. *Johns Hopkins Manual of Gynecology and Obstetrics.* 5th ed. Lippincott Williams & Wilkins; 2015:338.
10. Hatzichristou D, Rosen RC, Derogatis LR, et al. Recommendations for the clinical evaluation of men and women with sexual dysfunction. *J Sex Med.* 2010;7(1 Pt 2):337–348.
11. Platano G, Margraf J, Alder J, Bitzer J. Psychosocial factors and therapeutic approaches in the context of sexual history taking in men: a study conducted among Swiss general practitioners and urologists. *J Sex Med.* 2008;5(11):2533–2556.
12. Kruszka PS, Kruszka SJ. Evaluation of acute pelvic pain in women. *Am Fam Physician.* 2010;82(2):141–147.
13. Bettez M, Tu LM, Carlson K, et al. 2012 update: guidelines for adult urinary incontinence collaborative consensus document for the Canadian Urological Association. *Can Urol Assoc J.* 2012;6(5):354–363.
14. Markland AD, Vaughan CP, Johnson TM 2nd, Burgio KL, Goode PS. Incontinence. *Med Clin North Am.* 2011;95(3):539–554.
15. Holroyd-Leduc JM, Tannenbaum C, Thorpe KE, Straus SE. What type of urinary incontinence does this woman have? *JAMA.* 2008;299(12):1446–1456.
16. Wilson JF. In the clinic. Vaginitis and cervicitis. *Ann Intern Med.* 2009;151(5):ITC3-1–ITC3-16.
17. Eckert LO. Clinical practice. Acute vulvovaginitis. *N Engl J Med.* 2006;355(12):1244–1252.
18. Sexually Transmitted Infections Treatment Guidelines. Division of STD Prevention; National Center for HIV, Viral Hepatitis, STD, and TB Prevention; Centers for Disease Control and Prevention. Accessed January 1, 2024. https://www.cdc.gov/std/treatment-guidelines/default.htm
19. Jayson GC, Kohn EC, Kitchener HC, Ledermann JA. Ovarian cancer. *Lancet.* 2014;384(9951):1376–1388.
20. Tarnay CM, et al. "Urinary Incontinence & Pelvic Floor Disorders." In: DeCherney AH, et al. eds. *CURRENT Diagnosis & Treatment: Obstetrics & Gynecology,* 12th ed. McGraw-Hill Education, 2019. Accessed Januray 4, 2024. https://accessmedicine.mhmedical.com/content.aspx?bookid=2559§ionid=206964948
21. Southgate SJ, Herbst MK. Ultrasound of the urinary tract. In: *StatPearls.* StatPearls Publishing; January 16, 2023. Accessed October 14, 2024. https://www.statpearls.com/point-of-care/43410
22. Chan H. Noninvasive bladder volume measurement. *J Neurosci Nurs.* 1993;25(5):309–312.
23. Sung H, Ferlay J, Siegel RL, et al. Global Cancer Statistics 2020: GLOBOCAN estimates of incidence and mortality worldwide for 36 cancers in 185 countries. *CA Cancer J Clin.* 2021;71(3):209–249.
24. Siegel RL, Miller KD, Wagle NS, Jemal A. Cancer statistics, 2023. *CA Cancer J Clin.* 2023;73(1):17–48.
25. Surveillance Research Program. *SEER*Explorer: An interactive website for SEER cancer statistics.* National Cancer Institute. Updated July 31, 2023. Accessed October 26, 2023. https://seer.cancer.gov/statistics-network/explorer/
26. American Cancer Society. Risk Factors for Cervical Cancer. Accessed October 29, 2023. https://www.cancer.org/cancer/types/cervical-cancer/causes-risks-prevention/risk-factors
27. Meites E, Szilagyi PG, Chesson HW, Unger ER, Romero JR, Markowitz LE. Human papillomavirus vaccination for adults: updated recommendations of the Advisory Committee on Immunization Practices. *MMWR Morb Mortal Wkly Rep.* 2019;68(32):698–702.
28. Sawaya GF, Huchko MJ. Cervical cancer screening. *Med Clin North Am.* 2017;101(4):743–753.
29. U. S. Preventive Services Task Force, Curry SJ, Krist AH, et al. Screening for cervical cancer: US Preventive Services Task Force Recommendation Statement. *JAMA.* 2018;320(7):674–686.
30. Manson JE, Chlebowski RT, Stefanick ML, et al. Menopausal hormone therapy and health outcomes during the intervention and extended poststopping phases of the Women's Health Initiative randomized trials. *JAMA.* 2013;310(13):1353–1368.
31. U. S. Preventive Services Task Force, Mangione CM, Barry MJ, et al. Hormone therapy for the primary prevention of chronic conditions in postmenopausal persons: US Preventive Services Task Force Recommendation Statement. *JAMA.* 2022;328(17):1740–1746.
32. North American Menopause Society Advisory Panel. The 2022 hormone therapy position statement of The North American Menopause Society. *Menopause.* 2022;29(7):767–794.
33. O'Reilly N, Nelson HD, Conry JM, et al. Screening for urinary incontinence in women: a Recommendation From the Women's Preventive Services Initiative. *Ann Intern Med.* 2018;169(5):320–328.
34. Vaughan CP, Markland AD. Urinary incontinence in women. *Ann Intern Med.* 2020;172(3):ITC17–ITC32.
35. Daugirdas SP, Markossian T, Mueller ER, Durazo-Arvizu R, Cao G, Kramer H. Urinary incontinence and chronic conditions in the US population age 50 years and older. *Int Urogynecol J.* 2020;31(5):1013–1020.
36. Brown JS, Bradley CS, Subak LL, et al. The sensitivity and specificity of a simple test to distinguish between urge and stress urinary incontinence. *Ann Intern Med.* 2006;144(10):715–723.
37. Basra RK, Cortes E, Khullar V, Kelleher C. A comparison study of two lower urinary tract symptoms screening tools in clinical practice: the B-SAQ and OAB-V8 questionnaires. *J Obstet Gynaecol.* 2012;32(7):666–671.

38. Legro RS, Arslanian SA, Ehrmann DA, et al. Diagnosis and treatment of polycystic ovary syndrome: an Endocrine Society Clinical Practice Guideline. *J Clin Endocrinol Metab.* 2013;98(12):4565–4592.
39. Ehrmann DA. Polycystic ovary syndrome. *N Engl J Med.* 2005;352(12):1223–1236.
40. Brunham RC, Gottlieb SL, Paavonen J. Pelvic inflammatory disease. *N Engl J Med.* 2015;372(21):2039–2048.
41. US Preventive Services Task Force. Screening for cervical cancer: US Preventive Services Task Force recommendation statement. *JAMA.* 2018;320(7):674–686.
42. Huh WK, Ault KA, Chelmow D, et al. Use of primary high-risk human papillomavirus testing for cervical cancer screening: interim clinical guidance. *J Low Genit Tract Dis.* 2015;19(2):91–96.
43. Saslow D, Solomon D, Lawson HW, et al. American Cancer Society, American Society for Colposcopy and Cervical Pathology, and American Society for Clinical Pathology screening guidelines for the prevention and early detection of cervical cancer. *CA Cancer J Clin.* 2012;62(3): 147–172.
44. Fontham ETH, Wolf AMD, Church TR, et al. Cervical cancer screening for individuals at average risk: 2020 guideline update from the American Cancer Society. *CA Cancer J Clin.* 2020;70(5):321–346.
45. American College of Obstetricians and Gynecologists. Updated Cervical Cancer Screening Guidelines. Accessed October 28, 2023. https://www.acog.org/clinical/clinical-guidance/practice-advisory/articles/2021/04/updated-cervical-cancer-screening-guidelines

CHAPTER 25

Musculoskeletal System: Neck, Shoulders, and Upper Extremities

ANATOMY AND PHYSIOLOGY: GENERAL MUSCULOSKELETAL SYSTEM

The musculoskeletal system, an intricate network of bones, muscles, joints, and ligaments, is fundamental in providing structure and enabling movement in the human body. It encompasses the *vertebral spine*, a central pillar of support, and various *joints* that facilitate a wide range of physical activities. As you learn to examine the musculoskeletal system, focus on understanding the anatomy and its integration in facilitating movement. Emphasize not only the roles of individual joints but also the coordinated function of muscles, bones, and connective tissues throughout the entire system to appreciate how these components work together to enable various bodily movements.

Vertebral Spine

The *vertebral column*, or *spine*, is the central supporting structure of the neck, trunk, and back. The *concave curves* of the cervical and lumbar spine and the *convex curves* of the thoracic and sacrococcygeal spine help distribute upper body weight to the pelvis and lower extremities and cushion the concussive impact of walking or running (Fig. 25-1). Each region of the spine has unique characteristics (Box 25-1).

The vertebral column encases and protects the *spinal cord*, from which *spinal nerve roots* emerge. These nerve roots exit through the *intervertebral foramina* and are integral to the body's sensory and motor functions. The health and alignment of the vertebral column directly affect the spinal cord and nerve roots, with implications for neurologic function.

The complex mechanics of the spine reflect the coordinated action of vertebrae, intervertebral discs, ligaments, and muscles. The vertebral column contains *24 vertebrae* stacked on the sacrum and coccyx. A typical vertebra

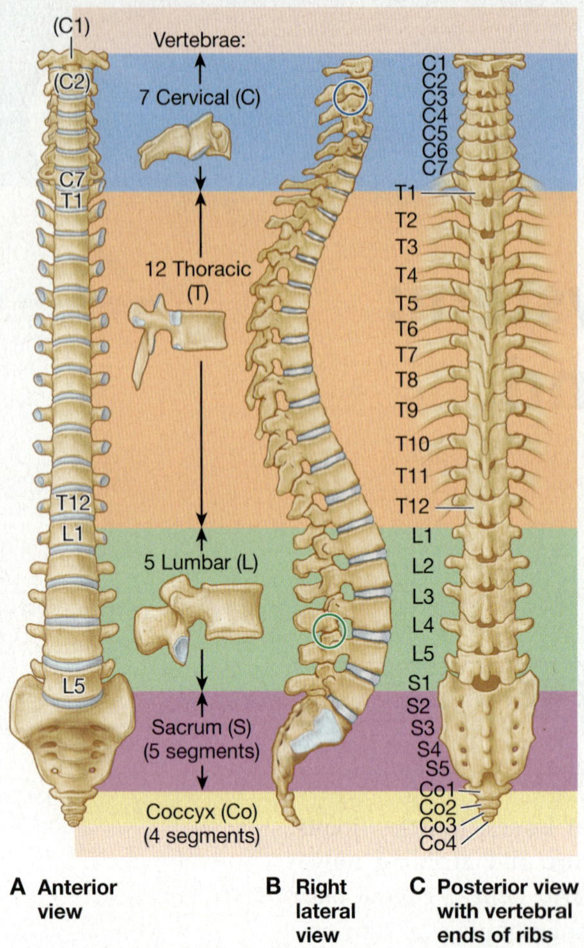

FIGURE 25-1. Three views of the vertebral columns. (Reprinted with permission from Moore KL, Dalley AF II, Agur AMR. *Clinically Oriented Anatomy.* 8th ed. Wolters Kluwer; 2018. Figure 2.1A-C.)

Box 25-1. Overview of Vertebral Spinal Regions

Vertebral Spine Region	General Function	Natural Curvature	Number of Vertebrae
Cervical	Designed for mobility, with smaller vertebrae and a greater range of motion	Lordotic (inward curve of the spine)	7
Thoracic	Provides stability with less flexibility, attached to the rib cage	Kyphotic (outward curve of the spine)	12
Lumbar	Bears the bulk of the body's weight, larger, robust vertebrae	Lordotic	5
Sacral	Provides a base for the pelvis, forms part of the pelvis	Kyphotic	5 (fused)
Coccygeal	Supports sitting, attachment site for ligaments and muscles	Kyphotic	3–5 (fused)

Box 25-2. Structural Components and Functions of the Vertebra

Component	Location/Description	Function
Vertebral body	Anteriorly positioned	Supports weight-bearing
Vertebral arch	Posteriorly located	Encloses the spinal cord
Spinous process	Projects posteriorly in the midline; bifid in the cervical spine	Serves as a muscular attachment site
Transverse processes	At the junction of the pedicle and the lamina; shorter in the cervical spine	Serve as muscular attachment sites
Articular processes (facets)	Two on each side of a vertebra, one facing up and one down, at the junction of the pedicles and laminae	Facilitate vertebral articulation
Intervertebral foramen	Formed by the inferior and superior articulating process of adjacent vertebrae	Provides a channel for spinal nerve roots
Transverse foramen	Present in the transverse process (cervical spine only)	Allows passage of the vertebral artery

contains sites for joint articulations, weight bearing, and muscle attachments as well as foramina for the spinal nerve roots to exit (Box 25-2).

The proximity of the spinal cord and spinal nerve roots to their bony vertebral casing and the intervertebral discs makes them vulnerable to disc herniation, impingement from degenerative changes in the vertebrae and facets, and trauma.

The flexibility of the spine is largely determined by the angle of the articular facet joints relative to the plane of the vertebral body. This varies at different levels of the spine, with the lower spine generally being less movable than the upper spine. The *intervertebral discs* between the vertebral bodies cushion movement and allow the vertebral column to curve, flex, and bend. These discs consist of a soft central core called the *nucleus pulposus* surrounded by a tough fibrous tissue, the *annulus fibrosis.*

Cervical Spine. The *cervical spine*, comprising the uppermost seven vertebrae (C1–C7) of the spinal column, is instrumental in supporting the head and facilitating diverse movements of the neck. This region is characterized by its high mobility, particularly in nodding and rotational movements, a feature enabled by the specialized design of the first two cervical vertebrae (Figs. 25-2 and 25-3): the *atlas* (C1) and the *axis* (C2).

Each cervical vertebra has a small body and larger vertebral foramen compared to other spinal regions, reflecting the balance between support and mobility (Figs. 25-4 and 25-5). The unique *transverse foramina* in these vertebrae allow passage for the vertebral arteries, vital for cerebral blood supply. The atlas and axis are distinctive: the atlas lacks a body and articulates with the occipital condyles, allowing for nodding motions, while the axis has a prominent dens (*odontoid process*) for pivotal head rotation.

The *cervical spinal nerves* (C1–C8), emerging from the vertebral column, form the *brachial plexus*, innervating the shoulders, arms, and hands.

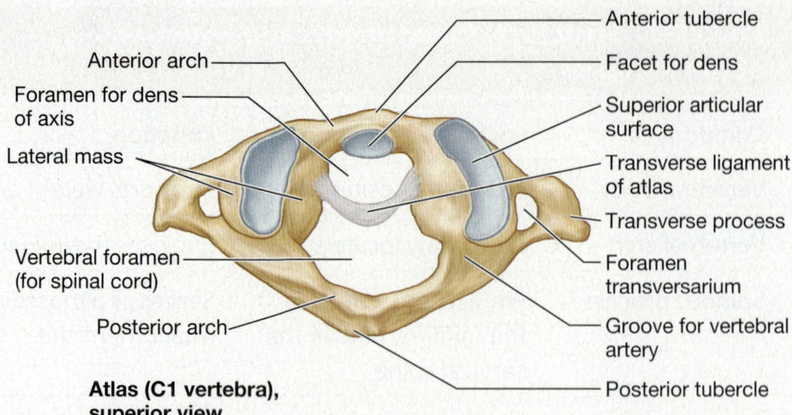

FIGURE 25-2. C1 vertebra: Atlas. (Reprinted with permission from Moore KL, Dalley AF II, Agur AMR. *Clinically Oriented Anatomy.* 8th ed. Wolters Kluwer; 2018. Figure 2.6B.)

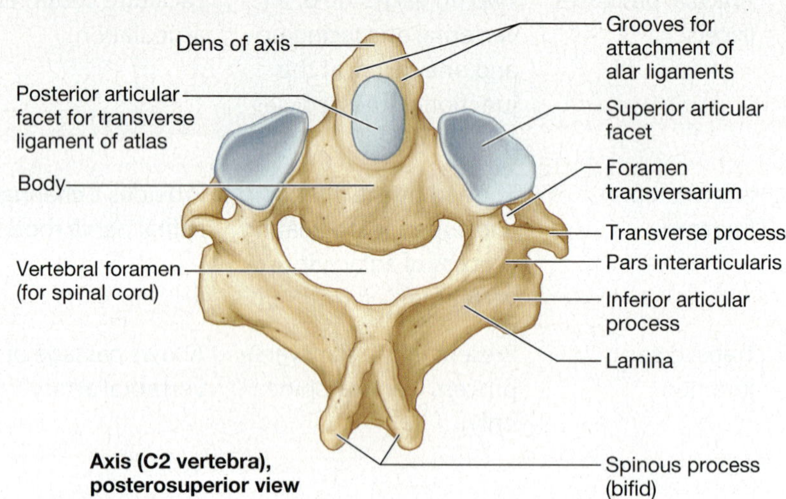

FIGURE 25-3. C2 vertebra: Axis. (Reprinted with permission from Moore KL, Dalley AF II, Agur AMR. *Clinically Oriented Anatomy.* 8th ed. Wolters Kluwer; 2018. Figure 2.6D.)

Thoracic Spine. The *thoracic spine*, also known as the *mid-back*, comprises T1 to T12. It extends from the base of the cervical spine to the lumbar spine. Unlike the highly flexible cervical spine, the 12 thoracic vertebrae are less mobile and primarily designed to provide stability and protection to vital organs. The thoracic spine plays a crucial role in protecting the heart, lungs, and other thoracic organs. Its stability also supports posture and provides a foundation for upper body movements.

Each thoracic vertebra has a unique structure, characterized by a vertebral body, spinous process, transverse processes, and *rib facets* (Fig. 25-6). The presence of *rib facets* on the vertebrae allows for the attachment of ribs, contributing to the structure and protection of the chest cavity.

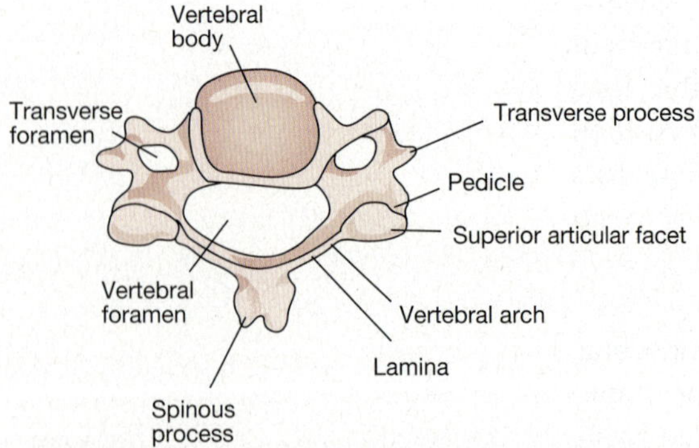

FIGURE 25-4. C4–C5 vertebrae coronal views.

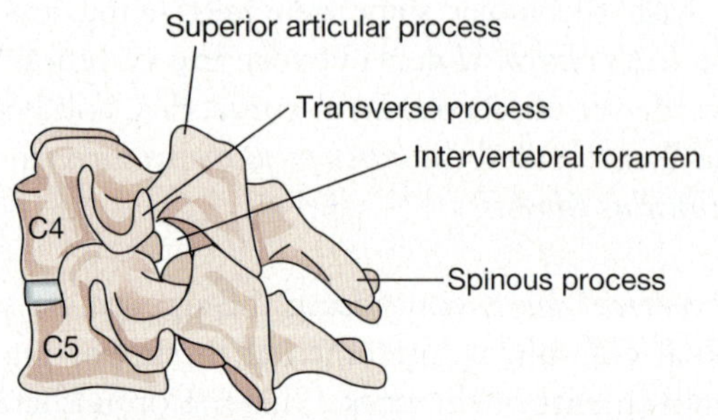

FIGURE 25-5. C4–C5 vertebrae lateral views.

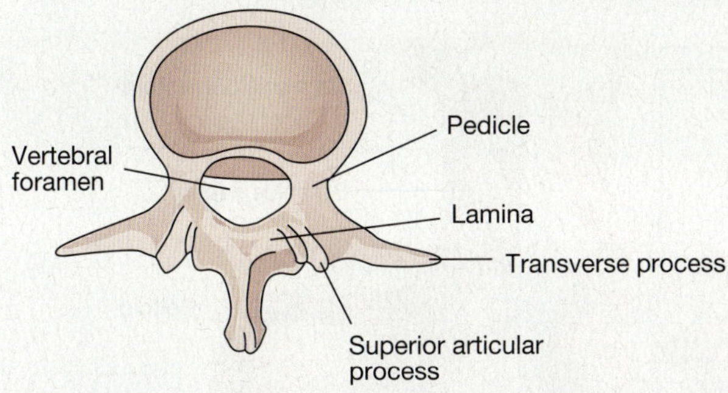

FIGURE 25-6. T12 vertebra coronal view.

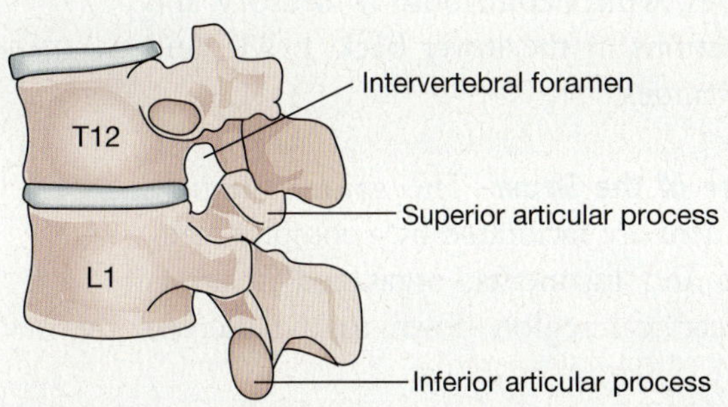

FIGURE 25-7. T12 and L1 vertebrae, lateral views.

Innervation of the thoracic spine is through the spinal nerves that exit between each pair of vertebrae. These nerves contribute to sensory and motor functions in the chest and upper abdominal regions.

Lumbar Spine. The *lumbar spine*, often referred to as the *lower back*, consists of L1 to L5. It is positioned below the thoracic spine and above the sacrum. The five lumbar vertebrae are the largest and strongest in the spine, designed to bear most of the body's weight and facilitate bending and twisting movements.

Each lumbar vertebra is characterized by a robust vertebral body, a thick and blunt spinous process, and robust transverse processes (Fig. 25-7). The structural features of the lumbar spine contribute to its weight-bearing capacity and flexibility.

The lumbar spine plays a pivotal role in providing stability and mobility to the lower back and trunk. It is responsible for maintaining an upright posture and facilitating various movements, such as bending forward (*flexion*), leaning backward (*extension*), and twisting (*rotation*).

Innervation of the lumbar spine is through the lumbar spinal nerves, which extend from the spinal cord and supply sensation and motor control to the lower back and lower extremities.

Sacrococcygeal Spine

The *sacrococcygeal spine*, also known as the sacrum and coccyx, comprises the lowest portion of the vertebral column. It consists of the *sacrum*, a triangular-shaped bone formed by the fusion of S1 to S5, and the *coccyx*, a small, tail-like structure at the base of the spine. The sacrum serves as a crucial junction point between the spine and the pelvis (Fig. 25-8).

The primary function of the sacrococcygeal spine is to provide support and stability to the pelvic region. It acts as an anchor for the hip bones (*ilium*) on either side, forming the *sacroiliac joints*. These joints play a vital role in transmitting the body's weight and forces from the spine to the pelvis and lower extremities.

Beyond its structural role, the sacrum also protects the sensitive nerves of the sacral canal, which continue as the *cauda equina* of the spinal cord. Innervation of the sacrococcygeal spine involves the *sacral*

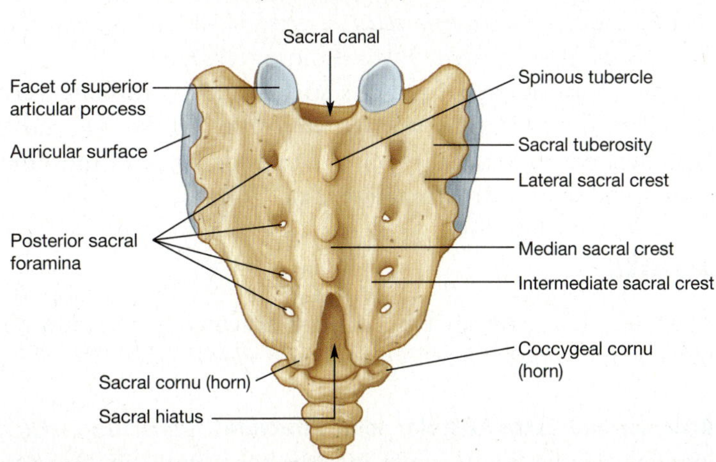

FIGURE 25-8. Sacrum and coccyx. (From the Anatomical Chart Company; Wolters Kluwer.)

spinal nerves, which contribute to sensory and motor functions in the lower back, pelvis, and lower extremities.

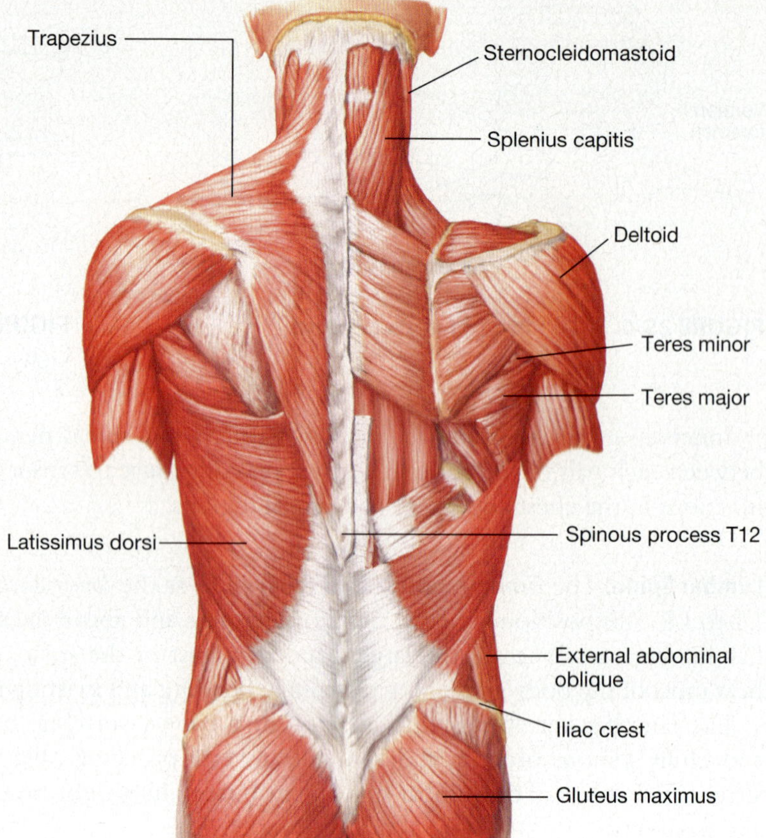

FIGURE 25-9. Muscles of the back.

Musculature of the Spine. The spine's support and movement are facilitated by a complex array of muscles and ligaments, organized in layers from the cervical region down to the sacrum (Fig. 25-9).

- Cervical region: At the top, the cervical spine is supported by muscles like the *sternocleidomastoid (SCM)* and *scalenes*, which assist in neck rotation and flexion. This region's stability and motion are further aided by intricate ligament networks.
- Thoracic region: Moving down to the thoracic spine, muscles such as the *erector spinae* and *intercostal muscles* contribute to maintaining posture and enabling controlled trunk rotation. Ligaments including the *ligamentum flavum* and *thoracolumbar fascia* provide additional structural support.
- Lumbar region: In the lower back, the lumbar spine is encased by the *lumbar erector spinae*, *psoas muscles*, and *abdominal muscles*, playing significant roles in trunk stability and movement. The lumbar region is structurally supported by the *anterior and posterior longitudinal ligaments* and the *supraspinous ligament*.
- Sacral region: The base of the spine, the sacrum, is stabilized by various ligaments, including the *sacroiliac* and *sacrococcygeal ligaments*, crucial for maintaining pelvic alignment.

Above all these, large, superficial muscles like the *trapezius* and *latissimus dorsi* form the outermost layer, attaching to each side of the spine. They overlie deeper muscle layers that attach to the head, neck, and spinous processes, such as the *splenius capitis*, *splenius cervicis*, and *sacrospinalis*, as well as smaller *intrinsic muscles* situated between the vertebrae.

This entire system of muscles and ligaments, running vertically down the spine, like the *paraspinal muscles* (*iliocostalis*, *longissimus*, and *spinalis*), ensures both flexibility and stability, enabling a wide range of movements while maintaining the spine's structural integrity.

Joints

There are three primary types of joint articulation allowing varying degrees of movement: *Synovial*, *cartilaginous*, and *fibrous joints* (Box 25-3).

Articular and Extra-Articular Joint Structures. *Articular structures*, which are integral to the joint itself, include the joint capsule, articular cartilage, synovium, synovial fluid, intra-articular ligaments, and juxta-articular bone.

Box 25-3. Types of Synovial Joints

Type of Joint	Description	Movement	Examples
Synovial			
Spheroidal (ball and socket) 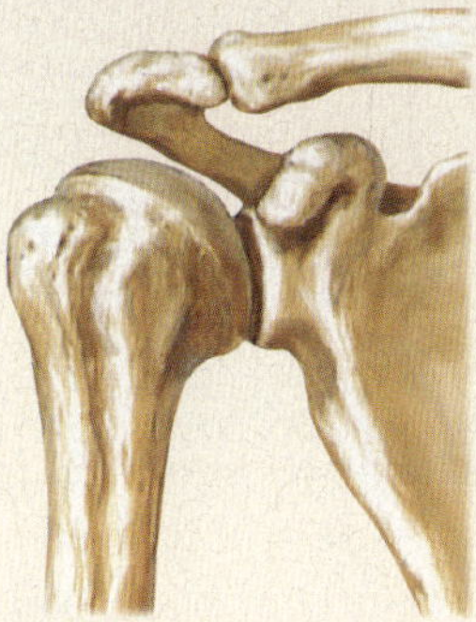	Rounded, convex surface fitting into a concave cavity; allows for a wide range of rotatory movements	Wide-ranging–flexion, extension, abduction, adduction, rotation, circumduction	Shoulder, hip
Hinge 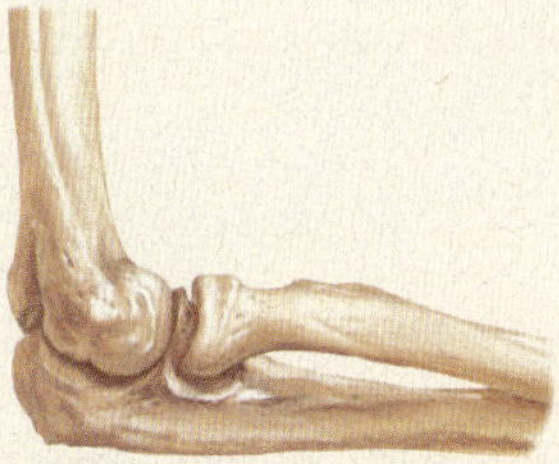	Flat, planar, or slightly curved surfaces; enable gliding motion exclusively in a single plane, mainly for flexion and extension movements	Motion in one plane; flexion, extension	Interphalangeal joints of hand and foot; elbow
Condylar 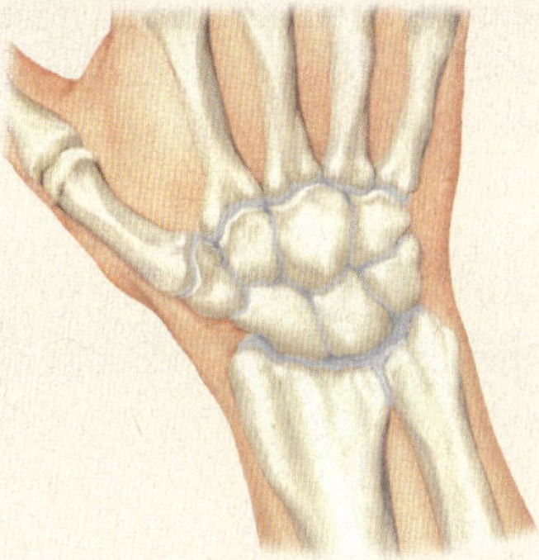	Convex or concave articulating surfaces; facilitate movements like flexion, extension, rotation, and coronal plane motions, with two articulating surfaces moving in conjunction	Movement of two articulating surfaces not dissociable	Knee; temporomandibular joint
Cartilaginous			
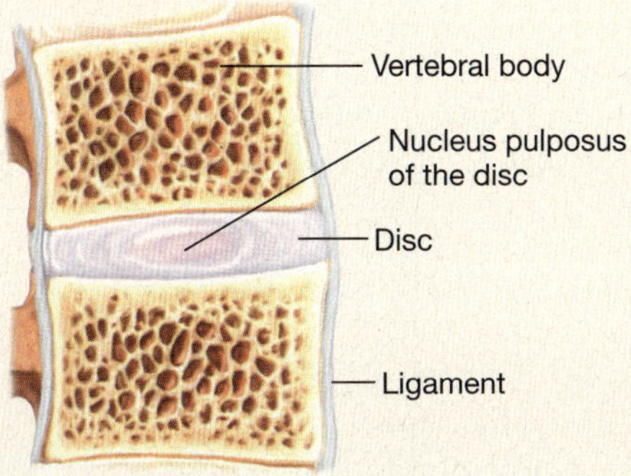	Fibrocartilaginous discs between bony surfaces, allowing limited movement and acting as shock absorbers; surfaces are covered with hyaline cartilage	Small amount of movement	Intervertebral joints, symphysis pubis, sternomanubrial joint

(continued)

Box 25-3. Types of Synovial Joints (*Continued*)

Type of Joint	Description	Movement	Examples
Fibrous			
	Bones joined by fibrous tissue or cartilage; allow almost no movement as bones are in near direct contact	No appreciable movement	Sutures of the skull

In certain cases, tendons or parts of tendons can also be categorized as intra-articular, being within the joint capsule.

Pathology of articular structures typically involves swelling and tenderness of the joint, crepitus, instability, "locking," or deformity and limits *both active and passive range of motion (ROM)* due to stiffness, mechanical blockage, or pain.[1]

Extra-articular structures are external to the joint capsule and are crucial for joint support and movement. Along with muscles, nonarticular bone, nerves, and the overlying skin, these include periarticular ligaments, tendons, bursae, fascia (Box 25-4).

Pathology involving extra-articular structures rarely causes intra-articular joint swelling, instability, or joint deformity. Extra-articular pain occurs from inflammation of bursae (**bursitis**), tendons (**tendinitis**), or tendon sheaths (**tenosynovitis**); from degeneration of tendons (**tendinosis**); or from *sprains* of ligaments or *strains* of muscle caused by stretching or tearing. It typically involves "point or focal tenderness in regions adjacent to articular structures" and limits *active ROM only.*[1]

Box 25-4. Nonarticular Joint Structures

Structure	Description
Ligaments	Tough, fibrous tissues that connect bones to other bones at joints; composed of dense bundles of collagen fibers, providing stability, and guiding joint movement while limiting excessive motion
Tendons	Specialized structures connecting muscle to bone, primarily made of type I collagen with large bundles of parallel fibers; elastic properties allow absorption of kinetic energy as potential energy during movement
Bursae	Disc-shaped synovial sacs that reduce friction during soft tissue movement; located between skin and bone or tendon, or adjacent to bones, ligaments, muscles, and tendons (e.g., prepatellar bursa of the knee and the subacromial/subdeltoid bursa of the shoulder)
Fascia	Band or sheet of connective tissue, primarily collagen, beneath the skin; attaches, stabilizes, encloses, and separates muscles and other internal organs to maintain structural integrity and coordinate body movements

HEALTH HISTORY: GENERAL APPROACH

Both the vertebral spine and joints are intricate structures comprising bones, ligaments, tendons, cartilage, nerves, bursae, and blood vessels. Each of these components can be susceptible to injury, compression, stretching, infection, and malignancies. A comprehensive history is vital in pinpointing which specific elements may be compromised or dysfunctional.[1]

Musculoskeletal Problems

Musculoskeletal problems range from pain, stiffness, and swelling to limitations in movement. Among these, joint pain (*arthralgia*) is often the most common reason for seeking health care. Regardless of the specific symptom, a similar, systematic approach is used for evaluation, requiring a diligent understanding of the underlying anatomy and function. Encourage specificity during your clinical interview, especially if the problem involves pain or discomfort, and ask the patient to point to the affected area if possible. A thorough exploration of each symptom's attributes, including context, associations, and chronology, is essential for you to build a comprehensive clinical picture (Box 25-5).

See Table 25-1, Patterns of Pain in and Around the Joints, pp. 830–831.

See Table 25-2, Systemic Manifestations of Musculoskeletal Disorders, p. 832.

Box 25-5. Clinical Attributes of Musculoskeletal Symptoms

Aspect	Description
Nature of problem	Determine the primary issue, such as pain, stiffness, swelling, weakness, or limitation in movement, guiding further diagnostic considerations.
Location	Identify if the symptom is localized to one joint (*monoarticular*), a few joints (*oligoarticular*), or multiple joints (*polyarticular*). The pattern of joint involvement can be crucial for diagnosis (Box 25-6).
Pattern of involvement	Assess if symptoms are constant or intermittent, symmetric or asymmetric, and whether they migrate or are stationary. This information is key to differentiating between various arthritic conditions.
Onset	Explore whether the onset was sudden or gradual, associated with a specific incident, or seemingly spontaneous. This distinction helps in differentiating between acute and chronic conditions.
Palliation/provocation	Understanding what actions or positions exacerbate or relieve symptoms can provide insights into the underlying causes.
Quality and severity	For pain or discomfort, describe the nature and severity, which helps in understanding the condition's impact on the patient's life.
Associated symptoms	Ask about the four cardinal features of inflammation—*swelling, warmth, redness*, in addition to *pain* (Box 25-7). Identifying these can help pinpoint the type of joint disorder.
Functional impact	Assess any changes in the ability to perform daily activities, to gauge the functional limitations caused by the symptoms.
Constitutional symptoms and systemic manifestations	These can be linked to specific joint disorders and provide valuable diagnostic information.
Family and medical history	Detailed family history can reveal genetic predispositions to certain musculoskeletal disorders.

Box 25-6. Possible Causes of Pain Based on Number of Joints Involved

Monoarticular	Oligoarticular/Pauciarticular	Polyarticular
Monoarticular arthritis	Infection (e.g., gonorrhea, rheumatic fever)	Rheumatoid arthritis
Focal joint injury	Osteoarthritis	Systemic lupus erythematosus
Extra-articular tissue (e.g., tendon, ligament, nerve)	Connective tissue disease	Psoriasis

Box 25-7. Assessing the Four Signs of Inflammation

Sign	Exam Technique	Clinical Implications
Swelling (*tumor*)	Palpate the joint area to assess for bogginess, doughiness, or fluid accumulation. Check for swelling in the synovial membrane, effusion in the joint space, and tenderness in bursae, tendons, or tendon sheaths.	Palpable swelling can be due to synovial membrane swelling (*synovitis*); *effusion* results in joint fluid accumulation; *tendinitis* involves tendon sheath tenderness.
Warmth (*calor*)	Use the backs of your fingers to feel the temperature of the involved joint. Compare it with the corresponding joint on the opposite side of the body or nearby tissues if both joints are affected.	Increased warmth in a joint may indicate inflammation, which can be seen in conditions like arthritis, tendinitis, bursitis, and osteomyelitis.
Redness (*rubor*)	Visually inspect the joint for redness, focusing particularly on more superficial joints like fingers, toes, and knees.	Redness is less common but can be seen in superficial joints. It may indicate acute inflammation as seen in septic arthritis, crystal-induced arthritis, and rheumatoid arthritis.[22,31–33]
Pain (*dolor*)	Gently palpate the joint and surrounding areas to locate specific points of tenderness. Focus on identifying the precise anatomic structure that is tender.	Redness over a tender joint suggests acute joint or synovium inflammation; diffuse tenderness could indicate arthritis or infection.

PHYSICAL EXAMINATION: GENERAL APPROACH

Keep the patient's baseline level of function in mind as you perform the musculoskeletal examination. During the general survey, assess the patient's general appearance, body proportions, and ease of movement. During this survey, visualize the underlying anatomy of the joints and recall pertinent elements of the history, for example, the mechanism of injury if there is trauma, and the time course of symptoms and specific functional limitation. As you watch the patient move, reflect on how the anatomy of the affected joint, muscle, tendon, or other soft tissue has been disturbed to result in what you see.[2]

As you begin your examination, remind yourself to be systematic. The approach can be divided into four broad sections best remembered by the mnemonic *IPROMS* ("*I promise...*") (Box 25-8). This includes:

Box 25-8. Examination Technique Framework Using IPROMS

Examination	Technique
Inspection (look)	Begin by checking if both sides of the joints look the same in terms of size, shape, and alignment. Look for any swelling, redness, or unusual deformities. Also, examine the skin for rashes, nodules, or muscle changes.
Palpation (feel)	Use your fingertips to feel around the joints, starting with less sensitive areas and progressing to more tender spots. Check for tenderness, warmth, swelling, and any irregularities in the joint structures. Pay attention to how the joint capsule and nearby tissues feel.
Range of motion (move)	Test the joint's movement by asking the patient to move it themselves (active). Then, gently move the joint yourself to see if there is any resistance, pain, or limited motion (passive). Make sure to compare both sides and note any differences or restrictions (see Box 25-9).
Special maneuvers (stress)	Use specific techniques to isolate and evaluate individual joints and soft tissues. These maneuvers often involve moving the joint in specific ways to reproduce symptoms or assess its stability and function.

- Inspection (*Look*): examining the body and its movements visually
- Palpation (*Feel*): examining the body by touch
- Range Of Motion (*Move*): assessing joints' movement capability
- Special maneuvers (*Stress*): performing specific tests or procedures to assess the function of a joint or soft tissue.

As a student learning these techniques, understanding the nuances of each step is key. These elements of the musculoskeletal examination—inspection, palpation, ROM, and special maneuvers—are integral to a comprehensive evaluation of the musculoskeletal system.

Inspection (Look)

A thorough visual examination starts by observing the patient's general posture, body symmetry, and any apparent deformities. Look for any curvature of the spine, muscle wasting, skin changes, or swelling that could indicate underlying pathologies. Note the alignment of the shoulders, hips, and knees. Visual clues often provide the first indication of musculoskeletal disorders.

Palpation (Feel)

Use your hands to explore the physical characteristics of joints, muscles, and surrounding tissues. Gently palpate around the spine and each joint to assess for tenderness, warmth, or irregularities, which could signify inflammation, injury, or other abnormalities. This tactile feedback is crucial in pinpointing areas of discomfort and understanding the underlying structures' condition.

Range of Motion (Move)

Evaluate the active and passive movements of each joint (Box 25-9). This comparison between active and passive movements can provide insights into the cause of joint issues, such as whether they stem from the muscles, the joints themselves, or neurologic problems.

Box 25-9. Comparison of Active and Passive Range of Motion

Both passive and active range of motion (ROM) serve important roles in the assessment of hip ROM, and each has its specific advantages. The choice between passive and active ROM depends on the clinical context and the goals of the assessment.

ROM	Purpose	Advantages	Limitations
Active	Evaluates the patient's ability to move the joint using their own muscle strength' provides information about muscle strength, joint function, and patient autonomy in movement	Helps in assessing the functional capacity of the joint, muscle coordination, and any pain experienced during movement; also useful in assessing the patient's willingness and ability to move the joint	Range can be limited by pain, muscle weakness, or lack of effort
Passive	Involves the examiner moving the joint without assistance from the patient; assesses the joint's mechanical limitations and integrity, independent of muscle strength	Can achieve a fuller range of motion and is particularly useful if the patient is unable or unwilling to move the joint actively; helps in identifying joint restrictions, capsular tightness, and potential ligament or cartilage issues	Does not provide information about muscle strength or the patient's functional ability

Special Maneuvers (Stress)

These specific tests isolate certain functions or structures within the joint or surrounding tissues. They can reproduce symptoms, assess ligament stability, and test the integrity of specific joint components. Each maneuver targets a particular aspect of joint function, providing valuable information for diagnosing specific conditions.

Other examination techniques include *testing for muscle strength* to aid in the assessment of joint function and ensuring *normal sensation* and *good distal pulses*. For these techniques, see Chapter 27, Nervous System, pp. 929–936 and 943–945, and Chapter 19, Peripheral Vascular System, pp. 550–556.

REGIONAL MUSCULOSKELETAL EXAMINATIONS

The following sections follow a top-down sequence, beginning with the jaw and moving into the upper extremities. The discussions of the hip, back and lower extremities are in Chapter 26, Musculoskeletal System: Lumbosacral Spine, Hips, and Lower Extremities, pp. 841–898. Each section reviews the anatomy and function of the joint and outlines a systematic approach to examining that area using the IPROMS framework.

ANATOMY: TEMPOROMANDIBULAR JOINT

The temporomandibular joint (TMJ) is the most active joint in the body, opening and closing, up to 2,000 times a day (Figs. 25-10 and 25-11). It is formed

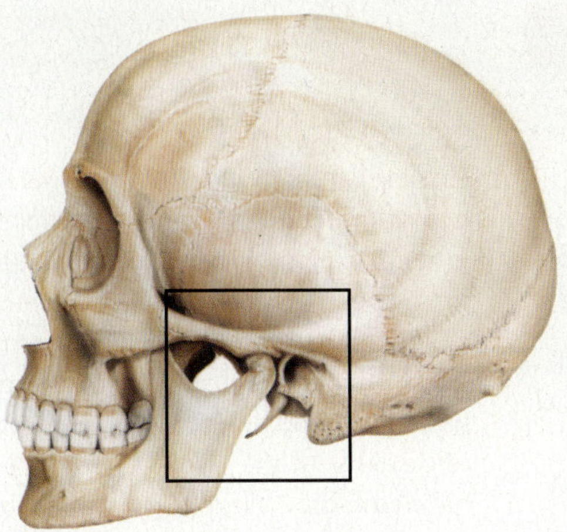

FIGURE 25-10. Area of temporomandibular joint in adult skull.

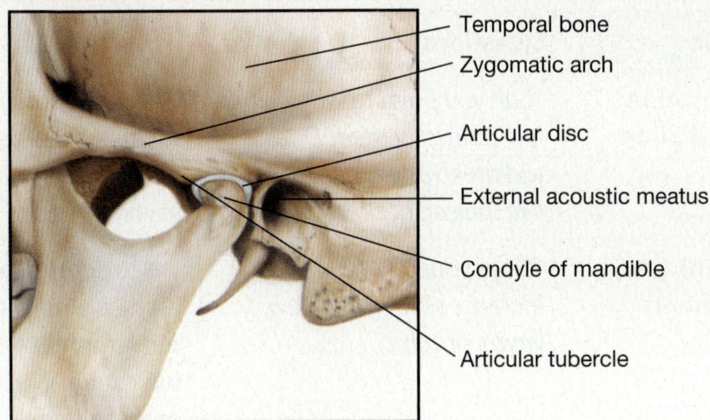

FIGURE 25-11. Temporomandibular joint, inset.

by the fossa and articular tubercle of the temporal bone and the condyle of the mandible and lies midway between the external acoustic meatus and the zygomatic arch.

The TMJ is a *condylar synovial joint* with a fibrocartilaginous disc that cushions the action of the condyle of the mandible against the synovial membrane and capsule of the articulating surfaces of the temporal bone. The *external pterygoids*, along with the *masseter*, *temporalis*, and *internal pterygoids*, collectively known as the *muscles of mastication*, are involved in the actions of opening, and closing the mouth. The *external (lateral) pterygoids* are the principal muscles opening the mouth (Fig. 25-12), while the *masseter*, the *temporalis*, and the *internal (medial) pterygoids* close the mouth and are innervated by cranial nerve V, the *trigeminal nerve* (see p. 923).

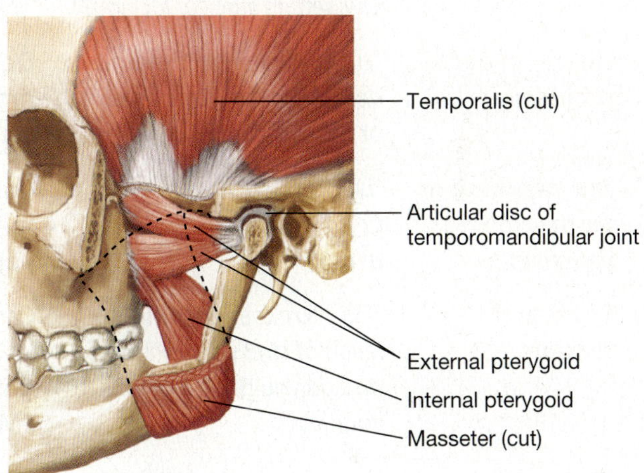

FIGURE 25-12. Muscles of mastication.

HEALTH HISTORY: GENERAL APPROACH

Common or Concerning Symptom

- Jaw pain

Jaw Pain

Jaw pain with clicking is a common issue that prompts patients to seek medical attention. An effective evaluation begins with the question, "*Can you describe your jaw pain and the clicking sounds?*" A thorough health history involves detailed inquiries about the characteristics, onset, pattern, and progression of the jaw pain and clicking as well as any accompanying symptoms (Box 25-10).

Box 25-10. Jaw Pain: High-Yield History Questions

Domain	Questions	Rationale
Pain location and radiation	*"Can you point to where your jaw pain is located? Does it radiate to any other areas like the ear, neck, or head?"*	Helps identify if pain is localized to the temporomandibular joint (TMJ) or involves other structures
Pain with jaw movements	*"Does your jaw pain increase when you chew, yawn, or talk?"*	Helps determine if the pain is associated with functional movements of the jaw, indicating TMJ dysfunction or muscle strain
Jaw sounds and sensations	*"Do you hear any clicking, popping, or grating sounds in your jaw? Do you feel your jaw getting stuck or locking?"*	Can indicate joint dysfunction or displacement within the TMJ
History of dental problems	*"Have you had any recent dental procedures, braces, or other dental issues?"*	Dental procedures and orthodontic treatments can impact TMJ health
Jaw clenching or teeth grinding (bruxism)	*"Do you clench your jaw or grind your teeth, especially at night?"*	Common contributors to TMJ disorders and jaw pain
Stress and tension	*"Do you experience high levels of stress or anxiety, and do you think it affects your jaw?"*	Can lead to unconscious jaw clenching or teeth grinding, exacerbating TMJ issues
Past jaw or facial injuries	*"Have you had any injuries to your face or jaw, like a hit or a fall?"*	Can lead to TMJ disorders or exacerbate existing jaw pain
Headache and ear symptoms	*"Do you experience headaches or ear-related symptoms like earaches or a feeling of fullness in the ears?"*	TMJ disorders can manifest as headaches or ear symptoms due to the close anatomic relationship

Possible causes include **TMJ disorders**, **dental infections** (bacterial infections in teeth or gums), **toothache** (often due to cavities or decay), **bruxism** (teeth grinding or clenching, often during sleep), **sinusitis** (inflammation of the sinuses, causing pressure and pain that can extend to the jaw), and **trigeminal neuralgia** (chronic pain condition affecting the trigeminal nerve in the face, leading to severe, sharp pain in the jaw area).[3,4]

TECHNIQUES OF EXAMINATION

Key Components of the Temporomandibular Joint Examination

I
- Inspect the face and temporomandibular joint (symmetry, swelling, redness, bulges).

P
- Palpate the temporomandibular joint.
- Palpate the muscles of mastication (masseter, temporalis, pterygoids).

ROM	▪ Assess temporomandibular joint range of motion (opening, closing, protrusion, retraction, side-to-side).
S	▪ None

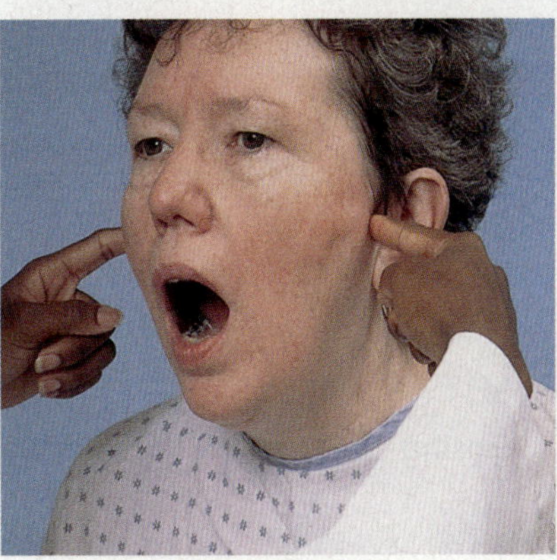

FIGURE 25-13. Palpating the TMJ while asking the patient to open and close their mouth.

Inspect the Face and Temporomandibular Joint

Inspect the face for symmetry. Inspect the TMJ for swelling or redness. Swelling may appear as a rounded bulge just anterior to the external auditory meatus.

Palpate the Temporomandibular Joint

To locate and palpate the joint, place the tips of your index fingers just in front of the tragus of each ear and ask the patient to open their mouth (Fig. 25-13). The fingertips should drop into the joint spaces as the mouth opens. Note any swelling or tenderness. Snapping or clicking may be felt or heard in normal people and is not necessarily a sign of pathology.

Palpable crepitus or clicking is present in poor occlusion, articular disc (meniscus) injury, and synovial swelling from trauma.[5,6]

Palpate the Muscles of Mastication

Palpate the *muscles of mastication* (see Fig. 25-12):

- *Masseters:* These are palpated externally at the angle of the mandible. To feel the masseter muscles, ask your patient to clench their teeth; the muscle will become more prominent and can be felt during both clenching and relaxation of the jaw.
- *Temporal muscles:* These are palpated externally at the temples. Similar to the masseters, ask your patient to clench their teeth to make the temporal muscles more noticeable and felt during clenching and relaxation.
- *Pterygoid muscles:* Palpation of the pterygoid muscles is challenging due to their location. The medial pterygoid can be approached internally in the oral cavity but is rarely palpated in routine exams. The lateral (external) pterygoid, located near the TMJ and deep within the upper jaw, is not accessible for direct palpation.

In temporomandibular disorders (TMD), there is pain and tenderness with palpation.

Assess Temporomandibular Joint Range of Motion

The TMJ has glide and hinge motions in its upper and lower portions, respectively. Grinding or chewing consists primarily of gliding movements in the upper compartments. Normally, as the mouth is opened wide, three fingers can be inserted between the incisors. During normal protrusion of the jaw, the bottom teeth can be placed in front of the upper teeth (Box 25-11).

Patients who are unable to close their mouths may have dislocated the TMJ, which can happen with extreme mouth opening or trauma.

Box 25-11. Range of Motion: Temporomandibular Joint

Movement	Examination Technique	Patient Instructions
Opening	Observe the range of jaw opening. Measure the distance between the upper and lower incisors at maximum opening. Normal opening is typically about 35–55 mm.	*"Open your mouth as wide as you can, like you're about to yawn."*
Closing	Note any deviations or asymmetry in the jaw's path as it closes. Assess for smoothness of movement and any sounds like clicking or popping.	*"Close your mouth gently, like you're slowly biting down on something soft."*
Protrusion	Observe the forward movement of the lower jaw. Check for the alignment of the lower teeth in front of the upper teeth and ensure smooth movement without deviations.	*"Stick out your lower jaw, like making an underbite face."* *"Push your bottom teeth out in front of your top teeth without opening your mouth."*
Retraction (retrusion)	Observe the backward movement of the lower jaw. Assess the patient's ability to pull the jaw straight back without shifting to either side.	*"Pull your lower jaw in, trying to hide your bottom teeth behind your top teeth."* *"Slide your chin backward, making a double chin."*
Side-to-side (laterotrusion)	Observe the lateral movement of the lower jaw to each side. Note ROM and any deviation or asymmetry in movement.	*"Gently move your jaw to the right and then to the left."* *"Without opening your mouth, shift your lower jaw to each side."*

ANATOMY: CERVICAL SPINE (NECK)

For information on the other vertebral spinal regions, refer to Chapter 26, Musculoskeletal System: Lumbosacral Spine, Hips, and Lower Extremities, pp. 841–898.

The *cervical spine*, which includes the upper part of the spinal column, is essential for supporting the head and allowing its movement (Fig. 25-14). Its functionality comes from the unique design of the cervical vertebrae, especially the atlas and axis, and the surrounding strong ligaments and muscles. This structure provides both stability and flexibility. Movement in the cervical spine is managed by various muscle groups, including the deep cervical flexors, upper trapezius, levator scapulae, and SCM muscles, which together facilitate neck movement and head rotation.

Review the details of the anatomy and biomechanics of the cervical spine on pp. 777–778.

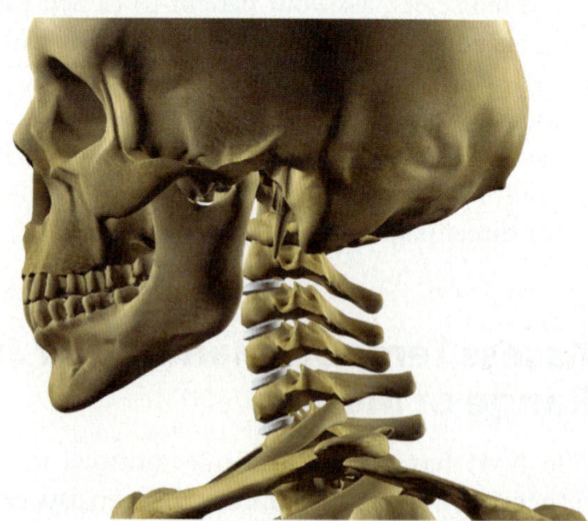

FIGURE 25-14. Lateral view of the cervical spine. (From LifeART image copyright © 2024 Lippincott Williams & Wilkins. All rights reserved.)

HEALTH HISTORY: GENERAL APPROACH

Common or Concerning Symptom

- Neck pain or stiffness

Neck Pain or Stiffness

Neck pain, medically referred to as *cervicalgia*, is a prevalent concern that brings patients into the clinical setting. A precise assessment begins with the inquiry, "Where is your neck pain located?" An in-depth health history should include detailed questioning about the nature, onset, pattern, and progression of the pain, as well as any related systemic symptoms (Box 25-12). Recall the set of health history domains for evaluating joint pain on pp. 783–784.

See Table 25-3, Pains in the Neck, p. 833.

Box 25-12. Neck Pain: High-Yield History Questions

Domain	Questions	Rationale
Location and radiation	*"Can you describe where your neck pain starts and if it spreads anywhere, like into your shoulders or down your arms?"*	Helps identify nerve involvement or muscular strain
Movement-related	*"Does moving your head in certain directions, like looking up or turning to the side, increase your pain?"*	Helps determine if pain is related to muscular strain, cervical spine issues, or nerve impingement
Onset and duration	*"When did your neck pain start, and how long have you been experiencing it?"*	Can help differentiate between acute injuries, chronic conditions, and postural issues
Effect of posture and position	*"Do certain positions or activities, like sitting at a computer or driving, make your neck pain worse or better?"*	Assists in assessing impact of posture and ergonomics (crucial in neck pain related to occupational or lifestyle factors)
Associated symptoms	*"Have you experienced any headache, numbness, or tingling in your arms or hands along with the neck pain?"*	Can indicate nerve involvement or tension-type headaches related to neck issues
Previous neck injuries or surgeries	*"Have you had any past injuries or surgeries to your neck?"*	Can be a significant factor in current neck pain and need to be considered for a comprehensive assessment
Sleeping habits and pillow use	*"How do you usually sleep, and what type of pillow do you use? Have you noticed your neck pain is related to your sleep?"*	Can influence neck pain, especially if causing abnormal neck positions during sleep
Stress and tension levels	*"Do you often feel stressed or tense, and do you think this affects your neck pain?"*	Can contribute to muscular tightness in the neck, leading to or exacerbating pain

Possible musculoskeletal causes include **cervical spondylosis** (age-related wear and tear affecting the spinal disks in the neck), **muscle strain** (often due to poor posture or overuse), **whiplash** (neck injury due to forceful, rapid back-and-forth movement of the neck), **cervical radiculopathy** (compression or irritation of a nerve in the neck, causing pain, numbness, or weakness radiating into the shoulder or arm), and **spinal stenosis** (narrowing of the spinal canal in the neck, leading to nerve compression and pain).

TECHNIQUES OF EXAMINATION

Key Components of the Cervical Spine (Neck) Examination

I	▪ Inspect the neck and posture (symmetry, deviation, atrophy, hypertrophy, position).
P	▪ Palpate the muscles of the neck (sternocleidomastoid, trapezius, scalenes, paraspinal muscles).
	▪ Palpate the neck and surrounding structures (cervical vertebrae, spinous process, facet joints, paraspinal muscles).
ROM	▪ Assess cervical spine (neck) range of motion (flexion, extension, rotation, lateral bending).
S	▪ Perform special maneuvers for the cervical spine, if indicated (Spurling test, facet loading maneuver).

Drape or gown the patient to expose the entire neck and upper shoulders. The patient should be seated or standing with arms at the sides. The head should be midline with shoulders even and relaxed.

Inspect the Neck and Posture

Begin by inspecting the cervical spine for any visible abnormalities or asymmetry. Ask the patient to sit or stand with their head in a neutral position. Pay attention to the alignment of the cervical spine. Look for any signs of deformity, swelling, or redness along the cervical spine, which may indicate underlying issues or injuries.

Neck stiffness can signal arthritis, muscle strain, or other underlying pathology that should be pursued. In some cases, headache may be present.

Viewing the patient from behind, identify the following (Fig. 25-15):

- *Spinous processes:* These are generally more prominent at the C7 and T1 levels. They become more evident when the patient flexes forward.
- *Paravertebral muscles:* Located on either side of the midline, these muscles should be assessed for symmetry and any signs of atrophy or hypertrophy.
- *Shoulder posture and scapular position:* Observe the overall posture of the shoulders and the position of the scapulae. Look for any asymmetry or deviations that might indicate underlying musculoskeletal issues.

In scoliosis, the spine undergoes a lateral and rotational curvature that results in the realignment of the head back to the midline, often leading to noticeable unequal shoulder heights.

Unequal shoulder heights also occur in "winging" of the scapula periscapular weakness. See Chapter 27, Nervous System, p. 952.

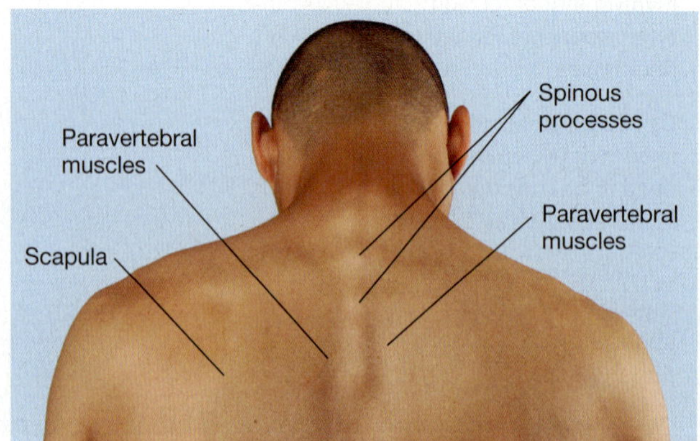

FIGURE 25-15. Surface anatomy of the neck, posterior view.

Palpate the Muscles of the Neck

Stand or sit behind or to the side of your patient. Proceed to palpate the neck muscles by gently feeling the *SCM muscles* on both sides of the neck, located just below the earlobes, and move downward along the neck. Use a gentle touch to assess for tenderness, tightness, or knots as you move downward along the neck.

Next, palpate the *trapezius muscles*, which extend from the neck to the shoulders. Feel for any muscle tension or discomfort. Finally, check the *scalene muscles* on the sides of the neck, again assessing for any tenderness or tightness. It is important to compare both sides for symmetry during this process.

Palpate the Neck and Surrounding Structures

Cervical Vertebrae. To assess the cervical spine's integrity and muscle tenderness, position yourself behind the patient, who is seated. Start by gently palpating along the *spinous processes of the cervical vertebrae*, beginning at the base of the skull (C1) and progressing down to the upper back (C7). Pay attention to any localized tenderness, irregularities, or misalignments.

Vertebral tenderness may raise concern for fracture, dislocation, underlying infection, or arthritis.

Facet Joints. Palpate the *facet joints* that lie between the cervical vertebrae 1 to 2 cm lateral to the spinous processes of C2 to C7. These joints lie deep to the trapezius muscle and may not be easily palpable unless the neck muscles are relaxed.

Tenderness occurs in arthritis, especially at the facet joints between C5 and C6. It can also result from muscle or fascial tightness related to poor neck or shoulder biomechanics, trauma (from cervical strain or "whiplash"), excessive loading of muscles (sometimes seen in weight lifters), or underlying altered mechanics from diseases like osteoarthritis (OA).

Paraspinal Muscles. Palpate the *paraspinal muscles* on both sides of the cervical spine. Begin at the base of the skull and move downward, feeling for muscle tension, knots, or areas of discomfort.

Assess Cervical Spine (Neck) Range of Motion

The neck is the most mobile portion of the spine, remarkable for its seven vertebrae supporting the 10- to 15-lb head. *Flexion* and *extension* occur primarily between the skull and C1 (atlas). *Rotation* primarily occurs at C1–C2 (axis). Finally, *lateral bending* primarily occurs at C2 to C7.

Limited ROM can be caused by stiffness from arthritis, pain from trauma, and muscle spasm.

Assess ROM and neck mobility while gently supporting the patient's head. Instruct the patient to perform neck movements (Box 25-13). Review the specific muscles responsible for each movement and their related patient instructions. Pay close attention to which of these movements, if any, reproduce the patient's symptoms, where those symptoms occur, and the characteristics of those symptoms.

Limited ROM generally signals underlying OA. However, sudden-onset limits in a patient's ROM generally warrant imaging, especially after trauma.

Box 25-13. Range of Motion: Cervical Spine (Neck)

Movement	Examination Technique	Patient Instructions
Flexion 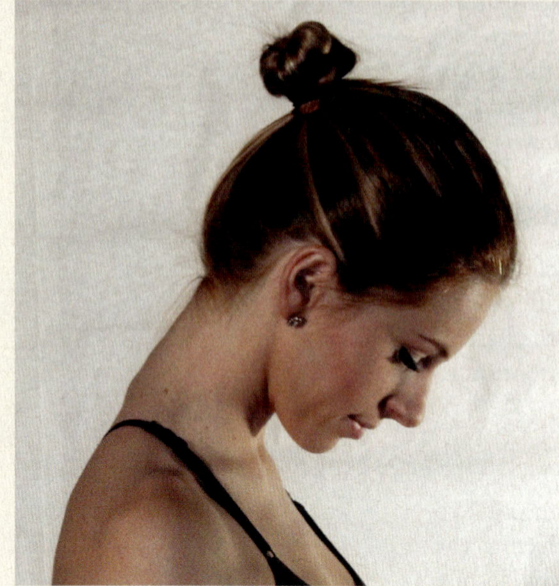	Observe and gently guide the patient's chin toward their chest. Note the ease of movement and any discomfort. Check the angle between the chin and chest, which typically should be close to touching.	*"Nod your head slowly, as if saying 'yes.'"* *"Try to touch your chin to your chest."*
Extension 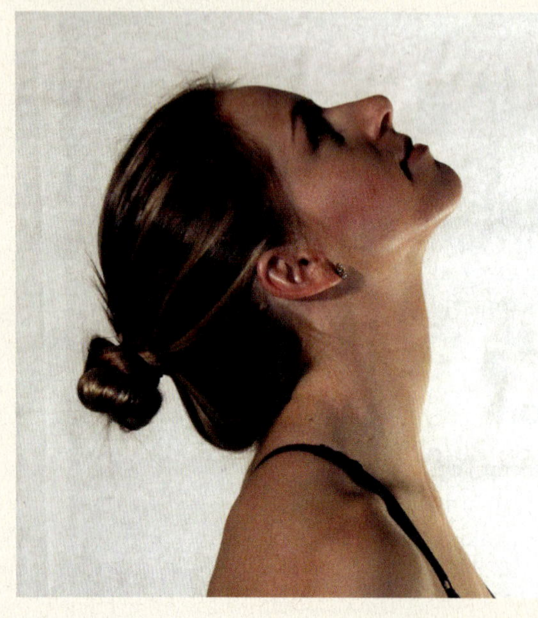	Assist the patient in tilting their head back to look at the ceiling. Observe the range and smoothness of backward head movement. Note the angle between their chin and neck.	*"Look up at the ceiling."* *"Lean your head back as far as is comfortable."*

Movement	Examination Technique	Patient Instructions
Rotation 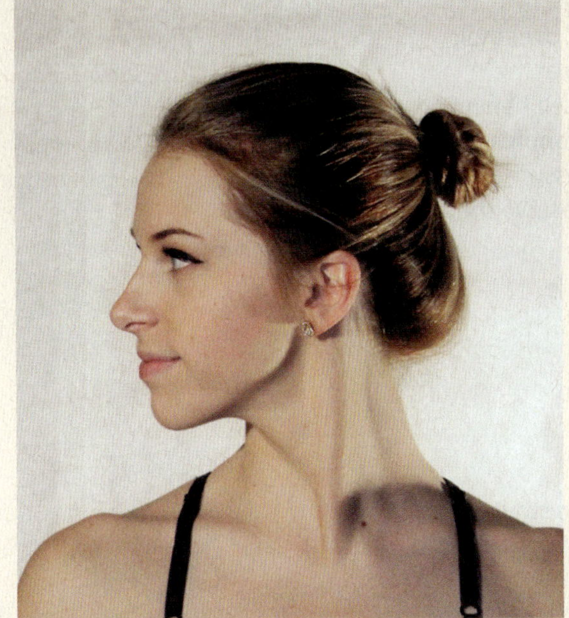	Hold the patient's shoulders steady to isolate neck movement. Observe as they turn their head to the right and left. Note the degree of rotation and any restrictions or pain.	*"Look to your right, then to your left, as if watching something move across the room."* *"Pretend you're trying to see directly behind you without moving your body."*
Lateral bending 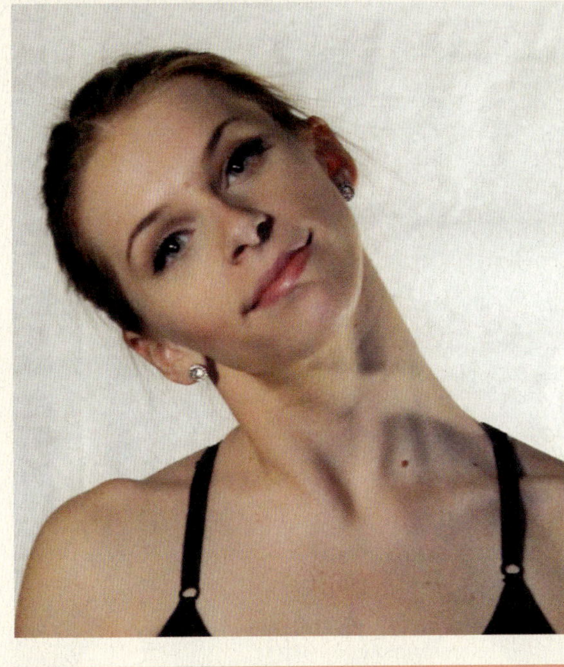	Monitor the patient's ability to tilt their head toward each shoulder. Ensure their shoulders remain level to accurately assess lateral bending. Note any limitations or pain on either side.	*"Try to touch your ear to your shoulder, without lifting your shoulder up."* *"Tilt your head to the side as if trying to listen to your shoulder."*

Reprinted with permission from Dadio GG, Nolan JA. *Clinical Pathways: An Occupational Therapy Assessment for Range of Motion & Manual Muscle Strength*. Wolters Kluwer; 2019. Figure 2-9A–D.

Box 25-14. Special Maneuvers: Cervical Spine (Neck)

Special Maneuver	Examination Technique	
Spurling test Structures assessed: cervical nerve roots 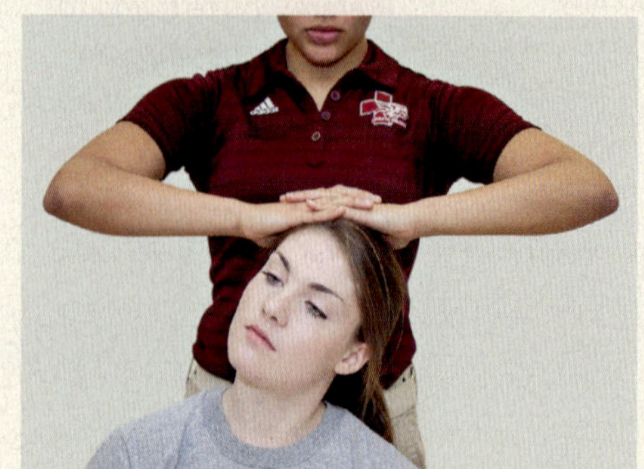	Have the patient look over their shoulder and then up at the ceiling. Position yourself behind the patient. Carefully apply gentle downward pressure on the patient's head. Observe the patient's response.	Spurling test is positive when the patient feels pain going down the arm on the same side the head is turned, indicating cervical nerve root involvement. Sensitivity varies from moderate to high (38% to 97%), with high specificity (89% to 100%).[7]
Facet loading maneuver Structures assessed: facet joint	Have the patient sit up straight. Ask the patient to move their head into extension and rotation. No downward pressure is applied. Observe the patient's response.	Localized pain or reproduced symptoms in the neck or shoulder on the side of rotation without radiation into the arm suggests facet joint involvement or irritation in the cervical spine.[8]

Reprinted with permission from Anderson MK. *Foundations of Athletic Training: Prevention, Assessment, and Management*. 6th ed. Wolters Kluwer; 2017. Figure 21-18.

Perform Special Maneuvers for the Cervical Spine (If Indicated)

In addition to the standard assessment, special maneuvers can help evaluate specific aspects of cervical spine function and identify potential issues (Box 25-14).

The pain referral patterns from the cervical facet joints can be intricate and sometimes overlapping. These patterns are crucial for clinicians to understand, as they assist in diagnosing the specific source of cervical pain (Fig. 25-16).

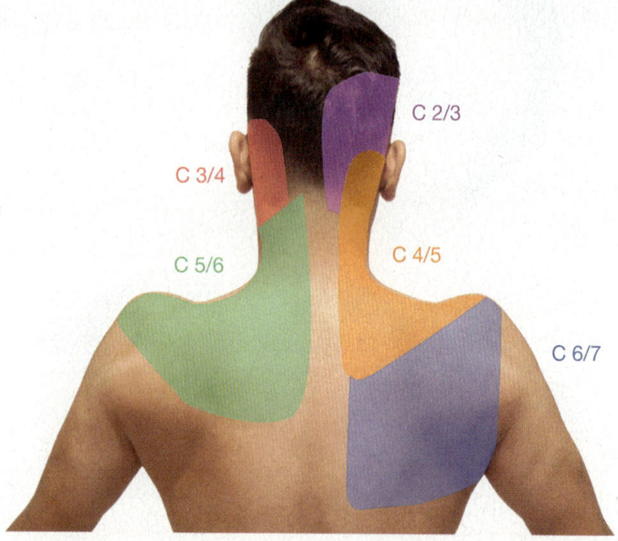

FIGURE 25-16. Posterior view of segmental maps showing pain referral patterns from the cervical facet joints (C2–3, purple; C3–4, red; C4–5, orange; C5–6, green; C6–7, blue). (Reprinted with permission from De Mesa C, Davis BA, Humphries M. Shoulder pain. In: De Mesa C, Sheth SJ, Keenan CR, McCarron RM, John J, eds. *Primary Care Pain Management*. Wolters Kluwer; 2020. Figure 16-6.)

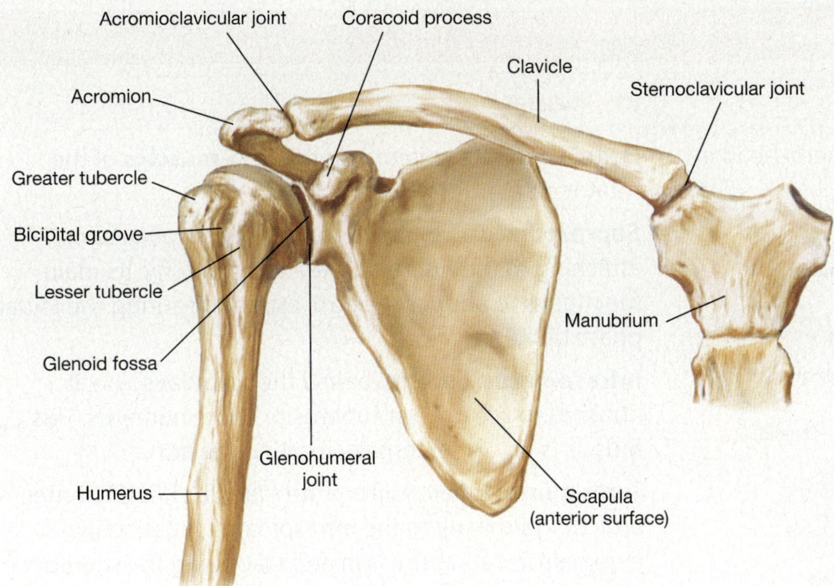

FIGURE 25-17. Anatomy of the right shoulder.

ANATOMY: SHOULDER

The *shoulder* derives its mobility from a complex interconnected structure of three joints called the *shoulder girdle.* The bony structures of the shoulder include the *humerus, clavicle,* and *scapula* (Fig. 25-17). The scapula is anchored to the axial skeleton by the *sternoclavicular joint* (often called the *scapulothoracic articulation* because it is not a true joint) and by the muscles that insert on it.

Stabilizing structures within the body can either be dynamic, like muscles, or static, such as bones, cartilage, and ligaments. An example is the shoulder, which is a complex assembly of three distinct joints and three groups of muscles (Boxes 25-15 and 25-16). These elements collectively contribute to the shoulder's stability and mobility.

Rotator cuff disorders are the most common cause of shoulder pain in primary care.

The principal bursa of the shoulder is the *subacromial subdeltoid bursa* that lies between the rotator cuff tendons and the acromion of the

Box 25-15. Shoulder Joint Articulations

Joint	Articulating Structures	Joint Type
Glenohumeral joint	Head of humerus with glenoid fossa of scapula	Ball-and-socket
Sternoclavicular joint	Medial end of clavicle with upper sternum	Saddle
Acromioclavicular joint	Lateral end of clavicle with acromion process of scapula	Plane

Box 25-16. Shoulder Muscle Groups

Muscle Group	Key Muscles
Scapulohumeral group: Stabilizes the humeral head in the scapular glenoid (Fig. 25-18) 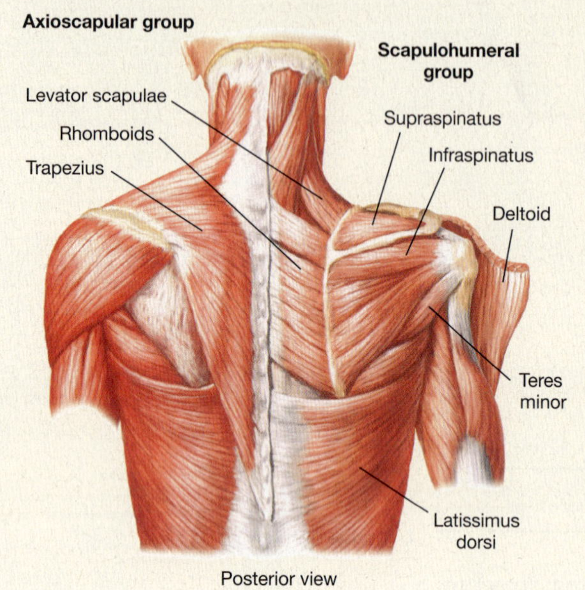 **FIGURE 25-18**	Deltoid and teres major and the **SITS muscles** of the rotator cuff: **Supraspinatus:** Originates above the scapular spine, attaching to the humerus' greater tuberosity. Its main function is to abduct the arm, especially during the initial phase of lifting. **Infraspinatus:** Located below the scapular spine, it attaches to the greater tuberosity of the humerus. This muscle is key for externally rotating the arm. **Teres minor:** Emerges from the scapula's lateral border, attaching similarly to the infraspinatus. It assists in externally rotating the arm and stabilizing the shoulder. **Subscapularis:** Arises from the scapula's anterior surface, attaching to the humerus' lesser tuberosity. It primarily rotates the arm internally and helps stabilize the shoulder joint.
Axioscapular group: Attaches the scapula to the trunk and performs various movements (see Fig. 25-18)	**Trapezius, rhomboids, serratus anterior, levator scapulae**. These muscles help in movements such as elevation, depression, protraction, retraction, and upward/downward rotation of the scapula.
Axiohumeral group: Attaches the humerus to the trunk and performs specific actions (Fig. 25-19) 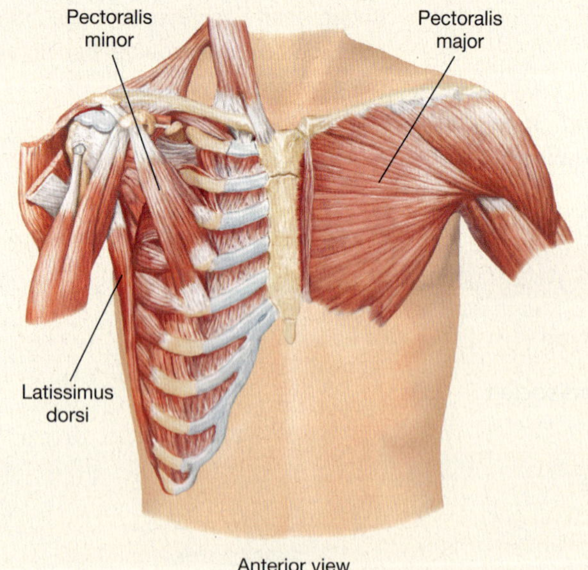 **FIGURE 25-19**	**Pectoralis major, pectoralis minor, latissimus dorsi.** These muscles are involved in movements like internal rotation, adduction, and extension of the humerus.

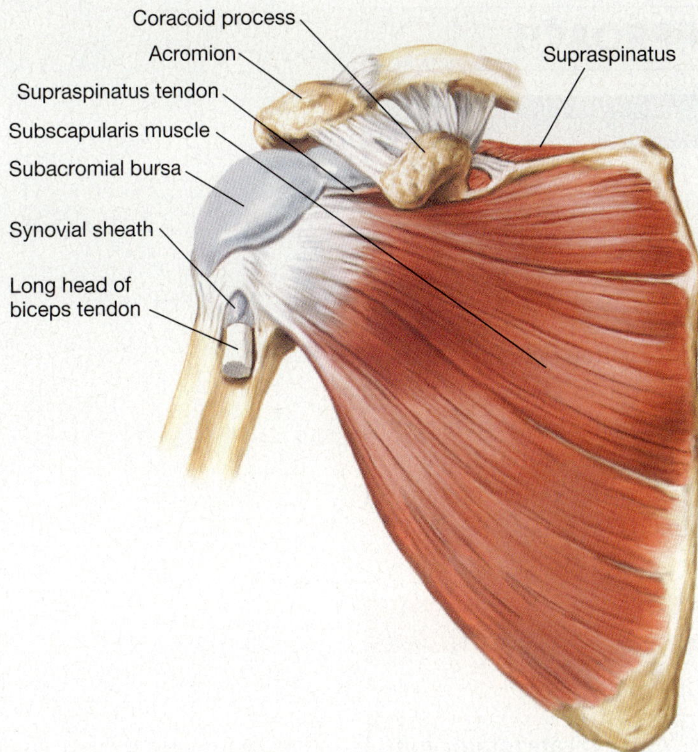

FIGURE 25-20. Anterior view of right shoulder showing insertions of the rotator cuff muscles, the tendon of the long head of the biceps in the bicipital groove, and bursae.

scapula, acromioclavicular (AC) joint, bicipital groove, and the deltoid muscle (Fig. 25-20). Abduction of the shoulder compresses this bursa and allows the rotator cuff to move smoothly under the scapula.

If the rotator cuff tendons or bursal surfaces are inflamed (*subacromial subdeltoid bursitis*), there may be tenderness just below the tip of the acromion, pain with abduction and external rotation, and loss of smooth active ROM.

A *fibrous articular capsule* formed by the tendon insertions of the rotator cuff and other capsular structures surrounds the glenohumeral joint. The loose fit of the capsule ensures the shoulder can move through a wide range of movement. The capsule is lined by a synovial membrane with two outpouchings—the *subscapular bursa* and the *synovial sheath* of the tendon of the long head of the biceps. The *tendon of the long head of the biceps* runs in the *bicipital groove* between the greater and lesser tubercles (see Fig. 25-20).

Inflammation of the fibrous capsule can lead to adhesion of the capsular tissues, causing pain and restricted ROM. This *adhesive capsulitis* or *frozen shoulder* results in restricted passive and active ROM.

HEALTH HISTORY: GENERAL APPROACH

Common or Concerning Symptom

- Shoulder pain

Shoulder Pain

Shoulder pain, a common symptom in clinical practice, often necessitates thorough evaluation. The initial step in its assessment involves asking, "*Can you pinpoint the exact location of your shoulder pain*?" A detailed health history is key, focusing on the pain's nature, onset, duration, and progression, along with any related systemic symptoms (Box 25-17). For a broader understanding of joint pain evaluation, review the health history domains on pages 783–784.

Box 25-17. Shoulder Pain: High-Yield History Questions

Domain	Questions	Rationale
Range of motion	*"Do you have difficulty lifting your arm above your head or reaching behind your back?"*	Can indicate rotator cuff issues or frozen shoulder, distinct from other joint problems
Pain with arm weight-bearing	*"Does your shoulder pain increase when you carry heavy objects or put weight on your arm?"*	Can suggest shoulder impingement or bursitis
Nighttime discomfort	*"Do you experience increased shoulder pain or discomfort when lying on the affected side or during the night?"*	Can indicate rotator cuff tears or bursitis
Joint instability	*"Have you ever felt like your shoulder is slipping out of place or experienced sudden weakness when using your arm?"*	Specific to issues like dislocations or labral tears
History of joint stiffness	*"Have you experienced prolonged periods of shoulder stiffness or inability to move your shoulder normally?"*	Stiffness especially after periods of immobility can indicate conditions like adhesive capsulitis (unique to shoulder)
Posture and alignment	*"Have you noticed any changes in the shape or alignment of your shoulder, such as drooping or protrusion?"*	Can indicate structural issues like dislocations or muscle atrophy

Possible causes include **rotator cuff tendinitis**, **shoulder impingement syndrome** (when the top of the shoulder blade puts pressure on the underlying soft tissues as the arm is lifted), **frozen shoulder**, **shoulder bursitis**, **shoulder dislocation or instability**, and **arthritis** (particularly OA, causing degeneration of the shoulder joint and pain).

Domain	Questions	Rationale
Pain radiating to arm	*"Do you feel the pain travel from your shoulder down to your arm or hand?"*	Can help distinguish shoulder-originating pain from other joint or nerve issues
Activity limitation	*"Are there specific activities or sports that you cannot perform due to your shoulder pain?"*	Can help distinguish from other joint issues

TECHNIQUES OF EXAMINATION

Ask the patient to disrobe appropriately, exposing the shoulder and upper extremity on the side being examined. Ensure the patient is comfortably seated or standing, depending on their preference and physical condition. Maintain good lighting to facilitate visual inspection.

See Table 25-4, Painful Shoulders, pp. 834–835.

Key Components of the Shoulder Joint Examination

I	■ Inspect the shoulder and associated structures (position, asymmetry, deformities, atrophy, fasciculations, swelling).
P	■ Palpate the shoulder and associated structures (clavicles, acromion, coracoid process, greater tubercle, SITS muscles, subacromial sub deltoid bursa, biceps tendon).
ROM	■ Assess shoulder range of motion (flexion, extension, abduction, adduction, and internal and external rotation).
S	■ Perform special maneuvers for the shoulder, if indicated (crossed body adduction test, Apley scratch test, pain provocation tests, strength tests, composite tests).

Inspect the Shoulder and Associated Structures

For the frontal inspection of the *anterior shoulder*, ask the patient to maintain an upright position, whether standing or seated, with their shoulder girdle in a neutral position. Their arms should be relaxed by their sides. Carefully observe the front of the shoulder and chest for any visible abnormalities, deformities, muscle atrophy, *fasciculations* (fine tremors of the muscles), or abnormal positioning in the anterior shoulder region.

Scoliosis may cause elevation of one shoulder. With anterior dislocation of the shoulder, the rounded lateral aspect of the shoulder appears flattened.[9]

Inspect the *clavicles*. Observe for any deformities, asymmetry, or abnormalities in clavicle alignment. Pay attention to the sternoclavicular joint where the clavicle connects to the sternum.

For inspection of the *posterior shoulder*, have the patient turn around to face away from you. Ask them to relax their arms and let them hang naturally. Inspect the back, with a focus on the *scapulae* and surrounding structures. Check for deformities, muscle atrophy, or other abnormalities in the posterior shoulder area.

Atrophy of the supraspinatus and infraspinatus with increased prominence of scapular spine can appear within 2 to 3 weeks of a rotator cuff tear.

Look for swelling of the joint capsule anteriorly or a bulge in the subacromial subdeltoid bursa under the deltoid muscle. Survey the entire upper extremity for color change, skin alteration, or unusual bony contours.

Swelling from synovial fluid accumulation is rare and must be significant before the glenohumeral joint capsule appears distended. Swelling in the AC joint is easier to detect as the joint is more superficial.

Palpate the Shoulder and Associated Structures

Clavicles. To palpate the clavicle, instruct the patient to sit or stand with their arms relaxed by their sides. Gently palpate the clavicle from the *sternoclavicular joint* near the base of the neck) to the *AC joint* near the shoulder (Fig. 25-21). Ask the patient to remain still and report any discomfort.

Acromion. With the patient in the same seated or standing position, begin by identifying the *acromion*, which is located at the outermost tip of the shoulder, forming the bony prominence that extends laterally (see Fig. 25-21). Place your fingers gently on the acromion's surface, using the pads of your fingertips. Start with light pressure and gradually increase if needed. While palpating, move your fingers in small circular motions or gentle strokes over the acromion. This helps you assess for any areas of tenderness, discomfort, or unusual sensations.

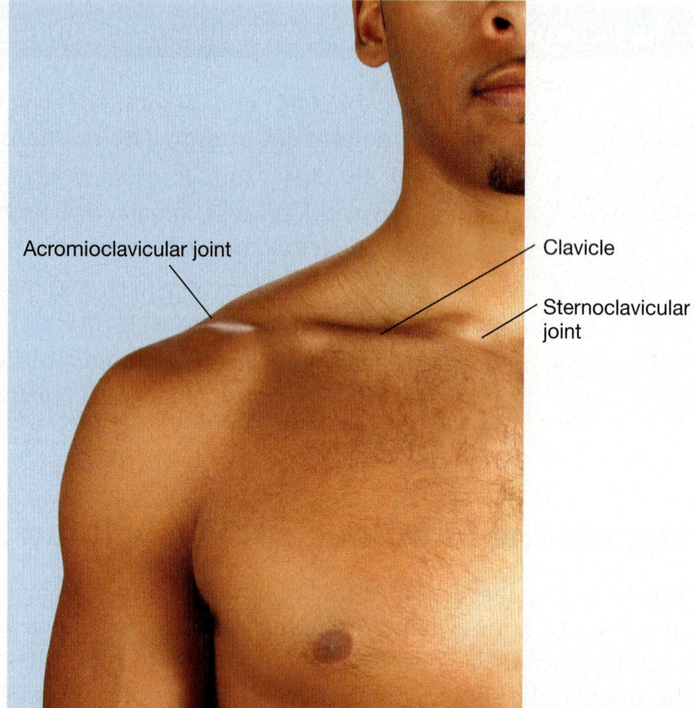

FIGURE 25-21. Surface anatomy of the shoulder, anterior view.

Coracoid Process. The *coracoid process* is a palpable bony prominence situated beneath the clavicle and anterior to the acromion, within the infraclavicular fossa region. Continue from the examination of the acromion by guiding your fingers slightly downward and medially with the patient's arm slightly flexed forward. This maneuver will help you locate the process as it moves in conjunction with the scapula. As you palpate, make small circular motions or gentle strokes over the coracoid process surface, systematically assessing for any tenderness, discomfort, or unusual sensations.

Greater Tubercle. Continue by palpating the *greater tubercle of the humerus*, a prominent landmark where the supraspinatus, infraspinatus, and teres minor muscles insert. This tubercle is best palpated by gently rotating the patient's upper arm internally and externally. As you palpate, examine for any tenderness, irregularities, or discomfort.

SITS Muscles. Position yourself standing or sitting at the patient's side.

- *Supraspinatus:* Begin by gently palpating the supraspinatus muscle, located directly under the acromion. It can be traced from its muscle belly above the scapular spine, extending posteriorly. To palpate this muscle effectively, especially its anterior part, you may need to gently extend the patient's shoulder (Fig. 25-22). This maneuver exposes the supraspinatus for easier palpation.
- *Infraspinatus:* Position yourself slightly behind the patient to palpate over the posterolateral aspect of the shoulder. This positioning allows for optimal access to the infraspinatus muscle which is located posteriorly and inferior to the supraspinatus.
- *Teres minor:* This muscle is situated just inferior to the infraspinatus. Due to its proximity to the infraspinatus and its less frequent involvement in rotator cuff pathology, isolating this muscle can be a challenge. Maintain your position behind the patient for the best approach to palpate this muscle.
- *Subscapularis:* To palpate the muscle, position yourself in front of the patient. This muscle inserts anteriorly on the medial side of the humerus, attaching to the lesser tuberosity. External rotation of the patient's shoulder may be necessary. This is best achieved by palpating medially to the biceps tendon, allowing you to access and evaluate the subscapularis muscle effectively.

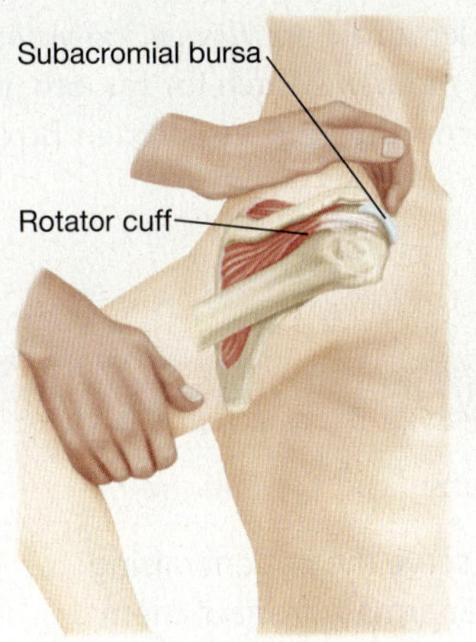

FIGURE 25-22. Palpating the SITS muscle insertions and subacromial bursa.

Tenderness over the SITS tendons and difficulty abducting the arm suggests tendinopathy or low-grade tearing, commonly of the supraspinatus. Inability to abduct the arm suggests high-grade or complete supraspinatus tear.

Subacromial Subdeltoid Bursa. To assess the *subacromial subdeltoid bursa*, passively extend the humerus by lifting the patient's elbow posteriorly. Carefully palpate the subacromial subdeltoid bursa, looking for any signs of tenderness or discomfort (see Fig. 25-22).

Localized tenderness in this position often indicates rotator cuff tendinopathy with the supraspinatus being the most commonly affected.

Biceps Tendon in the Bicipital Groove. Begin by identifying the *intertubercular bicipital groove*, also known as the *bicipital sulcus*, on the anterior aspect of the shoulder. This groove is situated between the greater tubercle and the lesser tubercle of the humerus. Ensure that the patient's arm being examined is in a neutral or slightly externally rotated position. This can be achieved by having them relax their arm by their side with the palm facing forward.

Gently palpate the biceps tendon within the intertubercular bicipital groove (Fig. 25-23). Start with light pressure and gradually increase if necessary. You can use the pads of your fingertips to assess the tendon's texture, size, and any areas of tenderness. While palpating, you may use different techniques to enhance the detection of the biceps tendon:

- Gently roll the tendon under your fingertips, feeling its movement within the groove.
- Rotate the patient's shoulder internally and externally to help you feel the tendon's position and movement more clearly.

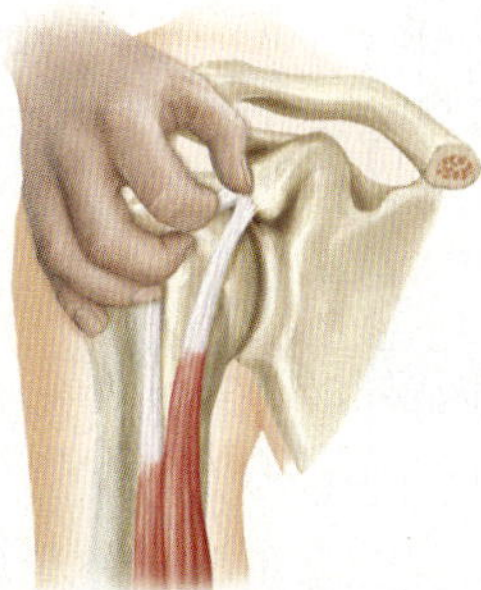

FIGURE 25-23. Palpating the long head of biceps along bicipital groove.

Assess Shoulder Range of Motion

The six cardinal movements of the shoulder girdle are *flexion, extension, abduction, adduction*, and *internal* and *external rotation*. Watch for smooth, fluid, and symmetric movement as the patient performs the motions listed in Box 25-18.

Restricted ROM occurs in bursitis, adhesive capsulitis, and rotator cuff tendinopathy or tears.

Box 25-18. Range of Motion: Shoulder Joint

Movement	Examination Technique	Patient Instructions
Flexion 180° 90° 0°	Observe the patient raising their arms in front of them and overhead. Note ROM and smoothness, and whether they can fully extend their arms without discomfort.	*"Raise your arms in front of you and overhead."* *"Raise your arm straight in front of you, like you're reaching to grab something off a high shelf."*
Extension 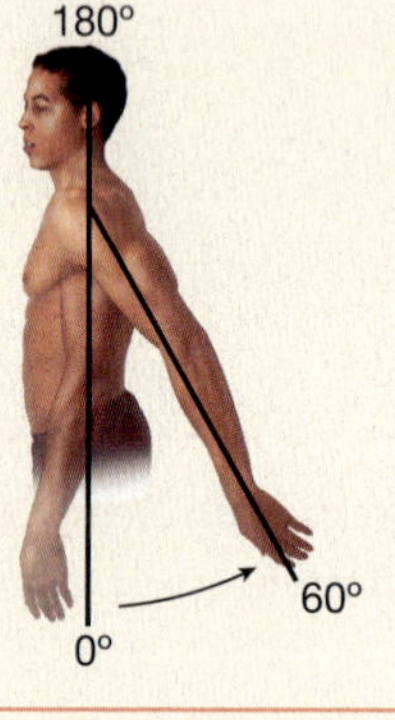	Watch as the patient moves their arm back behind their body. Check the extent of backward movement and any stiffness or pain.	*"Move your arm back behind you, like you're reaching for something in your back pocket."* *"Reach your arm back as if trying to touch the wall behind you."*
Abduction 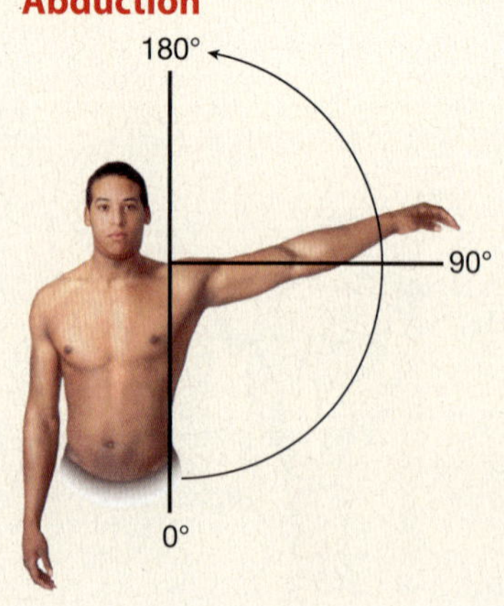	Monitor the patient raising their arms out to the side and then overhead. Assess their ability to lift their arms laterally up to or above shoulder height.	*"Raise your arms out to the side and then overhead, like making a big snow angel."*

Movement	Examination Technique	Patient Instructions
Adduction 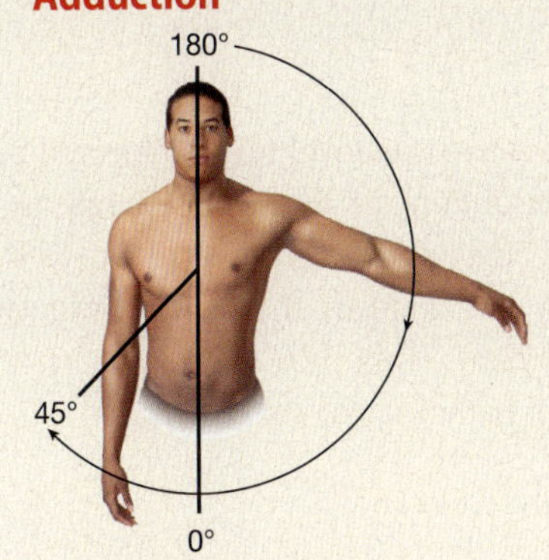	Have the patient lower their arm from a position of abduction (arm extended away from the body) back towards the midline of the body. Observe and assess the control, range, and any discomfort or restrictions in the movement as the arm moves inward towards the body.	*"Lower your arm down towards your side from an outstretched position, bringing it back close to your body."*
Internal rotation 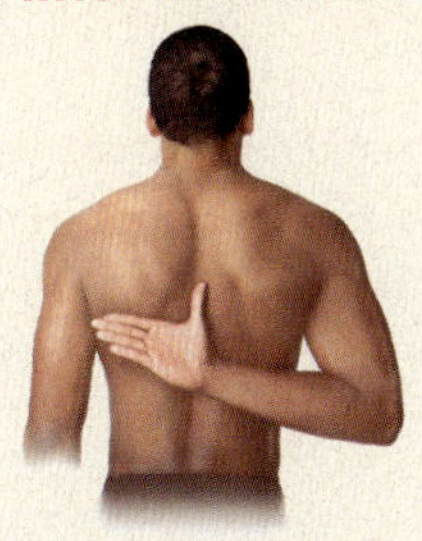	Observe the patient placing one hand behind their back. Note how high up the back they can reach and any limitations or discomfort.	*"Place one hand behind your back and try to touch your shoulder blade."* *"Reach up the middle of your back as if trying to scratch an itch you can't quite reach."*
External rotation 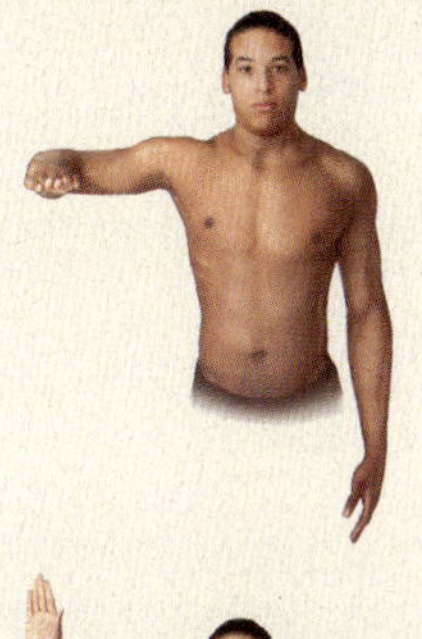 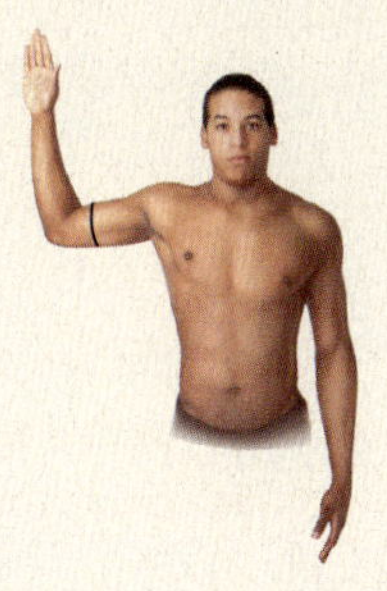	Ask the patient to raise their arm to shoulder level and bend their elbow so that the forearm is parallel to the ground. Have the patient rotate their forearm upward, toward the ceiling. Observe the range of motion, ease of movement, and note any signs of pain or restriction.	*"Raise your arm to shoulder level; bend your elbow and rotate your forearm toward the ceiling."* *"Place one hand behind your neck or head as if you are brushing your hair."*

Perform Special Maneuvers for the Shoulder (If Indicated)

Although performing these maneuvers takes supervision and practice, they increase the likelihood of identifying shoulder pathology. There are more than 150 different maneuvers for testing shoulder function, but few are well studied or validated. The maneuvers that have the best likelihood ratios (LRs) and the narrowest confidence intervals currently recommended are shown in Box 25-19.[10–12] In composite tests, the patient experiences either pain or weakness during the maneuver.

Box 25-19. Special Maneuvers: Shoulder Joint

Structures Assessed[9,10,12,34]	Special Maneuver	Examination Technique
Glenohumeral joint, acromioclavicular joint, and the muscles and tendons of the rotator cuff	**Crossover or crossed body adduction test** 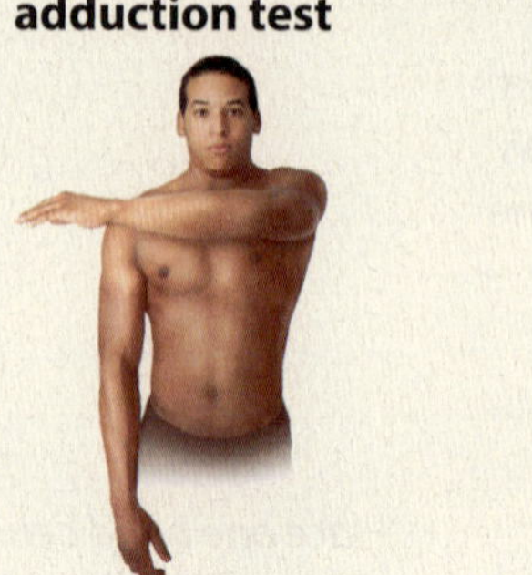 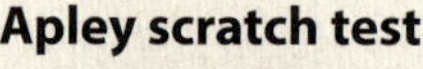	Position yourself in front of the patient who is seated or standing. Gently grasp their arm and carefully move it across their chest. Keep the arm horizontally adducted and internally rotated.
Rotator cuff muscles, particularly the supraspinatus muscle, and the mobility of the glenohumeral joint	**Apley scratch test** 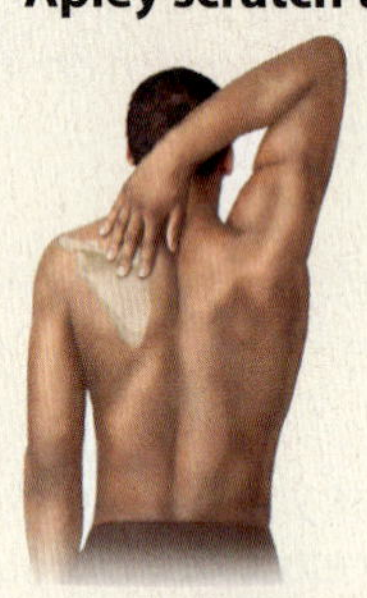	Start by asking the patient to reach behind their head with one hand and try to touch the opposite scapula. This assesses *abduction and external rotation* of the shoulder.
	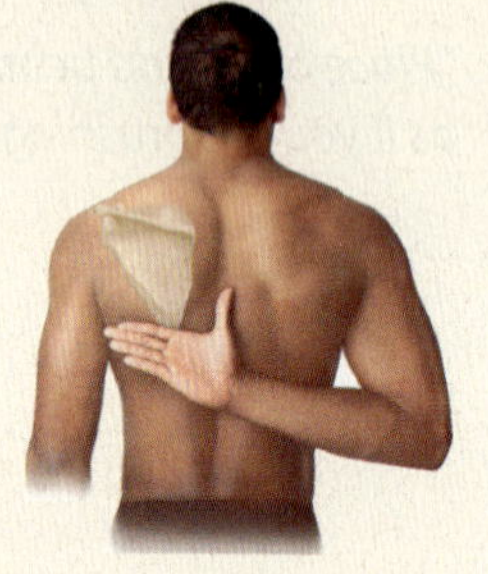	Next, instruct the patient to reach behind their back with the same hand and attempt to touch the opposite scapula, assessing *adduction and internal rotation*.
Pain Provocation Tests		
Assesses subacromial subdeltoid bursa and rotator cuff	**Painful arc test** 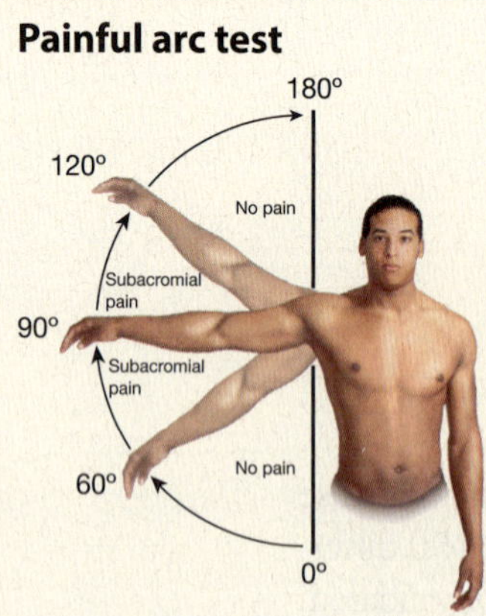	Ensure the patient is in a relaxed, seated or standing position. Ask them to raise their arm slowly and smoothly from a neutral position to the maximum overhead position.

A positive crossover test is indicated by pain during the maneuver, suggesting possible issues with the acromioclavicular (AC) joint or the coracoclavicular ligaments. This pain may point to AC joint pathology or instability.[13]

A positive Apley scratch test is marked by pain, restricted motion, or difficulty completing the movement, indicating possible shoulder joint instability or ligamentous laxity.

Pain or discomfort during the arc of motion indicates potential pathology involving the subacromial-subdeltoid bursa or the rotator cuff.

Structures Assessed[9,10,12,34]	Special Maneuver	Examination Technique	Examples of Abnormalities
Assesses internal structures of the shoulder, specifically the rotator cuff and subacromial space	**Neer impingement test** 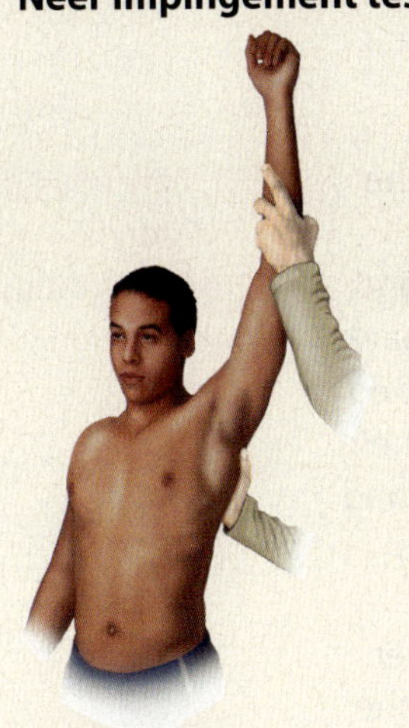	Position yourself in front of the patient, who is seated or standing position. Press on the scapula to prevent scapular motion with one hand and raise the patient's arm with the other. This compresses the greater tuberosity of the humerus against the acromion.	A positive Neer test is indicated by pain or discomfort during the maneuver, often suggesting subacromial impingement syndrome (most common) or a rotator cuff tear.
Assesses internal structures of the shoulder, including the rotator cuff	**Hawkins impingement test** 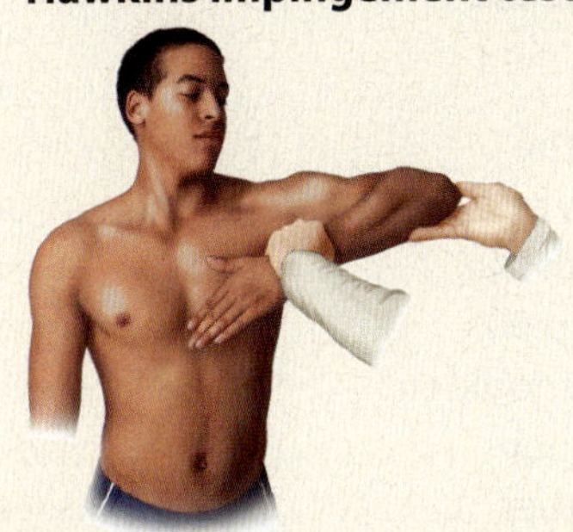	Position yourself in front of the patient who is seated or standing. Flex their shoulder and elbow to 90° with their palm facing down. Then, with one hand on their forearm and one on the arm, rotate the arm internally. This compresses the greater tuberosity against the supraspinatus tendon and coracoacromial ligament	A positive Hawkins or modified Hawkins-Kennedy test is indicated by pain or discomfort during the maneuver, often suggesting subacromial impingement syndrome (most common), rotator cuff pathology, or bicipital tendinitis.
	Modified Hawkins–Kennedy test	Starts similarly as the Hawkins test but instead of forcibly internally rotating the shoulder, the modified version allows for passive internal rotation by gently bringing the patient's forearm across their body. Observe their response for any pain or discomfort. These tests complement the Neer test in diagnosing rotator cuff issues.	

(*continued*)

Box 25-19. Special Maneuvers: Shoulder Joint (*Continued*)

Structures Assessed[9,10,12,34]	Special Maneuver	Examination Technique
Strength Tests		
Assesses function of the subscapularis muscle (internal rotation)	**Internal rotation lag test (lift-off test)** 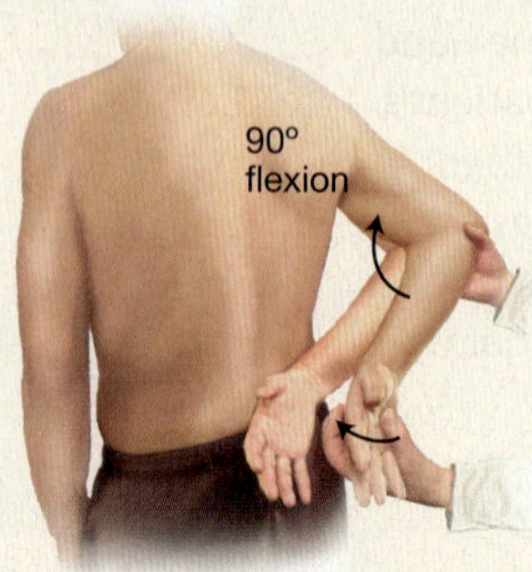	Standing behind the patient, bring the dorsum of their hand behind their low back with the elbow flexed to 90°. Then grip their wrist and lift the hand off the back, which further internally rotates the shoulder. Ask them to keep the hand in this position as you release the wrist.
Assesses function of the supraspinatus and infraspinatus muscles (external rotation)	**External rotation lag test** 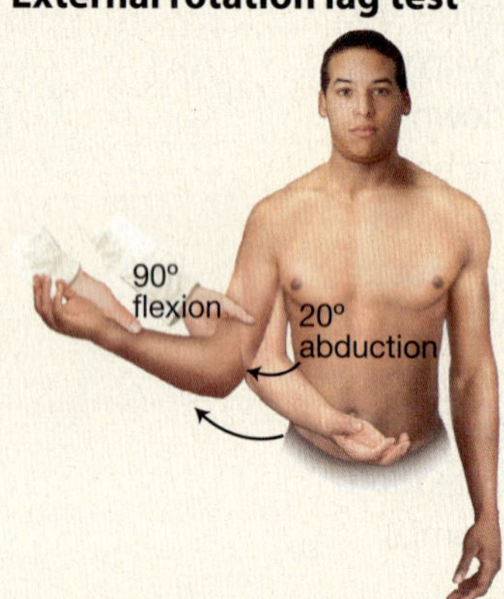	Gently hold the patient's arm at their side with the elbow bent to 90°. Rotate their shoulder outward so their forearm is either perpendicular to the body or as far out as they can comfortably go without pain. Let go of the arm and observe if they can maintain the position. Watch to see if their forearm falls toward the body instead of staying in place.
Assesses function of the supraspinatus muscle (abduction)	**Drop arm test** 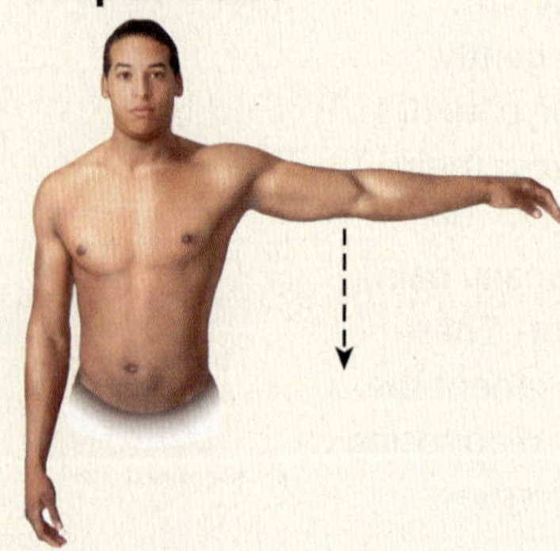	Ask the patient to fully abduct their arm to shoulder level, up to 90°, and lower it slowly. *Note that abduction above shoulder level, from 90° to 120°, reflects action of the deltoid muscle.*

If there is lag or weakness during internal rotation against resistance, it may indicate a subscapularis muscle tear or dysfunction.

A positive result for the external rotation lag test occurs when the patient is unable to maintain their arm in the externally rotated position after you release it, or when the arm lags or falls inward toward the body. This suggests potential issues with the supraspinatus or infraspinatus muscles, such as tears, weakness, or dysfunction.

If the patient is unable to control the arm's descent or experiences sudden dropping, it could indicate a supraspinatus tear or other rotator cuff pathology.

Structures Assessed[9,10,12,34]	Special Maneuver	Examination Technique	Examples of Abnormalities
Composite Tests			
Assesses function of the infraspinatus muscle (external rotation) and strength	**External rotation resistance test** 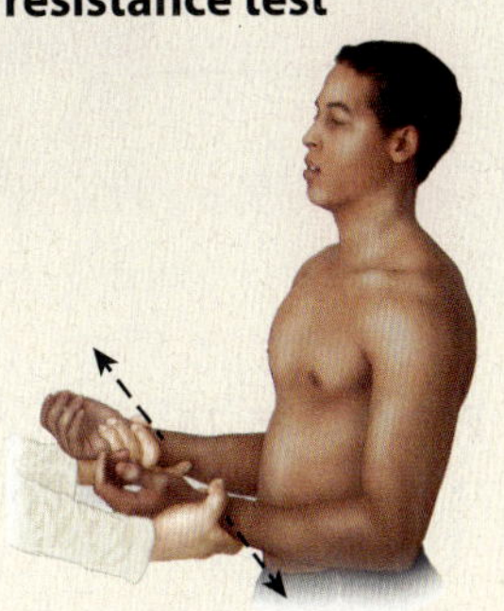	Ask the patient to adduct and flex their arm to 90°, with their thumbs turned up. Stabilize their elbow with one hand and apply pressure proximal to their wrist as they press the wrist outward in external rotation.	A positive result suggests potential issues with the infraspinatus muscle. It may indicate infraspinatus muscle weakness or pathology.
Assesses function of the supraspinatus muscle (abduction) and strength	**Empty can test** 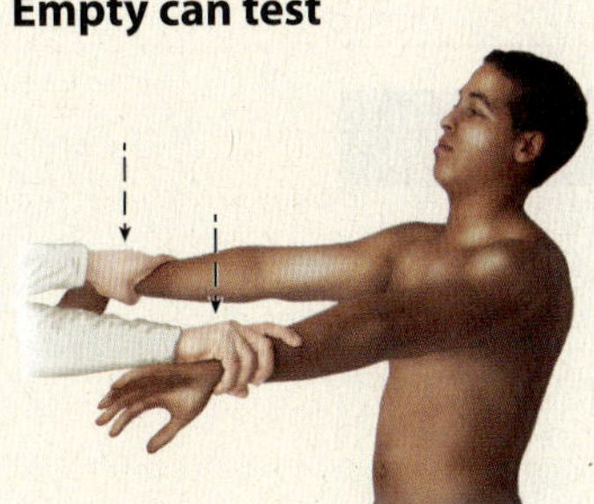	With the patient seated or standing, ask them to abduct and internally rotate their arm to 90° so that their thumb points downward (as if they are emptying the contents of a can - hence, the "empty can" position). Ask them to resist as you place downward pressure on their arm.	A positive empty can test indicates potential may suggest impingement or a partial tear of the supraspinatus tendon or muscle.

ANATOMY: ELBOW

The elbow helps position the hand in space and stabilizes the lever action of the forearm. The elbow joint is formed by the humerus and the two bones of the forearm, the radius and ulna (Fig. 25-24).

These bones have three articulations: the *ulnohumeral radiohumeral,* and *radioulnar joints.* All three share a large common articular cavity and an extensive synovial lining. These bones give rise to the three bony prominences of the elbow: the *medial and lateral epicondyles* of the humerus and the *olecranon process* of the ulna.

Muscles traversing the elbow include the *biceps brachii* (elbow flexion and forearm supination), the *brachialis* and *brachioradialis* (elbow flexion), the *triceps* (elbow extension), the *pronator teres* (forearm pronation), and the *supinator* (forearm supination). *The common extensor and flexor/pronator tendons* originate at the elbow before projecting into the forearm to assist with wrist and finger movement and with pronation of the forearm.

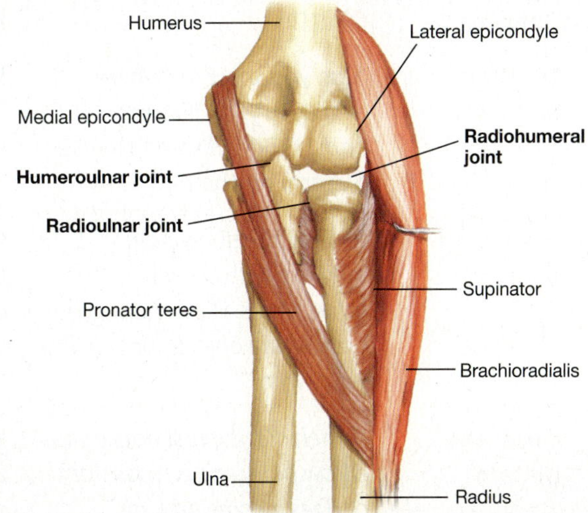

FIGURE 25-24. Anatomy of the left anterior elbow.

The *olecranon bursa* is the largest bursa in this region and lies between the olecranon process and the skin (Fig. 25-25). The bursa is not normally palpable but can swell and becomes tender when inflamed.

The *ulnar nerve* runs posteriorly in the ulnar groove between the medial epicondyle and the olecranon process. The *radial nerve* is adjacent to the lateral epicondyle and travels through the supinator muscle. On the ventral forearm, the *median nerve* is just medial to the brachial artery and biceps tendon in the antecubital fossa.

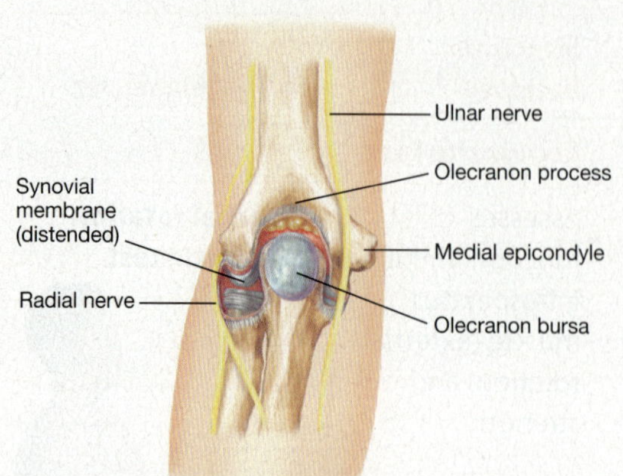

FIGURE 25-25. Left elbow, posterior view, revealing the olecranon bursa.

HEALTH HISTORY: GENERAL APPROACH

Common or Concerning Symptom

- Elbow pain

Elbow Pain

Elbow pain is a common reason for patients to seek consultation. To assess this, the first question to ask is, "Could you identify the exact area of your elbow pain?" The health history should focus on details such as the type, onset, pattern, and progression of the pain as well as any accompanying symptoms (Box 25-20). The health history domains for evaluating joint pain, as outlined on pages 783–784, provide a comprehensive framework.

Box 25-20. Elbow Pain: High-Yield History Questions

Domain	Questions	Rationale
Location and spread	*"Can you show me where exactly in your elbow the pain is? Does it spread to your forearm or wrist?"*	Helps identify specific tendons or nerves that may be affected
Movement-related	*"Does your elbow pain increase with certain movements, like bending your arm, lifting objects, or twisting your wrist?"*	Can suggest conditions like tennis elbow or golfer's elbow
Onset and pattern	*"When did you first notice your elbow pain, and is it constant or does it come and go?"*	Helps differentiate acute and chronic or repetitive strain injuries

Domain	Questions	Rationale
Activity and occupational impact	*"What kind of work do you do, and do you participate in any sports or hobbies that involve repetitive arm motions?"*	Can contribute to specific types of elbow pain, like tendonitis
Associated symptoms	*"Do you experience any numbness, tingling, or weakness in your hand or forearm along with the elbow pain?"*	Can indicate nerve involvement, such as in cubital tunnel syndrome
Previous injuries	*"Have you had any previous elbow injuries or surgeries?"*	Can be a significant factor in current elbow pain
Effect of rest or ice	*"Does resting, icing, or applying heat to your elbow affect your pain?"*	Can provide clues about inflammation and the nature of the injury
Stiffness and swelling	*"Do you notice any stiffness or swelling around your elbow joint?"*	Stiffness and swelling can be indicative of joint inflammation, bursitis, or other localized issues

Possible causes include **tennis elbow or lateral epicondylitis** (inflammation of the tendons that join the forearm muscles on the outside of the elbow, typically due to overuse), **golfer's elbow or medial epicondylitis** (affects the tendons on the inside of the elbow), **olecranon bursitis**, **elbow fractures**, **cubital tunnel syndrome** (pressure or stretching of the ulnar nerve), and **OA** in the elbow joint).

TECHNIQUES OF EXAMINATION

Key Components of the Elbow Joint Examination

I	■ Inspect the elbow joint (contour, asymmetry, nodules, swelling).
P	■ Palpate the elbow joint and adjoining structures (olecranon process, medial and lateral epicondyles, radial head, ulnar nerve).
ROM	■ Assess elbow range of motion (flexion, extension, pronation, supination).
S	■ Perform special maneuvers for the elbow joint, if indicated (Cozen and reverse Cozen test, Mill test, Maudsley test, golfer's elbow test, hook test).

Inspect the Elbow Joint

Ensure that your patient is seated comfortably with their arm relaxed. Support the patient's forearm with your opposite hand, maintaining the elbow flexed to about 70°. This relaxed position helps in better visualization and palpation. Identify the medial and lateral epicondyles and the olecranon process of the ulna. Inspect the contours of the elbow, including the extensor surface of the ulna and the olecranon process. Compare side to side to identify any subtle changes. Note any nodules or swelling.

See Table 25-5, Swollen or Tender Elbows, p. 836.

Palpate the Elbow Joint and Adjoining Structures

Olecranon Process. Start by palpating the olecranon process. Feel for warmth in the skin or around the joint that may suggest infection or underlying inflammation. Note any displacement of the olecranon process.

The olecranon is displaced posteriorly in posterior dislocation of the elbow and supracondylar fracture.

Epicondyles. Then press gently over the medial and lateral epicondyles to assess for tenderness (Fig. 25-26). Palpate the grooves between the epicondyles and the olecranon process, where the synovium is most easily examined. Normally the synovium and olecranon bursae are not palpable.

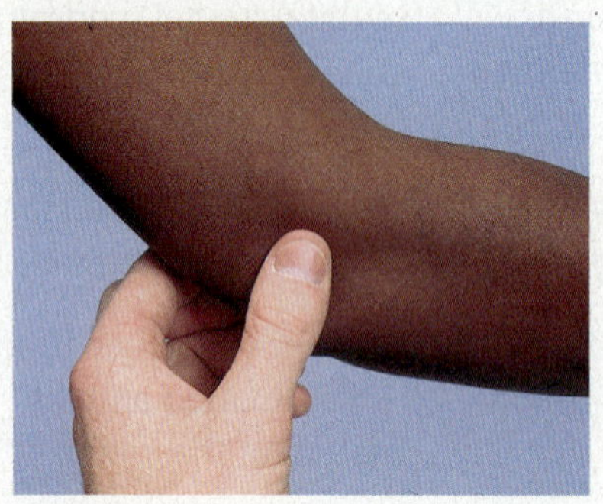

FIGURE 25-26. Palpating the epicondyles for tenderness.

Common extensor tendinopathy, also known as *lateral epicondylosis* or "tennis elbow," causes pain at the lateral epicondyle. Similarly, common flexor/pronator tendinopathy, known as *medial epicondylosis* or "golfer's elbow," results in pain at the medial epicondyle.

Radial Head. The radial head can be palpated approximately two fingerbreadths distal to the lateral epicondyle. Palpate it directly at rest and observe its movement during pronation and supination of the forearm.

Pay attention to any clicking or crepitus that may suggest underlying arthritis, loose body within the joint, or possible damage to the radial head.

Ulnar Nerve. The sensitive ulnar nerve can be palpated posteriorly between the olecranon process and the medial epicondyle (see Fig. 25-25).

Assess Elbow Range of Motion

ROM includes *flexion* and *extension* at the elbow and *pronation* and *supination* of the forearm, which also move the wrist and hand (Fig. 25-27). This should be done with the elbow by the side to ensure the patient does not use shoulder or scapular motion to compensate for restricted motion. Note the

Box 25-21. Range of Motion: Elbow Joint

Elbow Movement	Primary Muscles Affecting Movement	Patient Instructions
Flexion	Biceps brachii, brachialis, brachioradialis	*"Bend your elbow."*
Extension	Triceps brachii, anconeus	*"Straighten your elbow."*
Supination	Biceps brachii, supinator	*"Turn your palms up, as if carrying a bowl of soup."*
Pronation	Pronator teres, pronator quadratus	*"Turn your palms down."*

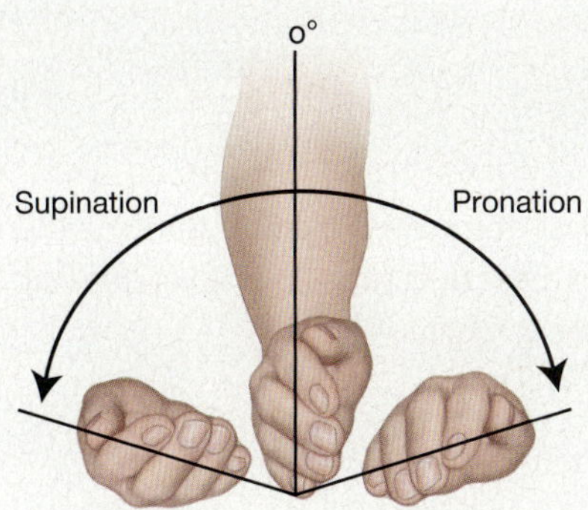

FIGURE 25-27. Elbow supination and pronation.

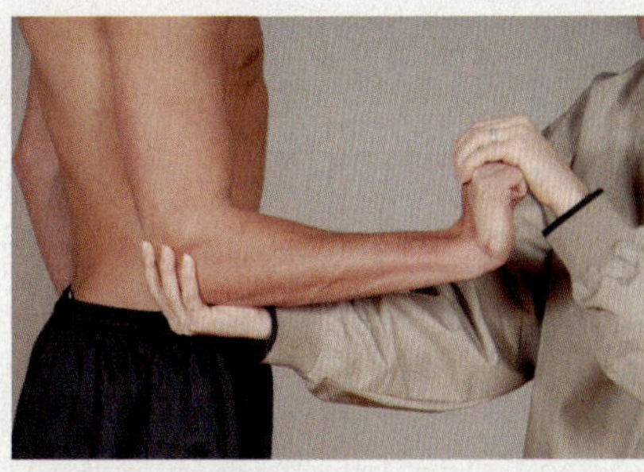

FIGURE 25-28. Cozen test for lateral epicondylitis or "tennis elbow." (Reprinted with permission from Anderson MK, Barnum M. *Foundations of Athletic Training: Prevention, Assessment, and Management.* 7th ed. Wolters Kluwer; 2022. Figure 20-24A.)

specific muscles responsible for each motion and the instructions to the patient (Box 25-21). Always compare movement side to side.

Perform Special Maneuvers for the Elbow Joint (If Indicated)

Three primary tests are used to confirm a diagnosis of lateral epicondylitis or "tennis elbow": the *Cozen test* (Fig. 25-28),[14] *Mill test*, and *Maudsley test.*[15] The two tests for medial epicondylitis reverse the Cozen and Mill tests (Box 25-22).

Box 25-22. Special Maneuvers: Elbow Joint

Special Maneuver	Structures Assessed	Examination Technique
Cozen test	Lateral epicondyle	Hold the patient's elbow steady with their forearm facing downward. Press gently on the bony part on the outside of the elbow. Ask the patient to lift their wrist up against your hand's resistance.
Mill test		Straighten the patient's elbow and bend their wrist downward while their forearm is facing downward.
Maudsley test		Ask the patient to lift their middle finger up against resistance, keeping their wrist straight and forearm in pronation.

Pain at the lateral elbow during any of these tests indicates *lateral epicondylitis* or "tennis elbow."

(continued)

Box 25-22. Special Maneuvers: Elbow Joint (*Continued*)

Special Maneuver	Structures Assessed	Examination Technique	
Reverse Cozen test	Medial epicondyle	Hold the patient's elbow with their palm facing upward. Ask them to bend their wrist and twist it downward against your resistance.	Pain at the medial elbow during either of these tests suggests *medial epicondylitis* or "golfer's elbow."
Golfer's elbow test		Passively extend the patient's elbow and wrist while maintaining the forearm in supination.	
Hook test	Distal biceps tendon	Ask the patient to bend their arm at the elbow and flex their biceps. Try to hook your finger under the tendon near the elbow crease.	Inability to hook the finger underneath the tendon suggests a possible complete rupture of the distal biceps tendon.

ANATOMY: WRIST AND HAND

The wrists and hands are intricate units comprising small, highly active joints that are used almost continuously during waking hours. This complex structure of numerous joints contributes significantly to the remarkable dexterity of the hands.

Wrist Structure

The *wrist* is formed by the distal ends of the *radius* and *ulna*, along with eight small *carpal bones* (Fig. 25-29). Key joints include the *radiocarpal (wrist) joint*, the distal *radioulnar joint*, and the *intercarpal joints*.

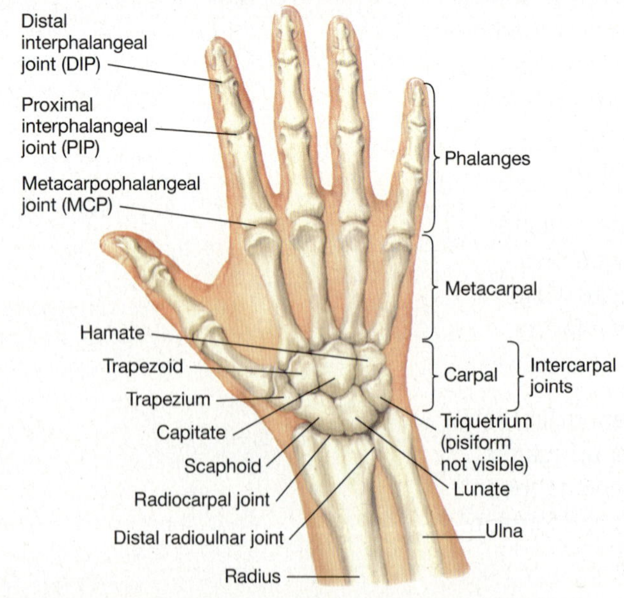

FIGURE 25-29. Anatomy of the right wrist and hand.

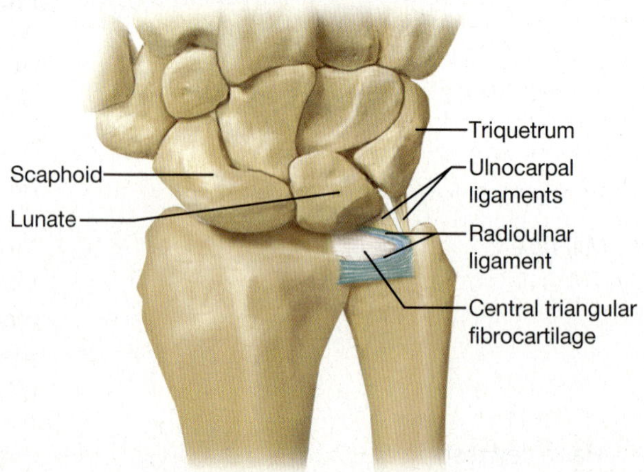

FIGURE 25-30. Triangular fibrocartilage complex (TFCC). (Reprinted with permission from Wiesel SW, ed. *Operative Techniques in Orthopaedic Surgery.* Wolters Kluwer Health/Lippincott Williams and Wilkins; 2011.)

The ulna, which does not directly articulate with the carpal row, is intricately connected to the carpal bones through the *triangular fibrocartilage complex (TFCC)*. The TFCC, a crucial structure in the wrist, not only bridges the ulna and carpal bones but also plays a vital role in radial and ulnar deviation as well as flexion and extension. This complex comprises the *articular disc, meniscus homologue, ulnocarpal ligaments, ulnar collateral ligament, and the extensor carpi ulnaris subsheath*, all of which work in concert to stabilize the ulnar aspect of the wrist (Fig. 25-30). Additionally, the joint capsule and synovial membrane collectively connect the radius to the ulna and to the proximal row of carpal bones, enhancing the wrist's overall stability and ROM.

The *carpal tunnel* is a channel beneath the palmar surface of the wrist and proximal hand. It contains the flexor tendons for the thumb and fingers as well as the *median nerve*.

Holding the tendons and tendon sheath in place is a transverse ligament, the *flexor retinaculum* (Fig. 25-31). The *median nerve* lies between the flexor retinaculum and the tendon sheath. The median nerve provides sensation to the palm and the palmar surface of the thumb, the second and third digits, and half of the fourth digit. It also innervates the thumb muscles of flexion, abduction, and opposition.

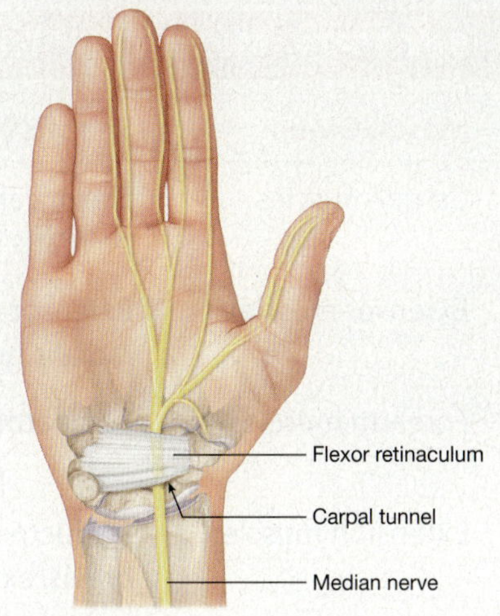

FIGURE 25-31. Carpal tunnel of the right hand.

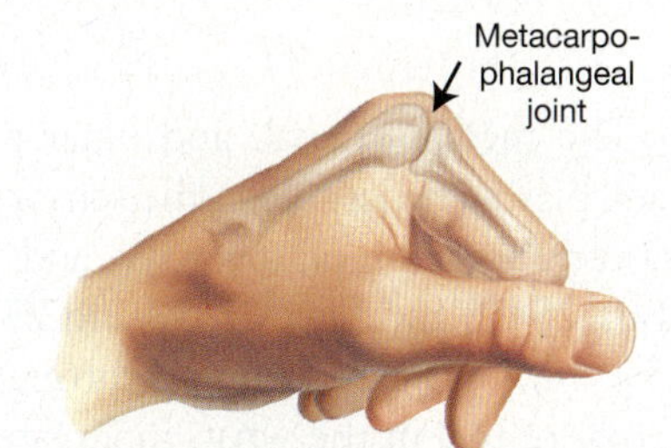

FIGURE 25-32. Metacarpophalangeal (MCP) joints.

Thumb arthritis, commonly seen as OA, primarily affects the first MCP joint.

Hand Structure

The metacarpal bones link the carpal bones to the fingers. Each *finger* comprises a *proximal, middle*, and *distal phalanx*, except for the thumb, which has only a proximal and distal phalanx. The hand's joints include the *metacarpophalangeal (MCP)* (Fig. 25-32), *proximal interphalangeal (PIP)*, and *distal interphalangeal (DIP) joints*.

Intrinsic muscles, tendons, tendon sheaths, and muscles play a vital role in the movement of the wrist and hand (Boxes 25-23 and 25-24).

Box 25-23. Intrinsic Muscles of the Hand and Their Functions

Muscle Group	Location in Hand	Specific Muscles	Function
Thenar eminence	Around the thumb	Abductor pollicis brevis, flexor pollicis brevis, opponens pollicis	Facilitates thumb flexion, abduction, and opposition
Hypothenar eminence	Around the fifth finger	Abductor digiti minimi, flexor digiti minimi brevis, opponens digiti minimi	Aids in abduction, flexion, and opposition of the fifth finger
Lumbricals	Attached to metacarpal bones	First through fourth lumbricals	Involved in flexion at the MCP joints and extension at the interphalangeal joints
Dorsal interossei	Attached to metacarpal bones	First through, fourth dorsal interossei	Involved in finger abduction
Palmar interossei	Attached to metacarpal bones	First through third palmar interossei	Involved in finger adduction

Box 25-24. Muscles and Tendons Affecting Wrist and Hand Movement

Muscle Group	Specific Muscles	Function
Carpal muscles	Flexor carpi radialis, flexor carpi ulnaris, palmaris longus	Facilitates wrist flexion
Extensor muscles	Extensor carpi radialis longus, extensor carpi radialis brevis, extensor carpi ulnaris	Enables wrist extension
Forearm muscles	Supinator, pronator teres, pronator quadratus	Powers supination and pronation of the forearm
Extension muscles	Abductor pollicis longus, extensor pollicis brevis, extensor pollicis longus	Controls thumb extension and abduction
Flexor and extensor muscles	Flexor digitorum superficialis, flexor digitorum profundus, extensor digitorum, extensor indicis	Controls flexion and extension of the fingers via tendons traveling in sheaths

The median, radial, and ulnar nerves each play a crucial role in the sensory and motor functions of the wrist and hand (Box 25-25 and Figs. 25-33 and 25-34). The *median nerve*, running through the carpal tunnel in the wrist, innervates the lateral palm and the palmar aspects of the thumb, index, middle, and half of the ring finger. It also controls some thumb muscles and aids in finger flexion. The *radial nerve*, less prone to compression, extends along the forearm to the wrist and primarily provides sensory input to the back of the hand and thumb. It also activates the extensor muscles in the forearm, crucial for extending the wrist and fingers. The *ulnar nerve*, travelling along the ulnar side of the forearm, is responsible for the sensation in the medial palm, little finger, and half of the ring finger as well as motor control of most intrinsic hand muscles, essential for fine motor skills.

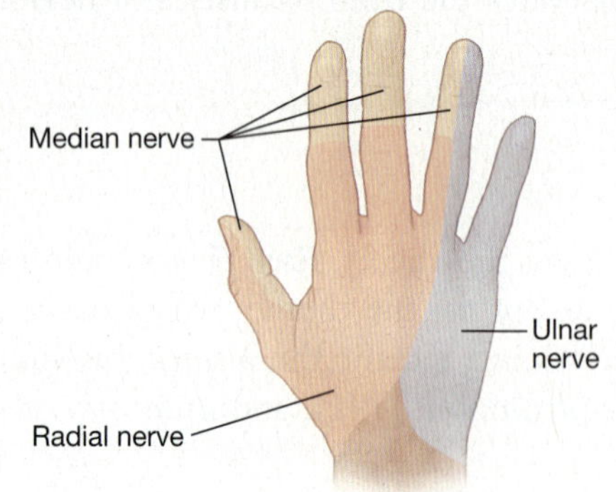

FIGURE 25-33. Peripheral innervation of the right hand (dorsum).

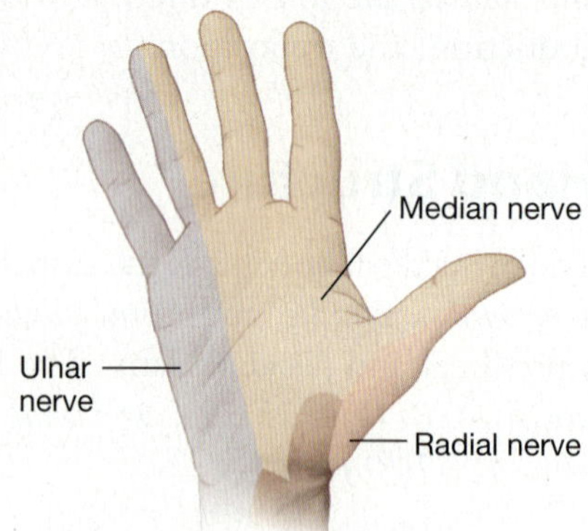

FIGURE 25-34. Peripheral innervation of the right hand (palmar).

Box 25-25. Nerve Innervation and Function in the Wrist and Hand

Nerve	Area of Innervation	Function
Median nerve	Thumb, index, middle, and part of ring finger	Critical in both sensory perception and motor control of the involved digits Involved in precise movements and grip strength
Radial nerve	Primarily back of hand and wrist	Essential for extension of the wrist and fingers Controls ability to lift hand and straighten fingers, playing a key role in hand and wrist positioning
Ulnar nerve	Little finger, adjacent half of ring finger, and some intrinsic hand muscles	Vital for fine motor skills, such as finger coordination and complex movements Also contributes to grip and ability to pinch objects between thumb and little finger

HEALTH HISTORY: GENERAL APPROACH

Common or Concerning Symptoms

- Wrist and hand pain

Wrist and Hand Pain

Evaluating wrist and hand pain starts with asking the patient, "*Can you point out the exact location of your pain?*" An in-depth health history focuses on the pain's type, beginning, course, and any symptoms that occur alongside it (Box 25-26). For a more general framework on joint pain assessment, see the health history domains listed on pages 783–784.

Box 25-26. Wrist and Hand Pain: High-Yield History Questions

Domain	Questions	Rationale
Location	*"Can you point to the exact area of your hand or wrist where you feel the most pain?"*	Helps pinpoint specific conditions related to different hand and wrist areas
Type of hand use	*"Does your pain worsen with specific hand movements, like gripping, twisting, or typing?"*	Can indicate possible overuse injuries or strain
Hand function changes	*"Have you noticed any changes in how well you can use your hand, like holding things tightly or moving your fingers easily?"*	Can detect functional impairments that may be associated with underlying musculoskeletal or neurologic conditions
Sensation alterations	*"Do you feel any numbness, tingling, or different sensations in your hand or fingers?"*	Can suggest nerve involvement or compression, common in conditions like carpal tunnel syndrome
Swelling or deformity	*"Have you seen any swelling, changes in color, or unusual shapes in your wrist or hand?"*	Looks for signs of inflammation, trauma, or degenerative changes that could influence diagnosis and treatment
Hobbies/ activities	*"Do you participate in any sports or recreational activities that may strain the elbow?"*	Can be a cause of elbow pain, such as overuse injuries in athletes

(continued)

Possible causes include **carpal tunnel syndrome** (compression of the median nerve in the wrist, leading to pain, numbness, and tingling in the hand), **arthritis** (including OA from wear and tear and RA from autoimmune disease), **tendinitis**, **ganglion cysts** (fluid-filled lumps near the joints or tendons of the wrist or hand), **De Quervain tenosynovitis** (inflammation of the tendons on the thumb side of the wrist, leading to pain and difficulty moving the thumb and wrist), and **fractures**.

Box 25-26. Wrist and Hand Pain: High-Yield History Questions (*Continued*)

Domain	Questions	Rationale
Effect of rest or activity	*"Does the pain in your hand change when you rest or when you move?"*	Differentiates between pain exacerbated by activity (e.g., overuse or mechanical issues) and pain relieved or unchanged by rest
Nighttime symptoms	*"Do you feel pain or discomfort in your wrist or hand when you sleep or first thing in the morning?"*	Can indicate carpal tunnel syndrome or inflammatory arthritis
Previous injuries	*"Have you ever hurt your hand or wrist before, or had any operations on them?"*	Can have long-term impacts on hand and wrist health, influencing current symptoms

TECHNIQUES OF EXAMINATION

Key Components of the Wrist Joint and Hand Examination

I	■ Inspect the wrist (asymmetry, position, movement, swelling, deformities, angulation, thickening, motion).
	■ Inspect the hand (position, movement, structure, swelling, deformities, wasting, asymmetry).
P	■ Palpate the wrist (distal radius and ulna, radial styloid, anatomic snuffbox, carpal bones).
	■ Palpate the hand (metacarpals, metacarpophalangeal joints, phalanges, proximal and distal interphalangeal joints tendons of the thumb and fingers).
ROM	■ Assess wrist, fingers, and thumb range of motion.
S	■ Perform special maneuvers for the wrist and hand, if indicated (hand strength test, Finkelstein test, thumb abduction test, thumb opposition test, Tinel sign, Phalen sign).

Inspect the Wrist

Begin by conducting a thorough inspection, comparing both of the patient's wrists side by side to identify any asymmetries or abnormalities. Pay attention to the position and movement of the wrist, ensuring that it moves smoothly and naturally. Look carefully for any swelling over the joints or signs of trauma on both the palmar and dorsal surfaces. Noting any deformities, angulation, or thickening of the flexor tendons is crucial in identifying potential issues. Observe the wrists in motion to assess for smooth, natural movement.

Guarded movement in the wrist could suggest an injury. Issues with the flexor tendons might lead to abnormal finger movements. Any misalignment in a finger could indicate an underlying fracture or joint injury.

Carefully inspect the palmar and dorsal surfaces of the wrist for any signs of swelling over the joints or indications of trauma.

Inspect the Hand

Inspection of the hand involves a thorough examination of its resting position, movement, and overall structure. When the patient's fingers are relaxed, they should be slightly flexed with the fingernail edges parallel. During flexion into a fist, fingers should point toward the scaphoid bone in the wrist.

Abnormal finger movement can signal flexor tendon damage. Misalignment of a finger suggests an underlying fracture or joint injury.

The palmar and dorsal surfaces of the hand should be inspected for any signs of swelling, trauma, deformities, or muscle wasting, particularly in the thenar and hypothenar eminences. Any asymmetry compared to the opposite side should be noted.

Dupuytren flexion contractures, which commonly affect the third, fourth, and fifth fingers, result from the thickening of the palmar fascia. Trigger digits, caused by stenosing tenosynovitis, are another condition to be aware of.[16]

For detailed descriptions of specific hand pathologies, refer to Table 25-6, Arthritis in the Hands, and Table 25-7, Swellings and Deformities of the Hands.

Observe the contours of the palm, namely the *thenar* and *hypothenar* eminences looking for any muscle wasting or asymmetry compared to the opposite side.

Thenar atrophy can occur in median nerve injury from carpal tunnel syndrome (sensitivity <50%; specificity >82%–99%).[17] In ulnar nerve injury, there is hypothenar atrophy.

Palpate the Wrist

Distal Radius and Ulna. Carefully feel the end points of the radius and ulna bones, located on the lateral and medial sides of the wrist, respectively. Also, palpate the distal radioulnar joint where these two bones meet. This area is crucial for detecting any abnormalities following injuries like falls (Fig. 25-35). Check for swelling, bogginess, or tenderness.

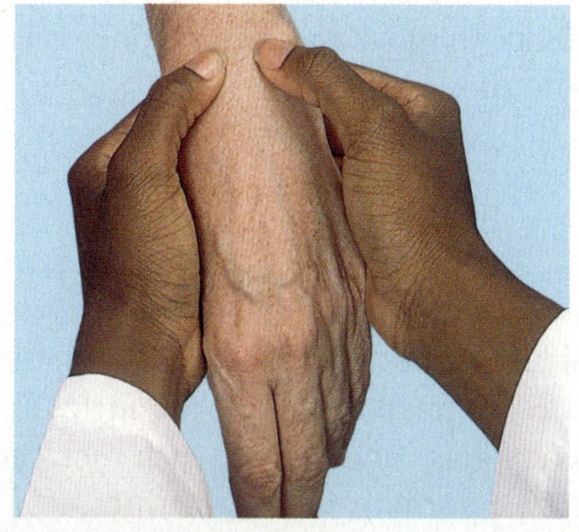

FIGURE 25-35. Palpating the distal radioulnar joint.

Tenderness or bony step-offs over the distal radius after a fall is suspicious for a distal radius fracture.

Use your thumbs to feel along the wrist joint's groove, covering both the volar and dorsal aspects. Identify any unusual swelling, stiffness, or tenderness, which can indicate joint pathology.

Radial Styloid and Anatomic Snuffbox. Palpate the *radial styloid bone* and the *anatomic snuffbox.* Start by locating the radial styloid process, a bony prominence found on the thumb side of the wrist at the distal end of the radius bone. Directly adjacent and just distal to this process is the anatomic snuffbox, a small, hollowed depression. This area is bordered by the tendons of the thumb, specifically the abductor pollicis longus and the extensor pollicis brevis.

Tenderness over the extensor and abductor tendons of the thumb at the radial styloid occurs in de Quervain tenosynovitis and gonococcal tenosynovitis. See Table 25-8, Tendon Sheath, Palmar Space, and Finger Infections, p. 839.

To make the anatomic snuffbox more visible and pronounced, ask the patient to move their thumb away from the palm of their hand (abduct the thumb). Once the snuffbox is visible, use your fingertips to gently palpate the area for tenderness (Fig. 25-36).

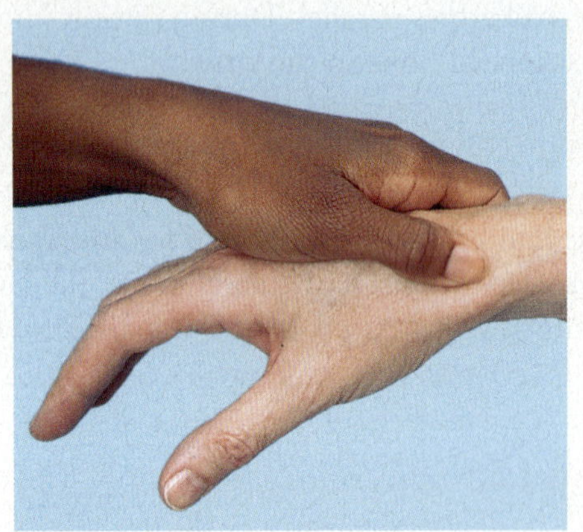

FIGURE 25-36. Palpating the anatomical snuffbox.

Tenderness in the "snuffbox" with wrist ulnar deviation and pain at the scaphoid tubercle, combined with the risk of avascular necrosis due to poor blood supply, strongly indicate a scaphoid fracture.[18]

Carpal Bones. Begin by having the patient extend their hand with the palm facing down. Gently support their hand with your nondominant hand. With your dominant hand, start palpating at the base of the wrist, where the radius and ulna meet the carpal bones. Use the pads of your fingers to apply gentle but firm pressure as you explore the wrist's bony landmarks.

Identify the proximal row of carpal bones, including the *scaphoid, lunate, triquetrum*, and *pisiform*. Move distally to palpate the second row of carpal bones, consisting of the *trapezium, trapezoid, capitate*, and *hamate* (see Figure 25-29). Pay attention to any tenderness, irregularities, or swelling that could indicate injury or pathology. Attempt to move the carpal bones relative to each other. There should be little to no movement.

Excessive movement of any carpal bones, especially when painful, suggests underlying ligament laxity or disruption.

Palpate the Hand

Metacarpals. With the patient's hand open and relaxed, palm facing upward, begin at the wrist and palpate distally along the length of each metacarpal bone. Start with the thumb's metacarpal, progressing toward the little finger. Use your thumb and index finger to gently grasp and palpate each metacarpal shaft and its base, assessing for tenderness, deformity, or irregularities.

Metacarpophalangeal Joints. Use your thumb to palpate each MCP joint just distal to and on each side of the extensor tendons as your index finger feels the head of the metacarpal in the palm (Fig. 25-37). Note any swelling, bogginess, or tenderness.

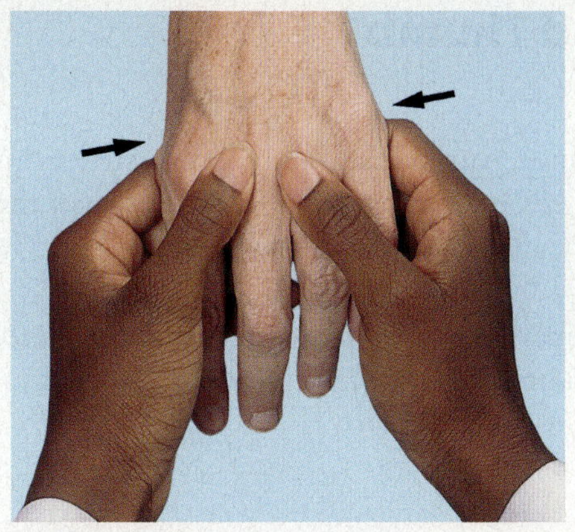

FIGURE 25-37. Palpating the metacarpophalangeal joints of the left hand.

The MCPs are often boggy or tender in RA but are rarely involved in OA. Focal tenderness after trauma may suggest underlying fracture.

Phalanges. To palpate the phalanges, ask the patient to relax their hand, either palm up or palm down. Starting with the thumb, palpate each phalanx, including the proximal, middle (except in the thumb, which has only two phalanges), and distal phalanges. Use a gentle, pinching motion with your thumb and index finger to palpate each bone, feeling for any asymmetry, swelling, or tenderness.

Proximal and Distal Interphalangeal Joints. Palpate the medial and lateral aspects of each PIP joint between your thumb and index finger, again checking for swelling, bogginess, bony enlargement, or tenderness. Using the same techniques, examine the DIP joints (Fig. 25-38).

Bouchard nodes in the PIPs are a classic sign of OA. *Heberden nodes*, which are more common than Bouchard nodes, are similar bony swellings that develop in the DIPs of patients with OA (Fig. 25-39).

Tendons of the Thumb and Fingers. Palpate along the tendons inserting on the thumb and fingers looking for tenderness, erythema, or inflammation. Examine for any focal thickening.

Tenderness and swelling occur in *tenosynovitis*. De Quervain tenosynovitis involves the extensor and abductor tendons of the thumb as they cross the radial styloid in the first dorsal compartment of the wrist.

FIGURE 25-38. Palpating the distal interphalangeal joints.

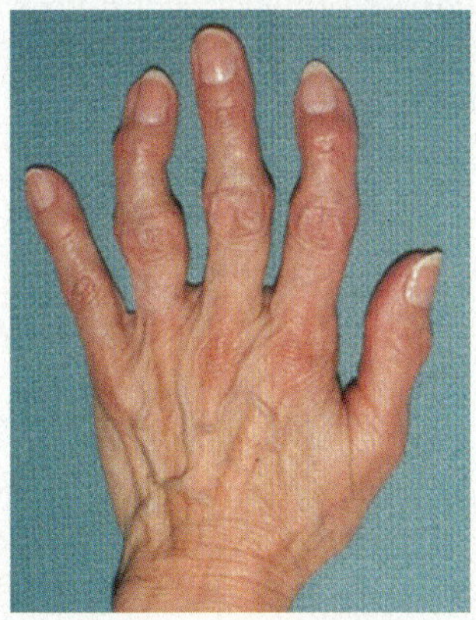

FIGURE 25-39. Heberden nodes (DIPs) and Bouchard nodes (PIPs) in a patient with classic hand osteoarthritis. (Modified with permission from Ballantyne JC, Fishman SM, Rathmell JP. *Bonica's Management of Pain.* 5th ed. Wolters Kluwer; 2019. Figure 34-3.)

Assess Wrist, Fingers, and Thumb Range of Motion

Wrist. During the wrist examination, guide your patient with clear instructions to assess all active ROM (Box 25-27). Always compare the ROM between the affected and unaffected sides to identify any abnormalities.

See Table 25-7, Swellings and Deformities of the Hands, p. 838.

Fingers. Evaluating the ROM of the fingers is an essential aspect of hand functionality assessment (Box 25-28). This involves the *flexor* and *extensor digitorum* as well as the *intrinsic muscles of the hand*.

Box 25-27. Range of Motion: Wrist

Movement	Examination Technique	Patient Instructions
Flexion 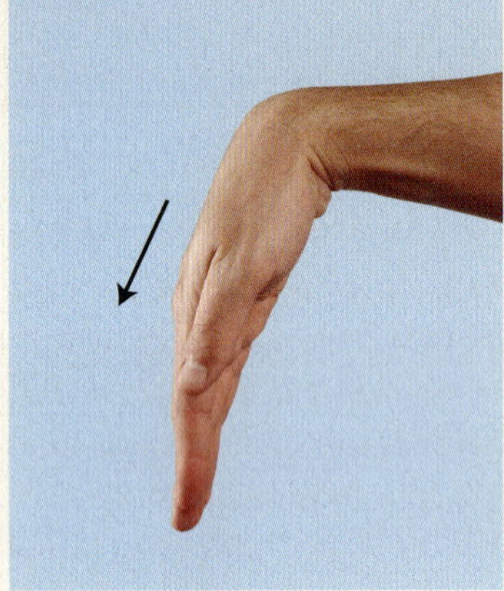 FIGURE 25-40	Observe the patient bending their wrist downward (Fig. 25-40). Assess the angle of flexion and note any stiffness or limitation in the movement.	*"Bend your wrist downward as if you're pushing something down with the palm of your hand."*
Extension 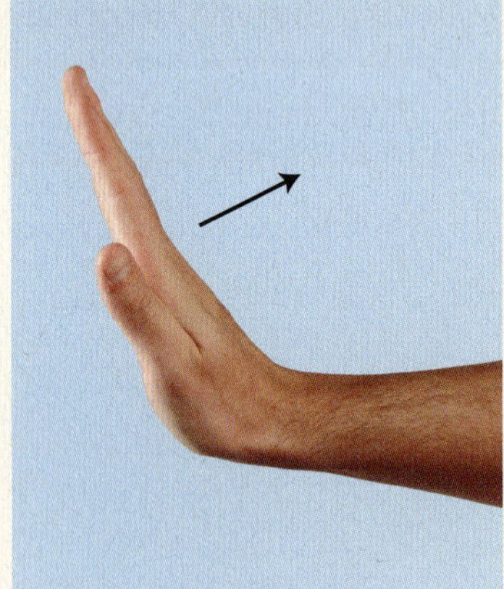 FIGURE 25-41	Watch as the patient bends their wrist upward (Fig. 25-41). Evaluate the extent of the upward bend and check for smoothness and symmetry in the movement.	*"Bend your wrist upward as if you're gesturing someone to stop with your palm facing outward."*

Movement	Examination Technique	Patient Instructions
Radial deviation FIGURE 25-42	Have the patient bend their wrist toward the thumb side (Fig. 25-42). Monitor the degree of lateral movement toward the radius bone and any discomfort.	*"Bend your wrist toward your thumb side."*
Ulnar deviation FIGURE 25-43	Observe the patient bending their wrist toward the fifth digit (pinky) side (Fig. 25-43). Check the extent of lateral movement toward the ulnar bone and note any pain or restriction.	*"Bend your wrist toward your pinky side."*
Circumduction	Watch the patient perform a circular motion with their wrist. Assess the fluidity and range of the circular movement and any unevenness or difficulty.	*"Rotate your wrist to draw a circle in the air with your fingertips."*

Box 25-28. Range of Motion: Hand (Metacarpophalangeal and Proximal and Distal Interphalangeal Joints)

Movement	Examination Technique	Patient Instructions
Combined finger flexion (full fist formation)	Observe the patient as they curl their fingers into a fist, flexing the MCP, PIP, and DIP joints together. Note the completeness of the fist and any discomfort.	*"Curl your fingers into a fist."*
Combined finger extension	Watch the patient as they extend all finger joints simultaneously. Evaluate the full extension of MCP, PIP, and DIP joints and the ability to spread the fingers wide.	*"Spread your fingers as wide as you can, straightening all joints."*
MCP joint flexion	Observe the patient flexing their MCP joints by bending their fingers toward their palm.	*"Bend your fingers at the base joints toward your palm."*
MCP joint extension	Watch the patient extend their MCP joints by straightening them.	*"Straighten your fingers at the base joints."*

(continued)

Box 25-28. Range of Motion: Hand (Metacarpophalangeal and Proximal and Distal Interphalangeal Joints) (*Continued*)

Movement	Examination Technique	Patient Instructions
MCP joint abduction 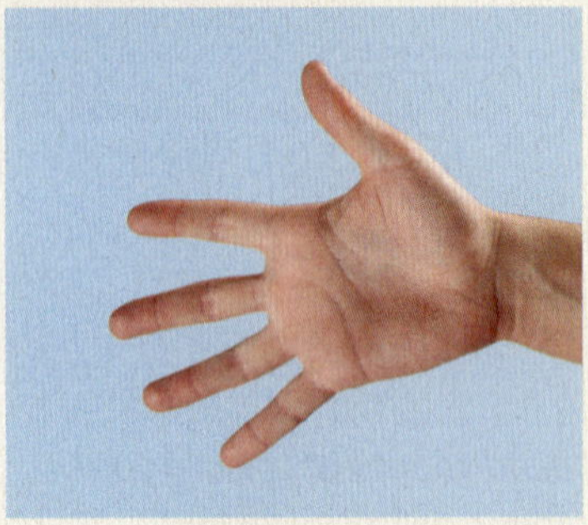 FIGURE 25-44	Have the patient move their fingers apart at the MCP joints (Fig. 25-44).	*"Move your fingers apart at the base of your fingers."*
MCP joint adduction 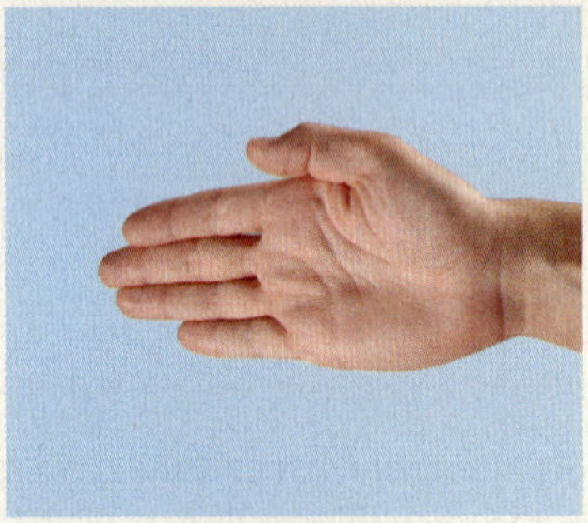 FIGURE 25-45	Observe the patient bringing their fingers together at the MCP joints (Fig. 25-45).	*"Bring your fingers together at the base of your fingers."*
PIP/DIP joint flexion 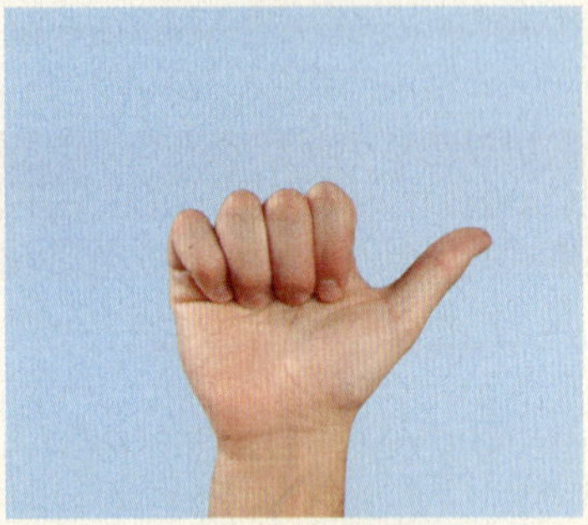 FIGURE 25-46	Stabilize the finger at the MCP joint and ask the patient to flex at the PIP and DIP joints (Fig. 25-46).	*"Bend your fingers at the middle and end joints, while I hold your finger at the base."*
PIP/DIP joint extension 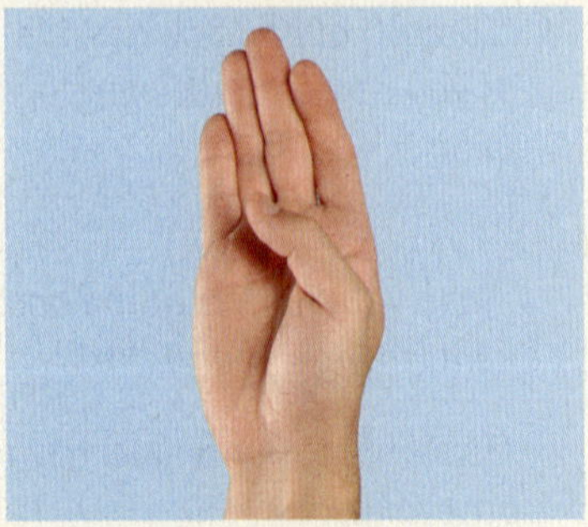 FIGURE 25-47	With the MCP joint stabilized, observe the patient extending at the PIP and DIP joints (Fig. 25-47).	*"Straighten your fingers at the middle and end joints, while I hold your finger at the base."*

Thumb. The thumb's ROM is vital for hand function, playing a key role in grip and precision handling of objects. The thumb has unique movements compared to the other fingers, including *flexion, extension, palmar abduction, radial abduction,* and *thumb adduction,* and *opposition* (Box 25-29). These movements are enabled by muscles like the *flexor pollicis longus, extensor pollicis brevis and longus,* and the *opponens pollicis.*

Box 25-29. Range of Motion: Thumb at Metacarpophalangeal, Interphalangeal, and Carpometacarpal Joints

Movement	Examination Technique	Patient Instructions
Thumb flexion at MCP and IP joints 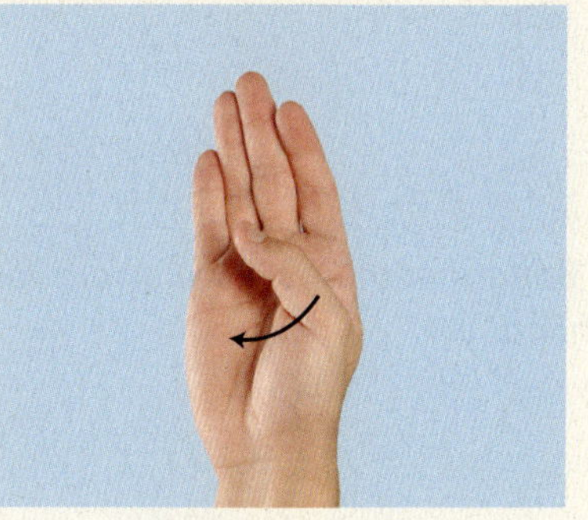 **FIGURE 25-48**	Observe the patient bending their thumb across their palm toward the pinky (Fig. 25-48). Note the range of motion and any difficulty in reaching the pinky or base of the little finger.	*"Bend your thumb across your palm toward your pinky."*
Thumb extension at MCP and IP joints 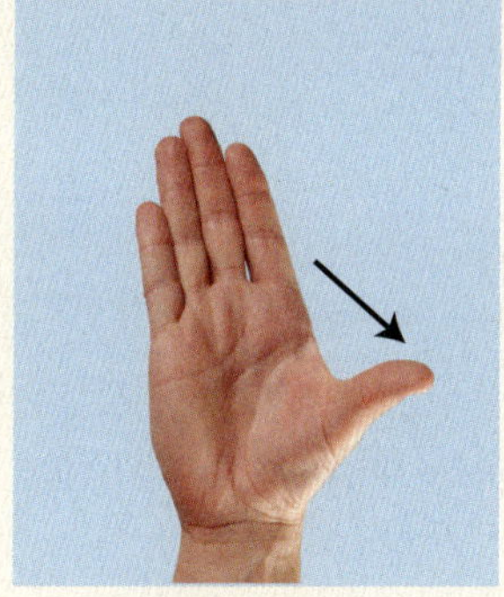 **FIGURE 25-49**	Watch the patient extend their thumb upward while their palm is facing forward (Fig. 25-49). Assess how high the thumb can be lifted, noting any stiffness or limitations.	*"With your palm facing you, lift your thumb up toward the ceiling."*
Palmar abduction at CMC joint 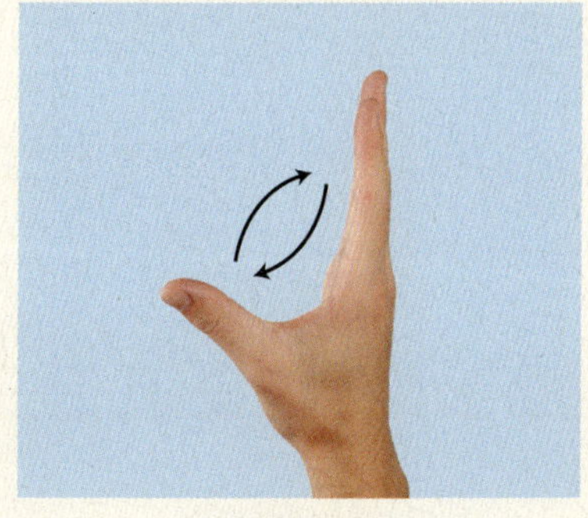 **FIGURE 25-50**	Have the patient move their thumb away from their hand perpendicular to the plane of the palm, forming an "L" shape (Fig. 25-50). Evaluate the angle between the thumb and the hand and note any difficulty in maintaining this position.	*"With your palm facing forward, lift your thumb upward, moving it away from the palm perpendicularly."*

(*continued*)

Box 25-29. Range of Motion: Thumb at Metacarpophalangeal, Interphalangeal, and Carpometacarpal Joints (*Continued*)

Movement	Examination Technique	Patient Instructions
Radial abduction at CMC joint 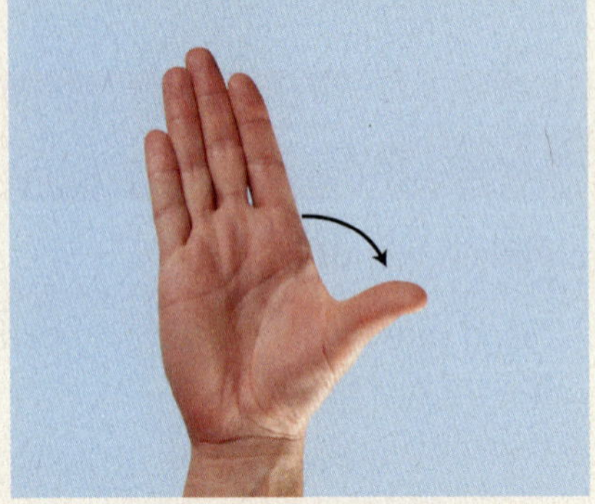 FIGURE 25-51	Instruct the patient to move their thumb laterally away from their index finger while keeping the palm facing forward. Observe the lateral movement (Fig. 25-51).	*"With your palm facing forward, slide your thumb outward, away from the hand, keeping it in line with the plane of the palm."*
Thumb adduction at CMC joint 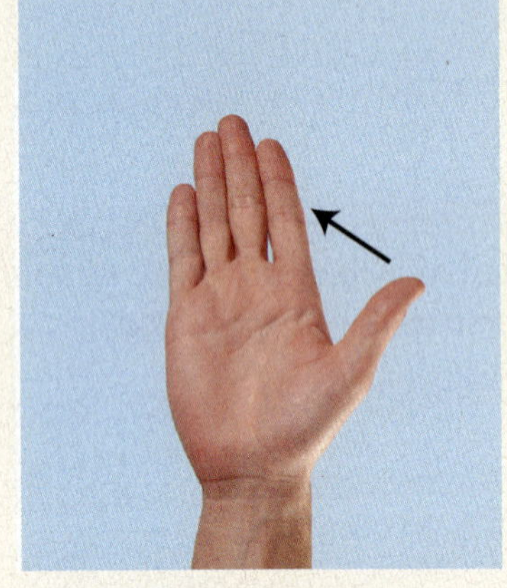 FIGURE 25-52	Observe the patient bringing their thumb back toward their hand (Fig. 25-52). Check the ease of this movement and whether the thumb can be brought close to or against the side of the hand.	*"Bring your thumb back toward your hand."*
Thumb opposition at CMC joint 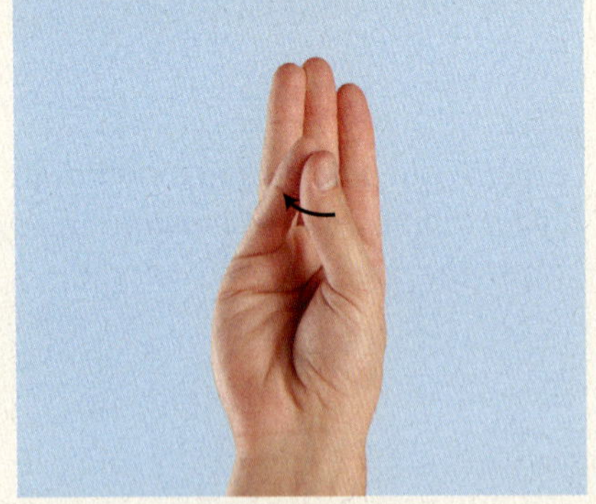 FIGURE 25-53	Monitor the patient touching the tip of their thumb to the tip of their pinky (Fig. 25-53). Assess their ability to make this contact and note if any other fingers are used to assist.	*"Touch the tip of your thumb to the tip of your pinky."*

Perform Special Maneuvers for the Wrist and Hand (If Indicated)

Among these, key tests include the *hand strength test*, *Finkelstein test*, and several maneuvers for identifying nerve entrapment neuropathies like *carpal tunnel syndrome* (Box 25-30).

Box 25-30. Special Maneuvers: Wrist and Hand

Special Maneuver	Structures Assessed	Examination Technique
Hand strength test FIGURE 25-54	Wrist joints, finger flexors, and intrinsic hand muscles	Ask the patient to grasp your second and third fingers tightly (Fig. 25-54). Then test finger abduction by having the patient spread their fingers and push inward against your second and fifth fingers.
Finkelstein test Tendon FIGURE 25-55	Tendons of the abductor pollicis longus and extensor pollicis brevis	Instruct the patient to grasp their thumb against the palm and then move the wrist into ulnar deviation (Fig. 25-55).
Thumb abduction test FIGURE 25-56	Median nerve in the carpal tunnel	Ask the patient to turn their hand palm up and raise their thumb straight up away from the palm, forming a 90° angle with the hand. Apply gentle downward resistance to the thumb (Fig. 25-56).

(*continued*)

Decreased grip strength indicates weakness of finger flexors and/or intrinsic hand muscles, which can be caused by arthritis, carpal tunnel syndrome, epicondylosis, cervical radiculopathy, or peripheral nerve disorders.

Pain during this maneuver suggests *de Quervain tenosynovitis*, an inflammation from overuse.

Weakness in thumb movements indicates median nerve involvement.[18,19]

Box 25-30. Special Maneuvers: Wrist and Hand (*Continued*)

Special Maneuver	Structures Assessed	Examination Technique	Examples of Abnormalities
Thumb opposition test	Median nerve, opponens pollicis muscle, and thenar muscles	Instruct the patient to touch their thumb to the tip of their little finger while you apply outward pressure against the base of their thumb (see Fig. 25-53).	
Tinel sign FIGURE 25-57	Median nerve in the carpal tunnel	Gently tap over the course of the median nerve as it runs through the carpal tunnel on the patient's wrist (Fig. 25-57).	Shooting pain or worsening numbness in the median nerve distribution during the Tinel sign, and numbness/tingling during the Phalen sign within 60 seconds, indicate carpal tunnel syndrome.[13,18,19]
Phalen sign FIGURE 25-58	Median nerve in the carpal tunnel	Ask the patient to flex their wrists maximally, either by holding their wrists in full flexion for 60 seconds or by pressing the backs of both hands together to form right angles (Fig. 25-58).	

RECORDING YOUR FINDINGS

When documenting musculoskeletal findings, use anatomic terminology that aligns with the structure and function of individual joints. Your documentation should include precise details regarding the location of any pathology or pain. Additionally, specify which movements elicit or replicate the patient's symptoms. This approach enhances the meaningfulness and informativeness of your assessment.

Recording the Musculoskeletal System Examination

"Full range of motion in all joints of the upper and lower extremities. No evidence of swelling or deformity."

OR

"Shoulder without evidence of deformities or asymmetries. Shoulder muscles without noticeable atrophy. Tenderness is noted in the area overlying the rotator cuff tendons. Limited range of motion with discomfort reported during forward flexion, pronounced restriction in external rotation with associated pain and restricted abduction, with the patient experiencing discomfort and guarding of the shoulder. Neer and Hawkins–Kennedy tests are positive."

Breaking down the physical examination documentation into specific sections highlights the crucial role of clinical observations in identifying diagnostic indicators. The findings described in the provided text are suspicious for a shoulder condition, and several possibilities should be considered:

- *Tenderness overlying rotator cuff tendons:* This suggests an issue with the rotator cuff, such as rotator cuff tendinopathy or inflammation.
- *Limited ROM:* Limited ROM, particularly with discomfort during forward flexion, pronounced restriction in external rotation, and restricted abduction, indicates a possible issue affecting the mobility of the shoulder joint.
- *Positive Neer and Hawkins–Kennedy tests:* This indicates a potential impingement syndrome in the shoulder. These tests are commonly used to assess for impingement of the rotator cuff tendons and subacromial bursa between the humerus and the acromion.

Based on these findings, a *rotator cuff–related pathology* is possible, which may include conditions like rotator cuff tendinopathy, rotator cuff tears, or subacromial impingement syndrome.

HEALTH PROMOTION AND COUNSELING: EVIDENCE AND RECOMMENDATIONS

This section on Health Promotion and Counseling, which covers osteoporosis including its burden of disease, risk factors, screening, and assessing fracture risk, can be found in Chapter 26, Musculoskeletal System: Lumbosacral Spine, Hips, and Lower Extremities, pp. 890–892.

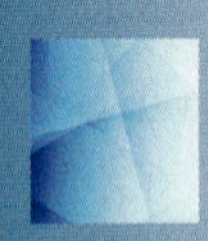

TABLE 25-1. Patterns of Pain in and Around the Joints

Problem	Process	Common Locations	Pattern of Spread	Onset	Progression and Duration
Rheumatoid Arthritis[20–22]	Chronic *synovial membrane* inflammation with secondary erosion of adjacent cartilage and bone and damage to ligaments and tendons	Hands—initially small joints (PIP and MCP joints), feet (MTP joints), wrists, knees, elbows, ankles	Symmetrically additive: progresses to other joints while persisting in initial joints	Usually insidious; human leukocyte antigen (HLA) and non-HLA genes account for >50% of risk of disease; involves proinflammatory cytokines	Often chronic (in >50%), with remissions and exacerbations
Osteoarthritis *(Degenerative Joint Disease)*[23]	Exact etiology is often unknown; leads to degeneration and progressive loss of joint *cartilage* with damage to underlying bone and abnormal formation of new bone at the cartilage and joint margins	Knees, hips, hands (distal, sometimes PIP joints), cervical and lumbar spine, and wrists (first carpometacarpal joint); also joints previously injured or diseased	Additive and asynchronous; may involve only one joint	Usually insidious; family history increases risk of disease; repetitive injury and obesity increase risk; surgical intervention is also a risk factor	Slowly progressive with temporary exacerbations after periods of increased use
Gouty Arthritis[24,25] *Acute Gout*	An inflammatory reaction to microcrystals of monosodium urate; more common in men (may have higher serum urate levels)	Base of the big toe (the first MTP joint), the instep or dorsa of feet, the ankles, knees, and elbows	Early attacks usually confined to one joint	Sudden; often at night; often after injury, surgery, fasting, or excessive food or alcohol intake but can be unprovoked	Occasional isolated attacks lasting days up to 2 wk; may get more frequent and severe and become polyarticular later in course
Chronic Tophaceous Gout	Multiple local accumulations of sodium urate nodules in the joints and other tissues (*tophi*), with or without inflammation	Feet, ankles, wrists, fingers, and elbows	Additive, not as symmetric as RA	Gradual with repeated attacks	Chronic symptoms with acute exacerbations
Polymyalgia Rheumatica[26]	Unclear etiology; occurs in those >50 y; more common in women; overlaps with giant cell arteritis	Muscles of the hip, shoulder, neck; symmetric		Insidious or abrupt, may appear overnight	Chronic but self-limiting
Fibromyalgia Syndrome[27]	Widespread musculoskeletal aching, pain, stiffness. Central pain sensitivity syndrome that may involve aberrant pain signaling and amplification	Multiple regions through the body evaluated with the Widespread Pain Index (WPI)	Shifts unpredictably or worsens in response to immobility, excessive use, or exposure to cold	Variable	Chronic, with "ups and downs"

Associated Symptoms				
Swelling	**Redness, Warmth, and Tenderness**	**Stiffness**	**Limitation of Motion**	**Generalized Symptoms**
Frequent swelling of synovial tissue in joints or tendon sheaths; also subcutaneous nodules	Tender, often warm, but seldom red	Prominent, often for an hour or more in the mornings, also after inactivity	Often develops; affected by associated joint contractures and subluxation, bursitis, and tendinopathy	Weakness, fatigue, weight loss, and low-grade fever are common
Joint effusions may be present, especially in the knees; bony enlargement may accentuate swollen appearance	Possibly tender, seldom warm, and rarely red. Inflammation may accompany disease flares and progression	Frequent but brief (usually 5–10 min), in the morning and with movement after inactivity	Often develops	Usually absent
Within and around involved joint	Exquisitely tender, hot, and red	Not evident	Motion is limited primarily by pain	Fever may be present so consider septic arthritis as well
Present as tophi in joints, bursae, and subcutaneous tissues; check ears and extensor surfaces for tophi	Tenderness, warmth, and redness may be present during exacerbations	Present	Present	Possibly fever; may develop renal failure and renal stones
Swelling and edema may be present over dorsum of hands, wrists, feet	Muscles often tender, but not warm or red	Prominent, especially in the morning	Pain restricts movement, especially in shoulders	Malaise, depression, anorexia, weight loss, fever
None	Tender points may be present in multiple locations throughout the musculoskeletal system'	Present, especially in the morning, often confused with inflammatory conditions	Absent, though stiffness is greater at the extremes of movement	Sleep disturbance, fatigue, cognitive issues, depression/anxiety, overlaps with other pain syndromes

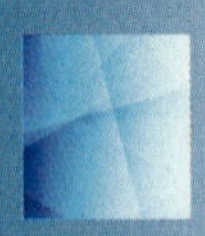

TABLE 25-2. Systemic Manifestations of Musculoskeletal Disorders

Musculoskeletal Disorder	Associated Systemic Manifestation
Systemic lupus erythematosus	Butterfly (*malar*) rash on the cheeks
Psoriatic arthritis	Scaly plaques, especially on extensor surfaces, and pitted nails
Dermatomyositis	Heliotrope rash on the upper eyelid
Gonococcal arthritis	Papules, pustules, or vesicles with reddened bases on the distal extremities
Lyme disease (erythema chronicum migrans)	Expanding erythematous "target" or "bull's eye" patch early in an illness
Sarcoidosis, Behçet disease (erythema nodosum)[28,29]	Painful subcutaneous nodules especially in pretibial area
Vasculitis	Palpable purpura
Serum sickness, drug reaction	Hives
Reactive arthritis (often with urethritis and/or uveitis)	Erosions or scaling on the penis and crusted scaling papules on the soles and palms
Arthritis of rubella	Maculopapular rash
Dermatomyositis, systemic sclerosis	Nailfold capillary changes
Hypertrophic osteoarthropathy	Clubbing of the fingernails (see p. 290)
Reactive arthritis, Behçet syndrome,[28,29] ankylosing spondylitis	Red, burning, and itchy eyes (conjunctivitis), eye pain and blurred vision (uveitis)
RA, IBD, vasculitis	Scleritis
Acute rheumatic fever or gonococcal arthritis	Preceding sore throat
RA (usually painless); Behçet disease	Oral ulcerations
RA; systemic sclerosis	Pneumonitis; interstitial lung disease
IBD, scleroderma, reactive arthritis from *Salmonella*, *Shigella*, *Yersinia*, *Campylobacter*	Diarrhea, abdominal pain, cramping
Reactive arthritis, gonococcal arthritis	Urethritis
Lyme disease with central nervous system involvement	Mental status change, facial or other weakness, sensory changes, radicular pain

IBD, inflammatory bowel disease; RA, rheumatoid arthritis.

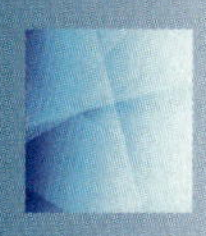

TABLE 25-3. Pains in the Neck

Patterns	Possible Causes	Physical Signs
Mechanical Neck Pain		
Aching pain in the cervical paraspinal muscles and ligaments with associated muscle spasm and stiffness and tightness in the upper back and shoulder, lasting up to 6 wk. No associated radiation, paresthesias, or weakness. Headache may be present.	Mechanism poorly understood, possibly sustained muscle contraction in the setting of weakness and poor biomechanics. Associated with poor posture, stress, poor sleep, poor head position during activities such as computer use, watching television, and driving.	Local muscle tenderness, pain on movement. No neurologic deficits. Possible trigger points in fibromyalgia. Torticollis if prolonged abnormal neck posture and muscle spasm.
Mechanical Neck Pain—Whiplash/Cervical Strain[8,30]		
Mechanical neck pain with aching paracervical pain and stiffness, often beginning the day after injury. Occipital headache, dizziness, malaise, and fatigue may be present. Chronic whiplash syndrome if symptoms last more than 6 mo (20–40% of injuries).	Musculoligamentous sprain or strain from forced hyperflexion/hyperextension injury to the neck, as in rear-end collisions.	Localized paracervical tenderness, decreased neck range of motion, perceived weakness of the upper extremities. Causes of cervical cord compression such as fracture, herniation, head injury, or altered consciousness are excluded.
Cervical Radiculopathy—From Nerve Root Compression[8,30]		
Sharp burning or tingling pain in the neck and one arm, with associated paresthesias and/or weakness that follow a neurologic (dermotomal/myotomal) pattern.	Dysfunction of cervical spinal nerve, nerve roots, or both from foraminal encroachment of the spinal nerve (~75%) or herniated cervical disc (~25%). Rarely from tumor, syrinx, or multiple sclerosis. Mechanisms may involve hypoxia of the nerve root and dorsal ganglion and release of inflammatory mediators.	*C7 nerve root affected most often (45–60%)*, with weakness in triceps and finger flexors, and extensors. C6 nerve root involvement also common with weakness in biceps, brachioradialis, and wrist extensors.
Cervical Myelopathy—From Cervical Cord Compression[8,30]		
Neck pain with bilateral weakness and paresthesias in both upper and lower extremities, often with urinary frequency. Hand clumsiness, palmar paresthesias, and gait changes may be subtle. Neck flexion often exacerbates symptoms.	Usually from cervical spondylosis, defined as cervical degenerative disc disease from spurs, degenerative thickening of the ligamentum flavum, and/or disc herniation; also from cervical stenosis from osteophytes, ossification of ligamentum flavum, and RA. Large central or paracentral disc herniation may also compress cord.	Hyperreflexia; clonus at the wrist, knee, or ankle; extensor plantar reflexes (positive Babinski signs); positive *Hoffman sign*: thumb/index flexion when the middle finger is flicked; and gait disturbances. May also see *Lhermitte sign:* neck flexion with resulting sensation of electrical shock radiating down the spine. Confirmation of cervical myelopathy warrants urgent neck immobilization and neurosurgical evaluation.

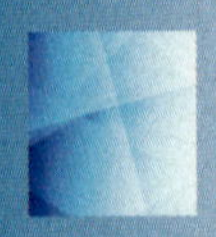

TABLE 25-4. Painful Shoulders

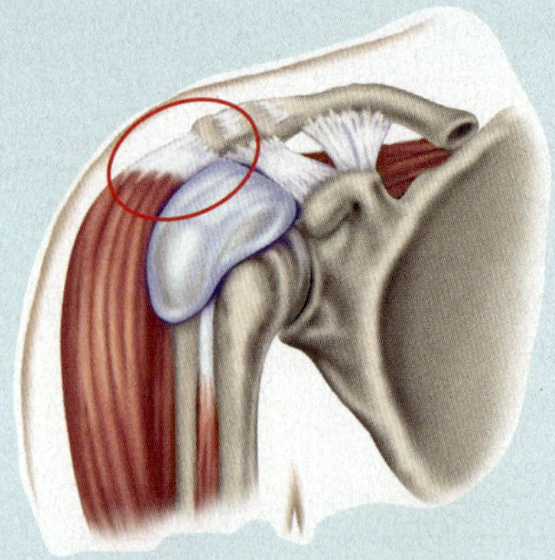

Rotator Cuff Tendinitis (Impingement Syndrome)

Repeated shoulder motion, for example, from throwing or swimming, can cause edema and hemorrhage followed by inflammation, most commonly involving the supraspinatus tendon. Acute, recurrent, or chronic pain may result, often aggravated by activity. Patients report sharp catches of pain, grating, and weakness when lifting the arm overhead. When the supraspinatus tendon is involved, *tenderness is maximal just below the tip of the acromion*. In older adults, bone spurs on the undersurface of the acromion may contribute to symptoms.

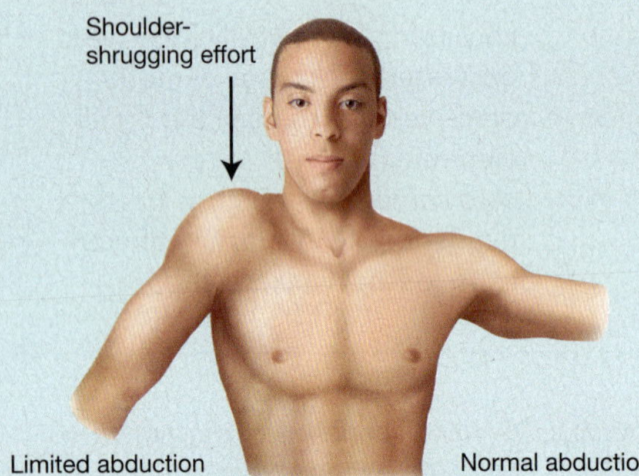

Rotator Cuff Tears

The rotator cuff muscles and tendons compress the humeral head into the concave glenoid fossa and strengthen arm movement—*the subscapularis in internal rotation, the supraspinatus in elevation, and the infraspinatus and teres minor in external rotation*. Injury from a fall, trauma, or repeated impingement against the acromion and the coracoacromial ligament may cause a partial- or full-thickness tear of tendons in the rotator cuff, especially in older patients. Patients complain of chronic shoulder pain, night pain, or catching and grating when raising the arm overhead. Weakness or tears of the tendons usually start in the supraspinatus tendon and progress posteriorly and anteriorly. Look for atrophy of the deltoid, supraspinatus, or infraspinatus muscles related to disuse from pain or retraction in the setting of a complete tear. Palpate anteriorly over the anterior greater tuberosity of the humerus to check for a defect in muscle attachment and below the acromion for crepitus during arm rotation. In a complete tear, active abduction and forward flexion at the glenohumeral joint are severely impaired, producing a characteristic shrug of the shoulder when trying to raise the arm and a positive "drop arm" test when trying to lower the arm (see p. 808).

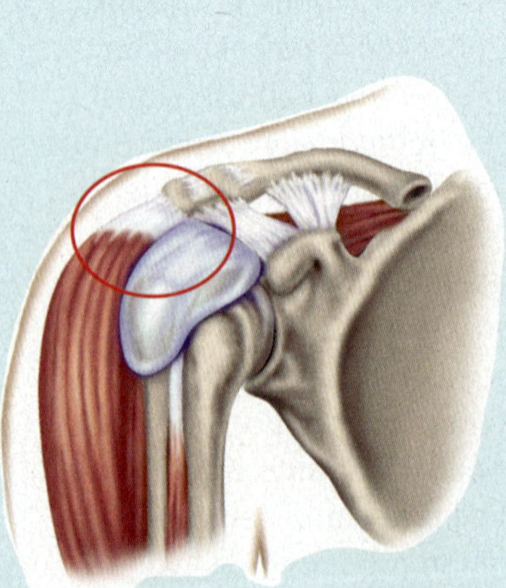

Calcific Tendinitis

Calcific tendinitis is a degenerative process in the tendon associated chronic tendon injury with improper healing that leads to the deposition of calcium salts. The supraspinatus tendon is usually involved. Acute disabling attacks of shoulder pain may occur, usually in patients ages ≥30 y, especially in individuals assigned female at birth. The arm is held close to the side, and all motions are severely limited by pain. Tenderness is maximal below the tip of the acromion when the supraspinatus is involved. The subacromial/subdeltoid bursa, which overlies the supraspinatus tendon, may also be inflamed. Chronic less severe pain may also occur.

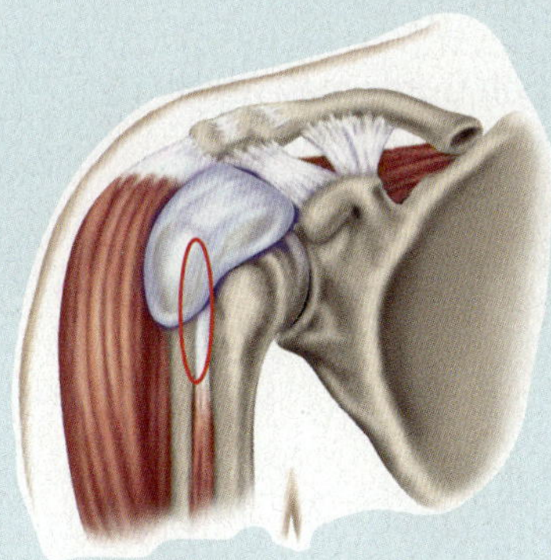

Bicipital Tendinitis

Inflammation of the long head of the biceps tendon and tendon sheath causes anterior shoulder pain resembling and often coexisting with rotator cuff tendinitis. Both conditions may involve impingement injury. Tenderness is maximal in the bicipital groove. Externally rotate and abduct the arm to separate this area from the subacromial tenderness of supraspinatus tendinitis. With the patient's arm at the side, elbow flexed to 90°, ask the patient to supinate the forearm against your resistance. Increased pain in the bicipital groove confirms this condition. Pain during resisted forward flexion of the shoulder with the elbow extended ("Speed test") is also characteristic.

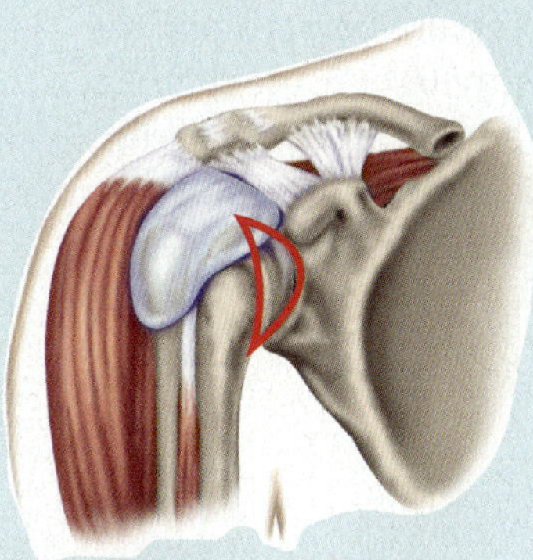

Adhesive Capsulitis (Frozen Shoulder)

Adhesive capsulitis refers to fibrosis of the glenohumeral joint capsule, manifested by diffuse, dull, aching pain in the shoulder and progressive restriction of active and passive range of motion, especially in external rotation, with localized tenderness. The condition is usually unilateral and occurs in people ages 40–60 y. There is often an antecedent disorder of the shoulder or another condition (such as myocardial infarction) that has decreased shoulder movements. The disorder may take 6 mo to 2 y to resolve. Stretching exercises and steroid injection may help.

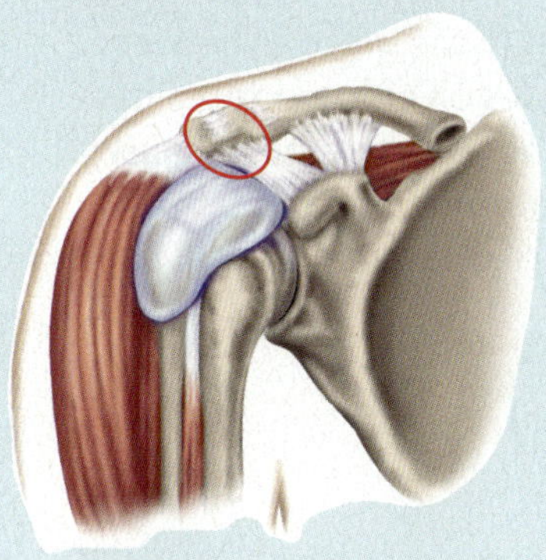

Acromioclavicular Arthritis

Acromioclavicular arthritis is relatively common, usually arising from prior direct injury to the shoulder girdle with resulting degenerative changes. Tenderness is localized over the acromioclavicular joint. Patients report pain with movements of the scapula and arm abduction. The cross-arm test may be positive.

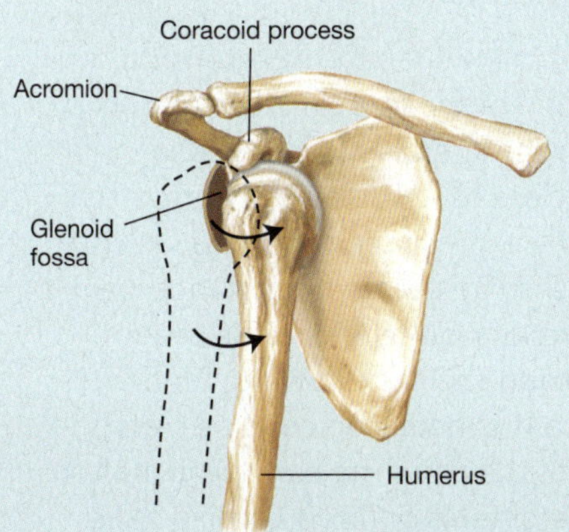

Anterior Dislocation of the Humerus

Shoulder instability from anterior subluxation or dislocation of the humerus usually results from a fall or forceful throwing motion. Recurrent episodes can become common unless treated or the precipitating motion avoided. The shoulder seems to "slip out of the joint" when the arm is abducted and externally rotated, causing a positive apprehension test for anterior instability when the examiner places the arm in this position. Any shoulder movement may cause pain, and patients hold the arm in a neutral position. The rounded lateral aspect of the shoulder appears flattened. Dislocations may also be inferior, posterior (relatively rare), and multidirectional.

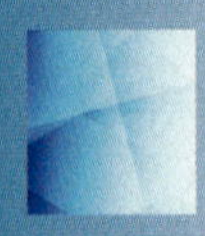

TABLE 25-5. Swollen or Tender Elbows

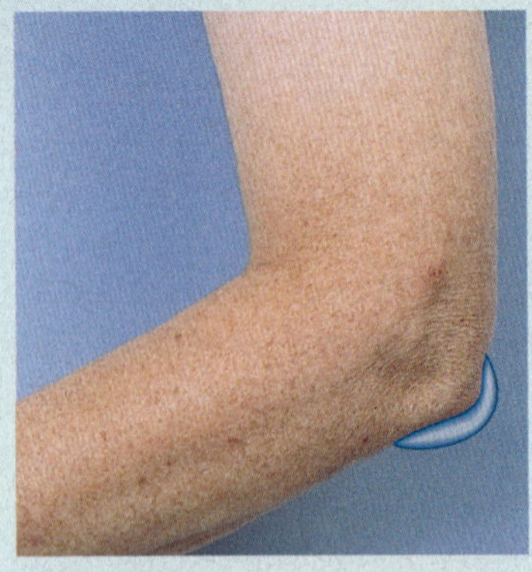

Olecranon Bursitis

Swelling and inflammation of the olecranon bursa may result from trauma, gout, or rheumatoid arthritis (RA). The swelling is superficial to the olecranon process and may reach 6 cm in diameter. Consider aspiration for both diagnosis and symptomatic relief.

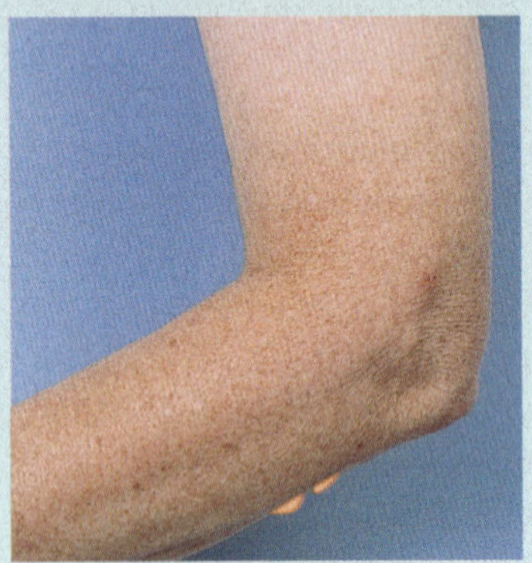

Rheumatoid Nodules

Subcutaneous nodules may develop at pressure points along the extensor surface of the ulna in patients with RA or acute rheumatic fever. They are firm and nontender. They are not attached to the overlying skin but may be attached to the underlying periosteum. They can develop in the area of the olecranon bursa, but often occur more distally.

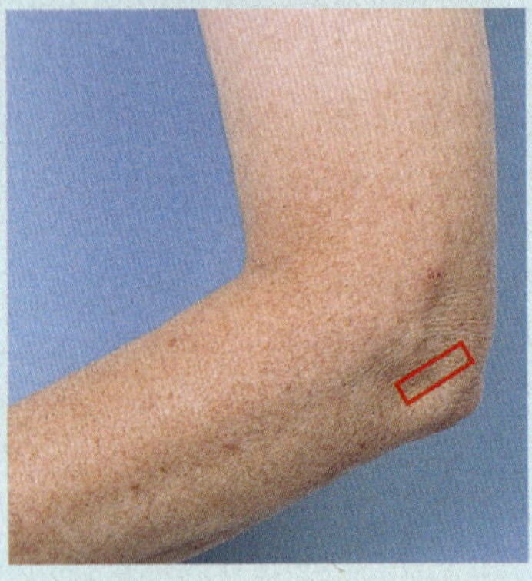

Arthritis of the Elbow

Synovial inflammation or fluid is felt best in the grooves between the olecranon process and the epicondyles on either side. Palpate for a boggy, soft, or fluctuant swelling and for tenderness. Causes include RA, gout and pseudogout, osteoarthritis, and trauma. Patients report pain, stiffness, and restricted motion.

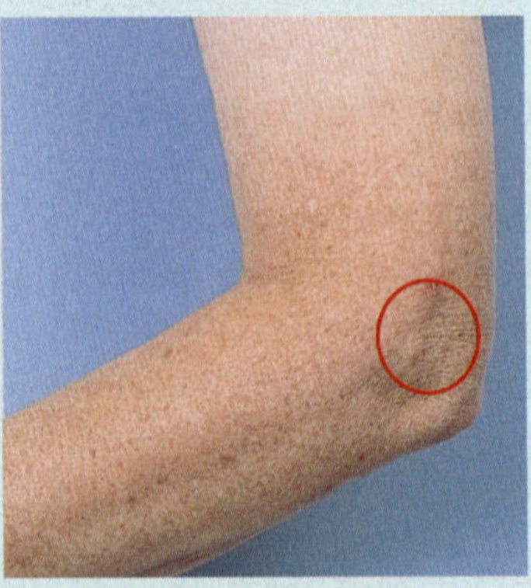

Epicondylitis

Lateral epicondylitis (tennis elbow) follows repetitive extension of the wrist or pronation–supination of the forearm. Pain and tenderness develop 1 cm distal to the lateral epicondyle and possibly in the extensor muscles close to it. The pain is most often caused by chronic tendinosis of the extensor carpi radialis brevis. When the patient tries to extend the wrist against resistance, pain increases. *Medial epicondylitis* (pitcher's, golfer's, or Little League elbow) follows repetitive wrist flexion such as throwing. Tenderness is maximal just lateral and distal to the medial epicondyle. Wrist flexion against resistance increases the pain. The pain is most often caused by tendinosis of the pronator teres or flexor carpi radialis.

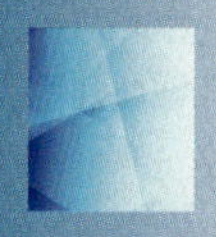

TABLE 25-6. Arthritis in the Hands

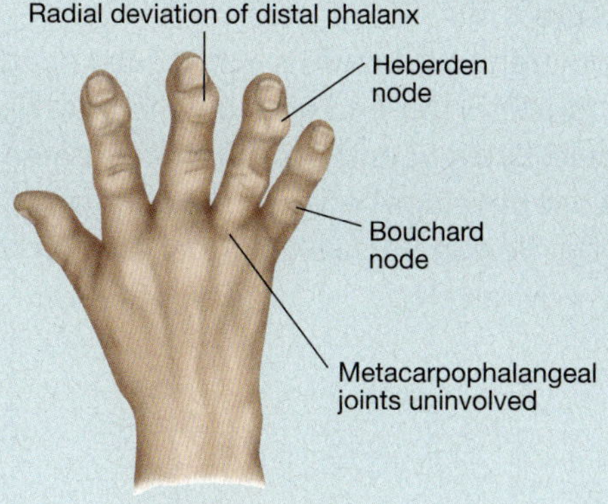

Osteoarthritis (Degenerative Joint Disease)

Heberden nodes on the dorsolateral aspects of the distal interphalangeal (DIP) joints from bony overgrowth of osteoarthritis (OA). Usually hard and painless, they affect middle-aged or older adults and are often associated with arthritic changes in other joints. Flexion and deviation deformities may develop. *Bouchard nodes* on the proximal interphalangeal (PIP) joints are less common. The metacarpophalangeal (MCP) joints are generally spared.

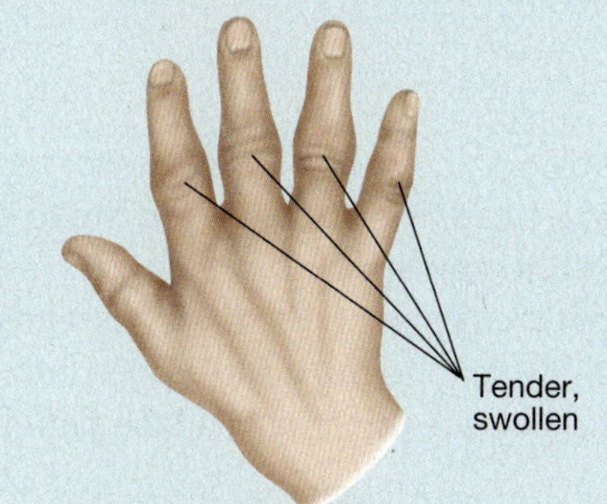

Acute Rheumatoid Arthritis

Tender, painful, stiff joints in *RA,* usually with symmetric involvement on both sides of the body. The DIP, MCP, and wrist joints are the most frequently affected. Note the fusiform or spindle-shaped swelling of the PIP joints in acute disease.

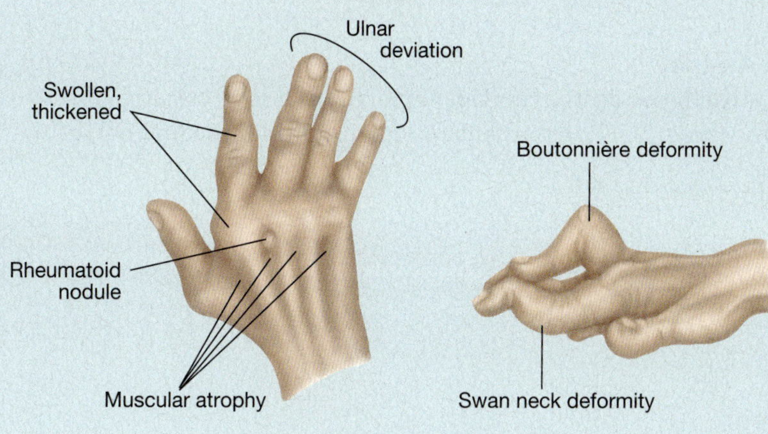

Chronic Rheumatoid Arthritis

In chronic disease, note the swelling and thickening of the MCP and PIP joints. Range of motion becomes limited, and fingers may deviate toward the ulnar side. The interosseous muscles atrophy. The fingers may show *"swan neck" deformities* (hyperextension of the PIP joints with fixed flexion of the DIP joints) related to inflammatory destruction of the joints and supporting ligaments. Less common is a *boutonnière deformity* (persistent flexion of the PIP joint with hyperextension of the DIP joint). Rheumatoid nodules are seen in the acute or the chronic stage.

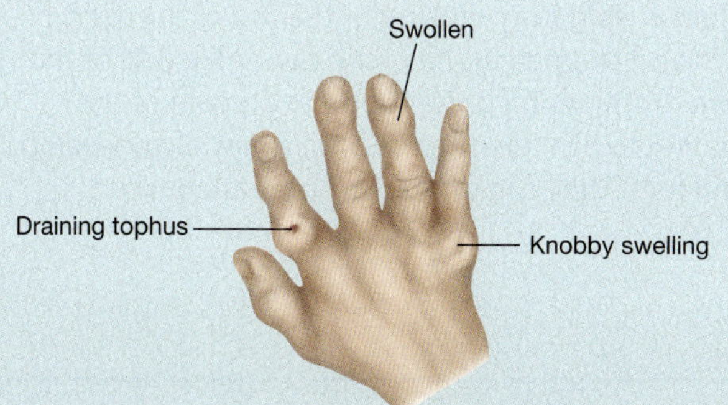

Chronic Tophaceous Gout[20]

Urate crystal deposits, often with surrounding inflammation, cause deformities in subcutaneous tissues, bursae, cartilage, and subchondral bone that mimic RA and OA. Joint involvement is usually less symmetric than in RA. Acute inflammation may be present. Knobby swellings around the joints ulcerate and discharge white chalk-like urates.

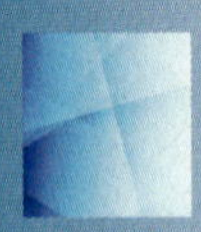

TABLE 25-7. Swellings and Deformities of the Hands

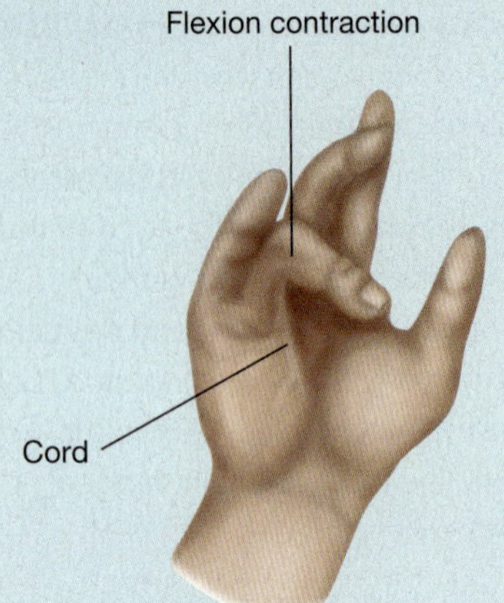

Dupuytren Contracture

The first sign of a Dupuytren contracture is a thickened band overlying the flexor tendon of the fourth finger and possibly the little finger near the distal palmar crease. Subsequently, the skin in this area puckers, and a thickened fibrotic cord develops between the palm and finger. Finger extension is limited, but flexion is usually normal. Flexion contracture of the fingers may gradually develop.

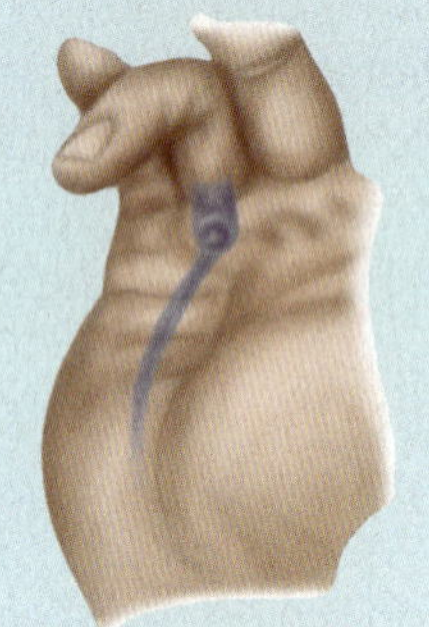

Trigger Finger

Trigger finger is caused by a painless nodule in a flexor tendon in the palm, near the metacarpal head. The nodule is too big to enter easily into the tendon sheath during extension of the fingers from a flexed position. With extra effort or assistance, the finger extends and flexes with a palpable and audible snap as the nodule pops into the tendon sheath. Watch, listen, and palpate the nodule as the patient flexes and extends the fingers.

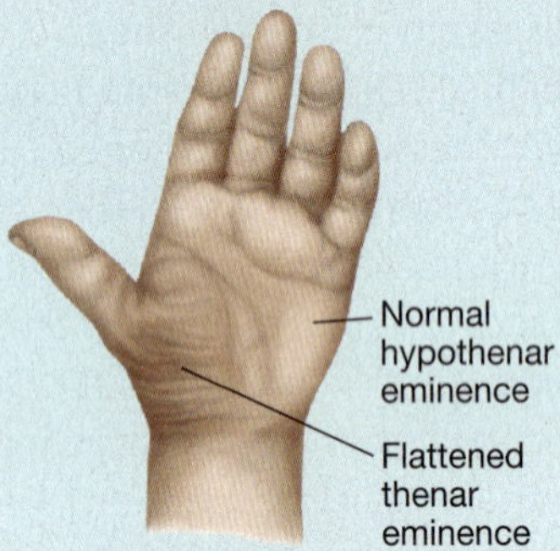

Thenar Atrophy

Thenar atrophy suggests a median nerve disorder such as carpal tunnel syndrome (see p. 928). Hypothenar atrophy suggests an ulnar nerve disorder.

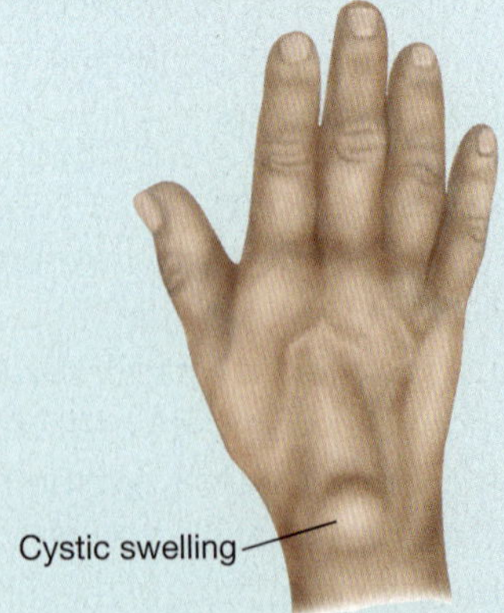

Ganglion

Ganglia are cystic, round, usually nontender swellings along tendon sheaths or joint capsules, frequently at the dorsum of the wrist. The cyst contains synovial fluid arising from erosion or tearing of the joint capsule or tendon sheath and trapped in the cystic cavity. Flexion of the wrist makes ganglia more prominent if present on the dorsum of the wrist with extension tending to obscure them. Ganglia may also develop on the hands, ankles, and feet. They can disappear spontaneously.

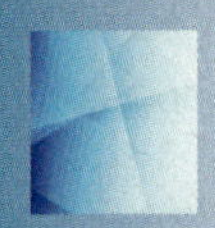

TABLE 25-8. Tendon Sheath, Palmar Space, and Finger Infections

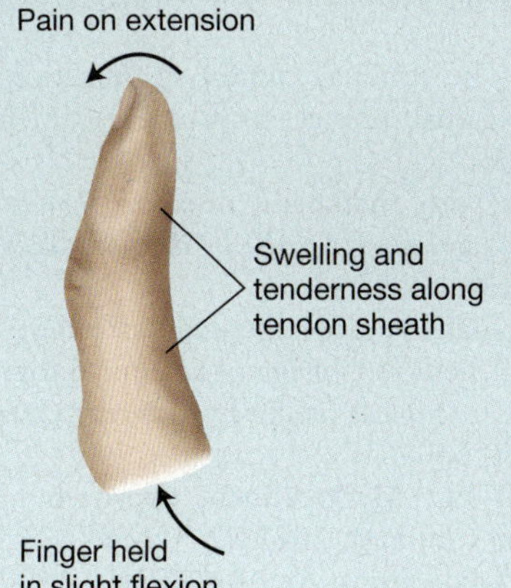

Acute Tenosynovitis

Inflammation of the flexor tendon sheaths, acute tenosynovitis, may follow local injury, overuse, or infection. Unlike arthritis, tenderness and swelling develop not in the joint but along the course of the tendon sheath. In the fingers, this often occurs from the distal phalanx to the level of the metacarpophalangeal joint. The finger is held in slight flexion since finger extension is very painful. Tenosynovitis can result from inflammation related to injury or irritation of the sheath or from infection. Causative infectious agents include *Staphylococcus* and *Streptococcus species,* disseminated gonorrhea, and *Candida albicans.*

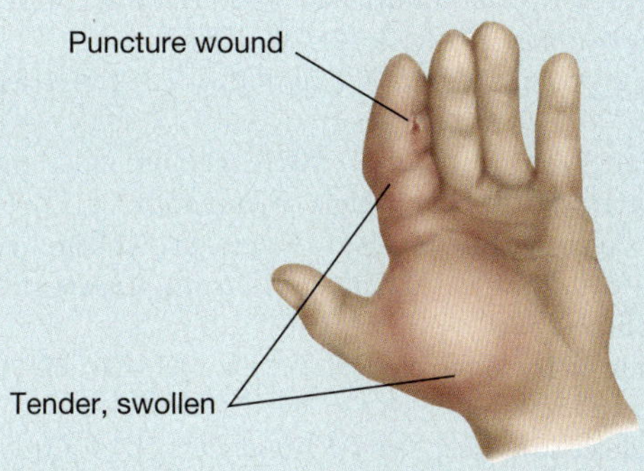

Acute Tenosynovitis and Thenar Space Involvement

Infectious tenosynovitis of the fingers may extend from the tendon sheath into the adjacent fascial spaces within the palm. Infections of the index finger and thenar space are illustrated. Early diagnosis and treatment are important.

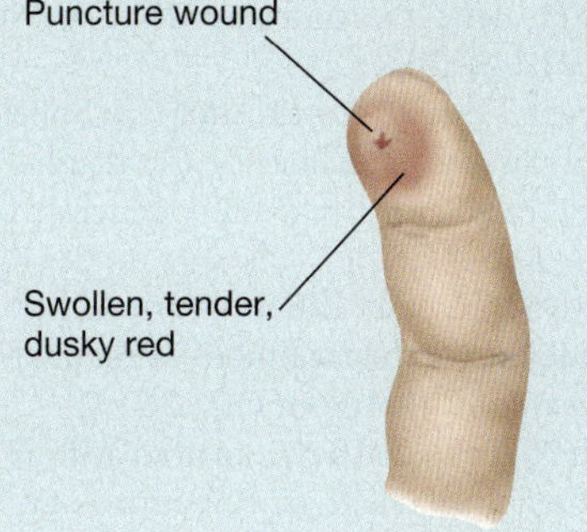

Felon

Injury to the fingertip may result in infection of the enclosed fascial spaces of the distal pulp or phalanx pad of the fingertip, usually from *Staphylococcus aureus.* Severe pain, localized tenderness, swelling, and dusky redness are characteristics. Early diagnosis and treatment, usually incision and drainage, are important for preventing abscess formation. If vesicles are present, consider herpetic whitlow instead, usually seen in health care workers exposed to herpes simplex virus in human saliva (rare when universal precautions are used).

REFERENCES

1. Cush JJ. Chapter 363: approach to articular and musculoskeletal disorders. In: Jameson JL, Fauci AS, Kasper DL, Hauser SL, Longo DL, Loscalzo J, eds. *Harrison's Principles of Internal Medicine.* 20th ed. McGraw-Hill Education; 2018.
2. Wilson CH. Chapter 164: the musculoskeletal examination. In: Walker HK, Hall WD, Hurst JW, eds. *Clinical Methods: The History, Physical, and Laboratory Examinations.* 3rd ed. Butterworths; 1990. Accessed February 18, 2024. https://www.ncbi.nlm.nih.gov/books/NBK272/
3. Durham J, Newton-John TRO, Zakrzewska JM. Temporomandibular disorders. *BMJ.* 2015;350:h1154.
4. Schiffman E, Ohrbach R, Truelove E, et al. Diagnostic criteria for temporomandibular disorders (DC/TMD) for clinical and research applications: recommendations of the International RDC/TMD Consortium Network and Orofacial Pain Special Interest Group. *J Oral Facial Pain Headache.* 2014; 28(1):6–27.
5. Appelboam A, Reuben AD, Benger JR, et al. Elbow extension test to rule out elbow fracture: multicentre, prospective validation and observational study of diagnostic accuracy in adults and children. *BMJ.* 2008;337:a2428.
6. Darracq MA, Vinson DR, Panacek EA. Preservation of active range of motion after acute elbow trauma predicts absence of elbow fracture. *Am J Emerg Med.* 2008;26(7):779–782.
7. Thoomes EJ, van Geest S, van der Windt DA, et al. Value of physical tests in diagnosing cervical radiculopathy: a systematic review. *Spine J.* 2018;18(1):179–189.
8. Onks CA, Billy G. Evaluation and treatment of cervical radiculopathy. *Prim Care.* 2013;40(4):837–848, vii-viii.
9. McGee SR. Chapter 55: examination of the musculoskeletal system—the shoulder. *Evidence-Based Physical Diagnosis.* 3rd ed. Elsevier/Saunders; 2012.
10. Whittle S, Buchbinder R. In the clinic. Rotator cuff disease. *Ann Intern Med.* 2015;162(1):ITC1–ITC16.
11. Jain NB, Luz J, Higgins LD, et al. The diagnostic accuracy of special tests for rotator cuff tear: the ROW Cohort Study. *Am J Phys Med Rehabil.* 2017;96(3):176–183.
12. Hanchard NC, Lenza M, Handoll HH, Takwoingi Y. Physical tests for shoulder impingements and local lesions of bursa, tendon or labrum that may accompany impingement. *Cochrane Database Syst Rev.* 2013;2013(4):CD007427.
13. McGee SR. *Evidence-Based Physical Diagnosis.* 5th ed. Elsevier; 2022:xii:705.
14. Ahmad Z, Siddiqui N, Malik SS, Abdus-Samee M, Tytherleigh-Strong G, Rushton N. Lateral epicondylitis: a review of pathology and management. *Bone Joint J.* 2013;95-B(9): 1158–1164.
15. Di Filippo L, Vincenzi S, Pennella D, Maselli F. Treatment, diagnostic criteria and variability of terminology for lateral elbow pain: findings from an overview of systematic reviews. *Healthcare (Basel).* 2022;10(6):1095.
16. Kenney RJ, Hammert WC. Physical examination of the hand. *J Hand Surg Am.* 2014;39(11):2324–2334; quiz 2334.
17. Kleopa KA. In the clinic. Carpal tunnel syndrome. *Ann Intern Med.* 2015;163(5):ITC1.
18. Sauvé PS, Rhee PC, Shin AY, Lindau T. Examination of the wrist: radial-sided wrist pain. *J Hand Surg Am.* 2014;39(10): 2089–2092.
19. D'Arcy CA, McGee S. The rational clinical examination. Does this patient have carpal tunnel syndrome? *JAMA.* 2000;283(23):3110–3117.
20. Approach to the patient with rheumatic disease. *Medical Knowledge Self-Assessment Program (MKSAP) 17 Rheumatology.* American College of Physicians; 2015.
21. Anderson J, Caplan L, Yazdany J, et al. Rheumatoid arthritis disease activity measures: American College of Rheumatology recommendations for use in clinical practice. *Arthritis Care Res (Hoboken).* 2012;64(5):640–647.
22. Davis JM 3rd, Matteson EL. My treatment approach to rheumatoid arthritis. *Mayo Clin Proc.* 2012;87(7):659–673.
23. Gelber AC. In the clinic. Osteoarthritis. *Ann Intern Med.* 2014; 161(1):ITC1–ITC16.
24. Mead T, Arabindoo K, Smith B. Managing gout: there's more we can do. *J Fam Pract.* 2014;63(12):707–713.
25. Neogi T. Clinical practice. Gout. *N Engl J Med.* 2011;364(5): 443–452.
26. Dejaco C, Singh YP, Perel P, et al. 2015 recommendations for the management of polymyalgia rheumatica: a European League Against Rheumatism/American College of Rheumatology collaborative initiative. *Arthritis Rheumatol.* 2015;67(10):2569–2580.
27. Clauw DJ. Fibromyalgia: a clinical review. *JAMA.* 2014; 311(15):1547–1555.
28. Davatchi F. Behcet's disease. *Int J Rheum Dis.* 2014;17(4): 355–357.
29. Hatemi G, Yazici Y, Yazici H. Behçet's syndrome. *Rheum Dis Clin North Am.* 2013;39(2):245–261.
30. Bono CM, Ghiselli G, Gilbert TJ, et al; North American Spine Society. An evidence-based clinical guideline for the diagnosis and treatment of cervical radiculopathy from degenerative disorders. *Spine J.* 2011;11(1):64–72.
31. Singh JA, Saag KG, Bridges SL Jr, et al. 2015 American College of Rheumatology Guideline for the treatment of rheumatoid arthritis. *Arthritis Rheumatol.* 2016;68(1):1–26.
32. Aletaha D, Neogi T, Silman AJ, et al. 2010 rheumatoid arthritis classification criteria: an American College of Rheumatology/ European League Against Rheumatism collaborative initiative. *Arthritis Rheum.* 2010;62(9):2569–2581.
33. Nagy G, van Vollenhoven RF. Sustained biologic-free and drug-free remission in rheumatoid arthritis, where are we now? *Arthritis Res Ther.* 2015;17(1):181.
34. Hermans J, Luime JJ, Meuffels DE, Reijman M, Simel DL, Bierma-Zeinstra SM. Does this patient with shoulder pain have rotator cuff disease? The Rational Clinical Examination systematic review. *JAMA.* 2013;310(8):837–847.

CHAPTER

26

Musculoskeletal System: Lumbosacral Spine, Hips, and Lower Extremities

ANATOMY: LUMBOSACRAL SPINE

A comprehensive and detailed guide to the general approach to history taking and physical examination of any musculoskeletal concern is presented in Chapter 25, Musculoskeletal System: Neck, Shoulders, and Upper Extremities, pp. 783–784.

Review the details of the anatomy of the entire vertebral spine in Chapter 25, Musculoskeletal System: Neck, Shoulders, and Upper Extremities, pp. 775–840.

The *lumbosacral spine*, comprising the lower part of the lumbar spine and the sacrum, is notable for its role in supporting the upper body's weight and providing a stable foundation for movement. This area's strength and stability, critical for supporting the body in various positions, come from the interlocking structure of the lumbar vertebrae and their articulation with the sacrum, the strong ligaments and muscles that support these structures, and the unique shape of the sacral bone (Fig. 26-1).

The movement of the lumbosacral area is governed by several muscle groups, each contributing to its stability and mobility (Fig. 26-2). These muscles include the large *paraspinal muscles* that run along the spine, the *abdominal muscles* that support the anterior aspect, and the *gluteal muscles* that connect to the sacrum and hips.

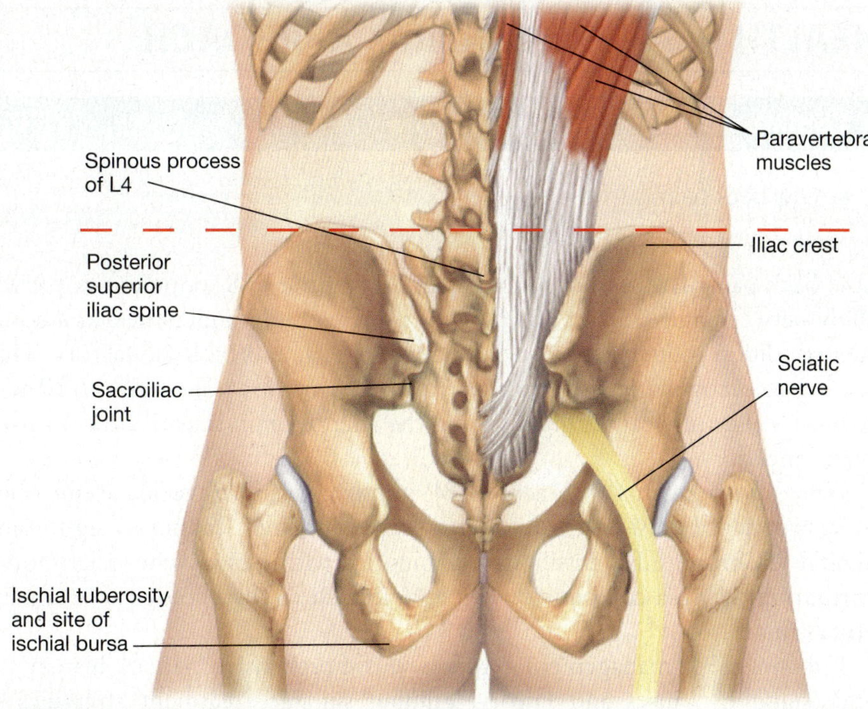

FIGURE 26-1. Lumbosacral spine and adjoining structures, posterior view. The dashed line marks the level of the iliac crest, aligning with L4.

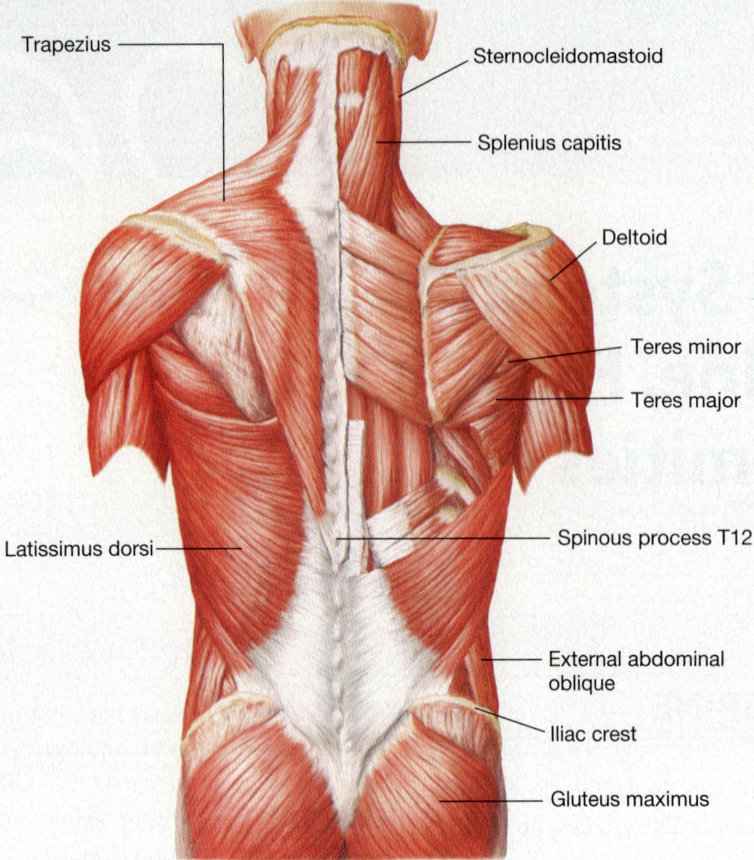

FIGURE 26-2. Muscles of the lower back, posterior view.

HEALTH HISTORY: GENERAL APPROACH

Common or Concerning Symptom

- Low back pain

Low back pain (LBP) affects more than 80% of the U.S. population, particularly between ages 35 and 55 years.[1] It is increasingly understood as a complex condition influenced by social, psychological, and biologic factors. This has led to recognizing *nociplastic pain*, a category for nonspecific LBP not linked to a specific cause, highlighting the role of brain sensitization in pain persistence.[2,3]

While most patients with acute LBP improve within 6 weeks, about one-third experience persistent pain after a year, sometimes leading to significant disability. Chronic LBP develops in a minority, with a biopsychosocial model attributing this to a combination of biological, social, psychological, and pain processing factors.[2,3]

Effective LBP management requires a comprehensive patient history to understand its causes and impact, guiding suitable treatment strategies 4 (Box 26-1).

Box 26-1. Low Back Pain: High-Yield History Questions

Domain	Questions	Rationale
Pain location and pattern	*"Can you describe where exactly in your lower back you feel the pain? Does it spread anywhere, like your legs or hips?"*	Helps identify specific lumbar spine issues or sciatic involvement
Movement-related pain	*"Does your back pain change when you move, bend, or lift objects? Are certain positions more comfortable?"*	Can indicate mechanical back issues, muscle strain, or disc problems
Onset and duration of pain	*"When did your low back pain begin, and how long has it been going on? Is it constant or intermittent?"*	*Acute:* can suggest sudden injury *Chronic:* can suggest long-term degeneration
Effect of posture and activity	*"Do certain activities or postures, like sitting for long periods or standing, worsen your back pain?"*	Identifies if occupational or lifestyle factors contribute to the pain, important for ergonomic or activity-related solutions
Associated symptoms	*"Do you experience any numbness, tingling, or weakness in your legs or feet along with the back pain?"*	Can indicate nerve involvement like sciatica or spinal stenosis
History of back injuries or surgeries	*"Have you had any previous injuries, treatments, or surgeries on your lower back?"*	Can help understand current symptoms and guiding treatment
Impact on daily activities	*"How does your back pain affect your daily routines, like walking, sleeping, or performing daily tasks?"*	Helps evaluate severity and functional implications
Lifestyle and exercise habits	*"Can you describe your general lifestyle and exercise habits? Do you have any regular physical activities or sedentary practices?"*	Play a significant role in low back health

Possible musculoskeletal causes include **lumbar strain** (stretch injury to the ligaments, tendons, and/or muscles of the lower back, often due to overuse, strain, or injury), **degenerative disc disease** (breakdown of spinal discs, leading to pain and stiffness), **herniated disc** (inner cushion of the spinal disc protrudes through the outer layer, pressing on nerves), **spinal stenosis** (narrowing of the spinal canal, which can put pressure on the nerves), **osteoarthritis of the spine** (wear and tear of the joints and discs in the neck and lower back), and **spondylolisthesis** (vertebra slips forward over the one below it).

Box 26-2 outlines crucial "red flags" in patients with acute LBP that suggest a potential need for imaging. These indicators help differentiate common musculoskeletal pain from serious conditions requiring immediate attention.

See Table 26-1, Low Back Pain, pp. 893–894, for serious causes of low back pain.

Box 26-2. Red Flags for Acute Low Back Pain Indicating Likely Need for Imaging

- Age <18 years or >65 years
- History of cancer
- Unexplained weight loss, fever, or recent decline in general health
- History of intravenous drug use or recent bacteremia
- Immunosuppression, HIV infection, current hemodialysis, or recent spinal procedure
- Long-term steroid therapy or risk factors for osteoporosis (see Box 26-24)
- Saddle anesthesia
- New bladder or bowel incontinence or new urinary retention
- Significant neurologic symptoms or progressive neurologic deficit

TECHNIQUES OF EXAMINATION

Key Components of the Lumbosacral Spine Examination

I	■ Inspect the gait (balance, posture, symmetry, stride, coordination, rhythm, stability, weakness). ■ Inspect the pelvic alignment (symmetry, tilting, lordotic curve, lateral curvatures).
P	■ Palpate the lumbosacral spine and adjoining structures (spinal processes, paraspinal muscles, sacroiliac joints, lumbosacral junction).
ROM	■ Assess lumbosacral spine range of motion (flexion, extension, lateral bending, rotation).
S	■ Perform special maneuvers on the lumbosacral spine joint, if indicated (straight leg raise or Laségue test, crossed straight leg raise test, flip test, lumbar flexion and extension test, FABER, thigh thrust test, sacroiliac compression test, sitting slump test).

Review the mnemonic IPROMS (Inspection, Palpation, Range Of Motion, and Special maneuvers) in Chapter 25, Musculoskeletal System: Neck, Shoulders, and Upper Extremities, pp. 784–786.

Observe the Gait

Careful observation of the patient's gait as they enter the room is a crucial first step. *Gait*, the manner in which a person walks, can reveal a lot about lumbar spine health and function.

See further discussion of gait assessment in Special Maneuvers and Techniques, Analyzing Gait on pp. 879–881.

During the *stance phase*, individuals with LBP may experience increased discomfort due to the weight-bearing stress on the lumbar spine. The spine's role in supporting and stabilizing the upper body becomes more pronounced during weight-bearing activities, often highlighting issues in the lumbar region. During the *swing phase*, the lumbar spine is less stressed compared to the stance phase. However, the need for lumbar stability and control during this phase can still highlight underlying back issues, especially with muscle weakness or imbalance.

Low back pain is often exacerbated during the weight-bearing stance phase of gait.

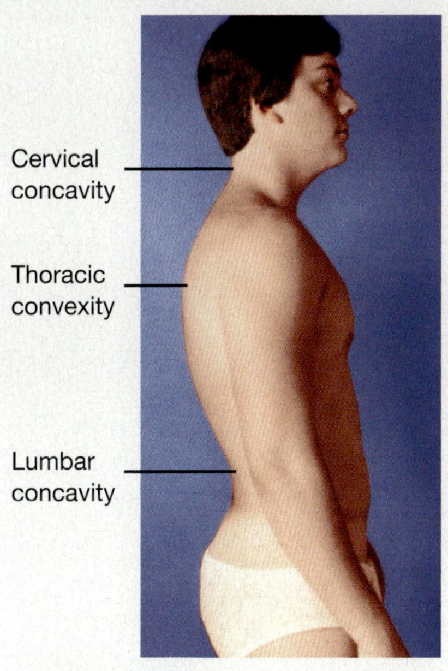

FIGURE 26-3. Inspecting lordotic curve from the side.

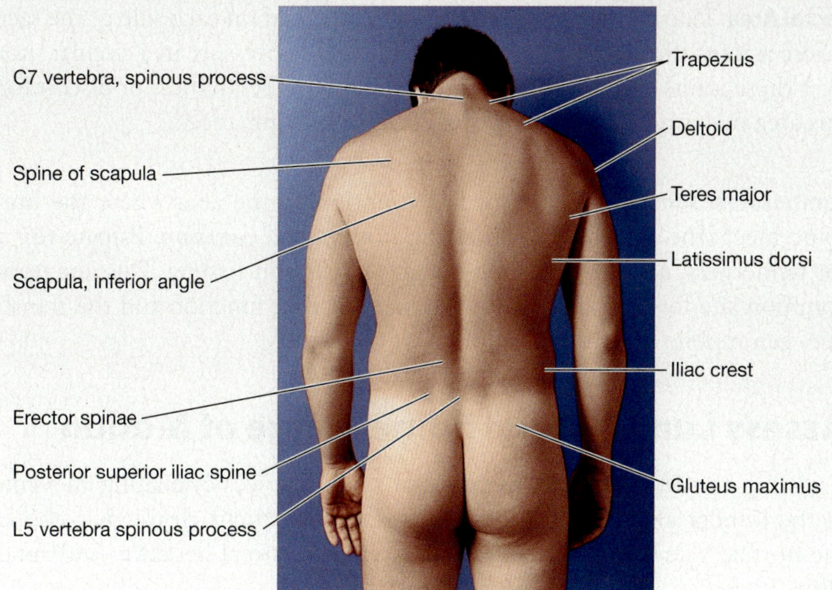

FIGURE 26-4. Inspecting the upright spine from behind.

Observe the Pelvic Alignment

When examining pelvic alignment, observe the patient from behind and from the side while they stand naturally with feet shoulder-width apart. Look for symmetry in the level of the iliac crests and the posterior superior iliac spines, noting any tilting that can indicate issues like leg length discrepancy or muscle imbalance. Additionally, assess changes in pelvic alignment during walking for dynamic insights.

Assess the Lordotic Curve. For the lordotic curve evaluation, observe the patient's lower back from the side (Fig. 26-3). Identify the natural inward curvature in the lumbar region and assess its depth.

Excessive curvature may indicate *hyperlordosis*, while a flattened curve could suggest a reduced lordotic angle, often seen in muscular strain or lumbar disc issues.

Next, examine the spine from behind. This view is essential for assessing symmetry and identifying any lateral curvatures or signs of scoliosis (Fig. 26-4). Look for any unevenness in the shoulders, waist creases, or any apparent asymmetry in the way the patient stands.

See Special Techniques and Maneuvers, Screening for Scoliosis, p. 883.

Palpate the Lumbosacral Spine and Adjoining Structures

Spinal Processes. Start at the top of the lumbar spine and palpate each *spinal process* down to the sacrum. Use the pads of your fingers to apply gentle pressure on each spinous process. Note any tenderness, swelling, or abnormalities, which could indicate issues like inflammation, injury, or degenerative changes.

Paraspinal Muscles. After examining the spinal processes, move laterally to palpate the *paraspinal muscles* on either side of the spine. Gently press and knead these muscles to assess their tone and look for areas of tenderness or spasm. Muscle tightness, spasms, or tenderness can indicate strain, overuse, or compensation for spinal abnormalities.

Sacral Area. Palpate the *sacroiliac (SI) joints*, located on each side of the sacrum where it joins the ilium of the pelvis. Apply gentle pressure in a circular motion over these joints and note any pain or tenderness. Tenderness or discomfort in this area may suggest SI joint dysfunction or inflammation.

Lumbosacral Junction. Pay particular attention to the area where the lumbar spine meets the sacrum, known as the *lumbosacral junction*. Palpate this area for tenderness, abnormalities, or changes in the soft tissues. This junction is a common site for LBP due to its high load-bearing function and the transition between mobile and more fixed parts of the spine.

Assess Lumbosacral Spine Range of Motion

Assessing the ROM of the lumbosacral spine involves evaluating movements in the lumbar and sacral regions. Instruct your patient clearly and check for the normal values of lumbar flexion, extension, lateral bending, and rotation (Box 26-3).[5]

Box 26-3. Range of Motion: Lumbosacral Spine

Movement	Examination Technique	Patient Instructions
Flexion	With the patient standing, ask them to bend forward and touch their toes. Note the degree of flexion and any discomfort.	*"Stand straight, then bend forward and try to touch your toes."*
Extension	Instruct the patient to bend backward from the waist while standing. Observe the extent and smoothness of the movement.	*"Stand straight, then arch your back and lean backward as far as you comfortably can."*

Movement	Examination Technique	Patient Instructions
Lateral bending	Have the patient stand and bend sideways at the waist, first to one side then the other. Assess for any asymmetry or limitation in movement.	*"Stand straight, then bend to the side, sliding your hand down your leg. Repeat on the other side."*
Rotation	Ask the patient to rotate their upper body while keeping their hips facing forward. This can be done standing or sitting.	*"Keep your hips facing forward and twist your upper body to one side and then the other."*

Each of these movements should be performed gently and within the limits of comfort. The lumbosacral spine typically allows for flexion 40° to 60°, extension 20° to 35°, lateral bending to each side 15° to 20°, and rotation to each side 3° to 18°. Note any deviations from these normal ranges as well as any pain or discomfort experienced during the movements.

Perform Special Maneuvers on the Lumbosacral Spine Joint (If Indicated)

Special maneuvers for the lumbosacral spine are essential examination techniques designed to assess the integrity and function of the lower back and surrounding structures. These maneuvers target different aspects of lumbosacral anatomy, offering a comprehensive assessment of spinal stability and mobility (Box 26-4).

Box 26-4. Special Maneuvers: Lumbosacral Spine

Special Maneuver	Structures Assessed	Examination Technique	
Straight leg raise (SLR) or Laségue test	Lumbosacral joint and nerve roots	With the patient lying supine, grasp their heel with one hand and lift the straight leg upward until pain or tension is felt in the hamstrings, then lower the leg until the pain or tension disappears. Next, dorsiflex the foot (Fig. 26-5).	Pain or sciatica symptoms during this test can indicate nerve root irritation or lumbar disc herniation.
Crossed straight leg raise test	Nerve roots, contralateral nerve tension	Perform the SLR on the unaffected leg.	Reproduction of sciatic pain on the symptomatic side may suggest nerve root irritation or a herniated disc.
Flip test	Sciatic nerve	With the patient seated, extend one leg at a time to stretch the sciatic nerve.	Pain or reproduction of sciatic symptoms indicates nerve root irritation.
Lumbar flexion and extension test	Lumbar spine	Ask the patient to bend forward and then backward from the waist. Observe for pain, limitation in movement, or asymmetry.	Pain or a significant limitation in movement during forward or backward bending of the waist may suggest underlying lumbar spine pathology, such as lumbar strain, discogenic pain, or facet joint dysfunction.
FABER (flexion, abduction, external rotation) or Patrick test	Sacroiliac joint, hip joint	Position the patient's leg so that their foot is on the opposite knee, forming a figure-four shape. Gently press down on the raised knee and opposite hip (Fig. 26-6).	Pain elicited in the SI area when the patient's leg is in a figure-four position (foot on opposite knee) indicates SI joint dysfunction, which can be caused by conditions like sacroiliitis or degenerative changes in the SI joints.
Thigh thrust test	Sacroiliac joint	With the patient lying supine, flex one hip to 90° and apply a gentle thrust along the axis of the femur.	Pain in the SI joint indicates possible pathology.
Distraction test	Facet joints	With the patient prone, apply pressure on their back to "distract" or pull apart the facet joints.	Pain relief points to facet joint pathology.
Sacroiliac compression test	Sacroiliac joint	With the patient prone or on their side, apply downward pressure on the spine.	Pain suggests facet joint or nerve root pathology.
Sitting slump test	Nerve roots, sciatic nerve	With the patient seated, ask them to slump forward, curving their spine. Their shoulders should round forward, and the head should bend toward the chest. Extend one knee while maintaining the slumped posture. Observe for any pain or discomfort. If there is no pain, dorsiflex the foot of the extended leg (Fig. 26-7).	Symptoms reproduced with neck flexion or foot dorsiflexion suggest nerve root impingement.

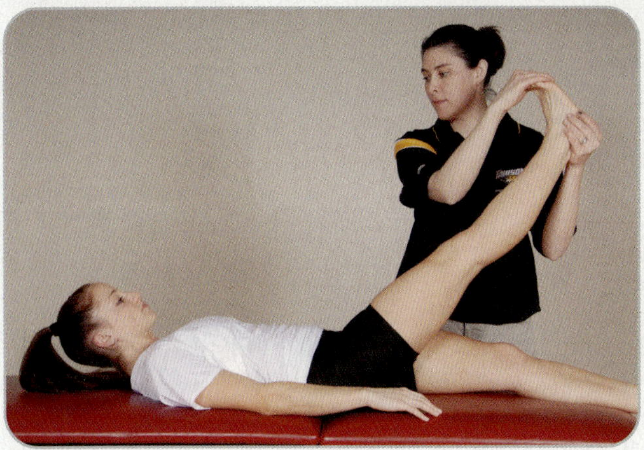

FIGURE 26-5. Straight leg raise (Laségue) test. (Reprinted with permission from Anderson MK, Barnum M. *Foundations of Athletic Training: Prevention, Assessment, and Management*. 7th ed. Wolters Kluwer; 2022. Figure 22-30.)

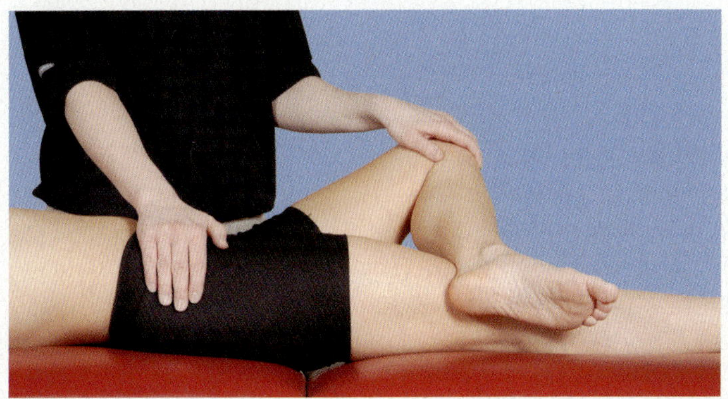

FIGURE 26-6. FABER or Patrick test. (Reprinted with permission from Anderson MK. *Foundations of Athletic Training: Prevention, Assessment, and Management*. 6th ed. Wolters Kluwer; 2017. Figure 16-19.)

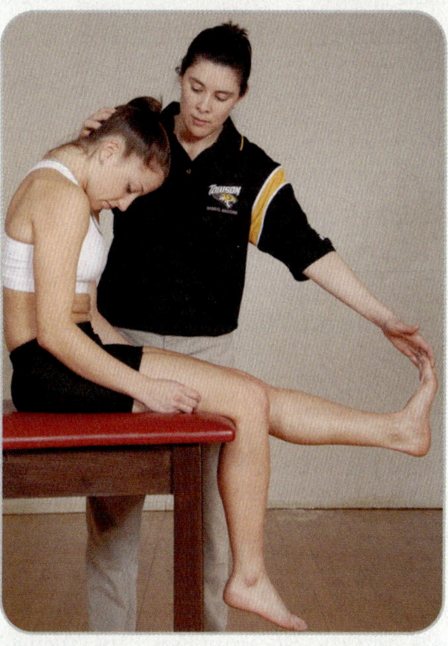

FIGURE 26-7. Sitting slump test. (Reprinted with permission from Anderson MK, Barnum M. *Foundations of Athletic Training: Prevention, Assessment, and Management*. 7th ed. Wolters Kluwer; 2022. Figure 22-29D.)

ANATOMY: HIP JOINT

The *hip joint* is notable for its strength, stability, and wide range of motion (ROM). This stability in spite its ROM, essential for weight bearing in different positions, arises from the deep fit of the head of the femur into the acetabulum, its strong fibrous articular capsule, and the powerful muscles that surround the joint and stabilize movement of the femur.

The hip joint is a ball-and-socket joint (Fig. 26-8). Note how the rounded head of the *femur* articulates with the cup-like cavity of the *acetabulum*. The hip joint lies just inferior to the middle third of the inguinal ligament. Review the bones of the pelvis—the *ilium*, the *ischium*, and the *pubis*—and the connection inferiorly at the *symphysis pubis* and posteriorly with the *sacrum*. Recognize that the *acetabulum* is a confluence of all three bones of the pelvis. The hip joint is not readily palpable because of the many overlying muscles and subcutaneous tissues.

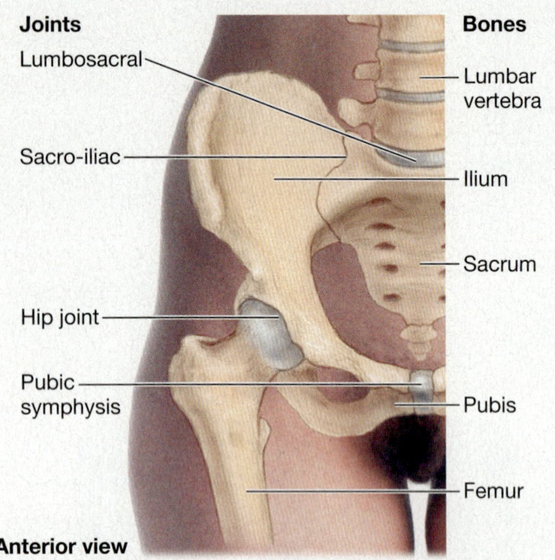

FIGURE 26-8. Joints and bones of pelvic girdle and hip. (Reprinted with permission from Moore KL, Agur AMR, Dalley AF II. *Essential Clinical Anatomy.* 4th ed. Wolters Kluwer Health/Lippincott Williams & Wilkins; 2011. Figure 5.44A.)

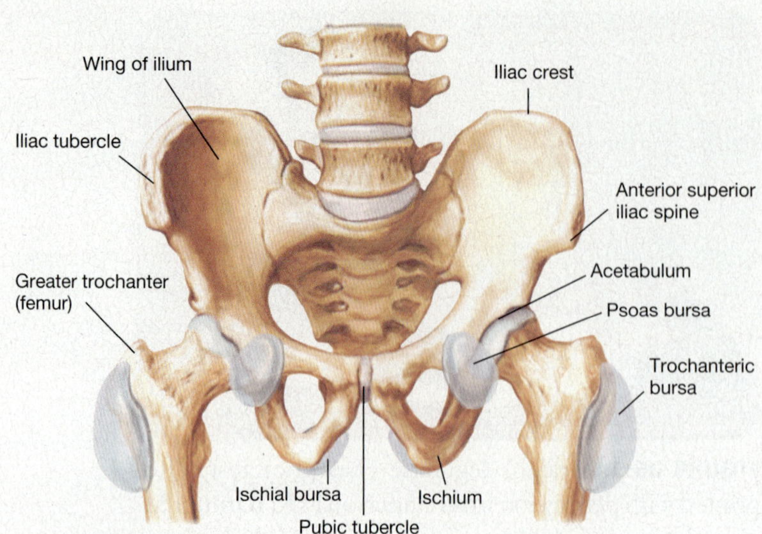

FIGURE 26-9. Anatomy of pelvis and hip, anterior view.

On the anterior surface of the hip, you can identify several key bony structures, including the *iliac crest* (at the level of L4), *iliac tubercle, anterior–superior iliac spine (ASIS), greater trochanter, pubic tubercle*, and *pubic symphysis* (Fig. 26-9).

Turning to the posterior surface of the hip, significant structures include the *posterior superior iliac spine* (at the level of S2), *greater trochanter, ischial tuberosity*, and the *SI joint* (Figs. 26-10 and 26-17).

The movement of the hip is governed by four robust muscle groups, each with a specific role in hip mobility (Box 26-5). Picture these groups as you examine patients and remember that each muscle must cross the joint line to move the femur in a given direction.

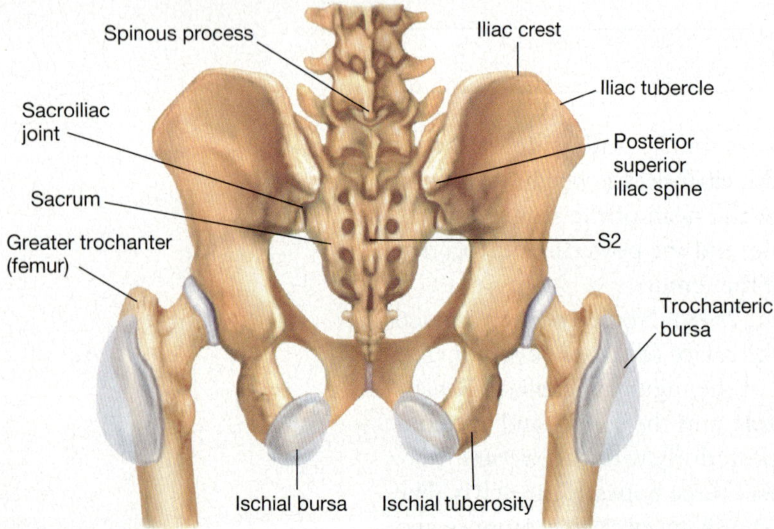

FIGURE 26-10. Anatomy of pelvis and hip with associated bursae, posterior view.

Box 26-5. Functional Classification of Hip Muscle

Muscle Group	Function	Included Muscles
Flexor	Hip flexion, muscles cross the anterior aspect of the hip	Iliopsoas, rectus femoris, pectineus, sartorius (Fig. 26-11).
Extensor	Hip extension, muscles cross the posterior aspect of the hip	Gluteus maximus, hamstrings, adductor magnus, gluteus medius (Fig. 26-12).
Adductor	Pulls the thigh toward the midline (*adducts*), muscles lie along the inside of the thigh and arise from the pubic ramus	Adductor longus, adductor brevis, adductor magnus, gracilis (Fig. 26-13).
Abductor	Pulls the thigh away from the midline (*abducts*) and stabilizes the pelvis during ambulation, muscles lie along the lateral aspect of the hip	Gluteus medius, gluteus minimus, tensor fasciae latae (Fig. 26-14).

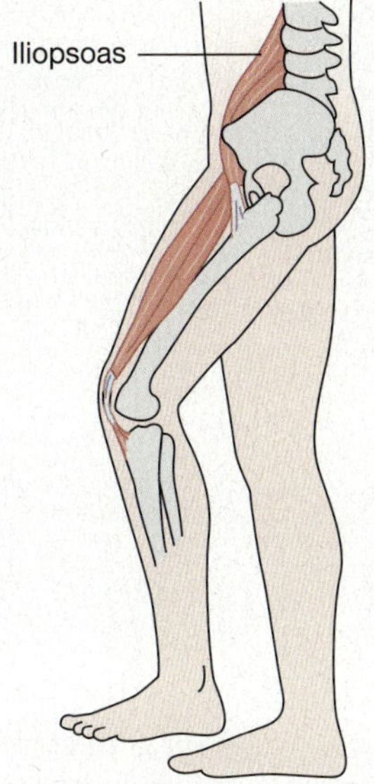

FIGURE 26-11. Flexor muscle group.

Gluteus maximus

Extensor Group

FIGURE 26-12. Extensor muscle group.

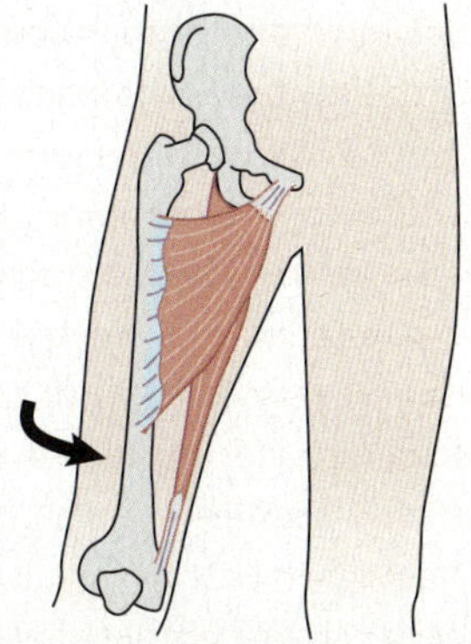

FIGURE 26-13. Adductor muscle group.

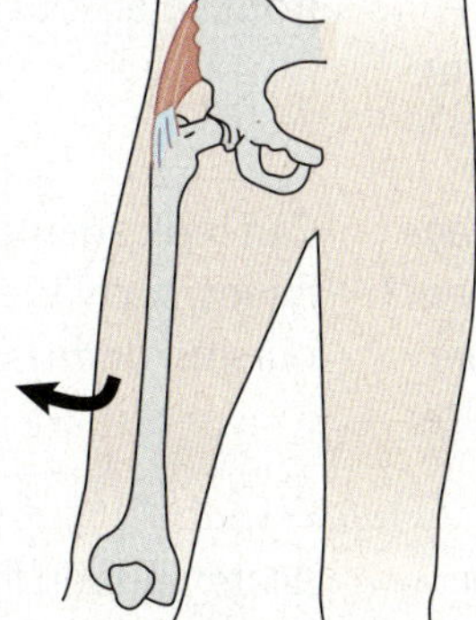

FIGURE 26-14. Abductor muscle group.

The hip joint itself is enclosed by a dense *articular capsule* that extends from the acetabulum to the femoral neck. This capsule plays a critical role in stabilizing the hip joint. Additionally, it receives reinforcement from three overlying ligaments and is lined with a synovial membrane, which contributes to joint lubrication.

Understanding the location and function of three principal hip bursae is important in the context of hip examinations. These include the *iliopsoas bursa* (*iliopectineal bursa*) anterior to the pelvis and hip joint, the *greater trochanteric bursa* (*subgluteus maximus bursa*) along the lateral aspect of the hip, and the *ischial* (*ischiogluteal*) bursa situated posteriorly, close to the sciatic nerve as shown in Figures 26-9 and 26-10.

HEALTH HISTORY: GENERAL APPROACH

Common or Concerning Symptom

- Hip pain

Hip pain is experienced across various age groups, commonly encountered in clinical practice. While it predominantly affects older adults due to degenerative conditions such as osteoarthritis, it is also prevalent among younger populations, including young athletes. In these younger patients, hip pain often arises from injuries, overuse, or developmental issues. Patients with hip pain typically report discomfort localized to the groin, thigh, or buttocks. As you perform the hip examination, remember that comprehensively assessing hip pain involves evaluating both mechanical and systemic causes (Box 26-6). Grasping these factors is key to determining the right treatment approaches.

Box 26-6. Hip Pain: High-Yield History Questions

Domain	Questions	Rationale
Pain location and pattern	*"Can you describe where exactly in your hip you feel the pain? Does it spread anywhere, like your legs or lower back?"*	Helps identify specific hip issues or radiating pain from adjacent structures.
Movement-related pain	*"Does your hip pain change when you move, walk, or sit? Are certain activities more comfortable or exacerbate the pain?"*	Can indicate mechanical issues, such as arthritis, bursitis, or muscle strain.
Onset and duration	*"When did your hip pain start, and how long has it been going on? Is it constant or does it come and go?"*	*Acute*: sudden injury *Chronic*: overuse, or degenerative conditions.

Possible causes include **osteoarthritis** (degeneration of the joint cartilage and underlying bone), **hip fractures** (typically due to falls or impacts), **bursitis** (inflammation of the fluid-filled sacs that cushion the hip joint), **tendinitis** (inflammation of the tendons around the hip, often due to overuse or strain), **hip labral tear** (tearing of the ring of cartilage around the socket of the hip joint), and **sciatica** (pain along the sciatic nerve, which can radiate from the lower back to the hip and down the leg).

Domain	Questions	Rationale
Effect of posture and activity	*"Do certain activities or positions, like sitting for long periods or climbing stairs, worsen your hip pain?"*	Can provide clues to the underlying cause of hip pain.
Associated symptoms	*"Do you experience any stiffness, clicking, or swelling in your hip joint? Any radiating pain down your leg or into your groin?"*	Stiffness or clicking may indicate conditions like osteoarthritis, while radiating pain could suggest nerve involvement.
History of back injuries or surgeries	*"Have you had any previous injuries, surgeries, or treatments on your hip? Any family history of hip conditions?"*	Past hip injuries or surgeries may contribute to current symptoms. Family history can provide insights into genetic predispositions to certain hip conditions.
Impact on daily activities	*"How does your hip pain affect your daily activities, such as walking, standing, or exercising? Do you have difficulty with specific movements?"*	Helps gauge severity and the need for intervention or lifestyle modifications.
Lifestyle and exercise habits	*"Can you describe your typical daily activities and exercise routine? Do you engage in regular physical activities or have sedentary habits?"*	Lifestyle factors may contribute to the development or exacerbation of hip pain.

TECHNIQUES OF EXAMINATION

Key Components of the Hip Joint Examination

I
- Inspect the hip joint (deformities, muscle asymmetry, atrophy, fasciculations, pelvic alignment, skin changes)

P
- Palpate the anterior hip landmarks (iliac crest, iliac tubercle, and anterior–superior iliac spine, greater trochanter, inguinal ligament and surrounding structures).
- Palpate the posterior hip landmarks (posterior–superior iliac spine, sacroiliac joint, ischial tuberosity)

ROM
- Assess hip joint range of motion (flexion extension, abduction, and adduction, external rotation, and internal rotation).

S
- Perform special maneuvers on the hip joint, if indicated (FADIR, DIRI, FABER, Kendall test, Thomas test)

Inspect the Hip Joint

Inspect the hip joint by having the patient stand upright or lie supine, with feet shoulder-width apart. Observe the anterior hip for deformities, muscle asymmetry, atrophy, fasciculations, pelvic alignment, and skin changes like discoloration or inflammation. Inspect the lateral hip for abnormalities around the greater trochanter. For the posterior hip, observe gluteal muscle bulk, sacroiliac joints, and skin changes. Note any bulging of the joint capsule and survey for discoloration or skin alterations. If relevant, assess gait and functional movement for abnormalities in hip motion (see gait assessment, pp. 879–881).

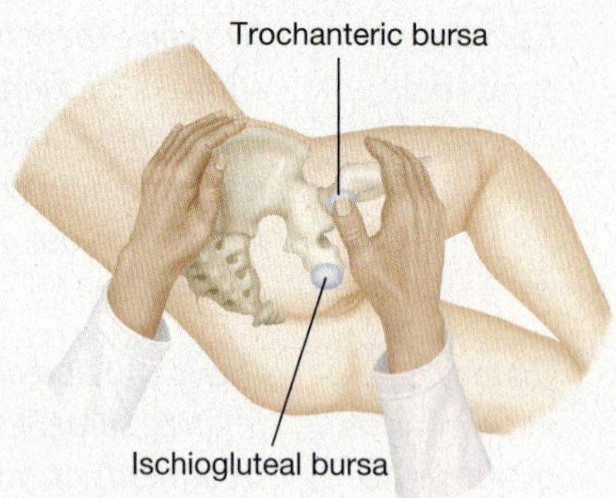

FIGURE 26-15. Palpating the trochanteric bursa.

Palpate the Anterior Hip Landmarks

Iliac Crest, Iliac Tubercle, and Anterior–Superior Iliac Spine. Begin by locating the *iliac crest* at the upper margin of the pelvis, usually at the level of the waist. Follow the downward anterior curve and locate the *iliac tubercle,* marking the widest point of the crest. Continue tracking downward to the *ASIS*, a prominent bony landmark.

Greater Trochanter of the Femur. Move your fingers laterally to the *greater trochanter* of the femur, usually where patients consider their hips to be and at the same level as the pubic symphysis. Be sure to palpate the anterior, superior, and posterior aspects of the greater trochanter since different tendinous attachments are found on each.[6] Also palpate the trochanteric bursa for any tenderness (Fig. 26-15).

Tenderness over the trochanter indicates greater trochanteric pain syndrome commonly caused by tendinopathy of the gluteus medius or minimus tendons or bursitis in inflammatory conditions.

Inguinal Ligament and Surrounding Structures. With the patient supine, ask them to place the heel of the leg being examined on the opposite knee. This position exposes the hip's anterior structures.

Then palpate along the *inguinal ligament*, which extends from the ASIS to the pubic tubercle. Along this path, you can also palpate the femoral pulse over the femoral triangle in the anterior groin (Fig. 26-16). The femoral nerve, artery, and vein bisect the overlying inguinal ligament with deep inguinal lymph nodes lying medially. The mnemonic **NAVEL** may help you remember the lateral-to-medial sequence of the femoral triangle's content: **N**erve–**A**rtery–**V**ein–**E**mpty space–**L**ymph node. Move your thumbs medially and inferiorly to the *pubic tubercle,* which lies at the same level as the greater trochanter.

Bulges along the ligament with Valsalva suggest an inguinal hernia. Pulsatile swelling suggests an aneurysm. Enlarged lymph nodes point to infection in the pelvis or lower extremity.

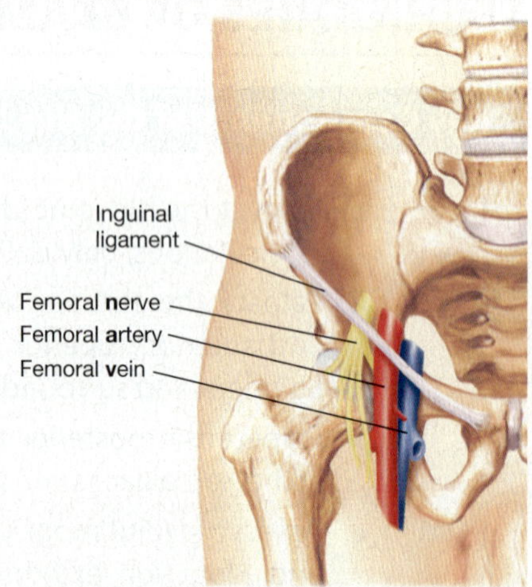

FIGURE 26-16. Inguinal ligament and the femoral triangle's contents: N-A-V-E-L.

Palpate the Posterior Hip Landmarks

Posterior–Superior Iliac Spine. Palpate the *posterior–superior iliac spine* (*PSIS*) just medial and inferior to the L5 spinous process. In some individuals, visible dimples over the PSIS may be present, serving as useful landmarks for orientation (Fig. 26-17).

Sacroiliac Joint. Once you have identified the PSIS, move your fingers downward in a vertical line toward the *SI joint.* The joint itself is rarely palpable, but the region may be tender in those with SI joint pain. Palpating this region requires a gentle yet firm touch to accurately assess for any tenderness or abnormalities.

Ischial Tuberosity. Reach your thumbs inferiorly from the base of the SI joint to palpate *ischial tuberosity* in the medial gluteal fold. Normally, the *ischiogluteal*

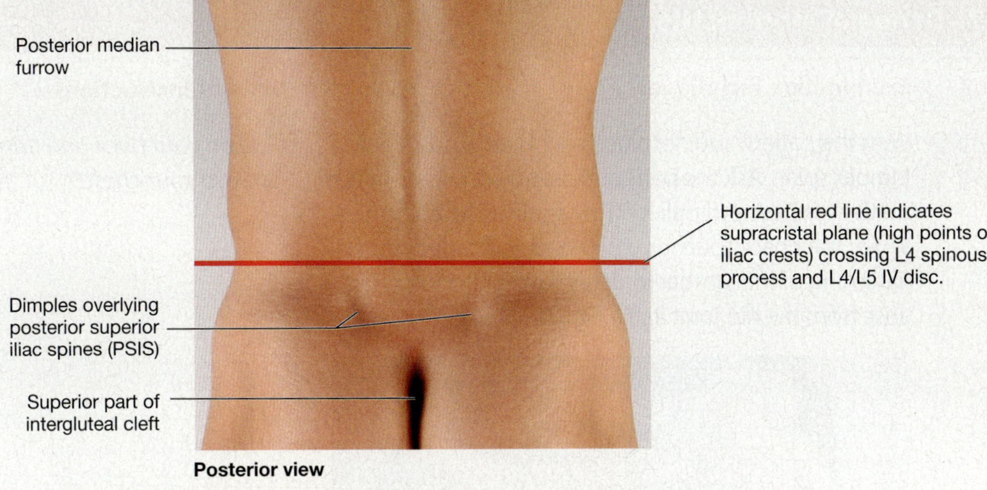

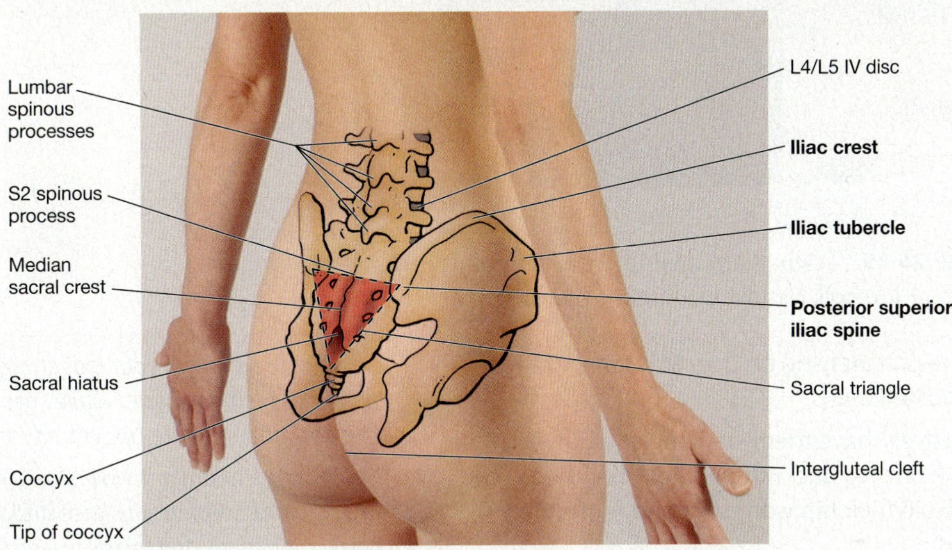

FIGURE 26-17. Surface anatomy of the hip joint and surrounding structures, posterior view. (Reprinted with permission from Agur AMR, Dalley AF II. *Moore's Essential Clinical Anatomy.* 6th ed. Wolters Kluwer; 2020. Figure SA2.2.)

bursa, over the ischial tuberosity, is not palpable unless inflamed (Fig. 26-18).

Look for tenderness in *ischiogluteal bursitis* or "weaver's bottom."

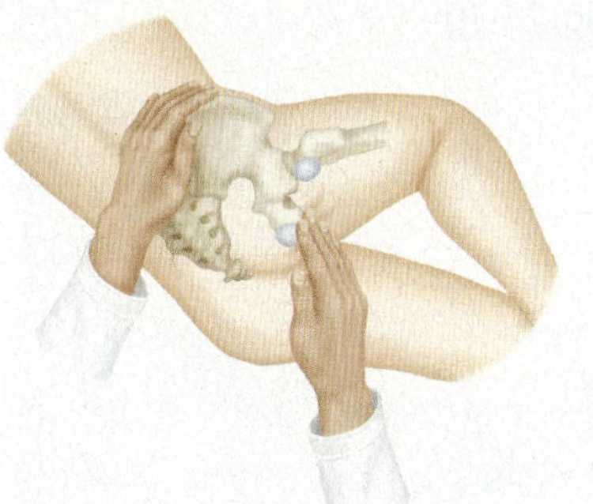

FIGURE 26-18. Palpating the ischiogluteal bursa.

Assess Hip Joint Range of Motion

Assess hip ROM and the specific muscles responsible for each movement. Review the instructions to the patient (Box 26-7). The choice between active and passive ROM in hip assessment should be based on the patient's specific needs, their ability to move the joint actively, and the clinical questions the assessment aims to answer. Normal values for hip flexion extension, abduction, and adduction are 130°, 15°, 45°, and 20°, respectively.[7–9]

Box 26-7. Range of Motion: Hip Joint

Movement	Examination Technique	Patient Instructions
Flexion	With the patient supine, place your hand under their lumbar spine. Ask the patient to bend each knee in turn up to the chest and pull it firmly against the abdomen. When their back touches your hand, indicating normal flattening of the lumbar lordosis, further flexion must arise from the hip joint itself (Fig. 26-19). 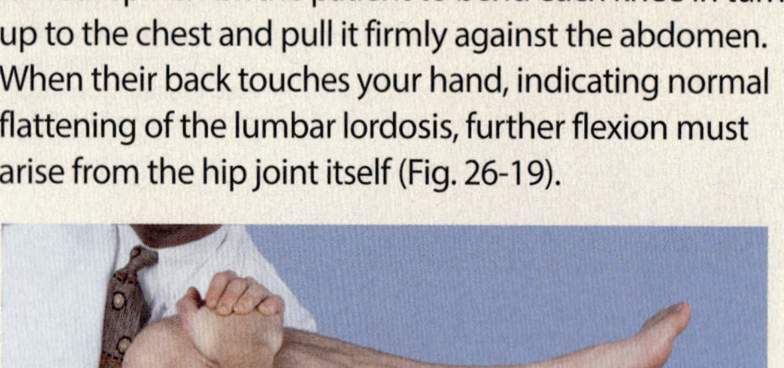 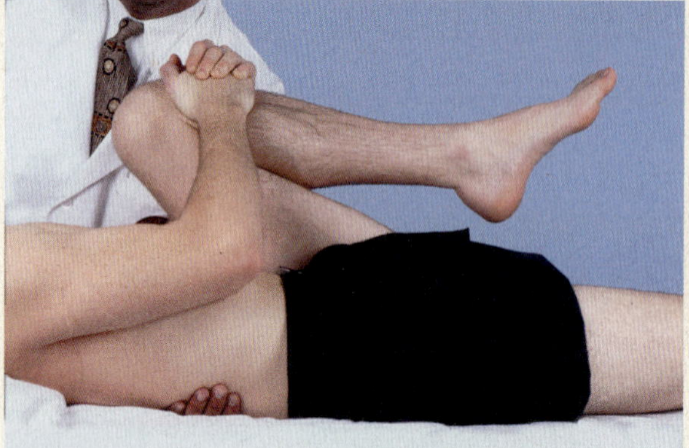 **FIGURE 26-19.** Testing hip flexion with flattening of lumbar lordosis against examiner's hand.	*"Lie on your back and bring your knee toward your chest."*
Extension	With the patient lying on their side, extend their thigh posteriorly. Alternatively, have them stand up straight. Ask them to move one leg backward without bending at the waist. Hold their hip with one hand for stability if needed.	*"Lie on your side with your legs straight. Now, lift your top leg backward while keeping your knee straight and your upper body steady."* *"Please stand up straight. Now, slowly move one leg backward, keeping your knee straight, your upper body steady and try not to lean forward."*
Abduction	With the patient lying supine, place one hand on the opposite ASIS to stabilize the pelvis. Instruct the patient to move their extended leg away from their body while keeping the knee straight, ensuring no pelvic movement (Fig. 26-20). 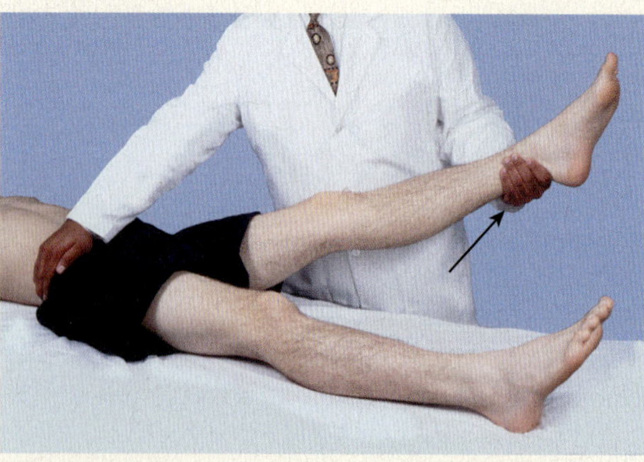 **FIGURE 26-20.** Testing left hip abduction (passive).	*"Lie on your back. I will place my hand on your pelvis to keep it stable. Now, move your leg to the side away from your body, keeping your knee straight."*

Movement	Examination Technique	Patient Instructions
Adduction	With the patient lying supine, place one hand on the opposite ASIS to stabilize the pelvis. Instruct the patient to move their extended leg medially across the body, over the opposite extremity, while keeping both hips flat on the table (Fig. 26-21). 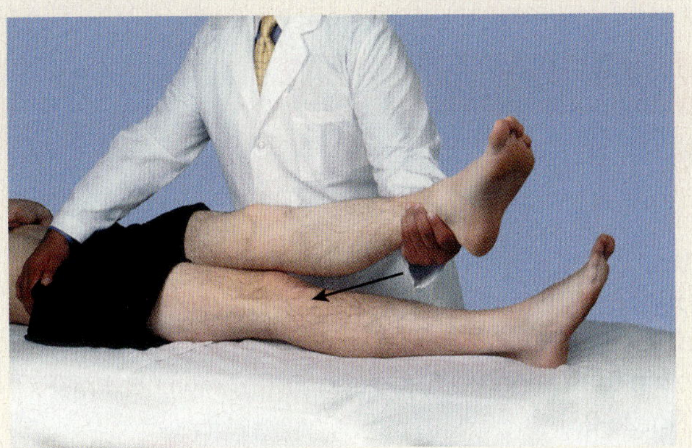 **FIGURE 26-21.** Testing left hip adduction (passive).	*"Lie on your back. I will place my hand on your pelvis to keep it stable. Now, move your leg across your body over the other leg, ensuring both hips stay on the table."*
External rotation	With the patient lying supine, flex their leg to 90° at the hip and knee while you stabilize their thigh with one hand and hold their leg in position. Instruct the patient to move their lower leg inward, causing the knee to rotate outward, to achieve external rotation at the hip (Fig. 26-22). 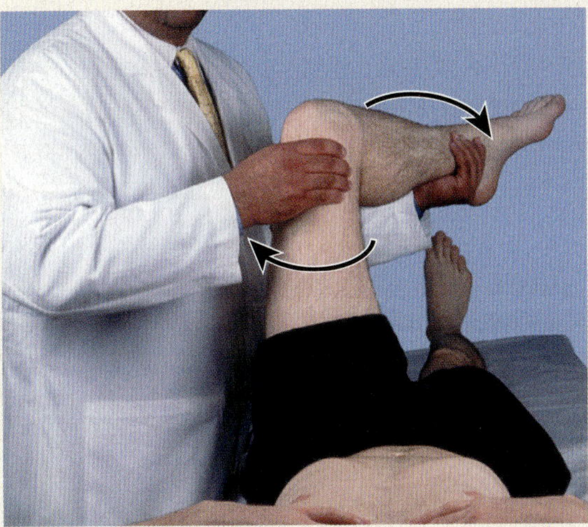 **FIGURE 26-22.** Testing external rotation of the left hip (passive).	*"Lie on your back. I will hold your leg at the hip and knee, bent to 90 degrees, and stabilize your thigh. Now, move your lower leg inward, so your knee rotates outward."*
Internal rotation	With the patient lying supine, flex their leg to 90° at the hip and knee while you stabilize their thigh with one hand and hold their leg in position. Instruct the patient to move their lower leg outward, causing the knee to rotate inward, to achieve *internal rotation* at the hip.	*"Lie on your back. I will hold your leg at the hip and knee, bent to 90 degrees, and stabilize your thigh. Now, move your lower leg outward, so your knee rotates inward."*

Perform Special Maneuvers on the Hip Joint (If Indicated)

Special maneuvers for the hip are a series of clinical examination techniques designed to isolate and test the integrity of the hip joint and surrounding structures.[10–12] Each maneuver targets different aspects of the hip anatomy, providing a comprehensive assessment of hip function and stability (Box 26-8).

Box 26-8. Special Maneuvers: Hip Joint

Special Maneuver	Structures Assessed	Examination Technique
Flexion, adduction, internal rotation (FADIR) maneuver	Hip joint	Position the patient supine and flex their hip to 90° with the thigh adducted. Then gradually internally rotate the hip to the end ROM, looking for pain (Fig. 26-23).
Scour test or dynamic internal rotatory impingement (DIRI) modification	Hip joint	Position the patient supine and flex their hip to 90°. Hold their knee in one hand and their ankle in the other while you adduct their thigh across their midline and gently internally rotate the hip. Then "scour" the hip by making small, circular movements with the thigh to reproduce painful symptoms (Fig. 26-24).
FABER (flexion, abduction, external rotation) or Patrick test	Groin strain	With the patient supine, position their leg into 90° of flexion and externally rotate and abduct it so that their ipsilateral ankle rests distal to the knee of the contralateral leg (see Fig. 26-6, p. 849).
Kendall test	Hip flexion contracture (rectus femoris)	The patient lies supine and flexes one hip by bringing the knee of the uninvolved leg to the chest, flattening the lumbar spine, while the tested leg hangs off the table. The thigh should lie flat on the table with the knee hanging freely (Fig. 26-25).
Thomas test	Hip flexion tightness (iliopsoas)	The patient sits at the table's edge, then lies back while bringing the uninvolved leg's knee to the chest to flatten the lower back. The tested leg remains extended at the table's edge. The thigh should stay flat on the table.

Pain with internal rotation suggests intra-articular pathology such as acetabular labral tears, femoroacetabular impingement (FAI), or hip osteoarthritis.

Pain or discomfort during the test indicates intra-articular pathology. The test accentuates the movements of the FADIR maneuver to reproduce painful symptoms.

Pain located in the groin area with the FABER test can indicate hip joint pathology, such as hip arthritis or a labral tear. This is also commonly seen in sports injuries involving forced abduction.

Targets the rectus femoris, which crosses the hip and knee. Key observations are whether the thigh stays flat and the knee hangs freely. Tightness is indicated if the thigh lifts or the knee extends.

Focuses on the iliopsoas, which only crosses the hip. The emphasis is on ensuring the thigh of the tested leg remains flat against the table when the patient brings the uninvolved knee to the chest, indicating whether iliopsoas tightness exists. The position of the knee itself is less emphasized than in the Kendall Test.

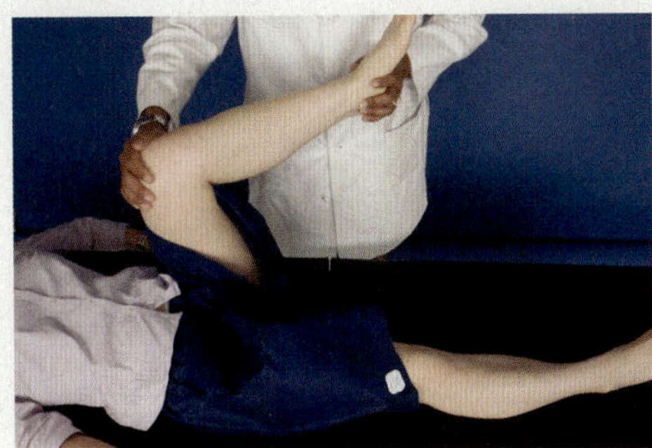

FIGURE 26-23. Impingement test (flexion, adduction, internal rotation [FADIR]) is performed with the hip in FADIR. (Reprinted with permission from Kim YJ, Novais E. *Hip Preservation Surgery in Children and Adolescents.* Wolters Kluwer; 2021. Figure 11-1.)

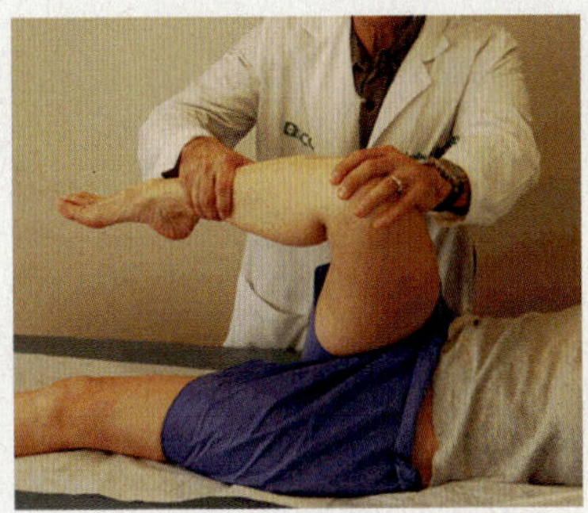

FIGURE 26-24. "Scouring" the hip in the scour test or DIRI modification. (Reprinted with permission from Wiesel SW. *Operative Techniques in Orthopaedic Surgery.* 2nd ed. Wolters Kluwer; 2016. Scour Test.)

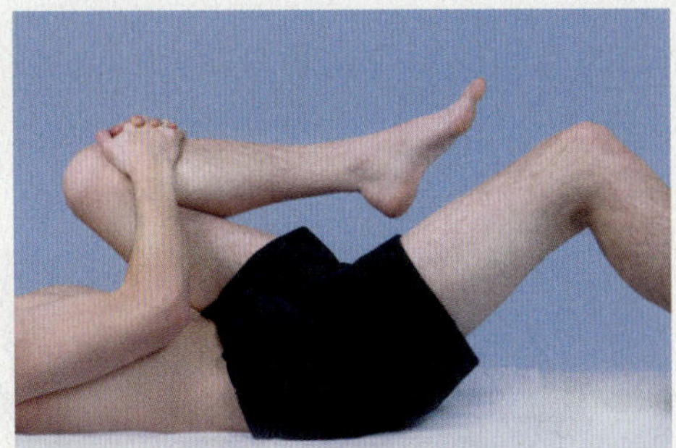

FIGURE 26-25. Positive flexion deformity of right hip (Kendall test).

ANATOMY: KNEE

The *knee joint* is the largest joint in the body. It is a hinge joint involving three bones: *femur, tibia,* and *patella* (*kneecap*). It has three articular surfaces or compartments: *between the medial femoral condyle and the tibia, between the lateral femoral condyle and the tibia,* and *between the femur and the patella.* Note how the two rounded condyles of the femur rest on the relatively flat *tibial plateau.*

The knee joint has no inherent stability, making it dependent on a complex of ligaments and tendons to hold the articulating femur and tibia in place. In combination with the lever action of the femur on the tibia, this can predispose the knee to injury.

Learn the bony landmarks in and around the knee to guide your examination (Box 26-9 and Figs. 26-26 to 26-28).

Box 26-9. Anatomic Landmarks of the Knee

Surface of the Knee	Anatomic Landmark	Description and Location
Medial surface	Adductor tubercle	Bony prominence on the femur, located on its medial aspect
	Medial epicondyle of the femur	Bony projection on the femur near the knee joint, on the inner side
	Medial condyle of the tibia	Inner part of the tibia that articulates with the femur
Anterior surface	Patella	Kneecap, situated on the front of the knee, embedded in the quadriceps tendon
	Patellar tendon	Extends from the patella below the knee, attaching to the tibial tuberosity
	Tibial tuberosity	Point where the patellar tendon attaches on the shinbone
Lateral surface	Lateral epicondyle of the femur	Bony prominence on the outer side of the femur, near the knee joint
	Lateral condyle of the tibia	Outer part of the tibia that articulates with the femur
	Head of the fibula	Located just below the knee joint, on the lateral side of the leg

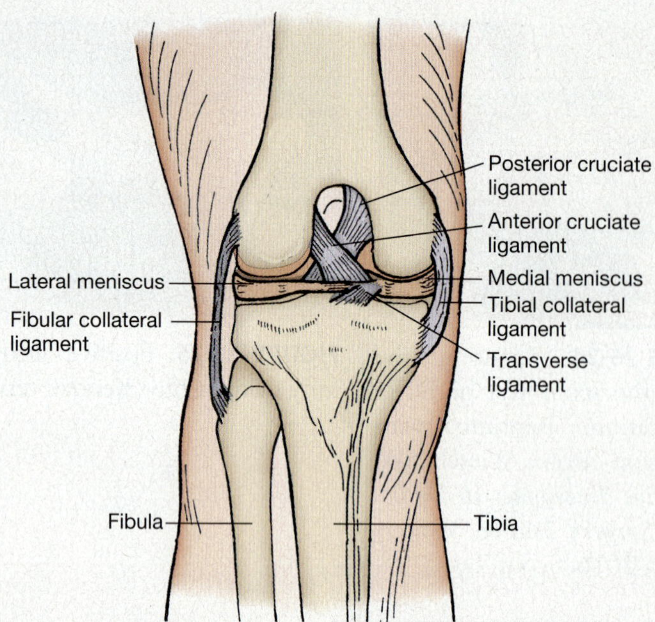

FIGURE 26-26. Anatomic landmarks of the right knee (patella removed), anterior view. (Reprinted with permission from Halliday NL, Chung HM. *BRS Gross Anatomy.* 9th ed. Wolters Kluwer; 2019. Figure 6-10.)

Two condylar *tibiofemoral joints* are formed by the convex curves of the medial and lateral condyles of the femur as they articulate with the concave condyles of the tibia. The third articular surface is the *patellofemoral joint.* The patella slides on the groove of the anterior aspect of the distal femur, called the *trochlear groove*, during flexion and extension of the knee.

Problems with patellar tracking can lead to anterior knee pain, arthritis, or patellar dislocation in severe cases.

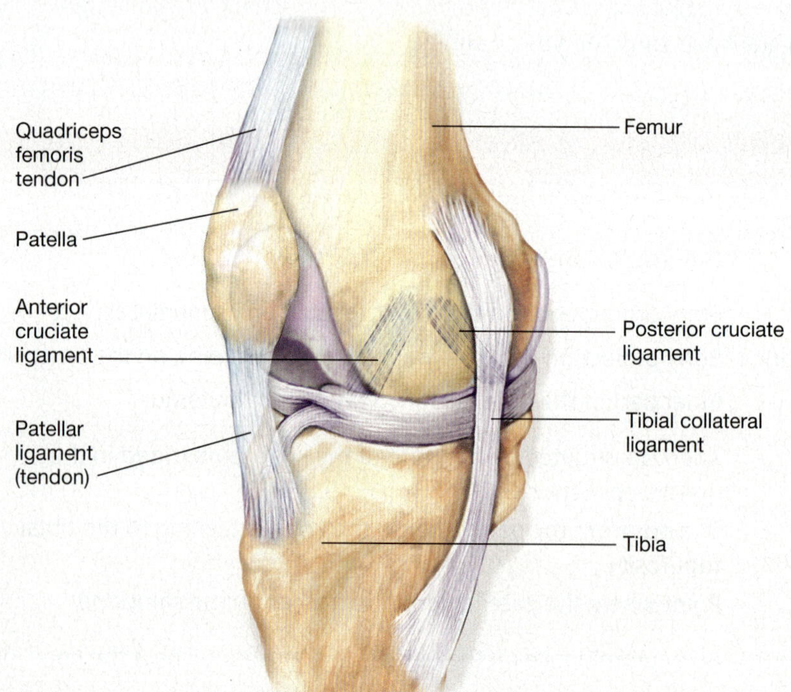

FIGURE 26-27. Anatomic landmarks of the right knee, oblique view. (From Anatomical Chart Company. Wolters Kluwer; 2005.)

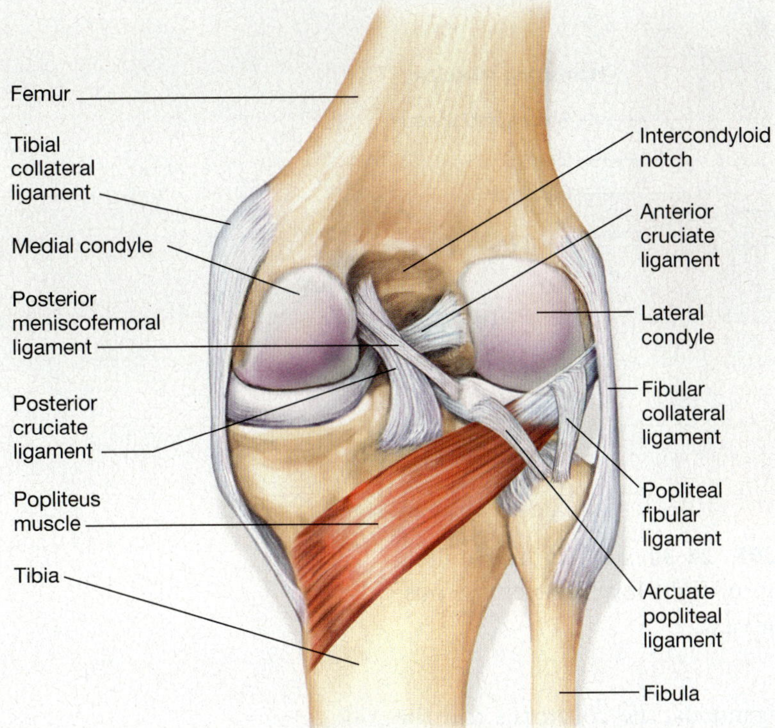

FIGURE 26-28. Anatomic landmarks of the right knee, posterior view. (From Anatomical Chart Company. Wolters Kluwer; 2005.)

Two powerful muscle groups move and stabilize the knee (Box 26-10). Both muscle groups have components that cross the hip joint and so act to flex and extend the hip as well as move the knee.

In persons with wide quadriceps (Q) angles (e.g., persons assigned female at birth and athletes in high-impact sports), the quadriceps contraction may exert a more lateral pull that can alter patellar tracking and may be a risk factor for anterior knee pain–related issues.

Box 26-10. Muscle Groups Moving and Stabilizing the Knee

Muscle Group	Components	Function	Location
Quadriceps femoris	Rectus femoris, vastus medialis, vastus lateralis, and vastus intermedius	Extends the knee	Covers the anterior, medial, and lateral aspects of the thigh (Fig. 26-29)
Hamstring muscles	Biceps femoris, semitendinosus, and semimembranosus	Flexes the knee	Located on the posterior aspect of the thigh (Fig. 26-30)

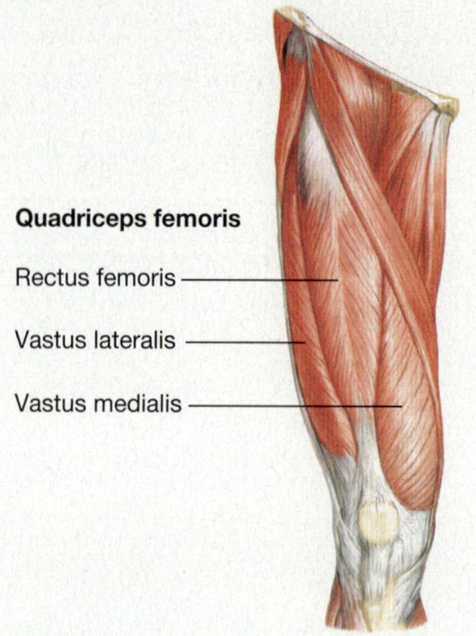

FIGURE 26-29. Quadriceps femoris muscle group of right lower extremity, anterior view.

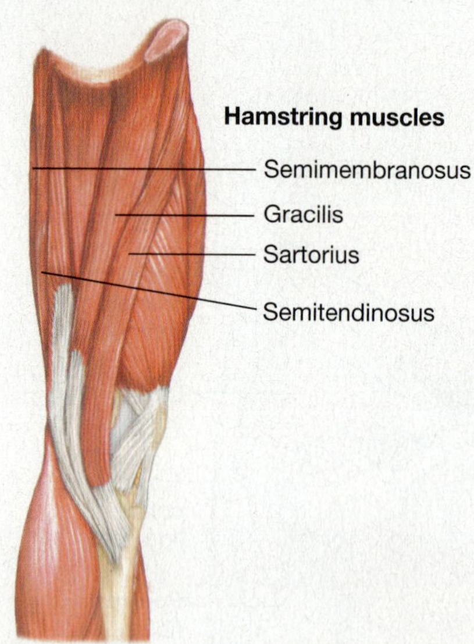

FIGURE 26-30. Hamstring muscle group of right lower extremity, posterior view.

The menisci and two important pairs of ligaments, the collaterals and the cruciates, are essential for knee stability (Box 26-11 and Fig. 26-31).

Note the concavities usually evident adjacent and superior to each side of the patella, known as the *infrapatellar space* (Fig. 26-32). Occupying these areas is the *synovial cavity of the knee*, one of the largest joint cavities in the body. It additionally contains the *infrapatellar fat pad* (also known as the *Hoffa fat pad*) and the *infrapatellar bursa*.

Box 26-11. Menisci and Ligaments with Their Specific Functions and Locations

Structure	Description	Function
Medial meniscus	Crescent-shaped fibrocartilaginous disc located on the medial side of the tibial plateau, allowing for contact with the medial femoral condyle	Cushions the action of the femur on the tibia and helps distribute force on the medial side of the knee
Lateral meniscus	Crescent-shaped fibrocartilaginous disc on the lateral side of the tibial plateau, complementing the lateral femoral condyle	Performs a similar cushioning and force distribution role on the lateral side of the knee
Medial collateral ligament (MCL)	Connects the medial femoral epicondyle to the medial condyle of the tibia and medial meniscus	Resists valgus stress (inward pressure) across the knee joint; broad and flat, not easily palpable
Lateral collateral ligament (LCL)	Connects the lateral femoral epicondyle to the head of the fibula	Resists varus stress (outward pressure) across the knee joint
Anterior cruciate ligament (ACL)	Crosses obliquely from the anteromedial tibia to the lateral femoral condyle	Prevents the tibia from sliding forward on the femur; *not clinically palpable*
Posterior cruciate ligament (PCL)	Crosses from the posterolateral tibia to the medial femoral condyle	Prevents the tibia from sliding backward on the femur; *not clinically palpable*

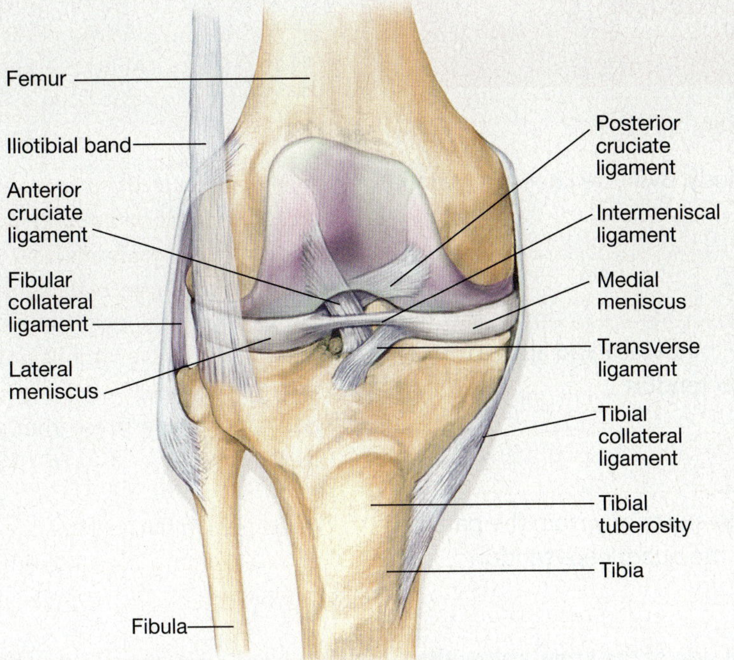

FIGURE 26-31. Right knee joint, anterior view (patella removed). (From Anatomical Chart Company. Wolters Kluwer; 2005.)

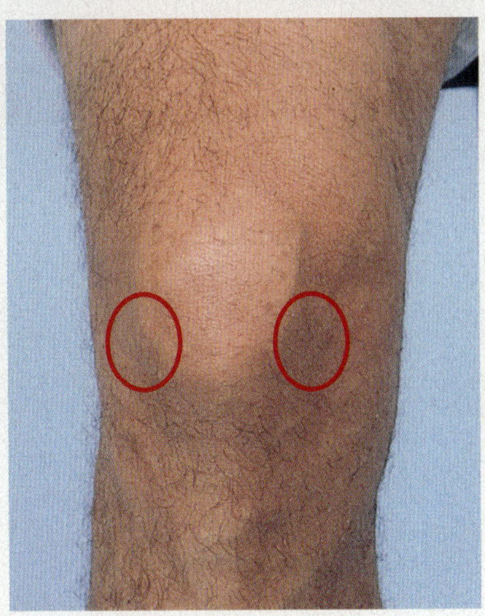

FIGURE 26-32. Infrapatellar spaces of the right knee occupied by the synovial cavity.

This cavity extends as the *suprapatellar recess* 6 cm above the upper border of the patella deep to the quadriceps muscle. This recess also lies in between the *suprapatellar* and *prefemoral fat pads.* The joint cavity covers the anterior, medial, and lateral surfaces of the knee as well as the condyles of the femur and tibia posteriorly.

Although the synovium is not normally palpable, these areas may become swollen and tender when the joint is inflamed or injured.

Several *bursae* lie near the knee (Box 26-12 and Fig. 26-33).

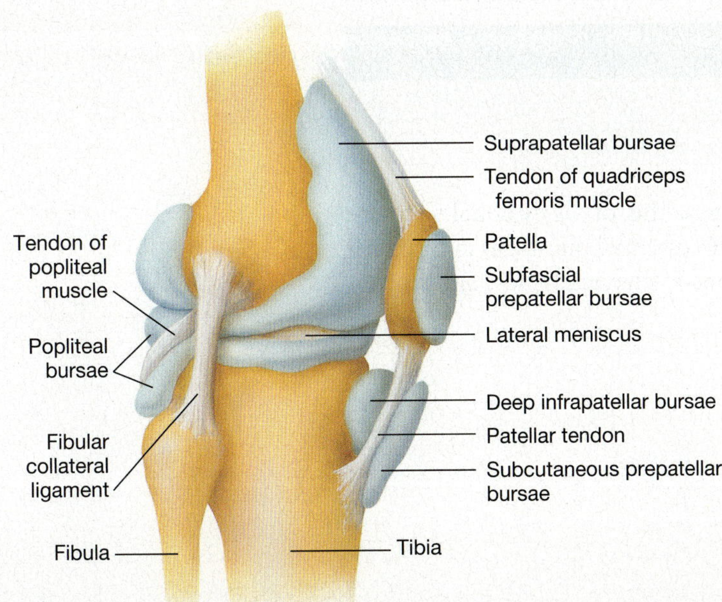

FIGURE 26-33. Right knee bursae. (From Anatomical Chart Company. Wolters Kluwer; 2005.)

Box 26-12. Bursae of the Knee: Location and Clinical Significance

Bursa	Location	
Prepatellar bursa	Anteriorly, over the kneecap (patella)	Inflammation leads to prepatellar bursitis, often associated with prolonged kneeling, commonly affecting individuals like carpet layers or gardeners.
Infrapatellar bursa	Below the patella and above the patellar tendon	This common site of inflammation in athletes is known as "jumper's knee" due to repetitive stress from activities like jumping.
Suprapatellar bursa	Extends superiorly from the patella under the quadriceps tendon	Inflammation can lead to knee stiffness and pain, often associated with overuse or injury.
Pes anserine bursa	Medial side of the knee, below the joint line	Bursitis here presents with medial knee pain, common in runners.
Gastrocnemio-semimembranosus bursa	Situated in the popliteal fossa at the back of the knee joint	Enlargement of this bursa leads to a *popliteal (Baker) cyst*, causing pain and restricted movement behind the knee.
Iliotibial band bursa	Lateral between the iliotibial band and the lateral femoral condyle	Inflammation causes lateral knee pain, common in runners and cyclists.

HEALTH HISTORY: GENERAL APPROACH

Common or Concerning Symptom

- Knee pain

When a patient presents with knee pain, a targeted history is essential to guide diagnosis and management. Box 26-13 provides essential questions tailored for knee pain evaluation, aiming to identify its onset, characteristics, and impact on function.

Box 26-13. Knee Pain: High-Yield Health History Questions

Domain	Questions	Rationale
Location	*"Can you specify where in the knee you feel the pain (front, back, inside, outside)?"*	Helps identify specific knee structures that might be involved, such as ligaments or menisci
Onset	*"Did your knee pain start suddenly or gradually increase over time?"*	*Sudden:* might indicate acute injury *Gradual:* could suggest a degenerative process
Relation to activity	*"Is the pain associated with certain activities, like climbing stairs, running, or sitting for long periods?"*	Can indicate patellofemoral pain syndrome, meniscal tears, or osteoarthritis
Mechanical symptoms	*"Do you experience locking, giving way, or popping in the knee?"*	Can suggest meniscal injuries or loose bodies within the joint
History of injury	*"Have you had any recent or past injuries to the knee?"*	Important for diagnosing ligament injuries or fractures
Swelling	*"Has your knee swelled up at any time? If so, was it immediate or did it develop over time?"*	*Immediate:* often indicates an acute injury *Delayed:* might be related to inflammation
Range of motion	*"Are you able to fully straighten or bend your knee without pain?"*	Limitations can indicate joint effusion, arthritis, or mechanical obstruction
Instability	*"Do you feel like your knee is unstable or unable to support your weight?"*	Can suggest ligamentous injury or weakness
Associated symptoms	*"Do you have any symptoms in your hips, ankles, or other joints?"*	Can indicate a systemic condition like rheumatoid arthritis or referred pain from the hip
Response to treatment	*"Have you tried any treatments, and have they helped?"*	Can aid in diagnosis and treatment planning

Possible causes include **osteoarthritis** (degeneration of joint cartilage and the underlying bone), **ligament injuries** (often due to sports-related activities), **meniscal tears** (injury to the shock-absorbing cartilage in the knee), **patellar tendinitis** (inflammation of the tendons connecting the kneecap to the shinbone, typically in athletes), **bursitis** (inflammation of the fluid-filled sacs that cushion the knee joint), and **iliotibial band syndrome** (inflammation of the ligament that runs down the outside of the thigh, leading to pain on the outside of the knee).

TECHNIQUES OF EXAMINATION

Key Components of the Knee Examination

I	■ Inspect the gait ■ Inspect the knee and surrounding structures (alignment, contours, atrophy, swelling).
P	■ Palpate the knee and adjoining structures (patella, patellar tendon, medial and lateral tibiofemoral joint and menisci, MCL, LCL, patellofemoral joint compartment, suprapatellar recess, knee bursae, popliteal fossa).
ROM	■ Assess knee joint range of motion (flexion, extension, medial rotation, and lateral rotation).
S	■ Perform special maneuvers on the hip joint, if indicated (McMurray test, Abduction or valgus stress test, adduction or varus stress test, anterior drawer sign, Lachman test, posterior drawer sign, patellar grind test).

Palpation and testing of the knee structures are especially helpful in diagnosis. The anterior cruciate ligament (ACL) and posterior cruciate ligament (PCL) are not palpable but are tested by special maneuvers.

Inspect the Gait

Inspect the *gait* for a smooth rhythmic flow as the patient enters the room. The knee should be extended at heel strike and mildly flexed at all other phases of swing and stance.

See further discussion of gait assessment in Special Techniques and Maneuvers, Analyzing Gait on pp. 879–881.

Stumbling or "giving way" of the knee during heel strike suggests quadriceps weakness or abnormal patellar tracking.

Inspect the Knee and Surrounding Structures

Check the alignment and contours of the knees including enlargement of the knee joint and any varus or valgus alignment. Observe for any atrophy of the quadriceps muscles.

Bow-legs (**genu varum**) and *knock-knees* (**genu valgum**) are common but may indicate underlying pathology. Patients with osteoarthritis may develop malalignment from cartilage loss and meniscal dysfunction.

Inspect the normal hollows around the patella. Loss of these hollows can be a sign of swelling in the knee joint and suprapatellar recess. Note any other swelling in or around the knee and which structure it may be related to.

Swelling directly over the patella occurs in prepatellar bursitis (housemaid's knee). Swelling over the tibial tubercle suggests infrapatellar or, if more medial, anserine bursitis.

Inspect the back of the knee in the popliteal fossa where a Baker cyst or bruising from tendon injury may be seen.

Palpate the Knee and Adjoining Structures

Ask the patient to sit on the edge of the examining table with their knees hanging relaxed in flexion or lie supine with knees flexed to 90°. In this position, bony landmarks are more visible, and the muscles, tendons, and ligaments are more relaxed, making them easier to palpate. Pay special attention to any areas of tenderness. Precisely localizing the structure causing pain helps narrow your differential diagnosis.

Bony enlargement at the joint margins, genu varum deformity, and stiffness lasting ≤30 minutes are typical findings in *osteoarthritis* (likelihood ratios [LRs] 11.8, 3.4, and 3.0, respectively).[13] Crepitus is also common but not diagnostic.

Medial Tibiofemoral Joint and Meniscus. Palpate the *medial tibiofemoral joint* and *medial meniscus* (Fig. 26-34). Facing the knee, place your thumbs in the soft tissue depressions on either side of the *patellar tendon*. Note that the inferior pole of the patella generally lies at the tibiofemoral joint line in this flexed position. Identify the groove of the *tibiofemoral joint* as you feel the edge of the tibial plateau. Follow it medially, noting any pain that is present.

A medial meniscus tear can manifest as joint line point tenderness. It is common after trauma and requires prompt evaluation.[14] Individuals with osteoarthritis (OA) may end up with chronic tears of the meniscus related to abnormal biomechanics and loading of the knee that do not require repair.

Medial Collateral Ligament. Palpate the *medial collateral ligament* (*MCL*). Medially, move your thumbs upward to palpate the *medial femoral epicondyle* where the MCL originates (see Fig. 26-30). It connects the medial epicondyle of the femur to the medial condyle and superior medial surface of the tibia (in flexion, the course may be more posterior than you anticipate). Move your

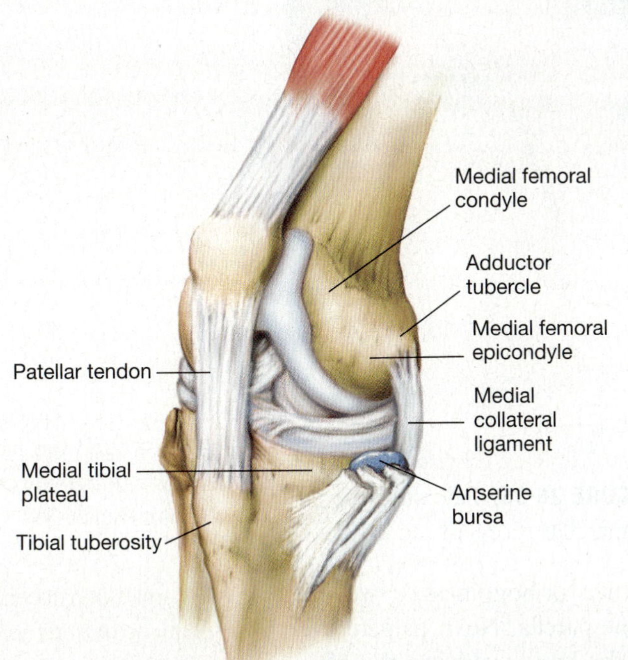

FIGURE 26-34. Structures in the medial compartment of the right knee.

thumbs downward along the general course this broad, flat ligament from its origin to insertion. Be aware that it may not be palpable.

MCL tenderness after injury is suspicious for an MCL tear. Lateral collateral ligament (LCL) injuries are less frequent. When either is injured, search for injury to the other ligaments and soft tissues of the knee that are also often affected.

Lateral Tibiofemoral Joint and Meniscus. Palpate the *lateral tibiofemoral joint* and *lateral meniscus* in the same position, starting at the patellar tendon and moving posteriorly along the tibial plateau. Pay attention to any areas of pain or tenderness.

Lateral Collateral Ligament. Palpate the *LCL*. The LCL originates on the lateral epicondyle of the femur and attaches to the fibular head. Ask the patient to cross one leg so that the ankle rests on the opposite knee and find the LCL as a firm cord that runs across the knee joint and attaches to the fibula.

Patella and Patellofemoral Joint Compartment. Palpate the *patellofemoral joint compartment*. Use your fingers to gently push the patella medially and feel along the medial edge of the patella. Then slide the patella laterally and feel along the lateral edge of the patella. Note any tenderness. Also note and increased or decreased movement of the patella

Significant movement of the patella suggests ligamentous laxity.

Pain and crepitus with knee flexion and extension arise from the roughened undersurface of the patella as it articulates with the femur. Crepitus during flexion and extension, along with restricted movement, may indicate patellofemoral osteoarthritis.[15,16]

Suprapatellar Recess. Palpate for any thickening or swelling in the *suprapatellar recess* and along the margins of the patella (Fig. 26-35). Start 10 cm above the superior border of the patella, well above the recess, and feel the soft tissues between your thumb and fingers. Note any muscular tenderness. Move your hand distally in progressive steps, trying to identify fluid or swelling in the recess if present.

Continue your palpation along the sides of the patella. Note any tenderness or increased warmth. Comparison to the other side can help identify swelling.

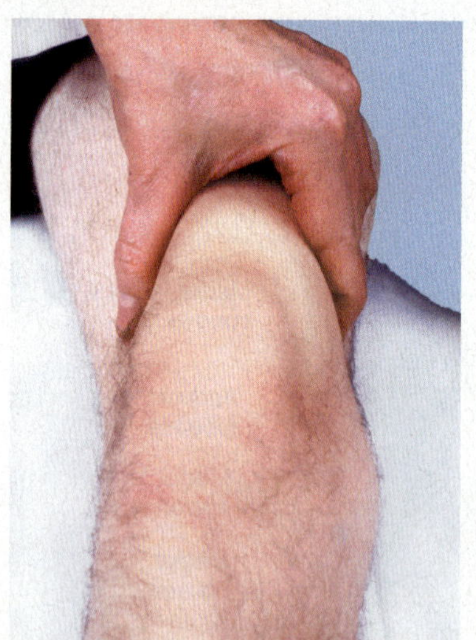

FIGURE 26-35. Palpating the suprapatellar recess of the left knee.

Swelling around the patella may point to synovial thickening or effusion of the knee joint (Fig. 26-36).

Knee Bursae. Check three key bursae around the knee for bogginess or swelling. Palpate the *prepatellar bursa* over the front of the patella. Next, palpate over the *anserine bursa* on the anteromedial side of the knee overlying the MCL insertion. Finally, on the posterior surface, with the patient's leg extended,

See examination techniques for gross assessment of knee joint effusions, in Special Techniques and Maneuvers, Detecting Knee Effusions, pp. 883–885.

Box 26-14. Range of Motion: Knee Joint

Movement	Examination Technique	Patient Instructions
Flexion	Have the patient sit or lie supine. Instruct them to bring their heel toward their buttocks, bending their knee. Assess the degree of flexion.	*"Sit or lie down and relax your leg. Please bend your knee, bringing your heel closer to your buttocks."*
Extension	With the patient supine, ask them to straighten their leg, lifting their heel off the table. Measure the angle of extension.	*"Lie on your back with your legs straight. Lift your heel off the table by straightening your knee as much as possible."*
Medial (internal) rotation	With the patient supine and knee flexed to 90°, ask them to rotate their lower leg inward, assessing the internal rotation of the knee.	*"Lie on your back with your knee bent. Rotate your foot inward as far as it feels comfortable."*
Lateral (external) rotation	With the patient supine and knee flexed to 90°, instruct the patient to rotate their lower leg outward to assess external rotation of the knee.	*"Lie on your back with your knee bent. Rotate your foot outward as far as it feels comfortable."*

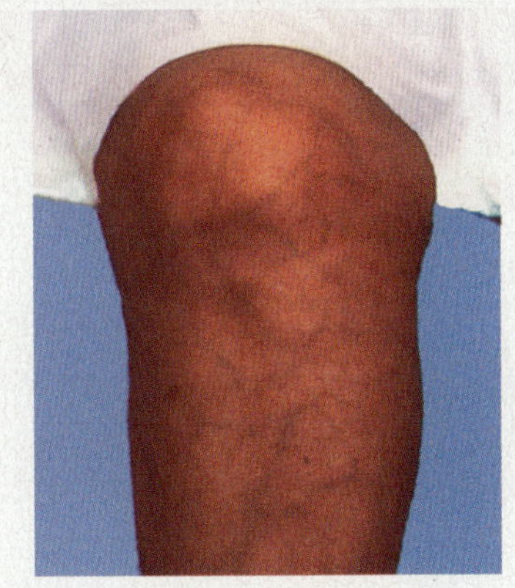

FIGURE 26-36. Effusion of the knee joint.

palpate the medial aspect of the *popliteal fossa* for swelling, like a Baker's cyst (see Fig. 26-33).

Assess Knee Range of Motion

The knee joint's ROM encompasses three main movements: flexion, extension, and rotation (Box 26-14). *Flexion* allows it to move from a fully straightened position (0°) to a bent position (up to 135°). *Extension* ranges from 0° to a slight hyperextension (about −5° to −10°). The knee also exhibits *rotation*, albeit to a lesser extent, when flexed. This includes *medial (internal) rotation* of about 10° to 30° and *lateral (external) rotation* of around 30° to 40°. These ROM values can vary based on individual factors like age and health.

Perform Special Maneuvers on the Knee Joint (If Indicated)

Special maneuvers in the knee are focused on testing ligamentous stability of the MCL, LCL, ACL, and PCL as well as the integrity of the medial and lateral menisci and the patellar tendon, particularly when there is a history of trauma or knee pain (Box 26-15).[13,17–20] Always examine both knees and compare findings.

Box 26-15. Special Maneuvers: Knee

Maneuver	Structures Assessed	Examination Technique	Examples of Abnormalities
McMurray test 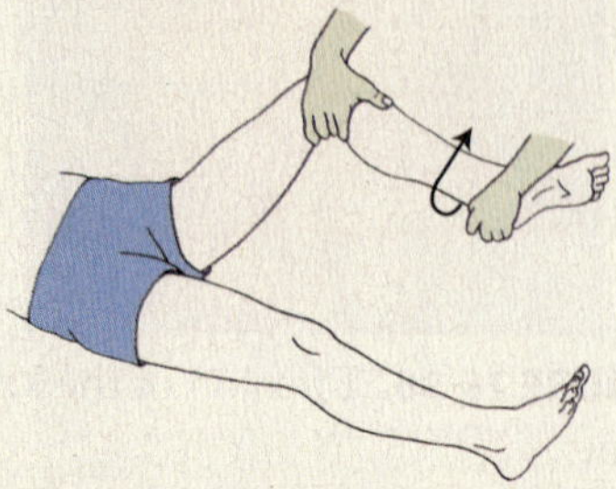	Medial and lateral meniscus	With the patient supine, grasp their heel, flex the knee, and rotate the lower leg externally, then extend it while applying valgus stress on the medial side. For the lateral meniscus, use internal rotation and varus stress.	A click or tenderness along the joint line during flexion and extension indicates a potential meniscus tear.[13]
Abduction (valgus) stress test 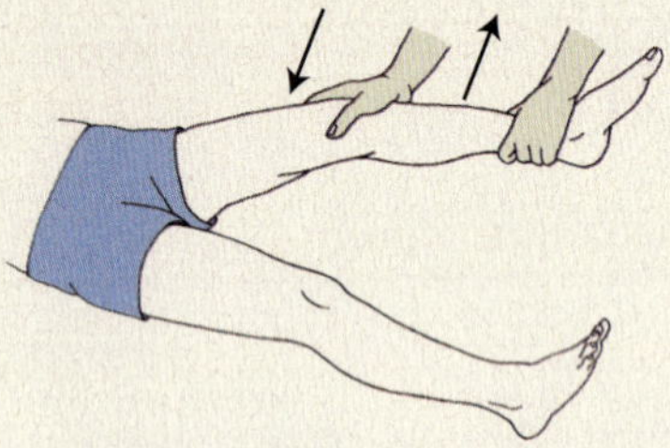	Medial collateral ligament (MCL)	With the patient supine and their knee slightly flexed, move the thigh 30° laterally, stabilize the femur, and apply valgus stress at the knee while pulling the ankle laterally.	Excessive widening of the joint or no endpoint suggests a ligament tear or sprain. Pain may indicate partial tear or sprain.[13]
Adduction (varus) stress test 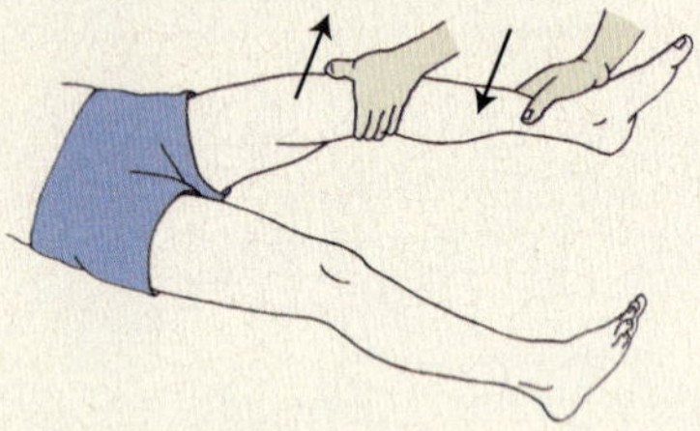	Lateral collateral ligament (LCL)	Position as for the valgus test, but apply varus stress by pushing laterally against the knee and pulling medially at the ankle.	Like the valgus test, excessive joint widening or lack of endpoint suggests a ligament tear or sprain, with pain indicating a partial tear or sprain.
Anterior drawer sign 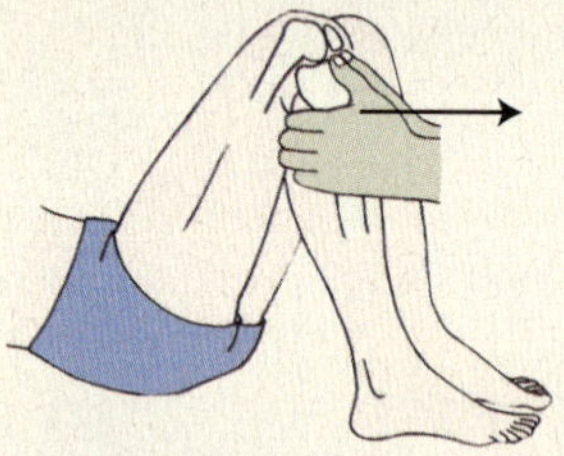	Anterior cruciate ligament (ACL)	With the patient supine and their hips and knees at 90°, draw the tibia forward and assess the movement compared to the opposite knee.	Excessive forward movement or lack of a firm endpoint suggests an ACL tear.[13]
Lachman test 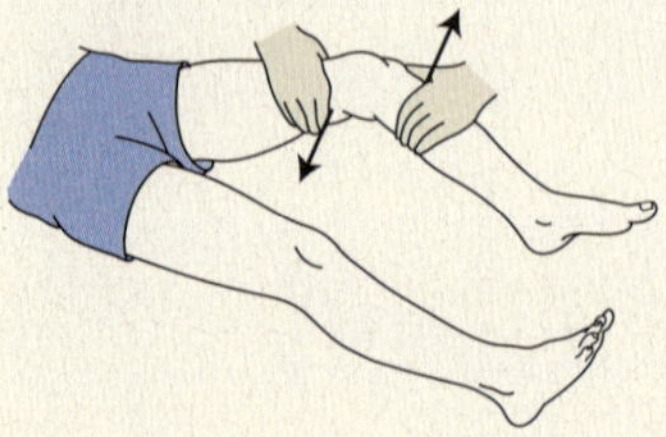		With the knee in 15° flexion, pull the tibia forward and push the femur back. Assess forward movement and endpoint firmness. *When done correctly, this test is more sensitive to an ACL tear than the anterior drawer sign.*	Similar to the anterior drawer sign, lack of a firm endpoint and excessive forward movement indicate an ACL tear.[13]

Maneuver	Structures Assessed	Examination Technique	
Posterior drawer sign	Posterior cruciate ligament (PCL)	Position as for the anterior drawer test, but push the tibia posteriorly. Observe the backward movement.	Excessive posterior movement of the tibia relative to the femur suggests a PCL tear.[13]
Patellar grind test	Patellofemoral joint	With the patient supine and their knee extended, compress the patella against the femur, move it medially and laterally, and ask the patient to contract their quadriceps.	Pain during compression and movement during quadriceps contraction suggests chondromalacia and patellofemoral pain syndrome.[15,16]

ACL tears are more frequent in certain populations, often associated with factors like increased ligamentous laxity, differences in ligament size, hormonal influences, and movement patterns. They often occur as noncontact injuries in sports that involve sudden deceleration with repeated landing and pivoting maneuvers such as basketball, soccer, football, volleyball, tennis, and gymnastics, and others. ACL injury prevention exercise programs have been well studied and are demonstrated to help prevent ACL tears.[21–23]

ANATOMY: ANKLE JOINT AND FOOT

The *ankle and foot* balance the body and absorb the impact of the heel strike and gait. Despite thick padding along the toes, sole, and heel and stabilizing bones, ligaments, and musculature at the ankles, the foot and ankle are frequent sites of sprain and bony injury.

The ankle is a hinge joint formed by the *tibia, fibula,* and *talus.* The tibia and fibula act as a mortise, or contoured recess, with the tibia and fibula cradling the talus medially and laterally to stabilize side-to-side movement.

The principal joints of the ankle are the *tibiotalar joint,* between the tibia and the talus, and the *subtalar (talocalcaneal) joint* (Fig. 26-37).

Note the principal landmarks of the ankle: the *medial malleolus,* the bony prominence at the distal end of the tibia, and the *lateral malleolus,* at the distal end of the fibula. Lodged under the talus and jutting posteriorly is the *calcaneus,* or heel bone.

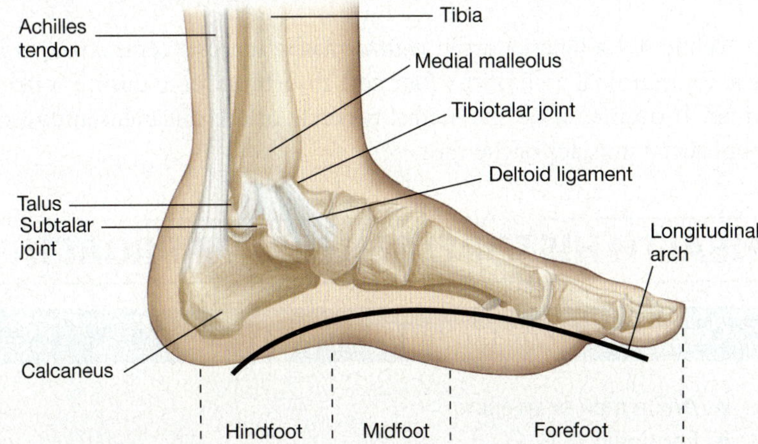

FIGURE 26-37. Anatomy of left ankle and foot, medial view.

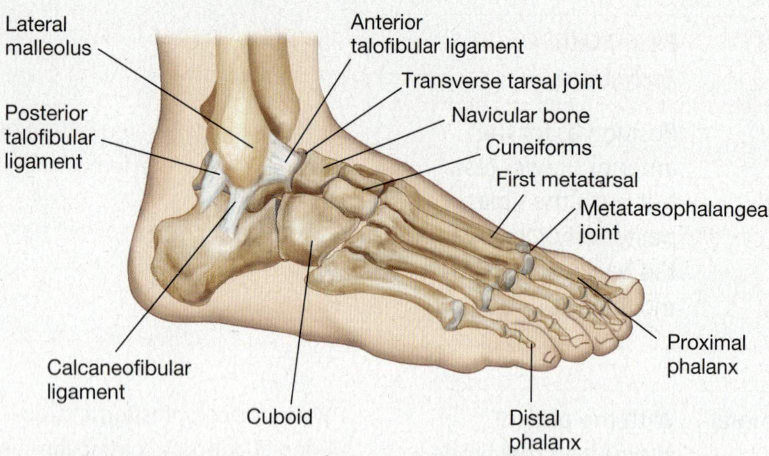

FIGURE 26-38. Anatomy of right ankle and foot, lateral view.

An imaginary line, the *longitudinal arch*, spans the foot, extending from the calcaneus of the hind foot along the tarsal bones of the midfoot (see cuneiform, navicular, and cuboid bones in Fig. 26-38) to the forefoot metatarsals and toes. The *heads of the metatarsals* are palpable in the ball of the foot. In the forefoot, identify the *metatarsophalangeal joints,* just proximal to the webs of the toes, and the *proximal interphalangeal* (*PIP*) and *distal interphalangeal* (*DIP*) *joints* of the toes.

The ankle can move in four ways: *plantar flexion*, *dorsiflexion*, *eversion*, and *inversion*. Most plantar flexion and dorsiflexion occur at the *tibiotalar joint*, while most eversion and inversion occur at the *subtalar* (*talocalcaneal*) *joint.*

Ligaments extend from each malleolus onto the foot. Medially, the triangle-shaped *deltoid ligament* fans out from the inferior surface of the medial malleolus to the talus and proximal tarsal bones, protecting against eversion stress.

Laterally, the *anterior talofibular ligament* (*ATFL*), the *calcaneofibular ligament* (*CFL*), and the *posterior talofibular ligament* (*PTFL*) protect against inversion stress (see Fig. 26-38). These three ligaments are weaker than the deltoid ligament and are at higher risk for injury from inversion injuries.

The ATFL is at the highest risk of injury during inversion ankle sprains and is often the first ligament to tear. The CFL is often involved next and involved in higher grade sprains that also affect the ATFL.

While not a ligament, the *plantar fascia* serves a central role in maintaining the longitudinal arch of the foot and absorbing force during walking and running. It originates on the medial tubercle of the calcaneus and inserts into the superficial muscles of the foot.

HEALTH HISTORY: GENERAL APPROACH

Common or Concerning Symptoms

- Ankle pain or swelling
- Foot pain

Ankle Pain or Swelling

Ankle pain can arise from various causes, ranging from acute injuries to chronic conditions. Accurate assessment requires specific questions to pinpoint the location, nature, and triggers of the pain (Box 26-16).

Box 26-16. Ankle Pain: High-Yield Health History Questions

Domain	Questions	Rationale
Specific location	*"Is the pain on the inside, outside, front, or back of the ankle?"*	Helps differentiate between conditions such as lateral ankle sprains and medial tibial stress syndrome
Character and quality	*"Does the pain feel like it's within the ankle joint, or does it feel more superficial, like in the tendons or skin?"*	Distinguishing joint pain from tendonitis or skin irritations can direct toward specific pathologies
Mechanical symptoms	*"Do you feel any catching, locking, or instability in your ankle?"*	*Instability:* may indicate ligamentous damage *Catching/locking:* could suggest osteochondral defects
Weight-bearing vs. Non–weight-bearing	*"Does the pain occur while standing or walking, or is it present even when you're at rest?"*	*Weight-bearing:* can be associated with structural issues *Rest pain:* might suggest inflammatory or neurologic conditions
Swelling and color changes	*"Did your ankle swell or change color with the onset of pain?"*	*Swelling/bruising:* often associated with trauma *Redness:* could indicate infection or gout
Timing and pattern	*"Does the pain come on suddenly with activity, or does it build up over time?"*	*Sudden, during activity:* might suggest acute injury *Gradual increase:* could indicate overuse

Possible causes include **ankle sprain** (injury to the ligaments due to twisting or turning the ankle), **ankle fracture** (breaks or cracks in the ankle bones, usually from impacts or falls), **arthritis** (joint inflammation, including OA from wear and tear, and rheumatoid arthritis from autoimmune disease), **tendinitis**, **gout** (formation of uric acid crystals in the joint, leading to painful swelling), and **complications from diabetes** (such as neuropathy, which involves nerve damage).

Foot Pain

Foot pain encompasses a wide array of conditions, each with unique presentations. A detailed health history is essential to identify the exact location and characteristics of the pain as well as factors that aggravate or alleviate it (Box 26-17).

Box 26-17. Foot Pain: High-Yield Health History Questions

Domain	Questions	Rationale
Precise location	*"Is the pain located in your heel, arch, ball of the foot, or toes?"*	Can indicate plantar fasciitis, metatarsalgia, or other localized foot conditions
Type of pain	*"Is the pain stabbing, burning, or throbbing?"*	*Stabbing:* may suggest plantar fasciitis *Burning:* could indicate neuropathy
Temporal pattern	*"Do you notice the pain more in the mornings or after periods of rest?"*	*Morning:* can be characteristic of plantar fasciitis *After rest:* might suggest arthritis
Activity-related pain	*"Are certain activities like running, jumping, or standing for long periods triggering your foot pain?"*	Identifies if pain is associated with high-impact activities or occupational stress
Footwear association	*"Does changing shoes or going barefoot affect your pain?"*	Lack of support can exacerbate conditions like flat feet or Achilles tendonitis
Changes in foot shape or skin	*"Have you noticed any new deformities, calluses, or skin changes in your foot?"*	*Structural:* may indicate bunions or hammertoes *Skin:* could suggest infections or calluses from pressure points

Possible causes include **plantar fasciitis** (inflammation of the plantar fascia, leading to heel pain and stiffness), **bunions** (bony bumps that form on the joint at the base of the big toe), **hammertoe** (abnormal bend in the middle joint of a toe, leading to pain and difficulty walking), **Achilles tendonitis** (inflammation of the Achilles tendon, causing pain at the back of the foot and above the heel), **metatarsalgia** (pain and inflammation in the ball of the foot), and **Morton neuroma** (thickening of tissue around the nerves leading to the toes, causing sharp pain and numbness).

TECHNIQUES OF EXAMINATION

Key Components of the Ankle Joint and Foot Examination

I
- Inspect the ankle and foot (deformities, asymmetry, swelling, skin changes, alignment, arches; skin: redness, bruises, cuts, blisters, ulcers, rashes; nails: color, thickness, fungal infection).

P
- Palpate the ankle, foot and surrounding structures (interphalangeal joints, metatarsophalangeal (MTP) joints, metatarsal heads, plantar surface, tarsometatarsal joints, navicular, cuboid bones, medial and lateral ankle ligaments, medial malleolus, lateral malleolus, subtalar joint, calcaneus, gastrocnemius and soleus muscles, Achilles tendon).

ROM
- Assess ankle and foot range of motion (dorsiflexion, plantarflexion, inversion, eversion).
- Assess toe range of motion (flexion, extension, abduction, adduction).

S
- Perform special maneuvers on the hip joint, if indicated (Anterior drawer test of the ankle, Talar tilt test, inversion/eversion test of the midfoot, metatarsophalangeal joint play or grind test, Thompson test or calf squeeze test).

Inspect the Ankle and Foot

Start with the patient seated or lying down, with their feet exposed for clear visibility.

Begin by observing the ankle and foot from a distance, looking for any gross deformities, asymmetry, swelling, or skin changes. Note the overall alignment of the foot in relation to the leg. Examine the toes for alignment and signs of deformities such as hammertoes or bunions.

Examine the skin over the entire foot and ankle. Look for signs of redness, bruises, cuts, blisters, or ulcers. Observe for any swelling around the joints, particularly the ankle joint. Pay special attention to areas under stress, like the heel or ball of the foot. Also, look for any signs of infection or rashes. Inspect the toenails for color, thickness, and signs of fungal infection.

Notice the arches of the feet—both the *medial (inner) and lateral (outer) arches.* Look for flat feet or high arches, which could indicate underlying structural issues.

See Table 26-2, Abnormalities of the Feet, p. 895, and Table 26-3, Abnormalities of the Toes and Soles, p. 896.

Palpate the Ankle, Foot and Surrounding Structures

Ensure that the patient's foot is relaxed. Starting with the toes, palpate each toe individually, assessing the *interphalangeal joints* for tenderness, swelling, or nodules. Move along to the *metatarsophalangeal* (*MTP*) *joints,* using a gentle, circular motion to palpate these areas.

Acute inflammation with tenderness and erythema of the first MTP joint is common in gout.

Progress to the *metatarsal heads,* applying slight pressure to identify any tenderness that could indicate stress fractures or Morton neuroma (Fig. 26-39). The *plantar surface* should also be palpated, checking for any plantar fascia tenderness that might suggest plantar fasciitis.

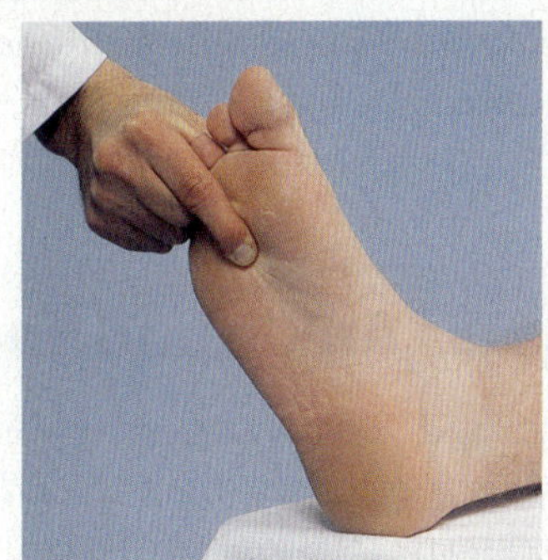

FIGURE 26-39. Palpating the metatarsal heads and grooves.

Next, move toward the midfoot, palpating the *tarsometatarsal joints,* the *navicular,* and the *cuboid bones.* This area can reveal pain associated with midfoot injuries or degenerative conditions. The *longitudinal* and *transverse arches* should also be assessed for integrity and tenderness.

As you approach the hindfoot, palpate for tenderness over the *medial and lateral ankle ligaments* and the *medial and lateral malleolus.* In trauma, the distal tips of the tibia and fibula, the navicular bone, and the base of the fifth metatarsal bone should also be palpated. This region is often involved in ankle sprains and fractures.

An inability to bear weight for four steps is suspicious for ankle fracture and warrants radiography (known as the *Ottawa ankle and foot rules*).[24–26]

Explore the *subtalar joint* by grasping the heel with one hand and the ankle with the other, gently moving the heel side to side to feel for any pain or resistance, which could suggest subtalar dysfunction.

Palpate the *heel.* Squeeze both sides of the *calcaneus* for tenderness. Palpate along the origin of the plantar fascia at the inferior and medial aspect of the calcaneus.

Calcaneal spurs commonly seen on x-rays are often not pathologic and do not change the diagnosis of plantar fasciopathy.[24]

Box 26-18. Range of Motion: Ankle Joint

Movement	Examination Technique	Patient Instructions
Dorsiflexion	With the patient seated or supine, stabilize their lower leg and dorsiflex their foot by bringing their toes up toward the shin. Assess the degree of dorsiflexion.	*"Sit or lie back with your leg straight. I will lift your foot upward. Let me know if there is any discomfort."*
Plantar flexion	From the same position, plantarflex their foot by pressing gently on the sole, moving their foot downward. Assess the degree of plantarflexion.	*"Relax your foot as I press down, pointing your toes away from you."*
Inversion	With the patient seated or lying, move the sole of their foot inward toward the midline of the body.	*"Keep your leg still while I turn the sole of your foot inward."*
Eversion	With the patient in the same position, move the sole of their foot outward, away from the midline of the body.	*"Relax as I turn the sole of your foot outward."*

Palpate the *gastrocnemius* and *soleus* muscles on the posterior lower leg. Their common tendon, the *Achilles*, is palpable from about the lower third of the calf to its insertion on the calcaneus.

Finally, focus on the Achilles tendon, which is prone to tendinitis or rupture. Palpate along its length from the calf musculature insertion to its insertion on the calcaneus. Feel for any gaps, thickening, nodules, or tenderness.

A defect in the muscles, tenderness, and swelling may signal a ruptured Achilles tendon.

Assess Ankle and Foot Range of Motion

Ankle and foot ROM incorporates several movements essential for weight bearing and locomotion: *dorsiflexion, plantarflexion, inversion, eversion*, and *toe movements* (Boxes 26-18 and 26-19).

Box 26-19. Range of Motion: Toes

Movement	Examination Technique	Patient Instructions
Toe flexion	With the patient seated or supine, flex their toes downward.	*"Curl your toes down as if you are grasping something with them."*
Toe extension	From the same position, extend their toes upward.	*"Try to spread your toes upward, away from the floor."*
Toe abduction	Have them spread their toes.	*"Spread your toes apart from each other as much as you can."*
Toe adduction	Instruct them to squeeze their toes together.	*"Bring your toes together as if you are pinching something between them."*

Perform Special Maneuvers on the Ankle and Foot (If Indicated)

Special maneuvers in the examination of the ankle and foot are primarily aimed at assessing the integrity and stability of the ligaments, tendons, and joints, especially in cases of trauma, pain, or instability. These maneuvers focus on structures like the Achilles tendon, the lateral ankle ligaments (including the ATFL, which is commonly injured), the deltoid ligament, and the integrity of the subtalar and midtarsal joints (Box 26-20). Always examine both ankles and feet for comparison.

Box 26-20. Special Maneuvers: Ankle Joint and Foot

Maneuver	Structures Assessed	Examination Technique
Anterior drawer test of the ankle	Anterior talofibular ligament (ATFL)	Grasp the anterior part of the patient's lower leg with one hand and the posterior portion of their heel with the other. Attempt to draw their heel forward under the tibia to feel for a hard endpoint (Fig. 26-40).
Talar tilt test	Calcaneofibular ligament (CFL) and subtalar (talocalcaneal) joint and	Stabilize the ankle, grasp the heel, and perform the talar tilt test by inverting and everting their foot (Figs. 26-41 and 26-42).
Inversion/eversion test of the midfoot	Transverse tarsal joint	Stabilize the heel and invert and evert their forefoot (Figs. 26-43 and 26-44).
Metatarsophalangeal joint play or grind test	Metatarsophalangeal joints	Move the proximal phalanx of each toe up and down.
Thompson test or calf squeeze test	Achilles tendon	With the patient prone and their knee and ankle flexed at 90° (or kneeling on a chair), squeeze the calf and observe for plantar flexion.

Excessive movement or lack of a hard end point suggests injury to the ATFL.

Pain during inversion indicates possible injury to the CFL. Pain in any direction may suggest arthritis; pain during ligament stretch suggests a sprain.

Discomfort or instability could indicate joint or ligament issues.

Pain may suggest acute synovitis. Instability occurs in chronic synovitis and claw-toe deformity.

Absent plantar flexion is a *positive test* for Achilles tendon rupture. Sudden severe pain "like a gunshot" with ecchymosis from the calf into the heel and a flat-footed gait with absent "toe-off" may all be present.

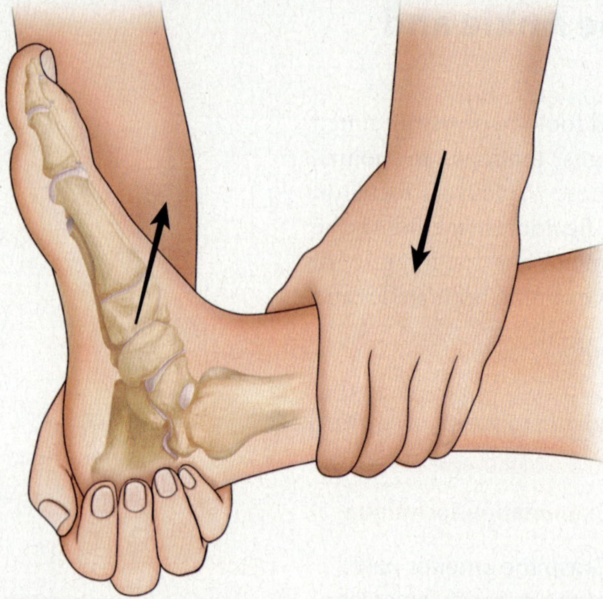

FIGURE 26-40. Anterior drawer test of the ankle: testing ATFL integrity.

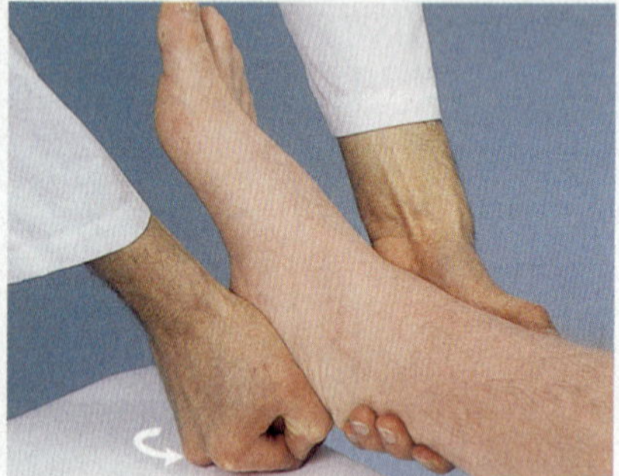

FIGURE 26-41. Talar tilt test: testing integrity of subtalar (talocalcaneal) joint by *inverting the heel.*

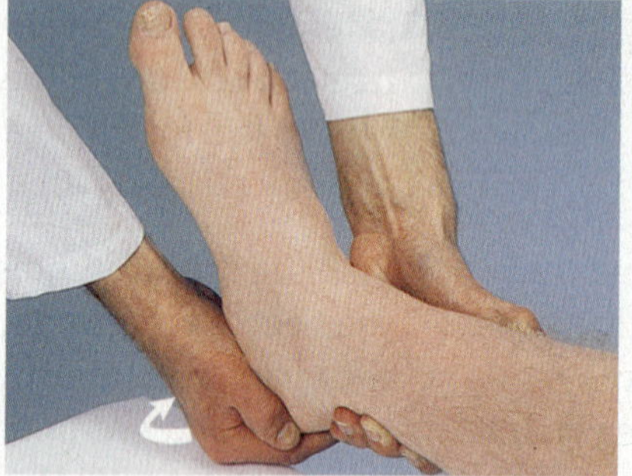

FIGURE 26-42. Talar tilt test: testing integrity of subtalar (talocalcaneal) joint by *everting the heel.*

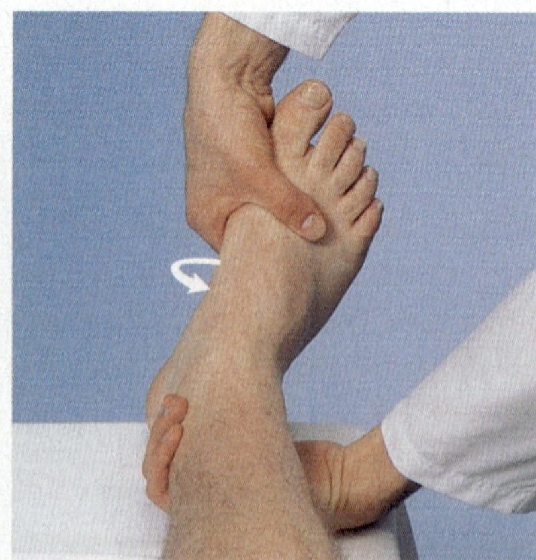

FIGURE 26-43. Inversion test: testing integrity of transverse tarsal joint by *inverting the forefoot.*

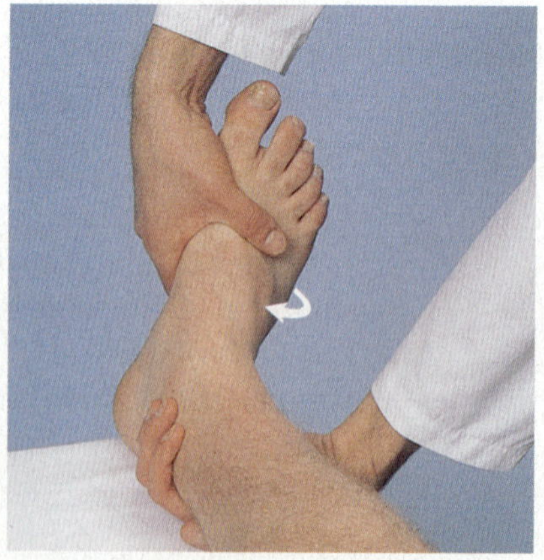

FIGURE 26-44. Inversion test: testing integrity of transverse tarsal joint by *everting the forefoot.*

SPECIAL TECHNIQUES AND MANEUVERS

Analyzing Gait

Gait, the manner or pattern in which a person walks, can reveal a lot about musculoskeletal health and function. A typical *gait cycle*, which is the sequence of movements occurring between the initial contact of one foot and the next contact of the same foot, consists of two distinct global phases:

Stance Phase. This phase occurs when the foot is on the ground, bearing the body's weight. It accounts for ~60% of the normal gait cycle and is further subdivided into subphases or stages (Fig. 26-45).

- *Heelstrike/contact stage:* First heel contact of lead leg to "toe-off" of contralateral leg; duration: 14% to 20%
- *Foot-flat/loading response stage:* First heel contact to first metatarsal head contact of lead leg; duration: 16% to 22%
- *Midstance stage:* Toe-off of contralateral leg to heel lift of lead leg; duration: 29% to 37%
- *Push-off/propulsive stage:* Heel lift to toe-off of lead leg; duration: 45% to 55%

Swing Phase. This phase occurs when the foot moves forward and does not bear weight, making up ~40% of the gait cycle.

As you prepare to conduct a gait analysis, start by positioning yourself to view the patient walking toward you, away from you, and across your field of vision. This multiangle approach is essential for a well-rounded assessment (Box 26-21).

Keep in mind that gait can be influenced by a variety of factors, including age, physical condition, underlying medical conditions, and even emotional state. Its analysis is as much about understanding your patient's health as it is about observing their walking pattern.

Measuring Leg Length

Discrepancies in leg length can be due to actual differences in bone length (structural) or alterations in the position of the pelvis and lower limbs (functional).

To measure leg length, the patient should be relaxed in the supine position and symmetrically aligned with legs extended. Take a measuring tape and place its end at the ASIS. Stretch the tape along the length of the leg, ensuring that

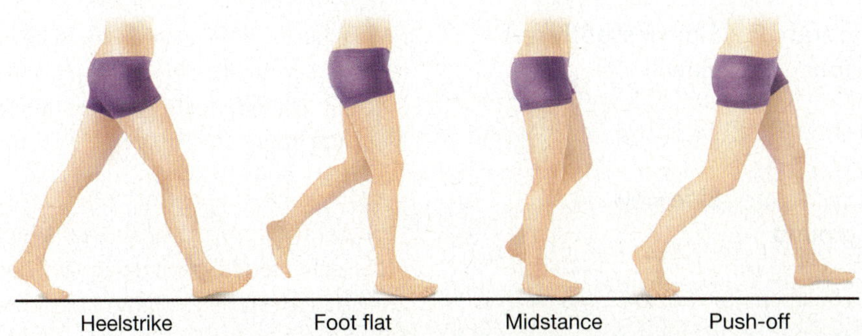

FIGURE 26-45. Stance phase of gait cycle.

Box 26-21. Components of Gait Assessment

Gait Component	Assessment Technique	Observation Viewpoint
Step length and stride length	Observe the distance between each footfall (step length) and the cycle of a complete step with the same foot (stride length). Look for equal and consistent distances (Fig. 26-46).	Side angle
Step width	Measure the space between the inside of the heels or feet. Assess if it is too wide or too narrow.	Front or back
Foot angle	Examine the angle at which each foot points relative to a straight line of walking. Check for inward or outward pointing.	Diagonal angle
Stance phase	Observe overall contact of the foot with the ground, including heel-to-toe roll.	Side view
Heelstrike/contact	Look at how the heel makes contact with the ground.	Side or diagonal view
Foot-flat/loading response	Watch the transition from heelstrike to the entire foot being flat.	Side view
Midstance	Focus on the body's weight distribution over the foot.	Rear or side view
Push-off/propulsive	Assess effectiveness and smoothness of the foot pushing off.	Side or slightly rear view
Swing phase	Examine the foot's movement off the ground and forward.	Side view

Uneven lengths could suggest limb discrepancies, arthritis, stroke, or muscular conditions; weakness often from neurologic issues.

Wider width may indicate hip weakness or balance disorders; narrower width often reflects spasticity, typical in cerebral palsy or stroke.

Inward pointing (pigeon-toed) results from tibial torsion or femoral anteversion; outward pointing (duck-footed) is due to hip issues or flat feet.

Dragging or shuffling might indicate Parkinson disease or foot drop; hesitance or instability could be due to knee or arthritic pain.

Forceful heelstriking suggests limited ankle flexibility; a soft heelstrike can indicate fear of pain from conditions like plantar fasciitis.

Transition issues may signal flatfoot deformity or tendon dysfunction; painful loading could be related to metatarsalgia or Morton neuroma.

Instability or misalignment could indicate knee osteoarthritis, hip dysfunction, or core weakness affecting stability.

Weakness during push-off could be due to toe conditions or forefoot pain; inefficient toe-off might suggest tendon dysfunction.

Reduced lift or abnormal trajectory can be due to stroke, hip flexor weakness, or muscular conditions; inadequate clearance suggests neuropathy or weakness.

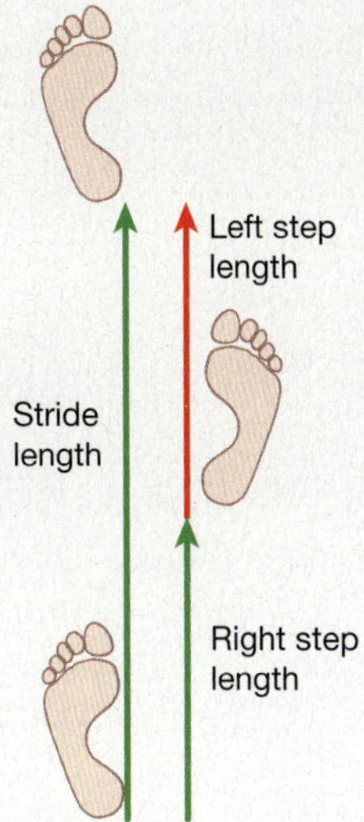

FIGURE 26-46. One stride length is equal to the sum of one right and left step length. (Reprinted with permission from Anderson MK. *Foundations of Athletic Training: Prevention, Assessment, and Management.* 6th ed. Wolters Kluwer; 2017. Figure 8-11A.)

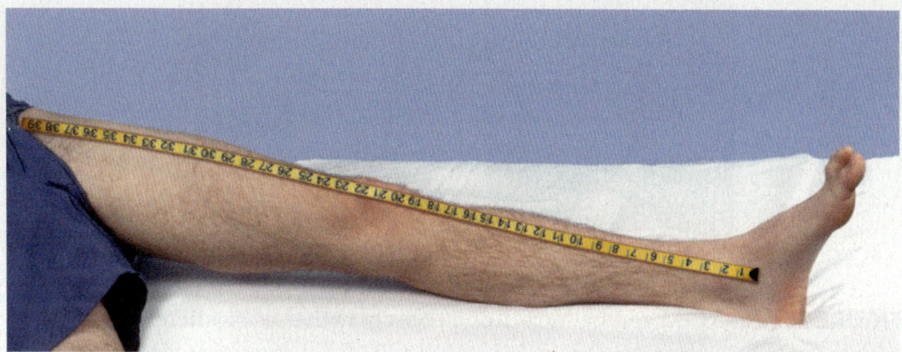

FIGURE 26-47. Measuring leg length from anterior superior iliac spine to medial malleolus.

it runs over the medial side of the knee (slightly above the knee joint) and down to the medial malleolus. The tape should remain in contact with the leg throughout its length (Fig. 26-47).

Measure to the nearest centimeter or millimeter for accuracy. Record the measurement for each leg separately. Ensure the patient's legs are in a neutral position and not rotated inward or outward, as this can affect the accuracy of the measurement. Additionally, repeat the measurement a few times to ensure consistency. Compare the measurements of both legs.

A difference of 1 cm or more may be clinically significant and warrants further investigation.

Measured leg length is the same in scoliosis in spite of the appearance of a leg-length discrepancy.

Describing Limited Joint Motion

Describing limited ROM involves observing and noting the reduced movement capacity of a joint, characterized by an inability to achieve full flexion, extension, or rotation compared to the typical functional scope of that joint. This limitation often presents as stiffness, discomfort during movement, or an observable shortfall in achieving the normal range.

The *goniometer* is still widely used for measuring ROM in degrees, appreciated for its simplicity and effectiveness (Fig. 26-48). However, newer tools like *digital goniometers* offer instant digital readings, and *inclinometers* are particularly useful for spinal assessments. Advanced motion analysis systems, employing sensors or cameras, are utilized mainly in research and specialized medical fields for detailed movement analysis.

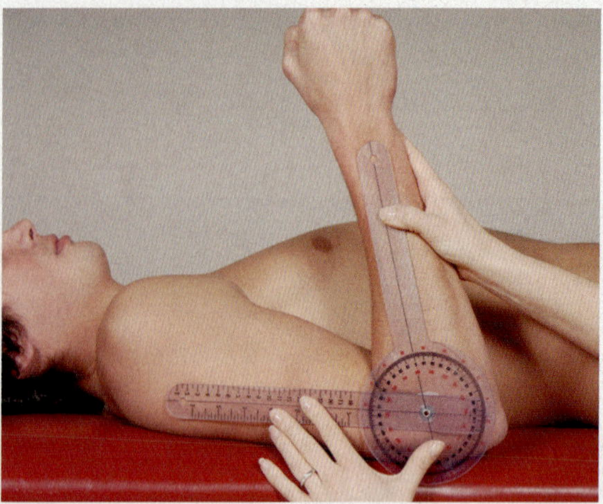

FIGURE 26-48. ROM can be measured precisely with a goniometer. (Reprinted with permission from Anderson MK, Parr GP. *Foundations of Athletic Training: Prevention, Assessment, and Management.* 5th ed. Wolters Kluwer Health/Lippincott Williams and Wilkins; 2013. Figure 5.4.)

In Figures 26-49 and 26-50, the red lines show the range of the patient's ROM, and the black lines show the normal range.

Observations may be described in several ways. The numbers in parentheses show abbreviated descriptions.

The elbow flexes from 45° to 90° (45° → 90°),

-or-

The elbow has a flexion deformity of 45° and can be flexed farther to 90° (45° → 90°).

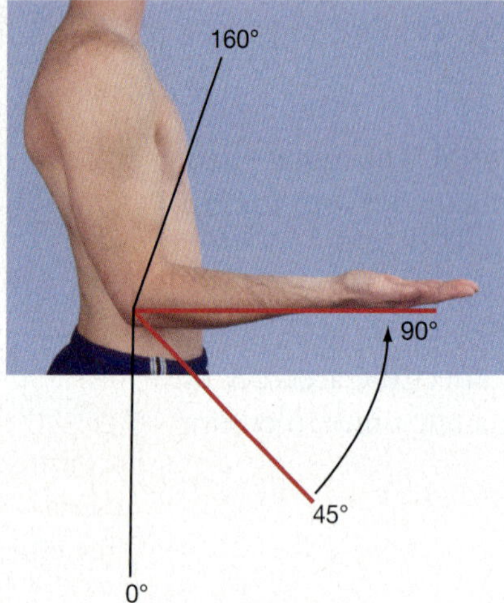

FIGURE 26-49. Normal (black) and patient's measured (red) ROM of elbow flexion.

Supination at elbow = 30° (0° → 30°)
Pronation at elbow = 45° (0° → 45°)

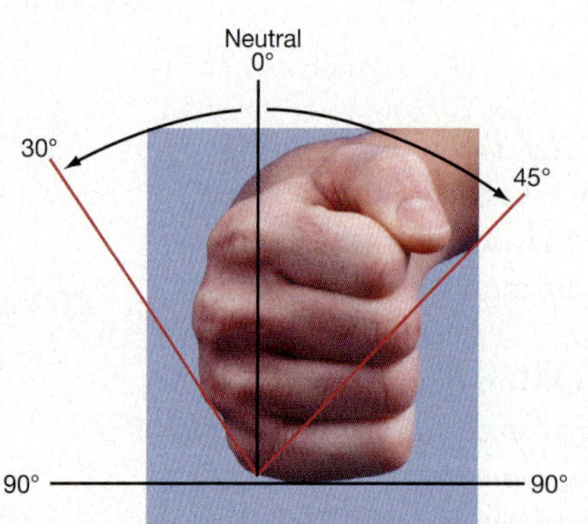

FIGURE 26-50. Normal (black) and patient's measured (red) ROM of elbow pronation and supination.

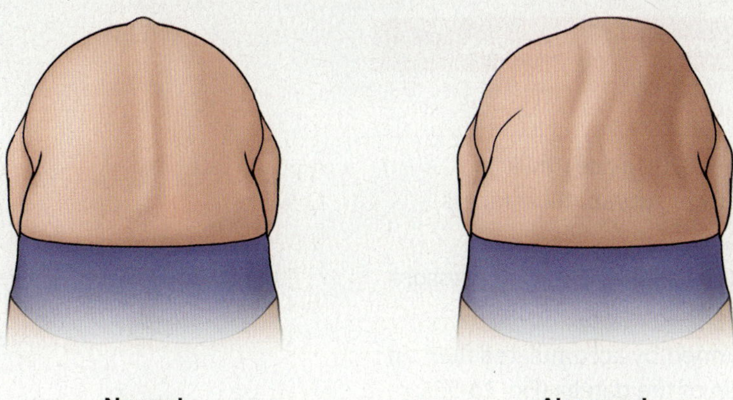

FIGURE 26-51. Adams forward bend test: back, bending away.

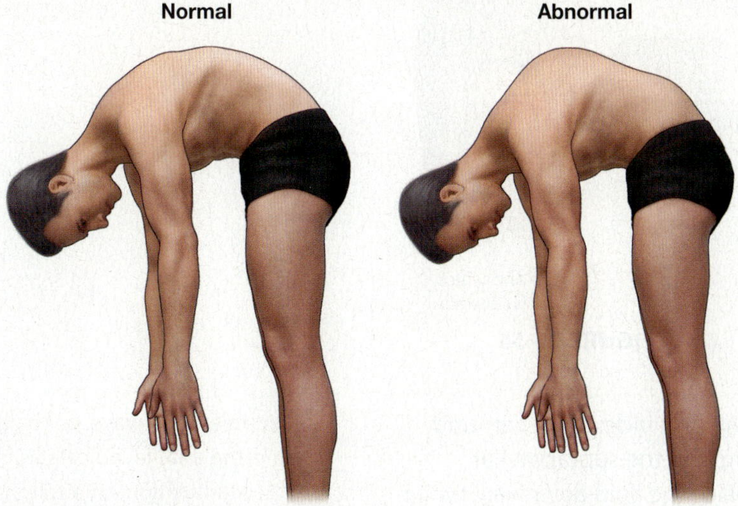

FIGURE 26-52. Adams forward bend test: side, in a bending position.

Screening for Scoliosis

The Adams test, also known as the *Adams forward bend test*, is used primarily to screen for scoliosis or abnormalities in spinal curvature. It is widely used due to its noninvasive nature and effectiveness in early detection of spinal issues, especially in growing children and adolescents.

Observe the patient from behind. Ask them to stand and then bend forward at the waist, with arms hanging freely and palms touching each other (Figs. 26-51 and 26-52). The feet should be together. Look for any asymmetry in the rib cage or the lower back. In a normal spine, the back appears symmetric, and the spine aligns in a straight line.

The appearance of a rib hump or a noticeable lateral curvature of the spine while the patient bends forward suggests scoliosis or other spinal deformities.

Detecting Knee Joint Effusions

Detecting knee effusions involves visual inspection and palpation to identify swelling and fluid accumulation within the knee joint. The following maneuvers (*bulge sign, balloon sign, and balloting of the patella*) help in detecting the presence, severity, and potential causes of fluid accumulation within the knee joint (Box 26-22).

Box 26-22. Special Maneuvers: Detecting Knee Effusions

Maneuver	Effusion Size	Examination Technique	Examples of Abnormalities
Bulge sign	Detects minor effusion	With knee extended, displace ("milk") fluid downward from suprapatellar recess (Fig. 26-53). Force fluid to lateral area by applying pressure on medial aspect of knee (Fig. 26-54). Tap the bulge formed by accumulated fluid on the lateral margin of the patella (Fig. 26-55).	A positive result, indicated by a medial bulge between the patella and femur, suggests a fluid accumulation in the knee joint often associated with inflammatory or degenerative conditions.[13]

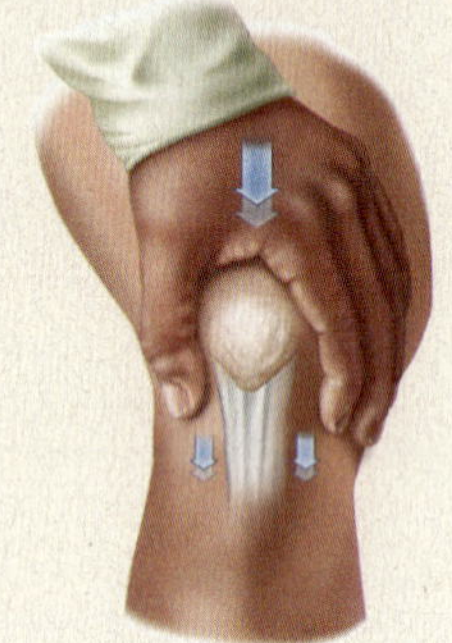

FIGURE 26-53

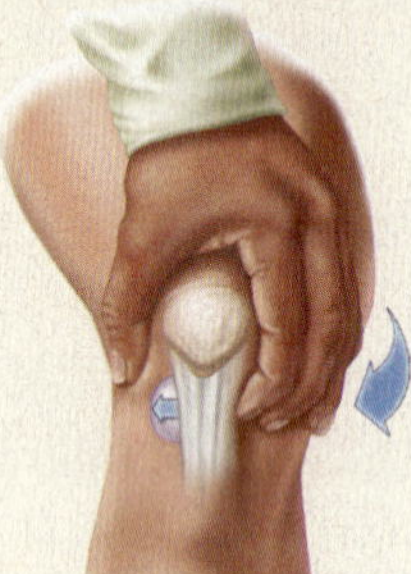

FIGURE 26-54

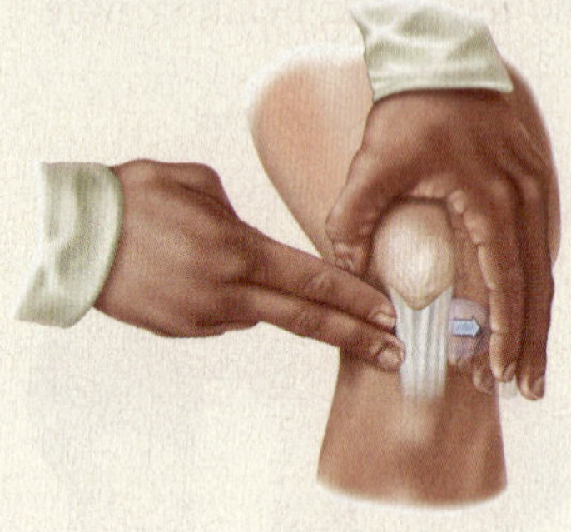

FIGURE 26-55

Maneuver	Effusion Size	Examination Technique	Examples of Abnormalities
Balloon sign	Detects moderate effusion	Place your thumb and index finger around the patella, compress the suprapatellar recess, and displace the fluid downward while compressing both sides of the knee to observe patella "balloon up." Feel for fluid next to the patella (Fig. 26-56).	A palpable fluid wave or "ballooning" around the patella indicates significant fluid accumulation, typically seen in severe cases like knee fractures or major inflammatory responses.

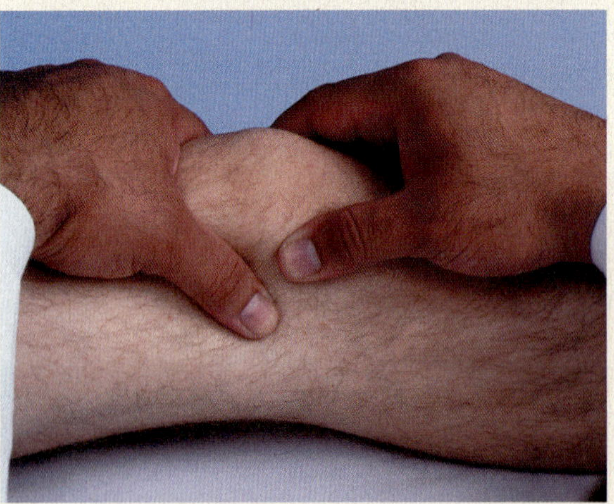

FIGURE 26-56

Maneuver	Effusion Size	Examination Technique
Balloting of the Patella	Detects large effusion	Compress the suprapatellar pouch and push sharply (balloting) the patella against femur in fluid-filled knee. Observe and feel for fluid movement (Fig. 26-57).

FIGURE 26-57

A fluid wave returning to the suprapatellar pouch upon compression suggests a considerable volume of fluid, indicative of significant knee pathology such as trauma, infection, or advanced joint disease.

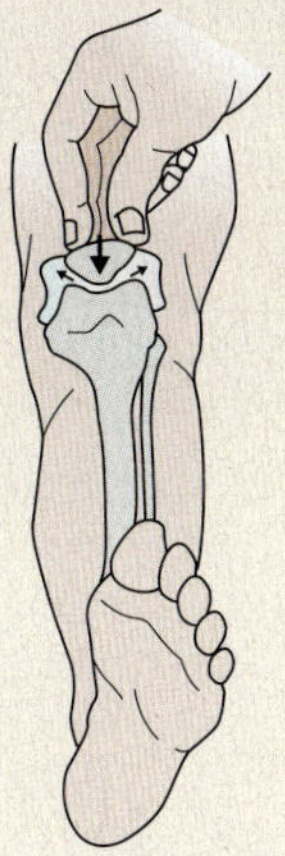

Modifications in Physical Examinations: Best Practices for Specialized Patient Populations

Musculoskeletal interventions, whether necessitated by trauma, disease, or degeneration, lead to changes in the physical examination. Box 26-23 guides you through the special considerations for patients with amputations, prosthetics, or joint replacements.

RECORDING YOUR FINDINGS

Use anatomic terms specific to the structure and function of individual joint problems to make your write-up of musculoskeletal findings more meaningful and informative. Describe the precise location of pathology or pain and which specific movements replicate it.

Recording the Musculoskeletal System Examination

"Full range of motion in all joints of the upper and lower extremities. No evidence of swelling or deformity."

OR

"Hand with Heberden nodes at the DIP joints, Bouchard nodes at PIP joints. Mild pain with flexion, extension, and rotation of both hips. Full range of motion in the knees, with moderate crepitus. No effusion but bony enlargement along the tibiofemoral joint line bilaterally. Both feet with hallux valgus at the first MTP joints."

OR

"Right knee with moderate effusion and tenderness over medial meniscus along the joint line. Moderate laxity of ACL on Lachman test. Moderate laxity with joint gapping noted on MCL stress testing. PCL and LCL intact with stress testing—no posterior drawer sign or tenderness with varus stress. Patellar tendon intact without tenderness with patient able to extend lower extremity without difficulty. Hamstring tendons with no tenderness to palpation. Good range of motion without significant pain in the hip and ankle. No other deformity or swelling."

Box 26-23. Musculoskeletal Examination in the Presence of Medical Devices, Conditions, or Procedures

	Patient with an Amputation	Patient with a Prosthetic Limb	Patient with a Joint Prosthesis
	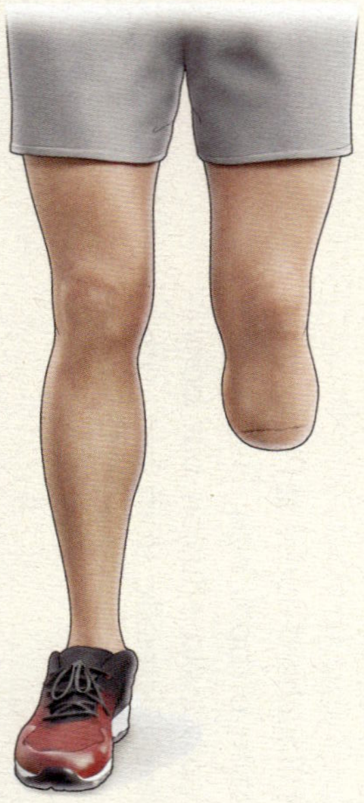	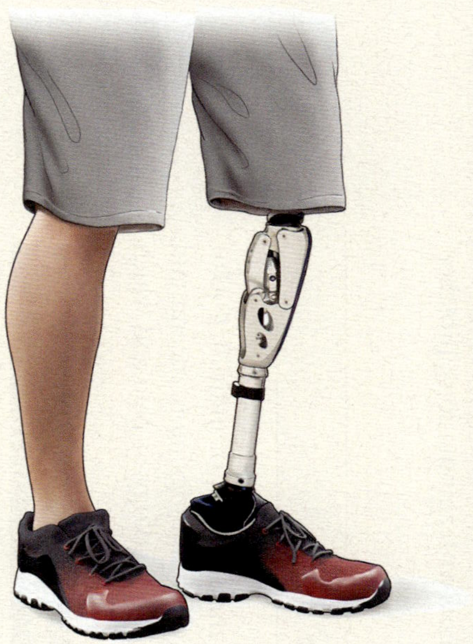	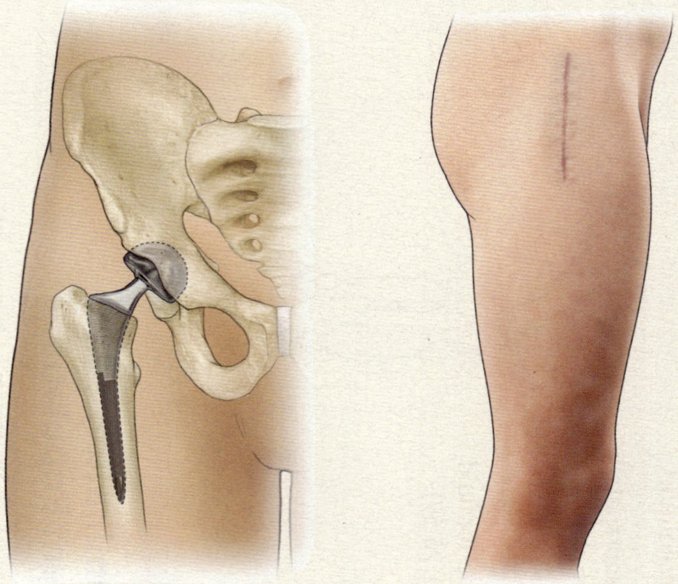
Device/ Condition	Removal of a limb or part of a limb, usually due to trauma, disease, or congenital conditions	Artificial device to replace or augment a missing or impaired part of the body, often a limb	Surgical procedure in which a damaged joint is replaced with an artificial implant, often made from metal, plastic, or ceramic materials
General Indication	Indicated following trauma, peripheral vascular disease, tumors, or severe infections that cannot be managed conservatively	To improve function and mobility, or for cosmetic reasons, after a limb has been amputated	Indicated for end-stage joint disease or damage that has not responded to conservative treatment, commonly due to osteoarthritis, rheumatoid arthritis, or trauma
General Location	Varies depending on the site of the amputation (e.g., above-knee, below-knee, arm)	Attached to the residual limb (stump); location varies based on which limb/ part is replaced	Common locations include the hip, knee, and shoulder; the elbow, wrist, and ankle are replaced much less commonly

Modification to the Physical Exam	1. Ask the patient to remove the prosthetic limb if one is present. 2. Inspect the stump for signs of skin irritation, breakdown, or ulcers. 3. Palpate gently to assess for warmth, fluctuance, tenderness, or bony spurs. 4. Evaluate the limb for proper hygiene and vascular status. 5. Ask about phantom limb sensations or pain. 6. Inquire about the patient's comfort and functional ability with the prosthesis, if one is present, and any changes in fit or function.	1. Ask the patient if they can remove the prosthesis for the exam. 2. Inspect the skin on the residual limb for pressure sores, irritation, or any other abnormalities. 3. Palpate the residual limb and stump, noting any tender areas or bony prominences. 4. Check the fit and alignment of the prosthesis. 5. Ask about the functionality of the prosthesis, any noises, or abnormal sensations (clicking, grinding), stability, and any recent changes in fit, function, or ROM.	1. Inspect the skin over the joint replacement for the presence of scars and for signs of inflammation or infection including erythema, edema, or a joint effusion. 2. Palpate around the joint for warmth, tenderness, or any abnormal fluid collections. 3. Inquire about pain or limitations before manipulating the joint. 4. Examine ROM but be gentle and cautious, understanding that there may be limitations compared to a natural joint. 5. Assess the neurovascular status of the limb distal to the prosthetic joint. 6. Inquire about the patient's comfort and functional ability with the prosthetic joint, any noises, or abnormal sensations (clicking, grinding), and any changes in ROM or function.

By analyzing the physical examination documentation into detailed sections, we emphasize the significant role that clinical observations play in pinpointing diagnostic clues. The findings described in the first note are suspicious for several potential musculoskeletal conditions:

- *Heberden nodes and Bouchard nodes:* These bony growths (osteophytes) typically develop in finger joints, specifically at the DIP joints for Heberden nodes and the PIP joints for Bouchard nodes. These findings indicate degenerative joint changes.
- *Mild pain in hips:* Mild pain during flexion, extension, and rotation of both hips could suggest hip joint issues, such as osteoarthritis or hip impingement.
- *Moderate crepitus in knees:* Moderate crackling or grating sounds or sensations in the knees may suggest cartilage degeneration, possibly due to osteoarthritis.
- *Bony enlargement along tibiofemoral joint line:* Bilateral bony enlargement may indicate osteoarthritis or other joint-related conditions affecting the knees.
- *Hallux valgus in feet:* Commonly known as a bunion, this is a deviation of the big toe toward the other toes.

These findings collectively raise suspicion for *osteoarthritis*, a degenerative joint disease that can affect multiple joints in the body.

The second patient note suggests findings pointing to potential issues related to the knee joint and surrounding structures:

- *Right knee with moderate effusion and tenderness over medial meniscus along the joint line:* These findings may indicate an injury or irritation of the medial meniscus, which is a cartilage structure in the knee joint. Effusion suggests inflammation.
- *Moderate laxity of ACL on Lachman test:* Lachman test results showing moderate laxity (looseness) of the ACL may suggest a partial or complete ACL tear.
- *Moderate laxity with joint gapping noted on MCL stress testing:* Moderate laxity and gapping during MCL stress testing could indicate an MCL injury.
- *PCL and LCL intact with stress testing—No posterior drawer sign or tenderness with varus stress:* The intact PCL and LCL are positive signs, and the absence of a posterior drawer sign and varus stress tenderness suggests these structures are not affected.
- *Patellar tendon intact without tenderness with patient able to extend lower extremity without difficulty:* These findings indicate a normal patellar tendon and the ability to extend the lower extremity without significant issues.
- *Hamstring tendons with no tenderness to palpation:* The absence of tenderness in the hamstring tendons suggests they are not inflamed or injured.
- *Good ROM without significant pain in the hip and ankle:* This is a positive finding, indicating that no significant mobility issues or pain in the hip and ankle joints exist.
- *No other deformity or swelling:* The absence of other deformities or swelling beyond the knee joint is reassuring.

Based on these findings, potential knee joint issues include *ACL and MCL injuries* as well as *meniscal involvement.*

POINT-OF-CARE ULTRASOUND EXAMINATION

Point-of-care ultrasound (POCUS) significantly enhances the diagnostic capabilities in musculoskeletal assessments by providing detailed visualization of joint structures, which is crucial for evaluating conditions like effusions or synovitis. This technique enables clinicians to identify and quantify joint fluid, offering insights that can refine diagnosis and treatment plans.

Detecting Joint Fluid

Physical Examination. The presence of joint swelling, pain with movement or palpation, and reduced ROM can indicate an effusion or synovitis. Joint fluid can result from various conditions, including trauma, infection, inflammatory diseases, or degenerative changes.

In the physical examination of the knee for joint fluid, you may encounter limitations, including subtle effusions that are difficult to detect through palpation alone and variations in patient anatomy that can obscure physical signs. Swelling, asymmetry, and signs of inflammation such as redness and warmth are common findings, but their presence can sometimes be subtle or nonspecific. The *bulge sign* (p. 884), indicating effusion and limitations in knee ROM, especially in extension, suggests fluid accumulation but might not quantify the extent accurately. The test for *ballottement* (p. 885), revealing a floating sensation of the patella, confirms fluid presence but not its cause. These limitations highlight the significant role of POCUS in knee evaluations, serving as a complement to physical examinations by providing a more detailed and comprehensive assessment of knee pathology.

Ultrasound Technique. The methodology for musculoskeletal POCUS involves precise probe manipulation to visualize the joint space clearly and identify pathologic findings such as fluid accumulation. This examination is typically performed with the patient in a position that best exposes the joint of interest, using a high-frequency linear probe for its superior resolution of superficial structures. Ultrasound settings should be adjusted to optimize the image quality for musculoskeletal examinations, typically employing a higher frequency and adjusting the gain as necessary.

Basic Ultrasound Setup	
Patient positioning	Supine with the knee slightly bent
Probe	High-frequency linear probe, ideal for superficial structures and detailed visualization of the joint space
Ultrasound setting	Musculoskeletal (MSK) mode, with adjustments to frequency and gain for optimal visualization of the joint space and surrounding structures

Detecting Knee Joint Fluid. Begin by positioning the ultrasound probe perpendicular to the knee's joint space, aligning the probe marker with a recognizable anatomic landmark for precise orientation (Fig. 26-58). Then, direct the scan toward the suprapatellar pouch, a common site for fluid collection. Applying gentle pressure with the probe helps evaluate the fluid's compressibility and volume.

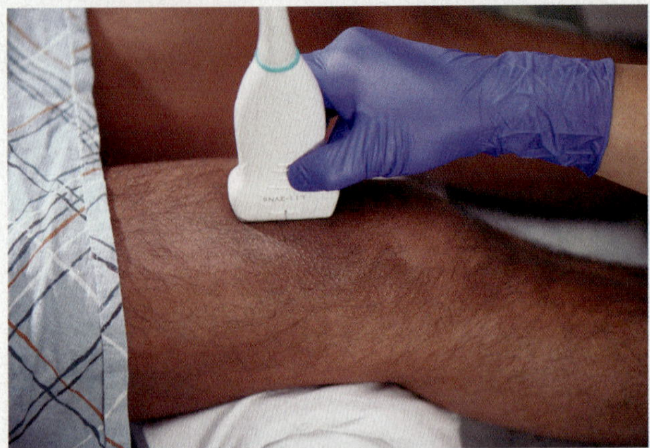

FIGURE 26-58. Probe positioning on a patient for knee joint evaluation.

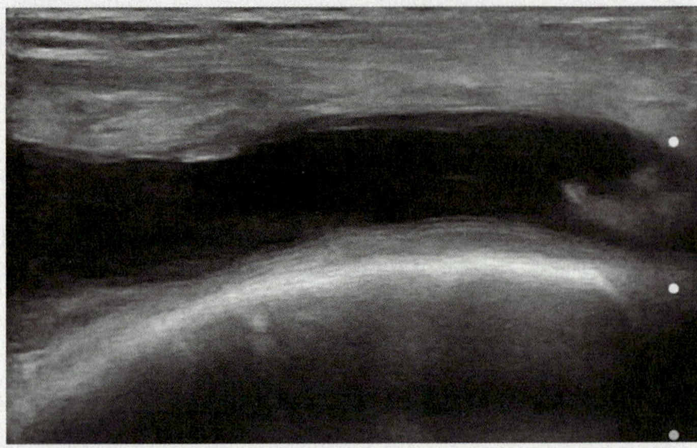

FIGURE 26-59. POCUS image of the knee showing fluid (dark area) above the kneecap bone (femur), indicating a knee effusion.

As you scan, identify areas that appear anechoic (completely black) or hypoechoic (dark grey), signaling the presence of fluid (Fig. 26-59). Adjusting the probe's angle and the applied pressure is essential to distinguish fluid from synovial thickening or other structures within the joint. On identifying fluid, freeze the imaging to measure the largest fluid pocket's dimensions with calipers, documenting the effusion's extent and aiding in the decision making for any interventions.

HEALTH PROMOTION AND COUNSELING: EVIDENCE AND RECOMMENDATIONS

Important Topics for Health Promotion and Counseling

- Osteoporosis: burden of disease and risk factors
- Osteoporosis: screening recommendations
- Osteoporosis: assessing fracture risk

In the following section, both traditional terms like "men," "women," "male," and "female" and inclusive terms such as "individuals assigned female at birth" and "individuals assigned male at birth" are used. This approach balances inclusivity with the need to accurately represent the original research.

Osteoporosis: Burden of Disease and Risk Factors

Osteoporosis, characterized by markedly decreased bone density, is a common U.S. health problem—12.6% of adults older than age 50 years have osteoporosis at the femoral neck or lumbar spine, including 19.6% of individuals assigned female at birth and 4.4% of individuals assigned male at birth.[27] Prevalence

Box 26-24. Risk Factors for Osteoporosis

- Postmenopausal status in individuals assigned female at birth
- Age ≥50 years
- Prior fragility fracture
- Low body mass index
- Low dietary calcium
- Vitamin D deficiency
- Tobacco and excessive alcohol use
- Immobilization
- Inadequate physical activity
- Osteoporosis in a first-degree relative, particularly with history of fragility fracture
- Clinical conditions such as hyperparathyroidism, thyrotoxicosis, celiac disease, inflammatory bowel disease, cirrhosis, chronic renal disease, organ transplantation, diabetes mellitus, HIV, hypogonadism, multiple myeloma, anorexia nervosa, and rheumatologic and autoimmune disorders
- Medications such as oral and high-dose inhaled corticosteroids, anticoagulants (long-term use), aromatase inhibitors for breast cancer, methotrexate, selected antiseizure medications, immunosuppressive agents, proton-pump inhibitors (long-term use), and androgen deprivation therapy for prostate cancer

increases with age, ranging from 5.1% among adults aged 50 to 59 years to 26.2% among adults aged 80 years and older.[28] Prevalence also varies by race and ethnicity; non-Hispanic Asian (18.4%) and Hispanic adults (14.5%) have the highest prevalence, while non-Hispanic Black adults (6.8%) have the lowest.[29] Approximately half of individuals experiencing menopause and 20% of older adults assigned male at birth sustain an osteoporosis-related fracture during their lifetime.[30] Vertebral and hip fractures increase risk of chronic pain, disability, and loss of independence. Hip fractures are associated with an estimated 21% to 30% risk of death in the year following the fracture, with higher mortality rate among individuals assigned male at birth.[30,31]

Each year in the United States, more than 2 million fractures are attributed to osteoporosis, leading to more than 400,000 hospitalizations and nearly 200,000 nursing home admissions.[30] More than 40% of adults ages 50 years and older are estimated to have *osteopenia*, defined as lower-than-normal bone mineral density (BMD) not meeting criteria for osteoporosis, representing well over 40 million people, including about 16 million individuals assigned male at birth.[27,28] Most fragility fractures actually occur among osteopenic adults. Common risk factors for osteoporosis are in Box 26-24.[30]

Osteoporosis: Screening Recommendations

In 2018, the U.S. Preventive Services Task Force (USPSTF) issued a grade B recommendation supporting osteoporosis screening for women ages 65 years and older and for younger women at increased risk.[31] The USPSTF found that bone measurement tests can accurately detect osteoporosis and predict the risk of osteoporotic fractures. Furthermore, the USPSTF found convincing evidence that treating osteoporosis with drug therapies, including antiresorptive

Box 26-25. World Health Organization Bone Density Criteria

- **Osteoporosis:** T score < −2.5 (>2.5 SDs below young adult mean)
- **Osteopenia:** T score between −1.0 and −2.5 (1.0–2.5 SDs below young adult mean)

agents (bisphosphonates, selective estrogen-receptor modulators, denosumab) and parathyroid hormone analogs, can reduce fractures in postmenopausal women.[32] However, the USPSTF found insufficient evidence about risks and benefits to recommend routine screening for men (I statement). The Bone Health and Osteoporosis Foundation does recommend screening all men ages 70 and older and selectively screening men ages 50 to 69 with clinical risk factors or a fracture after age 50.[30]

Measuring Bone Density. Bone strength depends on bone quality, bone density, and overall bone size. Because there is no direct way to measure bone strength, BMD—which provides roughly 60% of bone strength—is used as a reasonable surrogate. Dual-energy x-ray absorptiometry (DXA) scanning of the lumbar spine and femoral neck is the optimal standard for measuring BMD, diagnosing osteoporosis, and guiding treatment decisions. DXA measurement of BMD at the femoral neck is considered the best predictor of hip fracture.

Bone mass peaks by age 30 years. Bone loss from age-related declines in estrogen and testosterone is initially rapid, then slows and becomes continuous.

The World Health Organization (WHO) scoring criteria for *T scores* and *Z scores,* measured in standard deviations (SDs), are used worldwide (Box 26-25).[33] A *T Score* compares an individual's BMD to the average peak BMD of a healthy young adult of the same sex. A decrease of 1.0 SD is associated with a twofold increased risk for a fragility fracture.

Bone densitometry scoring also includes Z scores representing comparisons with age-matched controls. These measurements are useful for determining whether bone loss is caused by an underlying disease or condition rather than normal aging.

Osteoporosis: Assessing Fracture Risk

The USPSTF recommends using the *Fracture Risk Assessment (FRAX®)* calculator, which generates a 10-year osteoporotic fracture risk based on age; gender; weight; height; parental hip fracture history; use of glucocorticoids; presence of rheumatoid arthritis or conditions associated with secondary osteoporosis; current tobacco use; heavy alcohol use; and, when available, femoral neck BMD. The FRAX® calculator also provides a 10-year hip fracture risk (https://www.sheffield.ac.uk/FRAX/). This tool has been validated for African American, Hispanic, and Asian women in the United States and calculates fracture risks that are continent- and country specific.

A previous low-impact fracture from standing height or lower is the greatest risk factor for subsequent fracture.

Factors such as socioeconomic status, healthcare access, nutrition, and cultural influences can impact bone health outcomes and fracture risk. Differences in access to diagnostic tools, preventive care, and health behaviors across populations may contribute to variations in FRAX® risk assessments.

The USPSTF suggests using a *10-year osteoporotic fracture risk threshold of 8.4%* when considering BMD screening in women ages 50 to 64 years. Screening decisions for women in this age range should account for menopausal status, clinical judgment, and patient preferences and values.[31]

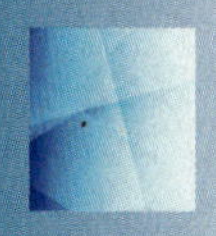

TABLE 26-1. Low Back Pain

Patterns	Possible Causes	Physical Signs
Mechanical Low Back Pain[1,34–38]		
Aching pain in the lumbosacral area; may radiate into the buttock or posterior thigh. Signifies anatomic or functional abnormality in absence of neoplastic, infectious, or inflammatory disease. Usually acute (<3 mo), idiopathic, benign, and self-limiting. Represents 97% of symptomatic low back pain. Commonly work related and occurring in patients 30–50 y. Risk factors include heavy lifting, poor conditioning, and obesity.	Often arises from muscle and ligament injuries (~70%) in the setting of underlying weakness and poor biomechanics. Can be age-related intervertebral disc or facet disease (~4%). Causes also include herniated disc (~4%), spinal stenosis (~3%), compression fractures (~4%), and spondylolisthesis (2%). SI joint pain should also be considered, especially if the buttock is involved.	Paraspinal muscle or facet tenderness, pain with back movement, loss of normal lumbar lordosis. Motor, sensory, and reflex findings are normal. In osteoporosis, check for thoracic kyphosis, percussion tenderness over a spinous process, or fractures in the thoracic spine or hip to evaluate for possible compression fracture.[39] Consider the SI joint if SI joint tests are positive.
Sciatica (Radicular Low Back Pain)[1,35,38,40]		
Shooting pain often below the knee, commonly into the lateral leg (L5) or posterior calf (S1). Typically accompanies low back pain, often with associated sensory abnormalities and weakness. Bending, sneezing, coughing, and straining can worsen the pain.	Sciatica is sensitive, ~95%, and specific, ~88%, for disc herniation. Usually from compression or traction of nerve root(s). More common in people ages ≥50 y. L5 and S1 roots are involved in ~95% of lumbar disc herniations. Compression from neoplastic conditions in <1% of cases. Tumor or significant midline disc herniation may cause bowel or bladder dysfunction with leg weakness called *cauda equina syndrome* (S2–S4) because it compresses the cauda equina. The SI joint can also cause a "pseudosciatica" with posterior thigh pain.	Leg weakness, absent or diminished reflexes, positive crossed straight-leg raise (pain in affected leg when healthy leg tested). Negative straight-leg raise makes diagnosis less likely. Ipsilateral straight-leg raise sensitive, about 65–98%, but not specific, about 10–60%. Seated slump test may also be used. Consider the SI joint if SI joint testing is positive.

(*continued*)

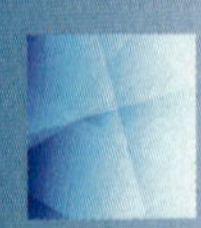

TABLE 26-1. Low Back Pain *(Continued)*

Patterns	Possible Causes	Physical Signs
Lumbar Spinal Stenosis[41,42]		
Neurogenic claudication with gluteal and/or lower extremity pain and/or fatigue that may occur with or without back pain. Pain is provoked by lumbar extension (as in walking uphill) due to reduced space in the lumbar spine from degenerative changes in the spinal canal. Positive LR is >6.0 if pain is absent when seated, improved with bending forward, or present in both buttocks and legs. Positive LR is <4.0 if gait is wide-based and Romberg test is abnormal.	Generally arises from confluent hypertrophic degenerative changes in the spine including arthritic facet hypertrophy, spondylolisthesis, degenerative disc changes (often with osteophyte formation), and thickening of the ligamentum flavum causing narrowing of the spinal canal centrally or in lateral recesses. More common after age 60 y.	Posture may be flexed forward to reduce symptoms with lower extremity weakness and hyporeflexia. Thigh pain may occur after 30 s of lumbar extension or short-duration walking. Straight-leg raise is usually negative.
Chronic Back Stiffness[43,44]	OA most common cause in older adults. Ankylosing spondylitis is an inflammatory polyarthritis more common in men younger than 40 y. Diffuse idiopathic hyperostosis (*DISH*) affects men more than women, usually age ≥50 y.	Findings depend on the underlying etiology. Decreased range of motion in the spine (flexion, extension, rotation).
Nocturnal Back Pain, Unrelieved by Rest[1]	Consider metastatic malignancy to the spine from cancer of the prostate, breast, lung, thyroid, and kidney, and multiple myeloma. Also, consider osteomyelitis and ankylosing spondylitis.	Loss of the normal lumbar lordosis, muscle spasm, limited anterior and lateral flexion. Lateral immobility of the spine, especially in thoracic area improves with exercise. Pain with percussion over the spine.
Pain Referred from the Abdomen or Pelvis		
Usually a deep, aching pain; the level varies with the source. Accounts for ~2% of low back pain.	Peptic ulcer, pancreatitis, pancreatic cancer, chronic prostatitis, endometriosis, dissecting aortic aneurysm, retroperitoneal tumor, and other causes.	Variable with the source. Local vertebral tenderness may be present. Spinal movements are not painful, and range of motion is not affected. Look for signs of the primary disorder.

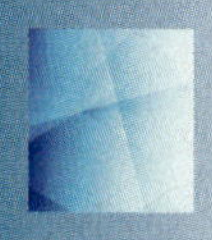

TABLE 26-2. Abnormalities of the Feet

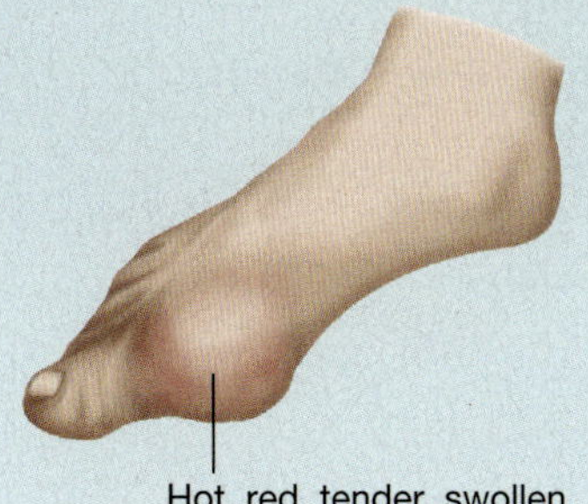

Acute Gouty Arthritis

The metatarsophalangeal joint of the great toe is the initial site of attack in 50% of acute gouty arthritis, although the ankle, tarsal, and knee joints are also commonly involved. The joint becomes painful, tender, and hot, with dusky red swelling that extends beyond the margin of the joint. It may be mistaken for a cellulitis.

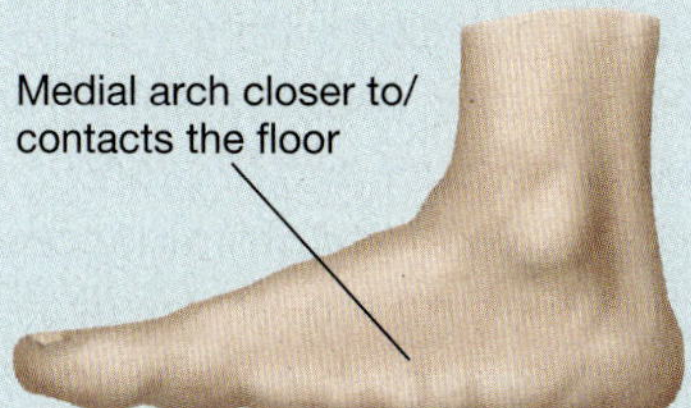

Flat Feet

Flat feet may be apparent only when standing. The longitudinal arch is flattened and approaches or touches the floor. The ankle is often in valgus positioning. Tenderness may be present from the medial malleolus down along the medial plantar surface of the foot. Flat feet may be a normal variant or arise from posterior tibial tendon dysfunction or prior foot injury. Inspect the shoes for excess wear on the inner sides of the soles and heels.

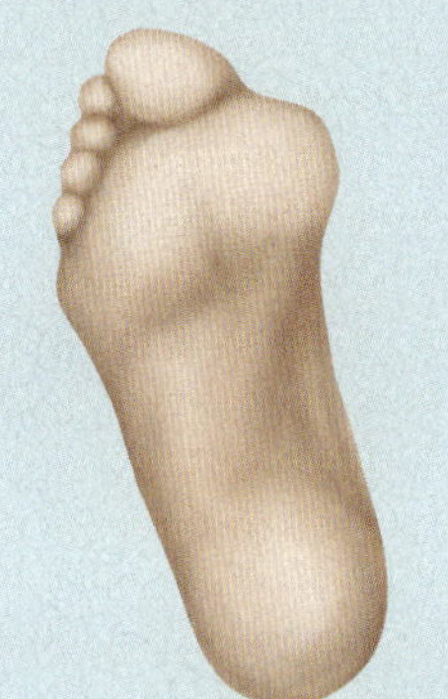

Hallux Valgus

Hallux valgus is a lateral deviation of the great toe relative to the metatarsal. The altered mechanics of the toe and increased prominence of the first MTP joint can lead to pain. Women are more likely to be affected than men.

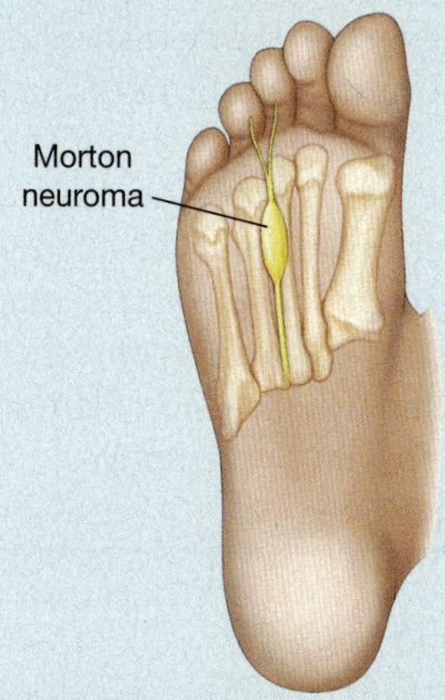

Morton Neuroma

Morton neuroma presents as hyperesthesia, numbness, aching, and burning radiating into the toes, most commonly the third and fourth toes. It results from perineural fibrosis of the common digital nerve due to repetitive nerve irritation or trauma (not a true neuroma). Check for symptom reproduction or a click with pressure on the plantar interspace while squeezing the metatarsals.

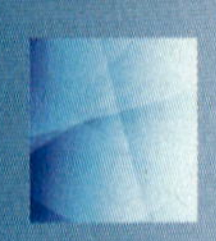

TABLE 26-3. Abnormalities of the Toes and Soles

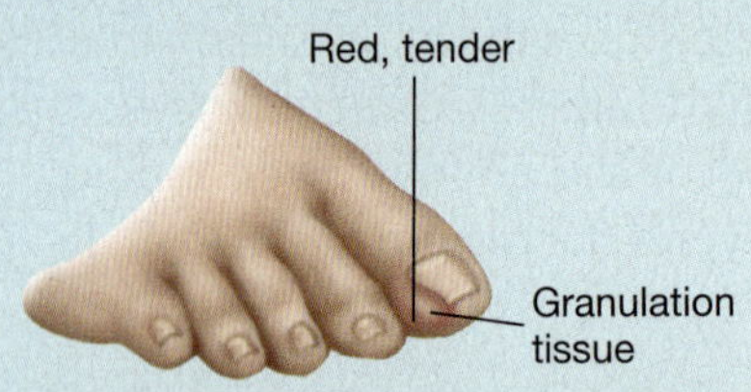

Ingrown Toenail

The edge of a toenail may grow into and injure the lateral nail fold, resulting in inflammation. This results in a tender, reddened, overhanging nail fold, sometimes with granulation tissue and purulent discharge. The great toe is most often affected.

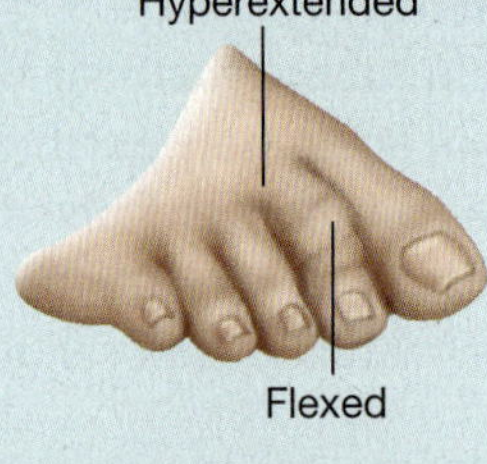

Hammer Toe

Usually involving the second toe, a hammer toe is characterized by hyperextension at the metatarsophalangeal joint with flexion at the proximal interphalangeal (PIP) joint. A corn frequently develops at the pressure point over the PIP joint.

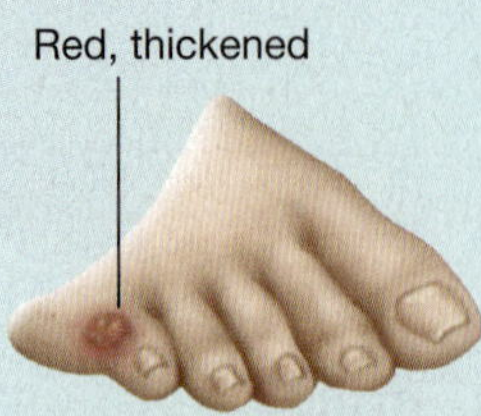

Corn

A corn is a painful conical thickening of skin with a hyperkeratotic core. It results from chronic pressure and friction, typically over bony prominences such as the fifth toe. When located in moist areas such as pressure points between the fourth and fifth toes, they are called *soft corns*.

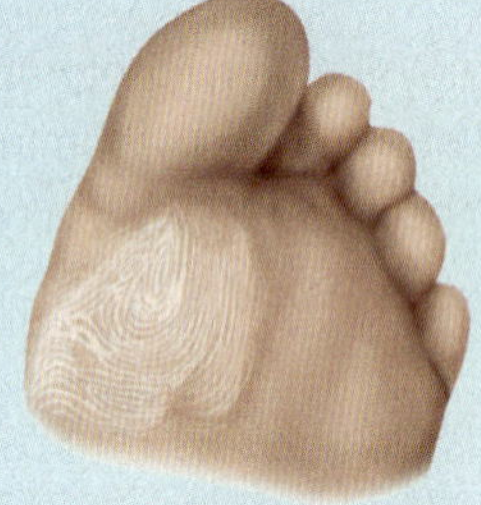

Callus

A callus is a diffuse area of thickened skin that develops in a region of chronic pressure or friction. A callus typically involves skin that is normally thick, such as the sole, and is usually painless. If a callus is painful, suspect an underlying plantar wart.

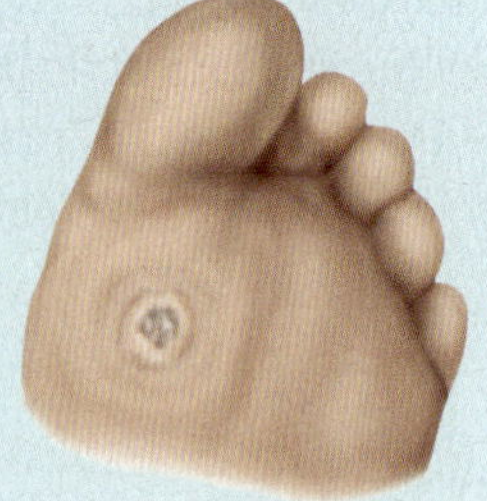

Plantar Wart

A plantar wart is a hyperkeratotic lesion caused by human papillomavirus. Located on the sole of the foot it often has characteristic small dark spots that give it a stippled appearance. Normal skin lines stop at the wart's edge. It is often tender if pinched side to side.

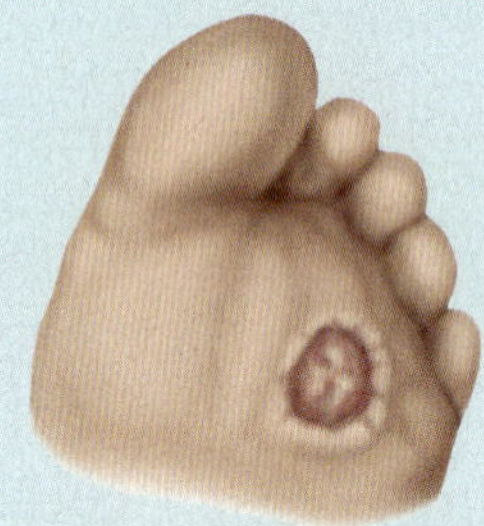

Neuropathic Ulcer

Neuropathic ulcers develop when pain sensation is diminished or absent, as in diabetic neuropathy, and are painless as a result. They may develop at pressure points on the feet or skin injury. Osteomyelitis may occur and amputation may ensue. Early detection of loss of sensation using a nylon filament can help with preventative strategies.

REFERENCES

1. Chou R. In the clinic. Low back pain. *Ann Intern Med.* 2014;160(11):ITC6-1–ITC6-16.
2. Knezevic NN, Candido KD, Vlaeyen JWS, Van Zundert J, Cohen SP. Low back pain. *Lancet.* 2021;398(10294):78–92.
3. Hartvigsen J, Hancock MJ, Kongsted A, et al; Lancet Low Back Pain Series Working Group. What low back pain is and why we need to pay attention. *Lancet.* 2018;391(10137):2356–2367.
4. Qaseem A, Wilt TJ, McLean RM, et al; Clinical Guidelines Committee of the American College of Physicians. Noninvasive treatments for acute, subacute, and chronic low back pain: a clinical practice guideline from the American College of Physicians. *Ann Intern Med.* 2017;166(7):514–530.
5. Metcalfe D, Perry DC, Claireaux HA, Simel DL, Zogg CK, Costa ML. Does this patient have hip osteoarthritis?: the rational clinical examination systematic review. *JAMA.* 2019; 322(23):2323–2333.
6. Thoomes EJ, van Geest S, van der Windt DA, et al. Value of physical tests in diagnosing cervical radiculopathy: a systematic review. *Spine J.* 2018;18(1):179–189.
7. Krebs DE, Goldvasser D, Lockert JD, Portney LG, Gill-Body KM. Is base of support greater in unsteady gait? *Phys Ther.* 2002;82(2):138–147.
8. Gelber AC. In the clinic. Osteoarthritis. *Ann Intern Med.* 2014;161(1):ITC1–ITC16.
9. Reiman MP, Goode AP, Hegedus EJ, Cook CE, Wright AA. Diagnostic accuracy of clinical tests of the hip: a systematic review with meta-analysis. *Br J Sports Med.* 2013;47(14): 893–902.
10. Frank RM, Slabaugh MA, Grumet RC, Bush-Joseph CA, Virkus WW, Nho SJ. Hip pain in active patients: what you may be missing. *J Fam Pract.* 2012;61(12):736–744.
11. Suarez JC, Ely EE, Mutnal AB, et al. Comprehensive approach to the evaluation of groin pain. *J Am Acad Orthop Surg.* 2013; 21(9):558–570.
12. Prather H, Harris-Hayes M, Hunt DM, Steger-May K, Mathew V, Clohisy JC. Reliability and agreement of hip range of motion and provocative physical examination tests in asymptomatic volunteers. *PM R.* 2010;2(10):888–895.
13. McGee SR. Chapter 57: examination of the musculoskeletal system—the knee. *Evidence-Based Physical Diagnosis.* 4th ed. Saunders; 2018.
14. Smith BE, Thacker D, Crewesmith A, Hall M. Special tests for assessing meniscal tears within the knee: a systematic review and meta-analysis. *Evid Based Med.* 2015;20(3):88–97.
15. Morelli V, Braxton TM Jr. Meniscal, plica, patellar, and patellofemoral injuries of the knee: updates, controversies and advancements. *Prim Care.* 2013;40(2):357–382.
16. Schiphof D, van Middelkoop M, de Klerk BM, et al. Crepitus is a first indication of patellofemoral osteoarthritis (and not of tibiofemoral osteoarthritis). *Osteoarthritis Cartilage.* 2014; 22(5):631–638.
17. Lester JD, Watson JN, Hutchinson MR. Physical examination of the patellofemoral joint. *Clin Sports Med.* 2014;33(3): 403–412.
18. Knutson T, Bothwell J, Durbin R. Evaluation and management of traumatic knee injuries in the emergency department. *Emerg Med Clin North Am.* 2015;33(2):345–362.
19. Karrasch C, Gallo RA. The acutely injured knee. *Med Clin North Am.* 2014;98(4):719–736.
20. Young C. In the clinic. Plantar fasciitis. *Ann Intern Med.* 2012;156(1 Pt 1):ITC1-1–ITC1-16.
21. Yu B, Garrett WE. Mechanisms of non-contact ACL injuries. *Br J Sports Med.* 2007;41(Suppl 1):i47–i51.
22. Donnell-Fink LA, Klara K, Collins JE, et al. Effectiveness of knee injury and anterior cruciate ligament tear prevention programs: a meta-analysis. *PLoS One.* 2015;10(12):e0144063.
23. Renstrom P, Ljungqvist A, Arendt E, et al. Non-contact ACL injuries in female athletes: an International Olympic Committee current concepts statement. *Br J Sports Med.* 2008;42(6): 394–412.
24. Papaliodis DN, Vanushkina MA, Richardson NG, DiPreta JA. The foot and ankle examination. *Med Clin North Am.* 2014; 98(2):181–204.
25. Tiemstra JD. Update on acute ankle sprains. *Am Fam Physician.* 2012;85(12):1170–1176.
26. Clauw DJ. Fibromyalgia: a clinical review. *JAMA.* 2014; 311(15):1547–1555.
27. Sarafrazi N, Wambogo EA, Sheperd JA. Osteoporosis or low bone mass in older adults: United States, 2017–2018. NCHS Data Brief, no 405. National Center for Health Statistics. Accessed February 18, 2024. https://www.cdc.gov/nchs/products/databriefs/db405.htm
28. Wright NC, Looker AC, Saag KG, et al. The recent prevalence of osteoporosis and low bone mass in the United States based on bone mineral density at the femoral neck or lumbar spine. *J Bone Miner Res.* 2014;29(11):2520–2526.
29. QuickStats: percentage* of adults aged >/=50 years with osteoporosis, (dagger) by Race and Hispanic origin (section sign)—United States, 2017–2018. *MMWR Morb Mortal Wkly Rep.* 2021;70(19):731.
30. LeBoff MS, Greenspan SL, Insogna KL, et al. The clinician's guide to prevention and treatment of osteoporosis. *Osteoporos Int.* 2022;33(10):2049–2102.
31. U. S. Preventive Services Task Force; Curry SJ, Krist AH, et al. Screening for osteoporosis to prevent fractures: US Preventive Services Task Force Recommendation Statement. *JAMA.* 2018;319(24):2521–2531.
32. Viswanathan M, Reddy S, Berkman N, et al. Screening to prevent osteoporotic fractures: updated evidence report and systematic review for the US Preventive Services Task Force. *JAMA.* 2018;319(24):2532–2551.
33. Kanis JA, McCloskey EV, Johansson H, Oden A, Melton LJ III, Khaltaev N. A reference standard for the description of osteoporosis. *Bone.* 2008;42(3):467–475.
34. Rozenberg S, Foltz V, Fautrel B. Treatment strategy for chronic low back pain. *Joint Bone Spine.* 2012;79(6):555–559.
35. Ropper AH, Zafonte RD. Sciatica. *N Engl J Med.* 2015; 372(13):1240–1248.
36. Davis MA, Onega T, Weeks WB, Lurie JD. Where the United States spends its spine dollars: expenditures on different ambulatory services for the management of back and neck conditions. *Spine (Phila Pa 1976).* 2012;37(19):1693–1701.
37. Balagué F, Mannion AF, Pellisé F, Cedraschi C. Non-specific low back pain. *Lancet.* 2012;379(9814):482–491.
38. Thawrani DP, Agabegi SS, Asghar F. Diagnosing sacroiliac joint pain. *J Am Acad Orthop Surg.* 2019;27(3):85–93.
39. Golob AL, Laya MB. Osteoporosis: screening, prevention, and management. *Med Clin North Am.* 2015;99(3):587–606.
40. McGee SR. Chapter 55: examination of the musculoskeletal system—the shoulder. *Evidence-Based Physical Diagnosis.* 3rd ed. Elsevier/Saunders; 2012.

41. Kreiner DS, Shaffer WO, Baisden JL, et al. An evidence-based clinical guideline for the diagnosis and treatment of degenerative lumbar spinal stenosis (update). *Spine J.* 2013;13(7): 734–743.
42. Suri P, Rainville J, Kalichman L, Katz JN. Does this older adult with lower extremity pain have the clinical syndrome of lumbar spinal stenosis? *JAMA.* 2010;304(23):2628–2636.
43. Raychaudhuri SP, Deodhar A. The classification and diagnostic criteria of ankylosing spondylitis. *J Autoimmun.* 2014; 48–49:128–133.
44. Assassi S, Weisman MH, Lee M, et al. New population-based reference values for spinal mobility measures based on the 2009–2010 National Health and Nutrition Examination Survey. *Arthritis Rheumatol.* 2014;66(9):2628–2637.

CHAPTER 27

Nervous System

ANATOMY AND PHYSIOLOGY

Accurate localization of lesions within the nervous system requires knowledge of its anatomy and organization. Begin by reviewing Figure 27-1.

The nervous system can be divided into the *central nervous system* (*CNS*) and the *peripheral nervous system* (*PNS*). The CNS comprises the brain and the spinal cord. The PNS includes the spinal nerves exiting the spinal cord, the peripheral nerves, and muscles.

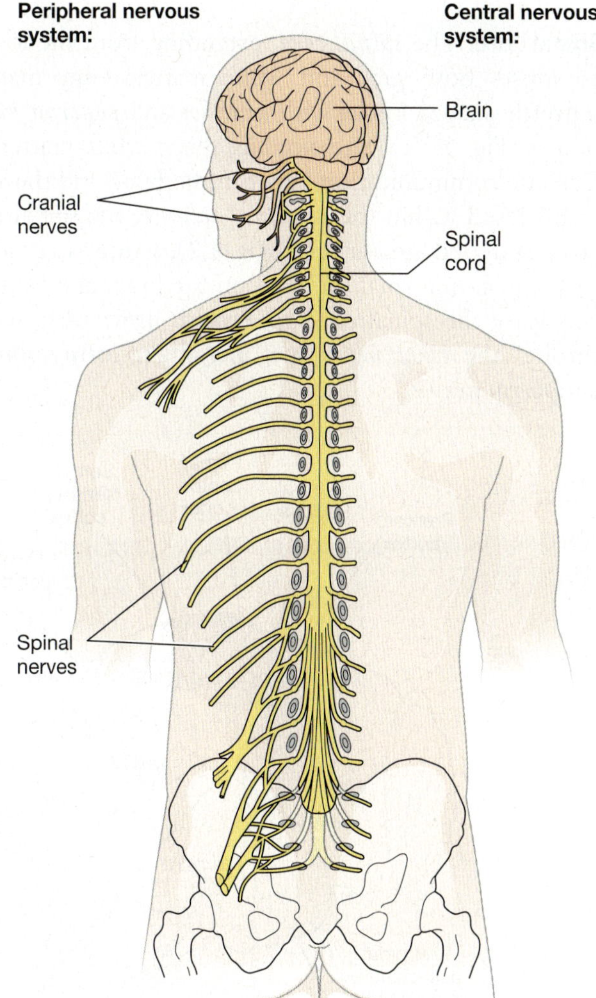

FIGURE 27-1. Central nervous system (CNS) and peripheral nervous system (PNS), coronal section. (Modified with permission from Cohen BJ, Hull KL. *Memmler's The Human Body in Health and Disease.* 14th ed. Jones & Bartlett Learning; 2019. Figure 9-1.)

Central Nervous System

Brain. The *brain*, an intricate network of neurons linked by axons, is primarily composed of the *cerebrum*, which divides into two cerebral hemispheres, further sectioned into the *frontal, parietal, temporal,* and *occipital lobes* (Fig. 27-2). The outer layer, known as the *cerebral cortex*, is made up of *gray matter*—clusters of neuron cell bodies. In contrast, *white matter* beneath consists of myelinated axons, enhancing the speed of nerve impulses.

Each cerebral cortex region specializes in distinct functions, such as speech comprehension, localized in part of the temporal lobe in the dominant hemisphere, typically the left (Fig. 27-3).

Beneath the cortex, the brain houses gray matter structures like the *basal ganglia*, crucial for movement, as well as the thalamus and hypothalamus. The *thalamus* acts as a relay for sensory information to the cortex, while the *hypothalamus* regulates vital functions and emotions, influencing the endocrine system via the *pituitary gland*. The *internal capsule*, a pathway of white matter, channels signals from the cortex to the brainstem and is vital for motor functions.

The brainstem, bridging the brain to the spinal cord, comprises the *midbrain, pons,* and *medulla*. It, along with the cerebral hemispheres and the *reticular activating system* in the upper brainstem, plays a pivotal role in maintaining consciousness. The *cerebellum*, positioned posterior to the brainstem and inferior to the cerebral hemispheres, is essential for coordinating movement and balance (see Fig. 27-2).

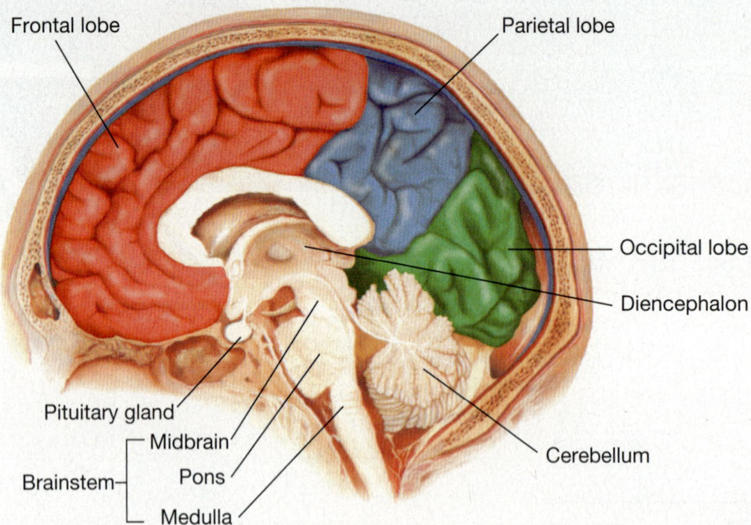

FIGURE 27-2. Right half of the brain, medial view.

Spinal Cord. The *spinal cord*, extending from the lower brainstem *(medulla)*, comprises both gray and white matter. Gray matter, characterized by its butterfly-shaped nuclei with *anterior* and *posterior horns*, houses neuronal cell bodies (Fig. 27-4). Surrounding this is white matter, composed of tracts that facilitate communication between the brain and the PNS.

Enclosed within the *vertebral column*, the spinal cord stretches to the first (L1) or second lumbar vertebrae (L2), acting as a crucial relay station for motor and sensory information between the brain and body (Fig. 27-5). Motor signals leave the spinal cord via *ventral nerve roots*, while sensory signals enter through the *dorsal nerve roots*, merging to form *spinal nerves* and subsequently *peripheral nerves*.

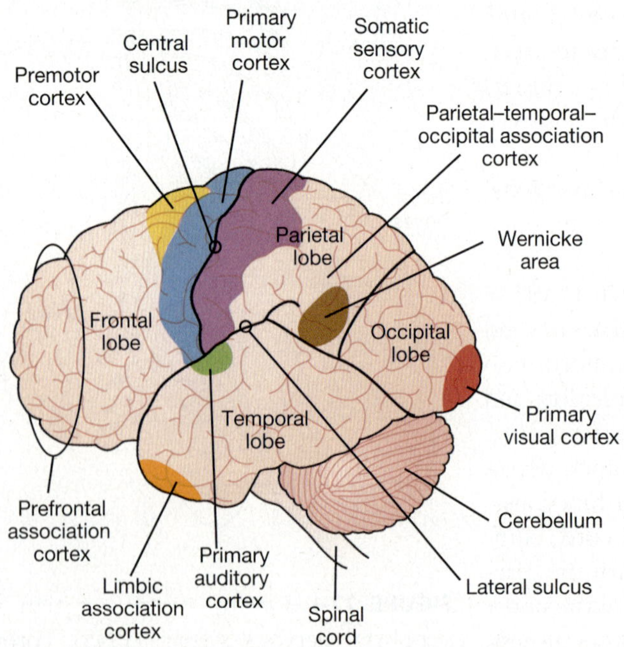

FIGURE 27-3. Regions of the cerebral cortex and selected functions. (Reprinted with permission from Rhoades RA, Bell DR. *Medical Physiology: Principles for Clinical Medicine*. 5th ed. Wolters Kluwer; 2018. Figure 7-12.)

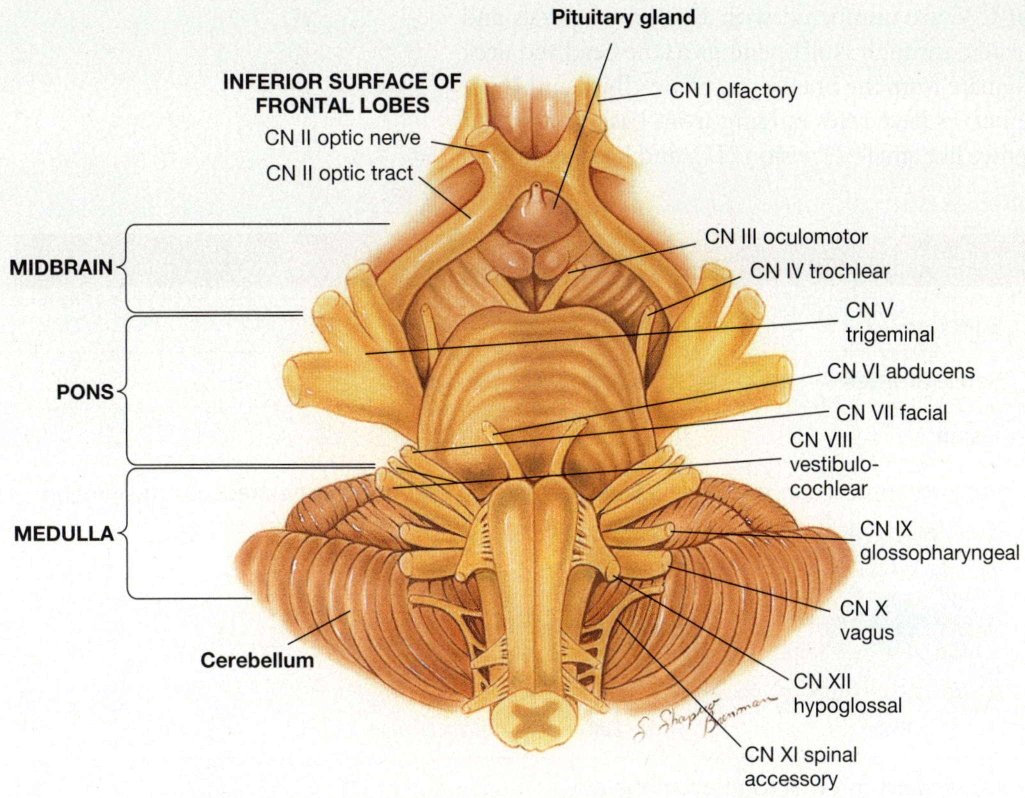

FIGURE 27-4. Cranial nerves, inferior surface of the brain.

Segmented into *cervical* (C1–C8), *thoracic* (T1–T12), *lumbar* (L1–L5), *sacral* (S1–S5), and *coccygeal* divisions, the spinal cord's girth is greatest in the cervical area, reflecting the density of nerve tracts serving both upper and lower limbs. The cord itself is shorter than the vertebral canal, with the lumbar and sacral nerve roots extending beyond the cord's termination at L1 or L2, spreading out in the *cauda equina*, reminiscent of a horse's tail.

To avoid injury to the spinal cord, most lumbar punctures are performed at the L3–L4 or L4–L5 vertebral interspaces.[1,2]

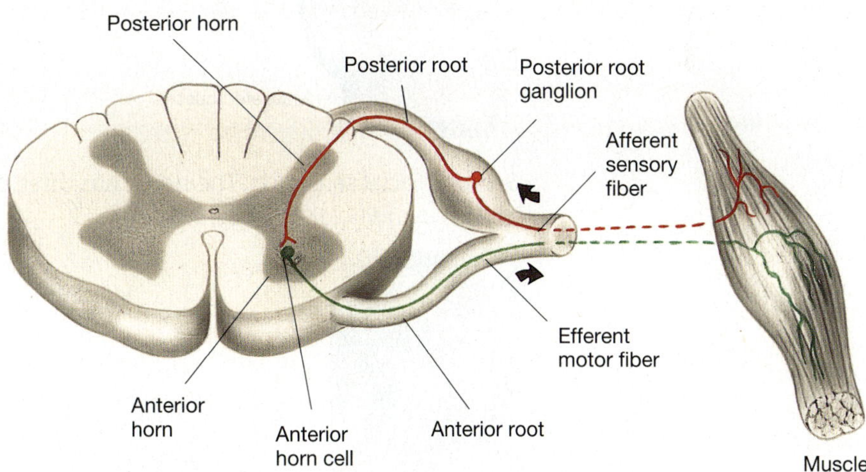

FIGURE 27-5. Spinal cord: cross section and the spinal reflex arc.

Peripheral Nervous System

The PNS encompasses *cranial nerves* (*CNs*) and *peripheral nerves*, extending to the heart, visceral organs, skin, and limbs. It integrates both the *somatic nervous system*, which controls muscle movements and sensory responses, and the *autonomic nervous system (ANS)*, which manages involuntary functions like digestion and blood pressure regulation. The ANS is further divided into the *sympathetic nervous system (SNS)*, activating organ functions during stress, and the *parasympathetic nervous system (PSNS)*, promoting energy conservation during rest.[3]

Cranial Nerves. The *12 pairs of CNs* are numbered with Roman numerals and extend from the brain and brainstem through skull openings to the head and neck (Box 27-1). CNs III to XII originate from the brainstem, while CNs I and II are direct brain extensions. These nerves have roles ranging from basic motor and sensory functions to specific senses like smell (I), vision (II), and hearing (VIII).

Box 27-1. Cranial Nerves

No.	Name	Function
I	Olfactory	Sense of smell
II	Optic	Vision
III	Oculomotor	Pupillary constriction, eyelid elevation (opening the eye), and most extraocular movements 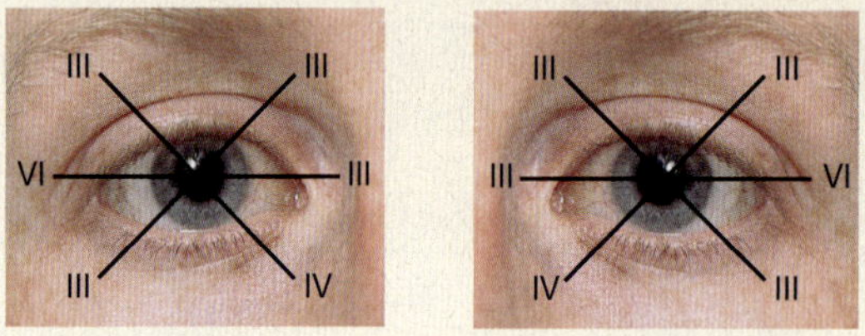 Right: III, III, VI, III, III, IV — Left: III, III, III, VI, IV, III
IV	Trochlear	Downward, internal rotation of the eye
V	Trigeminal	*Motor:* Temporal and masseter muscles (jaw clenching), lateral pterygoids (lateral jaw movement) 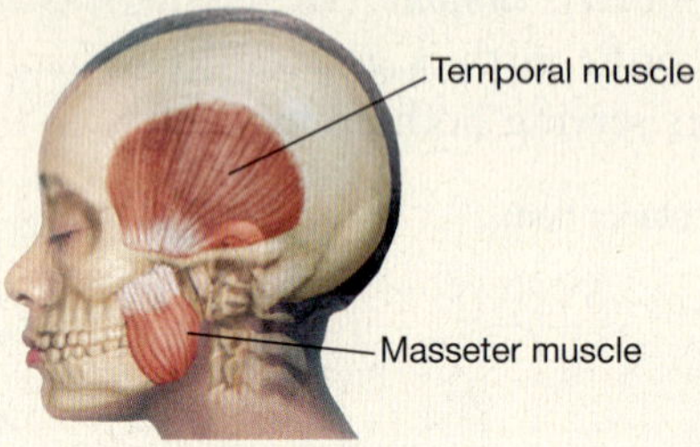 Temporal muscle; Masseter muscle *Sensory:* Facial sensation. The nerve has three divisions: (1) *ophthalmic*, (2) *maxillary*, and (3) *mandibular*. C2 = cervical spine 2. 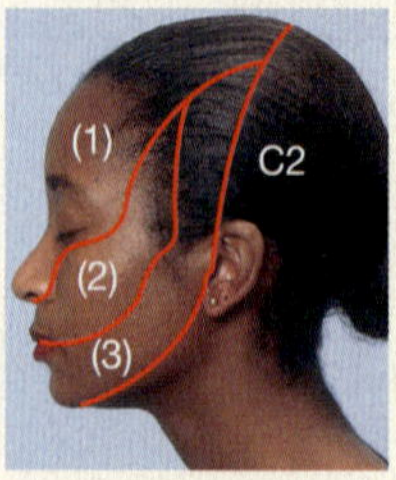 (1) (2) (3) C2
VI	Abducens	Lateral deviation of the eye
VII	Facial	*Motor:* Facial movements, including those of facial expression, closing the eye, and closing the mouth *Sensory:* Taste (salty, sweet, sour, and bitter) substances on the anterior two-thirds of the tongue and sensation from the ear
VIII	Vestibulocochlear	Hearing (*cochlear division*) and balance (*vestibular division*)

No.	Name	Function
IX	Glossopharyngeal	*Motor:* Pharynx *Sensory:* Posterior portions of the eardrum and ear canal, the pharynx, and the posterior tongue, including taste.
X	Vagus	*Motor:* Palate, pharynx, and larynx *Sensory:* Pharynx and larynx
XI	Spinal accessory	*Motor*: Sternocleidomastoid and trapezius
XII	Hypoglossal	*Motor*: Tongue

Peripheral Nerves. Peripheral nerves carry impulses to and from the spinal cord, with *31 pairs of spinal nerves* categorized as *8 cervical, 12 thoracic, 5 lumbar, 5 sacral,* and *1 coccygeal* (Fig. 27-6). Each nerve comprises an *ventral (anterior) nerve root* with motor fibers and a *dorsal (posterior) nerve root* with sensory fibers, merging to form a *spinal nerve* that connects with plexuses, giving rise to *peripheral nerves.* Spinal nerve fibers commingle with each other in the *brachial plexus* or the *lumbosacral plexus* outside the spinal column, from which peripheral nerves emerge. Most peripheral nerves contain both sensory (*afferent*) and motor (*efferent*) fibers.

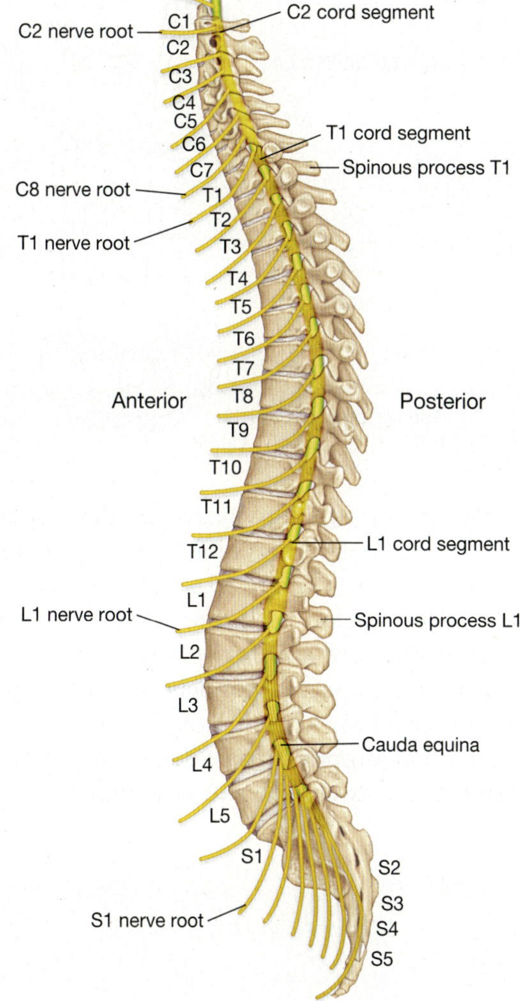

FIGURE 27-6. Spinal cord, lateral view.

Motor Pathways

Motor pathways involve the *corticospinal (pyramidal) system,* divided into upper and lower motor neurons. *Upper motor neurons* originate in the cerebral cortex's motor strip, with axons projecting to lower motor neurons via the *corticospinal tract.* This tract crosses sides at the medulla, allowing brain control over opposite body sides. *Lower motor neurons,* located in the spinal cord anterior horns or the brainstem for CNs, transmit impulses to muscles, facilitating contraction (Fig. 27-7).

Corticospinal tract fibers descend through the spinal cord after crossing sides, connecting with lower motor neurons located in the anterior horns, known as *anterior horn cells.* Lower motor neurons also exist in the brainstem, affecting CN motor functions. The *corticobulbar tract* involves upper motor neuron axons projecting to these brainstem neurons. Lower motor neuron axons carry impulses through cranial and spinal nerves to muscles, culminating in muscle contractions at the *neuromuscular junction (NMJ).*

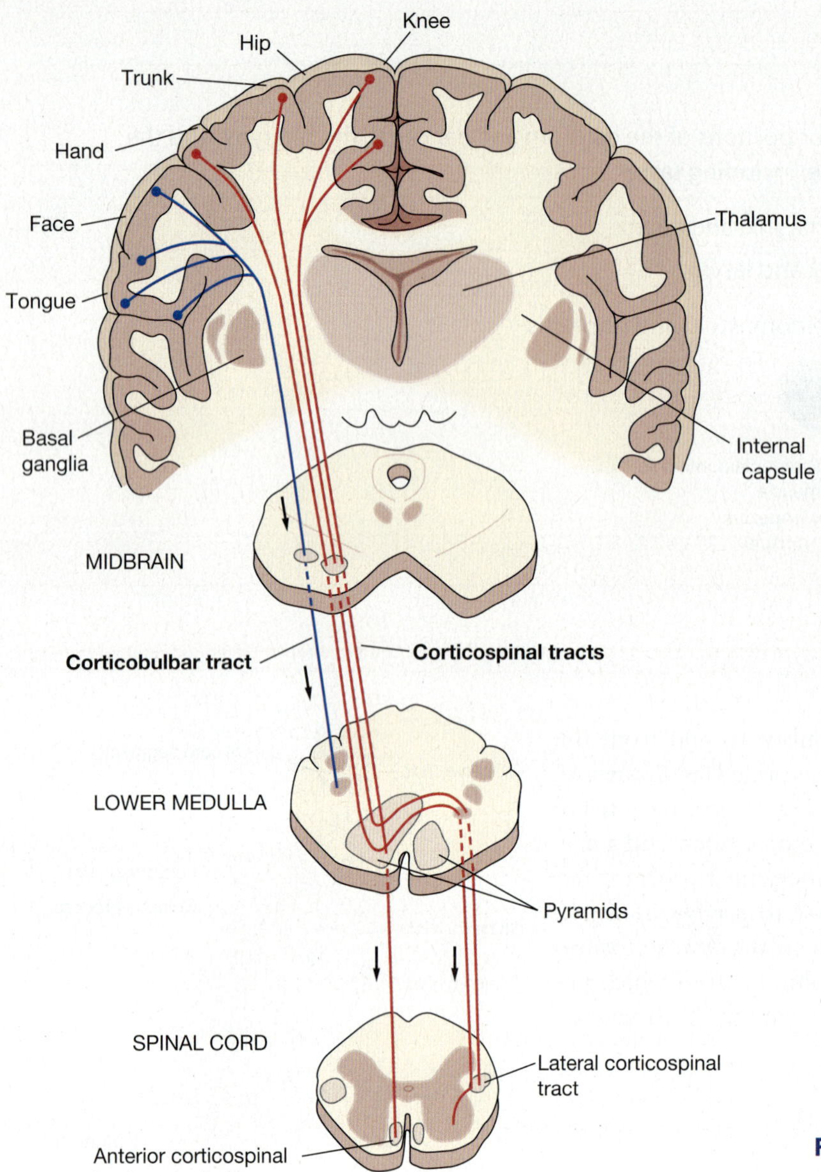

FIGURE 27-7. Motor pathways: corticospinal and corticobulbar tracts.

Motor function is regulated by three systems, including the *corticospinal tract*, which inhibits lower motor neurons (Box 27-2). Damage to upper motor neurons results in *increased muscle tone* and *hyperreflexia* due to the disinhibition of lower motor neurons. Conversely, damage to lower motor neurons leads to *decreased muscle tone, hyporeflexia, muscle atrophy, and fasciculations.* Characteristic upper motor neuron signs (increased muscle tone, hyperreflexia) and lower motor neuron signs (decreased muscle tone, hyporeflexia, fasciculations, and atrophy) can be demonstrated on neurologic examination to help distinguish between the two possibilities.

Weakness can result from damage to either UMNs and their corticospinal tract projections or LMNs and their extensions, including CNs, spinal nerve roots, or peripheral nerves.

UMNs rely on LMNs for movement execution; hence, LMN damage can cause segmental paralysis or weakness, regardless of UMN integrity. Corticospinal tract damage impairs or eliminates its functions below the injury level, affecting limb strength and fine motor skills.

UMN damage above their crossover in the medulla results in *contralateral* motor impairment, while damage below this point causes *ipsilateral* impairment.

Box 27-2. Control of Motor Function

- *Corticospinal (pyramidal) tract.* The corticospinal tracts mediate voluntary movement and integrate skilled, complicated, or delicate movements by stimulating selected muscular actions and inhibiting others. They synapse on lower motor neurons in the spinal cord which directly mediate movement. Damage to the corticospinal tract system causes *weakness.*
- *Basal ganglia system.* This complex system helps to maintain normal muscle tone and to control body movements, especially gross automatic movements such as walking. Damage to the basal ganglia can cause rigidity, slowness of movement (*bradykinesia*), involuntary movements, and/or disturbances in posture and gait.
- *Cerebellar system.* The cerebellum receives both sensory and motor input, coordinates motor activity, maintains equilibrium, and helps to control posture. Damage to the cerebellar system can impair coordination (*ataxia*), gait, and equilibrium, and decrease muscle tone. The cerebellum also helps coordinate eye movements and speech, so other signs like nystagmus or dysarthria may be seen.

Two auxiliary systems, the *basal ganglia* and *cerebellum*, indirectly modulate motor control facilitated by the corticospinal tract. Located deep within the cerebral hemispheres, the basal ganglia enhance voluntary movements and suppress involuntary ones. Meanwhile, the cerebellum, situated at the brain's base, coordinates movements and maintains posture by synthesizing visual, proprioceptive, and vestibular inputs with intended motor actions.

Disease of the basal ganglia system or cerebellar system does not cause paralysis but can be disabling.

Spinal Reflexes: Muscle Stretch Response

Muscle stretch reflexes involve both the CNS and PNS, more accurately described than the term "*deep tendon reflexes*" since tendons are not the primary focus. These *reflexes*, often monosynaptic and involving just two neurons (one sensory and one motor) across a single synapse, represent the most basic sensory–motor interaction. For a reflex to occur, the entire *reflex arc*—comprising sensory nerve fibers, spinal cord synapse, motor nerve fibers, NMJ, and muscle fibers—must be intact.

Tapping a tendon activates sensory fibers in the muscle, causing an impulse that travels to the spinal cord, synapses with a motor neuron, and triggers muscle contraction. Abnormal reflexes indicate potential lesions at specific spinal segments associated with those reflexes (Box 27-3).

Box 27-3. Muscle Stretch Reflexes

Reflex	Level
Triceps reflex	Cervical 6, 7
Brachioradialis (supinator) reflex	Cervical 5, 6
Biceps reflex	Cervical 5, 6
Knee reflex	Lumbar 2, 3, 4
Ankle reflex	Sacral 1

Sensory Pathways

Sensory impulses are critical for conscious sensation, body positioning, and regulating internal functions like blood pressure and respiration. They originate from sensory receptors in skin, muscles, and internal organs, traveling through peripheral nerves to the dorsal root ganglia, then centrally into the spinal cord. These impulses proceed to the brain's sensory cortex via two main pathways: the *spinothalamic tract*, carrying pain, temperature, and crude touch sensations with smaller, less myelinated neurons, and the *posterior columns*, conveying vibration, proprioception, and fine touch with larger, heavily myelinated neurons (Fig. 27-8).[4]

The peripheral component of the small-fiber *spinothalamic tract* arises in free nerve endings in the skin that register pain, temperature, and crude touch. Within one or two spinal segments from their entry into the cord, these fibers pass into the posterior horn and synapse with second-order neurons. The axons of these second-order neurons then cross to the opposite side and pass upward into the thalamus.

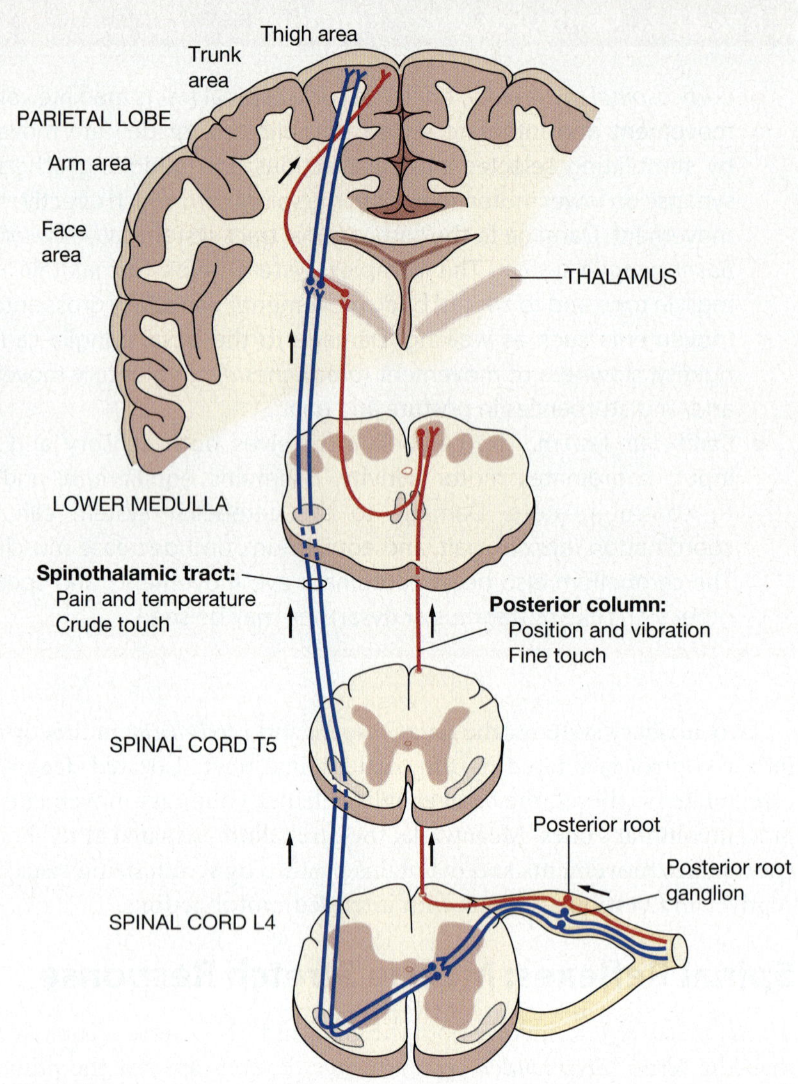

FIGURE 27-8. Sensory pathways: spinothalamic tract and posterior columns.

The *posterior column pathway* transmits from skin and joint receptors to the dorsal root ganglia, upward in the spinal cord to the medulla, where it crosses over and continues to the thalamus.

Patients with diabetes with small-fiber neuropathy report sharp, burning, or shooting foot pain, whereas those with large-fiber neuropathy experience numbness and tingling or even no sensation at all.[5,6]

See Table 27-1, Disorders of the Central and Peripheral Nervous Systems, pp. 965–966.

At the thalamus, basic sensation qualities are perceived; for detailed perception, impulses are relayed to the sensory cortex, where precise localization and discrimination occur.

Lesions in sensory pathways lead to specific sensory deficits: cortex damage affects fine discrimination without impacting basic sensations; posterior column damage impairs vibration and position sense; transverse spinal cord injury causes sensory loss, paralysis, and increased reflexes below the waist; partial spinal damage may spare crude and light touch due to bilateral impulse transmission.

Dermatomes. A *dermatome* is a band of skin innervated by the sensory root of a single spinal nerve. Knowledge of dermatomes helps you localize neurologic lesions to a specific level of the spinal cord, particularly in spinal cord injury. Dermatome and peripheral nerve patterns are illustrated in Figures 27-9 to 27-12, which reflect the international standard recommended by the American Spinal Injury Association.[7]

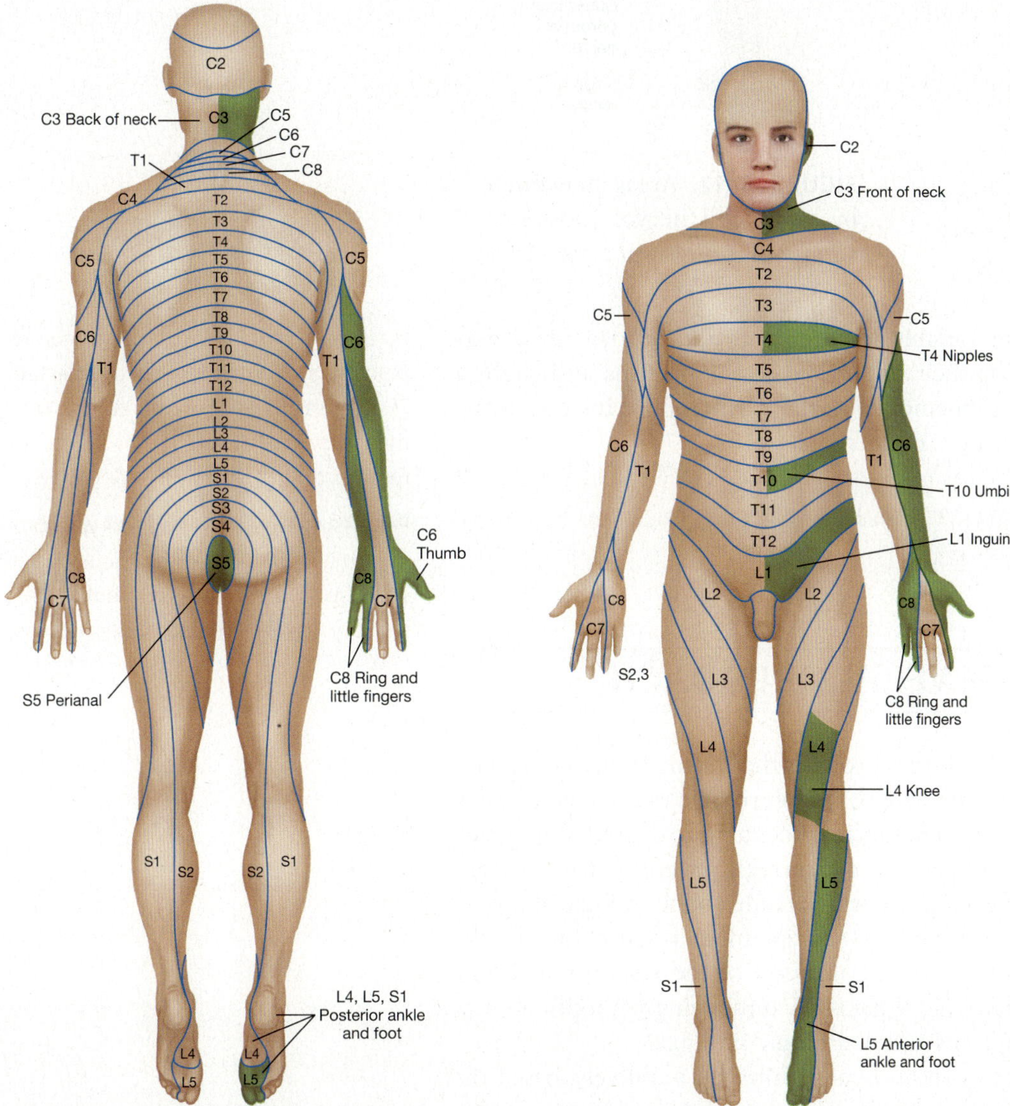

FIGURE 27-9. Dermatomes innervated by posterior roots (posterior view).

FIGURE 27-10. Dermatomes innervated by posterior roots (anterior view).

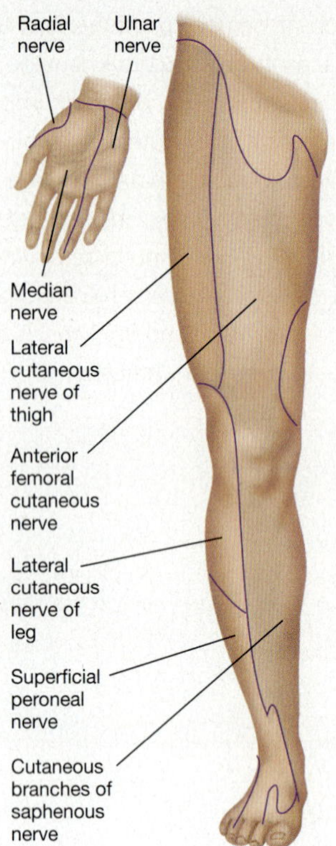

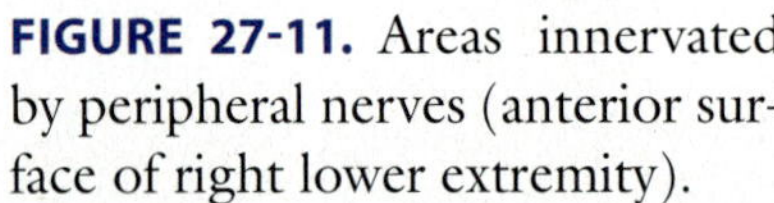

FIGURE 27-11. Areas innervated by peripheral nerves (anterior surface of right lower extremity).

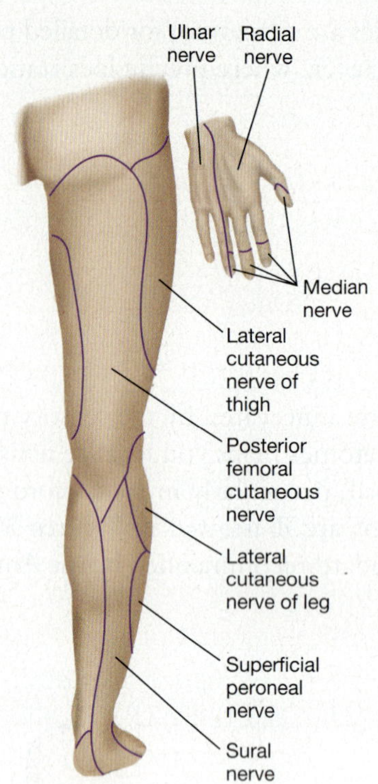

FIGURE 27-12. Areas innervated by peripheral nerves (posterior surface of right lower extremity).

Dermatome levels are more variable between individuals than these diagrams suggest. They overlap at their upper and lower margins and slightly across the midline. Do not try to memorize all the dermatomes. Instead, focus on learning the dermatomes shaded in green.

In spinal cord injury, all dermatomes below the level of injury can be affected. The sensory level may be several segments *lower* than the spinal lesion, for reasons that are not well understood.

Percussing for the level of vertebral pain may be helpful. In radiculopathy, damage to a spinal nerve root causes sensory loss limited to that dermatome.

HEALTH HISTORY: GENERAL APPROACH

For many of the body systems, the history provides the essential clues to diagnosis. While this is true for the nervous system, the neurologic examination allows you to assess all levels of nervous system function to a unique degree. With practice, you can obtain a history and perform a thorough yet efficient neurologic examination that enables you to detect the wide breadth of neurologic illness.

When neurologic disease is suspected, two complementary questions should guide your assessment: (1) What is the localization of the responsible lesion (or lesions) in the nervous system? (2) What is the underlying pathophysiology that explains the patient's symptoms and neurologic findings?

Questions about the patient's condition are addressed iteratively, based on responses during the interview, acknowledging that similar symptoms can arise from various pathologies. Reaching a neurologic diagnosis through this process requires practice.

The nervous system assessment starts immediately upon meeting the patient and is ongoing. Suspected abnormalities in mental status necessitate formal testing. Significant impairments in attention or memory, may render the patient's history unreliable, requiring critical information from other observers.

See Chapter 11, Cognition, Behavior, and Mental Status, pp. 205–217, techniques to conduct the formal mental status examination.

Symptom patterns help localize neurologic issues; determine if symptoms like weakness are unilateral or bilateral and affect proximal, distal, or all muscles. Probing for additional neurologic symptoms is essential, as patients might not link them directly, such as numbness in feet with walking difficulties. Identical symptoms can originate from various nervous system levels, including the brain, spinal cord, and peripheral structures. Neurologic diseases can manifest with positive symptoms like "pins-and-needles" sensation (*paresthesia*), and seizures or negative effects without noticeable symptoms, such as silent parietal lobe lesions.

The symptom's *onset* and *progression* are key to understanding its cause; sudden speech difficulties may indicate a stroke, while gradual changes might suggest a tumor. Transient symptoms, like those in transient ischemic attacks (TIAs) or multiple sclerosis, are critical but often underreported; asking about past symptoms can clarify the diagnosis.

Common or Concerning Symptoms

- Headache
- Dizziness or lightheadedness
- Weakness
- Numbness or abnormal or absent sensation
- Fainting and blacking out (near-syncope and syncope)
- Seizures
- Tremors or involuntary movements

Other common symptoms that may involve the nervous system are addressed in more detail in the following sections:

- Confusion (see Chapter 11, Cognition, Behavior, and Mental Status, p. 222)
- Memory loss (see Chapter 11, Cognition, Behavior, and Mental Status, pp. 204–205)
- Trouble speaking (see Table 27-2, Disorders of Speech, p. 968)
- Vision loss or blurred vision (see Chapter 14, Eyes, pp. 325–326)
- Difficulty walking (see Chapter 26, Musculoskeletal System: Lumbosacral Spine, Hips, and Lower Extremities, pp. 879–881 and Table 27-3, Abnormalities of Gait and Posture, p. 969)

Headache

Headaches, with a 30% lifetime prevalence in the general population, are predominantly tension-type, affecting half of all individuals.[8–10] Classified as *primary* (e.g., migraine, tension, cluster headaches) when no underlying disease is identified, or *secondary* when resulting from underlying conditions like meningitis or subarachnoid hemorrhage, obtaining a thorough history is essential since physical exams often appear normal (Box 27-4).[11–13] Any abnormal findings should prompt further investigation due to the potential for life-threatening secondary causes.

Common causes include **tension-type headaches** (dull, aching with forehead tightness), **migraines** (unilateral, pulsating with nausea or light sensitivity), **cluster headaches** (intense pain around one eye), **sinus headaches** (from sinus inflammation), **dehydration**, and **caffeine withdrawal**. Less frequent causes are **brain tumors** or **meningitis** (inflammation of the protective membranes covering the brain and spinal cord).

Box 27-4. Headache: High-Yield Health History Questions

Domain	Questions	Rationale
Location	*What is the location of your headache (e.g., one side, both sides, around the eyes, back of the head)?*	*Migraines:* typically affect one side of the head *Tension-type:* usually involve both sides *Cluster:* around the eyes *Occipital neuralgia:* back of the head[11,14] *Brain tumors and abscesses:* can cause focal or generalized pain, often worsening in the morning or with changes in position[15,16]
Quality	*How would you describe the pain (e.g., throbbing, pressure, stabbing)?*	*Throbbing:* often associated with migraines *Pressure:* typical for tension-type headaches *Stabbing:* can occur with cluster headaches or trigeminal neuralgia
Onset	*Did the headache start suddenly or gradually?*	*Sudden thunderclap headache:* medical emergency that could indicate a subarachnoid hemorrhage[17–19] *Gradual onset:* more common in migraines, tension-type headaches, and meningitis
Accompanying symptoms	*Are there any accompanying symptoms such as nausea, vomiting, fever, neck stiffness, visual changes, or sensitivity to light or sound?*	*Nausea, vomiting, and sensitivity to light or sound:* common with migraines or indicate increased intracranial pressure from a tumor or abscess *Visual changes:* could suggest migraine with aura or a more serious condition like stroke[14,20–22] *Gradual onset with fever and neck stiffness:* suggests meningitis
Triggers	*Do you have any triggers for your headache, like certain foods, stress, or changes in sleep?*	*Migraines:* can be triggered by various factors including foods, stress, hormonal changes, and sleep disturbances *Meningitis:* lack of specific triggers but with symptoms like fever and neck stiffness *Brain tumor or abscess:* continuous, unprovoked headaches worsening over time
Duration/ frequency	*How long do your headaches last, and how often do they occur?*	*Short duration, frequent:* cluster headaches *Longer duration, less frequent:* migraines *Persistent, progressive:* brain tumor or abscess
Medications	*Have you taken any medications for your headache, and have they been effective?*	Some drugs are particularly effective for specific types of headaches, such as triptans for migraines.[23] *Lack of response or worsening symptoms:* may suggest a more serious underlying condition like a brain tumor, abscess, or meningitis[24]
Family history	*Do you have a personal or family history of headaches or migraines?*	Can indicate a predisposition to migraines or other types of primary headache disorders[14,25]
Sleep disturbance	*Does your headache wake you up from sleep?*	Concerning for raised intracranial pressure, potentially due to a brain tumor or abscess

Look for important signs (red flags) that warn of headaches needing prompt investigation such as sudden onset "like a thunderclap," onset after age 50 years, and associated symptoms such as fever and stiff neck (Box 27-5).[12,27–29]

Migraine headache is often preceded by an aura or prodrome, and is highly likely if three of the five "**POUND**" features are present: **P**ulsatile or throbbing; **O**ne day duration, or lasts 4 to 72 hours if untreated; **U**nilateral; **N**ausea or vomiting; **D**isabling or intensity causing interruption of daily activity.[14,25]

Box 27-5. Headache Warning Signs

- Progressively frequent or severe over a 3-month period
- Sudden onset like a "thunderclap" or "the worst headache of my life"
- New onset after age 50 years
- Aggravated or relieved by change in position
- Precipitated by Valsalva maneuver or exertion
- Associated symptoms of fever, night sweats, or weight loss
- Presence of cancer, HIV infection, or pregnancy
- Recent head trauma
- Change in pattern from past headaches
- Lack of a similar headache in the past
- Associated papilledema, neck stiffness, or focal neurologic deficits

See Tables 27-4 and 27-5 on Primary Headaches and Secondary Headaches and Cranial Neuralgias on pp. 970–975.

Dizziness or Lightheadedness

As you learned in Chapter 15, Ears and Nose, *dizziness* and *lightheadedness* are common, somewhat vague, issues that prompt a more specific history and neurologic examination, with emphasis on detection of nystagmus and focal neurologic signs (Box 27-6).

Common causes include **benign positional vertigo** (dizziness with head movement changes); **dehydration**; **low blood pressure**, **anxiety**, or **stress** (leading to temporary light-headedness); **inner ear infections** (affecting balance); and **medication side effects.**

See Table 27-6, Syncope and Similar Disorders, pp. 976–977.

See Table 15-1, Dizziness and Vertigo, p. 384, in Chapter 15, Ears and Nose, for distinguishing symptoms and time course.

See Table 27-7, Types of Stroke, pp. 978–979.

Box 27-6. Dizziness or Lightheadedness: High-Yield Health History Questions

Domain	Questions	Rationale
Spinning sensation	*Do you feel like the room is spinning (vertigo), or is it more like a feeling of faintness?*	Can help distinguish between peripheral causes like benign paroxysmal positional vertigo (BPPV) and central causes or cardiovascular issues such as orthostatic hypotension
Positional changes	*Does your dizziness occur when you change positions, like sitting up from lying down?*	*Positional:* often associated with BPPV or orthostatic hypotension Nonpositional: consider vestibular neuronitis or Ménière disease if accompanied by hearing loss or tinnitus
Medications	*Are you currently taking any medications that might cause dizziness as a side effect?*	*Antihypertensives and diuretics:* can cause dizziness due to their effects on blood pressure or electrolyte balance *Absence of side effects:* suggests alternative cause
Hearing disturbances	*Do you have any hearing loss, ringing in the ears, or fullness in the ears along with your dizziness?*	*Hearing loss or tinnitus with dizziness:* suggests Ménière disease or acoustic neuroma[30] *Absence of these symptoms:* consider migraine-associated vertigo
Recent illness	*Have you had any recent illnesses, especially involving the head or ears?*	*Viral illness:* can lead to labyrinthitis or vestibular neuronitis, causing vertigo *Absence of illness:* points to vascular or neurologic causes
Associate or provoking symptoms	*Do you experience dizziness associated with certain activities or stress?*	*Activity or stress-induced:* could indicate psychogenic dizziness *Associated with palpitations:* cardiovascular cause (e.g., arrhythmia)
Precipitating events	*Does your dizziness get worse with head movements or when walking?*	*Worsening with head movements:* may indicate a vestibular or proprioceptive cause *Ataxia, diplopia, and dysarthria:* suspicious for vertebrobasilar TIA or stroke[31–36] *Present without specific triggers:* consider metabolic conditions (e.g., hypoglycemia)
Accompanying symptoms	*Have you had any other symptoms such as chest pain, shortness of breath, or palpitations along with dizziness?*	*Presence:* may point to a cardiovascular origin (e.g., arrhythmia or ischemia) *Absence:* consider neurologic or inner ear disorders

Weakness

Reports of weakness may have different meanings, including fatigue, apathy, drowsiness, or actual loss of strength. True motor weakness can arise from lesions affecting the CNS, a peripheral nerve, the NMJ, or a muscle.

Obtaining an accurate and detailed health history such as its time course and location is especially relevant (Box 27-7). Is it *proximal* (e.g., shoulder and/or hip girdle), *distal* (e.g., hands and/or feet), *symmetric* (e.g., same areas on both sides of the body), *asymmetric* (e.g., *focal* in a portion of the face or extremity, *monoparesis* in an extremity, *paraparesis* in both lower extremities, or *hemiparesis*, on one side of the body).

Neurologic causes include **myasthenia gravis** (autoimmune disorder causing varying degrees of muscle weakness), **Guillain–Barré syndrome** (rapid-onset muscle weakness caused by the immune system damaging the PNS), and **multiple sclerosis** (immune system attacks the protective covering of nerves, affecting muscle control). Other causes can be **amyotrophic lateral sclerosis** ([ALS] progressive nervous system disease causing loss of muscle control), **peripheral neuropathy** (damage to peripheral nerves affecting muscle strength), and **muscular dystrophies** (group of genetic diseases causing progressive weakness and loss of muscle mass).

Box 27-7. Weakness: High-Yield Health History Questions

Domain	Questions	Rationale
Persistence	*Is the weakness you are experiencing constant, or does it come and go?*	*Constant:* suggests a structural issue such as a brain or spinal cord lesion *Fluctuating:* could indicate a neuromuscular disorder like myasthenia gravis or periodic paralysis
Location	*Do you notice the weakness more in your arms and legs, or is it affecting your entire body?*	*Proximal (e.g., hips and shoulders):* can suggest myopathies or NMJ disorders *Distal:* might point to peripheral neuropathies or certain muscular dystrophies
Onset	*Did the weakness start suddenly, or has it been developing gradually over time?*	*Sudden onset:* can be seen in acute neurologic events such as stroke[31–36] or in inflammatory conditions like Guillain–Barré syndrome[37] *Gradual onset:* suggests a chronic process such as motor neuron disease or progressive muscular atrophy
Precipitating events	*Are there any specific activities or times of day when the weakness is more noticeable?*	*Diurnal variation:* characteristic of myasthenia gravis[38,39] *Morning only:* might be seen in inflammatory muscle diseases
Muscle pain or cramps	*Have you experienced any muscle pain, cramps, or changes in muscle size or shape?*	*Muscle pain and cramps:* can indicate myopathy *Changes in muscle size:* suggest atrophy, as seen in motor neuron disease, or hypertrophy in some dystrophic processes
Bulbar symptoms	*Are you experiencing any difficulties with breathing, swallowing, or changes in your voice?*	*Bulbar symptoms:* seen in neuromuscular disorders affecting the CNs, like myasthenic crisis or ALS

(*continued*)

Box 27-7. Weakness: High-Yield Health History Questions (*Continued*)

Domain	Questions	Rationale
Sensory changes	*Do you have any numbness, tingling, or loss of sensation along with the weakness?*	*Sensory changes:* point to peripheral neuropathy or central lesion affecting both sensory and motor pathways
Coordination issues	*Have you had any recent falls or difficulties with coordination?*	*Falls or coordination issues:* suggest cerebellar dysfunction or profound proximal weakness, as seen in polymyositis or dermatomyositis

To identify *proximal weakness*, ask about difficulty with movements such as combing hair, reaching up to a shelf, getting up out of a chair, or climbing stairs. To identify *distal weakness*, ask about hand strength when opening a jar or using scissors or buttoning buttons, or problems like tripping when walking.

Numbness or Abnormal or Absent Sensation

When assessing a patient reporting numbness, inquire further for a more precise description of their experience (Box 27-8). Ask whether they are experiencing a "pins and needles" sensation; known as *paresthesia*, have distorted sensations that are referred to as *dysesthesias*; or if they are noticing a reduction in sensitivity, termed *hypoesthesia*, or a complete absence of sensation, known as *anesthesia*.

Neurologic causes include **peripheral neuropathy** (damage to the peripheral nerves, leading to numbness, tingling, or weakness); **stroke** or **TIA; multiple sclerosis**, **spinal cord injuries**, and **diabetic neuropathy** (nerve damage due to high blood sugar levels leading to numbness or tingling); and **vitamin B12 deficiency** (which can affect nerve function, resulting in sensation changes).

Box 27-8. Numbness or Abnormal or Absent Sensation: High-Yield Health History Questions

Domain	Questions	Rationale
Location	*Is the numbness focused to a specific area or generalized throughout your body?*	*Localized:* suggests nerve entrapment or peripheral neuropathy *Generalized:* might indicate a systemic condition (e.g., diabetes or vitamin B12 deficiency)
Distribution	*Do you notice the numbness following a 'glove and stocking' pattern, like it covers your hands and feet?*	Typical for polyneuropathies, which often result from systemic diseases like diabetes, chronic alcohol use, or various toxic exposures[40,41]
Positional changes	*Does the numbness get worse or change with certain activities or positions?*	May suggest nerve compression syndromes, like carpal tunnel syndrome with wrist activities or meralgia paresthetica with prolonged standing
Motor weakness	*Have you noticed any changes in your muscle strength or difficulty with movement?*	Suggests a neurologic condition affecting both sensory and motor fibers, such as a cervical radiculopathy or motor neuron disease
Persistence	*Does the numbness come and go or is it constant?*	*Intermittent:* could be related to TIAs or seizures *Constant:* may suggest a chronic neuropathic process

Domain	Questions	Rationale
Bowel or bladder changes	*Are there any changes in bowel or bladder habits, or do you have back pain?*	Could indicate spinal cord pathology (e.g., herniated disc with nerve root compression or spinal stenosis)
Numbness at rest	*Do you experience numbness or tingling after being inactive for a while, or does it happen at night?*	*Nocturnal:* seen in conditions like carpal tunnel syndrome or restless legs syndrome
Associated symptoms	*Have you noticed any skin rashes or joint pain recently?*	Can point to a systemic inflammatory condition, like lupus or rheumatoid arthritis, affecting peripheral nerves

Fainting and Blacking Out (Near-Syncope and Syncope)

Patient reports of fainting or "passing out" are common and warrant a meticulous history to guide management and possible hospital admission (Box 27-9).[42] Begin by finding out whether the patient has actually lost consciousness (syncope). Seizures may be confused with syncope, but impairment of consciousness in seizure results from disordered neuronal firing rather than hypoperfusion of brain tissue.

Neurologic causes include **seizures** (sudden, uncontrolled electrical disturbances in the brain), **TIAs**, and **autonomic neuropathy** (damage to the nerves that regulate involuntary body functions, affecting blood pressure). Other neurologic triggers can be **vertebrobasilar insufficiency** (reduced blood flow in the arteries at the back of the brain) and **narcolepsy** (chronic sleep disorder with sudden sleep attacks and loss of muscle control).

Box 27-9. Near-Syncope and Syncope: High-Yield Health History Questions

Domain	Questions	Rationale
Positional changes	*Does the fainting occur when you stand up or change positions quickly?*	*On standing:* orthostatic hypotension from a sudden drop in blood pressure *No position change:* consider cardiac causes like arrhythmia[42]
Prodromal symptoms	*Before fainting, do you experience any warning signs like lightheadedness, nausea, or sweating?*	*Prodromal:* suggest vasovagal or reflex-mediated syncope *Absence:* might indicate a cardiac cause (e.g., arrhythmia)
Associated activities	*Are your fainting spells associated with any particular activity, like urination, defecation, or coughing?*	Known as situational syncope, which includes conditions like micturition syncope, defecation syncope, and cough syncope
Palpitations	*Have you noticed any palpitations or irregular heartbeats before fainting?*	*Palpitations:* may suggest arrhythmia *Absence:* consider noncardiac causes or silent arrhythmias
Associated symptoms	*Have you experienced any chest pain or shortness of breath prior to these episodes?*	Could indicate underlying cardiac condition like ischemic heart disease

(continued)

Box 27-9. Near-Syncope and Syncope: High-Yield Health History Questions (*Continued*)

Domain	Questions	Rationale
Medical history	*Do you have a history of heart disease or are you taking any cardiac medications?*	Increases risk due to arrhythmias,[43] structural heart disease, or medication side effects
Postictal symptoms	*After fainting, do you feel confused or have difficulty speaking or moving?*	May indicate a neurologic cause, such as seizure or TIA
Trauma history	*Have you had any recent head trauma, or do you experience headaches?*	*Head trauma:* suggests concussion *Headaches:* raises suspicion for a subarachnoid hemorrhage or other neurologic condition

Seizures

Patients reporting episodes of lost consciousness may indicate *seizures*, characterized by sudden, excessive cortical neuron discharges. Seizures are classified as *focal* or *generalized* based on their initial cortical focus and can be genetic, symptomatic with an identifiable cause, or idiopathic.[44] Witness accounts of the patient's condition before, during, and after the episode are crucial. A detailed history helps exclude other causes of unconsciousness and acute symptomatic seizures with clear explanations (Box 27-10).

Neurologic causes include **epilepsy** (abnormal brain activity causing two or more unprovoked seizures, loss of awareness), **brain tumors**, **stroke**, **traumatic brain injury** (which can alter brain function and lead to seizures), infections such as **meningitis** or **encephalitis** (inflammation of the brain or surrounding tissues that can affect brain function), and **autoimmune disorders**.

See Table 27-8, Seizure Disorders, pp. 980–981.

Box 27-10. Seizures: High-Yield Health History Questions

Domain	Questions	Rationale
Prior illness	*Have you had a fever or illness leading up to the seizure?*	*Febrile:* common in children and can occur with a rapid increase in body temperature *Absence:* consider *epilepsy* (two or more seizures that are not provoked by other illnesses or circumstances or other neurologic conditions)[45,46]
Triggers	*Did the seizure occur after a period of sleep deprivation, alcohol use, or missed meals?*	*Triggers:* can provoke seizures in susceptible individuals *Absence:* underlying seizure disorder more likely
Prodromal symptoms	*Have you noticed any unusual sensations or warnings before the seizure started?*	*Aura or prodrome:* can indicate a focal onset of a seizure before it generalizes, suggesting a specific region of brain involvement *Absence:* might suggest primary generalized seizure
Trauma history	*Do you have a history of head injury or neurologic disease?*	*History:* can increase risk due to scarring or damage to brain tissue *Absence:* idiopathic seizures or genetic causes may be explored

Domain	Questions	Rationale
Repetitive movements	*During the seizure, were there any repetitive movements, such as jerking or stiffening of limbs?*	*Stereotyped repetitive movements:* suggests a convulsive seizure, potentially a tonic–clonic type; tongue biting or bruising of limbs may also occur *Non-motor:* may have subtle features like behavioral arrest or automatisms
Associated symptoms	*Were there any changes in your breathing, color, or bowel/bladder control during the seizure?*	*Symptoms:* can indicate generalized tonic–clonic seizure *Absence:* nonconvulsive seizure (e.g., absence seizures)
Duration	*How long did the seizure last, and what was your condition immediately afterward?*	Duration and postictal state can help differentiate between seizure types and can indicate severity; prolonged confusion or sleepiness suggests a more significant impact on brain function
Medications	*Are you taking any medications that could lower the seizure threshold, or have you recently started or stopped any medications?*	*Medications/changes:* can lower seizure threshold or cause withdrawal seizures *Absence:* consider genetic or structural causes

Tremors or Involuntary Movements

Tremor, "a rhythmic oscillatory movement of a body part resulting from the contraction of opposing muscle groups," is the most common movement disorder.[47,48] It may be an isolated finding or part of a neurologic disorder.

Box 27-11. Tremors or Involuntary Movements: High-Yield Health History Questions

Domain	Questions	Rationale
Associated activities	*When do you notice the tremors or involuntary movements occurring—during rest or with activity?*	*Rest:* typical of Parkinson disease (PD) *Action/intention:* seen in cerebellar disorders[49,50] *Posture/movement:* consider essential tremor (high-frequency, bilateral, upper extremity tremor that occurs with both limb movement and sustained posture and subsides when the limb is relaxed; head, voice, and leg tremor may also be present)[48]
Location	*Are the tremors affecting a specific part of your body or are they generalized?*	*Focal:* suggest lesion in a specific part of the brain or peripheral nerve injury *Generalized:* could be due to a systemic condition or drug effect

(continued)

Neurologic causes include **Parkinson disease** (brain disorder leading to shaking, stiffness, and difficulty with balance and coordination), **essential tremor** (disorder causing rhythmic shaking, especially during voluntary movements), **Huntington disease** (genetic disorder causing the progressive breakdown of nerve cells in the brain, leading to involuntary movements), **dystonia** (condition causing involuntary muscle contractions and abnormal postures), **cerebellar ataxia** (damage to the cerebellum affecting coordination and leading to tremulous movement), and **drug-induced tremors**.

Distinct from these symptoms is **restless legs syndrome (RLS)**, present in 6% to 12% of the U.S. population, described as an unpleasant sensation in the legs, especially at night, that gets worse with rest and improves with movement of the symptomatic limb(s).[51–53] Reversible causes include pregnancy, renal disease, and iron deficiency.[59]

See Table 27-9, Tremors and Involuntary Movements, pp. 982–983.

Box 27-11. Tremors or Involuntary Movements: High-Yield Health History Questions (*Continued*)

Domain	Questions	Rationale
Family history	*Do you have a family history of tremors or neurologic diseases?*	*History:* could suggest a genetic disorder like essential tremor or Huntington disease if chorea is present *Absence:* may indicate acquired condition
Severity/ Persistence	*Have the tremors or movements been worsening over time, or are they intermittent?*	*Progressive:* could indicate degenerative disorder like PD *Intermittent:* may suggest a functional movement disorder or episodic ataxia
Accompanying symptoms	*Are the tremors or movements accompanied by rigidity, slowness, or trouble with balance?*	*Rigidity and bradykinesia:* characteristic of PD[49,50] *Balance:* consider ataxias or other cerebellar disorders.
Stimulant use	*Do you consume caffeine or other stimulants, and have you noticed any relation to the tremors?*	*Consumption:* can exacerbate or cause tremors *Nonconsumption:* consider idiopathic or pathologic causes.
Repetitive movements	*Are the involuntary movements repetitive and rhythmic, or are they more irregular and unpredictable?*	*Repetitive and rhythmic:* suggest tremor *Irregular, unpredictable:* could be myoclonus, tics, or chorea
Medications	*Have you started or stopped any medications that could be associated with these symptoms?*	Common with medications like lithium or certain antipsychotics; withdrawal from alcohol or benzodiazepines can also cause tremor

PHYSICAL EXAMINATION: GENERAL APPROACH

As you interview the patient, remember the dual goals of your assessment: *localizing the lesion(s)* and *identifying the underlying pathophysiology* (Box 27-11). Once again, these questions are answered iteratively as you learn about the patient from your neurologic findings. When you conduct the neurologic examination, adopt a fixed routine or examination sequence to minimize omission of one of its important components. Whether you perform a comprehensive or screening examination, organize your thinking into six categories: (1) mental status; (2) cranial nerves (CNs); (3) motor system; (4) reflexes; and (5) sensory system; (6) coordination, station and gait.[54]

See Box 4-11, Suggested Comprehensive (Head-to-Toe) Physical Examination Sequence in Chapter 4, Physical Examination, pp. 78–80.

As you refine your skills in performing neurologic examinations, you will learn to integrate them with other examination parts for efficiency. Start evaluating mental status during initial interviews and incorporate CN assessments with head and neck exams. Also, assess neurologic aspects in the limbs during peripheral and musculoskeletal examinations. However, always interpret and document your findings in terms of the nervous system as a whole.

TECHNIQUES OF EXAMINATION: MENTAL STATUS

Key Components of the Examination of the Nervous System: Mental Status

- Assess mental status (level of alertness, orientation, attention, language function, memory, calculation, visuo-spatial processing, abstract reasoning)

Assess Mental Status

Evaluating a patient's mental status is a critical component of the neurologic examination and plays a vital role in diagnosing and managing a wide range of psychiatric and neurologic conditions. It offers insight into the patient's cognitive, emotional, and psychological well-being. Through a comprehensive assessment, clinicians can identify changes in mental functions, detect abnormalities, and determine the appropriate course of treatment.

Box 27-12 outlines key aspects of the mental status examination. This structured approach ensures a thorough evaluation of the patient's mental health, aiding in accurate diagnosis and effective management.

Review the evaluation of mental status detailed in Chapter 11, Cognition, Behavior, and Mental Status, pages 205–217. This includes assessing alertness levels, language functions, memory, calculation skills, visuospatial processing capabilities, and abstract reasoning.

Box 27-12. Mental Status Examination Components

Component	What to Evaluate	Description
Level of alertness	Consciousness Attention Orientation	Assess the patient's basic state of wakefulness and responsiveness to external stimuli, as well as their ability to maintain attention and demonstrate awareness of their identity, location, time, and situation.
Language function	Fluency Comprehension Repetition Naming	Evaluate the patient's ability to produce speech (*fluency*), understand spoken and written language (*comprehension*), repeat words or phrases (*repetition*), and name objects or describe their use (*naming*).
Memory	Short-term Long-term	Test the patient's ability to recall recent events or information (*short-term memory*) and to remember information acquired in the past (*long-term memory*).
Calculation	Basic arithmetic More complex calculations	Assess the patient's ability to perform addition and subtraction and more complex calculations if appropriate.
Visuospatial processing	Copying shapes Navigating spaces	Examine the patient's ability to understand and interact with the spatial environment, including their ability to copy two-dimensional shapes and navigate or describe spatial relationships.
Abstract reasoning	Interpreting proverbs Problem-solving tasks	Test the patient's ability to think abstractly by interpreting the meaning of proverbs or solving problems that require understanding beyond the concrete details.

TECHNIQUES OF EXAMINATION: CRANIAL NERVES

Key Components of the Examination of the Nervous System: Cranial Nerves

- Test for cranial nerve I—Olfactory (sense of smell)
- Test for cranial nerve II—Optic (visual acuity, visual fields, fundoscopic exam)
- Test for cranial nerves II and III—Optic and Oculomotor (pupillary light reflex, pupil size and shape)
- Test for cranial nerves III, IV, and VI—Oculomotor, Trochlear, and Abducens (extraocular movements, eyelid elevation)
- Test for cranial nerve V—Trigeminal (facial sensation, jaw movement, corneal reflex with VII)
- Test for cranial nerve VII—Facial (facial movements, symmetry, taste for anterior 2/3 of tongue)
- Test for cranial nerve VIII—Vestibulocochlear (hearing and balance)
- Test for cranial nerves IX and X—Glossopharyngeal and Vagus (swallowing, palate elevation, gag reflex, voice quality)
- Test for cranial nerve XI—Spinal Accessory (shoulder shrug, head rotation against resistance)
- Test for cranial nerve XII—Hypoglossal (tongue movement, symmetry, strength)

Test for Cranial Nerve I—Olfactory

Test the *sense of smell* by presenting the patient with familiar nonirritating odors. First, make sure that each nasal passage is patent by compressing one side of the nose and asking them to sniff through the other. Then ask them to close both eyes. Occlude one nostril and test smell in the other with substances like coffee, soap, or vanilla. Avoid noxious odors like ammonia that might stimulate CN V. Ask the patient to identify each odor. Test smell on the other side. Normally the patient perceives odors on each side and identifies them correctly.

Loss of smell occurs in sinus conditions, head trauma, smoking, aging, use of cocaine, and *Parkinson disease.*

Test for Cranial Nerve II—Optic

Test Visual Acuity in Each Eye. To test visual acuity, use a Snellen chart to examine each eye separately, accurately assessing the patient's ability to read and distinguish fine details.

For a detailed discussion of the techniques for examining visual acuity, review Chapter 14, Eyes, pp. 328–329.

Inspect Optic Fundi with an Ophthalmoscope. Utilize an ophthalmoscope to examine the optic fundus of each eye, with a focus on identifying *papilledema* (indicative of increased intracranial pressure), *optic atrophy* (pallor signaling nerve fiber loss from conditions like optic neuritis or neurodegenerative diseases), and any signs of retinal vascular diseases like *hemorrhages* or *exudates*, which may reflect systemic issues with neurologic implications, including diabetes or hypertension.

For a detailed discussion of the techniques of fundoscopy, review Chapter 14, Eyes, pp. 335–339.

Test the Visual Fields by Confrontation. This test evaluates visual pathways and brain processing by having the examiner and patient cover opposite eyes and face each other. The examiner introduces stimuli at different peripheral points while the patient focuses on the examiner's eye.

See Table 14-2, Visual Field Defects, in Chapter 14, Eyes, p. 348.[55]

Test for Cranial Nerves II and III—Optic and Oculomotor

Inspect the Size and Shape of the Pupils. Compare one side with the other. *Anisocoria*, defined as a discrepancy greater than 0.4 mm in the diameter between one pupil and its counterpart, can be observed in as many as 38% of individuals without any health issues.

If the large pupil reacts poorly to light or anisocoria worsens in light, the large pupil has abnormal pupillary constriction, as seen in CN III palsy. Consider intracranial aneurysm if the patient is awake and transtentorial herniation if the patient is comatose.

Test Pupillary Reactions to Light. Evaluating pupillary responses to light involves shining a light into each eye and observing the pupils' constriction. This test helps identify neurologic function by assessing the direct and consensual light reflex pathways.

See Table 14-6, Pupillary Abnormalities, in Chapter 14, Eyes, p. 352.

Check Near Response: Constriction, Convergence, and Lens Accommodation. Examine pupillary constriction in *response to light* (pupillary constrictor muscle), *eye convergence* (medial rectus muscles) on focusing on a near object, and *lens accommodation* (ciliary muscle) for clear vision at varying distances. These assessments provide insights into the functioning of the optic nerve and neurologic pathways.

If anisocoria worsens in darkness, with normal pupillary reaction to light but abnormal pupillary dilation in one eye, this suggests Horner syndrome affecting sympathetic innervation.[56]

Test for Cranial Nerves III, IV, and VI—Oculomotor, Trochlear, and Abducens

Test Extraocular Movements. Test in the six cardinal directions of gaze and look for loss of conjugate movements in any of the six directions. Check convergence of the eyes. Ask patients if they experience *diplopia* when testing. Ask which direction of gaze makes the diplopia worse and inspect the eyes closely for asymmetric deviation of movement. Determine if the diplopia is *monocular* or *binocular* by asking the patient to cover one eye, and then the other.

See Chapter 14, Eyes, p. 334, for a more detailed discussion of testing extraocular movements.

See Table 14-7, Dysconjugate Gaze, p. 353. Binocular diplopia occurs in disorders that result in ocular misalignment including CN III, IV, and/or VI palsy internuclear ophthalmoplegia; myasthenia gravis; and eye muscle disorders including trauma and thyroid ophthalmopathy.[57]

Identify Nystagmus. Look for involuntary jerking movement of the eyes with quick and slow components. Note the direction of gaze in which it appears, the plane of the nystagmus (*horizontal*, *vertical*, *rotary*, or *mixed*), and the direction of the *fast* and *slow components* (as well as whether this changes directions). Nystagmus is named for the direction of the fast component (e.g., left-beating nystagmus). Ask the patient to fix their vision on a distant object and observe if the nystagmus increases or decreases.

See Table 27-10, Nystagmus, pp. 984–985. Nystagmus is seen in cerebellar disease (increases with retinal fixation, may be accompanied by ataxia and dysarthria), vestibular disorders (decreases with retinal fixation, is not direction-changing), and internuclear ophthalmoplegia.

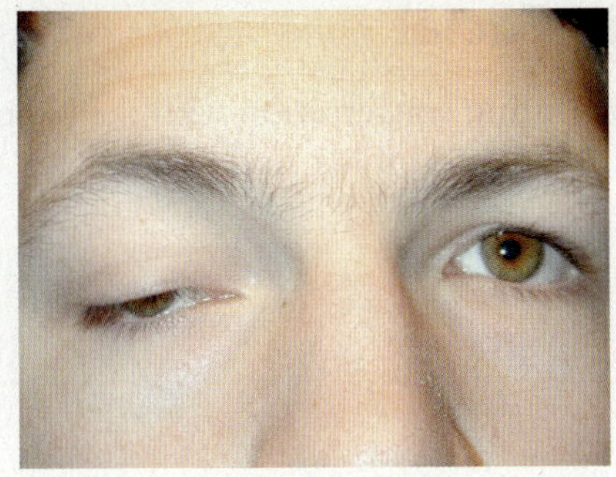

FIGURE 27-13. Right upper eyelid ptosis from cranial nerve III palsy. (Reprinted with permission from Savino PJ, Danesh-Meyer HV. *Wills Eye Hospital Color Atlas & Synopsis of Clinical Ophthalmology: Neuro-Ophthalmology*. 3rd ed. Wolters Kluwer; 2019. Figure 10-1A.)

Look for Ptosis. *Ptosis*, or drooping of the upper eyelids, is observed by identifying where on the eye the eyelid falls in relationship to the iris and pupil (Fig. 27-13). A slight difference in the width of the palpebral fissures is a normal variant in approximately a third of patients.

Ptosis is seen in CN III palsy, Horner syndrome (ptosis, miosis, forehead anhidrosis), and myasthenia gravis.

Test for Cranial Nerve V—Trigeminal

Palpate Temporal and Masseter Muscles (Motor). While palpating the temporal and masseter muscles in turn, *ask the patient to firmly clench their teeth* (Figs. 27-14 and 27-15). Note the strength of muscle contraction. Ask them to open and move the jaw from side to side.

Difficulty clenching the jaw or moving it to the opposite side suggests masseter and lateral pterygoid weakness, respectively. Jaw deviation during opening points to weakness on the deviating side.

Test Sensation in Face (Sensory). Begin by informing the patient of the procedure. To assess sensation across the three divisions of CN V, instruct the patient to close their eyes and focus on the specified areas in Figure 27-16.

Look for unilateral weakness in CN V pontine lesions, bilateral weakness in bilateral hemispheric disease.

For *light touch*, gently apply a fine cotton wisp to their skin and request a response to each contact. To evaluate *pain sensation*, use a new, sharp implement for each patient, such as a modified cotton swab, ensuring safety and preventing infection. Incorporate both sharp and blunt stimuli to differentiate between sharp and dull sensations, prompting the patient to compare the feeling on both sides.

Isolated sensory loss occurs in peripheral nerve disorders, including lesions of the trigeminal nerve (CN V).

Stroke can cause distinct patterns of sensory loss. Cortical or thalamic lesions can result in contralateral facial and body sensory loss; brainstem strokes can cause sensory loss to pain in the ipsilateral face but contralateral body.

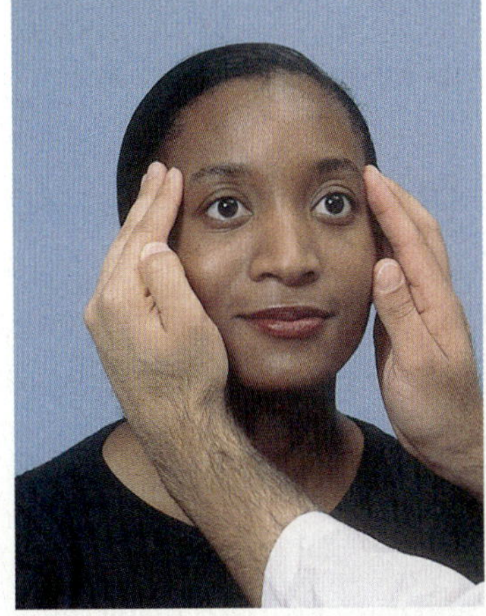

FIGURE 27-14. Palpating the temporal muscles.

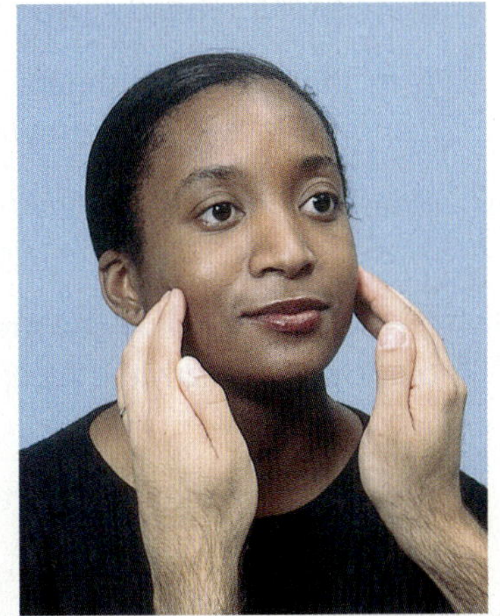

FIGURE 27-15. Palpating the masseter muscles.

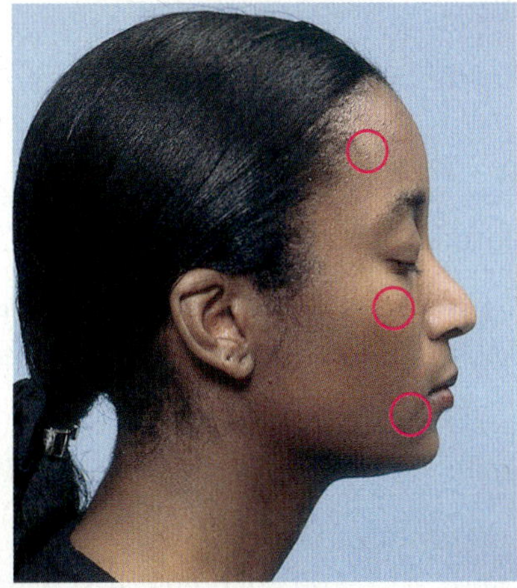

FIGURE 27-16. Areas for testing sensation of the three divisions of cranial nerve V.

Test for Cranial Nerve VII—Facial

Inspect the Face. Inspect both at rest and during conversation with the patient. Note any asymmetry, often visible in the nasolabial folds, and observe any tics or other abnormal movements.

Flattening of the nasolabial fold and drooping of the lower eyelid suggest facial weakness.

A peripheral injury to CN VII, as seen in Bell palsy, affects both the upper and lower face; a central lesion affects mainly the lower face. Loss of taste, hyperacusis, and increased or decreased tearing can also occur in Bell palsy.[58]

See Table 27-11, Types of Facial Paralysis, p. 986.

Test Muscles of Facial Expression. Ask the patient to perform a series of facial expressions as outlined in Box 27-13.

In unilateral facial paralysis, the mouth droops on the paralyzed side when the patient smiles or grimaces.

Patients with Parkinson's disease may exhibit decreased facial expressivity, known as *masked facies.* This is related to the *bradykinesia* that may be seen elsewhere in the body.

Test for Cranial Nerve VIII—Vestibulocochlear

Assess Gross Hearing with Whispered Voice Test. Ask the patient to cover the ear not being tested, or alternatively, the examiner can rub their fingers together near the opposite ear to mask any sound. Then, from a short distance, the examiner whispers a series of numbers into the ear being tested. The patient is asked to repeat the numbers back, allowing the examiner to gauge the patient's hearing acuity in each ear.[59]

See Whispered Voice Test for Auditory Acuity in Chapter 15, Ears and Nose, pp. 375–376.

Box 27-13. Assessment of Facial Muscle Function

Action	Patient Instructions	Rationale
Eyebrow lift	*"Try to raise both of your eyebrows as high as you can."*	Evaluates the function of the frontal belly of the occipitofrontalis muscle for forehead movement
Frown	*"Furrow your brows as if you are worried or concentrating hard."*	Tests the corrugator supercilii and procerus muscles, which are responsible for brow furrowing
Eye closure	*"Close your eyes as tightly as possible. Resist when I try to open them."*	Measures the strength and function of the orbicularis oculi muscles in eyelid closure (Fig. 27-17)
Teeth display	*"Open your mouth slightly and show both your upper and lower teeth."*	Checks the symmetry and strength of the muscles controlling the lips, particularly the zygomaticus major and minor and the orbicularis oris
Smile	*"Give a wide, genuine smile."*	Assesses the coordinated action of the zygomaticus, orbicularis oris, and buccinator muscles in facial expressions
Cheek puff	*"Puff out both cheeks with air, like you are blowing up a balloon."*	Tests the integrity of the facial nerves and muscles, particularly the buccinator muscle, in maintaining air pressure within the cheeks

Determine Hearing Loss with Tuning Fork Tests (Rinne and Weber, if Indicated). If hearing loss is present, determine if the loss is *conductive*, from impaired "air through ear" transmission, or *sensorineural*, from damage to the cochlear branch of CN VIII. To differentiate between these types, perform the *Rinne test to assess air and bone conduction*, and the *Weber test to evaluate sound lateralization*.

See techniques for Weber and Rinne tests in Chapter 15, Ears and Nose, pp. 375–377, and Table 15-4, Patterns of Hearing Loss, p. 388.

Excess cerumen, otosclerosis, and otitis media cause conductive hearing loss; *presbycusis* from aging is usually from sensorineural hearing loss.

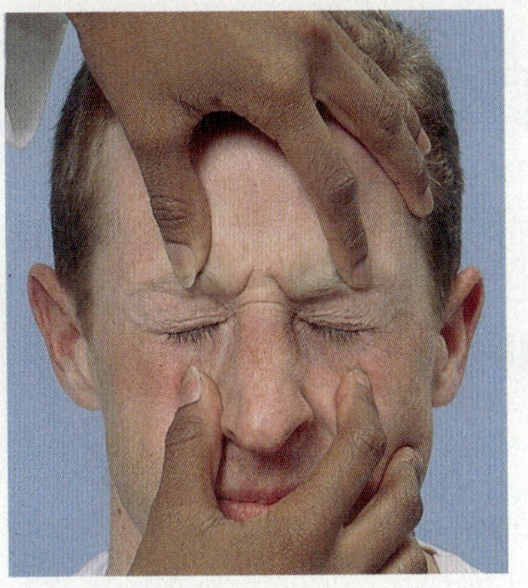

FIGURE 27-17. Testing the eyelid muscle strength.

Test for Cranial Nerves IX and X—Glossopharyngeal and Vagus

Assess Speech. Assess the patient's voice for hoarseness or a nasal quality. Hoarseness might point to vocal cord issues, while nasal speech can indicate problems with the soft palate's function.

Hoarseness occurs in vocal cord paralysis; nasal voice in paralysis of the palate.

Assess Swallowing and Palate/Uvula Movement. Assess swallowing difficulties by asking the patient to say *"ah"* or to simulate a yawn, allowing you to closely observe the movements of the soft palate and pharynx. Normally, *the soft palate should elevate symmetrically, the uvula should stay centered, and the sides of the posterior pharynx should converge medially*, akin to a closing curtain. Be mindful that a naturally slight curvature of the uvula, which can occur as a normal variation.

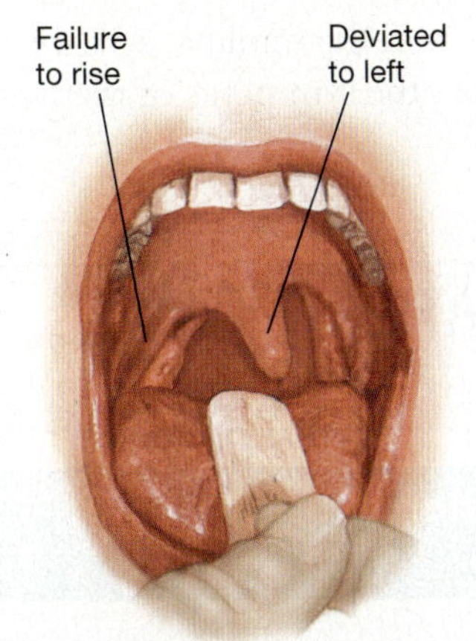

FIGURE 27-18. Weakness of the right palate leads to a deviation of the uvula to the left (unaffected side).

The palate fails to rise with a bilateral lesion of CN X. In unilateral paralysis, one side of the palate fails to rise and, together with the uvula, is pulled toward the normal side (Fig. 27-18).

Test for Cranial Nerve XI—Spinal Accessory

Test Trapezii Strength. Standing behind the patient, look for atrophy or small irregular twitching movements (fasciculations) in the trapezius muscles, and compare one side with the other. Ask the patient to shrug both shoulders upward against your hands (Fig. 27-19). Note the strength and contraction of the trapezii.

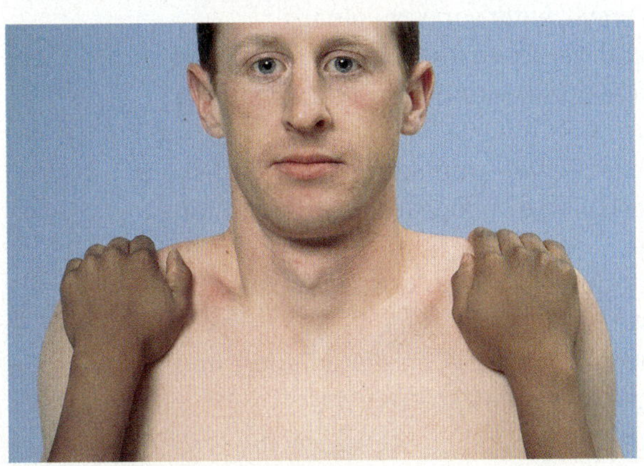

FIGURE 27-19. Testing trapezius strength.

In trapezius muscle paralysis, the shoulder droops, and the scapula is displaced downward and laterally.

Test Sternocleidomastoid Strength Against Resistance. Ask the patient to turn the head to each side against your hand. Observe the contraction of the opposite sternocleidomastoid (SCM) muscle and note the force of the movement against your hand (Fig. 27-20).

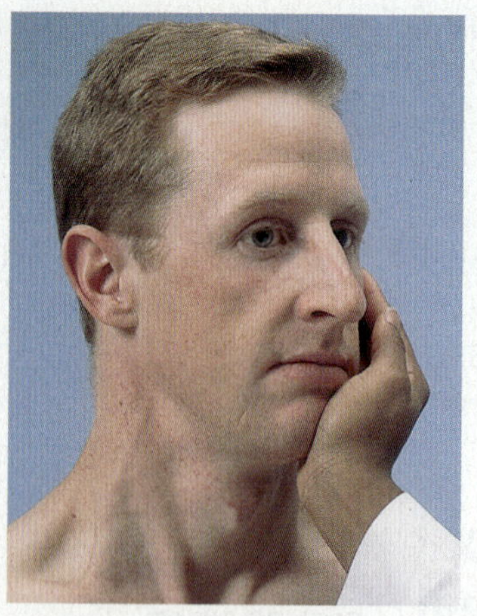

FIGURE 27-20. Testing sternocleidomastoid strength.

A supine patient with bilateral weakness of the SCM muscles has difficulty raising the head off the pillow.

Test for Cranial Nerve XII—Hypoglossal

Inspect and Test Tongue Movement. Inspect the patient's tongue as it lies resting on the floor of the mouth. Look for any atrophy or fasciculations. Some coarse, restless movements are normal.

Facial, tongue, pharyngeal, or laryngeal weakness can cause *dysarthria* but does not cause *aphasia*. Tongue atrophy and fasciculations can be seen in patients with ALS.

Then, with the patient's tongue protruded, look for asymmetry, atrophy, or deviation from the midline. Ask the patient to move the tongue from side to side and note the symmetry of the movement.

The protruded tongue deviates to the weak side. It deviates away from the side of the cortical lesion, and toward the side of a CN XII lesion.

TECHNIQUES OF EXAMINATION: MOTOR SYSTEM

Key Components of the Examination of the Nervous System: Motor System

- Assess the motor system for body position, involuntary movements, and muscle characteristics (bulk, tone, strength).
- Test shoulder abduction (C5, C6, axillary nerve—deltoid).
- Test elbow flexion (C5, C6, musculocutaneous nerve—biceps and brachioradialis) and extension (C6, C7, C8, radial nerve—triceps).
- Test wrist flexion (C7, C8, median nerve—flexor carpi radialis; ulnar nerve—flexor carpi ulnaris) and extension (C6, C7, C8, radial nerve—extensor carpi radialis longus and brevis, extensor carpi ulnaris).
- Test finger extension (C7, C8, radial nerve—extensor digitorum) and abduction (C8, T1, ulnar nerve—first dorsal interosseous and abductor digiti minimi).
- Test thumb abduction (C8, T1, median nerve—abductor pollicis brevis).
- Test hip flexion (L2, L3, L4, femoral nerve—iliopsoas) and extension (S1—gluteus maximus).
- Test knee flexion (L5, S1, S2, sciatic nerve—hamstrings) and extension (L2, L3, L4, femoral nerve—quadriceps).
- Test ankle dorsiflexion (L4, L5, peroneal nerve—tibialis anterior) and plantar flexion (S1, tibial nerve—gastrocnemius, soleus).

Assess the Motor System for Body Position, Involuntary Movements, and Muscle Characteristics

As you assess the motor system, focus on body position, involuntary movements, and characteristics of the muscles (*bulk, tone, and strength*). You can use this sequence for assessing overall motor function, or check each component in the arms, legs, and trunk in turn. If you detect an abnormality, identify the muscle(s) involved and determine if it is central or peripheral in origin. Learn which and nerve roots innervate the major muscle groups.

Body Position. Observe the patient's body position during movement and at rest.

Abnormal positions alert you to conditions such as mono- or hemiparesis from stroke. See Table 27-12, Abnormal Body Postures, p. 987.

Involuntary Movements. Watch for involuntary movements such as *tremors* (rhythmic, oscillating movements), *tics* (sudden, rapid, repetitive movements or vocalizations that are nonrhythmic), *chorea* (irregular, unpredictable, flowing movements), or *fasciculations* (brief, spontaneous contractions affecting a small number of muscle fibers). Tapping on the muscles with a reflex hammer can stimulate fasciculations if they are not seen at rest.

Noting their location, quality, rate, rhythm, and amplitude can help characterize the type of movement. Observe their relation to posture, activity, fatigue, emotion, and distraction.

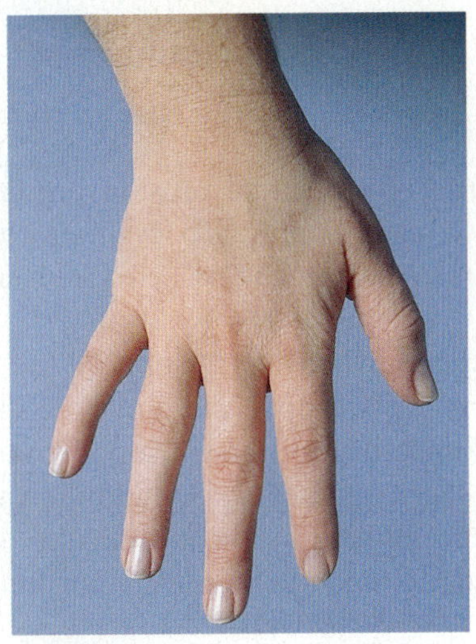

FIGURE 27-21. No interosseous atrophy—44-year-old person.

See Table 27-9, Tremors and Involuntary Movements, pp. 982–983.

Muscle Bulk. Inspect the size and contours of muscles. Flattened or concave appearances may indicate muscle bulk loss due to atrophy or wasting. Determine whether this process is unilateral or bilateral and whether it affects proximal or distal muscle groups.

When inspecting for atrophy, pay particular attention to the hands, shoulders, thighs, and calves. The spaces between the metacarpals, where the dorsal interosseous muscles lie, should be full or only slightly depressed (Fig. 27-21). The thenar and hypothenar eminences of the hands should be full and convex (Fig. 27-22). Mild atrophy of the hand muscles occurs in normal aging (Figs. 27-23 and 27-24).

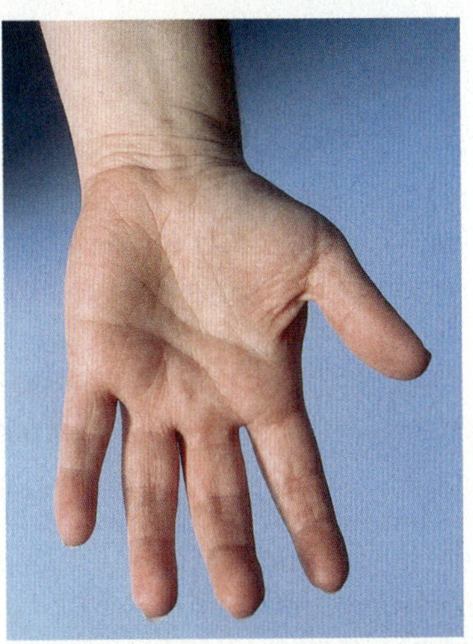

FIGURE 27-22. No hypothenar atrophy—44-year-old person.

Atrophy is a sign of lower motor neuron pathology and can be seen in motor neuron disease, diseases affecting the nerve roots exiting the spinal cord (radiculopathy), and peripheral neuropathy.

Flattening of the thenar and hypothenar eminences (seen in median and ulnar nerve damage, respectively) and furrowing between the metacarpals suggest atrophy.

In the Duchenne form of muscular dystrophy, weak muscles may exhibit *pseudohypertrophy*, an apparent increase in muscle bulk caused by increased fat and connective tissue replacing muscle.

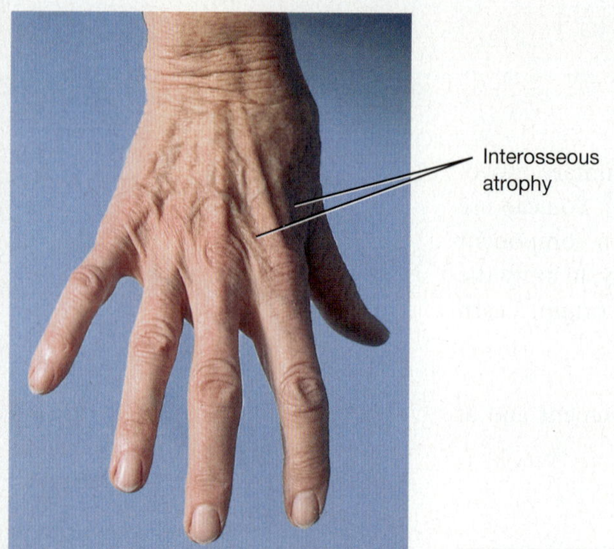

FIGURE 27-23. Interosseous atrophy—84-year-old person.

FIGURE 27-24. Hypothenar atrophy—84-year-old person.

Muscle Tone. *Muscle tone* refers to the slight residual tension present in a healthy, relaxed muscle with an intact nerve supply. To evaluate this, encourage the patient to fully relax before assessing the muscle's resistance to passive stretching.

For the upper limbs, gently hold the patient's hand, support the elbow, and smoothly flex and extend the fingers, wrist, elbow, and move the shoulder through a moderate range of motion. Similarly, for the legs, support the thigh with one hand, grasp the foot with the other, and flex and extend the knee and ankle on each side. Observe the resistance offered by the muscle during these movements, noting any increased resistance that could indicate tension in the patient.

Decreased resistance (*hypotonia*) suggests disease of the PNS or cerebellum or the acute stages of spinal cord injury. See Table 27-13, Disorders of Muscle Tone, p. 988.

If you suspect decreased resistance, hold the forearm, and gently shake the patient's forearm, and observe how freely the hand moves back and forth. Normal muscle tone allows for free movement but not complete floppiness.

Marked floppiness indicates muscle hypotonia or flaccidity, usually from a peripheral motor system disorder.

If resistance is increased, determine if it varies as you move the limb or persists throughout the full range of motion and if it persists in both directions, for example, during both flexion and extension (Box 27-14). Vary the speed at which you move the limb. Feel for any jerkiness in the resistance.

Box 27-14. Spasticity and Rigidity in Neurologic Conditions

Term	Characteristics	Commonly Associated With
Spasticity	Increased tone that is velocity-dependent and worsens at extremes of range; resistance increases with more rapid movement	Central diseases affecting the corticospinal tract
Rigidity	Increased tone that remains constant throughout the range of motion; not velocity-dependent	Central disorders affecting the basal ganglia, like Parkinson disease

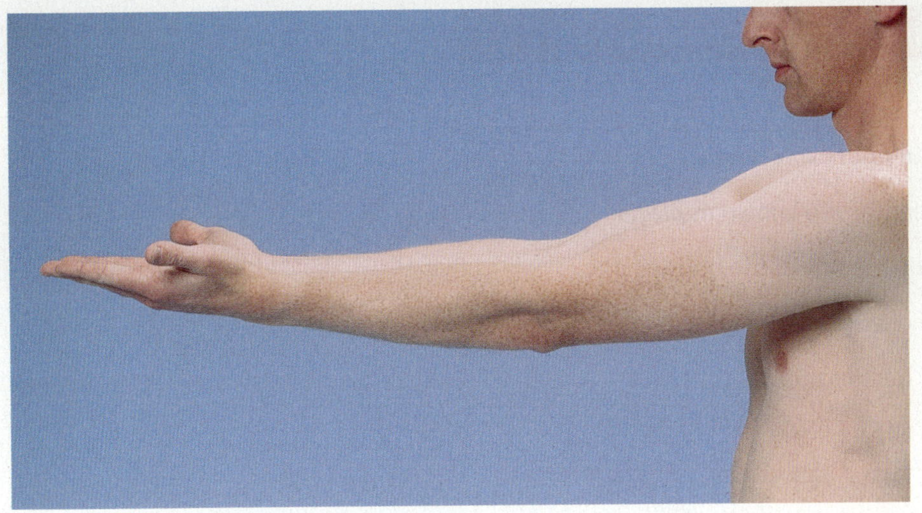

FIGURE 27-25. Testing for pronator drift.

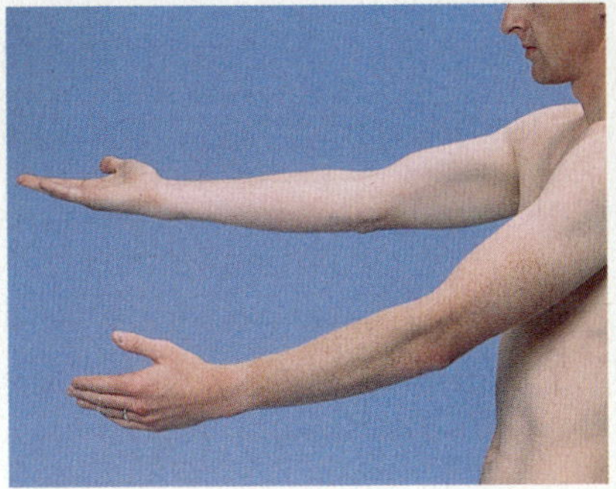

FIGURE 27-26. Positive test for pronator drift of left side.

Pronator Drift. Ask the patient to extend both arms straight forward with their palms facing upward (Fig. 27-25). Under normal conditions, patients are able to maintain this position without difficulty.

Pronator drift occurs when the forearm and palm turn inward and down (Fig. 27-26) and is both sensitive and specific for a corticospinal tract lesion in the contralateral hemisphere. The fingers may also abduct or flex.[60–63]

Next, instruct the patient to keep their arms extended and close their eyes, then briskly tap their arms downward. Normally, the arms should smoothly return to the horizontal position. This test evaluates their ability to maintain arm position and coordination in response to unexpected changes.

In loss of position sense, the arms may drift sideways or upward, potentially accompanied by writhing hand movements. Patients with this condition might not be aware of the arm displacement and, when prompted to correct it, may do so poorly.

In cases of cerebellar incoordination, when the arm is subjected to a positional change, such as in the pronator drift test, it may overshoot its original position on attempting to return to the starting posture and exhibit a bouncing movement both.

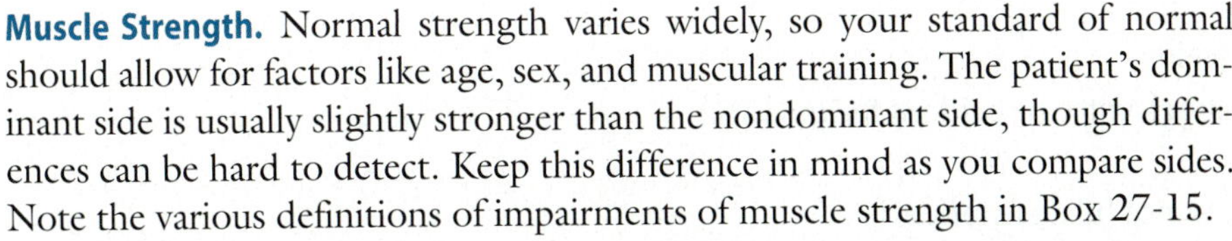

Muscle Strength. Normal strength varies widely, so your standard of normal should allow for factors like age, sex, and muscular training. The patient's dominant side is usually slightly stronger than the nondominant side, though differences can be hard to detect. Keep this difference in mind as you compare sides. Note the various definitions of impairments of muscle strength in Box 27-15.

Test muscle strength by asking the patient to actively resist your movement. Remember that a muscle is strongest when shortened, and weaker when lengthened. Give the patient the advantage as you try to overcome the resistance and judge true the muscle's true strength. During muscle strength tests, some patients may not be able to sustain effort, which can be attributed to factors such as pain, misunderstanding the instructions, an attempt to assist the examiner, or functional neurologic disorders. You must consider these variables to accurately interpret test results.

See Table 27-1, Disorders of the Central and Peripheral Nervous Systems, pp. 965–966.

Box 27-15. Definitions of Muscle Strength Impairment

Term	Definition
Paresis	Impaired strength or weakness
Paralysis	Absent strength, also known as *plegia*
Hemiparesis	Weakness of one side of the body
Hemiplegia	Paralysis of one side of the body
Paraplegia	Paralysis of both legs
Quadriplegia	Paralysis of all four limbs

To effectively assess and document muscle strength during a neurologic exam, a standardized scale ranging from 0 to 5 is used (Box 27-16). Many clinicians make further distinctions by adding plus or minus signs toward the stronger end of this scale. By adding a *"4+"* designation, clinicians can indicate a level of strength that is better than *"active movement against gravity and some resistance"* but still not equivalent to *"full resistance without evident fatigue."* Conversely, *"5–"* rating denotes a slight detectable weakness that does not meet the criteria for normal muscle strength (grade 5) yet is above the strength described by grade 4.

The subsequent sections detail techniques for evaluating the strength of specific major muscle groups. Note that a comprehensive neurologic screening may not necessitate examining every muscle outlined. When assessing muscle strength, compare the patient's muscle performance against your own similar muscle groups to ensure accurate and fair evaluation.

Focus solely on the muscle group under examination to avoid compensatory actions from other muscles. For instance, support the patient's upper arm during tests of elbow flexion and extension to isolate the movement and prevent involvement from the shoulder muscles. Keep the force focused on one joint at a time.

Box 27-16. Scale for Grading Muscle Strength

Muscle strength is graded on a 0 to 5 scale:

5—Active movement against full resistance without evident fatigue. This is normal muscle strength.

4—Active movement against gravity but not full resistance

3—Active movement against gravity is possible, but not against resistance.

2—Active movement of the body part with gravity eliminated (planar motion)

1—A barely detectable flicker or trace of contraction

0—No muscular contraction detected

Source: Medical Research Council. *Aids to the examination of the peripheral nervous system.* Bailliere Tindall, 1986. Used with the permission of the Medical Research Council.

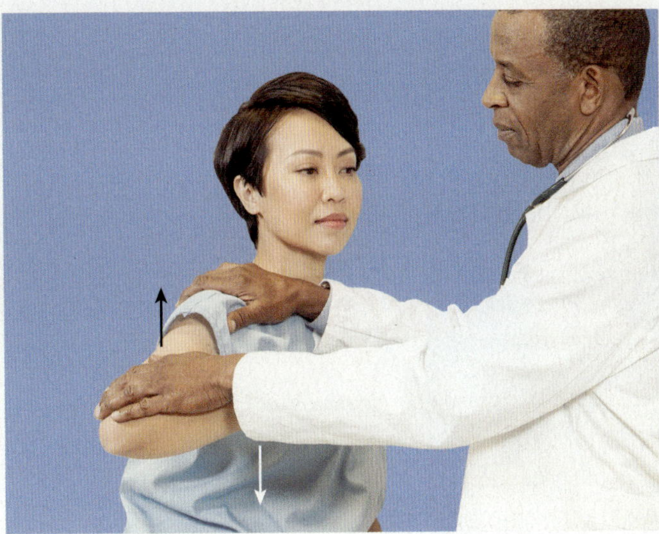

FIGURE 27-27. Testing shoulder abduction (C5, C6, axillary nerve—deltoid).

Additionally, information regarding spinal root innervations and the corresponding muscles is provided in parentheses. This is essential for more accurately pinpointing lesions within the spinal cord or PNS. For more detailed diagnostic procedures, refer to specialized neurology literature for advanced testing methods.

Test Abduction at the Shoulder

Shoulder Abduction (C5, C6, Axillary Nerve—Deltoid). Ask the patient to raise their arm from the side to shoulder level. Then apply firm, downward pressure on their upper arm while it is in an abducted position (Fig. 27-27). Both arms can be tested simultaneously to facilitate a direct comparison between sides.

Test Flexion and Extension at the Elbow

Elbow Flexion (C5, C6, Musculocutaneous Nerve—Biceps and Brachioradialis). Instruct the patient to flex the elbow by pulling against your hand (Fig. 27-28).

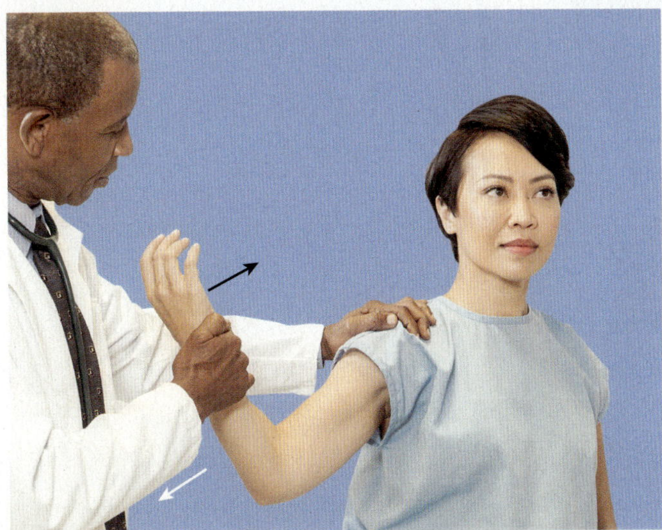

FIGURE 27-28. Testing elbow flexion (C5, C6, musculocutaneous nerve—biceps, brachioradialis).

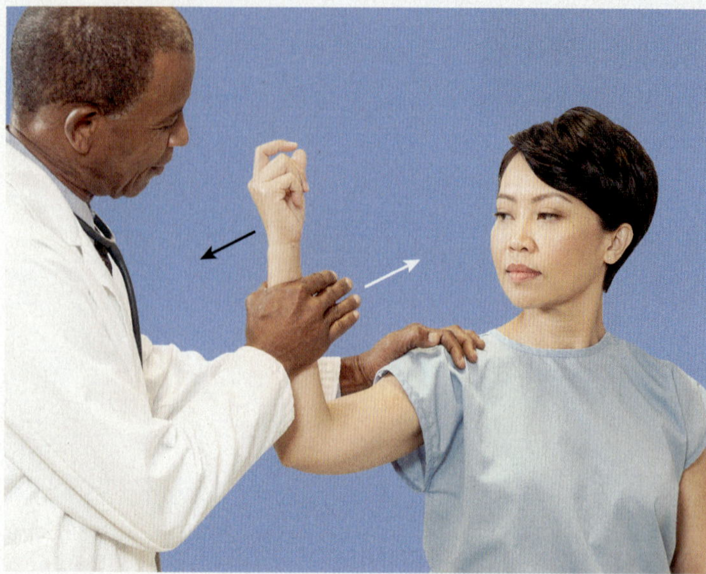

FIGURE 27-29. Testing elbow extension (C6, C7, C8, radial nerve—triceps).

Elbow Extension (C6, C7, C8, Radial Nerve—Triceps). Have the patient extend the elbow by pushing against your hand (Fig. 27-29).

Test Flexion and Extension at the Wrist

Wrist Flexion (C7, C8, Median Nerve—Flexor Carpi Radialis; Ulnar Nerve—Flexor Carpi Ulnaris). For flexion testing, have the patient bend their wrist forward with the palm facing down and fingers pointed toward the ground. Apply upward resistance against the palm or fingers to evaluate the strength of the wrist flexors.

Wrist Extension (C6, C7, C8, Radial Nerve—Extensor Carpi Radialis Longus and Brevis, Extensor Carpi Ulnaris). Instruct the patient either to clench their hand into a fist and resist as you apply downward pressure (Fig. 27-30). Or, ask them to extend their forearms with fingers straight and palms up, then press down on their palms.

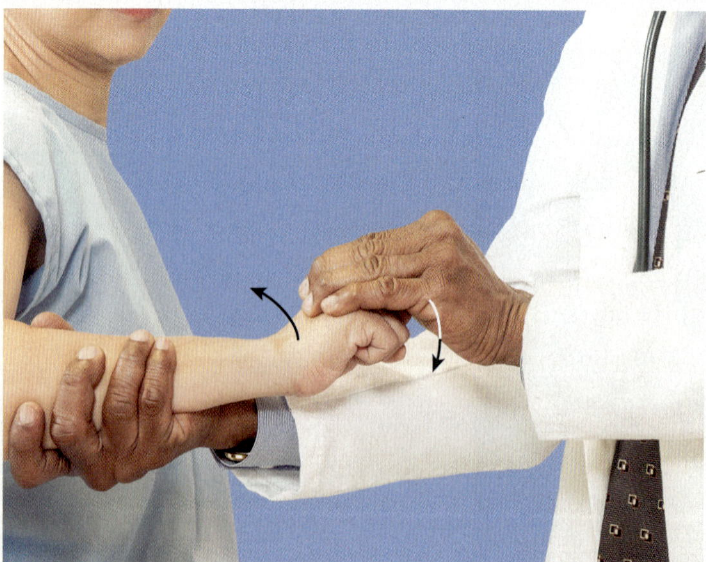

FIGURE 27-30. Testing wrist extension (C6, C7, C8, radial nerve—extensor carpi radialis longus and brevis, extensor carpi ulnaris).

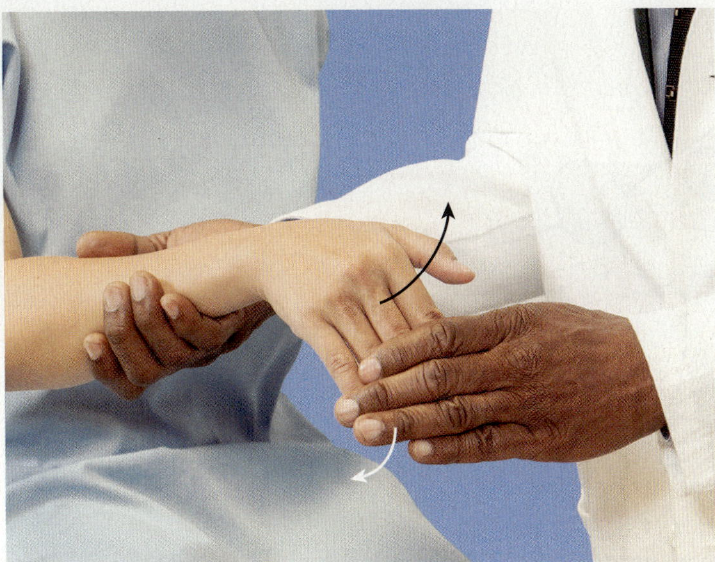

FIGURE 27-31. Testing finger extension (C7, C8, radial nerve—extensor digitorum).

Test Extension and Abduction of the Fingers

Finger Extension (C7, C8, Radial Nerve—Extensor Digitorum). Hold the patient's forearm or palm with one hand, and with the fingers of your other hand, press down on the patient's extended fingers (Fig. 27-31).

Wrist and finger extensor weakness can be caused by radial nerve injury, but may also be seen in stroke affecting the arm area of the motor cortex. Signs of upper vs. lower motor neuron dysfunction or weakness of other muscle groups can help differentiate.

Finger Abduction (C8, T1, Ulnar Nerve—First Dorsal Interosseous and Abductor Digiti Minimi). Place the patient's hand palm down or on its side with the fingers spread and extended. Then, ask the patient to resist as you attempt to push their fingers together (Fig. 27-32).

Weak finger abduction occurs in ulnar nerve disorders.

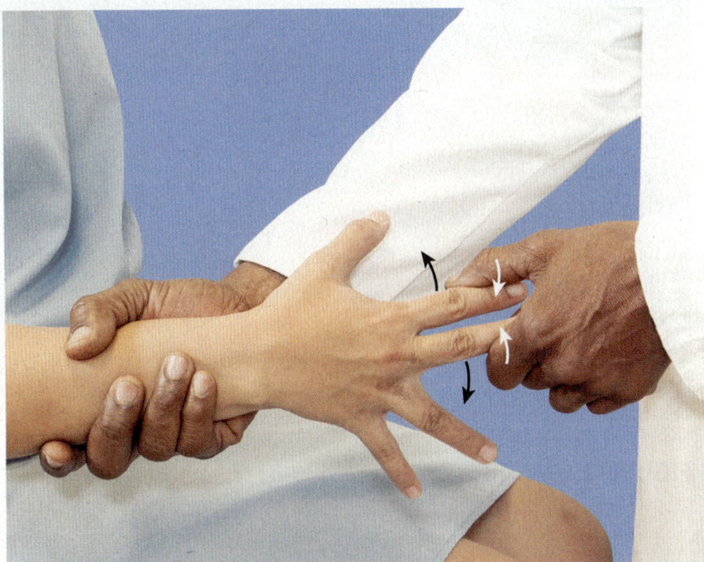

FIGURE 27-32. Testing finger abduction (C8, T1, ulnar nerve—first dorsal interosseous and abductor digiti minimi).

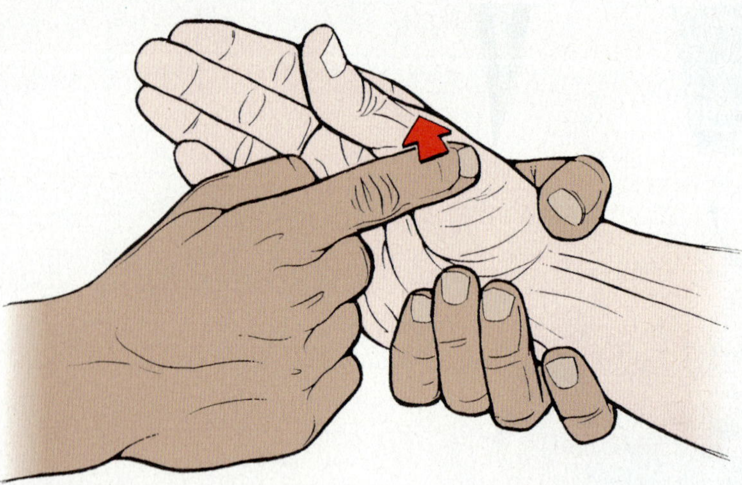

FIGURE 27-33. Testing abduction of the thumb (C8, T1, median nerve—abductor pollicis brevis). (MediClip image copyright © 2003 Lippincott Williams & Wilkins. All rights reserved.)

Test for Adduction and Abduction of the Thumb

Test Adduction of the Thumb (C8, T1, Ulnar Nerve—Adductor Pollicis). With the patient's forearm in a supinated position (palm facing upward), ask the patient to bring their thumb across the palm toward the base of the little finger. Apply resistance by attempting to pull the thumb away from the palm.

Test Abduction of the Thumb (C8, T1, Median Nerve—Abductor Pollicis Brevis). Place the patient's forearm in a position so that their palm is facing upward, fully supinated. Instruct the patient to extend the thumb upward toward the ceiling. Then, attempt to press the thumb directly down into the palm (Fig. 27-33).

Inspect for weak abduction of the thumb in median nerve disorders such as carpal tunnel syndrome (see Chapter 25, Musculoskeletal System: Neck, Shoulders, and Upper Extremities, pp. 827–828).

Test Flexion and Extension at the Hips

Hip Flexion (L2, L3, L4, Femoral Nerve—Iliopsoas). Whether the patient is seated or lying down, place your hand on the middle of their thigh. Instruct them to lift their leg against your resistance, as shown in Figure 27-34.

Hip Extension (S1—Gluteus Maximus). Ask the patient to lie on their stomach and then lift the leg off the bed. Apply downward pressure on the posterior thigh to assess resistance.

FIGURE 27-34. Testing hip flexion (L2, L3, L4, femoral nerve—iliopsoas).

Test Adduction and Abduction at the Hips

Hip Adduction (L2, L3, L4, Obturator Nerve—Adductors). With the patient either lying down on the bed or sitting, place your hands securely between their knees. Instruct the patient to press their legs together against your hands.

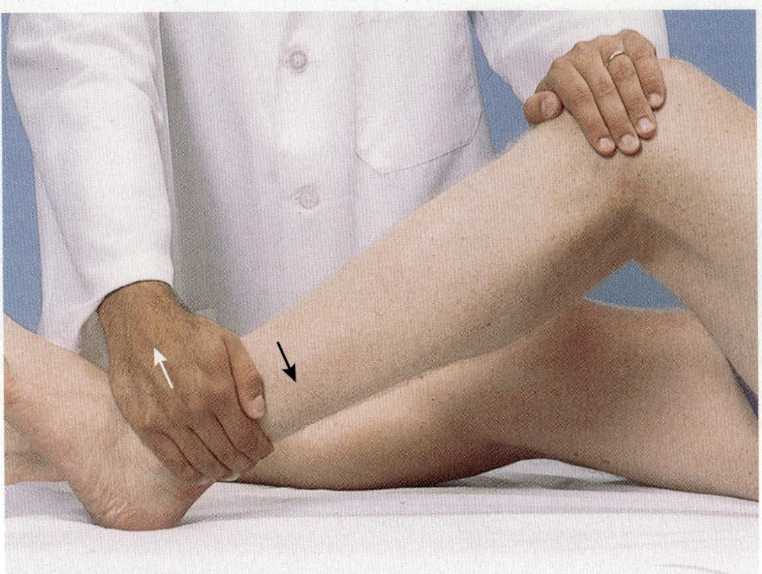

FIGURE 27-35. Testing knee flexion (L5, S1, S2, sciatic nerve—hamstrings).

Hip Abduction (L4, L5, S1—Gluteus Medius and Minimus). Position your hands firmly outside the patient's knees and ask them to spread both legs against your resistance. For a gravity-assisted assessment, have the patient lie on their side and raise the top leg upward.

Symmetric weakness of the proximal muscles suggests myopathy; symmetric weakness of distal muscles suggests polyneuropathy, or disorders of peripheral nerves.

Test Flexion and Extension at the Knee

Knee Flexion (L5, S1, S2, Sciatic Nerve—Hamstrings). While the patient remains supine, position their leg so the knee is bent, and the foot is on the bed. Ask the patient to resist as you attempt to straighten the leg (Fig. 27-35). To test this muscle against gravity, lie the patient prone.

Knee Extension (L2, L3, L4, Femoral Nerve—Quadriceps). With the patient lying on their back (supine), support their knee in a slightly bent position. Instruct them to straighten the leg against your hand (Fig. 27-36). Given the quadriceps

FIGURE 27-36. Testing knee extension (L2, L3, L4, femoral nerve—quadriceps).

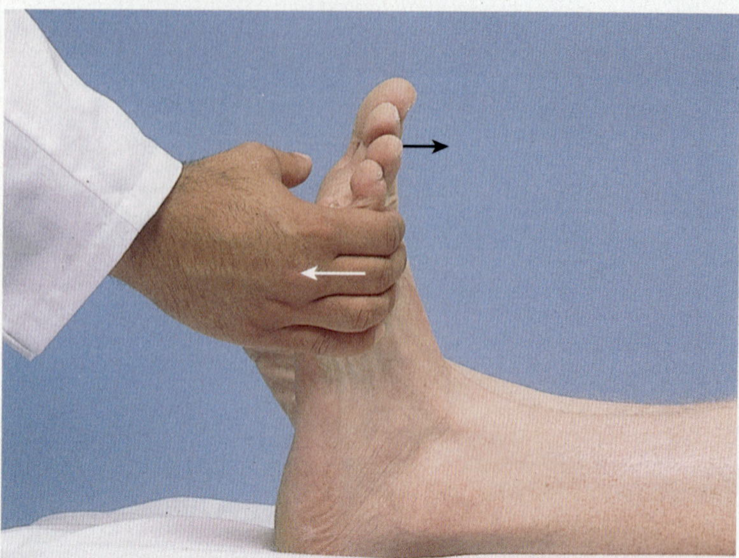

FIGURE 27-37. Testing ankle dorsiflexion (L4, L5, peroneal nerve—tibialis anterior).

muscle's strength, anticipate a strong effort. This test can also be conducted with the patient seated.

Test Dorsiflexion and Plantar Flexion of the Ankle

Ankle Dorsiflexion (L4, L5, Peroneal Nerve—Tibialis Anterior). Instruct the patient to pull their foot upward against your hand, assessing the strength of the tibialis anterior muscle (Fig. 27-37).

Plantar Flexion (S1, Tibial Nerve—Gastrocnemius, Soleus). Ask the patient to push their foot downward against your hand, testing gastrocnemius and soleus muscle strength (Fig. 27-38). Additionally, walking on heels evaluates ankle dorsiflexion, while walking on toes assesses plantar flexion capabilities.

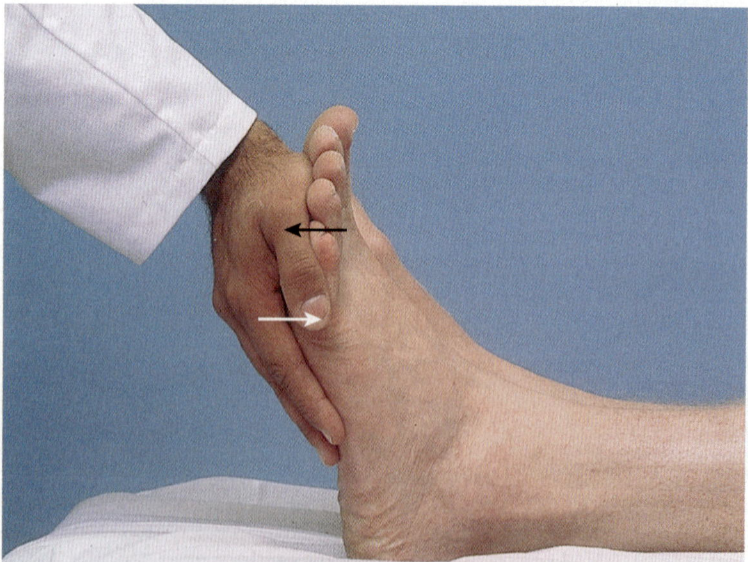

FIGURE 27-38. Testing plantar flexion (S1, tibial nerve—gastrocnemius, soleus).

TECHNIQUES OF EXAMINATION: REFLEXES

Key Components of the Examination of the Nervous System: Muscle Stretch Reflexes

- Elicit the biceps reflex (C5, C6).
- Elicit the triceps reflex (C6, C7).
- Elicit the brachioradialis reflex (C5, C6).
- Elicit the quadriceps (patellar) reflex (L2, L3, L4).
- Elicit the Achilles (ankle) reflex (primarily S1).
- Test for clonus.
- Assess plantar responses.
- Elicit cutaneous or superficial stimulation reflexes.

Eliciting the *muscle stretch reflexes* requires special handling of the reflex hammer. Select a properly weighted reflex hammer and learn the different uses of the pointed end and the flat end. For example, the pointed end is useful for striking small areas such as your finger as it overlies the biceps tendon.

Testing reflexes involves several key steps to ensure accuracy and consistency in your findings. First, ensure your patient is relaxed and position the limbs properly and symmetrically. This helps elicit a more natural reflex response.

The technique for eliciting reflexes varies based on the type of reflex hammer in use, but the underlying principle remains consistent: to deliver a quick, precise tap that effectively induces a reflex response without applying undue force.

- *Using a Thomas reflex hammer:* Hold the Thomas reflex hammer loosely between your thumb and index finger, allowing it to swing freely in an arc. This motion is facilitated by the flexibility in your wrist, ensuring the tap is swift and direct (Fig. 27-39). The key is to let the hammer do the work by using enough force to provoke a definite reflex response, but not so much that it causes discomfort or an exaggerated reflex.
- *Using a Queen square hammer:* Grip the lightweight handle of the queen square hammer near its end to maximize the pendulum effect when striking. The hammer's design itself ensures precision and control, allowing for a gentle tap on the tendon.

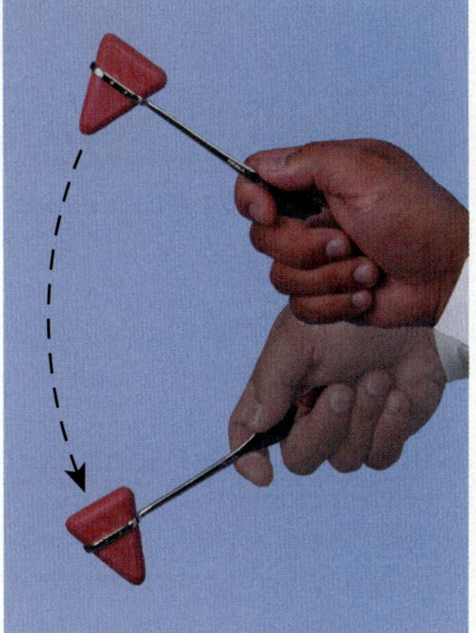

FIGURE 27-39. Proper use of a Thomas reflex hammer: Striking with a brisk relaxed swing.

Note the speed, force, and amplitude of the reflex response. Grade the response according to the scale comparing one side with the other. Reflexes are typically graded on a scale from 0 to 4 (Box 27-17).[64]

Hyperactive reflexes *(hyperreflexia)* occur in CNS lesions affecting the descending corticospinal tract. Look for associated upper motor neuron findings of weakness, spasticity, and/or a positive Babinski sign.

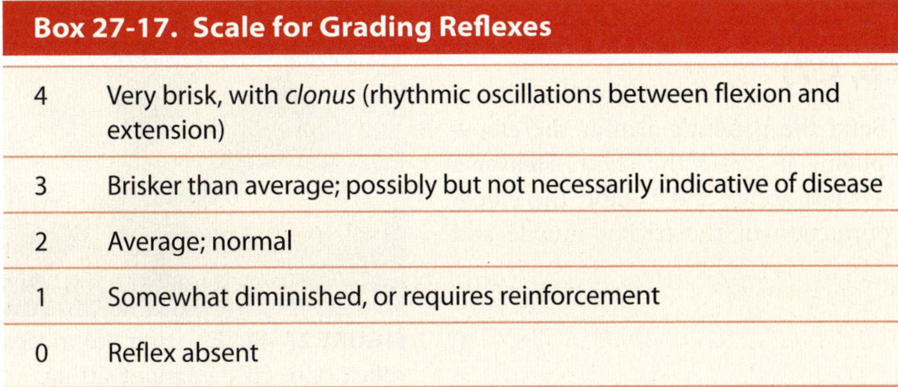

Box 27-17. Scale for Grading Reflexes

Grade	Description
4	Very brisk, with *clonus* (rhythmic oscillations between flexion and extension)
3	Brisker than average; possibly but not necessarily indicative of disease
2	Average; normal
1	Somewhat diminished, or requires reinforcement
0	Reflex absent

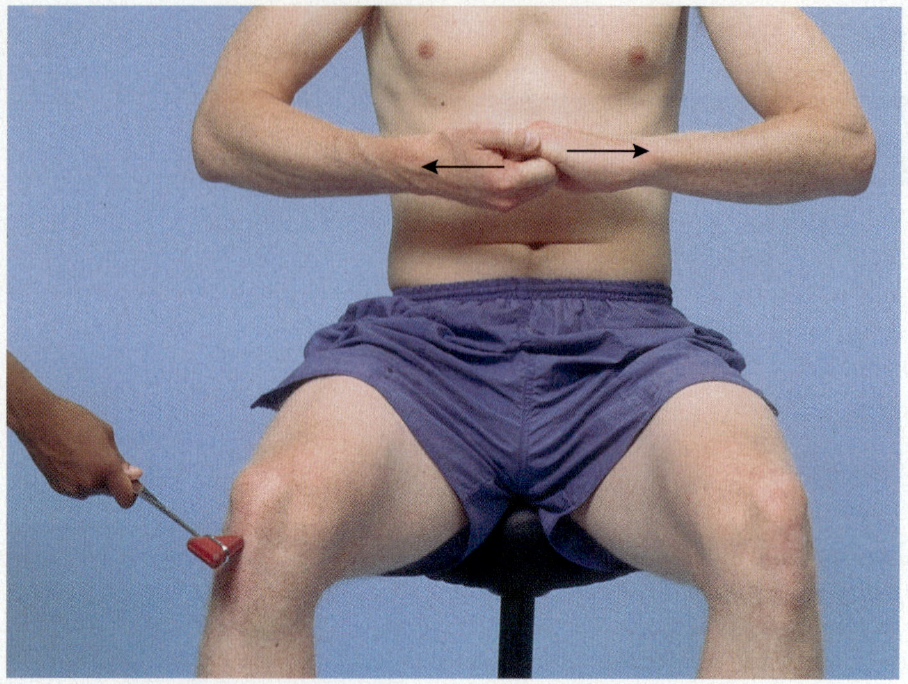

FIGURE 27-40. Reinforcing the quadriceps (patellar) reflex.

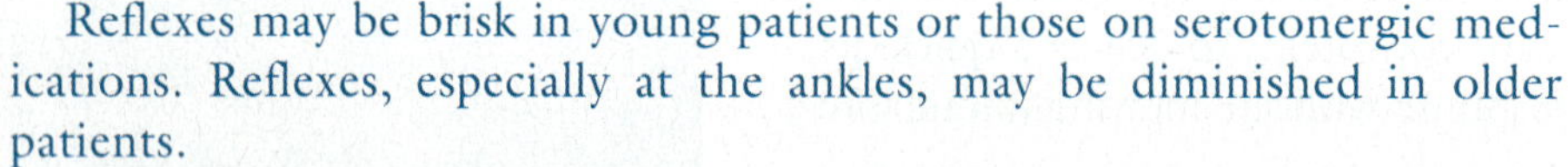

Reflexes may be brisk in young patients or those on serotonergic medications. Reflexes, especially at the ankles, may be diminished in older patients.

If a reflex appears diminished or absent, employ reinforcement by having the patient perform an isometric contraction of other muscles for up to 10 seconds to potentially increase reflex activity. For arm reflexes, this can be done by asking the patient to clench their teeth or squeeze their knees together. For leg reflexes, have the patient interlock their fingers and pull against each hand (Fig. 27-40). If using reinforcement is necessary to elicit a reflex, grade the response as a "1."

Elicit the Biceps Reflex (C5, C6)

The patient's elbow should be partially flexed and their forearm pronated with palm down. Place your thumb or finger firmly on the biceps tendon. Aim the strike with the reflex hammer directly through your digit toward the biceps tendon (Figs. 27-41 and 27-42). Observe flexion at the elbow and watch for and feel the contraction of the biceps muscle.

Elicit the Triceps Reflex (C6, C7)

The patient may be sitting or supine. Bend the patient's arm at the elbow with the palm facing the body, gently pulling it across the chest. Deliver a direct blow to the triceps tendon, located just above and behind the elbow (Figs. 27-43 and 27-44). Watch for contraction of the triceps muscle and extension at the elbow.

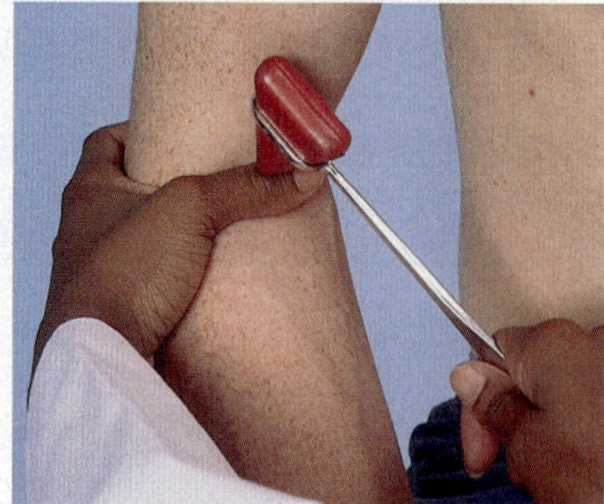

FIGURE 27-41. Eliciting the biceps reflex (C5, C6)—patient sitting.

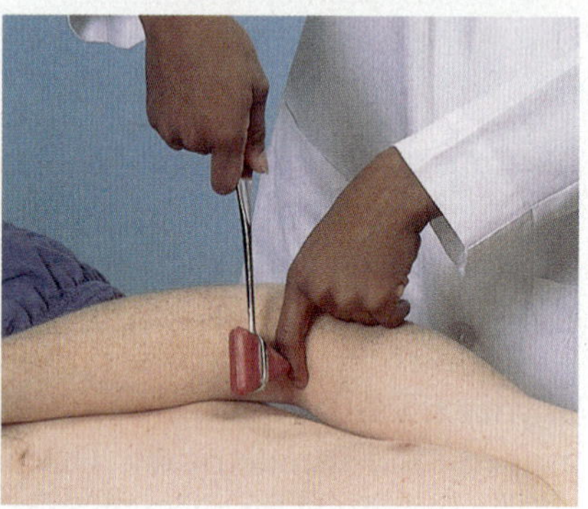

FIGURE 27-42. Eliciting the biceps reflex (C5, C6)—patient supine.

Hypoactive or absent reflexes (*hyporeflexia*) occur in PNS lesions affecting the spinal nerve roots, brachial or lumbosacral plexus, or peripheral nerves. Look for associated lower motor neuron findings of weakness, atrophy, and/or fasciculations.

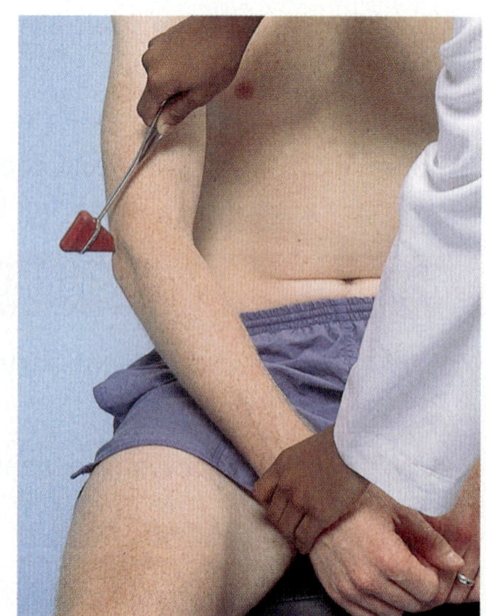

FIGURE 27-43. Eliciting the triceps reflex (C6, C7)—patient sitting.

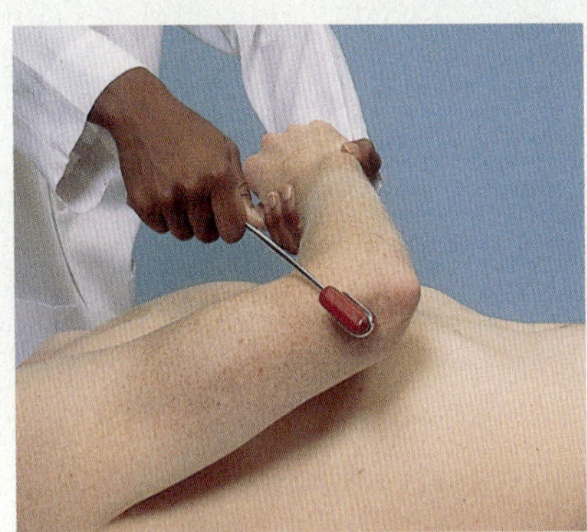

FIGURE 27-44. Eliciting the triceps reflex (C6, C7)—patient supine.

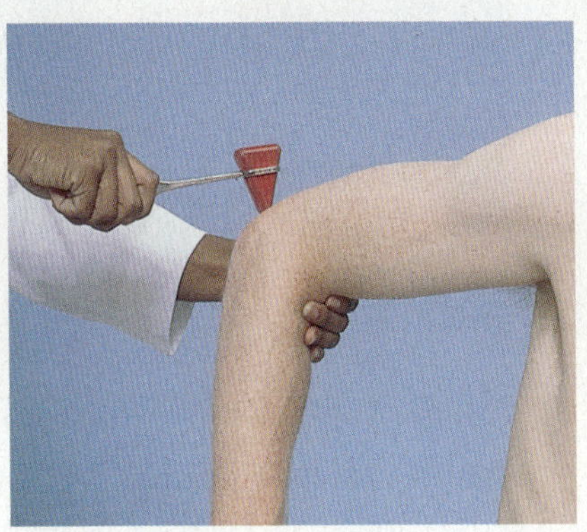

FIGURE 27-45. Eliciting the triceps reflex with the elbow supported.

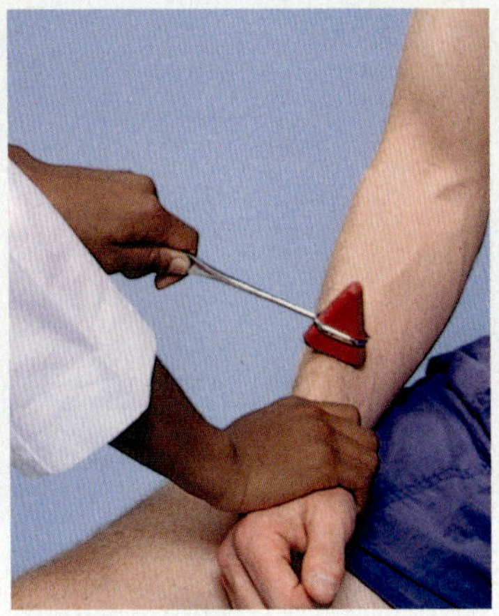

FIGURE 27-46. Eliciting the brachioradialis reflex (C5, C6).

If you have difficulty getting the patient to relax, try supporting their upper arm. Encourage them to allow their arm to dangle freely, as if it were weightless, before striking the triceps tendon (Fig. 27-45).

Elicit the Brachioradialis Reflex (C5, C6)

Position the patient's hand on their abdomen or lap, with the forearm slightly pronated. Use either the point or the flat edge of the reflex hammer to strike the radius approximately 2 to 4 inches above the wrist (Fig. 27-46). Observe for elbow flexion and forearm supination following the strike.

Elicit the Quadriceps (Patellar) Reflex (L2–L4)

The patient can be seated or lying down, with the knee flexed. Briskly tap the patellar tendon just below the patella (Fig. 27-47). Note contraction of the

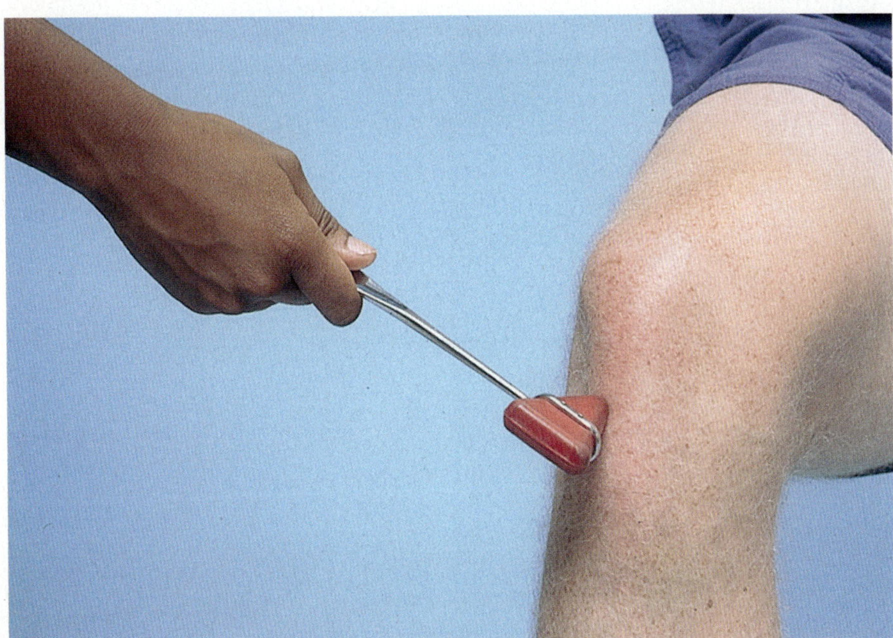

FIGURE 27-47. Eliciting the quadriceps/patellar (L2–L4) reflex—patient sitting.

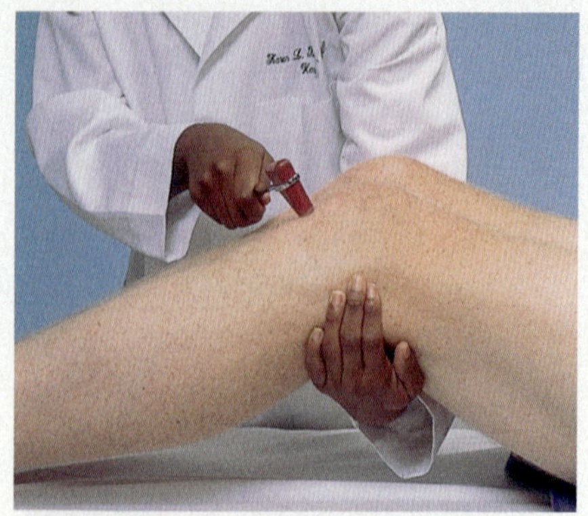

FIGURE 27-48. Eliciting the quadriceps/patellar (L2–L4) reflex—patient supine with both legs supported.

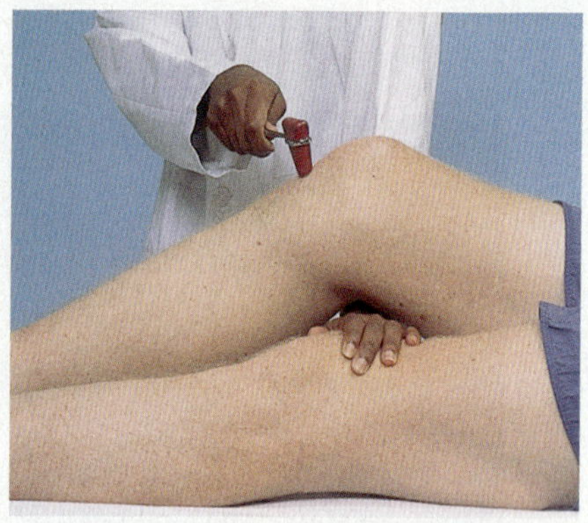

FIGURE 27-49. Eliciting the quadriceps/patellar (L2–L4) reflex—patient supine with one leg supported.

quadriceps with extension at the knee. Placing your hand on the patient's anterior thigh lets you feel this reflex.

For supine patients, there are two examination options: either support both knees simultaneously to assess slight differences between quadriceps reflexes, or place your supporting arm under the patient's leg if supporting both legs is uncomfortable (Figs. 27-48 and 27-49). Some patients find it easier to relax with this method.

Elicit the Achilles (Ankle) Reflex (Primarily S1)

If the patient is sitting, partially dorsiflex the foot at the ankle. Persuade the patient to relax. Strike the Achilles tendon and watch and feel for plantar flexion at the ankle (Fig. 27-50). Also note the speed of relaxation after muscular contraction.

The slowed relaxation phase of reflexes in *hypothyroidism* is often best detected during the ankle reflex.

When the patient is seated, dorsiflex the foot partially at the ankle and encourage relaxation. Strike the Achilles tendon and observe both visually and

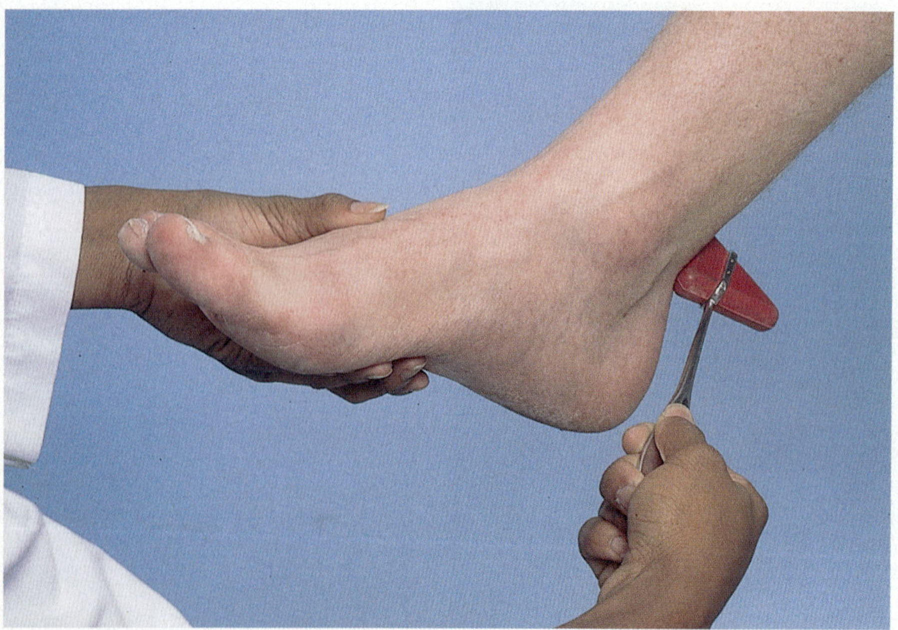

FIGURE 27-50. Eliciting the Achilles/ankle reflex (S1)—patient sitting.

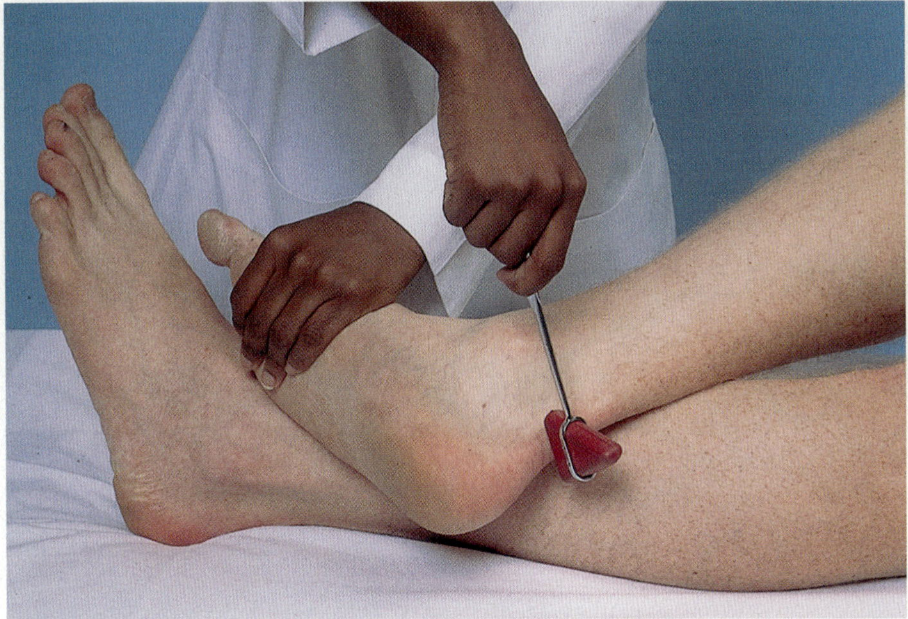

FIGURE 27-51. Eliciting the Achilles/ankle reflex (S1)—patient supine.

tactilely for plantar flexion at the ankle (Fig. 27-51). Take note of the speed of relaxation following muscular contraction.

Test for Clonus (if indicated)

If the patient's reflexes seem hyperactive, test for *ankle clonus.* Support their knee in a partially flexed position. With your other hand, dorsiflex and plantar flex their ankle a few times while encouraging them to relax, then sharply dorsiflex the ankle and maintain it in dorsiflexion (Fig. 27-52). Look and feel for rhythmic oscillations between ankle dorsiflexion and plantar flexion. Normally the ankle does not react to this stimulus and will remain held in dorsiflexion.

Sustained clonus points to CNS disease affecting the corticospinal tract.

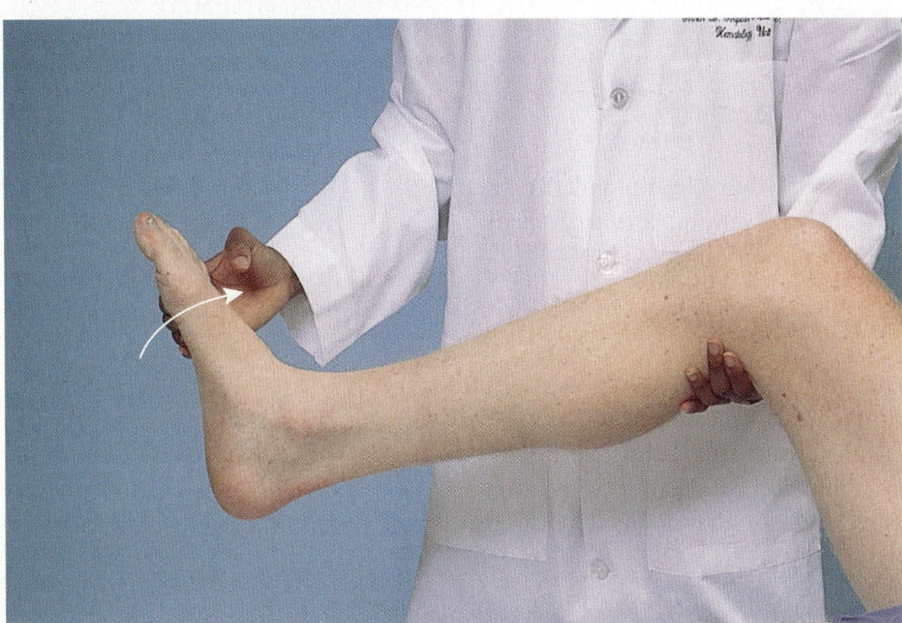

FIGURE 27-52. Testing for ankle clonus.

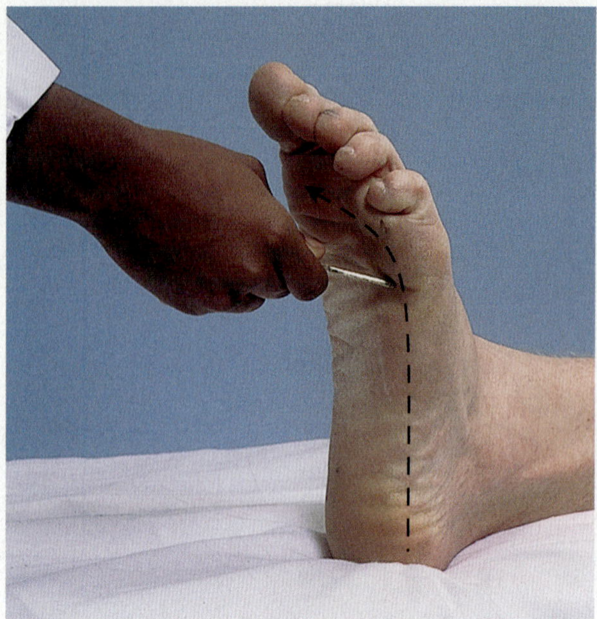

FIGURE 27-53. Testing the plantar response.

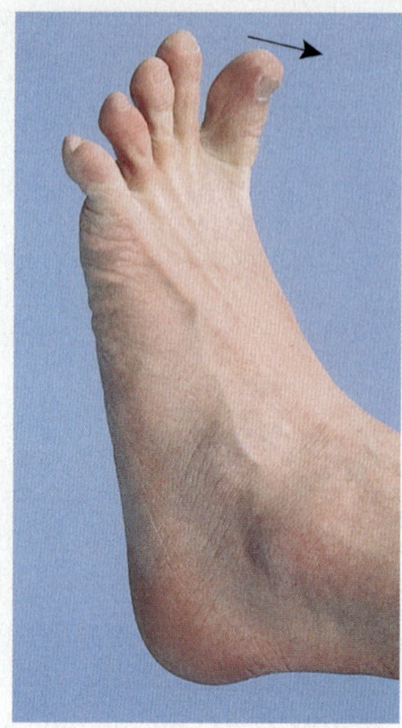

FIGURE 27-54. Abnormal plantar response (Babinski response). Note fanning the other toes apart and dorsiflexion of big toe.

There may be a few clonic beats if the patient is tense or has recently exercised. Clonus must be present for a reflex to be graded 4 (see p. 937).

Assess Plantar Responses

Plantar Response (Corticospinal Tract). Using a key or the wooden end of an applicator stick, stroke the lateral aspect of the sole from the heel to the ball of the foot, curving medially across the ball (Fig. 27-53). Use the lightest stimulus needed to provoke a response but increase firmness if necessary. Closely observe movement of the big toe, normally plantar flexion.

Abnormality can be reported as either an "extensor plantar response" or a *"positive Babinski response"* (Fig. 27-54), and indicates a CNS lesion affecting the corticospinal tract (sensitivity ~50%; specificity 99%).[65] The Babinski response can be transiently positive in unconscious states from drug or alcohol intoxication and during the postictal period following a seizure.

Some patients withdraw from this stimulus by flexing the hip and the knee. Hold the ankle, if necessary, to complete your observation. At times, it is difficult to distinguish withdrawal from a Babinski response.

Elicit Superficial Stimulation Reflex

Anal (Anocutaneous) Reflex (S2–S4). To assess the anal reflex, lightly stroke both sides of the anus with the smooth, blunt end of a cotton swab applicator. Observe for a reflexive contraction of the external anal sphincter. Placing a gloved finger inside the anus during the examination enhances the detection of this reflex contraction by providing direct feedback on the sphincter's response.

Loss of the anal (anocutaneous) reflex suggests a lesion in the S2–S3–S4 reflex arc, seen in cauda equina lesions.

TECHNIQUES OF EXAMINATION: SENSORY SYSTEM, COORDINATION, STATION, AND GAIT

Key Components of the Examination of the Nervous System: Sensory System, Coordination, Station, and Gait

- Assess sensation (pain, temperature, position, vibration, propioception, light touch, discriminative sensation).
- Test coordination (rapid alternating movements, and point-to-point movements).
- Perform gait assessment (casual, walk on toes and heels, tandem).
- Assess station (Romberg test).

Assess Sensation

To assess the sensory system effectively, your examination may encompass a variety of sensation types. These include:

- **Pain and/or temperature:** These sensations are primarily mediated through the *spinothalamic tracts*, essential for detecting potentially harmful stimuli and changes in external temperature.
- **Position and/or vibration and propioception:** These senses are conveyed through the *posterior columns.* They are essential for understanding the body's position in space (proprioception), sensing vibratory stimuli, and detecting the position of limbs without visual cues.
- **Light touch:** Sensations of light touch are processed through both the *spinothalamic tracts* and *posterior columns*, allowing for the detection of gentle contact with the skin.
- **Discriminative sensations:** This category includes more complex sensory experiences that not only depend on the basic sensory modalities mentioned but also require intricate processing by the sensory cortex. These sensations enable the recognition of texture, shape, and two-point discrimination.

Given that sensory testing can be fatiguing for patients, potentially leading to unreliable results, approach the examination with efficiency in mind. It is not necessary to assess every sensory modality in all patients. Instead, prioritize testing based on specific clinical indications:

By tailoring the sensory examination to each patient's unique symptoms and clinical presentation, you can maximize the efficiency of your assessment while minimizing discomfort and fatigue for the patient (Box 27-18).

Box 27-18. Tips for Detecting Sensory Deficits

Associated Sensations	Technique and Description
All sensations	■ Compare identical regions on both sides of the body, such as arms, legs, and trunk, to identify disparities. ■ Alter the speed of testing to avoid predictable patterns that could influence patient responses. ■ When sensory loss or hypersensitivity is found, delineate its extent by moving from areas of altered sensation toward normal sensation. ■ Pay extra attention to areas with motor or reflex anomalies. ■ Look for signs of nerve damage or poor blood supply, such as areas with abnormal sweating, skin atrophy, or cutaneous ulcers.
Pain and temperature	■ Assess pain and temperature variations from distal to proximal areas, focusing on shoulders (C5), inner and outer forearms (C6, T1), thumbs and little fingers (C6, C8), fronts of thighs (L3), ankle at the medial malleolus (L4), dorsum of the foot (L5), fifth toes (S1), and medial buttock (S3). ■ Prioritize examination of regions where numbness or pain is specifically reported.
Light touch	■ Compare light touch sensations from distal to proximal areas, mirroring the areas listed under "Pain and temperature." ■ Give priority to areas of reported numbness.
Position, vibration, and proprioception	■ Begin testing with fingers and toes; if these are normal, it typically indicates that more proximal areas are also normal.
Discriminative sensations	■ Evaluate the ability to recognize texture and shape and perform two-point discrimination in areas with intact basic sensations.

Assess Pain, Temperature, Light Touch, Vibration, and Proprioception. Before each of the following tests shown in Box 27-19, show the patient what you plan to do and explain how you would like them to respond. The patient's eyes should be closed during actual testing.

Box 27-19. Overview of Sensory Testing Techniques

Sensation Tested	Technique	Instructions to Patient
Pain	Use the stick portion of a broken cotton swab or another suitable tool. Alternate between blunt and pointed ends, applying the lightest pressure needed to feel sharp. Avoid heavy pricks that draw blood. Discard the device after use to prevent infection transmission.	*"With your eyes closed, please tell me if this feels sharp or dull. Now, does this feel the same as this?"*

Analgesia refers to absence of pain sensation. *Hypoalgesia* refers to decreased sensitivity to pain, whereas *hyperalgesia* refers to increased pain sensitivity.

Allodynia refers to the perception of non-painful stimuli such as light touch as being painful. This is sometimes seen in polyneuropathy.

Sensation Tested	Technique	Instructions to Patient
Temperature	Use a tuning fork warmed or cooled by running water. This test is often omitted if pain sensation is normal and conducted if there are sensory deficits.	*"With your eyes closed, can you tell me if this feels hot or cold?"*
Light touch	Touch the skin lightly with a fine wisp of cotton, avoiding pressure. Avoid testing calloused skin, which is relatively insensitive.	*"Close your eyes and let me know when you feel a touch. Can you compare this sensation to this one and tell me if they feel the same?"*
Vibration	Use a 128-Hz tuning fork. Tap the prongs on the heel of your hand and place the base over a distal interphalangeal joint (Fig. 27-55). If vibration sense is impaired, proceed to more proximal bony prominences.	*"Close your eyes and tell me what you feel. Now, let me know when you can no longer feel the vibration."*
Proprioception (joint position sense)	Gently grasp the patient's big toe between your thumb and index finger, carefully positioning your fingers along the sides of the toe to minimize additional tactile stimuli (Fig. 27-56). Visually demonstrate the movements of "up" and "down" before testing with the patient's eyes closed. Apply the same principles when testing the fingers.	*"With your eyes closed, tell me if your toe is moving up or down."*

Vibration sense is often the first sensation lost in a peripheral neuropathy and increases the likelihood of peripheral neuropathy 16-fold.[6] Posterior column disease, seen in tertiary syphilis or vitamin B_{12} deficiency, also causes loss of vibration sense.[66]

Loss of proprioception or position sense, like loss of vibration sense, is seen in tertiary syphilis, multiple sclerosis, or B_{12} deficiency from posterior column damage, and in diabetic neuropathy.

Assess Discriminative Sensations. Because discriminative sensations depend on touch and position sense, they are useful only when these sensations are either intact or only slightly impaired. During all the tests in Box 27-20, ensure the patient's eyes are closed to rely solely on their tactile and proprioceptive senses.

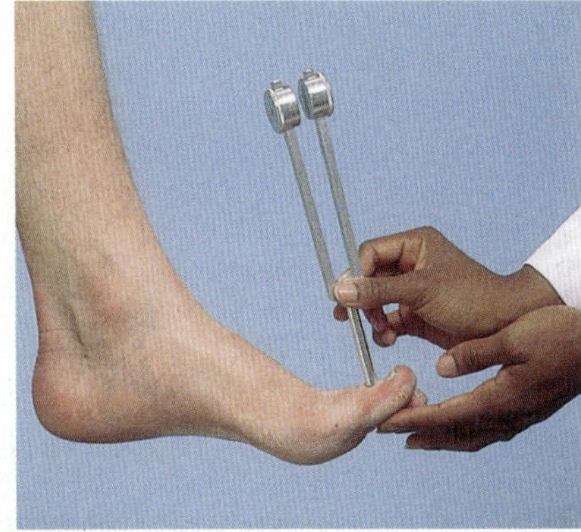

FIGURE 27-55. Testing vibration sense.

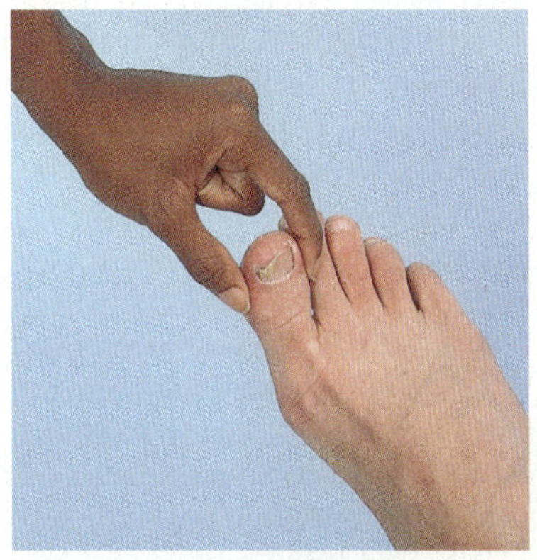

FIGURE 27-56. Testing joint position sense (proprioception).

Box 27-20. Sensory Examination Techniques: Discriminative Sensations

Sensory Test	Technique	Instructions to Patient
Stereognosis: ability to recognize an object by touch alone.	Place a familiar object (e.g., coin, paper clip, key, pencil, cotton ball) in the patient's hand. Observe if the patient can manipulate it skillfully and identify it within 5 seconds.	*"Please tell me what the object is by feeling it."*
Graphesthesia: ability to recognize writing on the skin purely by the sensation of touch.	Use the blunt end of a pen or pencil to draw a large number in the patient's palm (Fig. 27-57).	*"Tell me what number I am drawing on your palm."*
Point localization: ability to locate the point on the skin that has been touched.	Briefly touch a point on the patient's skin, then ask the patient to open their eyes and point to the place touched.	*"Point to where you felt my touch."*
Extinction: ability to perceive touch stimuli applied to two symmetrical areas of the body simultaneously.	Touch each arm individually, then touch corresponding areas on both arms simultaneously. Ask the patient to indicate where they felt the touch with each stimulus. Test the face and legs in the same manner if needed.	*"Tell me where you feel my touch."*

Astereognosis refers to the inability to recognize objects placed in the hand.

The inability to recognize numbers, or *agraphesthesia*, indicates a lesion in the sensory cortex.

Lesions of the sensory cortex impair the ability to localize points accurately.

In sensory neglect, stimuli on one side of the body are ignored despite intact primary sensory modalities. With extinction to double simultaneous stimulation, patients will correctly identify a tactile stimulus if the affected side is touched individually but will report touch only on the unaffected side if both sides are touched simultaneously.

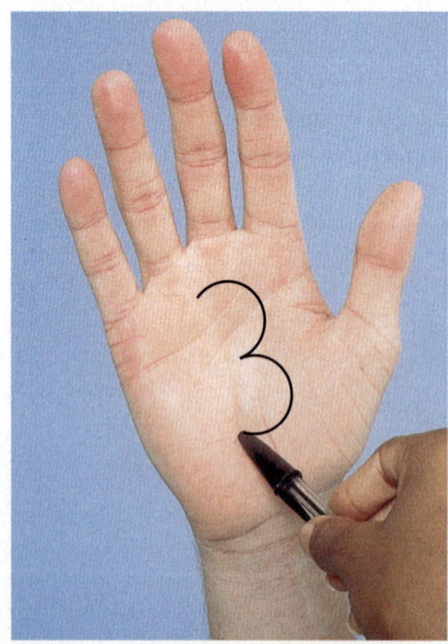

FIGURE 27-57. Testing discriminative sensation using number identification (graphesthesia).

Test Coordination (Rapid Alternating Movements)

The coordination of muscle movement requires four distinct yet interconnected areas of the nervous system to function in an integrated way:

- *Motor system:* This system is pivotal for muscle strength, providing the necessary force for movement.
- *Vestibular system:* Essential for maintaining balance, this system orchestrates the coordination of eye, head, and body movements, ensuring stability and orientation.
- *Sensory system:* Critical for discerning position sense, the sensory system allows the body to detect the position and movement of limbs, contributing to coordinated motion.
- *Cerebellar system:* The cerebellum plays a central role in integrating information from the motor, vestibular, and sensory systems to facilitate smooth, rhythmic movements and maintain steady posture.

Rapid Alternating Arm Movements. Show the patient how to strike one hand on their thigh, raise the hand, turn it over, and then strike the back of their hand down on the same place. Urge the patient to repeat these alternating movements as rapidly as possible (Fig. 27-58). Observe the speed, rhythm, and smoothness of the movements. Repeat with the other hand. The nondominant hand may perform less well.

In cerebellar disease, instead of alternating quickly, these movements are slow, irregular, and clumsy (*dysdiadochokinesis*).

Rapid Finger Tapping. Show the patient how to tap the distal joint of their thumb with the tip of their index finger, again as rapidly as possible (Fig. 27-59). Again, observe the speed, rhythm, and smoothness of the movements. The nondominant side often performs less well.

Cerebellar disease causes finger tapping to be imprecise, with an irregular rhythm. Upper motor neuron weakness and basal ganglia disease can also impair these movements, but not in the same manner. Movements will be slow and low amplitude.

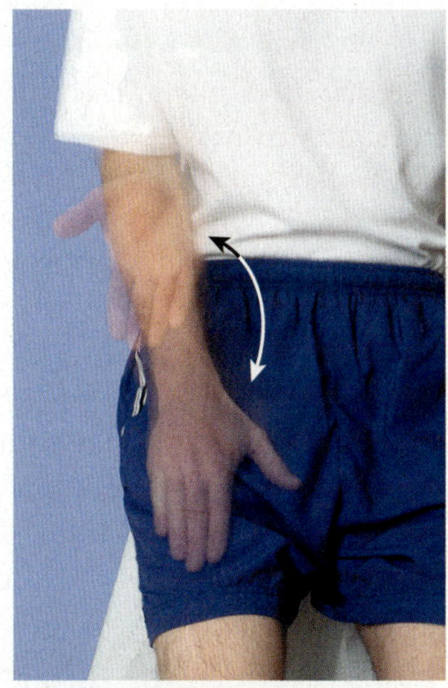

FIGURE 27-58. Testing coordination with rapid alternating arm movement.

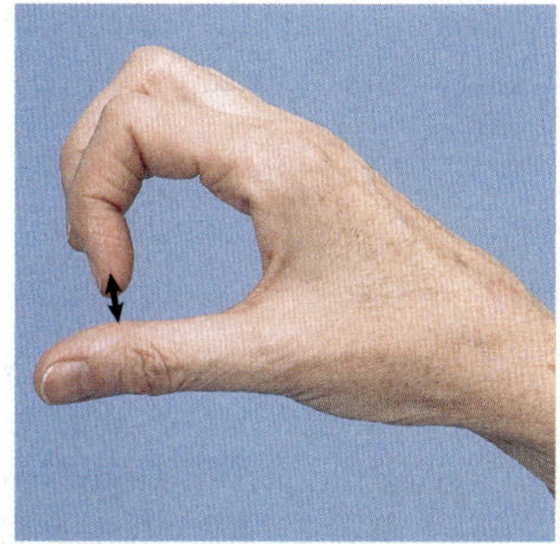

FIGURE 27-59. Testing coordination with rapid finger tapping.

Rapid Foot Tapping. Ask the patient to tap the ball of each foot in turn as quickly as possible on your hand or the floor. Note any slowness or awkwardness. Normally the feet do not perform as well as the hands.

Test Coordination (Point-to-Point Movements)

Finger-to-Nose Test. Ask the patient to alternately touch your index finger and their nose several times. Move your finger so that the patient must fully extend their arm to reach it, observing the accuracy and smoothness of movement and watching for any tremor.

In cerebellar disease, movements are clumsy, unsteady, and inappropriately variable in their speed, force, and direction. If the patient's finger over- or undershoots your finger, this is called *dysmetria*. An intention tremor may appear toward the end of the movement. See Table 27-9, Tremors and Involuntary Movements, pp. 982–983.

Next, hold your finger in a fixed position and instruct the patient to alternately touch their nose and your finger several times. After several repetitions, have them close both eyes and repeat the task. Perform this sequence on both sides. Typically, the patient successfully touches your finger with their eyes open or closed, relying on position sense, inner ear labyrinth, and cerebellar function for accurate movement.

If the accuracy of movement significantly worsens with eyes closed, this indicates a loss of position sense, also called *sensory ataxia*.

Heel-to-Shin Test. With the patient supine, ask the patient to place one heel on the opposite knee, then run it down the shin to the big toe (Fig. 27-60). Observe this movement for smoothness and accuracy. Repetition with the patient's eyes closed tests for position sense. Repeat on the other side.

In cerebellar disease, the heel may overshoot the knee (*dysmetria*), then oscillate from side to side down the shin (*intention tremor*). If position sense is absent, the heel lifts too high and the patient tries to look. With eyes closed, performance is poor.

Perform Gait Assessment

Casual Gait Assessment. Instruct the patient to rise from a sitting position without using their arms to push up, ensuring their arms are crossed across the chest to maintain balance. Then, have them walk across the room or down the hall, followed by a turn and return. Observe their posture, stance, balance, arm swing symmetry, and leg movements. Normally, balance remains intact, arms swing symmetrically at the sides, and turns are executed smoothly.

Difficulty rising from a chair suggests proximal weakness (extensors of the hip), weakness of the quadriceps (extensor of the knee), or both. See Box 30-12, Timed Get Up and Go Test in Chapter 30, Older Adults, pp. 11–76.

A wide-based, uncoordinated gait with reeling and instability is *ataxic*. Ataxia is seen in cerebellar disease, loss of position sense, and intoxication. Patients with Parkinson disease walk slowly with a stooped posture, shuffling short steps, and minimal arm-swing, See Table 27-3, Abnormalities of Gait and Posture, p. 969.

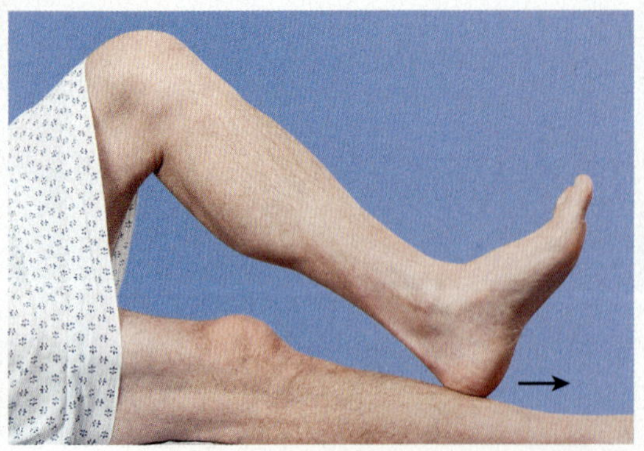

FIGURE 27-60. Testing coordination with heel-to-shin test. (Reprinted with permission from Weber JR, Kelley JH. *Health Assessment in Nursing*. 6th ed. Wolters Kluwer; 2018. Figure 25-22.)

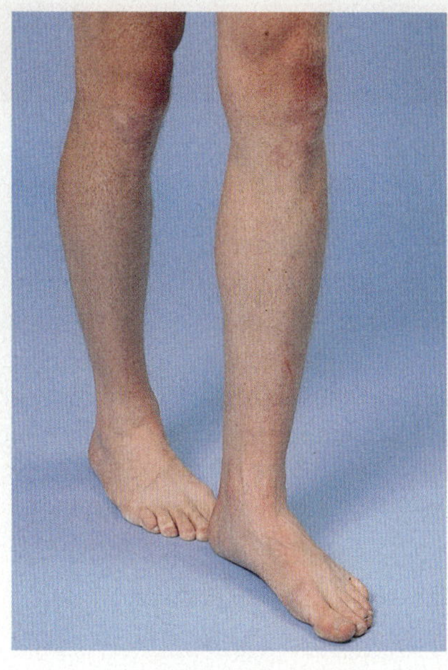

FIGURE 27-61. Testing tandem gait (heel-to-toe).

Tandem Gait Assessment. Ask the patient to walk in a straight line, placing one foot directly in front of the other, with the heel of the front foot touching the toes of the back foot. Instruct them to continue in this manner for a few steps. Observe their ability to maintain balance and coordination while walking heel to toe. Note any swaying, loss of balance, or inability to maintain the tandem position (Fig. 27-61).

Tandem walking may reveal ataxia that is not otherwise obvious.

Assess Station (Romberg Test)

This is a test of *position sense*, but since it requires the patient to be standing it is often performed alongside the gait assessment.

Ask your patient to stand with their feet together, arms by their sides, and eyes open. Ensure they are in a safe and stable environment, such as near a wall or with someone nearby to prevent falls. Ask the patient to maintain this position for about 30 seconds while you observe their balance and stability.

After the initial observation with eyes open, instruct the patient to close their eyes while maintaining the same stance. Again, observe the patient for approximately 30 seconds, noting any swaying, loss of balance, or other signs of instability. Compare their performance with eyes open versus eyes closed.

An increase in sway or loss of balance with eyes closed suggests a positive Romberg sign, indicating *sensory ataxia*. In *cerebellar ataxia*, the patient has difficulty standing with feet together whether the eyes are open or closed.

SPECIAL TECHNIQUES AND MANEUVERS

Detecting Meningeal Irritation

Perform the maneuvers in Box 27-21 whenever you suspect meningeal inflammation from meningitis or subarachnoid hemorrhage. Although these meningeal signs have low specificity, specificity is increased if other signs and symptoms (fever, recent onset of headache) suggestive of meningitis are present.[67]

Box 27-21. Physical Examination Maneuvers for Detecting Meningeal Irritation

Test Name	Technique	Patient Instructions	Normal Response
Nuchal rigidity	Ensure no injury or fracture to the cervical vertebrae or cord, often requiring radiologic evaluation. Then, with the patient supine, place your hands behind their head and flex their neck forward, if possible, until their chin touches their chest.	*"I'm going to gently flex your neck forward. Let me know if you feel any discomfort."*	Normally, the neck is supple, and the patient can easily bend the head and neck forward.
Brudzinski sign	As the neck is flexed, observe the hips and knees for any reaction (Fig. 27-62).	*"Relax as I flex your neck, and let me know if you feel any involuntary movement in your hips or knees."*	Normally, they should remain relaxed and motionless.
Kernig sign	Flex the patient's leg at both the hip and the knee, and then slowly extend the leg and straighten the knee (Fig. 27-63).	*"I'm going to flex your leg, and then slowly extend it. Please tell me if you feel any discomfort or pain, especially behind your knee."*	Discomfort behind the knee during full extension is normal but should not produce pain.
Jolt accentuation of headache (JAH)	Have the patient rotate their head side to side at a speed of two to three times per second.	*"Please rotate your head from side to side as if saying 'no' quickly. Let me know if this action worsens your headache."*	No increase in headache intensity when the patient rotates their head from side to side quickly.

Nuchal rigidity (neck stiffness with resistance to flexion) is found in approximately 84% of patients with acute bacterial meningitis and 21% to 86% of patients with subarachnoid hemorrhage.[68] It is most reliably present in severe meningeal inflammation, but its overall diagnostic accuracy is low.[69]

Flexion of both the hips and knees is a positive Brudzinski sign.

Pain and increased resistance to knee extension are a positive Kernig sign.[68–70]

Meningitis may be present in older adult patients in the absence of these signs, and in those without meningitis, the Kernig sign was positive in 12% and the Brudzinski sign was positive in 8%.[71,72]

Although a positive jolt accentuation of headache (JAH) strongly increases the possibility of meningitis, a negative result is not able to rule out the presence of acute meningitis.[73]

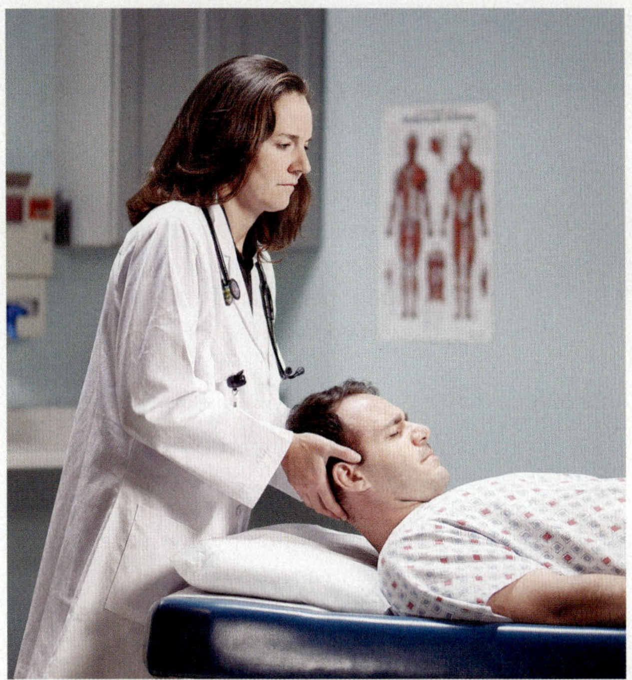

FIGURE 27-62. Testing for Brudzinski sign.

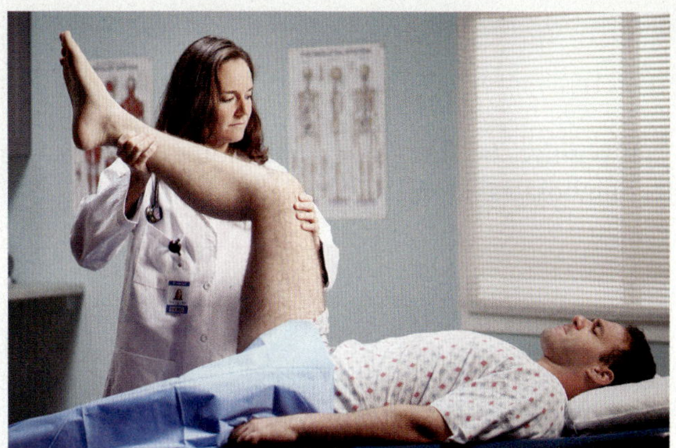

FIGURE 27-63. Testing for Kernig sign.

Assessing for Lumbosacral Radiculopathy

Straight Leg Raise. If the patient has low back pain that radiates down the thigh and leg, commonly called *sciatica* if in the sciatic nerve distribution, test *straight-leg raising* on each side in turn. Place the patient in the supine position. Raise the patient's relaxed and straightened leg, flexing the thigh at the hip (Fig. 27-64). Some examiners first raise the patient's leg with the knee flexed, then extend the leg.

See Table 26-1, Low Back Pain, pp. 893–894.

Compression of the spinal nerve root, as it passes through the vertebral foramen, causes a painful radiculopathy with associated muscle weakness and dermatomal sensory loss, commonly from a herniated disc. More than 95% of disc herniations in the lumbar spine occur at L4–L5 or L5–S1, where the spine angles sharply posterior. Look for ipsilateral leg wasting or weak ankle dorsiflexion, which makes the diagnosis five times more likely.[74]

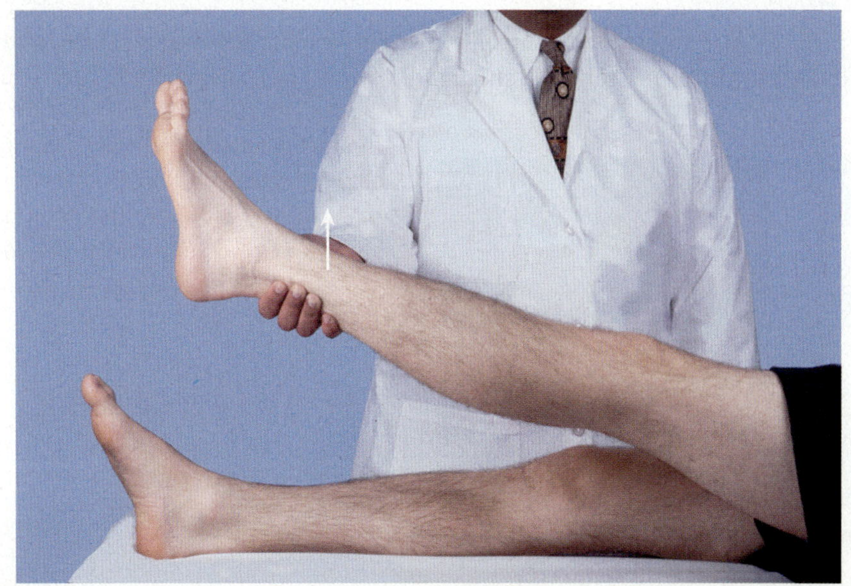

FIGURE 27-64. Testing for lumbosacral radiculopathy with the straight-leg raise.

Assess the degree of elevation at which pain occurs, the quality and distribution of the pain, and the effects of foot dorsiflexion. Tightness or discomfort in the buttocks or hamstrings is common during these maneuvers and should not be interpreted as "radiating pain" or a positive test.

Pain radiating into the ipsilateral leg is a positive straight leg test for lumbosacral radiculopathy. Foot dorsiflexion can further increase leg pain in lumbosacral radiculopathy, sciatic neuropathy, or both. Increased pain when the contralateral healthy leg is raised is a positive *crossed straight-leg raise sign.* These maneuvers stretch the affected nerve roots and sciatic nerve.

If positive, be sure to examine motor and sensory function and reflexes at the lumbosacral levels.

Sensitivity and specificity of positive ipsilateral straight-leg raise for lumbosacral radiculopathy in patients with sciatica are relatively low, with a likelihood ratio (LR) of only 1.5. For the crossed straight-leg raise, the LR is higher, 3.4.[74]

Detecting Asterixis (Flapping Tremor)

Ask the patient to "stop traffic" by extending both arms, with wrists dorsiflexed and fingers spread (Fig. 27-65). Observe for abnormal "flapping" tremor at the wrist. Watch for 30 seconds, encouraging the patient to maintain this position.

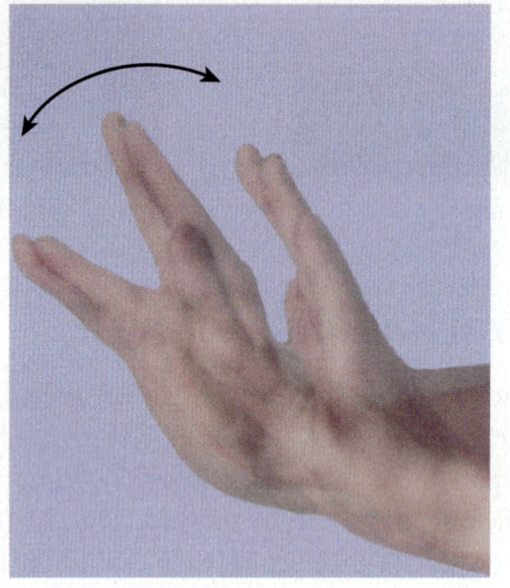

FIGURE 27-65. Testing for asterixis.

Sudden, brief loss of muscle tone manifest as nonrhythmic flexion of the hands and fingers followed by recovery indicates asterixis and suggests metabolic encephalopathy as seen in liver disease, uremia, and hypercapnia.

Asterixis is caused by abnormal function of the diencephalic motor centers that regulate agonist and antagonist muscle tone and maintain posture.[75]

Assessing Scapular Winging

Ask the patient to extend both arms and push against your hand or against a wall (Fig. 27-66). Observe the scapulae. Normally, they lie close to the thorax.

In winging, the medial border of the scapula juts backward (Fig. 27-67), suspicious of weakness of the trapezius or serratus anterior muscle (seen in muscular dystrophy) or injury to the long thoracic nerve. In very thin individuals, the scapulae may appear "winged" even when the musculature is intact.

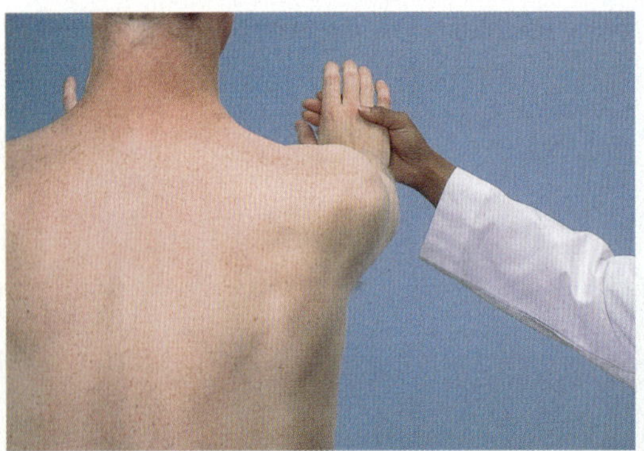

FIGURE 27-66. Testing for scapular winging.

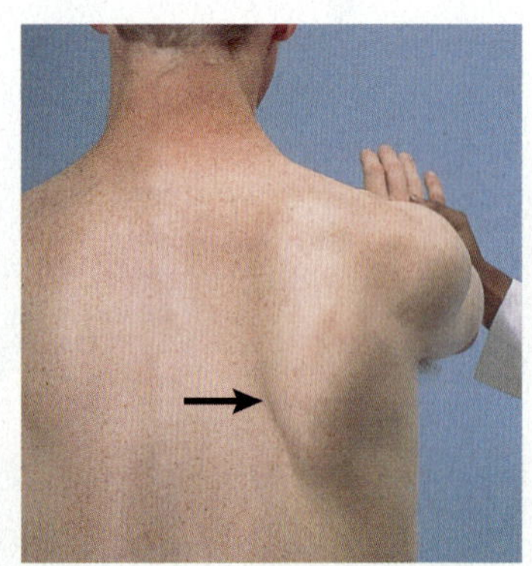

FIGURE 27-67. Scapular winging.

Evaluating Neurologic Status in Comatose Patients

Coma, a state of impaired arousal and awareness, signals a potentially life-threatening event affecting the two hemispheres, the brainstem, or both. Accurate assessment of the severity of the insult and its underlying cause is critical.[76–80] Although arousal and awareness are interrelated, "a change in one is not always associated with a similar change in the other."[81]

To systematically assess and document the neurologic status of comatose patients, clinicians utilize a series of evaluations and reflex tests. The usual sequence of history, physical examination, and laboratory evaluation does not apply. Boxes 27-22 through 27-24 outline key aspects of this neurologic evaluation, detailing specific tests and observations that are essential for a comprehensive assessment.

Box 27-22. Neurologic Evaluation of Comatose Patients

Area of Evaluation	Description and Precautions	Technique and Observations
Level of consciousness	Assess the patient's arousal level. Precise description and recording are crucial to avoid misleading terms.	Assess using clinical levels of consciousness (Box 27-23 and Fig. 27-68) and the Glasgow Coma Scale[82]; increase stimuli in a stepwise manner based on response.

(continued)

See Table 27-14, Glasgow Coma Scale, p. 989 and Table 27-15. Metabolic and Structural Coma, p. 990.

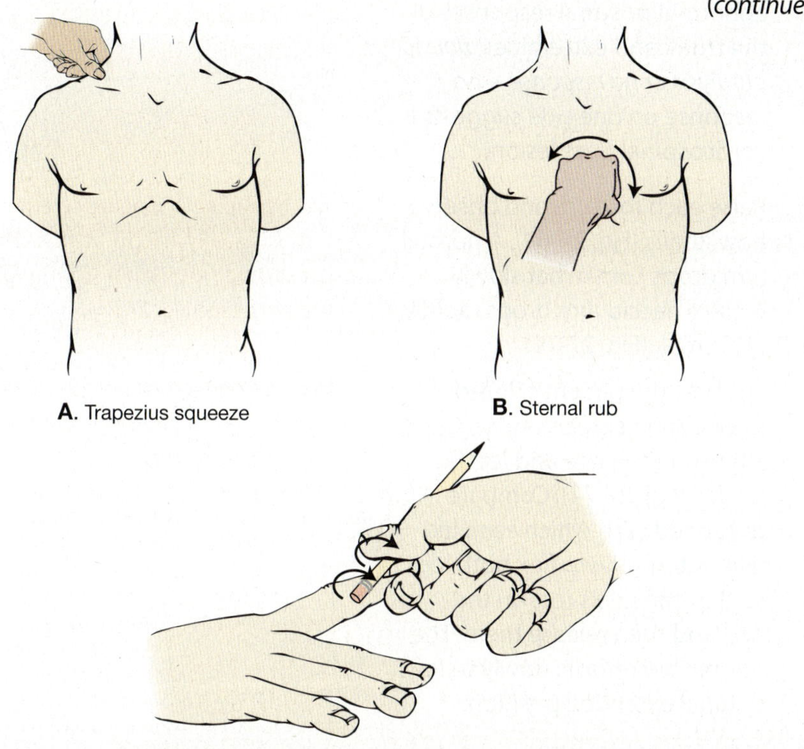

FIGURE 27-68. Maneuvers for testing arousal. **A.** Trapezius squeeze. **B.** Sternal rub. **C.** Nailbed pressure. (Modified with permission from Morton PG, Fontaine DK. *Critical Care Nursing: A Holistic Approach.* 11th ed. Wolters Kluwer; 2018. Figure 36-5.)

Box 27-22. Neurologic Evaluation of Comatose Patients (*Continued*)

Area of Evaluation	Description and Precautions	Technique and Observations
Respirations	Rate, rhythm, and pattern are observed due to their correlation with consciousness levels.	Observe respirations for abnormalities; note any irregularities.
Brainstem reflexes	Essential for assessing the health of the brainstem, these reflexes help localize causes of coma and inform prognosis (Box 27-24).	Perform tests for pupillary light reflex, ocular position and movement, oculocephalic reflex, oculovestibular reflex with caloric stimulation, corneal reflex, and gag reflex; note presence or absence of reflexes.
Posture and movement	Observes the patient's spontaneous movement or response to a painful stimulus, providing clues about brain function (See Fig. 27-68).	Apply a painful stimulus if necessary; categorize the movement response as *normal–avoidant*—the patient purposefully pushes the stimulus away or withdraws; *stereotypic*—the stimulus evokes abnormal postural responses of the trunk and extremities; *flaccid paralysis or no response*—no response on one side suggests a corticospinal tract lesion.
Muscle tone	Evaluates the resistance of muscles to passive movement, helping to assess the integrity of motor pathways.	Raise each forearm and observe how it falls (Fig. 27-69). A normal arm drops somewhat slowly while a flaccid arm drops rapidly, like a rock (Fig. 27-70) Support the patient's flexed knees. Then extend one leg at a time at the knee and let the leg fall (Fig. 27-71). Compare the speed with which each leg falls. Alternatively, flex both legs so that the heels rest on the bed and then release them. The normal leg returns slowly to its original extended position.

See Table 17-5, Abnormalities in Rate and Rhythm of Breathing, Chapter 17, Thorax and Lungs, p. 464.

See Table 27-12, Abnormal Body Postures, p. 987. Two stereotypic responses predominate in coma: decorticate rigidity and decerebrate rigidity.

The hemiplegia of acute cerebral infarction is usually flaccid at first. The limp hand drops to form a right angle with the wrist (see Fig. 27-71).

In acute hemiplegia, the flaccid leg falls rapidly into extension, with external rotation at the hip.

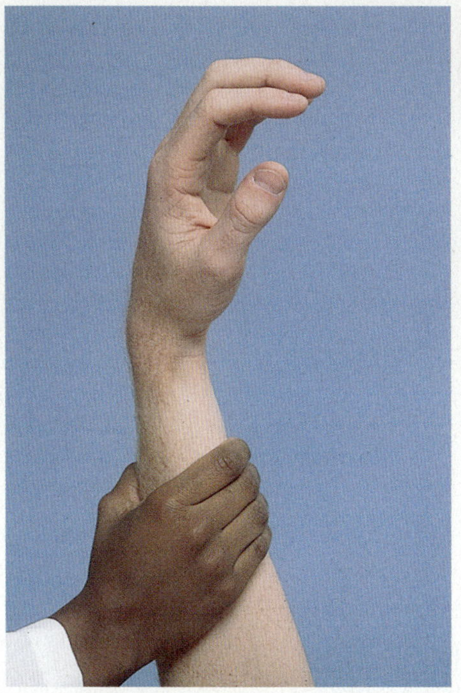

FIGURE 27-69. Testing muscle tone in the arm.

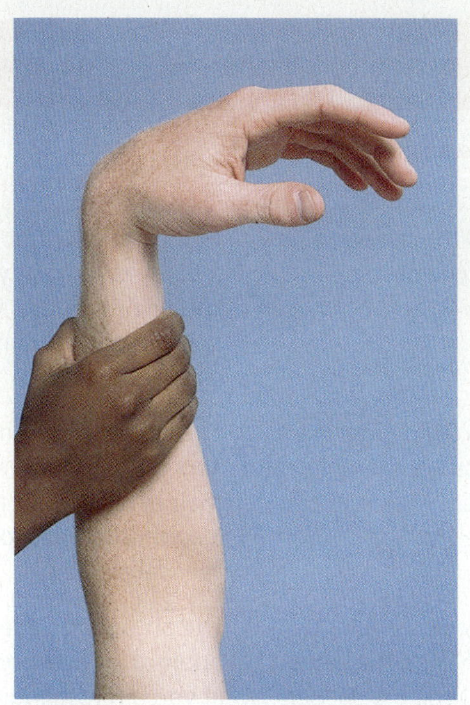

FIGURE 27-70. Arm tone flaccid. Note flexed wrist.

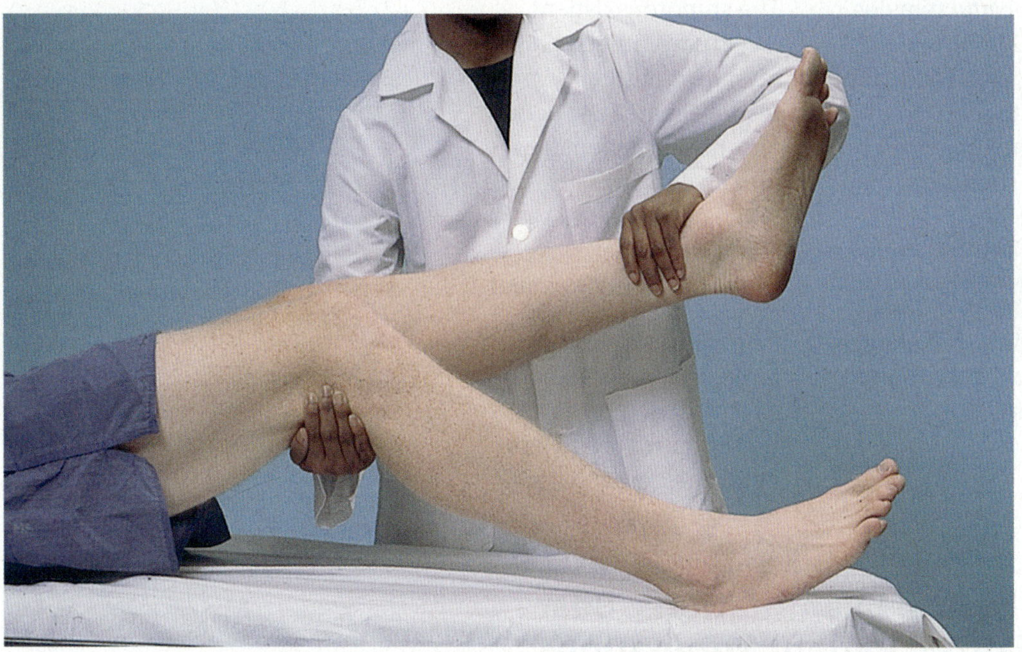

FIGURE 27-71. Testing muscle tone in the leg.

Box 27-23. Maneuvers for Testing Level of Consciousness (Arousal) and Expected Patient Response

Level	Maneuvers for Testing Arousal	Expected Patient Response
Alertness	Speak to the patient in a normal tone of voice.	The alert patient opens their eyes, looks at you, and responds fully and appropriately to stimuli (arousal intact).
Lethargy	Speak to the patient in a *loud voice*. For example, call the patient's name or ask, *"How are you?"*	The lethargic patient appears drowsy but opens their eyes and looks at you, responds to questions, and then falls asleep.
Obtundation	Apply *tactile* stimulus by gently shaking the patient as if awakening a sleeper.	The obtunded patient opens their eyes and looks at you but responds to you slowly and is somewhat confused. Alertness and interest in the environment are decreased.
Stupor	Apply a *painful* stimulus (see Fig. 27-68). For example, pinch a tendon, rub the sternum, or roll a pencil across a nail bed. (No stronger stimuli needed!)	The stuporous patient arouses from sleep only after painful stimuli. Verbal responses are slow or even absent. The patient lapses into an unresponsive state when the stimulus ceases. There is minimal awareness of self or the environment.
Coma	Apply repeated painful stimuli to the trunk and extremities.	A comatose patient remains unarousable with eyes closed. There is no evident response to inner need or external stimuli.

Modifications in Physical Examinations: Best Practices for Specialized Patient Populations

Effective management of patients with ventriculoperitoneal shunts or intrathecal catheters requires specific modifications in physical examinations (Box 27-25). These adjustments ensure accurate assessments of device functionality and patient health, which is crucial for detecting potential complications early.

Box 27-24. Brainstem Evaluation of Comatose Patients

Area of Evaluation	Description and Precautions	Technique and Observations
Pupillary light reflex (CN II, III)	Differentiates between structural and metabolic causes of coma by observing pupil reactions to light	Observe pupil size and reaction to light; note any asymmetry or absence of reaction.
Ocular position and movement (CN III, IV, VI)	Evaluates for gaze preference, which can indicate brainstem or hemispheric lesions	Observe eye position at rest and during horizontal deviation; check for gaze preference (Fig. 27-72).
Oculocephalic reflex (CN III, IV, VI, VIII)	Assesses brainstem function through eye movement in response to head turning (Fig. 27-73); ensure no neck injury exists before testing	Perform head turning to observe doll's eye movements; note the direction and presence of eye movement. In a comatose patient with an intact brainstem, as the head is turned in one direction, the eyes move toward the opposite side (*doll's eye movements*), as shown in Figure 27-74.
Oculovestibular reflex with caloric stimulation (CN III, IV, VI, VIII)	Tests brainstem function by observing eye movements in response to cold water irrigation in the ear; this test is usually not performed in an awake patient	Make sure the eardrums are intact and the ear canals clear. Administer ice water in the ear canal, observe for horizontal eye deviation; note the direction and presence of response.
Corneal reflex (CN V, VII)	Checks blink response to corneal stimulation, indicative of CN V and VII function	Touch the cornea with a fine wisp of cotton to elicit blink (Fig. 27-75). Observe and note any absence of blinking.
Gag reflex (CN IX, X)	Elicits a response from the back of the throat, indicating CN IX and X function	Stimulate the back of the throat lightly; observe and note the presence or absence of the gag reflex.

See Table 27-16, Pupils in Comatose Patients, p. 991.

In structural hemispheric lesions, the eyes "look at the lesion" in the affected hemisphere. In a unilateral pontine lesion or seizure affecting one hemisphere, the eyes "look away" from the affected side.

In a comatose patient with absent doll's eye movements, the eyes continue to look straight ahead, with no movement relative to head position. This is suspicious for a lesion of the midbrain or pons (Fig. 27-73).

No response to stimulation indicates brainstem injury.

Blinking is absent in both eyes in CN V lesions and on the side of weakness in lesions of CN VII.

Unilateral absence of this reflex suggests a lesion of CN IX, and perhaps CN X.

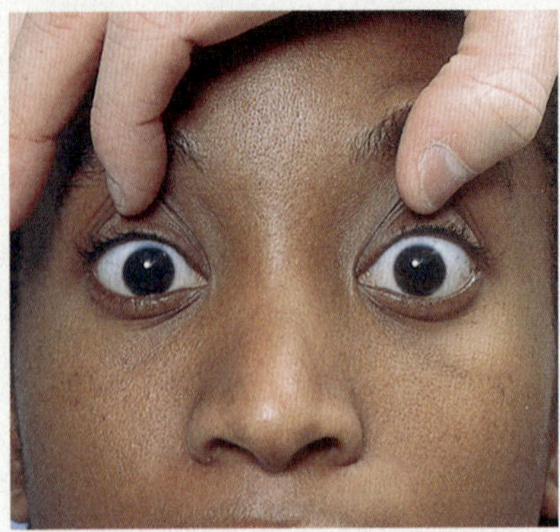

FIGURE 27-72. Ocular position and movement (CN III, IV, VI): Evaluate eye position at rest and check for gaze preference, which may indicate brainstem or hemispheric lesions.

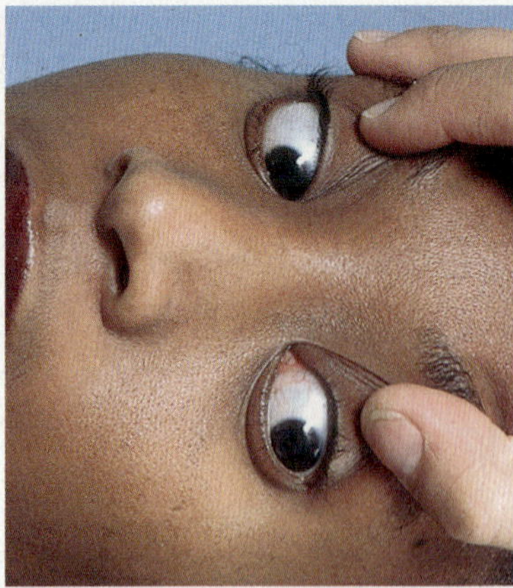

FIGURE 27-73. Oculocephalic reflex absent: The examiner gently turns the patient's head to the left. The eyes remain fixed and fail to move to the right (contralateral direction), suggesting brainstem dysfunction or impaired vestibulo-ocular reflex.

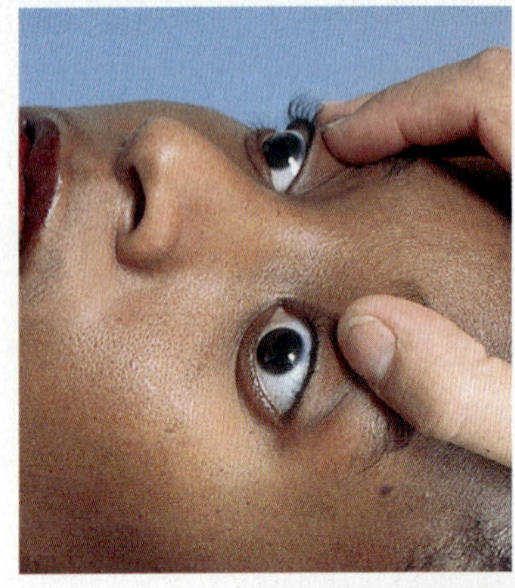

FIGURE 27-74. Oculocephalic reflex intact: The examiner gently turns the patient's head to the right. The eyes reflexively move to the left (contralateral direction), demonstrating doll's eye movement and an intact brainstem reflex.

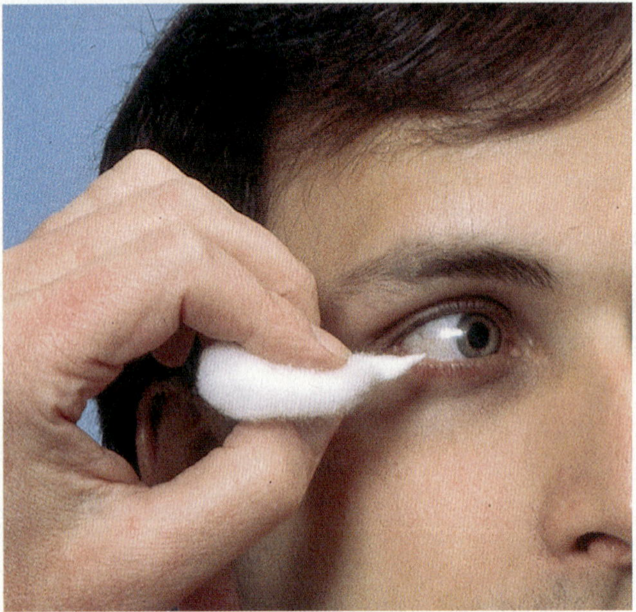

FIGURE 27-75. Testing the corneal reflex (cranial nerves V, VII).

Box 27-25. Neurologic Examination in the Presence of Medical Devices, Conditions, or Procedures

	Patient with a Ventriculoperitoneal Shunt	Patient with an Intrathecal Catheter or Pump
	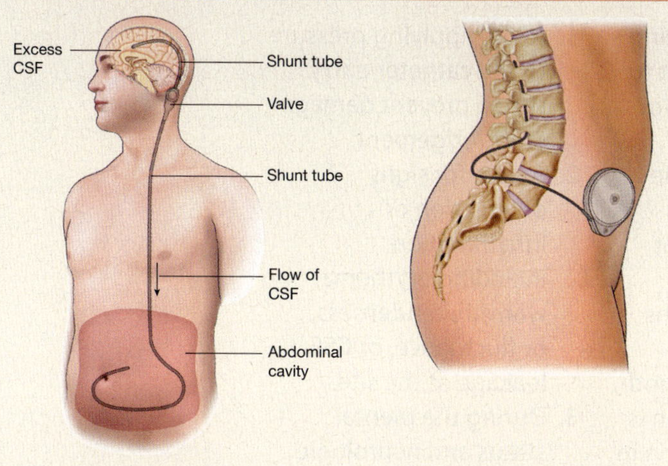	
Device/ Condition	Permanently implanted medical device that relieves pressure on the brain caused by excess cerebrospinal fluid (CSF) accumulation by rerouting it from the brain to the peritoneal cavity	Catheter inserted into the intrathecal space surrounding the spinal cord, typically for drug delivery
General Indication	Management of any disease process that can lead to hydrocephalus or increased intracranial pressure	Administration of medications (e.g., chemotherapy, medications for spasticity or intolerable pain) directly into the CSF surrounding the spinal cord
General Location	Shunt begins in one of the ventricles of the brain, extends subcutaneously down the neck and into the chest, and terminates in the peritoneal cavity; valve to regulate drainage may be present in the subcutaneous tissue of the scalp, behind the ear	Pump containing the medication is either implanted in the abdomen or low back or is located externally from the body, with a catheter extending into the intrathecal space, typically in the lumbar region but can be thoracic

(continued)

Box 27-25. Neurologic Examination in the Presence of Medical Devices, Conditions, or Procedures (*Continued*)

	Patient with a Ventriculoperitoneal Shunt	Patient with an Intrathecal Catheter or Pump
Modification to the Physical Exam	1. Be gentle when palpating the course of the shunt to prevent dislodgement or damage. 2. Assess the course of the shunt along the head and neck and the shunt valve (often located behind the ear) for signs of infection, including erythema, edema, warmth, or tenderness. Infection is a common complication in pediatric patients. 3. Assess for signs of shunt malfunction leading to elevated intracranial pressure, including increasing head circumference in infants, headache, vomiting, irritability, altered level of consciousness, focal neurologic deficits, or papilledema upon fundoscopic exam. 4. Always compare neurologic findings with baseline, if available.	1. Avoid applying pressure to the catheter entry site to prevent damage or dislodgement. 2. Assess for signs of infection or inflammation including erythema, warmth, tenderness, or fluctuance, or CSF leakage at the site. 3. During the mental status and neurologic exams, be observant for changes that might indicate drug toxicity, overdose, or withdrawal. 4. If an implanted pump is present, be gentle when palpating and inspect for signs of pump malfunction or infection. 5. Always assess the patient's pain level, muscle tone, and any other specific indicators related to the medication being administered.

RECORDING YOUR FINDINGS

Note that initially, you may use sentences to describe your findings; later you will use phrases. The style below contains phrases appropriate for most write-ups. Note the six components of the examination and write-up of the nervous system.

Recording the Nervous System Examination

"***Mental Status:*** Alert, relaxed, and cooperative. Thought process coherent. Oriented to person, place, and time. Speech is fluent, follows commands. Detailed cognitive testing deferred. ***Cranial Nerves:*** I—not tested; II through XII intact. ***Motor:*** Normal muscle bulk and tone. Strength 5/5 throughout. No pronator drift. ***Sensory:*** Pinprick, light touch, position, and vibration intact. Romberg—maintains balance with eyes closed. ***Reflexes:*** 2+ and symmetric with plantar reflexes downgoing. ***Coordination:*** Rapid alternating movements (RAMs), finger-to-nose (F⟶N), heel-to-shin (H⟶S) intact. ***Gait:*** Normal stance and stride."

OR

"***Mental Status:*** The patient is alert and tries to answer questions but has difficulty finding words. ***Cranial Nerves:*** I—not tested; II—visual acuity intact; visual fields full; II, III—pupils are equal and reactive to light. III, IV, VI—extraocular movements intact; V—temporal and masseter strength intact, corneal reflexes present; VII—prominent right facial droop and flattening of right nasolabial fold, left facial movements intact; VIII—hearing intact bilaterally to whispered voice; IX, X—gag intact; XI—strength of sternocleidomastoid and trapezius muscles 5/5; XII—tongue midline. ***Motor:*** Normal bulk. Spasticity in the right arm and right leg. Strength in right biceps, triceps, iliopsoas, gluteals, quadriceps, hamstring, and ankle flexor and extensor muscles 3/5; strength in comparable muscle groups on the left 5/5. Right pronator drift present. ***Sensory:*** decreased sensation to pinprick over right face, arm, and leg; intact on the left. Stereognosis and two-point discrimination not tested. Romberg—unable to test due to right leg weakness. ***Reflexes*** *(can record in two ways):*

	Biceps	Triceps	Brach	Knee	Ankle	Plantar
RT	++++	++++	++++	++++	++++	↑
LT	++	++	++	++	+	↓

OR

4+ 2+
4+ 2+
4+ 2+
4+
↑ 1+ 1+ ↓

Coordination: Unable to test on right due to right arm and leg weakness; RAMs, F⟶N, H⟶S intact on left. ***Gait:*** Patient unable to walk independently."

By meticulously dissecting each component of the examination, we can elucidate key findings indicative of focal neurologic dysfunction.

Mental status:

- *Difficulty in word retrieval:* Suggests possible expressive aphasia or cognitive impairment, indicative of cortical or subcortical dysfunction, such as a stroke or neurodegenerative disorder.

Cranial nerves:

- *Optic (II): Intact visual acuity and full visual fields:* Indicates preserved function of the optic nerve, ruling out primary visual pathway lesions.

- *Facial (VII): Prominent right facial droop and flattening of the right nasolabial fold:* Indicates CN VII palsy, commonly seen in peripheral facial nerve lesions like Bell palsy or central lesions involving the facial nucleus.
- *Vestibulocochlear (VIII): Bilateral intact hearing to whispered voice:* Indicates preserved function of the auditory nerve (CN VIII), ruling out significant sensorineural hearing loss.

Motor:

- *Spasticity noted in the right arm and leg:* Suggests upper motor neuron dysfunction, possibly due to a lesion in the corticospinal tract, such as a stroke.
- *Right pronator drift:* Indicative of motor weakness and asymmetry, likely secondary to the upper motor neuron lesion on the right side.

Coordination and Gait:

- *Inability to assess function on the right due to weakness:* Suggests cerebellar involvement, possibly from compression or dysfunction secondary to the primary lesion.

Sensory:

- *Decreased sensation to pinprick over the right face, arm, and leg:* Indicates sensory deficits on the right side, possibly related to a lesion in the thalamocortical pathways or the posterior column–medial lemniscus pathway.

Overall, these findings suggest a *focal neurologic deficit localized to the right hemisphere*, likely caused by an ischemic or hemorrhagic stroke or another structural lesion affecting the motor and sensory pathways. Further imaging studies such as MRI or CT scan of the brain would be warranted for accurate diagnosis and management.

HEALTH PROMOTION AND COUNSELING: EVIDENCE AND RECOMMENDATIONS

Important Topics for Health Promotion and Counseling

- Preventing cerebrovascular disease
- Aspirin chemoprophylaxis
- Screening for atrial fibrillation
- Screening for asymptomatic carotid artery stenosis

In the following section, both traditional terms like "men," "women," "male," and "female" and inclusive terms such as "individuals assigned female at birth" and "individuals assigned male at birth" are used. This approach balances inclusivity with the need to accurately represent the original research.

Preventing Cerebrovascular Disease

Stroke is an acute brain injury that can be caused by cerebrovascular ischemia (when there is blockage in blood vessels to the brain) or hemorrhage (when blood vessels rupture). Nearly 800,000 persons in the United States have a stroke each year, with more than 600,000 occurring as first-ever events.[83] Stroke is the fourth leading cause of death in the United States, killing about 140,000 persons each year. Stroke risk increases with age, although about 5% to 10% of strokes occur in persons ages 18 to 45 years. Compared to individuals assigned male at birth, those assigned female at birth have a higher lifetime risk of stroke, and stroke-related deaths are more common among this group, partly due to longer life expectancy.[84] Individuals from historically marginalized racial groups, such as African Americans, face a significantly higher risk of first ischemic stroke and stroke-related mortality compared to White individuals, highlighting the impact of systemic health disparities.[83] Stroke is a leading cause of long-term disability, and the total direct and indirect costs for stroke in the United States were estimated to be $56.5 billion.

Potentially modifiable risk factors for stroke, many of which are also risk factors for coronary artery disease, include tobacco use, blood pressure, diabetes, hyperlipidemia, physical inactivity, nutrition, and obesity. The U.S. Preventive Services Task Force (USPSTF) has issued guidelines addressing screening, counseling, and treatment for modifiable risk factors, including statin use for primary prevention of cardiovascular disease (Chapter 18, Cardiovascular System), tobacco smoking cessation (Chapter 7, Health Maintenance and Screening), screening for prediabetes and type 2 diabetes (Chapter 7, Health Maintenance and Screening), screening for high blood pressure (Chapter 18, Cardiovascular System), behavioral interventions for weight loss to prevent obesity-related morbidity and mortality (Chapter 10, General Survey, Vital Signs, and Pain), behavioral counseling interventions for healthy diet and physical activity for cardiovascular disease prevention (Chapter 18, Cardiovascular System), and screening and behavioral counseling for unhealthy alcohol use (Chapter 7, Health Maintenance and Screening).

Aspirin Chemoprophylaxis

The USPSTF found evidence that low-dose aspirin is associated with statistically significant risk reduction for nonfatal stroke and myocardial infarctions, although not for cardiovascular or all-cause mortality. Aspirin use was associated with increased risks for major gastrointestinal bleeding and intracranial bleeds. The risk of bleeding was noted be increased particularly among adults aged 60 and older. The USPSTF issued a grade C recommendation for aspirin use in the primary prevention of cardiovascular disease in adults ages 40 to 59 years with a 10-year cardiovascular disease risk at least 10%.[85] Cardiovascular risk can be estimated using the American College of Cardiology/American Heart Association (ACC/AHA) Pooled Cohort Equations.[86] Grade C implies that "decisions about initiating aspirin should be based on shared decision making between clinicians and patients about the potential benefits and harms." The recommended aspirin dose is 81 mg. The USPSTF issued a grade D recommendation against using aspirin for primary prevention of cardiovascular disease in persons ages 60 years and older.

Screening for Atrial Fibrillation

Atrial fibrillation is the most commonly treated arrhythmia and a major risk factor for stroke. Atrial fibrillation is often asymptomatic, although it can be detected with an electrocardiogram or with implantable or wearable devices. Anticoagulating patients with atrial fibrillation can significantly reduce the risk of stroke. However, the USPSTF found insufficient evidence to recommend for or against screening for atrial fibrillation (I statement).[87]

Screening for Asymptomatic Carotid Artery Stenosis

Carotid duplex ultrasound can accurately and safely detect significant (60% to 99%) carotid artery stenosis and is widely used for evaluating symptomatic patients. Although asymptomatic carotid artery stenosis is a stroke risk, it accounts for only a small proportion of ischemic strokes. Based on a systematic review, the USPSTF recommended against screening for asymptomatic carotid artery stenosis in the general adult population (grade D).[88] Studies have shown that carotid endarterectomy reduced the risk of stroke in asymptomatic patients with at least 50% to 60% carotid stenosis.[89] However, the estimated absolute 5-year overall risk reduction for stroke or death was small, and there was a 2% to 3% risk for perioperative stroke and death. Furthermore, the USPSTF found no evidence that ultrasound screening reduced the risk for ipsilateral stroke.

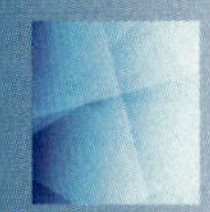

TABLE 27-1. Disorders of the Central and Peripheral Nervous Systems

Central Nervous System Disorders

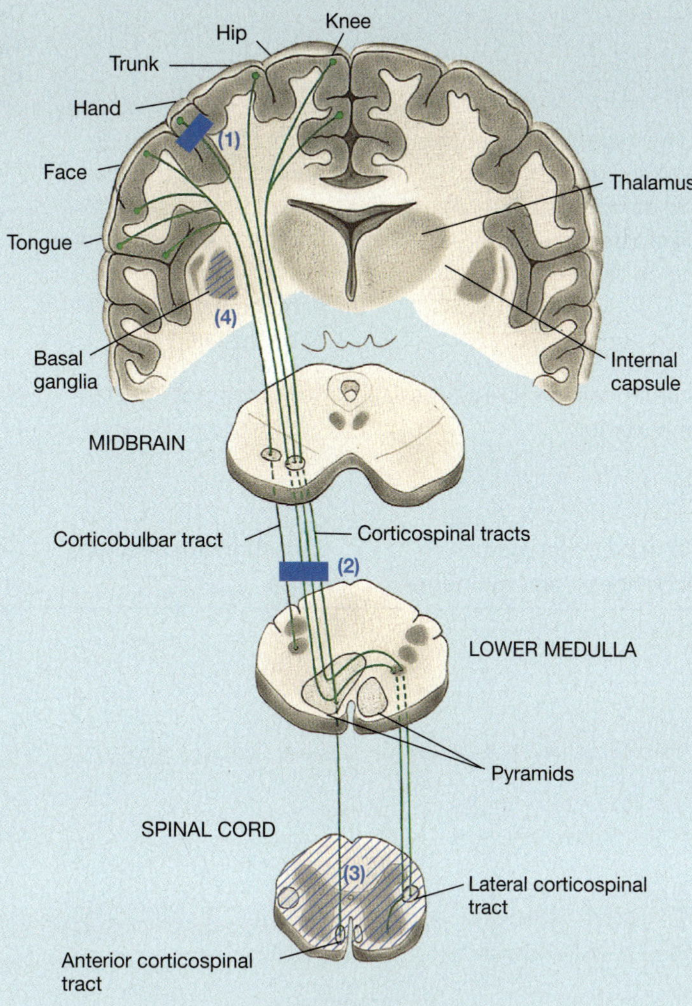

Location of Lesion	Typical Findings: Motor	Sensory	Deep Tendon Reflexes	Examples of Cause
Cerebral Cortex (1)	Chronic contralateral corticospinal-type weakness and spasticity; flexion is stronger than extension in the arm, plantar flexion is stronger than dorsiflexion in the foot, and the leg is externally rotated at the hip	Contralateral sensory loss in the face, limbs, and trunk on the same side as the motor deficits	↑	Cortical stroke
Brainstem (2)	Weakness and spasticity as above, plus cranial nerve (CN) deficits such as diplopia (from weakness of the extraocular muscles) and dysarthria	Variable depending on level of brainstem	↑	Brainstem stroke, multiple sclerosis plaque

(continued)

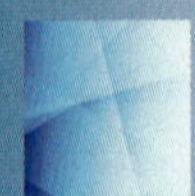

TABLE 27-1. Disorders of the Central and Peripheral Nervous Systems *(Continued)*

Location of Lesion	Typical Findings: Motor	Sensory	Deep Tendon Reflexes	Examples of Cause
Spinal Cord (3)	Weakness and spasticity as above, but often affecting both sides (when cord damage is bilateral), causing paraparesis or quadriparesis depending on the level of injury	Dermatomal sensory deficit on the trunk on one or both sides at the level of the lesion, and sensory loss from tract damage below the level of the lesion	↑	Trauma, spinal cord tumor
Subcortical Gray Matter: Basal Ganglia (4)	Slowness of movement (bradykinesia), rigidity, and tremor	Sensation not affected	Normal or ↓	Parkinsonism
Cerebellar (not illustrated)	Hypotonia, ataxia, nystagmus, dysdiadochokinesis, and dysmetria	Sensation not affected	Normal or ↓	Cerebellar stroke, brain tumor

Location of Lesion	Typical Findings: Motor	Typical Findings: Sensory	Typical Findings: Deep Tendon Reflexes	Examples of Cause
Peripheral Nervous System Disorders				
Anterior Horn Cell (1)	Weakness and atrophy in a segmental or focal pattern; fasciculations	Sensation intact	↓	Polio, amyotrophic lateral sclerosis
Spinal Roots and Nerves (2)	Weakness and atrophy in a root-innervated pattern; sometimes with fasciculations	Corresponding dermatomal sensory deficits	↓	Herniated cervical or lumbar disc
Peripheral Nerve—Mononeuropathy (3)	Weakness and atrophy in a peripheral nerve distribution; sometimes with fasciculations	Sensory loss in the pattern of that nerve	↓	Trauma, compression (e.g., carpal tunnel syndrome)
Peripheral Nerve—Polyneuropathy (4)	Weakness and atrophy more distal than proximal; sometimes with fasciculations	Sensory deficits, commonly in stocking-glove distribution	↓	Peripheral polyneuropathy of alcohol use disorder, diabetes
Neuromuscular Junction (5)	Fatigability more than weakness	Sensation intact	Normal	Myasthenia gravis
Muscle (6)	Weakness usually more proximal than distal; no fasciculations	Sensation intact	Normal or ↓	Muscular dystrophy

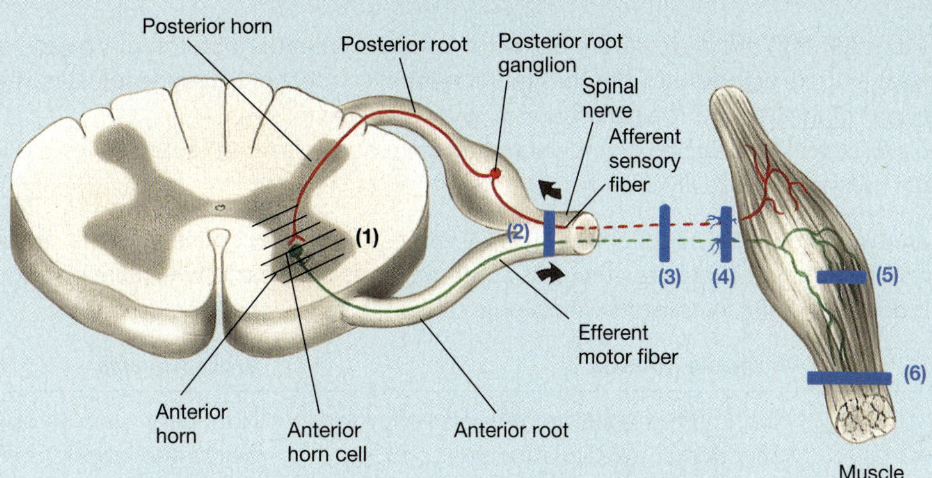

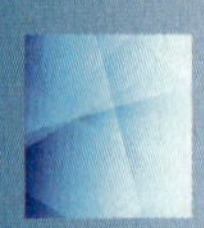

TABLE 27-2. Disorders of Speech

Disorders of speech fall into three groups affecting: (1) phonation of the voice, (2) the articulation of words, and (3) the production and comprehension of language.

- *Aphonia* refers to a loss of voice that accompanies disease affecting the larynx or its nerve supply. *Dysphonia* refers to less severe impairment in the volume, quality, or pitch of the voice. For example, a person may be hoarse or only able to speak in a whisper. Causes include laryngitis, laryngeal tumors, and unilateral vocal cord paralysis (CN X).
- *Dysarthria* refers to a defect in the muscular control of the speech apparatus (lips, tongue, palate, or pharynx). Words may be nasal, slurred, or indistinct, but the central symbolic aspect of language remains intact. Causes include motor lesions of the CNS or PNS, parkinsonism, and cerebellar disease.
- *Aphasia* refers to a disorder in producing or understanding language. It is often caused by lesions in the dominant cerebral hemisphere, usually the left.

Compared below are two common types of aphasia: (1) *Wernicke*, a fluent (receptive) aphasia, and (2) *Broca*, a nonfluent (or expressive) aphasia. There are other less common kinds of aphasia, which are distinguished by differing responses on the specific tests listed. Neurologic consultation is usually indicated.

	Wernicke Aphasia	Broca Aphasia
Qualities of Spontaneous Speech	Fluent; often rapid, voluble, and effortless. Inflection and articulation are good, but sentences lack meaning, and words are malformed (*paraphasias*) or invented (*neologisms*). The meaning of speech may be totally incomprehensible	Nonfluent; slow and broken, with few words and laborious effort. Inflection and articulation are impaired, but words are meaningful, with nouns, transitive verbs, and important adjectives. Small grammatical words are often dropped
Word Comprehension	Impaired	Fair to good
Repetition	Impaired	Impaired
Naming	Impaired	Impaired, though the patient recognizes objects
Reading Comprehension	Impaired	Fair to good
Writing	Impaired	Impaired
Location of Lesion	Posterior superior temporal lobe	Posterior inferior frontal lobe

Although it is important to recognize aphasia early in your encounter with a patient, integrate this information with your neurologic examination as you generate your differential diagnosis.

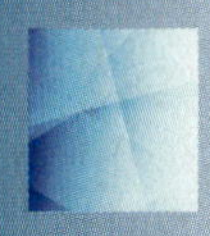

TABLE 27-3. Abnormalities of Gait and Posture

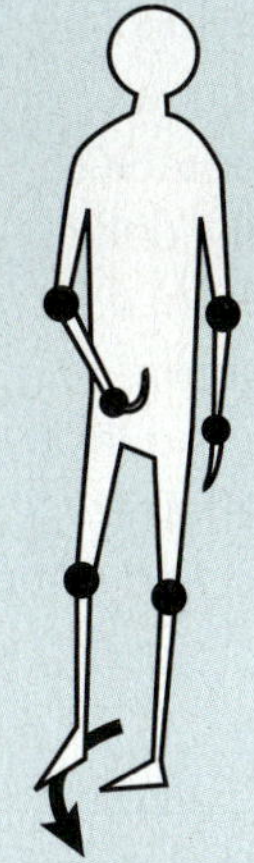

Spastic Hemiparesis

Spastic Hemiparesis

Seen in corticospinal tract lesions that cause poor control of flexor muscles during swing phase (for example, from stroke).

- Affected arm is flexed, immobile, and held close to the side, with elbow, wrists, and interphalangeal joints flexed.
- Affected leg extensors are spastic; ankles are plantar-flexed and inverted.
- Patients may drag toe, circle leg stiffly outward and forward (*circumduction*), or lean trunk to contralateral side to clear affected leg during walking.

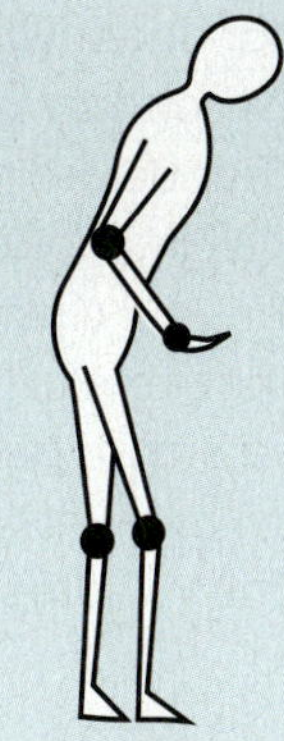

Parkinsonian Gait

Parkinsonian Gait

Seen in the basal ganglia defects of Parkinson disease.

- Posture is stooped, with flexion of head, arms, hips, and knees.
- Patients are slow getting started.
- Steps are short and shuffling, with involuntary hastening (*festination*).
- Arm swings are decreased, and patients turn around stiffly—"all in one piece."
- Postural control is poor (*anteropulsion* or *retropulsion*).

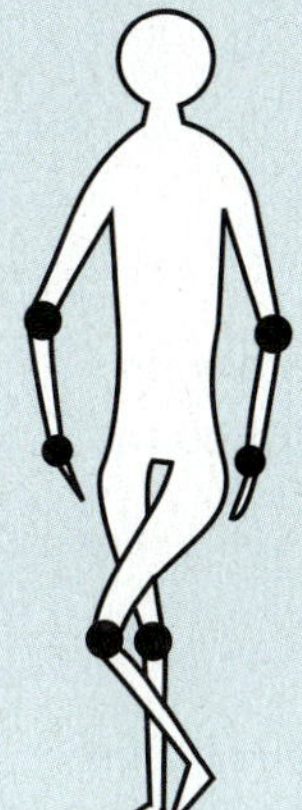

Scissors Gait

Seen in spinal cord disease, causing bilateral lower extremity spasticity, including adductor spasm.

- Gait is stiff. Patients advance each leg slowly, and the thighs tend to cross forward on each other at each step.
- Steps are short.
- Patients appear to be walking through water, and there may be compensating sway of the trunk away from the side of the advancing leg.
- Scissoring is seen in all spasticity disorders, most commonly cerebral palsy.

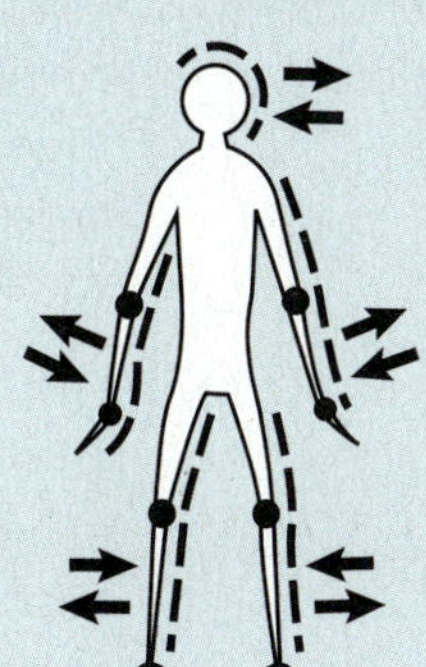

Cerebellar Ataxia

Seen in disease of the cerebellum or associated tracts.

- Gait is staggering and unsteady, with feet wide apart and exaggerated difficulty on turns.
- Patients cannot stand steadily with feet together, whether eyes are open or closed.
- Other cerebellar signs are present such as dysmetria, nystagmus, and intention tremor.

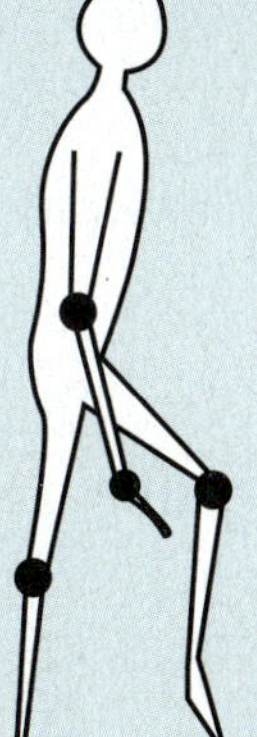

Steppage Gait

Steppage Gait

Seen in foot drop, usually secondary to peripheral nervous system disease.

- Patients either drag the feet or lift them high, with knees flexed, and bring them down with a slap onto the floor, appearing to be walking up stairs.
- Patients cannot walk on their heels.
- Gait may involve one or both legs.
- Tibialis anterior and toe extensors are weak.

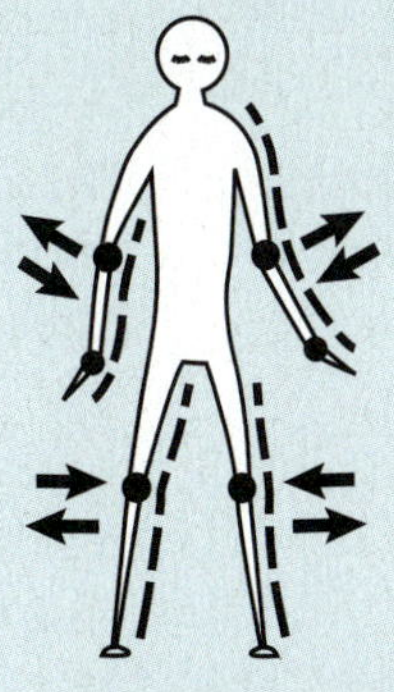

Sensory Ataxia

Sensory Ataxia

Seen in loss of position sense in the legs from polyneuropathy or posterior column damage.

- Gait is unsteady and wide based (with feet wide apart).
- Patients throw their feet forward and outward and bring them down, first on the heels and then on the toes, with a double tapping sound.
- Patients watch the ground for guidance when walking.
- With eyes closed, patients cannot stand steadily with feet together (positive Romberg sign), and the staggering gait worsens.

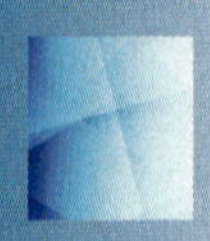

TABLE 27-4. Primary Headaches

Headaches are classified as *primary,* without underlying pathology, or *secondary*, with a serious underlying cause often warranting urgent attention. Secondary headaches are more likely to occur after age 50 with a sudden severe onset and should be ruled out before making the diagnosis of a primary headache.[3] About 90% of headaches are primary headaches and fall into four categories: tension, migraine, cluster, and chronic daily headache. The features of tension, migraine, and cluster headaches are highlighted below. *Chronic daily headache* is not a diagnosis, but a category containing pre-existing headaches that have been transformed into more pronounced forms of migraines, chronic tension-type headaches, and medication-overuse headaches and last more than 15 days a month for more than 3 mo.[90] Risk factors include obesity, >1 headache a week, caffeine ingestion, overuse of headache medications >10 days a month such as analgesics, ergots, and triptans, and sleep and mood disorders.

	Tension	Migraines	Cluster
Process	Process unclear—possibly heightened CNS pain sensitivity. Involves pericranial muscle tenderness; etiology also unclear	Neuronal dysfunction, possibly of brainstem origin, involving low serotonin level, spreading cortical depression and trigeminovascular activation; types: with aura; without aura; variants	Process unclear—possibly hypothalamic then trigemino-autonomic activation
Lifetime Prevalence	Most common headache (40%); prevalence ~50%	10% of headaches; prevalence 18% of U.S. adults; affects ~15% of individuals assigned female at birth, 6% of those assigned male at birth	<1%, more common in individuals assigned male at birth
Location	Usually bilateral; may be generalized or localized to the back of the head and upper neck or to the frontotemporal area	Unilateral in ~70%; bifrontal or global in ~30%	Unilateral, usually behind or around the eye or temple
Quality and Severity	Steady; pressing or tightening; nonthrobbing pain; mild to moderate intensity	Throbbing or aching, pain, moderate to severe in intensity; preceded by aura in up to 30%	Sharp, continuous, intense; severe in intensity
Timing			
Onset	Gradual	Fairly rapid, reaching a peak in 1–2 h	Abrupt; peaks within minutes
Duration	30 min to 7 days	4–72 h	15 min to 3 h
Course	Episodic; may be chronic	Recurrent—usually monthly, but weekly in ~10%; peak incidence early to midadolescence	Episodic, clustered in time, with several each day for 4–8 wk and then relief for 6–12 mo

	Tension	Migraines	Cluster
Associated Symptoms	Sometimes photophobia, phonophobia; scalp tenderness; nausea absent	Prodrome: nausea, vomiting, photophobia, phonophobia; aura in 30% usually; visual (flickering, zig-zagging lines)	Unilateral autonomic symptoms: lacrimation, rhinorrhea, miosis, ptosis, eyelid edema, conjunctival infection
Triggers/ Factors That Aggravate or Provoke	Sustained muscle tension, as in driving or typing; stress; sleep disturbances	Alcohol, certain foods, or stress may provoke; also menses, high altitude; aggravated by noise and bright light	During attack, sensitivity to alcohol may increase
Factors That Relieve	Possibly massage, relaxation	Quiet, dark room; sleep; sometimes transient relief from pressure on the involved artery	

Sources: Headache Classification Committee of the International Headache Society (IHS). The International Classification of Headache Disorders, 3rd edition (beta version). *Cephalalgia*. 2013;33(9):629–808; Lipton RB, Bigal ME, Steiner TJ, Silberstein SD, Olesen J. Classification of primary headaches. *Neurology*. 2004;63:427–435; Sun-Edelstein C, Bigal ME, Rapoport AM. Chronic migraine and medication overuse headache: clarifying the current International Headache Society classification criteria. *Cephalalgia*. 2009;29:445–452; Lipton RB, Stewart WF, Diamond S, Diamond ML, Reed M. Prevalence and burden of migraine in the United States: data from the American Migraine Study II. *Headache*. 2001;41:646–657; Fumal A, Schoenen J. Tension-type headache: current research and clinical management. *Lancet Neurol.* 2008;7:70–83; Nesbitt AD, Goadsby PJ. Cluster headache. *BMJ*. 2012;344:e2407.

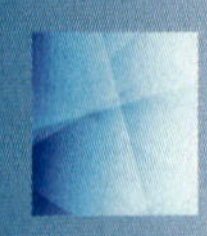

TABLE 27-5. Secondary Headaches and Cranial Neuralgias

Type	Process	Location	Quality and Severity
Secondary Headaches			
Analgesic Rebound	Withdrawal of medication	Previous headache pattern	Variable
Headaches from Eye Disorders			
■ ***Errors of Refraction (farsightedness and astigmatism, but not nearsightedness)***	Probably the sustained contraction of the extraocular muscles, and possibly of the frontal, temporal, and occipital muscles	Around and over the eyes; may radiate to the occipital area	Steady, aching, dull
■ ***Acute Glaucoma***	Sudden increase in intraocular pressure (see p. 355)	Pain in and around one eye	Steady, aching, often severe
Headache from Sinusitis	Mucosal inflammation of the paranasal sinuses	Usually frontal sinuses above the eyes or over the maxillary sinus	Aching or throbbing, severity variable; consider possible migraine
Meningitis	Viral or bacterial infection of the meninges surrounding the brain and spinal cord	Generalized	Steady or throbbing, very severe
Subarachnoid Hemorrhage—"Thunderclap Headache"	Bleeding from a ruptured cerebral saccular aneurysm; rarely from AV malformation, mycotic aneurysm	Generalized	Very severe, "the worst of my life"
Brain Tumor	Mass lesion causing displacement of or traction on pain-sensitive arteries and veins or pressure on nerves	Variable, including lobes of brain, cerebellum, brainstem	Aching, steady, dull pain that is worse upon awakening but improves after several hours

Timing			Associated Symptoms	Factors That Aggravate or Provoke	Factors That Relieve
Onset	**Duration**	**Course**			
Variable	Depends on prior headache pattern	Depends on frequency of "mini-withdrawals"	Depends on prior headache pattern	Fever, carbon monoxide, hypoxia, withdrawal of caffeine, other headache triggers	Depends on cause
Gradual	Variable	Variable	Eye fatigue, "sandy" sensations in eyes, redness of conjunctiva	Prolonged use of the eyes, particularly for close work	Rest of the eyes
Often rapid	Variable, may depend on treatment	Variable, may depend on treatment	Blurred vision, nausea, and vomiting; halos around lights, reddening of eye	Sometimes provoked by mydriatic drops	
Variable	Often daily, several hours at a time, persisting until treatment	Often daily in a repetitive pattern	Local tenderness, nasal congestion, discharge, and fever	May be aggravated by coughing, sneezing, or jarring the head	Nasal decongestants, antibiotics
Fairly rapid, usually <24 h; may be sudden onset	Variable, usually days	Viral: usually <1 wk; bacterial: persistent until treatment	Fever, stiff neck, photophobia, change in mental status	—	Immediate antibiotics until diagnosis of bacterial or viral
Sudden onset; can be less than a minute	Variable, usually days	Varies according to presenting severity and level of consciousness; worst if initial coma	Nausea, vomiting, loss of consciousness, neck pain. Possible prior neck symptoms from "sentinel leaks"	Rebleeding, ↑ intracranial pressure, cerebral edema	Subspecialty treatments
Variable	Often brief; depends on location and rate of growth	Intermittent but may progress in intensity over a period of days	Seizures, hemiparesis, field cuts, personality changes. Also nausea, vomiting, vision change, gait change	May be aggravated by coughing, sneezing, or sudden movements of the head	Subspecialty treatments

(*continued*)

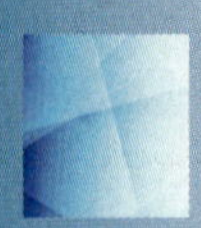

TABLE 27-5. Secondary Headaches and Cranial Neuralgias *(Continued)*

Type	Process	Location	Quality and Severity
Giant Cell (Temporal) Arteritis	Transmural lymphocytic vasculitis often involving multinucleated giant cells that disrupts the internal elastic lamina of large-caliber arteries	Localized near the involved artery, most often the temporal artery in those > age 50, individuals assigned female at birth > individuals assigned male at birth (2:1 ratio)	Throbbing, generalized, persistent; often severe
Postconcussion Headache	Follows mild acceleration–deceleration traumatic brain injury. May involve axonal, cerebrovascular autoregulatory, neurochemical injury	Often but not always localized to the injured area	Dull, aching, constant; may have features of tension and migraine headaches
Cranial Neuralgias			
Trigeminal Neuralgia (CN V)	Vascular compression of CN V, usually near entry to pons leading to focal demyelination, aberrant discharge. 10% with causative intracranial lesion	Cheek, jaws, lips, or gums; trigeminal nerve divisions 2 and 3 > 1	Shocklike, stabbing, burning; severe

Note: Blanks appear in this table when the categories are not applicable or not usually helpful in assessing the problem.

Sources: Headache Classification Committee of the International Headache Society (IHS). The International Classification of Headache Disorders, 3rd edition (beta version). *Cephalalgia*. 2013;33(9):629–808; Schwedt TJ, Matharu MS, Dodick DW. Thunderclap headache *Lancet Neurol.* 2006;5:621–631; Van de Beek D, de Gans J, Spanjaard L, Weisfelt M, Reitsma JB, Vermeulen M. Clinical features and prognostic factors in adults with bacterial meningitis. *N Engl J Med.* 2004;351:1849–1859; Salvarini C, Cantini F, Hunder GG. Polymyalgia rheumatica and giant-cell arteritis. *Lancet*. 2008;372:234–245; Smetana GW, Shmerling RH. Does this patient have temporal arteritis? *JAMA*. 2002;287:92–101; Ropper AH, Gorson KC. Clinical practice. Concussion. *N Engl J Med*. 2007;356:166–172; American College of Physicians. Neurology—MKSAP 16.

Timing			Associated Symptoms	Factors That Aggravate or Provoke	Factors That Relieve
Onset	Duration	Course			
Gradual or rapid	Variable	Recurrent or persistent over weeks to months	Tenderness over temporal artery, adjacent scalp; fever (in ~50%), fatigue, weight loss; new headache (~60%), jaw claudication (~50%), visual loss or blindness (~15%–20%), polymyalgia rheumatica (~50%)	Movement of neck and shoulders	Often steroids
Within 7 days of the injury up to 3 mo	Weeks to up to a year	Tends to diminish over time	Drowsiness, poor concentration, confusion, memory loss, blurred vision, dizziness, irritability, restlessness, fatigue	Mental and physical exertion, straining, stooping, emotional excitement, alcohol	Rest; medication
Abrupt, paroxysmal	Each jab lasts seconds but recurs at intervals of seconds or minutes	May recur daily for weeks to months then resolve; can be chronic progressive.	Exhaustion from recurrent pain	Touching certain areas of the lower face or mouth; chewing, talking, brushing teeth	Medication; neurovascular decompression

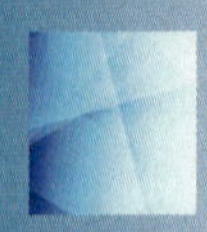

TABLE 27-6. Syncope and Similar Disorders

	Mechanism	Precipitating Factors	Predisposing Factors	Prodromal Manifestations	Postural Associations	Recovery
Vasovagal Syncope and **Vasodepressor Syncope**	For vasovagal syncope: reflex withdrawal of sympathetic tone and increased vagal tone causing drop in blood pressure and heart rate For vasodepressor syncope: same mechanism but no vagal surge or drop in heart rate Baroreflexes normal	Strong emotion such as fear or pain, prolonged standing, hot humid environment	Fatigue, hunger, preload reduction from dehydration, diuretics, vasodilators	Usually >10 s; palpitations, nausea, blurred vision, warmth, pallor, diaphoresis, light-headedness	Usually occurs when standing, at times when sitting	Prompt return of consciousness after lying down, but pallor, weakness, nausea, and slight confusion may persist for a time; most common type of syncope
Orthostatic Hypotension	Gravitationally mediated *redistribution and pooling of 300–800 mL blood* in the lower extremities and splanchnic venous system, caused by decreased venous return and an excessive fall in cardiac output, or by an inadequate vasoconstrictor mechanism (with inadequate release of norepinephrine)	Standing up	Aging; antihypertensive vasodilator drugs; prolonged bed rest central disorders: Parkinson disease, multiple system atrophy; dementia with Lewy bodies; peripheral neuropathy: diabetes, amyloidosis	Light-headedness, dizziness, cognitive slowing, fatigue; often none	Occurs soon after standing Supine hypertension is common	Prompt return to normal when lying down
	Hypovolemia, a diminished blood volume insufficient to maintain cardiac output and blood pressure	Standing up after hemorrhage or dehydration	Bleeding from the GI tract or trauma, potent diuretics, vomiting, diarrhea, polyuria	Light-headedness and palpitations (tachycardia) on standing up	Occurs soon after standing up	Improves with volume repletion
Cough Syncope	Neurally mediated, possibly from reflex vasodepressor-bradycardia response; cerebral hypoperfusion, increased CSF pressure also proposed	Severe paroxysm of coughing	COPD, asthma, pulmonary hypertension; typically occurs in overweight middle-aged patients	Often none except for cough; blurred vision, light-headedness may occur	May occur in any position	Prompt return to normal after a few seconds
Micturition Syncope	Vasovagal response, sudden hypotension proposed	Emptying the bladder after getting out of bed to void	Nocturia, usually in elderly or adult individuals assigned male at birth	Often none	Commonly just after (or during) voiding after standing up	Prompt return to normal
Cardiovascular Disorders						
Arrhythmias	Decreased cardiac output from cardiac ischemia, ventricular arrhythmias, prolonged QT syndrome, persistent bradycardia, intrafascicular block causing cerebral hypoperfusion; often sudden onset, sudden offset	Sudden change in rhythm to bradycardia or tachyarrhythmia	Ischemic or valvular heart disease, conduction abnormalities, pericardial disease, cardiomyopathy; aging decreases tolerance of abnormal rhythms	Palpitations, usually lasting <5 s; often none	May occur in any position	Prompt return to normal when arrhythmia resolves; most common cause of cardiac syncope; cardiogenic syncope has a 6-mo mortality >10%

	Mechanism	Precipitating Factors	Predisposing Factors	Prodromal Manifestations	Postural Associations	Recovery
Aortic Stenosis** and **Hypertrophic Cardiomyopathy	Vascular resistance falls with exercise, but cardiac output does not rise due to outflow obstruction	Exercise	Cardiac disorders	Chest pain, often none; onset is sudden	Occurs with or after exercise	Usually a prompt return to normal
Myocardial Infarction	Sudden arrhythmia or decreased cardiac output	Variable, often exertion	Coronary artery disease, coronary ischemia or vasospasm	Ischemic chest pain; may be silent	May occur in any position	Variable; related to time to diagnosis and treatment
Massive Pulmonary Embolism	Sudden hypoxia or decreased cardiac output	Variable, including prolonged bed rest, major surgery, clotting disorders, pregnancy	Deep vein thrombosis, bed rest, hypercoagulable states (systemic lupus erythematosus, cancer), protein S or C deficiency antithrombin III deficiency; estrogen therapy	Tachypnea, chest or pleuritic pain, dyspnea, anxiety, cough	May occur in any position	Related to time to diagnosis and treatment
Disorders Resembling Syncope						
Hypocapnia due to Hyperventilation	Constriction of cerebral blood vessels from hypocapnia induced by hyperventilation	Anxiety, panic disorder	Anxiety	Dyspnea, palpitations, chest discomfort, numbness, and tingling in hands and around the mouth lasting several minutes; consciousness is often maintained	May occur in any position	Slow improvement as hyperventilation ceases
Hypoglycemia	Insufficient glucose to maintain cerebral metabolism; epinephrine release contributes to symptoms; true syncope is uncommon	Variable, including fasting	Insulin therapy and a variety of metabolic disorders	Sweating, tremors, palpitations, hunger, headache, confusion, abnormal behavior, coma	May occur in any position	Variable, depending on severity and treatment
Functional Neurologic Symptom Disorder	Unknown mechanism Skin color, vital signs may be normal; sometimes with bizarre purposeful movements; usually occurs when other people present	Stress or trauma, psychological or physical Sometimes no precipitant identified	History of multiple somatic symptoms Often dissociative symptoms such as depersonalization, derealization, dissociative amnesia, or maladaptive personality traits; associated with past child abuse or neglect	Variable	A slump to the floor, often from a standing position, without injury	Variable; may be prolonged, often with fluctuating responsiveness and inconsistent neurologic findings

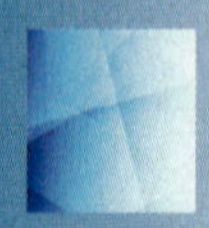

TABLE 27-7. Types of Stroke

Assessment of stroke requires careful history taking and a detailed physical examination, and should focus on three fundamental questions: What brain area and related vascular territory explain the patient's findings? Is the stroke ischemic or hemorrhagic? If ischemic, is the mechanism thrombosis or embolus?

Stroke is a medical emergency, and timing is of the essence. Answers to these questions are critical to patient outcomes and use of antithrombotic therapies.

In *acute ischemic stroke,* ischemic brain injury begins with a central core of very low perfusion and often irreversible cell death. This core is surrounded by an *ischemic penumbra* of metabolically disturbed cells that are still potentially viable, depending on the restoration of blood flow and duration of ischemia. Because most irreversible damage occurs in the first 3–6 h after onset of symptoms, achieving reperfusion as early as possible provides the best outcomes, with recovery in up to 50% of patients treated within 3 h in some studies.

Clinician performance in diagnosing stroke improves with training and experience. Understanding the pathophysiology of stroke takes dedication, expert supervision to improve techniques of neurologic examination, and perseverance. *This brief overview is intended to prompt further study and practice.* Accuracy in clinical examination is achievable, and more important than ever in determining patient therapy.[44,48,49] Review the discussion of stroke risk factors and primary prevention on pp. 962–964.

Clinical Features and Vascular Territories of Stroke

Clinical Finding	Vascular Territory	Additional Comments
Contralateral leg weakness	*Anterior circulation*—anterior cerebral artery (ACA)	The internal carotid arteries supply the anterior circulation, providing blood flow to the anterior and middle cerebral arteries
Contralateral face, arm > leg weakness, sensory loss, visual field loss, apraxia, aphasia (left middle cerebral artery [MCA]), or neglect (right MCA)	*Anterior circulation*—MCA	Largest vascular bed for stroke, so most common territory affected
Contralateral motor or sensory deficit without cortical signs (such as aphasia or neglect)	*Subcortical circulation*[a]—lenticulostriate deep-penetrating branches of MCA	Small vessel subcortical *lacunar infarcts* in internal capsule, thalamus, or brainstem. Five classical syndromes are seen: pure motor stroke (hemiplegia/hemiparesis), pure sensory stroke (hemianesthesia), ataxic hemiparesis, clumsy-hand/dysarthria syndrome, and mixed sensorimotor stroke
Contralateral visual field loss	*Posterior circulation*—posterior cerebral artery (PCA)	The paired vertebral arteries join to form the basilar artery, which supplies the posterior circulation. Bilateral PCA infarction causes cortical blindness but preserved pupillary light reaction.
Dysphagia, dysarthria, tongue/palate deviation, and/or ataxia with crossed sensory/motor deficits (= ipsilateral face with contralateral body)	*Posterior circulation*—Vertebral or basilar artery branches supplying the brainstem	
Oculomotor deficits and/or ataxia with crossed sensory/motor deficits	*Posterior circulation*—basilar artery	Complete basilar artery occlusion—"locked-in syndrome" with intact consciousness but with inability to speak and quadriplegia

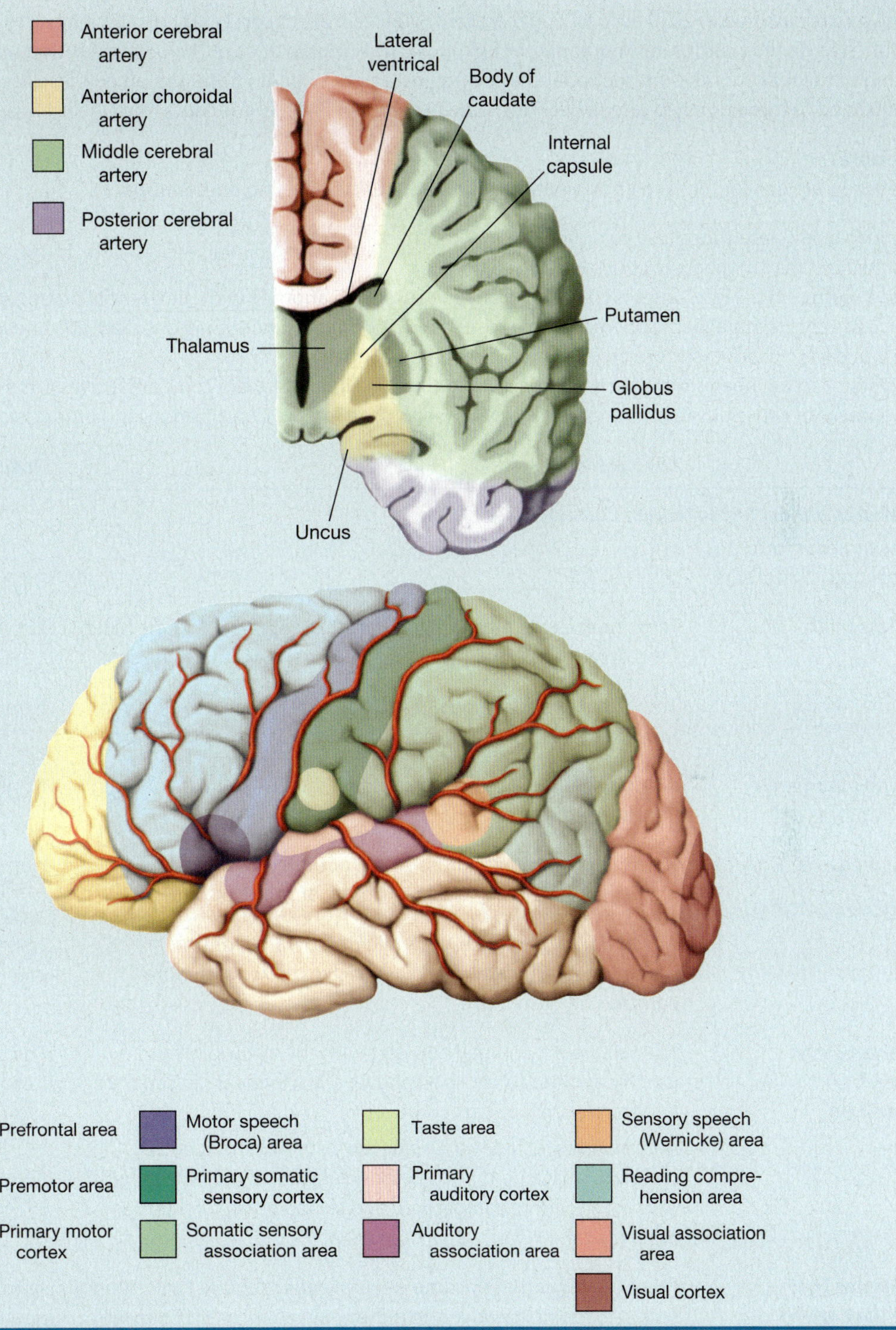

[a]Learn to differentiate cortical from subcortical involvement. *Subcortical or lacunar syndromes* do not affect higher cognitive function, language, or visual fields.

Source: Reproduced with permission from *Medical Knowledge Self-Assessment Program*, 14th edition (MKSAP 14), Neurology. American College of Physicians; 2006:52–68. Copyright © 2006 American College of Physicians.

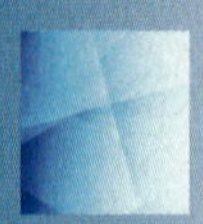

TABLE 27-8. Seizure Disorders

Seizures were reclassified in 2010 as *focal* or *generalized* to better reflect current medical science. Underlying causes should be identified as genetic, structural/metabolic, or unknown. The complexities of the reclassification scheme are best explored by turning to the report of the International League Against Epilepsy (ILAE) Commission on Classification and Terminology, 2005–2009 and to more detailed references. This table presents only basic concepts from the ILAE report.

Focal Seizures

Focal seizures "are conceptualized as originating within networks limited to *one hemisphere.*"

- They may be discretely localized or more widely distributed.
- Focal seizures may originate in subcortical structures.
- For each seizure type, ictal onset is *consistent* from one seizure to another, with preferential propagation patterns that can involve the contralateral hemisphere. In some cases, however, there is more than one network, and more than one seizure type, but each individual seizure type has a consistent site of onset."
- The distinction between simple partial and partial complex is eliminated, but clinicians are urged to recognize and describe "impairment of consciousness/awareness or other dyscognitive features, localization, and progression of ictal events."

Type	Clinical Manifestations	Postictal State
Focal Seizures without Impairment of Consciousness		
With observable motor and autonomic symptoms		
■ Jacksonian	Tonic then clonic movements that start unilaterally in the hand, foot, or face and spread to other body parts on the same side	Normal consciousness
■ Other motor	Turning of the head and eyes to one side, or tonic and clonic movements of an arm or leg without the Jacksonian spread	Normal consciousness
■ With autonomic symptoms	A "funny feeling" in the epigastrium, nausea, pallor, flushing, lightheadedness	Normal consciousness
With subjective sensory or psychic phenomena	Numbness, tingling; simple visual, auditory, or olfactory hallucinations such as flashing lights, buzzing, or odors	Normal consciousness
	Anxiety or fear; feelings of familiarity (déjà vu) or unreality; dreamy states; fear or rage; flashback experiences; more complex hallucinations	Normal consciousness
Focal Seizures with Impairment of Consciousness	The seizure may or may not start with the autonomic or psychic symptoms outlined above; consciousness is impaired, and the person appears confused Automatisms include automatic motor behaviors such as chewing, smacking the lips, walking about, and unbuttoning clothes; also more complicated and skilled behaviors such as driving a car	The patient may remember initial autonomic or psychic symptoms (which are then termed an *aura*), but is amnesic for the rest of the seizure. Temporary confusion and headache may occur
Focal Seizures That Become Generalized	Partial seizures that become generalized resemble tonic–clonic seizures (see next page); the patient may not recall the focal onset	As in a tonic–clonic seizure, described on the next page; two attributes indicate a partial seizure that has become generalized: (1) the recollection of an *aura,* and (2) a *unilateral* neurologic deficit during the postictal period

Generalized Seizures and Nonepileptic Seizures

Generalized seizures "are conceptualized as originating at some point within, and rapidly engaging, bilaterally distributed networks … that include cortical and subcortical structures, but do not necessarily include the entire cortex …"

- The location and lateralization are *not consistent* from one seizure to another.
- Generalized seizures can be asymmetric.
- They may begin with body movements, impaired consciousness, or both.
- If onset of tonic–clonic seizures begins after age 30 y, suspect either a partial seizure that has become generalized or a generalized seizure caused by a toxic or metabolic disorder.

Toxic and metabolic causes include withdrawal from alcohol or other sedative drugs, uremia, hypoglycemia, hyperglycemia, hyponatremia, drug toxicity, and bacterial meningitis.

Problem	Clinical Manifestations	Postictal (*Postseizure*) State
Generalized Seizures		
Tonic–Clonic (Grand Mal)[a]	The patient loses consciousness suddenly, sometimes with a cry, and the body stiffens into tonic extensor rigidity. Breathing stops, and the patient becomes cyanotic. A clonic phase of rhythmic muscular contraction follows. Breathing resumes and is often noisy, with excessive salivation. Injury, tongue biting, and urinary incontinence may occur.	Confusion, drowsiness, fatigue, headache, muscular aching, and sometimes the temporary persistence of bilateral neurologic deficits such as hyperactive reflexes and Babinski responses. The patient is amnestic about the seizure and aura.
Absence	A sudden brief lapse of consciousness, with momentary blinking, staring, or movements of the lips and hands but no falling. Two subtypes are: *typical absence*—lasts <10 s and stops abruptly; *atypical absence*—may last >10 s	No aura recalled. In typical absence, a prompt return to normal; in atypical absence, some postictal confusion
Myoclonic	Sudden, brief, rapid jerks, involving the trunk or limbs. Myoclonus has many potential causes, however, and is not always caused by seizure	Variable
Myoclonic Atonic (Drop Attack)	Sudden loss of consciousness with falling but no movements. Injury may occur	Either a prompt return to normal or a brief period of confusion
Nonepileptic Seizures (previously called pseudoseizures)		
May mimic seizures but are due to a conversion disorder (termed "Functional Neurologic Symptom Disorder" in *DSM-5*)	The movements may be complex and often do not follow a neuroanatomic pattern. Can sometimes be difficult to distinguish from epileptic seizure without EEG. It is not uncommon for a patient to have both epileptic and nonepileptic seizures.	Variable

[a] *Febrile convulsions* that resemble brief tonic–clonic seizures occur in infants and young children. They are usually benign but may also be the first manifestation of a seizure disorder.

Source: Adapted from Berg AT, Berkovic SF, Brodie MJ, et al. Revised terminology and concepts for organization of seizures and epilepsies: report of the ILAE Commission on Classification and Terminology, 2005–2009. *Epilepsia.* 2010;51(4):676–685. Copyright © 2010 International League Against Epilepsy. Reprinted by permission of John Wiley & Sons, Inc.

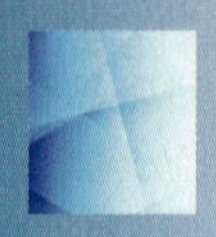

TABLE 27-9. Tremors and Involuntary Movements

Tremors

Tremors are rhythmic oscillatory movements, which may be roughly subdivided into three groups: resting (or static) tremors, postural tremors, and intention tremors.

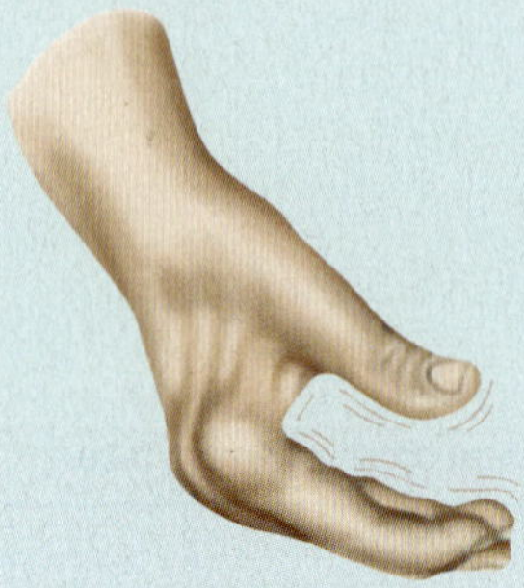

Resting (Static) Tremors

These tremors are most prominent at rest and may decrease or disappear with voluntary movement. Illustrated is the common, relatively slow, fine pill-rolling tremor of parkinsonism, about 5/s.

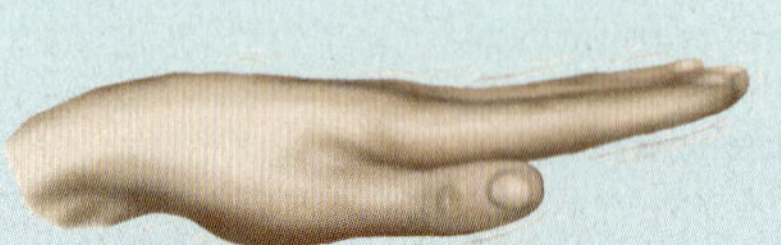

Postural Tremors

These tremors appear when the affected part is actively maintaining a posture. Examples include the fine rapid tremor of hyperthyroidism, the tremors of anxiety and fatigue, and benign essential (and often familial) tremor.

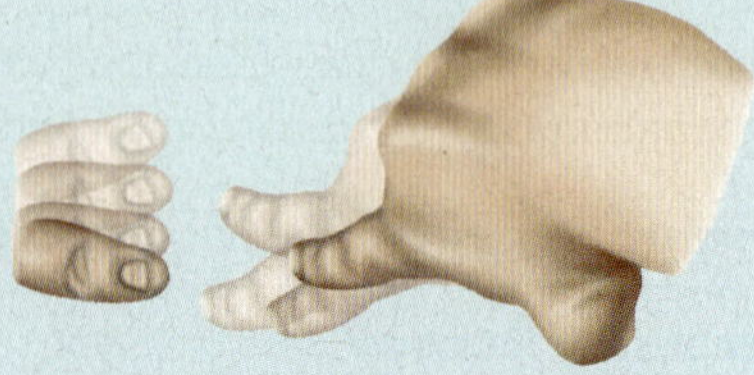

Intention Tremors

Intention tremors, absent at rest, appear with movement and get worse as the limb approaches the target. Seen in disorders affecting the cerebellum or its related tracts, such as multiple sclerosis or stroke.

Involuntary Movements

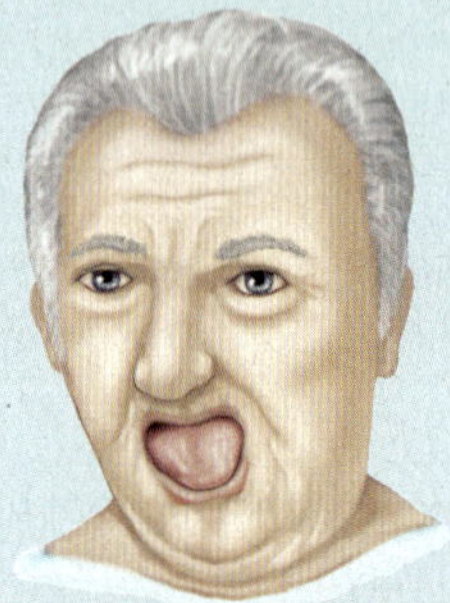

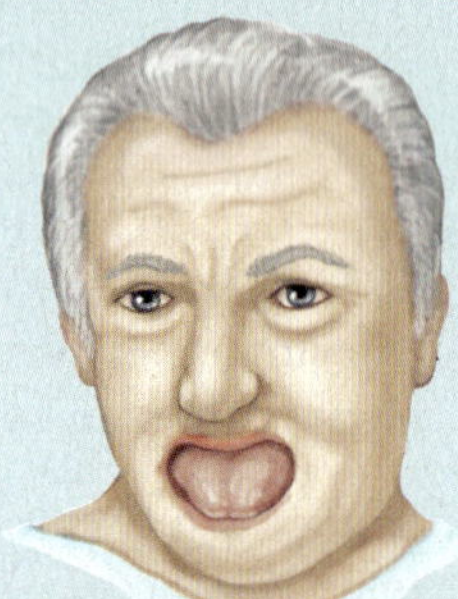

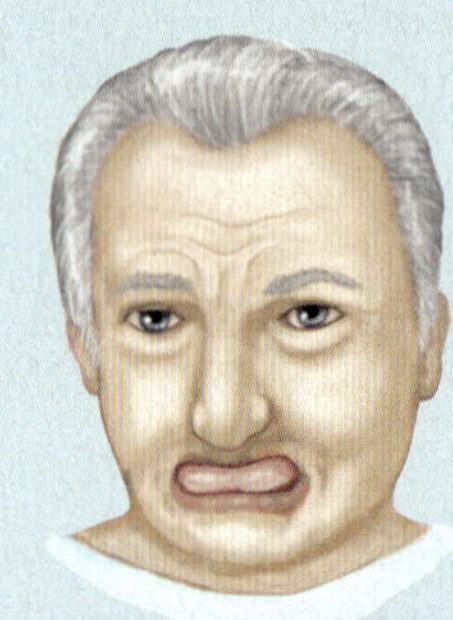

Oral–Facial Dyskinesias

Oral–facial dyskinesias are arrhythmic, repetitive, bizarre movements that chiefly involve the face, mouth, jaw, and tongue: grimacing, pursing of the lips, protrusions of the tongue, opening and closing of the mouth, and deviations of the jaw. The limbs and trunk are involved less often. These movements may be a late complication of antipsychotic or antiemetic drugs such as phenothiazines, termed *tardive* (late) dyskinesias. They also occur in long-standing psychoses, in some older adults, and in some edentulous persons.

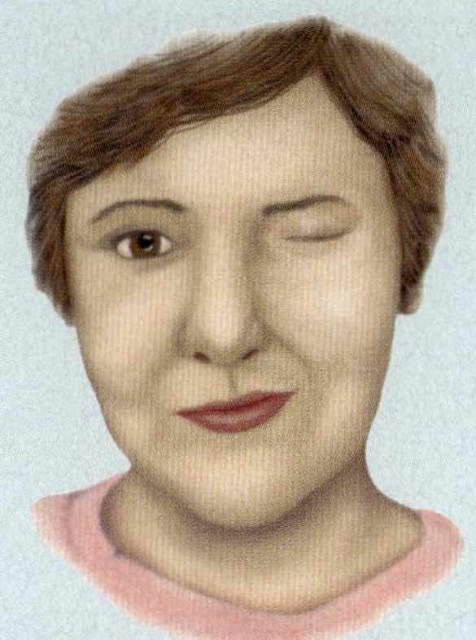

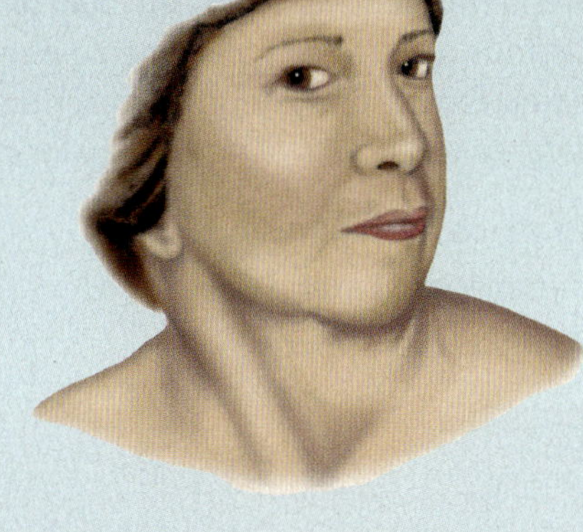

Tics

Tics are brief, repetitive, stereotyped, coordinated movements occurring at irregular intervals. Examples include repetitive winking, grimacing, and shoulder shrugging. Causes include Tourette syndrome and late effects of drugs such as phenothiazines.

Dystonia

Dystonia causes irregular movements resembling athetosis or tremor. These are often accompanied by abnormal postures that limit voluntary movement and can at times be painful. Examples include writer's cramp, blepharospasm, and as illustrated, spasmodic torticollis.

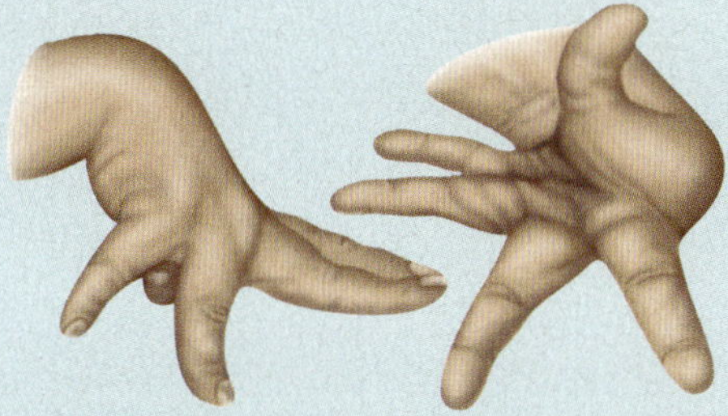

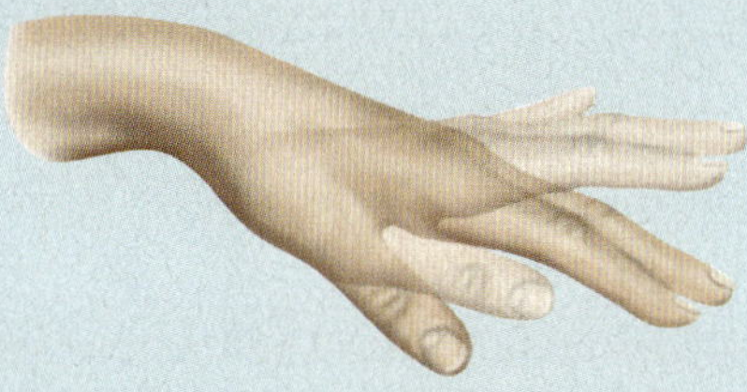

Athetosis

Athetoid movements are slower and more twisting and writhing than choreiform movements and have a larger amplitude. They most commonly involve the face and the distal extremities. Athetosis is often associated with spasticity. Causes include cerebral palsy.

Chorea

Choreiform movements are brief, rapid, jerky, irregular, and unpredictable. They occur at rest or interrupt normal coordinated movements. Unlike tics, they seldom repeat themselves. The face, head, lower arms, and hands are often involved. Causes include Sydenham chorea (with rheumatic fever) and Huntington disease.

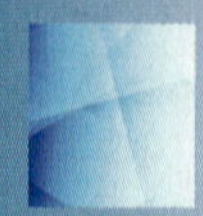

TABLE 27-10. Nystagmus

Nystagmus is a rhythmic oscillation of the eyes, analogous to a tremor in other parts of the body. It has multiple causes, including impairment of vision in early life, disorders of the labyrinth and the cerebellar system, and drug toxicity. Nystagmus occurs normally when a person watches a rapidly moving object (e.g., a passing train). Study the three characteristics of nystagmus described in this table so that you can correctly identify the type of nystagmus. Then refer to textbooks of neurology for differential diagnoses.

Direction of Gaze in which Nystagmus Appears

Example: Nystagmus on Right Lateral Gaze

Nystagmus Present (Right Lateral Gaze)

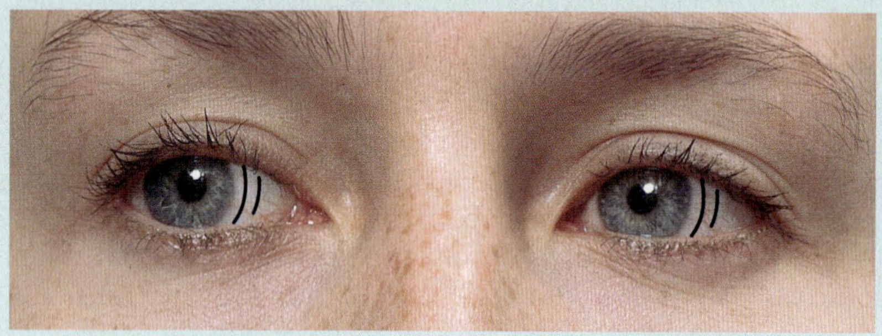

Although nystagmus may be present in all directions of gaze, it may appear or become accentuated only on deviation of the eyes (e.g., to the side or upward). On extreme lateral gaze, the normal person may show a few beats resembling nystagmus. Avoid making assessments in such extreme positions and *observe for nystagmus only within the field of full binocular vision.*

Nystagmus Not Present (Left Lateral Gaze)

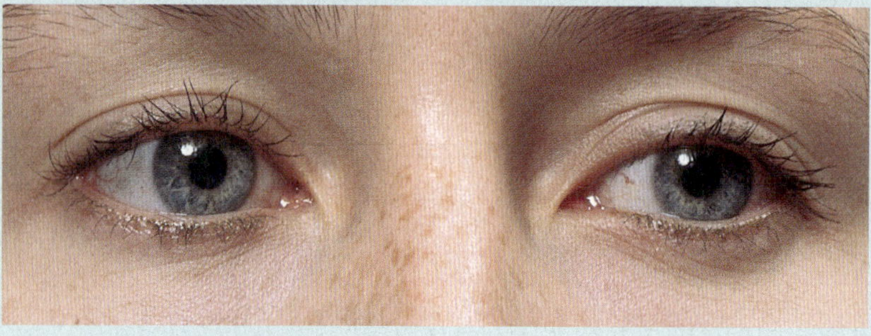

Direction of the Quick and Slow Phases

Example: Left-Beating Nystagmus—a Quick Jerk to the Left in Each Eye, then a Slow Drift to the Right

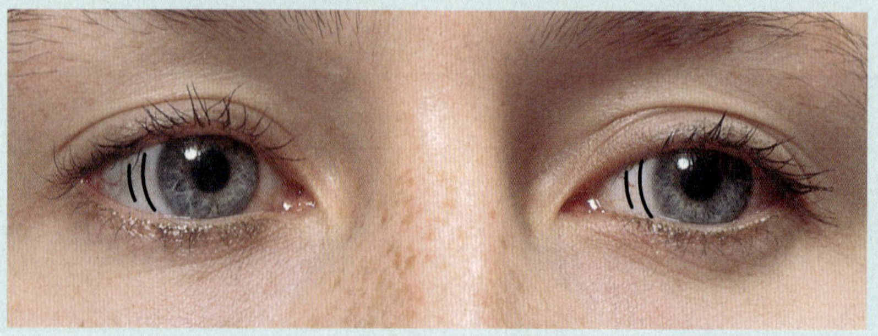

Nystagmus usually has both slow and fast movements but *is defined by its fast phase.*

For example, if the eyes jerk quickly to the patient's left and drift back slowly to the right, the patient is said to have *left-beating nystagmus.* Occasionally, nystagmus consists only of coarse oscillations without quick and slow components, described as *pendular.*

Plane of the Movements
Horizontal Nystagmus

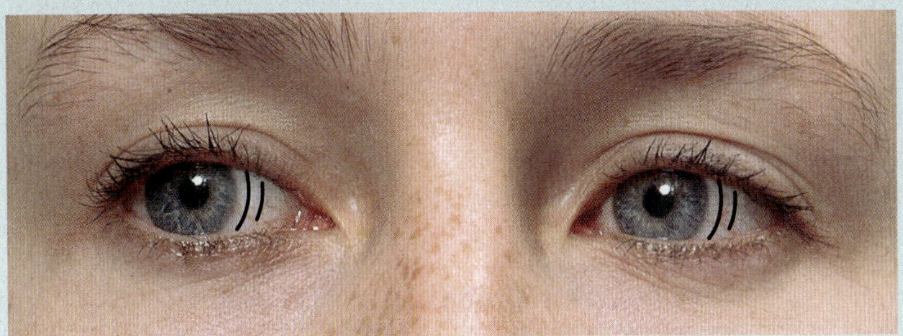

The movement of nystagmus may occur in one or more planes, namely horizontal, vertical, or rotary. It is the plane of the movements, not the direction of the gaze, that defines this variable.

Vertical Nystagmus

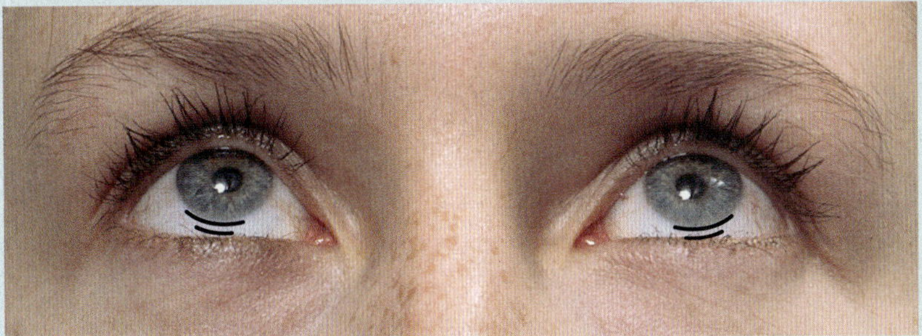

Rotary Nystagmus

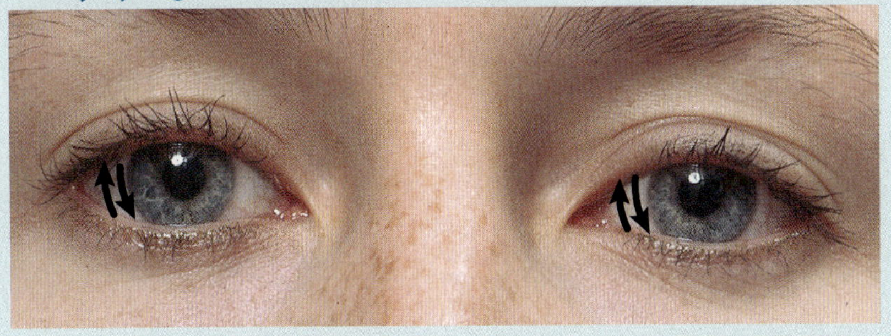

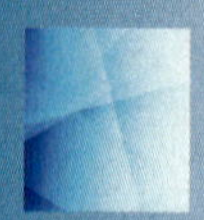

TABLE 27-11. Types of Facial Paralysis

Facial weakness or paralysis may result from either (1) a peripheral lesion of CN VII, the facial nerve, anywhere from its origin in the pons to its periphery in the face, or (2) a central lesion involving the upper motor neuron system between the cortex and the pons. A peripheral lesion of CN VII, exemplified here by a Bell palsy, is compared with a central lesion, exemplified by a left hemispheric cerebral infarction. These can be distinguished by their different effects on the upper portion of the face.

The lower portion of the face is normally controlled by upper motor neurons located on only one side of the cortex—the opposite side. *Left hemispheric damage to these pathways, as in stroke, weakens the right lower face.* The upper face, however, is controlled by pathways from both sides of the cortex. Even though the upper motor neurons on the left are destroyed, others on the right remain, and the right upper face continues to function fairly well.

CN VII—Peripheral Lesion

Peripheral nerve damage to CN VII paralyzes the entire right side of the face, including the forehead.

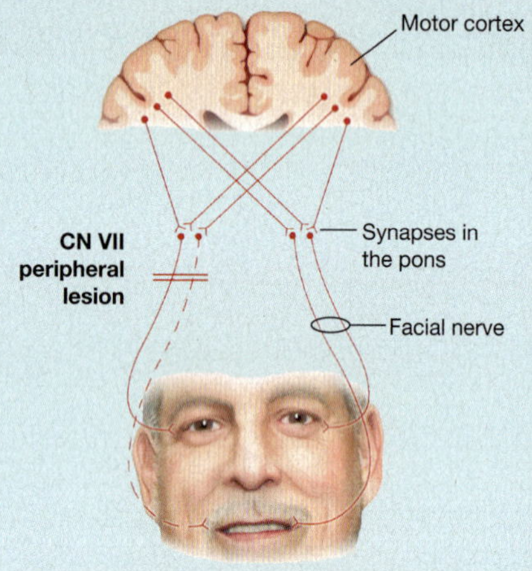

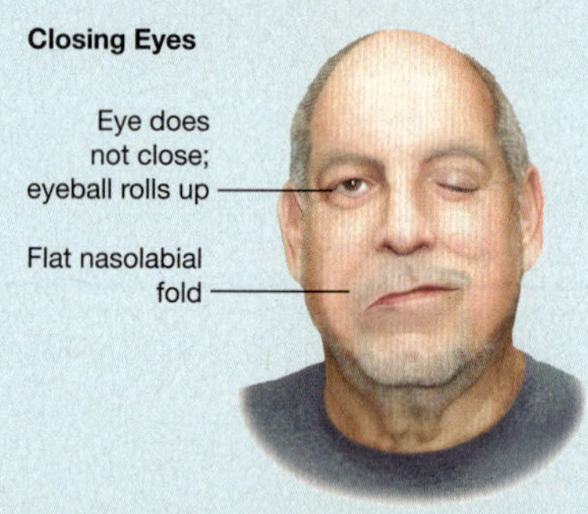

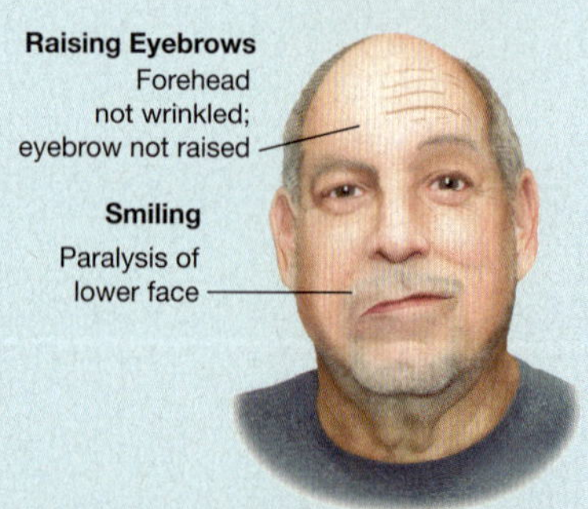

CN VII—Central Lesion

Central nerve damage to CN VII paralyzes the lower face but cortical innervation to the forehead is preserved.

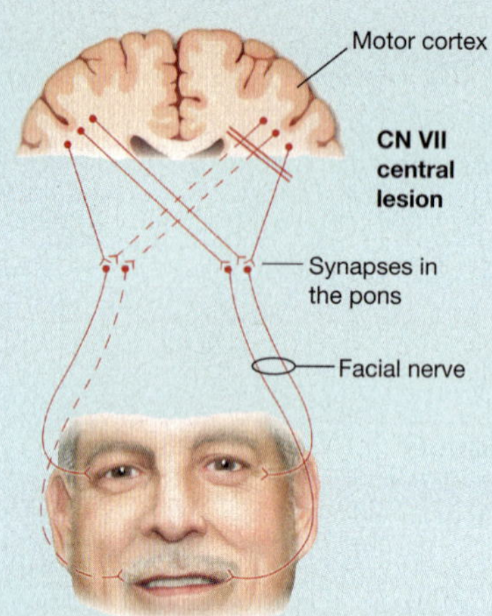

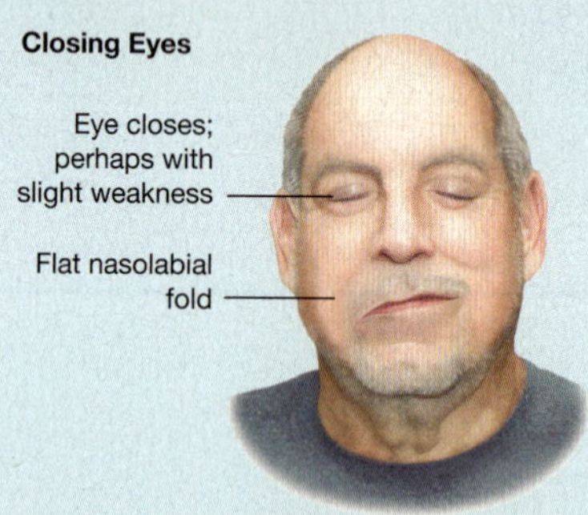

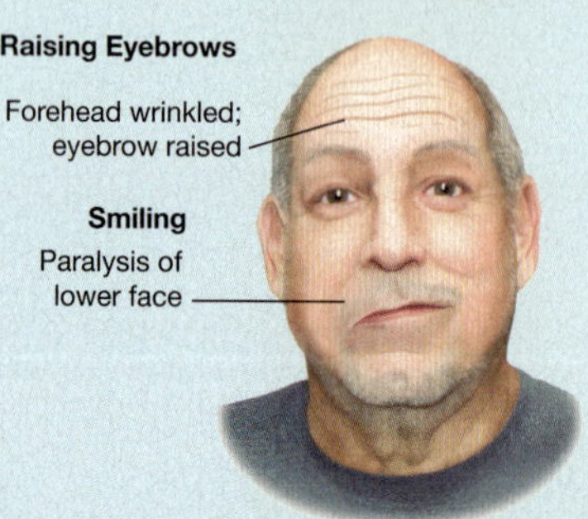

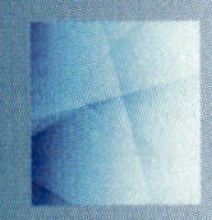

TABLE 27-12. Abnormal Body Postures

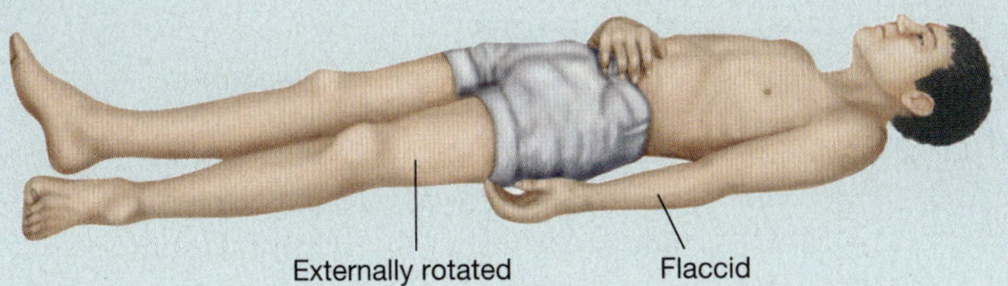

Hemiplegia (Early)

Sudden unilateral brain damage involving the corticospinal tract may produce a *hemiplegia* (one-sided paralysis), which is flaccid early in its course. Spasticity will develop later (see below). The paralyzed arm and leg are slack. They fall loosely and without tone when raised and dropped to the bed. Spontaneous movements or responses to noxious stimuli are limited to the opposite side. The leg may lie externally rotated. One side of the lower face may be paralyzed, and that cheek puffs out on expiration.

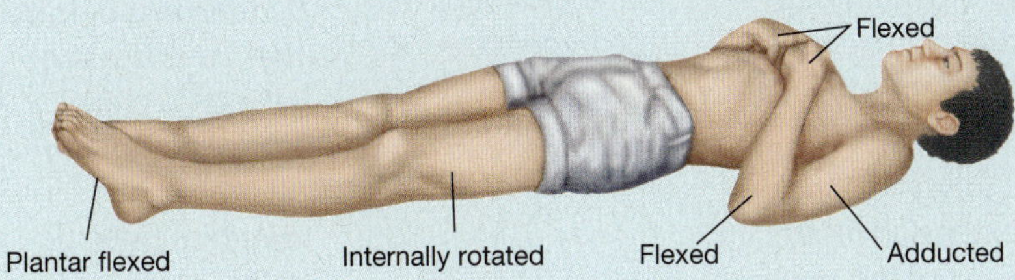

Decorticate Rigidity (Abnormal Flexor Response)

In *decorticate rigidity*, the upper arms are flexed tight to the sides with elbows, wrists, and fingers flexed. The legs are extended and internally rotated. The feet are plantar flexed. When seen bilaterally in a comatose patient, this implies a destructive lesion affecting the corticospinal tracts within or very near the cerebral hemispheres. This posture can also be seen unilaterally in a patient in the chronic recovery phase after a lesion of the corticospinal tract (chronic spastic hemiplegia), for example after stroke.

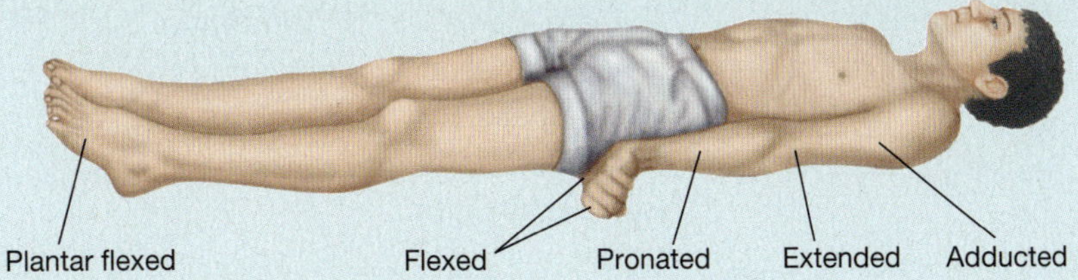

Decerebrate Rigidity (Abnormal Extensor Response)

In *decerebrate rigidity,* the jaws are clenched, and the neck is extended. The arms are adducted and stiffly extended at the elbows, with forearms pronated, wrists and fingers flexed. The legs are stiffly extended at the knees, with the feet plantar flexed. This posture may occur spontaneously or only in response to external stimuli such as light, noise, or pain. It is caused by a lesion in the diencephalon, midbrain, or pons, although may also arise from severe metabolic disorders such as hypoxia or hypoglycemia.

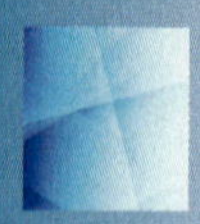

TABLE 27-13. Disorders of Muscle Tone

	Spasticity	Rigidity	Flaccidity (or Hypotonia)	Paratonia
Location of Lesion	Upper motor neuron or corticospinal tract systems	Basal ganglia system	Lower motor neuron system at any point from the anterior horn cell to the peripheral nerves, and in cerebellar disease	Both hemispheres, usually in the frontal lobes
Description	Increased muscle tone (*hypertonia*) is rate dependent. Tone increases when passive movement is rapid, and decreases when passive movement is slow. Tone is also greater at the extremes of the movement arc. During rapid passive movement, initial hypertonia may give way suddenly as the limb relaxes. This spastic "catch" and relaxation is known as "clasp-knife" resistance.	Increased resistance that persists throughout the movement arc, independent of rate of movement, is called *lead-pipe rigidity.* During flexion and extension of the wrist or forearm, a superimposed ratchet-like jerkiness is called *cogwheel rigidity* and can be due to underlying tremor.	Loss of muscle tone (*hypotonia*) causes the limb to be loose or floppy. The affected limbs may be hyperextensible or even flail-like. Flaccid muscles are often weak.	Sudden, irregular changes in tone accompany passive range of motion. Sudden loss of tone that increases the ease of motion is called *facilitatory paratonia, or mitgehen* (moving with). Sudden increase in tone making motion more difficult is called *oppositional paratonia, or gegenhalten* (holding against).
Common Cause	Stroke, especially late or chronic stage	Parkinsonism	Guillain–Barré syndrome; also initial phase of spinal cord injury (spinal shock) or stroke	Dementia

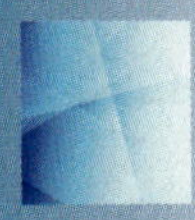

TABLE 27-14. Glasgow Coma Scale

Activity		Score
Eye Opening		
None	1 = Even to supraorbital pressure	
To pain	2 = Pain from sternum/limb/supraorbital pressure	
To speech	3 = Nonspecific response, not necessarily to command	
Spontaneous	4 = Eyes open, not necessarily aware	—
Motor Response		
None	1 = To any pain; limbs remain flaccid	
Extension	2 = Shoulder adducted, and shoulder and forearm internally rotated	
Flexor response	3 = Withdrawal response or assumption of hemiplegic posture	
Withdrawal	4 = Arm withdraws to pain, shoulder abducts	
Localizes pain	5 = Arm attempts to remove supraorbital/chest pressure	
Obeys commands	6 = Follows simple commands	—
Verbal Response		
None	1 = No verbalization of any type	
Incomprehensible	2 = Moans/groans, no speech	
Inappropriate	3 = Intelligible, no sustained sentences	
Confused	4 = Converses but confused, disoriented	
Oriented	5 = Converses and is oriented	—
		TOTAL (3–15)[a]

[a]**Interpretation:** Patients with scores of 3–8 usually are considered to be in a coma.

Source: Reprinted from Teasdale G, Jennett B. Assessment of coma and impaired consciousness. A practical scale. *Lancet*. 1974;304(7872):81–84. Copyright © 1974 Elsevier. With permission.

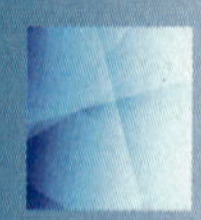

TABLE 27-15. Metabolic and Structural Coma

Although there are many causes of coma, most can be classified as either *structural* or *metabolic.* Findings vary widely in individual patients; the features listed are general guidelines rather than strict diagnostic criteria. Remember that *mental* disorders may mimic coma.

	Toxic—Metabolic	Structural
Pathophysiology	Arousal centers poisoned or critical substrates depleted	Lesion destroys or compresses brainstem arousal areas, either directly or secondary to more distant expanding mass lesions
Clinical Features		
■ Respiratory pattern	If regular, may be normal or hyperventilation If irregular, usually Cheyne–Stokes	Irregular, especially Cheyne–Stokes or ataxic breathing Also with selected stereotypical patterns like "apneustic" respiration (peak inspiratory arrest) or central hyperventilation
■ Pupillary size and reaction	Equal, reactive to light. If *pinpoint* from opiates or cholinergics, you may need a magnifying glass to see the reaction	Unequal or unreactive to light (fixed) *Midposition, fixed*—suggests midbrain compression
	May be unreactive if *fixed and dilated* from anticholinergics or hypothermia	*Dilated, fixed*—suggests compression of CN III from herniation
■ Level of consciousness	Changes *after* pupils change	Changes *before* pupils change
Examples of Cause	Uremia, liver failure, hyperglycemia, hypoglycemia, alcohol, drugs, hypothyroidism, anoxia, ischemia, meningitis, encephalitis, hyperthermia, hypothermia	Epidural, subdural, or intracerebral hemorrhage; large cerebral infarction; tumor, abscess; brainstem infarct, tumor, or hemorrhage; cerebellar infarct, hemorrhage, tumor, or abscess

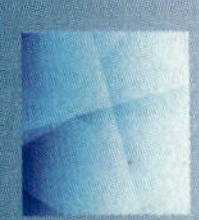

TABLE 27-16. Pupils in Comatose Patients

Pupillary size, equality, and light reactions are important signs in assessing the cause of coma and the region of the brain that is impaired. Keep in mind that unrelated pupillary abnormalities may precede coma, for example, from use of miotic drops for glaucoma or mydriatic drops for viewing the ocular fundi (not recommended when assessing a comatose patient).

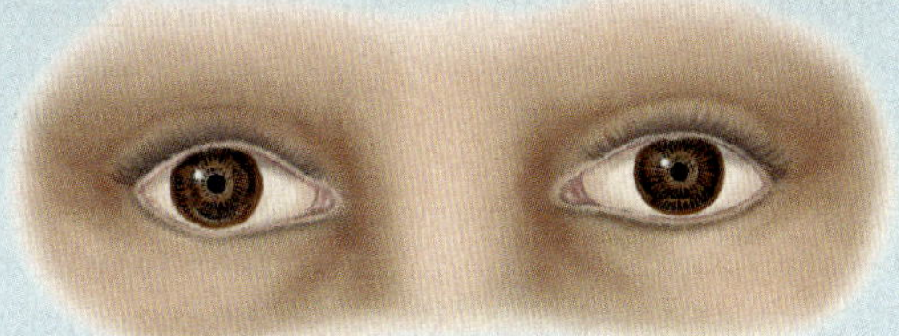

Small or Pinpoint Pupils

Bilaterally small pupils (1–2.5 mm) suggest damage to the sympathetic pathways in the hypothalamus, or metabolic encephalopathy, a diffuse failure of cerebral function that has many causes, including drugs. Light reactions are usually normal.

Pinpoint pupils (<1 mm) suggest a hemorrhage in the pons, or the effects of morphine, heroin, or other narcotics. The light reactions may be seen with a magnifying glass.

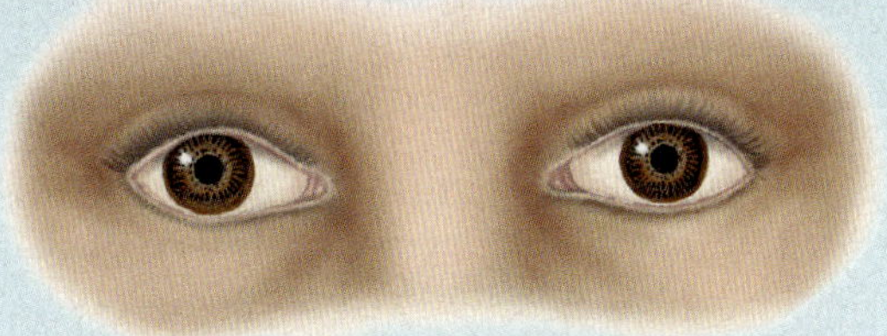

Midposition Fixed Pupils

Pupils that are in the *midposition or slightly dilated* (4–6 mm) and are *fixed to light* suggest structural damage in the midbrain.

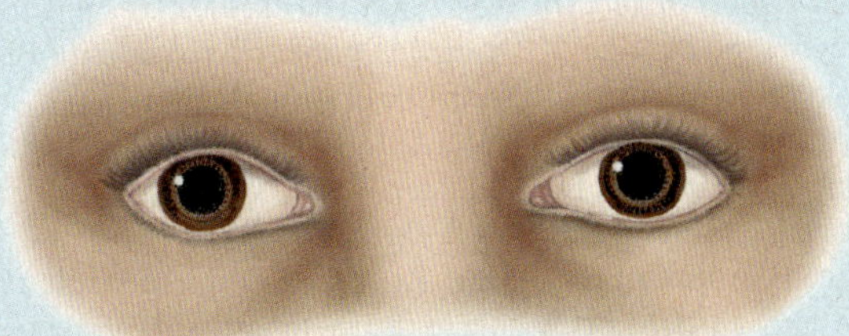

Large Pupils

Bilaterally fixed and dilated pupils may be due to severe anoxia and its sympathomimetic effects, as seen after cardiac arrest. They may also result from atropine-like agents, phenothiazines, or tricyclic antidepressants. *Bilaterally large reactive pupils* may be due to cocaine, amphetamine, LSD, or other sympathetic nervous system agonists.

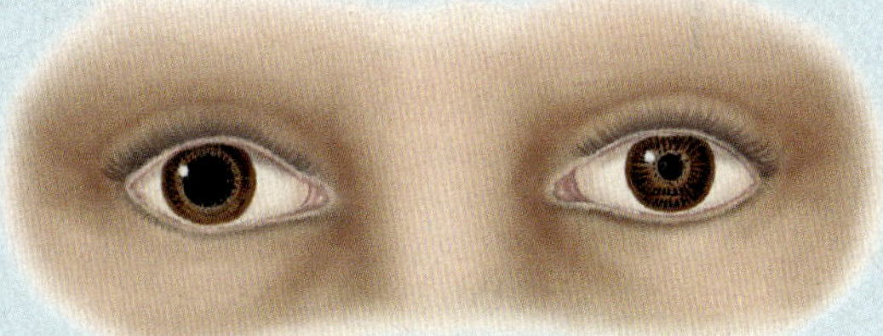

One Large Pupil

A pupil that is *fixed and dilated* warns of herniation of the temporal lobe, causing compression of the oculomotor nerve (CN III) and midbrain. A single large pupil can be seen in diabetic patients from infarction of CN III.

REFERENCES

1. Wright BL, Lai JT, Sinclair AJ. Cerebrospinal fluid and lumbar puncture: a practical review. *J Neurol.* 2012;259(8):1530–1545.
2. Straus SE, Thorpe KE, Holroyd-Leduc J. How do I perform a lumbar puncture and analyze the results to diagnose bacterial meningitis? *JAMA.* 2006;296(16):2012–2022.
3. National Institute of Neurological Disorders and Stroke. *Spinal Cord Injury.* U.S. Department of Health and Human Services, July 2024, Accessed March 18, 2024. https://www.ninds.nih.gov/health-information/disorders/spinal-cord-injury.
4. Chad DA, Stone JH, Gupta R. Case 14-2011—a woman with asymmetric sensory loss and paresthesias. *N Engl J Med.* 2011;364(19):1856–1865.
5. Dyck PJ, Herrmann DN, Staff NP, Dyck PJ. Assessing decreased sensation and increased sensory phenomena in diabetic polyneuropathies. *Diabetes.* 2013;62(11):3677–3686.
6. Kanji JN, Anglin RE, Hunt DL, Panju A. Does this patient with diabetes have large-fiber peripheral neuropathy? *JAMA.* 2010;303(15):1526–1532.
7. Hallett M. NINDS myotatic reflex scale. *Neurology.* 1993;43(12):2723.
8. Lipton RB, Bigal ME, Diamond M, Freitag F, Reed ML, Stewart WF. Migraine prevalence, disease burden, and the need for preventive therapy. *Neurology.* 2007;68(5):343–349.
9. Hazard E, Munakata J, Bigal ME, Rupnow MF, Lipton RB. The burden of migraine in the United States: current and emerging perspectives on disease management and economic analysis. *Value Health.* 2009;12(1):55–64.
10. Hale N, Paauw DS. Diagnosis and treatment of headache in the ambulatory care setting: a review of classic presentations and new considerations in diagnosis and management. *Med Clin North Am.* 2014;98(3):505–527.
11. Lipton RB, Bigal ME, Steiner TJ, Silberstein SD, Olesen J. Classification of primary headaches. *Neurology.* 2004;63(3):427–435.
12. Headache Classification Committee of the International Headache Society (IHS) The International Classification of Headache Disorders, 3rd edition. *Cephalalgia.* 2018;38(1):1–211.
13. Hainer BL, Matheson EM. Approach to acute headache in adults. *Am Fam Physician.* 2013;87(10):682–687.
14. MacGregor EA. Migraine. *Ann Intern Med.* 2017;166(7):ITC49–ITC64.
15. Omuro A, DeAngelis LM. Glioblastoma and other malignant gliomas: a clinical review. *JAMA.* 2013;310(17):1842–1850.
16. Brouwer MC, Tunkel AR, McKhann GM II, van de Beek D. Brain abscess. *N Engl J Med.* 2014;371(5):447–456.
17. D'Souza S. Aneurysmal subarachnoid hemorrhage. *J Neurosurg Anesthesiol.* 2015;27(3):222–240.
18. Mortimer AM, Bradley MD, Stoodley NG, Renowden SA. Thunderclap headache: diagnostic considerations and neuroimaging features. *Clin Radiol.* 2013;68(3):e101–e113.
19. Dilli E. Thunderclap headache. *Curr Neurol Neurosci Rep.* 2014;14(4):437.
20. Bushnell C, McCullough L. Stroke prevention in women: synopsis of the 2014 American Heart Association/American Stroke Association guideline. *Ann Intern Med.* 2014;160(12):853–857.
21. Sacco S, Ornello R, Ripa P, Pistoia F, Carolei A. Migraine and hemorrhagic stroke: a meta-analysis. *Stroke.* 2013;44(11):3032–3038.
22. Sacco S, Ricci S, Degan D, Carolei A. Migraine in women: the role of hormones and their impact on vascular diseases. *J Headache Pain.* 2012;13(3):177–189.
23. Dodick DW. Clinical practice. Chronic daily headache. *N Engl J Med.* 2006;354(2):158–165.
24. Schwedt TJ, Matharu MS, Dodick DW. Thunderclap headache. *Lancet Neurol.* 2006;5(7):621–631.
25. Gardner KL. Genetics of migraine: an update. *Headache.* 2006;46(1):S19–S24.
26. Detsky ME, McDonald DR, Baerlocher MO, Tomlinson GA, McCrory DC, Booth CM. Does this patient with headache have a migraine or need neuroimaging? *JAMA.* 2006;296(10):1274–1283.
27. Sun-Edelstein C, Bigal ME, Rapoport AM. Chronic migraine and medication overuse headache: clarifying the current International Headache Society classification criteria. *Cephalalgia.* 2009;29(4):445–452.
28. Fumal A, Schoenen J. Tension-type headache: current research and clinical management. *Lancet Neurol.* 2008;7(1):70–83.
29. Olesen J, Steiner T, Bousser MG, et al. Proposals for new standardized general diagnostic criteria for the secondary headaches. *Cephalalgia.* 2009;29(12):1331–1336.
30. Wipperman J. Dizziness and vertigo. *Prim Care.* 2014;41(1):115–131.
31. Siket MS, Edlow JA. Transient ischemic attack: reviewing the evolution of the definition, diagnosis, risk stratification, and management for the emergency physician. *Emerg Med Clin North Am.* 2012;30(3):745–770.
32. Cucchiara B, Kasner SE. In the clinic. Transient ischemic attack. *Ann Intern Med.* 2011;154(1):ITC11-15; quiz ITC1-16.
33. Karras C, Aitchison R, Aitchison P, Wang E, Kharasch M. Adult stroke summary. *Dis Mon.* 2013;59(5):210–216.
34. Nouh A, Remke J, Ruland S. Ischemic posterior circulation stroke: a review of anatomy, clinical presentations, diagnosis, and current management. *Front Neurol.* 2014;5:30.
35. Ishiyama G, Ishiyama A. Vertebrobasilar infarcts and ischemia. *Otolaryngol Clin North Am.* 2011;44(2):415–435.
36. Runchey S, McGee S. Does this patient have a hemorrhagic stroke? Clinical findings distinguishing hemorrhagic stroke from ischemic stroke. *JAMA.* 2010;303(22):2280–2286.
37. Yuki N, Hartung HP. Guillain-Barré syndrome. *N Engl J Med.* 2012;366(24):2294–2304.
38. Baggi F, Andreetta F, Maggi L, et al. Complete stable remission and autoantibody specificity in myasthenia gravis. *Neurology.* 2013;80(2):188–195.
39. Spillane J, Higham E, Kullmann DM. Myasthenia gravis. *BMJ.* 2012;345:e8497.
40. Yoo M, Sharma N, Pasnoor M, Kluding PM. Painful diabetic peripheral neuropathy: presentations, mechanisms, and exercise therapy. *J Diabetes Metab.* 2013;Suppl 10:005.
41. Gilron I, Baron R, Jensen T. Neuropathic pain: principles of diagnosis and treatment. *Mayo Clin Proc.* 2015;90(4):532–545.
42. Benditt DG, Adkisson WO. Approach to the patient with syncope: venues, presentations, diagnoses. *Cardiol Clin.* 2013;31(1):9–25.
43. Low PA, Tomalia VA. Orthostatic hypotension: mechanisms, causes, management. *J Clin Neurol.* 2015;11(3):220–226.
44. Epilepsy syndromes and their diagnosis. *Medical Knowledge Self-Assessment Program (MKSAP) 15 Neurology.* American College of Physicians; 2006:74.
45. Berg AT, Berkovic SF, Brodie MJ, et al. Revised terminology and concepts for organization of seizures and epilepsies:

report of the ILAE Commission on Classification and Terminology, 2005-2009. *Epilepsia.* 2010;51(4):676–685.
46. French JA, Pedley TA. Clinical practice. Initial management of epilepsy. *N Engl J Med.* 2008;359(2):166–176.
47. Elias WJ, Shah BB. Tremor. *JAMA.* 2014;311(9):948–954.
48. Benito-León J. Essential tremor: a neurodegenerative disease? *Tremor Other Hyperkinet Mov (NY).* 2014;4:252.
49. Connolly BS, Lang AE. Pharmacological treatment of Parkinson disease: a review. *JAMA.* 2014;311(16):1670–1683.
50. Jankovic J. Parkinson's disease: clinical features and diagnosis. *J Neurol Neurosurg Psychiatry.* 2008;79(4):368–376.
51. Wijemanne S, Jankovic J. Restless legs syndrome: clinical presentation diagnosis and treatment. *Sleep Med.* 2015;16(6):678–690.
52. Silber MH, Becker PM, Earley C, Garcia-Borreguero D, Ondo WG; Medical Advisory Board of the Willis-Ekbom Disease Foundation. Willis-Ekbom Disease Foundation revised consensus statement on the management of restless legs syndrome. *Mayo Clin Proc.* 2013;88(9):977–986.
53. Neurology clerkship core curriculum Guidelines. *American Academy of Neurology*, Oct. 2000, Accessed March 18, 2024. https://www.aan.com/globals/axon/assets/2770.pdf
54. McGee SR. Chapter 56: visual field testing. In: *Evidence-Based Physical Diagnosis.* 3rd ed. Elsevier/Saunders; 2012:513–520.
55. McGee SR. Chapter 20: the pupils. In: *Evidence-Based Physical Diagnosis.* 3rd ed. Elsevier/Saunders; 2012:176–178.
56. McGee SR. Chapter 57: nerves of the eye muscles. In: *Evidence-Based Physical Diagnosis.* 3rd ed. Elsevier/Saunders; 2012:521–531.
57. Zandian A, Osiro S, Hudson R, et al. The neurologist's dilemma: a comprehensive clinical review of Bell's palsy, with emphasis on current management trends. *Med Sci Monit.* 2014;20:83–90.
58. McGee SR. Chapter 22: hearing. In: *Evidence-Based Physical Diagnosis.* 3rd ed. Elsevier/Saunders; 2012:190.
59. Darcy P, Moughty AM. Images in clinical medicine. Pronator drift. *N Engl J Med.* 2013;369(16):e20.
60. Daum C, Aybek S. Validity of the "drift without pronation" sign in conversion disorder. *BMC Neurol.* 2013;13:31.
61. Stone J, Carson A, Duncan R, et al. Which neurological diseases are most likely to be associated with "symptoms unexplained by organic disease." *J Neurol.* 2012;259(1):33–38.
62. Stone J, Carson A, Sharpe M. Functional symptoms and signs in neurology: assessment and diagnosis. *J Neurol Neurosurg Psychiatry.* 2005;76(1):i2–i12.
63. Stabler SP. Clinical practice. Vitamin B12 deficiency. *N Engl J Med.* 2013;368(2):149–160.
64. Isaza Jaramillo SP, Uribe CS, García Jimenez FA, Cornejo-Ochoa W, Alvarez Restrepo JF, Román GC. Accuracy of the Babinski sign in the identification of pyramidal tract dysfunction. *J Neurol Sci.* 2014;343(1–2):66–68.
65. Forgie SE. The history and current relevance of the eponymous signs of meningitis. *Pediatr Infect Dis J.* 2016;35(7):749–751.
66. Kirshblum SC, Burns SP, Biering-Sorensen F, et al. International standards for neurological classification of spinal cord injury (revised 2011). *J Spinal Cord Med.* 2011;34(6):535–546.
67. McGee SR. Chapter 24: meninges. *Evidence-Based Physical Diagnosis.* 3rd ed. Elsevier/Saunders; 2012:210–214.
68. Thomas KE, Hasbun R, Jekel J, Quagliarello VJ. The diagnostic accuracy of Kernig's sign, Brudzinski's sign, and nuchal rigidity in adults with suspected meningitis. *Clin Infect Dis.* 2002;35(1):46–52.
69. Ward MA, Greenwood TM, Kumar DR, Mazza JJ, Yale SH. Josef Brudzinski and Vladimir Mikhailovich Kernig: signs for diagnosing meningitis. *Clin Med Res.* 2010;8(1):13–17.
70. Geiseler PJ, Nelson KE. Bacterial meningitis without clinical signs of meningeal irritation. *South Med J.* 1982;75(4):448–450.
71. Puxty JA, Fox RA, Horan MA. The frequency of physical signs usually attributed to meningeal irritation in elderly patients. *J Am Geriatr Soc.* 1983;31(10):590–592.
72. Afhami S, Dehghan Manshadi SA, Rezahosseini O. Jolt accentuation of headache: can this maneuver rule out acute meningitis? *BMC Res Notes.* 2017;10(1):540.
73. McGee SR. Chapter 62: disorders of the nerve roots, plexuses, and peripheral nerves. *Evidence-Based Physical Diagnosis.* 3rd ed. Elsevier/Saunders; 2012:607–609.
74. Mendizabal M, Silva MO. Images in clinical medicine. Asterixis. *N Engl J Med.* 2010;363(9):e14.
75. Edlow JA, Rabinstein A, Traub SJ, Wijdicks EF. Diagnosis of reversible causes of coma. *Lancet.* 2014;384(9959):2064–2076.
76. Moore SA, Wijdicks EF. The acutely comatose patient: clinical approach and diagnosis. *Semin Neurol.* 2013;33(2):110–120.
77. Wijdicks EFM. *The Comatose Patient.* 2nd ed. Oxford University Press; 2014.
78. Henry TR, Ezzeddine MA. Approach to the patient with transient alteration of consciousness. *Neurol Clin Pract.* 2012;2(3):179–186.
79. Pope JV, Edlow JA. Avoiding misdiagnosis in patients with neurological emergencies. *Emerg Med Int.* 2012;2012:949275.
80. Brown EN, Lydic R, Schiff ND. General anesthesia, sleep, and coma. *N Engl J Med.* 2010;363(27):2638–2650.
81. Teasdale G, Jennett B. Assessment of coma and impaired consciousness: a practical scale. *Lancet.* 1974;2(7872):81–84.
82. Sandroni C, Geocadin RG. Neurological prognostication after cardiac arrest. *Curr Opin Crit Care.* 2015;21(3):209–214.
83. Tsao CW, Aday AW, Almarzooq ZI, et al; American Heart Association Council on Epidemiology and Prevention Statistics Committee and Stroke Statistics Subcommittee. Heart Disease and Stroke Statistics-2023 Update: a report from the American Heart Association. *Circulation.* 2023;147(8):e93–e621.
84. GBD 2016 Lifetime Risk of Stroke Collaborators; Feigin VL, Nguyen G, Cercy K, et al. Global, regional, and country-specific lifetime risks of stroke, 1990 and 2016. *N Engl J Med.* 2018;379(25):2429–2437.
85. US Preventive Services Task Force; Davidson KW, Barry MJ, Mangione CM, et al. Aspirin use to prevent cardiovascular disease: US Preventive Services Task Force Recommendation Statement. *JAMA.* 2022;327(16):1577–1584.
86. Goff DC Jr., Lloyd-Jones DM, Bennett G, et al; American College of Cardiology/American Heart Association Task Force on Practice Guidelines. 2013 ACC/AHA guideline on the assessment of cardiovascular risk: a report of the American College of Cardiology/American Heart Association Task Force on Practice Guidelines. *Circulation.* 2014;129(25):S49–73.

87. US Preventive Services Task Force; Davidson KW, Barry MJ, Mangione CM, et al. Screening for atrial fibrillation: US Preventive Services Task Force Recommendation Statement. *JAMA.* 2022;327(4):360–367.
88. US Preventive Services Task Force; Krist AH, Davidson KW, Mangione CM, et al. Screening for asymptomatic carotid artery stenosis: US Preventive Services Task Force Recommendation Statement. *JAMA.* 2021;325(5):476–481.
89. Guirguis-Blake JM, Webber EM, Coppola EL. screening for asymptomatic carotid artery stenosis in the general population: updated evidence report and systematic review for the US Preventive Services Task Force. *JAMA.* 2021;325(5): 487–489.
90. Bhimraj A. Acute community-acquired bacterial meningitis in adults: an evidence-based review. *Cleve Clin J Med.* 2012;79(6): 393–400.

UNIT 3 Special Populations

CHAPTER 28

Children: Infancy Through Adolescence

INTRODUCTION

Chapter Content Guide

- General Principles of Child Development
- Surveillance of Development
- Key Components of Health Promotion
- Sections
  - Newborns and Infants
  - Preschool and School-Age Children
  - Adolescents

Section Organization:

- Health History: General Approach
- Surveillance of Development
- Physical Development
- Cognitive and Language Development
- Social and Emotional Development
- Physical Examination: General Approach
- Techniques of Examination
- Recording Your Findings
- Health Promotion and Counseling: Evidence and Recommendations

This chapter covers clinical assessments for pediatric age groups: *newborns* (0 to 28 days), *infants* (1 month to 1 year), *preschool-age children* (1 to 5 years), *school-age children* (6 to 11 years), and *adolescents* (12 to 18 years), as illustrated in Figures 28-1 to 28-3. It starts with general principles of development and health promotion, then addresses each age group in separate sections, discussing history taking, development surveillance, examination techniques, and health counseling.

Inexperienced examiners may feel intimidated when handling a tiny infant or an upset child, especially under the watchful eyes of anxious caregivers. The examination sequence should vary based on the child's age and comfort

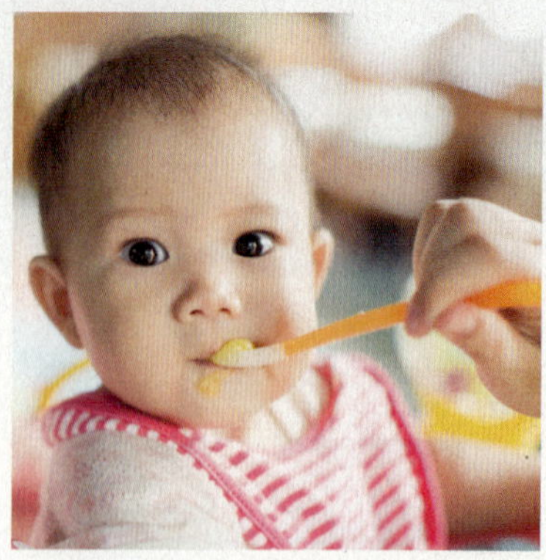

FIGURE 28-1. Infants (1 month to 1 year) undergo rapid growth and require careful observation of feeding habits and developmental milestones.

FIGURE 28-2. School-age children (6 to 11 years) develop literacy, reasoning, and independence, key aspects of developmental surveillance.

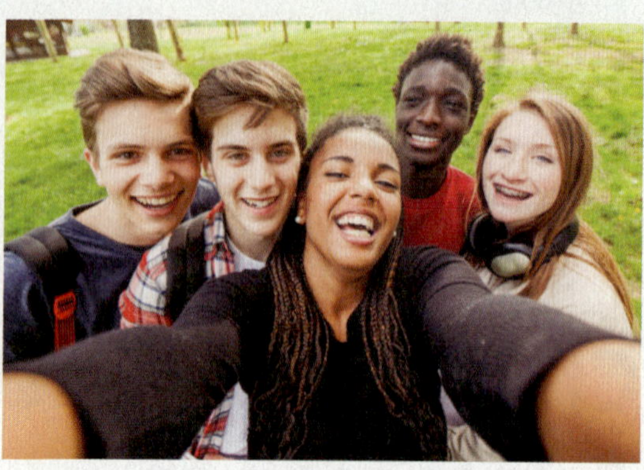

FIGURE 28-3. Adolescents (12 to 18 years) experience social and emotional growth, emphasizing the importance of age-appropriate health counseling and examination techniques.

level, performing less invasive maneuvers early and potentially distressing ones near the end. For example, auscultate the heart and lungs early, and examine the ears, mouth, and abdomen near the end. If the child reports pain in one area, examine that area last. While initially challenging, you may eventually enjoy almost all pediatric encounters.

GENERAL PRINCIPLES OF CHILD DEVELOPMENT

Childhood is a period of remarkable physical, cognitive, and social growth, the greatest in a person's lifetime (Fig. 28-4). Within a few years, children's weight increases 20-fold, and they acquire sophisticated language and reasoning, develop complex social interactions, and progress toward becoming adults (Box 28-1). Understanding typical physical, cognitive, and social development aids in effective interviews and physical examinations and helps distinguish typical from atypical findings.[1–3]

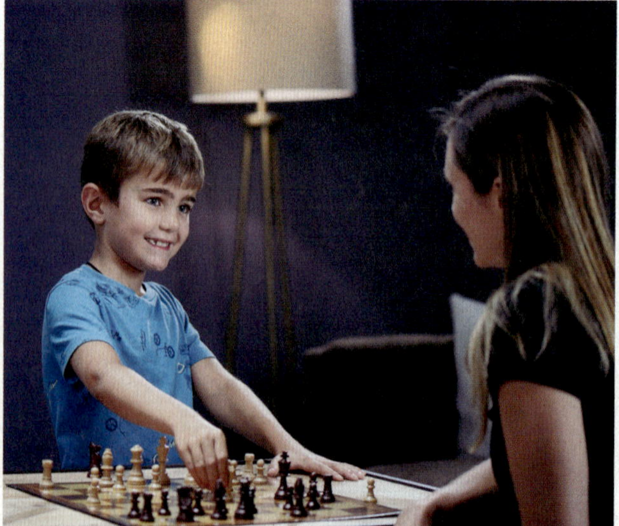

FIGURE 28-4. Interactive play fosters social and cognitive development during childhood.

Box 28-1. General Principles of Child Development

Principle 1: Typical development follows a predictable pathway governed by the maturing brain.	■ Age-specific milestones characterize development as normal or abnormal. ■ Evaluations determine the child's position along a developmental trajectory. ■ Milestones are achieved in a predictable order.
Principle 2: The range of typical development is wide.	■ Children mature at different rates. ■ Physical, cognitive, and social development should fall within the broad range of typical development for their age.
Principle 3: Various factors affect child development and health.	■ Chronic illnesses, child abuse, poverty, exposure to violence, and adverse childhood experiences (ACEs) can cause physical abnormalities or alter development. ■ Children with physical or cognitive disabilities may follow unique developmental trajectories that differ from typical age-specific patterns (Fig. 28-5). ■ Children with Down syndrome and other genetic syndromes have their own growth curves and health surveillance guidelines.
Principle 4: Developmental level affects clinical history and physical examination.	■ Interviewing a 5-year-old differs from interviewing an adolescent. Adapt the evaluation to the child's developmental level.[4]

Loss of milestones is always concerning.

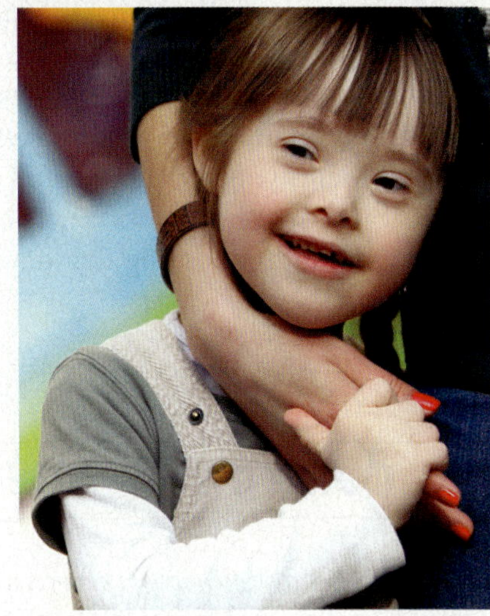

FIGURE 28-5. Children with Down syndrome and other selected genetic syndromes follow unique growth curves and specific health surveillance guidelines from the American Academy of Pediatrics (AAP).

SURVEILLANCE OF DEVELOPMENT

A child's development follows a predictable path, achieving sequential milestones. Developmental assessment maps a child's status compared to peers, using direct observation and input from caregivers and validated screeners.[5–9] Pediatric clinicians evaluate five critical domains: *physical* (gross and fine motor skills), *cognitive*, *language*, and *social-emotional*.

- **Physical:** *gross motor skills* include walking, sitting, or transferring positions; *fine motor skills* include manipulating objects for eating, drawing, or playing[10,11]; delays in physical milestones often prompt clinical visits
- **Cognitive:** measures the child's problem-solving abilities through intuition, perception, and reasoning, both verbal and nonverbal,[7] and involves the ability to retain and apply information appropriately[10,11]
- **Language:** involves the ability to articulate, receive, and express information, including nonverbal communication like waving and nodding;

skills develop through word combinations influenced by environmental interactions[10,11]

- **Social and emotional:** encompasses the child's ability to form and maintain relationships, regulate emotions and behaviors, and respond to others; includes self-help skills in activities of daily living such as feeding, dressing, and toileting[10,11]

The American Academy of Pediatrics (AAP) recommends using age-appropriate standardized screening instruments to assess these domains, which should complement comprehensive developmental exams.[12] Widely validated tools include the *Ages and Stages Questionnaire (ASQ)*,[13,14] *Early Language Milestone Scale (ELM Scale-2)*,[15–17] *Modified Checklist for Autism in Toddlers (MCHAT)*,[16] *Parents' Evaluation of Developmental Status (PEDS)*,[18] and *Survey of Well-Being of Young Children (SWYC)*.[19]

Clinicians should periodically use these instruments during preventive health visits, as they are more effective than observation and physical exams alone in identifying developmental delays. Suspected delays warrant further evaluation. Use validated screeners covering all five domains to identify delays and at-risk children, noting that development can change due to environmental factors.[20]

If a cooperative child fails a screening, precise testing is necessary.

KEY COMPONENTS OF HEALTH PROMOTION

The saying "*an ounce of prevention is worth a pound of cure*," is especially true for children. Pediatric clinicians prioritize health supervision and promotion. National and international guidelines emphasize disease detection and prevention, identifying risk factors, and promoting overall well-being.[21–23]

Every interaction with a child and family is an opportunity for health promotion. From the interview to the physical examination, think of your interactions as an opportunity for three important tasks: the identification of risk factors, the detection of clinical problems, and the promotion of health (Fig. 28-6). Provide age-appropriate guidance on development, identify stressors, and promote resilience through suggestions on activities and developmental strategies. Advise caregivers about upcoming developmental stages and strategies to encourage their child's development. Caregivers are key to health promotion, implementing advice given by clinicians. The AAP provides guidelines for *health supervision visits*, with additional needs for children with chronic illnesses or high-risk circumstances (see www.healthychildren.org).

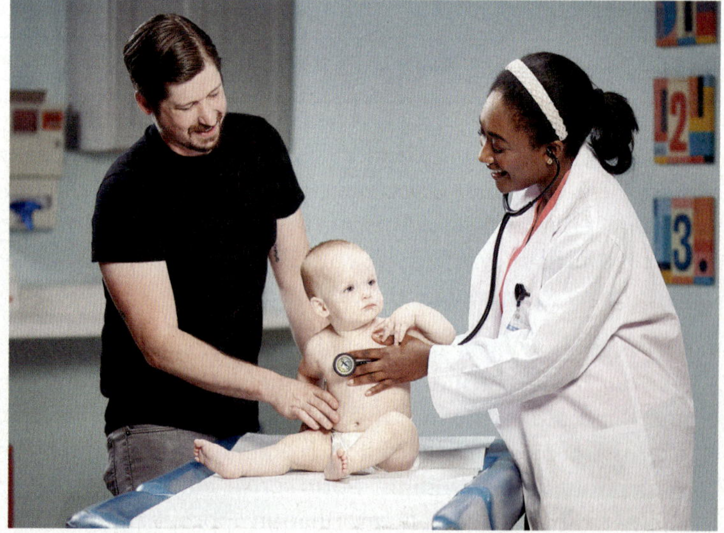

FIGURE 28-6. Infant exams focus on health promotion, immunizations, and early guidance.

Integrate physical findings with health promotion, demonstrating the link between healthy behaviors and physical health. For example, *Bright Futures* recommends screening for obesity starting at age 2 years and providing family-centered support to facilitate healthy eating and exercise.[24] Immunizations are crucial for health promotion, with updated guidelines from the U.S. Centers for Disease Control and Prevention ([CDC] see www.cdc.gov) and the AAP.[25,26]

National guidelines recommend age-specific screening procedures (Fig. 28-7), with detailed AAP recommendations available at https://www.aap.org/en/practice-management/care-delivery-approaches/periodicity-schedule/.[27] Anticipatory guidance, which covers a wide range of health topics, including safety and injury prevention, is also essential.[22,27] Key areas cover a broad range of topics, from clinical to developmental, social, and emotional health to safety and injury prevention (Box 28-2).

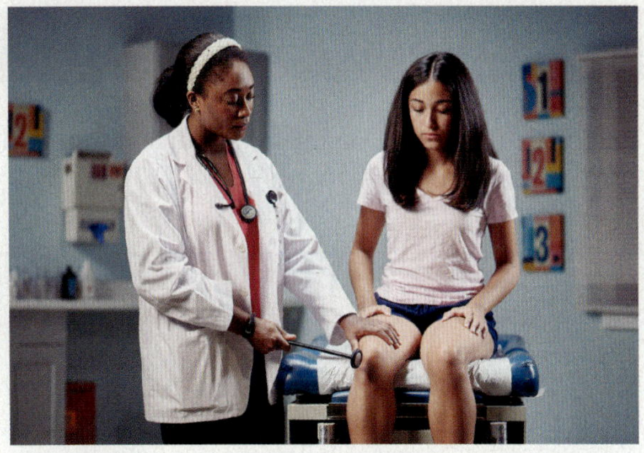

FIGURE 28-7. Adolescent exams emphasize screening, risk detection, and anticipatory guidance.

Box 28-2. Key Components of Pediatric Health Promotion

1. Age-appropriate developmental achievement of the child
    - Physical (maturation, growth, puberty)
    - Motor (gross and fine motor skills)
    - Cognitive (developmental milestones, language, school performance)
    - Emotional (self-regulation, mood, self-efficacy, self-esteem, independence)
    - Social (social competence, self-responsibility, integration with family and community, peer interactions)
2. Health supervision visits
    - Periodic assessment of physical, developmental, socio-emotional, and oral health
    - More frequent visits for children with special health care needs
3. Integration of physical examination findings with health promotion
4. Immunizations
5. Screening procedures
6. Oral health
7. Anticipatory guidance[22,25]
    - Healthy habits
    - Nutrition and healthy eating
    - Safety and prevention of injury
    - Physical activity
    - Sexual development and sexuality
    - Self-responsibility, efficacy, and healthy self-esteem
    - Family relationships (interactions, strengths, supports)
    - Positive caregiving strategies
    - Reading aloud with the child, interactive play or "time in"
    - Emotional and mental health
    - Oral health
    - Recognition of illness
    - Sleep
    - Screen time
    - Prevention of risky behaviors
    - School and vocation
    - Peer relationships
    - Community interactions
8. Partnership among health care provider, child/adolescent, and family

NEWBORNS AND INFANTS

The first year of life, or infancy, is divided into the *neonatal period* (the first 28 days) and the *postneonatal period* (29 days to 1 year).

HEALTH HISTORY: GENERAL APPROACH

The *newborn assessment*, typically performed within 12 to 24 hours after delivery, is a key opportunity to engage with the family, understand the pregnancy history, and observe family interactions. It allows providers to demonstrate the newborn's abilities and model positive interactions. Caregivers, while joyful, may be exhausted and anxious. Addressing their concerns and empathizing with their anxieties is essential.

The initial visit balances history-taking and anticipatory guidance, making it a natural conversation. Experienced clinicians can comfort and build strong bonds with families by being empathetic and calm. The visit is also ideal for discussing potential stressors and caregiving goals. During the exam, emphasize building caregiver–child relationships through interactive communication, known as "serve and return," which promotes brain development. Key components of the health history are detailed in Box 28-3.

Box 28-3. Key Components of the Health History for the Newborn Visit[21]

Questions and concerns from family

- Questions about the newborn, home environment, prenatal course, or delivery
- Concerns about physical features
- Concerns and questions about newborn care

Prenatal history, labor, and delivery

- Pregnancy history, complications, prenatal diagnoses
- Physical and mental health of the birthing parent and partner (if applicable)
- Use of tobacco, alcohol, or drugs during pregnancy
- Labor and delivery experience or complications
- History of prior pregnancies and other children in the household

Neonatal course prior to the visit

- Health and well-being of the birthing parent and others in the family or support network
- Feeding plans, including breastfeeding or chestfeeding, bottle feeding, or both

Neonatal history

- General well-being and any specific issues of concern
- Cultural or personal beliefs impacting care

Family history

- Comprehensive medical and genetic history, if time permits

Social history

- Social determinants (living situation, concerns about food, housing, utilities, relationships, adults involved in caring for the newborn, support network, exposure to violence, financial concerns, stressors)
- Any social concerns from family or caregivers
- Siblings, other household members, babysitter, or other caregivers

Caregivers' observation of the newborn's behavior and activity

- What the newborn has been able to do so far
- Level of activity, bonding, and attachment

Feeding and nutrition

- Type of feeding (breastfeeding/chestfeeding, formula, combination), how feeding is going

Sleeping, stooling, urination

- Frequency and color of stools and urine
- Sleep patterns, duration, and how the newborn falls asleep

Safety

- Car safety seats
- Safe sleep practices

Anticipatory guidance for newborn care

- Illness prevention
- Dressing appropriately, protection against heat, pets, and ensuring a safe home environment
- Care of newborn's body (umbilical cord, penis including circumcision decision, etc.)
- Information on upcoming visits, when to seek advice

Source: Adapted from Bright Futures.

SURVEILLANCE OF DEVELOPMENT

Monitoring and supporting infant development are crucial. Boxes 28-4 and 28-5 outline key aspects of physical, cognitive, language, and social and emotional development in newborns and infants.

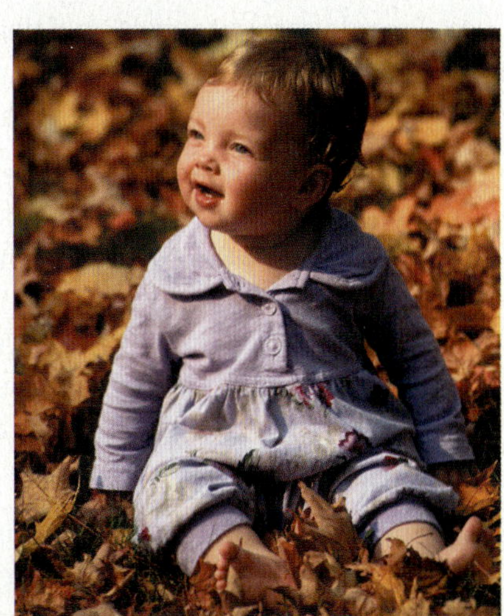

FIGURE 28-8. Sitting up while leaning on hands is a typical developmental milestone for a 6-month-old.

Box 28-4. Surveillance of Development: Newborns and Infants

Physical Development

- Newborns can fix on and follow human faces. Neurologic development progresses from head to trunk to arms and legs, before hands and fingers.
- Physical growth during infancy is rapid. Typical milestones include sitting up at 6 months and tripling weight by 1 year (Fig. 28-8).[28]

(*continued*)

Box 28-4. Surveillance of Development: Newborns and Infants (*Continued*)

- *Tummy time* supports neck, arm, and core strength needed for sitting and standing.
- Activity and exploration are crucial for learning through manipulation of the environment.
- Updated developmental milestones for 2022 include:
  - 3 months: lifting the head, batting at objects
  - 6 months: rolling over, reaching for objects, laughing, sitting with support
  - Older infants: transferring objects from hand to hand, crawling, standing with support, playing with objects by banging and grabbing
  - 1 year: pulling to stand and first steps often after the first year (Fig. 28-9)[5,29,30]

Health Care Approaches

- Regularly monitor growth.
- Provide guidance on tummy time.
- Provide early intervention for delayed milestones.

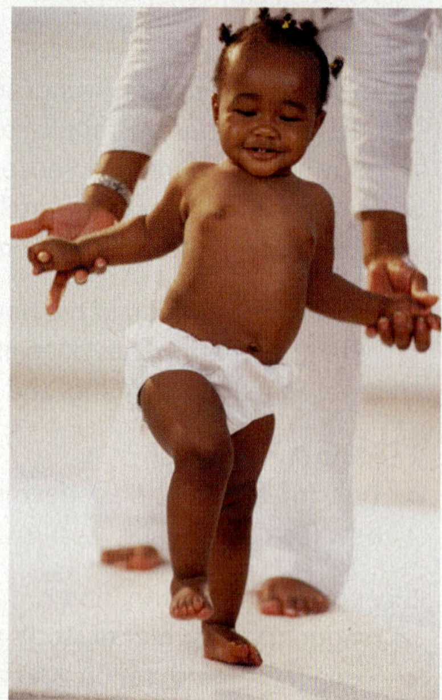

FIGURE 28-9. Children often take their first steps after 1 year.

Cognitive and Language Development

- Interaction with caregivers fosters understanding; talking, singing, and reading stimulate cognitive development.
- Infants learn cause-and-effect and object permanence by manipulating objects.
- By 9 months, infants imitate sounds, recognize their name, and seek comfort from caregivers during exams.
- Language progresses from cooing at 4 months to babbling at 9 months and saying "mama" or "dada" by 1 year.[31]

Health Care Approaches

- Encourage caregiver interaction through talking, singing, reading.
- Monitor cognitive and language milestones.
- Provide early intervention if delays noted.

If infants are not making age-appropriate sounds, consider testing for hearing deficits.

Social and Emotional Development

- By 1 month, infants recognize a caregiver's voice; by 2 months, they smile; key tasks include bonding, attachment, and developing trust.
- *Temperament* varies among infants, and the environment influences social development.
- Observe infant–caregiver interactions during assessments.
- If developmental skills plateau or are out of sequence, evaluate for developmental disabilities like autism or cerebral palsy.

Health Care Approaches

- Support caregiver-infant bonding.
- Observe interactions with caregivers.
- Evaluate for developmental disabilities if skills plateau.

Evaluate infants or toddlers with plateaued or out-of-sequence skills for developmental disabilities.

Box 28-5. Developmental Milestones: Birth to 12 Months[5]

Age	Gross/Fine Motor	Social/Emotional	Language/ Communication	Cognitive
2 months	■ Holds head up when on tummy _________ ■ Opens hands briefly	■ Calms down when spoken to or picked up ■ Looks at your face ■ Seems happy to see you ■ Smiles when you talk or smile	■ Makes sounds other than crying ■ Reacts to loud sounds	■ Watches you as you move ■ Looks at a toy for several seconds ■ Follows face
4 months	■ Sits with support, no head lag _________ ■ Hands predominantly open ■ Reaches for objects ■ Holds a toy in hand	■ Smiles to get your attention ■ Chuckles when you try to make them laugh ■ Looks at you, moves, or makes sounds to engage	■ Makes cooing sounds like "ooo" and "aahh" ■ Makes sounds back when you talk ■ Turns head toward the sound of your voice	■ If hungry, opens mouth when hungry (sees breast or bottle) ■ Looks at hands with interest
6 months	■ Rolls from front to back ■ Pushes up with straight arms when on tummy ■ Sits propped on hands ■ Reaches for objects with a raking grasp with one hand _________ ■ Transfers objects between hands	■ Knows familiar people ■ Likes to look at themselves in the mirror ■ Laughs when engaged	■ Takes turns making sounds with you ■ Blows "raspberries" (sticks tongue out and blows) ■ Makes squealing noises ■ Understands when being told "no"	■ Puts objects in mouth to explore them ■ Closes lips to show they do not want more food
9 months	■ Gets into sitting position by themselves ■ Sits without support _________ ■ Uses fingers to "rake" food toward themselves ■ Grasps objects using the thumb and fingers, keeping the object away from the palm (radial-digital grasp)	■ Is fearful around strangers ■ Shows several facial expressions ■ Reacts when you leave ■ Smiles or laughs when you play peek-a-boo	■ Makes different sounds like "mamama" and "bababa" ■ Lifts arms to be picked up ■ Looks when you call their name	■ Looks for objects when dropped out of sight ■ Bangs two objects together
12 months	■ Pulls up to stand ■ Walks, holding onto furniture _________ ■ Drinks from cup without a lid, as you hold it ■ Picks things up between thumb finger (pincer grasp)	■ Plays games like pat-a-cake ■ Waves "bye-bye"	■ Calls a parent or caregiver "mama" or "dada" or another special name ■ Understands "no"	■ Puts something in a container ■ Looks for things they see you hide

Source: Zubler JM, Wiggins LD, Macias MM, et al. Evidence-informed milestones for developmental surveillance tools. *Pediatrics*. 2022;149(3):e2021052138.

PHYSICAL EXAMINATION: GENERAL APPROACH

Newborns

Examining newborns immediately after birth is crucial for assessing their general condition, developmental status, and detecting congenital abnormalities. A comprehensive pediatric exam is usually performed within 24 hours of birth. Subsequent exams occur regularly or when the infant is ill (Fig. 28-10).

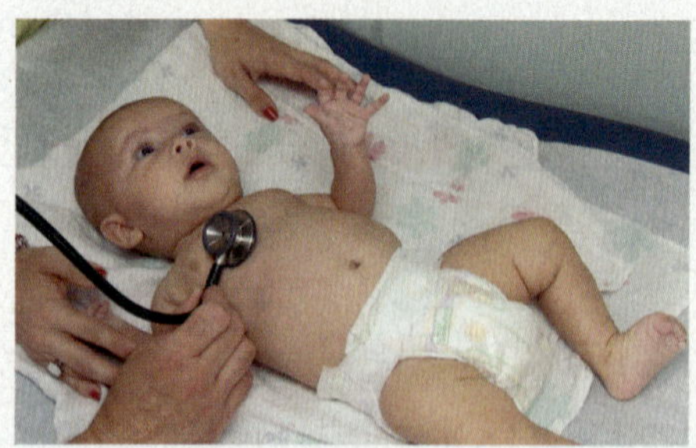

FIGURE 28-10. Infant exam evaluates growth, detects abnormalities, and involves caregivers in understanding health milestones.

Conducting the exam in front of the caregivers and narrating findings allows engagement and education about the newborn's development (Box 28-6).

Asking caregivers to point out concerns can help identify subtle abnormalities like birthmarks, skin tags, asymmetries, dimples, and abnormal movements.

Research by Dr. T. Berry Brazelton and others highlights the wide range of abilities in newborns (Box 28-7).[32] Demonstrating the newborn's abilities, such as quieting when spoken to softly and following a face with their eyes, can delight caregivers.

Reassure caregivers by stating normal findings and offering support for feeding techniques. Newborns are most responsive 1 to 2 hours after feeding. Start the exam with the newborn swaddled, undressing gradually to minimize stimulation. If the newborn becomes agitated, use a pacifier or let the newborn suck on your gloved finger. Reswaddle as needed to complete the exam.

Newborns not demonstrating expected behaviors may have neurologic conditions, drug withdrawal, or serious illness.

Box 28-6. Tips for Examining Newborns

- Examine the newborn in the presence of caregivers.
- Swaddle and then undress the newborn as the examination proceeds.
- Dim the lights and rock the newborn to encourage the eyes to open.
- Observe feeding, if possible, including breastfeeding, chestfeeding or bottle feeding.
- Demonstrate calming maneuvers to caregivers (e.g., swaddling).
- Observe and teach caregivers about transitions as the newborn arouses.
- Typical sequence for the examination of the newborn:
  - Careful observation before (and during) the examination
  - Heart
  - Lungs
  - Femoral pulses
  - Head, neck, and clavicles
  - Ears and mouth
  - Hips
  - Abdomen and genitourinary system
  - Lower extremities, upper extremities, back
  - Eyes, whenever they are spontaneously open or at end of examination
  - Skin, as you go along
  - Neurologic system

Box 28-7. What a Newborn Can Do

Core Elements[32]

Newborns have various behavioral states such as quiet sleep, active sleep, non–alert-waking, alert waking, active waking, and fussing and crying. Newborns are unique individuals and marked differences exist in temperament, personality, behavior, and learning. Newborns use all five senses (e.g., looking at human faces and turning to a caregiver's voice). Newborns interact dynamically with caregivers.

Examples of Complex Newborn Behavior

Habituation	Ability to selectively and progressively shut out negative stimuli (e.g., a repetitive sound)
Attachment	Reciprocal, dynamic process of interacting and bonding with the caregiver
State regulation	Ability to modulate the level of arousal in response to different degrees of stimulation (e.g., self-consoling)
Perception	Ability to regard faces, turn to voices, quiet in presence of singing, track colorful objects, respond to touch, and recognize familiar scents

Infants

Start with the infant sitting or lying in the caregiver's lap (Fig. 28-11). If the infant is tired, hungry, or ill, have the caregiver hold the infant against their chest. Ensure appropriate toys or familiar objects are nearby. A hungry infant may need feeding before the exam (Box 28-8).

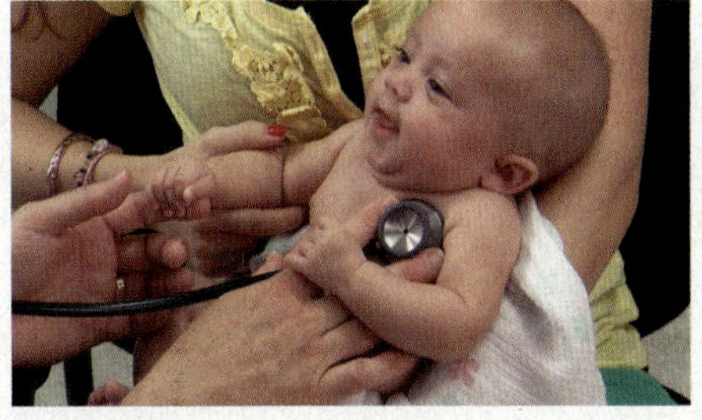

FIGURE 28-11. Start the examination while the child is still on the caregiver's lap.

Some neurologic conditions can be assessed during the general examination by evaluating the infant's tone and extremity movements.

Box 28-8. Tips for Examining Infants

- Approach the infant gradually, using a toy or object for distraction.
- Perform as much of the examination as possible with the infant in the caregiver's lap.
- Speak softly to the infant or mimic the infant's sounds to attract attention.
- If the infant is cranky, make sure they are well fed before proceeding.
- Ask a caregiver about the infant's strengths to elicit useful developmental and caregiving information.
- Do not expect to do a head-to-toe examination in a specific order. Work with what the infant gives you and save the mouth and ear examination for last.

Close observation of an awake infant can reveal tone abnormalities, skin color issues, jaundice, cyanosis, and respiratory problems. Observe caregiver–infant interactions, noting positive behaviors such as pride in the caregiver's face.

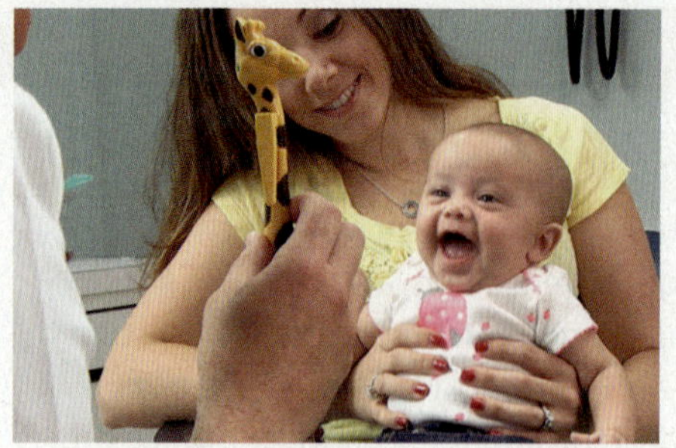

FIGURE 28-12. Children can have fun during the developmental examination.

Observing the infant's interactions with the caregiver can reveal issues such as developmental delay, language delay, hearing deficits, and inadequate caregiver-infant bonding. These observations may also identify maladaptive nurturing patterns due to caregiver mental health or limited social support.

Use developmentally appropriate methods such as *distraction* and *play* to examine the infant, employing methods like moving objects, flashing lights, toys, peek-a-boo, tickling, or noise (Fig. 28-12).

If the infant cannot be distracted or engaged, consider possible visual or hearing deficits.

TECHNIQUES OF EXAMINATION: NEWBORNS AND INFANTS

Apgar Score

Assess the Apgar Score. The Apgar score evaluates a newborn immediately after birth,[26] assessing five components to classify neurologic recovery from birth stress and cardiopulmonary adaptation to extrauterine life. Score each newborn at 1 and 5 minutes after birth on a 3-point scale (0, 1, or 2) for each component, with total scores ranging from 0 to 10. Continue scoring at 5-minute intervals until the score exceeds 7 (Box 28-9). If the 5-minute Apgar score is 8 or more, proceed to a more comprehensive examination.[28]

Example of Apgar score calculation for a newborn with hypoxia:

- Heart rate = 110 [2]
- Respiratory effort = slow, irregular [1]
- Muscle tone = some flexion of arms/legs [1]
- Reflex irritability = grimace [1]
- Color = blue, pale [0]

Apgar score = 5

Gestational Age and Birth Weight

Determine Gestational Age and Birth Weight. Classify newborns by gestational age and birth weight to predict clinical problems and morbidity (Box 28-10).[26] *Gestational age* is determined by specific neuromuscular signs and physical characteristics. The *Ballard Scoring System*[30] estimates gestational age within 2 weeks, even in extremely premature infants, with instructions for assessing neuromuscular and physical maturity included in Figure 28-13.

Preterm infants are at risk for short-term complications like respiratory and cardiovascular issues and long-term sequelae such as neurodevelopmental problems.

Late preterm infants face fewer complications but still significant risks.

Post-term infants have increased risks of perinatal mortality or morbidity, including asphyxia and meconium aspiration.

Box 28-9. Apgar Scoring System

	Assigned Score		
Clinical Sign	**0**	**1**	**2**
Heart rate	Absent	<100	>100
Respiratory effort	Absent	Slow and irregular	Good; strong
Muscle tone	Flaccid	Some flexion of the arms and legs	Active movement
Reflex irritability[a]	No responses	Grimace	Vigorous cry, sneeze, or cough
Color	Blue, pale	Pink body, blue extremities	Pink all over
1-Minute Apgar Score		**5-Minute Apgar Score**	
8–10	Normal	8–10	Normal
5–70–4	Some nervous system depression Severe depression, requiring immediate resuscitation	0–7	High risk for subsequent central nervous system and other organ system dysfunction

[a]Reaction to suction of nares with bulb syringe.

Box 28-10. Classification by Gestational Age and Birth Weight

Gestational Age Classification	Gestational Age
Extremely preterm	<28 weeks
Very preterm	28–31 weeks
Moderate to late term	32–36 weeks
Term	37–41 weeks
Post-term	≥42 weeks
Birth Weight Age Classification	**Weight**
Extremely low birth weight	<1,000 g
Very low birth weight	<1,500 g
Low birth weight	<2,500 g
Normal birth weight	≥2,500 g

The New Ballard Score for Determining Gestational Age in Weeks

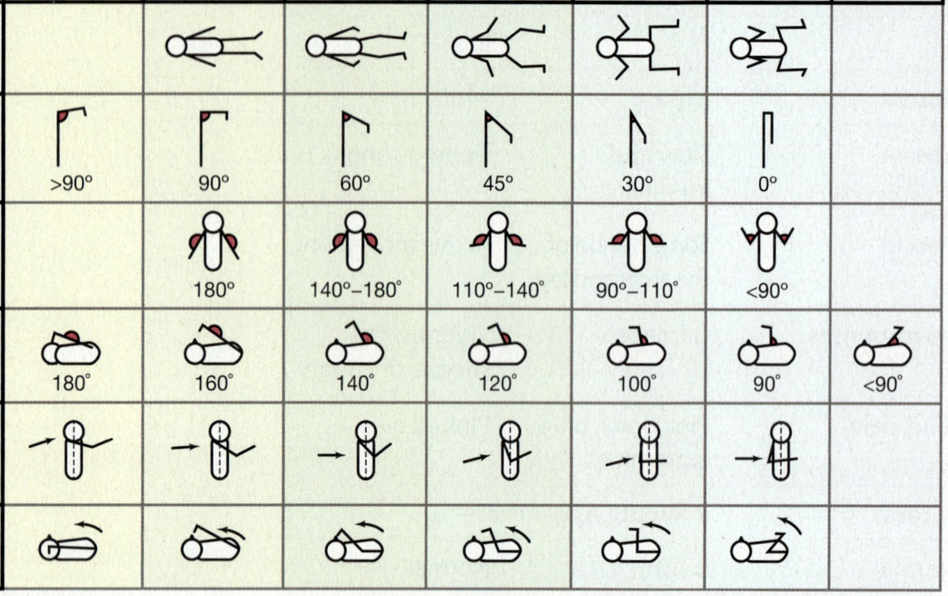

Neuromuscular Maturity

	−1	0	1	2	3	4	5
Posture							
Square window (wrist)	>90°	90°	60°	45°	30°	0°	
Arm recoil		180°	140°–180°	110°–140°	90°–110°	<90°	
Popliteal angle	180°	160°	140°	120°	100°	90°	<90°
Scarf sign							
Heel to ear							

Physical Maturity

	−1	0	1	2	3	4	5
Skin	Sticky friable transparent	Gelatinous red, translucent	Smooth pink, visible veins	Superficial peeling and/or rash, few veins	Cracking pale areas rare veins	Parchment deep cracking no vessels	Leathery cracked wrinkled
Lanugo	None	Sparse	Abundant	Thinning	Bald areas	Mostly bald	
Plantar surface	heel — toe 40–50 mm: −1 <40 mm: −2	>50 mm no crease	Faint red marks	Anterior transverse crease only	Creases anterior 2/3	Creases over entire sole	
Breast	Imperceptible	barely preceptible	flat areola no bud	Stippled areola 1–2-mm bud	Raised areola 3–4-mm bud	Full areola 5–10-mm bud	
Eye/ear	Lids fused loosely: −1 Tightly: −2	Lids open, pinna flat stays folded	Slightly curved pinna; soft, slow recoil	Well-curved pinna; soft, but ready recoil	Formed and firm instant recoil	Thick cartilage, ear stiff	
Genitals male	Scrotum flat, smooth	Scrotum empty, faint rugae	Testes in upper canal, rare rugae	Testes descending, few rugae	Testes down, good rugae	Testes pendulous, deep rugae	
Genitals female	Clitoris prominent, labia flat	Prominent clitoris, small labia minora	Prominent clitoris, enlarging minora	Majora and minora equally prominent	Majora large, minora small	Majora cover clitoris and minora	

Maturity Rating

Score	Weeks
−10	20
−5	22
0	24
5	26
10	28
15	30
20	32
25	34
30	36
35	38
40	40
45	42
50	44

FIGURE 28-13. Sum of the scores for all of the neuromuscular and physical maturity items provides an estimate of gestational age in weeks, using the maturity rating scale at the lower right potion of the figure. (Redrawn from Ballard JL, Khoury JC, Wedig K, Wang L, Eilers-Walsman BL, Lipp R. New Ballard Score, expanded to include extremely premature infants. *J Pediatr*. 1991;119(3):417–423. Copyright © 1991 Elsevier. With permission.)

Box 28-11. Newborn Classifications

Category	Abbreviation	Percentile
Small for gestational age	SGA	<10th
Appropriate for gestational age	AGA	10th–90th
Large for gestational age	LGA	>90th

Box 28-11 provides a classification of newborns based on their gestational age and birth weight, categorizing them as Small for Gestational Age (SGA), Appropriate for Gestational Age (AGA), or Large for Gestational Age (LGA). Figure 28-14 illustrates intrauterine growth curves, marking the 10th and 90th percentiles, and visually defines these categories of maturity in relation to gestational age and birth weight, helping identify deviations from expected growth patterns.

Large-for-gestational age (LGA) infants may experience birth difficulties, including injuries. Infants of individuals with diabetes are often LGA and may have metabolic abnormalities and congenital anomalies like heart disease.

Hypoglycemia is common among LGA newborns, leading to jitteriness, irritability, cyanosis, and other health issues.

Small-for-gestational-age (SGA) infants may result from fetal, placental, or maternal factors, with maternal smoking linked to SGA. These infants are at risk for hypoglycemia and hypothermia.

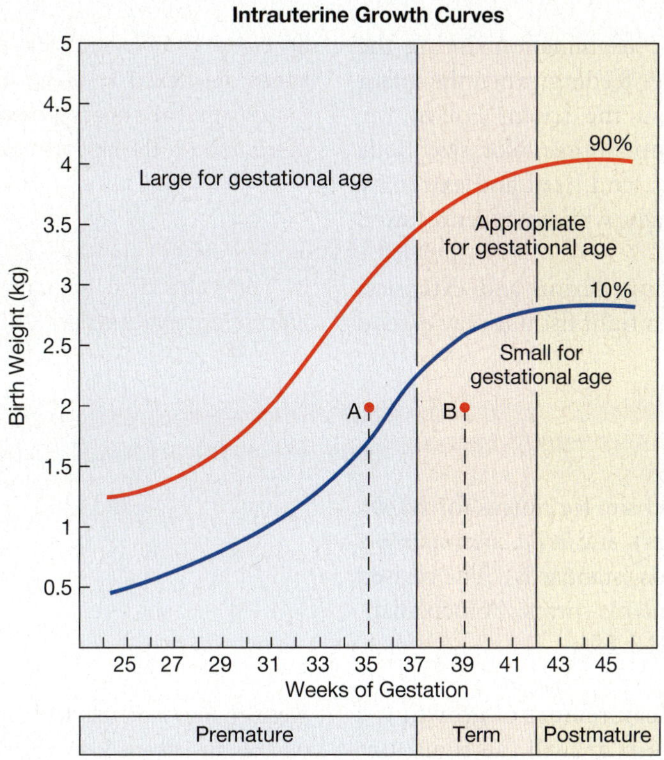

FIGURE 28-14. Level of intrauterine growth based on gestational age and birth weight of liveborn, single infant. Point A represents a premature infant; point B indicates an infant of similar birth weight who is mature but SGA. (Adapted from Sweet YA. Classification of the low-birth-weight infant. In: Klaus MH, Fanaroff AA, eds. *Care of the High-Risk Neonate.* 3rd ed. WB Saunders; 1986. Copyright © 1986 Elsevier. With permission.) More recent sex-specific Fenton growth charts have been published. (Fenton TR, Kim JH. A systematic review and meta-analysis to revise the Fenton growth chart for preterm infants. *BMC Pediatr.* 2013;13:1–3.)

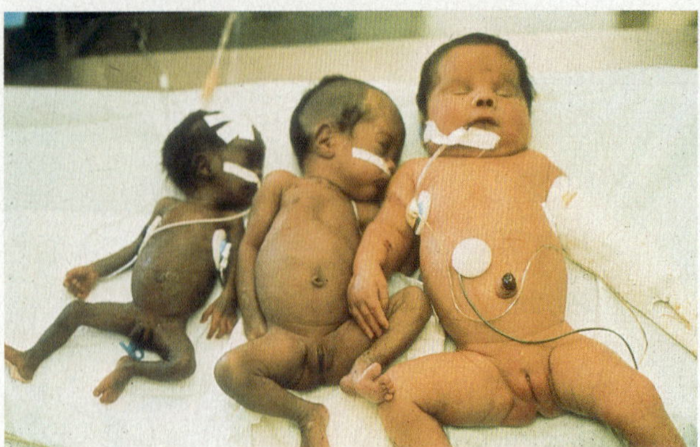

FIGURE 28-15. Infants who are small, average, and large for their gestational age.

The three infants in Figure 28-15, all born at 32 weeks, weighed 600 g (SGA), 1,400 g (AGA), and 2,750 g (LGA), each with different mortality rates.

Preterm infants are prone to respiratory distress syndrome, apnea, patent ductus arteriosus (PDA) with left-to-right shunt, and infection.

General Survey

Conduct a General Survey. Perform a comprehensive examination during the newborn's first day of life. Wait until 1 to 2 hours after feeding, when the infant is most responsive, and have the caregivers stay in the room. Follow the sequence in Box 28-6. Observe the undressed newborn, noting color, size, body proportions, nutritional status, posture, respirations, and head and extremity movements. Most full-term newborns lie symmetrically, with limbs semi-flexed and legs partially abducted at the hips.

In *breech infants* (buttock first), the knees are flexed in utero; in a *frank breech infant,* the knees are extended in utero. In both, the hips are flexed.

Note spontaneous motor activity, with alternating flexion and extension between arms and legs. Fingers are usually flexed in a tight fist but may extend in slow posturing movements.

By 4 days after birth, tremors at rest signal central nervous system (CNS) disease.

Somatic Growth

Refer to the World Health Organization (WHO) website for norms for *height, weight, body mass index* ([BMI] starting at age 2 years), and *head circumference* (https://www.who.int/tools/child-growth-standards/standards). The revised Fenton growth charts for preterm infants are also available (https://bmcpediatr.biomedcentral.com/articles/10.1186/1471-2431-13-59).

Measure Length, Weight, and Head Circumference. Measurement of growth is a key indicator of infant health. Deviations from normal growth can signal underlying problems. Compare growth parameters to age- and sex-specific norms and previous readings to identify trends. Confirm abnormalities by repeating measurements. Use consistent techniques and, if possible, the same scales for measuring height and weight (Box 28-12).

Variations beyond 2 standard deviations or outside the 3rd and 97th percentiles warrant further evaluation, as they can be early indicators of chronic childhood diseases (see examples in https://www.who.int/tools/child-growth-standards/standards).

The most important tools for assessing somatic growth are the growth charts, published by the National Center for Health Statistics (www.cdc.gov/nchs)[34] and the WHO (https://www.who.int/tools/child-growth-standards/standards).[35] These charts include height, weight, and head circumference for children up

A sudden or significant change in growth may indicate systemic disease or inappropriate excess weight gain due to overfeeding.

Box 28-12. Measurement Guidelines for Infant and Child Growth Metrics

Metric and Technique	Significance
Length ■ For children <2 years, use a measuring board or tray (Fig. 28-16). ■ Place the child on the board lying on their back. An assistant should hold the child still with hips and knees extended. ■ Tape measures are inaccurate for infants unless an assistant helps.	Tracks growth and helps identify potential endocrine disorders using velocity growth curves 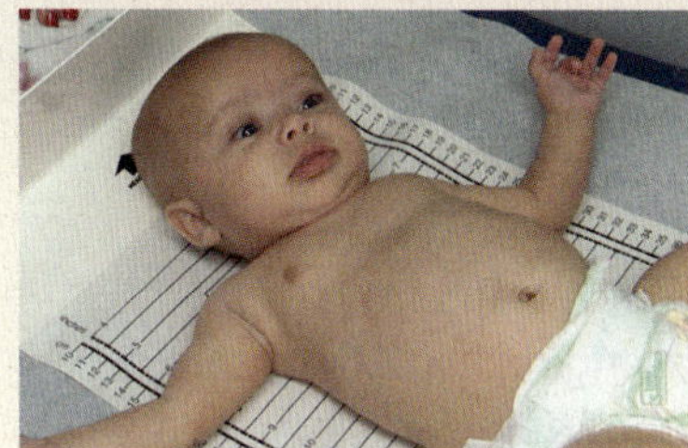 **FIGURE 28-16** Measuring infant length using a board with hips and knees extended.
Weight ■ Use an infant scale and, if possible, the same scale for each measurement. ■ Infants should be undressed or only in a diaper.	Monitors weight gain and can indicate growth faltering if weight falls below expected percentiles or drops significantly on growth charts
Head circumference ■ Measure during the first 2 years of life and any age if needed. ■ Use a flexible, nonstretchable measuring tape. ■ Place the tape just above the eyebrows and ears, around the largest part of the back of the head (Fig. 28-17).	Assesses brain and skull development; unusual measurements might indicate underlying medical conditions 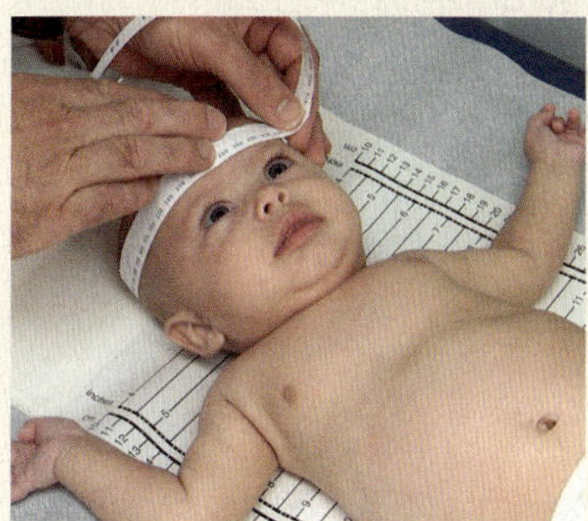 **FIGURE 28-17** Measuring head circumference with a flexible tape above the eyebrows and ears.

Reduced growth velocity, indicated by a drop in height percentile, may indicate a chronic condition such as neurologic, renal, cardiac, gastrointestinal, or endocrine disorders.

Growth faltering is defined as either (a) weight-for-length or BMI less than expected, or (b) weight dropping two percentile lines on a growth curve. Causes include psychosocial issues, family conditions, and various diseases.[33]

Microcephaly (small head size) may be familial or caused by premature suture closure, chromosomal abnormalities, congenital infections, maternal metabolic disorders, or neurologic issues. *Macrocephaly* (large head size, >95th percentile or 2 SD above the mean) can result from hydrocephalus, intracranial hemorrhage, brain tumors, or inherited syndromes, with familial megaloencephaly being benign.

to 36 months and height and weight for children 2 to 18 years. These growth charts have percentile lines, indicating the percentage of children above and below the child's measurement by chronologic age. Comparison with normal standards is essential because growth velocity is normally less during the second year than during the first year. Special charts are available for preterm infants and those with conditions like Down or Turner syndrome.

The AAP, National Institutes of Health (NIH), and CDC recommend using the 2006 WHO for children 0 to 23 months[34] and CDC charts for children 2 to 19 years.

Vital Signs

Measure the Viral Signs. Measure the infant's vital signs—blood pressure, pulse rate, respiratory rate, and temperature (Box 28-13). Regularly assess pain using standardized scales.

See pain severity assessment in Chapter 10, General Survey, Vital Signs, and Pain, pp. 186–188.

Box 28-13. Vital Signs Assessment in Infants

Measurement Technique	Clinical Considerations
Blood pressure (BP)	
■ Place the cuff on the upper arm or leg, ensuring the infant is calm, lying down, or securely held. Use an automatic device for accurate readings.	■ Obtaining accurate BP readings in infants is challenging (Fig. 28-18) but important for high-risk infants. ■ Routine BP measurements should begin after age 3 years. ■ Systolic BP gradually increases throughout childhood (e.g., at birth, the 5th, 50th, and 95th percentiles are 57, 59, and 82 mm Hg, respectively, and by 6 months, they rise to 85, 103, and 120 mm Hg).
Pulse rate	
■ Palpate the femoral arteries in the inguinal area or the brachial arteries in the antecubital fossa, or auscultate the heart.	■ Accurate measurement may be difficult in squirming infants. ■ More sensitive to illness, exercise, and emotion than in adults.
Respiratory rate	
■ Observe the chest and abdomen for at least 60 seconds while they are calm or asleep, noting the rate, pattern, and any signs of distress such as retractions or nasal flaring. ■ Infants have diaphragmatic breathing with minimal thoracic excursion.	■ *Newborns:* 30–68 breaths/min (1st and 99th percentiles, Box 28-14) ■ *Infants* 25–60 breaths/min[36] ■ Respiratory rate may vary considerably from moment to moment in the newborn, with alternating periods of rapid and slow breathing (*periodic breathing*). ■ Sleeping rate is most reliable; it can be up to 10 breaths/min faster during active sleep compared to quiet sleep. ■ Fever can increase respiratory rate by up to 10 breaths/min per °C

Sustained hypertension may indicate renal artery disease, congenital renal malformations, or coarctation of the aorta.

See pp. 1054–1056 for more on blood pressure cuff size and placement for children.

Tachycardia: may be sinus tachycardia or paroxysmal supraventricular tachycardia ([PSVT] if too rapid to count, usually >220/min in infants).

Bradycardia: possible causes include drug ingestion, hypoxia, intracranial/neurologic conditions, or heart block.

See Table 28-1, Abnormalities in Heart Rhythm, p. 1102 and Table 28-2, Abnormalities in Blood Pressure, p. 1102.

Tachypnea: can be a sign of upper or lower respiratory disease; cutoffs: >60/min (birth–2 months), >50/min (2–12 months)

Rapid, shallow breaths: may indicate cyanotic cardiac disease, metabolic acidosis, or pulmonary/neurologic diseases

Measurement Technique	Clinical Considerations
Temperature	
■ In infants under 3 months, a fever (≥38.0 °C or ≥100.4 °F) may indicate a serious infection and is considered an emergency. Febrile infants in this age group should have their temperature assessed rectally for accuracy.[37] ■ Place the infant prone, and separate the buttocks with the thumb and forefinger on one hand and with the other hand gently insert a well-lubricated rectal thermometer to a depth of 2–3 cm (Fig. 28-19). Keep the thermometer in place for at least 2 minutes.	■ *Infants:* Rectal temperature is most accurate. Auditory canal temperature is accurate. Axillary and thermal-tape skin temperatures are inaccurate. ■ Average rectal temperature is >99 °F (37.2 °C) until after age 3 years ■ Excessive bundling may elevate skin temperature but not usually core temperature. ■ May have temperature instability (high or low) due to sepsis, metabolic abnormality, or other serious conditions
Capillary refill time (CRT)	
■ Press finger for 5 seconds with moderate pressure; time the number of seconds it takes for the finger to regain its original color	■ Not a vital sign, but a helpful indicator ■ *Infants >1 week old:* <2 seconds

Prolonged: >3–4 seconds, a "red flag" for potential serious illness; high specificity but varying/low sensitivity[38]

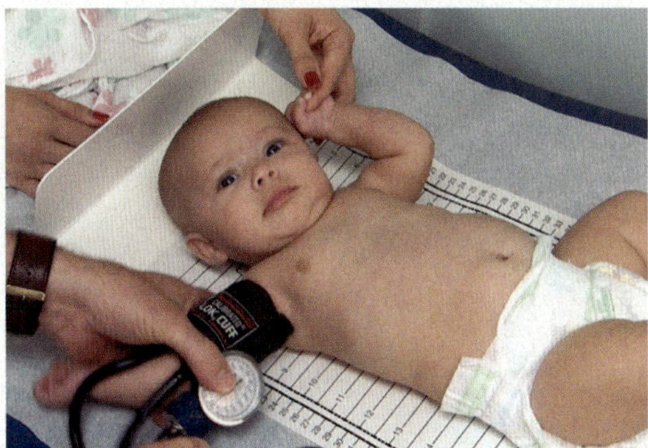

FIGURE 28-18. Measuring blood pressure in infants using a properly sized cuff.

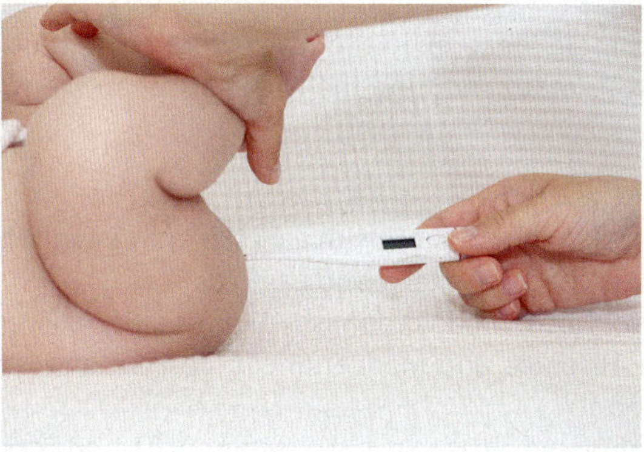

FIGURE 28-19. Rectal thermometers are the most accurate tool for infants.

Box 28-14. Heart Rates of Healthy Infants from Birth to 1 Year[36]

Age	Average Heart Rate (per minute)	Range (1st to 99th percentile) per minute
Birth–1 month	140	90–165
1–6 months	130	80–175
6–12 months	115	90–170

Source: Fleming S, Thompson M, Stevens R, et al. Normal ranges of heart rate and respiratory rate in children from birth to 18 years of age: a systematic review of observational studies. *Lancet*. 2011;377(9770):1011–1018.

Skin

Inspect the Skin. Examine the skin of the newborn or infant carefully to identify both normal markings and potentially abnormal ones (Box 28-15). Box 28-16 demonstrates normal markings. The newborn's skin has a unique characteristic texture and appearance. The texture is soft and smooth because it is thinner than the skin of older children.

Some newborns with polycythemia have a "ruddy" or purplish color.

Box 28-15. Newborn Skin Conditions and Observations on Inspection

Lanugo and vernix caseosa

- Fine downy hair (*lanugo*) covers the body, especially shoulders and back, and is shed within weeks; more prominent in premature infants
- Hair thickness on the head varies and is not predictive of later growth; this hair is shed within months and replaced with new hair
- Cheesy, white material (*vernix caseosa*) covers the body, protecting against maceration and infection, and moisturizing the fetus for birth

Vasomotor changes

- Cooling or chronic heat exposure can produce a bluish mottled appearance (*cutis marmorata*) on the trunk, arms, and legs, lasting for months and resolving with warming

Pigmentation

- Melanin affects skin color: infants with dark skin may initially have lighter skin except in nail beds, genitalia, and ear folds
- *Dermal melanocytosis* (dark or bluish pigmentation) is common in African, Asian, Hispanic, and Mediterranean descent and usually fades by late childhood
- Document pigmented areas to avoid concerns about bruising

Cyanosis

- Healthy newborns progress from slight cyanosis to pinkness within 10 minutes after birth; higher hematocrits make cyanosis easier to observe
- Check inside the mouth, tongue, and conjunctivae for cyanosis
- *Acrocyanosis*: blue hands and feet at birth, common in the first days (see Box 28-16)

If acrocyanosis persists beyond 8 hours or with warming, consider cyanotic congenital heart disease. See central cyanosis discussion on p. 1028.

- *Harlequin dyschromia*: transient cyanosis of half of the body or an extremity due to temporary vascular instability
- *Central cyanosis*: involves lips, tongue, and sublingual tissues, along with hands and feet

Jaundice

- *Physiologic jaundice* appears on day 2 or 3, peaks at day 5, and usually disappears within a week, although it may persist longer in infants who are breastfed or chestfed (see Box 28-16)
- Jaundice progresses from head to toe, with more intense yellow on the upper body
- Inadequate intake jaundice is common and should resolve by 10–14 days; persistent jaundice requires evaluation
- Physical examination cannot reliably predict bilirubin level; examine skin in natural daylight and apply pressure to observe yellowish blanching (Fig. 28-20)

Jaundice within the first 24 hours may indicate hemolytic disease. Late-appearing jaundice or jaundice beyond 2 to 3 weeks suggests biliary obstruction or liver disease.

Vascular markings

- Common benign marking: "*salmon patches*" (nevus simplex, "flame nevi," telangiectatic nevus, capillary hemangioma) are flat, irregular, light pink patches (see Box 28-16)
- Common on the nape of the neck ("*stork bite*") and on upper eyelids, forehead, or upper lip ("*angel kisses*"), often resolving by age 1 year and covered by the hairline
- They are not true nevi and result from distended capillaries

Edema

- Swelling over hands, feet, lower legs, pubis, and sacrum, usually disappears within a few days

Desquamation

- Superficial skin peeling, noticeable 24–36 hours after birth, especially in post-term infants, lasting 7–10 days

Birth trauma

- Note any signs of birth trauma; bruises should prompt a careful neurologic examination

A unilateral dark, purplish "port wine stain" over the ophthalmic branch of the trigeminal nerve may signal *Sturge–Weber syndrome*, associated with seizures, hemiparesis, glaucoma, and intellectual disability.

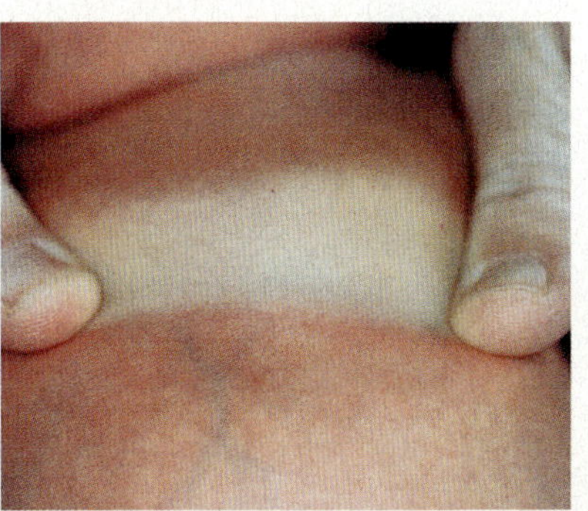

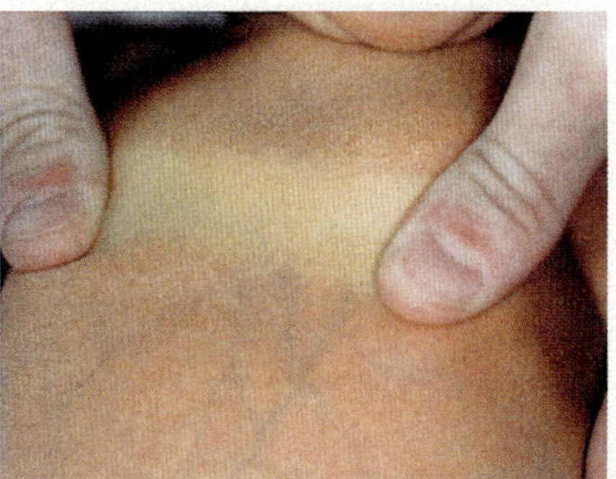

FIGURE 28-20. Pressing the red color from the skin allows better recognition of the yellow (**left**) or jaundice (**right**). (Reprinted with permission from Fletcher MA. *Physical Diagnosis in Neonatology*. Lippincott-Raven; 1998.)

Palpate the Skin. Palpate the newborn's skin to assess hydration (*turgor*). Roll a fold of skin on the abdomen between your thumb and forefinger. Well-hydrated skin returns to normal immediately; delayed return (*tenting*) indicates dehydration.

Significant edema of the hands and feet in a newborn female (plus a webbed neck) suggests Turner syndrome. Dehydration is common, usually due to insufficient intake or diarrhea.

Identify four common dermatologic conditions in newborns—miliaria rubra, erythema toxicum, transient neonatal pustular melanosis, and milia (see Box 28-17). None are clinically significant.

Box 28-16. Newborn Skin Findings

Common Nonpathologic Conditions

Acrocyanosis

This bluish discoloration usually appears in the palms and soles.

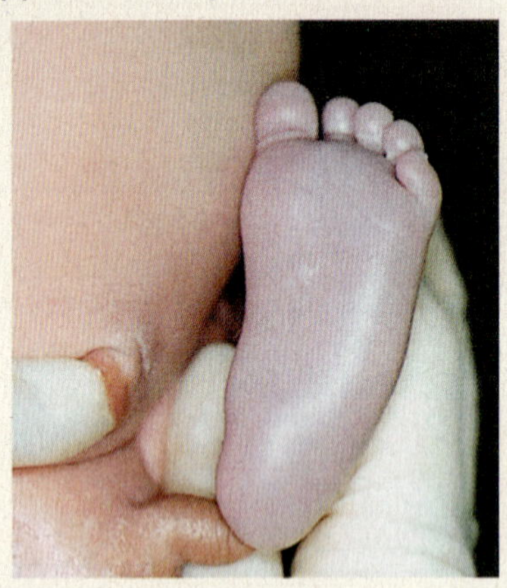

Jaundice

Physiologic jaundice occurs during days 2–5 of life and progresses from head to toe as it peaks.

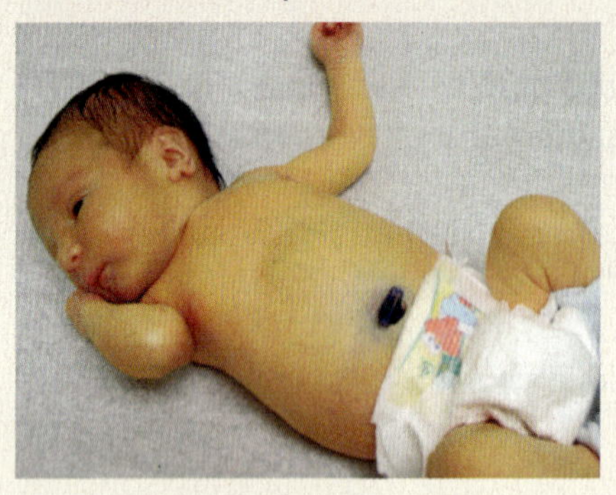

Cyanotic congenital heart disease can present with severe acrocyanosis, which persists despite warming.

Extreme jaundice may signify a hemolytic process or biliary or liver disease.

Common Benign Rashes

Miliaria Rubra

Scattered erythematous papules, vesicles, or pustules, usually on the face, neck and trunk, result from obstruction of the sweat gland ducts; this condition disappears spontaneously within weeks.

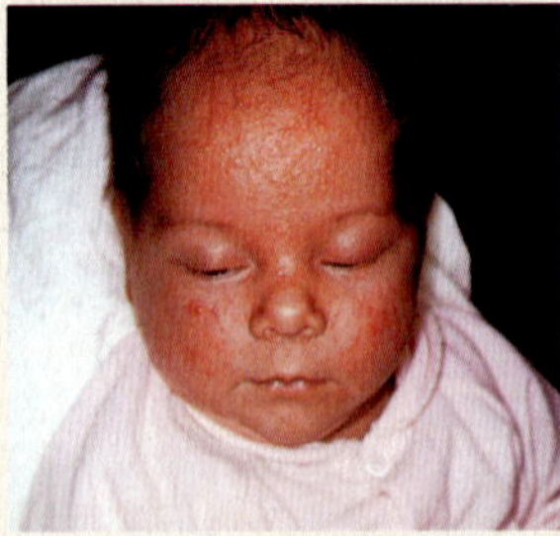

Erythema Toxicum

Usually appearing on days 1–3, this rash consists of erythematous macules with central pinpoint pustules on an erythematous base, scattered diffusely over the entire body. These lesions are of unknown etiology but disappear within 1 week of birth.

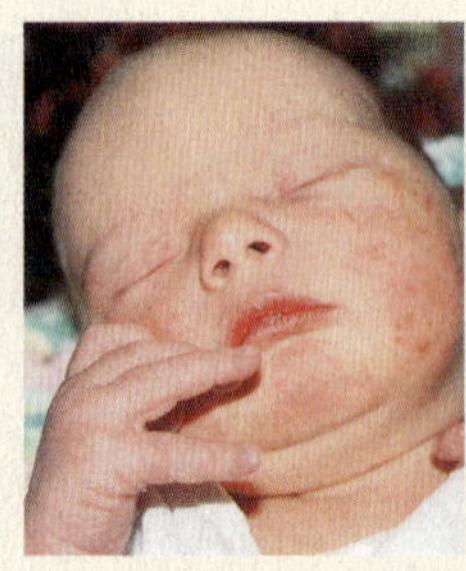

Both erythema toxicum and pustular melanosis may resemble the vesiculopustular rash of herpes simplex or *Staphylococcus aureus* skin infection.

Transient Neonatal Pustular Melanosis
Seen more commonly in infants with darker skin tones, the rash presents at birth as some combination of pustules, scale, and hyperpigmented macules.

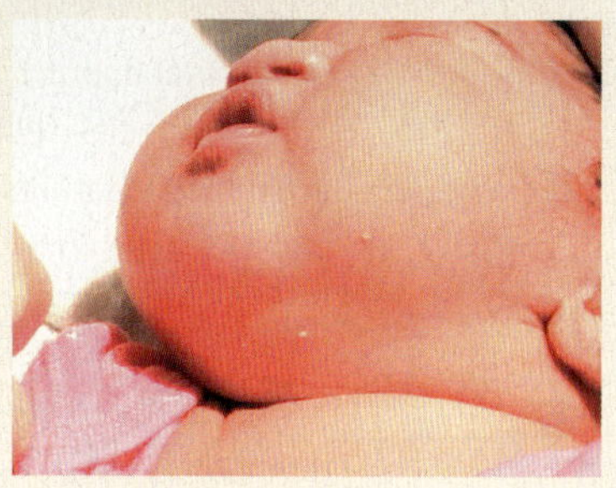

Milia
Pinhead-sized white, pearly papules, without surrounding erythema, on the chin, and forehead. Milia usually appear within the first few weeks and disappears over several weeks.

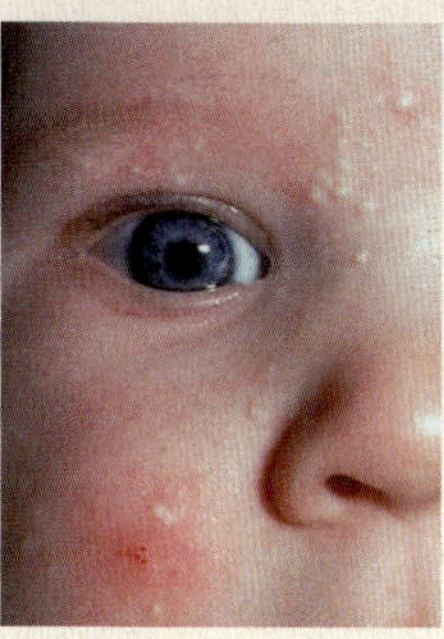

Benign Birthmarks

Eyelid Patch
This birthmark fades, usually within the first year of life.

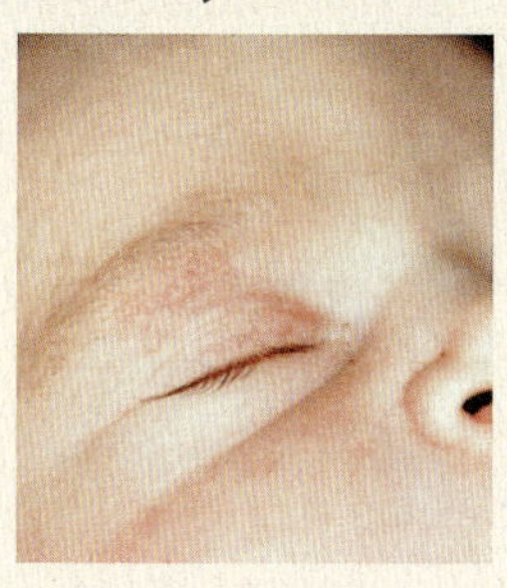

Salmon Patch
Also called the "*stork bite*," or "*angel kiss*," this splotchy pink mark fades with age, although not completely.

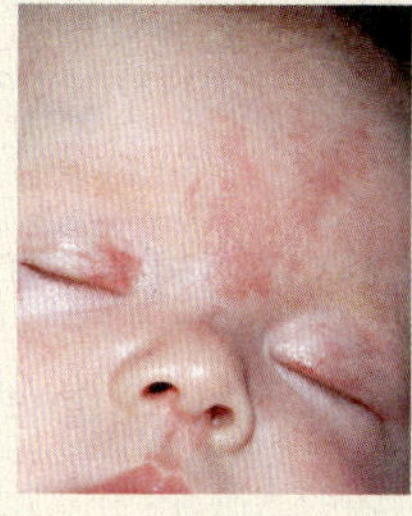

Café-au-lait Spots
These light-brown pigmented lesions usually have borders and are uniform appearance. They are noted in >10% of infants with darker skin tones.

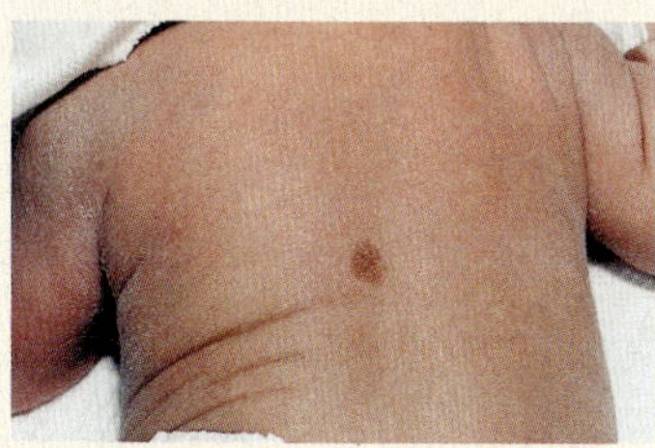

Isolated lesions are benign, but multiple lesions with sharp borders may indicate neurofibromatosis.

Congenital Dermal Melanocytosis
These are more common among infants with darker skin tones. Note them so that they are not mistaken for bruises.

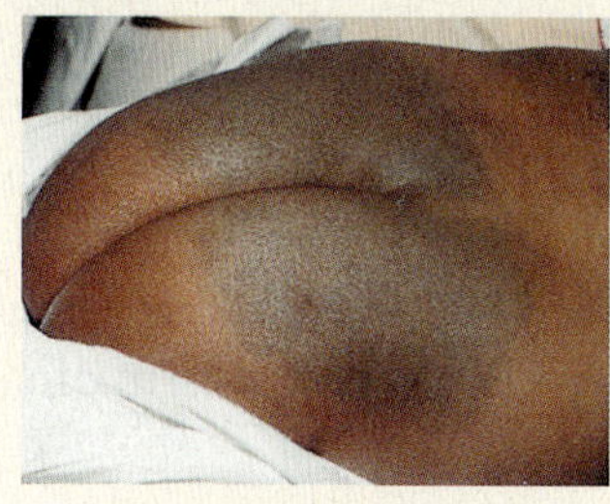

See Table 28-3, Common Skin Rashes and Skin Findings in Newborns and Infants, p. 1103.

Sources of photos: *Jaundice*—Reprinted with permission from Chung EK, Atkinson-McEvoy LR, Lai NL, Terry M. *Visual Diagnosis and Treatment in Pediatrics*. 3rd ed. Wolters Kluwer; 2015. Figure 7-7; *Milia*—Reprinted with permission from Burkhart CN, Morrell D. *VisualDx: Essential Pediatric Dermatology*. Wolters Kluwer Health/Lippincott Williams & Wilkins; 2010. Figure 4-87; *Salmon patch*—Reprinted with permission from Goodheart HP, Gonzalez ME. *Goodheart's Photoguide to Common Pediatric and Adult Skin Disorders*. 4th ed. Wolters Kluwer; 2016. Figure 1-8.

Box 28-17. Evaluating a Newborn with Possible Abnormal Facies

Carefully review the history, especially:
- Family history
- Pregnancy and prenatal history
- Perinatal history

Note abnormalities on other parts of the physical examination, especially:
- Growth
- Development
- Other dysmorphic somatic features

Perform measurements (and plot percentiles), especially:
- Head circumference
- Height
- Weight

Consider the three mechanisms of facial dysmorphogenesis:
- Deformations from intrauterine constraint
- Disruptions from amniotic bands or fetal tissue
- Malformations from intrinsic abnormality in face/head or brain

Examine the biological parents and siblings:
- Similarities to a biological parent may be reassuring (e.g., large head) but may also be an indication of a familial condition

Try to determine whether the facial features fit a recognizable syndrome, comparing with:
- References (including measurements) and pictures of syndromes
- Tables/databases of combinations of features

Most developmental and genetic syndromes with abnormal facies also have other abnormalities in other organ systems.

An infant with congenital hypothyroidism may have distinct facial features and other abnormal facial features (see Table 28-7, Diagnostic Facies in Infancy and Childhood, pp. 1107–1108).

A child with abnormal shape or length of palpebral fissures:

- Upslanting palpebral fissures: Commonly associated with Down syndrome.
- Downslanting palpebral fissures: Often observed in Noonan syndrome
- Short palpebral fissures: Frequently linked to fetal alcohol spectrum disorders (FASD).

See Table 28-7, Diagnostic Facies in Infancy and Childhood, pp. 1107–1108.

Head

At birth, an infant's head may seem large relative to the body, accounting for one-fourth of body length and one-third of body weight. By adulthood, these proportions change to one-eighth and 1/10, respectively.

Sutures separate the skull bones, intersecting at *fontanelles*. The *anterior fontanelle*, 4 to 6 cm at birth, typically closes by 18 months in 80% of infants and by 22 months in 90%.[39] The *posterior fontanelle*, 1 to 2 cm at birth, usually closes by 2 months. Overlapping cranial bones (*molding*) from birth canal passage disappear within 2 days.

Enlarged fontanelles may indicate congenital hypothyroidism. Delayed closure can be due to hypothyroidism, megalocephaly, increased intracranial pressure, rickets, or other conditions.

Examine the Sutures. Sutures should feel like thin troughs between bone plates, with fontanelles as soft concavities (Fig. 28-21).

Bony ridges along sutures may indicate *craniosynostosis,* often with asymmetric head shape and/or microcephaly due to lack of brain growth or metabolic abnormalities.

See Table 28-6, Abnormalities of the Head, p. 1106.

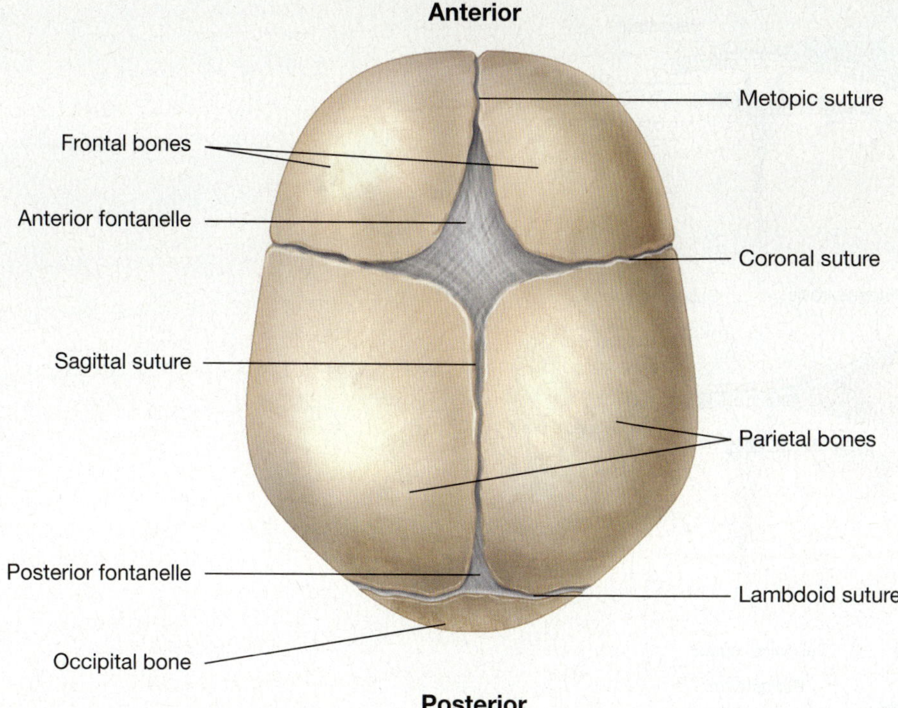

FIGURE 28-21. Sutures, bony plates, and fontanelles in a normal newborn skull.

Assess Fontanelle Fullness and Tension. Examine fontanelle fullness and tension, reflecting intracranial pressure. A soft, flat fontanelle is normal; intermittent fullness during crying or vomiting is also normal. Pulsations are usually normal. Palpate the fontanelle with the infant lying down to rule out dehydration.

A bulging, tense fontanelle may indicate increased intracranial pressure from bleeding, infections, neoplastic disease, or hydrocephalus.

A depressed fontanelle suggests dehydration.

Inspect the Scalp Veins. Inspect the scalp veins carefully to assess for dilatation.

Scalp veins dilatation indicates long-standing increased intracranial pressure.

Evaluate Skull Symmetry. Carefully assess skull symmetry. Premature infants' heads are often long and narrow (*dolichocephaly/scaphocephaly*), usually normalizing within 1 to 2 years. *Caput succedaneum* (swollen scalp) from birth pressure resolves in 1 to 2 days (Fig. 28-22). *Cephalohematoma* from birth trauma resolves within 3 weeks. *Subgaleal hemorrhage* is a rare emergency, appearing right after birth. *Positional plagiocephaly* refers to asymmetry from lying on one side, usually resolving with increased activity and varied positioning (Fig. 28-23).

These should be differentiated from **craniosynostosis**, which involves premature closure of a suture (see Table 28-6).

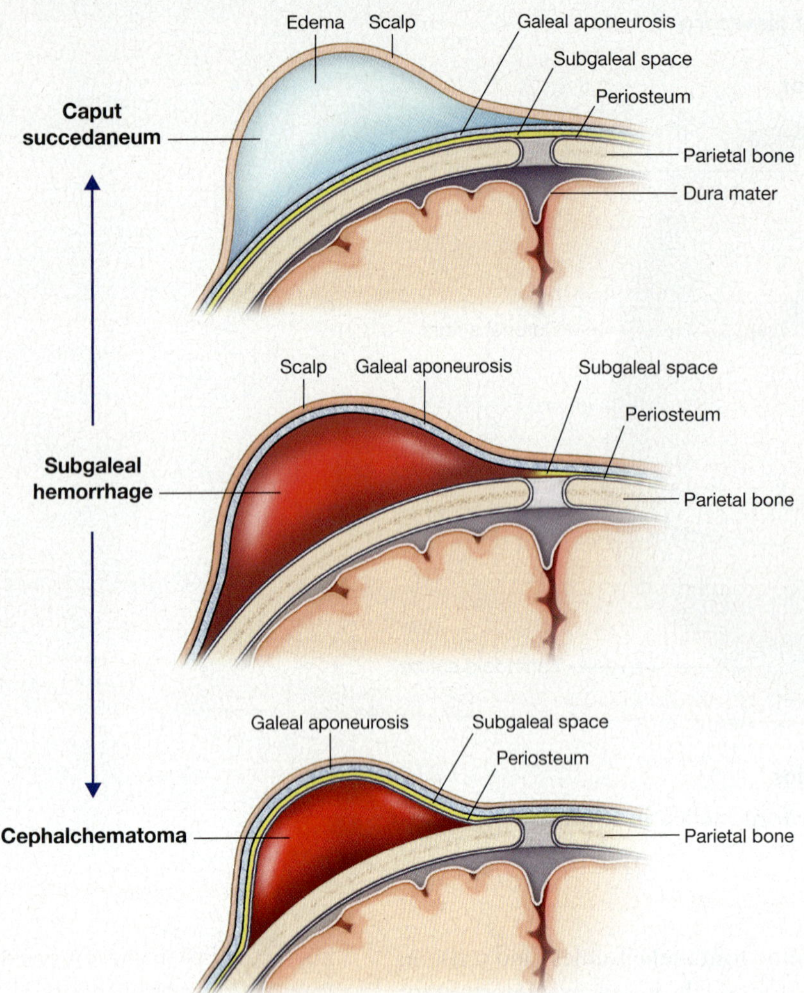

FIGURE 28-22. Comparison of caput succedaneum (scalp edema crossing sutures), subgaleal hemorrhage (bleeding in the subgaleal space), and cephalhematoma (subperiosteal blood, confined by sutures).

Interestingly, the current trend to have newborns sleep on their backs to reduce the risk for sudden infant death syndrome (SIDS) has resulted in more cases of *positional plagiocephaly* (Fig. 28-23), which can result in an asymmetric head with occipital flattening (*plagiocephaly*) or flattening of the occiput symmetrically with widening of the head (*brachycephaly*). This condition can be prevented by frequent repositioning (providing "tummy time" when the infant is awake).

Plagiocephaly may also reflect pathology such as lack of stimulation of the infant. *Torticollis* (tightening of the sternocleidomastoid [SCM] muscle from injury during birth) is another common cause of positional plagiocephaly. The recommended treatment for this condition is physical therapy to stretch the neck muscle involved and restore full range of motion (ROM).

Measure Head Circumference. Measure head circumference using techniques in Box 28-12, pp. 1011.

Assess Facial Symmetry. Examine the face for symmetry and compare with biological parents. Identify specific syndromes with systematic assessment (Box 28-17).[40]

Micrognathia or *mandibular hypoplasia* (small chin) may indicate syndromes like Pierre Robin.

Facial asymmetry may reflect nerve palsy from congenital disorders, birth trauma, infection, or other causes.

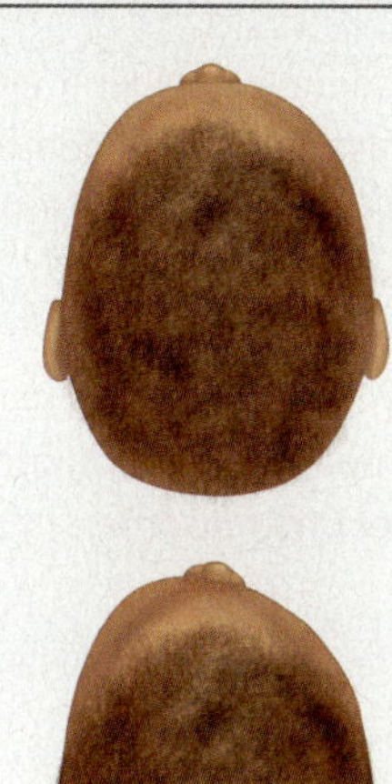

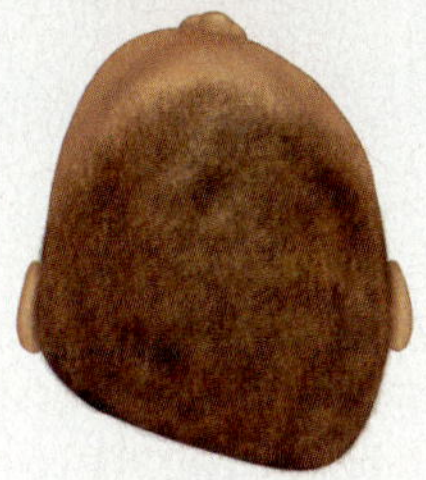

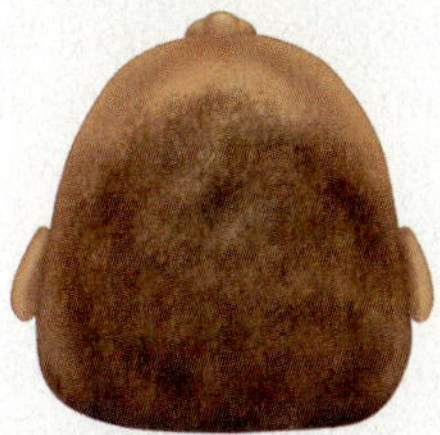

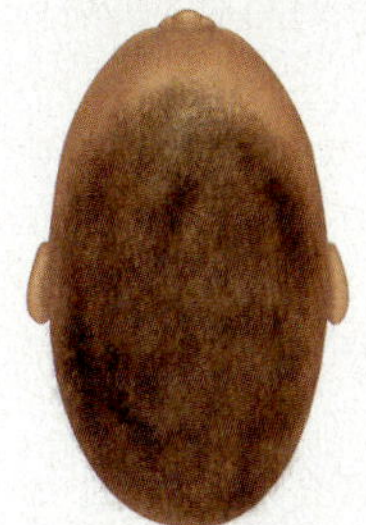

FIGURE 28-23. Four common head shapes of newborns.

Check for Chvostek Sign. Percuss the cheek to check for *Chvostek sign*, which is present in some metabolic disturbances and occasionally in healthy infants. Percuss at the top of the cheek just below the zygomatic bone in front of the ear, using the tip of your index or middle finger.

A positive Chvostek sign produces facial grimacing from repeated muscle contractions, seen in hypocalcemic tetany, tetanus, and hyperventilation-induced tetany.

Eyes

To examine the eyes of infants, use tricks to encourage cooperation. Small colorful toys can help as fixation devices. Newborns may follow a bright light or your face during an alert period. Some can turn their heads 90° to each side.

Inspect the Eyes. Newborns keep their eyes closed except during brief awake periods. If you try to separate their eyelids, they will tighten them more. Use subdued lighting, as bright light causes infants to blink. Awaken the infant gently and support in a sitting position to help the eyes open.

A newborn who cannot open an eye may have congenital ptosis due to birth trauma or cranial nerve III palsy.

Subconjunctival hemorrhages are common in neonates born via vaginal delivery and resolve within a few weeks.

Assess Eye Movements. Hold the infant upright and rotate yourself with the infant in one direction. This usually causes the eyes to open, allowing examination of sclerae, pupils, irises, and extraocular movements (Fig. 28-24). When rotation stops, the eyes look in the opposite direction after a few nystagmoid movements.

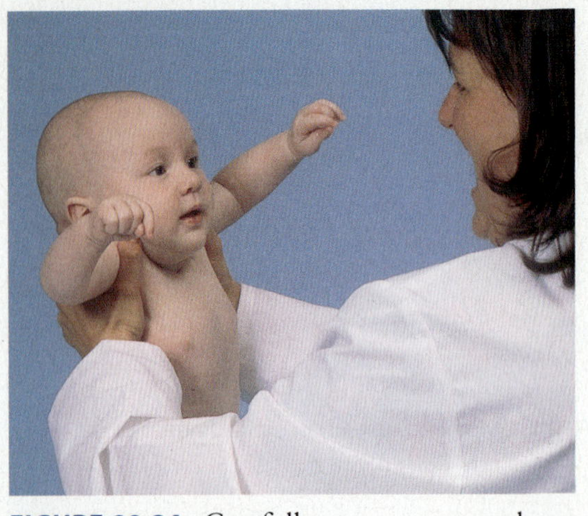

FIGURE 28-24. Carefully assess gaze and eye movements.

Nystagmus (wandering or shaking eye movements) persisting after 2 months or the described maneuver may indicate poor vision or CNS disease.

Failure to gaze or follow your face may indicate visual impairment from congenital cataracts or other disorders.

Look for Doll's Eye Reflex. During the first 10 days of life, the eyes may stare in one direction if just the head is turned without moving the body.

Alternating convergent or divergent strabismus persisting beyond 3 months, or persistent strabismus of any type, may indicate ocular motor weakness or another abnormality in the visual system. Intermittent strabismus generally resolves, but if not by 3 months, consult a pediatric ophthalmologist.

Check for Abnormalities in Sclerae and Pupils. Newborns' eyes may be edematous from the birth process. Look for congenital problems in the sclera and pupils. Observe pupillary reactions to light, noting initial asymmetry that should resolve over time. Inspect irises for abnormalities.

Colobomas represent defects in the iris and may be associated with vision loss and genetic disorders.

Brushfield spots (seen with an ophthalmoscope) are a ring of white specks in the iris strongly suggestive of Down syndrome.

See Table 28-8, Abnormalities of the Eyes, Ears, and Mouth, p. 1109.

Examine the Conjunctiva. Examine the conjunctiva for swelling or redness. Most newborn nurseries use an antibiotic eye ointment to help prevent gonococcal eye infection. This sometimes causes temporary swelling around the eyes.

Persistent ocular discharge and tearing may indicate dacryocystitis, congenital glaucoma, neonatal conjunctivitis, or nasolacrimal duct obstruction.

Assess Vision Indirectly. You cannot measure visual acuity in newborns or infants directly. Use visual reflexes to assess vision: direct and consensual pupillary constriction, *optic blink reflex*, and response to quick movement of an object. Visual acuity sharpens during the first year as the ability to focus improves[96] (Box 28-18).

Failure to progress along visual milestones may indicate delayed visual maturation or abnormal vision.

Box 28-18. Visual Milestones of Infancy

Birth	Blinks, may regard face
1 month	Fixes on objects
1½–2 months	Coordinated eye movements
3 months	Eyes converge, infant reaches toward a visual stimulus
12 months	Acuity around 20/60–20/80

Perform the Ophthalmoscopic Examination. A thorough ophthalmoscopic examination is difficult in infants but may be needed if abnormalities are noted. Examine the red reflex with the ophthalmoscope at 0 diopters from about 10 inches away. The reflex should be bright and symmetric.

Congenital glaucoma and birth trauma may cause corneal cloudiness.

A dark light reflex can result from cataracts or other disorders. A white retinal reflex (*leukokoria*) is abnormal and may indicate cataract, retinal detachment, chorioretinitis, or retinoblastoma.

Examine the optic disc area as you would for an adult. In infants, the optic disc is difficult to visualize but is lighter in color with less macular pigmentation. The foveal light reflection may not be visible. Small retinal hemorrhages may occur in healthy newborns.

Papilledema is rare in infants because the fontanelles and open sutures accommodate increased intracranial pressure.

Extensive hemorrhages may suggest severe anoxia, subdural hematoma, subarachnoid hemorrhage, or trauma.

Ears

Physical examination of an infant's ears can detect structural problems, otitis media, and hearing loss. The goals are to determine the position, shape, and features of the ear and to detect abnormalities.

Examine the Ears. Assess ear position in relation to the eyes. An imaginary line from the inner and outer canthi of the eyes should cross the pinna; if below, the infant has low-set ears.

Small, incompletely developed, or low-set auricles may indicate congenital defects, especially renal disease.

Perform the Otoscopic Examination. Check the ear canal's patency. A small skin tag, cleft, or pit found just forward of the tragus represents a remnant of the *first branchial cleft* and usually has no significance. The ear canal is directed downward; pull the auricle gently downward and outward for the best view of the eardrum. The tympanic membrane's light reflex is diffuse and will become cone-shaped over several months.

Otoscopic techniques are detailed on pp. 1059–1060.

Acute otitis media (see p. 1109) can occur in infants.

Assess Hearing. Universal hearing tests for newborns are common, but assess hearing through developmental indicators.

Acoustic Blink Reflex. The acoustic blink reflex occurs in response to a sudden sharp sound. You can produce it by snapping your fingers or using a bell, beeper, or other noisemaking device approximately 1 foot from the infant's ear. Be sure you are not producing an airstream that may cause the infant to blink (Box 28-19). This reflex may be difficult to elicit during the first 2 to 3 days of life. After it is elicited several times within a brief period, the reflex disappears, a phenomenon known as *habituation*. This crude test of hearing certainly is not diagnostic.

Perinatal problems increasing the risk for hearing defects include low birth weight, anoxia, ototoxic medications, congenital infections, severe hyperbilirubinemia, and meningitis.

Nose

The most important component of the examination of the infant nose is to *test for patency of these nasal passages.* Infants are obligate nasal breathers.

Test Nasal Patency. Assess nasal patency by gently occluding each nostril while holding the infant's mouth closed. Do not occlude both nostrils simultaneously.

The nasal passages in newborns may be obstructed in *choanal atresia.* It can be assessed by passing a feeding tube through each nostril into the posterior pharynx.

Box 28-19. Signs that an Infant Can Hear

Age	Sign
0–2 months	Startle response and blink to a sudden noise Calming down with soothing voice or music
2–3 months	Change in body movements in response to sound Change in facial expression to familiar sounds Turning eyes and head to sound
3–4 months	Turning to listen to voices and conversation
6–7 months	Appropriate language development

Inspect the Nose. Ensure the nasal septum is midline. Maxillary and ethmoid sinuses are present at birth but small. Palpation of newborn sinuses is not helpful.

Mouth and Pharynx

Inspect the Mouth. Use a tongue depressor and flashlight to inspect the mouth and pharynx (Fig. 28-25). A caregiver can help stabilize the infant's head and arms. Palpate the hard palate to ensure it is intact. *Epstein pearls* and petechiae are common findings and usually resolve within months. Older infants produce a lot of saliva and drool frequently.

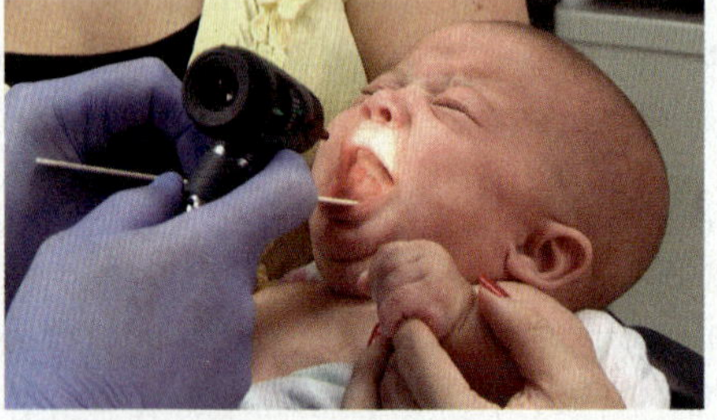

FIGURE 28-25. Caregiver assistance helps with oral assessment.

A congenital fissure of the palate is a *cleft palate*.

Inspect the Tongue. The frenulum varies in tightness; limiting protrusion of the tongue (*ankyloglossia* or *tongue tie*). A tight frenulum may also lead to feeding difficulties with either breast or bottle.

A prominent, protruding tongue may signal congenital hypothyroidism, Down syndrome, or Beckwith–Wiedemann syndrome.

You will often see a whitish covering on the tongue. If this coating is from milk, it can be easily removed by scraping or wiping it away. Use a tongue depressor or your gloved finger to wipe away the coating.

Oral candidiasis (*thrush*) has white plaques that are difficult to wipe away, with an erythematous raw base. See Table 28-8, Abnormalities of the Eyes, Ears, and Mouth, p. 1109.

Check Teeth. Tooth eruption varies widely. A general rule is one tooth per month of age between 6 and 26 months, up to 20 primary teeth.

Natal teeth, present at birth, can be early eruptions or part of syndromes.

Inspect the Pharynx. The pharynx is best seen while the infant is crying. Avoid eliciting strong gag reflex by not sticking a tongue depressor more than two thirds of the way over the tongue. Tonsils are not prominent in infants but grow with age.

Supernumerary teeth are usually dysmorphic and shed within days but are removed to prevent aspiration.

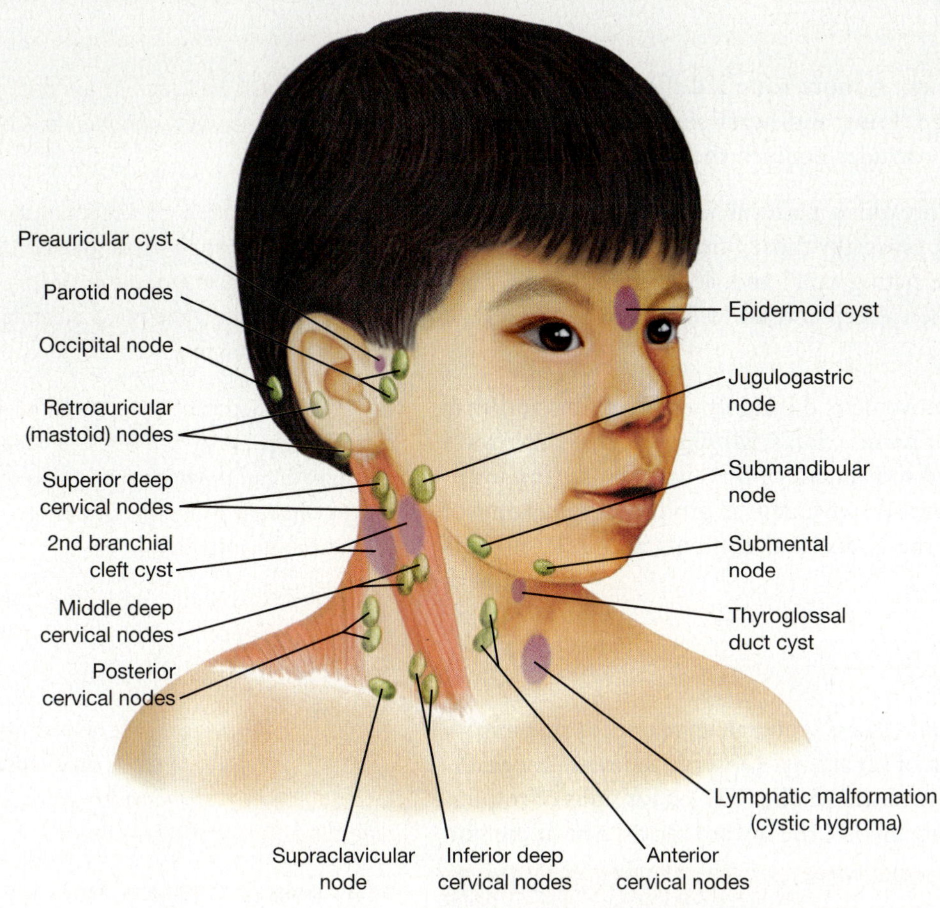

FIGURE 28-26. Lymph nodes and cysts of the head and neck.

Evaluate the Cry. Listen for a vigorous cry. Observe its strength, pitch, and response to stimulation, noting any abnormalities such as weak, high-pitched, or absent cries that may indicate underlying issues.

Weak cry: Indicates respiratory compromise, neuromuscular weakness, or vocal cord paralysis.

High-pitched cry: Associated with increased intracranial pressure, hypoglycemia, or cri-du-chat ("cry of the cat") syndrome (also known as 5p-syndrome).

Absent cry: Suggests severe illness, asphyxia, or significant neurological impairment.

Neck

Palpate the Neck. Palpate lymph nodes and check for masses like congenital cysts (Fig. 28-26). The thyroid cartilage and trachea should be in the correct position. Palpate while infants are lying supine.

Branchial cleft cysts appear as small dimples or openings anterior to the midportion of the SCM muscle.

Congenital torticollis, or a "wry neck," results from bleeding into the SCM muscle during delivery.

Inspect the Clavicles. Palpate for fractures, looking for breaks in contour, tenderness, crepitus, and limited arm movement.

Clavicle fractures may occur during birth, particularly during difficult deliveries.

Thorax and Lungs

Inspect the Thorax. The infant's thorax is more rounded than an adult's, with a thin chest wall and pliant rib cage. Lung and heart sounds are transmitted clearly. The xiphoid process often protrudes beneath the skin.

Common chest wall variants are *pectus excavatum* and *pectus carinatum,* p. 465.

Inspect Breathing Patterns. Inspect breathing patterns when the infant is calm. Observe for 60 seconds. Newborns, especially those born prematurely, may exhibit "*periodic breathing*," with alternating rapid and slow rates. Normal rates are 30 to 40 breaths per minute when asleep and 40 to 60 when awake.

Apnea, or cessation of breathing for >20 seconds, is often accompanied by bradycardia and may indicate respiratory or CNS causes, and rarely a cardiopulmonary condition.

Healthy infants show little rib movement during quiet breathing and may display *thoracoabdominal paradox* or *paradoxical breathing*, which is the inward movement of the chest and outward movement of the abdomen during inspirations (*abdominal breathing*). Outward movement is produced by descent of the diaphragm, which compresses the abdominal contents and in turn shifts the lower ribs outward.

Airway obstruction or lower respiratory disease can cause *Hoover sign* (seesaw breathing) in which the abdomen moves outward while the chest moves inward during inspiration.

Children with muscle weakness may exhibit paradoxical breathing at several years of age.

Visually Inspect Respiratory Function. Assess general appearance, respiratory rate, color, breath sounds, and work of breathing. Observe the nose, especially during feeding, as infants are obligate nasal breathers. Look for signs of respiratory distress (Box 28-20). *Retractions* involve the inward movement of the skin

Pulmonary diseases increase respiratory effort, while cardiac diseases may cause tachypnea without increased work of breathing ("peaceful tachypnea").

Nasal flaring, which reduces airway resistance, along with grunting and tachypnea, can indicate upper or lower airway pathology, including lower respiratory infections such as bronchiolitis and pneumonia.

Acute stridor is likely a serious condition. Causes include laryngotracheobronchitis (croup), epiglottitis, bacterial tracheitis, foreign body, hemangioma, or a vascular ring.

Box 28-20. Observing Respiration

Type of Assessment	Specific Observable Pathology
General appearance	Inability to feed or smile Lack of consolability
Respiratory rate	Tachypnea (see p. 1012), bradypnea, apnea
Color	Pallor or cyanosis
Nasal component of breathing	Nasal flaring (enlargement of both nasal openings during inspiration)
Audible breath sounds	Grunting (repetitive, short expiratory sound) Wheezing (musical expiratory sound) Stridor (high-pitched, usually inspiratory noise) Obstruction (lack of or diminished breath sounds)
Work of breathing	Nasal flaring (enlargement of both nares during inspiration) Head bobbing (head movement due to accessory muscle use) Grunting (expiratory noises) Retractions (chest indrawing): Supraclavicular (above clavicles) Intercostal (between the ribs) Substernal (at xiphoid process) Subcostal (just below the costal margin)

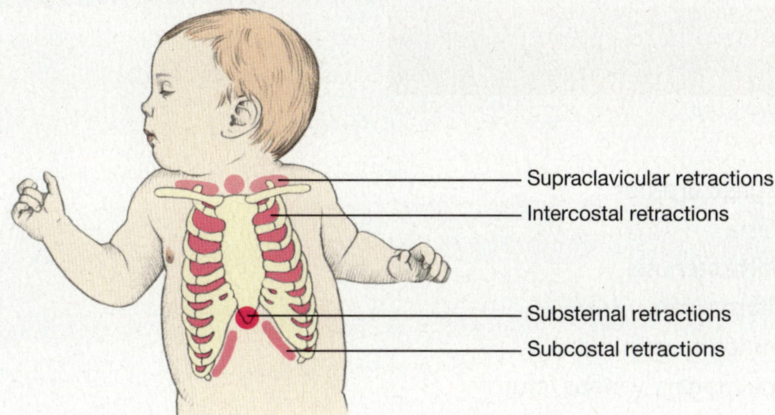

FIGURE 28-27. Anatomic locations of retractions (chest indrawing).

between the ribs during inspiration, primarily driven by diaphragm movement with little assistance from thoracic muscles (Fig. 28-27).

Palpate the Chest. The infant's chest is hyperresonant throughout, making it difficult to detect abnormalities on palpation or percussion. *Percussion is least helpful.* Although challenging, try to assess *tactile fremitus* by palpation. Place your hand or fingertips over each side of the chest during vocalizations and feel for symmetry in the transmitted vibrations.

Infants have excellent transmission of sounds throughout the chest. Any abnormalities of tactile fremitus or on percussion suggest pathology.

Auscultate Breath Sounds. Infant breath sounds are louder and harsher due to the proximity of the stethoscope to the sound origin. *Distinguishing upper airway sounds from chest sounds can be challenging* (Box 28-21). Upper airway sounds, usually heard during inspiration, are transmitted symmetrically and arise from extrathoracic sources like the trachea or larynx. Higher inspiratory flow rates produce turbulent flow and appreciable sounds. Expiratory sounds, often asymmetric and arising from intrathoracic sources, are loudest over the site of pathology. Hold the stethoscope just above the infant's mouth and nose to differentiate upper from lower airway sounds.

Wheezes commonly occur from asthma and less commonly from bronchiolitis.

Rhonchi occur with upper respiratory infections.

Crackles can be heard with pneumonia and bronchiolitis.

Upper respiratory infections, while not serious, can produce loud inspiratory sounds transmitted to the chest.

Box 28-21. Distinguishing Upper Airway from Lower Airway Sounds in Infants

Technique	Upper Airway	Lower Airway
Compare sounds from nose/stethoscope	Same sounds	Often different sounds
Listen to type of sounds	Harsh and loud	Variable
Note symmetry (left vs. right; upper vs. lower)	Symmetric	Often asymmetric
Inspiratory vs. expiratory	Almost always inspiratory	Often has expiratory phase
Hold stethoscope above infant's mouth	Inspiratory sounds remain loud	Often quieter than by auscultation of the chest

Box 28-22. Cardiac Causes of Central Cyanosis in Infants and Children

Age of Onset	Potential Cardiac Cause
Immediately at birth or within a few days	Transposition of the great arteries Pulmonary valve atresia Severe pulmonary valve stenosis Possibly Ebstein malformation Additional conditions (often within days): Total anomalous pulmonary venous return Hypoplastic left heart syndrome Truncus arteriosus (sometimes) Single ventricle variants
Weeks, months, or years of life	All of the above plus: Pulmonary vascular disease with atrial, ventricular, or great vessel shunting (right-to-left shunting)

Evaluate Breath Sound Patterns. Breath sound pattern refers to the distribution, timing, and quality of breath sounds across the chest during auscultation. In a normal pattern, breath sounds are louder at the apex and symmetrical across the chest.

Unilateral diminished sounds suggest pneumothorax, pleural effusion, or lobar collapse on the affected side.

Biphasic sounds, involving both inspiratory and expiratory components, indicate severe airway obstruction.

Transmitted upper airway sounds occur when inspiratory sounds from the upper airways are louder than expected over the chest, often caused by an upper respiratory infection.

Heart

Inspect for Cyanosis. Before examining the heart, check for cyanosis, particularly *central cyanosis* involving the lips, tongue, and sublingual tissues (Box 28-22). The best area to check is the tongue and oral mucosa, not the nail beds, lips, or the extremities. The distribution of cyanosis should be evaluated. *Acrocyanosis* in the newborn, which spares the oral mucosa, is discussed on pages 1016 and 1111. An oximetry reading will confirm desaturation.

Central cyanosis is *always abnormal* and may indicate congenital cardiac abnormalities or respiratory diseases. Cardiac causes of central cyanosis involve right-to-left shunting and various congenital cardiac lesions.[41] See Table 28-10, Cyanosis in Children, p. 1111.

Assess Noncardiac Findings. Evaluate the infant's nutritional state, responsiveness, irritability, and fatigue, as these can indicate cardiac disease. Noncardiac findings are often present in infants with cardiac disease (Box 28-23).

The combination of tachypnea, tachycardia, and hepatomegaly suggests heart failure.

Box 28-23. Noncardiac Findings Commonly Present in Infants with Cardiac Disease

Poor feeding	Sweating with feeding	Poor overall appearance
Failure to thrive	Hepatomegaly	Tachypnea

Palpate the Precordium. Palpate the chest wall along the precordium to assess heart volume changes. A hyperdynamic precordium indicates a significant volume change. The *point of maximal cardiac impulse (PMI)* is not always palpable in infants and can be affected by respiratory patterns, a full stomach, and the infant's position. The PMI is usually an interspace higher in infants due to the horizontal position of the heart.

A *"rolling" heave* at the left sternal border suggests increased right ventricular work, while the same motion near the apex indicates left ventricular work.

Thrills indicating turbulence within the heart or great vessels, are best felt with the palm or base of the fingers. They have a rough, vibrating quality (Fig. 28-28).

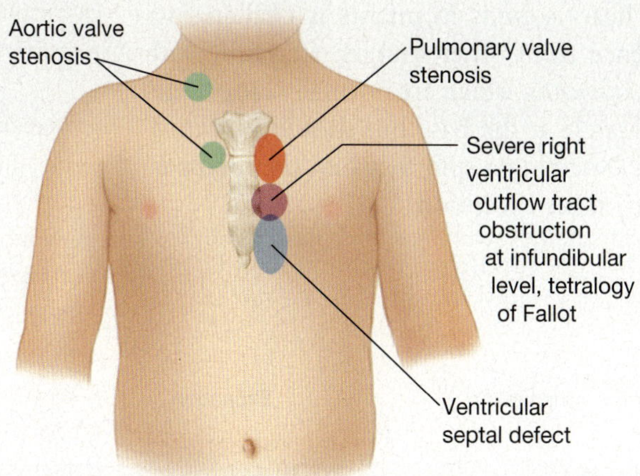

FIGURE 28-28. Location of thrills in infants and children.

Patent ductus arteriosus (PDA) is associated with a hyperdynamic precordium and bounding distal pulses.

Visible and palpable chest pulsations suggest a hyperdynamic state from increased metabolic rate or inefficient pumping due to a cardiac defect.

Auscultate Heart Rhythm. Auscultate the heart rhythm in infants, as it is easier than feeling peripheral pulses. In older children, assess the rhythm either way (Box 28-24). Infants and children often have a normal sinus dysrhythmia, with the heart rate increasing on inspiration and decreasing on expiration.

The most common abnormal dysrhythmia in infants is *supraventricular tachycardia (SVT)*, characterized by a sustained and regular heart rate around ≥220 beats per minute. The child may appear healthy, pale, or moderately ill.

Ventricular premature contractions generally occur in otherwise healthy infants but can be associated with cardiac disease, electrolyte, or metabolic disturbances.

Box 28-24. Characteristics of Normal Variants of Heart Rhythms in Children

Characteristics	Atrial Premature Contractions (APCs) or Ventricular Premature Contractions (VPCs)	Normal Sinus Dysrhythmias
Age group most commonly affected	Neonates (may occur at any time)	After infancy and throughout childhood
Relation to breathing (respiration)	No correlation	Strong correlation: Increases with inspiration, decreases with expiration
Effect of exercise on tachycardia	Abnormal beats are eliminated during exercise	Irregular rhythm may become more noticeable post-exercise but resolves at rest
Characteristic of rhythm	Isolated skipped or missed beats	Gradually faster with inspiration and suddenly slower with expiration
Number of abnormal beats	Typically single, isolated beats	Multiple beats, often occurring in repetitive cycles
Clinical significance	Benign in nature	Always benign (by definition)

Many neonates and some older children have premature atrial or ventricular beats, often described as "skipped" beats. These can usually be eradicated by increasing the intrinsic sinus rate through exercise, such as crying in an infant or jumping in an older child. In healthy children, these beats are usually benign and rarely persist.

Auscultate Heart Sounds. Auscultating heart sounds in infants is challenging due to their rapid nature and interference from other sounds. Carefully and systematically evaluate the *S_1 and S_2 heart sounds*, which are normally crisp. The second sound (S_2) is usually heard separately at the base but should fuse into a single sound during deep expiration. Detecting a split S_2 when the infant is quiet or asleep is usually reassuring, with some exceptions.

Distant heart tones suggest pericardial effusion.

Pathologic arrhythmias in children can result from structural cardiac lesions, drug ingestion, metabolic abnormalities, endocrine disorders, serious infections, postinfectious states, or conduction disturbances without structural heart disease.

Listen for the intensity of A_2 (aortic component) and P_2 (pulmonic component). A_2 is normally louder than P_2 at the base (Fig. 28-29).

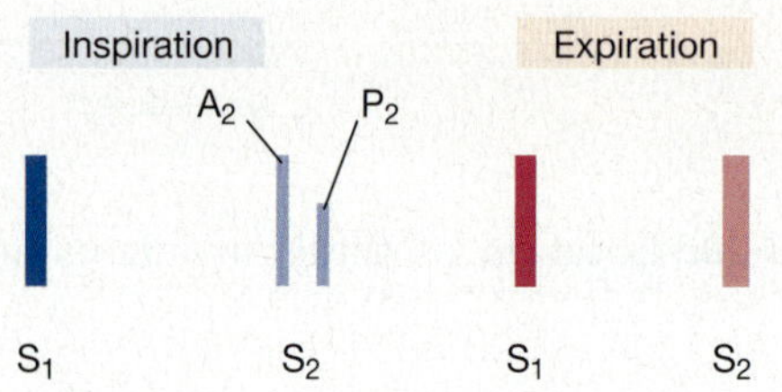

FIGURE 28-29. Healthy heart sounds in infants.

A louder-than-normal P_2 suggests pulmonary hypertension or an atrial septal defect (ASD).

Persistent splitting of S_2 may indicate a right ventricular volume load or cardiac lesions associated with pulmonary hypertension.

Third heart sounds (S_3), low-pitched early diastolic sounds, are frequently heard and are normal. A *fourth heart sound (S_4)*, occurring just before S_1, is less common in children.

A high-intensity S_3, or a gallop, indicates underlying pathology.

An S_4 suggests decreased ventricular compliance and heart failure.

A widely split S_2 varying with respiration and occurring with a normal heart rate and rhythm, may mimic a gallop but is not pathologic.

A true *gallop rhythm* (tachycardia plus a loud S_3, S_4, or both) indicates heart failure due to poor ventricular function.

Characterize Heart Murmurs. Evaluating heart murmurs in children involves noting their location, timing, intensity, and quality. If well-characterized, diagnosis is often clinical, but tools like the electrocardiogram (ECG), chest x-ray, and echocardiography may confirm findings. Many serious cardiac malformations present with additional signs and symptoms beyond the murmur.

Noncardiac findings associated with cardiac disease increase the likelihood that a murmur is pathologic.

Most children will have *functional* (benign) murmurs, identifiable by specific qualities and lack of associated abnormalities. Benign murmurs occur without other signs and indicate normal growth.[42–44] Box 28-25 characterizes two *benign* heart murmurs in infants according to their locations and key characteristics.

Pathologic murmurs of congenital heart disease can be present at birth or appear later. See Table 28-11, Congenital Heart Murmurs, on pp. 1112–1114.

In some infants, a soft, ejection murmur heard in the axilla and back indicates *benign peripheral pulmonary stenosis*, usually disappearing by age 1.

A pulmonary flow murmur with other signs of disease may indicate conditions like Williams syndrome or congenital rubella syndrome, differing from benign peripheral pulmonary stenosis.

Box 28-25. Two Common Benign Murmurs in Infants

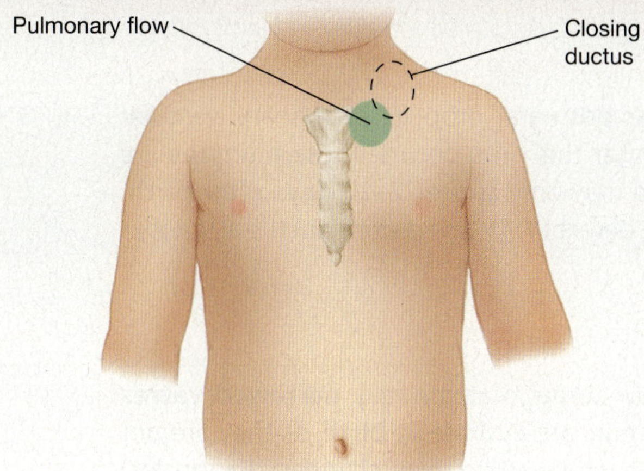

Typical Age	Benign Murmur	Relation to S_1 and S_2	Description and Location
Newborn	*Closing ductus*		Harsh, ejection (crescendo) systolic murmur that, as patent ductus arteriosus closes, becomes continuous Upper left sternal border
Newborn–1 year	*Peripheral pulmonary flow murmur*	S_1 S_2	Soft, ejection, systolic Upper left sternal border, radiating to lung fields and axillae

When detecting a murmur, note all qualities to distinguish between pathologic and benign ones. Understanding physiologic changes aids in this distinction (Box 28-26).

A newborn with a heart murmur and central cyanosis likely has congenital heart disease and requires urgent evaluation. See Table 28-11, Congenital Heart Murmurs, pp. 1112–1114.

Peripheral Vascular System

The major branches of the aorta can be assessed by evaluating *peripheral pulses.* All neonates should have their pulses evaluated during their newborn examination.

Palpate the Peripheral Pulses. In neonates and infants, the *brachial artery pulse* in the antecubital fossa is easier to feel than the *radial artery pulse* at the wrist. Both *temporal arteries* should be felt just in front of the ear.

Palpate the *femoral pulses*, located midline just below the inguinal crease, between the iliac crest and the symphysis pubis. Take your time to find femoral pulses; they can be difficult to detect in active infants. Use the pads of your index and middle finger together. Flexing the infant's thighs on the abdomen may help.

Absence or diminution of femoral pulses indicates *coarctation of the aorta*. If femoral pulses are undetectable, measure blood pressures in one lower and both upper extremities. Normally, lower extremity blood pressure is slightly higher than in the upper extremities. If equal or lower in the leg, coarctation is likely present.

Box 28-26. Physiologic Basis for Selected Pathologic Heart Murmurs

Change in Pulmonary Vascular Resistance

- Murmurs dependent on the postnatal drop in pulmonary vascular resistance become audible after this drop occurs. These murmurs are often **inaudible at birth** and may only appear **7–10 days after birth.** **Examples:** ventricular septal defect (VSD) and patent ductus arteriosus (PDA).

Obstructive Lesions

- Caused by normal blood flow through abnormally **narrowed valves** or outflow tracts. These murmurs are **audible at birth**, as they are not dependent on pulmonary vascular resistance changes. **Examples:** pulmonic stenosis and aortic stenosis.

Pressure Gradient Differences

- Murmurs caused by **high-pressure gradients** between heart chambers or valves. These murmurs are **audible at birth** because of the already existing pressure differences between the chambers. **Example:** atrioventricular valve regurgitation

Changes Associated with Growth of Children

- Some murmurs become audible later due to changes in **normal blood flow patterns** with growth. Certain obstructive defects or shunt-related murmurs appear later as anatomy or compliance evolves over time. **Examples:** aortic stenosis - may not be heard until adolescence or adulthood, despite being congenital; atrial septal defect (ASD) - pulmonary flow murmur often appears ≥1 year due to increased right ventricular compliance and shunting.

Palpate lower extremity pulses using your index or middle finger. The *dorsalis pedis* and *posterior tibial pulses* may be difficult to feel unless an abnormality is present (Fig. 28-30). Normal pulses should have a sharp rise and be firm and well localized.

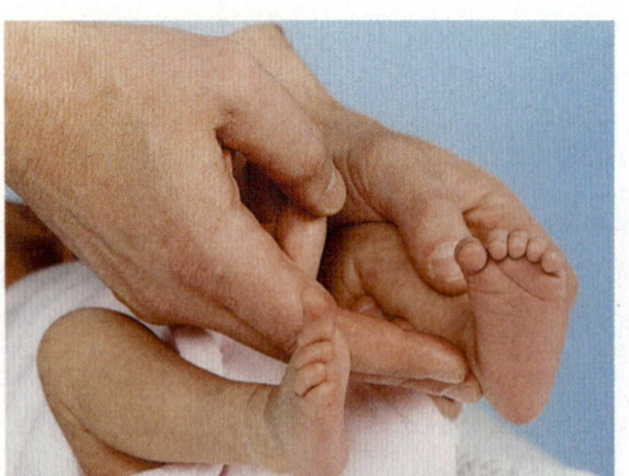

FIGURE 28-30. Palpating pulses in the lower extremity.

A weak or thready pulse may reflect myocardial dysfunction and heart failure, especially with tachycardia.

Pulses in the feet of neonates and infants are often faint, but conditions like PDA or truncus arteriosus can cause full pulses.

Breasts

The breasts of newborns, regardless of sex, are often enlarged due to maternal estrogen effect, lasting several months. They may also be engorged with a white liquid, sometimes called *neonatal milk*, which may last 1 to 2 weeks.

In *premature thelarche*, breast development occurs, typically between 6 months and 2 years, without other signs of puberty or hormonal abnormalities.

Abdomen

Inspect the Abdomen. Inspect the infant's abdomen while they are lying supine, preferably asleep. The abdomen is protuberant due to underdeveloped abdominal muscles. You will easily notice blood vessels and intestinal peristalsis.

Inspect the newborn's *umbilical cord* to detect abnormalities, noting the presence of two thick-walled arteries and one larger, thin-walled vein at the 12 o'clock position.

A single umbilical artery may indicate congenital anomalies or be isolated.

The umbilicus may have a long cutaneous portion (*umbilicus cutis*) covered with skin and an amniotic portion (*umbilicus amnioticus*) covered by a firm gelatinous substance, *Wharton jelly*. The amniotic portion dries up and falls off within 2 weeks, while the cutaneous portion retracts to be flush with the abdominal wall.

An umbilical granuloma at the base of the navel is pink granulation tissue formed during healing.

Inspect the area around the umbilicus for redness or swelling. The abdominal skin around the umbilicus should be the same color as the infant's abdomen.

Infection of the umbilical stump (*omphalitis*) presents with periumbilical edema and erythema.

Umbilical hernias, caused by a defect in the abdominal wall, may be prominent with increased intra-abdominal pressure and usually resolve by age 5. *Diastasis recti*, a benign condition, involves separation of the rectus abdominis muscles and resolves during early childhood.

Auscultate the Abdomen. Auscultate a quiet infant's abdomen to hear musical bowel sounds by placing your stethoscope on the infant's abdomen.

Percuss the Abdomen. Percuss the abdomen as you would for an adult, noting greater tympanitic sounds due to air swallowing. Percussion helps determine the size of organs and detect masses. To relax the infant, hold their legs flexed at the knees and hips with one hand and palpate the abdomen with the other. A soother (pacifier or dummy) may also help.

A silent, tympanic, distended, and tender abdomen suggests peritonitis.

Palpate the Liver. Gently palpate the liver, starting low in the abdomen and moving upward. The liver edge is typically felt 1 to 3 cm below the right costal margin. Simultaneous percussion and auscultation can help assess liver size (Box 28-27).[45]

Causes of hepatomegaly include hepatitis, storage diseases, vascular congestion, and late presentation of biliary obstruction.

Palpate the Spleen. The spleen, felt under the left costal margin, is soft with a sharp edge and rarely extends more than 1 to 2 cm below the margin.

Splenomegaly can be due to infections, hemolytic anemias, infiltrative disorders, inflammatory or autoimmune diseases, and portal hypertension.

Box 28-27. Liver Size in Healthy Term Newborns

By palpation and percussion[97]	Mean, 5.9 ± 0.7 cm
Projection below right costal margin	Mean, 2.5 ± 1.0 cm

Palpate Other Abdominal Structures. You may note pulsations in the epigastrium from the *aorta*. Rarely, you can palpate the *kidneys* by placing your fingers in front and behind each kidney. Identify normal structures first, then use palpation to detect abnormal masses.

Abnormal abdominal masses can be related to the *kidney* (e.g., hydronephrosis), *bladder* (e.g., urethral obstruction), *bowel* (e.g., stool from Hirschsprung disease or intussusception), and tumors.

Pyloric stenosis, presenting around age 4 to 6 weeks, may be felt as a 2-cm firm mass ("olive-like") in the right upper quadrant or midline. Peristaltic waves may be visible during feeding.

Penis, Testes, and Scrotum

Inspect the genitalia with the infant supine noting the appearance of the penis, testes, and scrotum.

Inspect the Penis. The *foreskin (prepuce)* covers the glans penis and is nonretractable at birth but may retract enough to visualize the external urethral meatus. Gradually, the foreskin becomes retractable over months to years. Check the location of the urethral meatus to ensure it does not open on the underside of the penis.

Inspect the *shaft of the penis* for surface abnormalities, ensuring it appears straight without ventral curvature.

The rate of circumcision has declined in North America and varies worldwide. Health benefits include a reduced risk of urinary tract infections (UTI), sexually transmitted infections (STIs), and the need for future circumcision. Risks include bleeding, infection, and urethral meatal stenosis. The decision should be made by caregivers based on their religious, ethical, and cultural beliefs and understanding of current medical evidence.[46]

Hypospadias refers to the abnormal location of the urethral orifice on the ventral surface of the penis. A fixed, downward bowing is called chordee or ventral curvature, which may accompany hypospadias (see Table 28-12, Common Abnormalities in the Genitourinary Anatomy Associated with Testes and Penises, p. 1115).

Micropenis is a normally structured penis with stretched length <1.9 cm.

Inspect the Scrotum. Inspect the scrotum for *rugae*, which should be present by 40 weeks' gestation. Scrotal edema may occur for several days postbirth due to maternal estrogen effects.

Palpate the Testes. Palpate the *testes* in the scrotal sacs, moving downward from the external inguinal ring. If a testis is in the inguinal canal, gently milk it downward into the scrotum. The newborn's testes should be about 10 mm in width and 15 mm in length, typically lying in the scrotal sacs. Examine the testes for swelling within the scrotal sac and over the inguinal ring.

The incidence of undescended testes (*cryptorchidism*) is about 30% among premature infants, 3% among term neonates, and 1% by age 1 year. An undescended testicle often results in an underdeveloped and tight scrotum (see Table 28-12, Common Abnormalities in the Genitourinary Anatomy Associated with Testes and Penises, p. 1115).

Assess for Scrotal Masses. If swelling is detected in the scrotal sac, differentiate it from the testis. Note if the size changes with increased abdominal pressure (e.g., crying). Check if your fingers can trap the mass in the scrotal sac, apply gentle pressure to reduce its size, and note any tenderness or *transillumination* (Fig. 28-31).

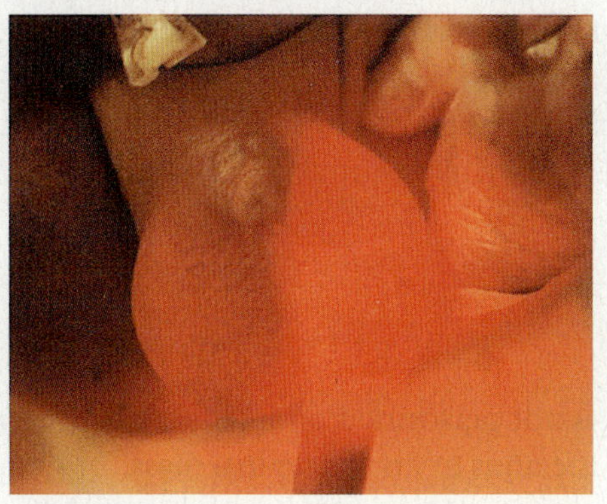

FIGURE 28-31. Transillumination of a hydrocele. (Reprinted with permission from Fletcher MA. *Physical Diagnosis in Neonatology.* Lippincott-Raven; 1998.)

Hydroceles and inguinal hernias are common scrotal masses in newborns, often coexisting and more common on the right side. *Hydroceles*, which can be reducible (communicating) or nonreducible (noncommunicating), are typically transilluminable and resolve by 18 months (Fig. 28-31). *Hernias* are usually reducible, do not transilluminate unless large, and do not resolve on their own. A thickened spermatic cord (*silk sign*) may be noted.

Vulva and Vagina

Examine the External Genitalia. With the infant supine, inspect the genitalia. In newborns the genitalia are prominent due to maternal estrogen effects, which decreases during the first year. The *labia majora* and *minora* are dull pink in lighter-skinned infants and may be hyperpigmented in darker-skinned infants. A milky white vaginal discharge, sometimes blood-tinged, is common in the first few weeks due to hormonal withdrawal and is not a cause for concern.

Ambiguous genitalia, involving atypical development of external genitalia, is a rare condition caused by endocrine disorders such as congenital adrenal hyperplasia.

Inspect the Labia and Clitoris. Systematically examine the structures, including the clitoris size; labia majora color and size; and any rashes, bruises, or lesions (Fig. 28-32).

Labial adhesions, which are thin and attach the labia minora to each other at the midline, occur frequently and often disappear without treatment.

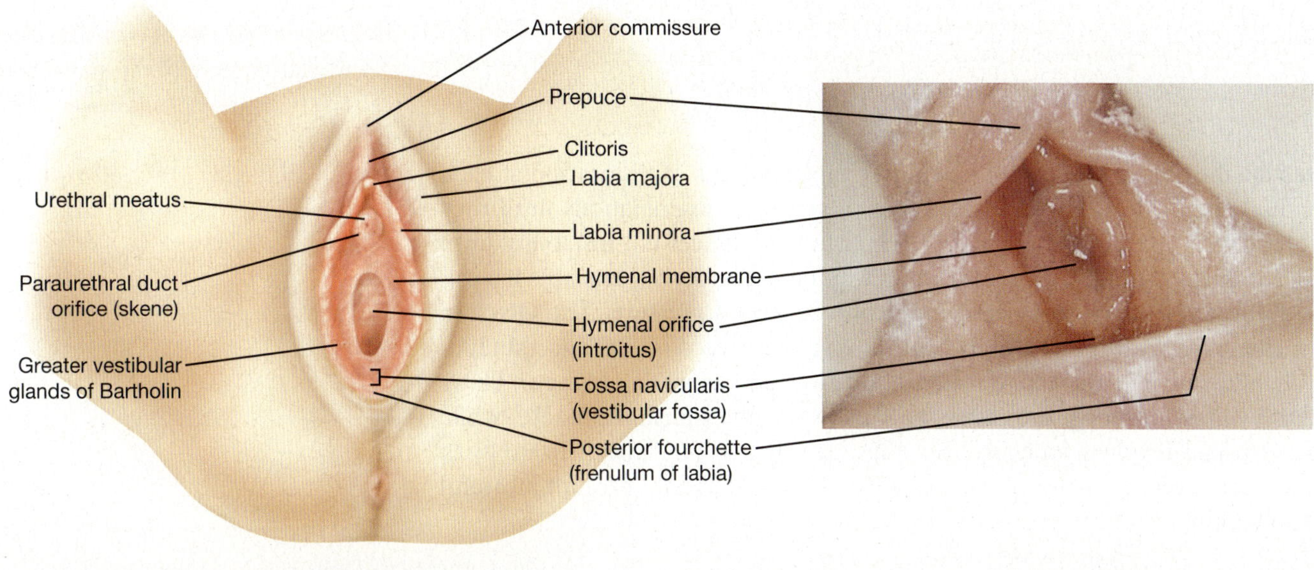

FIGURE 28-32. External genitalia of prepubertal individual with female anatomy. The photo at the right shows the highly estrogenized hymen of a newborn with thickening and hypertrophy of hymenal tissue.

Inspect the Urethral Orifice, Labia Minora, and Hymen. Separate the labia majora at their midpoint with the thumb of each hand (Figs. 28-83 and 28-84). Inspect the urethral orifice and labia minora. Assess the *hymen*, which, in newborns and infants, is thickened and avascular with a central orifice covering the *vaginal opening*. Note any discharge.

An imperforate hymen may be noted at birth.

Rectum and Anus

In general, a digital rectal examination is not performed on infants or children unless there is a question of patency of the anus or an abdominal mass. In such cases, flex the infant's hips and fold the legs to the head. Use a lubricated and gloved pinky finger for the examination.

A common cause of blood in the stool of infants is an *anal fissure*, a superficial break in the surface of the anus and observable with the naked eye.

Musculoskeletal System

Significant changes in the musculoskeletal system occur during infancy. Much of the examination focuses on detecting congenital abnormalities in the hands, spine, hips, legs, and feet. Combine the musculoskeletal examination with the neurologic and developmental examination. Use IPROMS (**I**nspection, **P**alpation, **R**ange **O**f **M**otion, and **S**pecial maneuvers) to assess the musculoskeletal system (see Chapter 25, Musculoskeletal System: Neck, Shoulders, and Upper Extremities, pp. 784–786).

Inspection can reveal gross deformities such as dwarfism, congenital abnormalities of extremities or digits, and amniotic bands.

Examine the Hands. The newborn's hands are typically clenched due to the palmar grasp reflex (p. 1041). Help the infant extend their fingers and inspect for defects. Palpate along the clavicle for lumps, tenderness, or crepitus, which may indicate a fracture from a difficult birth.

Skin tags, remnants of digits, *polydactyly* (extra fingers), or *syndactyly* (webbed fingers) are congenital defects noted at birth.

Examine the Spine. Inspect the spine for major defects and subtle abnormalities like pigmented spots, hairy patches, or deep pits. Palpate the spine in the lumbosacral region for vertebral deformities.

Major defects like *meningomyeloceles* are often detected by ultrasound before birth. *Spina bifida occulta* may be associated with defects of the spinal cord causing severe neurologic dysfunction.

Examine the Hips. Examine the newborn's hips for signs of dislocation at each examination.[47,48] All infants should receive serial hip examinations until they are walking. Use the Barlow and Ortolani tests to detect hip instability until age 2 months. The Barlow test evaluates whether an intact but unstable hip can be dislocated posteriorly by applying gentle backward pressure. The Ortolani test then assesses whether a dislocated hip can be reduced into the acetabulum by gently opening the hip through abduction and upward pressure. Think of the motions during the tests: the Barlow involves pushing 'back,' while the Ortolani involves 'opening' the hips. A soft audible "click" heard with these maneuvers does not prove a dislocated hip but should prompt a careful examination.

Developmental dysplasia of the hip is important to detect early for better outcomes.

Perform the Barlow Test. Place the infant supine with their hips and knees flexed to 90 degrees, positioning your index fingers over the greater trochanters and thumbs on the medial aspect of the thighs (Fig. 28-33). Gently apply

A positive Barlow sign indicates a potentially dislocatable hip, requiring follow-up or referral.

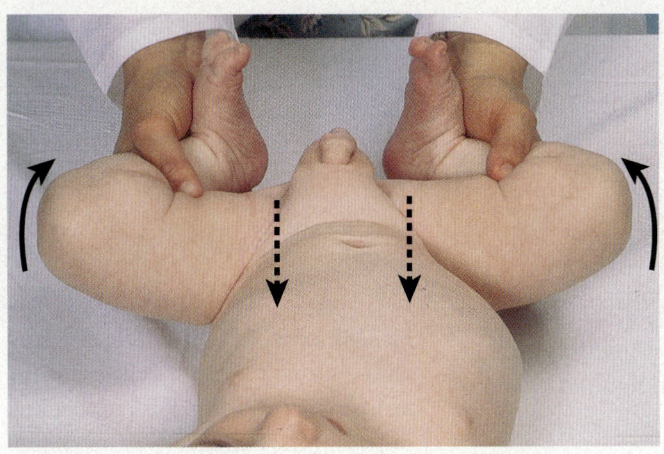

FIGURE 28-33. Starting position for the Barlow test. Hips and knees flexed to 90°. Thumbs stabilize thighs medially; index fingers on greater trochanters. Black arrows indicate stabilization; dashed arrows show direction of gentle posterior pressure.

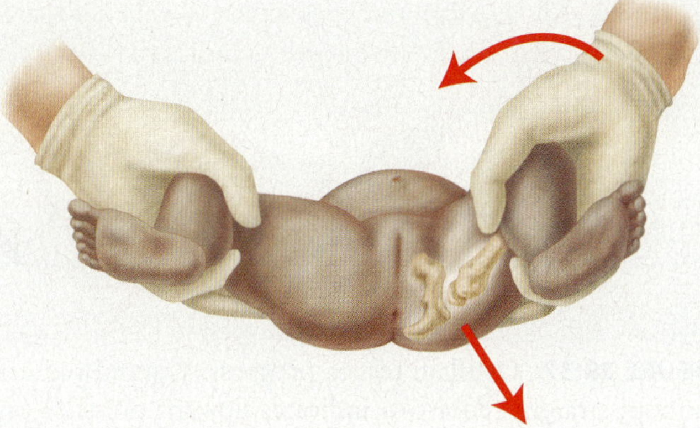

FIGURE 28-34. Barlow test in progress. Straight red arrow shows posterior pressure by thumbs; curved red arrow indicates adduction of thighs. Tests for femoral head dislocation from the acetabulum.

posterior pressure to the hip joint while adducting the thigh toward the midline (Fig. 28-34). Feel for any movement of the femoral head as it dislocates posteriorly, which would indicate hip instability (Fig. 28-35).

Perform the Ortolani Test. Keeping the infant in the same position, maintain your hands as placed for the Barlow test (Fig. 28-36). Abduct both hips simultaneously while lifting upward with your fingers on the greater trochanters (Fig. 28-37). This maneuver assesses for the reduction of a posteriorly dislocated femoral head back into the acetabulum. Feel or listen for a "clunk," which indicates successful reduction and confirms prior dislocation.

A "clunk" felt during the Ortolani test indicates a positive sign for hip dysplasia.

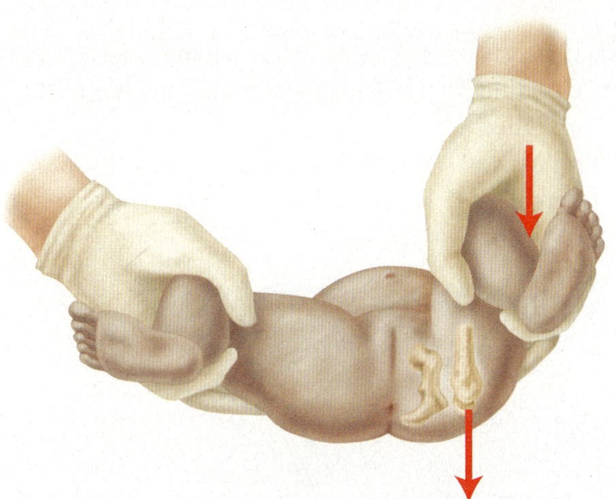

FIGURE 28-35. Barlow test, ending position. Straight red arrows indicate posterior and downward pressure applied by thumbs to confirm hip instability.

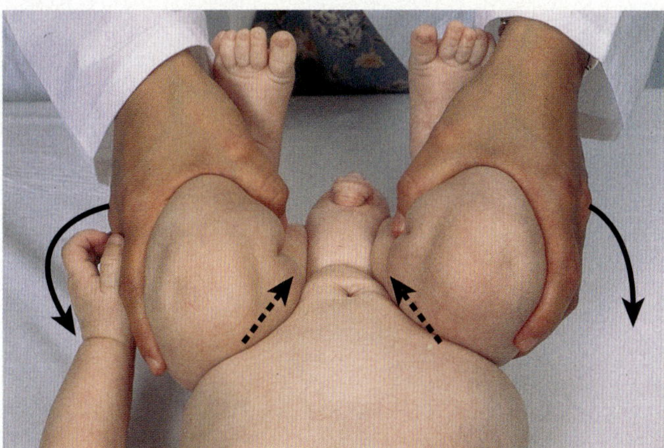

FIGURE 28-36. Starting position for the Ortolani test. Hips and knees flexed to 90°. Thumbs stabilize thighs; index fingers on greater trochanters. Black arrows indicate stabilization; dashed arrows show upward force during abduction.

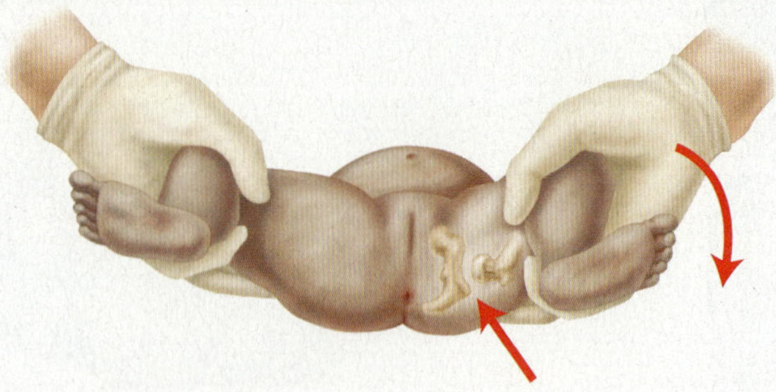

FIGURE 28-37. Ortolani test in progress. Curved red arrow shows abduction motion; straight red arrow indicates upward pressure on the femoral head to reduce dislocation.

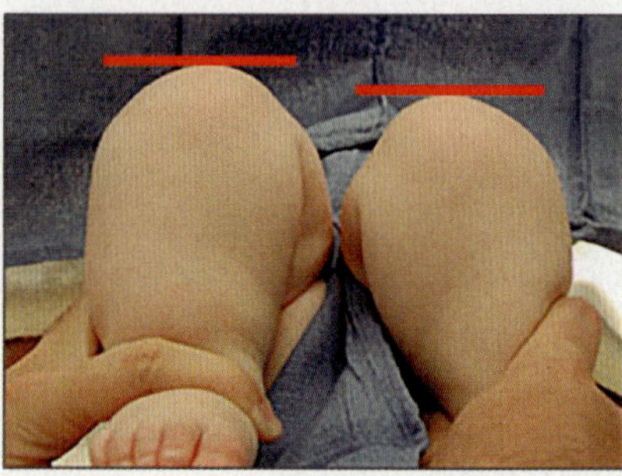

FIGURE 28-38. Positive Galeazzi sign with shortening of the left femur, in an infant with left hip dislocation. (Reprinted with permission from Storer SK, Skaggs DL. Developmental dysplasia of the hip. *Am Fam Physician.* 2006;74(8):1310–1316. Copyright © 2006 American Academy of Family Physicians. All Rights Reserved.)

Test for Femoral Shortening. Use the *Galeazzi or Allis sign* to test for femoral shortening. Place the feet together with knees flexed and sacrum flat on the table, noting any difference in knee heights (Fig. 28-38).

Examine the Legs. Assess the symmetry, bowing, and torsion of the legs. There should be no discrepancy in leg length. Most newborns are *bowlegged* (*varus*), reflecting their curled-up intrauterine position. Some infants exhibit twisting or *torsion* of the tibia inwardly or outwardly on its longitudinal axis. Tibial torsion usually corrects itself by age 4 after weight-bearing months.[47]

Severe bowing can be due to rickets or Blount disease, while tibial torsion occurs with deformities of the feet or hips.

Inspect the Feet. Examine the feet for deformities. At birth, foot deformities are common and often result from intrauterine positioning. Begin by inspecting the natural alignment of the feet in a neutral position (Figs. 28-39). These deformities should be flexible and correctable to a neutral position. Gently move the foot to an overcorrected position to assess flexibility (Fig. 28-40). Scratch or stroke along the outer edge to see if the foot assumes a normal position.

True deformities of the feet do not return to the neutral position even with manipulation.

The newborn foot has several benign features that may initially cause concern. The foot appears flat due to a plantar fat pad and often shows inversion, elevating the outer margin. Some infants have forefoot adduction without inversion, called *metatarsus adductus*, which requires close follow-up. Others have adduction of the entire foot. In all these normal variants, the position can be easily corrected to neutral and even beyond without resistance. They usually resolve within 1 to 2 years.

See Table 28-13, Common Musculoskeletal Findings in Young Children, p. 1115.

The most common severe congenital foot deformity is *talipes equinovarus* or *clubfoot.*

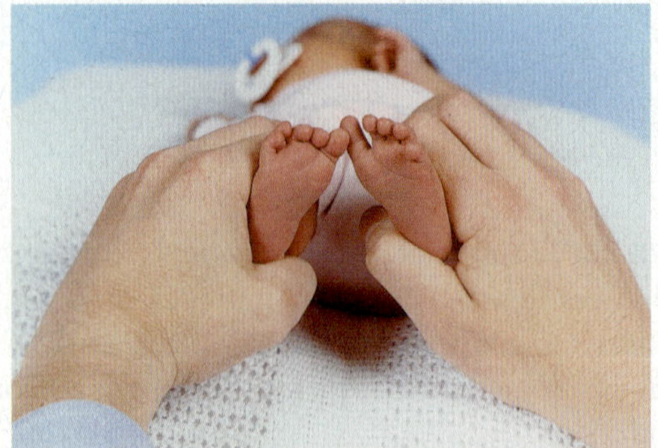

FIGURE 28-39. Assessing the alignment of the feet.

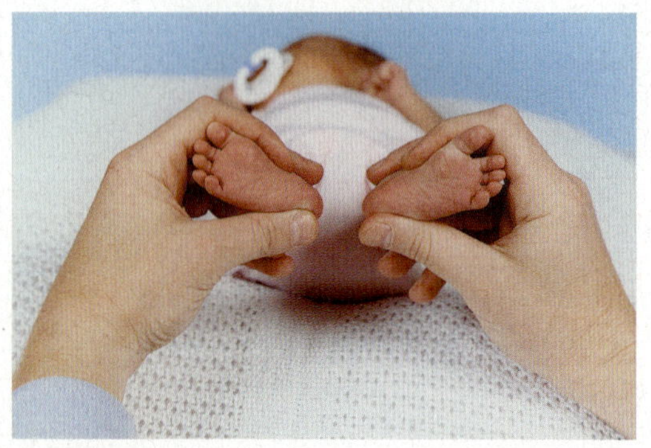

FIGURE 28-40. Assessing flexibility by overcorrecting the feet.

Nervous System

The examination of the nervous system in infants includes techniques specific to this age group. Unlike many adult neurologic abnormalities that produce asymmetric localized findings, abnormalities in infants often present as developmental issues. Thus, the neurologic and developmental examinations should be conducted together.

Severe neurologic disease signs in infants include extreme irritability; persistent posture asymmetry; constant head-turning; persistent, marked extension of the head, neck, and extremities (*opisthotonus*); severe flaccidity; limited pain response; and sometimes seizures.

The neurologic screening examination for newborns should assess *mental status, gross motor function, tone, cry, deep tendon reflexes (DTRs)*, and *primitive reflexes*. More detailed examinations are indicated if abnormalities are suspected.[49,50]

Subtle neonatal behaviors like fine tremors, irritability, and poor self-regulation may indicate opioid withdrawal.

Assess Mental Status. Assess the mental status of newborns by observing their activities during alert periods (see Box 28-6, p. 1004).

Persistent irritability may indicate neurologic insult or metabolic, infectious, or environmental conditions such as drug withdrawal.

Assess Motor Function and Tone. Observe the infant's position at rest and test resistance to passive movement. Assess tone by moving each major joint through its ROM, noting any spasticity or flaccidity. Hold the infant in your hands to determine if the tone is normal, increased, or decreased. An infant with normal tone responds to vertical suspension and does not "slip through the hands" (Fig. 28-41). Increased or decreased tone may indicate intracranial disease, often accompanied by other signs.

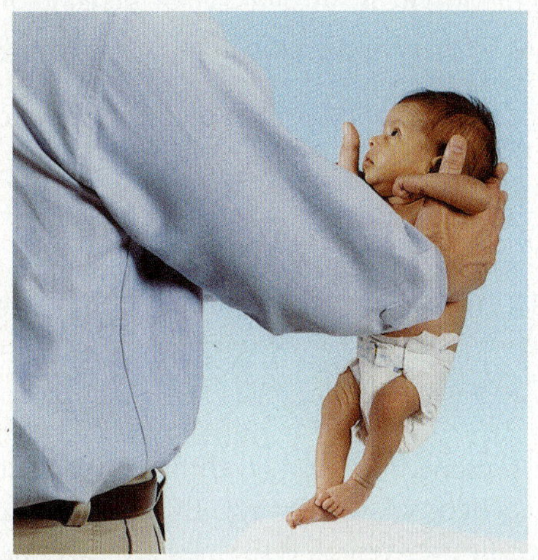

FIGURE 28-41. Assessing motor tone.

Newborns with hypotonia often lie in a frog-leg position. Hypotonia can be caused by CNS abnormalities and motor unit disorders.

The *scarf sign* (elbow passes midline when the arm is extended) suggests hypotonia.

Assess Sensory Function. Test sensory function by flicking the infant's palm or sole. Observe for withdrawal, arousal, and change in facial expression. Do not use a pin to test for pain.

If changes in facial expression or cry follow a painful stimulus but no withdrawal occurs, weakness or paralysis may be present.

Test Cranial Nerves. Test the cranial nerves of the newborn or infant using strategies in Box 28-28.

Abnormalities in cranial nerves can suggest intracranial lesion, hemorrhage, or congenital malformations.

Congenital facial nerve palsy can result from birth trauma or developmental defects.

Dysphagia, or difficulty in swallowing, can be due to injury to cranial nerves IX, X, and XII.

Box 28-28. Strategies to Assess Cranial Nerves in Newborns and Infants

Cranial Nerve	Function	Strategy
I	Smell	Very difficult to test
II	Vision	Have infant regard your face and look for facial response and tracking
II, III	Response to light	Darken room, raise infant to sitting position to open eyes Use light and test for *optic blink reflex* (blink in response to light) Use otoscope light (without speculum) to assess pupillary responses
III, IV, VI	Extraocular movements	Observe how well the infant tracks your smiling face (or a bright light) and whether the eyes move together
V	Sensation and strength	Test rooting reflex (see Box 28-29) Test sucking reflex (watch infant suck breast, bottle, or pacifier) and strength of suck
VII	Facial expressions	Observe infant crying and smiling; note facial symmetry
VIII	Hearing	Test acoustic blink reflex (blinking of both eyes in response to a loud noise) Observe tracking in response to sound
IX, X	Swallowing Gag reflex	Observe coordination during swallowing Test for gag reflex
XI	Shoulder symmetry	Observe symmetry of shoulders
XII	Tongue movements	Observe coordination of sucking, swallowing, and tongue thrusting

Elicit Deep Tendon Reflexes. DTRs are present but may be difficult to elicit and vary in intensity due to immature corticospinal pathways. Exaggerated or absent reflexes have little diagnostic significance unless responses are extreme or asymmetric.

A progressive increase in DTRs during the first year of life may indicate CNS disease such as cerebral palsy, especially if coupled with increased tone. Central hypotonia followed by progressively increased tone is another common presentation.

Decreased DTRs could suggest lower motor neuron disease.

Use the same techniques as for adults, substituting your index or middle finger for the reflex hammer (Fig. 28-42). The triceps, brachioradialis, and abdominal reflexes are difficult to elicit before age 6 months.

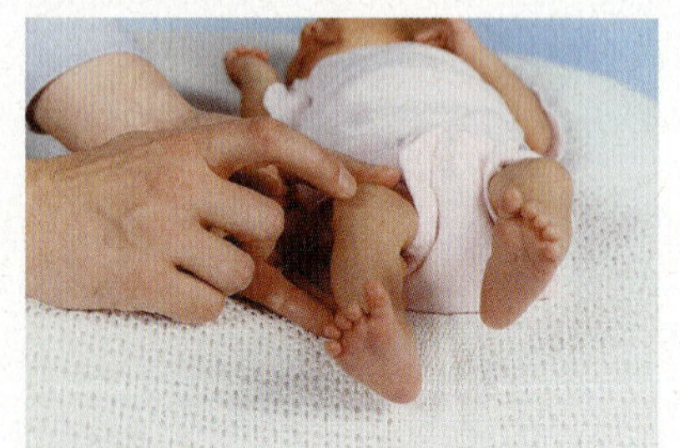

FIGURE 28-42. Assessing deep tendon reflexes with finger.

As in adults, asymmetric reflexes suggest a lesion of the peripheral nerves or spinal segment or can be due to an intracranial lesion.

The *anal reflex* or *"anal wink"* is present at birth and is important to elicit if a spinal cord lesion is suspected.

An absent anal reflex suggests loss of innervation of the external sphincter muscle due to a spinal cord abnormality.

The Babinski response to plantar stimulation (dorsiflexion of big toe and fanning of other toes) is positive in newborns and may persist for several months.

A positive Babinski persisting for many months may signal a corticospinal tract abnormality.

To elicit the *ankle reflex* in an infant, grasp the malleolus and abruptly dorsiflex the ankle (Fig. 28-43). Rapid, rhythmic plantar flexion (*ankle clonus*) up to 10 beats is normal in newborns.

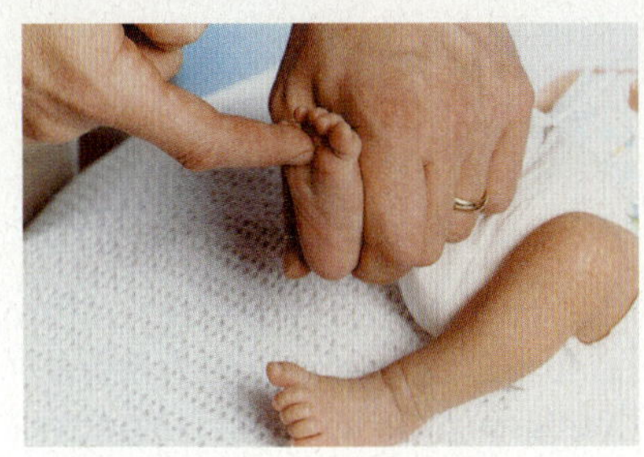

FIGURE 28-43. Assessing ankle reflexes.

Continuous contractions (*sustained ankle clonus*) suggest CNS disease.

Irritability, jitteriness, tremors, hypertonicity, and hyperactive reflexes may indicate *neonatal abstinence syndrome* (NAS) from maternal substance use or hypoglycemia. NAS from opioid use can include these signs along with autonomic signs, poor feeding, and seizures.

Assess Primitive Reflexes. Evaluate the developing CNS by assessing *infantile automatisms* or *primitive reflexes*, which develop during gestation, are generally present at birth, and disappear at defined ages (Box 28-29). Abnormalities in these reflexes suggest neurologic disease and require further investigation.[51]

Signs of a neurologic or developmental abnormality include primitive reflexes that are absent at the appropriate age, present longer than normal, or are asymmetric or associated with posturing or twitching.

Box 28-29. Primitive Reflexes

Primitive Reflex	Technique	Abnormality
Asymmetric Tonic Neck Reflex (ATNR) Birth to 2–3 months 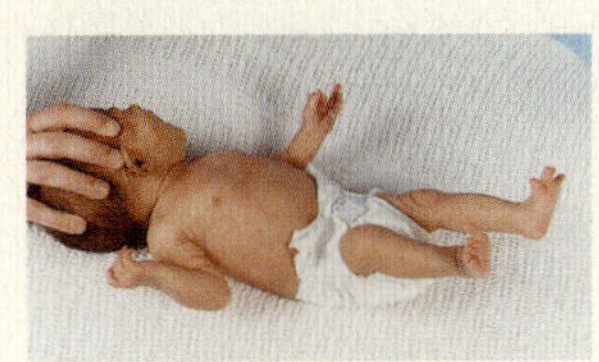	With the infant supine, turn their head to one side. The arms/legs on the side to which head is turned will extend, while the opposite arm/leg will flex. Repeat on the other side.	Absence suggests a transverse spinal cord lesion or injury. Persistence >4 months suggests a developmental problem.
Palmar Grasp Reflex Birth to 3–4 months 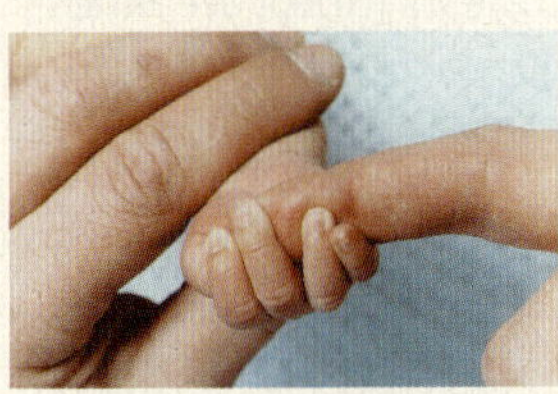	Place your fingers into the infant's hands and press against the palmar surfaces. The infant will flex all fingers to grasp your fingers.	Persistence >4–6 months suggests pyramidal tract dysfunction.

(*continued*)

Box 28-29. Primitive Reflexes (*Continued*)

Primitive Reflex	Technique	Abnormality
Rooting Reflex Birth to 3–4 months 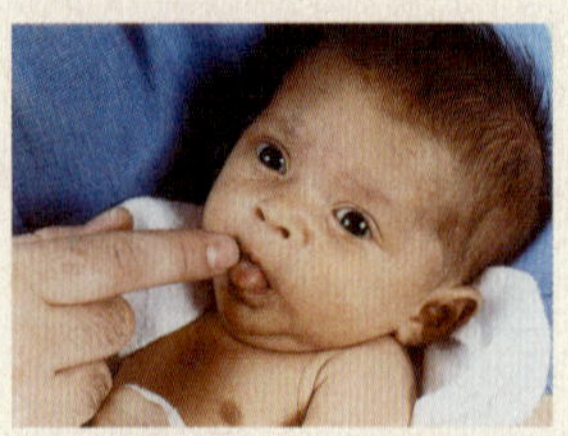	Stroke the perioral skin at the corners of the mouth. Their mouth will open, and the infant will turn their head toward the stimulated side and suck.	Absence indicates severe CNS disease. Persistence >4 months suggests neurologic disease; >6 months strongly suggests it.
Trunk Incurvation (Galant) Reflex Birth to 3–4 months 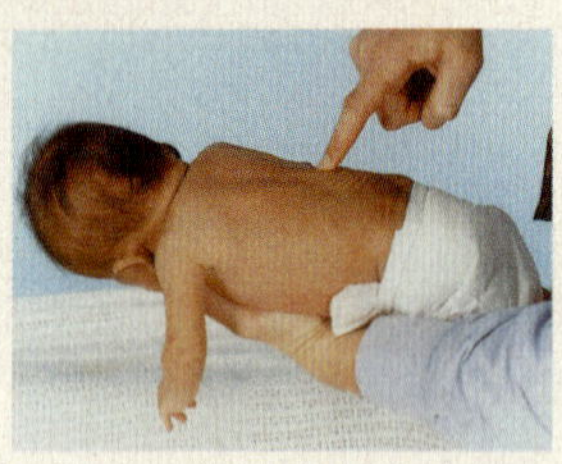	Support the infant prone and stroke one side of the back 1 cm from midline, from shoulder to buttocks. Their spine will curve toward the stimulated side.	Absence suggests a transverse spinal cord lesion. Persistence may indicate delayed development.
Moro Reflex (Startle Reflex) Birth to 4 months 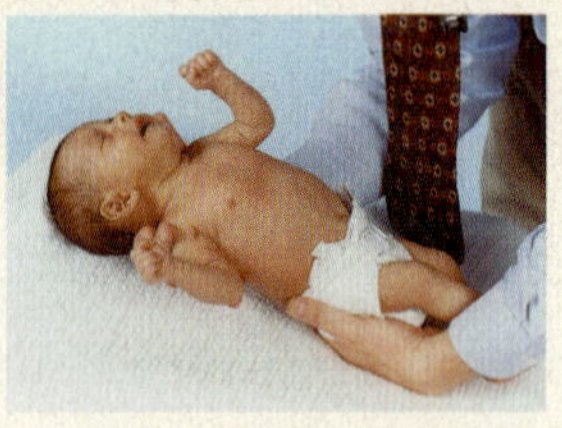	Hold the infant supine, supporting their head, back, and legs. Abruptly lower the entire body about 1 foot. The arms will abduct and extend, hands will open, and legs will flex. The infant may cry.	Asymmetric response suggests fracture or brachial plexus injury. Persistence >4 months suggests central nervous system development issues and sometimes predicts cerebral palsy.
Plantar Grasp Reflex Birth to 6–8 months 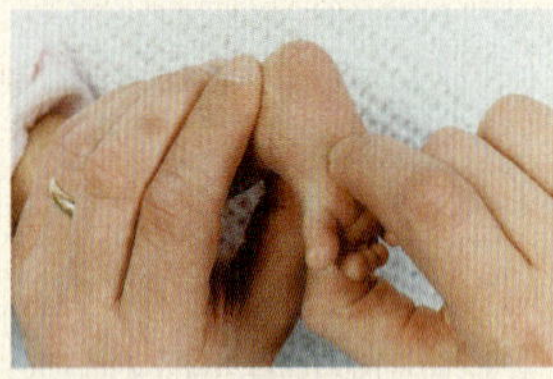	Touch the sole at the base of their toes. Their toes will curl.	Persistence >8 months suggests pyramidal tract dysfunction.
Landau Reflex 3–24 months 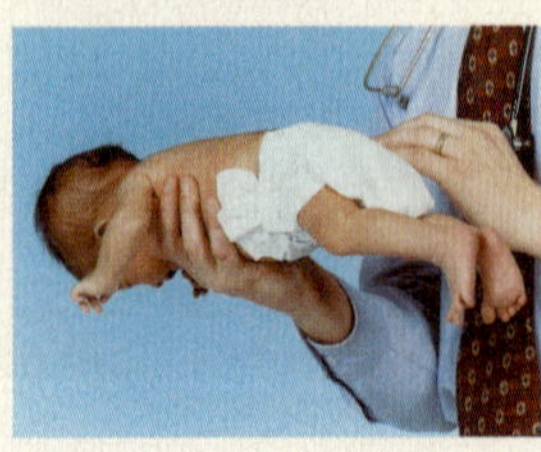	Suspend the infant prone with one hand. Their head will lift, and their spine will straighten.	Absence suggests motor weakness or neurologic dysfunction.

Primitive Reflex	Technique	Abnormality
Positive Support Reflex Birth or 2 months until 6 months 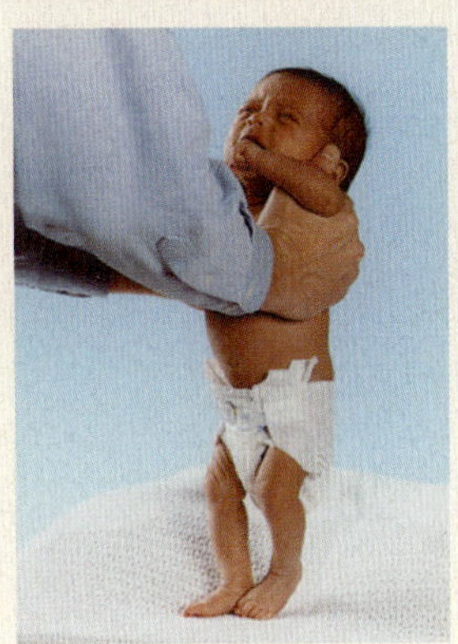	Hold the infant around the trunk and lower until their feet touch a flat surface. Their hips, knees, and ankles will extend, and the infant will stand up, partially bearing weight, sagging after 20–30 seconds.	Absence suggests hypotonia or flaccidity.
Placing and Stepping Reflexes Birth (best after 4 days; variable age to disappear) 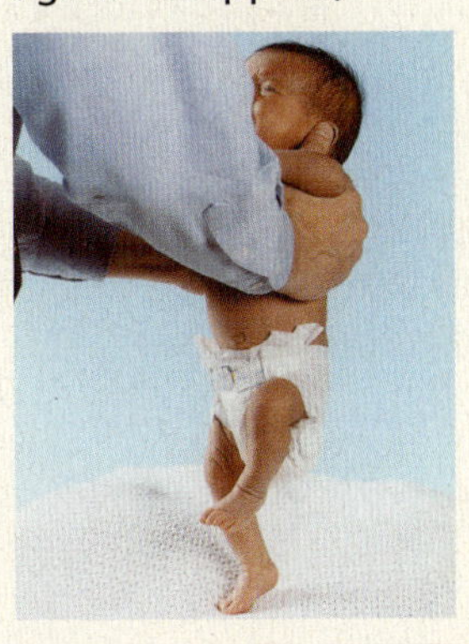	Hold the infant upright as in the positive support reflex. Have one sole touch the tabletop. Their hip and knee of that foot will flex, and the other foot will step forward. Alternate stepping will occur.	Absence suggests paralysis or hypotonia. Breech delivery may result in absence of placing reflex.
Parachute Reflex 8 months and does not disappear 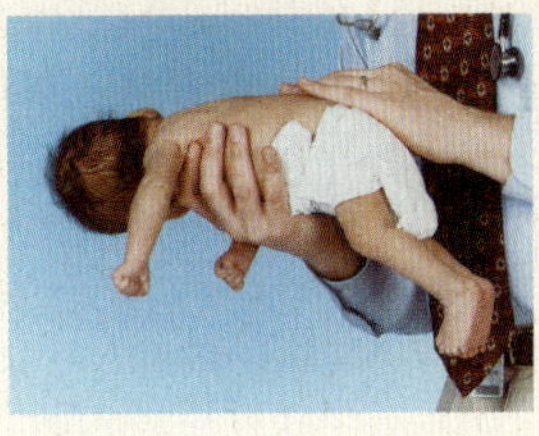	Suspend the infant prone and slowly lower their head toward a surface. Their arms and legs will extend in a protective fashion.	Delay in appearance may predict future delays in motor development. Asymmetry may indicate upper extremity issues.

Conduct the Developmental Assessment. By observing and playing with the infant, you can conduct both a developmental screening examination and an assessment for gross motor and fine motor achievements (Box 28-30). Infants with developmental delays may show abnormalities on the neurologic examination, as much of the examination is based on age-specific norms.

Look for *weakness* by observing sitting, standing, and transitions. Note *posture* (station) during sitting or standing. Assess fine motor development in older infants similarly, combining the neurologic and developmental examination. Key milestones include the development of the pincer grasp, the ability to manipulate objects, and tasks like building a tower of blocks or scribbling. Fine and gross motor development progresses from proximal to distal.

Many causes of developmental delay exist but often no cause is identified. Etiologies include *prenatal* (genetic, CNS, congenital hypothyroidism), *perinatal* (preterm, asphyxia, infection, trauma), and *postnatal* (trauma, infection, toxin, abuse).

Box 28-30. Abnormalities Detected While Observing Play

Behavioral[a]

Poor caregiver–child interactions

Conflicts between siblings

Concerns about caregiving approaches to discipline

Signs of a challenging temperament

Developmental

Gross motor skills delay

Fine motor skills delay

Language delay (expressive or receptive)

Delay in social or emotional tasks

Social or Environmental

Caregiver stress, depression

Risk for abuse or neglect

Neurologic

Weakness

Abnormal posture

Spasticity

Clumsiness

Attentional challenges, hyperactivity

Traits associated with autism

Musculoskeletal

Structural abnormalities

[a]Note: The child's behavior during the visit may not represent typical behavior, but your observations may serve as a springboard for discussion with caregivers.

Since some neurologic abnormalities produce deficits or slow cognitive and social development, assess the infant's cognitive and social/emotional development alongside the neurologic and developmental examination.

Refer to the developmental milestones in Box 28-5 on p. 1003 and standardized developmental screening instruments to identify age-specific developmental tasks to evaluate.

Developmental delay across more than one domain (e.g., motor plus cognitive) suggests more severe disease.

RECORDING YOUR FINDINGS

The clinical record format is the same for children and adults, although the sequence of the physical exam may vary. Document findings in the traditional written or electronic format, starting with sentences and progressing to phrases. This style includes phrases suitable for most write-ups. Note any atypical findings and modifications for caregiver reports.

The structure and sequence of the write-up for newborn or infant exams are similar to those for young children. Use the example on pp. 1078–1081 and the key history elements in Box 28-3 on pp. 1000–1001 as guides.

HEALTH PROMOTION AND COUNSELING: EVIDENCE AND RECOMMENDATIONS

The AAP and the group Bright Futures[22] recommend health supervision visits for infants younger than age 1 year at the following ages: birth; 3 to 5 days; by 1 month; and at 2, 4, 6, 9, and 12 months (Fig. 28-44). This is called the *Infant Periodicity Schedule*. Health supervision visits provide opportunities to answer caregivers' questions, assess the infant's growth and development, perform a comprehensive physical examination, and provide anticipatory guidance. Age-appropriate anticipatory guidance includes healthy habits and behaviors, social competence of caregivers, caregiving techniques, family relationships, and community interactions.

Regular visits provide an opportunity to plot a course for healthy and successful development. Infants generally are well during these visits, enhancing the quality of the experience. Caregivers are usually receptive to suggestions about health promotion, which can have major, long-term influences on the child and family. Strong interviewing skills are necessary as you discuss strategies to optimize the health and well-being of their infants. Adjust the content to the appropriate developmental level of the infant. As an exercise, review the critical components of a health supervision visit for a 6-month-old in Box 28-31.

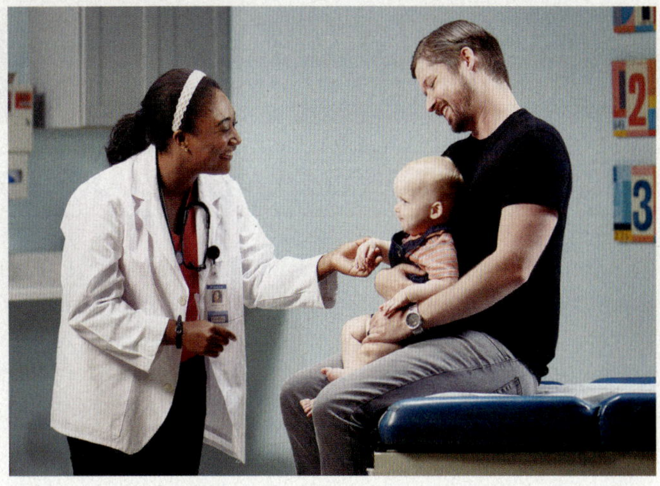

FIGURE 28-44. Regular health supervision serves many purposes.

Box 28-31. Components of a Health Supervision Visit for a 6-Month-Old

Discussions with Caregivers

Address caregivers' concerns/questions

Provide advice tailored to the infant and family's needs

Obtain social history, including caregiving environment and dynamics

Assess development, nutrition, sleep, elimination, safety, oral health, family relationships, stressors, caregiving beliefs, community factors

Developmental Assessment

Use a standardized developmental instrument to measure milestones

Assess milestones by history

Assess milestones by examination

Physical Examination

Perform a comprehensive examination, including growth parameters and percentiles for age

Screening Tests

Assess vision and hearing

Screen for social risk factors

Immunizations

Follow the schedule provided by the American Academy of Pediatrics (AAP) or U.S. Centers for Disease Control and Prevention (CDC)

Anticipatory Guidance

Healthy Habits and Behaviors

Injury and illness prevention

Use infant seat, watch for rolling, caution on walkers, poisons, tobacco exposure

Nutrition

Feeding human milk (via breastfeeding, chestfeeding, or expressed milk) or formula, with iron and vitamin D supplementation if needed. Introduce solids safely, avoid juice, and take precautions to prevent choking or overfeeding.

Oral health

Avoid bottles at bedtime, ensure fluoride use, and introduce brushing

Caregiver–Infant Interaction

Encourage activities that promote development, such as talking, reading, singing, music, and play

Family Dynamics

Support caregiver well-being (e.g., time for self-care, babysitters, or other support systems)

Community Resources

Provide guidance on childcare, community resources, and support networks

PRESCHOOL-AGE AND SCHOOL-AGE CHILDREN

HEALTH HISTORY: GENERAL APPROACH

Children typically come with a parent or caregiver. Even when alone in the examination room, they are usually there at their caregiver's request, who often waits outside. When interviewing a child, consider both the child's and the caregiver's needs and perspectives. Building rapport and effective communication with families is crucial for accurate diagnosis and successful treatment (Box 28-32).

Box 28-32. Techniques for Building Rapport and Effective Communication with Families

Best Practices	Examples of Communication
Establishing Rapport ■ Greet and establish rapport with everyone present (Fig. 28-45). ■ Refer to the child by name to create a personalized connection. ■ Ask about the role or relationship of all adults and children present. ■ Address caregivers formally (e.g., *"Mr. Smith"* or *"Ms. Smith"*). ■ Clarify the household structure with questions like, *"Who else lives in the home?"* or *"Do you live together?"* ■ Avoid assumptions about family involvement (e.g., do not assume separated or non-residential caregivers are uninvolved). ■ Use eye contact and playful engagement, and talk about the child's interests. ■ Calm and connect with anxious children by spending time at the beginning.	Clinician to family: ■ *"Tell me [patient's name]'s relationship to everyone here."* ■ *"Who else lives in the home?"* or *"Do you live together?"* 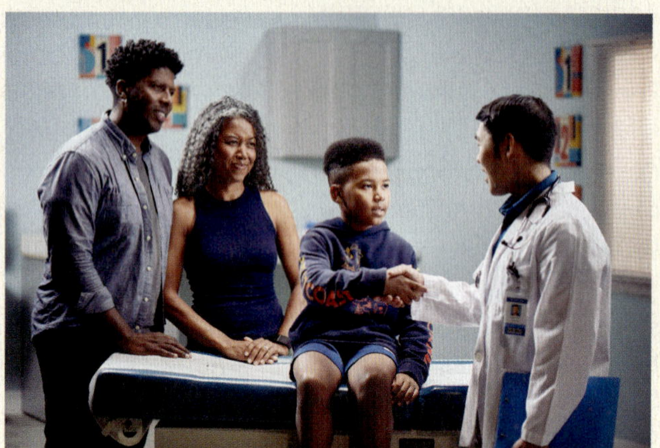 **FIGURE 28-45** Greeting the child to build rapport with the family.
Working With Families ■ Start with the child for information, then confirm with caregivers. ■ Ask open-ended questions followed by specifics. ■ Observe family interactions for valuable insights into dynamics and relationships. ■ Build trust through empathy active listening, and understanding each family's unique context. ■ Partner with caregivers, recognizing them as experts in their child's needs and experiences.	Clinician to child: ■ *"Are you sick? . . . Tell me about it."* ■ *"Your mom tells me that you get stomachaches. Tell me about them."* ■ *"Show me where you get the pain. What does it feel like?"* ■ *"Is it sharp like a pinprick, or does it ache?"* ■ *"Does it stay in the same spot, or does it move around?"* ■ *"What helps make it go away? What makes it worse?"* ■ *"What do you think causes it?"*

Best Practices	Examples of Communication
Multiple Agendas ■ Each individual in the room, including the clinician, may have differing views on the issue and its resolution (Fig. 28-46). ■ Discover as many of these perspectives and agendas as possible. Family members who are not present (e.g., the absent parent, caregiver, or grandparent) may also have concerns. Ask about those concerns, too. ■ Balance these concerns with clinical observations and provide education about the range of normal development.	Clinician to family member: ■ *"If [patient's name]'s father were here today, what questions or concerns would he have?"* Clinician to caregiver: ■ *"Have you discussed this with other family members or anyone else?"* ■ *"What do they think?"* 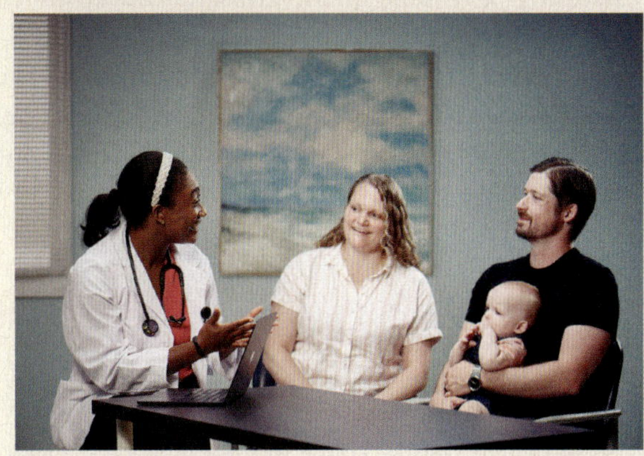 **FIGURE 28-46** Addressing varied concerns with the family.
Family as a Resource ■ Recognize caregivers as experts in their child's care and collaborate as a consultant. ■ Respect cultural, socioeconomic, and family practice variations. ■ Support caregivers and avoid judgmental comments. ■ Acknowledge the challenges of caregiving and praise successes.	Clinician to caregiver: ■ *"You are doing such a wonderful job with [patient name]. Being a caregiver takes so much work, and [patient's name]'s behavior here today clearly shows your efforts. We might have some suggestions for you at the end of the visit."* Clinician to child: ■ *"[Patient name], you are so lucky to someone really special taking care of you!"*
Hidden Agendas: ■ As with adults, the stated concern may not relate to the real reason the caregiver has brought the child to see you. ■ The presented issue may serve as a bridge to deeper concerns. ■ Foster trust by creating a welcoming atmosphere and using open-ended, facilitating questions to encourage honesty.	Clinician to caregiver: ■ *"Do you have any other concerns about [patient name]?"* ■ *"Was there anything else that you wanted to tell/ask me today?"*

SURVEILLANCE OF DEVELOPMENT: EARLY CHILDHOOD, 1 TO 4 YEARS

During early childhood (ages 1 to 4), children are usually accompanied by their parents or caregivers for health assessments. Even if the child is alone in the consultation, the caregiver's presence and input are crucial. These interactions typically arise from caregivers' concerns about their child's development and well-being.

When assessing a young child, consider developmental milestones and behavioral cues as well as the caregiver's insights (Box 28-33). Effective communication and trust-building with both the child and the family are essential for accurate evaluation and treatment planning. Strategies to engage families and address their concerns can significantly enhance the quality of care.

Distinguish between isolated delays in one aspect of development (e.g., motor coordination or language) and more generalized delays in several components. The latter is more likely to reflect global neurologic disorders such as cognitive disability from many etiologies.

Box 28-33. Surveillance of Development: Early Childhood (1 to 4 Years)

Physical Development

- Rate of physical growth slows by approximately half after infancy.
- After 2 years, toddlers gain about 2–3 kg and grow 5 cm per year.
- Children become leaner and develop more adult-like body proportions.
- Gross and fine motor skills develop quickly:
  - Most children walk by 15–18 months, run well by 2 years, and pedal a tricycle and jump by 4 years.
  - Fine motor skills develop through neurologic maturation and play (Fig. 28-47).
  - An 18-month-old scribbles, a 2-year-old draws lines, a 3-year-old copies a circle, and a 4-year-old can draw a simple person and start to copy simple capital letters.

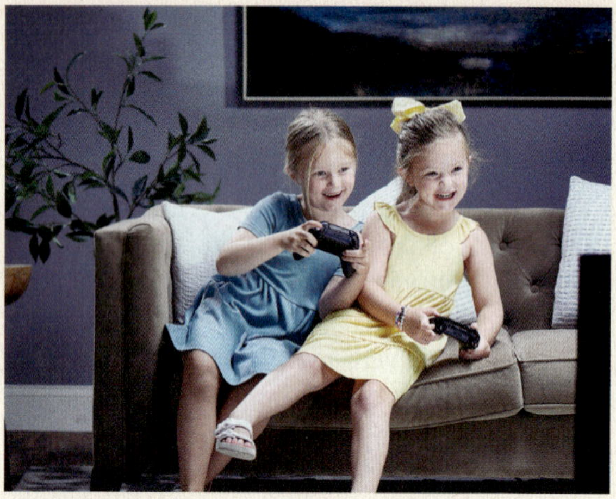

FIGURE 28-47. Fine motor skills develop along with cognition.

Health Care Approaches

- Regular monitoring of growth parameters (weight, height)
- Guidance on physical activity and motor skill development
- Nutritional counseling to support healthy growth
- Encouragement of age-appropriate play activities to enhance motor skills

Cognitive and Language Development

- Toddlers transition from sensorimotor learning to symbolic thinking.
- They solve simple problems, remember songs, and engage in imitative play.
- Language development is rapid:
  - An 18-month-old with 10–20 words becomes a 2-year-old who speaks in 3-word sentences, and a 3-year-old who converses well.
  - By age 4 years, preschoolers form complex sentences.
- They remain preoperational and have not yet developed sustained logical thought processes.
- Assess fine motor coordination, cognition, and language by asking children older than 3 years to draw a picture or copy objects and then discuss their pictures.

Health Care Approaches

- Monitor language milestones and provide early intervention if delays are noticed.
- Encouraging cognitive development through interactive play and problem-solving activities.
- Support caregivers to promote language-rich environments.

Social and Emotional Development

- Socio-emotional skills develop rapidly:
  - Toddlers begin to engage in pretend play, parallel play, and imitative play.
  - They become imaginative and develop new intellectual pursuits (Fig. 28-48).
  - A drive for independence emerges.
- Toddlers are impulsive and have poor self-regulation, commonly leading to temper tantrums.
- Self-regulation is an important developmental task with a wide range of what is considered typical.

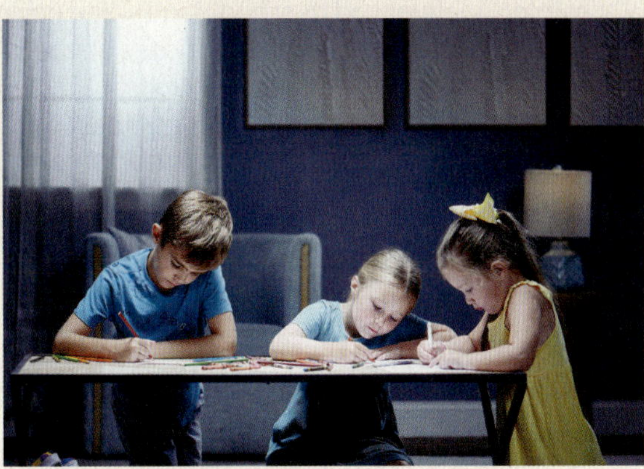

FIGURE 28-48. Individual personalities of young children emerge as their intellect grows.

Health Care Approaches

- Provide guidance for caregivers on managing temper tantrums and promoting emotional regulation.
- Encourage social interactions with peers through playgroups and structured activities.
- Support developing independence while ensuring safety.

SURVEILLANCE OF DEVELOPMENT: MIDDLE CHILDHOOD, 5 TO 10 YEARS

During middle childhood (ages 5 to 10), children undergo significant physical, cognitive, and emotional development (Box 28-34). This stage is marked by goal-directed exploration, increased physical and cognitive abilities, and achievements through trial and error. Health evaluations often involve the child and a parent or caregiver, although children at this age can provide more personal input due to their growing independence.

Box 28-34. Surveillance of Development: Middle Childhood (5 to 10 Years)

Physical Development

- Growth is steady with improved strength and coordination (Fig. 28-49).
- Be aware of limitations in children with disabilities or chronic illnesses.
- Participation in activities increases physical abilities.

Health Care Approaches

- Regularly monitor growth and physical development.
- Encourage physical activity.
- Support children with physical disabilities or chronic illnesses.

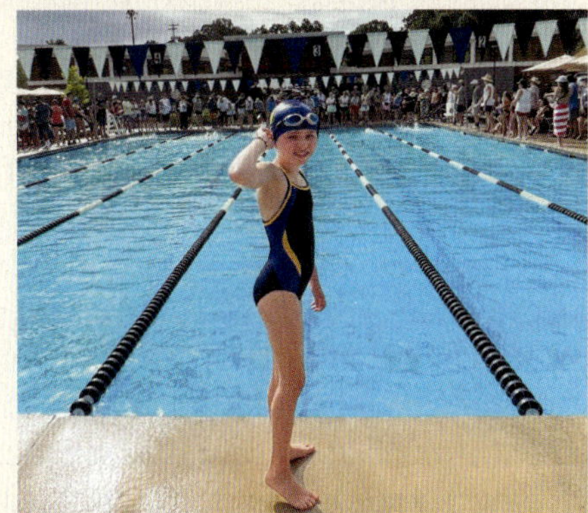

FIGURE 28-49. Physical abilities rapidly progress in early childhood.

(continued)

Box 28-34. Surveillance of Development: Middle Childhood (5 to 10 Years) (*Continued*)

Cognitive and Language Development

- Children become *"concrete operational"* with limited logic and complex learning.
- Learning is influenced by school, family, and environment (Fig. 28-50).
- Major task is developing *self-efficacy* or the child's belief in their ability to thrive in different situations.
- Language becomes increasingly complex.
- School performance is a key indicator of cognitive development.

Health Care Approaches

- Monitor school performance and cognitive milestones.
- Encourage a stimulating learning environment.
- Support children with learning difficulties.

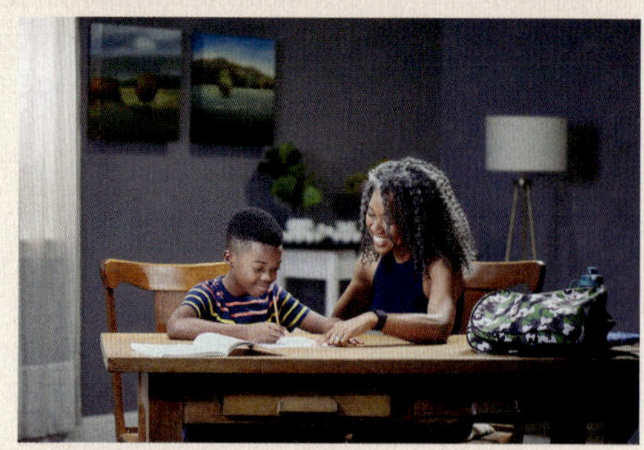

FIGURE 28-50. Cognitive development is shaped by family relationships.

Social and Emotional Development

- Increasing independence, initiating activities, and valuing achievements are seen.
- Self-esteem and social "fit" within family, school, and peers develop.
- Guilt and poor self-esteem may emerge.
- Moral development remains simple and concrete with a clear sense of "right and wrong."

Health Care Approaches

- Encourage social interactions and activities.
- Support emotional regulation and self-esteem.
- Provide guidance on moral and ethical behavior.

When evaluating children in this age range, consider their increasing autonomy and ability to communicate their experiences and concerns. The caregiver's role remains crucial, as their observations and insights offer a comprehensive view of the child's health and development. Establishing strong rapport with both the child and caregiver is essential for accurate information gathering and ensuring the child feels comfortable and understood.

PHYSICAL EXAMINATION: GENERAL APPROACH

An important aspect of examining children is that caregivers are usually watching and participating, allowing you to observe the caregiver–child interaction. Note whether the child displays age-appropriate behaviors. Assess the "goodness of fit" between caregivers and child. Some abnormal interactions may result from the unnatural setting of the examination room, while others may indicate interactional problems. Observing the child's interactions with caregivers and the child's unstructured play in the examination room can reveal abnormalities in physical, cognitive, and social development or issues with the caregiver–child relationship. This also provides opportunities for gentle education and anticipatory guidance. Follow the guidelines of trauma-informed care discussed at the beginning of this section.

Healthy toddlers may initially be alarmed by the examiner. Some will be uncooperative but most eventually warm up. If this behavior persists or is not developmentally appropriate, an underlying behavioral or developmental issue may be present. Older, school-age children typically have more self-control and prior experience with clinicians and are generally cooperative with the examination (Box 28-35).

Box 28-35. Assessing Children: Younger and Older

Assessing Younger Children

- Avoid physical struggles, crying, or a distraught caregiver; successfully managing this is part of the "art of medicine" in pediatrics.
- Gain the child's confidence and alleviate fears from the start.
- Tailor your approach to the visit's circumstances.
- Offer a cleaned toy or book to build rapport, especially during health supervision visits.
- Keep the child dressed during the interview to minimize apprehension and observe natural interactions with caregivers.
- Engage children by asking simple questions about their illness or toys, complimenting their appearance or behavior, telling a story, or playing a simple game (Fig. 28-51).
- If the child is shy, focus on the caregiver to let the child warm up gradually.
- Help anxious caregivers relax by suggesting they read or play with the child.
- When examining siblings, start with the oldest to set a positive example.
- Approach the child pleasantly and explain each step of the examination.
- Maintain conversation with the family to provide a distraction.
- For toddlers (9–15 months) with stranger anxiety, avoid quick approaches and direct eye contact initially.
- Keep the toddler in the caregiver's lap for most of the examination.
- Perform physical exams with the child in the caregiver's lap; expose only the body part being examined if they resist undressing.
- Patience, distraction, play, flexibility in the order of the exam, and a caring but firm approach are key to examining young children (Fig. 28-52).

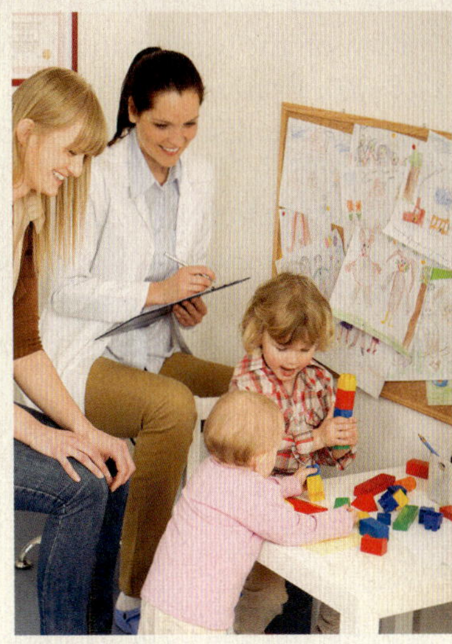

FIGURE 28-51. Engaging children in play is sometimes part of the assessment.

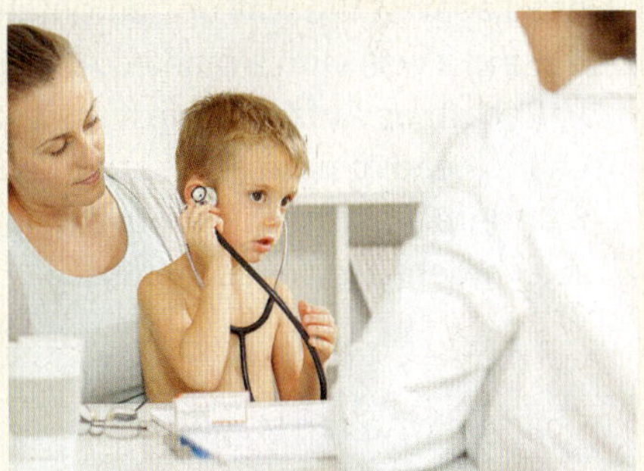

FIGURE 28-52. Familiarizing the child with the equipment and procedures can reduce anxiety in children.

Assessing Older Children

- Examining school-age children usually poses fewer difficulties.
- Address unpleasant memories from previous clinical encounters.
- Many children are modest; provide gowns and leave underwear in place as long as possible.
- Consider leaving the room while the child changes with their caregiver's help (Fig. 28-53).
- Some children may prefer certain siblings or family members to leave the room, but most are comfortable having a caregiver, regardless of gender, present.
- Caregivers of children younger than 11 should stay with them during the exam. Follow your setting's chaperone policy.

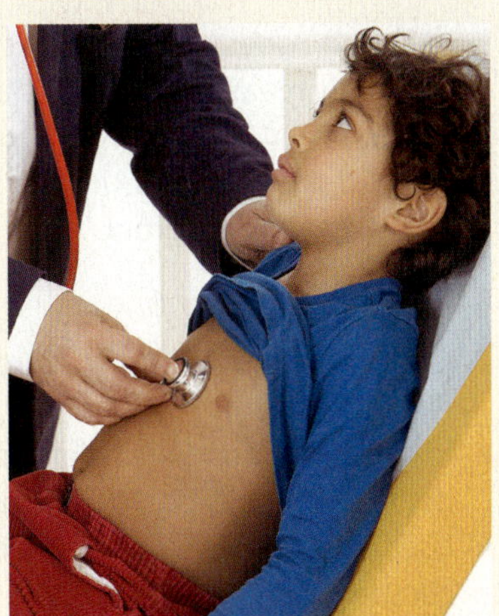

FIGURE 28-53. Clinicians need to be aware of older children's developing modesty.

TECHNIQUES OF EXAMINATION

The order of the examination now begins to follow that used for adults (Box 28-36). Examine painful areas last and forewarn children about areas you are going to examine. If a child resists part of the examination, you can return to it at the end.

Reassure caregivers that resistance to examination is developmentally appropriate. Some caregivers may respond by scolding the child, which can inadvertently worsen the situation. Involve caregivers in the examination. Learn which techniques and approaches work best and are most comfortable for you.

Box 28-36. Somatic Growth Patterns in Children

Technique	Significance
Height	
▪ For children age >2 years, measure standing height using wall-mounted stadiometers. ▪ Have the child stand with heels, back, and head against the wall or stadiometer. ▪ If using a wall with a marked ruler, place a flat board or surface against the top of the child's head at right angles to the ruler. ▪ Stand-up weight scales with a height attachment are not accurate.	▪ Tracks linear growth ▪ After age 2 years, children should grow ≥5 cm per year; during puberty, growth velocity increases
Weight	
▪ Children who can stand should be weighed in a gown or clothing without shoes on a stand-up scale. ▪ Use the same scales across successive visits for comparability.	▪ Monitors weight gain and identifies potential growth issues
Head Circumference	
▪ Generally measure until the child reaches 24 months. ▪ After 24 months, measure if suspecting a genetic or CNS disorder.	▪ Assesses brain and skull development
Body Mass Index for Age	
▪ Use age- and sex-specific charts to assess BMI (Box 28-39). ▪ BMI measurements are helpful for early detection of obesity in children age >2 years. ▪ Use the same scales for accuracy and comparability. ▪ Inform caregivers about their child's BMI and the impact of healthy eating and physical activity.	▪ Helps in early detection of obesity ▪ Obesity often begins before age 6–8 years

Short stature, height <5th percentile, can be a normal variant (e.g., familial short stature and constitutional delay) or caused by chronic diseases (e.g., growth hormone deficiency; endocrine, gastrointestinal, renal, and metabolic diseases; and genetic syndromes).

Etiologies for insufficient caloric intake causing poor growth (in weight and height) include psychosocial, gastrointestinal, and endocrine disorders.

Weight percentiles help identify undernutrition, overnutrition, and growth disorders.

Unusual measurements may indicate underlying medical conditions.

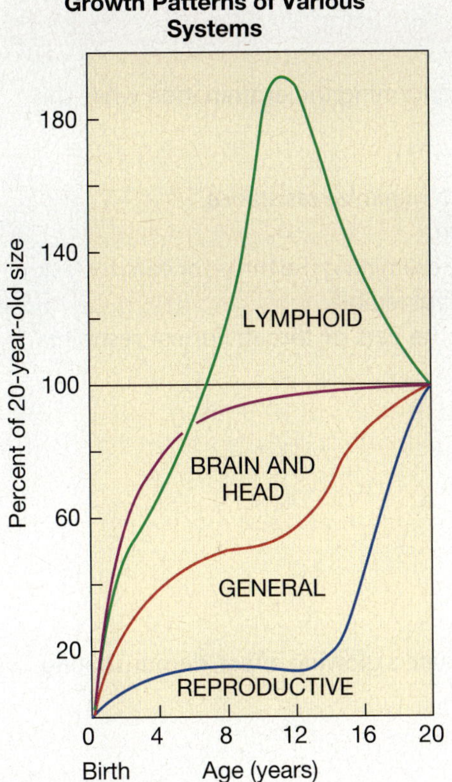

FIGURE 28-54. Growth patterns of various systems.

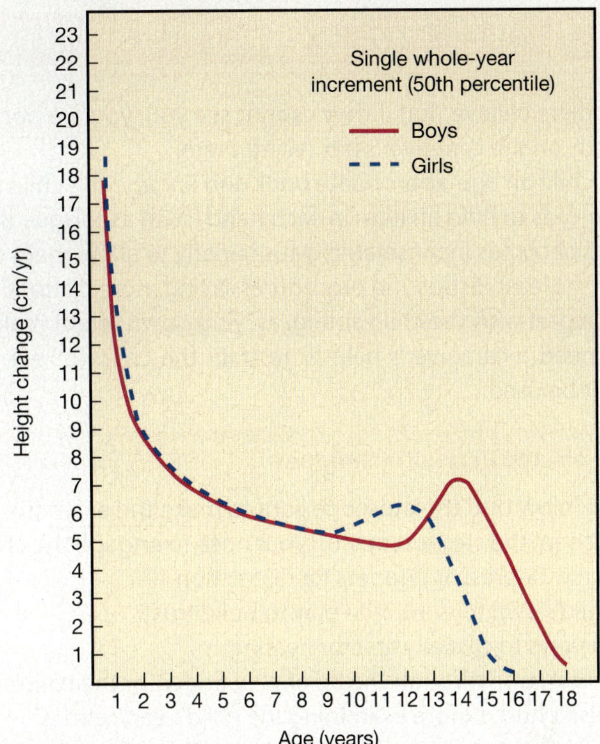

FIGURE 28-55. Velocity curves for length and height for boys and girls based on intervals of 1 year. (Reprinted from Lowrey GH. *Growth and Development of Children*. 8th ed. Year Book Medical; 1986. Copyright © 1986 Elsevier. With permission.)

Somatic Growth

Figures 28-54 and 28-55 demonstrate somatic growth patterns in children (Box 28-37).

Box 28-37. Tips for Examining Young Children (1- to 4-Year-Olds)

Useful Strategies for Examination

- Have the caregiver help you facilitate the examination (e.g., removing clothing, holding child on lap). Try to be at the child's eye level.
- Use a reassuring voice throughout the examination.
- Let the child see and touch the examination tools you will be using.
- First examine the child's toy or teddy bear, or even the caregiver, then move on to the child.
- Allow the child to participate in the examination (e.g., by moving the stethoscope). Then gently guide them back to complete the areas that were missed.
- Ask a toddler who keeps pushing you away to *"hold your hand."* Then encourage them to "help you" with the examination.
- Avoid asking permission to examine a body part because you will do the examination anyway. Instead, ask the child which ear or which part of the body he or she would like you to examine first.
- Make a game out of the examination! For example, *"Let's see how big your tongue is!"* or *"Is there a toy hiding in your ear? Let's see!"*

(continued)

Box 28-37. Tips for Examining Young Children (1- to 4-Year-Olds) (*Continued*)

- Some toddlers believe that if they cannot see you, you are not there. Try performing the examination while the child stands on the caregiver's lap, facing them.
- Hand the child an age-appropriate book and engage the child in reading.
- Ask 2-year-olds to hold an item in each hand (such as tongue depressors), to minimize resistance.
- If the child becomes inconsolable, pause briefly to allow them to calm down.
- Start with the least distressing procedures saving more distressing ones, like examining the throat or ears, for last.
- Begin each part with the child sitting, as lying down might make them feel vulnerable.
- You may need a caregiver's help to restrain the child for examination of the ears or throat. Formal restraints should not be used.

Engaging Tools and Playful Techniques

- Pretend to "blow out" the otoscope light to make the exam fun.
- Playfully "beep" the stethoscope on your nose to engage the child.
- Make tongue-depressor puppets for distraction.
- Use the child's own toys into the play to build trust.
- Jingle your keys to casually test for hearing.
- Shine the otoscope through the tip of your finger (or the child's finger) to create a glowing effect, demonstrating that it doesn't hurt, before examining the child's ears with it.
- Offer age-appropriate toys and books during the visit.
- Use a fun toy attached to the stethoscope to make it less intimidating.

Note: Make sure to clean toys and your stethoscope between patients.

Vital Signs

Accurate measurement of vital signs is crucial in pediatric care, as it provides essential information about a child's health status. This includes measuring blood pressure, pulse rate, respiratory rate, and temperature, each requiring specific techniques to ensure accuracy (Box 28-38).

Box 28-38. Vital Signs Assessment in Children

Measurement Technique	Clinical Significance
Blood Pressure (BP)	
■ The most frequent cause of elevated BP in children is often an improperly performed examination, usually due to an incorrect cuff size. ■ Measure BP with the child calm; use automatic or manual cuffs with appropriate cuff size. ■ The bladder length of the cuff should encircle 80–100% of the child's arm circumference.	■ Hypertension in childhood, often coexisting with obesity, is more common than previously thought and should be managed appropriately. ■ AAP defines normal, elevated, and high BP with measurements on at least three separate occasions (Box 28-40).[52]

Obesity increases the prevalence of hypertension.

Measurement Technique	Clinical Significance
▪ The cuff's width-to-arm circumference ratio should be 0.45–0.55 (Fig. 28-56). ▪ First Korotkoff sound indicates systolic pressure; disappearance of sounds indicates diastolic pressure. ▪ If needed, use palpation to determine the systolic BP, remembering that the reading obtained is ~10 mm Hg lower by palpation than by auscultation. ▪ If the BP is initially elevated, measure again at the end of the examination; leave the cuff on the arm (deflated) and repeat later.	▪ Avoid falsely labeling a child or adolescent as having hypertension due to the stigma, potential activity limitations, and possible treatment side effects. ▪ Anxiety or "white-coat hypertension" is a common cause of elevated BP readings.
Pulse Rate	
▪ Measure heart rate over a 60-second interval. ▪ For older children, use the same technique as adults.	▪ Average heart rates and normal ranges vary by age (Box 28-41).
Respiratory Rate	
▪ Observe chest wall movements for two 30-second intervals or over 1 minute before stimulating the child. ▪ Direct auscultation or placing the stethoscope in front of the mouth can be used to count respirations but may be falsely elevated if the child is agitated. ▪ For older children, use the same technique as adults.	▪ Respiratory rate ranges from 20–40 breaths/min during early childhood and 15–25 during late childhood, reaching adult levels around age 15 years.[36] ▪ The commonly accepted standard for tachypnea in children aged >1 year is a respiratory rate >40 breaths/min.
Temperature	
▪ Use auditory canal temperature recordings for quick and comfortable readings.	▪ For children <3 years who appear very ill with a fever, evaluate for serious infections such as sepsis, UTI, or pneumonia.

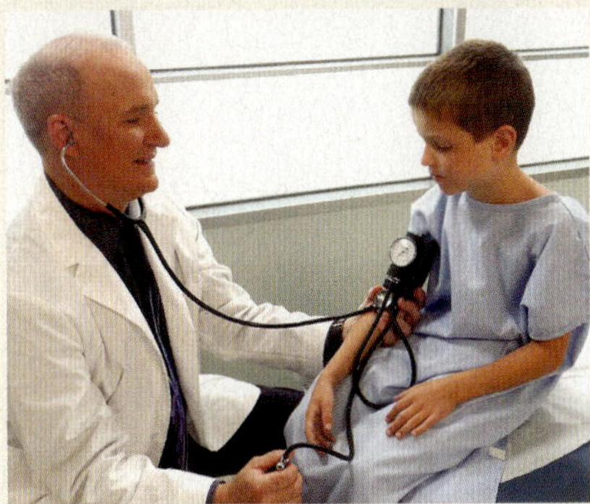

FIGURE 28-56 Ensuring accurate blood pressure measurement by using the correct cuff size and technique.

Sinus bradycardia is defined as a heart rate <60 beats/min in children >3 years.

The best single physical finding for ruling out pneumonia is an *absence of tachypnea*.

Children <3 years with fever should be evaluated for serious infections.

Box 28-39. Interpreting Body Mass Index in Children

Group	BMI for Age
Underweight	<5th percentile
Healthy weight	5th–85th percentile
Overweight	85th–95th percentile
Obese	≥95th percentile

Most children with exogenous obesity are tall for their age, while children with endocrine causes of obesity tend to be short.

Among U.S. children, 19% have a BMI in the 95th percentile or greater. If obesity prevalence continues, 57% of children will have obesity by age 35.

Long-term morbidity from childhood obesity affects many organ systems. Prevention, early detection, and aggressive management are needed.

Transient hypertension can be caused by medications for asthma (e.g., prednisone) and ADHD (e.g., methylphenidate).

Sustained hypertension[52] may result from primary or secondary causes, including obesity, renal, endocrine, or neurologic disease.

Box 28-40. Updated Definitions of Blood Pressure Categories and Stages[52]

	For Children Ages 1 to <13 years	For Children Ages ≥13 years
Normal	<90th percentile	<120/<80 mm Hg
Elevated	≥90th percentile to <95th percentile or 120/80 mm Hg to <95th percentile (whichever is lower)	120/<80 to 129/<80 mm Hg
Stage 1 hypertension	≥95th percentile to <95th percentile + 12 mm Hg, or 130/80 to 139/89 mm Hg (whichever is lower)	130/80 to 139/89 mm Hg
Stage 2 hypertension	≥95th percentile + 12 mm Hg, or ≥140/90 mm Hg (whichever is lower)	≥140/90 mm Hg

Source: Reproduced with permission from Flynn JT, Kaelber DC, Baker-Smith CM, et al. Clinical practice guideline for screening and management of high blood pressure in children and adolescents. *Pediatrics*. 2017;140(3):e20171904. Copyright © 2017 American Academy of Pediatrics.

Box 28-41. Average Heart Rate of Children at Rest[36]

Age (Years)	Average Rate (Median)	Range (1st to 99th percentile)
1–2	110–120	88–155
2–6	100–110	65–140
6–10	75–90	52–130

Source: Fleming S, Thompson M, Stevens R, et al. Normal ranges of heart rate and respiratory rate in children from birth to 18 years of age: a systematic review of observational studies. *Lancet*. 2011; 377(9770):1011–1018.

Skin

After a child's first year of life, the techniques of examination are the same as those for the adult.

See Chapter 12, Skin, Hair, and Nails. Also see Table 28-5, Common Skin Lesions during Childhood, p. 1105.

Head

When examining the head and neck, tailor your examination to the child's stage of growth and development. Even before touching the child, carefully observe *head shape and symmetry* and presence of *abnormal facies.* Abnormal facies may not be apparent until later in childhood; therefore, examine both the face and the head of all children closely.

See Table 28-7, Diagnostic Facies in Infancy and Childhood, pp. 1107–1108.

Fetal alcohol syndrome can cause abnormal facies (p. 1107), microcephaly, and developmental delay.

Eyes

The key components of the eye exam for young children are assessing conjugate gaze, evaluating the red reflex (Fig. 28-57 and see section under newborn eye exam, p. 1023), and testing visual acuity in each eye.

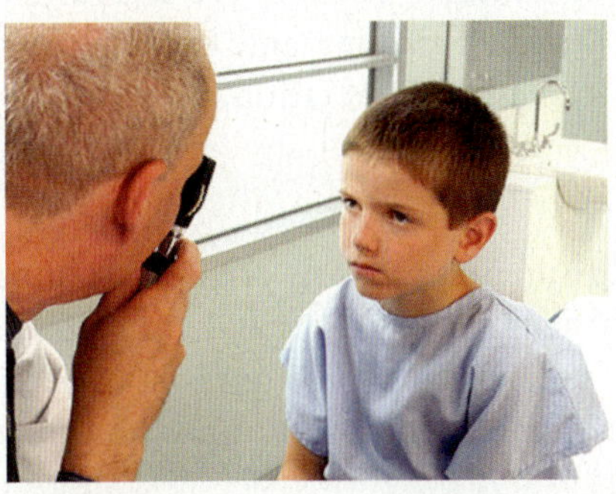

FIGURE 28-57. Examing the red reflex on a young child using an opthlamoscope.

Assess Conjugate Gaze. See methods from Chapter 14 to assess eye position, alignment, and extraocular muscle function. The *corneal light reflex test* and the *cover–uncover test* are especially useful.

Anisometropia (different refractive errors in each eye) can lead to *amblyopia*, or reduced vision, which can become permanent if not corrected early.

Perform the cover–uncover test (Fig. 28-58) as a game, asking the child to watch your nose or tell if you are smiling while you cover one eye. Watch for eye deviation when uncovered, then repeat for the other eye.

Strabismus is indicated by movement of either eye when uncovered.

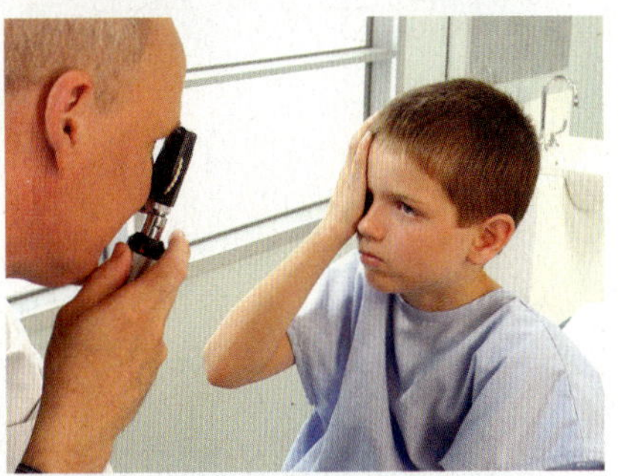

FIGURE 28-58. Conducting an eye examination using an ophthalmoscope, while the child participates in a cover-uncover test to assess eye alignment.

Strabismus (Table 28-8 Abnormalities of the Eyes, Ears, and Mouth, p. 1109) requires treatment to prevent amblyopia. Common forms are nasal ("eso") or temporal ("exo") deviations. Latent strabismus ("phoria") occurs when fixation is disrupted, while manifest strabismus ("tropia") is always present.

Box 28-42. Visual Acuity Development

Age	Visual Acuity
3 months	Eyes converge, infant reaches for objects
12 months	–20/200
Younger than 4 years	~20/40
4 years and older	~20/30 or better

Test Visual Acuity. For children under 3, assess fixation preference by alternately covering each eye. A child with normal vision will not object, while a child with poor vision in one eye will resist covering the good eye. Refer to an optometrist if you have doubts about visual acuity (Box 28-42). In all tests of visual acuity, ensure both eyes show the same result to avoid amblyopia.

Reduced visual acuity is more likely in children born prematurely or with neurologic or developmental disorders. Any difference in visual acuity between eyes is abnormal by age 5. Near vision problems can lead to reading difficulties, headaches, and school issues.

For children 4 and older, use an eye chart with optotypes (characters or symbols). If they don't know letters or numbers, use pictures or the "E" chart. Most children can indicate the direction the "E" is pointing (Figs. 28-59 and 28-60).[53]

Myopia is the most common visual disorder in children and can be easily detected.

Assess Visual Fields. For infants and young children, test one eye at a time with the child on the caregiver's lap. Hold the head midline and bring a toy into view from behind. Turn it into a game for better cooperation.

Ears

Properly Position the Child for the Exam. Examining the ear canal and tympanic membrane in young children can be challenging as they may be sensitive and fearful. With practice, you can master this technique. It is often best to perform this exam at the end as children may need brief restraint.

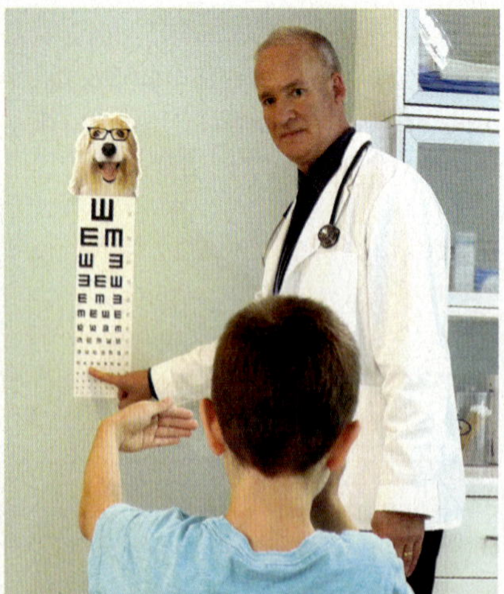

FIGURE 28-59. Child reading an E chart during a visual acuity test, covering one eye for accuracy.

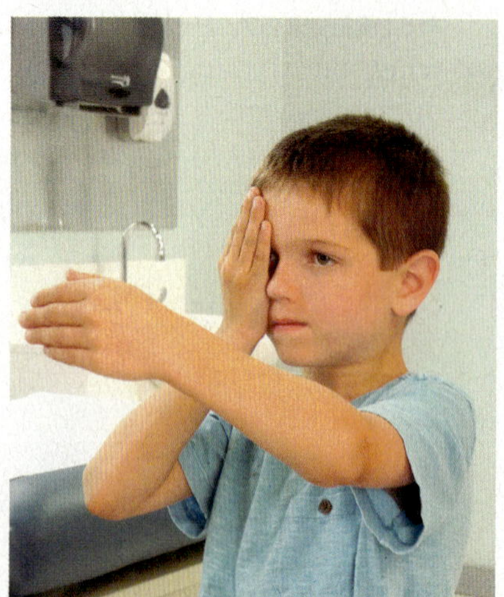

FIGURE 28-60. Child indicates the direction of the E during a visual acuity test.

Ask the caregiver about their preferred positioning for the child. The two common positions are lying down with gentle restraint or sitting on the caregiver's lap depending on the child's comfort level.

- **Sitting on caregiver's lap**: Position the child's legs between the caregiver's legs. The caregiver can use one arm to secure the child's body and the other hand to steady the head by placing it gently on the child's forehead.
- **Supine position**: The caregiver holds the child's arms either extended or close to the sides to limit motion (Figs. 28-61 and 28-62).

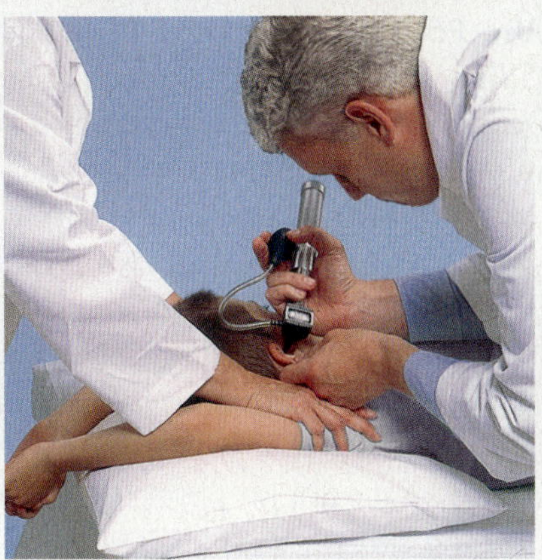

FIGURE 28-61. Gently examining the right ear while holding the otoscope in the right hand and pulling the auricle with the left hand.

Perform an Otoscopic Examination. Make the otoscopic exam a game to allay fears, such as pretending to find an imaginary object in the ear (Box 28-43). Gently place and withdraw the otoscopic speculum into the ear so the child gets used to the procedure. Show the child the speculum does not hurt by letting them touch it and shine a light through your finger.

Hold the head and gently pull the pinna (auricle) upward while holding the otoscope with your other hand (Box 28-44). If you cannot visualize the tympanic membrane, try pulling the pinna backward and downward. Inspect the area behind the pinna, over the mastoid bone.

With otitis externa (but not otitis media), movement of the pinna elicits pain.

With acute mastoiditis, the auricle may protrude forward and outward, and the area over the mastoid bone is red, swollen, and tender.

Many students have difficulty visualizing a child's tympanic membrane. In young children, the external auditory canal is directed upward and backward from the outside, so pull the auricle upward, outward, and backward for the best view. Use one hand to press the child's head and pull up on the auricle, and the other hand to position the otoscope.

Acute otitis media is common in childhood. Symptoms include a red, bulging tympanic membrane, a dull or absent light reflex, and diminished movement on pneumatic otoscopy. Purulent material may also be present behind the tympanic membrane. The most useful diagnostic symptom is ear pain combined with these signs.[54–57] See Table 28-8, Abnormalities of the Eyes, Ears, and Mouth, p. 1109.

Box 28-43. Tips for Conducting the Otoscopic Examination

- Use the otoscope at the best angle with the largest possible speculum for better visualization and less discomfort.
- A small speculum may not provide a seal for pneumatic otoscopy.
- If using a pneumatic otoscope, do not apply too much pressure, which may hurt or upset the child.
- Insert the speculum ¼–½ inch into the canal.
- Identify key landmarks and assess for abnormalities of the tympanic membrane.
- Remove cerumen if it is blocking your view, using one of the following:
  - Flushing the ears
  - Special plastic curettes (ensure the child's head is stabilized to avoid injury).
  - Moistened microtipped cotton swab if not totally occluded
  - Specialized ear-cleaning instruments.

Use Pneumatic Otoscopy (If Indicated). Some clinicians use a pneumatic otoscope to assess the mobility of the tympanic membrane by varying the pressure in the external auditory canal. This requires a patient who remains still. Squeezing the bulb introduces or removes air, causing the tympanic membrane to move (see Figs. 28-61 and 28-62).

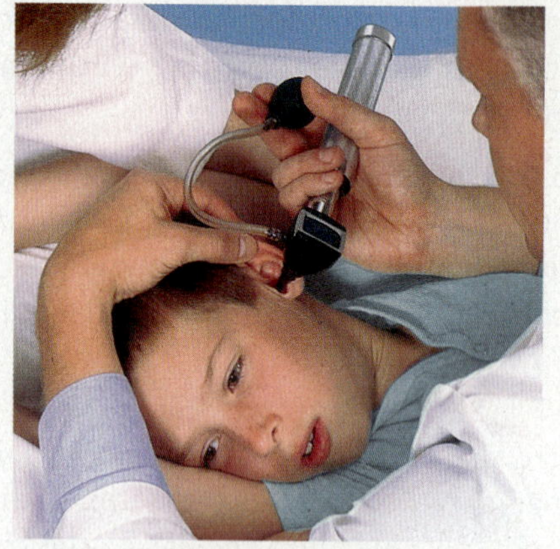

FIGURE 28-62. Examining the left ear while holding the otoscope in the right hand and pulling the auricle with the left hand.

Acute otitis media may cause a ruptured tympanic membrane, resulting in pus in the auditory canal, which obstructs the view of the tympanic membrane.

If the tympanic membrane does not move perceptibly, the child likely has a middle ear effusion or an air leak.

A child with acute otitis media may flinch due to pain from the air pressure.

Box 28-44. Methods for Holding the Otoscope

Upward/Lateral Handle Method

Commonly used in adults, the otoscope handle points upward or laterally while you pull up on the auricle (see Figs. 28-61 and 28-62).

Downward Handle Method

The handle of the otoscope points down toward the child's feet, preferred by many clinicians due to the angle of the auditory canal in children (Figs. 28-63 and 28-64).

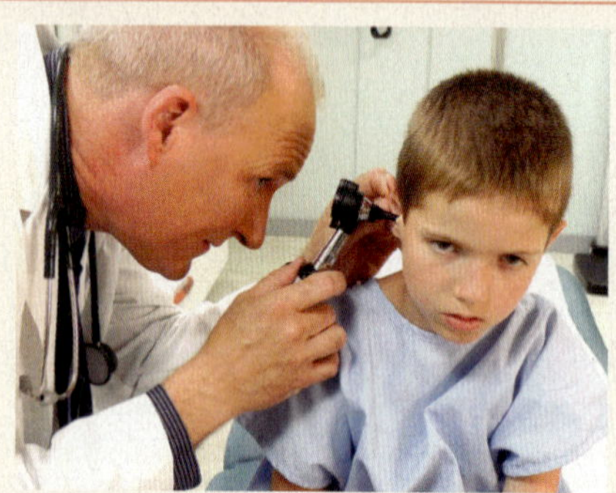

FIGURE 28-63. Examining the right ear while holding the otoscope in the right hand and pulling the auricle with the left hand.

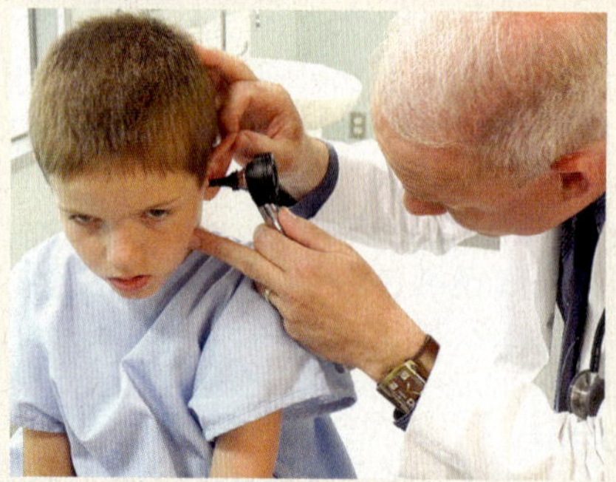

FIGURE 28-64. Examining the left ear with the otoscope in the left hand while pulling the auricle upward with the right hand, aligning with the child's auditory canal anatomy.

Perform a Gross Hearing Test. In very young children, use the *whispered voice test*. Stand behind the child, cover one ear canal, and rub the tragus. Whisper letters, numbers, or words and have the child repeat them, then test the other ear.[58]

Younger children who fail these screening maneuvers or have speech delays should have audiometric testing for possible hearing deficits or central auditory processing disorders.

Up to 15% of school-age children have at least mild hearing loss, emphasizing the importance of screening.[58]

Children can have conductive, sensorineural, and mixed conductive and sensorineural hearing loss.

Causes of *conductive hearing loss* include congenital abnormalities, ossicular abnormalities, cerumen impaction, trauma, otitis media, and tympanic membrane perforation.

Causes of *sensorineural hearing loss* include genetic, hereditary congenital infections, structural variants of the inner ear, ototoxic drugs, trauma, and some infections such as meningitis.

Formal hearing testing is necessary for accurate detection of hearing deficits in young children, and children as young as 6 months can undergo behavioral hearing tests. For older children, use formal hearing test methods (Box 28-45). Concerns about hearing loss should lead to a referral to an audiologist.

AAP recommends that all children older than 4 years have a full-scale acoustic screening test using standardized equipment (Figs. 28-65 and 28-66).[22] Even though a normal hearing screen at birth is reassuring, some hearing loss can be acquired with age, affecting language and development. Test the entire acoustic range, including the speaking range (500 to 8,000 Hz). Box 28-47 shows one classification of hearing ranges.

Box 28-45. Hearing Ranges on Formal Acoustic Screening Tests

Normal hearing	0–20 dB
Mild hearing loss	21–40 dB
Moderate hearing loss	41–60 dB
Severe hearing loss	61–90 dB
Profound hearing loss	>90 dB

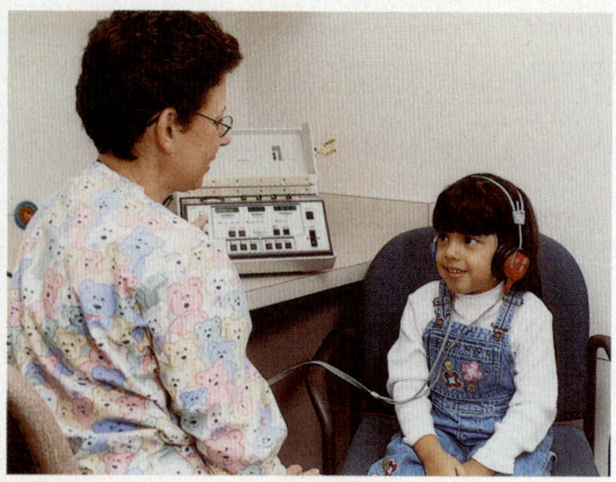

FIGURE 28-65. Standardized testing equipment provides more precise metrics.

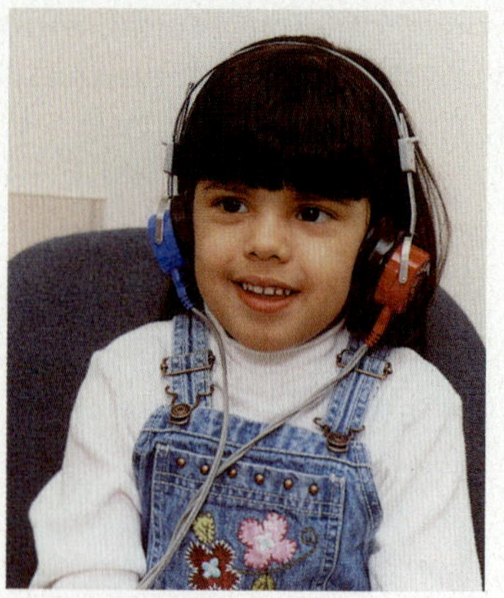

FIGURE 28-66. Children often enjoy a full-scale acoustic screening test.

Nose and Sinuses

Inspect the Nose. Use a large speculum on your otoscope to inspect the anterior portion of the nose, noting the color and condition of the nasal mucous membranes, septal deviation, and the presence of polyps (Fig. 28-67).

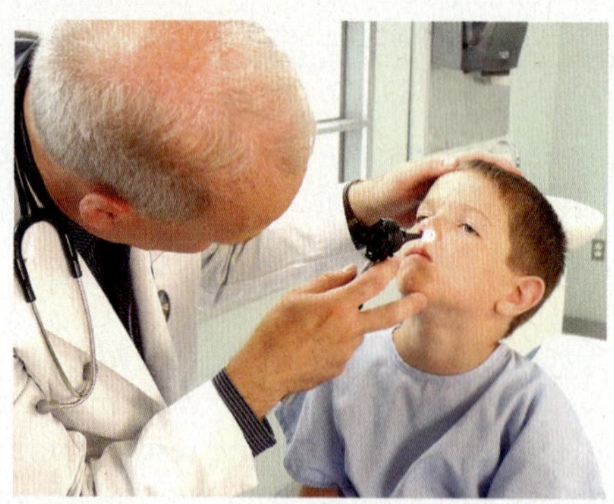

FIGURE 28-67. Nasal inspection of children.

Pale, boggy nasal mucous membranes indicate allergic rhinitis. Purulent rhinitis is common in viral infections.

Examine the Sinuses. Sinuses develop at varying ages (Box 28-46).[59] Older children's sinuses can be palpated or percussed for tenderness.[60] Transillumination of younger children's paranasal sinuses is not reliable for diagnosing sinusitis or fluid presence.

Foul-smelling, purulent, unilateral discharge suggests a foreign body.

Nasal polyps are gray/yellow growths inside the nares.

Sinusitis symptoms include purulent rhinorrhea for >10 days, worsening course, or severe symptoms with high fever and purulent rhinorrhea for >3 days.[61]

Box 28-46. Age of Pneumatization of Sinuses in Children

Sinus	Age of Pneumatization
Ethmoid	Birth
Maxillary	Birth to several years
Sphenoid	5–6 years
Frontal	7–8 years (continues until adolescence)

Mouth and Pharynx

Examine the mouth and pharynx last, as it may require caregiver's assistance to gently restrain the child. Healthy children are more likely to cooperate with this examination than sick children, especially if the sick child sees the tongue depressor or has had previous experience with throat cultures. Have the child say "ahhh" to view the posterior pharynx without a tongue depressor (Fig. 28-68).

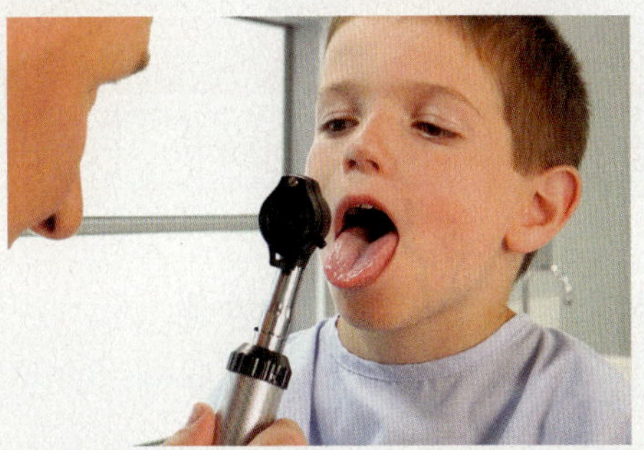

FIGURE 28-68. Children generally imitate well enough to allow you to inspect the back of their mouths.

Inspect the Pharynx. Use a tongue depressor if necessary, pushing down and slightly forward while the child says "ahhh." In resistant children, slip the depressor between the teeth and cheek, then turn it horizontally to push down on the tongue.

Inspect the Teeth. Check for timing and sequence of eruption, number, character, condition, and position. Abnormal enamel may indicate disease. Inspect the upper teeth by having the child look up with the mouth wide open ("lift the lip" technique, Fig. 28-69).

Dental caries (cavities) is the most common health problem in children. They are particularly prevalent in populations living in impoverished areas and can cause both short-term and long-term problems.[62] Cavities are highly preventable and can be treated with dental visits.

Dental caries are caused by bacterial activity. Cavities are more likely among young children who have prolonged bottle-feeding ("nursing-bottle caries").

See Table 28-9, Abnormalities of the Teeth, Pharynx, and Neck, p. 1110, for different stages of caries.

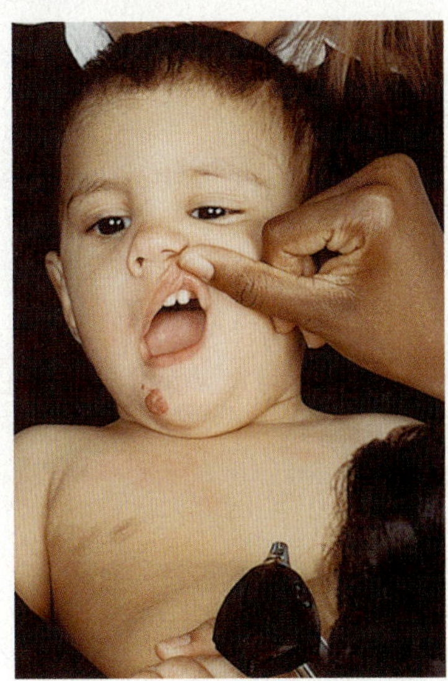

FIGURE 28-69. Lift the lip to check for dental caries.

Teeth staining can be intrinsic or extrinsic. Intrinsic stains, which cannot be polished off, may result from tetracycline use before age 8 (yellow, gray, or brown), liver disease ("green stain"), or fluorosis (white stain). Extrinsic stains, like iron preparation (black stain) or fluoride (white stain), can be polished off (see Table 28-9, Abnormalities of the Teeth, Pharynx, and Neck, p. 1110).

Box 28-47 displays the common pattern of tooth eruption. In general, lower teeth erupt a bit earlier than upper teeth.

Box 28-47. Tooth Types and Age of Eruption

Tooth Type	Approximate Age of Eruption[53] Primary (months)	Permanent (years)
Central incisor	5–8	6–8
Lateral incisor	5–11	7–9
Cuspids	24–30	11–12
First bicuspids	—	10–12
Second bicuspids	—	10–12
First molars	16–20	6–7
Second molars	24–30	11–13
Third molars	—	17–22

Source: Lunt RC, Law DB. A review of the chronology of eruption of deciduous teeth. *J Am Dent Assoc.* 1974;89(4):872–879.

Delayed tooth eruption can result from genetic disorders or systemic diseases.

Look for abnormalities in tooth position, such as malocclusion, *maxillary protrusion* (*overbite*), and *mandibular protrusion* (*underbite*). Demonstrate these by asking the child to bite down while parting the lips. Normally, the lower teeth are within the arch of the upper teeth.

Malocclusion and misalignment of teeth can be from thumb sucking, excess pacifier use, hereditary conditions, or premature loss of primary teeth.

Inspect the Tongue. Carefully inspect the tongue, including the underside (Fig. 28-70). Most children will happily stick their tongue out at you and move it from side to side.

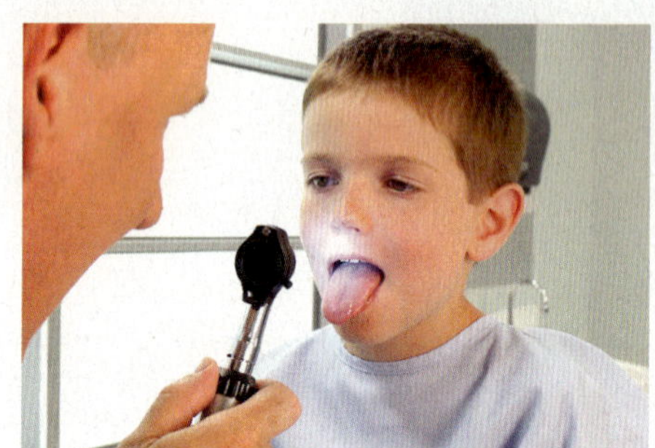

FIGURE 28-70. Inspect all parts of the tongue.

A *geographic tongue* is a benign but chronic condition in which part of the tongue has a rough, map-like appearance, varying over time due to a benign inflammatory process.[63]

Common abnormalities include coated tongue in viral infections and "*strawberry tongue*" from strep throat, scarlet fever, or (rarely) Kawasaki disease.

Some young children have a *tight frenulum*. Have the child touch their tongue to the roof of their mouth to diagnose this condition, which usually does not require treatment unless it interferes with eating or speech.

Children who are severely "tongue-tied" might have a speech impediment.

Examine the Tonsils. Note the size, position, symmetry, and appearance of the tonsils. Tonsillar tissue peaks in growth between 2 and 10 years (see Fig. 28-54, p. 1053). Tonsil size varies and is often categorized by the percent of the width of the posterior oropharynx they reduce (<25%, 50%, etc.). They often appear more obstructive than they are.

Streptococcal pharyngitis typically produces white or yellow exudates on the tonsils or posterior pharynx, a beefy-red uvula, and palatal petechiae[64]; see Table 28-9, Abnormalities of the Teeth, Pharynx, and Neck, p. 1110.

Tonsils in children usually have deep crypts on their surfaces, often with white concretions or food particles protruding, which does not indicate disease.

A peritonsillar abscess is suggested by erythema and asymmetric protrusion of one tonsil, pain, difficulty opening the mouth (*trismus*), and lateral displacement of the uvula.

Box 28-48. Voice Changes—Clues to Underlying Abnormalities

Voice Change	Possible Abnormality
Hypernasal speech	Submucosal cleft palate
Nasal voice plus snoring	Adenoidal hypertrophy
Hoarseness plus cough	Viral infection (croup)
"Hot potato speech"	Tonsillitis

Tonsillitis can be caused by bacteria like *Streptococcus* and *Staphylococcus* and by viruses. The "hot potato" voice is accompanied by enlarged tonsils with exudates.

Enlarged tonsils and adenoids coupled with the rise in childhood obesity have resulted in many children who snore and have obstructive sleep apnea.

Look for clues of a submucosal cleft palate such as notching of the posterior margin of the hard palate or a bifid uvula. Because the mucosa is intact, the underlying defect is easily missed but needs referral to otolaryngology.

Note the quality of the child's voice, as certain abnormalities can change its pitch and quality (Box 28-48).

Abnormal breath odor may help lead to a specific diagnosis.

Halitosis (bad breath) in a child can be caused by upper respiratory, pharyngeal, or mouth infection; foreign body in the nose; sinusitis; dental disease; and gastroesophageal reflux.

Neck

Beyond infancy, the techniques for examining the neck are the same as for adults.

Palpate Lymph Nodes. Lymphadenopathy is uncommon during infancy but very common in childhood. The lymphatic system peaks at 12 years, and cervical or tonsillar lymph nodes reach their peak size between 8 and 16 years (see Fig. 28-54).

Lymphadenopathy is usually caused by viral or bacterial infections (see Table 28-9, Abnormalities of the Teeth, Pharynx, and Neck, p. 1110).

Most enlarged lymph nodes in children are due to infections (mostly viral, but sometimes bacterial) and not malignancy. Differentiating normal lymph nodes from abnormal ones or congenital cysts of the neck is important.

Malignancy is more likely if the node is >2 cm, hard, or fixed to the skin or underlying tissues (i.e., not mobile) and accompanied by serious systemic signs such as weight loss.

Figure 28-26 on p. 1025 demonstrates the typical anatomical locations of lymph nodes and congenital cysts of the neck.

Assess Neck Mobility. Ensure that the neck is supple and mobile in all directions. This is particularly important when the head is held asymmetrically or when CNS disease, such as meningitis, is suspected.

In young children, it may be difficult to differentiate low posterior cervical lymph nodes from supraclavicular lymph nodes, which are always abnormal and raise suspicion for an abdominal malignancy.

In children, *nuchal rigidity* is a more reliable indicator of meningeal irritation than *Brudzinski* or *Kernig* signs, which have low sensitivity for detecting meningitis.

To detect nuchal rigidity in older children, ask the child to sit upright with their legs extended on the examining table and touch their chin to their chest (*chin-to-chest maneuver*). Younger children can be persuaded to flex their necks by following a small toy or light beam.

Alternatively, you can test for nuchal rigidity with the child lying on the examining table. Nearly all children with nuchal rigidity will appear extremely sick, irritable, and difficult to examine. The incidence of bacterial meningitis has decreased significantly due to routine vaccinations.

Nuchal rigidity is marked resistance to head movement in any direction, suggesting meningeal irritation from meningitis, bleeding, tumor, or other causes. These children are extremely irritable, difficult to console, and may exhibit "paradoxical irritability"—increased irritability when being held.

When meningeal irritation is present, the child may assume the *tripod position (see Fig. 28-72)*. and be unable to perform the chin-to-chest maneuver.

See Table 28-14, Power of Prevention: Vaccine-Preventable Diseases, pp. 1116–1117.

Thorax and Lungs

As children age, the lung examination becomes similar to that for adults. Cooperation is critical.

Auscultation is often easiest when a child feels secure, such as when sitting in a caregiver's lap or being held close, allowing for a relaxed and effective examination (Fig. 28-71). Let a child who seems fearful of the stethoscope play with it before it touches their chest.

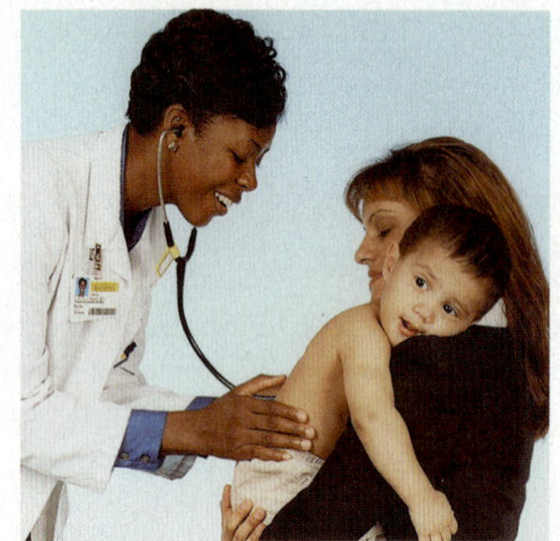

FIGURE 28-71. Young children are easiest to auscultate when held by a caregiver.

With *upper* airway obstruction like croup, inspiration is prolonged and accompanied by stridor, cough, or rhonchi. With *lower* airway obstruction like asthma, expiration is prolonged and often accompanied by wheezing or cough

Young children often hold their breath when asked to *"take deep breaths,"* complicating auscultation. It is easier to let preschoolers breathe normally. Demonstrate to older children how to take quiet, deep breaths and make it a game. For a forced expiratory maneuver, ask the child to blow out imaginary birthday candles or use pinwheels (Fig. 28-72).

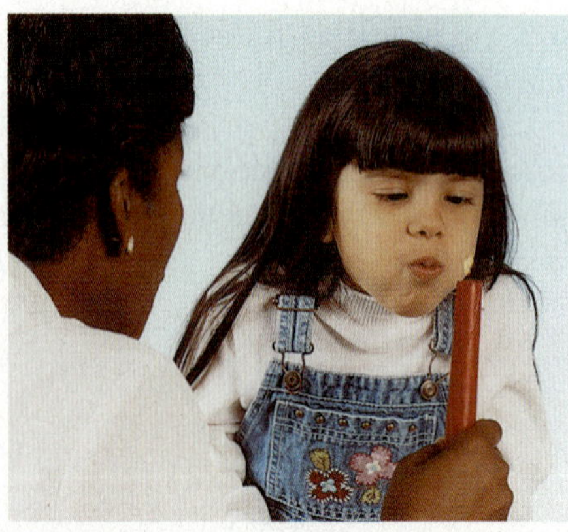

FIGURE 28-72. Getting a child to perform a forced expiration.

Pneumonia in young children generally manifests with fever, tachypnea, dyspnea, and increased work of breathing.

Upper respiratory infections due to viruses present similarly in children and adults; children generally appear well without lower respiratory signs.

Acute asthma may present with expiratory wheezing and a prolonged expiratory phase due to reversible bronchospasm. Wheezing may be heard without a stethoscope and is apparent on auscultation. Expiratory wheeze from lower airway bronchospasm can be accompanied by inspiratory rhonchi from upper airway congestion.[65,66]

Older children are usually cooperative for the respiratory examination, allowing you to perform maneuvers such as palpating for *fremitus* and auscultating for 'E to A' changes indicative of *egophony*. (Fig. 28-72). As children grow, assessing the work of breathing, nasal flaring, and grunting becomes less helpful for detecting respiratory pathology. Palpation, percussion, and auscultation gain importance in examining the thorax and lungs.

Assess the relative proportion of time spent on inspiration versus expiration. The normal ratio is about 1:2. Prolonged inspirations or expirations indicate disease location, and the degree of prolongation and effort, or "work of breathing," relates to disease severity.

Children in respiratory distress may assume a "*tripod position*," leaning forward to optimize airway patency (Fig. 28-73). This position can also be caused by pharyngeal obstruction.

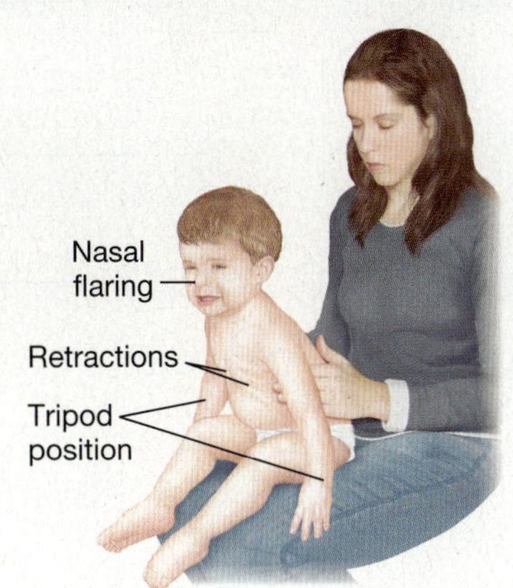

FIGURE 28-73. Child in respiratory distress.

Children showing signs of respiratory distress must be managed emergently. Possible causes include upper airway obstruction (such as epiglottitis or bacterial tracheitis), bacterial or viral lower respiratory infections, and foreign-body obstruction.

Heart and Vascular System

The examination of the heart and vascular system in infants and children is similar to that in adults. A child's fearfulness or inability to cooperate can make the examination difficult, while their desire to play can make it easier and more productive. Use your knowledge of the child's developmental stage and some helpful techniques (Box 28-49).

Auscultate for Benign Murmurs. Preschool and school-age children often have benign murmurs (Fig. 28-74 and Box 28-50).

Murmurs without recognizable features of common benign murmurs in young children may indicate underlying heart disease and should be thoroughly evaluated by a pediatric cardiologist.

Pathologic murmurs indicating cardiac disease (e.g., aortic stenosis and mitral valve disease) can first appear after infancy and during childhood.

Box 28-49. Techniques to Enhance Your Cardiac Examination in Young Children

Young children (2–4 years)

- Start by examining the child's arm or caregiver's arm first with your stethoscope to build familiarity.
- Allow the child touch and explore your stethoscope briefly to ease anxiety.
- Examine the child while they are on their caregiver's lap, turning them to face you as needed.
- Provide the child something to hold in each hand, preventing them from pushing you away
- Distract the child with a low-volume video on a smartphone or tablet.
- Maintain light, engaging conversation to hold their attention, pausing briefly to listen as they may forget the examination is happening.

Older children (5–10 years)

- Explain what you plan to do in simple, age-appropriate language.
- Remind the child that the stethoscope might be cold
- Say *"shhh"* very gently with a smile, to encourage quietness in a reassuring way.
- Ask the child to breathe normally during the examination.

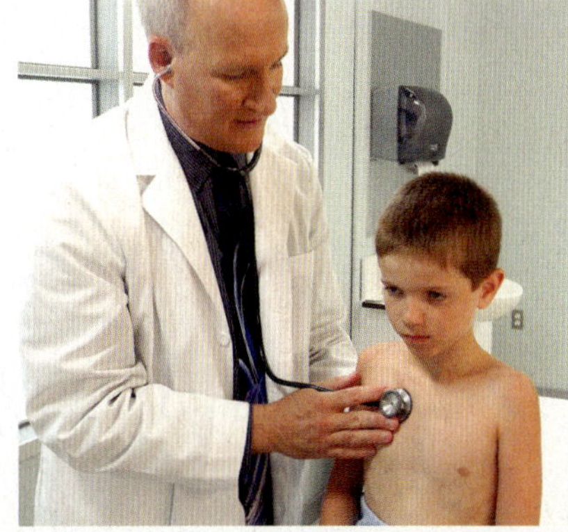

FIGURE 28-74. Auscultating for murmurs.

Box 28-50. Location and Characteristics of Benign Murmurs in Children

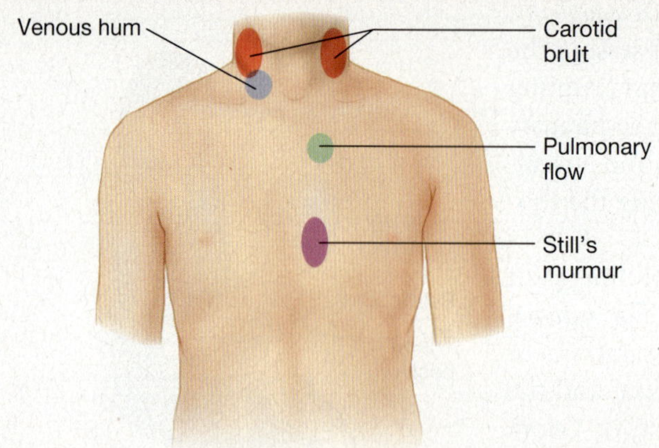

Typical Age	Relation to S_1 and S_2	Key Characteristics and Response to Maneuvers
Preschool or early school age	*Still murmur*	■ Most common benign murmur ■ Grade I–II/VI, musical, vibratory, multiple overtones, early and midsystolic ■ Located along mid/lower left sternal border; also over the carotid arteries ■ Carotid artery compression will usually cause the precordial murmur to disappear; diminishes when sitting or standing, louder when lying down[43] **PE Maneuver:** ■ May be accentuated with increased cardiac output (e.g., from fever or exercise)
Preschool or early school age	*Venous hum*	■ Soft, hollow, continuous, louder in diastole ■ Heard just above or below the clavicle ■ Has the same quality as breath sounds and is frequently overlooked[43] **PE Maneuver:** ■ Can be eliminated by maneuvers affecting venous return (e.g., lying supine or jugular venous compression)
Preschool and later	*Carotid bruit*	■ Early and midsystolic, slightly harsh, usually louder on left ■ Heard in the carotid area or just above the clavicles ■ May be heard alone or with Still murmur **PE Maneuver:** ■ Eliminated by carotid compression
Preschool and school age	*Pulmonary flow murmur* S_1 S_2	■ Grade I–II/VI, soft systolic crescendo–decrescendo ■ Located on the left upper sternal border **PE Maneuver:** ■ Like the Still murmur, louder when lying down, quieter when sitting or standing

Measure Blood Pressure in Extremities. Measure blood pressure in both arms and one leg once to check for possible coarctation of the aorta. After ruling out coarctation, measure only the right arm blood pressure.

In coarctation of the aorta the blood pressure is lower in the legs than in the arms.

Abdomen

Inspect the Abdomen. Toddlers and young children commonly have protuberant abdomens, most apparent when upright. The examination can follow the same order as for adults, but you may need to distract the child during the examination.

In exaggerated "pot-belly" appearance may indicate malabsorption (e.g., celiac disease), cystic fibrosis, or constipation; in regions with limited resources, it can signal nutritional deficiencies (e.g., kwashiorkor) or intestinal parasites.

The increasing prevalence of childhood obesity has resulted in many children having larger abdomens, making the examination more challenging, but the steps remain the same.

Palpate the Abdomen. Most children are ticklish when you first place your hand on their abdomen. This reaction often disappears if you distract the child with conversation and place your whole hand flush on the abdominal surface for a few moments without probing. For very sensitive children who tighten their abdominal muscles, start by placing the child's hand under yours. Eventually, you can remove the child's hand and palpate the abdomen freely.

Flexing the knees and hips can help relax the child's abdominal wall (Fig. 28-75). Palpate lightly in all areas first, then deeply, leaving the site of potential pathology for last.

Constipation, a common condition in childhood, can cause a protuberant abdomen. The abdomen is often tympanitic on percussion, and stool may be felt on palpation.

Abdominal pain from acute gastroenteritis is common. Despite the pain, the physical examination is usually normal except for increased bowel sounds on auscultation and mild tenderness on palpation.

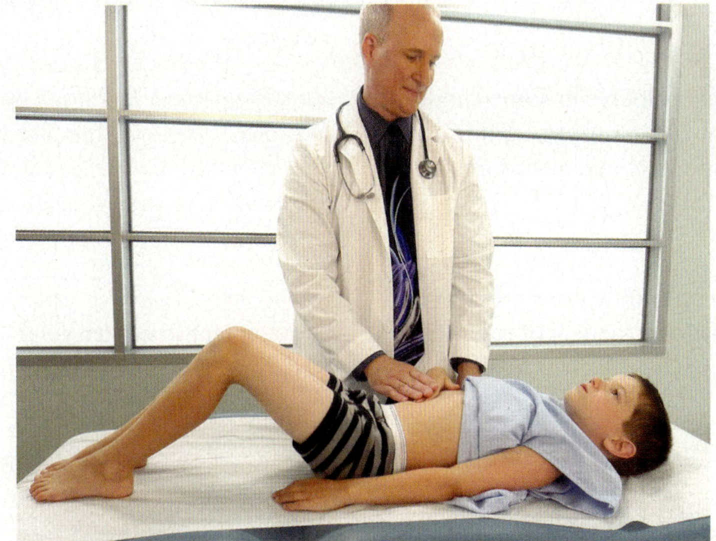

FIGURE 28-75. Flexing the knees and hips to relax the abdominal wall during palpation.

Box 28-51. Expected Liver Span in Children (Measured by Percussion)

Age in Years	Mean Estimated Liver Span (cm)	
	Assigned Male at Birth	Assigned Female at Birth
2	3.5	3.6
3	4.0	4.0
4	4.4	4.3
5	4.8	4.5
6	5.1	4.8
8	5.6	5.1
10	6.1	5.4

Palpating for abdominal tenderness in an older child is the same as in adults, though causes of abdominal pain differ, covering a wide spectrum of acute and chronic diseases. Localization of tenderness helps pinpoint the abdominal structures likely causing the pain.

In acute appendicitis, check for *involuntary rigidity, rebound tenderness, Rovsing sign, or positive psoas or obturator sign.* Other causes include gastroenteritis, constipation, and gastrointestinal obstruction.[67]

Measure the Liver Span. Palpate the *liver edge* and measure its span using percussion techniques as you would in an adult. Expected liver spans by percussion are shown in Box 28-51.

Hepatomegaly in young children is unusual and can be caused by cystic fibrosis, parasites, fatty liver, hepatitis, and tumors. If accompanied by splenomegaly, consider portal hypertension, storage diseases, chronic infections, and malignancy.

Palpate the Spleen. The *spleen*, like the liver, may be palpable in some children. It is soft with a sharp edge and projects downward like a tongue from under the left costal margin. The spleen is moveable and rarely extends more than 1 to 2 cm below the costal margin.

Splenomegaly can be caused by infections, hematologic disorders like hemolytic anemias, infiltrative disorders, inflammatory or autoimmune diseases, and congestion from portal hypertension.

Palpate the Other Abdominal Structures. You will commonly note pulsations in the epigastrium caused by the *aorta*, felt most easily to the left of the midline on deep palpation.

An abdominal mass felt on palpation may represent stool from constipation, a distended bladder, or a serious condition like a tumor.

Penis and Scrotum

The genital examination can be anxiety-provoking for older children and caregivers. It is important to perform the examination to detect abnormalities and reassure caregivers when findings are normal. Always have an appropriate chaperone, such as a caregiver, present during the genital examination. Students should generally be accompanied by experienced clinicians to ensure proper technique and provide support.

Inspect the Penis. The size in prepubertal children has little significance unless abnormally large or small. In children with obesity, the fat pad over the symphysis pubis may partially obscure the penis.

In precocious puberty, the penis and testes are enlarged with signs of pubertal changes due to excess androgens, which can be caused by conditions like adrenal or pituitary tumors.

Palpate the Scrotum and Testes. Palpation may cause the testis to retract into the inguinal canal (*cremasteric reflex*), appearing undescended. Examine the child when relaxed to minimize this reflex. Have the child lie down, and with warm hands, palpate the lower abdomen, working downward toward the scrotum along the inguinal canal to minimize retraction.

If the testis can be detected in the scrotum, it is considered descended, even if it frequently moves to the inguinal canal. A retractile testis can be brought into the scrotum and stays there, whereas an undescended testis quickly returns to the inguinal canal.

Cryptorchidism requires surgical correction and should be differentiated from a retractile testis.

A painless scrotal mass in a young child is usually due to a hydrocele or a non-incarcerated inguinal hernia. Other rare causes include a varicocele or tumor.

A painful testicle requires urgent consultation and treatment.

Possible causes of a painful testicle include infection such as epididymitis or orchitis, torsion of the testicle, or torsion of the appendix testis.

Elicit the Cremasteric Reflex. Gently stroke upward or downward along the medial aspect of the thigh. The testis on the side being stroked will move upward.

Examine Inguinal Canal. Examine the inguinal canal as you would for adults, noting any swelling that may reflect an inguinal hernia. Have the child increase abdominal pressure by pretending to blow a balloon or fill up their cheeks and blow, noting whether a bulge in the inguinal canal increases with Valsalva.

Testicular torsion most commonly occurs between ages 12 to 18 but can occur at any age including before birth.

Inguinal hernias in older children present as they do in adult males with swelling in the inguinal canal, particularly following a Valsalva maneuver.

Vulva and Surrounding Structures

Always have a caregiver or appropriate chaperone present during the examination of the vulva and surrounding structures. This exam can cause anxiety for both the child and caregivers, so it is important to identify any abnormalities and reassure them if findings are normal. Explain to the child, according to their developmental stage, which parts will be examined and that it is a routine part of the check-up to help alleviate anxiety.

The genital examination is consistent from late infancy to adolescence. Use a calm, gentle approach with a developmentally appropriate explanation. A bright light source is essential. Most children can be examined in the supine, frog-leg position.

If the child is reluctant, having the caregiver sit on the examination table with them, or performing the examination with the child sitting in the caregiver's lap can be helpful (Fig. 28-76). Avoid using footrests, as these may frighten the child. Conduct the examination efficiently and systematically.

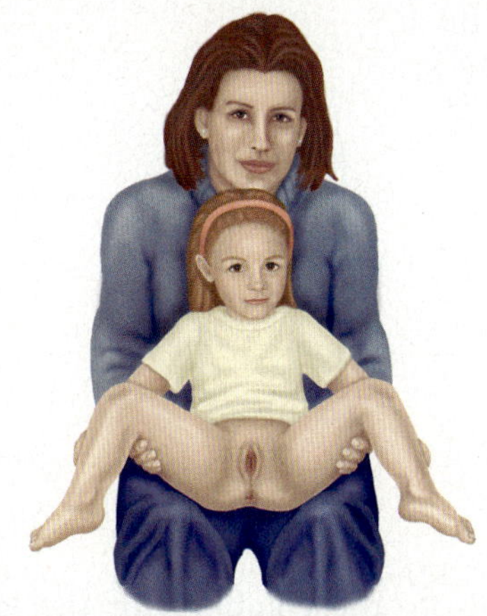

FIGURE 28-76. Positioning the caregiver behind the child provides support and facilitates a calm, secure environment for the examination.

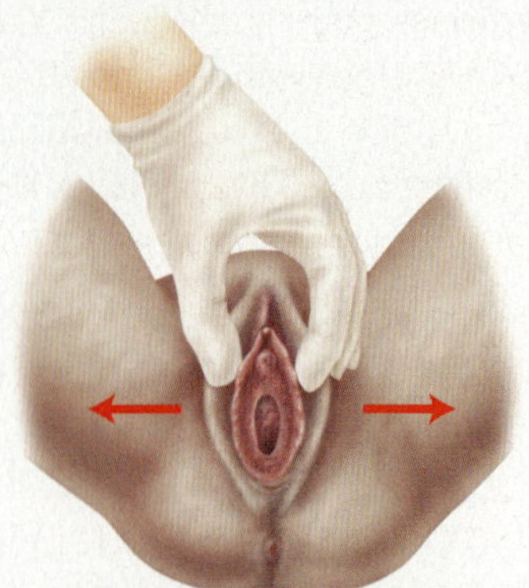

FIGURE 28-77. Visualizing genital structures by gently separating the labia majora with one hand.

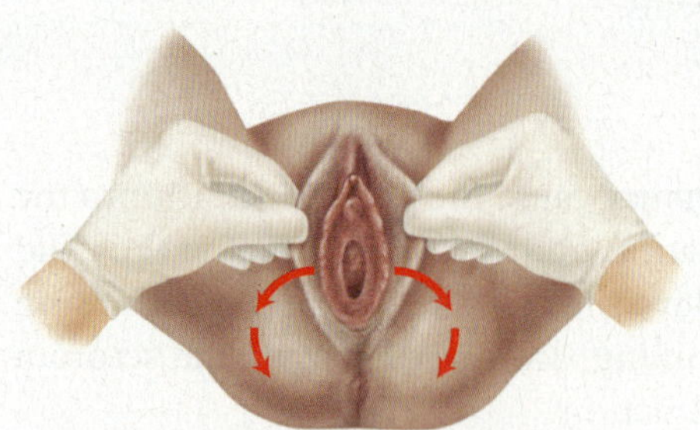

FIGURE 28-78. Applying lateral and outward traction on the labia majora with both hands for enhanced visualization.

Examine the Vulva. Inspect the external genitalia for pubic hair; clitoris size; labia majora color and size; and the presence of rashes, bruises, or other lesions. After infancy, the labia majora and minora flatten, and the hymenal membrane becomes thin, translucent, and vascular, with easily identifiable edges.

If a thorough genital exam is needed, visualize the structures by separating the labia with your fingers (Fig. 28-77). You can also grasp the labia between your thumb and index finger of each hand, separating the labia majora with gentle traction laterally and toward you to view the inner structures (Fig. 28-78). Labial adhesions or fusion of the labia minora are normal findings in prepubertal children. The finding of vaginal bleeding is worrisome and warrants further evaluation.

Pubic hair age <7 years is considered precocious adrenarche and requires evaluation.

Vulvovaginal pruritus and erythema can be caused by irritants, bubble baths, masturbation, pinworms, and infections like *Candida* and STIs.

Rashes can result from irritation, sweating, and infections.

Vaginal discharge can be from perineal irritation, foreign body, nonspecific vulvovaginitis, *Candida*, pinworms, or STI from abuse.

Precocious puberty may lead to the onset of menses in a young child.

Purulent, profuse, malodorous, and blood-tinged discharge should be evaluated for the presence of infection, foreign body, or trauma.

Note the condition of the labia minora, urethra, hymen, and proximal vagina. If you cannot visualize the hymen edges, ask the child to take a deep breath to relax the abdominal muscles.

Sexual abuse is unfortunately common; up to a fifth of women report some history of abuse as a child, with varying severity.[68]

Avoid touching the hymenal edges as they are sensitive. Examine for discharge, labial adhesions, lesions, estrogenization, hymenal variations, and hygiene. A thin, white discharge (leukorrhea) can be normal. A speculum examination is contraindicated in a prepubertal child unless there is suspicion of severe trauma or foreign body; it should be performed by an expert.

Abrasions or signs of trauma of the external genitalia can be from benign causes such as masturbation, irritants, or accidental trauma but should also raise the possibility of sexual abuse.

The hymen in infants and young girls can have various configurations (Box 28-52). The physical examination may reveal mounds, notches, and tags on the hymen that may all be normal variants. The size of the vaginal orifice can vary with age and with examination technique. Therefore, there is no correlation between the size of the vaginal orifice and whether or not the patient has been sexually assaulted.[69]

Physical signs strongly suggestive of abuse include lacerations, ecchymoses, newly healed scars, lack of hymenal tissue from 3 to 9 o'clock, and healed hymenal transections. Other concerning signs are purulent discharge and herpetic lesions.

Box 28-52. Normal Configurations of the Hymen in Prepubertal and Adolescent Individuals

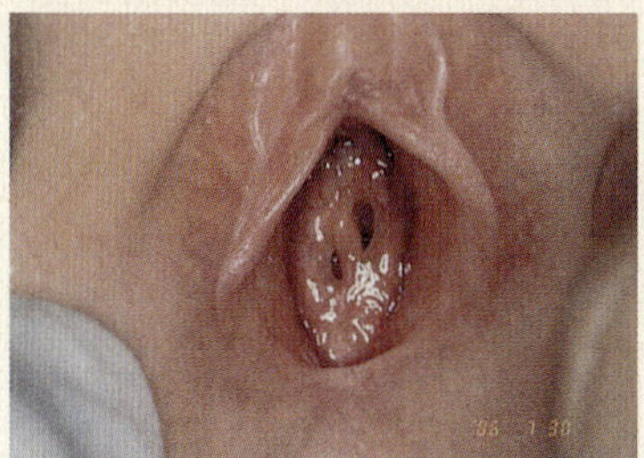

A septate hymen resulting in two orifices; gentle traction is needed to visualize the two openings

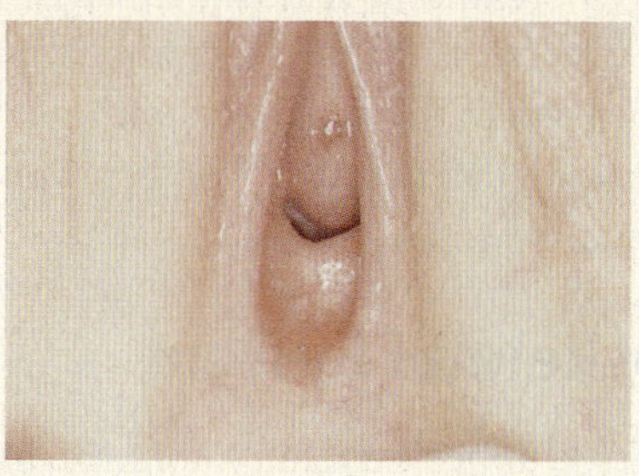

A crescent-shaped hymen (does not encircle the vaginal orifice; borders the lower part of the vaginal orifice and extends to the posterior and lateral margins of the hymenal ring)

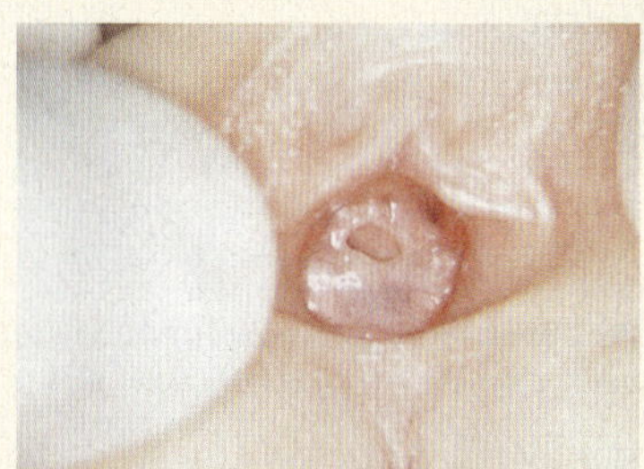

An annular hymen surrounds the orifice), visible with labial traction

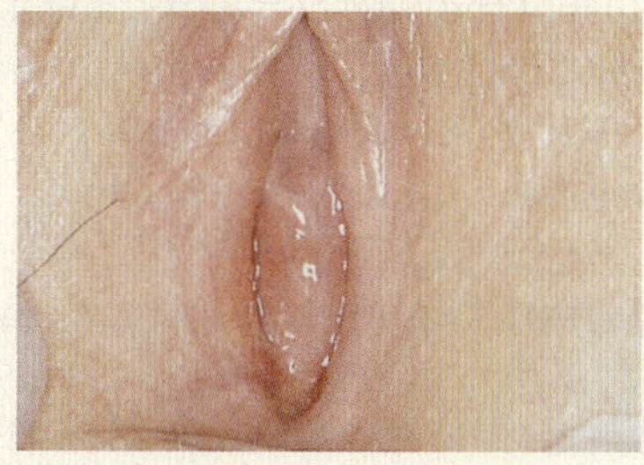

Redundant labial tissue suggesting estrogen effect; may require greater traction or a knee–chest position to fully visualize the hymenal orifice; if unable to locate an orifice, consider evaluating for an imperforate hymen

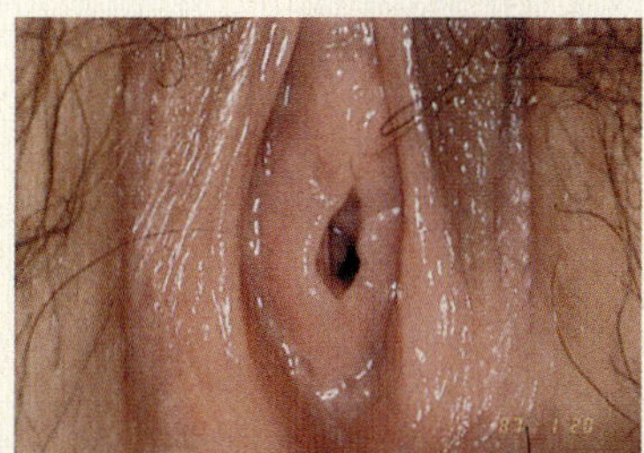

12-year-old individual with annular hymen and hormonal influence of puberty, causing thickened, pink tissue

Source of photos: Reprinted with permission from Reece R, Ludwig S, eds. *Child Abuse: Medical Diagnosis and Management*. 2nd ed. Lippincott Williams & Wilkins; 2001.

The physical examination may reveal signs that suggest *sexual abuse,* and the examination is particularly important if there are suspicious clues in the history. Even with known abuse, most examinations will be unremarkable; a normal genital examination does not rule out sexual abuse. If the hymenal edges are smooth and uninterrupted, the hymen is probably normal, but this does not rule out abuse, as the hymen can heal over 7 to 10 days.

Without a plausible history of accidental injury, findings suggestive of sexual abuse include acute lacerations or bruising of the labia, penis, scrotum, perineum, or posterior forchette; bruising, petechiae, or abrasions of the hymen; vaginal laceration; or perianal bruising or laceration.[69]

Rectum and Anus

The rectal examination is not routine but should be performed when certain types of intra-abdominal, pelvic, or perirectal disease are suspected. For young children, the examination can be done in the side-lying or lithotomy position, with the lithotomy position is often less intimidating and more practical for visualization. Have the child lie on their back with knees and hips flexed and legs abducted. Drape from the waist down and provide frequent reassurance. Ask the child to breathe in and out through their mouth to relax. Spread the buttocks and observe the anus. Use a lubricated, gloved index finger, even in small children. Palpate the abdomen with your other hand to distract the child and note abdominal structures. The prostate gland is not palpable in prepubescent children.

Anal skin tags can be present in inflammatory bowel disease but are often incidental findings when located in the midline.

Tenderness during a rectal exam usually indicates an infectious or inflammatory cause, such as an abscess or appendicitis.

Musculoskeletal System

In older children, upper extremity abnormalities are rare without injury.

Toddlers may develop *nursemaid's elbow* or subluxation of the radial head from a tugging injury, holding their arms slightly flexed at the elbows.

Observe Posture and Movement. Young children typically have increased lumbar concavity, decreased thoracic convexity, and a protuberant abdomen. Observe the child standing and walking barefoot, touching their toes, rising from sitting, running a short distance, and picking up objects. Detect most abnormalities by watching from the front and behind.

Assess Leg Alignment. During early infancy, a normal progression from bowleggedness (Fig. 28-79) begins to disappear at about 18 months, often transitioning to knock-knees. The *knock-knee pattern* (Fig. 28-80) is usually maximal by age 3 years and corrects by age 7 years.

Severe bowing of the legs (*genu varum*) may be physiologic and resolve spontaneously. Extreme or unilateral bowing may indicate pathologic causes like rickets or tibia vara (*Blount disease*).

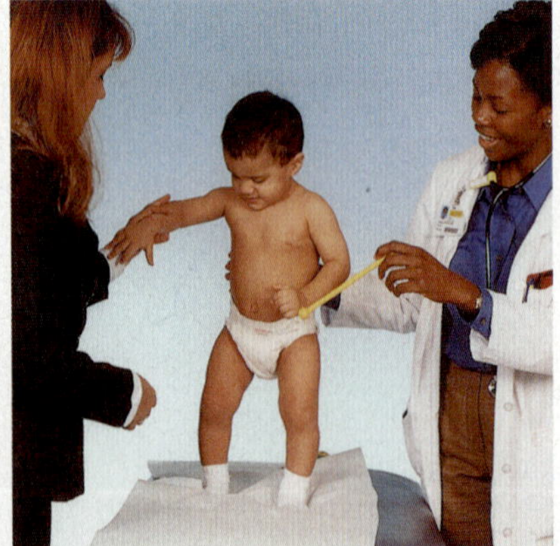

FIGURE 28-79. Bowleggedness (*genu varus*) is normal in early childhood.

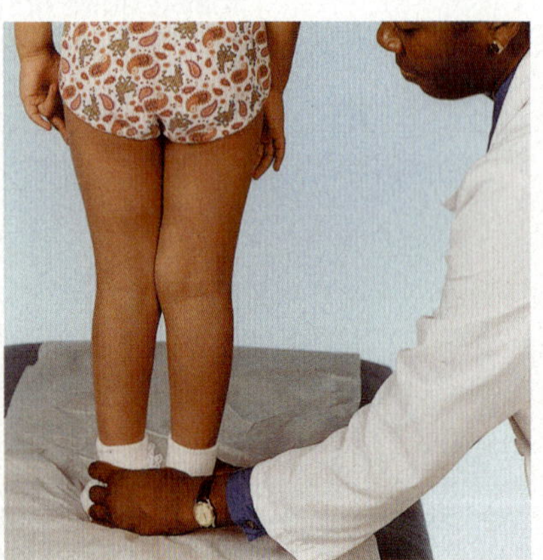

FIGURE 28-80. Knock-knee (*genu valgus*) is considered normal ages 3–7 years.

Check for Tibial Torsion. Assess tibial torsion by having the toddler lie prone with their knees flexed to 90°, noting the thigh–foot axis (normal is +10° to +15°). A negative thigh–foot angle indicates internal tibial torsion (Fig. 28-81). Check the symmetry of the malleoli position.

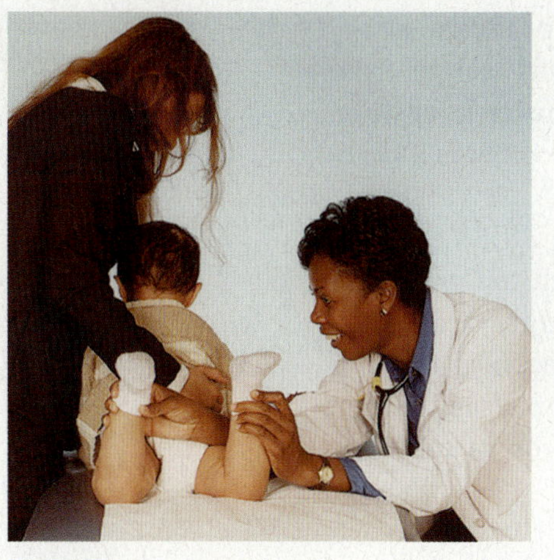

FIGURE 28-81. Checking for tibial torsion.

The most common lower extremity pathology in childhood is *injury from accidents*. Fractures are common due to incompletely developed bones and growth plates, and frequent play injuries. Joint injuries, sprains, and strains are also common.

A chronic limp in childhood could be caused by juvenile idiopathic arthritis, Blount disease, hip disorders like avascular necrosis of the hip, leg-length discrepancy, spinal disorders, or (rarely) malignancy.

Inspect for Femoral Torsion. Inspect for femoral torsion by observing the child's gait and the alignment of the feet during walking. Medial femoral torsion (or femoral anteversion) presents as an inward twisting of the femur resulting in toeing in by the child after age 3 to 4 years; this tends to resolve by 8 to 10 years of age, although mild toeing in may persist into adulthood.

Screen for Scoliosis. Inspect any child who can stand for scoliosis using techniques described on pp. 1097–1098.

Determine Leg Shortening. Determine any leg shortening that may accompany hip disease through one of several methods (Box 28-53).

Box 28-53. Methods for Assessing Leg Shortening

Method	Description
Galeazzi test	■ The test can be used to determine leg shortening (discussed in detail on page 1038).
Distance comparison	■ Compare the distance from the anterior superior spine of the ilium to the medial malleolus on each side. ■ Ensure the hips are level and straighten the legs for precise measurement. ■ Straighten the child by pulling gently on their legs. ■ Compare the levels of the medial malleoli with each other. ■ Put a small ink dot over the prominent malleoli and touch them together for a direct measure.
Iliac crest comparison	■ Have the child stand straight. ■ Place your hands horizontally over the iliac crests from behind. ■ Note any small discrepancies. ■ If you suspect leg-length discrepancy, place a book under the shorter leg; if this equalizes the iliac crests, a leg-length discrepancy is likely.

Test for Hip Disease. Test for severe hip disease by observing from behind as the child shifts weight from one leg to the other. A pelvis that remains level when weight is shifted from one foot to the other is a *negative Trendelenburg sign* (Fig. 28-82).[70]

A *positive Trendelenburg sign* (Fig. 28-83), indicative of severe hip disease, occurs when the pelvis tilts toward the unaffected hip during weight-bearing on the affected side. This tilt happens because the gluteus medius and minimus muscles are weak and cannot hold the pelvis level, resulting in a drop of the non–weight-bearing leg.

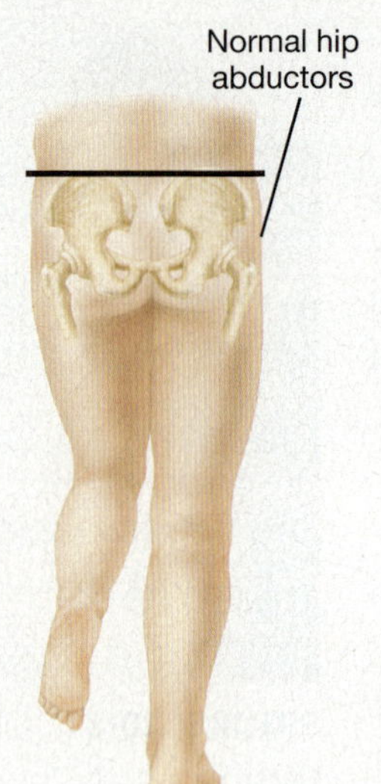

FIGURE 28-82. Trendelenburg test showing a negative result. The pelvis remains level when the child lifts one leg off the ground, indicating normal hip abductor strength.

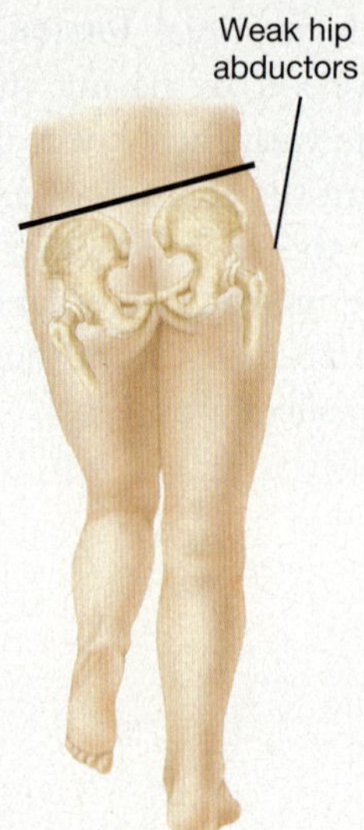

FIGURE 28-83. Trendelenburg test showing a positive result. The pelvis dips on the side of the lifted leg, suggesting weakness in the contralateral hip abductors.

Nervous System

Beyond infancy, the neurologic examination includes components evaluated in adults. Combine the neurologic and developmental assessment into a game to assess optimal development and neurologic performance.

Children with spastic diplegias may have hypotonia as infants and then excessive tone with spasticity, scissoring, and clenched fists as toddlers and young children.

Use a validated developmental screen for preschool children. Children usually enjoy this component. Many neurologic conditions in children are accompanied by developmental abnormalities. For children older than 3 years, ask them to draw a picture or copy objects to simultaneously test fine motor coordination, cognition, and language.

Problems with social interaction, verbal and nonverbal communication, restricted interests, and repetitive behaviors could be signs of autism.

Test Sensation. Use a cotton ball or tickling to test sensation with the child's eyes closed. Do not use pinpricks.

Distinguish between isolated delays in one aspect of development (e.g., coordination or language) and generalized delays in several components, which may indicate global neurologic disorders with various etiologies.

Evaluate Gait, Strength, and Coordination. Observe the child's gait while they walk and run. Note any asymmetries, weakness, tripping, or clumsiness. Follow developmental milestones for maneuvers such as heel-to-toe walking (Fig. 28-84), hopping, and jumping. Use a toy to test upper extremity coordination and strength. If concerned about strength, have the child lie on the floor and stand up, closely observing the stages.

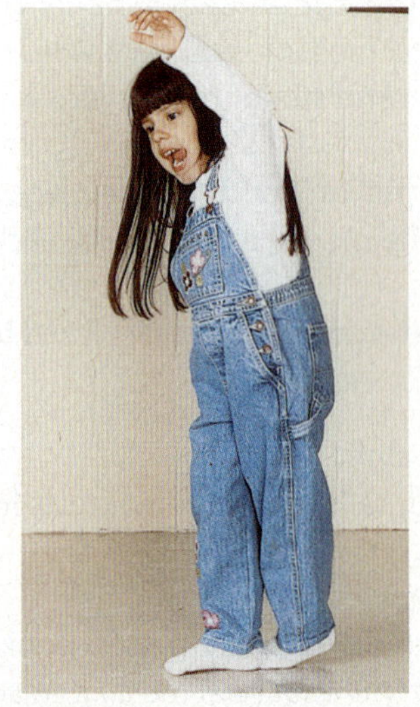

FIGURE 28-84. Heel-to-toe walking is a coordination milestone.

In children with an uncoordinated gait, distinguish orthopedic causes from neurologic abnormalities like cerebral palsy, ataxia, or neuromuscular conditions.

In certain forms of muscular dystrophy, children will rise to standing by rolling over prone and pushing off the floor with their arms while keeping their legs extended (*Gower sign*).

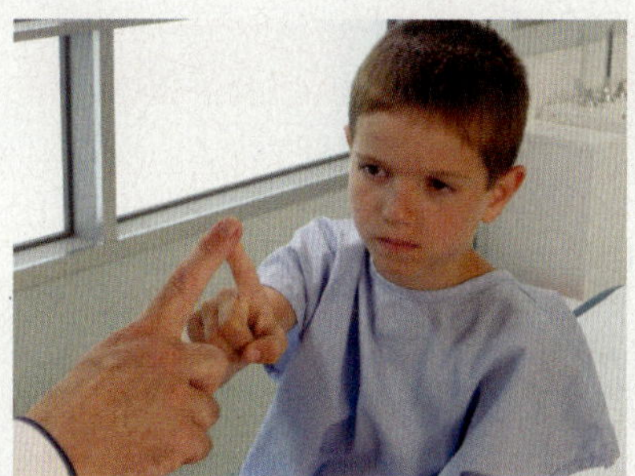

FIGURE 28-85. Finger-to-nose test—first have the child touch your finger.

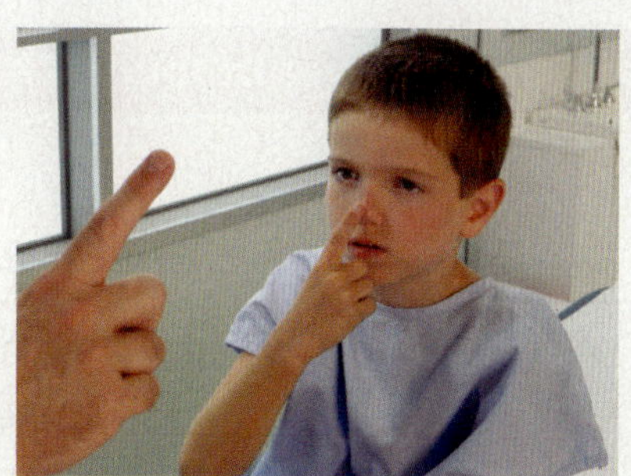

FIGURE 28-86. Then have the child touch their nose.

Check Hand Preference. Hand preference is usually demonstrated by age 2 years. If a younger child has a clear hand preference, check for weakness in the nonpreferred upper extremity.

Elicit Deep Tendon Reflexes. Test DTRs as in adults. Demonstrate the reflex hammer on the child's hand, assuring them it will not hurt. Have the child keep their eyes closed during the exam to prevent tensing.

Children with mild cerebral palsy may have both slightly increased tone and hyperreflexia.

Assess Cerebellar Function. Test cerebellar function using finger-to-nose and rapid alternating movements of the hands or fingers (Figs. 28-85 and 28-86). Children older than 5 years should be able to tell right from left, allowing for right–left discrimination tasks as done in adults.

Children with attention-deficit/hyperactivity disorder (ADHD) may have difficulty cooperating with the neurologic and developmental examination due to problems focusing. High-energy levels, fidgetiness, and difficulty in structured situations are common. Conditions like anxiety may have similar manifestations, warranting a complete history and physical examination.

Assess Cranial Nerves. Assess cranial nerves using developmentally appropriate strategies (Box 28-54).

Localizing neurologic signs are rare in children but can be caused by trauma, brain tumor, intracranial bleed, or infection. Increased intracranial pressure can cause cranial nerve abnormalities, papilledema, and altered mental status.

Children with meningitis, encephalitis, or cerebral abscess may have cranial nerve abnormalities along with altered consciousness and other signs.

Facial nerve palsy can be congenital, but it is often caused by infection or trauma.

RECORDING YOUR FINDINGS

The format of the clinical record is the same for both children and adults. Although the sequence of the physical examination may vary, convert your clinical findings into the same order of the traditional written or electronic

Box 28-54. Strategies to Assess Cranial Nerves in Young Children

Cranial Nerve	Function	Assessment
I	Smell	Testable in older children using familiar scents (e.g., vanilla or coffee).
II	Vision	Assess visual acuity with a Snellen chart after age 3 years for visual acuity. Test visual fields as for an adult; the caregiver may need to hold the child's head
III, IV, VI	Extraocular movements	Have the child track a light or an object (toy preferable); caregiver may need to hold the child's head
V	Sensation and chewing	Play a game with a soft cotton ball to test sensation Have the child clench their teeth and chew or swallow some food
VII	Facial expression	Have the child "make faces" or imitate you as you make faces (including moving your eyebrows) and observe symmetry and facial movements
VIII	Hearing and balance	Perform auditory testing after age 4 years; whisper a word or command behind the child's back and have the child repeat it Assess balance in older children.
IX, X	Swallowing and gag reflex	Ask the child stick the tongue out and "*say "ah"*." Observe movement of the uvula and soft palate Test the gag reflex if needed.
XI	Shoulder and neck strength	Have the child push your hand away with their head Have the child shrug their shoulders while you push down with your hands to *"see how strong you are"*
XII	Tongue movement	Ask the child to stick out their tongue and move it side to side.

format. Initially, you may use sentences to describe your findings; later you will use phrases. The style here contains phrases appropriate for most write-ups.

Recording the Pediatric Examination

4/19/2025

Eli Abraham Nolan is an active, 26-month-old boy accompanied by his father, Matthew Nolan, who is concerned about his development and behavior.

Source: Father.

Chief Concern: Slow development and difficult behavior.

History of Present Illness: Eli appears to be developing more slowly than his older sister did. He uses single words and simple phrases, rarely combines words, and appears frustrated with not being able to communicate. People understand less than a quarter of his speech. Physical development seems normal to the mother: he can throw a ball, kick, scribble, and dress himself well. He has had no head trauma, chronic illnesses, seizures, or regression in his milestones.

Eli's dad is also concerned about his behavior. Eli is extremely stubborn, frequently has tantrums, gets angry easily (especially with his older sister), throws objects, bites, and physically strikes others when he doesn't get his way. His behavior seems worse around his father who reports that he is "fine" at his childcare center. He moves from one activity to another with an inability to sit still to read or play a game. Of note, he is sometimes affectionate and cuddly. He does make eye contact and plays normally with toys. He has no unusual movements.

Eli is selective eater preferring energy-dense, low-nutrient foods such as junk food and little else. He will not eat fruits or vegetables and drinks large amounts of juice and soda. His father has tried everything to get him to eat healthy food, to no avail.

The family has been under substantial stress during the past year because Eli's father has been unemployed. Although Eli now has Medicaid insurance, the parents are uninsured.

Eli sleeps through the night.

Medications. One multivitamin daily.

Past Medical History

Pregnancy. Uneventful. Dad reduced tobacco use to a half-pack a day and consumed alcohol at times. He states that he does not use of other drugs or any infections.

Newborn Period. Born vaginally at 40 weeks; left the hospital in 2 days. Birth weight 2.5 kg (5 lb, 8 oz). Dad does not know why Eli was small at birth.

Illnesses. Only minor illnesses; no hospitalizations.

Accidents. Required sutures last year for a facial laceration secondary to a fall on the road. He did not lose consciousness and had no sequelae.

Preventive Care. Eli has had regular preventive check-ups. At the last appointment 6 months ago, his regular physician said that Eli was a bit behind on some developmental milestones and suggested a childcare center that she knew was excellent as well as increased parental attention to reading, speaking, playing, and stimulation. Immunizations are up to date. His lead level was elevated mildly last year, and Dad reports that he had "low blood." No dental visit yet.

Family History

Strong family history of diabetes (two grandparents, none with diabetes as children) and hypertension. No familial history of childhood developmental, psychiatric, or chronic illnesses.

Developmental History: Sat (6 months), crawled (9 months), and walked (13 months). First words ("mama" and "car") said at 1 year.

Social History: Eli lives with his parents, Matthew Nolan and Wesley Anne Nolan, who are married, and his older sister, Lucille Reneé (5 years old), in a rented apartment. Dad has had intermittent work for a year, and Mom works part-time as a restaurant server.

Mom had depression during Eli's first year and attended some counseling but stopped (lack of money for visits or medications). She gets support from her mother who lives 30 minutes away, and many friends.

Dad describes a loving and intact family. They eat dinner together daily, limit screen time, read to both children, and play at a nearby park.

Environmental Exposures. Both parents smoke (outside the house).

Safety. Dad reports this as a major concern: he can barely leave Eli out of his sight without him "getting into something." He fears he will run under a car; the family is thinking of fencing in their small yard. Eli sits in his car seat most of the time; smoke detectors work in the home. Dad's guns are locked; medications are in a cabinet in the parents' bedroom.

Review of Systems

General. No major illnesses.

Skin. Dry and itchy. Last year he was prescribed hydrocortisone for it.

Head, Eyes, Ears, Nose, and Throat (HEENT). Head: No trauma. *Eyes:* Vision fine. *Ears:* Multiple infections in the past year. Frequently ignores parents' requests; they can't tell if this is purposeful, or if he can't hear well. *Nose:* Often runny; Dad wonders about allergies. *Mouth*: Brushes teeth sometimes (a frequent source of dispute); no tooth pain.

Neck. No lumps. Glands in neck seem large.

Respiratory. Frequent cough and whistle in chest. Dad cannot identify trigger; it resolves. He can run around all day without being tired.

Cardiovascular. No known heart disease. He had a murmur when younger, but it went away.

Gastrointestinal. Appetite and eating habits described above. Regular bowel movements. He is in the process of toilet training and wears pull-up diapers at night but not at childcare.

Urinary. Good stream. No prior urinary tract infections.

Genital. Normal.

Musculoskeletal. Very active; never gets tired. Minor bumps.

Neurologic. Walks and runs well; seems coordinated for age. No stiffness, seizures, or fainting. His memory seems great, but attention span is poor.

Psychiatric. Generally, seems happy. Cries easily; bounces back and forth from trying to be independent to needing cuddling and comforting.

Physical Examination

General Appearance: Eli is an active and energetic toddler. He plays with the reflex hammer, pretending it is a truck. He appears closely bonded with his father, looking at him occasionally for comfort. He seems concerned that Eli will break something. His clothes are clean.

Vital Signs. Ht 90 cm (90th percentile). Wt 16 kg (>95th percentile). BMI 19.8 (>95th percentile). Head circumference 50 cm (75th percentile). BP 108/58. Heart rate 90 beats/min and regular. Respiratory rate 30/min; varies with activity. Temperature (ear) 37.5 °C. No obvious pain.

Skin. Normal except for bruises on the anterior aspects of his legs, and patchy, dry skin over external surface of elbows.

HEENT. Head: Normocephalic; no lesions. *Eyes:* Difficult to examine because he won't sit still. Symmetric with normal extraocular movements. Pupils 4 to 5 mm, and symmetrically reactive to light. Discs difficult to visualize; no hemorrhages noted. *Ears:* Normal pinna; no external abnormalities. Normal external canals and tympanic membranes. *Nose:* Normal nares; septum midline. *Mouth:* Several darkened teeth (inside surface of upper incisors). One clear cavity on upper right incisor. Tongue normal. Cobblestoning of posterior pharynx; no exudates. Tonsils large but adequate gap (1.5 cm) between them. No allergic shiners.

Neck. Supple, midline trachea, no thyroid palpable.

Lymph Nodes. Easily palpable (1.5–2 cm), firm, mobile anterior cervical lymph nodes bilaterally. Small (0.5 cm) nodes in inguinal canal bilaterally. All lymph nodes mobile and nontender.

Lungs. Good expansion. No tachypnea or dyspnea. Congestion audible but seems to be upper airway (louder near mouth, symmetric). No rhonchi, rales, or wheezes. Clear to auscultation.

Cardiovascular. PMI in 4th or 5th interspace and midsternal line. Normal S_1 and S_2. No murmurs or abnormal heart sounds. Normal femoral pulses; dorsalis pedis pulses palpable bilaterally. Capillary refill brisk.

Breasts. Normal, with some fat under both.

Abdomen. Protuberant but soft; no masses or tenderness. Liver span 2 cm below right costal margin and not tender. Spleen and kidneys not palpable. Bowel sounds present.

Genitalia. Tanner I circumcised penis; no pubic hair, lesions, or discharge. Testes descended, difficult to palpate because of active cremasteric reflex. Normal scrotum both sides.

Musculoskeletal. Normal range of motion of upper and lower extremities and all joints. Spine straight. Gait normal.

Neurologic. Mental Status: Happy, cooperative, active child. *Developmental:* Gross motor—Jumps and throws objects. Fine motor—Imitates vertical line. Language—Does not combine words; single words only, three to four noted during examination. Personal–social—Washes face, brushes teeth, and puts on shirt. Overall—Normal, except for language, which appears delayed. *Cranial Nerves:* Intact, although several difficult to elicit. *Cerebellar:* Normal gait; good balance. *Deep tendon reflexes:* Normal and symmetric throughout with downgoing toes. *Sensory:* Deferred.

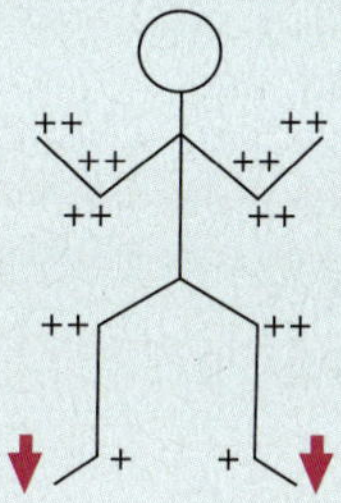

By analyzing the physical examination documentation into detailed sections, we emphasize the significant role that clinical observations play in pinpointing diagnostic clues. The findings described in this note are suspicious for several potential developmental and behavioral conditions:

- Developmental delays:
  - *Language:* Eli uses only single words and simple phrases, rarely combines words, and is often frustrated due to communication difficulties. People understand <25% of his speech, suggesting a significant language delay.
  - *Physical development:* Despite his language delay, Eli's physical development appears normal. He can throw a ball, kick, scribble, and dress himself, indicating that his gross and fine motor skills are within normal limits for his age.

- Behavioral concerns:
  - *Tantrums and aggression:* Eli is described as extremely stubborn, frequently having tantrums, getting angry easily, and displaying aggressive behaviors such as throwing objects, biting, and striking others. These behaviors seem worse around his father, suggesting possible environmental or relational factors contributing to his behavior.
  - *Attention and activity level:* Eli moves quickly from one activity to another and cannot sit still to read or play a game, indicating potential issues with attention span and hyperactivity.
  - *Picky eating:* Eli is an extremely picky eater, consuming large quantities of junk food and refusing fruits and vegetables. This dietary pattern can impact his overall nutrition and health.
- Social and environmental factors:
  - *Family stress:* The family has been under substantial stress due to the father's unemployment. Eli is on Medicaid, but his parents are uninsured, which might limit access to additional resources or interventions.
  - *Parental support:* Despite the stress, the father describes a loving and intact family environment, with regular family dinners, limited screen time, and engagement in activities like reading and playing at the park.

Physical examination findings:

- *Growth parameters:* Eli's height (90 cm) is in the 90th percentile, and his weight (16 kg) and BMI (19.8) are both above the 95th percentile, indicating that he is overweight for his age.
- *Skin:* He has dry and itchy skin with bruises on the anterior aspects of his legs, which may be consistent with his active nature and possible dietary deficiencies.
- *HEENT:* The presence of several darkened teeth and a cavity indicates poor dental hygiene, potentially linked to his high intake of sugary foods and drinks.
- *Lymph nodes:* Enlarged, firm, and mobile anterior cervical lymph nodes suggest possible recurrent infections or a reactive process.
- *Respiratory:* Frequent cough and whistling in the chest, with no identified triggers, raise the possibility of respiratory issues like asthma or allergies.
- *Cardiovascular:* Normal heart sounds, no murmurs, normal pulses, and capillary refill, indicating no immediate cardiovascular concerns.
- *Neurologic:* Normal reflexes and coordination for his age, but attention span and language skills are notably delayed.

These findings collectively raise suspicion for several potential developmental and behavioral conditions. Eli's significant language delay suggests a need for early intervention with speech therapy. His behavioral symptoms, such as difficulty sitting still and frequent tantrums, indicate possible *ADHD*. His poor dietary habits and reliance on junk food could lead to *nutritional deficiencies* affecting his overall health and development. Additionally, his aggressive and oppositional behaviors may point to an underlying *behavioral disorder*, potentially exacerbated by family stress.

A comprehensive developmental evaluation and possible referral to a pediatric neurologist or psychologist are recommended to further assess and address Eli's developmental and behavioral needs.

HEALTH PROMOTION AND COUNSELING: EVIDENCE AND RECOMMENDATIONS

Children 1 to 4 Years

The AAP and Bright Futures schedules recommend health supervision visits at 12, 15, 18, and 24 months, with annual visits at ages 3 and 4.[36,40] A visit at 30 months is also recommended to assess development.

During these visits, clinicians address caregivers' concerns; evaluate growth and development; perform a comprehensive physical exam; and provide anticipatory guidance on healthy habits, social competence, family relationships, and community interactions. This is a critical age for preventing childhood obesity, as many children begin their trajectory toward obesity after age 2.

Also assess the child's development. Standardized developmental screening instruments are recommended to measure different dimensions of development, as problems may not be identified through general history and examination.[71,72] Differentiating typical developmental behavior from potential behavioral or mental health concerns is crucial.

Box 28-55 demonstrates the major components of a health supervision visit for a 3-year-old, focusing on health promotion. These health promotion issues can also be addressed during other visits, even when the child is mildly ill.

Box 28-55. Components of a Health Supervision Visit for a 3-Year-Old

Discussions with Parents or Caregivers

- Address any concerns[21]
- Offer tailored advice on childcare, school readiness, and social engagement.
- Major topic areas: development, nutrition, safety, oral health, family relationships, and community support.

Developmental Assessment

- Evaluate milestones: gross and fine motor, personal–social, language, and cognitive
- Use a validated developmental screener

Physical Examination

- Conduct a thorough examination, including growth parameters with percentiles for age

Screening Tests

- Vision (formal testing starting at age 3 years), hearing (formal testing starting at age 4 years), hematocrit and lead levels (if high risk); screen for social risk factors and needs

Immunizations

- Follow the most recent American Academy of Pediatrics schedule

(continued)

Box 28-55. Components of a Health Supervision Visit for a 3-Year-Old (*Continued*)

Anticipatory Guidance

Healthy Habits and Behaviors

- Discuss injury and illness prevention: car seats, poison prevention, avoiding tobacco exposure, supervision, water safety, and firearm safety
- Promote nutrition and exercise: assess for obesity risk, encourage healthy meals and snacks.
- Emphasize oral health: encourage brushing teeth and visiting the dentist.

Caregiver-Child Interaction

- Promote shared activities such as reading, play, and limiting screen time.

Family Relationships

- Explore family routines and discuss trusted childcare or babysitting arrangements.

Community Interaction

- Provide information about local childcare and other supportive resources.

Children 5 to 10 Years

The AAP and Bright Futures recommend annual health supervision visits during this period.[21] These visits provide opportunities to assess the child's physical, mental, and developmental health; the caregiver–child relationship; peer relationships; and school performance (Fig. 28-87).

Health promotion should be incorporated into all interactions with children and families. Older children enjoy talking directly with the examiner. Include the child in conversations using age-appropriate language and concepts. Discuss the child's school experiences, peer interactions, and other cognitive and social activities.

Focus on healthy habits such as good nutrition, exercise, reading, stimulating activities, healthy sleep hygiene, screen time, and safety. About 20% of children have some type of chronic physical, developmental, or mental condition.[73] These children should be seen more frequently for monitoring, disease management, and preventive care (Fig. 28-88).

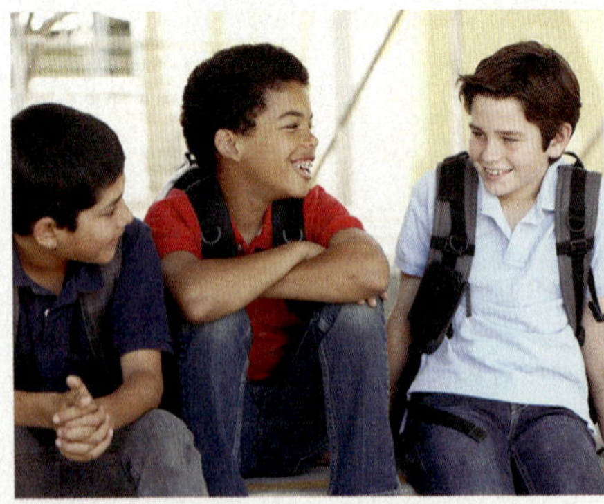

FIGURE 28-87. Peer relationships and mental health are essential aspects of development for children aged 5 to 10 years, offering opportunities to build emotional resilience and social skills.

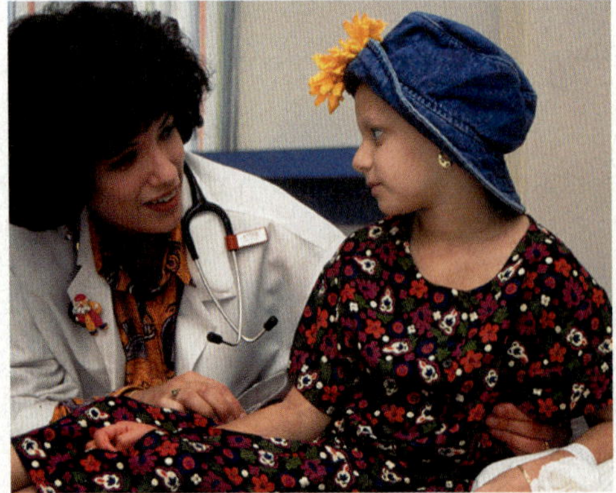

FIGURE 28-88. Establishing rapport with children who have chronic conditions can enhance trust and improve their overall health outcomes.

For all children, health promotion involves assessing and promoting the family's overall health.

The specific components of the health supervision visit for older children are similar to those for younger children. Emphasize school performance, appropriate and safe sports and activities, and healthy peer relationships.

ADOLESCENTS

HEALTH HISTORY: GENERAL APPROACH

The key to successfully examining adolescents is creating a comfortable and confidential environment. This approach makes the examination more relaxed and informative. Box 28-56 highlights essential actions for approaching adolescents regarding their health history. By implementing these actions, you can effectively engage with them, ensuring a thorough and meaningful health history that addresses both their physical and emotional well-being.

Box 28-56. Approaches to Adolescent Health History: Key Actions and Considerations

Consider Cognitive and Social Development

- Consider the teen's cognitive and social development when addressing privacy, caregiver involvement, and confidentiality.

Build Trust

- Building trust is vital.
- Show genuine interest in the adolescent early and maintain it for effective communication (Fig. 28-89).
- Focus on the adolescent rather than their problems to encourage openness.

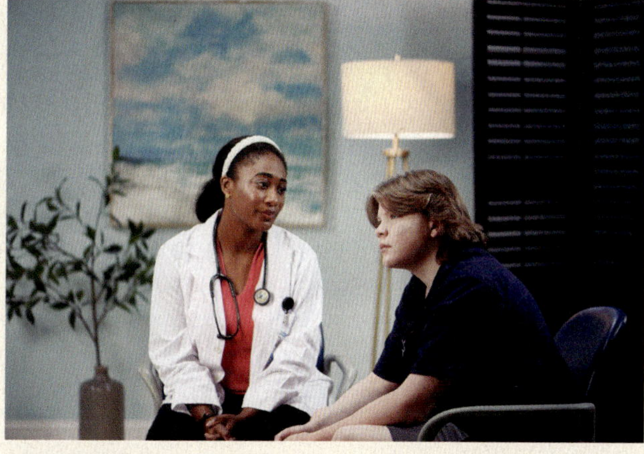

FIGURE 28-89. Building trust with adolescents is essential for fostering open communication and addressing their unique cognitive and social development needs.

Use Effective Interview Techniques

- Start with specific questions to build rapport and get the conversation going.
- Initially, you may need to talk more to engage the adolescent.
- Chat informally about friends, school, hobbies, and family.
- Avoid using silence or asking about feelings directly.
- Use summarization and transitional statements, and explain each step of the physical examination to engage the youth.
- Once rapport is established, shift to open-ended questions and ask about any concerns or questions the adolescent may have.
- Prompt adolescents to discuss anything else they might have in mind, as they often hesitate to bring up sensitive topics.
- Use phrases like, *"teens your age often have questions about..."*

(*continued*)

Box 28-56. Approaches to Adolescent Health History: Key Actions and Considerations (*Continued*)

Recognize Developmental Stages

- Be cautious with early developers who may appear older and late developers who may seem younger.
- Adolescents' behavior is related to their developmental stage and not necessarily to chronologic age or physical maturation.

Ensure Confidentiality

- Explain to caregivers and adolescents the importance of some degree of independence and confidentiality in health care.
- Begin asking caregivers to leave the room for part of the interview around ages 11–12 to prepare for future visits.
- Make it clear that confidentiality is not unlimited. State explicitly that you may need to act on information if there are safety concerns. Examples: *"I will not tell your parents what we talk about unless you give me permission, or I am concerned about your safety. For example, if you were to talk to me about hurting yourself or someone else and I thought that you really were at risk to follow through, I would need to discuss it with others to help you."*
- Familiarize yourself with local laws regarding confidentiality, reproductive care, and adolescents' rights.

Involve Caregivers Appropriately

- Before the caregiver leaves, obtain a relevant clinical history and clarify their agenda for the visit.
- When alone with the adolescent, ask for their agenda and reassure them about confidentiality.
- Encourage adolescents to discuss sensitive issues with their caregivers and offer to help facilitate the conversation.
- Assess the caregivers' perspective and obtain the young person's consent before involving the caregiver further.

HEEADSSS Assessment

Obtaining an adequate psychosocial history from an adolescent offers you the ability to contextualize their lives. Since most adolescents have minimal clinical problems, most of their medical issues stem from risky behaviors. The HEEADSSS assessment is a good guide.[74] The acronym stands for **H**ome environment, **E**ducation and employment, **E**ating, peer-related **A**ctivities, **D**rugs, **S**exuality, **S**uicide/depression, and **S**afety from injury and violence.[74–76] It is analogous to the "review of systems" and is a valuable tool for assessing the physical, emotional, and social well-being of adolescents (Box 28-57).[76] The information you gather can then be used to provide appropriate support for your patient.

Box 28-57. HEEADSSS Assessment

Category	Sample Question Topics
Home environment	Who lives with you? How long have you lived there? Own room? What are relationships like at home? Recent moves or running away?
Education and employment	School/grade performance—any recent changes? Suspension, termination, dropping out? Favorite/least favorite class? Safety at school? Work outside of school?

Category	Sample Question Topics
Eating	Likes and dislikes about your body? Any recent changes in your weight or appetite? Any worries about weight? Worries about having food to eat?
Activities	With peers and family? Faith and religious activities? Clubs, sports activities? Electronic media? History of arrests, acting out, crime?
Drugs and alcohol	Use of tobacco, vaping, alcohol, or drugs by peers, by teen, by family members? Which drugs?
Sexuality	Gender identity, sexual attraction? Degree and types of sexual experience and acts? Number of partners? Intimate partner violence? Sexually transmitted infections, contraception, pregnancy/abortion?
Suicide, depression, and self-harm	Have you thought about hurting yourself or someone else? Have you lost interest in things that you used to really enjoy?
Safety from injury and violence	History of accidents, physical or sexual abuse, or bullying? Concerns about online activities? Violence in home, school, or neighborhood? Access to firearms? Seatbelt use? Ridden with someone who was drunk or high? Any violence in school? Where you live? Ever been picked on or bullied? Ever felt the need to protect yourself?

Source: Used with permission of SLACK Incorporated from Smith GL, McGuinness TM. Adolescent psychosocial assessment: the HEEADSSS. *J Psychosoc Nurs Ment Health Serv*. 2017;55(5):24–27; permission conveyed through Copyright Clearance Center, Inc.

SURVEILLANCE OF DEVELOPMENT: 11 TO 20 YEARS

Interview and examination techniques vary widely depending on the adolescent's physical, cognitive, and social/emotional levels of development. Box 28-58 demonstrates common developmental tasks or achievements of adolescence, typical characteristics you might note during the history, and helpful health care approaches. Note the wide variability of ages at which adolescents go through these stages.

Box 28-58. Surveillance of Development: 11 to 20 Years

Physical Development

- Adolescence marks the transition from childhood to adulthood.
- Physical changes typically begin around age 10 in those assigned female at birth and age 11 in those assigned male at birth.
- Most assigned females typically complete pubertal development by age 14, while assigned males typically do so by age 16.
- The age of onset and duration of puberty vary widely, although the stages follow the same sequence in all adolescents.
- Early adolescents are often preoccupied with these physical changes (Fig. 28-90).

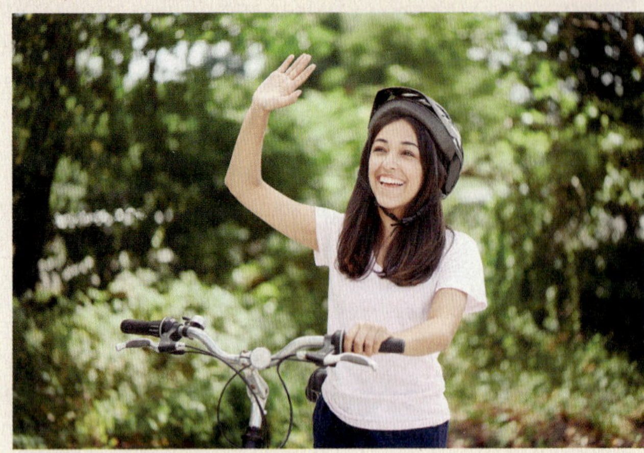

FIGURE 28-90. Promoting physical activity and safety is an important aspect of adolescent health supervision.

Health Care Approaches

- Regularly monitor growth and development milestones.
- Provide guidance on managing physical changes and puberty.
- Provide support for body image and self-esteem.

Cognitive Development

- Adolescents undergo significant cognitive changes, progressing from concrete to formal operational thinking.
- They acquire the ability to reason logically, think abstractly, and consider the future implications of their actions.
- Cognitive development varies widely; many adolescents exhibit impulsivity and not future-oriented.
- Values, beliefs, and judgment grow increasingly sophisticated.
- Brain development, especially in the prefrontal cortex, continues into the 20s.

Health Care Approaches

- Encourage critical thinking and problem-solving skills.
- Support educational and career planning.
- Monitor for impulsive behaviors and provide appropriate guidance.

Social and Emotional Development

- Adolescence involves a transition from family-dominated influences to increased autonomy and peer influence (Fig. 28-91).
- Adolescents often navigate identity, independence, and intimacy, which can lead to stress, health challenges, and risk-taking behaviors.
- These years present opportunities for health promotion and prevention.

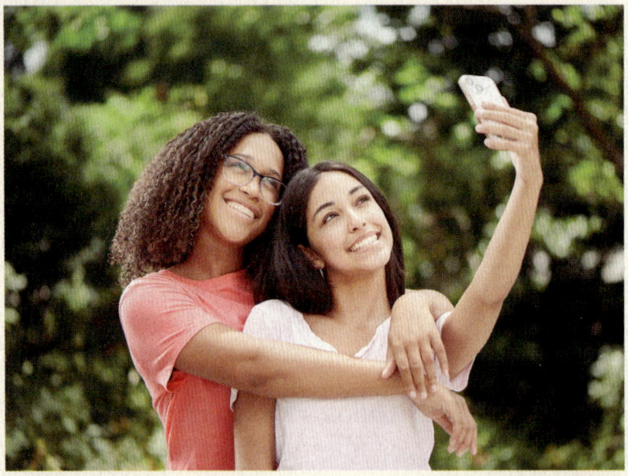

FIGURE 28-91. Encouraging healthy peer relationships supports emotional and social development during adolescence.

Health Care Approaches

- Encourage healthy peer relationships and social activities.
- Support emotional regulation and identity formation.
- Provide guidance to avoid high-risk behaviors and foster overall health.

Gender and Sexual Identity Formation among Adolescents

Discussing sexuality and gender can be challenging for adolescents, who may struggle with gender identity, sexual orientation, and self-image. Clinicians must create a welcoming, supportive, confidential, and nonjudgmental environment to facilitate these discussions.

Recent data from the CDC's 2021 Youth Risk Behavior Survey (YRBS) found that 12% of high school students identified as lesbian, gay, or bisexual, and 3.2% were unsure of their sexual orientation. Although the 2021 YRBS did not include a question on transgender identity, the 2016 survey indicated that 1.8% of students identified as transgender.[77,78] The 2022 Minnesota Student Survey showed that 11% of students in 8th grade or higher identified as transgender, genderfluid, nonbinary, two-spirit, or unsure or chose not to answer the gender question. This marks a significant increase from previous years.

Mental health challenges are prevalent among these students, with 63% reporting long-term mental health, behavioral, or emotional problems, a trend worsened by the COVID-19 pandemic.[79,80] LGBTQ+ youth value the opportunity to discuss their gender and sexuality with their clinician but often delay disclosure until a strong, trusting relationship is established. Only 35% of LGBTQ+ youth reported that their clinician knew their LGBTQ+ identity.[81–83] Emphasizing confidentiality is essential, as disclosing a teenager's sexual or gender identity to parents or caregivers without consent can result in harm.[84]

It is important to affirm that being LGBTQ+ is a natural variation of human identity and is not inherently linked to high-risk behaviors or poor health outcomes. However, LGBTQ+ youth often face discrimination, stigma, and rejection, which can lead to psychological distress and increased vulnerability to high-risk behaviors. These challenges may include ostracism, bullying, parental or caregiver rejection, abuse, and homelessness, contributing to health disparities in mental health, suicide risk, substance use, and higher rates of STIs.[77]

Clinicians should actively screen for signs of bullying, depression, and suicide risk while supporting adolescents in identifying their strengths and talents.[21] With proper guidance and affirmation, LGBTQ+ youth can thrive, build resilience, and develop healthy sexual and gender identities without a significant increase in high-risk behaviors compared to their peers.[85]

PHYSICAL EXAMINATION: GENERAL APPROACH

As in middle childhood, modesty is important among adolescents. The patient should remain dressed until the examination begins (Fig. 28-92). Leave the room while the patient puts on a gown. Not all adolescents are willing to wear a gown, so partially uncovering as the examination proceeds to preserve modesty is important. Most adolescents older than 13 years prefer to be examined without a caregiver in the room, but this depends on the patient's developmental level, familiarity with the examiner, relationship with the caregiver, and culture. Ask younger adolescents and their caregivers about their preferences.

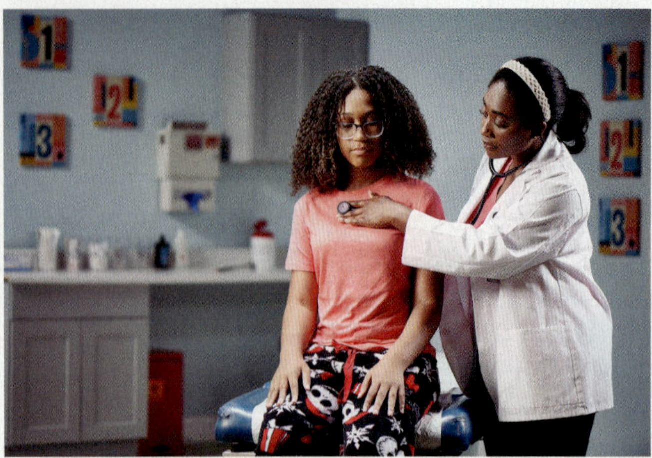

FIGURE 28-92. Adolescents may require a patient-centered approach during examinations, including discussions about clothing and privacy preferences.

It is safest to have a chaperone in the room, regardless of patient gender, when examining a patient's breasts or genitalia. Discuss the issue of chaperones with patients and caregivers, and record the shared decision in the clinical chart. This practice is required in some U.S. states and many organizations.[86]

TECHNIQUES OF EXAMINATION

The sequence and content of the physical examination of the adolescent are similar to those in the adult (Box 28-59). Keep in mind, however, issues unique to adolescents such as puberty, growth, development, family and peer relationships, sexuality, healthy decision making, and high-risk behaviors.

Box 28-59. Techniques of Adolescent Examination

Organ/System	Details	Examples of Abnormalities
Somatic growth: height and weight	▪ Adolescents should wear gowns to be weighed or remove shoes and heavy clothing, especially if being evaluated for weight loss. ▪ Use the same scale for serial weights and heights.	Obesity and eating disorders (anorexia, bulimia, and avoidant/restrictive food intake disorder [ARFID]) are major public health problems. Regular weight assessments, monitoring for complications, and promoting healthy choices are crucial.
Vital signs	Ongoing evaluations of blood pressure are important for adolescents[73]: ▪ Average heart rate (10–14 years): 85 beats/min (range: 55–115 beats/min) ▪ Average heart rate (15+ years): 60–100 beats/min ▪ Percentiles for blood pressure are shown on p. 1056.	Causes of hypertension include primary hypertension, renal disease, and drug use.

Organ/System	Details
Skin	■ Examine for acne, blemishes, warts, and moles. ■ Focus on the face and back for acne. ■ Counsel on excessive ultraviolet exposure, need for sunscreen, and tanning risks. ■ Counsel older adolescents to begin performing a regular self-examination of the skin, as shown on p. 258.
HEENT	■ Examination methods are similar to adults. ■ Regular visual acuity testing is important.
Thorax and lungs	■ Examination techniques are the same as for adults.
Breasts	■ Breast changes are among the first visible signs of puberty. ■ Generally, over a 4-year period, the breasts progress through five stages, called *Tanner stages* or *sexual maturity rating* (*SMR*) stages (Box 28-60). ■ Breast buds enlarge, changing contour and darkening the areola coinciding with the development of pubic hair and other secondary sexual characteristics, as shown on p. 1094. ■ Menarche usually occurs during breast stage 3 or 4. ■ Historically, the onset of breast development and pubic hair has ranged from 8–13 years (average 11 years), but some studies suggest lowering the age cutoff to 7.[87–89] ■ Breast development varies by age, race, and ethnicity; ~10% of individuals experience different development rates, leading to temporary asymmetry. Reassurance that this usually resolves is helpful.[87,89] ■ In individuals assigned male at birth, breasts consist of a small nipple and areola. During puberty, about one third develop a breast bud ≥2 cm in diameter, usually in one breast. Those who are obese may develop substantial breast tissue.

(continued)

Adolescent acne tends to resolve eventually but often benefits from proper treatment. It tends to begin during middle to late puberty.

See Table 28-4, "Warts, Lesions That Resemble Warts, and Other Raised Lesions," on p. 1104.

Persistent fever, sore throat, swollen tonsils, and cervical lymphadenopathy may indicate streptococcal pharyngitis or infectious mononucleosis.

Breast buds (pea-size firm masses inferior to the nipple) are common in early puberty and are benign.

Breast asymmetry is common in adolescents, particularly when adolescents are between Tanner stages 2 and 4 and usually resolves on its own.

The American Cancer Society and USPSTF no longer recommend breast self-examinations for individuals of any age to screen for breast cancer.[90] Some professional organizations advise providing instructions for self-examination or breast self-awareness.

Gynecomastia (enlarged breasts) in adolescents assigned male at birth, on one or both sides, often resolves within a few years.

Breast masses or nodules, usually *benign fibroadenomas* or cysts, in adolescent assigned female at birth are usually benign but should always be evaluated.[91]

Box 28-59. Techniques of Adolescent Examination (*Continued*)

Organ/System	Details
Heart	■ Examination techniques are the same as for adults. ■ Benign pulmonary flow murmurs are common in adolescents and have the following characteristics: grade I–II/VI, soft, nonharsh (Box 28-61). The pulmonary closure sound should have normal intensity. Splitting of S_2 should cease during expiration. Adolescents with a benign pulmonary ejection murmur will have normal intensity and normally split S_2.
Abdomen	■ Techniques are the same as for adults. ■ Palpate the liver; liver size approaches adult size during puberty. Nonpalpable liver suggests no hepatomegaly. ■ If you can palpate the lower edge, use light percussion to assess liver span.
Genitalia (Assigned Male at Birth)	■ Examination is similar to that of adults. Pubertal changes follow a well-established sequence. ■ Assign a sexual maturity rating; the five Tanner stages of sexual development involve changes in the penis, testes, and scrotum (Box 28-62). ■ Puberty typically begins with testes enlargement at ages 9–13.5 years (Fig. 28-93). Next, pubic hair appears, along with progressive enlargement of the penis.[92] These changes generally take about 3 years (range: 1.8–5 years). ■ Inspect the penis for sores and discharge as you would in an adult. ■ In uncircumcised adolescents, the foreskin should be easily retractable by adolescence; this is also an opportunity to discuss normal hygiene practices.
Genitalia (Assigned Female at Birth)	■ External examination is similar to that of school-age children. ■ If a pelvic examination is clinically necessary, it should follow the same technique as for adults, but indications for pelvic exams in adolescents are now much more stringent. ■ When performing a pelvic examination, a full explanation of the steps; demonstration of instruments; and a gentle, reassuring approach are necessary. A chaperone must be present. ■ An adolescent's first pelvic examination should be performed by an experienced health care provider. ■ The first visible sign of puberty is usually the appearance of breast buds, although pubic hair sometimes appears earlier.

A pulmonary flow murmur with a fixed split-second heart sound suggests right-heart volume load like an ASD.

The pulmonary flow murmur may also be heard in the presence of volume overload from any cause such as chronic anemia and following exercise. It may persist into adulthood.

Hepatomegaly in teens may be from infections such as hepatitis or infectious mononucleosis, inflammatory bowel disease, or tumors.

Splenomegaly with sore throat and fever may indicate infectious mononucleosis.

Delayed puberty is suspected if no signs by age 14. The most common cause is constitutional delay, often familial.

Nocturnal or daytime ejaculation begins around SMR 3, but penile discharge may indicate an STI.

Vaginal discharge in young adolescents can be from various causes like STIs, bacterial vaginosis, or foreign body.

Pubertal development prior to the normal age range may signify *precocious puberty*. *Premature adrenarche* is usually benign, but may occasionally be associated with polycystic ovary syndrome, insulin resistance, and metabolic syndrome.

Organ/System	Details
	■ Initial signs of puberty are hymenal thickening and redundancy secondary to estrogen, widening of the hips, and beginning of a height spurt (Fig. 28-94). ■ Assign a sexual maturity rating, independent of chronologic age. ■ The assessment of sexual maturity is based on both growth of pubic hair (Box 28-63) and the development of breasts.[88] Counsel them about this sequence and their current stage.
Rectum and anus	■ Examination is the same as for adults. ■ Routine rectal examination is not recommended unless there is a particular concern.
Musculoskeletal system	■ Evaluations for scoliosis and screening for sports participation are common (see pp. 1098–1100). ■ Other examination segments are the same as for adults.
Nervous system	■ Examination is similar to that of adults. ■ Assess developmental achievement according to age-specific milestones, as described on p. 1088.

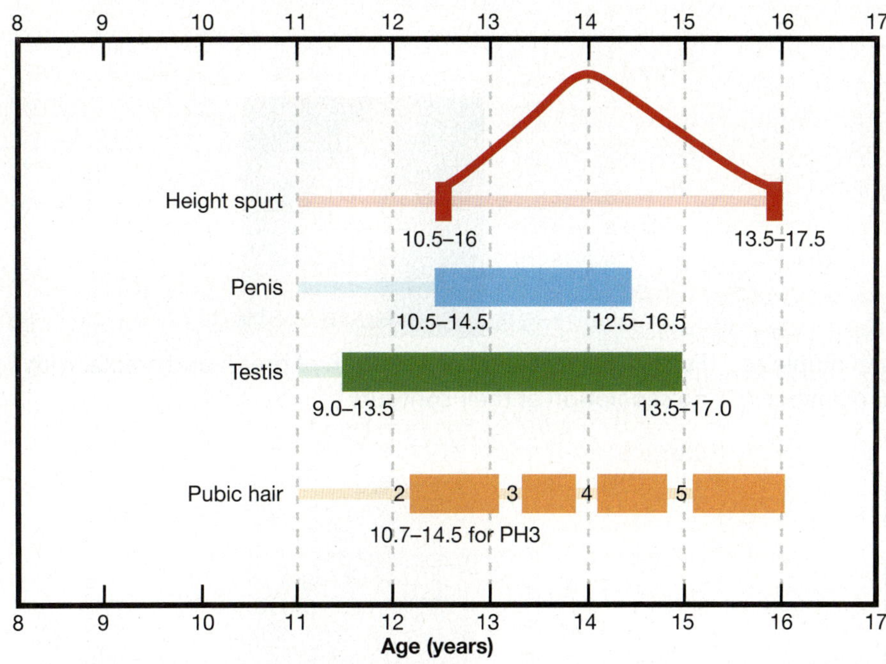

Numbers below the bars indicate the ranges in age within which the changes occur.

FIGURE 28-93. Pubertal milestones in adolescents with testosterone-driven development: This graph shows the timing of height spurts, penile growth, testicular development, and pubic hair stages (PH2–PH5) in relation to age.

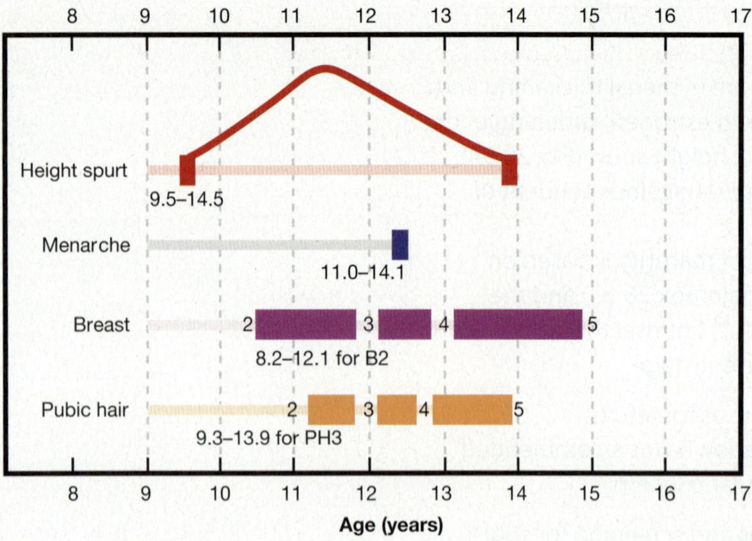

FIGURE 28-94. Pubertal milestones in adolescents with estrogen-driven development: The graph illustrates the timing of height spurts, menarche, breast development (stages B2–B5), and pubic hair stages (PH2–PH5) in relation to age.

Box 28-60. Sexual Maturity Ratings: Breasts (Estrogen-Driven Development)

Stage 1

Preadolescent: elevation of nipple only

Stage 2

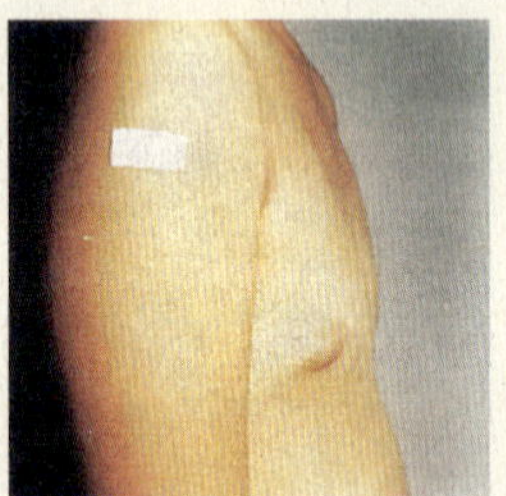

Breast bud stage: elevation of breast and nipple as a small mound; enlargement of areolar diameter

Stage 3

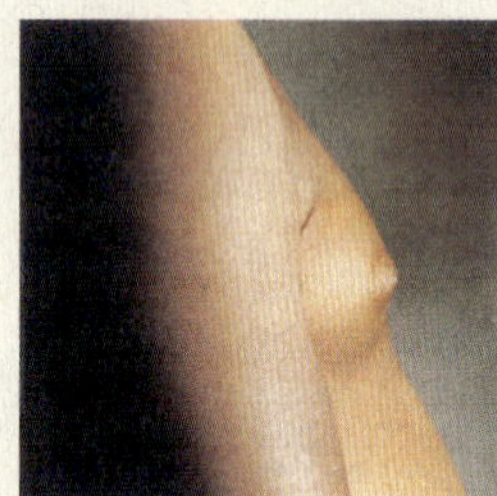

Further enlargement of elevation of breast and areola, with no separation of their contours

Stage 4

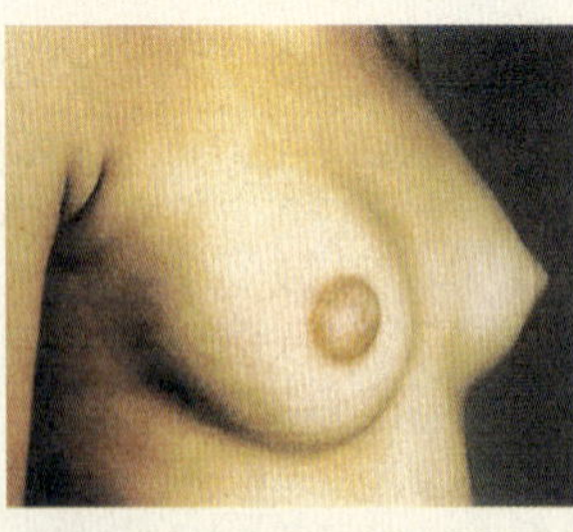

Projection of areola and nipple to form a secondary mound above the level of breast

Stage 5

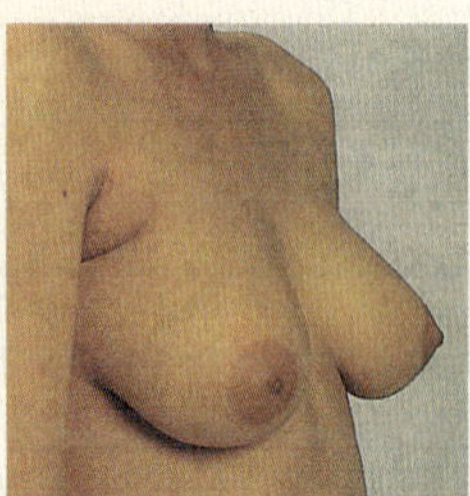

Mature stage: projection of nipple only; areola has receded to general contour of the breast (although in some individuals the areola continues to form a secondary mound)

Source: Photos used with permission of American Academy of Pediatrics—Books from Herman-Giddens ME, Bourdony CJ. *Assessment of Sexual Maturity Stages in Girls*. American Academy of Pediatrics, 1995; permission conveyed through Copyright Clearance Center, Inc.

Box 28-61. Location and Characteristics of Pulmonary Flow Murmur in Adolescents

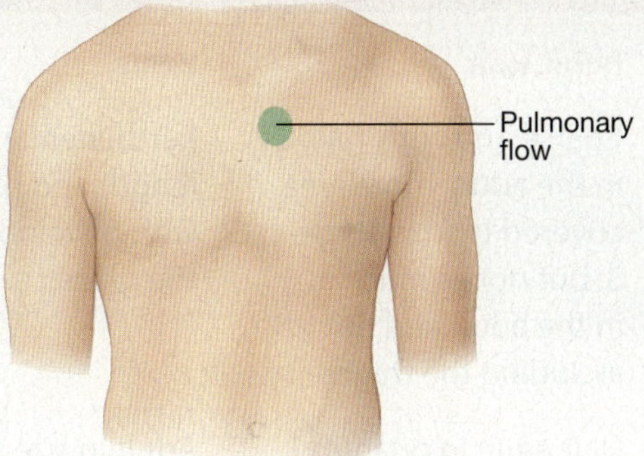

Typical Age	Name	Relation to S_1 and S_2	Description and Location
Older child, adolescence, and later	*Pulmonary flow murmur*	S_1 S_2	Grade I–II/VI soft, nonharsh Ejection in timing Upper left sternal border Normal P_2

Box 28-62. Sexual Maturity Rating: Pubic Hair, Penis, Testes and Scrotum (Testosterone-Driven Development)

In assigning sexual maturity rating in individuals undergoing testosterone-driven puberty, observe each of the three characteristics separately because they may develop at different rates. Record two separate ratings: pubic hair and genital. If the penis and testes differ in their stages, average the two into a single figure for the genital rating. These photos demonstrate pubertal development in an uncircumcised male genitalia.

	Pubic Hair	Penis	Testes and Scrotum
Stage 1	Preadolescent—no pubic hair except for the fine body hair (vellus hair) similar to that on the abdomen	Preadolescent—same size and proportions as in childhood	Preadolescent—same size and proportions as in childhood
Stage 2	Sparse growth of long, slightly pigmented, downy hair, straight or only slightly curled, chiefly at the base of the penis	Slight or no enlargement	Testes larger; scrotum larger, somewhat reddened, and altered in texture
Stage 3	Darker, coarser, curlier hair spreading sparsely over the pubic symphysis	Larger, especially in length	Further enlarged

(*continued*)

Box 28-62. Sexual Maturity Rating: Pubic Hair, Penis, Testes and Scrotum (Testosterone-Driven Development) (*Continued*)

	Pubic Hair	Penis	Testes and Scrotum
Stage 4	Coarse and curly hair, as in the adult; more area covered than in stage 3, but not as much as in the adult and not yet including the thighs	Further enlarged in length and breadth, with development of the glans	Further enlarged; scrotal skin darkened
Stage 5	Hair adult in quantity and quality, spreads to the medial surfaces of the thighs but not up over the abdomen	Adult in size and shape	Adult in size and shape

Source: Photos reprinted from Wales JKH, Wit JM, Rogol AD. *Pediatric Endocrinology and Growth*. 2nd ed. W.B. Saunders; 2003. Copyright © 2003 Elsevier. With permission.

Box 28-63. Sexual Maturity Ratings: Pubic Hair (Estrogen-Driven Development)

Stage 1

Preadolescent—no pubic hair except for the fine body hair (vellus hair) similar to that on the abdomen

Stage 2

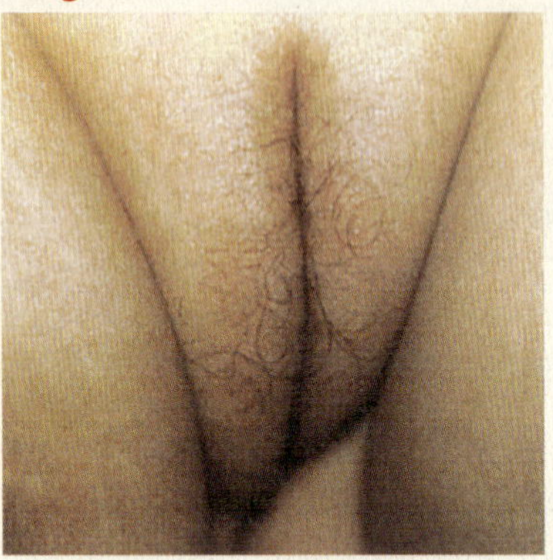

Sparse growth of long, slightly pigmented, downy hair, straight or only slightly curled, chiefly along the labia

Stage 3

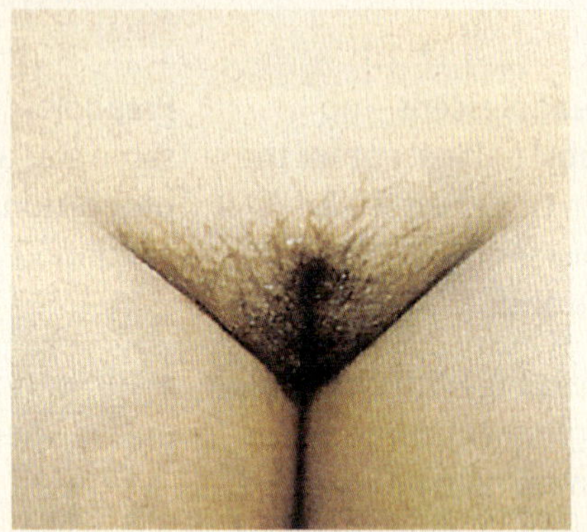

Darker, coarser, curlier hair, spreading sparsely over the pubic symphysis

Amenorrhea in adolescence can be *primary* (no menarche by age 16 years) or *secondary* (cessation of menses in an adolescent who had previously menstruated). While primary amenorrhea is usually due to anatomic or genetic causes, secondary amenorrhea can be due to a variety of etiologies such as stress, excessive exercise, and eating disorders.

Delayed puberty (no breasts or pubic hair development by age 12 years) in an adolescent individuals below the third percentile in height may be from Turner syndrome or chronic disease. The two most common causes of delayed sexual development in an extremely thin adolescent individuals are anorexia nervosa and chronic disease.

Obesity in individuals assigned female at birth can be associated with early onset of puberty.

Stage 4

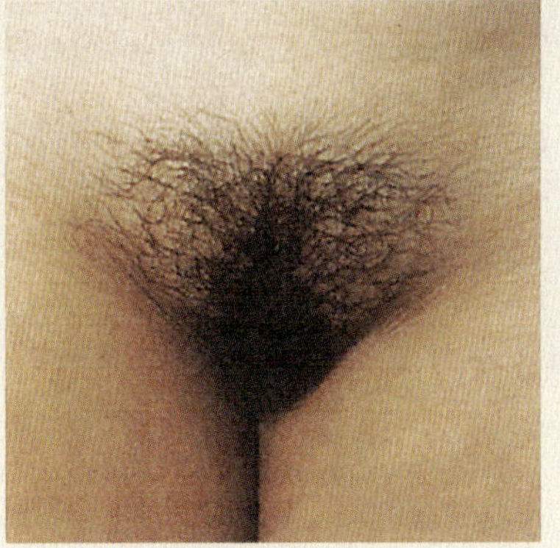

Coarse and curly hair as in adults; more area covered than in stage 3 but not as much as in the adult and not yet including the thighs

Stage 5

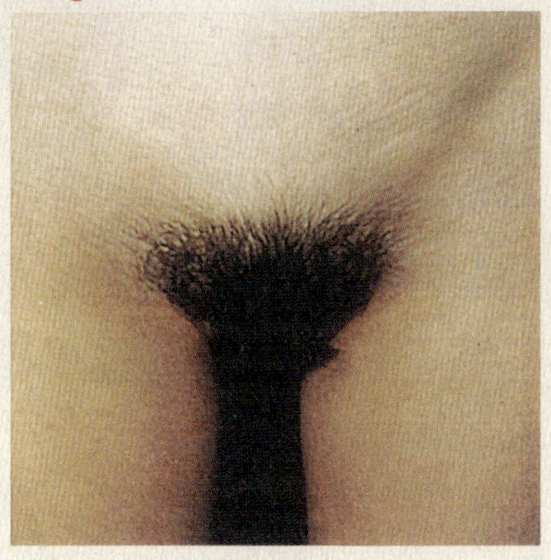

Hair adult in quantity and quality, spreads on the medial surfaces of the thighs but not up over the abdomen

Source: Photos used with permission of American Academy of Pediatrics—Books from Herman-Giddens ME, Bourdony CJ. *Assessment of Sexual Maturity Stages in Girls*. American Academy of Pediatrics, 1995; permission conveyed through Copyright Clearance Center, Inc.

SPECIAL TECHNIQUES AND MANEUVERS

Assessing for Scoliosis

Examine the patient standing to assess shoulder, scapula, and hip symmetry. Have the patient bend forward with knees straight and head down (*Adams forward bend test*) to check for asymmetry.

Use a scoliometer to measure scoliosis (Fig. 28-95). Place the scoliometer over the spine at the point of maximum prominence, ensuring the spine is parallel to the floor. Move it along the spine to find the maximal prominence. An angle greater than 7° is concerning and may warrant a specialist referral. Sensitivity and specificity of the Adams forward bend test and scoliometer vary with the examiner's skill and experience. Smartphone apps that mimic a scoliometer can provide convenient assessments.

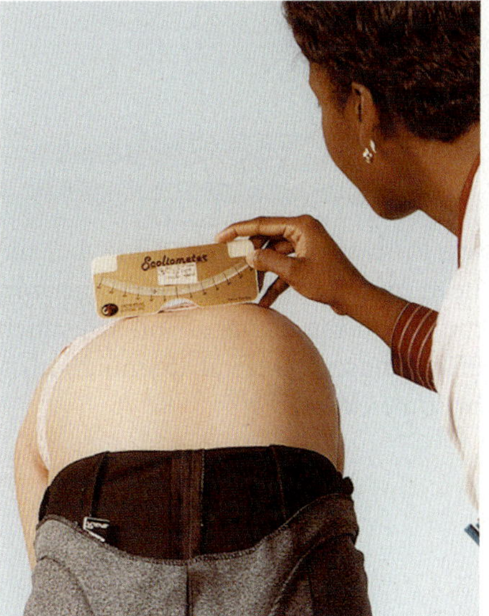

FIGURE 28-95. Measure and record scoliosis with a scoliometer.

Scoliosis in young children is rare; mild scoliosis in older children occurs in 2% to 4% of adolescents. It appears as an asymmetrical rise in the thoracic or lumbar region.

Types of scoliosis include idiopathic (75% of cases, mostly in females, usually detected in early adolescence), neuromuscular, and congenital. The right hemithorax is generally more prominent in idiopathic scoliosis.

You can also use a plumb line to assess back symmetry. Place the top of the plumb line at C7 and have the patient stand straight (Fig. 28-96). The plumb line should extend to the gluteal crease.

Scoliosis is more common among children and adolescents with neurologic or musculoskeletal abnormalities. Apparent scoliosis, including an abnormal plumb line test, can be caused by a leg-length discrepancy (p. 1075).

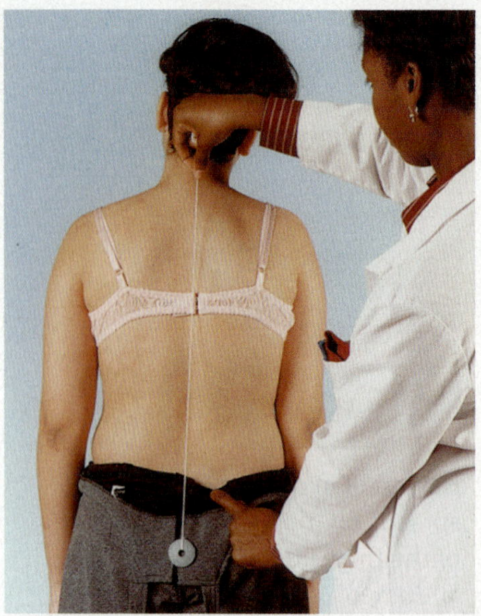

FIGURE 28-96. Measuring scoliosis with a plumb line.

Conducting Sports Preparticipation Physical Evaluation

Millions of children and adolescents participate in organized sports and often require medical clearance. Start with a thorough medical history focusing on cardiovascular risk factors, prior surgeries, injuries, other medical problems, and family history. A complete history is the most sensitive and specific part of the evaluation for detecting risk factors or abnormalities that could preclude sports participation.[93]

This evaluation is often one of the few times a healthy adolescent will see a clinician, so include screening questions and anticipatory guidance (see Health Promotion and Counseling, pp. 1100–1101). Perform a general physical examination, with special attention to the heart and lungs, and include vision and hearing screening. Conduct a thorough musculoskeletal examination, looking for weakness, limited ROM, and evidence of previous injury.

Important risk factors for sudden cardiovascular death during sports include episodes of dizziness or palpitations, prior syncope (particularly if associated with exercise), or family history of sudden death or cardiomyopathy in young or middle-age relatives.

During the examination, carefully assess for cardiac murmurs and wheezing in the lungs. If the adolescent has had head injuries or a concussion, perform a focused neurologic examination and consider using a concussion assessment tool. A 2-minute preparticipation screening musculoskeletal examination, as shown in Box 28-64, is recommended by some experts.[94,95]

Box 28-64. Screening Musculoskeletal Examination for Sports

Position and Instruction to Patient

Step 1: Stand straight, facing forward. Note for any asymmetry or swelling of joints.

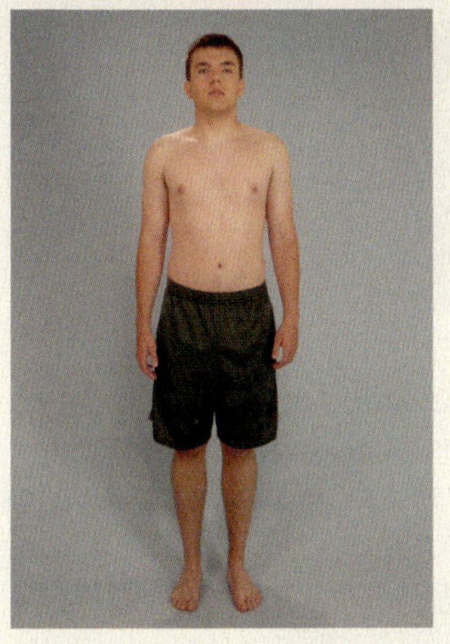

Step 2: Move neck in all directions. Note for any loss of range of motion (ROM).

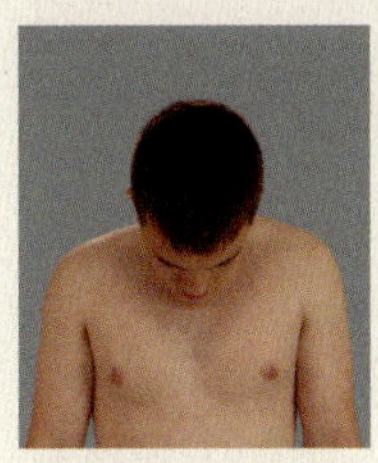

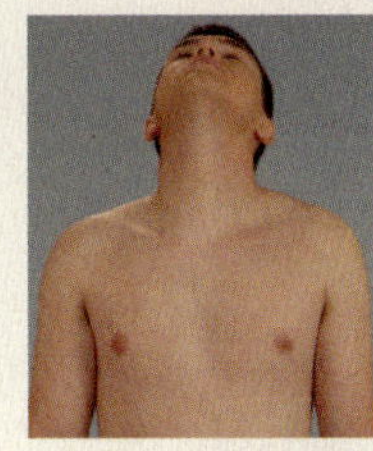

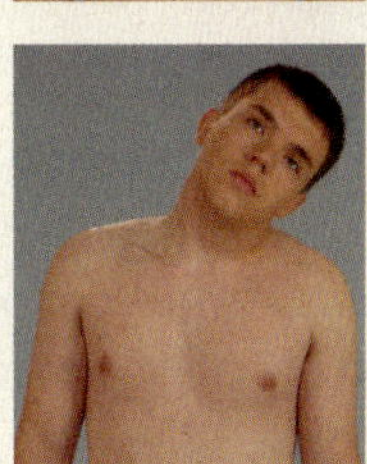

Step 3: Shrug shoulders against resistance. Note for any weakness of shoulder, neck, or trapezius muscles.

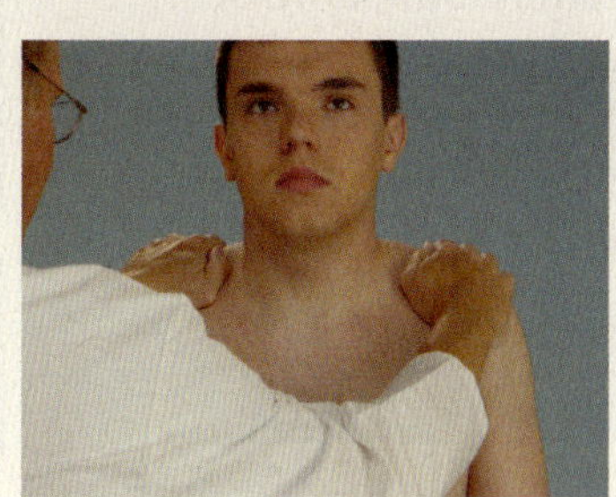

Step 4: Hold arms out to the side against resistance, and actively raise arms over the head. Note any loss of strength of deltoid muscle.

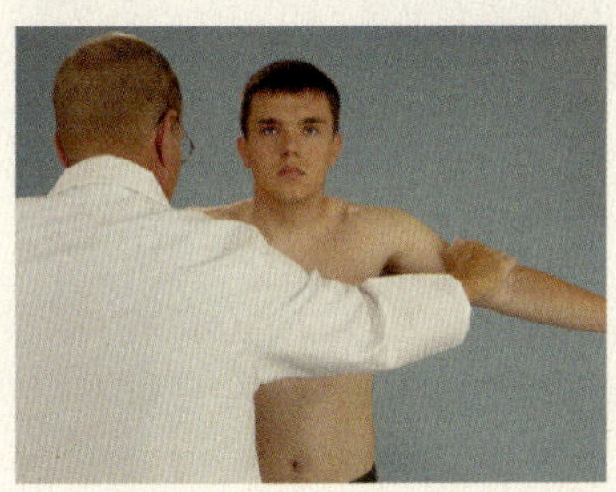

Step 5: Hold arms out to side with elbows bent 90°; raise and lower arms. Note any loss of external rotation and injury of glenohumeral joint.

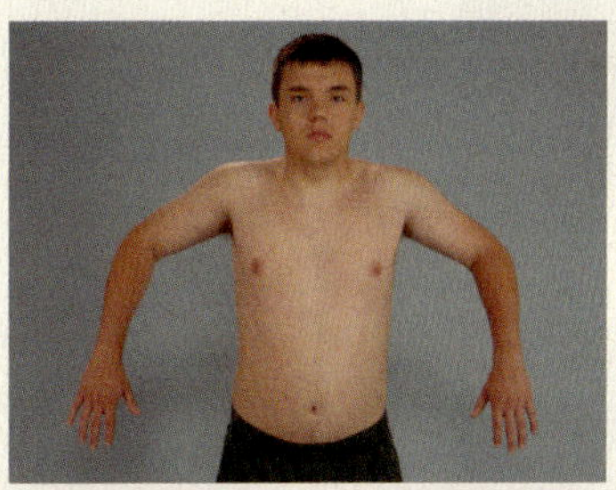

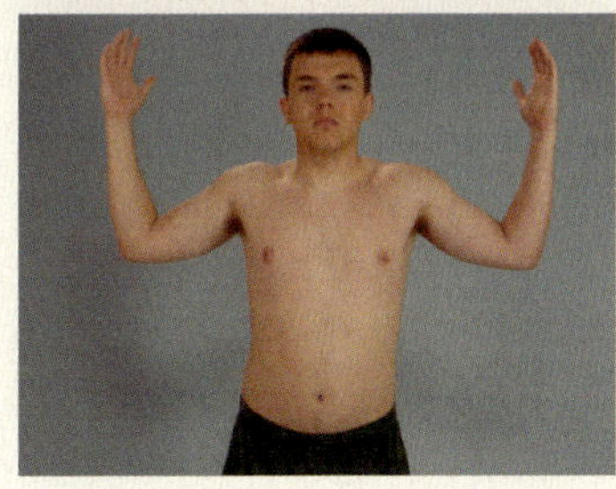

Step 6: Hold arms out, completely bend, and straighten elbows (should be able to easily touch the shoulder). Note any reduced ROM of elbow.

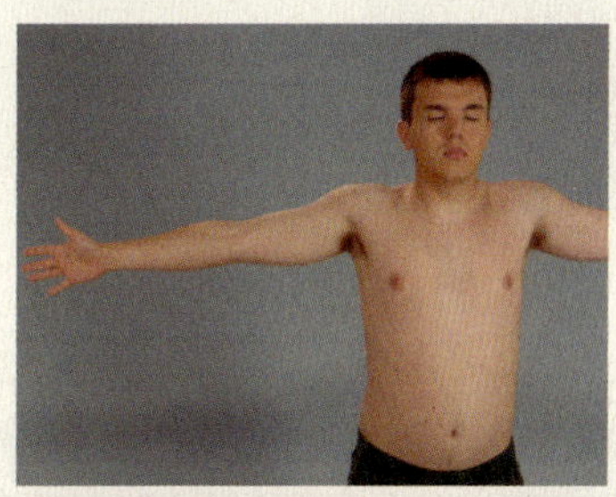

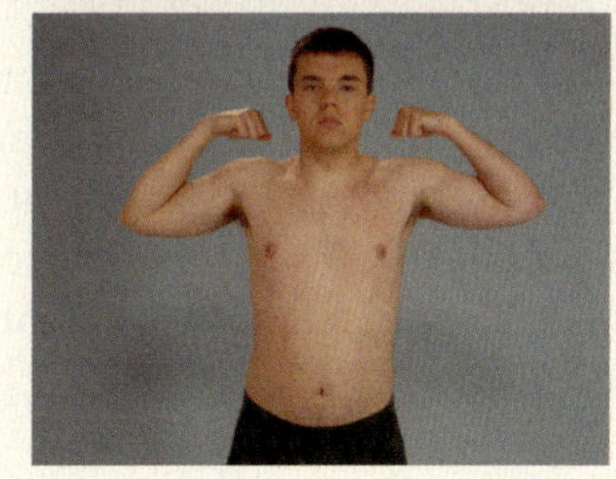

(continued)

Box 28-64. Screening Musculoskeletal Examination for Sports (*Continued*)

Step 7: Hold arms down, bend elbows 90°, and pronate and supinate forearms. Note any reduced ROM from prior injury to forearm, elbow, or wrist.

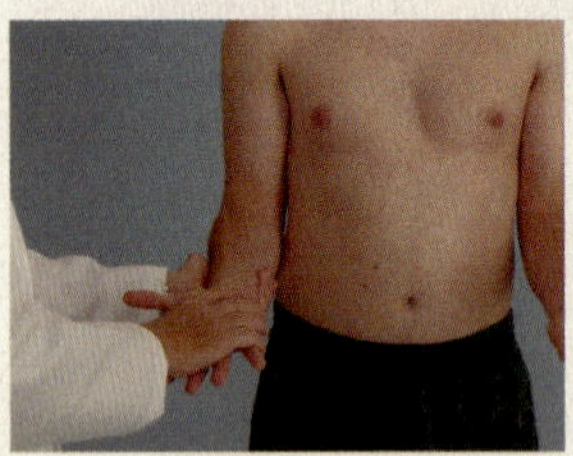

Step 8: Make a fist, clench, and then spread fingers. Note protruding knuckle, reduced ROM of fingers from prior sprain or fracture.

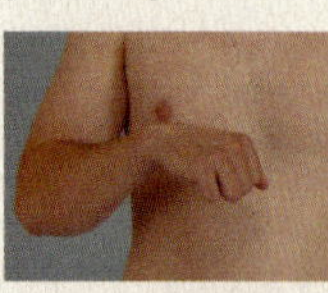

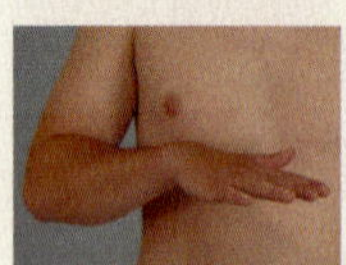

Step 9: Squat and duck-walk for four steps forward. Note inability to fully flex knees and difficulty standing up from prior knee or ankle injury.

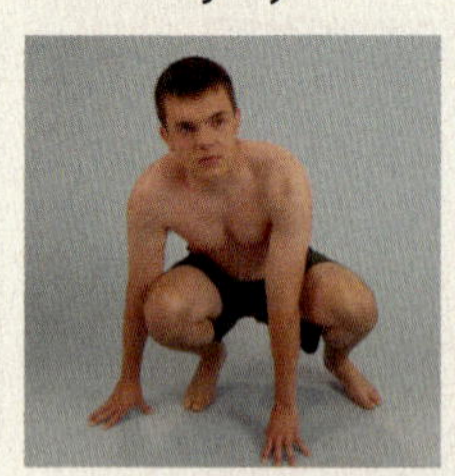

Step 10: Stand straight with arms at sides, facing back. Check whether shoulders, scapula, and hips are even. Note any asymmetry from scoliosis, leg-length discrepancy, or weakness from prior injury.

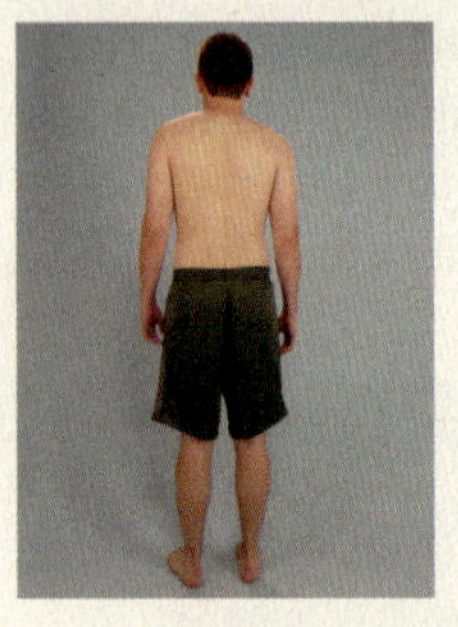

Step 11: Bend forward with knees straight and touch toes. Note any asymmetry from scoliosis and twisting of back from low back pain.

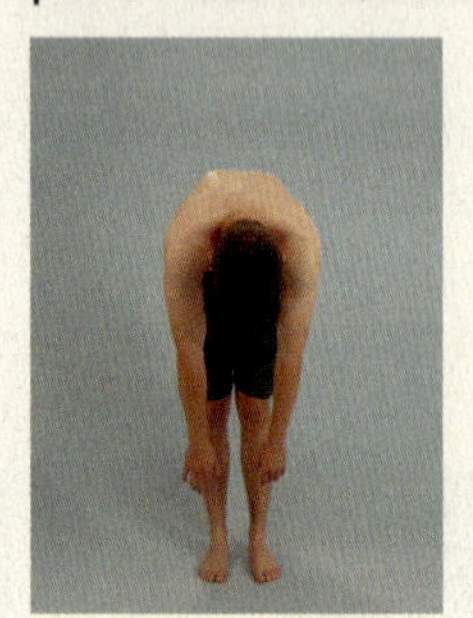

Step 12: Stand on heels and rise to the toes. Note any wasting of calf muscles from prior ankle or Achilles tendon injury.

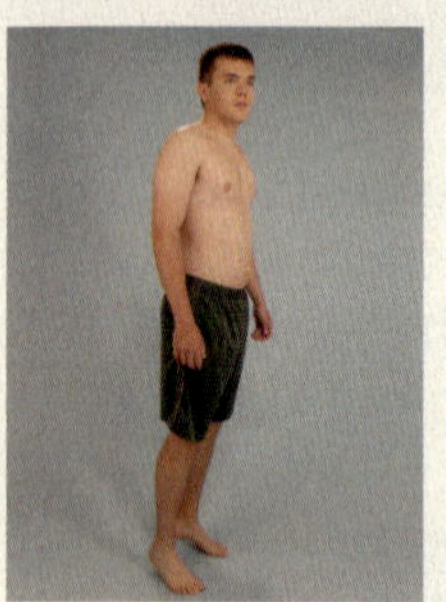

RECORDING YOUR FINDINGS

The clinical record format is the same for both children and adults. Although the sequence of the physical examination may vary, convert your findings into the traditional written or electronic format order. The history and physical examination write-up for adolescents mirrors that of adults or younger children (pp. 1078–1081). Include key elements of the HEEADSSS evaluation in the history section.

HEALTH PROMOTION AND COUNSELING: EVIDENCE AND RECOMMENDATIONS

The AAP recommends annual health supervision visits for adolescents.[21] Include health promotion in all encounters with youth. Adolescents with chronic problems or high-risk behaviors may need additional visits for health promotion and anticipatory guidance.

Many adult chronic diseases have roots in childhood or adolescence. Obesity, cardiovascular disease, substance use (including drugs, tobacco, or alcohol), and mental health challenges like depression are influenced by experiences and behaviors established during these formative years. For instance, many adults with obesity were affected by it as adolescents, and almost all adults who use tobacco began their habits before age 18. Effective health promotion can help adolescents develop healthy habits and lifestyles, reducing the risk of chronic health problems (Fig. 28-97).

Confidential issues like mental health, substance use, sexual health, and eating behaviors should be addressed privately with adolescents. Use self-completed screening questionnaires before the visit to facilitate comprehensive assessment of risk factors, streamline the discussion, and ensure privacy. This approach saves time and allows for a focused discussion on specific behaviors during the visit. The AAP's Bright Futures provides guidelines for preventive services for adolescents (Box 28-65).[21]

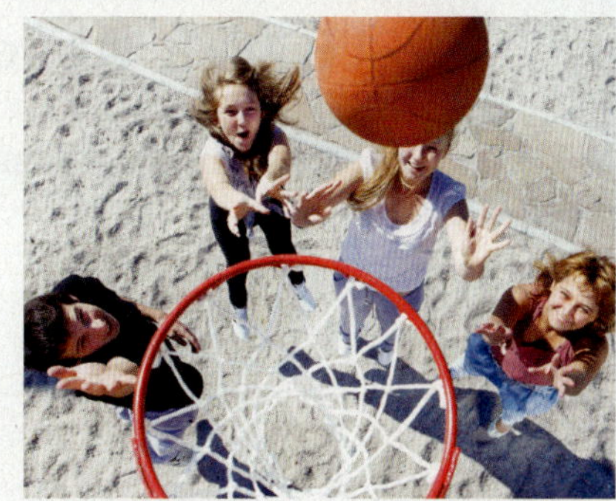

FIGURE 28-97. Inquire about and encourage adolescents to participate in healthy activities.

Box 28-65. Components of a Health Supervision Visit for Adolescents Ages 11–18 Years

Discussions with Parents or Caregivers

- Address concerns and questions.
- Provide guidance about supervision, encouraging progressively responsible decision making
- Ask about school, activities, social interactions
- Assess the adolescent's behaviors and habits, mental health

Discussions with Adolescent

- *Social and Emotional:* mental health, friendships family, gender identity, pronouns preferred by the adolescent
- *Physical Development:* puberty, body image, and self-concept.
- *Behaviors and Habits:* nutrition, exercise, TV or computer screen time, substance use (e.g., drugs, alcohol, tobacco, vaping), and sleep hygiene.
- *Relationships and Sexual Health:* dating, sexual activity, sexual orientation, and addressing unwanted sexual experiences
- *Family Functioning:* relations with parents, caregivers and siblings
- *School and Future Goals*: Academic performance, strengths, extracurricular activities, and career aspirations.

Physical Examination

- Perform a careful examination; note growth parameters, sexual maturity ratings

Screening Tests

- Vision and hearing, blood pressure; consider hematocrit screening for individuals who menstruate; point of care testing for sexually transmitted infections as appropriate; assess emotional health and risk factors (using a validated instrument)

Immunizations

- Follow the schedule from the American Academy of Pediatrics

Anticipatory Guidance—Teen

- *Promote Healthy Habits and Behaviors:*
  - Injury and illness prevention
    - Seat belts, avoiding impaired driving, helmets, sun, firearm safety.
  - Nutrition
    - Healthy eating habits, obesity prevention
  - Oral health:
    - Regular dental visits and proper hygiene.
  - Physical activity and limiting screen time.
- *Sexual Health*:
  - Emphasize confidentiality, safer sex practices, contraception if needed
- *High-Risk Behaviors*:
  - Discuss prevention strategies, peer relationships, family communication, and boundary-setting.
- *Social Development*:
  - Encourage involvement in school, community activities, and future planning.

Anticipatory Guidance—Parent or Caregiver

- Foster positive interactions, support, safety, setting appropriate boundaries, model healthy behaviors, encourage gradual responsibility

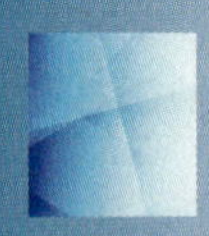

TABLE 28-1. Abnormalities in Heart Rhythm

Supraventricular Tachycardia

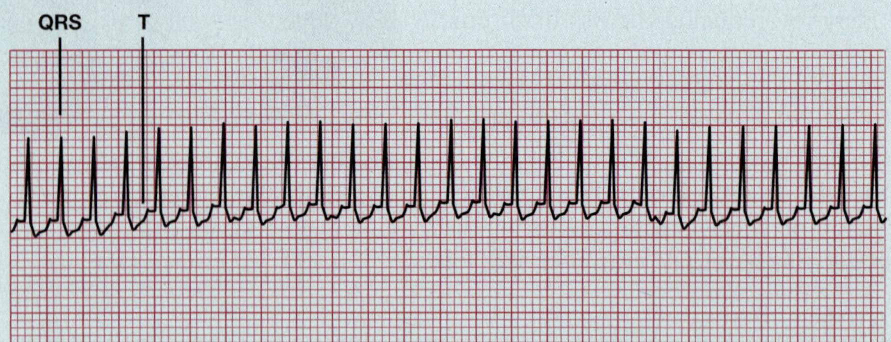

Paroxysmal supraventricular tachycardia (PSVT) is the most common dysrhythmia in children. Some infants with SVT look well or may be somewhat pale with tachypnea but have a heart rate of ≥220 beats/min or higher. Others are ill and in cardiovascular collapse. P waves have different morphology or are not seen.

SVT in infants is usually sustained, requiring clinical therapy for conversion to a normal rate and rhythm. In older children, it is more likely to be truly paroxysmal, with episodes of varying duration and frequency.

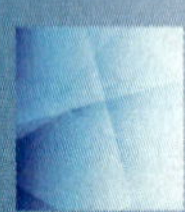

TABLE 28-2. Abnormalities in Blood Pressure

Hypertension in Childhood—Typical Example

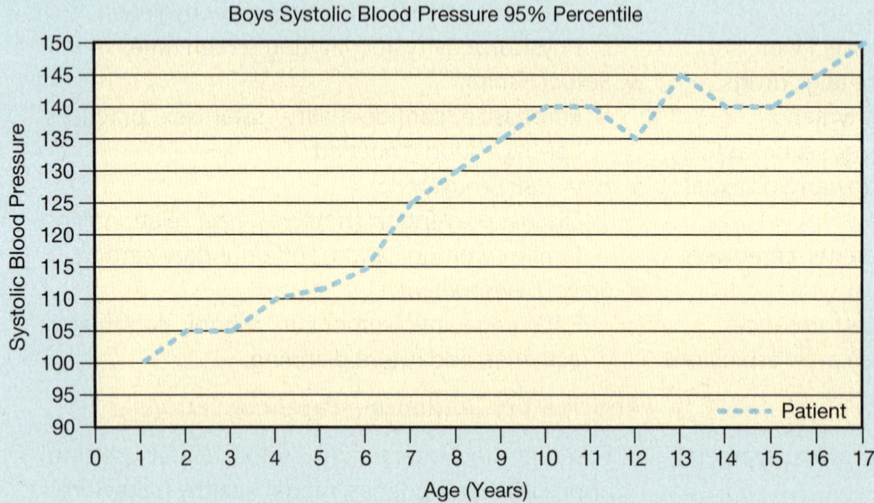

Hypertension can start in childhood.[36] Although elevated blood pressure in young children is more likely to have a renal, cardiac, or endocrine cause, older children and adolescents with hypertension are most likely to have primary or essential hypertension.

This child developed hypertension, and it "tracked" into adulthood. Children tend to remain in the same percentile for blood pressure as they grow. This tracking of blood pressure continues into adulthood, supporting the concept that adult essential hypertension often begins during childhood.

The consequences of untreated hypertension can be severe and include cardiac, renal, and visual sequelae.

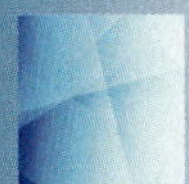

TABLE 28-3. Common Skin Rashes and Skin Findings in Newborns and Infants

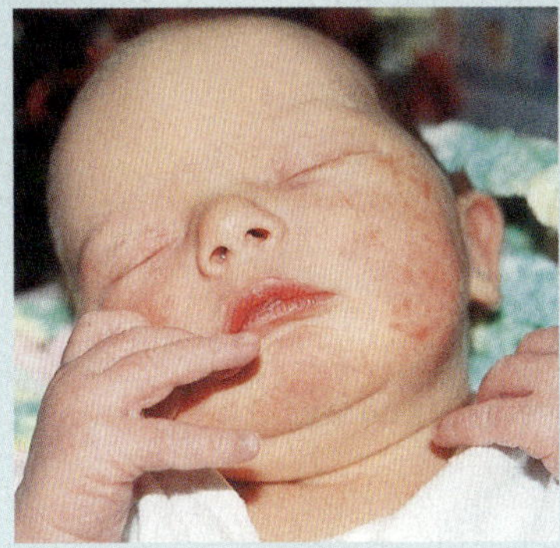

Erythema Toxicum
These common yellow or white pustules are surrounded by a red base.

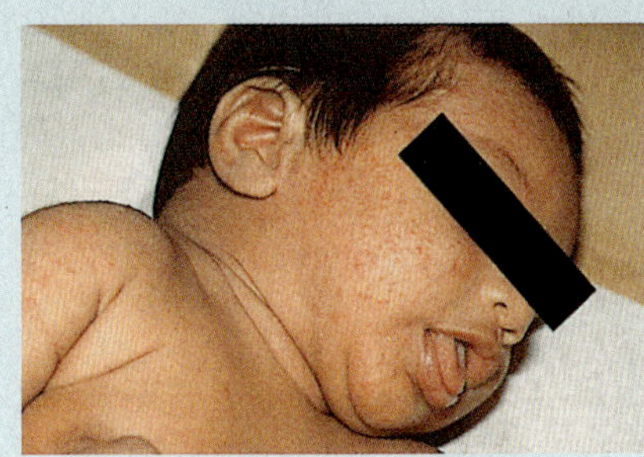

Neonatal Acne
Red pustules and papules are most prominent over the cheeks and nose of some newborns.

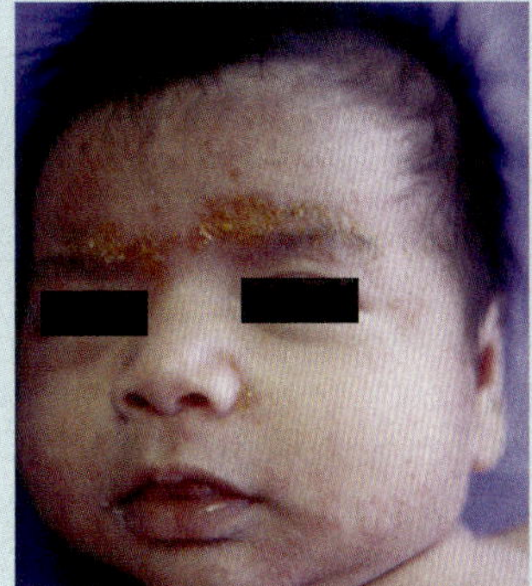

Seborrhea
Salmon red, scaly, and yellow, greasy eruption on the face, neck, axilla, diaper area, and behind ears.

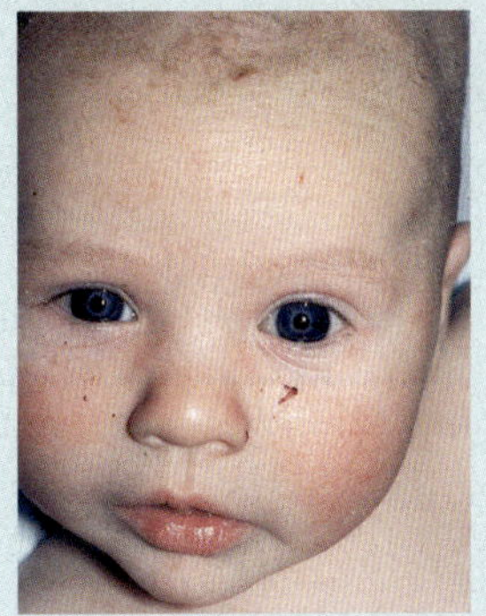

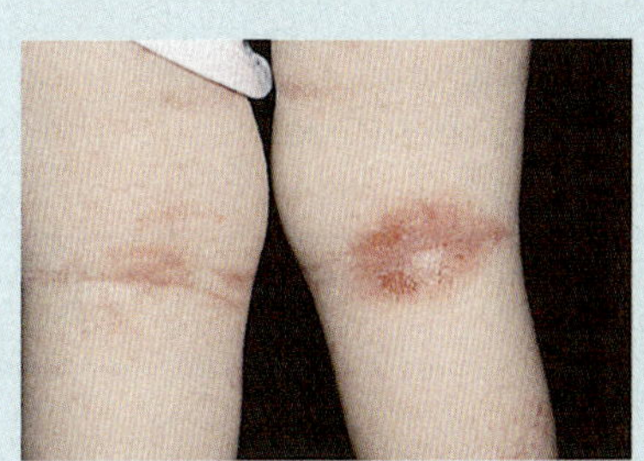

Atopic Dermatitis (Eczema)
Erythema, scaling, dry skin, and intense itching characterize this condition, often appearing on face and flexure surfaces.

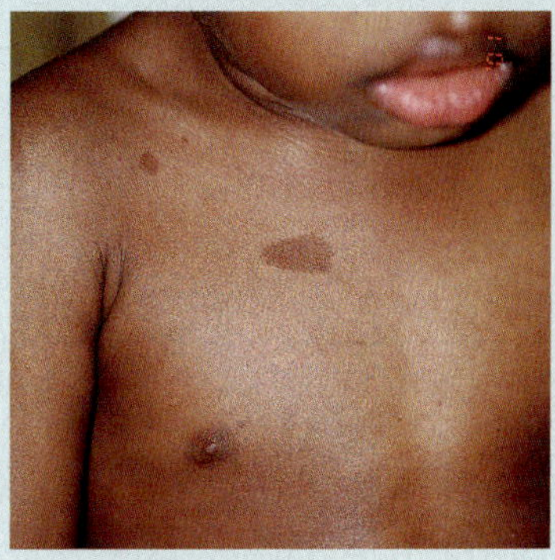

Neurofibromatosis
Characteristic features include >5 café-au-lait spots and axillary and groin freckling.

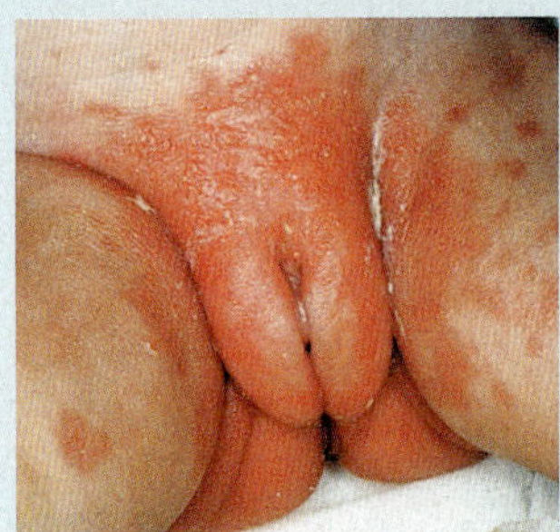

Candidal Diaper Dermatitis
This bright red rash involves the intertriginous folds, with small "satellite lesions" along the edges.

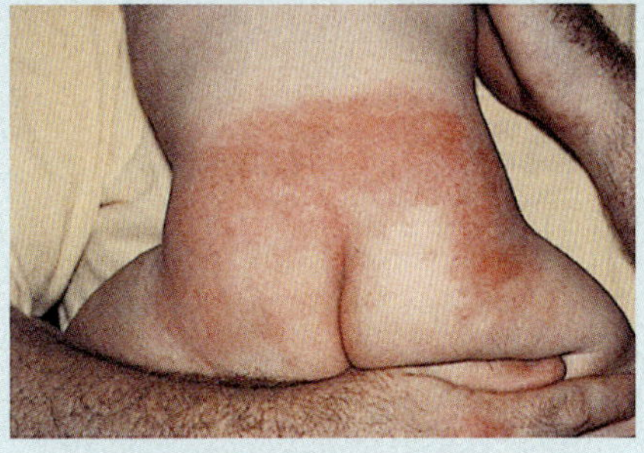

Contact Diaper Dermatitis
This irritant rash is secondary to diarrhea or irritation and is noted along the diaper contact areas.

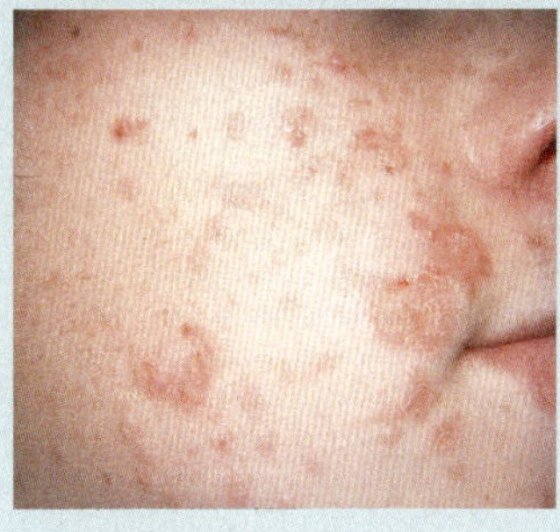

Impetigo
This infection is due to bacteria and can appear bullous or crusty and yellowed with some pus and is often around the face.

Sources of photos: *Erythema Toxicum*—Reprinted with permission from Bowden VR, Greenberg CS. *Children and Their Families: The Continuum of Nursing Care*. 3rd ed. Wolters Kluwer Health/Lippincott Williams & Wilkins; 2014. Figure 25-7; *Seborrhea*—Reprinted with permission from Salimpour RR, Salimpour P, Salimpour P. *Photographic Atlas of Pediatric Disorders and Diagnosis*. Wolters Kluwer Health/Lippincott Williams & Wilkins; 2014:283; *Atopic Dermatitis*—Reprinted with permission from Goodheart HP. *Goodheart's Photoguide of Common Skin Disorders*. 2nd ed. Lippincott Williams & Wilkins; 2003. Figure 2-9 and Goodheart HP. *Goodheart's Photoguide of Common Skin Disorders*. 2nd ed. Lippincott Williams & Wilkins; 2003. Figure 2-11; *Impetigo*—Reprinted with permission from Fleisher GR, Ludwig W, Baskin MN. *Atlas of Pediatric Emergency Medicine*. Lippincott Williams & Wilkins; 2004. Figure 11-30.

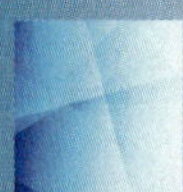

TABLE 28-4. Warts and Lesions that Resemble Warts, and Other Raised Lesions

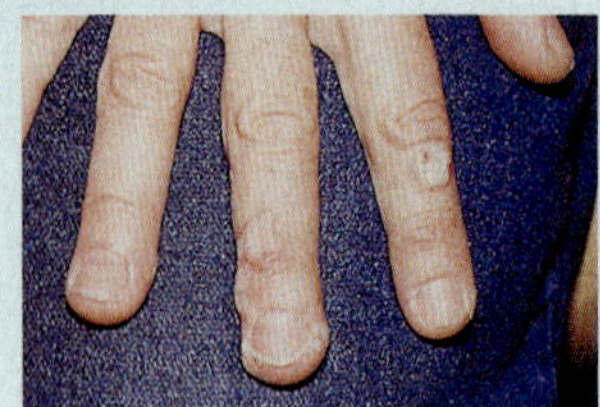

Verruca Vulgaris
Dry, rough warts on hands

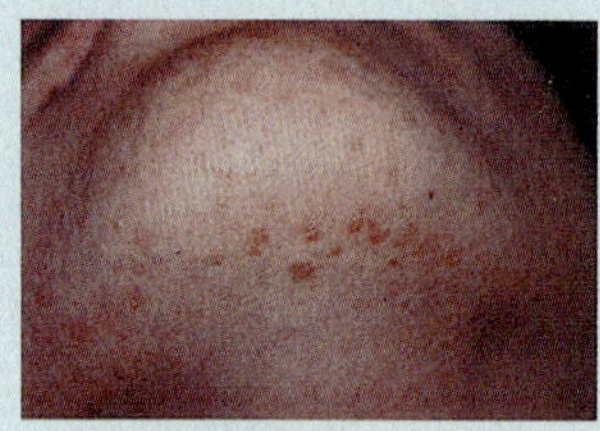

Verruca Plana
Small, flat warts

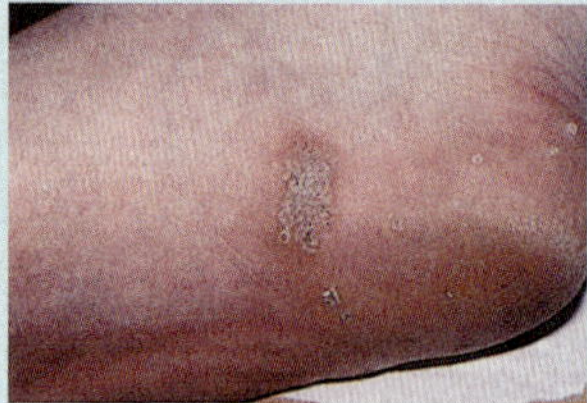

Plantar Warts
Tender warts on feet

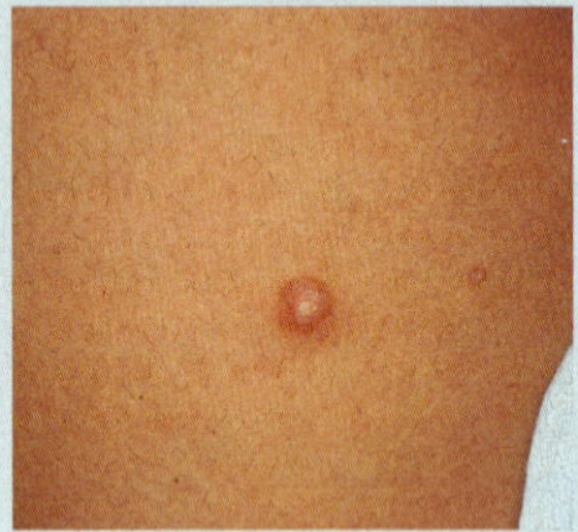

Molluscum Contagiosum
Dome-shaped, fleshy lesions with central umbilication.

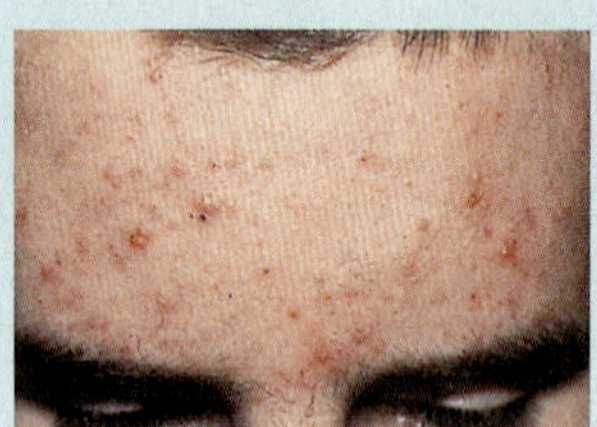

Adolescent Acne
Open comedones (blackheads) and closed comedones (whiteheads) shown at the left, and inflamed pustules (right).

Source of photos: *Molluscum Contagiosum*—Reprinted with permission from Fleisher GR, Ludwig W, Baskin MN. *Atlas of Pediatric Emergency Medicine*. Lippincott Williams & Wilkins; 2004. Figure 6-25.

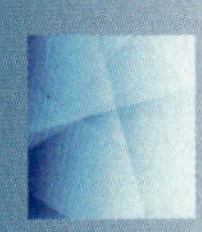

TABLE 28-5. Common Skin Lesions during Childhood

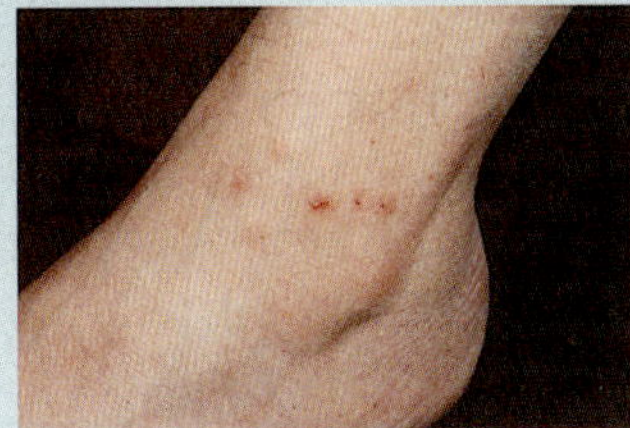

Insect Bites
Intensely pruritic, red, distinct papules characterize these lesions.

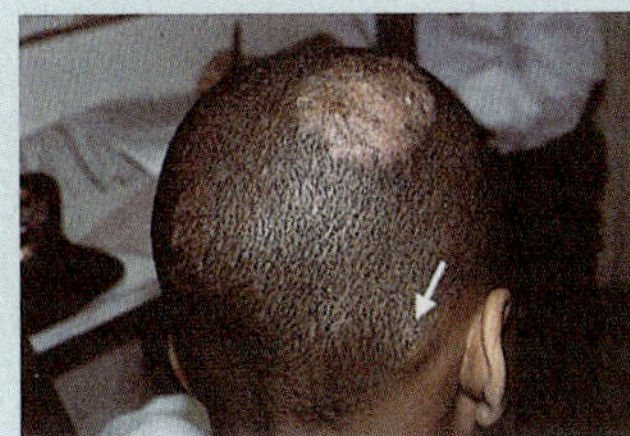

Tinea Capitis
Scaling, crusting, and hair loss are seen in the scalp, along with a painful plaque (kerion) and occipital lymph node (*arrow*).

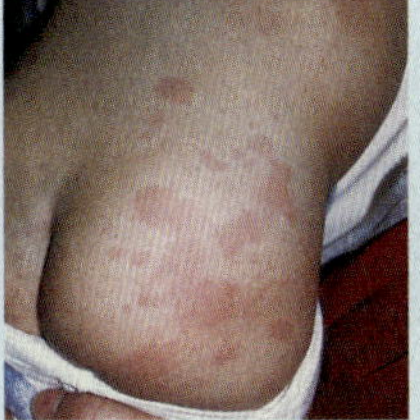

Urticaria (Hives)
This pruritic, allergic sensitivity reaction changes shape quickly.

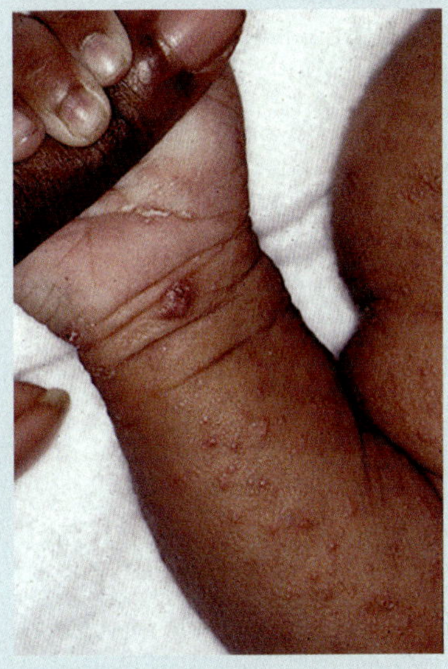

Scabies
Intensely itchy papules and vesicles, sometimes burrows, most often on extremities.

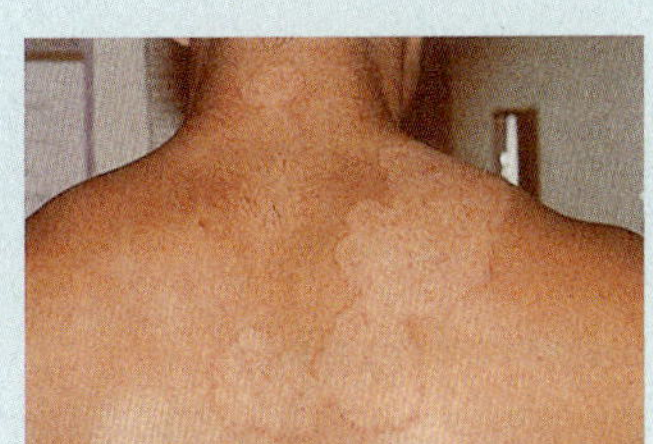

Tinea Corporis
This annular lesion has central clearing and papules along the border.

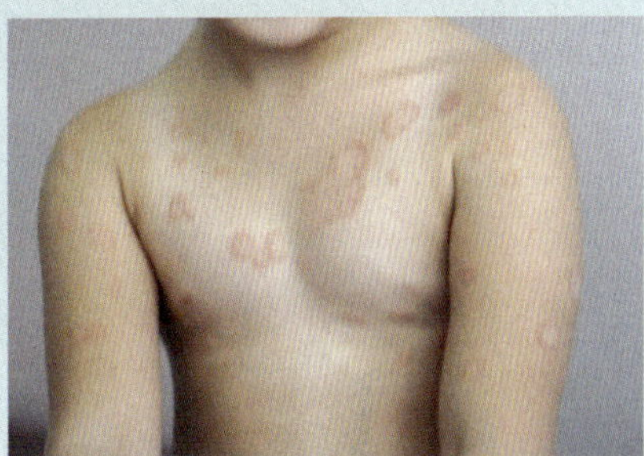

Pityriasis Rosea
Oval lesions on trunk, in older children, often in a "Christmas-tree" pattern, sometimes a herald patch (large patch that appears first).

Sources of photos: *Bites*, *Tinea Capitis*, and *Tinea Corporis*—Reprinted with permission from Goodheart HP, Gonzalez ME. *Goodheart's Photoguide to Common Pediatric and Adult Skin Disorders*. 4th ed. Wolters Kluwer; 2016. Figures 9-11, 18-8, and 29-2; *Urticaria*—Reprinted with permission from Chung EK, Atkinson-McEvoy LR, Lai NL, Terry M. *Visual Diagnosis and Treatment in Pediatrics*. 3rd ed. Wolters Kluwer; 2015. Figure 64-1; *Scabies*—Courtesy of Ronald W. Cotliar, MD; *Pityriasis Rosea*—Reprinted with permission from Salimpour RR, Salimpour P, Salimpour P. *Photographic Atlas of Pediatric Disorders and Diagnosis*. Wolters Kluwer Health/Lippincott Williams & Wilkins; 2014:244.

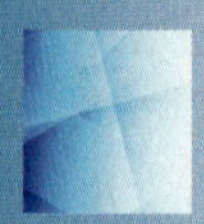

TABLE 28-6. Abnormalities of the Head

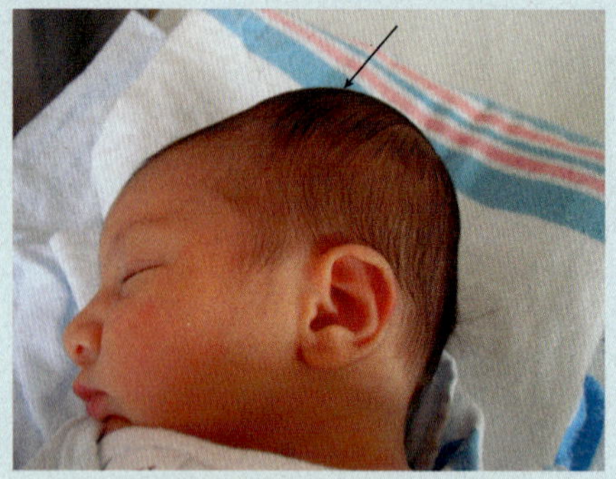

Cephalohematoma

Although not present at birth, cephalohematomas appear within the first 24 h from subperiosteal hemorrhage involving the outer table of one of the cranial bones. The swelling, shown at the *arrow,* does not extend across a suture though it is occasionally bilateral following a difficult birth. The swelling is initially soft, then develops a raised bony margin within a few days from calcium deposits at the edge of the periosteum. It tends to resolve within several weeks.

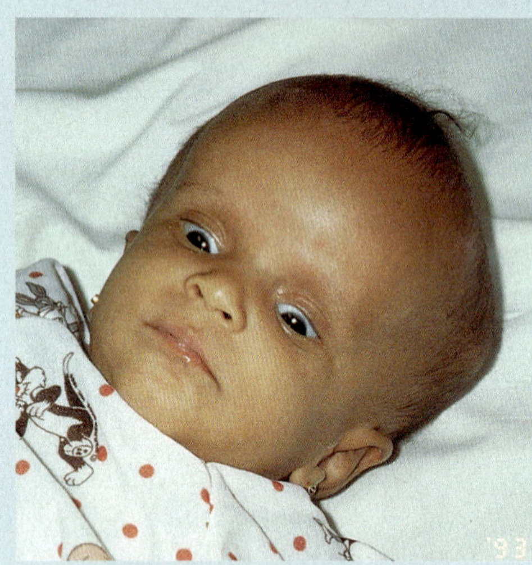

Hydrocephalus

In hydrocephaly, the anterior fontanelle is bulging, and the eyes may be deviated downward revealing the upper sclerae and creating the *setting sun* sign, as shown on the left.

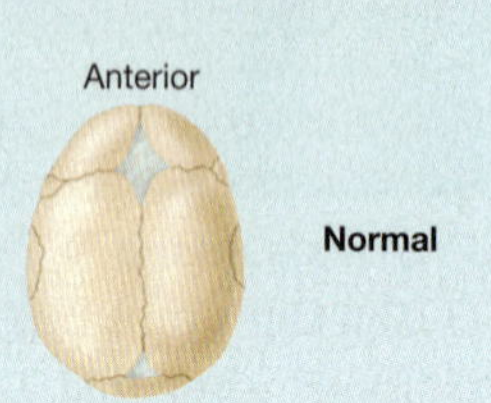

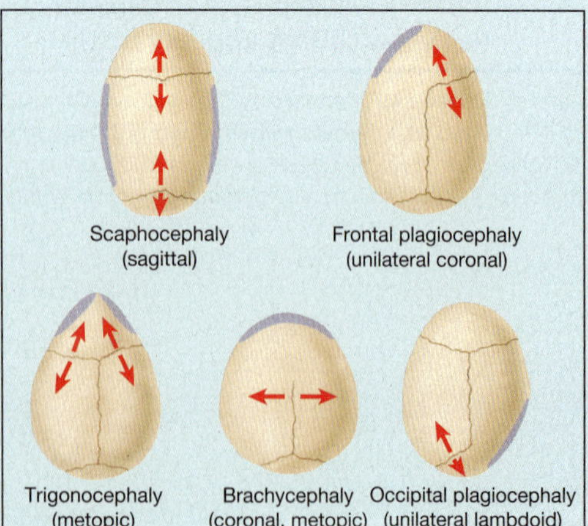

Craniosynostosis

Craniosynostosis is a condition of premature closure of one or more sutures of the skull. This results in an abnormal growth and shape of the skull because growth will occur across sutures that are not affected but not across sutures that are affected.

The figures demonstrate different skull shapes associated with the various types of craniosynostosis. The prematurely closed suture line is noted by the absence of a suture line in each figure. Scaphocephaly and frontal plagiocephaly are the most common forms of craniosynostosis. The *blue shading* shows areas of maximal flattening. The *red arrows* show the direction of continued growth across the sutures, which is normal.

Sources of photos: *Cephalohematoma*—Reprinted with permission from Chung EK, Atkinson-McEvoy LR, Lai NL, Terry M. *Visual Diagnosis and Treatment in Pediatrics*. 3rd ed. Wolters Kluwer; 2015. Figure 2-6; *Hydrocephalus*—Reprinted with permission from Fleisher GR, Ludwig W, Baskin MN. *Atlas of Pediatric Emergency Medicine*. Lippincott Williams & Wilkins; 2004. Figure 14.4.

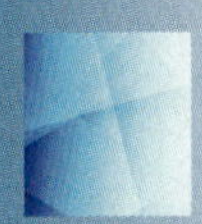

TABLE 28-7. Diagnostic Facies in Infancy and Childhood

Fetal Alcohol Syndrome

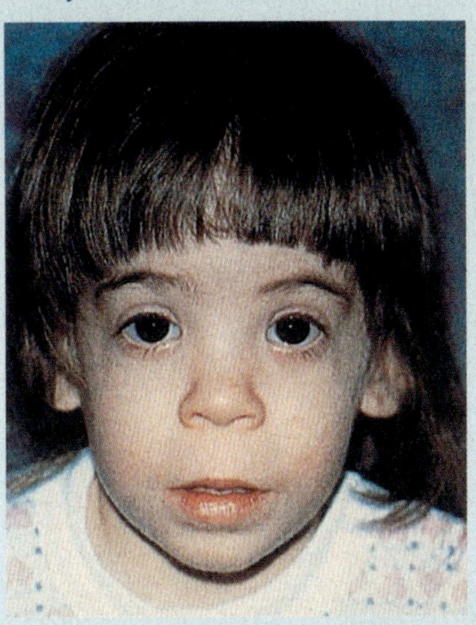

Infants born to individuals with alcohol use disorder are at risk for growth deficiency, microcephaly, and intellectual disability. Facial features include short palpebral fissures, a wide and flattened philtrum, and thin lips.

Congenital Hypothyroidism

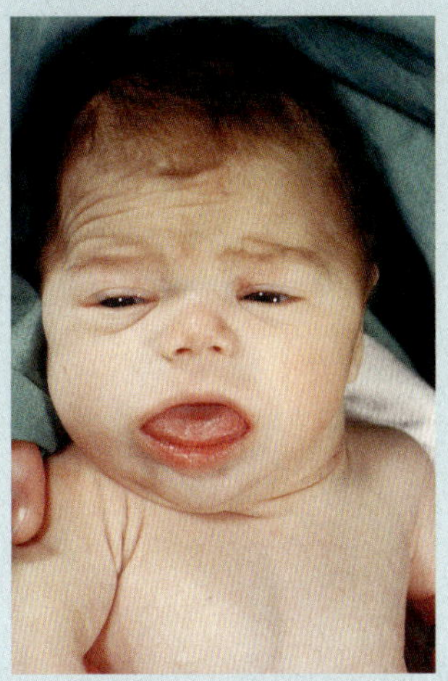

Children with congenital hypothyroidism often have distinct facial features, a low-set hairline, sparse eyebrows, and an enlarged tongue. Other signs include a hoarse cry, umbilical hernia, dry and cold extremities, myxedema, mottled skin, and intellectual disability. As most infants with congenital hypothyroidism show no physical signs, newborn screening is common.

Congenital Syphilis

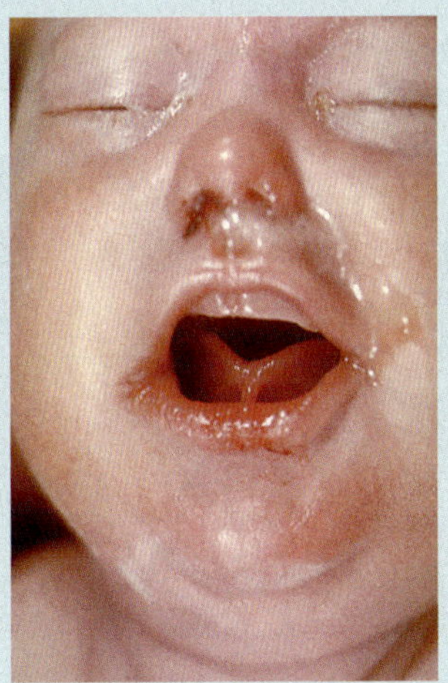

In utero infection by *Treponema pallidum* after week 16 of gestation affects nearly all fetal organs and has a high mortality rate if untreated. Surviving infants show signs within the first month, including frontal bone bulging, saddle nose, snuffles, circumoral rash, rhagades, saber shins, and Hutchinson teeth (see p. 413).

Facial Nerve Palsy

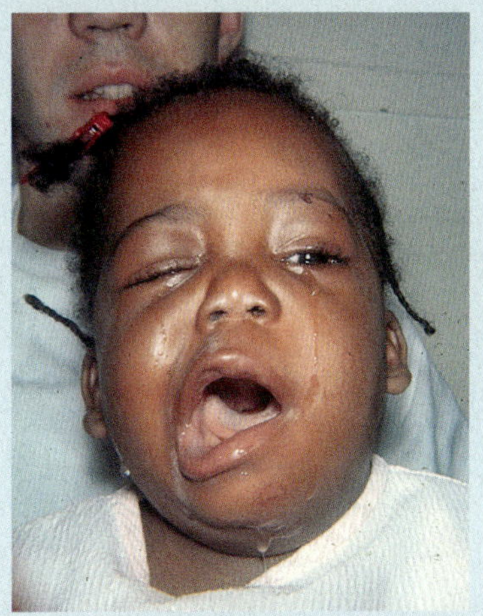

Peripheral facial nerve paralysis can result from birth injury, otitis media, or unknown causes (Bell palsy). Signs include a flattened nasolabial fold and an inability to close the eye on the affected side, which is accentuated during crying. Most children fully recover.

(*continued*)

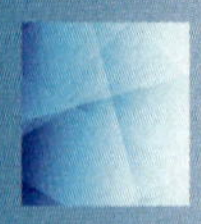

TABLE 28-7. Diagnostic Facies in Infancy and Childhood *(Continued)*

Down Syndrome

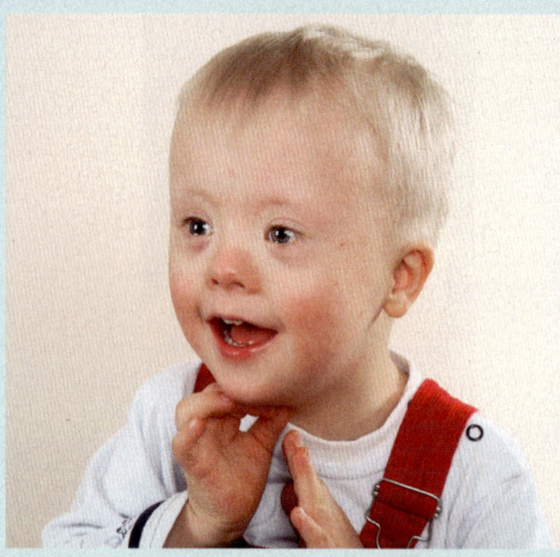

Children with Down syndrome (trisomy 21) typically have a small, rounded head, flattened nasal bridge, oblique palpebral fissures, prominent epicanthal folds, small low-set ears, and a large tongue. Associated features include hypotonia, transverse palmar creases, incurving of the fifth fingers (*clinodactyly*), Brushfield spots (see p. 1109), and cognitive impairment.

Nonaccidental Trauma

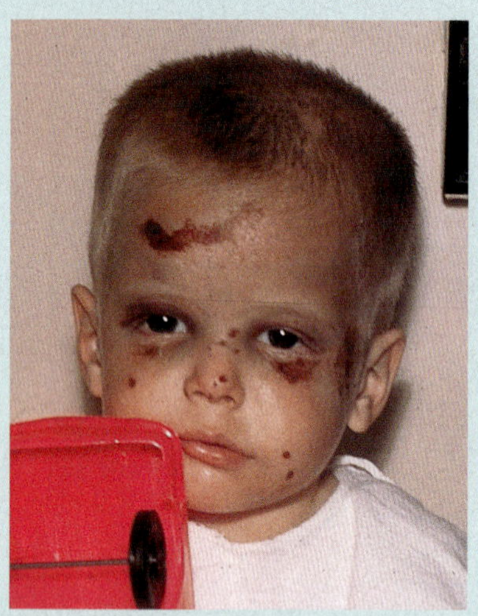

Physically abused children may show *old and new bruises* on the head and face, bruises in unusual locations (e.g., axilla, groin), fractures at different healing stages, and skin lesions that match the shape of the implements used (e.g., hand, belt buckle, rope, cigarette).

Perennial Allergic Rhinitis

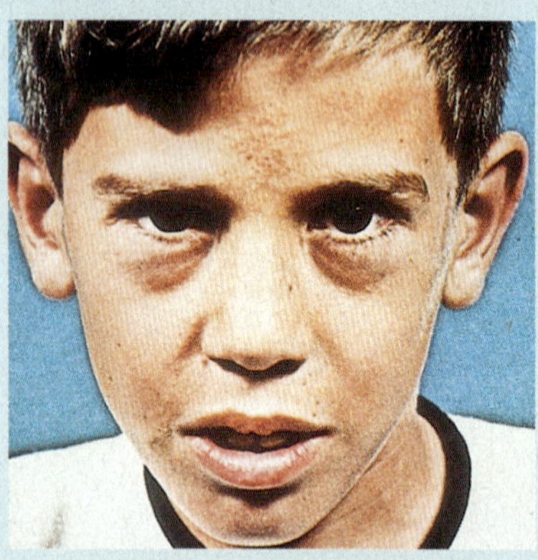

Children with perennial allergic rhinitis often breathe through their mouths and have edema and darkening under the eyes ("allergic shiners"). They may also exhibit the "allergic salute" (pushing the nose upward) and grimacing due to nasal itching and obstruction.

Hyperthyroidism

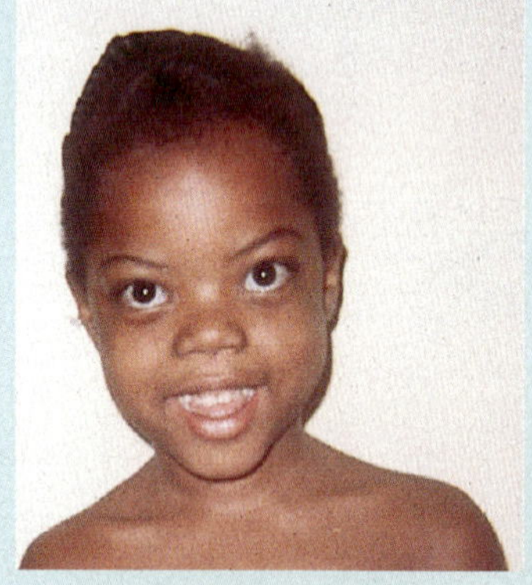

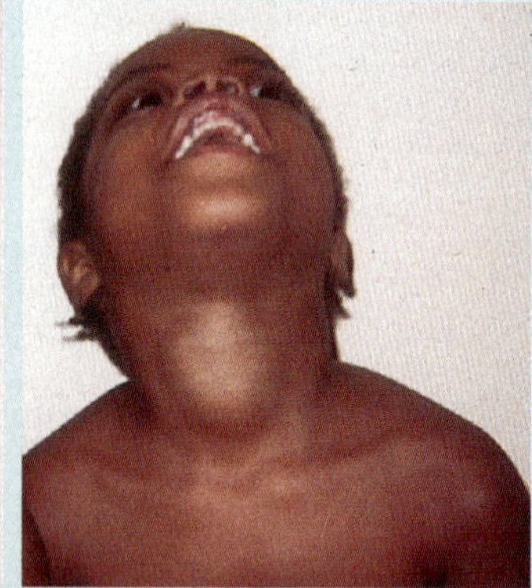

Thyrotoxicosis (Graves disease) affects about 2 per 1,000 children under 10 years old. Symptoms include tachycardia, hypermetabolism, and accelerated growth. Facial characteristics in affected children include "staring" eyes and goiter.

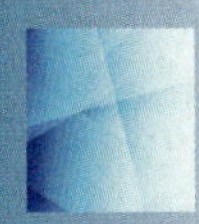

TABLE 28-8. Abnormalities of the Eyes, Ears, and Mouth

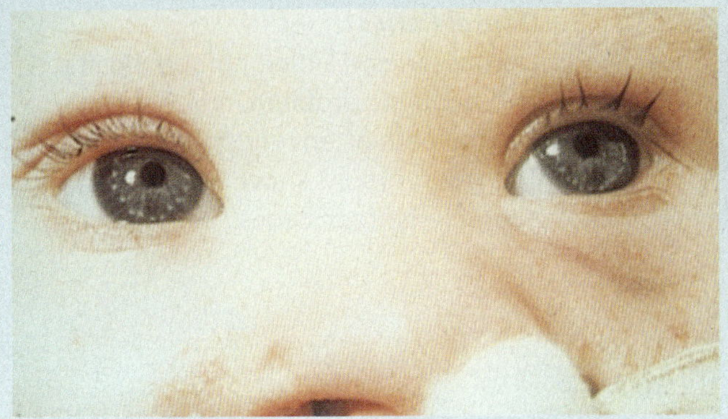

Brushfield Spots

These abnormal speckling spots on the iris suggest Down syndrome.

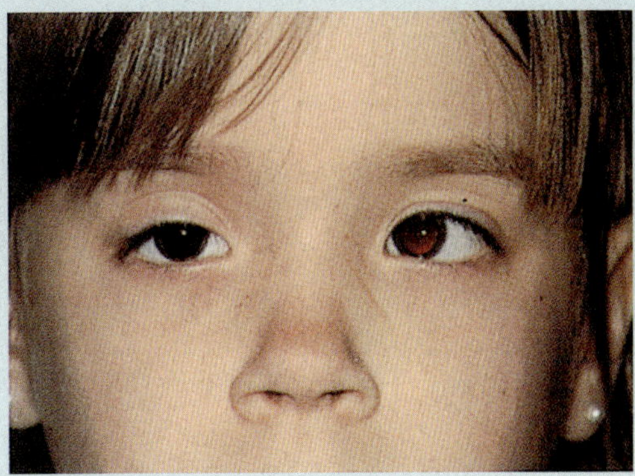

Strabismus

Strabismus, or misalignment of the eyes, can lead to visual impairment. Esotropia, shown here, is an inward deviation.

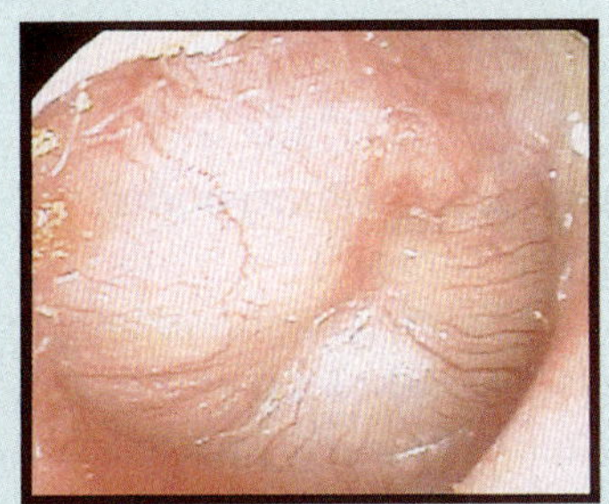

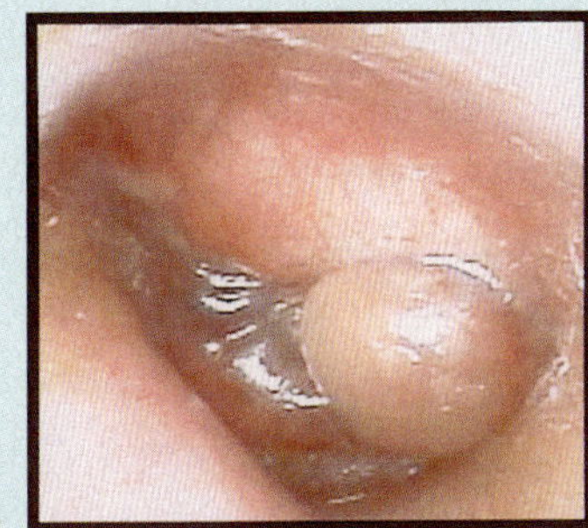

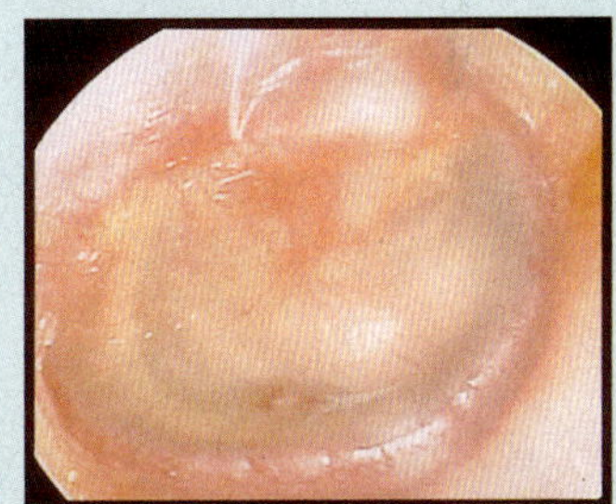

Otitis Media

Otitis media is one of the most common conditions in young children. The spectrum of otitis media is shown here. **A:** Typical acute otitis media with a red, distorted, bulging tympanic membrane in a highly symptomatic child. **B:** Acute otitis media with bullae formation and fluid visible behind the tympanic membrane. **C:** Otitis media with effusion, showing a yellowish fluid behind a retracted and thickened tympanic membrane. Often you can no longer visualize the normal landmarks such as the light reflex and handle of the malleus.

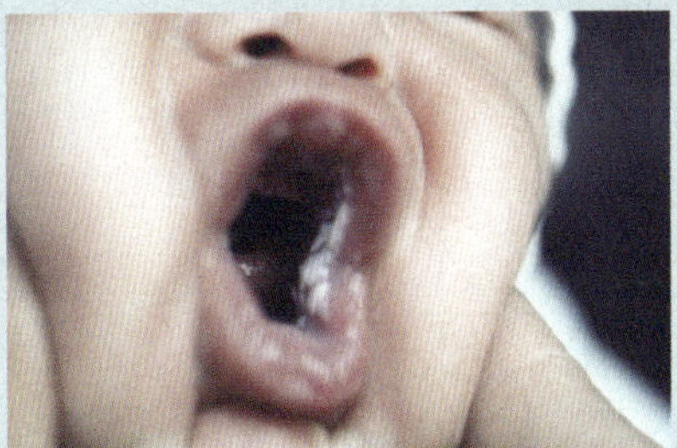

Oral Candidiasis ("Thrush")

This infection is common in infants. The white plaques do not rub off.

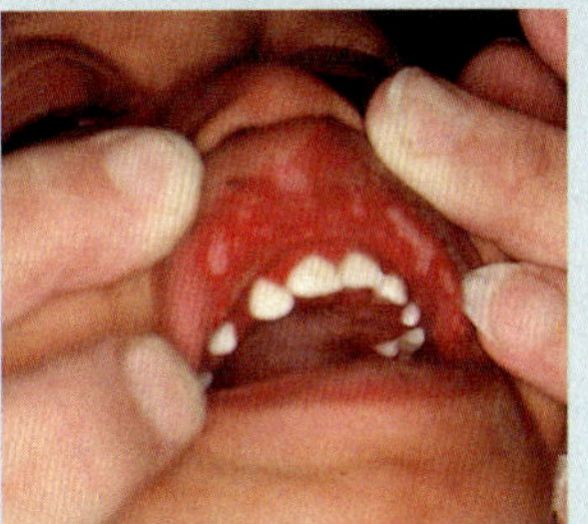

Herpetic Stomatitis

Tender ulcerations on the oral mucosa are surrounded by erythema.

Sources of photos: *Otitis Media*—Courtesy of Alejandro Hoberman, Children's Hospital of Pittsburgh, University of Pittsburgh; *Thrush*—Reprinted with permission from Salimpour RR, Salimpour P, Salimpour P. *Photographic Atlas of Pediatric Disorders and Diagnosis.* Wolters Kluwer Health/Lippincott Williams & Wilkins; 2014:304; *Herpetic Stomatitis*—Reprinted with permission from Fleisher GR, Ludwig W, Baskin MN. *Atlas of Pediatric Emergency Medicine.* Lippincott Williams & Wilkins; 2004. Figure 11-7B.

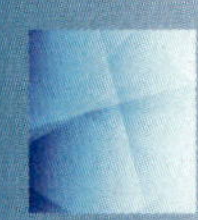

TABLE 28-9. Abnormalities of the Teeth, Pharynx, and Neck

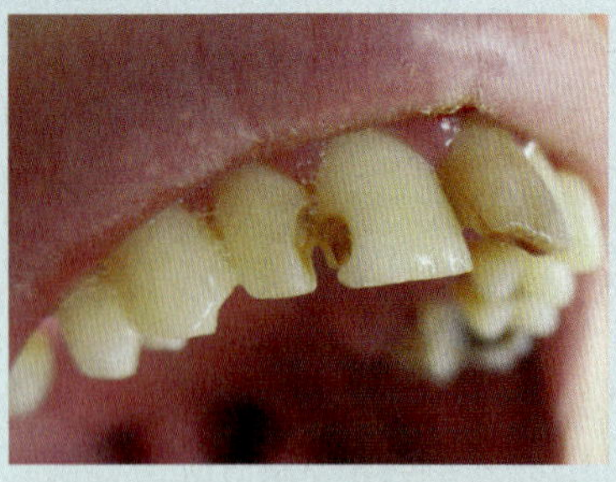

Dental caries (early childhood caries [ECC])

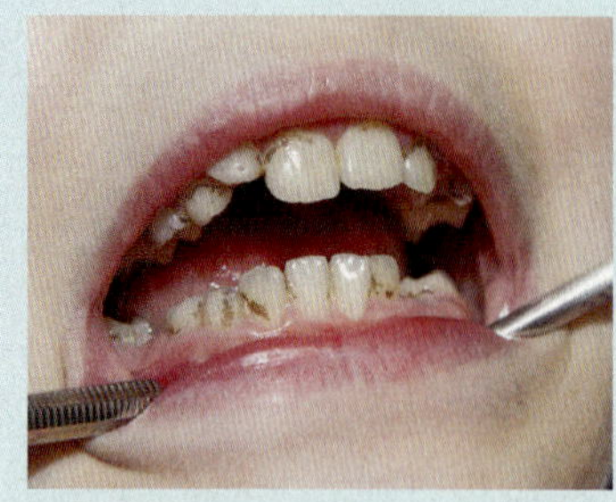

Severe ECC

Dental Caries

Dental caries is a major global health and pediatric problem. White spots on the teeth often reflect early caries. The photographs show different characteristics of caries.

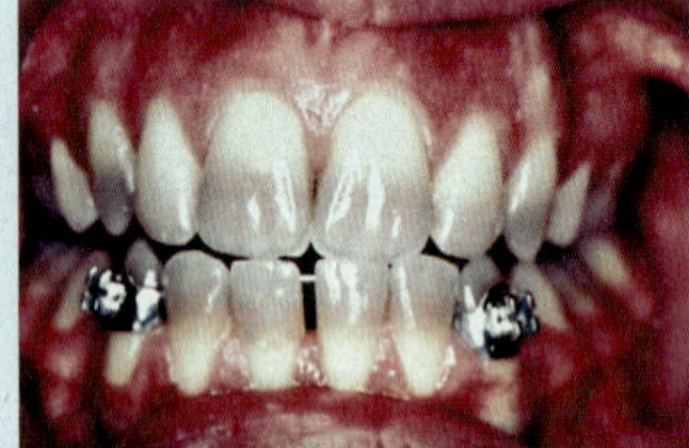

Staining of the Teeth

Various causes can lead to staining of the teeth of children, including intrinsic stains such as tetracycline (*left*) or extrinsic stains such as poor oral hygiene (carious lesions shown in previous figures). Extrinsic stains can be removed.

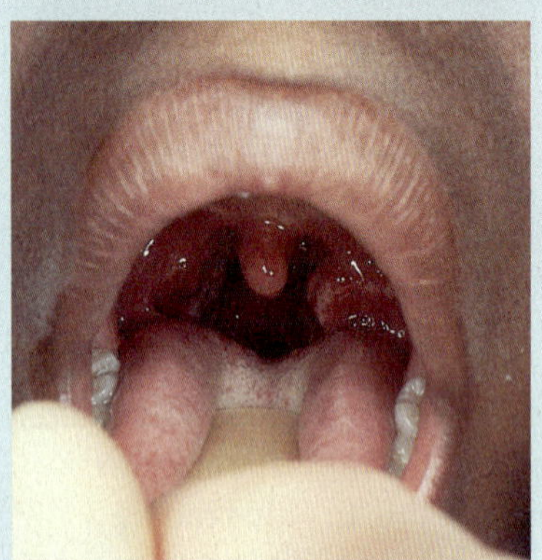

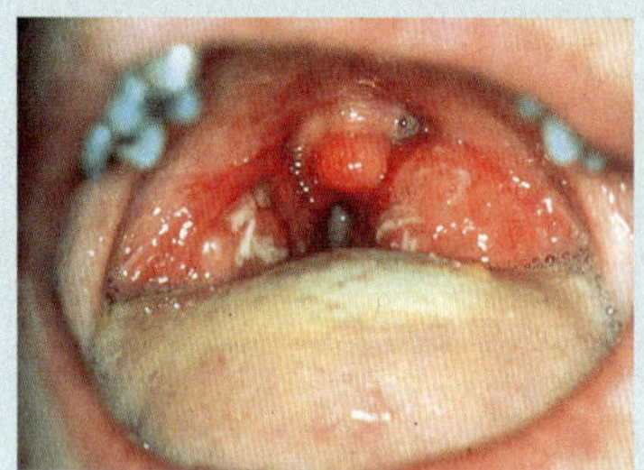

Streptococcal Pharyngitis ("Strep Throat")

This common childhood infection has a classic presentation of erythema of the posterior pharynx and palatal petechiae. A foul-smelling exudate is also commonly noted.

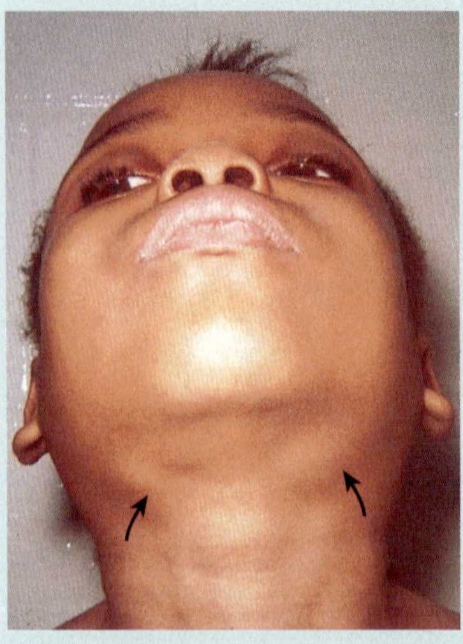

Lymphadenopathy

Enlarged and tender cervical lymph nodes are common in children. The most likely causes are viral and bacterial infections. Lymph node enlargement can be bilateral (*left*).

Sources of photos: *Dental Caries*—Reprinted with permission from Sherman SC, Cico SJ, Nordquist E, Ross C, Wang E. *Atlas of Clinical Emergency Medicine*. Wolters Kluwer; 2016. Figure 5-6; *Staining of the Teeth*—Used with permission from Shutterstock. By Maliutina Anna.

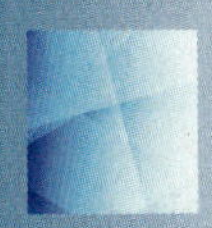

TABLE 28-10. Cyanosis in Children

It is important to recognize cyanosis. The best location to examine is the mucous membranes. Cyanosis is a "raspberry" color, whereas normal mucous membranes should have a "strawberry" color. Try to identify the cyanosis in these photographs before reading the captions.

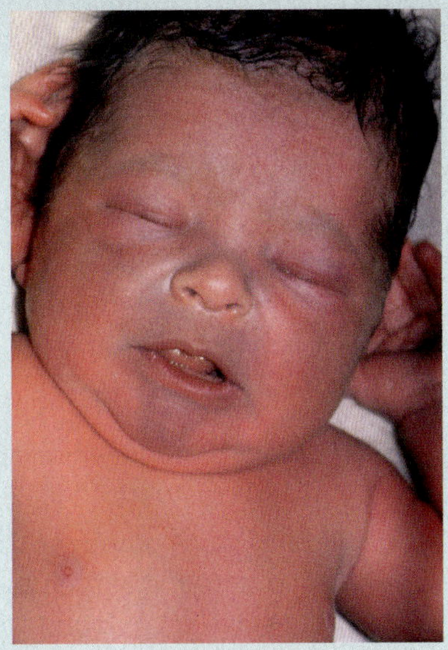

Generalized Cyanosis
This infant has total anomalous pulmonary venous return and an oxygen saturation level of 80%.

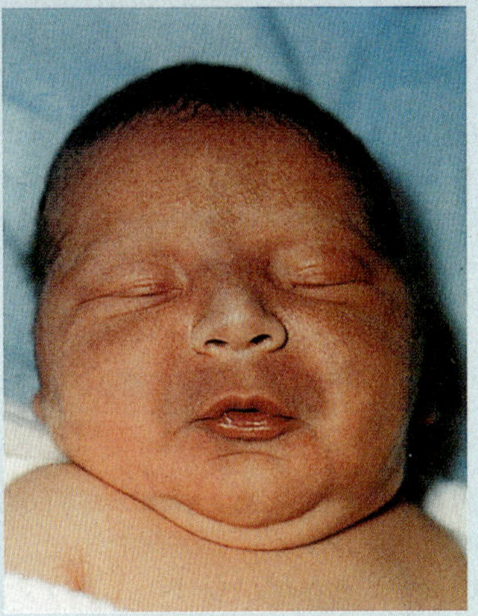

Perioral Cyanosis
This infant has mild cyanosis above the lips, but the mucous membranes remain pink.

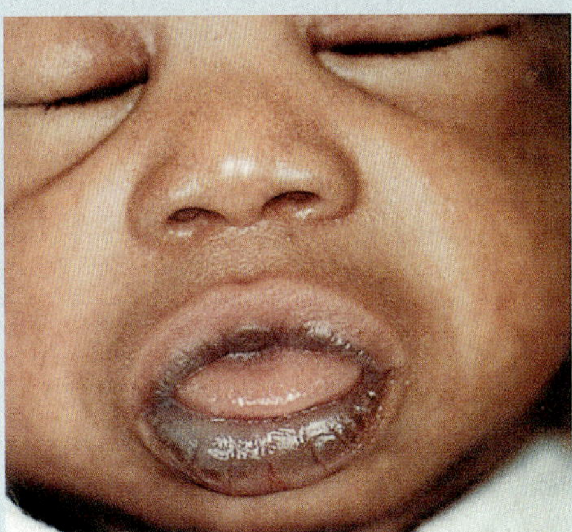

Bluish Lips, Giving Appearance of Cyanosis
Normal pigment deposition in the vermilion border of the lips gives them a bluish hue, but the mucous membranes are pink.

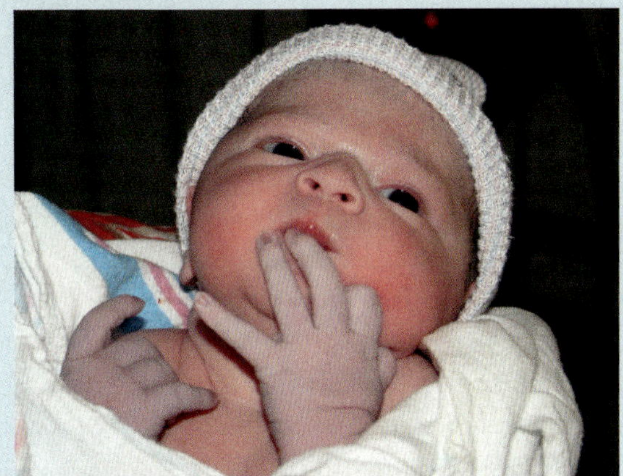

Acrocyanosis
A newborn with acrocyanosis, evident as bluish discoloration of the hands and fingers, while the face and lips remain pink. This is a normal finding in the first 24–48 hours of life due to immature peripheral circulation.

Sources of photos: *Perioral Cyanosis, Bluish Lips, Giving Appearance of Cyanosis*—Reprinted with permission from Fletcher MA. *Physical Diagnosis in Neonatology*. Lippincott-Raven; 1998; *Acrocyanosis*—Reprinted with permission from Kyle T, Carman S. *Essentials of Pediatric Nursing*. 3rd ed. Wolters Kluwer; 2017.

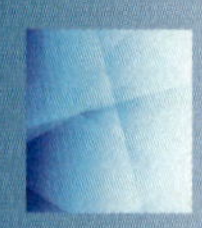

TABLE 28-11. Congenital Heart Murmurs

Some heart murmurs reflect underlying heart disease. If you understand their physiologic causes, you will more readily be able to identify and distinguish them from innocent heart murmurs. Obstructive lesions result when blood flows through under-sized valves or narrowed vessels. Because this problem does not depend on the drop in pulmonary vascular resistance following birth, these murmurs are audible at birth. Defects with left-to-right shunts, on the other hand, depend on the drop in pulmonary vascular resistance that occurs shortly after birth. High-pressured shunts such as ventricular septal defect, patent ductus arteriosus, and persistent truncus arteriosus may not be heard until ≥1 wk after birth; the murmur gets louder as peripheral vascular resistance drops. Low-pressured left-to-right shunts, such as atrial septal defects, may not be heard until age ≥1 y. Many children with congenital cardiac defects have combinations of defects or variations of abnormalities, so findings on cardiac examination may not follow these classic patterns. This table shows a limited selection of the more common murmurs, starting with murmurs that appear in the newborn period.

Congenital Defect and Mechanism	Characteristics of the Murmur	Associated Findings
Pulmonary Valve Stenosis		
Usually a normal valve annulus with fusion of some or most of the valve leaflets, restricting flow across the valve ***Mild*** ***Severe*** 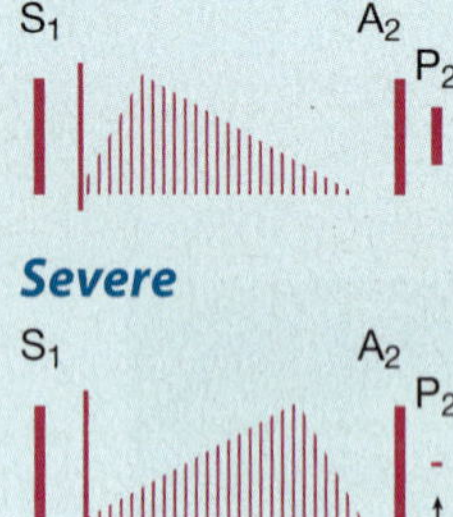 	*Location.* Upper left sternal border *Radiation.* In mild degrees of stenosis, the murmur may be heard over the course of the pulmonary arteries in the lung fields *Intensity.* Increases in intensity and duration as the degree of obstruction increases *Quality.* Ejection, peaking later in systole as the obstruction increases	Usually a prominent ejection click in early systole Pulmonary component of the second sound at the base (P_2) becomes delayed and softer, disappearing as obstruction increases; inspiration may increase murmur; expiration may increase click Growth usually normal Newborns with severe stenosis may be cyanotic from right-to-left atrial shunting and rapidly develop heart failure as the ductus arteriosus closes
Aortic Valve Stenosis		
Usually a bicuspid valve with progressive obstruction, but may occur as a result of a dysplastic valve or damage from rheumatic fever or degenerative disease 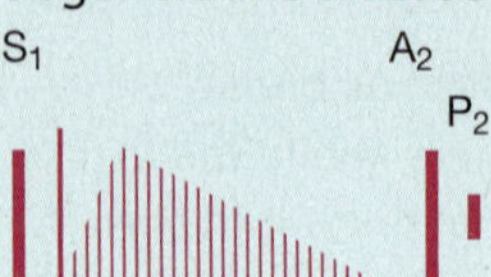 	*Location.* Midsternum, upper right sternal border *Radiation.* To the carotid arteries and suprasternal notch; may also be a thrill *Intensity.* Varies, louder with increasingly severe obstruction *Quality.* An ejection, often harsh, systolic murmur	May be an associated ejection click Aortic closure sound may be increased in intensity; a diastolic murmur of aortic valve regurgitation (not shown in the diagram) may be present; newborns with severe stenosis may have weak or absent pulses and severe heart failure; may not be audible until adulthood even though the valve is congenitally abnormal

Congenital Defect and Mechanism	Characteristics of the Murmur	Associated Findings
Tetralogy of Fallot Complex defect with ventricular septal defect (VSD), infundibular and usually valvular right ventricular outflow obstruction, malrotation of the aorta, and right-to-left shunting at ventricular septal level *With Pulmonic Stenosis* 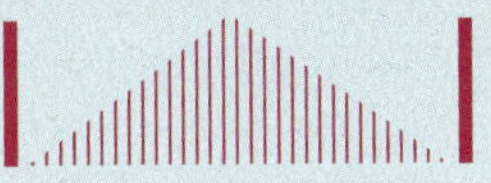 *With Pulmonic Atresia* 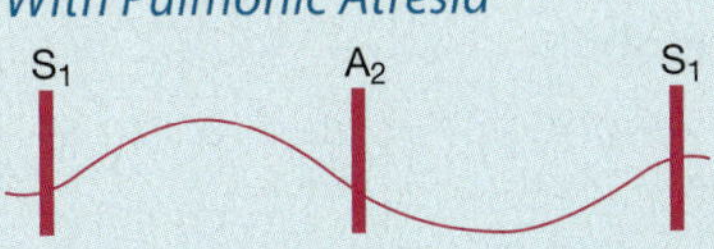	*General.* Variable cyanosis, increasing with activity *Location.* Mid-to-upper left sternal border; if pulmonary atresia, the continuous murmur of ductus arteriosus flow at upper left sternal border or in the back *Radiation.* Little, to upper left sternal border, occasionally to lung fields *Intensity.* Usually grade III–IV *Quality.* Systolic ejection murmur	Normal pulses Pulmonary closure sound usually not heard; may have abrupt hypercyanotic spells with sudden increase in cyanosis, air hunger, altered level of awareness Failure to gain weight with persistent and increasingly severe cyanosis Long-term persistence of cyanosis accompanied by clubbing of fingers and toes Persistent hypoxemia leads to polycythemia (accentuates cyanosis)
Transposition of the Great Arteries Severe defect with failure of rotation of the great vessels, leaving the aorta to arise from the right ventricle (RV) and the pulmonary artery from the left ventricle (LV)	*General.* Intense generalized cyanosis *Location.* No characteristic murmur; if present, it may reflect an associated defect such as VSD *Radiation and Quality.* Depends on associated abnormalities	Single loud second sound of the anterior aortic valve Frequent rapid development of heart failure Frequent associated defects as described at left
Ventricular Septal Defect Blood going from a high-pressure LV through a defect in the septum to the lower-pressure RV creates turbulence, usually throughout systole *Small to Moderate* 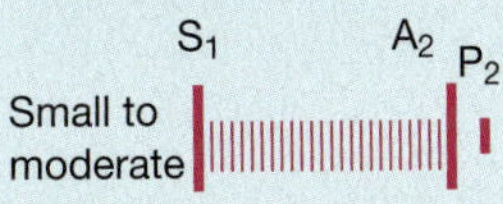	*Location.* Lower left sternal border *Radiation.* Little *Intensity.* Variable, only partially determined by the size of the shunt; small shunts with a high-pressure gradient may have very loud murmurs; large defects with elevated pulmonary vascular resistance may have no murmur; grade II–IV/VI with a thrill if grade IV/VI or higher *Quality.* Pansystolic, usually harsh, may obscure S_1 and S_2 if loud enough	With large shunts, a low-pitched middiastolic murmur of relative mitral stenosis may be heard at the apex As pulmonary artery pressure increases, pulmonic component of the second sounds at the base increases in intensity; when pulmonary artery pressure equals aortic pressure there may be no murmur and P_2 will be very loud In low-volume shunts, growth is normal In larger shunts, heart failure may occur by 6–8 wk; poor weight gain, poor feeding Associated defects are frequent

(*continued*)

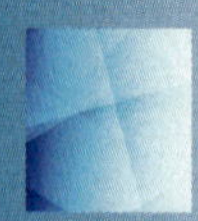

TABLE 28-11. Congenital Heart Murmurs *(Continued)*

Congenital Defect and Mechanism	Characteristics of the Murmur	Associated Findings
Patent Ductus Arteriosus Continuous flow from aorta to pulmonary artery throughout the cardiac cycle when ductus arteriosus does not close after birth *Small to Moderate* 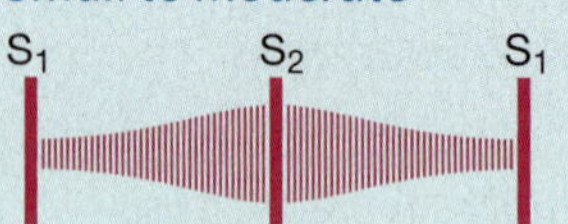 	*Location.* Upper left sternal border and to left *Radiation.* Sometimes to the back *Intensity.* Varies depending on size of the shunt, usually grade II–III/VI *Quality.* Hollow, sometimes machinery-like murmur continuous throughout the cardiac cycle, although occasionally almost inaudible in late diastole, uninterrupted by the heart sounds, louder in systole	Full to bounding pulses Noticed at birth in the premature infant who may have bounding pulses, a hyperdynamic precordium, and an atypical murmur Noticed later in the full-term infant as pulmonary vascular resistance falls May develop heart failure at 4–6 wk if large shunt Poor weight gain related to size of shunt Pulmonary hypertension affects murmur as above
Atrial Septal Defect Left-to-right shunt through an opening in the atrial septum, possible at various levels 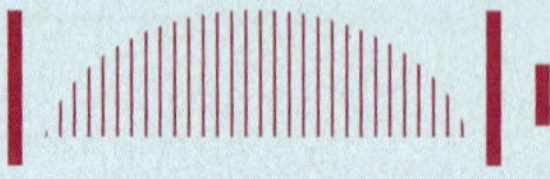 	*Location.* Upper left sternal border *Radiation.* To the back *Intensity.* Variable, usually grade II–III/VI *Quality.* Ejection but without the harsh quality	Widely split S_2 throughout all phases of respiration, normal intensity Usually not heard until >1 y Gradual decrease in weight gain as shunt increases Decreased exercise tolerance, subtle, not dramatic Heart failure is rare

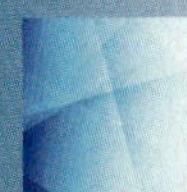

TABLE 28-12. Common Abnormalities in the Genitourinary Anatomy Associated with Testes and Penises

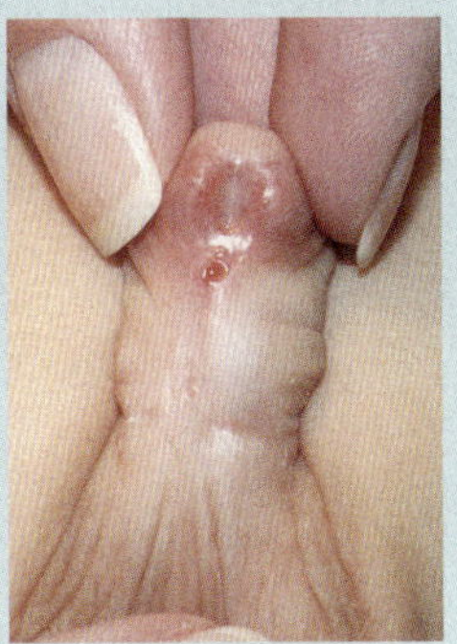

Hypospadias

Hypospadias is the most common congenital penile abnormality. The urethral meatus opens abnormally on the ventral surface of the penis. One form is shown; more severe forms involve openings on the lower shaft or scrotum.

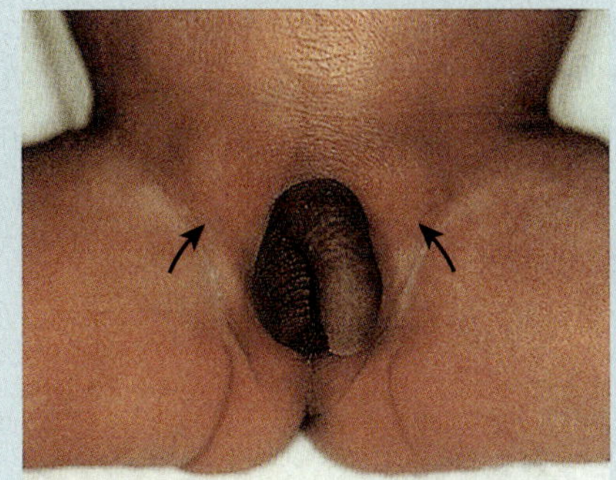

Undescended Testicle

Distinguish between undescended testes (with testes in the inguinal canals—see *arrows*), from highly retractile testes from an active cremasteric reflex.

Sources of photos: *Hypospadias*—Courtesy of Warren Snodgrass, MD, Hypospadias Specialty Center; *Undescended Testicle*—Reprinted with permission from Fletcher MA. *Physical Diagnosis in Neonatology*. Lippincott-Raven; 1998.

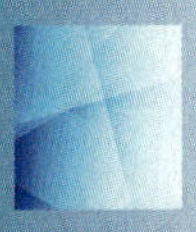

TABLE 28-13. Common Musculoskeletal Findings in Young Children

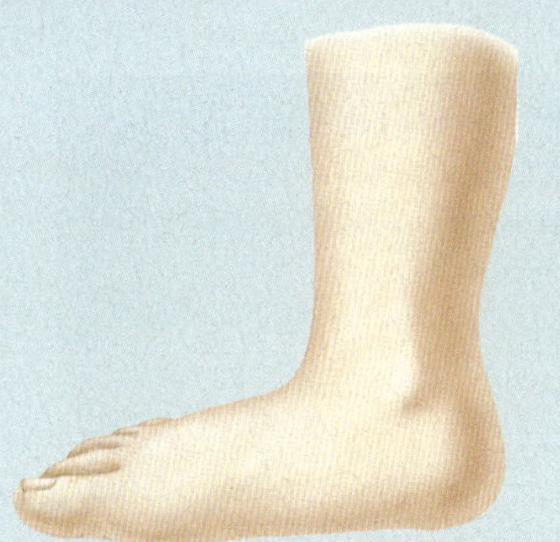

Flat feet or *pes planus* from laxity of the soft tissue structures of the foot

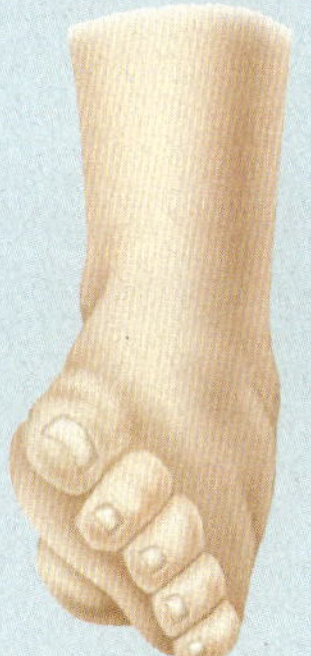

Inversion of the foot (*varus*)

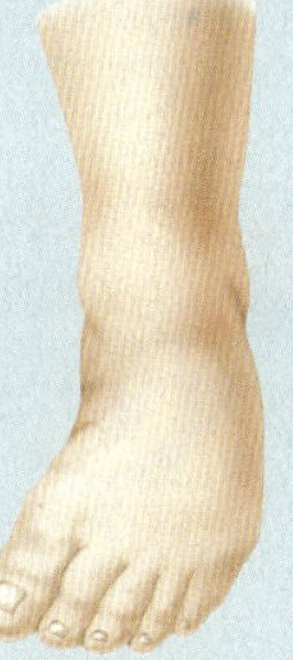

Metatarsus adductus; the forefoot is adducted and not inverted

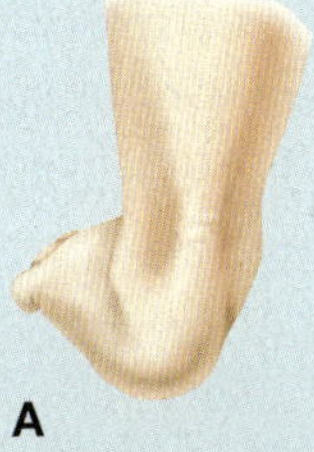

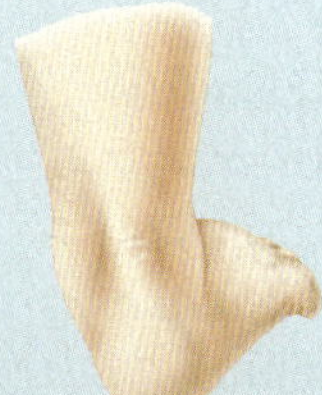

A

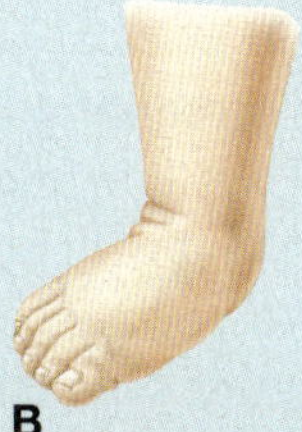

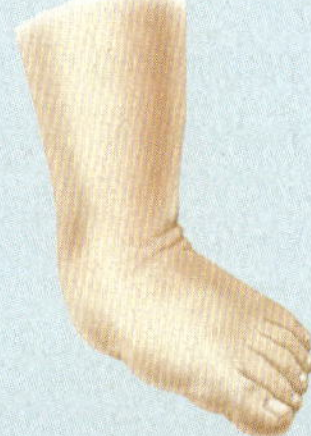

B

Pronation. **A:** When viewed from behind, hindfoot is everted. **B:** When viewed from the front, forefoot is everted and abducted.

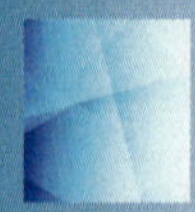

TABLE 28-14. Power of Prevention: Vaccine-Preventable Diseases

Childhood vaccines have been named the single most important clinical intervention in the world in terms of influence on public health. Because of vaccinations, we hope you will never see many of these conditions, but you should be able to identify them. Try to identify the diseases before reading the captions.

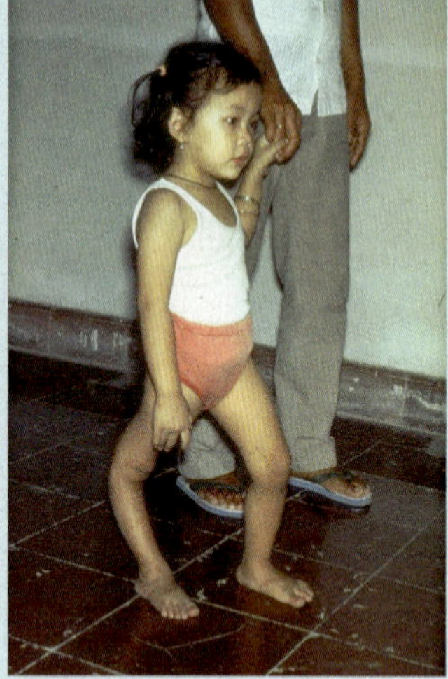

Polio
Child with residual paralysis and muscle atrophy of the lower limb, characteristic of post-polio syndrome, a sequela of poliomyelitis.

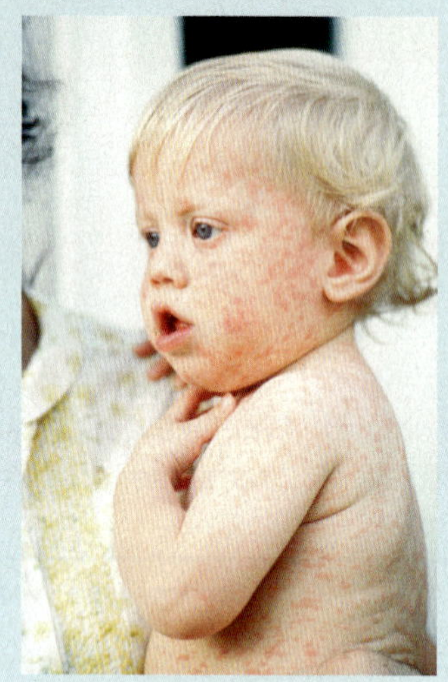

Measles
Child with a widespread maculopapular rash characteristic of measles (rubeola), accompanied by conjunctivitis and respiratory symptoms, which are hallmark features of the disease.

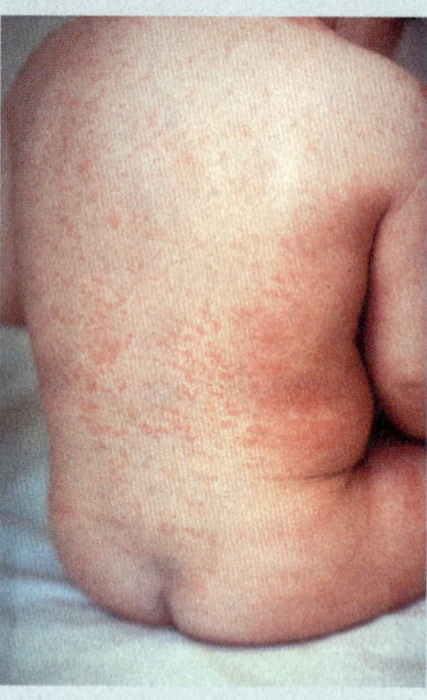

Rubella
Infant with a fine, pink maculopapular rash characteristic of rubella, beginning on the face and spreading to the trunk and extremities.

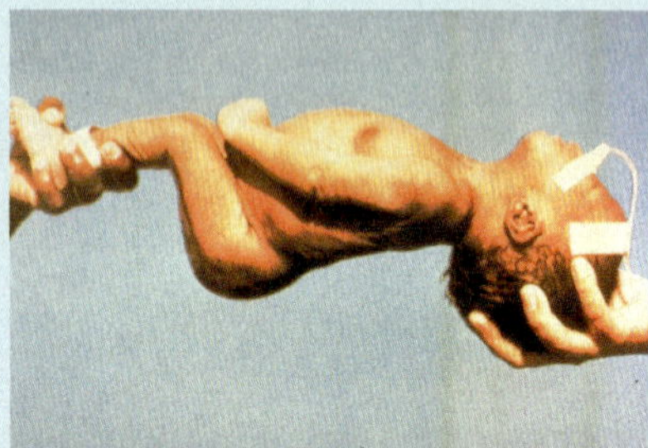

Tetanus
Neonate with severe opisthotonos due to neonatal tetanus, characterized by generalized muscle rigidity and arching of the back, a hallmark of tetanus infection.

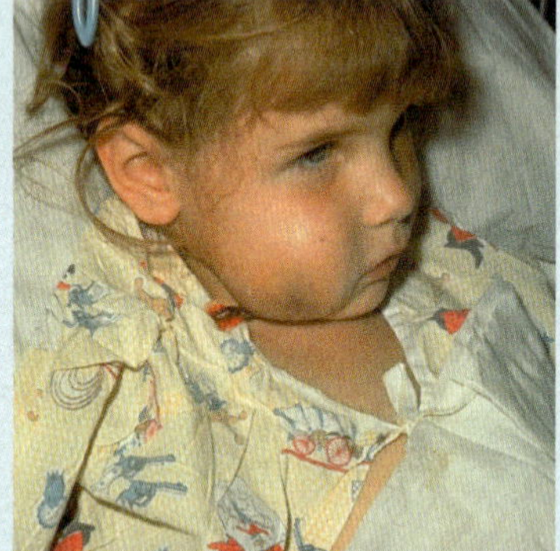

***Haemophilus Influenzae* Type b**
Child presenting with unilateral facial swelling and erythema consistent with buccal cellulitis, often associated with *Haemophilus influenzae* type b infection.

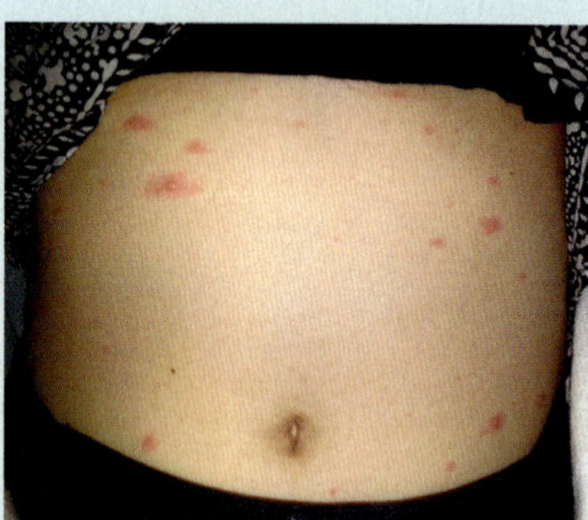

Varicella
Abdomen displaying classic vesicular lesions in various stages of healing, characteristic of varicella (chickenpox).

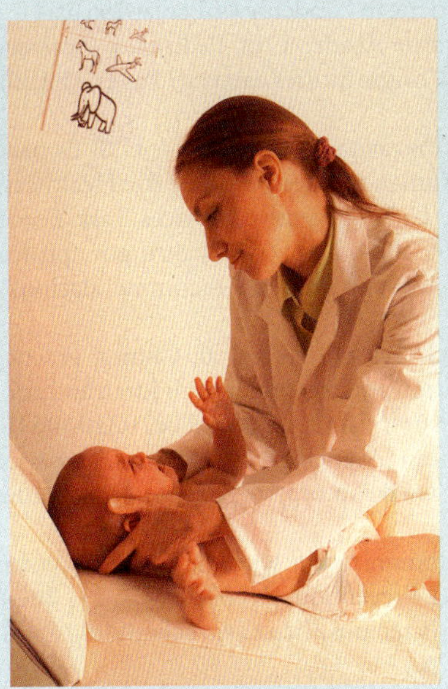

Meningococcemia
Clinician assessing an infant for nuchal rigidity, a key sign of meningitis, which can result from meningococcemia.

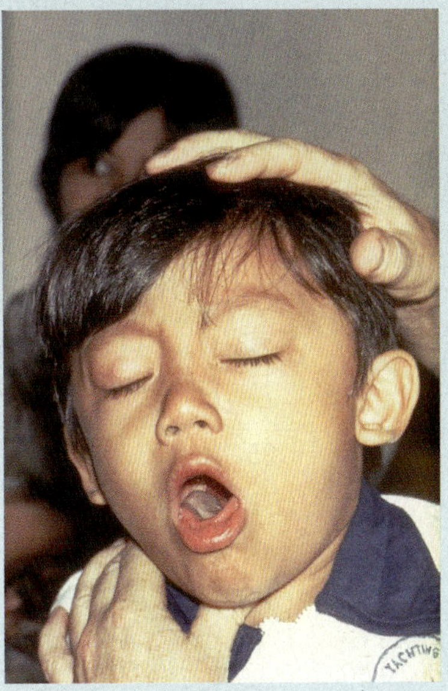

Pertussis
Child exhibiting a paroxysmal coughing episode characteristic of pertussis (whooping cough), often followed by a high-pitched 'whoop' sound during inspiration.

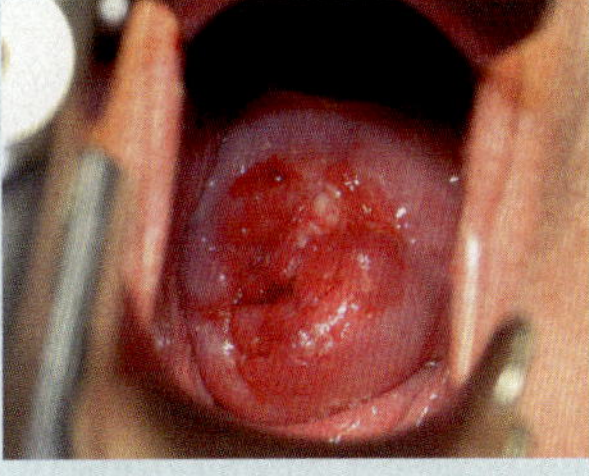

Human papillomavirus (HPV)
HPV-associated lesions in the cervix (top) and oropharynx (bottom). These images demonstrate the widespread impact of HPV infection, contributing to cancers in both the anogenital region and the head and neck. Vaccination is critical for preventing HPV-related malignancies.

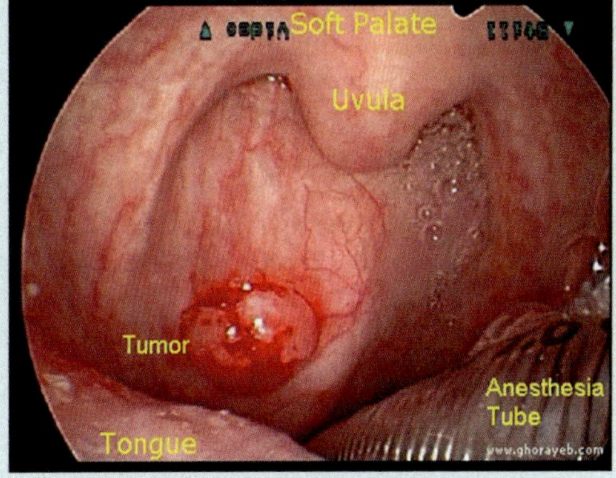

Oropharyngeal Cancer. Sequela of HPV

Sources of photos: *Polio*—Courtesy of World Health Organization; *Haemophilus influenzae*—Courtesy of Children's Immunization Project, St. Paul, Minnesota; *Tetanus*—Courtesy of Centers for Disease Control and Prevention. *Pertussis*—Courtesy of Centers for Disease Control and Prevention; *Varicella*—Reprinted with permission from Kaffenberger J, Flowers RH, Zlotoff BJ, Wick MR. Cutaneous viral infections. In: Gru AA, Wick MR, Mir A, Zlotoff B, Dehner LP, eds. *Pediatric Dermatopathology and Dermatology*. Wolters Kluwer; 2019. Figure 19-8; *Cervical Cancer*—Reprinted with permission from Anderson DM, Lee J, Elkas JC. Cervical and vaginal cancer. In: Berek JS, ed. *Berek & Novak's Gynecology*. 16th ed. Wolters Kluwer; 2020. Figure 38-1; *Oropharyngeal Cancer*—Reprinted with permission from Béchara Y. Ghorayeb, MD, Houston, Texas.

REFERENCES

1. Carey WB, Crocker AC, Coleman WL, Elias ER, Feldman HM. *Developmental-Behavioral Pediatrics.* 4th ed. Saunders; 2009.
2. Levine MD, Carey WB, Crocker AC. *Developmental-Behavioral Pediatrics.* 3rd ed. Saunders; 1999.
3. American Academy of Pediatrics Section on developmental and behavioral pediatrics. Voigt RG, Macias MM, Myers SM, Tapia CD, eds. *Developmental and Behavioral Pediatrics.* 2nd ed. American Academy of Pediatrics; 2018.
4. Dixon SD, Stein MT. *Encounters with Children: Pediatric Behavior and Development.* 4th ed. Mosby; 2005.
5. Zubler JM, Wiggins LD, Macias MM, et al. Evidence-informed milestones for developmental surveillance tools. *Pediatrics.* 2022;149(3):e2021052138.
6. Scharf RJ, Scharf GJ, Stroustrup A. Developmental milestones. *Pediatr Rev.* 2016;37(1):25–37; quiz 38, 47.
7. Rydz D, Shevell MI, Majnemer A, Oskoui M. Developmental screening. *J Child Neurol.* 2005;20(1):4–21.
8. Squires J, Nickel RE, Eisert D. Early detection of developmental problems: strategies for monitoring young children in the practice setting. *J Dev Behav Pediatr.* 1996;17(6):420–427.
9. Gilbride KE. Developmental testing. *Pediatr Rev.* 1995;16(9):338–345.
10. Wolraich ML, ed. *Disorders of Development and Learning.* 3rd ed. BC Decker; 2003.
11. First LR, Palfrey JS. The infant or young child with developmental delay. *N Engl J Med.* 1994;330(7):478–483.
12. Council on Children With Disabilities; Section on Developmental Behavioral Pediatrics; Bright Futures Steering Committee; Medical Home Initiatives for Children With Special Needs Project Advisory Committee. Identifying infants and young children with developmental disorders in the medical home: an algorithm for developmental surveillance and screening. *Pediatrics.* 2006;118(1):405–420.
13. ASQ3. *Ages & Stages Questionnaires®*, Third Edition (ASQ® -3). https://agesandstages.com/products-pricing/asq3
14. Bricker DD, Squires J, Mounts L, et al. *Ages & Stages Questionnaires (ASQ): A Parent-Completed, Child-Monitoring System.* 2nd ed. Paul H. Brookes Publishing Co; 1999.
15. Drotar D, Stancin T, Dworkin PH, Sices L, Wood S. Selecting developmental surveillance and screening tools. *Pediatr Rev.* 2008;29(10):e52–e58.
16. Robins DL, Fein D, Barton ML, Green JA. The Modified Checklist for Autism in Toddlers: an initial study investigating the early detection of autism and pervasive developmental disorders. *J Autism Dev Disord.* 2001;31(2):131–144.
17. Coplan J, Gleason JR. Test-retest and interobserver reliability of the Early Language Milestone Scale, second edition. *J Pediatr Health Care.* 1993;7(5):212–219.
18. Glascoe FP. *Collaborating with Parents: Using Parents' Evaluation of Developmental Status to Detect and Address Developmental and Behavioral Problems.* Ellsworth & Vandermeer Press; 1998.
19. Perrin EC, Sheldrick C, Visco Z, Mattern K. *The Survey of Well-Being of Young Children (SWYC) User's Manual.* Tufts Medical Center; 2016. https://pediatrics.tuftsmedicalcenter.org/the-survey-of-wellbeing-of-young-children/manual-training-resources
20. Newacheck PW, Strickland B, Shonkoff JP, et al. An epidemiologic profile of children with special health care needs. *Pediatrics.* 1998;102(1):117–123.
21. Hagan JF Jr, Shaw JS, Duncan PM, eds. *Bright Futures: Guidelines for Health Supervision of Infants, Children, and Adolescents.* 4th ed. American Academy of Pediatrics; 2017.
22. Bright Futures. American Academy of Pediatrics. Accessed May 19, 2024. https://brightfutures.aap.org/Pages/default.aspx
23. *The Guide to Clinical Preventive Services 2014.* U.S. Department of Health and Human Services; Agency for Healthcare Research and Quality; U.S. Preventive Services Task Force; 2014. Accessed May 19, 2024. http://www.ahrq.gov/professionals/clinicians-providers/guidelines-recommendations/guide
24. Hampl SE, Hassink SG, Skinner AC, et al. Clinical practice guideline for the evaluation and treatment of children and adolescents with obesity. *Pediatrics.* 2023;151(2):e2022060640.
25. Immunizations. American Academy of Pediatrics. Accessed May 19, 2024. https://www.aap.org/en/patient-care/immunizations/
26. Child and adolescent immunization schedule by age. Centers for Disease Control and Prevention. Accessed May 21, 2024. https://www.cdc.gov/vaccines/hcp/imz-schedules/child-adolescent-age.html
27. Pediatrics AAP. Preventive Care/Periodicity Schedule. Accessed May 21, 2024. https://www.aap.org/en/practice-management/care-delivery-approaches/periodicity-schedule/
28. Johnson CP, Blasco PA. Infant growth and development. *Pediatr Rev.* 1997;18(7):224–242.
29. Colson ER, Dworkin PH. Toddler development. *Pediatr Rev.* 1997;18(8):255–259.
30. Crotty JE, Martin-Herz SP, Scharf RJ. Cognitive development. *Pediatr Rev.* 2023;44(2):58–67.
31. Coplan J. Normal speech and language development: an overview. *Pediatr Rev.* 1995;16(3):91–100.
32. Brazelton TB. Working with families: opportunities for early intervention. *Pediatr Clin North Am.* 1995;42(1):1–9.
33. Tang MN, Adolphe S, Rogers SR, Frank DA. Failure to thrive or growth faltering: medical, developmental/behavioral, nutritional, and social dimensions. *Pediatr Rev.* 2021;42(11):590–603.
34. Grummer-Strawn LM, Reinold C, Krebs NF. Use of World Health Organization and CDC growth charts for children aged 0–59 months in the United States. *MMWR Recomm Rep.* 2010;59(RR09):1–15.
35. Wright CM, Williams AF, Elliman D, et al. Using the new UK-WHO growth charts. *BMJ.* 2010;340:c1140.
36. Fleming S, Thompson M, Stevens R, et al. Normal ranges of heart rate and respiratory rate in children from birth to 18 years of age: a systematic review of observational studies. *Lancet.* 2011;377(9770):1011–1018.
37. Herzog LW, Coyne LJ. What is fever? Normal temperature in infants less than 3 months old. *Clin Pediatr (Phila).* 1993;32(3):142–146.
38. Fleming S, Gill P, Jones C, et al. The diagnostic value of capillary refill time for detecting serious illness in children: a systematic review and meta-analysis. *PLoS One.* 2015;10(9):e0138155.
39. Pindrik J, Ye X, Ji BG, Pendleton C, Ahn ES. Anterior fontanelle closure and size in full-term children based on head

computed tomography. *Clin Pediatr (Phila)*. 2014;53(12): 1149–1157.
40. Fong CT. Clinical diagnosis of genetic diseases. *Pediatr Ann.* 1993;22(5):277–281.
41. Lees MH. Cyanosis of the newborn infant: recognition and clinical evaluation. *J Pediatr*. 1970;77(3):484–498.
42. Callahan CW Jr, Alpert B. Simultaneous percussion auscultation technique for the determination of liver span. *Arch Pediatr Adolesc Med.* 1994;148(8):873–875.
43. Frank JE, Jacobe KM. Evaluation and management of heart murmurs in children. *Am Fam Physician*. 2011;84(7):793–800.
44. Reiff MI, Osborn LM. Clinical estimation of liver size in newborn infants. *Pediatrics.* 1983;71(1):46–48.
45. Burger BJ, Burger JD, Bos CF, Obermann WR, Rozing PM, Vandenbroucke JP. Neonatal screening and staggered early treatment for congenital dislocation or dysplasia of the hip. *Lancet.* 1990;336(8730):1549–1553.
46. American Academy of Pediatrics Task Force on Circumcision. Circumcision policy statement. *Pediatrics.* 2012;130(3): 585–586.
47. Scherl SA. Common lower extremity problems in children. *Pediatr Rev.* 2004;25(2):52–62.
48. Zafeiriou DI. Primitive reflexes and postural reactions in the neurodevelopmental examination. *Pediatr Neurol.* 2004; 31(1):1–8.
49. Luiz DM, Foxcroft CD, Stewart R. The construct validity of the Griffiths scales of mental development. *Child Care Health Dev.* 2001;27(1):73–83.
50. Ashby AT, Beier AD. Review of pediatric neurologic history and age-appropriate neurologic examination in the office. *Pediatr Clin North Am.* 2021;68(4):707–714.
51. Aylward GP. Developmental screening and assessment: what are we thinking? *J Dev Behav Pediatr*. 2009;30(2):169–173.
52. Flynn JT, Kaelber DC, Baker-Smith CM, et al. Clinical practice guideline for screening and management of high blood pressure in children and adolescents. *Pediatrics.* 2017; 140(3):e20171904.
53. Shamis DJ. Collecting the "facts": vision assessment techniques: pearls and pitfalls. *Am Orthopt J.* 1996;46(1):7–13.
54. Blomgren K, Pitkäranta A. Current challenges in diagnosis of acute otitis media. *Int J Pediatr Otorhinolaryngol.* 2005; 69(3):295–299.
55. Coker TR, Chan LS, Newberry SJ, et al. Diagnosis, microbial epidemiology, and antibiotic treatment of acute otitis media in children: a systematic review. *JAMA*. 2010;304(19): 2161–2169.
56. Rothman R, Owens T, Simel DL. Does this child have acute otitis media? *JAMA*. 2003;290(12):1633–1640.
57. Jamal A, Alsabea A, Tarakmeh M, Safar A. Etiology, diagnosis, complications, and management of acute otitis media in children. *Cureus.* 2022;14(8):e28019.
58. Pirozzo S, Papinczak T, Glasziou P. Whispered voice test for screening for hearing impairment in adults and children: systematic review. *BMJ*. 2003;327(7421):967.
59. American Academy of Pediatrics Subcommittee on Management of Sinusitis and Committee on Quality Improvement. Clinical practice guideline: management of sinusitis. *Pediatrics.* 2001;108(3):798–808.
60. Wolf AM, Wender RC, Etzioni RB, et al; American Cancer Society Prostate Cancer Advisory Committee. American Cancer Society guideline for the early detection of prostate cancer: update 2010. *CA Cancer J Clin.* 2010;60(2):70–98.
61. Wald ER, Applegate KE, Bordley C, et al; American Academy of Pediatrics. Clinical practice guideline for the diagnosis and management of acute bacterial sinusitis in children aged 1 to 18 years. *Pediatrics.* 2013;132(1):e262–e280.
62. Tinanoff N, Reisine S. Update on early childhood caries since the surgeon general's report. *Acad Pediatr.* 2009;9(6):396–403.
63. Assimakopoulos D, Patrikakos G, Fotika C, Elisaf M. Benign migratory glossitis or geographic tongue: an enigmatic oral lesion. *Am J Med.* 2002;113(9):751–755.
64. Ebell MH, Smith MA, Barry HC, Ives K, Carey M. Does this patient have strep throat? *JAMA*. 2000;284(22):2912–2918.
65. Akinbami LJ, Moorman JE, Liu X. Asthma prevalence, health care use, and mortality: United States, 2005–2009. *Natl Health Stat Report.* 2011;32:1–14.
66. Centers for Disease Control and Prevention (CDC). Most recent National Asthma data. Accessed May 19, 2024. https://www.cdc.gov/asthma/most_recent_national_asthma_data.htm
67. Ashcraft KW. Consultation with the specialist: acute abdominal pain. *Pediatr Rev*. 2000;21(11):363–367.
68. Euser S, Alink LR, Stoltenborgh M, Bakermans-Kranenburg MJ, van IJzendoorn MH. A gloomy picture: a meta-analysis of randomized controlled trials reveals disappointing effectiveness of programs aiming at preventing child maltreatment. *BMC Public Health.* 2015;15:1068.
69. Kellogg ND, Farst KJ, Adams JA. Interpretation of medical findings in suspected child sexual abuse: an update for 2023. *Child Abuse Negl.* 2023;145:106283.
70. Bruce RW Jr. Torsional and angular deformities. *Pediatr Clin North Am.* 1996;43(4):867–881.
71. Ogden CL, Carroll MD, Kit BK, Flegal KM. Prevalence of obesity and trends in body mass index among US children and adolescents, 1999–2010. *JAMA*. 2012;307(5):483–490.
72. Polfuss ML, Duderstadt KG, Kilanowski JF, Thompson ME, Davis RL, Quinn M. Childhood obesity: evidence-based guidelines for clinical practice-part one. *J Pediatr Health Care.* 2020;34(3):283–290.
73. Ingelfinger JR. The child or adolescent with elevated blood pressure. *N Engl J Med.* 2014;371(11):1075.
74. Goldenring JM, Cohen E. Getting into adolescent heads. *Contemp Pediatr*. 1988;5(7):75–90.
75. Goldenring JM, Rosen DS. Getting into adolescent heads: an essential update. *Contemp Pediatr.* 2004;21:64–90.
76. Smith GL, McGuinness TM. Adolescent psychosocial assessment: the HEEADSSS. *J Psychosoc Nurs Ment Health Serv.* 2017;55(5):24–27.
77. Kann L, McManus T, Harris WA, et al. Youth risk behavior surveillance—United States, 2017. *MMWR Surveill Summ.* 2018;67(8):1–114.
78. Centers for Disease Control and Prevention (CDC). Youth risk behavior surveillance—United States, 2021. Accessed June 8, 2024. https://www.cdc.gov/healthyyouth/data/yrbs/index.htm
79. Rider GN, McMorris BJ, Gower AL, Coleman E, Eisenberg ME. Health and care utilization of transgender and gender nonconforming youth: a population-based study. *Pediatrics.* 2018;141(3):e20171683.
80. MN Department of Health. 2022 Minnesota Student Survey. Accessed June 8, 2024. https://www.health.state.mn.us/data/mchs/surveys/mss/index.html
81. Hoffman ND, Freeman K, Swann S. Healthcare preferences of lesbian, gay, bisexual, transgender and questioning youth. *J Adolesc Health.* 2009;45(3):222–229.

82. Meckler GD, Elliott MN, Kanouse DE, Beals KP, Schuster MA. Nondisclosure of sexual orientation to a physician among a sample of gay, lesbian, and bisexual youth. *Arch Pediatr Adolesc Med.* 2006;160(12):1248–1254.
83. Baams L, Kaufman TML. Sexual orientation and gender identity/expression in adolescent research: two decades in review. *J Sex Res.* 2023;60(7):1004–1019.
84. Arreola S, Neilands T, Pollack L, Paul J, Catania J. Childhood sexual experiences and adult health sequelae among gay and bisexual men: defining childhood sexual abuse. *J Sex Res.* 2008;45(3):246–252.
85. Spigarelli MG. Adolescent sexual orientation. *Adolesc Med State Art Rev.* 2007;18(3):508–518, vii.
86. American Academy of Pediatrics Committee on Practice and Ambulatory Medicine. Use of chaperones during the physical examination of the pediatric patient. *Pediatrics.* 2011;127(5): 991–993.
87. Biro FM, Galvez MP, Greenspan LC, et al. Pubertal assessment method and baseline characteristics in a mixed longitudinal study of girls. *Pediatrics.* 2010;126(3):e583–e590.
88. Herman-Giddens ME, Slora EJ, Wasserman RC, et al. Secondary sexual characteristics and menses in young girls seen in office practice: a study from the Pediatric Research in Office Settings network. *Pediatrics.* 1997;99(4):505–512.
89. Biro FM, Greenspan LC, Galvez MP, et al. Onset of breast development in a longitudinal cohort. *Pediatrics.* 2013;132(6): 1019–1027.
90. Oeffinger KC, Fontham ET, Etzioni R, et al. Breast cancer screening for women at average risk: 2015 guideline update from the American Cancer Society. *JAMA.* 2015;314(15): 1599–1614.
91. ACOG Committee on Adolescent Healthcare. ACOG Committee Opinion no. 350, November 2006: breast concerns in the adolescent. *Obstet Gynecol.* 2006;108(5):1329–1336.
92. Herman-Giddens ME, Steffes J, Harris D, et al. Secondary sexual characteristics in boys: data from the Pediatric Research in Office Settings Network. *Pediatrics.* 2012;130(5):e1058–e1068.
93. McCrory P, Meeuwisse WH, Aubry M, et al. Consensus statement on concussion in sport: the 4th International Conference on Concussion in Sport, Zurich, November 2012. *J Athl Train.* 2013;5(4):255–279.
94. Metzl JD. Preparticipation examination of the adolescent athlete: part 1. *Pediatr Rev.* 2001;22(6):199–204.
95. Metzl JD. Preparticipation examination of the adolescent athlete: part 2. *Pediatr Rev.* 2001;22(7):228–239.
96. Hyvärinen L, Walthes R, Jacob N, Chaplin KN, Leonhardt M. Current understanding of what infants see. *Curr Ophthalmol Rep.* 2014;2(4):142–149.
97. American Academy of Pediatrics Committee on Quality Improvement, Subcommittee on Developmental Dysplasia of the Hip. Clinical practice guideline: early detection of developmental dysplasia of the hip. *Pediatrics.* 2000;105(4): 896–905.

CHAPTER 29

Pregnant Persons

ANATOMY AND PHYSIOLOGY

Anatomic Changes

During pregnancy, the body undergoes remarkable changes to support the developing fetus. Changes in the breasts, abdomen, and urogenital tract are the most visible signs of pregnancy (Fig. 29-1). These physiologic adaptations are crucial for supporting pregnancy, highlighting the body's incredible capacity to nurture and protect the developing fetus.

Table 29-1, Physiologic Changes in Normal Pregnancy, pp. 1152–1154. Also, review the anatomy and physiology of these body systems in Chapter 20, Breasts and Axillae; Chapter 21, Abdomen; and Chapter 24, Pelvis and Genitourinary System: Vulva, Vagina, Uterus, and Adnexa.

External Abdomen. The skin over the abdomen stretches, often leading to purplish stretch marks (*striae gravidarum*) and a brownish black vertical line known as the *linea nigra* (Fig. 29-2). As the pregnancy progresses, increased tension on the abdominal wall can cause the rectus abdominis muscles to separate at the midline, a condition called *diastasis recti*, making fetal parts potentially palpable in severe cases.

Uterus. The uterus undergoes significant changes during pregnancy to accommodate the growing fetus. It transforms in both size and position, starting from about 70 g at conception and increasing to nearly 1,100 g at delivery, capable of holding between 5 and 20 L of fluid.[1] Initially, in the first trimester, the uterus remains within the pelvis, resembling an inverted pear and may retain its *anteverted* (forward-leaning), *retroverted* (backward-leaning), or *retroflexed* (backward-bent) posture.

By the second trimester, around 12 to 14 weeks, the gravid uterus becomes externally palpable as it expands into a more globular shape and rises beyond the pelvic brim. This growth propels the uterus into a predominantly anteverted position due to the enlarging fetus, which begins to exert pressure on the bladder, resulting in more frequent urination. Concurrently, the intestines are displaced laterally and superiorly to accommodate the uterus, and there is a slight uterine dextrorotation to make room for the rectosigmoid structures on the left side of the pelvis.

The uterus stretches its own supporting ligaments, causing "round ligament pain" in the lower quadrants.

This dextrorotation leads to greater discomfort on the right side as well as increased right-sided hydronephrosis.[1]

Growth patterns of the gravid uterus are shown in Figure 29-3, demonstrating the correlation between gestational age and measurable fundal height. Sagittal depictions of the gravid abdomen during each trimester appear in Figures 29-4 to 29-6.

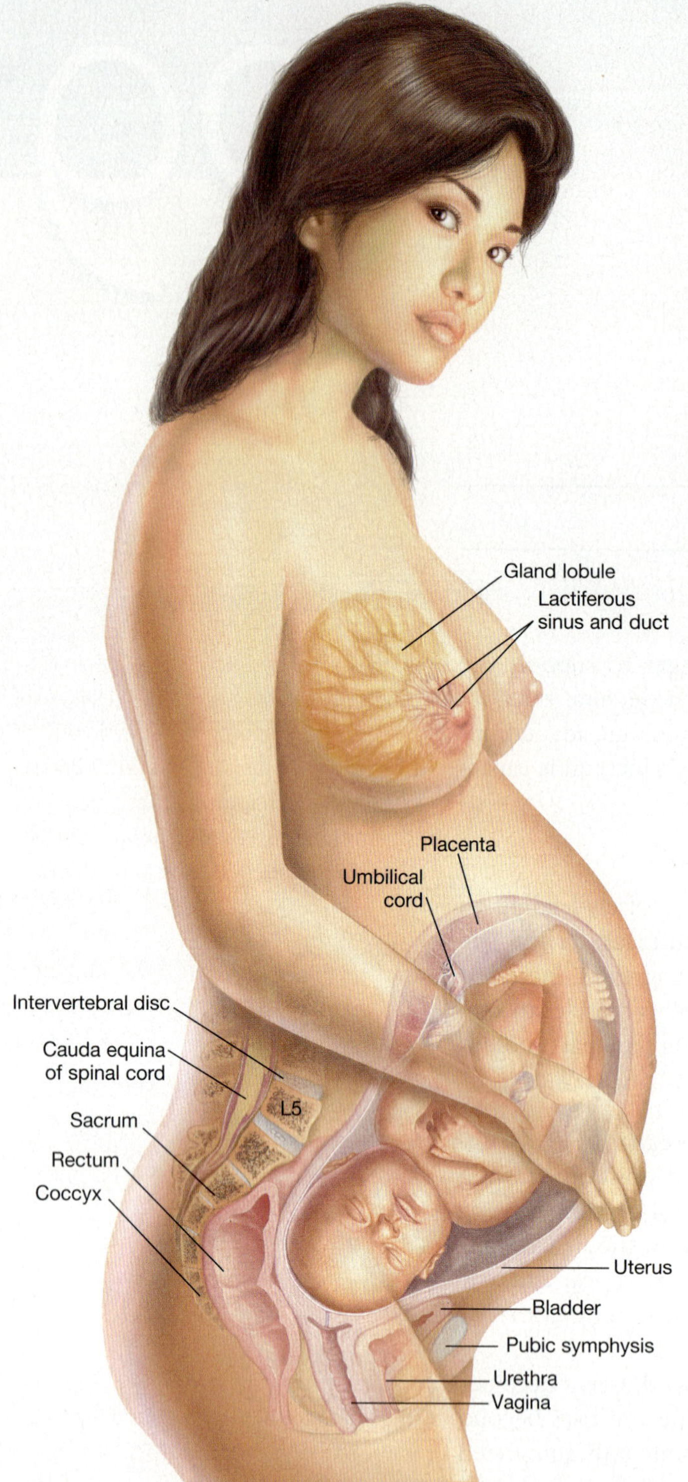

FIGURE 29-1. Pregnant person with breast and uterine changes. Anatomic relation of uterus with near-term infant to nearby structures also shown.

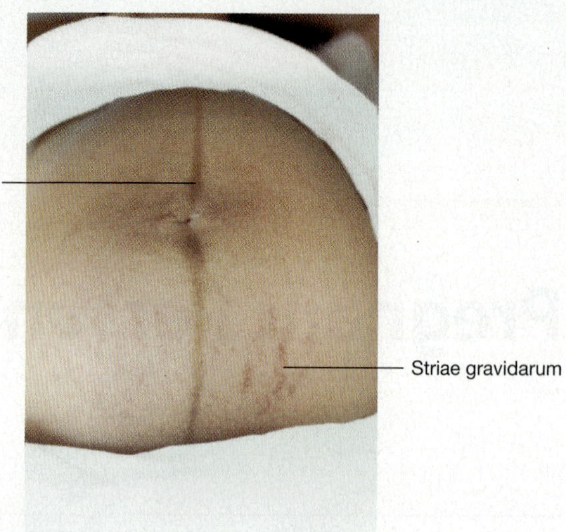

FIGURE 29-2. Striae gravidarum or "stretch marks" and linea nigra in the abdomen.

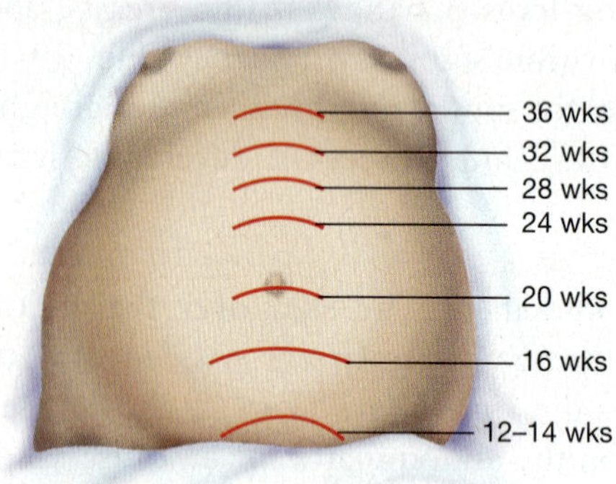

FIGURE 29-3. Uterine fundal height by weeks of pregnancy.

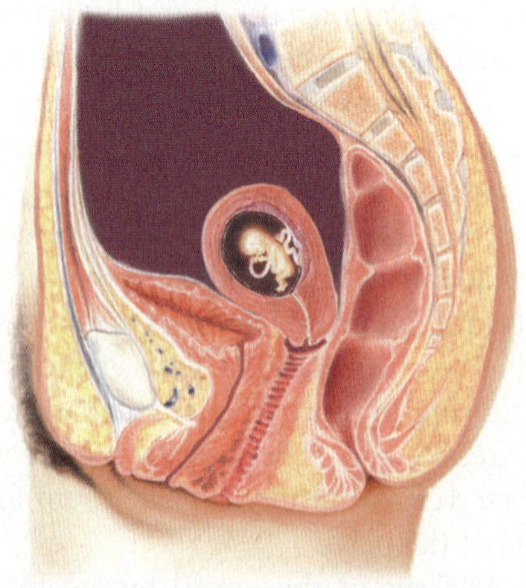

FIGURE 29-4. Sagittal depiction of the gravid abdomen during first trimester (1 to 12 weeks).

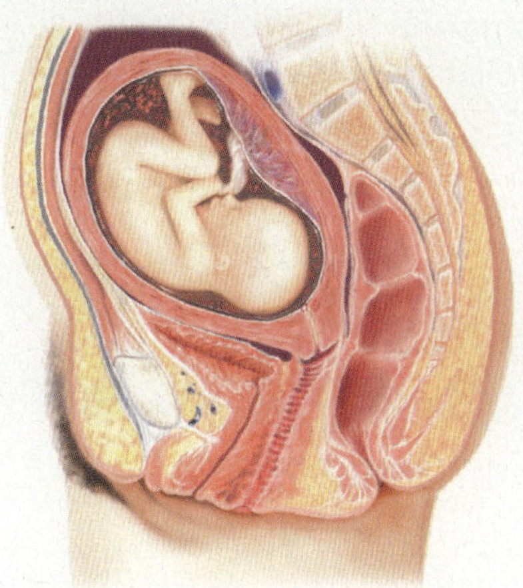

FIGURE 29-5. Sagittal depiction of the gravid abdomen during second trimester (13 to 26 weeks).

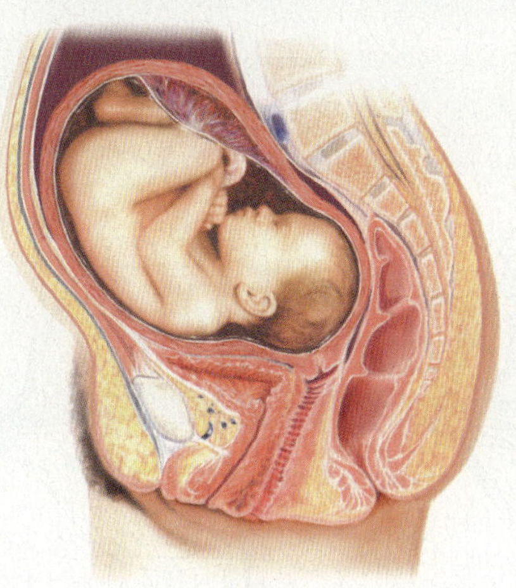

FIGURE 29-6. Sagittal depiction of the gravid abdomen during third trimester (27 to 40 weeks).

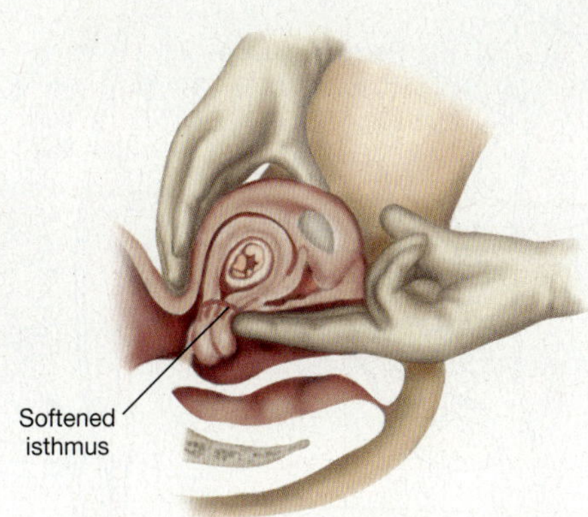

FIGURE 29-7. Hegar sign, palpable softening of the cervical isthmus.

Vagina. In the pelvis, increased vascularity changes the color of the vagina and cervix to a bluish hue, a phenomenon known as the *Chadwick sign*. The vaginal walls become more rugated due to thicker mucosa and loosened connective tissue, with normal vaginal secretions becoming thicker and more profuse, a condition referred to as *leukorrhea of pregnancy*. These changes, including a proliferation of *Lactobacillus acidophilus*, which lowers the vaginal pH, protect against some infections.

These changes may potentially increase susceptibility to conditions like vaginal candidiasis.

Cervix. The cervix softens and changes color to a bluish or cyanotic shade ~1 month after conception, a reflection of increased vascularity, edema, and glandular hyperplasia.[1] *Hegar sign* is the palpable softening of the *cervical isthmus*, the portion of the uterus that narrows into the cervix (Fig. 29-7). This is part of cervical remodeling that facilitates dilation during delivery, with copious secretions forming a mucus plug that protects against pathogens until expelled at delivery.

Adnexa. Early in pregnancy, the corpus luteum may be palpable on the ovary, disappearing as the placenta takes over hormonal support.

Breasts. The breasts undergo moderate enlargement due to increased vascularity and glandular hyperplasia, becoming more nodular by the end of the first trimester (Fig. 29-8). Nipples enlarge and darken, with Montgomery glands becoming more pronounced and the venous pattern more visible. Breasts may begin secreting colostrum, a nutrient-rich precursor to milk, during the second and third trimesters, accompanied by increased breast tenderness. Breast tenderness may make them more sensitive during examination.

Physiologic Hormonal Changes

Pregnancy brings numerous physiologic changes, primarily driven by hormonal fluctuations (Box 29-1). These hormonal changes support the pregnancy and cause noticeable anatomic alterations. For example, the basal metabolic rate rises by 15% to 20%, leading to increased energy needs across the trimesters.[1]

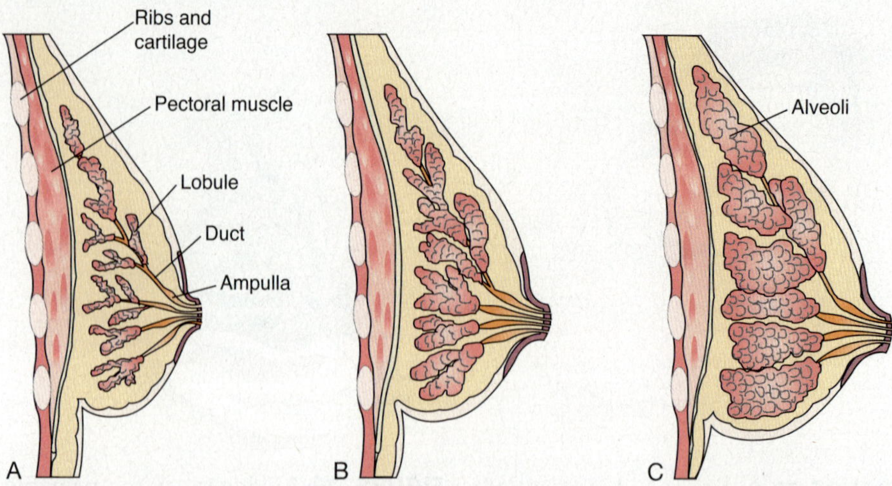

FIGURE 29-8. Comparison of the nonpregnant, nonlactating, adult breast (**A**); pregnant breast (**B**); and lactating breast (**C**). In **C**, note the increased size of the overall breast, as well as its ducts and lobules. (Reprinted with permission from Evans RJ, Evans MK, Brown YMR. *Canadian Maternity, Newborn, and Women's Health Nursing*. 2nd ed. Wolters Kluwer; 2015. Figure 21-3.)

Box 29-1. Physiological Hormonal Changes in Pregnancy

Hormone	Effect on Pregnancy
Estrogen	Promotes endometrial growth, enlarges the pituitary gland, increases prolactin output,[1] and contributes to a hypercoagulable state, increasing the risk of thromboembolic events[2]
Progesterone	Increases tidal volume and alveolar minute ventilation, causes respiratory alkalosis and shortness of breath,[3] decreases gastrointestinal motility, and relaxes ureters and the bladder[1]
Human chorionic gonadotropin (hCG)	Maintains pregnancy, stabilizes the endometrium in early pregnancy, and supports progesterone synthesis[4]; pregnancy tests measure for two of its five variants
Placental growth hormone	Influences fetal growth, development of preeclampsia,[1] and contributes to insulin resistance, raising the risk of developing gestational diabetes mellitus[5–7]
Thyroid function	Increases thyroid-binding globulin, cross-stimulates thyroid-stimulating hormone receptors by β-hCG, leading to slight increases in serum T_3 and T_4 levels, representing a physiologic euthyroid state[8]
Relaxin	Aids in the remodeling of reproductive tract connective tissue and increases renal hemodynamics and serum osmolality; does not significantly affect peripheral joint laxity during pregnancy
Erythropoietin	Increases erythrocyte mass but is accompanied by a greater increase in plasma volume, causing physiologic anemia and helping protect against blood loss during childbirth

HEALTH HISTORY: GENERAL APPROACH

Prenatal visits are critical for providing medical care and improving outcomes for both the pregnant individual and the fetus. These appointments should focus on addressing any symptoms of concern, evaluating the health of both the pregnant person and the fetus, and offering guidance for the remainder of the pregnancy. Pregnant individuals commonly attend visits with partners or family members for support. However, it is important to also have private conversations with the pregnant individual to discuss sensitive topics such as obstetric history, feelings about the pregnancy, substance use, sexually transmitted infections (STIs), and intimate partner violence (IPV). Initial health histories should be taken with the individual fully clothed to ensure comfort and privacy.

Initial Prenatal Visit

Prenatal care aims to enhance health and minimize risks for pregnant individuals and their fetuses. The initial prenatal visit's objectives include assessing the health of the pregnant person and fetus, confirming the pregnancy, estimating gestational age, planning ongoing care, and discussing the pregnant person's expectations and concerns. These visits should start early in pregnancy but can be adapted based on when the individual first seeks care. Subsequent visits monitor health changes, review pregnancy-related examination findings, and provide counseling and preventive screenings.

Confirming Pregnancy. Confirming the pregnancy through a urine test is usually the first step, followed by determining the last menstrual period (LMP) and possibly an ultrasound to establish the gestational age. These methods help verify the pregnancy and its viability early on.

Determining Gestational Age and Expected Date of Delivery. Accurate dating is crucial for managing the pregnancy effectively. It helps in reassuring about the pregnancy's progress, scheduling appropriate screenings, and preparing for labor and delivery (Box 29-2).

Box 29-2. Determining Gestational Age and the Expected Date of Delivery

- ***Gestational age.*** To establish gestational age, count the number of weeks and days from the first day of the LMP. If the actual date of conception is known (as with in vitro fertilization), a conception age 2 weeks less than the menstrual age can be used to calculate *menstrual age* (i.e., a corrected or adjusted LMP dating) to establish dating. Counting this menstrual age from the LMP, although biologically distinct from date of conception, is the standard means of calculating fetal age, yielding an average pregnancy length of 40 weeks.
- ***Expected date of delivery (EDD).*** The EDD is 40 weeks from the LMP. Using the *Naegele rule*, EDD can be estimated by taking the LMP, adding 7 days, subtracting 3 months, and adding 1 year. For example:
  - LMP = November 26, 2025
  - +7 days = December 2, 2025
  - −3 months = September 2, 2025
  - +1 year = September 2, 2026 = EDD

(continued)

Box 29-2. Determining Gestational Age and the Expected Date of Delivery (*Continued*)

- ***Tools for calculations.*** Pregnancy wheels and online calculators are commonly used to calculate the EDD. However, pregnancy wheels vary widely in quality and accuracy. Online calculators may be more reliable but should be checked for accuracy before routine use.
- ***Limitations on pregnancy dating.*** Patient recall of the LMP is highly variable. Even when this date is accurate, the LMP can be affected by hormonal contraceptives, menstrual irregularities, and variations in ovulation that result in atypical cycle lengths. LMP dating should be checked against physical examination markers such as fundal height, and any wide discrepancies should be clarified by ultrasound evaluation. In clinical practice, dating by ultrasound is widespread, regardless of the certainty of the LMP, even though this approach is not currently endorsed by national guidelines.

Symptoms Associated with Pregnancy. A thorough review of symptoms, including missed periods, breast tenderness, nausea, vomiting, fatigue, and urinary frequency, helps in monitoring the pregnancy's progress and addressing any concerns early (Box 29-3).

Box 29-3. Common Concerns during Pregnancy and Their Explanations

Common Concerns	Trimester	Explanation
Abdominal pain (lower)	Second	Rapid growth causes tension and stretching of the round ligaments that support the uterus, causing sharp or cramping pain with movement or position change.
Abdominal striae	Second or third	Stretching of the skin and tearing of the collagen in the dermis contribute to thin, usually pink, bands, or *striae gravidarum* (stretch marks) that may persist or fade over time after delivery.
Amenorrhea (missed periods)	All	High levels of estrogen, progesterone, and hCG build up the endometrium and prevent menses, causing a missed period, which is often the first noticeable sign of pregnancy.
Backache	All	Hormonally induced relaxation of the pelvic ligaments contributes to musculoskeletal aches. Lordosis required to balance the gravid uterus contributes to lower back strain. Breast enlargement may contribute to upper backaches.
Breast tenderness/ tingling	First	Pregnancy hormones stimulate the growth of breast tissue, which causes swelling and possible aching, tenderness, and tingling. Increased blood flow can make delicate veins more visible beneath the skin.

Common Concerns	Trimester	Explanation
Constipation	All	Constipation results from slowed gastrointestinal transit due to hormonal changes, dehydration from nausea and vomiting, and the supplemental iron in prenatal vitamins.
Contractions	Third	Irregular and unpredictable uterine contractions (*Braxton Hicks* contractions) are rarely associated with labor. Contractions that become regular or painful should be evaluated for onset of labor.
Edema	Third	Decreased venous return, obstruction of lymphatic flow, and reduced plasma colloid oncotic pressure commonly cause lower extremity edema. However, sudden severe edema and hypertension may signal preeclampsia.
Fatigue	First/third	Fatigue is related to the rapid change in energy requirements, sedative effects of progesterone, changes in body mechanics due to the gravid uterus, and sleep disturbance.
Heartburn	All	Progesterone relaxes the lower esophageal sphincter, allowing gastric contents to reflux into the esophagus. The gravid uterus also exerts physical pressure against the stomach with increasing gestational age, contributing to reflux symptoms.[1]
Hemorrhoids	All	Hemorrhoids may be caused by constipation, decreased venous return from increasing pressure in the pelvis, compression by fetal parts, and changes in activity level during pregnancy.
Loss of mucus plug	Third	Passage of the mucus plug is common during labor but may occur prior to the onset of contractions. As long as regular contractions, bleeding, or loss of fluid is not occurring, loss of the mucus plug is unlikely to trigger the onset of labor.
Nausea and/or vomiting	First	This is poorly understood but appears to reflect hormonal changes, slowed gastrointestinal peristalsis, alterations in smell and taste, and sociocultural factors. Up to 75% of pregnant persons experience nausea in pregnancy.[9]

Hyperemesis gravidarum is vomiting with weight loss of >5% of prepregnancy weight.

(*continued*)

Box 29-3. Common Concerns during Pregnancy and Their Explanations (*Continued*)

Common Concerns	Trimester	Explanation
Urinary frequency	All	Increases in blood volume and filtration rate through the kidneys result in increased urine production, while pressure from the gravid uterus reduces potential space for the bladder. Dysuria or suprapubic pain should be investigated for urinary tract infection.
Vaginal discharge	All	Asymptomatic milky white discharge (*leukorrhea*) results from increased secretions from vaginal and cervical epithelia due to vasocongestion and hormonal changes. Any foul-smelling or pruritic discharge should be investigated.

Concerns and Attitudes toward Pregnancy. Understanding how the pregnant individual feels about the pregnancy is vital. Discuss their support system, any concerns or fears, and plans for the pregnancy in a supportive and nonjudgmental manner, acknowledging diverse family structures and circumstances.

Current Health Status and Previous Medical History. A comprehensive review of the individual's health history, including any conditions that could affect the pregnancy, is essential. This includes prior abdominal surgeries; hypertension; diabetes; and any other significant health issues such as cardiac disorders including childhood surgery for congenital heart disease, asthma, autoimmune disorders, hypercoagulability states from lupus anticoagulant or anticardiolipin antibodies, mental health disorders such as postpartum depression, human immunodeficiency virus (HIV), STIs, and abnormal Pap smears.

Previous Obstetric History. Discussing previous pregnancies, their outcomes, and any complications encountered provides valuable insights into potential risks or considerations for the current pregnancy. A terminology system for pregnancy outcomes is widely used in health care to document reproductive histories inclusively. *Gravidity* indicates the total number of pregnancies an individual has experienced, while *parity* denotes the number of pregnancies reaching viable gestational age (≥24 weeks), irrespective of the outcome being a live birth or stillbirth. For instance, an individual described as "gravida 2, para 2" (G2P2) has had two pregnancies, both of which resulted in deliveries after 24 weeks. A "gravida 2, para 0" (G2P0) individual has had two pregnancies, with neither reaching 24 weeks.

Parity is detailed further into categories of *term deliveries, preterm deliveries, abortions* (inclusive of spontaneous and induced terminations), and *living children* (*TPAL*). For example, an individual with two losses before 20 weeks, three children delivered at term, and a current pregnancy is G6P3023. In the case of multiples (e.g., twins), the pregnancy is counted once in the gravidity and parity categories, except in the count of living children, where each child is counted. Thus, a first pregnancy resulting in twins delivered at term is G1P1002. This system ensures a consistent and inclusive approach to documenting and discussing reproductive history.

Risk Factors Affecting the Health of the Pregnant Individual and the Fetus. Screening for lifestyle factors (tobacco, alcohol, or drug use) and environmental exposures, assessing nutritional status, and identifying any sources of stress or history of abuse are critical for optimizing prenatal care.

Family Medical History of the Pregnant Individual and Any Biologic Contributors. Collecting information on the genetic and health history of the pregnant individual and any biologic contributors can help identify potential hereditary conditions or risks to the fetus.

Considerations for Genetic Screening and Testing for Chromosomal Abnormalities. Offering and discussing options for genetic screening and testing for chromosomal abnormalities and specific genetic disorders helps in making informed decisions about the pregnancy, such as trisomies 21, 18, and 13 and sex-chromosome abnormalities.[10–12]

Intentions Regarding Infant Feeding. Exploring the benefits of breastfeeding or chestfeeding and offering support and education can boost the likelihood of successful infant feeding, providing health benefits for both the infant and the pregnant individual.[13–15]

Considerations for Contraception after Childbirth. Initiate this discussion early, as postpartum contraception reduces the risk of unintended pregnancy and shortened interpregnancy intervals, which are linked to increases in adverse pregnancy outcomes.[16,17] Plans for contraception will depend on the patient's preferences, clinical history, and decision about infant feeding.

Concluding the Initial Visit. Reaffirm your support for the pregnant person's health and address any questions. Emphasize the importance of regular prenatal care and outline the schedule for future visits.

Subsequent Prenatal Visits

While the ideal number of prenatal visits is not definitively set, they typically occur monthly up to 28 weeks' gestation, every 2 weeks until 36 weeks, then weekly until birth. Update and document the medical history at each visit, paying close attention to fetal movements, contractions, fluid leakage, and any bleeding.[18] Physical examination findings at every visit should include vital signs (especially blood pressure and weight), fundal height, verification of fetal heart rate (FHR), and determination of fetal position and activity, as described later in Techniques of Examination. At each visit, the urine should be tested for infection, glucose, and protein.

PHYSICAL EXAMINATION: GENERAL APPROACH

Physical examinations during pregnancy are focused and tailored to the individual's needs, with a comprehensive exam including breast and pelvic assessments typically conducted at the first prenatal visit. Patients' comfort with various parts of this examination may vary due to personal experiences or cultural considerations, which should be respectfully explored and accommodated.

Ensuring the comfort and privacy of the pregnant individual is paramount, taking into account personal and cultural preferences. If others are present, confirm if the individual prefers them to stay or leave during the exam. For those unfamiliar with pelvic exams, a detailed explanation of the process can aid in cooperation and ease any discomfort. Modesty concerns should be carefully balanced with the necessity of a thorough examination.

To facilitate the examination, especially of the breasts and abdomen, use a front-opening gown. Ensure that all equipment and examination tables are suitable for individuals of varying body sizes and consider suggesting that the patient empties their bladder before beginning, particularly prior to a pelvic exam.

TECHNIQUES OF EXAMINATION

Key Components of the Examination of the Pregnant Individual

- Position the pregnant individual.
- Prepare the examining equipment.
- Conduct a general inspection.
- Measure height, weight, and vital signs.
- Inspect the head and neck.
- Inspect, percuss, and auscultate the thorax and lungs.
- Examine the heart.
- Examine the breasts.
- Examine the abdomen.
- Examine the external genitalia.
- Inspect the internal genitalia.
- Examine the internal genitalia.
- Consider examining the anus, rectum, and rectovaginal septum.
- Examine the extremities.

Position the Pregnant Individual

In the early stages of pregnancy, individuals can be examined while lying down. In later stages, a semi-sitting position with bent knees or a slight leftward tilt is preferred to enhance comfort and prevent pressure on major blood vessels from the growing uterus (Fig. 29-9). Pregnant individuals should avoid lying flat for extended periods. Most of the examination, except for the pelvic exam, can be conducted while sitting or lying on their side.

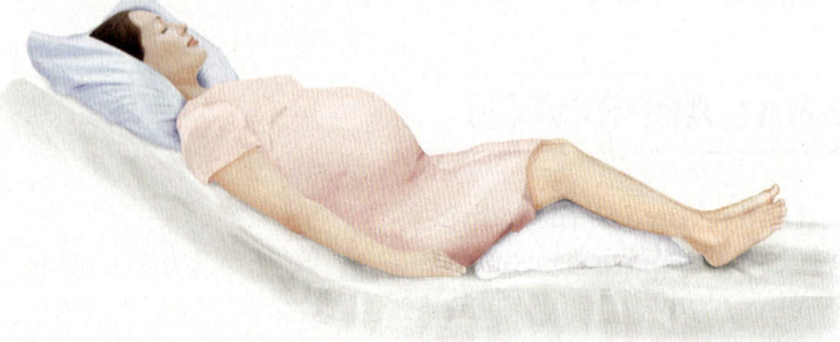

FIGURE 29-9. Semi-sitting position of the pregnant person for examination.

Box 29-4. Equipment for Examining the Pregnant Person

- *Gynecologic speculum and lubrication:* Due to vaginal wall relaxation during pregnancy, a larger-than-usual speculum may be needed in multiparous patients.
- *Sampling materials:* Because of the increased vascularity of vaginal and cervical structures, the cervical brush may cause bleeding that interferes with Pap smear samples, so the "broom" sampling device is preferred during pregnancy. Use additional swabs as needed to screen for STIs, group B strep, and wet mount preparations.
- *Tape measure:* A plastic or paper tape measure is used to assess the size of the uterus after 20 gestational weeks.
- *Doppler fetal monitor and gel:* This handheld device is applied externally to the gravid abdomen to assess fetal heart tones after 10 weeks' gestation.

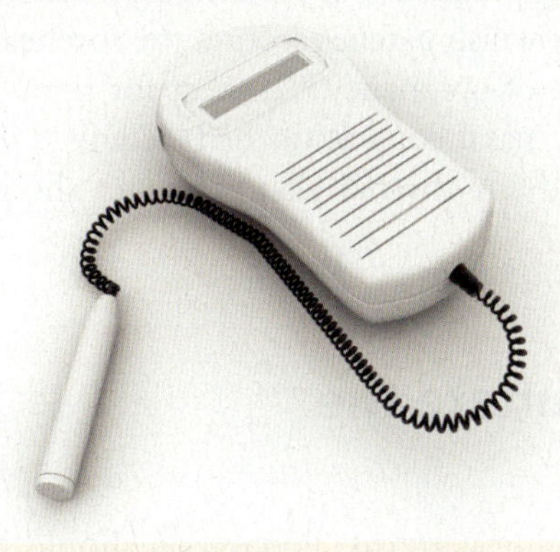

Handheld Doppler monitor.

During the exam, if the individual feels lightheaded while sitting, encourage sitting upright and taking time when standing. The examination should be conducted efficiently to maintain comfort.

Compression interferes with venous return from the lower extremities and pelvic vessels, causing the patient to feel dizzy and faint, also known as *supine hypotension*.

Prepare the Examining Equipment

Before starting the examination, make sure to approach the patient with a comforting touch and movements. Warm your hands and use firm, yet gentle palpation. Maintain continuous contact with the abdominal surface, primarily using the sensitive palmar surfaces of your fingertips. Gather all necessary equipment in advance to facilitate a smooth examination process (Box 29-4).

Conduct a General Inspection

Observe the pregnant individual as soon as they enter the examination room. Pay attention to their general appearance, mood, and mobility. Look for signs of discomfort, distress, or difficulty in moving. These observations offer an initial insight into their health status, including emotional and nutritional states.

Be vigilant for signs that may indicate underlying conditions, such as preeclampsia or thyroid disorders.

Measure Height, Weight, and Vital Signs

Measure the patient's height and weight accurately at the initial visit and use these metrics to calculate their body mass index (BMI). These measurements are crucial for assessing nutritional status and identifying potential risks associated with different weight categories during pregnancy. They guide dietary recommendations, physical activity advice, and monitoring strategies to support a healthy pregnancy outcome.

Weight loss due to nausea and vomiting that exceeds 5% of prepregnancy weight is considered excessive, representing *hyperemesis gravidarum,* and can lead to adverse pregnancy outcomes.

At every visit, measure blood pressure using an appropriately sized cuff and the correct technique, referencing the *Eighth Joint National Committee* (*JNC8*) (see p. 182) guidelines for normal ranges.[19] Additionally, count the respiratory rate for a full minute to ensure accuracy, noting any deviations from the norm.

Hypertensive disorders, affecting 5% to 10% of all pregnancies, can affect virtually every organ system, so all elevations in blood pressure must be closely monitored.[20]

See section Hypertensive Disorders of Pregnancy, p. 1143.

Inspect the Head and Neck

During the examination, focus on identifying pregnancy-specific changes such as *chloasma* or *melasma*, which are irregular brownish patches around the forehead, cheeks, nose, and jaw, known as the "mask of pregnancy." Inspect for signs of pallor or jaundice in the eyes and note any nasal congestion or bleeding. Oral health, particularly the gums and teeth, and any thyroid gland changes should also be assessed.

Modest symmetric enlargement due to glandular hyperplasia and increased vascularity is normal. However, thyroid enlargement, goiters, and nodules are abnormal and require investigation.

Inspect, Percuss, and Auscultate the Thorax and Lungs

Inspect the thorax for contours and breathing patterns. Percussion should be used to observe diaphragmatic elevation that may be seen as early as the first trimester. Auscultate for clear breath sounds without wheezes, rales, or rhonchi.

Examine the Heart

Palpate the apical impulse, which may be rotated upward and to the left toward the fourth intercostal space by the enlarging uterus. Listen for a venous hum or a continuous mammary souffle ("a puff of air," pronounced ***soo-fuhl***) often found during pregnancy due to increased blood flow through the breast vasculature. It is commonly heard during late pregnancy or lactation and is strongest in the second or third intercostal space at the sternal border bilaterally.

Assess for murmurs, which may signal anemia or be related to the physiologic increase in circulating blood volume. A diastolic murmur in pregnancy is never normal and should be investigated further. See also Chapter 18, Cardiovascular System, pp. 472–538.

Examine the Breasts

The breast examination should note symmetry, color changes, and the presence of Montgomery glands (Fig. 29-10). Normal changes include a marked venous pattern and darkened nipples and areolae.

Bloody or purulent discharge should not be attributed to pregnancy and requires immediate investigation. See also Chapter 20, Breasts and Axillae, pp. 583–584.

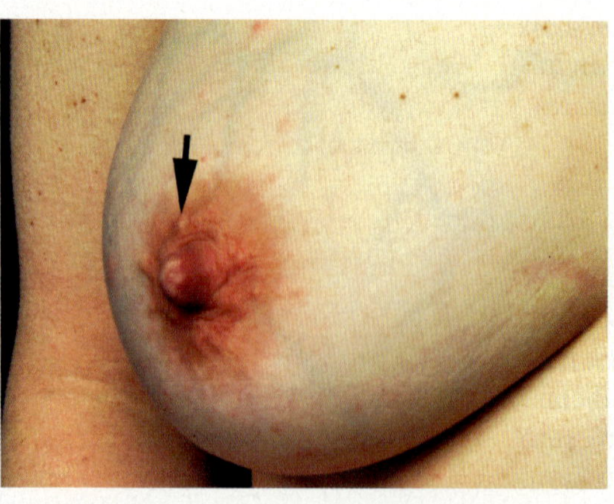

FIGURE 29-10. Hypertrophic areolar sebaceous glands (Montgomery glands). These can be seen in up to 36% of pregnant women and typically resolve postpartum. (Reprinted with permission from Kroumpouzos G. *Text Atlas of Obstetric Dermatology*. Wolters Kluwer Health/Lippincott Williams & Wilkins; 2014. Figure 7-1.)

Compress each nipple between your thumb and index finger; colostrum may express from the nipples during later trimesters. Reassure the individual that this is normal and that they may also experience "*let down*," a spontaneous mild leakage often accompanied by a cramping sensation in the breast during a hot shower or orgasm in the third trimester.

Examine the Abdomen

To conduct an abdominal examination, assist the patient into a semi-sitting position with their knees flexed. This position is conducive to a thorough examination (see Fig. 29-9).

Inspect the Abdomen. Inspect the abdomen for striae, scars, size, shape, and contour. Purplish *striae* and a *linea nigra* are normal in pregnancy (see Fig. 29-2).

Cesarean scars on the abdomen might not align with the orientation of the scar on the uterus, an important consideration when evaluating the appropriateness of vaginal delivery after a cesarean section.

Palpate the Abdomen. When palpating the abdomen, expect to feel the mass of the gravid uterus, which is a normal finding. Palpate for fetal movement, typically felt by the examiner externally after 24 gestational weeks and by the pregnant individual between 18 and 24 weeks, known as "*quickening*."

If fetal movement is not detected after 24 weeks, it may indicate a miscalculation of gestational age, fetal demise, severe morbidity, or a false pregnancy. Confirming fetal health and gestational age with an ultrasound is crucial in such cases.

Assess Uterine Contractility. Assess uterine contractility by feeling for irregular contractions, which can start as early as 12 weeks and may be triggered by palpation in the third trimester. The abdomen might feel tense or firm during contractions, making it difficult to palpate fetal parts; relaxation follows these contractions.

Regular uterine contractions at <37 weeks, with or without pain and bleeding, are abnormal and suggest preterm labor.

Measure the Fundal Height. Measure the fundal height if gestational age is above 20 weeks. Using a tape measure, start from the pubic symphysis, placing the "zero" end at the bone you can firmly feel there, and extend the tape to the very top of the uterine fundus (Fig. 29-11). Though subject to error between 16 and 36 weeks, measurement of the *fundal height in centimeters* should roughly equal the number of weeks of gestation. This widely used technique may underdetect newborns who are small for gestational age.[21–23]

A fundal height >4 cm larger or smaller than expected warrants further investigation for conditions such as multiple gestation, large fetus, low amniotic fluid, or fetal anomalies through ultrasound.

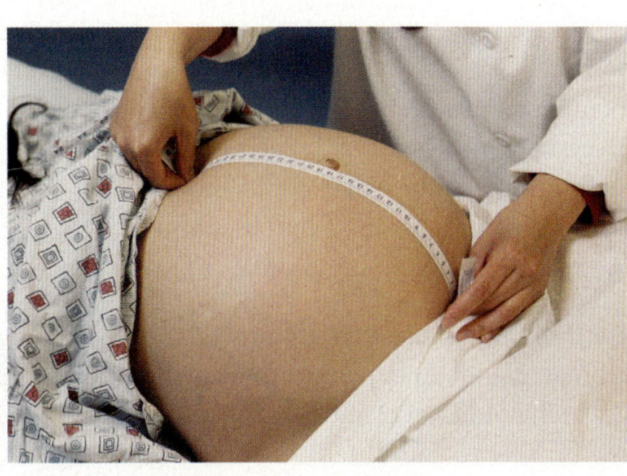

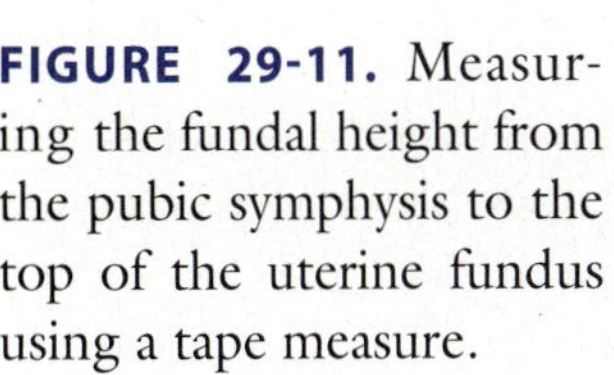

FIGURE 29-11. Measuring the fundal height from the pubic symphysis to the top of the uterine fundus using a tape measure.

Auscultate Fetal Heart Tones. Auscultate fetal heart tones using a Doppler fetal monitor, typically audible from as early as 10 to 12 weeks' gestation. Note that detection timing may vary across different body types, including in individuals with higher body mass, which could slightly delay audible detection.

Inaudible fetal heart tones could suggest less advanced gestation than estimated, fetal demise, a false pregnancy, or an observational error. Always investigate these situations with a formal ultrasound.

Location. The location of fetal heart tones changes throughout pregnancy. From 10 to 18 weeks' gestation, tones are best detected along the midline of the lower abdomen. Beyond this period, the optimal location shifts to over the back or chest, depending on the fetal position; Leopold maneuvers can assist in determining this (see Special Techniques, pp. 1137–1139).

Hearing more than one fetal heart tone, especially with varying rates after 24 weeks, suggests the possibility of multiple gestations.

Rate. The *FHR* typically ranges between 110 and 160 beats/min. A rate of 60 to 90 beats/min is usually maternal, thus an appropriate FHR should be confirmed.

Sustained dips in FHR, or *"decelerations,"* have a wide differential diagnosis but always warrant investigation, at least by formal FHR monitoring.

Rhythm. FHR should vary from beat to beat, particularly later in pregnancy, indicating increased fetal activity. Difficulty in assessing this variability with a Doppler warrants the use of formal FHR monitoring for a more accurate evaluation.

Lack of beat-to-beat variability is challenging to discern with a handheld Doppler and signifies the need for formal monitoring to ensure fetal well-being.

Examine the External Genitalia

For this portion of the examination, carefully assist the patient into a supine position with their feet placed in footrests. This position ensures both patient comfort and the effectiveness of the examination. Minimize the duration in this position to prevent supine hypotension syndrome, caused by uterine compression of the vena cava and aorta. Prioritize gathering all necessary examination tools before beginning. This not only streamlines the process but also reduces patient anxiety by avoiding interruptions.

Inspect the External Genitalia. Begin with a comprehensive visual examination of the external genitalia, noting any changes such as the relaxation of the vaginal introitus or enlargement of the labia and clitoris, which are normal physiologic changes during pregnancy. Additionally, palpate gently to assess the texture and any abnormalities. Specific conditions to identify include:

- *Labial varicosities:* These can become particularly pronounced and painful during pregnancy, resulting from increased venous pressure.

Labial varicosities that arise during pregnancy can become tortuous and painful. Cystoceles and rectoceles may be pronounced due to the muscle relaxation of pregnancy. Lesions and sores occur with herpes simplex infection.

- *Cystoceles and rectoceles:* Look for and document any evidence of prolapse, which may become more noticeable due to pregnancy-induced muscle relaxation.
- *Lesions or sores:* Carefully inspect for any abnormalities that could indicate infections, paying close attention to symptoms indicative of herpes simplex infection.

Palpate the Greater Vestibular Glands (Bartholin) and the Paraurethral Glands (Skene). Gently palpate the greater vestibular glands and paraurethral glands for signs of tenderness or cyst formation, which could necessitate further evaluation and treatment.

See also Chapter 24, Pelvis and Genitourinary System: Vulva, Vagina, Uterus, and Adnexa, p. 754.

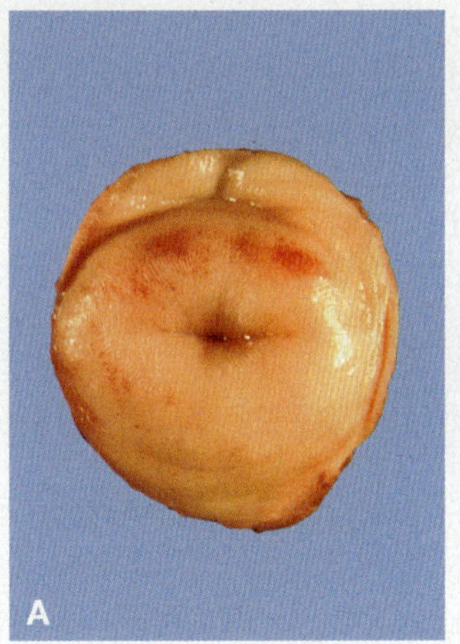

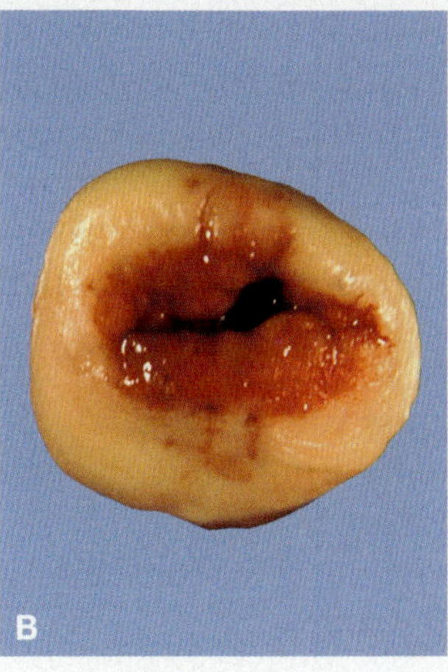

FIGURE 29-12. Typically, the external os in a nulliparous cervix appears as a circular dot (**A**), and in a parous cervix, the opening is wider and more slit-like and gaping (**B**). (Reprinted with permission from Reichert RA. *Diagnostic Gynecologic and Obstetric Pathology: An Atlas and Text.* Wolters Kluwer Health/ Lippincott Williams & Wilkins; 2012. Figure 3-1.)

Inspect the Internal Genitalia

Relaxation of the perineal and vulvar structures during pregnancy may minimize, but not eliminate, discomfort from the speculum examination. The increased vascularity of vaginal and cervical structures promotes friability, so insert and open the speculum gently to prevent tissue trauma and bleeding. During the third trimester, perform this examination only when necessary, as descent of the fetal parts into the pelvis can make the examination very uncomfortable.

Review the pelvic examination using a speculum in Chapter 24, Pelvis and Genitourinary System: Vulva, Vagina, Uterus, and Adnexa, pp. 748–750.

Inspect the Cervix for Color, Shape, and Closure. Carefully insert and open the speculum, ensuring to minimize discomfort. Observe the external os appearance, which can vary among individuals based on their birthing history (Fig. 29-12). Examine the cervix for its color, shape, and any indicators of *ectropion* or lacerations.

A pink cervix suggests a nonpregnant state. Cervical erosion, erythema, discharge, or irritation suggests cervicitis, and warrants investigation for STIs.

Assess Vaginal Health. Inspect the vaginal walls as you withdraw the speculum. Check for color, relaxation, rugae, and discharge. Normal findings include bluish color, deep rugae, and increased milky white discharge (*leukorrhea*).

Abnormal discharges should prompt further investigation for possible infections impacting pregnancy.

Examine the Internal Genitalia

Performing the bimanual examination is often easier during pregnancy due to pelvic floor relaxation. Avoiding sensitive urethral structures, insert two lubricated fingers into the introitus, palmar side down, with slight pressure downward on the perineum. Maintaining downward pressure on the perineum, gently turn the fingers palmar side up.

Evaluate the Cervix. Because of softening during pregnancy, or *Hegar sign* (see Fig. 29-7), the cervix may be difficult to identify. Warn patients that this exam may cause cramping and pressure. The cervix may feel irregular if Nabothian cysts or healed lacerations from prior deliveries are present.

- *Estimate cervical length.* Gently palpate from the cervical tip to the lateral fornix to assess the length. Typically, <34 to 36 weeks' gestation, the cervix maintains a length of ≥3 cm, indicating standard progression of pregnancy.

Cervical opening or shortening (*cervical effacement*) <37 weeks may indicate preterm labor.

- *Palpate the cervical os.* Examine the cervix only when necessary because palpation is very uncomfortable. Encourage the patient to draw their heels as close to their buttocks as possible, which naturally shortens the vagina. The external os might be slightly open in individuals who have given birth before, allowing a fingertip to pass through. However, the internal os generally remains closed until the later stages of pregnancy, irrespective of the number of previous births.

Assess the Uterus. With your internal fingers placed at either side of the cervix and your external hand on the patient's abdomen, use your internal fingers to gently lift their uterus upward toward your abdominal hand. Hold the fundal portion of the uterus between your two hands and assess the uterine size, keeping in mind the contours of the gravid uterus at various gestational intervals (see Fig. 29-3). Palpate for shape, consistency, and position.

Anomalies in the shape or size of the uterus, such as a bicornuate uterus or the presence of fibroids, require careful monitoring and possibly additional imaging to assess their impact on pregnancy progression.

Palpate the Right and Left Adnexa. Palpate the adnexa for masses or tenderness that might suggest ectopic pregnancy, ovarian cysts, or other gynecologic conditions.

Adnexal tenderness or masses early in gestation require ultrasound evaluation to rule out ectopic pregnancy. Acute pelvic inflammatory disease is rare in pregnancy, especially after the first trimester, because the adnexa are sealed by the gravid uterus and mucus plug.

Consider Examining the Anus, Rectum, and Rectovaginal Septum

The rectal examination is not standard in prenatal care unless concerning symptoms like rectal bleeding or masses or conditions compromise the rectovaginal septum. Rectal examination may help you assess the size of a retroverted or retroflexed uterus, but transvaginal ultrasound provides superior information.

Hemorrhoids often become engorged late in pregnancy; they may be painful, bleed, or thrombose.

Examine the Extremities

Ask the patient to resume sitting or to lie on their left side.

Inspect the Legs for Varicose Veins. Begin with a visual examination of both legs, from the thighs down to the feet, looking for enlarged, twisted veins that typically appear raised and are blue or dark purple. Varicose veins are more common on the lower legs due to pressure on the veins in the pelvic area.

Varicose veins may begin or worsen during pregnancy.

Palpate the Extremities for Edema in the Pretibial, Ankle, and Pedal Distributions. Although several scales exist based on the extent of edema or the time it takes for a skin indentation to rebound, it is more prudent to describe and record your observation as you would any skin examination finding. Physiologic edema is common in advanced stages of pregnancy, during hot weather, and in individuals who stand for extended periods due to decreased venous return from the lower extremities.

Unilateral severe edema with calf tenderness warrants prompt evaluation for DVT. Hand or facial edema >20 gestational weeks is nonspecific for preeclampsia but should be investigated.[24,25]

Elicit Knee and Ankle Deep Tendon Reflexes. Assessing knee and ankle deep tendon reflexes is vital for monitoring changes in neurologic and vascular health in pregnancy.

In pregnancy, heightened reflexes might indicate increased nervous system excitability, often associated with conditions like preeclampsia.

Review the technique of eliciting the knee and ankle reflexes in Chapter 27, Nervous System, pp. 939–941.

SPECIAL TECHNIQUES

Leopold Maneuvers

Leopold maneuvers are used to determine the fetal position in the maternal abdomen beginning in the second trimester; accuracy is greatest after 36 weeks' gestation (Fig. 29-13).[26] Although less accurate for assessing fetal growth,[27] these examination findings help determine readiness for vaginal delivery by assessing:

- Upper and lower fetal pole, namely, the proximal and distal fetal parts
- Maternal side where the fetal back is located
- Descent of the presenting part into the maternal pelvis
- Extent of flexion of the fetal head
- Estimated size and weight of the fetus (this advanced skill will not be addressed further here)

Note that not all findings are truly diagnostic, and ultrasound may be required to conclusively determine fetal position.

Common deviations include *breech presentation* (parts other than the head, such as buttocks or foot, present at the maternal pelvis), and lack of engagement of the presenting part in the maternal pelvis at term. If discovered prior to term, breech presentations may sometimes be corrected by rotational maneuvers.

First Maneuver (Upper Fetal Pole). Stand at the patient's side, facing their head. Palpate the uppermost part of the gravid uterus gently, with your fingertips together, to determine what fetal part is located at the fundus, which is the "upper fetal pole" (Fig. 29-14).

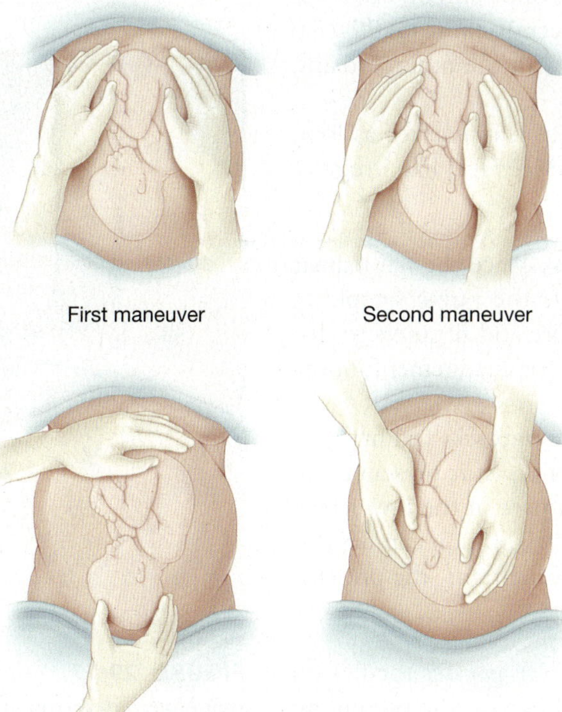

FIGURE 29-13. Leopold maneuvers for determining fetal position after 36 weeks' gestation. (Reprinted with permission from Casanova R, Chuang A, Goepfert AR, et al. *Beckmann and Ling's Obstetrics and Gynecology.* 8th ed. Wolters Kluwer; 2019. Figure 9-7.)

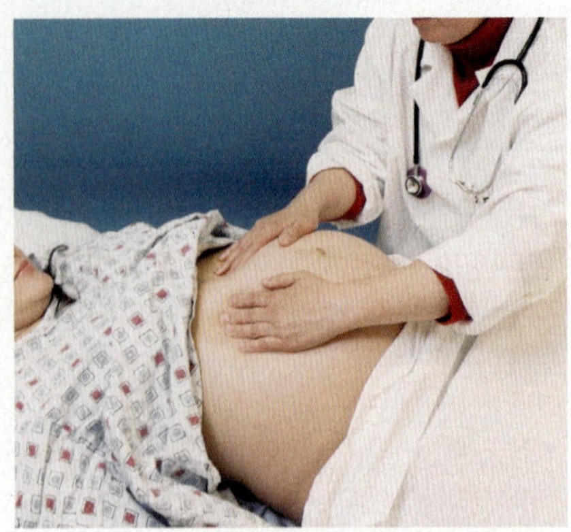

FIGURE 29-14. First Leopold maneuver: determination of what is in the fundus. (Reprinted with permission from Weber JR, Kelley JH. *Health Assessment in Nursing*. 6th ed. Wolters Kluwer; 2018. Figure 29-13.)

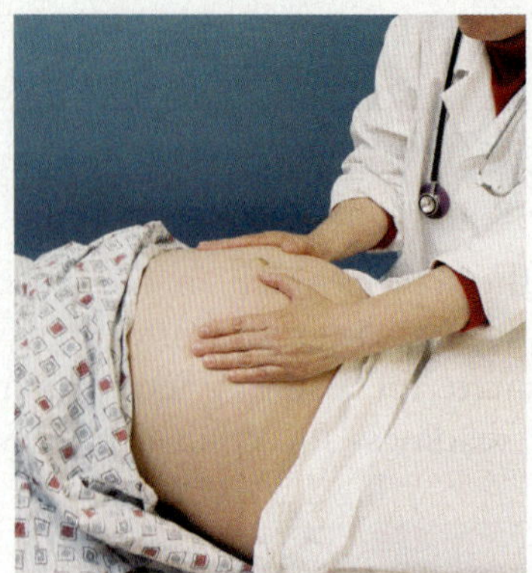

FIGURE 29-15. Second Leopold maneuver: evaluation of the fetal back and extremities. (Reprinted with permission from Weber JR, Kelley JH. *Health Assessment in Nursing*. 6th ed. Wolters Kluwer; 2018. Figure 29-14.)

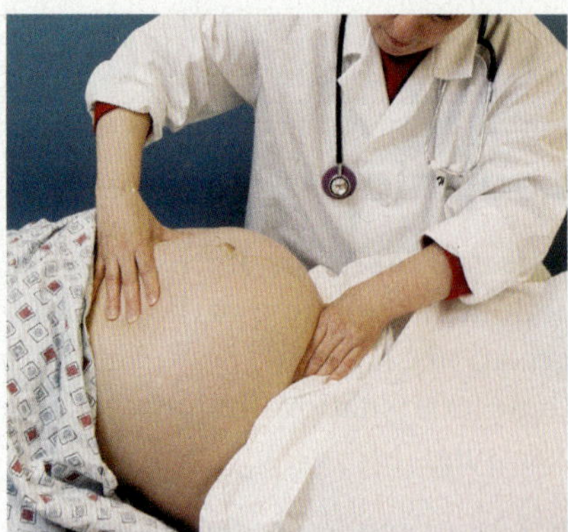

FIGURE 29-16. Third Leopold maneuver: palpation of the presenting part above the symphysis. (Reprinted with permission from Weber JR, Kelley JH. *Health Assessment in Nursing*. 6th ed. Wolters Kluwer; 2018. Figure 29-15.)

The fetal buttocks are usually at the upper fetal pole; they feel firm but irregular and less globular than the head. The fetal head feels firm, round, and smooth. Occasionally, neither part is easily palpated at the fundus, such as when the fetus is transverse.

Second Maneuver (Sides of the Maternal Abdomen). Place one hand on each side of the patient's abdomen, holding the fetal body between them (Fig. 29-15). Steady the uterus with one hand and palpate the fetus with the other, looking for the back on one side and extremities on the other.

By 32 weeks' gestation, the fetal back has a smooth, firm surface as long or longer than the examiner's hand. The fetal arms and legs feel like irregular bumps. The fetus may kick if awake and active.

Third Maneuver (Lower Fetal Pole and Descent into Pelvis). Place the flat palmar surfaces of your fingertips on the fetal pole just above the pubic symphysis (Fig. 29-16). Palpate the presenting fetal part for texture and firmness to distinguish the head from the buttocks. Judge the descent, or engagement, of the presenting part into the maternal pelvis.

Again, the fetal head feels very firm and globular; the buttocks feel firm but irregular and less globular than the head. In a *vertex* or *cephalic* presentation, the fetal head is the presenting part. If the most distal part of the lower fetal pole cannot be palpated, it is usually engaged in the pelvis. If you can depress the tissues over the maternal bladder without touching the fetus, the presenting part is proximal to your fingers.

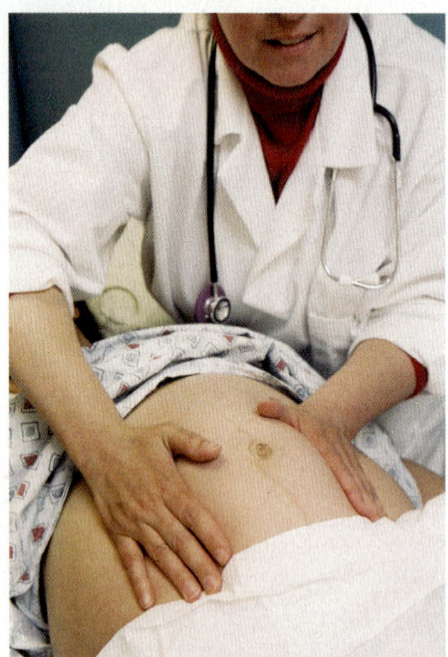

FIGURE 29-17. Fourth Leopold maneuver: determination of the direction and degree of flexion of the head. (Reprinted with permission from Weber JR, Kelley JH. *Health Assessment in Nursing*. 6th ed. Wolters Kluwer; 2018. Figure 29-16.)

Fourth Maneuver (Flexion of the Fetal Head). This maneuver assesses the flexion or extension of the fetal head, presuming that the fetal head is the presenting part in the pelvis. Facing the patient's feet with your hands positioned on either side of the gravid uterus, identify the fetal front and back sides (Fig. 29-17). Using one hand at a time, slide your fingers down each side of the fetal body until you reach the "cephalic prominence," that is, where the fetal brow or occiput juts out.

If the cephalic prominence juts out along the line of the fetal back, the head is extended. If the cephalic prominence juts out along the line of the fetal anterior side, the head is flexed.

RECORDING YOUR FINDINGS

Typically, the record for a pregnant patient follows a standard order: age, Gs and Ps, weeks of gestation, means of determining gestational age (ultrasound vs. LMP), chief concern, chief pregnancy complications, and important history and examination findings. Two sample write-ups are given below.

See nomenclature for pregnancy outcomes pp. 1128–1129.

Recording the Physical Examination of the Pregnant PERSON

"32-year-old G3P1102 at 18 weeks' gestation by LMP presents to establish prenatal care. Pregnancy complicated by closely spaced pregnancies, prior iatrogenic preterm birth for preeclampsia, and prior cesarean delivery. Patient does not yet note fetal movement; denies contractions, vaginal bleeding, and leakage of fluids. On external examination, low-transverse cesarean scar is evident; fundus is palpable just below umbilicus. On internal examination, cervix is open to fingertip at the external os but closed at the internal os; cervix is 3 cm long; uterus enlarged to size consistent with 18-week gestation. Speculum examination shows leukorrhea with positive Chadwick sign. FHR by Doppler is 140–145 beats/min."

OR

"21-year-old G1P0 at 33 weeks' gestation as determined by 19-week ultrasound presents with chief concern of decreased fetal movement. Pregnancy complicated by rare prenatal visits and unhoused status. Patient reports minimal fetal movement over the last 24 hours; denies contractions, vaginal bleeding, or leakage of fluid. On external exam, a nontender gravid abdomen with no scars is noted; fundus is measured at 32 cm; fetus is vertex but not engaged in pelvis by Leopold maneuvers. On internal examination, cervix is closed, long, and high; speculum examination shows thin gray discharge with clue cells on wet mount. FHR by Doppler is 155–160 beats/min."

Dissecting the clinical presentation and examination findings of a 21-year-old G1P0 at 33 weeks' gestation highlights the importance of detailed clinical observation in diagnosing and managing pregnancy-related complications. The patient's background, including infrequent prenatal visits and unhoused status, adds complexity to her care. Key findings from the examination provide essential insights:

- *Decreased fetal movement:* The patient's primary concern of diminished fetal movement over the last 24 hours is a critical symptom, warranting immediate evaluation for fetal well-being.
- *Gravid abdomen without scars:* The absence of scars indicates no previous abdominal surgeries, including cesarean deliveries, which can affect current pregnancy management and delivery approach.
- *Fundal height at 32 cm:* This measurement is slightly below the expected 33 cm for gestational age, suggesting a potential discrepancy in fetal growth that needs further assessment.

- *Vertex presentation not engaged:* Determined through Leopold maneuvers, this finding is typical for the gestational age, but engagement status warrants monitoring as the patient approaches term.
- *Closed, long, high cervix:* This indicates no imminent signs of labor. The cervix's condition is reassuring but requires continued observation in the context of decreased fetal movement.
- *Thin, gray discharge with clue cells on wet mount:* Suggests bacterial vaginosis (BV), a condition associated with increased risks for preterm labor, warranting treatment.
- *FHR 155 to 160 BPM:* This falls within the normal range for gestational age, suggesting current fetal well-being despite the patient's decreased perception of movement.

In summary, the patient's presentation raises concerns for *potential fetal growth restriction* (suggested by the fundal height slightly below what is expected for gestational age) and BV, against a backdrop of decreased fetal movement. While the normal FHR provides some reassurance, the context demands a comprehensive approach to assess and ensure fetal well-being, address the identified BV, and closely monitor for any signs of preterm labor.

HEALTH PROMOTION AND COUNSELING: EVIDENCE AND RECOMMENDATIONS

Important Topics for Health Promotion and Counseling

- Screening for infectious diseases
- Genetic testing and aneuploidy screening
- Screening for medical conditions associated with pregnancy
- Intimate partner violence screening
- Rh(D) incompatibility screening
- Screening and counseling for unhealthy behaviors
- Screening for healthy weight and weight gain in pregnancy
- Interventions to prevent perinatal depression
- Breastfeeding
- Immunizations in pregnancy
- Preventive medicine
- Unintended pregnancy

In the following section, both traditional terms like "men," "women," "male," and "female" and inclusive terms such as "individuals assigned female at birth" and "individuals assigned male at birth" are used. This approach balances inclusivity with the need to accurately represent the original research.

Screening for Infectious Diseases

Screening for Hepatitis B Virus Infection. Infants born to individuals with hepatitis B virus (HBV) infection are at risk for perinatal transmission. This exposure is associated with an increased risk for chronic liver infection, which can lead to cirrhosis and hepatocellular cancer. The U.S. Centers for Disease Control and Prevention (CDC) estimated that nearly 21,000 infants were at risk for perinatal transmission in 2017 because they were born to persons with an HBV infection.[28] The U.S. Preventive Services Task Force (USPSTF) issued a grade A recommendation to screen all pregnant persons with a hepatitis B surface antigen (HBsAg) test at their first prenatal visit.[29] The test should be ordered even if the person was previously vaccinated or tested.

The American College of Obstetricians and Gynecologists (ACOG) also recommends testing for HBsAg and anti–hepatitis C antibody if they do not have documented negative test results.[30] Persons who have evidence of HBV infection in pregnancy are eligible for treatment to decrease viral load and reduce the risk of perinatal transmission. Vaccination is recommended for pregnant persons lacking immunity to hepatitis B. High-risk patients (multiple sexual partners, STI treatment in pregnancy, injection drug use, or a sexual or household contact with chronic HBV) should be retested at the time of delivery. The pediatric team should treat neonates whose mothers are HbsAg-positive with hepatitis B vaccination and hepatitis B immune globulin (HBIG) to prevent vertical transmission.

Screening for Syphilis Infection. The U.S. rates of primary and secondary syphilis in persons of reproductive age have been markedly increasing in the past decade, particularly among American Indian/Alaska Native, non-Hispanic Black, and Asian/Pacific Islander persons.[31–33] Untreated syphilis infections in pregnancy are associated with stillbirths, prematurity, neonatal death, and congenital syphilis (from transmitting the spirochete *Treponema pallidum* to the fetus). Congenital syphilis can cause serious comorbidities, including neurosyphilis, bony deformities, blindness, and deafness. Cases of congenital syphilis have been increasing over the past decade and currently affect an estimated 1 in every 1,300 live births. Treating the infected pregnant person with parenteral benzathine penicillin G reduces the risks for these outcomes, particularly when treatment is administered earlier in pregnancy.

The USPSTF issued a grade A recommendation to screen early for syphilis in all pregnant persons.[34] Serologic testing includes nontreponemal tests, such as the Venereal Disease Research Laboratory (VDRL) or the rapid plasma reagin (RPR), and a treponemal test such as fluorescent treponemal antibody absorption (FTA-ABS). Either test can be used first for persons without a history of syphilis, but confirmatory testing is required because false-positive results are common during pregnancy. The CDC recommends screening pregnant persons at 28 weeks and at delivery if they are at increased risk for acquiring syphilis during pregnancy, including misusing drugs, having an STI during pregnancy, having multiple/new sex partners, and having a sex partner with an STI.[35] Testing for syphilis is also recommended for persons delivering a stillborn infant. Infants born to birthing parents with syphilis should undergo nontreponemal testing and be clinically evaluated for congenital syphilis.[31] The decision to treat the infant should be based on the clinical presentation, serologic testing of the birthing parent and infant, and whether the birthing parent was treated.[33]

Screening for HIV Infection. The rate of perinatal HIV transmission has substantially declined since the early 1990s, with maternal-to-child transmission rates now lower than 1% due to the combination of receiving antiretroviral therapy (ART) prenatally and during labor and delivery, elective cesarean deliveries, and forgoing breastfeeding.[36] Because these interventions are effective in preventing perinatal HIV transmission, the USPSTF has issued a grade A recommendation to screen for HIV infection in all pregnant persons, including those presenting in labor or at delivery with an unknown HIV status.[37] The CDC recommends HIV screening at the initial prenatal visit, with patient refusal of HIV testing documented in the health record (i.e., an "opt-out" approach).[38]

High-risk populations should be rescreened in the third trimester, ideally before 36 weeks' gestation. For those who were not screened during pregnancy, rapid HIV testing is recommended during the delivery admission. The CDC recommends testing for HIV infection using an FDA-approved antigen/antibody immunoassay that detects HIV-1 and HIV-2 antibodies and the HIV-1 p24 antigen.[39] If the screen is positive, confirmatory testing should be performed with an HIV-1/HIV-2 antibody differentiation immunoassay. Specimens with nonreactive or indeterminate results on the differentiation immunoassay should be further tested with an HIV-1 nucleic acid test to differentiate an acute HIV-1 infection from a false-positive result.

Bacteriuria Screening. Asymptomatic bacteriuria is present in 2% to 10% of pregnant persons.[40] Pyelonephritis, which occurs in 1% to 2% of pregnancies, is associated with complications such as septicemia, adult respiratory distress syndrome, and anemia as well as adverse pregnancy outcomes, including low birth weight and preterm births.

The USPSTF found adequate evidence that treating pregnant persons for asymptomatic bacteriuria reduced the risk of developing pyelonephritis.[41] They issued a grade B recommendation to screen pregnant persons for asymptomatic bacteriuria by culturing a clean-catch midstream urine sample in early pregnancy. The ACOG recommends that patients with a positive screening urine culture (colony counts >100,000 CFU/mL) be treated with antibiotics for 5 to 7 days.[40] There is insufficient evidence to recommend whether to repeat screening after a negative initial culture result or after treating asymptomatic bacteriuria.

Genetic Testing and Aneuploidy Screening

ACOG recommends offering screening or diagnostic testing (with chorionic villus sampling or amniocentesis) for *aneuploidy* (extra or missing chromosomes) to all pregnant persons, regardless of age or other risk factors.[42] Counseling about screening and testing should occur early during the pregnancy and be part of a shared decision-making discussion that addresses the risk for having a fetal genetic disorder. Risk factors include older parental age, parental carriers of chromosomal rearrangement, parental aneuploidy, a previous child with a structural birth defect, or parental carriers of a genetic disorder (e.g., Tay–Sachs disease, cystic fibrosis, sickle cell disease).

Screening for Medical Conditions Associated with Pregnancy

Screening for Gestational Diabetes. *Gestational diabetes*, which affects 6% to 9% of U.S. pregnancies, is defined as diabetes that develops during pregnancy.[43,44] The prevalence of gestational diabetes is lowest among non-Hispanic White persons and higher among Hispanic, non-Hispanic Black, American Indian/Alaska Native, and Asian/Pacific Islander persons. The risk for gestational diabetes is increased among pregnant persons who are obese or older.

Gestational diabetes is associated with risks, including undergoing cesarean delivery, preeclampsia, preterm delivery, and developing diabetes later in life. Fetal and neonatal risks associated with gestational diabetes include stillbirth, macrosomia (birth weight >4 kg), large-for-gestational-age (LGA) infants, shoulder dystocia, birth injury, neonatal hypoglycemia and hyperbilirubinemia, and neonatal intensive care (NICU) admissions. Treatment, including lifestyle changes and antidiabetic medications, has been shown to reduce risks for cesarean and preterm deliveries, perinatal death, excessive fetal growth, shoulder dystocia, birth injuries, and NICU admissions.[45]

The USPSTF issued a grade B recommendation to screen for gestational diabetes in all asymptomatic pregnant persons at 24 weeks' gestation or later.[43] The most common testing performed in the United States is a two-step screening. A 50-g oral glucose tolerance test (OGTT) followed by a 1-hour blood glucose measurement is performed between weeks 24 and 28. Persons with a positive screen then undergo a 100-g, 3-hour diagnostic OGTT. Blood glucose levels are checked at baseline (fasting) and after 1, 2, and 3 hours. Gestational diabetes is diagnosed when two or more values are abnormal.

Screening for Hypertensive Disorders of Pregnancy. Hypertensive disorders of pregnancy (HDP) include chronic hypertension, gestational hypertension, preeclampsia, and eclampsia.[46] *Chronic hypertension* is high blood pressure before pregnancy or before 20 weeks' gestation. *Gestational hypertension* is systolic blood pressure at least 140 mm Hg and/or diastolic blood pressure at least 90 mm Hg on two occasions after 20 weeks' gestation. *Preeclampsia* is defined by either new-onset gestational hypertension or severe hypertension and at least one of the following additional features: proteinuria, thrombocytopenia, renal insufficiency, impaired liver function, pulmonary hypertension, or new-onset refractory headaches. Up to half of pregnant persons with gestational hypertension eventually meet criteria for preeclampsia.[46] *Eclampsia* is characterized by new-onset tonic–clonic, focal, or multifocal seizures. HDP affects 1 in 7 U.S. hospital deliveries and is a leading cause of pregnancy-related deaths.[47] The prevalence of HDP in hospital deliveries was highest among non-Hispanic Black and American Indian/Native Alaskan persons and persons ages 35 years and older. Adverse outcomes for the fetus and newborn include fetal growth restriction, low birth weight, and stillbirth.[48] ACOG recommends definitively managing severe preeclampsia and eclampsia by inducing early labor for vaginal delivery or performing a cesarean delivery.[46]

The USPSTF found adequate evidence that treating eclampsia reduces risks for maternal and fetal morbidity and mortality. They issued a grade B recommendation to screen for hypertensive disorders during pregnancy with blood pressure measurements.[48]

Screening for Iron Deficiency. The estimated prevalence of iron deficiency and anemia among U.S. pregnant persons is about 18% and 5%, respectively.[49] Rates of iron deficiency increase throughout pregnancy because increasing amounts of iron are needed to support maternal erythrocyte mass, fetal red blood cell (RBC) production, and fetoplacental growth. Observational studies suggest that iron deficiency is associated with low birth weight, premature birth, and infant mortality.

The USPSTF found insufficient evidence to recommend screening pregnant individuals who do not have symptoms of iron deficiency anemia (I statement).[50] However, ACOG recommends screening all pregnant individuals for anemia.[51]

A omplete blood count, which includes hemoglobin, hematocrit, and mean corpuscular volume (MCV), is recommended in the first trimester and at 24 to 28 weeks' gestation. Patients with anemia should be evaluated for iron deficiency by measuring serum iron, total iron-binding capacity, transferrin saturation, ferritin, and free erythrocyte protoporphyrin levels.

Screening for Perinatal Depression

Perinatal depression is defined as depressive episodes occurring during pregnancy and the postpartum period (first 12 months).[52] An estimated 15% to 20% of pregnant persons experience depression during pregnancy, and 10% experience postnatal depression.[53] American Indian/Alaska Native and Asian/Pacific Islander persons have higher reported rates of postpartum depression.[54] Risk factors for depression during pregnancy include past history of depression, anxiety, history of sexual or physical abuse, IPV, unplanned or unwanted pregnancy, stressful life events, low level of social and financial support, low socioeconomic status, pregestational and gestational diabetes, tobacco use, and complications during pregnancy.[55]

Postpartum depression is associated with depression and anxiety during pregnancy; stressful life events; breastfeeding/chestfeeding problems; and complications with childbirth, including preterm birth and/or admission to a NICU. Depression during pregnancy is associated with suicide and self-harm and increased risks of preterm birth and low birth weight.[53] Postpartum depression may interfere with parent–infant bonding; cause doubts about parenting abilities; and be associated with thoughts of death, suicide, and self-harm or harming the infant.[56] Perinatal depression is also associated with childhood adverse outcomes, including cognitive and behavioral problems, attention-deficit/hyperactivity disorder, and autism.[53]

The USPSTF found adequate evidence that screening for perinatal depression and psychotherapy for depression results in improved health outcomes; however, there was inadequate evidence to make recommendations about pharmacotherapy.[57] The USPSTF issued a grade B recommendation to screen for major depressive disorders, including for pregnant and postpartum persons.[58] They further noted that it was reasonable to assess for depression throughout pregnancy and during the postpartum period. ACOG recommends that clinicians screen individuals at least once during the perinatal period for depression and anxiety symptoms using a standardized, validated tool.[55] Additionally, ACOG recommends that clinicians assess mood and emotional well-being at a comprehensive postpartum visit, with subsequent referrals to behavioral health resources as needed.

Commonly used screening tools for perinatal depression include the Edinburgh Postnatal Depression Scale (EPDS)[59] and the Patient Health Questionnaire-9 (PHQ-9).[60] The *EPDS* consists of 10 self-reported items, takes less than 5 minutes to complete, has been translated into 50 different languages, has a low required reading level, and is easy to score. The EPDS includes anxiety symptoms, which are a prominent feature of perinatal mood disorders, and excludes constitutional symptoms of depression, such as changes in sleeping patterns, that are common in pregnancy and the postpartum period. The EPDS has relatively high sensitivity and specificity. The *PHQ-9* is a brief 9-item questionnaire focused on the nine diagnostic criteria for *Diagnostic and Statistical Manual of Mental Health Disorders*-IV depressive disorders. The PHQ-9 is one of the most validated tools in mental health and can assist clinicians with diagnosing depression and monitoring treatment response.

Intimate Partner Violence Screening

Pregnancy is a time of increased risk from IPV. Pre-existing patterns of abuse may intensify from verbal to physical abuse or from mild to severe physical abuse. During pregnancy, 1 in 10 individuals experiences some form of abuse, which has been associated with delayed prenatal care, preterm delivery, low infant birth weight, and even death of the birthing parent and fetus.[61,62] Prevalence of abuse is higher among pregnant persons who are teenage, American Indian/Alaska Native, non-Hispanic Black, and have less than 12 years of education.[63]

The USPSTF issued a grade B recommendation to screen individuals assigned female at birth of reproductive age for IPV and to provide support services.[64] The USPSTF suggests several screening instruments, including the Humiliation, Afraid, Rape, Kick (HARK); Hurt/Insult/Threaten/Scream (HITS); Extended Hurt/Insult/Threaten/Scream (E-HITS); Partner Violence Screen (PVS); and Woman Abuse Screening Tool (WAST).[65] HARK includes four questions that assess emotional and physical IPV in the past year. HITS includes four items that assess the frequency of IPV, and E-HITS includes an additional question assessing the frequency of sexual violence. PVS includes three items that assess physical abuse and current safety. WAST includes eight items that assess physical and emotional IPV. The sensitivity of these instruments ranged from 64% to 87%, and the specificity ranged from 80% to 95%.

ACOG recommends universal screening of all individuals assigned female at birth for domestic violence without regard to socioeconomic status, including pregnant individuals at the first prenatal visit and at least once each trimester.[61] Screening should occur in private and safe settings with the pregnant person alone. For a nonjudgmental approach, ACOG recommends using framing and confidentiality statements and then asking screening questions. Examples are listed in Box 29-5.

Box 29-5. ACOG Screening Approach for Intimate Partner Violence[61]

Framing Statement

"We've started talking to all of our patients about safe and healthy relationships because it can have such a large impact on your health."

Confidentiality Statement

"Before we get started, I want you to know that everything here is confidential, meaning that I won't talk to anyone else about what is said unless you tell me that... (insert the laws in your state about what is necessary to disclose)."

Sample Screening Questions

"Has your current partner ever threatened you or made you feel afraid?"

"Has your partner ever hit, choked, or physically hurt you?"

"Has your partner ever forced you to do something sexually that you did not want to do, or refused your request to use condoms?

Source: Reprinted with permission from ACOG Committee opinion no. 518: intimate partner violence. *Obstet Gynecol*. 2012;119(2 Pt 1):412–417. Copyright © 2012 by The American College of Obstetricians and Gynecologists.

Box 29-6. National Domestic Violence Hotline

Website: www.thehotline.org
1–800–799-SAFE (7233)
TTY for hearing impaired: 1–800–787–3224

Watch for clues of abuse such as frequent last-minute appointment changes; partners who refuse to leave the patient alone during the visit; signs of depression, substance abuse, mental health problems; new or recurrent STIs; and bruises or other injuries. Patients may take several visits before acknowledging abuse due to fear about safety and reprisal.

If the pregnant person acknowledges abuse, ask about the best way for you to help. The person may set limits on sharing information. Accept decisions about how to handle the situation safely, with the caveat that if children are involved, you may be required to report harmful behaviors to the authorities. Provide patients with resource materials that include safety procedures and lists of shelters, counseling centers, hotline numbers, and other trusted local referrals (Box 29-6). Plan future appointments at more frequent intervals. Finally, complete as thorough a physical examination as the patient permits and document all injuries with photographs or body maps.

Rh(D) Incompatibility Screening

Rh(D) incompatibility occurs when an Rh(D)-negative person is pregnant with an Rh(D)-positive fetus. In the absence of preventive measures, a small proportion of these pregnancies will result in alloimmunization, in which the pregnant person develops Rh(D) antibody. In subsequent pregnancies, the maternal antibody can cross into the fetal circulation, increasing the risk of fetal anemia, hydrops fetalis, and fetal death.

The USPSTF issued a grade A recommendation for Rh(D) blood typing and anti-Rh(D) antibody testing at the first prenatal visit. If the antibody screen is positive, the antibody should be identified, and a titer obtained. ACOG recommends repeating laboratory testing with each pregnancy and testing for ABO blood group in case there would be need for urgent transfusion in late pregnancy or with delivery. The USPSTF issued a grade B recommendation for repeating Rh(D) antibody testing at 24 to 28 weeks for all unsensitized Rh(D)-negative pregnant persons unless the biological co-parent is known to be Rh(D)-negative. A dose of Rh(D) immunoglobulin is then recommended for all unsensitized pregnant persons. Additionally, a dose of Rh(D) immunoglobulin should be administered to Rh(D)-negative persons who are not known to be sensitized within 72 hours of delivery when the infant is Rh(D) positive.[66,67]

Screening and Counseling for Unhealthy Behaviors

Tobacco Use. Tobacco use during pregnancy is associated with increased risks for miscarriage, preterm birth, and low birth weight.[68] Infants exposed to tobacco during pregnancy and after birth are at increased risk for sudden infant death syndrome and lung damage. The USPSTF issued a grade A recommendation for clinicians to "ask all pregnant persons about tobacco use, advise them to stop using tobacco, and provide behavioral interventions for cessation to pregnant persons who use tobacco."[69] However, evidence is insufficient to assess the balance of benefits and harms of offering e-cigarettes or pharmacotherapy, including nicotine replacement therapy, varenicline, and bupropion sustained-release, to support cessation efforts in pregnant persons (I statement).

Alcohol Use. Alcohol use during pregnancy is an important preventable risk for miscarriage, stillbirth, and developmental disabilities known as fetal alcohol spectrum disorders.[70] ACOG states that there is no safe amount or type of alcohol during pregnancy and that persons trying to get pregnant should not drink alcohol.[71] The USPSTF issued a grade B recommendation to screen for unhealthy alcohol use in adults, including pregnant persons, and offer brief behavioral counseling interventions for those engaged in risky or hazardous drinking.[72]

Drug Use. Using opiates, marijuana, or stimulants during pregnancy can lead to adverse pregnancy outcomes, including miscarriage/spontaneous abortion, placental abruption, preterm birth, and low birth weight.[73] Adverse effects on infants include risks for cognitive deficits, sudden infant death syndrome, and neonatal abstinence syndrome. ACOG strongly discourages pregnant persons from using marijuana, illicit drugs, or misusing prescription medications.[74] The USPSTF issued a grade B recommendation to ask all adults, including pregnant persons, about unhealthy drug use so that clinicians can offer or refer patients for appropriate care.[75]

Counseling for Healthy Weight and Weight Gain in Pregnancy

Weight gain should be closely monitored during pregnancy, as poor birth outcomes are associated with both excess and inadequate weight gain. In 2020, ACOG affirmed the 2009 weight gain guidelines from the National Academy of Medicine (Box 29-7).[76,77] Recommended weight gain during pregnancy

Box 29-7. Recommendations for Total and Rate of Weight Gain during Pregnancy, by Prepregnancy Body Mass Index, 2009

Prepregnancy Weight Category (BMI)[a]	Recommended Total Weight Gain (pounds) Singlet Gestation	Recommended Total Weight Gain (pounds) Twin Gestations	Recommended Rates of Weight Gain in the 2nd and 3rd Trimesters
	Range	Range	Pounds/week: Mean (range)
Underweight, or <18.5 kg/m²	28–40	–	1.0 (1–1.3)
Normal weight, or 18.5–24.9 kg/m²	25–35	37–54	1.0 (0.8–1.0)
Overweight, or 25.0–29.9 kg/m²	15–25	31–50	0.6 (0.5–0.7)
Obese, or >30 kg/m²	11–20	25–42	0.5 (0.4–0.6)

[a]Calculate Your Body Mass Index, National Heart, Lung, and Blood Institute at http://www.nhlbi.nih.gov/health/educational/lose_wt/BMI/bmicalc.htm

depends on baseline BMI and whether there are twin gestations. Data are insufficient to make weight gain recommendations for pregnant persons with triplet or higher gestations.

Pregnancy outcomes associated with excess weight gain include gestational diabetes, HDP, cesarean deliveries, and preterm birth; associated infant outcomes include macrosomia, being large for gestational age, birth injury, and hypoglycemia.[78] Low gestational weight gain is associated with adverse effects on infant birth weight and preterm birth. In 2015, more than half of U.S. pregnant persons had a prepregnancy BMI categorized as obese or overweight.[79] More than half of the pregnant persons who were overweight or obese before pregnancy exceeded recommended weight gain, while about 30% of those who were underweight gained less weight than recommended.[80] Prepregnancy obesity rates are higher among American Indian/Alaska Native, Black, and Hispanic persons compared to non-Hispanic White persons.[81]

Behavioral change counseling interventions have been associated with reduced gestational weight gain and lowered risks for gestational diabetes and emergency cesarean deliveries. Interventions were also associated with decreased risk for macrosomia and LGA infants.[81] In 2021, the USPSTF issued a grade B recommendation that clinicians offer adolescent and adult pregnant persons behavioral counseling interventions to promote healthy weight gain and prevent excessive weight gain during pregnancy.[82] Interventions, which can be provided by diverse practitioners in a variety of settings and delivery methods, should generally begin at the end of the first trimester or early in the second trimester. ACOG highlights the importance of addressing weight gain, diet, and exercise at the initial visit and throughout pregnancy.[76] Obtain weights at each visit and plot the results so that they are easy for you and your patient to review and discuss.

Interventions to Prevent Perinatal Depression

See also Chapter 11, Cognition, Behavior, and Mental Status, pp. 218–219.

The epidemiology, risk factors, and harms of perinatal depression are described in the Screening for Perinatal Depression section (p. 1144). The USPSTF[58] and ACOG[55] both recommend screening during pregnancy and postpartum to identify persons with perinatal depression. The USPSTF further issued a grade B recommendation to provide counseling interventions for pregnant persons at risk for depression or postpartum depression.[83] Evidence from controlled trials demonstrates that counseling interventions, including cognitive behavioral therapy and interpersonal therapy, are associated with a lower likelihood of developing perinatal depression.[84] The USPSTF suggests a pragmatic approach of targeting preventive interventions to pregnant persons with "a history of depression, current depressive symptoms (that do not reach a diagnostic threshold), low income or adolescent or single parenthood, recent IPV, or mental health-related factors such as elevated anxiety symptoms or a history of significant negative life events."

Breastfeeding or Chestfeeding

Breastfeeding or chestfeeding provides health benefits for children and parents.[85] Breastfeeding or chestfeeding during infancy and childhood is associated with reduced risks of acute otitis media, asthma, gastrointestinal infections, obesity, type 1 diabetes, and sudden infant death syndrome. It also offers health benefits, including lowered risks for breast and ovarian cancer, hypertension, and type 2 diabetes. However, breastfeeding or chestfeeding rates are low.[86] According to the CDC, only 83% of infants born in 2020 were ever breastfed, and only 1 in 4 were exclusively breastfed or chestfed through 6 months. Fewer infants born to non-Hispanic Black parents were ever breastfed or chestfed compared to those born to Asian, non-Hispanic White, or Hispanic parents.[87] The USPSTF found evidence that interventions, including one-on-one counseling from a health professional, peer support, and formalized educational programs, increased the likelihood of initiating and continuing exclusive breastfeeding or chestfeeding at 6 months. The USPSTF issued a grade B recommendation to provide interventions during pregnancy and after delivery to support these feeding practices.[88]

Immunizations in Pregnancy

The CDC Advisory Committee on Immunization Practices (ACIP) and ACOG recommend administering a Tdap vaccination during each pregnancy to protect against pertussis, ideally at 27 to 36 weeks' gestation, regardless of the prior immunization history. Other vaccinations routinely recommended for every pregnancy include inactivated influenza vaccine (if pregnant during flu season), respiratory syncytial virus (at weeks 32 to 36 if pregnant during September to January), and COVID-19 (if not up to date). If medically indicated, hepatitis A, hepatitis B, meningococcal conjugate, polio, and pneumococcal polysaccharide vaccines can safely be given during pregnancy. The following vaccinations should be avoided during pregnancy: human papillomavirus, live attenuated influenza vaccine, varicella, and measles/mumps/rubella. All nonimmune persons should be immunized for rubella (MMR) and varicella *immediately* after pregnancy and before discharge from the health facility.[89,90]

Preventive Medications

Multivitamin and Mineral Supplementation. ACOG recommends prenatal vitamin and mineral supplements that include folic acid, vitamin D, calcium, iron, iodine, choline, omega-3 fatty acids, B vitamins, and vitamin C.[91]

Folate deficiency in pregnancy is associated with neural tube defects (NTDs) in the developing fetus. Although folic acid is obtained from foods such as leafy greens, legumes, and whole grains and from food fortification (in the United States), folic acid requirements increase during pregnancy, and dietary sources may not be sufficient to prevent NTDs.[92] Multiple studies have shown that folic acid supplementation reduces the risk of NTDs.[93]

The USPSTF issued a grade A recommendation that persons who are planning to become pregnant or who could become pregnant take a daily supplement containing 0.4 mg (400 μg) to 0.8 mg (800 μg) of folic acid.[94] Supplementation should be initiated at least 1 month before conception and continued through the first trimester. ACOG recommends a daily folic acid supplementation of 4 mg (4,000 μg) for persons with a high risk of NTDs, such as those with a previously affected pregnancy.[91]

Iron requirements increase dramatically during pregnancy because iron is needed with advancing gestation to support the erythrocyte mass of the pregnant individual, fetal RBC production, and fetoplacental growth. Iron deficiency anemia during pregnancy can be associated with increased risk for low birth weight, preterm births, and infant mortality. ACOG recommends that all pregnant persons begin a daily low-dose (27 mg) supplement of iron in the first trimester.[51] ACOG also recommends screening for iron deficiency anemia (see Iron Deficiency Screening, pp. 1143–1144) and considering parenteral iron therapy for "those who cannot tolerate or do not respond to oral iron or for those with severe anemia deficiency later in pregnancy."

Aspirin for Preeclampsia. The Screening for Hypertensive Disorders of Pregnancy section describes preeclampsia and the potential adverse maternal and fetal outcomes (p. 1143). High-risk factors for preeclampsia include preeclampsia in a previous pregnancy, multifetal gestation, chronic hypertension, type 1 or type 2 diabetes before pregnancy, kidney disease, and autoimmune disease.[95] Moderate-risk factors include nulliparity, obesity, family history of preeclampsia, age 35 years or older, lower income, Black race (due to social factors), in vitro conception, and personal history reasons such as a greater than 10-year interval between pregnancies.

The USPSTF found good-quality evidence from randomized trials showing that daily low-dose aspirin for high-risk persons prevented preeclampsia and reduced complications for both the pregnant individual and the fetus. They issued a grade B recommendation to use a daily 81-mg dose of aspirin after 12 weeks' gestation to persons who are at high risk for preeclampsia and have no contraindications to taking aspirin.[95] The risk determination is based on the pregnant person having least one high-risk factor or at least two moderate-risk factors.

Unintended Pregnancy

Teen birth rates in the United States declined by more than 50% in the past decade, although substantial racial/ethnic and geographic disparities exist.[96] In 2019, the birth rates for teens who are non-Hispanic black, Hispanic, and American Indian/Alaska Native were more than double the rate for teens who are non-Hispanic White.[97]

More than 40% of U.S. pregnancies are unintended, including about 70% of pregnancies in teens ages 15 to 19 years.[96] Counsel persons who can become pregnant about the timing of ovulation in the menstrual cycle and how to plan or prevent pregnancy. Be familiar with the numerous options for contraception and their effectiveness (Box 29-8).

Box 29-8. Types of Family Planning Methods[98]

Methods	Types of Contraception
Natural	Fertility awareness/periodic abstinence, withdrawal, lactation
Barrier	External (male) condom, internal (female) condom, diaphragm, cervical cap, sponge
Implantable	Intrauterine devices (IUDs), subdermal implant of levonorgestrel
Pharmacologic/hormonal	Spermicide, oral contraceptives (estrogen and progesterone; progestin only), estrogen/progesterone injectables and patch, hormonal vaginal contraceptive ring, emergency contraception
Surgery (permanent)	Tubal ligation, vasectomy

Source: Centers for Disease Control and Prevention. Contraception. Accessed February 2, 2024. https://www.cdc.gov/reproductivehealth/contraception/

Failure rates are lowest for the subdermal implant, IUD, sterilization in individuals assigned female at birth, and vasectomy at less than 0.8% per year (<1 pregnancy/100 women/year) and highest for external (male) and internal (female) condoms, withdrawal, sponge in parous indivuduals, diaphragms, and spermicides, ranging from 13% to more than 20% per year (≥20 pregnancies/100 women/year). Fertility awareness–based methods are associated with failure rates range from 2% to 23%. Failure rates for injectables, oral contraceptives, the patch, and vaginal rings range from 4% to 7% per year (4 to 7 pregnancies/100 women/year).[98]

Take the time to understand the individual's or partners' concerns and preferences and respect these preferences whenever possible. Continued use of a preferred method is superior to a more effective method that is abandoned. For teenagers, a confidential setting eases discussion of topics that may seem private and difficult to explore.

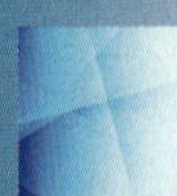

TABLE 29-1. Normal Anatomic and Physiologic Changes in Pregnancy

Organ System	Organ of Interest	Change in Normal Pregnancy	Clinical Relevance
Vital signs	Heart rate	↑ (Progresses throughout gestation)	
	Blood pressure	↓ (Nadir in second trimester)	
	Respiratory rate	←→	
	Oxygen saturation	←→	
Skin	Skin	Increased cutaneous blood flow	Dissipation of excess heat due to increased metabolism
		Hyperpigmentation	
		Spider angiomas and palmar erythema	Unclear clinical significance, likely related to hyperestrogenemia
	Hair	Scalp hair thickening	
		Hirsutism	Unclear clinical significance; severe hirsutism with signs of virilization should be investigated
Respiratory	Lungs	↑ Oxygen consumption 20%	Shifts CO_2 from fetus to maternal circulation
		↓ Arterial pCO_2	ABGs demonstrate respiratory alkalosis
		↑ Ventilation	Aids in CO_2 removal
		↓ TLV, RV, FRC	
		↑ TV, minute ventilation	
		↓ Pulmonary vascular resistance	
		←→ Lung compliance	
	Diaphragm	Diaphragm elevated 4 cm	Diaphragmatic elevation and increased minute ventilation contribute to sensation of dyspnea in pregnancy
Cardiovascular	Heart	↑ Cardiac output up to 50%	Related to both increased pulse and stroke volume Further augmented by ~20% in multifetal gestations
		Heart displaced left and upward	Appearance of cardiomegaly on imaging
		Exaggerated split S_1	Systolic murmurs are common, ≤90% of pregnant patients
		Hyperdynamic LV function	
	Peripheral vasculature	↓ Systemic vascular resistance	↑ Venous pooling and postural hypotension.
		↓ BP (diastolic > systolic)	↑ Dependent edema and varicose veins
		↓ Venous flow in the lower extremities due to compression by the gravid uterus	Predisposes to thrombosis

Organ System	Organ of Interest	Change in Normal Pregnancy	Clinical Relevance
Gastrointestinal	Stomach	↓ Gastric emptying	Contributes to nausea, acid reflux
		↓ Esophageal sphincter tone	
	Intestinal tracts, large and small	Displaced superiorly and laterally	Appendicitis may present atypically
		↓ Motility	Contributes to hemorrhoids, constipation
	Hepatobiliary tree	←→ Liver size	
		↑ Hepatic blood flow	
		↓ Serum albumin concentration	
		↓ Gallbladder motility	
			↑ Biliary stasis and incidence of cholesterol gallstones, cholecystitis
			↑ Risk of cholestasis
Hematologic	Plasma	↑ Circulating volume 40–45%	Provision of nutrients to the fetus/placenta, protection against impaired venous return
	Blood	↑ Erythrocyte production and volume	Protection against blood loss during parturition
		↑ Reticulocyte count	Unclear clinical significance—related to hemodilution and ↑ consumption
		↑ Iron turnover	Leads to iron deficiency anemia, pica
		↓ Hemoglobin and hematocrit	
		↑ Leukocytosis	
		↓ Platelets	Increased risk of epistaxis, nasal congestion
		↑ Inflammatory markers (CRP, ESR)	Unreliable markers of inflammation
	Coagulation	↑ Clotting factors (except factors XI and XIII)	
		↑ Fibrinogen	Maintains balance of coagulation and fibrinolysis—overall hypercoagulable state
		↓ Protein C and total protein S	
		↑ Fibrinolysis and ↑D-dimer	D-Dimer is an unreliable marker of thrombotic risk

(*continued*)

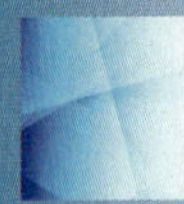

TABLE 29-1. Normal Anatomic and Physiologic Changes in Pregnancy *(Continued)*

Organ System	Organ of Interest	Change in Normal Pregnancy	Clinical Relevance
Urinary	Bladder	Hyperplasia of bladder muscle and connective tissue	↑ Urinary frequency and incontinence
		Elevation of trigone	
		↑ Bladder pressure	
	Ureters	Laterally displaced and compressed	Contributes to hydronephrosis, more commonly right-sided
		↑ Dilation and relaxation	
	Kidneys	↑ Renin–angiotensin–aldosterone system	Maintains BP first trimester; hypertension does not result in normal pregnancy due to angiotensin II refractoriness as pregnancy progresses
			Contributes to urinary frequency
		↑ Kidney size	
		↑ GFR and plasma flow	
		↓ Serum creatinine	Cr >0.9 mg/dL should be evaluated
		↑ Creatinine clearance 30%	
Musculoskeletal	Spine	Lumbar lordosis	Shifts center of gravity to accommodate the gravid uterus; may contribute to low back pain
		Pelvic joint relaxation—symphysis pubis, sacroiliac and sacrococcygeal joints	Pubic symphysis separation >1 cm may cause significant pain and gait disturbance

ABG, arterial blood gases; *Cr*, creatinine; *CRP*, c-reactive protein; *ESR*, erythrocyte sedimentation rate; *LV*, left ventricle; *BP*, blood pressure; *TLV*, total lung volume; *RV*, residual volume; *FRC*, functional residual capacity; *TV*, tidal volume; CO_2, carbon dioxide; *GFR*, glomerular filtration rate.

Source: Chapter 2: Maternal anatomy, Chapter 4: Maternal physiology. In: Cunningham FG, Leveno KJ, Bloom SL, et al., eds. *Williams Obstetrics*. 25th ed. McGraw-Hill Education; 2018.

REFERENCES

1. Chapter 2: Maternal anatomy, Chapter 4: Maternal physiology. In: Cunningham FG, Leveno KJ, Bloom SL, et al., eds. *Williams Obstetrics*. 25th ed. McGraw-Hill Education; 2018.
2. ACOG Practice Bulletin No. 196 summary: thromboembolism in pregnancy. *Obstet Gynecol*. 2018;132(1):243–248.
3. McCormack MC, Wise RA. Respiratory physiology in pregnancy. In: Bourjeily G, Rosene-Montella K, eds. *Pulmonary Problems in Pregnancy*. Humana Press; 2009. Accessed March 18, 2024. https://link.springer.com/chapter/10.1007/978-1-59745-445-2_2
4. Nwabuobi C, Arlier S, Schatz F, Guzeloglu-Kayisli O, Lockwood CJ, Kayisli UA. hCG: biological functions and clinical applications. *Int J Mol Sci*. 2017;18(10):2037.
5. Noctor E, Dunne FP. Type 2 diabetes after gestational diabetes: the influence of changing diagnostic criteria. *World J Diabetes*. 2015;6(2):234–244.
6. Kim C, Newton KM, Knopp RH. Gestational diabetes and the incidence of type 2 diabetes: a systematic review. *Diabetes Care*. 2002;25(10):1862–1868.
7. American Diabetes Association. 13. Management of diabetes in pregnancy: standards of medical care in diabetes—2018. *Diabetes Care*. 2018;41(Suppl 1):S137–S143.
8. Patton PE, Samuels MH, Trinidad R, Caughey AB. Controversies in the management of hypothyroidism during pregnancy. *Obstet Gynecol Surv*. 2014;69(6):346–358.
9. Committee on Obstetric Practice. ACOG Practice Bulletin No. 189: nausea and vomiting of pregnancy. *Obstet Gynecol*. 2018;131(1):e15–e30.
10. Committee on Practice Bulletins—Obstetrics; Committee on Genetics; Society for Maternal-Fetal Medicine. Practice Bulletin No. 162: prenatal diagnostic testing for genetic disorders. *Obstet Gynecol*. 2016;127(5):e108–e122.
11. Practice Bulletin No. 163: screening for fetal aneuploidy. *Obstet Gynecol*. 2016;127(5):e123–e137.
12. FAQs: carrier screening. American College of Obstetricians and Gynecologists. Accessed March 18, 2024. https://www.acog.org/womens-health/faqs/carrier-screening
13. Lord SJ, Bernstein L, Johnson KA, et al. Breast cancer risk and hormone receptor status in older women by parity, age of first birth, and breastfeeding: a case-control study. *Cancer Epidemiol Biomarkers Prev*. 2008;17(7):1723–1730.
14. Ursin G, Bernstein L, Lord SJ, et al. Reproductive factors and subtypes of breast cancer defined by hormone receptor and histology. *Br J Cancer*. 2005;93(3):364–371.
15. Final recommendation statement: breastfeeding: primary care interventions. U.S. Preventive Services Task Force. Accessed March 18, 2024. https://www.uspreventiveservicestaskforce.org/Page/Document/RecommendationStatementFinal/breastfeeding-primary-care-interventions
16. DeFranco EA, Ehrlich S, Muglia LJ. Influence of interpregnancy interval on birth timing. *BJOG*. 2014;121(13):1633–1640.
17. Thiel de Bocanegra H, Chang R, Howell M, Darney P. Interpregnancy intervals: impact of postpartum contraceptive effectiveness and coverage. *Am J Obstet Gynecol*. 2014;210(4):311.e1–311.e8.
18. American Academy of Pediatrics; American College of Obstetricians and Gynecologists. *Guidelines for Perinatal Care*. 8th ed. 2017. Accessed March 18, 2024. https://www.acog.org/clinical-information/physician-faqs/-/media/3a22e153b67446a6b31fb051e469187c.ashx
19. Task Force on Hypertension in Pregnancy. Hypertension in pregnancy: report of the American College of Obstetricians and Gynecologists' Task Force on Hypertension in Pregnancy. *Obstet Gynecol*. 2013;122(5):1122–1131.
20. Chapter 40: Hypertensive disorders, Chapter 50: Chronic hypertension. In: Cunningham FG, Leveno KJ, Bloom SL, et al., eds. *Williams Obstetrics*. 25th ed. McGraw-Hill Education; 2018.
21. Pay AS, Wiik J, Backe B, Jacobsson B, Strandell A, Klovning A. Symphysis-fundus height measurement to predict small-for-gestational-age status at birth: a systematic review. *BMC Pregnancy Childbirth*. 2015;15:22.
22. White LJ, Lee SJ, Stepniewska K, et al. Estimation of gestational age from fundal height: a solution for resource-poor settings. *J R Soc Interface*. 2012;9(68):503–510.
23. Robert Peter J, Ho JJ, Valliapan J, Sivasangari S. Symphysial fundal height (SFH) measurement in pregnancy for detecting abnormal fetal growth. *Cochrane Database Syst Rev*. 2015;(9):CD008136.
24. Powe CE, Levine RJ, Karumanchi SA. Preeclampsia, a disease of the maternal endothelium: the role of antiangiogenic factors and implications for later cardiovascular disease. *Circulation*. 2011;123(24):2856–2869.
25. Chen CW, Jaffe IZ, Karumanchi SA. Pre-eclampsia and cardiovascular disease. *Cardiovasc Res*. 2014;101(4):579–586.
26. Kirkham C, Harris S, Grzybowski S. Evidence-based prenatal care: part I. General prenatal care and counseling issues. *Am Fam Physician*. 2005;71(7):1307–1316.
27. Goetzinger KR, Odibo AO, Shanks AL, Roehl KA, Cahill AG. Clinical accuracy of estimated fetal weight in term pregnancies in a teaching hospital. *J Matern Fetal Neonatal Med*. 2014;27(1):89–93.
28. Centers for Disease Control and Prevention. HBV Infection. Accessed February 11, 2024. https://www.cdc.gov/hepatitis-b/hcp/perinatal-provider-overview/clinical-testing-guidelines.html. Accessed September 10, 2024.
29. U.S. Preventive Services Task Force; Owens DK, Davidson KW, Krist AH, et al. Screening for hepatitis B virus infection in pregnant women: U.S. Preventive Services Task Force Reaffirmation Recommendation Statement. *JAMA*. 2019;322(4):349–354.
30. Viral hepatitis in pregnancy: ACOG Clinical Practice Guideline No. 6. *Obstet Gynecol*. 2023;142(3):745–759.
31. Stafford IA, Workowski KA, Bachmann LH. Syphilis complicating pregnancy and congenital syphilis. *N Engl J Med*. 2024;390(3):242–253.
32. Centers for Disease Control and Prevention. Syphilis. Accessed September 10, 2024. https://www.cdc.gov/sti/about/about-stis-and-pregnancy.html.
33. Cooper JM, Sánchez PJ. Congenital syphilis. *Semin Perinatol*. 2018;42(3):176–184.
34. U.S. Preventive Services Task Force; Curry SJ, Krist AH, Owens DK, et al. Screening for syphilis infection in pregnant women: U.S. Preventive Services Task Force Reaffirmation Recommendation Statement. *JAMA*. 2018;320(9):911–917.
35. Workowski KA, Bachmann LH, Chan PA, et al. Sexually Transmitted Infections Treatment Guidelines, 2021. *MMWR Recomm Rep*. 2021;70(4):1–187.
36. Nesheim SR, FitzHarris LF, Mahle Gray K, Lampe MA. Epidemiology of perinatal HIV transmission in the United States in the era of its elimination. *Pediatr Infect Dis J*. 2019;38(6):611–616.

37. U.S. Preventive Services Task Force; Owens DK, Davidson KW, Krist AH, et al. Screening for HIV infection: U.S. Preventive Services Task Force Recommendation Statement. *JAMA.* 2019;321(23):2326–2336.
38. Branson BM, Handsfield HH, Lampe MA, et al. Revised recommendations for HIV testing of adults, adolescents, and pregnant women in health-care settings. *MMWR Recomm Rep.* 2006;55(RR-14):1–17.
39. National Center for HIV/AIDS Viral Hepatitis and TB Prevention (U.S.). 2018 Quick reference guide: Recommended laboratory HIV testing algorithm for serum or plasma specimens. Accessed February 6, 2024. https://stacks.cdc.gov/view/cdc/50872
40. Urinary tract infections in pregnant individuals. *Obstet Gynecol.* 2023;142(2):435–445.
41. U.S. Preventive Services Task Force; Owens DK, Davidson KW, et al. Screening for asymptomatic bacteriuria in adults: U.S. Preventive Services Task Force Recommendation Statement. *JAMA.* 2019;322(12):1188–1194.
42. Practice Bulletin No. 162: prenatal diagnostic testing for genetic disorders. *Obstet Gynecol.* 2016;127(5):e108–e122.
43. U.S. Preventive Services Task Force; Davidson KW, Barry MJ, Mangione CM, et al. Screening for gestational diabetes: U.S. Preventive Services Task Force Recommendation Statement. *JAMA.* 2021;326(6):531–538.
44. ACOG Practice Bulletin No. 190: gestational diabetes mellitus. *Obstet Gynecol.* 2018;131(2):e49–e64.
45. Pillay J, Donovan L, Guitard S, et al. Screening for gestational diabetes: updated evidence report and systematic review for the U.S. Preventive Services Task Force. *JAMA.* 2021; 326(6):539–562.
46. Gestational hypertension and preeclampsia: ACOG Practice Bulletin, Number 222. *Obstet Gynecol.* 2020;135(6): e237–e260.
47. Ford ND, Cox S, Ko JY, et al. Hypertensive disorders in pregnancy and mortality at delivery hospitalization—United States, 2017–2019. *MMWR Morb Mortal Wkly Rep.* 2022;71(17):585–591.
48. U.S. Preventive Services Task Force; Barry MJ, Nicholson WK, Silverstein M, et al. Screening for hypertensive disorders of pregnancy: U.S. Preventive Services Task Force Final Recommendation Statement. *JAMA.* 2023;330(11): 1074–1082.
49. Cantor AG, Bougatsos C, McDonagh M. Routine iron supplementation and screening for iron deficiency anemia in pregnancy. *Ann Intern Med.* 2015;163(5):400.
50. Siu AL, U.S. Preventive Services Task Force. Screening for iron deficiency anemia and iron supplementation in pregnant women to improve maternal health and birth outcomes: U.S. Preventive Services Task Force Recommendation Statement. *Ann Intern Med.* 2015;163(7):529–536.
51. Anemia in pregnancy: ACOG Practice Bulletin, Number 233. *Obstet Gynecol.* 2021;138(2):e55–e64.
52. ACOG Committee Opinion No. 757: Screening for Perinatal Depression. *Obstet Gynecol.* 2018;132(5):e208–e212.
53. Howard LM, Khalifeh H. Perinatal mental health: a review of progress and challenges. *World Psychiatry.* 2020;19(3): 313–327.
54. Ko JY, Rockhill KM, Tong VT, Morrow B, Farr SL. Trends in Postpartum Depressive Symptoms—27 States, 2004, 2008, and 2012. *MMWR Morb Mortal Wkly Rep.* 2017;66(6): 153–158.
55. Screening and diagnosis of mental health conditions during pregnancy and postpartum: ACOG Clinical Practice Guideline No. 4. *Obstet Gynecol.* 2023;141(6):1232–1261.
56. National Institutes of Mental Health. Perinatal Depression. Accessed February 10, 2024. https://www.nimh.nih.gov/health/publications/perinatal-depression
57. O'Connor EA, Perdue LA, Coppola EL, Henninger ML, Thomas RG, Gaynes BN. Depression and suicide risk screening: updated evidence report and systematic review for the U.S. Preventive Services Task Force. *JAMA.* 2023;329(23):2068–2085.
58. U.S. Preventive Services Task Force; Barry MJ, Nicholson WK, Silverstein M, et al. Screening for depression and suicide risk in adults: U.S. Preventive Services Task Force Recommendation Statement. *JAMA.* 2023;329(23):2057–2067.
59. Cox JL, Holden JM, Sagovsky R. Detection of postnatal depression. Development of the 10-item Edinburgh Postnatal Depression Scale. *Br J Psychiatry.* 1987;150:782–786.
60. Kroenke K, Spitzer RL, Williams JB. The PHQ-9: validity of a brief depression severity measure. *J Gen Intern Med.* 2001; 16(9):606–613.
61. ACOG Committee Opinion No. 518: Intimate partner violence. *Obstet Gynecol.* 2012;119(2 Pt 1):412–417.
62. Alhusen JL, Ray E, Sharps P, Bullock L. Intimate partner violence during pregnancy: maternal and neonatal outcomes. *J Womens Health (Larchmt).* 2015;24(1):100–106.
63. Chisholm CA, Bullock L, Ferguson JEJ 2nd. Intimate partner violence and pregnancy: epidemiology and impact. *Am J Obstet Gynecol.* 2017;217(2):141–144.
64. U.S. Preventive Services Task Force; Curry SJ, Krist AH, Owens DK, et al. Screening for intimate partner violence, elder abuse, and abuse of vulnerable adults: U.S. Preventive Services Task Force Final Recommendation Statement. *JAMA.* 2018;320(16):1678–1687.
65. Feltner C, Wallace I, Berkman N, et al. *Screening for Intimate Partner Violence, Elder Abuse, and Abuse of Vulnerable Adults: An Evidence Review for the U.S. Preventive Services Task Force.* 2018. *U.S. Preventive Services Task Force Evidence Syntheses, formerly Systematic Evidence Reviews.*
66. U.S. Preventive Services Task Force. Rh(D) Incompatibility: Screening. Accessed January 26, 2024. https://www.uspreventiveservicestaskforce.org/uspstf/recommendation/rh-d-incompatibility-screening
67. Practice Bulletin No. 181: Prevention of Rh D Alloimmunization. *Obstet Gynecol.* 2017;130(2):e57–e70.
68. Centers for Disease Control and Prevention. Smoking During Pregnancy. Accessed February 7, 2024. https://www.cdc.gov/tobacco/basic_information/health_effects/pregnancy/index.htm
69. U.S. Preventive Services Task Force; Krist AH, Davidson KW, Mangione CM, et al. Interventions for Tobacco Smoking Cessation in Adults, Including Pregnant Persons: U.S. Preventive Services Task Force Recommendation Statement. *JAMA.* 2021;325(3):265–279.
70. Centers for Disease Control and Prevention. Alcohol Use During Pregnancy. Accessed February 6, 2024. https://www.cdc.gov/alcohol-pregnancy/about/index.html
71. American College of Obstetricians and Gynecologists. Alcohol and Pregnancy. Accessed February 6, 2024. https://www.acog.org/womens-health/infographics/alcohol-and-pregnancy
72. U.S. Preventive Services Task Force; Curry SJ, Krist AH, Owens DK, et al. Screening and behavioral counseling interventions to reduce unhealthy alcohol use in adolescents and

adults: U.S. Preventive Services Task Force Recommendation Statement. *JAMA*. 2018;320(18):1899–1909.
73. Forray A, Foster D. Substance use in the perinatal period. *Curr Psychiatry Rep*. 2015;17(11):91.
74. American College of Obstetricians and Gynecologists. Tobacco, Alcohol, Drugs, and Pregnancy. Accessed February 5, 2024. https://www.acog.org/womens-health/faqs/tobacco-alcohol-drugs-and-pregnancy
75. U.S. Preventive Services Task Force; Krist AH, Davidson KW, Mangione CM, et al. Screening for unhealthy drug use: U.S. Preventive Services Task Force Recommendation Statement. *JAMA*. 2020;323(22):2301–2309.
76. American College of Obstetricians and Gynecologists. ACOG Committee Opinion no. 548: weight gain during pregnancy. *Obstet Gynecol*. 2013;121(1):210–212.
77. Institute of Medicine and National Research Council Committee to Reexamine IOM Pregnancy Weight Guidelines. *Weight Gain During Pregnancy: Reexamining the Guidelines*. National Academies Press; 2009.
78. Goldstein RF, Abell SK, Ranasinha S, et al. Association of gestational weight gain with maternal and infant outcomes: a systematic review and meta-analysis. *JAMA*. 2017;317(21):2207–2225.
79. Deputy NP, Dub B, Sharma AJ. Prevalence and trends in prepregnancy normal weight - 48 States, New York City, and District of Columbia, 2011–2015. *MMWR Morb Mortal Wkly Rep*. 2018;66(51–52):1402–1407.
80. Centers for Disease Control and Prevention. QuickStats: Gestational weight gain among women with full-term, singleton births, compared with recommendations—48 States and the District of Columbia, 2015. Accessed February 11, 2024. https://blogs.cdc.gov/nchs/2016/10/14/3272/
81. Cantor AG, Jungbauer RM, McDonagh M, et al. Counseling and behavioral interventions for healthy weight and weight gain in pregnancy: evidence report and systematic review for the U.S. Preventive Services Task Force. *JAMA*. 2021;325(20):2094–2109.
82. U.S. Preventive Services Task Force; Davidson KW, Barry MJ, Mangione CM, et al. Behavioral counseling interventions for healthy weight and weight gain in pregnancy: U.S. Preventive Services Task Force Recommendation Statement. *JAMA*. 2021;325(20):2087–2093.
83. U.S. Preventive Services Task Force; Curry SJ, Krist AH, Owens DK, et al. Interventions to prevent perinatal depression: U.S. Preventive Services Task Force Recommendation Statement. *JAMA*. 2019;321(6):580–587.
84. O'Connor E, Senger CA, Henninger ML, Coppola E, Gaynes BN. Interventions to prevent perinatal depression: evidence report and systematic review for the U.S. Preventive Services Task Force. *JAMA*. 2019;321(6):588–601.
85. Centers for Disease Control and Prevention. Breastfeeding. Why It Matter. Accessed February 8, 2024. https://www.cdc.gov/breastfeeding/about-breastfeeding/why-it-matters.html
86. Centers for Disease Control and Prevention. Results: Breastfeeding Rates. National Immunization Survey-Child. Accessed February 8, 2024. https://www.cdc.gov/breastfeeding/data/nis_data/results.html
87. Centers for Disease Control and Prevention. Breastfeeding. Facts. Accessed February 12, 2024. https://www.cdc.gov/breastfeeding/data/facts.html
88. U.S. Preventive Services Task Force; Bibbins-Domingo K, Grossman DC, Curry SJ, et al. Primary care interventions to support breastfeeding: U.S. Preventive Services Task Force Recommendation Statement. *JAMA*. 2016;316(16):1688–1693.
89. ACOG Committee Opinion No. 741: Maternal Immunization. *Obstet Gynecol*. 2018;131(6):e214–e217.
90. Murthy N, Wodi AP, Cineas S, Ault KA. Advisory Committee on Immunization Practices. Recommended Adult Immunization Schedule, United States, 2023. *Ann Intern Med*. 2023;176(3):367–380.
91. American College of Obstetricians and Gynecologists. Nutrition During Pregnancy. Accessed February 5, 2024. https://www.acog.org/womens-health/faqs/nutrition-during-pregnancy#:~:text=When%20you%20are%20pregnant%20you,first%2012%20weeks%20of%20pregnancy.
92. Greenberg JA, Bell SJ, Guan Y, Yu YH. Folic acid supplementation and pregnancy: more than just neural tube defect prevention. *Rev Obstet Gynecol*. 2011;4(2):52–59.
93. Viswanathan M, Urrutia RP, Hudson KN, Middleton JC, Kahwati LC. Folic acid supplementation to prevent neural tube defects: updated evidence report and systematic review for the U.S. Preventive Services Task Force. *JAMA*. 2023;330(5):460–466.
94. U.S. Preventive Services Task Force; Barry MJ, Nicholson WK, Silverstein M, et al. Folic acid supplementation to prevent neural tube defects: U.S. Preventive Services Task Force Reaffirmation Recommendation Statement. *JAMA*. 2023;330(5):454–459.
95. U.S. Preventive Services Task Force; Davidson KW, Barry MJ, Mangione CM, et al. Aspirin use to prevent preeclampsia and related morbidity and mortality: U.S. Preventive Services Task Force Recommendation Statement. *JAMA*. 2021;326(12):1186–1191.
96. Rossen LM, Hamilton BE, Abma JC, Gregory ECW, Beresovsky V, Resendez AV. *Updated methodology to estimate overall and unintended pregnancy rates in the United States*. 2023. *Vital and health Statistics Series 2, Data evaluation and methods research*. https://stacks.cdc.gov/view/cdc/124395. Accessed September 10, 2024.
97. Centers for Disease Control and Prevention. About Teen Pregnancy. Accessed February 2, 2024. https://www.cdc.gov/reproductive-health/teen-pregnancy/. Accessed September 10, 2024
98. Centers for Disease Control and Prevention. Contraception. Accessed September 10, 2024. https://www.cdc.gov/contraception/index.html.

CHAPTER

30

Older Adults

ADDRESSING THE CHALLENGES OF GLOBAL AGING

Globally, people are living longer, with most individuals now expecting to live into their 60s and beyond (Fig. 30-1). This trend is universal, with significant growth in both the size and proportion of older populations worldwide.[1] By 2030, one in six people globally will be age 60 years or older. In the United States, the older adult population is projected to double to 98 million by 2060, comprising nearly 24% of the total population.[2,3] The "oldest-old" group, those aged 85 and above, is expected to reach 20 million by 2060. This demographic shift highlights the imperative for societies worldwide to not only extend life span but also enhance the "health span" of the aging population. The goal is to empower older adults to maintain their functionality and enjoy vibrant, active lives within their communities.

Chapter Content Guide

- Defining the Older Adult
- Caring for Older Adults: Clinical Considerations
- Communicating Effectively with Older Adults

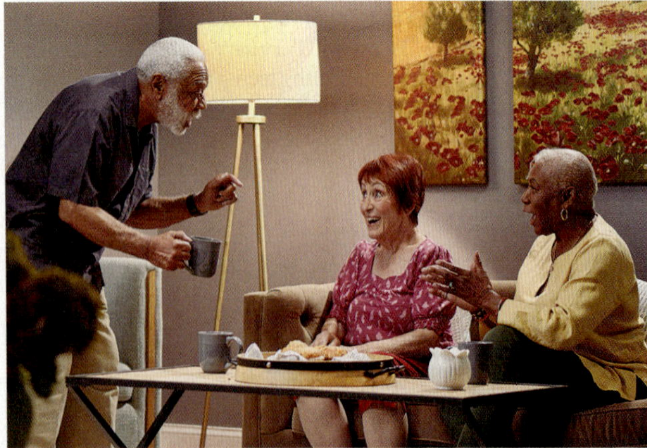

FIGURE 30-1. Older adults maximizing health span can enjoy rich, active lives.

Box 30-1. Defining Aging: Usual, Pathologic, and Successful Aging

Primary (usual): inevitable changes that occur with aging, such as a slower metabolism, reduced muscle mass, and decreased skin elasticity, which are not indicative of disease

Secondary (pathologic): atypical changes that signify diseases or health conditions, like Alzheimer disease or osteoporosis, underscoring the importance of differentiating these from primary aging in clinical assessments

Successful: goes beyond the absence of disease to include maintaining physical and cognitive function, engagement in social and productive activities, and achieving a good quality of life

- Geriatric 5Ms
- Health History: Applying the 5Ms Framework
- Adjusting Physical Examination Techniques For Older Adults
- Geriatric Assessment: Applying the 5Ms Framework
- Health Promotion and Counseling: Evidence and Recommendations

DEFINING OLDER ADULTHOOD

Older adults are typically aged 65 years and older. However, aging is a highly individualized process that varies significantly, influenced by factors such as physical activity, mental health, and social networks (Box 30-1).[4] While chronologic age provides a guideline, the assessment of an older adult should be tailored to their unique physical, cognitive, and social characteristics.[5–7] This individualized approach allows for more meaningful patient engagement and better alignment with their health priorities and preferences.

This chapter uses the term "older adult" for persons 65 years and older over terms such as "senior," "aged," or "elderly."[8] Society's preferences for words and terms change too often, too fast, and too arbitrarily to make definitive recommendations about usage.[9] Take the time to find out which term your older adult patients prefer.

ANATOMIC AND PHYSIOLOGIC CHANGES IN OLDER ADULTS

Understanding the anatomic and physiologic changes that accompany aging is crucial for making accurate diagnoses, creating effective treatment plans, and providing personalized care to older adults (Box 30-2). Recognizing these normal changes will help you avoid misinterpreting signs of aging as pathological conditions.[10] Key areas to focus on include the increased risk of cardiovascular diseases due to arterial stiffness, changes in skin elasticity and bone

Box 30-2. Anatomic and Physiologic Changes in Older Adults

System	Changes
General survey	■ Older adults may present with notable physical changes including decreased height due to vertebral compression (Fig. 30-2), increased waist circumference, and changes in skin texture. ■ Overall energy levels may decrease, and their general demeanor may reflect the cumulative effects of chronic conditions.
Mental status	■ Risk of depression, anxiety, and loneliness increases due to social, physical, and psychological factors. ■ Cognitive decline can affect memory, problem solving, and language skills.
Vital signs	■ Systolic blood pressure increases due to arterial stiffness; diastolic may plateau or decrease,[12] leading to a widened pulse pressure. ■ Resting heart rate remains relatively unchanged, but the maximal heart rate declines, affecting exercise tolerance.[13] ■ Temperature regulation becomes less efficient, with older adults feeling colder more easily.
Skin	■ Skin becomes thinner, less elastic, and more prone to damage and bruising due to a decrease in collagen and subcutaneous fat. ■ Age spots (*solar lentigines*) and keratoses become more common (Fig. 30-3). ■ Wound healing is slower, and the risk of skin infections and ulcers increases.

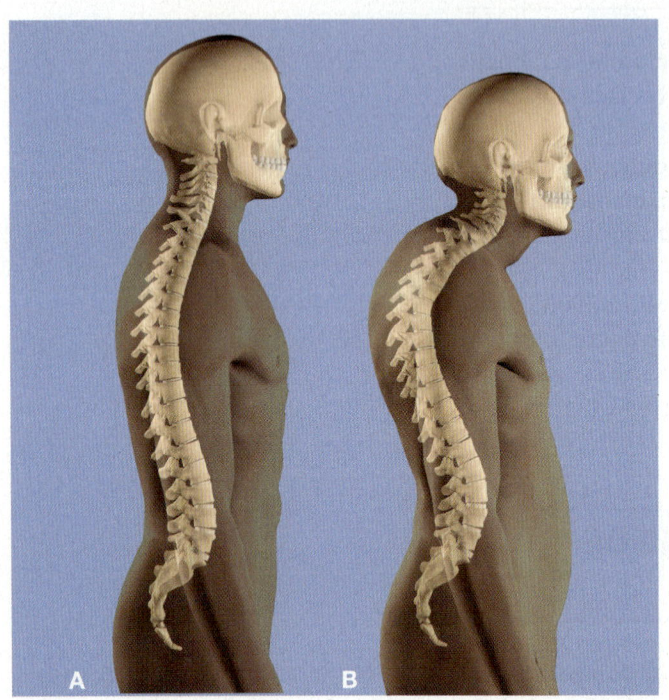

FIGURE 30-2. Aging changes in the vertebral column. **A.** Normal spinal column. **B.** Kyphosis. (Source: LifeART image copyright © 2019 Lippincott Williams & Wilkins. All rights reserved.)

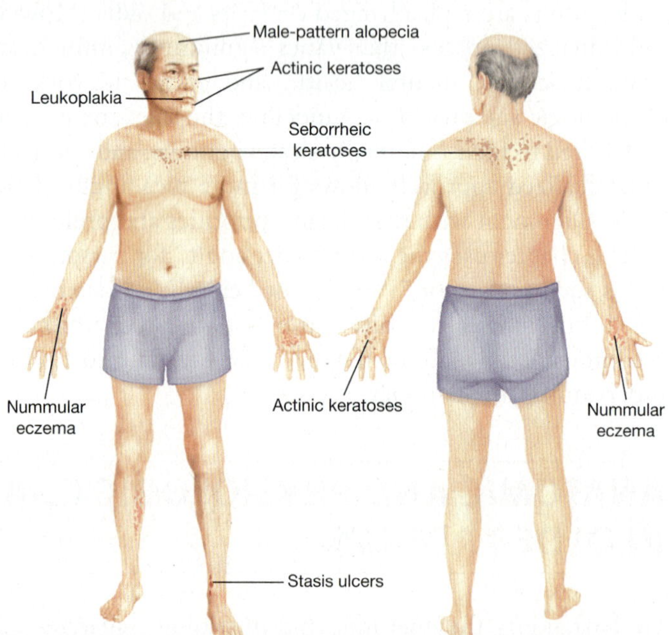

FIGURE 30-3. Skin and hair changes in older adults.

System	Changes
Head, eyes, ears, nose, and throat	■ Visual acuity declines with *presbyopia*, (Fig. 30-4) cataracts, and age-related macular degeneration increasing in prevalence. ■ Hearing loss (*presbycusis*) affects high-frequency sounds initially. ■ Oral health issues like gum disease, tooth loss, and dry mouth (*xerostomia*) become more common. ■ Sense of taste may diminish, and difficulty swallowing (*dysphagia*) may occur.
Breasts and axillae	■ Glandular tissue is replaced by fat, leading to changes in breast size and elasticity. Some males may develop gynecomastia.
Thorax and lungs	■ Lung elasticity decreases, and chest wall stiffness increases, reducing lung capacity and efficiency.[14] ■ Risk of respiratory infections increases due to decreased ciliary and immune function. ■ Pulmonary reserve diminishes, affecting tolerance to exercise and respiratory stresses.
Cardiovascular system	■ Heart may increase in size, particularly the left ventricle, leading to potential issues with heart function. ■ Arterial stiffness contributes to hypertension. ■ Electrical conduction system can degenerate, increasing arrhythmia risks.[15] ■ Systolic murmurs become more common due to valvular heart diseases like aortic sclerosis or mitral valve prolapse.[15]
Peripheral vascular system	■ Decreased elasticity of the blood vessels contributes to peripheral artery disease and chronic venous insufficiency.[14] ■ Lymphatic drainage efficiency may decline, leading to edema.

(continued)

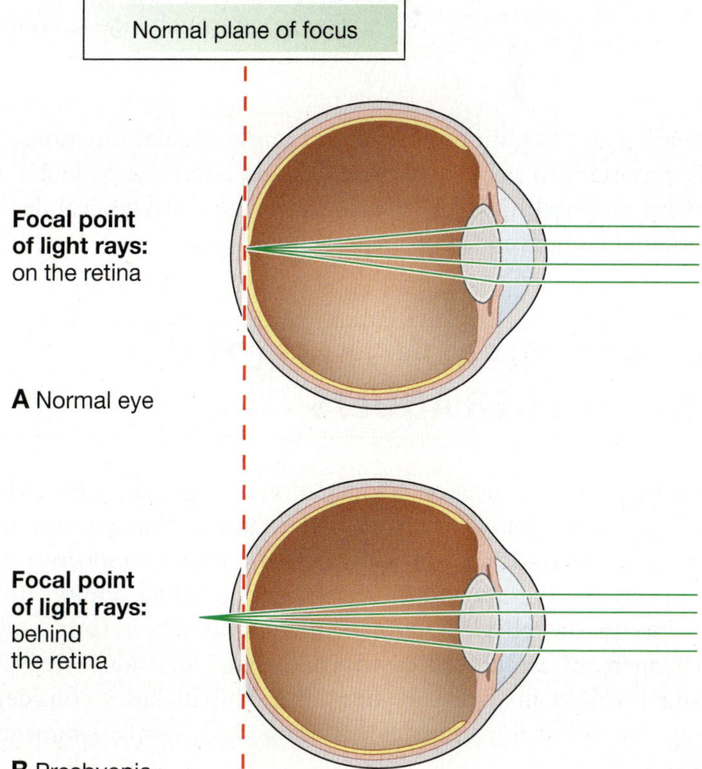

FIGURE 30-4. Refractive changes with aging. **A.** Normal. **B.** Presbyopia. With age, the lens stiffens and can no longer cause rays from near objects to converge on the retina. Rays converge behind the retina. (Reprinted with permission from McConnell TH. *The Nature of Disease: Pathology for the Health Professions.* 2nd ed. Wolters Kluwer Health/Lippincott Williams & Wilkins; 2014. Figure 25-5.)

Box 30-2. Anatomic and Physiologic Changes in Older Adults (*Continued*)

System	Changes
Gastrointestinal system	▪ Decreased saliva production can affect digestion and oral health. ▪ Esophageal motility may decrease, and the risk of gastroesophageal reflux disease (GERD) increases. ▪ Gastric emptying slows, and risk of peptic ulcer disease increases. ▪ Liver size and blood flow decrease, affecting drug metabolism. ▪ Constipation becomes more common due to reduced gut motility.
Genitourinary system: penis, scrotum, and prostate	▪ Prostate enlargement is common, affecting urination.[16] ▪ Libido and erectile function may decrease due to lower testosterone levels and vascular changes.[14] ▪ Testicular atrophy can occur, along with a reduction in sperm quality.
Genitourinary system: vulva, vagina, uterus, and adnexa	▪ Postmenopausal changes include vaginal dryness, atrophy, and increased pH leading to a higher risk of infections. ▪ Pelvic floor muscles may weaken, increasing the risk of prolapse and incontinence.[17] ▪ Ovarian reserve decreases, and the endometrium may thin, affecting reproductive health.[18]
Musculoskeletal system	▪ Bone density decreases, raising the risk of fractures (*osteoporosis*). ▪ Muscle mass and strength decline (*sarcopenia*), and joint cartilage wears down, increasing osteoarthritis risks. ▪ Risk of falls increases due to decreased balance and proprioception. ▪ Joint range of motion may decrease.
Nervous system	▪ Cognitive functions may slow, and risk of neurodegenerative diseases such as Alzheimer disease increases. ▪ Peripheral neuropathy becomes more common, affecting sensation. ▪ Sleep patterns change to lighter and more fragmented sleep.

density, and alterations in renal and cardiovascular functions.[11] As a student, it is important to assess how these changes affect the patient's overall functional status and health, which is essential for informed clinical decision making and offering compassionate, patient-centered care.

COMMUNICATING EFFECTIVELY WITH OLDER ADULTS

Effective communication is foundational when caring for older adults, considering the physiologic, sensory, and cognitive changes that accompany aging. As a future clinician you will need to create a supportive environment that respects the dignity and life experiences of older adults (Box 30-3). Adjustments in the physical setup of the health care setting and the manner of engagement are critical to ensuring that older adults feel heard, respected, and involved in their care decisions. This includes considerations for hearing and vision impairments and using clear, simple language free of medical jargon.[19]

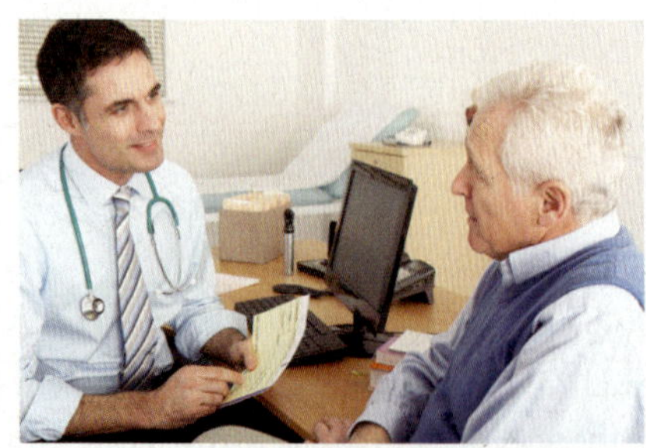

FIGURE 30-5. Conducting the health interview fully facing the patient and at eye level.

Box 30-3. Optimizing Patient Encounters with Older Adults

Aspect	Details
Adjust the environment	■ Ensure the room temperature is comfortable, reflecting the older patient's decreased ability to regulate body temperature. ■ Increase ambient lighting in the consultation area to help compensate for diminished vision, ensuring it is bright enough to facilitate reading and task completion without causing glare. ■ Arrange for seating that reduces the need for unnecessary movement, considering mobility challenges. ■ Eliminate obstacles and ensure clear pathways to accommodate those with walking aids or wheelchairs.
Direct communication	■ Maintain eye contact and use facial expressions and gestures (visual cues) to enhance communication (Fig. 30-5). ■ Speak clearly, slowly, and in a tone that is easy to follow, allowing time for the patient to process the information and respond. ■ Use simple language and avoid medical jargon to ensure that the patient fully understands the conversation. ■ Validate the patient's feelings and concerns through active listening, showing empathy and understanding.
Hearing considerations	■ Before starting the conversation, inquire about the patient's hearing preferences and adjust your speaking volume accordingly. ■ Position yourself so that light is on your face, not behind you, to facilitate lip-reading for patients who rely on visual cues. ■ Use written materials or visual aids to support verbal communication, ensuring that these materials are in large, readable fonts. ■ Regularly check in with the patient to confirm understanding, inviting questions and clarifications.
Visit format and content	■ Begin the visit by discussing the patient's primary concerns and objectives to ensure that their most pressing issues are addressed. ■ Encourage patients to bring a list of medications, symptoms, and questions to the visit to help structure the conversation and ensure that all relevant topics are covered. ■ Integrate life review or storytelling into the visit, as discussing past experiences can provide valuable context for current health issues and treatment preferences. ■ Focus on building a therapeutic relationship, emphasizing collaboration and respect for the patient's autonomy and preferences.
Efficient and considerate assessment	■ Tailor the assessment to the patient's specific health status, avoiding unnecessary tests that may cause stress or discomfort. ■ Engage family members or caregivers in the discussion when appropriate, ensuring a holistic understanding of the patient's health and social context. ■ Prioritize the most critical assessments for the beginning of the visit when the patient is most alert and able to participate fully.[20] ■ Provide clear, written summaries of discussions, decisions, and care plans, ensuring the patient and their caregivers fully understand the next steps.

Box 30-4. Geriatric 5Ms

Mind	Evaluate cognitive function and mental health, including memory, decision making, and screening for conditions like dementia, depression, and anxiety.
Mobility	Assess physical ability and functional mobility, including gait, balance, strength, range of motion, mobility aids, and fall risk.
Medications	Review the medication regimen, including prescription drugs, over-the-counter (OTC) medications, and supplements, to identify interactions and optimize therapy.
Multicomplexity	Understand the interplay of multiple health issues, their treatments, and their impact on overall health and well-being.
Matters Most	Discuss the individual's values, preferences, and goals of care, aligning treatment with their priorities and quality of life.

GERIATRIC 5Ms

The Geriatric 5Ms framework has emerged as a pivotal approach in health care for older adults, providing a structured method to address their unique needs and complexities.[21] Developed through clinical expertise, research findings, and patient-centered principles, the framework consists of five key domains: *Mind*, *Mobility*, *Medications*, *Multicomplexity*, and *Matters Most* (Box 30-4). These domains are crucial for understanding and addressing the health concerns of older adults, allowing you to deliver tailored interventions that optimize health outcomes and overall well-being.

The Geriatric 5Ms serve not only to enhance the history taking, physical examination, and assessment of older adults but also complements traditional methods by focusing on aspects especially relevant to the aging population.

HEALTH HISTORY: APPLYING THE 5Ms FRAMEWORK

Effective history taking in older adults using the Geriatric 5Ms framework involves a thorough understanding of their unique health care needs, including their medical conditions, cognitive function, mental health, mobility, and medication management. Equally important is your ability to show empathy and create an environment where your older adult patients feel comfortable sharing their experiences and concerns.

Mind

When you assess cognitive function and mental health, ask about any changes in memory, mood, and social behavior, which can significantly impact your patients' overall well-being (Box 30-5).

Box 30-5. Mind: High-Yield Health History Questions

Questions	Rationale
Have you noticed any changes in your memory or thinking skills?	Early signs of dementia include forgetfulness and difficulty with complex tasks
How is your mood on most days?	Persistent sadness or low mood might indicate depression
Do you find pleasure in activities you previously enjoyed?	Loss of interest is a common symptom of depression
Have you experienced any changes in your sleep patterns?	Can be indicative of depression or anxiety disorders
Have you had any thoughts of harming yourself or others?	Warrant immediate attention and intervention for safety
Do you often feel anxious or on edge?	Can be a sign of an anxiety disorder, which often coexists with depression or other psychiatric conditions
Have you noticed any changes in your social behavior or interests?	Withdrawal can be an early sign of dementia or an indicator of depression
Do you struggle with concentration or decision making?	Can be symptoms of both depression and cognitive decline
Have you been diagnosed with any psychiatric conditions in the past, or are there any family members with such diagnoses?	Can increase the risk of similar conditions
Have you experienced any traumatic events recently or in the past?	May lead to post-traumatic stress disorder (PTSD) and other mental health issues
How would you describe your energy levels throughout the day?	Variations can indicate depression or other mental health conditions
Have you noticed any changes in your appetite or weight?	Can be symptoms of depression or anxiety disorders

Mobility

When assessing mobility, focus on understanding the physical abilities and limitations of your older adult patients. Ask questions about their ability to perform daily activities, any recent falls, and the use of mobility aids (Box 30-6). This information is vital for tailoring interventions that improve their independence and quality of life.

Box 30-6. Mobility: High-Yield Health History Questions

Questions	Rationale
How would you describe your ability to perform daily activities, such as walking, climbing stairs, or carrying groceries?	Can indicate mobility issues or the risk of falls.
Have you experienced any falls in the past year? If so, how many and under what circumstances?	Falls are significant indicators of mobility problems
Do you use any aids or devices to assist with mobility (e.g., cane, walker, wheelchair)?	May provide insight into the severity of mobility issues and the individual's adaptation strategies
Have you noticed any changes in your balance or coordination recently?	May increase fall risk and indicate problems with the vestibular system or neurologic conditions
Do you experience any pain or discomfort while moving or at rest?	Can significantly affect mobility and quality of life
Are there any activities you avoid due to difficulty moving or fear of falling?	Can indicate mobility issues impacting quality of life
How would you rate your level of physical activity on a typical day?	May help gauge their mobility and identify potential areas for improvement
Have you had any recent surgeries or medical conditions that have affected your mobility?	Can directly impact mobility
Do you experience any swelling, numbness, or tingling in your legs or feet?	May indicate circulatory or neurologic issues that could affect mobility
Have you noticed any muscle weakness or difficulty in controlling your movements?	Can be signs of neurologic conditions or muscular disorders affecting mobility
How confident do you feel moving around in different environments (e.g., home, outdoors, public spaces)?	Can indicate how mobility issues are managed and the effectiveness of any interventions
Are there any environmental factors at home or work that make mobility challenging?	May help in planning modifications to enhance mobility and independence

Medications

Review all medications your patient is taking,—including prescription drugs, OTC products, and supplements. Be mindful of *polypharmacy* in which a patient is taking five or more medications. This ensures effective management to optimize health outcomes and minimize risks. As you review your patient's medications, critically assess each medication's necessity, aiming toward *deprescribing*, which is the systematic reduction or cessation of medications that are no longer beneficial or necessary (Box 30-7).

Box 30-7. Medications: High-Yield Health History Questions

Questions	Rationale
Can you list all the medications you are currently taking, including OTC drugs and supplements?	Helps identify polypharmacy risks, potential drug interactions, and opportunities to streamline medication regimens
Have you experienced any side effects from your medications?	Crucial for adjusting medication plans to enhance safety and effectiveness
How do you manage your medication schedule?	May reveal adherence challenges or opportunities for simplification
Have you stopped taking any medications recently? If so, why?	Can indicate issues with side effects, cost, or perceived ineffectiveness
Do you have any difficulties with taking your medications, such as swallowing pills?	May impact adherence and effectiveness, necessitating adjustments to the medication regimen
Have you noticed any changes in your symptoms or conditions since starting or changing medications?	May indicate medication effectiveness or the need for adjustment
Do you use any alternative therapies or remedies in addition to your prescribed medications?	Alternative therapies can interact with medications, affecting safety and efficacy
How do you obtain your medications? (e.g., pharmacy, mail order)	Can influence adherence and the potential for running out of critical prescriptions
Have you had any hospitalizations or emergency visits related to medication issues?	Can signal serious medication problems or adverse events
Do you have any concerns or questions about your current medication regimen?	Can improve adherence and satisfaction with treatment and provide education on medication use
Have you received any medication reviews from a healthcare professional in the past year?	Can prevent polypharmacy and optimize medication regimens for safety and efficacy
Are there any medications you believe are no longer necessary or effective?	Can guide discussions about the necessity and effectiveness of each medication, potentially reducing polypharmacy

Multicomplexity

Managing multiple chronic conditions and their treatments is a significant aspect of caring for older adults. Your role is to understand how these conditions interact and affect their daily life and overall health (Box 30-8).

Box 30-8. Multicomplexity: High-Yield Health History Questions

Questions	Rationale
Can you list all the chronic conditions you have been diagnosed with?	Important for managing care effectively and avoiding conflicting treatments
How do these conditions affect your daily life and activities?	Can guide prioritization of care interventions to improve quality of life
Are you currently receiving treatment for all these conditions?	Key to managing multicomplexity and avoiding the undertreatment of any one condition
Have you experienced any side effects or challenges with your current treatments?	Can help optimize treatment plans and mitigate the negative impacts of polypharmacy
How do you manage your medication regimen for these conditions?	May reveal potential for simplification or support needs to enhance adherence
Have you ever felt overwhelmed by managing these conditions?	Can prompt support interventions, such as case management or counseling, to assist with the complexities of care
Do your conditions affect each other in any way?	Can inform a more cohesive and integrated approach to management, exacerbations, and complications
How do you prioritize your health care appointments and treatments?	May help align health care provision with the patient's most pressing needs and preferences
Have you noticed any changes in your symptoms or the effectiveness of your treatment over time?	Crucial for timely adjustments in care plans to address evolving needs
Do you face any barriers in accessing care or treatments for your conditions?	Allows for targeted interventions to improve access to necessary care and resources
How do you coordinate care among your different health care providers?	Essential in managing multiple chronic conditions
What are your main concerns or goals in managing these conditions?	Ensures that treatment plans are patient-centered and focused on achieving the best possible outcomes

Matters Most

Engaging in meaningful discussions about personal values, preferences, and care goals is crucial, particularly regarding end-of-life care preferences and the role of palliative and life-sustaining measures (Fig. 30-6). By focusing on what matters most, you can ensure that their care aligns with their priorities, enhancing both quality of life and care (Box 30-9).

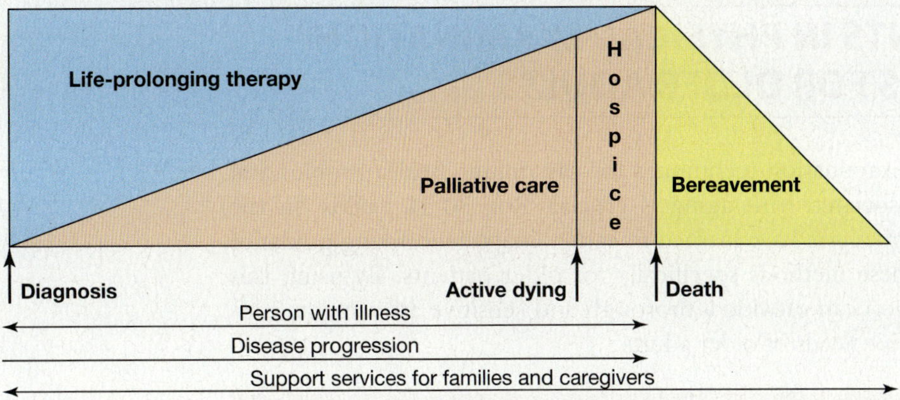

FIGURE 30-6. The place of palliative care within the course of illness. (Reprinted with permission from Burggraf V, Kim KY, Knight AL. *Healthy Aging: Principles and Clinical Practice for Clinicians.* Wolters Kluwer Health; 2015. Figure 29-1.)

Box 30-9. Matters Most: High-Yield Health History Questions

Questions	Rationale
What are your most important health care goals right now?	Helps tailor care to meet specific needs and desires, ensuring alignment with patient values
How do you prefer to receive information about your health? (e.g., detailed information, general overview)	Allows for better communication and helps ensure that patients are fully informed and comfortable with decisions
Have you thought about the type of care you would want at the end of your life?	Ensures that care plans are consistent with the patient's wishes, even if they become unable to communicate them later
Do you have an advance directive or living will?	Critical for understanding and respecting the patient's wishes regarding health care interventions and end-of-life care
Who would you like to make healthcare decisions on your behalf if you are unable to do so?	Ensures that decisions are made by someone who understands the patient's values and desires
Are there any specific treatments or interventions you would not want?	Prevents unwanted treatments and respects the patient's autonomy
How do you feel about the quality of life versus the length of life?	Helps clarify the patient's values regarding life-sustaining treatments and aggressive interventions in the context of terminal illness
What are your thoughts on hospice care or palliative care?	Helps ensure that care aligns with the patient's wishes for comfort and quality of life at the end stages
Are you particularly afraid of or concerned about anything regarding your health or treatments?	Can guide care planning and provide reassurance and support tailored to the patient's emotional needs
How important is it for you to remain independent in your daily activities?	Helps in planning care that aligns with patient values
Are any religious or spiritual beliefs important to you in your care?	Crucial in providing holistic and person-centered care
What brings you joy and how can we help support that in your care?	Can greatly enhance the patient's quality of life and satisfaction with their care

ADJUSTMENTS IN PHYSICAL EXAMINATION TECHNIQUES FOR OLDER ADULTS

Adjusting physical examination techniques for the unique health profiles and physical changes associated with aging is crucial. Box 30-10 builds on the examination techniques you have learned in earlier chapters, offering guidance on how to adapt these methods specifically for older patients. By using this tailored approach, you can provide a thorough and sensitive assessment, considering the distinctive needs of older adults.

Box 30-10. Adaptations for Physical Examination in Older Adults

System	Modifications in Physical Examination Maneuvers
General survey	▪ Carefully observe the patient's posture, gait, and overall physical condition to identify signs of frailty or potential nutritional deficiencies. ▪ Assist patients during transitions between positions to ensure comfort and safety, allowing extra time for these movements to accommodate any physical limitations.
Vital signs	▪ Ensure the blood pressure cuff fits properly to avoid measurement errors (see pp. 176–179).[22–25] Measure blood pressure in both seated and standing positions to assess for *orthostatic hypotension*, defined as a drop in SBP of ≥20 mm Hg or DBP of ≥10 mm Hg within 3 min of standing. ▪ Incorporate assessments of pulse oximetry and temperature, paying attention to variations that may indicate circulatory or thermoregulatory changes associated with aging.[26–29]
Skin	▪ Perform a detailed examination of the skin under adequate lighting, checking for bruises, pressure injuries in high-risk areas, and other signs of skin breakdown. ▪ Assess hydration by examining skin turgor and be gentle when handling skin to avoid causing tears or injuries. ▪ Regularly check for signs of skin cancers, especially in sun-exposed areas.
Hair and hails	▪ Examine the scalp for hair distribution, texture changes, and any signs of scalp diseases such as scarring alopecia. ▪ Evaluate nails for changes in color, shape, and texture, noting any abnormalities that could indicate nutritional issues or systemic diseases.

For adults aged ≥60 years, the eighth Joint National Committee (JNC8) recommends blood pressure target of ≤150/90 mm Hg but notes that if treatment results in SBP <140 mm Hg and is "well tolerated without adverse effects to health or quality of life", treatment does not need to be adjusted.[39]

Alopecia, or hair loss, can be diffuse, patchy, or total. Male and female pattern hair loss is normal with aging.

System	Modifications in Physical Examination Maneuvers
Head and neck	■ Look for signs of oral cancers and check dental health for decay or gum disease. ■ Assess the thyroid gland with gentle palpation to accommodate decreased neck mobility in older patients.[30] ■ Be cautious during palpation of the temporal arteries to avoid discomfort, especially in patients at risk for temporal arteritis.
Eyes	■ Note any structural changes such as atrophy of periorbital fat leading to sunken eyes. Check for conditions like senile ptosis and complications from eyelid malposition such as *entropion* or *ectropion*.[31,32] ■ Use ophthalmoscopic examination to check for common age-related conditions such as cataracts, glaucoma, and macular degeneration.[33] ■ Account for slower pupil dilation and possible complications from age-related vision loss (*presbyopia).*
Ears	■ Adapt otoscopic examination techniques for older adults who may have increased earwax accumulation or narrowed ear canals. ■ Assess hearing using techniques sensitive to age-related hearing loss (*presbycusis*), which may affect the patient's ability to follow verbal instructions during the exam.[34]
Nose	■ Inspect the nasal cavity for mucosal dryness, polyps, or any signs of infection, taking care to be gentle due to the increased risk of nasal bleeding in older adults.
Oral cavity and teeth	■ Look for signs of oral cancers, note any ulcers or infections, and assess the overall dental health including gum disease and tooth decay.[35,36] ■ Discuss symptoms of dry mouth (*xerostomia*), which is common among older adults, and can significantly impact dental health and comfort.
Thorax and lungs	■ Observe respiratory effort and listen for abnormal breath sounds like crackles or wheezes, which may indicate underlying cardiac or pulmonary conditions.[37] ■ Note any changes in chest wall dynamics that could affect breathing.

(continued)

An increased cup-to-disc ratio suggests primary open-angle glaucoma (POAG), caused by irreversible optic neuropathy and leading to loss of peripheral and central vision and blindness (Fig. 30-7).[40,41]

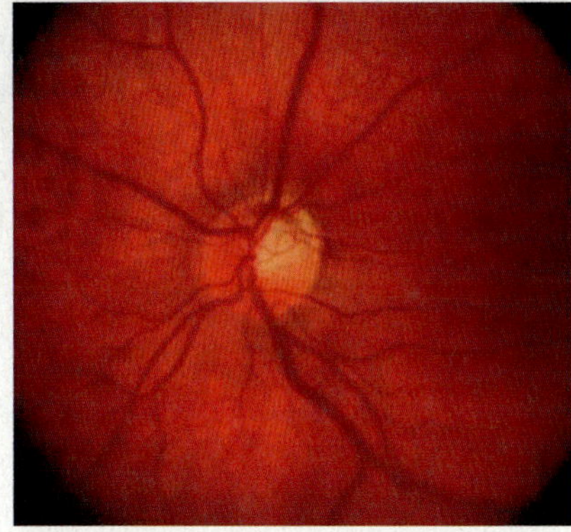

FIGURE 30-7. Fundus with increased cup-to-disc ratio ("disc cupping") due to glaucoma.

Macular degeneration causes poor central vision and blindness (Fig. 30-8).[42] Types include dry atrophic (more common but less severe) and wet exudative, or neovascular.

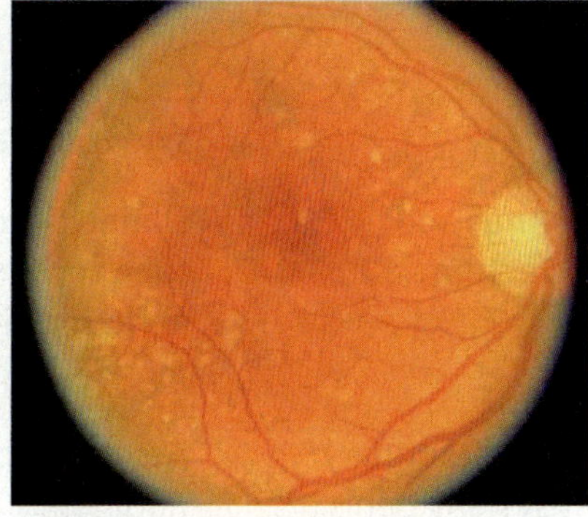

FIGURE 30-8. Fundus with age-related macular degeneration. Notice the "drusen spots" located centrally.

Box 30-10. Adaptations for Physical Examination in Older Adults (*Continued*)

System	Modifications in Physical Examination Maneuvers
Breasts and axillae	▪ Inspect for any abnormalities such as masses, skin changes, or nipple discharge. Consider changes in breast tissue composition that may affect palpation findings and screening outcomes.
Cardiovascular system	▪ Use auscultation techniques to carefully evaluate heart sounds and murmurs, adapting positioning and stethoscope use to maximize acoustic detection.[37] ▪ Monitor for any signs of cardiac arrhythmias or vascular abnormalities.
Peripheral vascular system	▪ Check for signs of venous insufficiency or peripheral arterial disease (PAD), such as varicosities, ulcerations, or color changes in the extremities. ▪ Assess pulse quality and perform the ankle–brachial index (ABI) test if necessary to quantify vascular compromise.
Abdomen	▪ Palpate the abdomen gently, checking for areas of tenderness or organomegaly, and be particularly cautious around the aortic region to detect any signs of an aneurysm.
Anus and rectum	▪ During the digital rectal exam, assess sphincter tone and check for any rectal masses or abnormalities. Be aware of potential decreases in muscle tone due to aging.
Genitourinary system: penis, scrotum, and prostate	▪ Assess the prostate gland for size, consistency, and nodules. ▪ Examine the scrotum and testicles for any signs of masses, asymmetry, or other abnormalities.
Genitourinary system: vulva, vagina, uterus, and adnexa	▪ Conduct pelvic exams with sensitivity, using lubricant and appropriate speculum size to minimize discomfort, especially in cases of vaginal atrophy.[38] ▪ Check for signs of pelvic organ prolapse and discuss symptoms of urinary incontinence or other postmenopausal issues affecting quality of life.

A systolic crescendo–decrescendo murmur heard in the second right interspace suggests either aortic sclerosis or aortic stenosis. Aortic sclerosis is more common, occuring in up to 40% of community-dwelling older adults, while aortic stenosis affects 2% to 3% of this population. Both conditions are associated with an increased risk of cardiovascular disease and mortality.[43,44]

Diminished or absent pulses are present in PAD with an ABI <0.9. The ABI has a sensitivity of 70% and specificity of 90%. Notably, 30% to 60% of patients with PAD report no leg symptoms.[45] See Chapter 19, Peripheral Vascular System, Ankle–Brachial Index, p. 557.

System	Modifications in Physical Examination Maneuvers
Musculoskeletal system	■ Inspect and palpate joints for signs of arthritis or other degenerative changes, being careful to adjust the force of palpation in patients with osteoporosis. ■ Assess range of motion while supporting the patient to avoid strain. ■ Perform specialized maneuvers like the Timed Get Up and Go test to evaluate balance and gait safely (p. 1176).
Nervous system	■ Assess cognitive functions using tools like the Mini-Cog or Montreal Cognitive Assessment, allowing extra time for responses, and simplifying instructions. ■ Evaluate mood with tools like the Geriatric Depression Scale, and systematically test cranial nerves and sensory responses to identify any deficits.

Abnormalities of gait and balance, especially widening of base, slowing, and lengthening of stride, and difficulty turning, are correlated with risk for falls.[46,47]

Tremor, rigidity, akinesia, and postural instability (TRAP) are the most common features of Parkinson disease (PD).[48] The tremor in PD is slow frequency, occurs at rest, has a "pill-rolling" quality, and is aggravated by stress and inhibited during sleep or movement.

See Tables 11-8, Screening for Dementia: The Mini-Cog, p. 232, and 11-9, Screening for Dementia: Montreal Cognitive Assessment (MoCA), p. 233.

See Table 11-5, Screening for Depression: Geriatric Depression Scale, p. 228.

GERIATRIC ASSESSMENT: APPLYING THE 5Ms FRAMEWORK

When conducting physical examination for older adults, your approach goes beyond the basic assessments typically conducted in younger populations, exploring physical, psychological, functional, and social domains. This holistic approach, integrating the Geriatric 5Ms framework, helps you gain a deeper understanding of an older adult patient's health status and preferences (Box 30-11). It aids in the development of targeted interventions that enhance functioning and quality of life, ensuring that care and management are comprehensively tailored to meet the individual needs of older adults.

Mind

The Mind component of the Geriatric 5Ms emphasizes the significance of cognitive and mental health assessments in caring for older adults. Conducting a

Box 30-11. Geriatric Assessment Using the 5Ms Framework

Mind
- Assess cognitive function
- Observe for signs of confusion
- Screen for depression, anxiety, and other mental health conditions

Mobility
- Review activities of daily living
- Evaluate gait, balance, and strength
- Determine need for mobility aids
- Assess fall risk

Medications
- Manage polypharmacy and consider deprescribing
- Ensure optimal prescribing
- Monitor for adverse medication effects

Multicomplexity
- Recognize atypical presentations of diseases
- Evaluate for geriatric syndromes

Matters most
- Provide individualized care
- Engage in shared decision making
- Enhance quality of life
- Facilitate advance care planning
- Reduce unnecessary interventions

thorough evaluation of cognitive function and mental health is pivotal for spotting conditions that may impact your patient's quality of life, decision-making capacity, and overall health.

Assess Cognitive Function. Cognitive assessments play a vital role in detecting conditions such as dementia. Although the Mini-Mental State Examination (MMSE) has been a standard tool, its use is restricted by copyright issues. Alternative recommended tests include the Mini-Cog, the Montreal Cognitive Assessment (MoCA), and the St. Louis University Mental Status Exam (SLUMS).[49] These tools help in identifying various cognitive impairments, with the Mini-Cog focusing on memory and clock-drawing tasks, and the MoCA providing a broader evaluation of cognitive functions.[50]

See Tables 11-3, Neurocognitive Disorders: Delirium and Dementia, p. 226; 11-8, Screening for Dementia: The Mini-Cog, p. 232; 11-9, Screening for Dementia: Montreal Cognitive Assessment (MoCA), p. 233; and 11-10, Screening for Cognitive Impairment and Dementia: Saint Louis University Mental Status Exam (SLUMS), p. 234.

Observe for Signs of Confusion. Pay attention to signs of confusion, memory loss, and altered mental status. Observing your patient's conversational ability, response appropriateness, and memory recall provides insight into their cognitive function. Inconsistencies or challenges in managing familiar tasks may indicate cognitive impairments. One of the more common screening tests for delirium is the *Confusion assessment method (CAM).*

See Box 11-20, Confusion Assessment Method (CAM) Diagnostic Algorithm, p. 222.

Screen for Depression, Anxiety, and Other Mental Health Conditions. Depression and anxiety are prevalent but often underdiagnosed in older adults. Make it a habit to use screening tools like the Geriatric Depression Scale (GDS), Generalized Anxiety Disorder-7 (GAD-7) questionnaire, and Patient Health Questionnaire-9 (PHQ-9) is crucial. These tools aid in detecting mental health conditions that significantly affect your patient's well-being and are manageable with appropriate interventions.

See Tables 11-5, Screening for Depression: Geriatric Depression Scale, p. 228; 11-6, Screening for Depression: Patient Health Questionnaire (PHQ-9), pp. 229–230; and 11-7, Screening for Anxiety Disorders: GAD-7, p. 231.

Mobility

As you assess mobility in older adults, focus on evaluating gait, balance, strength, and the use of mobility aids. Effective assessment of mobility helps in tailoring interventions that improve independence and reduce the risk of falls, crucial for maintaining quality of life in older adults.

Review Activities of Daily Living. Start by evaluating both basic and instrumental activities of daily living. These include the *basic activities of daily living (ADLs)*, which consist of six essential self-care tasks—*bathing, dressing, toileting, transferring, maintaining continence,* and *feeding.* Then, progressing to more complex activities, the *instrumental activities of daily living (IADLs)—using the telephone, shopping, preparing food, housekeeping, doing laundry, transportation, taking medicine,* and *managing finances,* helps gauge an older adult's level of independence and functional capacity.

Review the ADLs and IADLs in Chapter 3, Health History, p. 52.

Evaluate Gait, Balance, and Strength. Effective mobility in older adults hinges on three interconnected aspects: *gait, balance, and strength.*

- *Gait analysis:* Observe walking patterns to detect potential issues like arthritis.
- *Balance evaluation:* Assess how well your patient maintains their center of gravity to identify fall risks.
- *Strength assessment:* Focus on lower-body strength crucial for daily activities. Recognizing weaknesses in these areas is vital for preventing mobility impairments and falls.

Given the intertwined nature of gait, balance, and strength in mobility, several performance-based assessment tools have been developed to evaluate these components collectively (Box 30-12).

Determine Need for Mobility Aids. *Mobility aids* are devices designed to assist individuals with walking or improve their mobility. Common aids include canes, walkers, and wheelchairs (Fig. 30-9). It involves ensuring these aids are correctly fitted and that your older adult patient is adequately trained in their use to improve mobility and safety (Box 30-13).

Box 30-12. Commonly Used Performance-Based Assessment Tools for Gait, Balance, and Strength

Step	Timed Up and Go (TUG) Test	Berg Balance Scale
Components	Inherently evaluates gait speed, balance (especially during the turn), and strength.	Consists of 14 tasks of varying difficulty. While it is a balance-focused test, many tasks require strength.
When to use	Provides indirect insights into balance and lower-body strength, as these are necessary to perform the test efficiently.	Primarily assesses balance but also touches on the strength needed for maintaining positions and the control required for safe movement, indirectly related to gait.
Sample script to introduce the tool	*"We're going to do a simple test where you'll stand up from a chair, walk a short distance, turn around, walk back, and sit down. It helps us assess your mobility."*	*"This test includes different tasks like standing up from a chair, standing on one leg, and reaching forward. It helps us see how well you balance and move."*
Materials needed	Chair with armrests, stopwatch, a marked 3-meter (or 10-foot) course.	Chair, stopwatch, various objects for tasks (e.g., a step, cones), scoring sheet.
Administration	Measure the time it takes for the individual to complete the sequence of actions from starting seated to returning to the seated position.	Administer the 14 balance tasks, observing and recording the individual's ability to perform each task, noting any difficulties or inability to complete tasks.
Scoring	Record the time taken to complete the test.	Each task is scored on a scale, usually from 0 (unable to perform) to 4 (performs task independently).
Interpretation	Longer times suggest potential mobility issues, requiring further assessment or intervention.	Lower scores indicate balance impairments, which may inform fall risk assessments and need for therapeutic interventions.

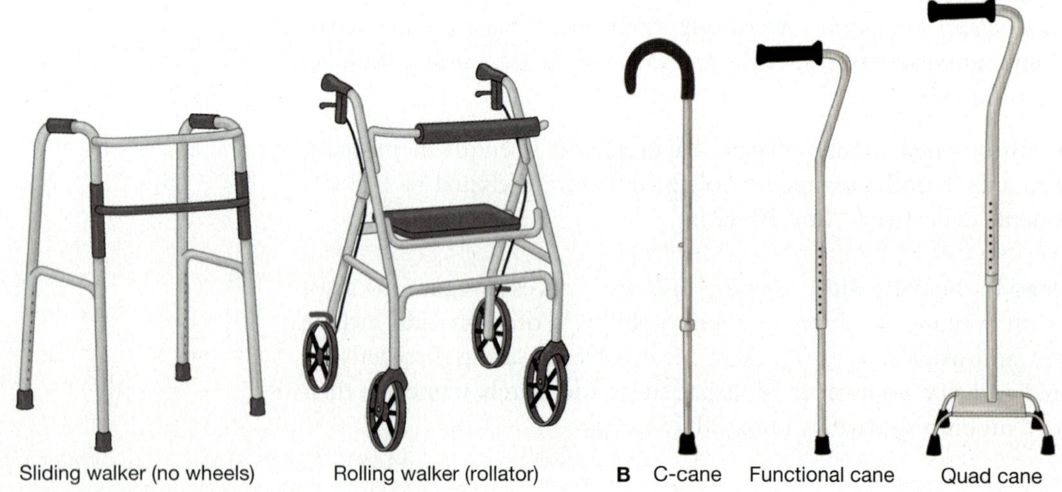

FIGURE 30-9. Commonly used assistive mobility devices. (Reprinted with permission from Hinkle JL, Cheever JH. *Brunner & Suddarth's Textbook of Medical-Surgical Nursing*. 14th ed. Wolters Kluwer; 2018. Figure 10-3.)

Box 30-13. Selecting Assistive Mobility Devices

Device	Description	Indication
Standard cane	A handheld device with a single tip that provides stability and balance during walking; often made of lightweight materials with adjustable height options	For individuals needing slight balance or walking support, typically the first aid used postinjury or in early physical rehabilitation
Quad cane	A cane with a base featuring four small feet, providing greater stability than a standard cane; adjustable in height and made of durable materials	Ideal for those who require more support than a single-point cane but less than a walker
Walker (without wheels or with two wheels)	A sturdy, four-legged device designed to provide stability. Walkers without wheels require the user to lift it slightly for movement, offering maximum stability. Walkers with two wheels have wheels on the front legs for forward movement while the rear legs without wheels provide friction and stability	Suitable for individuals needing significant walking support. Walkers without wheels are ideal for those requiring maximum stability, while walkers with two wheels are better for users who need moderate support and easier forward mobility
Walker with four wheels (rollator)	A fully wheeled walker typically equipped with a padded seat, handlebars, and brakes; designed for smooth mobility across various surfaces	Ideal for those with the strength to control a fully wheeled device; requires substantial support but also prioritizes independence and ease of mobility over different terrains
Wheelchair	A chair mounted on wheels, available in manual or electric-powered versions, designed for individuals unable to walk or with significant walking limitations	For individuals with severe mobility impairments or when long-distance mobility is required, reflecting a permanent or long-term limitation
Mobility scooter	An electric-powered vehicle with a comfortable seat, foot platform, and handlebars or a steering wheel; designed for outdoor use and covering longer distances	For individuals with chronic limitations who retain some mobility and upper body strength but need assistance for long distances, especially outdoors

Assessing Height. Correct device height is crucial for effectiveness and comfort:

- *Canes:* Top of the cane should reach the wrist crease when the user stands upright to ensure optimal support.
- *Walkers and rollators:* Handles should align with the user's wrist crease for proper posture and balance.
- *Crutches:* Ensure a 1- to 2-inch gap between the top of the crutches and the armpit, with handgrips at wrist crease height.

Considering Handedness and Device Use. Adjust canes and crutches to accommodate one-sided weaknesses or injuries. Consider the device's intended indoor or outdoor use, frequency of use, ease of transportation and storage, and suitability for different terrains to ensure it meets your patient's needs.

Assess Fall Risk. Fall risk assessment is vital for identifying potential hazards that could lead to falls, significantly impacting an older adult's life. This involves examining environmental factors, medication side effects, and physical or cognitive impairments. By identifying potential risks, you can implement strategies to minimize falls and improve your patient's safety.

See Interventions for Falls Prevention in Community-Dwelling Older Adults, pp. 1189–1190.

Medications

As you care for older adults, conducting a thorough review of all medications is imperative due to the increased risk of adverse drug reactions in this population.[51,52] This includes prescriptions, OTC medications, and supplements. The review helps in optimizing the medication regimen, reducing polypharmacy,[52,53] and ensuring that each medication is necessary and beneficial.[54]

Manage Polypharmacy and Consider Deprescribing. Widely used tools to identify potential issues like drug interactions, adverse effects, and opportunities for optimization include the *American Geriatrics Society (AGS) Beers Criteria*, which is a guideline to help improve the safety of prescribing medications for older adults.[55,56] It lists potentially inappropriate medications that should be avoided in older populations due to their risk of causing adverse effects. *STOPP/START Criteria (Screening Tool of Older Persons' potentially inappropriate Prescriptions/Screening Tool to Alert doctors to Right Treatment)* is another resource for identifying potentially inappropriate medications and highlights omissions in treatment for older adults (Box 30-14).

Ensure Optimal Prescribing. Clinical decision support systems (CDSS) use algorithms and integrate with electronic health records (EHRs) to provide tailored medication recommendations.[57,58] They alert you to potential interactions and dosing errors, enhancing care quality. Disease-specific guidelines help standardize treatment based on evidence, especially for chronic conditions prevalent in older adults.

Box 30-14. Tools for Medication Review for Older Adults

Step	Beers Criteria	STOPP Criteria	START Criteria
When to use	To identify drugs with a higher risk of adverse effects in this population	To check for overmedication, inappropriate prescriptions, or harmful interactions	To determine essential medications absent in the regimen, especially for prevention and chronic conditions
How to use	Match the patient's current medications against the list and noting any that are flagged by the criteria.	Identify inappropriate, interacting, or redundant medications in the patient's list.	Check for necessary treatments that may be missing from the patient's regimen, crucial for treatment optimization.
Interpretation	Consider the patient's health, comorbidities, and risk factors to decide on stopping, substituting, or adjusting doses.	Review each medication, weighing the pros and cons of modification based on the patient's specific health details.	Evaluate missing treatments, considering their potential benefits against the patient's overall health and preferences.

Monitor for Adverse Medication Effects. EHR systems include tools to track adverse drug events, collecting data on negative outcomes to enable quick pattern identification and timely intervention.[59] Encouraging patients to keep medication diaries also aids in monitoring side effects and medication use.

Multicomplexity

Addressing multicomplexity involves managing multiple chronic conditions and their interconnected impacts on your older adult's health. This requires a nuanced understanding of how various health issues interplay and affect the overall well-being of the patient.

Recognize Atypical Presentations of Diseases. Older adults often exhibit signs and symptoms that diverge from the classic descriptions found in textbooks. This variance is largely due to the physiologic changes of aging, compounded by the presence of multiple comorbidities. Your ability to identify these atypical presentations is critical for making accurate diagnoses and providing appropriate care (Box 30-15).

Box 30-15. Atypical Presentations of Diseases in Older Adults

Condition	Typical Presentations	Atypical Presentations
Dehydration	Signs include thirst and dry mucous membranes	This may present with confusion, falls, or acute kidney injury, as older adults may not feel or express thirst traditionally.
Depression	Often manifests as sadness or despair	Older adults may show a loss of interest in activities, weight loss, or neglect of personal care instead of expressing sadness.
Diabetes mellitus	Characterized by polyuria, polydipsia, and polyphagia	Symptoms may be less pronounced. Hypoglycemia can present with confusion or behavioral changes.
Gastrointestinal (GI) bleeding	Presents with overt bleeding or abdominal pain	Presentation can be nonspecific, such as weakness, dizziness, or postural hypotension, which might not directly suggest GI bleeding.
Hyperthyroidism	Symptoms include heat intolerance, palpitations, and sweating	Older individuals might show instead nonspecific signs like atrial fibrillation, weight loss, or fatigue.
Hypothyroidism	Typically causes fatigue, constipation, dry skin, and cold intolerance	Symptoms can be subtle and easily attributed to aging or other conditions, complicating diagnosis.
Infections (urinary tract infection, pneumonia)	Characterized by fever and localized signs such as pain or cough	Older adults may present instead with general symptoms like confusion or a decline in functional status.
Myocardial infarction	Commonly presents with chest pain or discomfort	This may present as fatigue, shortness of breath, syncope, or confusion, which can lead to delayed diagnosis.
Stroke	Symptoms include sudden numbness or weakness on one side of the body, confusion, and trouble speaking or walking	Older adults might experience more subtle signs such as unexplained falls or isolated dizziness, making early recognition challenging.

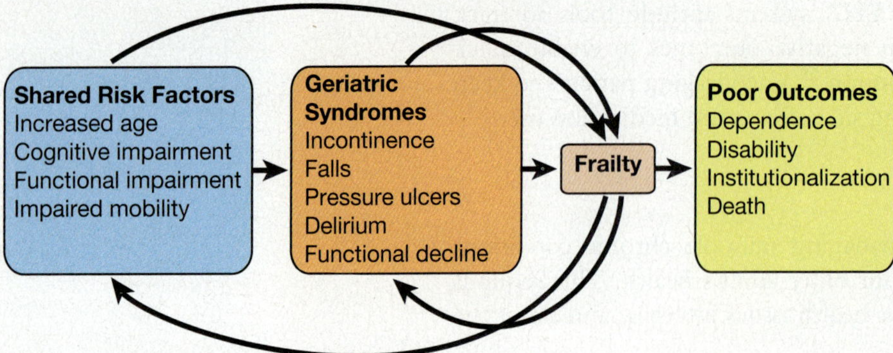

FIGURE 30-10. Interaction between geriatric syndromes and age-related risk factors resulting in poor outcomes.

Evaluate for Geriatric Syndromes. A *geriatric syndrome* is "a multifactorial condition that involves the interaction between identifiable situation-specific stressors and underlying age-related risk factors, resulting in damage across multiple organ systems" (Fig. 30-10).[60] These syndromes are strongly linked to functional decline.[61] Experts state that "evaluating functional status, frailty, and other geriatric syndromes while simultaneously addressing individual disease processes is at the heart of geriatric approach to primary care."[62] Recognizing these syndromes is especially important because they may cluster in patterns unfamiliar or unexpected to the patient (Box 30-16).

Matters Most

Understanding what matters most to your older patients is essential for aligning care with their values and preferences. This involves engaging in meaningful conversations about their goals for care, preferences for treatments, and their definitions of quality of life. This aspect of the 5Ms emphasizes the importance of patient-centered care that respects and prioritizes the personal preferences and values of the older adult.

Provide Individualized Care. Older adults often present with complex health needs and diverse life experiences, necessitating personalized care. What matters most to each individual significantly shapes their health outcomes and quality of life. For one patient, this might mean maintaining independence in daily activities, managing pain to tolerable levels, or prioritizing life-prolonging treatments.

Engage in Shared Decision Making. Focusing on what matters most to the patient, you can actively engage in shared decision making. This collaborative process includes the patient and often family members in health care decisions, ensuring that treatments and care plans resonate with the patient's values, preferences, and goals.

Enhance Quality of Life. For many older adults, improving quality of life is a paramount concern, often taking precedence over life-extending interventions. *Quality of life* encompasses an individual's overall well-being, including physical, mental, emotional, and social functioning. It extends beyond physical health to include the degree of satisfaction or happiness that individuals experience in their lives. By understanding what is most important to your older adult patients, you can prioritize interventions that boost their well-being and life satisfaction.

Box 30-16. Geriatric Syndromes and Assessment Tools

Geriatric Syndrome	Description	Validated Assessment Tools
Delirium	Rapid-onset medical condition characterized by confusion, disturbed concentration, and cognitive dysfunction, often resulting from a physical illness, medication, or surgery	Confusion Assessment Method (CAM), p. 222, Delirium Observation Screening Scale (DOSS)[63–66]
Dementia	Chronic or progressive syndrome marked by deterioration in cognitive function beyond what might be expected from normal aging, affecting memory, thinking, orientation, comprehension, calculation, learning capacity, language, and judgment	Mini-Mental State Examination (MMSE); Montreal Cognitive Assessment (MoCA) p. 233; Mini-Cog, p. 232; Saint Louis University Mental Status Exam (SLUMS), p. 234[49,50,62,67–73]
Depression	Common mental disorder among older adults, characterized by persistent sadness and a lack of interest or pleasure in previously rewarding or enjoyable activities	Geriatric Depression Scale (GDS), p. 228, Patient Health Questionnaire-9 (PHQ-9), pp. 229–230[74–80]
Falls	Contributes to considerable morbidity and mortality	Timed Up and Go (TUG) test, p. 1176; Berg Balance Scale; Fall Risk Assessment Tool (FRAT)[81–85]
Frailty	Characterized by increased vulnerability to external stressors and diminished strength, endurance, and physiologic function, which increases the risk of adverse health outcomes	Fried Frailty Criteria, Frailty Index, Edmonton Frail Scale[86,87]
Urinary or fecal incontinence	Characterized by involuntary leakage of urine or feces	Bladder Diary, Incontinence Severity Index, Overactive Bladder Symptom Score[88]
Malnutrition	Characterized by deficiency, excess, or imbalance of energy, protein, and other nutrients causes measurable adverse effects on tissue/body form (body shape, size, and composition) and function and clinical outcome	Mini Nutritional Assessment (MNA), Geriatric Nutritional Risk Index (GNRI)[89]
Polypharmacy	Can increase the risk of adverse drug reactions and interactions	Beers Criteria for Potentially Inappropriate Medication Use in Older Adults, p. 1178; STOPP/START criteria, p. 1178[56,90]
Pressure ulcers	Localized injuries to the skin and/or underlying tissue, usually over a bony prominence, as a result of pressure, or pressure in combination with shear	Braden Scale for Predicting Pressure Ulcer Risk, Pressure Ulcer Scale for Healing (PUSH)[91]
Sensory impairment	Diminished or lack of ability to see, hear, or maintain balance, impacting ability to communicate and navigate environments effectively	Snellen Chart for vision, p. 328; Pure-tone audiometry for hearing[92,93]

Facilitate Advance Care Planning. Discussing and understanding a patient's preferences for future health care, including end-of-life care, is crucial in aligning care with what matters most to them. This guides advance care planning, ensuring that interventions correspond with the patient's wishes, particularly in scenarios in which they may be unable to make decisions themselves. Advance directive documents serve as essential tools in this process, allowing patients to clearly express their healthcare preferences clearly and ensuring these preferences are honored (Box 30-17).

See Advance Care Planning in Chapter 2, Interviewing, Communication, and Interpersonal Skills, pp. 32–34.

Reduce Unnecessary Interventions. By centering care around your older patient's goals and preferences, you can avoid unnecessary or unwanted medical interventions. This not only respects your patient's autonomy but also can prevent potential harm from overtreatment.

Box 30-17. Understanding Advance Directives

Type	Purpose	Key Features
Living will	To outline the types of medical treatments and life-sustaining measures an individual wants or does not want	▪ Specifies wishes regarding medical treatment in specific scenarios ▪ Does not name a health care proxy
Durable power of attorney for healthcare	To designate a person (a *health care proxy*) to make health care decisions on the patient's behalf if they are unable to do so	▪ Appoints a trusted person to make medical decisions ▪ The proxy's authority can be as broad or as limited as the individual decides
DNR (Do not resuscitate)	Indicates that the individual does not want to have cardiopulmonary resuscitation (CPR) if their heart stops beating or they stop breathing	▪ Specifically addresses the wish to avoid CPR, which includes chest compressions, defibrillation, and administration of life-saving medications ▪ Must be signed by a physician to be valid and often needs to be reviewed and renewed periodically
DNI (Do not intubate)	Specifies that the individual does not want to be placed on a mechanical ventilator to assist with breathing if they are unable to breathe on their own	▪ Focuses specifically on the wish to avoid mechanical ventilation, which may include the use of a breathing tube and ventilator ▪ Can be part of a broader advance directive or a standalone order, depending on the jurisdiction ▪ Like the DNR, it must be signed by a physician and clearly communicated to all health care providers involved in the patient's care
Physician orders for life-sustaining treatment (POLST) or medical orders for scope of treatment (MOST)	For seriously ill or frail individuals, to outline a plan for end-of-life care based on their wishes, including treatments they want or do not want	▪ Converts patient wishes into medical orders ▪ Covers a range of treatments, including resuscitation, hospitalization, and antibiotics ▪ Must be reviewed and signed by a health care provider

HEALTH PROMOTION AND COUNSELING: EVIDENCE AND RECOMMENDATIONS

Important Topics for Health Promotion and Counseling in the Older Adult

- When to Screen
- Immunizations
- Cancer Screening
- Elder Abuse
- Household Safety for Falls Prevention
- Screening for Neurocognitive Disorders (See Chapter 11, Cognition, Behavior, and Mental Status, pp. 220–222.)

In the following section, both traditional terms like "men," "women," "male," and "female" and inclusive terms such as "individuals assigned female at birth" and "individuals assigned male at birth" are used. This approach balances inclusivity with the need to accurately represent the original research.

When to Screen

As more adults live into their 80s and beyond, decisions about offering preventive care become more complex. Although there is relative consensus about immunization recommendations and the importance of assessing older adults for geriatric syndromes such as urinary incontinence and fall risk, disease-specific screening can be problematic.[94] The risks for harm from screening tests and disease treatments increase with age and with comorbidities. The evidence base for offering screening in older adults, particularly those with declining health status and multiple morbidities, is limited because clinical prevention trials usually enroll younger (<75 years) and healthier participants. Furthermore, the aging population is physiologically heterogeneous, and predicting long-term health trajectories to identify those who will benefit from interventions is difficult when based on age alone.[95] A 75-year-old female with no comorbidities and low frailty has a 14.7-year life expectancy. Meanwhile, a 75-year-old female with high comorbidities and frailty has only a 7.1-year life expectancy. Accordingly, decisions about disease-specific screening and preventive services should be individualized, based on the person's overall health and estimated life expectancy rather than age alone.[94,96]

In Figure 30-11, the vertical axis shows the health status distribution of the population aged 65 years and older, and the horizontal bars show the variation in the importance of offering specific screening and preventive services.

The American Geriatrics Society recommends a set of guiding principles for addressing medical decisions in older adults with multimorbidity.[97]

1. Elicit and incorporate patient (and family/caregiver) preferences into medical decision making.
2. Recognize the limitations of the evidence base and interpret and apply the medical literature specifically for this population.

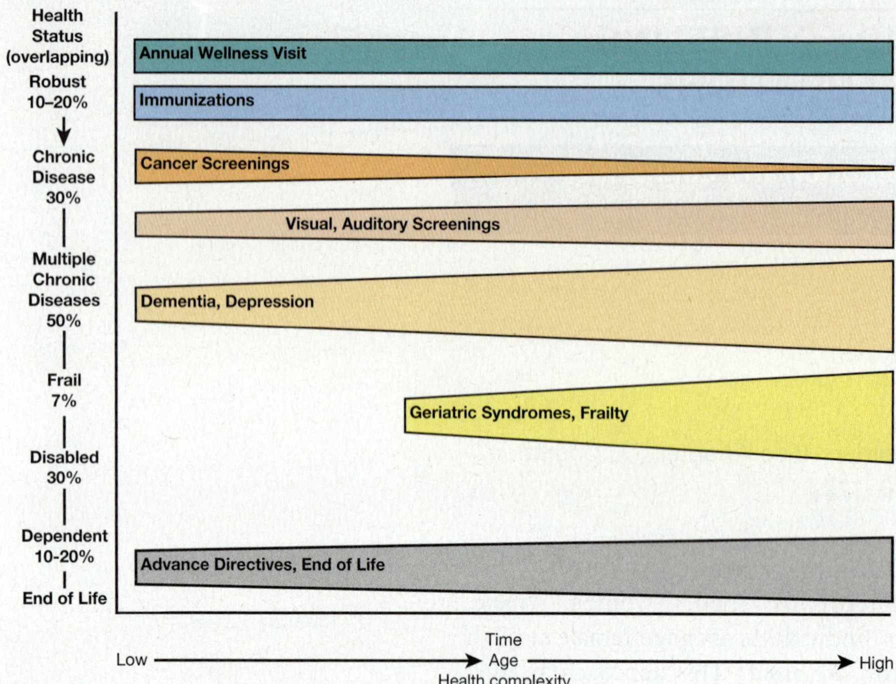

FIGURE 30-11. Older adults: relative role of screening and preventive services according to functional status. (From Nicholas JA, Hall WJ. Screening and preventive services for older adults. *Mt Sinai J Med.* 2011;78(4):498–508. Copyright © 2011 Mount Sinai School of Medicine. Reprinted by permission of John Wiley & Sons, Inc.)

3. Frame clinical management decisions within the context of harms, burdens, benefits, and prognosis (e.g., remaining life expectancy, functional status, and quality of life).
4. Consider treatment complexity and feasibility when making clinical management decisions.
5. Use strategies for choosing therapies that optimize benefit, minimize harm, and enhance quality of life.

If life expectancy is short, give priority to treatment that benefits the patient in the time that remains. Consider avoiding screening if it overburdens older adults who have multiple clinical problems, shortened life expectancy, or dementia. Tests that help with prognosis and planning may still be warranted even if the patient does not want to pursue treatment.

Immunizations

Many vaccines are routinely recommended for older adults in the United States (Box 30-18). For the most up-to-date recommendations, consult the updated annual guidelines and contraindications provided by the U.S. Centers for Disease Control and Prevention (CDC) through the annual immunization schedules from the Advisory Committee on Immunization Practices (ACIP) or at http://www.cdc.gov/vaccines.

See Chapter 7, Health Maintenance and Screening, Immunization Guidelines for Adults, pp. 132–135.

Box 30-18. Older Adult Immunizations, 2024[98]

- **COVID-19:** All individuals aged 6 months and older should receive the 2024–2025 COVID-19 vaccine. Adults aged 65 and older, as well as those who are immunocompromised, may receive a second dose 6 months after their initial vaccination.
- **Influenza vaccination:** Adults aged ≥65 years should receive one high-dose quadrivalent inactivated influenza vaccine annually.
- **Respiratory syncytial virus (RSV) vaccine:** Adults aged 75 and older should receive one dose of any FDA-approved RSV vaccine. For adults aged 60–74, vaccination is recommended based on shared decision-making, particularly for those with conditions that increase their risk of severe RSV disease (e.g., chronic lung or heart disease).
- **Tetanus, diphtheria, and acellular pertussis (Tdap or Td):** Administer one dose of Tdap to older adults who previously did not receive the vaccine as an adult or child. A Tdap or Td vaccine booster should be offered every 10 years.
- **Varicella:** Administer two doses to older adults without evidence of immunity to varicella 4–8 weeks apart
- **Zoster recombinant:** Administer two doses of recombinant zoster vaccine (RZV) 2–6 months apart to adults aged >50 years regardless of past episode of herpes zoster or receipt of zoster vaccine live (ZVL).
- **Pneumococcal vaccination:** Adults aged ≥50 years who have never been vaccinated for pneumococcal pneumonia can receive one dose of PCV21, PCV20 (conjugated vaccine), or PCV15 (conjugate vaccine). If PCV15 is used, it should be followed by one dose of PPSV23 (polysaccharide vaccine) at least 1 year later. Recommendations for those who previously received a pneumococcal vaccine depend on their vaccination history and specific medical conditions. For guidance, refer to the ACIP adult immunization schedule[98] or download the free CDC mobile app: https://www.cdc.gov/digital-social-media-tools/mobile/applications/cdcgeneral/promos/cdcmobileapp.html
- **Hepatitis B vaccine:** Adults aged ≥60 years with risk factors (chronic liver disease, HIV, sexual exposure, injection drug use, percutaneous or mucosal risk for exposure to blood, incarceration, travel to countries with intermediate or higher endemic hepatitis B and adults aged ≥60 years with diabetes should receive this, based on shared decision making.

Source: Murthy N, Wodi AP, McNally VV, Daley MF, Cineas S; Advisory Committee on Immunization Practices. Recommended adult immunization schedule, United States, 2024. *Ann Intern Med.* 2024;177(2):221–237.

Cancer Screening

Guidelines often recommend discontinuing cancer screening at age 75 or when life expectancy is less than 10 years because elderly and frail adults face the harms of screening, particularly false-positive results, complications from diagnostic procedures and treatments, overdiagnosis, and overtreatment without being likely to derive any survival benefit. A useful tool for assessing life expectancy is e-prognosis (https://eprognosis.ucsf.edu). This tool estimates 10-year life expectancy based on age, comorbidities, health behaviors, and frailty and specifically addresses whether an older adult would likely benefit from breast or colorectal cancer screening. The U.S. Preventive Services Task Force (USPSTF) recommendations which address an upper age for cancer screening are summarized in Box 30-19.

Box 30-19. Screening Recommendations for Older Adults: U.S. Preventive Services Task Force

- **Breast cancer (2016)[99]:** Recommends mammography every 2 years for women aged 40–74 years (grade B) and cites insufficient evidence for screening women aged ≥75 years (I statement).
- **Cervical cancer (2018)[100]:** Recommends *against* routine screening for women age <65 years if they have had adequate recent screening with normal Pap smears and are not otherwise at high risk for cervical cancer (grade D).
- **Colorectal cancer (2021)[101]:** Recommends screening for colorectal cancer in adults aged **45–75 years** (Grade A for ages 50–75; Grade B for ages 45–49). Available strategies and screening intervals include colonoscopy every 10 years, computed tomography (CT) colonography every 5 years, annual fecal immunochemical test, annual high-sensitivity fecal occult blood test (FOBT), fecal DNA test every 1 or 3 years, or flexible sigmoidoscopy every 5 years. Recommends that routine screening for adults aged 76–85 years be an individualized decision that considers the patient's overall health, previous screening history, and preferences due to moderate certainty that the net benefit is small (grade C).
- **Prostate cancer (2018)[102]:** Recommends that prostate-specific antigen (PSA)-based screening for prostate cancer for men aged 55–69 years be an individualized decision in a patient who discusses with their clinician the potential benefits and harms from screening and clarifies their values and preferences. This recommendation is based on moderate certainty that the net benefit of screening is small (grade C). Recommends *against* PSA-based screening for prostate cancer in men aged ≥70 years due to evidence that expected harms are greater than expected benefits (grade D).
- **Lung cancer (2021)[103]:** For adults aged 50–80 years with a 20-pack-year smoking history, and those who currently smoke or have quit within the past 15 years, recommends annual screening with low-dose CT (grade B). Screening should be *discontinued* once a person reaches age 81, has not smoked for 15 years, or develops a health problem that substantially limits life expectancy or the ability or willingness to have curative lung surgery.

Many experts, however, feel that clinical judgment and informed patient preference should supersede age-cutoff guidelines in making screening decisions for older adults.[104–106] Walter and Covinsky developed a useful conceptual framework for individualized cancer screening decision making in older adults that incorporates the patient's characteristics and preferences.[104]

1. *Estimate life expectancy and cancer risk.* Decisions are initially approached by quantitatively estimating life expectancy, the risk of cancer death from a screen-detectable cancer, and potential screening outcomes using data from the medical literature.
2. *Consider patient values and preferences.* The next component of the framework is considering the estimated benefits and harms through the lens of the patient's values and preferences.
3. *Present benefits and harms.* After determining life expectancy and the risk of dying from a screen-detectable cancer, clinicians next present the benefits

and harms of screening. Benefits can be expressed as absolute risk reductions or its reciprocal, the number needed to screen (NNS). The NNS can be used to show how the intersection of age and life expectancy markedly impacts benefit; patients with less than a 5-year life expectancy are unlikely to benefit from cancer screening. The harms of cancer screening in older adults arise from complications from diagnostic procedures performed to evaluate false positive results, the overdiagnosis and overtreatment of indolent cancers, and the psychological distress of undergoing screening and being diagnosed with cancer.

4. *Elicit patient preferences.* The final step in the decision-making process is eliciting the patient's values and preferences for the various potential outcomes of screening. Lee and colleagues proposed also looking at the lag-time to benefit from cancer screening in the context of life expectancy. Screening should be recommended if life expectancy substantially exceeds the lag-time to benefit and discouraged if lag-time to benefit substantially exceeds life expectancy.[105] When the lag-time and life expectancy are similar, screening decisions should be based on patient preferences.

Unfortunately, older adults with limited life expectancy are often overscreened.[96,106,107] Patients want screening because they tend to overestimate the benefit of screening and underestimate the potential harms; clinicians may also overestimate the benefit of screening and find it difficult to discuss stopping screening or to accurately estimate life expectancy. Effective strategies to help clinicians communicate about risk include using visual displays of data (see eprognosis.ucsf.edu), weighing for patients the relative benefits of screening for cancer versus prioritizing life-extending treatment for known comorbidities, and engaging the patient using the framework for individualized decision-making process described above.

The American College of Physicians, which views screening from more of a public health perspective, identified high- and low-value screening strategies for older adults that factor in health benefits, frequency of screening, and harms and costs (Box 30-20).

Elder Abuse

Elder abuse is defined as "an intentional act or lack of action by a caregiver or another person in a relationship involving an expectation of trust that causes or creates a risk of harm to an older adult."[110] Harms include physical abuse, sexual abuse, emotional/psychological abuse, neglect, and financial abuse/exploitation. The 1-year prevalence of abuse among U.S. community-residing older adults has been estimated to be about 10%.[111–113] However, the prevalence of abuse is thought to be underestimated due to the patient's fear of reprisal, physical or cognitive inability to report, and unwillingness to expose the abuser, many of whom are family members. The strongest risk factors for being abused include functional disability, cognitive impairment, poor physical or mental health, and low income. The risk for elder abuse is lower among those with higher levels of social support and more extensive social networks. Elder abuse is associated with adverse health outcomes, including increased mortality risk, nursing home placement, and psychological distress.[114]

In its 2018 review, the USPSTF found no valid, reliable screening tools in the primary care setting to identify abuse of older or vulnerable adults without recognized signs and symptoms of abuse and therefore cited insufficient evidence

Box 30-20. High- and Low-Value Screening for Five Types of Cancer in Older Adults[108,109]

Cancer Type	High-Value Strategies (recommended)	Low-Value Strategies (not recommended
Breast	**Women aged 65–74 years:** Biennial mammography screening if life expectancy is ≥10 years	**Women aged ≥75 years:** Screening is not recommended for those with a life expectancy <10 years or who have significant comorbidities
Cervical	**Women aged >65 years:** No screening if they have had adequate prior negative results and are not at high risk	**Women aged >65 years:** Screening is unnecessary if adequate prior negative screening has been performed
Colorectal	**Adults aged 65–75 years:** Screening with fecal immunochemical test (FIT) annually or colonoscopy every 10 years for those in good health with a life expectancy ≥10 years	**Adults aged >75 years:** Screening is not recommended for those with a life expectancy <10 years or who have significant comorbidities
Prostate	**Men aged 65–69 years:** Shared decision-making for PSA testing in those with a life expectancy ≥10 years after discussing benefits and harms	**Men aged ≥70 years:** PSA screening is not recommended due to low net benefit

PSA, prostate-specific antigen.

Sources: Wilt TJ, Harris RP, Qaseem A; High Value Care Task Force of the American College of Physicians. Screening for cancer: advice for high-value care from the American College of Physicians. *Ann Intern Med.* 2015;162(10):718–725; Qaseem A, Harrod CS, Crandall CJ, et al. Screening for colorectal cancer in asymptomatic average-risk adults: a guidance statement from the American College of Physicians (version 2). *Ann Intern Med.* 2023;176(8): 1092–1100.

See further discussions about screening breast cancer in Chapter 20, Breasts and Axillae, pp. 595–599; colorectal cancer in Chapter 21, Abdomen, p. 653–654; cervical cancer in Chapter 24, Pelvis and Genitourinary System: Vulva, Vagina, Uterus, and Adnexa, pp. 759–760, and prostate cancer in Chapter 23, Pelvis and Genitourinary System: Penis, Scrotum, and Prostate, pp. 712–713.

for recommending screening (I statement).[114] However, the USPSTF identified risk factors for elder abuse, including "isolation and lack of social support, functional impairment, and poor physical health." While routine screening was not recommended, the USPSTF noted that most clinicians have never asked about elder abuse. Clinicians should be aware of risk factors for elder abuse and be able to recognize signs and symptoms of abuse (Box 30-21).[115] Resources for addressing elder abuse include Adult Protective Services (https://www.napsanow.org/help-in-your-area), the National Center on Elder Abuse (https://ncea.acl.gov/interventions#gsc.tab=0), and long-term care ombudsmen (https://theconsumervoice.org/get_help).[115]

Box 30-21. Spotting the Signs of Elder Abuse

- Appearing depressed, confused, agitated, or withdrawn
- Isolation from family and friends
- Unexplained bruises, burns, cuts, pressure marks, or scars
- Appearing dirty, underfed, dehydrated, over- or undermedicated, or not receiving needed care for medical problems
- Developing preventable conditions such as bedsores
- Recent changes in banking or spending patterns

Household Safety and Falls Prevention

Approximately 30% of adults aged 65 and older fall each year.[116] About 75% of the falls occur at home, either inside or outside.[117,118] Fall-related injuries usually occur with walking, engaging in vigorous activity, and climbing stairs. Most falls are caused by slipping, tripping, or loss of balance. The most common reasons for emergency department visits or being hospitalized following a fall are hip fractures and head injuries, which can adversely impact survival, daily function, and independence.[118,119] Encourage older adults to adopt corrective measures for poor lighting, chairs at awkward heights, slippery or irregular surfaces, and environmental hazards (Box 30-22).

Box 30-22. Home Safety Tips for Older Adults[122,123]

- Install bright lighting and lightweight curtains or shades.
- Install handrails and lights on all staircases. Pathways and walkways should be well-lit.
- Remove items that cause tripping like papers, books, clothes, and shoes from stairs and walkways.
- Remove or secure small throw rugs and other rugs with double-sided tape.
- Wear shoes both inside and outside the house. Avoid bare feet and wearing slippers.
- Store medications safely.
- Keep commonly used items in cabinets that are easy to reach without using a step stool.
- Install grab bars and nonslip mats or safety strips in baths and showers.
- Repair faulty plugs and electrical cords.
- Install smoke alarms and have a plan for escaping fire.
- Secure all firearms.
- Have a clinical alert device/system for calling a universal emergency number such as 911 or emergency contacts.

Sources: Health in Aging Foundation. Tip Sheet: Home Safety Tips for Older Adults. Accessed February 26, 2024. https://www.healthinaging.org/tools-and-tips/tip-sheet-home-safety-tips-older-adults

Centers for Disease Control and Prevention. What You Can Do To Prevent Falls. Accessed February 28, 2024. https://www.cdc.gov/steadi/pdf/STEADI-Brochure-WhatYouCanDo-508.pdf

Preventing Falls. In 2020, 14 million U.S. adults aged ≥65 years reported falling during the previous year, and there were nearly 39,000 fall-related deaths.[120] Falls and fall-related deaths were higher among adults aged ≥85 years compared to younger age groups. While a higher proportion of women reported falls than did men, women had a lower rate of fall-related deaths. Falls are the leading cause of fatal and nonfatal injuries among older adults and accounted for an estimated 3 million emergency room visits and more than 950,000 hospitalizations in 2018.[121] The annual medical costs attributed to fatal and nonfatal falls in older adults are more than $50 billion.[116] Risk factors for falls include increasing age, impaired gait and balance, postural hypotension, loss of strength, medication use, comorbid illnesses, depression, cognitive impairment, environmental hazards, and visual deficits.

The USPSTF issued a grade B recommendation in 2018 to provide exercise or physical therapy to prevent falls among at-risk community-dwelling adults aged 65 and older.[85]

The USPSTF recommends personalized decision making (grade C) regarding multifactorial fall-prevention interventions for at-risk community-dwelling adults aged 65 and older.[85] This begins with comprehensively assessing modifiable fall risk factors and then offering appropriately targeted multidisciplinary interventions. The USPSTF recommends against daily vitamin D supplementation to prevent falls (grade D).

REFERENCES

1. World Report on Ageing and Health. *World Health Organization*; 2015. Accessed May 11, 2024. https://www.who.int/publications/i/item/9789241565042
2. Older Americans 2020: Key Indicators of Well-Being. *Federal Interagency Forum on Aging-Related Statistics*; 2020. Accessed May 11, 2024. https://agingstats.gov/docs/LatestReport/OA20_508_10142020.pdf
3. Health, United States, 2013: With Special Feature on Prescription Drugs. *National Center for Health Statistics, Centers for Disease Control and Prevention, U.S. Department of Health and Human Services*; 2014. Accessed May 11, 2024. http://www.cdc.gov/nchs/data/hus/hus13.pdf#018
4. Sabia S, Singh-Manoux A, Hagger-Johnson G, Cambois E, Brunner EJ, Kivimaki M. Influence of individual and combined healthy behaviours on successful aging. *CMAJ*. 2012;184(18):1985–1992.
5. Davy C, Bleasel J, Liu H, Tchan M, Ponniah S, Brown A. Effectiveness of chronic care models: opportunities for improving healthcare practice and health outcomes: a systematic review. *BMC Health Serv Res*. 2015;15:194.
6. Partnership for Health in Aging Workgroup on Interdisciplinary Team Training in Geriatrics. Position statement on interdisciplinary team training in geriatrics: an essential component of quality health care for older adults. *J Am Geriatr Soc*. 2014;62(5):961–965.
7. Bodenheimer T, Wagner EH, Grumbach K. Improving primary care for patients with chronic illness. *JAMA*. 2002;288(14):1775–1779.
8. Quinlan N, O'Neill D. "Older" or "elderly"–are medical journals sensitive to the wishes of older people? *J Am Geriatr Soc*. 2008;56(10):1983–1984.
9. Dahmen NS, Cozma R. *Media Takes: On Aging*. International Longevity Center - USA; Aging Services of California; 2009. Accessed May 11, 2024. https://www.ilc-alliance.org/wp-content/uploads/publication-pdfs/Media_Takes_On_Aging.pdf
10. US Preventive Services Task Force. Screening for intimate partner violence, elder abuse, and abuse of vulnerable adults: US Preventive Services Task Force final recommendation statement. *JAMA*. 2018;320(16):1678–1687.
11. Frontera WR. Physiologic changes of the musculoskeletal system with aging: a brief review. *Phys Med Rehabil Clin N Am*. 2017;28(4):705–711.
12. Smith WCS. Hypertension in the elderly: an opportunity to improve health. *J R Coll Physicians Edinb*. 1999;29:211–213.
13. Kane RL, Ouslander JG, Abrass IB, Resnick B. Chapter 3: evaluating the geriatric patient. *Essentials of Clinical Geriatrics*. 7th ed. McGraw-Hill Education LLC; 2013.
14. Kevorkian RT, Morley JE. Chapter 3: the physiology of ageing. In: Sinclair AJ, Morley JE, Vellas B, eds. *Pathy's Principles and Practice of Geriatric Medicine*. 5th ed. Wiley-Blackwell; 2012:33.
15. Otto CM, Lind BK, Kitzman DW, Gersh BJ, Siscovick DS. Association of aortic-valve sclerosis with cardiovascular mortality and morbidity in the elderly. *N Engl J Med*. 1999;341(3):142–147.
16. Hollingsworth JM, Wilt TJ. Lower urinary tract symptoms in men. *BMJ*. 2014;349:g4474.
17. Gorina Y, Schappert S, Bercovitz A, Elgaddal N, Kramarow E. *Prevalence of Incontinence Among Older Americans*. National

Center for Health Statistics; 2014;3(36):1–33. Vital Health Statistics. Accessed May 11, 2024. http://www.cdc.gov/nchs/data/series/sr_03/sr03_036.pdf

18. Morley JE, Tolson DT. Chapter 9: sexuality and ageing. In: Sinclair AJ, Morley JE, Vellas B, eds. *Pathy's Principles and Practice of Geriatric Medicine.* 5th ed. Wiley-Blackwell; 2012:93.
19. O'Keeffe J. *Creating a Senior Friendly Physical Environment in Our Hospitals.* Regional Geriatric Assessment Program of Ottawa. Accessed May 11, 2024. https://www.rgpeo.com/wp-content/uploads/2020/05/creating-a-senior-friendly-physical-environment.pdf
20. Rosen SL, Reuben DB. Geriatric assessment tools. *Mt Sinai J Med.* 2011;78(4):489–497.
21. Tinetti M, Huang A, Molnar F. The Geriatrics 5M's: a new way of communicating what we do. *J Am Geriatr Soc.* 2017;65(9):2115.
22. Kitzman DW, Taffet G. Chapter 74: effects of aging on cardiovascular structure and function. In: Halter JB, Ouslander JG, Tinetti ME, Studenski S, High KP, Asthana S, eds. *Hazzard's Geriatric Medicine and Gerontology.* 6th ed. McGraw-Hill Companies, Inc; 2009.
23. Freeman R, Wieling W, Axelrod FB, et al. Consensus statement on the definition of orthostatic hypotension, neurally mediated syncope and the postural tachycardia syndrome. *Clin Auton Res.* 2011;21(2):69–72.
24. Vijayan J, Sharma VK. Neurogenic orthostatic hypotension - management update and role of droxidopa. *Ther Clin Risk Manag.* 2015;11:915–923.
25. Sathyapalan T, Aye MM, Atkin SL. Postural hypotension. *BMJ.* 2011;342:d3128.
26. James PA, Oparil S, Carter BL, et al. 2014 evidence-based guideline for the management of high blood pressure in adults: report from the panel members appointed to the Eighth Joint National Committee (JNC 8). *JAMA.* 2014;311(5): 507–520.
27. Krakoff LR, Gillespie RL, Ferdinand KC, et al. 2014 hypertension recommendations from the eighth joint national committee panel members raise concerns for elderly black and female populations. *J Am Coll Cardiol.* 2014;64(4): 394–402.
28. Benetos A, Rossignol P, Cherubini A, et al. Polypharmacy in the aging patient: management of hypertension in octogenarians. *JAMA.* 2015;314(2):170–180.
29. Bangalore S, Gong Y, Cooper-DeHoff RM, Pepine CJ, Messerli FH. 2014 Eighth Joint National Committee panel recommendation for blood pressure targets revisited: results from the INVEST study. *J Am Coll Cardiol.* 2014;64(8): 784–793.
30. Papaleontiou M, Haymart MR. Approach to and treatment of thyroid disorders in the elderly. *Med Clin North Am.* 2012;96(2):297–310.
31. Perlmuter LC, Sarda G, Casavant V, Mosnaim AD. A review of the etiology, associated comorbidities, and treatment of orthostatic hypotension. *Am J Ther.* 2013;20(3):279–291.
32. Carter SR. Eyelid disorders: diagnosis and management. *Am Fam Physician.* 1998;57(11):2695–2702.
33. Addis VM, DeVore HK, Summerfield ME. Acute visual changes in the elderly. *Clin Geriatr Med.* 2013;29(1):165–180.
34. Bagai A, Thavendiranathan P, Detsky AS. Does this patient have hearing impairment? *JAMA.* 2006;295(4):416–428.
35. Friedman PK, Kaufman LB, Karpas SL. Oral health disparity in older adults: dental decay and tooth loss. *Dent Clin North Am.* 2014;58(4):757–770.
36. Yellowitz JA, Schneiderman MT. Elder's oral health crisis. *J Evid Based Dent Pract.* 2014;14(Suppl):191–200.
37. Gibson PG, McDonald VM, Marks GB. Asthma in older adults. *Lancet.* 2010;376(9743):803–813.
38. Miller KL, Baraldi CA. Geriatric gynecology: promoting health and avoiding harm. *Am J Obstet Gynecol.* 2012;207(5): 355–367.
39. Gillespie LD, Robertson MC, Gillespie WJ, et al. Interventions for preventing falls in older people living in the community. *Cochrane Database Syst Rev.* 2012;(9):CD007146.
40. Wang JJ, Baker ML, Hand PJ, et al. Transient ischemic attack and acute ischemic stroke: associations with retinal microvascular signs. *Stroke.* 2011;42(2):404–408.
41. Vajaranant TS, Wu S, Torres M, Varma R. The changing face of primary open-angle glaucoma in the United States: demographic and geographic changes from 2011 to 2050. *Am J Ophthalmol.* 2012;154(2):303–314.e3.
42. Ratnapriya R, Chew EY. Age-related macular degeneration-clinical review and genetics update. *Clin Genet.* 2013;84(2): 160–166.
43. Coffey S, Cox B, Williams MJ. The prevalence, incidence, progression, and risks of aortic valve sclerosis: a systematic review and meta-analysis. *J Am Coll Cardiol.* 2014;63(25 Pt A): 2852–2861.
44. Manning WJ. Asymptomatic aortic stenosis in the elderly: a clinical review. *JAMA.* 2013;310(14):1490–1497.
45. McDermott MM. Lower extremity manifestations of peripheral artery disease: the pathophysiologic and functional implications of leg ischemia. *Circ Res.* 2015;116(9): 1540–1550.
46. Panel on Prevention of Falls in Older Persons; American Geriatrics Society and British Geriatrics Society. Summary of the updated American Geriatrics Society/British Geriatrics Society clinical practice guideline for prevention of falls in older persons. *J Am Geriatr Soc.* 2011;59(1):148–157.
47. Moyer VA. Prevention of falls in community-dwelling older adults: U.S. Preventive Services Task Force recommendation statement. *Ann Intern Med.* 2012;157(3):197–204.
48. Frank C, Pari G, Rossiter JP. Approach to diagnosis of Parkinson disease. *Can Fam Physician.* 2006;52(7): 862–868.
49. Seitz DP, Chan CC, Newton HT, et al. Mini-Cog for the detection of dementia within a primary care setting. *Cochrane Database Syst Rev.* 2021;7(7):CD011415.
50. Cummings-Vaughn LA, Chavakula NN, Malmstrom TK, Tumosa N, Morley JE, Cruz-Oliver DM. Veterans Affairs Saint Louis University Mental Status examination compared with the Montreal Cognitive Assessment and the Short Test of Mental Status. *J Am Geriatr Soc.* 2014;62(7):1341–1346.
51. Centers for Disease Control and Prevention. *Percent of U.S. Adults 55 and Over with Chronic Conditions.* Published September 2009. Accessed November 24, 2024. https://www.cdc.gov/nchs/data/health_policy/adult_chronic_conditions.pdf
52. Wooten JM. Rules for improving pharmacotherapy in older adult patients: part 1 (rules 1-5). *South Med J.* 2015;108(2): 97–104.

53. Wooten JM. Rules for improving pharmacotherapy in older adult patients: part 2 (rules 6-10). *South Med J.* 2015;108(3): 145–150.
54. Redmond P, Grimes TC, McDonnell R, Boland F, Hughes C, Fahey T. Impact of medication reconciliation for improving transitions of care. *Cochrane Database Syst Rev.* 2018; 8:CD010791.
55. American Geriatrics Society 2015 Beers Criteria Update Expert Panel. American Geriatrics Society 2015 Updated Beers Criteria for potentially inappropriate medication use in older adults. *J Am Geriatr Soc.* 2015;63(11):2227–2246.
56. 2019 American Geriatrics Society Beers Criteria® Update Expert Panel. American Geriatrics Society 2019 Updated AGS Beers Criteria® for potentially inappropriate medication use in older adults. *J Am Geriatr Soc.* 2019;67(4):674–694.
57. Linkens A, Kurstjens D, Zwietering NA, et al. Clinical decision support systems in hospitalized older patients: an exploratory analysis in a real-life clinical setting. *Drugs Real World Outcomes.* 2023;10(3):363–370.
58. Abdellatif A, Bouaud J, Nghiem D, Lafuente-Lafuente C, Belmin J, Seroussi B. Clinical decision support systems in nursing homes: a scoping review. *Stud Health Technol Inform.* 2020;270:542–546.
59. Harris Y, Hu DJ, Lee C, Mistry M, York A, Johnson TK. Advancing medication safety: establishing a national action plan for adverse drug event prevention. *Jt Comm J Qual Patient Saf.* 2015;41(8):351–360.
60. Carlson C, Merel SE, Yukawa M. Geriatric syndromes and geriatric assessment for the generalist. *Med Clin North Am.* 2015;99(2):263–279.
61. Koroukian SM, Warner DF, Owusu C, Given CW. Multimorbidity redefined: prospective health outcomes and the cumulative effect of co-occurring conditions. *Prev Chronic Dis.* 2015;12:E55.
62. Strandberg TE, Pitkälä KH, Tilvis RS, O'Neill D, Erkinjuntti TJ. Geriatric syndromes–vascular disorders? *Ann Med.* 2013;45(3):265–273.
63. Ellis G, Marshall T, Ritchie C. Comprehensive geriatric assessment in the emergency department. *Clin Interv Aging.* 2014;9:2033–2043.
64. Wong CL, Holroyd-Leduc J, Simel DL, Straus SE. Does this patient have delirium? Value of bedside instruments. *JAMA.* 2010;304(7):779–786.
65. Vasilevskis EE, Han JH, Hughes CG, Ely EW. Epidemiology and risk factors for delirium across hospital settings. *Best Pract Res Clin Anaesthesiol.* 2012;26(3):277–287.
66. Marcantonio ER. In the clinic. Delirium. *Ann Intern Med.* 2011;154(11):ITC6-1–ITC6-16.
67. Tsoi KK, Chan JY, Hirai HW, Wong SY, Kwok TC. Cognitive tests to detect dementia: a systematic review and meta-analysis. *JAMA Intern Med.* 2015;175(9):1450–1458.
68. Roalf DR, Moberg PJ, Xie SX, Wolk DA, Moelter ST, Arnold SE. Comparative accuracies of two common screening instruments for classification of Alzheimer's disease, mild cognitive impairment, and healthy aging. *Alzheimers Dement.* 2013;9(5):529–537.
69. Langa KM, Levine DA. The diagnosis and management of mild cognitive impairment: a clinical review. *JAMA.* 2014; 312(23):2551–2561.
70. Liew TM, Feng L, Gao Q, Ng TP, Yap P. Diagnostic utility of Montreal Cognitive Assessment in the Fifth Edition of Diagnostic and Statistical Manual of Mental Disorders: major and mild neurocognitive disorders. *J Am Med Dir Assoc.* 2015;16(2):144–148.
71. Borson S, Scanlan JM, Chen P, Ganguli M. The Mini-Cog as a screen for dementia: validation in a population-based sample. *J Am Geriatr Soc.* 2003;51(10):1451–1454.
72. Nasreddine ZS, Phillips NA, Bédirian V, et al. The Montreal Cognitive Assessment, MoCA: a brief screening tool for mild cognitive impairment. *J Am Geriatr Soc.* 2005;53(4): 695–699.
73. Moyer VA. Screening for cognitive impairment in older adults: U.S. Preventive Services Task Force recommendation statement. *Ann Intern Med.* 2014;160(11):791–797.
74. Sheikh JI, Yesavage JA. Geriatric Depression Scale (GDS): recent evidence and development of a shorter version. *Clinical Gerontologist.* 1986;5(1–2):165–173.
75. Kroenke K, Spitzer RL, Williams JB. The Patient Health Questionnaire-2: validity of a two-item depression screener. *Med Care.* 2003;41(11):1284–1292.
76. Kroenke K, Spitzer RL, Williams JB. The PHQ-9: validity of a brief depression severity measure. *J Gen Intern Med.* 2001;16(9):606–613.
77. Sheikh JI, Yesavage JA, Brooks JO III, et al. Proposed factor structure of the Geriatric Depression Scale. *Int Psychogeriatr.* 1991;3(1):23–28.
78. O'Connor E, Rossom RC, Henninger M, et al. Screening for Depression in Adults: An Updated Systematic Evidence Review for the U.S. Preventive Services Task Force: Evidence Syntheses, No. 128. Agency for Healthcare Research and Quality (US); 2016.
79. Siu AL, Force USPST, Bibbins-Domingo K, et al. Screening for depression in adults: US Preventive Services Task Force Recommendation Statement. *JAMA.* 2016;315(4): 380–387.
80. Brink TL, Yesavage JA, Lum O, Heersema PH, Adey M, Rose TL. Screening tests for geriatric depression. *Clin Gerontol.* 1982;1(1):37–43.
81. Podsiadlo D, Richardson S. The timed "Up & Go": a test of basic functional mobility for frail elderly persons. *J Am Geriatr Soc.* 1991;39(2):142–148.
82. Stevens JA, Phelan EA. Development of STEADI: a fall prevention resource for health care providers. *Health Promot Pract.* 2013;14(5):706–714.
83. Bergen G, Stevens MR, Burns ER. Falls and fall injuries among adults aged ≥65 years - United States, 2014. *MMWR Morb Mortal Wkly Rep.* 2016;65(37):993–998.
84. Josephson KR, Fabacher DA, Rubenstein LZ. Home safety and fall prevention. *Clin Geriatr Med.* 1991;7(4):707–731.
85. US Preventive Services Task Force, Grossman DC, Curry SJ, et al. Interventions to prevent falls in community-dwelling older adults: US Preventive Services Task Force recommendation statement. *JAMA.* 2018;319(16):1696–1704.
86. Lam JYJ, Barras M, Scott IA, Long D, Shafiee Hanjani L, Falconer N. Scoping review of studies evaluating frailty and its association with medication harm. *Drugs Aging.* 2022; 39(5):333–353.
87. McIsaac DI, MacDonald DB, Aucoin SD. Frailty for perioperative clinicians: a narrative review. *Anesth Analg.* 2020; 130(6):1450–1460.
88. Todhunter-Brown A, Hazelton C, Campbell P, Elders A, Hagen S, McClurg D. Conservative interventions for treating urinary incontinence in women: an Overview of Cochrane systematic reviews. *Cochrane Database Syst Rev.* 2022;9(9):Cd012337.

89. Dent E, Hoogendijk EO, Visvanathan R, Wright ORL. Malnutrition screening and assessment in hospitalised older people: a review. *J Nutr Health Aging*. 2019; 23(5):431–441.
90. O'Mahony D, Cherubini A, Guiteras AR, et al. STOPP/START criteria for potentially inappropriate prescribing in older people: version 3. *Eur Geriatr Med*. 2023;14(4): 625–632.
91. Smet S, Probst S, Holloway S, Fourie A, Beele H, Beeckman D. The measurement properties of assessment tools for chronic wounds: a systematic review. *Int J Nurs Stud*. 2021; 121:103998.
92. Jaiswal A, Gupta S, Paramasivam A, et al. Continuum of care for older adults with concurrent hearing and vision impairment: a systematic review. *Innov Aging*. 2022;7(1):igac076.
93. Chou R, Bougatsos C, Jungbauer R, et al. U.S. Preventive Services Task Force Evidence Syntheses, formerly Systematic Evidence Reviews. *Screening for Impaired Visual Acuity in Older Adults: A Systematic Review for the US Preventive Services Task Force*. Agency for Healthcare Research and Quality (US); 2022.
94. Nicholas JA, Hall WJ. Screening and preventive services for older adults. *Mt Sinai J Med*. 2011;78(4):498–508.
95. Schoenborn NL, Blackford AL, Joshu CE, Boyd CM, Varadhan R. Life expectancy estimates based on comorbidities and frailty to inform preventive care. *J Am Geriatr Soc*. 2022;70(1):99–109.
96. Schoenborn NL, Huang J, Sheehan OC, Wolff JL, Roth DL, Boyd CM. Influence of age, health, and function on cancer screening in older adults with limited life expectancy. *J Gen Intern Med*. 2019;34(1):110–117.
97. Boyd C, Smith CD, Masoudi FA, et al. decision making for older adults with multiple chronic conditions: executive summary for the American Geriatrics Society Guiding Principles on the care of older adults with multimorbidity. *J Am Geriatr Soc*. 2019;67(4):665–673.
98. Murthy N, Wodi AP, McNally VV, Daley MF, Cineas S, Advisory Committee on Immunization P. Recommended Adult Immunization Schedule, United States, 2024. *Ann Intern Med*. 2024;177(2):221–237.
99. U.S. Preventive Services Task Force. Screening for breast cancer: U.S. Preventive Services Task Force Draft Recommendation Statement. *Ann Intern Med*. Published online May 9, 2023. Accessed February 28, 2024. https://www.uspreventiveservicestaskforce.org/uspstf/recommendation/breast-cancer-screening
100. U. S. Preventive Services Task Force, Curry SJ, Krist AH, et al. Screening for cervical cancer: US Preventive Services Task Force Recommendation Statement. *JAMA*. 2018;320(7): 674–686.
101. U. S. Preventive Services Task Force, Davidson KW, Barry MJ, et al. Screening for colorectal cancer: US Preventive Services Task Force Recommendation Statement. *JAMA*. 2021;325(19):1965–1977.
102. U. S. Preventive Services Task Force, Grossman DC, Curry SJ, et al. Screening for prostate cancer: US Preventive Services Task Force Recommendation Statement. *JAMA*. 2018; 319(18):1901–1913.
103. U. S. Preventive Services Task Force, Krist AH, Davidson KW, et al. Screening for lung cancer: US Preventive Services Task Force Recommendation Statement. *JAMA*. 2021; 325(10):962–970.
104. Walter LC, Covinsky KE. Cancer screening in elderly patients: a framework for individualized decision making. *JAMA*. 2001;285(21):2750–2756.
105. Lee KT, Harris RP, Schoenborn NL. Individualized approach to cancer screening in older adults. *Clin Geriatr Med*. 2018;34(1):11–23.
106. Kotwal AA, Walter LC. Cancer screening in older adults: individualized decision-making and communication strategies. *Med Clin North Am*. 2020;104(6):989–1006.
107. Kotwal AA, Walter LC, Lee SJ, Dale W. Are we choosing wisely? Older adults' cancer screening intentions and recalled discussions with physicians about stopping. *J Gen Intern Med*. 2019;34(8):1538–1545.
108. Wilt TJ, Harris RP, Qaseem A, High value care Task Force of the American College of P. Screening for cancer: advice for high-value care from the American College of Physicians. *Ann Intern Med*. 2015;162(10):718–725.
109. Qaseem A, Harrod CS, Crandall CJ, et al. Screening for colorectal cancer in asymptomatic average-risk adults: a guidance statement From the American College of Physicians (Version 2). *Ann Intern Med*. 2023;176(8):1092–1100.
110. Hall JE, Karch DL, Crosby AE. *Elder Abuse Surveillance: Uniform Definitions and Recommended Core Data Elements For Use in Elder Abuse Surveillance, Version 1.0*. National Center for Injury Prevention and Control, Centers for Disease Control and Prevention. Accessed February 28, 2024. https://www.cdc.gov/violenceprevention/pdf/ea_book_revised_2016.pdf
111. Centers for Disease Control and Prevention. *About Abuse of Older Persons*. Accessed February 28, 2024. https://www.cdc.gov/elder-abuse/about/index.html
112. Pillemer K, Burnes D, Riffin C, Lachs MS. Elder abuse: global situation, risk factors, and prevention strategies. *Gerontologist*. 2016;56(Suppl 2):S194–S205.
113. Acierno R, Hernandez MA, Amstadter AB, et al. Prevalence and correlates of emotional, physical, sexual, and financial abuse and potential neglect in the United States: the National Elder Mistreatment Study. *Am J Public Health*. 2010;100(2):292–297.
114. U. S. Preventive Services Task Force, Curry SJ, Krist AH, et al. Screening for intimate partner violence, elder abuse, and abuse of vulnerable adults: US Preventive Services Task Force Final Recommendation Statement. *JAMA*. 2018; 320(16):1678–1687.
115. National Institute on Aging. Elder Abuse. Accessed February 28, 2024. https://www.nia.nih.gov/health/elder-abuse/elder-abuse
116. Florence CS, Bergen G, Atherly A, Burns E, Stevens J, Drake C. Medical costs of fatal and nonfatal falls in older adults. *J Am Geriatr Soc*. 2018;66(4):693–698.
117. Timsina LR, Willetts JL, Brennan MJ, et al. Circumstances of fall-related injuries by age and gender among community-dwelling adults in the United States. *PLoS One*. 2017;12(5): e0176561.
118. Choi NG, Choi BY, DiNitto DM, Marti CN, Kunik ME. Fall-related emergency department visits and hospitalizations among community-dwelling older adults: examination of health problems and injury characteristics. *BMC Geriatr*. 2019;19(1):303.
119. Centers for Disease Control and Prevention. Facts About Falls. Accessed February 27, 2024. https://www.cdc.gov/falls/facts.html

120. Kakara R, Bergen G, Burns E, Stevens M. Nonfatal and fatal falls among adults aged ≥65 Years—United States, 2020-2021. *MMWR Morb Mortal Wkly Rep.* 2023; 72(35):938–943.
121. Moreland B, Kakara R, Henry A. Trends in nonfatal falls and fall-related injuries among adults aged ≥65 Years—United States, 2012–2018. *MMWR Morb Mortal Wkly Rep.* 2020;69(27):875–881.
122. Health in Aging Foundation. Tip Sheet: Home Safety Tips for Older Adults. Accessed February 26, 2024. https://www.healthinaging.org/tools-and-tips/tip-sheet-home-safety-tips-older-adults
123. Centers for Disease Control and Prevention. What You Can Do To Prevent Falls. Accessed February 28, 2024. https://www.cdc.gov/steadi/pdf/STEADI-Brochure-WhatYouCanDo-508.pdf

Index

Note: Page numbers followed by f *indicate figures; those followed by* b *indicate in-chapter boxed material; those followed by* t *indicate end-of-chapter tables. Items related to children, adolescents, and older adults can be found listed under those entries as well as the specific anatomic area.*

A

C

D

E

F

H

J

K

L

Q

R

S

U

V